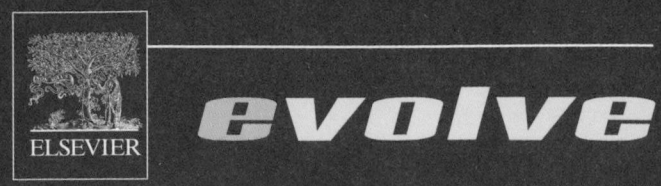

http://evolve.elsevier.com/Lehne/

- **Audio Drug Glossary**
  Listen to audio clips for each drug listed in Appendix B: Pronunciation of Generic Names of the Top 200 Prescribed Drugs in 2002.

- **Lehne's *Pharmacology for Nursing Care UPDATES***
  A carefully researched newsletter that covers the latest new drugs, drug alerts, and important advances in therapeutics. Available in an online version that can be searched by chapter or by drug name, as well as a downloadable, printable version that you can read while commuting, on study breaks, etc.

- **WebLinks**
  An exciting resource that lets you link to hundreds of Web sites carefully chosen to supplement the content of the textbook. The WebLinks are regularly updated, with new ones added as they develop.

- ***Mosby's DrugConsult* Internet Edition**
  Basic-level access to this comprehensive database of the most current, unbiased, accurate, and reliable drug information available. Includes Drug Updates, free information on the top 200 drugs by prescription, and Online Extras, including new drug approvals, safety notices, new drug indications, and links to pharmaceutical manufacturers for more information.

- **Canadian Drug Names**
  A comprehensive and up-to-date list of trade names for drugs commonly prescribed in Canada.

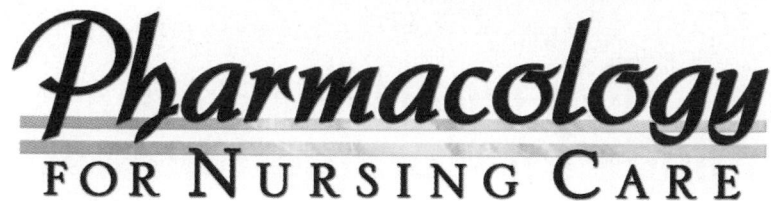

Study Guide to Accompany
Pharmacology for Nursing Care, 5th Edition

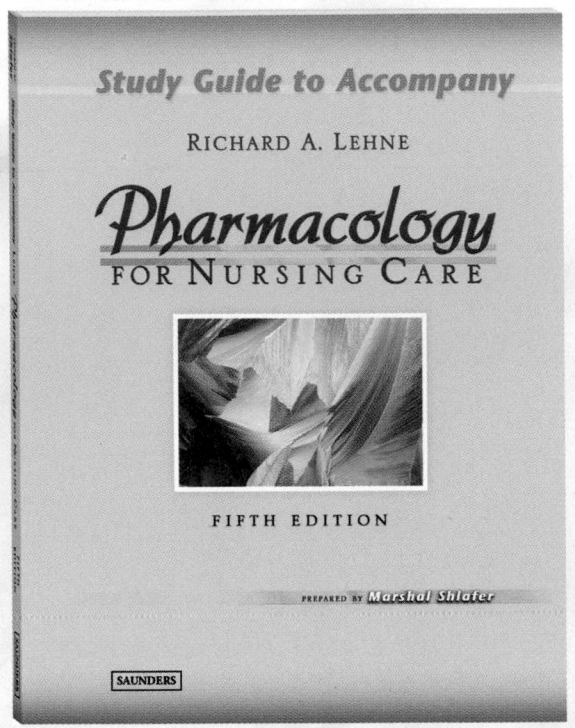

MARSHAL SHLAFER, PhD

Professor, Department of Pharmacology
University of Michigan Medical School
Ann Arbor, Michigan

This exceptional new study guide – completely
rewritten for the 5th edition – applies the unique
teaching style and educational expertise of renowned
educator Marshal Shlafer to Lehne's engaging
textbook, for a study tool that is second to none.
Features a wealth of learning activities, including
Key Terms, Critical Thinking Questions, and true-to-life
Case Studies that will help you get the most out of the
Lehne textbook, ensure that you have mastered the
content, and prepare for the NCLEX exam. *Answer
Guidelines* are provided on the EVOLVE website.

November 2003 • Approx. 280 pp. • ISBN: 0-7216-0128-6

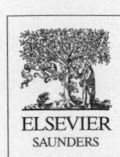

NMX-621

Pharmacology
FOR NURSING CARE

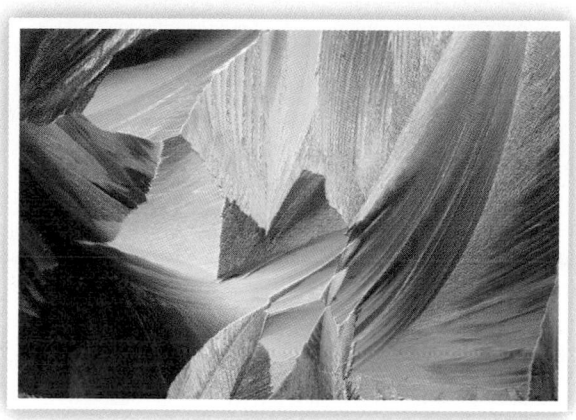

FIFTH EDITION

RICHARD A. LEHNE, PhD

formerly
Lecturer, University of Arizona College of Nursing
Lecturer, University of Virginia School of Nursing
Research Assistant Professor, Department of Pharmacology
University of Virginia School of Medicine
Charlottesville, Virginia

IN CONSULTATION WITH

Linda A. Moore, EdD, RN, APRN, BC (GNP/ANP), MSCN
Associate Professor of Nursing
Adult Health Nursing
School of Nursing
University of North Carolina at Charlotte;
Nurse Practitioner
Multiple Sclerosis Center
Carolinas HealthCare Systems
Charlotte, North Carolina

Leanna J. Crosby, DNSc, G/ANP-C
Nurse Practitioner in Primary Care
Southern Arizona Veterans Administration
Healthcare System;
Adjunct Associate Professor
College of Nursing
University of Arizona
Tucson, Arizona

Diane B. Hamilton, PhD, RN
Professor
School of Nursing
Western Michigan University
Kalamazoo, Michigan

SAUNDERS
An Imprint of Elsevier

SAUNDERS
An Imprint of Elsevier

11830 Westline Industrial Drive
St. Louis, Missouri 63146

PHARMACOLOGY FOR NURSING CARE   ISBN 0-7216-9843-3
Copyright © 2004, Saunders. All rights reserved.

NOTICE

Pharmacology is an ever-changing field. Standard safety precautions must be followed, but as new research and clinical experience broaden our knowledge, changes in treatment and drug therapy may become necessary or appropriate. Readers are advised to check the most current product information provided by the manufacturer of each drug to be administered to verify the recommended dose, the method and duration of administration, and contraindications. It is the responsibility of the licensed prescriber, relying on experience and knowledge of the patient, to determine dosages and the best treatment for each individual patient. Neither the publisher nor the editor assumes any liability for any injury and/or damage to persons or property arising from this publication.

Previous editions copyrighted 2001, 1998, 1994, 1990.

International Standard Book Number 0-7216-9843-3

Executive Editor: Robin Carter
Managing Editor: Lee Henderson
Publishing Services Manager: Catherine Albright Jackson
Project Manager: Celeste Clingan
Designer: Teresa McBryan Breckwoldt
Cover Design: Paul M. Fry

Cover Art: The cover art is a photomicrograph of crystalline carbamazepine (Tegretol, others), a drug with multiple uses, including suppression of seizures, relief of neuropathic pain, and stabilization of mood in patients with bipolar disorder.

Printed in the United States of America

Last digit is the print number: 9   8   7   6   5   4   3   2

Dedicated
to

Nancy

Who has enriched my life in
ways I could not have imagined

Thank you, Nance,

for

bringing flowers to the yard,
top-notch pots to the kitchen,
and the concept of fashion to my outdated wardrobe;

and for

teaching me about horses and ponies,
and tractors and Bush Hogs,
and barn dogs and Jack Russell terriers;

and for

introducing me to Ashley and Gentry,
and Gordon and Helen,
and everyone else in your close-knit and welcoming family;

and, most especially, for

sharing your warmth at night,
your dreams in the morning,
and your trust and love all day long.

About the Author

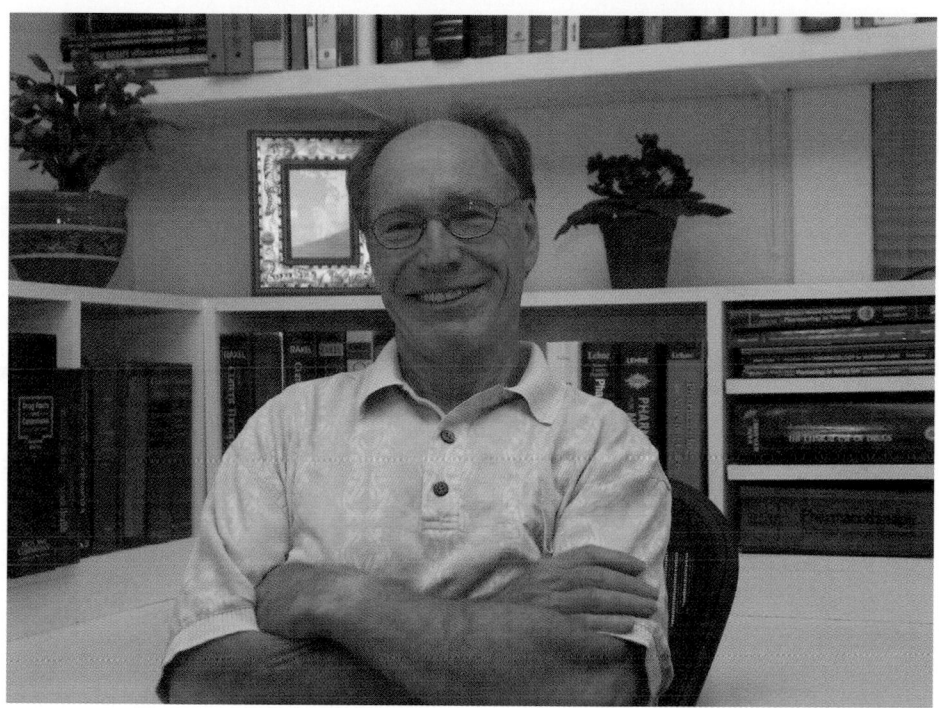

Richard A. Lehne, PhD, received his BA from Drew University and his PhD in pharmacology from George Washington University. His involvement in nursing education began 24 years ago at the University of Virginia School of Nursing, where he taught undergraduate and graduate pharmacology courses and was voted best teacher by his students. He has also taught at the University of Arizona in both the School of Nursing and School of Pharmacy. For the past 18 years, most of his time has been devoted to creating and revising this book. Dr. Lehne (rhymes with zany or rainy) lives in Charlottesville, VA, where he likes to bike (as age, weather, and editors permit), practice cooking (it's like being back in the lab, but more fun), and help Nancy (his SO) conduct equestrian shows at her farm (he now knows the difference between a horse and a pony, sort of). Oh yes, and he's still waiting (wistfully) for the neighbor's roosters to discover migration.

Consultants

Linda A. Moore, EdD, RN, APRN, BC (GNP/ANP), MSCN, is an Associate Professor of Nursing at the University of North Carolina at Charlotte and a Nurse Practitioner in the Multiple Sclerosis Center of Carolinas HealthCare Systems. She received her BSN from Duke University and her MSN and EdD from the University of Virginia. Her teaching responsibilities encompass courses for undergraduate (RN to BSN) and graduate students. Her major clinical and research interests are multiple sclerosis, cardiovascular nursing, and gerontologic nursing. Dr. Moore is a member of the North Carolina Nurses' Association, Sigma Theta Tau, and the International Organization of Multiple Sclerosis Nurses.

Leanna J. Crosby, DNSc, G/ANP-C, received her diploma in nursing from St. Luke's Hospital School of Nursing, her baccalaureate and master's degrees from the University of Virginia, and her doctorate in nursing science from Catholic University of America. Also, she completed the adult nurse practitioner program at the University of Virginia and the gerontologic nurse practitioner program at the University of Arizona. Dr. Crosby has done extensive research in chronic rheumatoid disease, and has taught physiology and pathophysiology to a generation of appreciative graduate and undergraduate students. Currently, she is working as a nurse practitioner within the Department of Veteran Affairs, Southern Arizona Veterans Administration Healthcare System, and is an Adjunct Associate Professor at the University of Arizona College of Nursing. Dr. Crosby is a member of the American Nurses Association, Sigma Theta Tau, and the Arizona Nurses' Association, and serves on the Arizona State Board of Nursing Advanced Practice Committee. In addition, she serves as the VISN 18 (Arizona, Texas, and New Mexico) coordinator for the Advanced Practice Nursing Network. At the local level, she is Membership Chair for the Southern Arizona Nurse Practitioner Association, a member of the Professional Standards Board for Nursing at the Southern Arizona VA Medical Center, and Chair of the Tucson VA IACUC Animal Research Committee.

Diane B. Hamilton, PhD, RN, received her BA from Northwestern University, her BSN from West Texas State University, her MA in Community Mental Health and Gerontologic Nursing from the University of Iowa, and her PhD in Psychosocial Nursing and Nursing History from the University of Virginia. She has extensive experience in psychiatric nursing, including serving as Attending Nurse at the Institute of Psychiatry of the Medical University of South Carolina. She has taught psychiatry and behavioral science to medical students, and gerontology, community health, psychiatric nursing, and nursing history to nursing students. Currently, she is a Professor in the School of Nursing at Western Michigan University, where she teaches psychiatric nursing and nursing history and does nursing history research. Dr. Hamilton is a member of the American Nurses Association, the American Association of the History of Nursing, the American Association for the History of Medicine, the American Association of University Women, and Sigma Theta Tau. In addition, Dr. Hamilton is a recipient of the Best of *Image* Award in nursing history, the Lavinia Dock Award for historical scholarship, the Best Investigator Award from the University of Rochester, the Golden Apple Teaching Award from the Medical University of South Carolina and the Distinguished Scholar Award from Western Michigan University.

Preface to the Fifth Edition

OVERVIEW OF THE BOOK

Welcome to the fifth edition of *Pharmacology for Nursing Care,* the pharmacology text that students like to read, really. This edition, like the first four, was written to be a true textbook—that is, a book that focuses on essentials and downplays secondary details. To give the book focus, three primary techniques are employed: (1) teaching through prototypes, (2) use of large print for essential information and small print for secondary information, and (3) limiting discussion of adverse effects and drug interactions to ones that are of particular clinical significance. Also, key points are summarized at the end of each chapter. To reinforce the relationship between pharmacologic knowledge and nursing practice, nursing implications are integrated into the body of each chapter. In addition, to provide rapid access to nursing content, nursing implications are summarized at the end of most chapters, using a nursing process format. As in prior editions, this edition emphasizes conceptual material, thereby reducing rote memorization, promoting comprehension, and increasing reader friendliness. For a description of the book's classic distinguishing features, please refer to the Preface to the First Edition, which follows on page XI.

NEW IN THIS EDITION

Pharmacology for Nursing Care has been revised cover to cover. All chapters have been updated and two new chapters and one new appendix have been added. Topics with significantly expanded coverage include medication errors, adverse drug reactions, Parkinson's disease, pain management, diabetes, hypertension, cholesterol-lowering drugs, hormone replacement therapy, and therapy of viral infections. This edition introduces a host of new drugs and six new Special Interest Topics. In addition, new treatment guidelines have been added, and older guidelines have been updated.

New Drugs

More than 100 new drugs and formulations have been added. Important among these are atomoxatine [Strattera], the first nonstimulant for attention deficit-hyperactivity disorder; aripiprazole [Abilify], the first dopamine system stabilizer for psychosis; ezetimibe [Zetia], the first drug to block cholesterol absorption; teriparatide [Forteo], the first drug to significantly increase bone formation; and enfuvirtide [Fuzeon], the first fusion inhibitor for HIV infection.

New Chapters

This edition has two new chapters. Chapter 102 (Drugs for the Ear) focuses primarily on otitis media, one of the most common disorders of childhood. Otitis externa is also discussed.

Chapter 106 (Potential Weapons of Biologic, Radiologic, and Chemical Terrorism) focuses primarily on potential bacterial and viral weapons (e.g., anthrax, small pox). Biotoxins, chemicals (nerve agents, mustard gas), and radiologic weapons are discussed as well.

Restructured Content

Our coverage of neurodegenerative disorders now appears in a subsection of its own in Unit V, entitled "Drugs for Neurdegenerative Disorders." This subsection includes separate chapters on drugs for Parkinson's disease (Chapter 21) and drugs for Alzheimer's disease (Chapter 22). Likewise, the coverage of anticancer drugs has now been split into two chapters: Chapter 98, Anticancer Drugs I: Cytotoxic Agents and Chapter 99, Anticancer Drugs II: Hormones, Hormone Antagonists, Biologic Response Modifiers, and Other Anticancer Drugs.

New Special Interest Topics

This edition has 25 boxes on Special Interest Topics, which address issues that I find especially engaging and hope you will too. Some boxes discuss cutting-edge therapies, some discuss ongoing controversies, some discuss topics of general interest, and some discuss issues featured in the popular press. Titles of the six new boxes are:

- *Has the Placebo Lost Its Effect?*
- *Postpartum Depression*
- *Isolated Systolic Hypertension: The Real Killer of Aging Americans*
- *And the Best Drug Is . . . The Cheap One!*
- *Attention Ladies: Digoxin May Be Hazardous to Your Health*
- *Face Time with Botox*

A complete list of Special Interest Topics appears on the inside back cover of the book.

New Appendix

Because drug names are often hard to pronounce, we've added a pronunciation guide—Appendix B—for the 200 most widely prescribed drugs in 2002. Sound files to accompany Appendix B are available online at *evolve.elsevier.com/Lehne/.*

New Feature: Full-Color Printing

For the first time, *Pharmacology for Nursing Care* is printed in full color. The most obvious impact is on the figures: All new figures were drawn in full color, and full color was added to all existing figures. Color has also been used to enhance headings and other design elements. Why did we switch to full color? Primarily to facilitate learning. Of course, we also think the extra color makes the book look better.

ONLINE RESOURCES FOR STUDENTS

To accompany this edition, we have four online resources: Content Updates, an Audio Drug Glossary, WebLinks, and a list of important Canadian drug names. All of these resources are available at *evolve.elsevier.com/Lehne/*.

Content Updates

Pharmacology undergoes steady and sometimes rapid evolution. Important new drugs are introduced each year, uses for older drugs change, and previously unknown toxicities of available drugs may be revealed. As a result, a pharmacology text can quickly become dated. To keep this text current, we are providing *"Pharmacology for Nursing Care* UPDATES" online. Each update will focus on new drugs, drug alerts, and important advances in therapeutics. Content is keyed to chapters in the book. Issues can be searched by chapter number and by drug name. All content can be downloaded and printed.

Audio Drug Glossary

The Audio Drug Glossary contains sound files that pronounce the generic names of the 200 most commonly prescribed drugs. As discussed in Chapter 3, if drugs were assigned generic names whose pronunciation was obvious, a glossary such as this would be unnecessary. I look forward to the day when that's the case.

WebLinks

The WebLinks provided on the Evolve website represent a large and dynamic library of links to drug-related web sites, keyed to the table of contents of this edition. The links are reviewed and edited frequently to ensure being current.

ANCILLARIES

Instructor's Resource (CD-ROM, Online)

The Instructor's Resource for the fifth edition is available on CD-ROM (ISBN 0-7216-0257-6) and online. It has four components: Instructor's Manual, Test Bank, Image Collection, and PowerPoint Collection.

- The Instructor's Manual is completely new, and emphasizes creative learning strategies to help students apply knowledge of pharmacology to nursing practice. The manual includes Teaching Strategies, Web Research Activities, Critical Thinking Case Studies, and an Open-Book Quiz for each chapter. Answers to the Open-Book Quizzes and Answer Guidelines for the Critical Thinking Case Studies are also provided.
- The Test Bank provides 750 NCLEX-style questions presented in versatile ExamView software, which allows faculty to customize paper-based or online exams through an easy-to-use, intuitive interface. For each question, we indicate the correct answer, nursing process step, NCLEX client-needs category, and cognitive type.
- The Image Collection contains every illustration from the book—about 150 all told, most in full color. The images

are presented in electronic format to facilitate classroom projection or online teaching.
- The PowerPoint Collection consists of nearly 600 text slides, which have been revised and updated for this edition. The slides may be used as-is, or adapted for classroom use or online presentation.

To obtain these resources, contact your Saunders-Elsevier Educational Sales Representative. If you don't know who your rep is, you can find out by checking the Sales Rep Locator at *us.elsevierhealth.com/replocator.jsp* or by calling Saunders-Elsevier Faculty Support at 1-800-222-9570.

Pharmacology Instruction Online

Our new online learning tool—*Pharmacology Online to Accompany Lehne: Pharmacology for Nursing Care,* fifth edition (ISBN 0-7216-0250-9)—consists of ready-to-use modules that work hand-in-hand with the textbook. The package features nine in-depth, case-based modules that promote "learning by doing," and cover such major topics as pharmacokinetics, pharmacodynamics, basic principles of neuropharmacology, and hypertension. In addition, the package has additional modules that address key topics through a variety of engaging, interactive learning activities. All modules can be customized to meet unique teaching needs. For more information, contact your Saunders-Elsevier sales representative, who can be identified by calling 1-800-222-9570 or logging on to *us.elsevierhealth.com/replocator.jsp.*

Study Guide

The *Study Guide* (ISBN 0-7216-0128-6) is completely new. It was created by Marshal Shlafer, PhD, a gifted teacher and writer from the University of Michigan. The *Study Guide* features innovative learning activities for each chapter of the text, delivered in a clever and engaging style that will help students learn essential content and prepare for licensure exams.

Mosby's Drug Consult

All faculty and students using *Pharmacology for Nursing Care,* fifth edition, are entitled to free basic-level access to *Mosby's Drug Consult Internet Edition,* a resource with information on new drug approvals, new indications for existing drugs, and drug safety notices. To access this resource, log on to *mosbysdrugconsult.com.*

YOUR COMMENTS ARE WELCOME

I'd like to hear from you. All feedback is welcome. Suggestions for improving the book are especially helpful, as are reports of mistakes (small or large) that you may spot. Of course, I'd also like to hear from readers who simply have something nice to say. You can reach me by e-mail at *lehne@adelphia.net* or by U.S. postal service care of Saunders-Elsevier.

Richard A. Lehne

Preface to the First Edition

Pharmacology pervades all phases of nursing practice and relates directly to patient care and patient education. Yet, despite its importance, pharmacology remains an area with which students, practicing nurses, and teachers are often uneasy. Much of this ill ease stems from traditional approaches to the subject, in which memorizing details takes precedence over understanding. In this text, the opposite approach is used. Here, the guiding principle is to establish a basic understanding of drugs, after which secondary details can be learned as needed.

I wrote this text with two major objectives. First, I want to help nursing students establish a knowledge base in the basic science of drugs. Second, I want to demonstrate how that knowledge can be directly applied in providing patient care and patient education. To achieve these goals, I have used several innovative techniques, which are described below.

Laying Foundations in Basic Principles. Understanding drugs requires a strong foundation in basic pharmacologic principles. To establish this foundation, major chapters are dedicated to the following topics: basic principles that apply to all drugs (Chapters 4 through 8), basic principles of drug therapy across the life-span (Chapters 9 through 11), basic principles of neuropharmacology (Chapter 12), basic principles of antimicrobial chemotherapy (Chapter 79), and basic principles of cancer chemotherapy (Chapter 97).

Reviewing Physiology and Pathophysiology. To understand the actions of a drug, we must first understand the biologic systems that the drug influences. For all major drug families, relevant physiology and pathophysiology are reviewed. In almost all cases, reviews are presented at the beginning of each chapter, rather than in a systems review at the beginning of a unit. This juxtaposition of pharmacology, physiology, and pathophysiology is designed to facilitate understanding of the relationships among these subjects.

Teaching Through Prototypes. Within each drug family, we can usually identify one agent whose features characterize all members of the group. Such a drug can be viewed as a prototype. Because other family members are very similar to the prototype, to know the prototype is to know the basic properties of all family members.

The benefits of teaching through prototypes can be appreciated with an example. Let's consider the nonsteroidal anti-inflammatory drugs (NSAIDs), a family that includes aspirin, ibuprofen [Motrin, others], naproxen [Naprosyn, Anaprox], celecoxib [Celebrex], and more than 20 other drugs. Traditionally, information on these drugs is presented in a series of paragraphs describing each drug in turn. When attempting to study from such a list, students are likely to learn many drug names and little else; the important concept of similarity among family members is easily lost. In this text, the family prototype—aspirin—is discussed first and in depth. After this,

instruction is completed by pointing out the relatively minor ways in which individual NSAIDs differ from aspirin. Not only is this approach more efficient than the traditional approach, but also is more effective, in that similarities among family members are emphasized.

Large Print and Small Print: A Way to Focus on Essentials. Pharmacology is exceptionally rich in detail. There are many drug families, each with multiple members and each member with its own catalogue of indications, contraindications, adverse effects, and drug interactions. This abundance of detail confronts teachers with the difficult question of what to teach, and confronts students with the equally difficult question of what to study. Attempts to answer these questions can frustrate teachers and students alike. Even worse, in the presence of myriad details, basic concepts can be obscured.

To help focus on essentials, this text employs two sizes of type. Large type is intended to say, "On your first exposure to this topic, this is the core of information you should learn." Small type is intended to say, "Here is additional information that you may want to learn after mastering the material in large type." As a rule, large print is reserved for prototypes, basic principles of pharmacology, and reviews of physiology and pathophysiology. Small print is used for secondary information about the prototypes and for discussion of drugs that are not prototypes. This technique allows the book to contain a large body of detail without having that detail cloud the big picture. Furthermore, because the technique highlights essentials, it minimizes questions about what to teach and what to study.

The use of large and small print is especially valuable for discussing adverse effects and drug interactions. Most drugs are associated with many adverse effects and interactions. As a rule, however, only a few of these are noteworthy. In traditional texts, practically all adverse effects and interactions are presented, creating long and tedious lists. In this text, those few adverse effects and interactions that are especially characteristic are highlighted through presentation in large print; the remainder are noted briefly in small print. The net result? Rather than overwhelming students with a long and forbidding list, this text delineates a moderate body of information that's truly important, and thereby greatly facilitates comprehension.

Nursing Implications: Demonstrating the Application of Pharmacology to Nursing Practice. The principal reason for asking a nursing student to learn pharmacology is to enhance his or her ability to provide patient care and education. To show students how pharmacologic knowledge can be applied to nursing practice, nursing implications are *integrated into the body of each chapter.* That is, as specific drugs and drug families are discussed, the nursing implications inherent in the pharmacologic information are discussed side-by-side with the basic science. To facilitate access to nursing information, nursing implications are also *summarized at the end of most chapters*. These summaries serve to reinforce the information presented in the main text.

In chapters that are especially brief or that address drugs that are infrequently used, summaries of nursing implications have been omitted. However, even in these chapters, nursing implications are incorporated into the chapter body.

A Note About Drug Therapy. Throughout this text, as we discuss specific drug families (e.g., beta-adrenergic blockers), we discuss the clinical applications of those drugs. Similarly, in chapters that focus on specific diseases (e.g., Parkinson's disease, hypertension), we indicate which drugs are generally considered most appropriate for treatment. However, it is important to note that clinical applications of individual drugs often change over time: A drug may acquire new indications that are not discussed here, or it may cease to be used for indications that *are* discussed here. Likewise, drug therapy of specific diseases is continually evolving: As clinical experience expands and superior drugs are developed, the list of preferred drugs can change. Accordingly, although the drug therapies presented in this text reflect a general consensus on what

is considered best *today*, these therapies may not be considered best a few years from now—and, in therapeutic areas where there is controversy or where change is especially rapid, the treatments discussed here may be considered inappropriate by some clinicians right now.

About Dosage Calculations. Unlike many nursing pharmacology texts, this one has no section on dosage calculation. Why this departure from tradition? First, adequate discussion of this important subject simply isn't feasible in a text dedicated to the basic science of drugs; the amount of space that can be allotted is too small. Second, thanks to the availability of several excellent publications on the subject (e.g., Drug Calculations, 7th Edition: Process & Problems for Clinical Practice), there is no need to include this information in a pharmacology text.

Ways to Use This Textbook. Because of its focus on essentials, this text is especially well suited to serve as the primary text for a course dedicated specifically to pharmacology. In addition, the book's focused approach makes it a valuable resource for pharmacologic instruction within an integrated curriculum and for self-directed learning by students, teachers, and practitioners.

Richard A. Lehne

Acknowledgments

I want to begin by thanking everyone involved at my extended publishing family, which now encompasses W.B. Saunders, Mosby, and Elsevier Health Sciences. Since 1985, these good people have given me support, encouragement, and guidance, along with the latitude to write the book I wanted to. For this edition, five individuals deserve special mention:

- Robin Carter, now executive publisher (formerly my acquisitions editor), embodies a refreshing blend of strength, warmth, and humor. In addition, she has conflict resolution skills to rival those of Jimmy Carter. Her only fault? Owing to a lamentable instability, at times she's been downright hard to find (over the past few years, publishing's gift to realtors has lived in no fewer than four locations: Philadelphia, Tucson, Phoenix, and, [now permanently?] St. Louis).

- Lee Henderson, the project's managing editor, did more than I'll likely ever know. He lined up reviewers, kept track of my progress, provided support as needed, and attended to the myriad details that precede and follow production. However, perhaps his greatest contribution was to ensure that my stress level never dropped to the tolerable range (by calling at least twice a day to remind me that being even a teeny bit more on schedule would be highly appreciated). Oh, did I mention that Lee's not only good at his job, but also a very likable guy with whom I've enjoyed working for two editions?

- Marie Thomas, Lee's editorial assistant, had the unglamorous (but nonetheless essential) job of receiving, logging, and photocopying nearly 2000 pages of manuscript, so that other members of the team would have grist for their mills She also filled in for Lee whenever duty called. More importantly, Marie shared her compassion, insight, and keen wit, thereby making the few dark hours of this project considerably brighter.

- Celeste Clingan coordinated production and Catherine Jackson (Celeste's boss) kept a watchful eye on the process. More about them in a moment.

When the manuscript was nearly done (or so I thought), the book went into production, a painstaking process that carries a high risk of frayed nerves, strained relationships, and perforated ulcers—but not this time! Everyone involved contributed superb work, for which I am warmly and hugely grateful. How good was their work? So good that I hope the entire team will reconvene for the next edition (a sentiment I've never expressed before). And why was this team so good? Credit and appreciation go entirely to Catherine Jackson—publishing services manager—who used her considerable influence and experience to secure the best people available. Also, whenever *big* problems arose, Catherine brokered a solution. I want to extend special thanks to Celeste Clingan, our project manager. Throughout production, she remained cheerful, enthusiastic, surprisingly calm, and remarkably accommodating (we even conspired to make design changes on the fly, but don't tell anyone). Of greatest importance, she did everything necessary to ensure that the book in your hand would meet her high standards of quality. Of course, Celeste could not have accomplished all this without the hard work of other team members— especially the incomparable Diane Wilson, who typeset the *entire* book, including tables, flawlessly. Amazing. (If you've never been an author protecting your book from typesetters, you cannot fully appreciate just how grateful I am to Diane.) Finally, I want to thank Cindy Geiss, who colorized the artwork that was carried over from the fourth edition, and created most of the new art for this edition.

And then there's Jeanne Allison. It was Jeanne's job to make sure the artwork actually got done (you know those artists). Also, it seemed that whenever Lee failed to make his daily phone calls, Jeanne would take up the slack, making deft but gentle thrusts with a poke-the-author stick of her own.

I want to thank two contributors, Alfred J. Rémillard, PhD and Alan P. Agins, PhD. Fred Rémillard created the appendix on Canadian drug information for the first edition of this book, and has revised it for each subsequent edition. For the fourth edition of this book, Alan Agins (along with yours truly) created the chapter on herbal supplements, which served as the foundation for the updated version that appears in this edition.

I am grateful for the helpful suggestions offered by five reviewers: Betty Ferrell, PhD, FAAN, who reviewed Chapter 28 (Pain Management in Patients with Cancer); Eugenia Fulcher, RN, BSN, EdD, CMA, Robert Fulcher, RPh, BSPL, and Natasha Leskovsek, RN, MBA, MPM, JD, who reviewed Chapter 57 (Drugs Related to Hypothalamic and Pituitary Function) and Chapter 62 (Drug Therapy of Infertility); and Joseph Schwartzman, MD, who reviewed *all* of the chapters on antimicrobial drugs.

Last, but surely not least, I want to thank all members of the Saunders/Mosby educational sales force, whose professionalism and determination have contributed immeasurably to the book's success.

Rich Lehne

Detailed Table of Contents

III   DRUG THERAPY ACROSS THE LIFESPAN

IV   PERIPHERAL NERVOUS SYSTEM DRUGS

IX   WOMEN'S HEALTH

XIX ALTERNATIVE THERAPY

XX TOXICOLOGY

APPENDIXES

Orientation to Pharmacology

If you are like most students reading this text, by this point in your life you've been hitting the books for 15 years or more and have probably asked yourself, "What's the purpose of all this education?" In the past your question may have lacked a satisfying answer. Happily, now you have one: The reason you've spent most of your life in school was to get ready to study pharmacology!

There's good reason why you haven't approached pharmacology before now. Pharmacology is a science that draws on information from multiple disciplines, including anatomy, physiology, psychology, chemistry, and microbiology. Consequently, before you could begin your study of pharmacology, you had to become familiar with these other sciences. Now that you've established the requisite knowledge base, you're finally ready to learn about drugs.

FOUR BASIC TERMS

At this point it will help to define four basic terms: *drug, pharmacology, clinical pharmacology,* and *therapeutics.* As we go through these definitions, we will also discuss the principal kinds of information this text will focus on.

Drug. A drug is defined as *any chemical that can affect living processes.* By this definition, virtually all chemicals can be considered drugs, since, when given in large enough amounts, all chemicals will have some effect on life. Clearly, it is beyond the scope of this text to consider all compounds that fit the definition of a drug. Accordingly, rather than studying all drugs, we will limit discussion to those drugs that have therapeutic applications.

Pharmacology. Pharmacology can be defined as *the study of drugs and their interactions with living systems.* Given this

definition, the science of pharmacology can claim a huge body of knowledge as its own. Under our definition, pharmacology encompasses the study of the physical and chemical properties of drugs as well as their biochemical and physiologic effects. In addition, pharmacology includes knowledge of the history, sources, and uses of drugs as well as knowledge of drug absorption, distribution, metabolism, and excretion. Since pharmacology encompasses such a broad spectrum of information, it would be inappropriate (not to mention impossible) to address the entire scope of pharmacology in this text. Consequently, we will restrict consideration to information that is clinically relevant.

Clinical Pharmacology. Clinical pharmacology is defined as *the study of drugs in humans.* This discipline includes the study of drugs in *patients* as well as in *healthy volunteers* (during new drug development). Since clinical pharmacology encompasses all aspects of the interaction between drugs and people, and since our primary interest is the use of drugs to treat patients, clinical pharmacology includes some information that will be outside the scope of this text.

Therapeutics. Therapeutics, also known as *pharmacotherapeutics,* is defined as *the use of drugs to diagnose, prevent, or treat disease or to prevent pregnancy.* Alternatively, therapeutics can be defined simply as *the medical use of drugs.*

In this text, therapeutics will be our principal concern. That is, discussions will focus largely on the basic science information needed to understand the use of drugs as therapeutic agents. This information should help you understand how drugs produce their effects—both therapeutic and adverse; the reasons for giving a particular drug to a particular patient; and the rationale underlying selection of dosage, route, and schedule of administration. In addition, knowledge of pharmacology will help you understand the strategies employed to promote beneficial drug effects and to minimize undesired effects. It is my hope that, by applying this knowledge, you will provide optimal patient care and education. It is also my hope that your knowledge of pharmacology will render working with medications less mysterious and therefore more gratifying.

PROPERTIES OF AN IDEAL DRUG

If we were developing a new drug, we would want that drug to be as good as possible. In order to approach perfection, our new drug should have certain properties, such as *effectiveness and safety.* In the discussion below, we consider the characteristics that an ideal drug might possess. I must stress, however, that the ideal medication exists only in theory; in reality, *there is no such thing as a perfect drug.* The truth of this statement will become apparent as we consider the properties that an ideal drug should have.

The Big Three: Effectiveness, Safety, and Selectivity

The three most important characteristics that any drug can have are effectiveness, safety, and selectivity.

Effectiveness. An effective drug is one that elicits the responses for which it is given. *Effectiveness is the most important property a drug can have.* Regardless of its other virtues, if a drug is not effective—that is, if it doesn't do anything useful—there is no justification for giving it. Current U.S. law requires that all new drugs be proved effective prior to release for marketing.

Safety. A safe drug is defined as one that cannot produce harmful effects—even if administered in very high doses and for a very long time. *There is no such thing as a safe drug.* All drugs have the ability to cause injury, especially with higher doses. The chances of producing adverse effects can be reduced by proper drug selection and proper dosing. However, the risk of adverse effects can never be eliminated. The following examples illustrate this point:

- Certain anticancer drugs (e.g., cyclophosphamide, methotrexate), at usual therapeutic doses, always increase the risk of serious infection.
- Opioid analgesics (e.g., morphine, meperidine), at high therapeutic doses, can cause potentially fatal respiratory depression.
- Aspirin and related drugs, when taken chronically in high therapeutic doses, can cause life-threatening gastric ulceration, perforation, and bleeding.

Clearly, drugs are not safe. This fact may explain why the Greeks chose the word *pharmakon,* which can be translated as *poison,* as a name for these compounds.

Selectivity. A selective drug is defined as one that elicits only the response for which it is given. A selective drug would not produce side effects. *There is no such thing as a selective drug: All medications cause side effects.* Common examples include the drowsiness that can be caused by many antihistamines; the morning sickness, cramps, and depression that can be caused by oral contraceptives; and the sexual dysfunction (e.g., impotence, anorgasmia) commonly caused by fluoxetine [Prozac] and related antidepressants.

Additional Properties of an Ideal Drug

Reversible Action. For most drugs, it is important that effects be reversible. That is, in most cases, we want drug actions to subside within an appropriate time. General anesthetics, for example, would be useless if patients never woke up. Likewise, it is unlikely that oral contraceptives would find widespread acceptance if they caused permanent sterility. For a few drugs, most notably antibiotics and anticancer agents, reversibility is not a desirable characteristic; with these compounds, we want their toxicity to target cells to endure.

Predictability. It would be very helpful if, prior to drug administration, we could know with certainty just how a given patient will respond. Unfortunately, since each patient is unique, the accuracy of such predictions cannot be guaranteed. Accordingly, in order to maximize the chances of eliciting desired responses, we must tailor therapy to the individual.

Ease of Administration. An ideal drug should be simple to administer: the route should be convenient, and the number of doses per day should be low. Diabetic patients, who face a lifetime of multiple insulin injections each day, are not likely to judge this drug ideal. Likewise, drugs that require intravenous infusion are rarely considered ideal by the nurse who must set up the infusion apparatus and monitor its function.

In addition to convenience, ease of administration has two other benefits: (1) it can enhance patient adherence and (2) it can decrease errors in drug administration. Patients are more likely to adhere to a dosing schedule that consists of once-a-day administration than to one that requires several daily doses. Similarly, hospital personnel are less likely to commit medication errors when administering oral drugs than when preparing and administering intravenous formulations.

Freedom from Drug Interactions. When a patient is taking two or more drugs, those drugs can interact with one another. These interactions may either augment or reduce drug responses. For example, respiratory depression caused by diazepam [Valium], which is normally minimal, can be greatly *intensified* by alcohol. Conversely, the antibacterial effects of tetracycline can be greatly *reduced* by taking iron or calcium supplements. Because of the potential for interactions among drugs, when a patient is taking more than one agent, the possible impact of drug interactions must be considered. An ideal drug would not interact with other agents. Unfortunately, few medicines are devoid of significant interactions.

Low Cost. An ideal drug would be easy to afford. The cost of drugs can be a substantial financial burden. As an extreme example, 1 year of therapy with human growth hormone (somatrem) costs between $10,000 and $20,000. More commonly, expense becomes a significant factor when a medication must be taken chronically. For example, people with hypertension, arthritis, or diabetes must take medications lifelong. The cumulative expense of such treatment can be huge—even for drugs of moderate price.

Chemical Stability. Some drugs lose effectiveness during storage. Others, which may be stable on the shelf, can rapidly lose effectiveness when put into solution (e.g., in preparation for infusion). These losses in efficacy result from chemical instability. Because of chemical instability, stocks of certain drugs must be periodically discarded. An ideal drug would retain its activity indefinitely, both on the shelf and in solution.

Possession of a Simple Generic Name. Generic names of drugs are usually complex, and therefore difficult to remember and pronounce. As a rule, the trade name for a drug is simpler than its generic name. Examples of drugs that have complex generic names and simple trade names include sildenafil [Viagra], acetaminophen [Tylenol], and ciprofloxacin [Cipro]. Since generic names are preferable to trade names (for reasons discussed in Chapter 3), an ideal drug should have a generic name that is easy to recall and pronounce.

Because No Drug Is Ideal . . .

From the preceding, we can see that available medications are not ideal. No drug is safe. All drugs produce side effects. Drug responses may be difficult to predict and altered by drug interactions. Drugs may be expensive, unstable, and hard to administer. Because medications are not ideal, all members of the healthcare team must exercise care to promote therapeutic effects and minimize drug-induced harm.

THE THERAPEUTIC OBJECTIVE

The objective of drug therapy is to provide maximum benefit with minimum harm. If drugs were ideal, we could achieve this objective with relative ease. However, since drugs are not ideal, we must exercise skill and care if treatment is to result in more good than harm. As detailed in Chapter 2, you, as a nurse, have a critical responsibility in achieving the therapeutic objective. In order to meet this responsibility, you must understand drugs. The primary purpose of this text is to help you gain that understanding.

FACTORS THAT DETERMINE THE INTENSITY OF DRUG RESPONSES

Multiple factors determine how an individual will respond to a prescribed dose of a particular drug (Fig. 1–1). By understanding these factors, you will be able to think rationally about how drugs produce their effects. As a result, you will be able to contribute maximally to achieving the therapeutic objective.

Our ultimate concern when administering a drug is the intensity of the response. Working our way up from the bottom of Figure 1–1, we can see that the intensity of the response is determined ultimately by the concentration of the drug at its sites of action. As the figure suggests, the primary determinant of this concentration is the administered dose. When administration is performed correctly, the dose that was given will bear a close relationship to the dose that was prescribed. The steps leading from prescribed dose to intensity of the response are considered below.

Administration

Dosage size and the route and timing of administration are important determinants of drug responses. Accordingly, the prescribing clinician will consider these variables with care. Unfortunately, because of poor patient compliance and med-ication errors by hospital staff, drugs are not always administered as prescribed. The result may be toxicity (if the dosage is too high) or treatment failure (if the dosage is too low). To help minimize errors caused by poor compliance, you should give patients complete instruction about their medication and how to take it.

Medication errors made by hospital staff may result in a drug being administered by the wrong route, in the wrong dose, or at the wrong time; the patient may even be given the wrong drug. These errors can be made by pharmacists, physicians, and nurses. Any of these errors will detract from achieving the therapeutic objective.

Pharmacokinetics

Pharmacokinetic processes determine how much of an administered dose gets to its sites of action. There are four major pharmacokinetic processes: (1) drug absorption, (2) drug distribution, (3) drug metabolism, and (4) drug excretion. Collectively, these processes can be thought of as the *impact of the body on drugs*. The pharmacokinetic processes are discussed at length in Chapter 4.

Pharmacodynamics

Once a drug has reached its site of action, pharmacodynamic processes determine the nature and intensity of the response. Pharmacodynamics can be thought of as the *impact of drugs on the body*. In most cases, the initial step leading to a response is the binding of a drug to its receptor. This drug-receptor interaction is followed by a sequence of events that ultimately results in a response. As indicated in Figure 1–1, the patient's "functional state" can influence pharmacodynamic processes. For example, a patient who has developed tolerance to morphine will respond less intensely to a particular dose than will a patient who lacks tolerance. Placebo (psychologic) effects also help determine the responses that a drug elicits. Pharmacodynamics is discussed at length in Chapter 5.

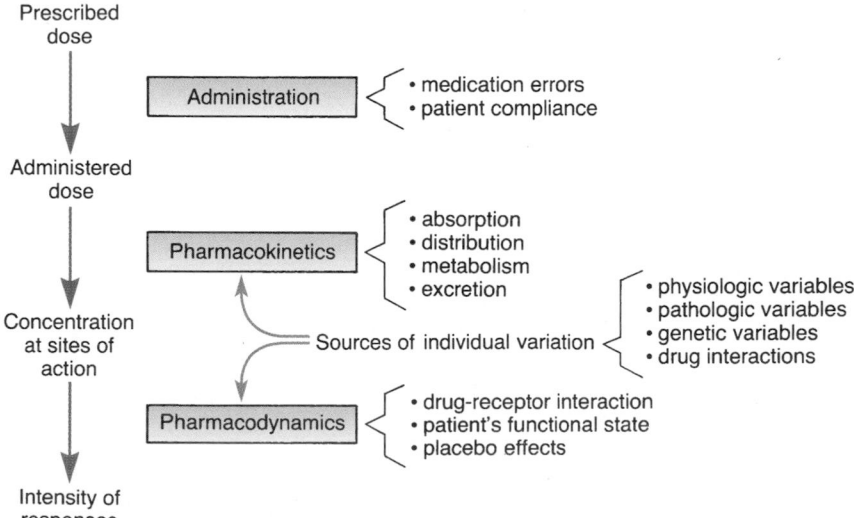

Figure 1–1 ■ **Factors that determine the intensity of drug responses.** (Adapted from Koch-Weser J. Drug therapy: Serum drug concentrations as therapeutic guides. N Engl J Med 1972;287:227.)

Sources of Individual Variation

Characteristics unique to each patient can influence pharmacokinetic and pharmacodynamic processes and, by doing so, can help determine the patient's response to a drug. As indicated in Figure 1–1, sources of individual variation include drug interactions; physiologic variables (e.g., age, gender, weight); pathophysiologic variables (especially diminished function of the kidneys and liver, the major organs of drug elimination); and genetic variables. Genetic factors can alter the metabolism of drugs and can predispose the patient to unique drug reactions. Because individuals differ from one another, no two patients will respond identically to the same drug regimen. Accordingly, if the therapeutic objective is to be achieved, it is essential that drug therapy be matched to the individual. Individual variation in drug responses is the subject of Chapter 8.

SUMMARY

Whenever medicines are used, our goal is to promote desired effects and minimize adverse effects. In order to achieve this objective, we need to understand pharmacokinetics and pharmacodynamics, the principal determinants of drug responses. In addition, we must account for potential sources of individual variation in drug responses. When all of these considerations are made, the regimen will be tailored to the individual, and hence should produce maximum benefit with minimum harm.

⣿ KEY POINTS

- The most important properties of an ideal drug are effectiveness, safety, and selectivity.
- If a drug is not effective, it should not be used.
- There is no such thing as a safe drug: All drugs can cause harm.
- There is no such thing as a selective drug: All drugs can cause side effects.
- The objective of drug therapy is to provide maximum benefit with minimum harm.
- Because all patients are unique, drug therapy must be tailored to each individual.

Application of Pharmacology in Nursing Practice

My principal goal in this chapter is to answer the question "Why should a nursing student learn about drugs?" By addressing this question, I hope to give you some extra motivation to study pharmacology. Why? Because I have known many students who, at the beginning of a pharmacology course, question the value of learning the material. Hopefully, when you complete the chapter, you will be convinced that understanding drugs is essential for nursing practice and, therefore, that putting time and effort into learning about drugs will be a worthwhile investment. If you are already convinced that understanding pharmacology is important, then just scan the chapter quickly. However, if you are skeptical, then read the chapter carefully. Hopefully, doing so will help you see the light, and thereby boost your motivation for the job ahead.

EVOLUTION OF NURSING RESPONSIBILITIES REGARDING DRUGS

At one time, a nurse's responsibility regarding medications focused mainly on the *Five Rights of Drug Administration,* namely, give the *right drug* to the *right patient* in the *right dose* by the *right route* at the *right time.* Clearly, the Five Rights are important. However, although these basics are essential, much more is required if the therapeutic objective is to be achieved. The Five Rights guarantee only that a drug will be administered as prescribed. Correct administration, without additional interventions, cannot ensure that treatment will result in maximum benefit and minimum harm.

The limitations of the Five Rights can be illustrated with this analogy: The nurse who sees his or her responsibility as being over following correct drug administration would be like a baseball pitcher who felt that his responsibility was over once he had thrown the ball toward the batter. As the pitcher must be ready to respond to the consequences of the interaction between ball and bat, the nurse must be poised to respond to the consequences of the interaction between drug and patient. Put another way, although both the nurse and the pitcher have a clear obligation to deliver their respective "pills" in the most appropriate fashion, proper delivery is only the beginning of their responsibilities: *Important events will take place after the "pill" is delivered, and these must be responded to.* Like the pitcher, the nurse can respond rapidly and effectively only by anticipating (knowing in advance) what the possible reactions to the pill might be.

In order to anticipate possible reactions, both the nurse and the pitcher require certain kinds of knowledge. Just as the pitcher must understand the abilities of the opposing batter, the nurse must understand the patient and the disorder for which he or she is being treated. As the pitcher must know the most appropriate pitch (e.g., fast ball, curve, slider) to deliver in specific circumstances, the nurse must know what medications are appropriate for the patient and must check to ensure that the medication ordered is among them. Conversely, as the pitcher must know what pitches *not* to throw at a particular batter, the nurse must know what drugs are *contraindicated* for the patient. As the pitcher must know the most likely outcome after the ball and bat interact, the nurse must know the probable consequences of the interaction between drug and patient.

Although this analogy is not perfect (the nurse and patient are on the same team, whereas the pitcher and batter are not), it does help us appreciate that the nurse's responsibility extends well beyond the Five Rights. Consequently, in addition to the limited information needed to administer drugs in accordance with the Five Rights, you must acquire a broad base of pharmacologic knowledge so as to contribute fully to achieving the therapeutic objective.

In drug therapy today, nurses, together with physicians and pharmacists, participate in a system of checks and balances designed to promote beneficial effects and minimize harm. Nurses are especially important within this system because it is the nurse—not the physician—who follows the patient's status most closely. As a result, you are likely to be the first member of the healthcare team to observe and evaluate drug responses, and to intervene if required. In order to observe and evaluate drug responses, and in order to intervene rapidly and appropriately, you must know *in advance* the responses that a medication is likely to elicit. Put another way, in order to provide professional care, you must understand drugs; the stronger your knowledge of pharmacology, the more you will be able to *anticipate* drug responses and not simply react to them after the fact.

Within our system of checks and balances, the nurse has an important role as patient advocate. It is your responsibility to detect mistakes made by pharmacists and physicians—and mistakes *will* be made. For example, the physician may overlook potential drug interactions, or may be unaware of alterations in the patient's status that would preclude use of a particular drug, or may select the correct drug but may order an inappropriate dosage or route of administration. Since it is the nurse who actually administers drugs, the nurse is the last person to check medications prior to administration. Consequently, you are the patient's last line of defense against medication errors. It is ethically and legally unacceptable for you to administer a drug that is harmful to the patient—even though the medication has been prescribed by a licensed physician and dispensed by a licensed pharmacist: In your role as patient advocate, you must protect the patient against medication errors made by other members of the healthcare team. In serving as patient advocate, it is impossible to know too much about drugs.

APPLICATION OF PHARMACOLOGY IN PATIENT CARE

The two major areas in which you can apply pharmacologic knowledge are patient care and patient education. Patient care is considered in this section. Patient education is considered in the following section. In discussing the applications of pharmacology in patient care, we will focus on seven aspects of drug therapy: (1) preadministration assessment, (2) dosage and administration, (3) evaluating and promoting therapeutic effects, (4) minimizing adverse effects, (5) minimizing adverse interactions, (6) making PRN decisions, and (7) managing toxicity.

Preadministration Assessment

All drug therapy begins with assessment of the patient. Assessment has three basic goals: (1) collecting baseline data needed to evaluate therapeutic and adverse responses, (2) identifying high-risk patients, and (3) assessing the patient's capacity for self-care. The first two goals are highly specific for each drug. Accordingly, we cannot achieve these goals without understanding pharmacology. The third goal applies generally to all drugs; hence, it does not usually require specific knowledge of the drug you are about to give. Preadministration assessment is discussed further under *Application of the Nursing Process in Drug Therapy.*

Collecting Baseline Data. Baseline data are needed to evaluate drug responses, both therapeutic and adverse. For example, if we plan to give a drug to lower blood pressure, we must know the patient's blood pressure prior to treatment. Without such baseline data, we would have no way of determining the effectiveness of our drug. Similarly, if we are planning to give a drug that can damage the liver, we need to obtain baseline liver function test counts in order to evaluate this potential toxicity. Obviously, in order to collect appropriate baseline data, we must first know the effects that our drug is likely to produce.

Identifying High-Risk Patients. Multiple factors can predispose an individual patient to adverse reactions from specific drugs. Important predisposing factors are pathophysiology (especially liver and kidney dysfunction), genetic factors, drug allergies, pregnancy, old age, and extreme youth.

Patients with penicillin allergy provide a dramatic example of those at risk: Giving penicillin to these people can kill them. Accordingly, whenever treatment with penicillin is under consideration, we must determine if the patient has had an allergic reaction to a penicillin in the past. If the patient has a history of penicillin allergy, an alternative antibiotic should be employed. If there is no effective alternative, facilities for managing a severe reaction should be in place before the drug is administered.

From the preceding example, we can see that, when we are planning drug therapy, we must identify patients who are at high risk of reacting adversely. The tools for identification are the patient history, physical examination, and laboratory tests. Of course, if identification is to be successful, you must know what to look for (i.e., you must know the factors that can increase the risk of severe reactions to the drug in question). Once the high-risk patient has been identified, we can take steps to reduce the risk. We might select an alternative drug, or, if no alternative is available, we can at least prepare in advance to manage a possible reaction.

Dosage and Administration

Earlier, we noted the Five Rights of Drug Administration and agreed on their importance. Although you can implement the Five Rights without a detailed knowledge of pharmacology, having such knowledge can help reduce your contribution to medication errors. Some examples will illustrate this point:

■ Certain drugs have more than one indication, and dosage may differ depending on which indication the drug is used for. Aspirin, for example, is given in low doses to relieve pain and in high doses to suppress inflammation (e.g., in patients with arthritis). If you don't know about these differences, you may administer too much aspirin to the patient with pain or too little to the patient with inflammation.

■ Many drugs can be administered by more than one route, and dosage may differ depending upon the route selected. Morphine, for example, may be administered by mouth or by injection (e.g., subcutaneous, intramuscular, intravenous). Oral doses are generally much larger than injected doses. Accordingly, if a large dose intended for oral use were to be mistakenly administered by injection, the result could prove fatal. The nurse who understands the pharmacology of morphine is unlikely to make this error.

■ Certain intravenous agents can cause severe local injury if the line through which they are being infused becomes extravasated. Accordingly, when such drugs are given, special care must be taken to prevent extravasation. The infusion must be monitored closely, and, if extravasation occurs, corrective steps must be taken immediately to minimize harm. The nurse who doesn't understand these drugs will be unprepared to work with them safely.

The following basic guidelines can help ensure correct administration:

■ Read the medication order carefully. If the order is unclear, verify it with the prescribing physician.
■ Verify the identity of the patient by comparing the name on the wristband with the name on the drug order or administration record.
■ Read the medication label carefully. Verify the identity of the drug, the amount of drug (per tablet, volume of liquid, etc.), and its suitability for administration by the intended route.
■ Verify dosage calculations.
■ Implement any special handling the drug may require.
■ Don't administer any drug if you don't understand the reason for its use.

Evaluating and Promoting Therapeutic Effects

Evaluating Therapeutic Responses. Evaluation is one of the most important aspects of drug therapy. After all, this is the process that tells us whether or not our drug is doing anything useful. Because the nurse follows the patient's status most closely, the nurse is in the best position to evaluate therapeutic responses.

In order to make an evaluation, you must know the rationale for treatment and the nature and time course of the intended response. If you lack this knowledge, you will be unable to evaluate the patient's progress. When beneficial responses develop as hoped for, ignorance of expected effects might not be so bad. However, when desired responses do not occur, it may be essential to identify the failure quickly, since timely implementation of alternative therapy may be needed.

When evaluating responses to a drug that has more than one application, you can do so only if you know the specific indication for which the medication is being used. Nifedipine, for example, is given for two cardiovascular disorders: hypertension and angina pectoris. When the drug is used to treat hypertension, you should monitor for a reduction in blood pressure. In contrast, when this drug is used to treat angina, you should monitor for a reduction in chest pain. Clearly, if you are to make the proper evaluation, you must understand the reason for drug use.

Promoting Compliance. Drugs can be of great value to patients, but only if they are taken correctly. Drugs that are self-administered in the wrong dose, by the wrong route, or at the wrong time cannot produce maximum benefit—and may

even prove harmful. Obviously, successful therapy requires active and informed participation by the patient. By educating patients about the drugs they are taking, you can help elicit the required participation.

Implementing Nondrug Measures. Drug therapy can often be enhanced by nonpharmacologic measures. Examples include (1) enhancing drug therapy of asthma through breathing exercises, biofeedback, and emotional support; (2) enhancing drug therapy of arthritis through exercise, physical therapy, and rest; and (3) enhancing drug therapy of hypertension through weight reduction, smoking cessation, and sodium restriction. As a nurse, you may provide these supportive measures directly, through patient education, or by coordinating the activities of other healthcare providers.

Minimizing Adverse Effects

All drugs have the potential to produce undesired effects. Common examples include gastric erosion caused by aspirin, sedation caused by antihistamines, hypoglycemia caused by insulin, and excessive fluid loss caused by diuretics. When drugs are employed properly, the incidence and severity of such effects can be reduced. Measures to reduce adverse effects include identifying high-risk patients through the patient history, ensuring proper administration through patient education, and forewarning patients about activities that might precipitate an adverse reaction.

When untoward effects cannot be avoided, discomfort and injury can often be minimized by appropriate intervention. For example, timely administration of glucose will prevent brain damage from insulin-induced hypoglycemia. In order to help reduce adverse effects, you must know the following about the drugs you're working with:

■ The major adverse effects that the drug can produce
■ The time when these reactions are likely to occur
■ Early signs that an adverse reaction is developing
■ Interventions that can minimize discomfort and harm

Minimizing Adverse Interactions

When a patient is taking two or more drugs, those drugs may interact with one another to diminish therapeutic effects or intensify adverse effects. For example, the ability of oral contraceptives to protect against pregnancy can be reduced by concurrent therapy with phenobarbital (an antiseizure drug), and the risk of thromboembolism from oral contraceptives can be increased by smoking cigarettes.

As a nurse, you can help reduce the incidence and intensity of adverse interactions in several ways. These include taking a thorough drug history, advising the patient to avoid over-the-counter drugs that can interact with the prescribed medication, monitoring for adverse interactions *known* to occur between the drugs the patient is taking, and being alert for as-yet *unknown* interactions.

Making PRN Decisions

A PRN medication order is one in which the nurse has discretion regarding how much drug to give and when to give it. (PRN is an abbreviation that stands for *pro re nata,* a Latin phrase meaning *as needed* or *as the occasion arises.*) PRN orders are most common for hypnotics (sleeping pills). In order to implement a PRN order rationally, you must know the reason for drug use and be able to assess the patient's medication needs. Clearly, the better your knowledge of pharmacology, the better your PRN decisions are likely to be.

Managing Toxicity

Some adverse drug reactions are extremely dangerous; if toxicity is not diagnosed early and responded to quickly, irreversible injury or death can result. In order to minimize harm, you must know the early signs of toxicity and the procedure for toxicity management.

APPLICATION OF PHARMACOLOGY IN PATIENT EDUCATION

In most cases, it is the nurse's responsibility to educate patients about medications. In your role as educator, you must give the patient the following information:

- Drug name and therapeutic category (e.g., penicillin: antibiotic)
- Dosage size
- Dosing schedule
- Route and technique of administration
- Expected therapeutic response and when it should develop
- Nondrug measures to enhance therapeutic responses
- Duration of treatment
- Method of drug storage
- Symptoms of major adverse effects, and measures to minimize discomfort and harm
- Major adverse drug-drug and drug-food interactions
- Whom to contact in the event of therapeutic failure, severe adverse reactions, or severe adverse interactions

In order to communicate this information effectively and accurately, you must first understand it. That is, to be a good drug educator, you must know pharmacology.

In the discussion below, we will consider the relationship between patient education and the following aspects of drug therapy: dosage and administration, promoting therapeutic effects, minimizing adverse effects, and minimizing adverse interactions.

Dosage and Administration

Drug Name. The patient should know the name of the medication he or she is taking. If the drug has been prescribed by trade name, the patient should be given its generic name too. This information will reduce the risk of overdose that can result when a patient fails to realize that two prescriptions that bear different names actually contain the same medicine.

Dosage Size and Schedule of Administration. Patients must be told how much drug to take and when to take it. For some medications, dosage must be adjusted by the patient. Insulin provides a good example. For insulin therapy to be truly successful, the patient must adjust doses to accommodate alterations in caloric intake. How to make this adjustment is taught by the nurse.

With PRN medications, the schedule of administration is not fixed. Rather, these drugs are taken as conditions require. For example, some people with asthma experience exercise-induced bronchospasm. To minimize such attacks, these individuals can take supplementary medication prior to anticipated exertion. It is your responsibility to teach patients when PRN drugs should be taken.

The patient should know what to do if a dose is missed. With oral contraceptives, for example, if one dose is missed, the omitted dose should be taken together with the next scheduled dose. However, if three or more doses are missed, a new cycle of administration must be initiated.

Some patients have difficulty remembering whether or not they have taken their medication. Possible causes include mental illness, advanced age, and complex regimens. To facilitate accurate dosing, you can provide the patient with a pill box that has separate compartments for each day of the week, and then teach him or her to load the compartments weekly. To determine if they have taken their medicine, patients can simply examine the box.

Technique of Administration. Patients must be taught how to administer their drugs. This is especially important for routes that may be unfamiliar (e.g., sublingual for nitroglycerin) and for techniques that are difficult (e.g., subcutaneous injection of insulin). Patients taking oral medications may require special instructions. For example, some oral preparations must not be chewed or crushed; some should be taken with fluids; and some should be taken with meals, whereas others should not. Careful attention must be paid to the patient who, because of disability (e.g., visual or intellectual impairment, limited manual dexterity), may find self-medication difficult.

Duration of Drug Use. Just as patients must know when to take their medicine, they must know when to stop. In some cases (e.g., treatment of acute pain), patients should discontinue drug use as soon as symptoms subside. In other cases (e.g., treatment of hypertension), patients should know that therapy will probably continue lifelong. For other conditions (e.g., gastric ulcers), medication may be prescribed for a specific time interval, after which the patient should return for re-evaluation.

Drug Storage. Certain medications are chemically unstable and hence deteriorate rapidly if stored improperly. Patients who are using unstable drugs must be taught how to store them correctly (e.g., under refrigeration, in a light-proof container). All drugs should be stored where children can't reach them.

Promoting Therapeutic Effects

In order to participate fully in achieving the therapeutic objective, patients must know the nature and time course of expected beneficial effects. With this knowledge, patients can help evaluate the success or failure of treatment. By recognizing treatment failure, the informed patient will be able to seek timely implementation of alternative therapy.

With some drugs, such as those used to treat depression and schizophrenia, beneficial effects are delayed, taking weeks or months to develop. Awareness that treatment may not produce immediate results allows the patient to have realistic expectations and helps reduce anxiety about therapeutic failure.

As noted above, nondrug measures can complement drug therapy. For example, although drugs are useful in managing adult-onset diabetes, exercise and caloric restriction are at least as important. Teaching the patient about nondrug measures can greatly increase the chances of success.

Minimizing Adverse Effects

Knowledge of adverse drug effects will enable the patient to avoid some adverse effects and minimize others through early detection. The following examples should underscore the value of educating patients about the undesired drug effects:

- Insulin overdose can cause blood glucose levels to drop precipitously. Early signs of hypoglycemia include sweating and increased heart rate. The patient who has been taught to recognize these early signs can respond by ingesting glucose-rich foods, thereby restoring blood sugar to a safe level. In contrast, the patient who fails to recognize evolving hypoglycemia and does not ingest glucose may become comatose, and may even die.
- Many anticancer drugs predispose patients to acquiring serious infections. The patient who is aware of this possibility can take steps to avoid contagion (e.g., avoiding contact with people who have an infection; avoiding foods likely to contain pathogens). In addition, the informed patient is in a position to notify the physician at the first sign that an infection is developing, thereby allowing rapid treatment. In contrast, the patient who has not received adequate education is at increased risk of illness or death from an infectious disease.
- Some side effects, although benign, can be disturbing if they occur without warning. For example, rifampin (a drug for tuberculosis) imparts a harmless red-orange color to urine, sweat, saliva, and tears. Your patient will appreciate knowing about this effect in advance.

Minimizing Adverse Interactions

Patient education can help avoid hazardous drug-drug and drug-food interactions. For example, phenelzine (an antidepressant) can cause dangerous elevations in blood pressure if taken in combination with certain drugs (e.g., amphetamines) or certain foods (e.g., figs, avocados, most cheeses). Accordingly, it is essential that patients taking phenelzine be given explicit and emphatic instruction regarding the drugs and foods they must avoid.

APPLICATION OF THE NURSING PROCESS IN DRUG THERAPY

The nursing process is a conceptual framework that nurses employ to guide healthcare delivery. In this section we consider how the nursing process can be applied in drug therapy.

Review of the Nursing Process

Before discussing the nursing process as it applies to drug therapy, we need to review the process itself. Since you are probably familiar with the process already, this review will be brief.

In its simplest form, the nursing process can be viewed as a cyclic procedure that has five basic steps: (1) assessment, (2) analysis (including nursing diagnoses), (3) planning, (4) implementation, and (5) evaluation.

Assessment. Assessment consists of collecting data about the patient. These data are used to identify actual and potential health problems. The database established during assessment provides a foundation for subsequent steps in the process. Important methods of data collection are the patient interview, medical and drug-use histories, the physical examination, observation of the patient, and laboratory tests.

Analysis: Nursing Diagnoses. In this step, the nurse analyzes the database to determine actual and potential health problems. These problems may be physiologic, psychologic, or sociologic. Each problem is stated in the form of a *nursing diagnosis,* which can be defined as an actual or potential health problem that nurses are qualified and licensed to treat.

A complete nursing diagnosis consists of two statements: (1) a statement of the patient's actual or potential health problem, followed by (2) a statement of the problem's probable cause or risk factors. Typically, the statements are separated by the phrase *related to,* as in this example of a drug-associated nursing diagnosis: "noncompliance with the prescribed regimen [the problem] related to inability to self-administer medication [the cause]."

Planning. In the planning step, the nurse delineates specific interventions directed at solving or preventing the problems identified in analysis. The plan must be individualized for each patient. When creating a care plan, the nurse must define goals, set priorities, identify nursing interventions, and establish criteria for evaluating success. In addition to nursing interventions, the plan should include interventions performed by other healthcare providers. Planning is an ongoing process that must be modified as new data are gathered.

Implementation (Intervention). Implementation begins with carrying out the interventions identified during planning. Some interventions are collaborative while others are independent. Collaborative interventions require a physician's order, whereas independent interventions do not. In addition to carrying out interventions, implementation involves coordinating actions of other members of the healthcare team. Implementation is completed by observing and recording the outcomes of treatment. Records should be thorough and precise.

Evaluation. This step is performed to determine the degree to which treatment has succeeded. Evaluation is accomplished by analyzing the data collected during implementation. Evaluation should identify those interventions that should be continued, those that should be discontinued, and potential new interventions that should be implemented. Evaluation completes the initial cycle of the nursing process and provides the basis for beginning the cycle anew.

Applying the Nursing Process in Drug Therapy

Having reviewed the nursing process itself, we can now discuss the process as it pertains to drug therapy. Recall that the overall objective in drug therapy is to produce maximum benefit with minimum harm. To accomplish this, we must take into account the unique characteristics of each patient. That is, we must individualize therapy. The nursing process is well suited to help us do this. As the discussion below indicates, in order to apply the nursing process in drug therapy, you must first have a solid knowledge base in pharmacology. You will also see that applying the nursing process to drug therapy is, in large part, an exercise in common sense.

Preadministration Assessment

Preadministration assessment establishes the baseline data needed to tailor drug therapy to the individual. By identifying the variables that can affect an individual's responses to drugs, we can adapt treatment so as to maximize benefits and minimize harm. Preadministration assessment has four basic goals:

- Collection of baseline data needed to evaluate therapeutic responses
- Collection of baseline data needed to evaluate adverse effects
- Identification of high-risk patients
- Assessment of the patient's capacity for self-care

The first three goals are specific to the particular drug being used. Accordingly, in order to achieve these goals, you must know the pharmacology of the drug under consideration. The fourth goal applies more or less equally to all drugs—although this goal may be more critical for some drugs than others.

Important methods of data collection include interviewing the patient and family, observing the patient, physical examination, laboratory tests, the patient's medical history, and the patient's drug history. The drug history should include prescription drugs, over-the-counter drugs, herbal medications, and drugs taken for nonmedical purposes (alcohol, nicotine, caffeine, illicit drugs). Prior adverse drug reactions should be noted, including drug allergies and idiosyncratic reactions.

Baseline Data Needed to Evaluate Therapeutic Effects. Drugs are administered to achieve a desired response. In order to know if we have produced that response, we need to establish baseline measurements of the parameter that therapy is directed at changing. For example, if we are giving a drug to lower blood pressure, we need to know what the patient's blood pressure was prior to treatment. Without this information, we have no basis for determining the effect of our drug. And if we can't determine whether or not a drug is working, there's little justification for giving it. From the above example, it should be obvious that, in order to know what baseline measurements to make, you must first know the reason for drug use. This knowledge comes from studying pharmacology.

Baseline Data Needed to Evaluate Adverse Effects. All drugs have the ability to produce undesired effects. In practically all cases, the adverse effects that a particular drug can produce are known. In many cases, development of an adverse effect will be completely obvious in the absence of any baseline data. For example, we don't need special baseline data to know that hair loss following cancer chemotherapy was caused by the drug. However, in other cases, baseline data are needed to determine whether or not an adverse effect has occurred. For example, some drugs can impair liver function. In order to know if a drug has disrupted liver function, we need to know the state of liver function prior to drug use. With-

out this information, we can't tell from later measurements whether apparent liver dysfunction was pre-existing or caused by the drug. Clearly, in cases like this, baseline data are needed. As noted earlier, knowing what data to collect comes directly from your knowledge of the drug under consideration.

Identification of High-Risk Patients. Because of his or her individual characteristics, a particular patient may be at high risk of experiencing an adverse response to a particular drug. Just which individual characteristics will predispose a patient to an adverse reaction depends on the drug under consideration. For example, if a drug is eliminated from the body primarily by renal excretion, an individual with impaired kidney function will be at risk of having this drug accumulate to a toxic level. Similarly, if a drug is eliminated by the liver, an individual with impaired liver function will be at risk of having that drug accumulate to a toxic level. The message here is that, in order to identify the patient at risk, you must know the pharmacology of the drug to be administered.

Multiple factors can increase the patient's risk of adverse reactions to a particular drug. Impaired liver and kidney function were just mentioned. Other factors include age, body composition, pregnancy, diet, genetic heritage, other drugs being used, and practically any pathophysiologic condition. These factors are discussed at length in Chapter 6 (Drug Interactions), Chapter 7 (Adverse Drug Reactions and Medication Errors), Chapter 8 (Individual Variation in Drug Responses), Chapter 9 (Drug Therapy During Pregnancy and Breast-Feeding), Chapter 10 (Drug Therapy in Pediatric Patients), and Chapter 11 (Drug Therapy in Geriatric Patients).

When identifying factors that put the patient at risk, you should distinguish between factors that put the patient at extremely high risk versus factors that put the patient at moderate or low risk. The terms *contraindication* and *precaution* can be used for this distinction. A *contraindication* is defined as a pre-existing condition that precludes use of a particular drug under all but the most desperate circumstances. For example, a previous severe allergic reaction to penicillin (which can be life threatening) would be a contraindication to using penicillin again—unless the patient has a life-threatening infection that cannot be controlled with other antibiotics. A *precaution*, by contrast, can be defined as a pre-existing condition that significantly increases the risk of an adverse reaction to a particular drug, but not to a degree that is life threatening. For example, a previous mild allergic reaction to penicillin would constitute a precaution to using this drug again. That is, the drug may be used, but greater than normal caution must be exercised. Preferably, an alternative drug would be selected.

Assessment of the Patient's Capacity for Self-Care. If drug therapy is to succeed, the outpatient must be willing and able to self-administer medication as prescribed. Accordingly, his or her capacity for self-care must be assessed. If assessment reveals that the patient is incapable of self-medication, alternative care must be arranged.

Multiple factors can affect the capacity for self-care and the probability of adhering to the prescribed regimen. Patients with reduced visual acuity or limited manual dexterity may be unable to self-medicate, especially if the technique of administration is complex. Patients with limited intellectual ability may be incapable of understanding or remembering what they are supposed to do. Patients with severe mental illness (e.g., depression, schizophrenia) may lack the understanding or motivation needed to self-medicate. Some patients may lack the money to pay for drugs. Others may fail to take medications as prescribed because of individual or cultural attitudes toward drugs. Among geriatric patients, the most common cause for failed self-medication is a conviction that the drug was simply not needed in the dosage prescribed. A thorough assessment will identify all of these factors, thereby enabling you to account for them when formulating nursing diagnoses and the patient care plan.

Analysis and Nursing Diagnoses

With respect to drug therapy, the analysis phase of the nursing process has three objectives. First, you must judge the appropriateness of the prescribed regimen. Second, you must identify potential health problems that the drug might cause. Third, you must determine the patient's capacity for self-care.

As the last link in the patient's chain of defense against inappropriate drug therapy, the nurse must analyze the data collected during assessment to determine if the proposed treatment has a reasonable likelihood of being effective and safe. This judgment is made by considering the medical diagnosis, the known actions of the prescribed drug, the patient's prior responses to the drug, and the presence of contraindications to the drug. You should question the drug's appropriateness if (1) the drug has no actions that are known to benefit individuals with the patient's medical diagnosis, (2) the patient failed to respond to the drug in the past, (3) the patient had a serious adverse reaction to the drug in the past, or (4) the patient has a condition or is using a drug that contraindicates the prescribed drug. If any of these conditions apply, you should consult with the prescribing physician to determine if the drug should be given.

Analysis must identify potential adverse effects and drug interactions. This is accomplished by synthesizing knowledge of the drug under consideration and the data collected during assessment. Knowledge of the drug itself will indicate adverse effects that practically all patients are likely to experience. Data on the individual patient will indicate additional adverse effects and interactions to which the particular patient is predisposed. Once potential adverse effects and interactions have been identified, pertinent nursing diagnoses can

be easily formulated. For example, if treatment is likely to cause respiratory depression, an appropriate nursing diagnosis would be "impaired gas exchange related to drug therapy." Table 2–1 presents additional examples of nursing diagnoses that can be readily derived from your knowledge of adverse effects and interactions that treatment may cause.

Analysis must characterize the patient's capacity for self-care. The analysis should indicate potential impediments to self-care (e.g., visual impairment, reduced manual dexterity, impaired cognitive function, insufficient understanding of the prescribed regimen) so that these factors can be addressed in the care plan. To varying degrees, nearly all patients will be unfamiliar with self-medication and the drug regimen. Accordingly, a nursing diagnosis applicable to almost every patient is "deficient knowledge related to the drug regimen."

Planning

Planning consists of defining goals, establishing priorities, identifying specific interventions, and establishing criteria for evaluating success. Good planning will allow you to promote beneficial drug effects. Of equal or greater importance, good planning will allow you to anticipate adverse effects—rather than react to them after the fact.

Defining Goals. In all cases, the goal of drug therapy is to produce maximum benefit with minimum harm. That is, we want to employ drugs in such a way as to maximize therapeutic responses while preventing or minimizing adverse reactions and interactions. The objective of planning is to formulate ways to achieve this goal.

Setting Priorities. This requires knowledge of the drug under consideration and the patient's unique characteristics—and even then, setting priorities can be difficult. Highest priority is given to life-threatening conditions (e.g., anaphylactic shock, ventricular fibrillation). These may be drug induced or the result of disease. High priority is also given to reactions that cause severe, acute discomfort and to reactions that can result in long-term harm. Since we cannot manage all problems simultaneously, less severe problems must wait until the patient and care provider have the time and resources to address them.

TABLE 2–1 ■ Examples of Nursing Diagnoses That Can Be Derived From Knowledge of Adverse Drug Effects		
Drug	**Adverse Effect**	**Related Nursing Diagnosis**
Amphetamine	CNS stimulation	Disturbed sleep pattern related to drug-induced CNS excitation
Aspirin	Gastric erosion	Pain related to aspirin-induced gastric erosion
Atropine	Urinary retention	Urinary retention related to drug therapy
Bethanechol	Stimulation of GI smooth muscle	Bowel incontinence related to drug-induced increase in bowel motility
Clonidine	Impotence	Sexual dysfunction related to drug-induced impotence
Cyclophosphamide	Reduction in white blood cell counts	Risk for infection related to drug-induced neutropenia
Digoxin	Dysrhythmias	Ineffective tissue perfusion related to drug-induced cardiac dysrhythmias
Furosemide	Excessive urine production	Deficient fluid volume related to drug-induced diuresis
Gentamicin	Damage to the eighth cranial nerve	Disturbed sensory perception: hearing impairment related to drug therapy
Glucocorticoids	Thinning of the skin	Impaired skin integrity related to drug therapy
Haloperidol	Involuntary movements	Low self-esteem related to drug-induced involuntary movements
Nitroglycerin	Hypotension	Risk for injury related to dizziness caused by drug-induced hypotension
Propranolol	Bradycardia	Decreased cardiac output related to drug-induced bradycardia
Warfarin	Spontaneous bleeding	Risk for injury related to drug-induced bleeding

CNS = central nervous system, GI = gastrointestinal.

Identifying Interventions. The heart of planning is identification of nursing interventions. These interventions can be divided into four major groups: (1) drug administration, (2) interventions to enhance therapeutic effects, (3) interventions to minimize adverse effects and interactions, and (4) patient education (which encompasses information in the first three groups).

When planning drug administration, you must consider dosage size and route of administration as well as less obvious factors, including timing of administration with respect to meals and with respect to administration of other drugs. Timing with respect to side effects is also important. For example, if a drug causes sedation, it may be desirable to give the drug at bedtime, rather than in the morning or during the day.

Nondrug measures can help promote therapeutic effects and should be included in the plan. For example, drug therapy of hypertension can be combined with weight loss (in obese patients), salt restriction, and smoking cessation.

Interventions to prevent or minimize adverse effects are of obvious importance. When planning these interventions, you should distinguish between reactions that develop quickly and reactions that are delayed. A few drugs can cause severe adverse reactions (e.g., anaphylactic shock) shortly after administration. When planning to administer such a drug, you should ensure that facilities for managing possible reactions are immediately available. Delayed reactions can often be minimized, if not avoided entirely. The plan should include interventions to do so.

Well-planned patient education is central to success. The plan should account for the patient's capacity to learn, and it should address the following: technique of administration, dosage size and timing, duration of treatment, method of drug storage, measures to promote therapeutic effects, and measures to minimize adverse effects. Patient education is discussed at length above.

Establishing Criteria for Evaluation. The need for objective criteria by which to measure desired drug responses is obvious: Without such criteria we could not determine if our drug was doing anything useful. As a result, we would have no rational basis for making dosage adjustments or for deciding how long treatment should last. If the drug is to be used on an outpatient basis, follow-up visits for evaluation should be planned.

Implementation

Implementation of the care plan in drug therapy has four major components: (1) drug administration, (2) patient education, (3) interventions to promote therapeutic effects, and (4) interventions to minimize adverse effects. These critical nursing activities are discussed at length above.

Evaluation

Over the course of drug therapy, the patient must be evaluated for (1) therapeutic responses, (2) adverse drug reactions and interactions, (3) compliance (adherence to the prescribed regimen), and (4) satisfaction with treatment. How frequently evaluations are performed depends on the expected time course of therapeutic and adverse effects. Like assessment, evaluation is based on laboratory tests, observation of the patient, physical examination, and patient interviews. The conclusions drawn during evaluation provide the basis for modifying nursing interventions and the drug regimen.

Therapeutic responses are evaluated by comparing the patient's current status with the baseline data. In order to evaluate treatment, you must know the reason for drug use, the criteria for success (as defined during planning), and the expected time course of responses (some drugs act within minutes, whereas others may take weeks or even months to produce beneficial effects).

The need to anticipate and evaluate adverse effects is self-evident. To make these evaluations, you must know which adverse effects are likely to occur, how they are manifested, and their probable time course. The method of monitoring is determined by the expected effect. For example, if hypotension is expected, blood pressure is monitored; if constipation is expected, bowel function is monitored; and so on. Since some adverse effects can be fatal in the absence of timely detection, it is impossible to overemphasize the importance of monitoring and being prepared for rapid intervention.

Evaluation of compliance is desirable in all patients—and is especially valuable when therapeutic failure occurs or when adverse effects are unexpectedly severe. Methods of evaluating compliance include measurement of plasma drug levels, interviewing the patient, and counting pills. The evaluation should determine if the patient understands when to take medication, what dosage to take, and the technique of administration.

Patient satisfaction with drug therapy increases quality of life and promotes compliance. If the patient is dissatisfied, an otherwise effective regimen may not be taken as prescribed. Factors that can cause dissatisfaction include unacceptable side effects, inconvenient dosing schedule, difficulty of administration, and high cost. When evaluation reveals dissatisfaction, an attempt should be made to alter the regimen to make it more acceptable.

Use of a Modified Nursing Process Format to Summarize Nursing Implications in This Text

Throughout this text, nursing implications are *integrated into the body of each chapter.* The reason for integrating nursing information with basic science information is to reinforce the relationship between pharmacologic knowledge and nursing practice. In addition to being integrated, nursing implications are *summarized at the end of most chapters.* The purpose of the summaries is to provide a concise and readily accessible reference on patient care and patient education related to specific drugs and drug families.

The format employed for summarizing nursing implications reflects the nursing process (Table 2–2). However, as you can see, we have modified the headings somewhat. This was done to accommodate the needs of pharmacology instruction and to keep the summaries concise. The components of the format are discussed below.

Preadministration Assessment. This section summarizes the information you should have before giving a drug. Each section begins by stating the reason for drug use. This is followed by a summary of the baseline data needed to evaluate therapeutic and adverse effects. After this, contraindications and precautions are summarized, under the heading *Identifying High-Risk Patients.*

Implementation: Administration. This section summarizes routes of administration, guidelines for dosage adjust-

TABLE 2–2 ■ Modified Nursing Process Format for Summaries of Nursing Implications
Preadministration Assessment
Therapeutic Goal
Baseline Data
Identifying High-Risk Patients
Implementation: Administration
Routes
Administration
Implementation: Measures to Enhance Therapeutic Effects
Ongoing Evaluation and Interventions
Summary of Monitoring
Evaluating Therapeutic Effects
Minimizing Adverse Effects
Minimizing Adverse Interactions
Managing Toxicity

since nursing diagnoses can be readily formulated from one's knowledge of pharmacology, and since a long list of diagnoses would dilute the impact of other important information, we decided to omit nursing diagnoses from the summaries.

Planning has not been used as a heading for three reasons. First, planning applies primarily to the overall management of the disorder for which a particular drug is being used—and much less to the drug itself. Second, since planning is discussed at length and more appropriately in nonpharmacology nursing texts, such as those on medical-surgical nursing, there is no need to repeat this information here. Third, most planning is done with the aid of standardized nursing care plans—either computerized or in print format. These standardized plans are sufficient for most drug-related planning. Please note, however, that although we don't have a separate heading for planning, critical issues in planning are nonetheless included.

ment, and special considerations in administration, such as timing with respect to meals, preparation of intravenous solutions, and unusual techniques of administration.

Implementation: Measures to Enhance Therapeutic Effects. This section addresses issues such as diet modification, measures to increase comfort, and ways to promote adherence to the prescribed regimen.

Ongoing Evaluation and Interventions. This section summarizes nursing implications that relate to drug responses, both therapeutic and undesired. As indicated in Table 2–2, the section has five subsections: (1) summary of monitoring, (2) evaluating therapeutic effects, (3) minimizing adverse effects, (4) minimizing adverse interactions, and (5) managing toxicity. The monitoring section summarizes the physiologic and psychologic parameters that must be monitored in order to evaluate therapeutic and adverse responses. The section on therapeutic effects summarizes criteria and procedures for evaluating therapeutic responses. The section on adverse effects summarizes the major adverse reactions that should be monitored for and presents interventions to minimize harm. The section on adverse interactions summarizes the major drug interactions to be alert for and gives interventions to minimize them. The section on toxicity describes major symptoms of toxicity and treatment.

Patient Education. This topic does not have a section of its own. Rather, patient education is integrated into the other sections. That is, as we summarize the nursing implications that relate to a particular topic, such as drug administration or a specific adverse effect, patient education related to that topic is discussed concurrently. This integration is done to promote clarity and efficiency of communication. In order to make this important information stand out, it appears in colored type.

What About Diagnosis and Planning? These headings are not used in the summaries. There are several reasons for the omission, the dominant one being efficiency of communication.

Nursing diagnoses have been left out because they are extremely numerous and largely self-evident. Yes, we could have included a list of diagnoses for each drug. However, since nursing diagnoses derive from drug effects, and since all drugs cause many effects (primarily adverse), the list of diagnoses for each drug would be very long. Accordingly,

SUMMARY

We began this chapter by asking, "Why should a nursing student learn pharmacology?" To answer the question, we explored the applications of pharmacology in nursing practice. We observed that nursing responsibilities regarding drugs go far beyond the Five Rights of Drug Administration. We observed also that the nurse has a critical role as patient advocate, serving as the patient's last line of defense against medication errors. We then discussed the many ways in which pharmacologic knowledge can be put to practical use in patient care and patient education. We saw that, by applying knowledge of pharmacology, you can have a positive influence on virtually all aspects of drug therapy, thereby helping to maximize benefits and minimize harm. Hopefully, your appreciation of the importance of pharmacology in nursing practice, coupled with your desire to provide optimal patient care, will provide the motivation you will need to develop an in-depth understanding of drugs.

⸚ KEY POINTS

- Nursing responsibilities with regard to drugs extend far beyond the Five Rights of Drug Administration.
- You are the patient's last line of defense against medication errors.
- Your knowledge of pharmacology has a wide variety of practical applications in patient care and patient education.
- By applying your knowledge of pharmacology, you will make a large contribution to achieving the therapeutic objective of maximum benefit with minimum harm.
- Application of the nursing process in drug therapy is directed at individualizing treatment, which is critical to achieving the therapeutic objective.
- The goal of preadministration assessment is to gather data needed for (1) evaluation of therapeutic and adverse effects, (2) identification of high-risk pa-

tients, and (3) assessment of the patient's capacity for self-care.

■ The analysis and diagnosis phase of treatment is directed at (1) judging the appropriateness of the prescribed therapy, (2) identifying potential health problems treatment might cause, and (3) characterizing the patient's capacity for self-care.

■ Planning is directed at (1) defining goals, (2) establishing priorities, and (3) establishing criteria for evaluating success.

■ In the evaluation stage, the objective is to evaluate (1) therapeutic responses, (2) adverse reactions and interactions, (3) patient compliance, and (4) patient satisfaction with treatment.

Drug Regulation, Development, Names, and Information

In this chapter we complete our introduction to pharmacology by considering five diverse but important topics. These are (1) drug regulation, (2) new drug development, (3) the annoying problem of drug names, (4) over-the-counter drugs, and (5) sources of drug information.

LANDMARK DRUG LEGISLATION

The history of drug legislation in the United States reflects an evolution in our national posture toward regulating the pharmaceutical industry. That posture has changed from one of minimal control to one of extensive control. For the most part, increased regulation has been beneficial, resulting in safer and more effective drugs.

The first American law to regulate drugs was the *Federal Pure Food and Drug Act* of 1906. This law was very weak: Its only requirement was that drugs be *free of adulterants.* The law said nothing about drug safety and effectiveness.

The *Food, Drug and Cosmetic Act,* passed in 1938, was much stronger than the Pure Food and Drug Act and was the first legislation to regulate drug safety. The motivation behind the 1938 law was a tragedy in which more than 100 people died following use of a new medication. The lethal preparation contained an antibiotic (sulfanilamide) plus a solubilizing agent (diethylene glycol). Tests revealed that the solvent was the cause of death. (Diethylene glycol is commonly used as automotive antifreeze.) To reduce the chances that such a tragedy might happen again, Congress required that all new drugs undergo testing for toxicity. The results of these tests were to be reviewed by the *Food and Drug Administration* (FDA), and only those drugs judged to be safe would receive FDA approval for marketing.

The next major drug legislation was the *Harris-Kefauver Amendments* to the Food, Drug and Cosmetic Act, passed in 1962. This law was created in response to the thalidomide tragedy that occurred in Europe in the early 1960s. Thalidomide is a sedative now known to cause birth defects. Because the drug was used widely by pregnant women, thousands of infants were born with phocomelia, a rare birth defect characterized by the gross malformation or complete absence of arms or legs. This tragedy was especially poignant in that it resulted from nonessential drug use: The women who took thalidomide could have done very well without it. Thalidomide was not a problem in the United States because the drug had been withheld by the FDA (see Box 104–1).

Because of the European experience with thalidomide, the Harris-Kefauver Amendments sought to strengthen all aspects of drug regulation. One of the bill's major provisions was to require proof of *effectiveness* before a new drug could be marketed. Remarkably, this was the first law to demand that drugs actually be of some benefit. The new act also required that all old drugs that had been introduced between 1932 and 1962 undergo testing for effectiveness; any drug that failed to prove useful would be withdrawn. Lastly, the Harris-Kefauver Act established rigorous procedures for testing new drugs. These procedures are discussed below under *New Drug Development.*

In 1970, Congress passed the *Controlled Substances Act* (Title II of the Comprehensive Drug Abuse Prevention and Control Act). This legislation set rules for the manufacture and distribution of drugs considered to have potential for abuse. One provision of the law defines categories into which controlled substances are placed. These categories are named Schedules I, II, III, IV, and V. Drugs in Schedule I have no accepted medical use in the United States and are deemed to have a high potential for abuse. Examples include heroin, mescaline, and lysergic acid diethylamide (LSD). Drugs in Schedules II through V have accepted medical applications but also have the potential for abuse. The abuse potential of these agents becomes progressively less as we proceed from Schedule II to Schedule V. The Controlled Substances Act is discussed further in Chapter 37 (Drug Abuse: Basic Considerations).

In 1992, FDA regulations were changed to permit accelerated approval of drugs for acquired immunodeficiency syndrome (AIDS) and cancer. Under the new guidelines, a drug could be approved for marketing prior to completion of Phase III trials (see below), provided that rigorous follow-up studies were performed. The rationale for this change was that the unknown risks associated with early approval are balanced by the need for more effective drugs.

The *Food and Drug Administration Modernization Act* of 1997 called for widespread changes in FDA regulations. Implementation is in progress. For health professionals, five provisions of the Act are of particular interest:

- The fast track system created for AIDS drugs and cancer drugs now includes drugs for other serious and life-threatening illnesses.
- Manufacturers who plan to stop making a drug must inform patients at least 6 months in advance, thereby giving patients time to find another source of the drug.
- The FDA can now require drug companies to test drugs in children. The information produced will allow drug therapy in young patients to be more rational. (In the past, drugs were not tested in children. Hence, pediatricians lacked reliable information upon which to base therapeutic decisions.)
- A clinical trial database will be established for drugs directed at serious or life-threatening illnesses. These data will allow clinicians and patients to make informed decisions about using experimental drugs.
- Drug companies can now give physicians journal articles and certain other information regarding "off-label" uses of drugs. (An "off-label" use is a use that has not been evaluated by the FDA.) Prior to the new act, physicians were allowed to prescribe a drug for an off-label use, but the manufacturer was not allowed to promote the drug for that use—even if promotion was limited to providing potentially helpful information. In return for being allowed to give physicians journal articles regarding off-label uses, manufacturers must promise to do research to support the claims made in the articles.

NEW DRUG DEVELOPMENT

The development and testing of new drugs is an expensive and lengthy process, requiring from 6 to 12 years for completion. It is estimated that, for every 5000 compounds that enter testing, only one emerges as a new product. Estimates of the cost of developing a new drug range from $200 million to $800 million.

Rigorous procedures for testing have been established so that newly released drugs might be both safe and effective. Unfortunately, although testing can determine effectiveness, it cannot guarantee that a new drug will be safe: Significant adverse effects may evade detection during testing only to become apparent once a new drug has been released for general use.

The Randomized Controlled Trial

Randomized controlled trials (RCTs) are the most reliable way to objectively assess drug therapies (and all other therapeutic interventions). Accordingly, RCTs are used to evaluate all new drugs. RCTs have three distinguishing features: use of controls, randomization, and blinding. All three serve to minimize the influence of personal bias on trial results.

Use of Controls. When a new drug is under development, we want to know how it compares with a standard drug used for the same disorder, or perhaps how it compares with no treatment at all. In order to make these comparisons, some subjects in the RCT are given the new drug and some are given either (1) a standard treatment or (2) a placebo (i.e., an inactive compound formulated to look like the experimental drug). Subjects receiving either the standard drug or the placebo are referred to as *controls*. Controls are important because they help us determine if the new treatment is more effective (or less effective) than standard treatments, or at least if the new treatment is better (or worse) than no treatment at all. Likewise, controls allow us to compare the safety of the new drug with that of the old drug, a placebo, or both.

Randomization. In an RCT, subjects are randomly assigned to either the control group or the experiment group (i.e., the group receiving the new drug). The purpose of randomization is to prevent allocation bias, which results when subjects in the experimental group are different from those in the control group. For example, in the absence of randomization, researchers could load the experimental group with patients who have mild disease and load the control group with patients who have severe disease. In this case, any differences in outcome may well be due to the severity of the disease rather than differences in treatment efficacy. And even if researchers try to avoid bias by purposely assigning subjects who appear similar to both groups, allocation bias can result from *unknown* factors that can influence outcome. By assigning subjects randomly to the control and experimental groups, all factors—known and unknown, important and unimportant—should be equally represented in both groups. As a result, the influences of these factors on outcome should tend to cancel each other out, leaving differences in the treatments as the best explanation for any differences in outcome.

Blinding. A blinded study is one in which the people involved do not know to which group—control or experimental—individual subjects have been randomized. If only the subjects have been "blinded," the trial is referred to as *single blind*. If the researchers as well as the subjects are kept in the dark, the trial is referred to as *double blind*. Of the two, double-blind trials are the more objective. Blinding is accomplished by administering the experimental drug and the control compound (either placebo or comparison drug) in identical formulations (e.g., green capsules) that bear a numeric code. At the end of the study, the code is accessed to reveal which subjects were controls and which received the experimental drug. When subjects and researchers are not blinded, their preconceptions about the benefits and risks of the new drug can readily bias study results. Hence, blinding is done to minimize the impact of personal bias.

Stages of New Drug Development

The testing of new drugs has two principal steps: *preclinical testing* and *clinical testing*. Preclinical tests are performed in animals. Clinical tests are done in humans. The steps in drug development are outlined in Table 3–1.

Preclinical Testing

Preclinical testing is required before a new drug may be tested in humans. During preclinical testing, drugs are evaluated for *toxicities, pharmacokinetic properties,* and *potentially useful biologic effects*. Preclinical tests may take 1 to 5 years. When sufficient preclinical data have been gathered, the drug developer may apply to the FDA for permission to begin testing in hu-

TABLE 3–1 ░░▪ Steps in New Drug Development

Preclinical Testing (in animals)
   Toxicity
   Pharmacokinetics
   Possible Useful Effects
              ↓
 Investigational New Drug (IND) Status
              ↓
 Clinical Testing (in humans)
   Phase I
       Subjects: normal volunteers
       Tests: metabolism and biologic effects
   Phase II
       Subjects: patients
       Tests: therapeutic utility and dosage range
   Phase III
       Subjects: patients
       Tests: safety and effectiveness
 Conditional Approval of New Drug Application (NDA)
              ↓
 Phase IV: Postmarketing Surveillance

mans. If the application is approved, the drug is awarded *Investigational New Drug* status and clinical trials may commence.

Clinical Testing

Clinical trials occur in four phases, and may take 2 to 10 years to complete. The first three phases are done before a new drug is marketed. The fourth phase is done after marketing has begun.

Phase I. Phase I trials are usually conducted in *normal volunteers*. However, if a drug is likely to have severe side effects, as many anticancer drugs do, the trial is done in volunteer patients who have the disease under consideration. Phase I testing has two goals: evaluation of drug metabolism and determination of effects in humans.

Phases II and III. In these trials, drugs are tested in *patients*. The objective is to determine therapeutic effects, dosage range, and safety. During Phase II and Phase III trials, only 500 to 5000 patients receive the drug; of these, only a few hundred take it for more than 3 to 6 months. Upon completing Phase III, the drug manufacturer applies to the FDA for conditional approval of a *New Drug Application*. If conditional approval is granted, Phase IV may begin.

Phase IV: Postmarketing Surveillance. In Phase IV, the new drug is released for general use, permitting observation of its effects in a large population. Frequently, new adverse effects are revealed. The success of Phase IV depends largely on voluntary reporting by prescribing physicians.

Limitations of the Testing Procedure

It is important for nurses and other healthcare professionals to appreciate the limitations of the drug development process. Two problems are of particular concern. First, until recently, information on drug use in women and children has been limited. Second, new drugs are likely to have adverse effects that were not detected during clinical trials.

Limited Information in Women and Children

Women. Until recently, very little drug testing was done in women. In almost all cases, women of child-bearing age were excluded from early clinical trials. The rationale for excluding women was concern for fetal safety. Unfortunately, FDA policy took this concern to an extreme, effectively barring all women of child-bearing age from Phase I and Phase II trials—even if the women were not pregnant and were using adequate birth control. The only women allowed to participate in early clinical trials were those with a life-threatening illness that might respond to the drug under study.

Because of limited drug testing in women, we don't know with precision how women will respond to drugs. We don't know if beneficial effects in women will be equivalent to those seen in men. Nor do we know if adverse effects will be equivalent to those in men. We don't know how timing of drug administration with respect to the menstrual cycle will affect beneficial and adverse responses. We don't know if drug disposition (absorption, distribution, metabolism, and excretion) will be the same in women as in men. Furthermore, of the various drugs that might be used to treat a particular illness, we don't know if the ones that are most effective in men will also be most effective in women. Lastly, we don't know about the safety of drug use during pregnancy.

During the 1990s, the FDA issued a series of guidelines mandating participation of women (and minorities) in trials of new drugs. In addition, the FDA revoked a 1977 guideline that barred women from most trials. Because of these changes, the proportion of women in trials of most new drugs now equals the proportion of women in the population. The data generated since the implementation of the new guidelines have been reassuring: most gender effects have been limited to pharmacokinetics, and more importantly, for most drugs, gender has shown little impact on efficacy, safety, or dosage. However, although the new guidelines are an important step forward, even with them, it will take a long time to close the gender gap in our knowledge of drugs.

Children. Until recently, children, like women, had been excluded from clinical trials of drugs. As a result, information on dosage, therapeutic responses, and adverse effects in children has been limited. As noted above, the FDA can now force drug companies to conduct clinical trials in children. However, it will still be a long time before we have the information needed to use drugs safely and effectively in young patients.

Failure to Detect All Adverse Effects

The testing procedure cannot detect all adverse effects before a new drug is released. There are three reasons for this problem: (1) during clinical trials a relatively small number of patients are given the drug; (2) because these patients are carefully selected, they do not represent the full spectrum of individuals who will eventually take the drug; and (3) patients in trials take the drug for a relatively short time. Because of these unavoidable limitations in the testing process, effects that occur infrequently, effects that take a long time to develop, and effects that occur only in certain types of patients may go undetected. Hence, despite our best efforts, when a new drug is released, it may well have adverse effects of which we are as yet unaware.

The hidden dangers in new drugs are illustrated by the data in Table 3–2. This table presents information on nine drugs

TABLE 3–2 ■ Some New Drugs That Were Withdrawn From the U.S. Market for Safety Reasons

Drug	Indication	Year Introduced/ Year Withdrawn	Months on the Market	Reason for Withdrawal
Rapacuronium [Raplon]	Neuromuscular blockade	1999/2001	19	Bronchospasm, unexplained fatalities
Alosetron* [Lotronex]	Irritable bowel syndrome	2000/2000	9	Ischemic colitis, severe constipation, deaths have occurred
Troglitazone [Rezulin]	Type 2 diabetes	1999/2000	12	Fatal liver failure
Grepafloxacin [Raxar]	Infection	1997/1999	19	Severe cardiovascular events, including seven deaths
Bromfenac [Duract]	Acute pain	1997/1998	11	Severe hepatic failure
Mibefradil [Posicor]	Hypertension, angina pectoris	1997/1998	11	Inhibits drug metabolism, causing toxic accumulation of many drugs
Dexfenfluramine [Redux]	Obesity	1996/1997	16	Valvular heart disease
Flosequinan [Manoplax]	Heart failure	1992/1993	4	Increased hospitalization; decreased survival
Temafloxacin [Omniflox]	Infection	1992/1992	4	Hypoglycemia; hemolytic anemia, often associated with renal failure, hepatotoxicity, and coagulopathy

*Alosetron was returned to the market on June 7, 2002, marking the first time the Food and Drug Administration has reapproved use of a drug that had been withdrawn for safety reasons. There are now restrictions on who can prescribe the drug and who can use it.

that were withdrawn from the U.S. market soon after receiving FDA approval. In all cases, the reason for withdrawal was a serious adverse effect that went undetected in clinical trials. Admittedly, only a few hidden adverse effects are as severe as the ones in the table. Hence, most do not necessitate drug withdrawal. Nonetheless, the drugs in the table should serve as a strong warning about the unknown dangers that a new drug may harbor.

Because adverse effects may go undetected, when working with a new drug, you should be especially watchful for previously unreported drug reactions. If a patient taking a new drug begins to show unusual symptoms, it is prudent to suspect that the new drug may be the cause—even though the symptoms are not yet mentioned in the literature.

Exercising Discretion Regarding New Drugs

When thinking about prescribing a new drug, the clinician would do well to follow this guideline: *Be neither the first to adopt the new nor the last to abandon the old.* Recall that the therapeutic objective is to produce maximum benefit with minimum harm. To achieve this objective, we must balance the inherent risks in giving a drug against its potential benefits. As a rule, new drugs have actions very similar to those of older agents. That is, it is rare for a new drug to be able to do something that an older drug can't do already. Consequently, the need to treat a particular disorder seldom constitutes a compelling reason to select a new drug over an agent that has been available for years. Furthermore, new drugs generally present greater risks than the old ones. As noted above, at the time of its introduction, a new drug is likely to have adverse effects that have not yet been reported, and these effects may prove very bad for some patients. In contrast, older, more familiar drugs are less likely to cause unpleasant surprises. Consequently, when we weigh the benefits of a new drug against its risks, it is likely that the benefits will be insufficient to justify the risks—especially when an older drug, whose properties are well known, would probably provide adequate

treatment. Accordingly, when it comes to the use of new drugs, it is usually better to adopt a wait-and-see policy, letting more adventurous clinicians discover the hidden dangers that a new drug may harbor.

DRUG NAMES

The topic of drug names is important and confusing. The topic is important because the names we employ affect our ability to communicate about medicines. The subject is confusing because we have evolved a system in which any drug can have a large number of names.

In approaching the discussion of drug names, we begin by defining the types of names that drugs have. After that we consider (1) the complications that arise from assigning multiple names to a drug, and (2) the benefits of using just one name: the generic (nonproprietary) name.

The Three Types of Drug Names

Drugs have three types of names: (1) a chemical name, (2) a generic or nonproprietary name, and (3) a trade or proprietary name. Examples of these names appear in Table 3–3. All of the names in the table are for the same drug, a compound most familiar to us under the trade name *Tylenol*.

Chemical Name. The chemical name constitutes a description of a drug using the nomenclature of chemistry. As you can see from the example in Table 3–3, a drug's chemical name can be long and complex. Because of their complexity, chemical names are inappropriate for everyday use. For example, few people would communicate using the chemical term *N*-acetyl-*para*-aminophenol when a more simple generic name (*acetaminophen*) or trade name (e.g., *Tylenol*) could be used.

Generic Name. The generic name of a drug is assigned by the United States Adopted Names Council. Each drug has only one generic name. The generic name is also known as the *nonproprietary* name. Generic names are less complex than chemical names but typically more complex than trade

TABLE 3–3 ▪ The Three Types of Drug Names

Type of Drug Name	Examples
Chemical Name	*N*-Acetyl-*para*-aminophenol
Generic Name (nonproprietary name)	Acetaminophen
Trade Name (proprietary name)	Acephen, Aceta, Anacin-3, Apacet, Arthritis Pain Formula Aspirin Free, Aspirin Free Pain Relief, Banesin, Bromo Seltzer, Dapa, Datril, Dolane, Dorcol Children's Fever and Pain Reducer, Feverall, Genapap, Genebs, Halenol, Liquiprin Elixir, Meda Tab, Myapap, Neopap, Oraphen-PD, Panadol, Panex, Panex 500, Phenaphen Caplets, Snaplets-FR Granules, St. Joseph Aspirin-Free for Children, Suppap-325, Tapanol Extra Strength, Tempra, Tylenol

The chemical, generic, and trade names listed are all names for the drug whose structure is pictured in this table. This drug is most familiar to us as Tylenol, one of its trade names.

TABLE 3–4 ▪ Generic Names and Trade Names of Some Common Drugs

Generic Name	Trade Name
Acetaminophen	Tylenol
Ciprofloxacin	Cipro
Fluoxetine	Prozac
Furosemide	Lasix
Ibuprofen	Motrin
Sildenafil	Viagra

names. For reasons presented below, generic names are preferable to trade names for general use.

Trade Name. Trade names, also known as proprietary or brand names, are the names under which a drug is marketed. These names are created by drug companies with the intention that they be easy for nurses, physicians, pharmacists, and consumers to recall and pronounce. Since any drug can be marketed in different formulations and by multiple companies, the number of trade names that a drug can have is large. By way of illustration, Table 3–3 gives the 31 trade names, including Tylenol, that exist for the drug whose generic name is *acetaminophen*.

Trade names must be approved by the FDA. The review process tries to ensure that no two trade names are too similar. In addition, trade names cannot imply unlikely efficacy—which may explain why sibutramine (a new diet pill) is named *Meridia* rather than something more suggestive, like *Fat-B-Gone* or *PoundsOff*.

Which Name To Use, Generic or Trade?

We employ drug names in two ways: (1) for written and oral communication about medicines and (2) for labeling medication containers. In both cases, accurate communication is imperative. For communication to be accurate, when we read or hear a drug name, we must know what compound that name is referring to. We can't know what's in a pill if we don't know what the name on its bottle means. Likewise, we can't communicate orally about drugs if the names we employ go unrecognized. Clearly, if we are to communicate accurately, name recognition is essential. As discussed below, name

recognition would be facilitated through universal use of generic names.

The Little Problems with Generic Names

In almost all cases, the generic name for a drug is longer and more complicated than its trade name. This fact is illustrated in Table 3–4, which compares the generic and trade names for six common drugs. A simple analysis reveals that the average generic name in the table has 4.3 syllables. In contrast, the average trade name has only 2.3 syllables. That is, the generic names are nearly twice as long as the trade names.

Because generic names are more complex than trade names, generic names can be more difficult to remember and pronounce. As an exercise, try pronouncing the names in Table 3–4. While trade names like *Motrin* and *Prozac* roll off the tongue with ease, their generic counterparts—*ibuprofen* and *fluoxetine*—tend to tie the tongue in knots.

Why is it that generic names are more complicated than trade names? One reason is that the pharmaceutical industry has an important role in establishing generic names. When a pharmaceutical company has developed a new drug, that company submits a suggested generic name to the United States Adopted Names Council, the body responsible for assigning a drug its generic name. As a rule, the Council adopts the name the company suggests. Since, from a marketing perspective, it is to the company's advantage to have a product whose trade name is more easily recognized than its generic name, it seems unlikely that a company will suggest a simple, euphonious generic name. Also contributing to the complexity of generic names are the guidelines established by the Council for naming drugs.

The Big Problems with Trade Names

A Single Drug Can Have Multiple Trade Names. The principal objection to trade names is their vast number. Although a drug can have only one generic name, it can have unlimited trade names. As the number of trade names for a single drug expands, the burden of name recognition becomes progressively heavier. By way of illustration, the drug whose generic name is acetaminophen has trade names that number in excess of 30 (see Table 3–3). Although most clinicians will recognize this drug's generic name, few are familiar with all the trade names. As we can see, recalling a single generic name—even if it's complex—is still easier than recalling a host of trade names for the same drug. Accordingly, if generic names were employed universally, accurate communication would be facilitated. Conversely, using multiple trade names does nothing but create confusion.

By clouding communication about drugs, use of trade names can result in "double medication," with potentially disastrous results. Because patients frequently see more than one physician, it is possible for a patient to be given prescriptions for the same drug by two different doctors. If those prescriptions are written for different brand names, then the two bottles the patient receives will be labeled with different names. Consequently, although both bottles contain the same drug, the patient may be unaware of this fact. If both medications are taken as prescribed, excessive dosing will result. However, if generic names had been used, both labels would bear the same name, thereby informing the patient that both bottles contain the same drug. Given this information, the patient is likely to consult the prescribing physicians to determine if both prescriptions should be honored.

The Same Trade Name Can Be Used for Different Products. As indicated in Table 3–5, products that have very similar trade names can actually contain very different drugs. For example, although the two Monistat products have nearly identical trade names, they actually contain two different drugs. Confusion would be avoided by simply labeling these products *miconazole* and *tioconazole,* rather than *Monistat 1* and *Monistat 3.*

The problem becomes even more complex for products that contain two or more drugs. When such combination products are referred to by trade name, the name is unlikely to indicate either the number of drugs present or their identity. Referring to Table 3–5, there is nothing about the trade name *Excedrin Tablets* to suggest that the product bearing this name consists of three different drugs: aspirin, acetaminophen, and caffeine. Moreover, there is nothing in the trade names *Excedrin Tablets* and *Excedrin P.M.* to tell us that these two products have different compositions. By discarding the trade names and labeling one product *acetaminophen plus aspirin plus caffeine* and the other *acetaminophen plus diphenhydramine,* we could eliminate any confusion.

The two 4-Way products listed in Table 3–5 further illustrate the potential for trade names to be misleading. If nothing else, the name *4-Way* suggests that the product contains more than one drug. In fact, the name seems to imply the presence of *four* drugs. However, this implication is not correct: Neither 4-Way preparation is composed of four drugs. One preparation—*4-Way Long-Lasting Nasal Spray*—contains only one drug. The other preparation—*4-Way Fast-Acting Nasal Spray*—contains three drugs. Furthermore, please note that these similarly named products are, in fact, completely different; they have no ingredients in common. Hence, in the case of these 4-Way products, we can see that the trade name cannot be taken to mean either (1) the presence of four different drugs or (2) that these preparations that bear similar names have the same composition. Had generic names been employed to label these products, there could be no confusion about their makeup.

Perhaps the most disturbing aspect of trade names is illustrated by the reformulation of *Ex-Lax,* a well-known laxative product. In 1999, the manufacturer of Ex-Lax switched the active ingredient in Ex-Lax from phenolphthalein to senna (in response to concerns that phenolphthalein might cause cancer). However, although the active ingredient changed, the brand name did not. As a result, new bottles of Ex-Lax contain a drug that is completely different from the one found in bottles of Ex-Lax produced in 1998. This example illustrates an important point: Manufacturers can reformulate brand-name products whenever they want—without changing the name at all.

TABLE 3–5 ■ Some Pharmaceutical Products That Share the Same Trade Name	
Product Name	**Drugs in the Product**
Monistat 1	Miconazole
Monistat 3	Tioconazole
Tavist	Clemastine
Tavist Sinus	Acetaminophen + pseudoephedrine
Excedrin Tablets	Acetaminophen + aspirin + caffeine
Excedrin P.M.	Acetaminophen + diphenhydramine
4-Way Long-Lasting Nasal Spray	Oxymetazoline
4-Way Fast-Acting Nasal Spray	Phenylephrine + naphazoline + pyrilamine

Hence, there is no guarantee that the brand-name product you buy today contains the same drug as did the brand-name product you bought last week, last month, or last year.

In the spring of 1999, the FDA issued a ruling that will help reduce the confusion created by trade names—but only for over-the-counter (OTC) drugs. When the ruling is implemented, generic names for the drugs in OTC products will be clearly and prominently listed on the label, using a standardized format.

What If Peas Were Marketed Like Drugs?

Given the problems that trade names create, why do we use trade names at all? We use trade names because the pharmaceutical industry wants them. Why? Because trade names give this industry a unique and powerful tool with which to market its products. As we shall see, the extent to which trade names are exploited to promote drug sales is without parallel in the marketing of any other product.

To understand the immense marketing value that trade names have for drug companies, it will be helpful to consider the marketing of a product that is not a drug. Take peas, for example. All companies that sell peas use the same name—*peas*—to identify their product. When we buy peas, no matter whose, all pea packages say "PEAS" in big letters on the label. Pea packages even have a picture of peas to help us identify what's inside. Consequently, when we choose a package of peas, we know with certainty what we're buying.

When we want to compare different *brands* of peas, the task is easy. Company A's peas are easily distinguished from those of company B or company C by the presence of a company name on the label. Consequently, thanks to the way peas are marketed, we have no trouble understanding (1) just what we are buying and (2) who made it. As a result, we can easily select the product we want from the manufacturer we like best.

Now let's consider what we could expect if peas were marketed like drugs. Under the new system, pea packages would have no pictures of peas on them. Nor would pea packages proclaim "PEAS" in big letters to help us identify their contents. Instead, pea packages would be emblazoned with trade names—like *Vegi-P* or *Producin* or *NuPod-500's.* If peas were marketed using trade names, when we went shopping for peas we'd be obliged to read a lot of fine print to find the product we wanted. And once we finally did turn up a package with peas in it—for example, the one labeled *NuPod-500's*—we'd probably buy NuPod-500's for life, it being too much trouble to figure out which of the other packages with meaningless names on them also contain peas. From the point of view of the people who sell NuPod-500's, this technique of marketing by trade names is a terrific arrangement. Consumers will be loyal to their product not because that product is better or cheaper than someone else's, but because product labeling with trade names makes it very difficult to identify the competition so that comparisons can be made. Fortunately, we don't allow this kind of marketing for peas. When we shop for peas, we demand that all pea packages bear the word *peas*—not *Vegi-P* or *NuPod-500's* or any other trade name. Why we permit medicines to be marketed in any less informative a manner is a disturbing question.

When we consider that drugs, unlike peas, cannot be identified by simple observation, the use of trade names for marketing becomes especially unsettling. With peas, once we open the package, we no longer need the label to identify the contents. We know what peas look like. Hence, even if peas were marketed like drugs, we would not be completely dependent upon labeling to identify the product. With drugs we have no options: Since we cannot identify a drug by looking at it, we cannot escape reliance on package labeling to inform us about the medicine inside. It is ironic that a product whose label is so essential for identification can be marketed under a system that employs multiple trade names, thereby making product identification needlessly and dangerously difficult.

Generic Products Versus Brand-Name Products

To complete our discussion of drug names, we need to address two questions: (1) Do significant differences exist between different brands of the same drug? and (2) If such differences do exist, do they justify the use of trade names? The answer to both questions is NO!

Are Generic Products and Brand-Name Products Therapeutically Equivalent? When a new drug comes to market, it is sold under a trade name by the company that developed it. When that company's patent expires, other companies can produce the drug and market it under its generic name. Our question, then, is, "Are the generic formulations equivalent to the brand-name formulation produced by the original manufacturer?"

Because all equivalent products—generic or brand name—contain the same dose of the same drug, the only concern with generic formulations is the rate and extent of their absorption. For a few drugs (e.g., phenytoin, warfarin), a slight increase in absorption can result in toxicity, and a slight decrease can result in therapeutic failure. Hence, for these agents, a small difference in absorption can be important. Until recently, there was concern that generic formulations of these drugs were not as safe or reliable as the brand-name formulation. However, there is no well-documented evidence to support this concern. Hence, it is reasonable to conclude that *all FDA-approved generic products are therapeutically equivalent to their brand-name counterparts.* A list of FDA-approved generic equivalents is available on the Internet at *www.fda.gov/cder/ob/default.htm.*

Would a Difference Between Brand-Name and Generic Products Justify the Use of Trade Names? Even if generic formulations *were* significantly different from brand-name formulations, this would not justify using trade names to identify preferred products. If physicians want to prescribe a drug made by a particular company, they needn't resort to trade names to do so; their preference can be indicated simply by including the manufacturer's name on the prescription. As with peas, if we prefer a particular brand (e.g., BIRDS EYE), that's what we ask for. We haven't found it necessary to create a complicated system of alternative names for peas in order to distinguish one brand from another. On the contrary, common sense tells us that such a system of trade names would make it more difficult—not easier—for us to clearly communicate our needs. Perhaps some day we will market medicines with as much common sense as we use for vegetables.

Conclusion Regarding Generic Names and Trade Names

In the preceding discussion, we considered the advantages and disadvantages associated with trade names and generic names. We noted that, although generic names may be long, this disadvantage is more than offset by the fact that each drug has only one generic name. In contrast, the sole virtue of trade names—ease of recall and pronunciation—is far outweighed by the problems that stem from the existence of multiple trade names for a single drug. Multiple trade names can impede name recognition and can thereby promote medication errors and miscommunication about drugs. With generic names, the opposite is achieved: facilitation of communication and promotion of safe and effective drug use. Clearly, generic names are preferable to trade names. Accordingly, until such time as trade names are outlawed, the least we can do is actively discourage their use. In this text, generic names are employed for routine discussion. Although trade names are presented, they are not emphasized. We may eventually see the day when trade names are abandoned and generic names are employed universally. On that day, efforts to achieve the therapeutic objective will receive a significant boost.

OVER-THE-COUNTER DRUGS

Over-the-counter (OTC) drugs are defined as drugs that can be purchased without a prescription. These agents are used for a wide variety of complaints, including mild pain, motion sickness, allergies, colds, constipation, and heartburn. Whether a drug is available by prescription or over the counter is ultimately determined by the FDA.

OTC drugs are an important part of healthcare. When used properly, these agents can provide relief from many ailments while saving consumers the expense and inconvenience of visiting a prescriber. The following facts underscore how important the OTC market is:

- Americans spend about $20 billion annually on OTC drugs.
- OTC drugs account for 60% of all doses administered.
- Forty percent of Americans take at least one OTC drug every 2 days.
- Four times as many illnesses are treated by a consumer using an OTC drug as by a consumer visiting a physician.
- With most (60% to 95%) illnesses, initial therapy consists of self-care, including self-medication with an OTC drug.
- The average home medicine cabinet contains 24 OTC preparations.

Some drugs that were originally sold only by prescription are now sold over the counter. Since the 1970s, over 60 prescription drugs have been switched to OTC status. About 50 more are under FDA consideration for the change. Because of this process, more and more highly effective drugs are becoming directly available to consumers. Unfortunately, most consumers lack the knowledge needed to choose the most appropriate drug from among the steadily increasing options.

In 1999, the FDA issued a regulation that will give OTC drugs standardized labels that are informative and easy to understand. The new labels, titled *Drug Facts,* will be written in plain language and will have a user-friendly format. The type will be big enough to read. Active ingredients will be listed first, followed by uses, warnings, directions, and inactive ingredients. This information should help consumers select drugs that can provide the most benefit with the least risk. Implementation of the regulation will take several years.

In contrast to some texts, which discuss all OTC drugs in a single chapter, this text discusses OTC drugs throughout. Why? Because this format allows presentation of OTC drugs in their proper pharmacologic and therapeutic contexts. I believe this makes more sense than lumping these drugs together solely because they can be purchased without a prescription.

SOURCES OF DRUG INFORMATION

There is much more to pharmacology than we can address in this text. When you need additional information, the sources discussed below should help.

People

Clinicians and Pharmacists. Nurses and other clinicians can be invaluable sources of information about medicines. Pharmacists know a great deal about drugs and are usually eager to share their expertise.

Poison Control Centers. Poison control centers are located throughout the country. These centers are accessible by telephone, permitting rapid access to information about medicines and toxic compounds. Appendix F lists the names, addresses, and telephone numbers of the certified regional poison control centers in the United States.

Pharmaceutical Sales Representatives. Pharmaceutical sales representatives (drug representatives) can be useful sources of drug information. These people know their own products very well, and they can provide detailed, authoritative information about them. Keep in mind, however, that the ultimate job of the drug representative is sales—not education. Because their objective is sales, drug representatives may fail to volunteer negative information about their product. Likewise, they are unlikely to point out superior qualities in a competing drug. (Is a Chevrolet salesperson going to extol the virtues of a Ford?) Such a lack of complete candor does not mean that drug representatives are unethical; they are simply doing their job. However, since full disclosure may be inconsistent with successful sales, the drug representative may not be your best source of information—

especially if you are trying to establish an unbiased comparison between the representative's product and a drug from a competing manufacturer.

Published Information

The publications described below are general references. These works cover a broad range of topics but in limited depth. Accordingly, these references are most useful as initial sources of information. If more detail is needed, specialty publications should be consulted. Some important drug references, including the ones described below, are listed in Table 3–6.

Text-like Books

Goodman & Gilman's The Pharmacological Basis of Therapeutics is the classic text/reference on pharmacology used by medical students and practicing physicians. As its name implies, this book focuses on the basic science information that underlies drug use—and not on therapeutics per se. New editions are released about every 4 to 5 years.

Pharmacotherapy: A Pathophysiologic Approach is a comprehensive text on drug therapy. Each chapter focuses on the treatment of a specific disorder. To facilitate understanding of drug therapy, the book presents thorough reviews of pathophysiology.

Applied Therapeutics: The Clinical Use of Drugs is another comprehensive text on drug therapy, with each chapter focusing on a specific disorder. However, this book is different from the others in that it employs a case-study approach to presenting content on pharmacology and therapeutics.

TABLE 3–6 ■ Some Important Drug References

General Information on Drug Actions, Pharmacokinetics, Therapeutics, Adverse Effects, and Drug Interactions

Goodman and Gilman's The Pharmacological Basis of Therapeutics, 10th ed. Hardman JG, et al. (eds). McGraw-Hill, New York, 2001

Pharmacotherapy: A Pathophysiologic Approach, 5th ed. DiPiro JT, et al. (eds). Elsevier Science Publishing, New York, 2002

Applied Therapeutics: The Clinical Use of Drugs, 7th ed. Koda-Kimble MA, Young LY (eds). Applied Therapeutics, Inc., Vancouver, WA, 2001

Detailed Information on Specific Drugs and Drug Families

AHFS Drug Information. McEvoy GK (ed). American Society of Hospital Pharmacists, Bethesda, MD (updated annually)

Drug Facts and Comparisons, Loose-leaf ed. Facts and Comparisons, St. Louis (updated monthly)

Physicians' Desk Reference. Medical Economics Data Production Co., Montvale, NJ (updated annually)

United States Pharmacopeia Drug Information (USP DI): Drug Information for the Health Care Professional. The United States Pharmacopeial Convention, Inc., Rockville, MD (updated bimonthly)

Very Current Information

The Medical Letter. The Medical Letter, Inc., New Rochelle, NY (published bimonthly)

Prescriber's Letter. Therapeutic Research Center, Stockton, CA (published monthly)

Newsletters

The Medical Letter on Drugs and Therapeutics is a bimonthly publication that gives current information on drugs. A typical issue discusses two or three agents. Discussions consist of a summary of data from clinical trials plus a conclusion regarding the drug's therapeutic utility. The conclusions can be a valuable guide when deciding whether or not to use a new drug.

Prescriber's Letter is a monthly publication with very current information. Unlike *The Medical Letter*, which usually focuses on just two or three drugs, this newsletter addresses (briefly) most major drug-related developments—from new drugs to FDA warnings to new uses of older agents. In addition, subscribers can access an Internet site that provides expanded information on all topics addressed in the monthly letter.

Reference Books

The *Physicians' Desk Reference*, also known as the PDR, is a reference work financed by the pharmaceutical industry. The information on each drug is identical to the information on its package insert. In addition to textual content, the PDR has a pictorial section for product identification. The PDR is updated annually.

Drug Facts and Comparisons is a comprehensive reference that contains monographs on virtually every drug marketed in the United States. Information is provided on drug actions, indications, warnings, precautions, adverse reactions, dosage, and administration. In addition to describing the properties of single medications, the book lists the contents of most combination products sold in this country. Indexing is by generic name and by trade name. *Drug Facts and Comparisons* is available in a loose-leaf format (updated monthly) and a hard-cover format (published annually).

A number of drug references have been compiled expressly for nurses. All of these address topics of special interest to the nurse, including information on administration, assessment, evaluation, and patient education. Representative nursing drug references include *Nurse's Drug Handbook* and *Mosby's Drug Guide for Nurses*.

The Internet

The Internet can be a valuable source of drug information. However, since anyone, regardless of qualifications, can post information, not everything you find will be accurate. Accordingly, you need to exercise discretion when searching for information. A list of reliable drug-related information is available online at *evolve.elsevier.com/Lehne/*.

⠶ KEY POINTS

- The Food, Drug and Cosmetic Act of 1938 was the first legislation to regulate drug safety.
- The Harris-Kefauver Amendments, passed in 1962, were the first legislation to demand that drugs actually be of some benefit.
- The Controlled Substances Act, passed in 1970, set rules for the manufacture and distribution of drugs considered to have potential for abuse.
- Development of a new drug is an extremely expensive process that takes years to complete.
- The randomized controlled trial is the most reliable way to objectively assess drug therapy.
- Drug testing in Phase II and Phase III clinical trials is limited to a relatively small number of subjects, most of whom take the drug for a relatively short time.
- Since women and children have been excluded from drug trials in the past, our understanding of drugs in these people is limited.
- When a new drug is released for general use, it may well have adverse effects that have not yet been detected. Consequently, when working with a new drug, you should be especially watchful for previously unreported drug reactions.
- Drugs have three types of names: a chemical name, a generic or nonproprietary name, and a trade or proprietary name.
- Each drug has only one generic name but can have many trade names.
- Generic names facilitate communication and therefore are good. In contrast, trade names confuse communication and should be outlawed. (Even science authors are allowed to voice an opinion now and then.)
- Over-the-counter (OTC) drugs are defined as drugs that can be purchased without a prescription.
- Since the job of the drug representative is sales and not education, this person may not be your best source of drug information—especially if you are trying to establish an unbiased comparison between the representative's product and a drug from a competing manufacturer.
- As pharmacology students, you should know that *Goodman & Gilman's The Pharmacological Basis of Therapeutics* (aka *G & G*) is the classic text/reference on pharmacology.

Pharmacokinetics

The term *pharmacokinetics* is derived from two Greek words: *pharmakon* (drug or poison) and *kinesis* (motion). As this derivation implies, pharmacokinetics is the study of drug movement throughout the body. Pharmacokinetics also includes drug metabolism and drug excretion.

There are four basic pharmacokinetic processes: *absorption, distribution, metabolism,* and *excretion* (Fig. 4–1). Absorption is defined as the movement of a drug from its site of administration into the blood. Distribution is defined as drug movement from the blood to the interstitial space of tissues and from there into cells. Metabolism (biotransformation) is defined as enzymatically mediated alteration of drug structure. Excretion is the

movement of drugs and their metabolites out of the body. The combination of metabolism plus excretion is called *elimination.* The four pharmacokinetic processes, acting in concert, determine the concentration of a drug at its sites of action.

APPLICATION OF PHARMACOKINETICS IN THERAPEUTICS

By applying knowledge of pharmacokinetics to drug therapy, we can help maximize beneficial effects and minimize harm. Recall that the intensity of the response to a drug is directly related to the concentration of the drug at its site of action. To maximize beneficial effects, we must achieve concentrations that are high enough to elicit desired responses; to minimize harm, we must avoid unnecessarily high concentrations. This balance is achieved by selecting the most appropriate route, dosage, and dosing schedule. The only way we can rationally choose the most effective route, dosage, and schedule is by considering pharmacokinetic factors.

As a nurse, you will have ample opportunity to apply knowledge of pharmacokinetics in clinical practice. For example, by understanding the reasons behind selection of route, dosage, and dosing schedule, you will be less likely to commit medication errors than will the nurse who, through lack of this knowledge, administers medications by blindly following physicians' orders. Also, as noted in Chapter 2, physicians do make mistakes. Accordingly, you will have occasion to question or even challenge physicians regarding their selection of dosage, route, or schedule of administration. In order to alter a physician's decision, you will need a rational argument to support your position. To present that argument, you will need to understand pharmacokinetics.

Knowledge of pharmacokinetics can increase job satisfaction. Working with medications is a significant component of nursing practice. If you lack knowledge of pharmacokinetics, drugs will always be somewhat mysterious and, as a result, will be a potential source of ill ease. By helping to demystify drug therapy, knowledge of pharmacokinetics can decrease some of the stress of nursing practice and can increase intellectual and professional satisfaction.

A NOTE TO CHEMOPHOBES

Before we proceed to the heart of this chapter, some advance notice (and encouragement) are in order for chemophobes (students who fear chemistry) who are reading this text. Since drugs are chemicals, we cannot discuss pharmacology meaningfully without occasionally talking about chemistry. This chapter has some chemistry in it. In fact, the chemistry

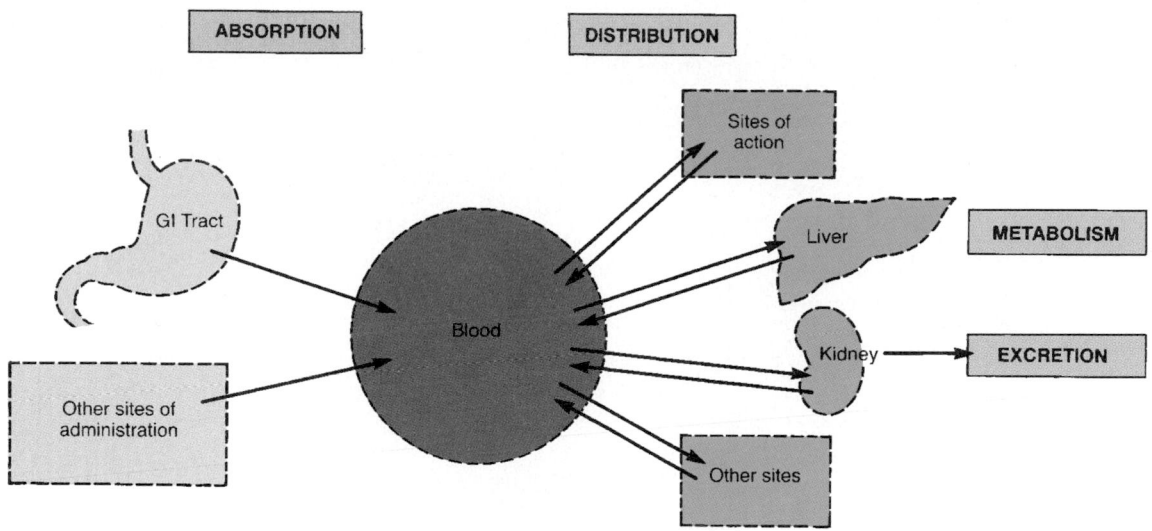

Figure 4–1 ■ **The four basic pharmacokinetic processes.**
Dotted lines represent membranes that must be crossed as drugs move throughout the body.

presented here is the most difficult in the book. Accordingly, once you've worked your way through this chapter, the chapters that follow will be a relative breeze. Since the concepts addressed here are fundamental, and since they reappear frequently, all students, including chemophobes, are encouraged to learn this material now—regardless of the effort required.

I also want to comment on the chemical structures that appear in the book. Structures are presented only to illustrate and emphasize concepts. They are not intended for memorization, and they are certainly not intended for exams. So, relax, look at the pictures, and focus on the concepts they are trying to help you grasp.

PASSAGE OF DRUGS ACROSS MEMBRANES

All four phases of pharmacokinetics—absorption, distribution, metabolism, and excretion—involve drug movement. To move throughout the body, drugs must cross membranes. Drugs must cross membranes to enter the blood from their site of administration. Once in the blood, drugs must cross membranes to leave the vascular system and reach their sites of action. In addition, drugs must cross membranes to undergo metabolism and excretion. Accordingly, the factors that determine the passage of drugs across biologic membranes have a profound influence on all aspects of pharmacokinetics.

Membrane Structure

Biologic membranes are composed of layers of individual cells. The cells composing most membranes are very close to one another—so close, in fact, that drugs must usually pass *through* cells, rather than between them, in order to cross the membrane. Hence, the ability of a drug to cross a biologic membrane is determined primarily by its ability to pass through single cells. The major barrier to passage through a cell is the cytoplasmic membrane (the membrane that surrounds every cell).

The basic structure of the cell membrane is depicted in Figure 4–2. As indicated, the basic membrane structure consists of a double layer of molecules known as *phospholipids*. Phospholipids are simply lipids (fats) that contain an atom of phosphate.

In Figure 4–2, the phospholipid molecules are depicted as having a round head (the phosphate-containing component) and two tails (long-chain hydrocarbons). The large objects embedded in the membrane represent protein molecules. These proteins serve a variety of functions.

Three Ways to Cross a Cell Membrane

The three most important ways by which drugs cross cell membranes are (1) passage through channels or pores, (2) passage with the aid of a transport system, and (3) direct penetration of the membrane itself. Of the three, direct penetration of the membrane is most common.

Channels and Pores

Very few drugs cross membranes via channels or pores. The channels in membranes are extremely small (approximately 4 angstroms). Consequently, only the smallest of compounds (molecular weight less than 200) can use these holes as a route of transit. Agents with the ability to cross membranes via channels include small ions, such as potassium and sodium.

Transport Systems

Transport systems are carriers that can move drugs from one side of the cell membrane to the other. Some transport systems require the expenditure of energy; others do not. All transport systems are selective: They will not carry just any drug. Whether or not a transporter will carry a particular drug depends upon the drug's structure.

Transport systems are an important means of drug transit. For example, certain orally administered drugs could not be absorbed unless there were transport systems to move them across the membranes that separate the lumen of the intestine from the blood. A number of drugs could not reach intracellular sites of

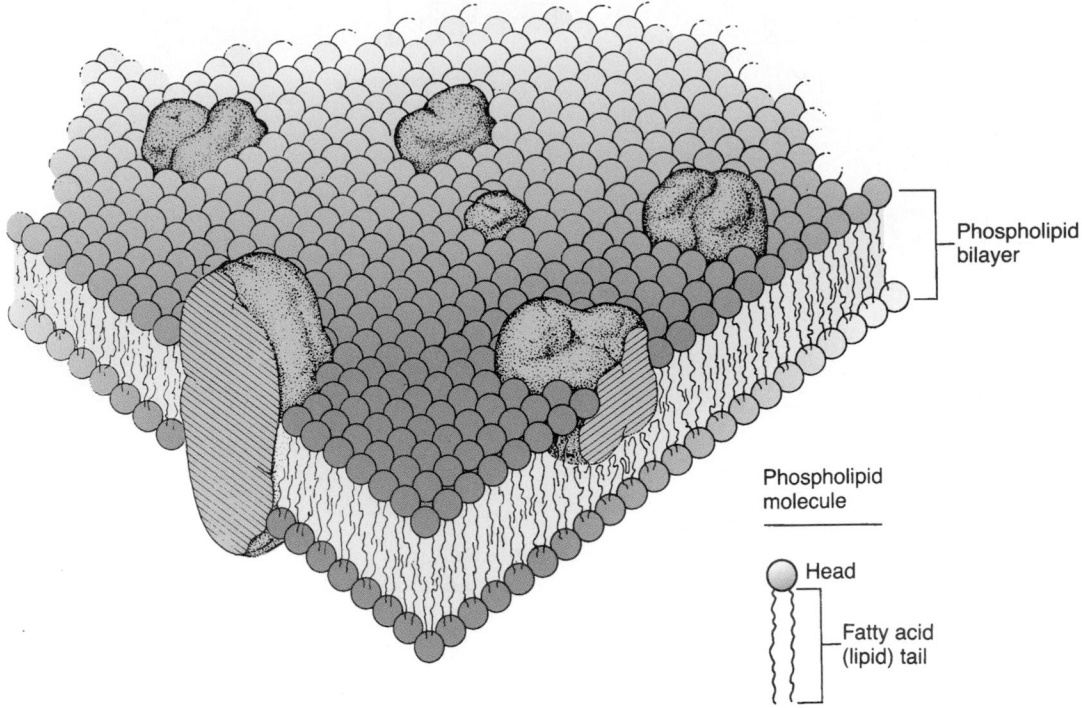

Phospholipid bilayer

Phospholipid molecule

○ Head

Fatty acid (lipid) tail

Figure 4–2 ■ Structure of the cell membrane.
The cell membrane consists primarily of a double layer of phospholipid molecules. The large globular structures represent protein molecules imbedded in the lipid bilayer. (Modified from Singer SJ, Nicolson GL. The fluid mosaic model of the structure of cell membranes. Science 1972;175:720.)

action without a transport system to move them across the cell membrane. Renal excretion of many drugs would be extremely slow were it not for transport systems in the kidney that can pump drugs from the blood into the renal tubules.

Direct Penetration of the Membrane

For most drugs, movement throughout the body is dependent on their ability to penetrate membranes directly. This is because (1) most drugs are too large to pass through channels or pores and (2) most drugs lack transport systems to help them cross all of the membranes that separate drugs from their sites of action, metabolism, and excretion.

In order to directly penetrate membranes, a drug must be *lipid soluble* (lipophilic). Recall that membranes are composed primarily of lipids. Consequently, if a drug is to penetrate a membrane, it must be able to dissolve into the lipids that compose the membrane.

Certain kinds of molecules are *not* lipid soluble and therefore cannot penetrate membranes. This group consists of *polar molecules* and *ions.*

Polar Molecules

Polar molecules are molecules with uneven distribution of electrical charge. That is, positive and negative charges within the molecule tend to congregate separately from one another. Water is the classic example. As depicted in Figure 4–3A, the electrons (negative charges) in the water molecule spend more time in the vicinity of the oxygen atom than in the vicinity of the two hydrogen atoms. As a result, the area around the oxy-

gen atom tends to be negatively charged, whereas the area around the hydrogen atoms tends to be positively charged. Kanamycin (Fig. 4–3B), an antibiotic, is an example of a polar drug. The hydroxyl groups, which attract electrons, give kanamycin its polar nature.

Although polar molecules have an uneven *distribution* of charge, they have no *net* charge. Polar molecules have an equal number of protons (which bear a single positive charge) and electrons (which bear a single negative charge). As a result, the positive and negative charges balance each other exactly, and the molecule as a whole has neither a net positive charge nor a net negative charge. Molecules that *do* bear a net charge are called *ions.* These are discussed below.

There is a general rule in chemistry that states: "like dissolves like." In accord with this rule, polar molecules will dissolve in *polar* solvents (such as water) but will not dissolve in *nonpolar* solvents (such as oil). Table sugar provides a common example. I'm sure you've observed that sugar, a polar compound, readily dissolves in water but does not dissolve in salad oil, butter, and other lipids, which are nonpolar compounds. Just as sugar is unable to dissolve in lipids, polar drugs are unable to dissolve in the lipid bilayer of the cell membrane.

Ions

Ions are defined as molecules that have a *net electrical charge* (either positive or negative). Except for very small molecules, *ions are unable to cross membranes.*

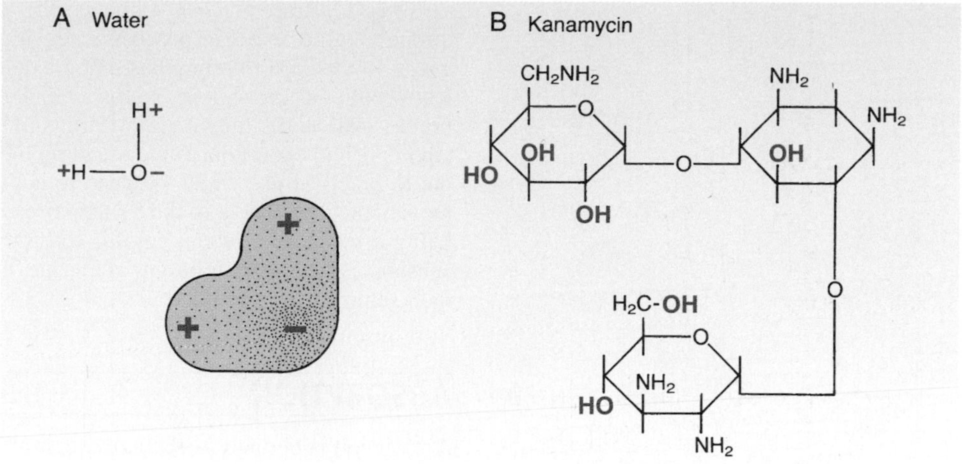

Figure 4–3 ■ Polar molecules.
A, Stippling shows the distribution of electrons within the water molecule. As indicated, water's electrons spend more time near the oxygen atom than near the hydrogen atoms, making the area near the oxygen atom somewhat negative and the area near the hydrogen atoms more positive. *B,* Kanamycin is a polar drug. The —OH groups of kanamycin attract electrons, thereby causing the area around these groups to be more negative than the rest of the molecule.

Quaternary Ammonium Compounds

Quaternary ammonium compounds are molecules that contain at least one atom of nitrogen and *carry a positive charge at all times.* The constant charge on these compounds results from atypical bonding to the nitrogen. In most nitrogen-containing compounds, the nitrogen atom bears only three chemical bonds. In contrast, the nitrogen atoms of quaternary ammonium compounds have four chemical bonds (Fig. 4–4A). It is because of the fourth bond that quaternary ammonium compounds always carry a positive charge. Because of the charge, these compounds are unable to cross most membranes.

Tubocurarine (Fig. 4–4B) is a representative quaternary ammonium compound. In purified form, tubocurarine is employed as a muscle relaxant for surgery and other procedures. A crude preparation—curare—is used by South American Indians as an arrow poison. When employed for hunting, tubocurarine (curare) produces paralysis of the diaphragm and other skeletal muscles, causing death by asphyxiation. Interestingly, even though meat from animals killed with curare is laden with poison, it can be eaten with no ill effect. Why can this poison be ingested safely? Because tubocurarine, being a quaternary ammonium compound, cannot cross membranes, and therefore cannot be absorbed from the intestine; as long as it remains in the lumen of the intestine, curare can do no harm. As you might gather, when tubocurarine is used clinically, it cannot be administered by mouth; instead, it must be injected. Once in the bloodstream, tubocurarine has ready access to its sites of action on the surface of muscles.

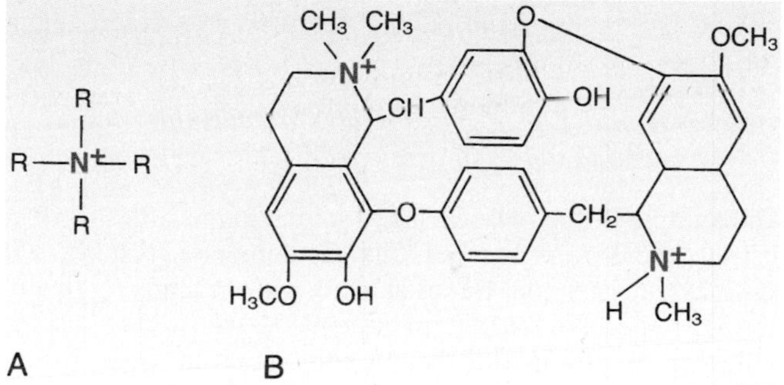

pH-Dependent Ionization

Unlike quaternary ammonium compounds, which always carry a charge, certain drugs can exist in either a charged or uncharged form. Many drugs are either weak organic acids or weak organic bases. Weak acids and bases can exist in charged and uncharged forms. Whether a weak acid or base will carry a charge is determined by the pH of the surrounding medium.

Figure 4–4 ■ Quaternary ammonium compounds.
A, The basic structure of quaternary ammonium compounds. Because the nitrogen atom has bonds to four organic radicals, quaternary ammonium compounds always carry a positive charge. Because of this charge, quaternary ammonium compounds are not lipid soluble and cannot cross most membranes. *B,* Tubocurarine is a representative quaternary ammonium compound. Note that tubocurarine contains two "quaternized" nitrogen atoms.

A review of acid-base chemistry will be helpful. An acid is defined as a compound that can give up a hydrogen ion (proton). Put another way, *an acid is a proton donor.* A base is defined as a compound that can take on a hydrogen ion. That is, *a base is a proton acceptor.* When an acid gives up its proton, which is positively charged, the acid itself becomes negatively charged. Conversely, when a base accepts a proton, the base becomes positively charged. These reactions are depicted in Figure 4–5, which uses aspirin as an example of an acid and amphetamine as an example of a base. Because the process of an acid giving up a proton or a base accepting a proton converts the acid or base into a charged particle (ion), the process for either an acid or a base is termed *ionization.*

Figure 4–5 ▪ Ionization of weak acids and weak bases. The extent of ionization of weak acids (*A*) and weak bases (*B*) depends on the pH of their surroundings. The ionized (charged) forms of acids and bases are not lipid soluble and do not readily cross membranes. Note that acids ionize by giving up a proton and that bases ionize by taking on a proton.

The extent to which a weak acid or weak base becomes ionized is determined in part by the pH of its environment. The following rules apply:

▪ *Acids tend to ionize in basic (alkaline) media.*
▪ *Bases tend to ionize in acidic media.*

An example of the pH-dependent ionization of a drug will illustrate the significance of this phenomenon. Aspirin will serve as our example. Being an acid, aspirin tends to give up its proton (become ionized) in basic media. Conversely, aspirin will keep its proton and remain nonionized in acidic media. Hence, when aspirin is in the stomach (an acidic medium), most of the aspirin molecules remain nonionized. Because aspirin molecules are nonionized in the stomach, they can be absorbed across the membranes that separate the stomach from the bloodstream. When aspirin molecules pass from the stomach into the small intestine, where the environment is relatively alkaline, they change to their ionized form. As a result, absorption of aspirin from the intestine is impeded.

Ion Trapping (pH Partitioning)

Because the ionization of drugs is pH dependent, when the pH of the fluid on one side of a membrane differs from the pH of the fluid on the other side, drug molecules will tend to accumulate on the side where the pH most favors their ionization. Accordingly, since acidic drugs tend to ionize in basic media, and since basic drugs tend to ionize in acidic media, *when there is a pH gradient between two sides of a membrane,*

▪ *Acidic drugs will accumulate on the alkaline side.*
▪ *Basic drugs will accumulate on the acidic side.*

The process whereby a drug accumulates on the side of a membrane where the pH most favors its ionization is referred to as *ion trapping* or *pH partitioning*. Figure 4–6 shows the steps of ion trapping using aspirin as an example.

Since ion trapping can influence the movement of drugs throughout the body, the process is not simply of academic interest. Rather, ion trapping has practical clinical implications. Knowledge of ion trapping helps us understand drug absorption as well as the movement of drugs to sites of action, metabolism, and excretion. Understanding of ion trapping can be put to practical use when we need to actively influence drug movement. Poisoning is the principal example: By manipulating urinary pH, we can employ ion trapping to draw toxic substances from the blood into the urine, thereby accelerating their removal from the body.

ABSORPTION

Absorption is defined as *the movement of a drug from its site of administration into the blood.* The *rate* of absorption determines how *soon* effects will begin. The *amount* of absorption helps determine how *intense* effects will be.

Factors Affecting Drug Absorption

The rate at which a drug undergoes absorption is influenced by the physical and chemical properties of the drug itself and by physiologic and anatomic factors at the site of absorption.

Rate of Dissolution. Before a drug can be absorbed, it must first dissolve. Hence, the rate of dissolution helps determine the rate of absorption. Drugs in formulations that allow rapid dissolution have a faster onset than drugs formulated for slow dissolution.

Surface Area. The surface area available for absorption is a major determinant of the rate of absorption. The larger the surface area, the faster absorption will be. For this reason, orally administered drugs are usually absorbed from the small intestine rather than from the stomach. (Recall that the small intestine, because of its lining of microvilli, has an extremely large surface area, whereas the surface area of the stomach is relatively small.)

Blood Flow. Drugs are absorbed most rapidly from sites where blood flow is high. This is because blood containing newly absorbed drug will be replaced rapidly by drug-free blood, thereby maintaining a large gradient between the concentration of drug outside the blood and the concentration of drug in the blood. The greater this concentration gradient, the more rapid absorption will be.

Lipid Solubility. As a rule, highly lipid-soluble drugs are absorbed more rapidly than drugs whose lipid solubility is low. This is because lipid-soluble drugs can readily cross the membranes that separate them from the blood, whereas drugs of low lipid solubility cannot.

pH Partitioning. pH partitioning can influence drug absorption. Absorption will be enhanced when the difference between the pH of plasma and the pH at the site of administration is such that drug molecules will have a greater tendency to be ionized in the plasma.

Characteristics of Commonly Used Routes of Administration

The routes of administration that are used most commonly fall into two major groups: *enteral* (via the gastrointestinal tract) and *parenteral*. The literal definition of *parenteral* is

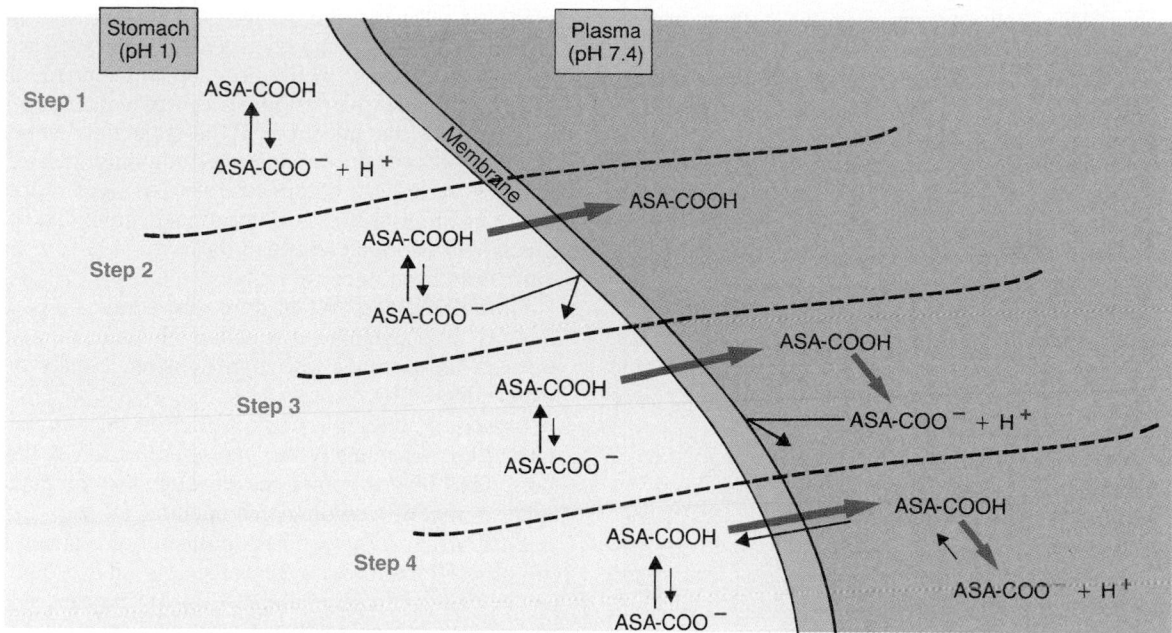

Figure 4–6 ■ Ion trapping of drugs.
This figure demonstrates ion trapping using aspirin as an example. Because aspirin is an acidic drug, it will be nonionized in acid media and ionized in alkaline media. As indicated, ion trapping causes molecules of orally administered aspirin to move from the acidic (pH 1) environment of the stomach to the more alkaline (pH 7.4) environment of the plasma, thereby causing aspirin to accumulate in the blood. In the figure, aspirin (acetylsalicylic acid) is depicted as ASA with its COOH (carboxylic acid) group attached.

Step 1, Once ingested, ASA dissolves in the stomach contents, after which some ASA molecules give up a proton and become ionized. However, most of the ASA in the stomach remains nonionized. Why? Because the stomach is acidic, and acidic drugs don't ionize in acidic media.

Step 2, Since most ASA molecules in the stomach are nonionized (and therefore lipid soluble), most ASA molecules in the stomach can readily cross the membranes that separate the stomach lumen from the plasma. Because of the concentration gradient that exists between the stomach and the plasma, nonionized ASA molecules will begin moving into the plasma. (Note that, because of their charge, ionized ASA molecules cannot leave the stomach.)

Step 3, As the nonionized ASA molecules enter the relatively alkaline environment of the plasma, most give up a proton (H^+) and become negatively charged ions. ASA molecules that become ionized in the plasma cannot diffuse back into the stomach.

Step 4, As the nonionized ASA molecules in the plasma become ionized, more nonionized molecules will pass from the stomach to the plasma to replace them. This passage occurs because the laws of diffusion demand equal concentrations of diffusible substances on both sides of the membrane. Since only the nonionized form of ASA is able to diffuse across the membrane, it is this form that the laws of diffusion will attempt to equilibrate. Nonionized ASA will continue to move from the stomach to the plasma until the amount of ionized ASA in plasma has become large enough to prevent conversion of newly arrived nonionized molecules into the ionized form. Equilibrium will then be established between the plasma and the stomach. At equilibrium, there will be equal amounts of nonionized ASA in the stomach and plasma. However, on the plasma side, the amount of ionized ASA will be much larger than on the stomach side. Since there are equal concentrations of nonionized ASA on both sides of the membrane but a much higher concentration of ionized ASA in the plasma, the total concentration of ASA in plasma will be much higher than in the stomach.

outside the gastrointestinal tract. However, in common parlance, the term *parenteral* is used to mean *by injection.* The principal parenteral routes are *intravenous, subcutaneous,* and *intramuscular.*

For each of the major routes of administration—oral (PO), intravenous (IV), intramuscular (IM), and subcutaneous (SC)—

the pattern of drug absorption (i.e., the rate and extent of absorption) is unique. Consequently, the route by which a drug is administered will significantly affect both the time of onset and the intensity of effects. Why do patterns of absorption differ between routes? Because the barriers to absorption associated with each route are different. In the discussion below, we examine these barriers and their influence on absorption pattern. In addition, as we discuss each major route, we will consider its clinical advantages and disadvantages.

Intravenous

Barriers to Absorption. When a drug is administered IV, there are no barriers to absorption. Recall that absorption is defined as the movement of a drug from its site of administration into the blood. Since IV administration puts a drug directly into the blood, all barriers are bypassed.

Absorption Pattern. Intravenous administration results in "absorption" that is both instantaneous and complete. Intravenous "absorption" is instantaneous in that drug enters the blood directly. "Absorption" is complete in that virtually all of the administered dose reaches the blood.

Advantages. Rapid Onset. Intravenous administration results in rapid onset of drug action. Although rapid onset is not always important, it is clearly beneficial in emergencies.

Control. Since the entire dose is administered directly into the blood, we have precise control over levels of drug in the blood. This contrasts with the other major routes of administration, and especially with oral administration (see below).

Use of Large Fluid Volumes. The IV route is the only parenteral route that permits the use of large volumes of fluid. Some drugs that require parenteral administration are poorly soluble in water and therefore must be dissolved in a large volume. Because of the physical limitations presented by soft tissues (e.g., muscle, subcutaneous tissue), injection of large volumes at these sites is not feasible. In contrast, the amount of fluid that can be infused into a vein, although limited, is nonetheless relatively big.

Use of Irritant Drugs. Certain drugs, because of their irritant properties, can be administered only by the IV route. A number of anticancer drugs, for example, are very chemically reactive. If present in high concentrations, these agents can cause severe local injury. However, when administered through a freely flowing IV line, these drugs are rapidly diluted in the blood, thereby minimizing the risk of injury.

Disadvantages. High Cost, Difficulty, and Inconvenience. Intravenous administration is expensive, difficult, and inconvenient. The cost of IV administration sets and their set-up charges can be substantial. Setting up an IV line takes time and special training. Because of the difficulty involved, most patients are unable to self-administer IV drugs, and therefore must depend on a healthcare professional. Because patients are tethered to lines and bottles, their mobility is limited. In sharp contrast, oral administration is easy, convenient, and cheap.

Irreversibility. More important than cost or convenience, IV administration can be *dangerous*. Once a drug has been injected, there is no turning back; the drug is in the body and cannot be retrieved. Hence, if the dose is excessive, avoiding harm may be impossible.

To minimize risk, IV drugs should be injected slowly (over 1 minute or more). Since all of the blood in the body is circulated about once every minute, by injecting a drug over a 1-minute interval, we cause it to be diluted in the largest volume of blood possible. By doing so, we can avoid drug concentrations that are unnecessarily—or even dangerously—high.

Performing IV injections slowly has the additional advantage of reducing the risk of toxicity to the central nervous system (CNS). When a drug is injected into the antecubital vein of the arm, it takes about 15 seconds for the drug to reach the brain. Consequently, if the dose is sufficient to cause CNS toxicity, signs of toxicity may become apparent 15 seconds after starting the injection. If the injection is being done slowly (e.g., over a 1-minute interval), only 25% of the total dose will have been administered when signs of toxicity appear. If administration is discontinued immediately, adverse effects will be much less than they would have been had the entire dose been injected.

Fluid Overload. When drugs are administered in a large volume, fluid overload can occur. This can be a significant problem for patients with hypertension, kidney disease, or heart failure.

Infection. Infection can occur from injecting a contaminated drug. Fortunately, the risk of infection is much lower today than it was before the development of modern techniques for sterilizing drugs intended for IV use.

Embolism. Intravenous administration carries a risk of embolism (blood vessel blockage at a site distant from the point of administration). Embolism can be caused in several ways. First, insertion of an IV needle can injure the venous wall, leading to formation of a thrombus (clot); embolism can result if the clot breaks loose and becomes lodged in another vessel. Second, injection of hypotonic or hypertonic fluids can destroy red blood cells; the debris from these cells can produce embolism.

Lastly, injection of drugs that are not fully dissolved can cause embolism. Particles of undissolved drug are like small grains of sand, which can become embedded in blood vessels and cause blockage. Because of the risk of embolism, you should check IV solutions prior to administration to ensure that drugs are in solution. If the fluid is cloudy or contains particles, the drug is not dissolved and must not be administered.

The Importance of Reading Labels. Not all formulations of the same drug are appropriate for IV administration. Accordingly, it is essential to read the label before giving a drug IV. Two examples will illustrate the importance of this admonition. The first is insulin. Only one preparation of insulin, labeled *insulin injection,* can be administered safely IV. Insulin injection is a clear solution formulated for IV use. With one exception, all other insulin preparations are *particulate suspensions.* These preparations are intended for SC administration only. Because of their particulate nature, these preparations could prove fatal if given IV. By checking the label, inadvertent IV injection of particulate insulin can be avoided.

Epinephrine provides our second example of the importance of reading the label before giving a drug IV. Epinephrine, which stimulates the cardiovascular system, can be injected by several routes (IM, IV, SC, intracardiac, intraspinal). It must be noted, however, that a solution prepared for use by one route will differ in concentration from a solution prepared for use by other routes. For example, whereas solutions intended for *subcutaneous* administration are *concentrated,* solutions intended for *intravenous* use are *dilute.* If a solution prepared for SC use were to be inadvertently administered IV, the result could prove *fatal.* (Intravenous administration of concentrated epinephrine could overstimulate the heart and blood vessels, causing severe hypertension, cerebral hemorrhage, stroke, and death.) The take-home message is that simply giving the *right drug* is not sufficient; you must also be sure that the formulation and concentration are *appropriate for the intended route.*

Intramuscular

Barriers to Absorption. When a drug is injected IM, the only barrier to absorption is the *capillary wall.* In capillary beds that serve muscles and most other tissues, there are "large" spaces between the cells that compose the capillary wall (Fig. 4–7). Drugs can pass through these spaces with ease, and need not cross cell membranes to enter the bloodstream. Accordingly, like IV administration, IM administration presents no significant barriers to absorption.

Absorption Pattern. Drugs administered IM may be absorbed rapidly or slowly. The rate of absorption is determined largely by two factors: (1) water solubility of the drug and (2) blood flow to the site of injection. Drugs that are highly soluble in water will be absorbed rapidly (within 10 to 30 minutes), whereas drugs that are poorly soluble will be absorbed slowly. Similarly, absorption will be rapid from sites where blood flow is high, and slow where blood flow is low.

Advantages. The IM route can be used for parenteral administration of *poorly soluble drugs.* Recall that drugs must be dissolved if they are to be administered IV. Consequently, the IV route cannot be used for poorly soluble compounds. In contrast, since little harm will come from depositing a suspension of undissolved drug in the interstitial space of muscle tissue, the IM route is acceptable for drugs whose water solubility is poor.

A second advantage of the IM route is that we can use it to administer *depot preparations* (preparations from which the drug is absorbed slowly over an extended time). Depending on the depot formulation, the effects of a single injection may persist for days, weeks, or even months. For example, *benzathine penicillin G,* a depot preparation of penicillin, can re-

lease therapeutically effective amounts of penicillin for a month or more following a single IM injection. In contrast, a single IM injection of penicillin G itself would be absorbed and excreted in less than 1 day. The obvious advantage of depot preparations is that they can greatly reduce the number of injections required during long-term therapy.

Disadvantages. The major drawbacks of IM administration are discomfort and inconvenience. Intramuscular injection of some preparations can be painful. Also, IM injections can cause local tissue injury and possibly nerve damage (if the injection is done improperly). Like all other forms of parenteral administration, IM injections are less convenient than oral administration.

Subcutaneous

The pharmacokinetics of SC administration are nearly identical to those of IM administration. As with IM administration, there are no significant barriers to absorption: Once a drug has been injected SC, it readily enters the blood by passing through the spaces between cells of the capillary wall. As with IM administration, blood flow and drug solubility are the major determinants of how fast absorption takes place. Because of the similarities between SC and IM administration, these routes have similar advantages (suitability for poorly soluble drugs and depot preparations) and drawbacks (discomfort, inconvenience, potential for injury).

Oral

In the discussion below, the abbreviation PO is used in reference to oral administration. This abbreviation stands for *per os,* a Latin phrase meaning *by way of the mouth.*

Barriers to Absorption. Following oral administration, drugs may be absorbed from the stomach or the intestine. In either case, there are two barriers to cross: (1) the layer of *epithelial cells* that lines the GI tract, and (2) the *capillary wall.*

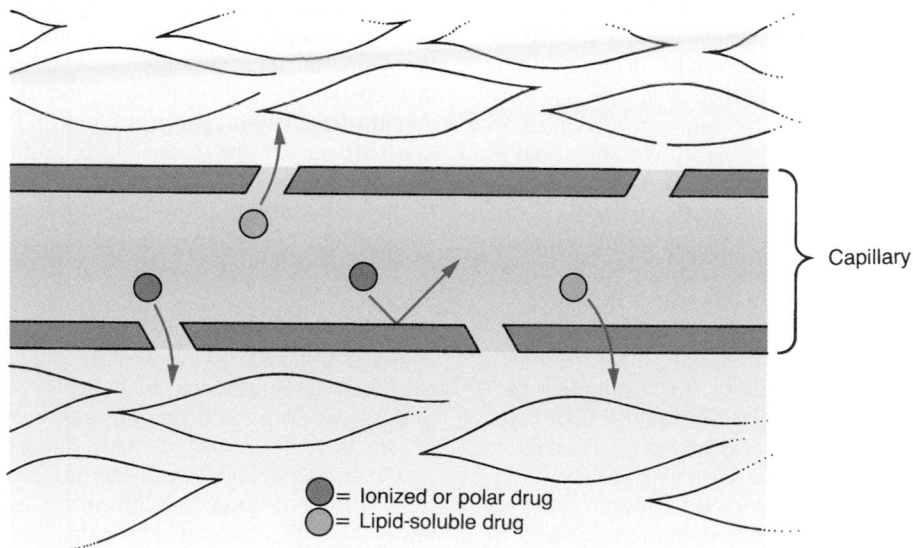

Figure 4–7 ■ Drug movement at typical capillary beds.
In most capillary beds, "large" gaps exist between the cells that compose the capillary wall. Drugs and other molecules can pass freely into and out of the bloodstream through these gaps. As illustrated, lipid-soluble compounds can also pass directly through the cells of the capillary wall.

Since the walls of the capillaries that serve the GI tract offer no significant resistance to absorption, the major barrier to absorption is the GI epithelium. To cross this layer of tightly packed cells, drugs must pass *through* cells rather than between them.

Absorption Pattern. Because of multiple factors, the rate and extent of drug absorption following oral administration can be *highly variable.* Factors that can influence absorption include (1) solubility and stability of the drug, (2) gastric and intestinal pH, (3) gastric emptying time, (4) food in the gut, (5) coadministration of other drugs, and (6) special coatings on the drug preparation.

Advantages. Oral administration is easy, convenient, and inexpensive. (By inexpensive, we don't mean that oral drugs themselves are inexpensive, but rather that there is no cost for the process of administration.) Because of its relative ease, oral administration is the preferred route for self-medication.

Although absorption of oral drugs can be highly variable, this route is still *safer than injection.* With oral administration, there is no risk of fluid overload, infection, or embolism. Furthermore, since oral administration is potentially reversible, whereas injections are not, oral administration is much safer. Recall that with parenteral administration there is no turning back: Once a drug has been injected, there is little we can do to prevent absorption and subsequent effects. Therefore, when giving drugs parenterally, we must live with the consequences of our mistakes. In contrast, if need be, there are steps we can take to prevent absorption following inappropriate oral administration. For example, by inducing either emesis (vomiting) or catharsis (rapid emptying of the small intestine and bowel) or both, we can remove orally administered drugs from the body before there has been sufficient time for absorption. In addition, we can prevent harm from orally administered drugs by giving activated charcoal, a compound that adsorbs drugs while they are still in the GI tract; once drugs are adsorbed onto the charcoal, they cannot be absorbed into the bloodstream. Our ability to prevent the absorption of orally administered drugs gives PO medications a safety factor that is unavailable with drugs given by injection.

Disadvantages. Variability. The major disadvantage of PO therapy is that absorption can be highly variable. That is, a drug administered to patient A may be absorbed rapidly and completely, whereas the same drug given to patient B may be absorbed slowly and incompletely. This variability makes it difficult to control the concentration of a drug at its sites of action, and therefore makes it difficult to control the onset, intensity, and duration of responses.

Inactivation. Oral administration can lead to inactivation of certain drugs. Penicillin G, for example, can't be taken orally because it would be destroyed by stomach acid. Similarly, insulin can't be taken orally because it would be destroyed by digestive enzymes. Some drugs can't be taken orally because they would undergo rapid inactivation by hepatic enzymes as they pass through the liver on their way from the GI tract to the general circulation. This phenomenon, known as the "first-pass effect," is discussed later.

Patient Requirements. Oral drug administration requires a conscious, cooperative patient. Drugs cannot be administered PO to comatose individuals or to individuals who, for whatever reason (e.g., psychosis, seizure, obstinacy, nausea), are unable or unwilling to swallow medication.

Local Irritation. Some oral preparations cause local irritation of the GI tract, which can result in discomfort, nausea, and vomiting.

Comparing Oral Administration with Parenteral Administration

Because of ease, convenience, and relative safety, *oral administration is generally preferred to parenteral administration.* However, there are situations in which parenteral administration is clearly superior. Parenteral administration may be indicated in emergencies when rapid onset is required. Parenteral administration is desirable when plasma drug levels must be tightly controlled. (Because of variable absorption, oral administration does not permit tight control of plasma drug levels.) Parenteral administration is preferred for those drugs that would be destroyed by gastric acidity or digestive enzymes if given orally (e.g., insulin, penicillin G). Drugs such as the quaternary ammonium compounds, which cannot cross membranes, require parenteral administration to produce systemic effects. Parenteral administration is also required for drugs that would cause severe local injury if administered by mouth (e.g., certain anticancer agents). In addition, parenteral administration is indicated when the prolonged effects of a depot preparation are desired. Lastly, parenteral therapy is superior to oral therapy for patients who cannot or will not take drugs orally.

Pharmaceutical Preparations for Oral Administration

There are several kinds of "packages" (formulations) into which a drug can be put for oral administration. Three such formulations—*tablets, enteric coatings,* and *sustained-release preparations*—are discussed below.

Before we discuss drug formulations, it will be helpful to define two terms: *chemical equivalence* and *bioavailability.* Drug preparations are considered *chemically equivalent* if they contain the same amount of the identical chemical compound (drug). Preparations are considered equal in *bioavailability* if the drug they contain is absorbed at the same rate and to the same extent. Please note that it is possible for two formulations of the same drug to be chemically equivalent while differing in bioavailability.

Tablets. A tablet is a mixture of a drug plus binders and fillers, all of which have been compressed together. Tablets made by different manufacturers can differ in their rates of disintegration and dissolution, causing differences in bioavailability. As a result, two tablets that contain the same amount of the same drug can differ with respect to onset and intensity of effects.

Enteric-Coated Preparations. Enteric-coated preparations consist of drugs that have been covered with a material designed to dissolve in the intestine but not the stomach. Materials used for enteric coatings include fatty acids, waxes, and shellac. Since enteric-coated preparations release their contents into the intestine and not the stomach, these preparations are employed for two general purposes: (1) to protect drugs from acid and pepsin in the stomach and (2) to protect the stomach from drugs that can cause gastric discomfort.

The primary disadvantage of enteric-coated preparations is that absorption can be even more variable than with standard tablets. Since gastric emptying time can vary from minutes up to 12 hours, and since enteric-coated preparations cannot be absorbed until they leave the stomach, variations in gastric emptying time can alter time of onset. Furthermore, enteric coatings sometimes fail to dissolve, thereby allowing medication to pass through the GI tract without being absorbed at all.

Sustained-Release Preparations. Sustained-release formulations are capsules filled with tiny spheres that contain the actual drug; the spheres have coatings that dissolve at variable rates. Since some spheres dissolve more slowly than others, drug is released steadily throughout the day. The primary advantage of sustained-release preparations is that they permit a reduction in the number of daily doses. These formulations have the additional advantage of producing relatively steady drug levels over an extended time (much like giving a drug by infusion). The major disadvantages of sustained-release formulations are high cost and the potential for variable absorption.

Additional Routes of Administration

Drugs can be administered by a number of routes in addition to those already discussed. Drugs can be applied *topically* for local therapy of the skin, eyes, ears, nose, mouth, and vagina. In a few cases, topical agents (e.g., nitroglycerin, nicotine, testosterone) are formulated for *transdermal* absorption into the systemic circulation. Some drugs are *inhaled* to elicit local effects in the lung, especially in the treatment of asthma. Other inhalational agents (e.g., volatile anesthetics, oxygen) are used for their systemic effects. *Rectal suppositories* may be employed for local effects or for effects throughout the body. *Vaginal suppositories* may be employed to treat local disorders. For management of some conditions, drugs must be given by *direct injection into a specific site* (e.g., heart, joints, nerves, CNS). The unique characteristics of these routes are addressed throughout the book as we discuss specific drugs that employ them.

DISTRIBUTION

Distribution is defined as *the movement of drugs throughout the body*. Drug distribution is determined by three major factors: blood flow to tissues, the ability of a drug to exit the vascular system, and, to a lesser extent, the ability of a drug to enter cells.

Blood Flow to Tissues

In the first phase of distribution, drugs are carried by the blood to the tissues and organs of the body. The rate at which drugs are delivered to a particular tissue is determined by blood flow to the tissue. Since most tissues are well perfused, regional blood flow is rarely a limiting factor in drug distribution.

There are two pathologic conditions—abscesses and tumors—in which low regional blood flow can affect drug therapy. An abscess is a pus-filled pocket of infection that has no internal blood vessels. Because abscesses lack a blood supply, antibiotics cannot reach the bacteria within. Accordingly, if drug therapy is to be effective, the abscess must first be surgically drained.

Solid tumors have a limited blood supply. Although blood flow to the outer regions of tumors is relatively high, blood flow becomes progressively lower toward the core. As a result, we cannot achieve high drug levels deep within tumors. Limited blood flow is a major reason why solid tumors are resistant to drug therapy.

Exiting the Vascular System

After a drug has been delivered to an organ or tissue via the blood, the next phase of distribution is to exit the vasculature. Since most drugs do not produce their effects within the blood, the ability to leave the vascular system is an important determinant of drug actions. Exiting the vascular system is also necessary for drugs to undergo metabolism and excretion. Drugs in the vascular system leave the blood at capillary beds.

Typical Capillary Beds

Most capillary beds offer no resistance to the departure of drugs. That is, in most tissues, drugs can leave the vasculature by passing through pores in the capillary wall. Since drugs pass *between* capillary cells rather than *through* them, movement into the interstitial space is not impeded. The exit of drugs from a typical capillary bed is depicted in Figure 4–7.

The Blood-Brain Barrier

The term *blood-brain barrier* refers to the unique anatomy of capillaries in the CNS. As shown in Figure 4–8, there are *tight junctions* between the cells that compose the walls of most capillaries in the CNS. These junctions are so tight that they prevent drug passage. Consequently, in order to leave the blood and reach sites of action within the brain, a drug must be able to pass *through* cells of the capillary wall. Only drugs that are *lipid soluble* or have a *transport system* can cross the blood-brain barrier to a significant degree.

The presence of the blood-brain barrier is a mixed blessing. The good news is that the barrier protects the brain from injury by potentially toxic substances. The bad news is that the barrier can be a significant obstacle to therapy of CNS disorders. The barrier can, for example, impede access of antibiotics to CNS infections.

The blood-brain barrier is not fully developed at birth. As a result, newborns are much more sensitive than older children or adults to medicines that act on the brain. Likewise, neonates are especially vulnerable to CNS poisons.

Placental Drug Transfer

The membranes of the placenta separate the maternal circulation from the fetal circulation (Fig. 4–9). *The membranes of the placenta do NOT constitute an absolute barrier to the passage of drugs.* The same factors that determine the movement of drugs across other membranes determine the movement of drugs across the placenta. Accordingly, lipid-soluble, nonionized compounds readily pass from the maternal bloodstream into the blood of the fetus. In contrast, compounds that are ionized, highly polar, or protein bound (see below) are largely excluded.

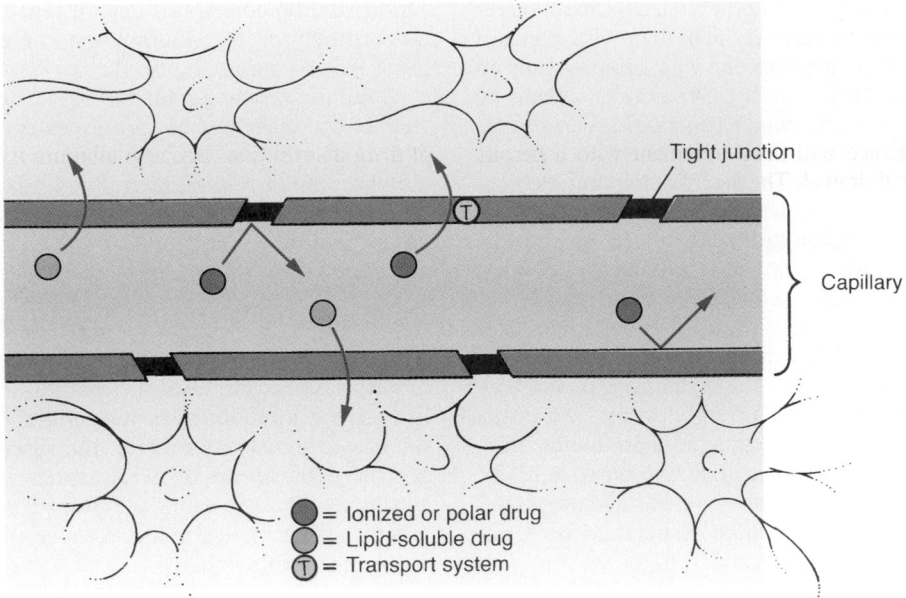

Figure 4–8 ■ **Drug movement across the blood-brain barrier.**
Tight junctions between cells that compose the walls of capillaries in the CNS prevent drugs from passing between cells to exit the vascular system. Consequently, in order to reach sites of action within the brain, a drug must pass directly through cells of the capillary wall. To do this, the drug must be lipid soluble or be able to use an existing transport system.

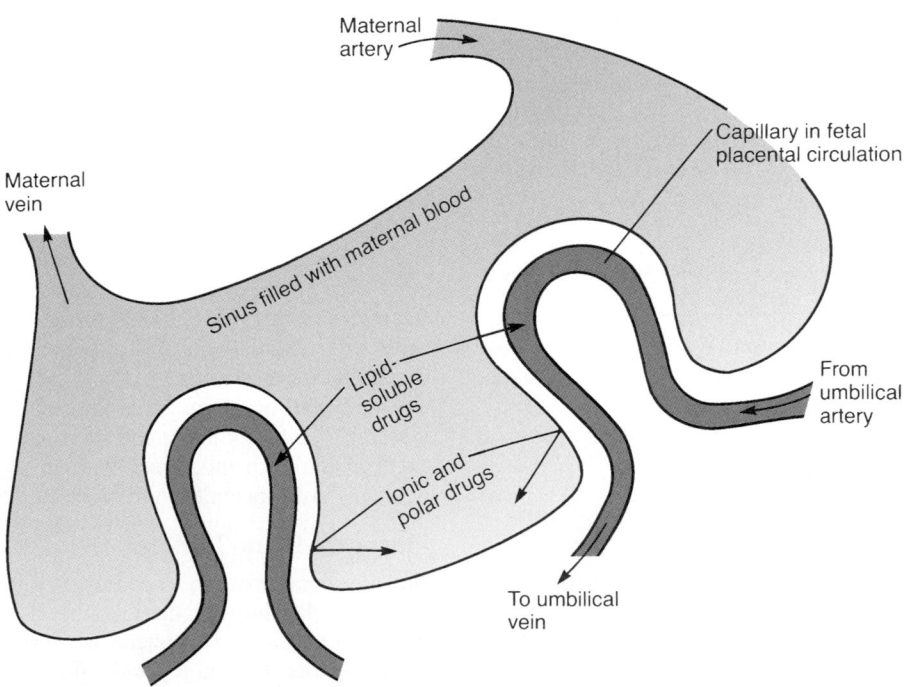

Figure 4–9 ■ **Placental drug transfer.**
To enter the fetal circulation, drugs must cross membranes of the maternal and fetal vascular systems. Lipid-soluble drugs can readily cross these membranes and enter the fetal blood, whereas ions and polar molecules are prevented from reaching the fetal blood.

Drugs that have the ability to cross the placenta can cause serious harm. Some compounds can cause birth defects, ranging from low birth weight to mental retardation to gross malformations. (Recall the thalidomide experience.) If a pregnant woman is a habitual user of opioids (e.g., heroin), her child will be born drug dependent, and hence will need treatment with a heroin substitute to prevent withdrawal. The use of respiratory depressants (anesthetics and analgesics) during delivery can depress respiration in the neonate; infants exposed to respiratory depressants must be monitored until breathing has normalized.

Protein Binding

Drugs can form reversible bonds with various proteins in the body. Of all the proteins to which drugs can bind, *plasma albumin* is the most important. Albumin is the most abundant protein in plasma. Like other proteins, albumin is a large molecule, having a molecular weight of 69,000. Because of its size, *albumin always remains within the bloodstream:* Albumin is too large to squeeze through pores in the capillary wall, and no transport system exists by which it might leave.

Figure 4–10*A* depicts the binding of drug molecules to albumin. Note that the drug molecules are much smaller than albumin. (The molecular mass of the average drug is about 300 to 500 compared with 69,000 for albumin.) As indicated by the two-way arrows, binding between albumin and drugs is *reversible*. As a result, a drug may exist either *bound* or *unbound* (free).

For drugs with the ability to bind with plasma albumin, only some molecules will be bound at any moment. The percentage of drug molecules that are bound is determined by the strength of the attraction between albumin and the drug. For example, the attraction between albumin and warfarin (an anticoagulant) is strong, causing nearly all (99%) of the warfarin molecules in plasma to be bound, leaving only 1% free. For

gentamicin (an antibiotic), the ratio of bound to free is quite different; since the attraction between gentamicin and albumin is relatively weak, less than 10% of the gentamicin molecules in plasma are bound, leaving more than 90% free.

An important consequence of protein binding is restriction of drug distribution. Because albumin is too large to leave the bloodstream, drug molecules that are bound to albumin cannot leave either (Fig. 4–10*B*). As a result, bound molecules cannot reach their sites of action, metabolism, or excretion.

In addition to restricting the distribution of drugs, protein binding can be a source of drug interactions. As suggested by Figure 4–10*A*, each molecule of albumin has only a few sites to which drug molecules can bind. Because the number of binding sites is limited, drugs with the ability to bind albumin will compete with one another for binding sites. As a result, one drug can displace another from albumin, causing the free concentration of the displaced drug to rise. By increasing levels of free drug, competition for binding can increase the intensity of drug responses. If the intensity increases excessively, toxicity can result.

Entering Cells

Some drugs must enter cells to reach their sites of action, and practically all drugs must enter cells to undergo metabolism and excretion. The factors that determine the ability of a drug to cross cell membranes are the same factors that determine the passage of drugs across all other membranes, namely, lipid solubility, the presence of a transport system, or both.

As discussed in Chapter 5, many drugs produce their effects by binding to receptors located on the external surface of the cell membrane. Obviously, these drugs do not need to cross the cell membrane in order to act.

METABOLISM

Drug metabolism, also known as *biotransformation*, is defined as *the enzymatic alteration of drug structure*. Most drug metabolism takes place in the liver.

Hepatic Drug-Metabolizing Enzymes

Most drug metabolism that takes place in the liver is performed by the *hepatic microsomal enzyme system*, also known as the *P450 system*. The term *P450* refers to *cytochrome P450*, a key component of this enzyme system.

It is important to appreciate that cytochrome P450 is not a single molecular entity, but rather a group of 12 closely related enzyme families. Three of the cytochrome P450 (CYP) families—designated CYP1, CYP2, and CYP3—metabolize drugs. The other nine families metabolize endogenous compounds (e.g., steroids, fatty acids). Each of the three P450 families that metabolize drugs is itself composed of multiple forms, each of which metabolizes only certain drugs. To identify the individual forms of cytochrome P450, we use designations such as CYP1A2, CYP2D6, and CYP3A4, indicating specific members of the CYP1, CYP2, and CYP3 families, respectively. I mention this nomenclature only so that it will be familiar when you come across it in your reading. This information is not intended for memorization.

A **Reversible Binding of a Drug to Albumin**

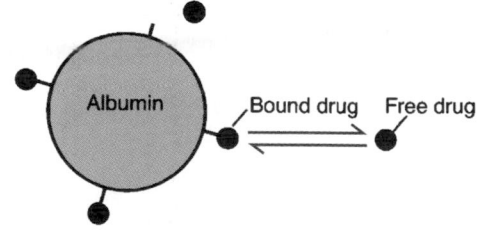

B **Retention of Protein-Bound Drug Within the Vasculature**

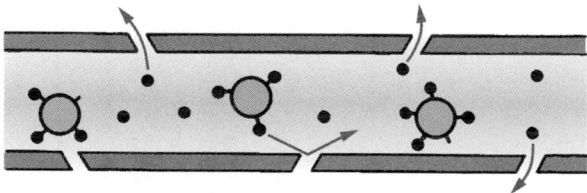

Figure 4–10 ■ Protein binding of drugs.
A, Albumin is the most prevalent protein in plasma and the most important of the proteins to which drugs bind. *B,* Only unbound (free) drug molecules can leave the vascular system. Bound molecules are too large to fit through the pores in the capillary wall.

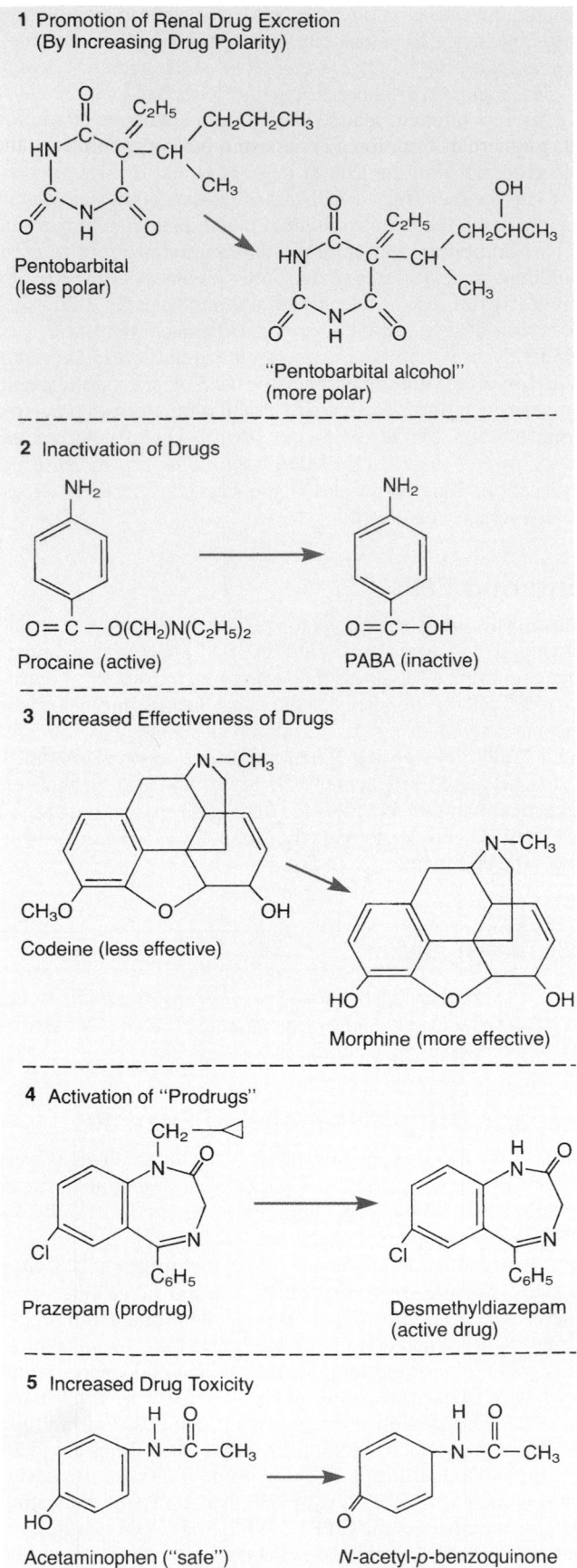

1 Promotion of Renal Drug Excretion
(By Increasing Drug Polarity)

Pentobarbital
(less polar)

"Pentobarbital alcohol"
(more polar)

2 Inactivation of Drugs

Procaine (active)

PABA (inactive)

3 Increased Effectiveness of Drugs

Codeine (less effective)

Morphine (more effective)

4 Activation of "Prodrugs"

Prazepam (prodrug)

Desmethyldiazepam
(active drug)

5 Increased Drug Toxicity

Acetaminophen ("safe")

N-acetyl-p-benzoquinone
(hepatotoxic)

Figure 4–11 ■ Therapeutic consequences of drug metabolism. (See text for details.)

Hepatic microsomal enzymes are capable of catalyzing a wide variety of reactions that employ drugs as substrates. Some of these reactions are illustrated in Figure 4–11. As these examples indicate, drug metabolism doesn't always result in the breakdown of drugs into smaller molecules; drug metabolism can also result in the synthesis of a molecule that is larger than the parent drug.

Therapeutic Consequences of Drug Metabolism

Drug metabolism has five possible consequences of therapeutic significance: (1) accelerated renal excretion of drugs, (2) drug inactivation, (3) increased therapeutic action, (4) activation of prodrugs, and (5) increased or decreased toxicity. Figure 4–11 depicts reactions that illustrate these consequences of metabolism.

Accelerated Renal Drug Excretion. The most important consequence of drug metabolism is promotion of renal drug excretion. As discussed in the next section, the kidney, which is the major organ of drug excretion, is unable to excrete drugs that are highly lipid soluble. By converting lipid-soluble drugs into more polar (less lipid-soluble) compounds, drug metabolism makes it possible for the kidney to excrete many drugs. For certain highly lipid-soluble drugs (e.g., thiopental), complete renal excretion would take years were it not for their conversion into more polar compounds by drug-metabolizing enzymes.

Drug Inactivation. Drug metabolism can convert pharmacologically active compounds to inactive forms. This process is illustrated by the conversion of procaine (a local anesthetic) into *para*-aminobenzoic acid (PABA), an inactive metabolite (see Fig. 4–11).

Increased Therapeutic Action. Metabolism can increase the effectiveness of some drugs. This consequence of metabolism is illustrated by the conversion of codeine into morphine (see Fig. 4–11). The analgesic activity of morphine is so much greater than that of codeine that formation of morphine may account for virtually all the pain relief that occurs following codeine administration.

Activation of Prodrugs. A *prodrug* is a compound that is pharmacologically inactive as administered and then undergoes conversion to its active form within the body. Activation of a prodrug is illustrated by the metabolic conversion of prazepam into desmethyldiazepam (see Fig. 4–11). (Prazepam is a close relative of diazepam, a drug familiar to us under the trade name Valium.)

Increased or Decreased Toxicity. By converting drugs into inactive forms, metabolism can decrease toxicity. Conversely, metabolism can increase the potential for harm by converting relatively safe compounds into forms that are toxic. Increased toxicity is illustrated by the conversion of acetaminophen [Tylenol, others] into a hepatotoxic metabolite (see Fig. 4–11). It is this product of metabolism, and not acetaminophen itself, that causes injury when acetaminophen is taken in overdose.

Special Considerations in Drug Metabolism

Several factors can influence the rate at which drugs are metabolized. These must be accounted for in drug therapy.

Age. The drug-metabolizing capacity of infants is limited. The liver does not develop its full capacity to metabolize drugs until about 1 year after birth. *During the time prior to hepatic maturation, infants are especially sensitive to drugs, and care must be taken to avoid injury.*

Induction of Drug-Metabolizing Enzymes. Some drugs act on the liver to increase rates of drug metabolism. For example, when phenobarbital is administered for several days, it can cause the drug-metabolizing capacity of the liver to double. Phenobarbital increases metabolism by causing the liver to synthesize drug-metabolizing enzymes. This process of stimulating enzyme synthesis is known as *induction.*

Induction of drug-metabolizing enzymes can have two therapeutic consequences. First, by stimulating the liver to produce more drug-metabolizing enzymes, a drug can increase the rate of its own metabolism, thereby necessitating an increase in its dosage to maintain therapeutic effects. Second, induction of drug-metabolizing enzymes can accelerate the metabolism of other drugs used concurrently, necessitating an increase in their dosages.

First-Pass Effect. The term *first-pass effect* refers to the rapid hepatic inactivation of certain oral drugs. When drugs are administered orally, they are absorbed from the GI tract and carried directly to the liver via the hepatic portal circulation. If the capacity of the liver to metabolize a drug is extremely high, that drug can be completely inactivated on its first pass through the liver. As a result, no therapeutic effects will occur. To circumvent the first-pass effect, a drug that undergoes rapid hepatic metabolism is often administered parenterally. This permits the drug to temporarily bypass the liver, thereby allowing it to reach therapeutic levels in the systemic blood.

Nitroglycerin is the classic example of a drug that undergoes such rapid hepatic metabolism that it is largely without effect following oral administration. However, when administered sublingually (under the tongue), nitroglycerin is very active. Sublingual administration is effective because it permits nitroglycerin to be absorbed through the oral mucosa directly into the systemic circulation. Once in the circulation, the drug is carried to its sites of action prior to passage through the liver. Hence, therapeutic action can be exerted before the drug is exposed to hepatic enzymes.

Nutritional Status. Hepatic drug-metabolizing enzymes require a number of co-factors to function. In the malnourished patient, these co-factors may be deficient, causing drug metabolism to be compromised.

Competition Between Drugs. When two drugs are metabolized by the same metabolic pathway, they may compete with each other for metabolism, and thereby decrease the rate at which one or both agents are metabolized. If metabolism is depressed enough, a drug can accumulate to dangerous levels.

EXCRETION

Drug excretion is defined as *the removal of drugs from the body.* Drugs and their metabolites can exit the body in urine, bile, sweat, saliva, breast milk, and expired air. The most important organ for drug excretion is the kidney.

Renal Drug Excretion

The kidneys account for the majority of drug excretion. When the kidneys are healthy, they serve to limit the duration of action of many drugs. Conversely, if renal failure occurs, both the duration and intensity of drug responses may increase.

Steps in Renal Drug Excretion

Urinary excretion of drugs is the net result of three processes: (1) glomerular filtration, (2) passive tubular reabsorption, and (3) active tubular secretion (Fig. 4–12).

Glomerular Filtration. Renal excretion begins at the glomerulus of the kidney tubule. The glomerulus consists of a capillary network surrounded by Bowman's capsule; small pores perforate the capillary walls. As blood flows through the glomerular capillaries, fluids and small molecules—including drugs—are forced through the pores of the capillary wall. This process, called glomerular filtration, moves drugs from the blood into the tubular urine. Blood cells and large molecules (e.g., proteins) are too big to pass through the capillary pores and therefore do not undergo filtration. Because large molecules are not filtered, drugs bound to albumin remain behind in the blood.

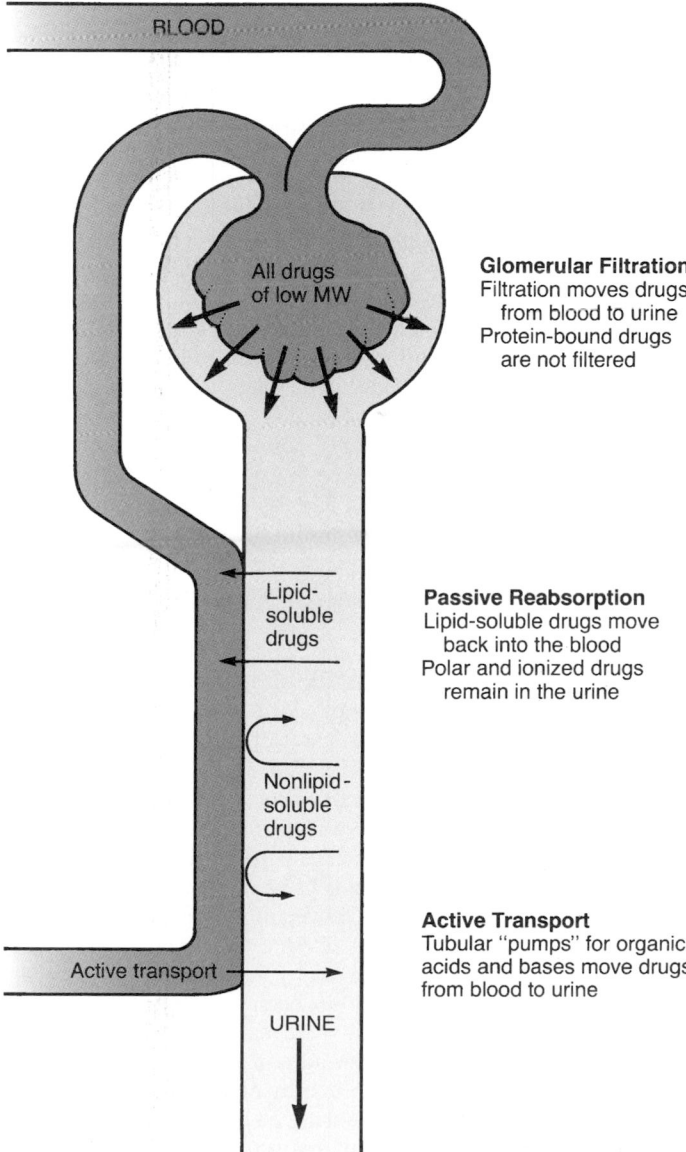

Figure 4–12 ■ **Renal drug excretion.** (Redrawn from Binns TB [ed]. Absorption and Distribution of Drugs. Edinburgh, Churchill Livingstone, 1964.)

Passive Tubular Reabsorption. As depicted in Figure 4–12, the vessels that deliver blood to the glomerulus return to proximity with the renal tubule at a point distal to the glomerulus. At this distal site, drug concentrations in the blood are lower than drug concentrations in the tubule. This concentration gradient acts as a driving force to move drugs from the lumen of the tubule back into the blood. Since lipid-soluble drugs can readily cross the membranes that compose the tubular and vascular walls, *drugs that are lipid soluble undergo passive reabsorption from the tubule back into the blood.* In contrast, drugs that are not lipid soluble (ions and polar compounds) remain in the urine to be excreted. By converting lipid-soluble drugs into more polar forms, drug metabolism reduces passive reabsorption of drugs and thereby accelerates their excretion.

Active Tubular Secretion. There are active transport systems in the kidney tubules that pump drugs from the blood to the tubular urine. The tubules have two classes of pumps, one for organic acids and one for organic bases. These pumps have a relatively high capacity and play a significant role in excreting certain compounds.

Factors That Modify Renal Drug Excretion

pH-Dependent Ionization. The phenomenon of pH-dependent ionization can be used to accelerate renal excretion of drugs. Recall that passive tubular reabsorption is limited to lipid-soluble compounds. Since ions are not lipid soluble, drugs that are ionized at the pH of tubular urine will remain in the tubule and be excreted. Consequently, by manipulating urinary pH in such a way as to promote the ionization of a drug, we can decrease passive reabsorption back into the blood and thereby hasten the drug's elimination. This principle has been employed to promote the excretion of poisons as well as medications that have been taken in toxic doses.

The treatment of aspirin poisoning provides an example of how manipulation of urinary pH can be put to therapeutic advantage. When children have been exposed to toxic doses of aspirin, they can be treated, in part, by giving an agent that elevates urinary pH (i.e., makes the urine more basic). Since aspirin is an acidic drug, and since acids tend to ionize in basic media, elevation of urinary pH causes more of the aspirin molecules present in urine to become ionized. As a result, less drug is passively reabsorbed and hence more is excreted.

Competition for Active Tubular Transport. Competition between drugs for active tubular transport can delay their renal excretion, thereby prolonging effects. The active transport systems of the renal tubules can be envisioned as motor-driven revolving doors that carry drugs from the plasma into the renal tubules. These "revolving doors" can carry only a limited number of drug molecules per unit time. Accordingly, if there are too many molecules present, some must wait their turn. Because of competition, if we administer two drugs at the same time, and if both drugs use the same transport system, excretion of each will be delayed by the presence of the other.

Competition for transport has been employed clinically to prolong the effects of drugs that normally undergo rapid renal excretion. For example, when administered alone, penicillin is rapidly cleared from the blood by active tubular transport. Excretion of penicillin can be delayed by concurrent administration of probenecid, an agent that is removed from the blood by the same tubular transport system that pumps penicillin. Hence, if a large dose of probenecid is administered, renal excretion of penicillin will be delayed while the transport system is occupied with moving the probenecid. By delaying penicillin excretion, probenecid prolongs antibacterial effects.

Age. The kidneys of newborns are not fully developed. Until their kidneys reach full capacity (a few months after birth), infants have a limited capacity to excrete drugs. This must be accounted for when medicating an infant.

Nonrenal Routes of Drug Excretion

In most cases, excretion of drugs by nonrenal routes has minimal clinical significance. However, in certain situations, nonrenal excretion can have important therapeutic and toxicologic consequences.

Breast Milk

Drugs taken by breast-feeding women can undergo excretion into milk. As a result, breast-feeding can expose the nursing infant to drugs. The factors that influence the appearance of drugs in breast milk are the same factors that determine the passage of drugs across membranes. Accordingly, lipid-soluble drugs will have ready access to breast milk, whereas drugs that are polar, ionized, or protein bound will not enter in significant amounts. Because infants may be harmed by compounds excreted in breast milk, it is recommended that nursing mothers avoid all drugs. If a woman must take medication, she should consult with her prescriber to ensure that the drug will not reach concentrations in her milk that are high enough to harm her baby.

Other Nonrenal Routes of Excretion

The *bile* is an important route of excretion for certain drugs. Recall that bile is secreted into the intestine and then leaves the body in the feces. In some cases, drugs entering the intestine in bile may undergo reabsorption back into the portal blood. This reabsorption, referred to as *enterohepatic recirculation,* can substantially prolong a drug's sojourn in the body.

The *lungs* are the major route by which volatile anesthetics are excreted.

Small amounts of drugs can appear in *sweat* and *saliva.* These routes have little therapeutic or toxicologic significance.

TIME COURSE OF DRUG RESPONSES

To achieve the therapeutic objective, we must control the time course of drug responses. We need to regulate the time at which drug responses start, the time they are most intense, and the time they cease. Since the four pharmacokinetic processes—absorption, distribution, metabolism, and excretion—determine how much drug will be at its sites of action at any given time, these processes are the major determinants of the time course over which drug responses take place. Having discussed the individual processes that contribute to determining the time course of drug action, we are now prepared to discuss the time course itself.

Plasma Drug Levels

In most cases, the time course of drug action bears a direct relationship to the concentration of a drug in the blood. Hence, before discussing the time course per se, we will review several important concepts related to plasma drug levels.

Clinical Significance of Plasma Drug Levels

Clinicians frequently monitor plasma drug levels in efforts to regulate drug responses. When measurements indicate that drug levels are inappropriate, these levels can be adjusted up or down by changing dosage, the timing of administration, or both.

The practice of regulating plasma drug levels in order to control drug responses should seem a bit odd, given that (1) drug responses are related to drug concentrations at *sites of action* and that (2) the site of action of most drugs is not in the blood. The question arises, "Why adjust plasma levels of a drug when what really matters is the concentration of that drug at its sites of action?" The answer begins with the following observation: More often than not, it is a practical impossibility to measure drug concentrations at sites of action. For example, when a patient with epilepsy takes phenytoin (an anticonvulsant), we cannot routinely draw samples from inside the skull to see if brain levels of the medication are adequate for seizure control. Fortunately, in the case of phenytoin and most other drugs, it is not necessary to measure drug concentrations at actual sites of action in order to have an objective basis for adjusting dosage. Experience has shown that, for most drugs, *there is a direct correlation between therapeutic and toxic responses and the amount of drug present in plasma.* Therefore, although we can't usually measure drug concentrations at sites of action, we can determine plasma drug concentrations that, in turn, are highly predictive of therapeutic and toxic responses. Accordingly, the dosing objective is commonly spoken of in terms of achieving a specific plasma level of a drug.

Two Plasma Drug Levels Defined

Two plasma drug levels are of special importance: (1) the minimum effective concentration and (2) the toxic concentration. These levels are depicted in Figure 4–13 and defined below.

Minimum Effective Concentration. The minimum effective concentration (MEC) is defined as *the plasma drug level below which therapeutic effects will not occur.* Hence, to be of benefit, a drug must be present in concentrations at or above the MEC.

Toxic Concentration. Toxicity occurs when plasma drug levels climb too high. The plasma level at which toxic effects begin is termed the *toxic concentration.* Doses must be kept small enough so that the toxic concentration is not reached.

Therapeutic Range

As indicated in Figure 4–13, there is a range of plasma drug levels, falling between the MEC and the toxic concentration, that is termed the *therapeutic range.* When plasma levels are within the therapeutic range, there is enough drug present to produce therapeutic responses but not so much that toxicity results. *The objective of drug dosing is to maintain plasma drug levels within the therapeutic range.*

The width of the therapeutic range is a major determinant of the ease with which a drug can be used safely. Drugs that have a narrow therapeutic range are difficult to administer safely. Conversely, drugs that have a wide therapeutic range can be administered safely with relative ease. Acetaminophen, for example, has a relatively wide therapeutic range: The toxic concentration is about 30 times greater than the MEC. Because

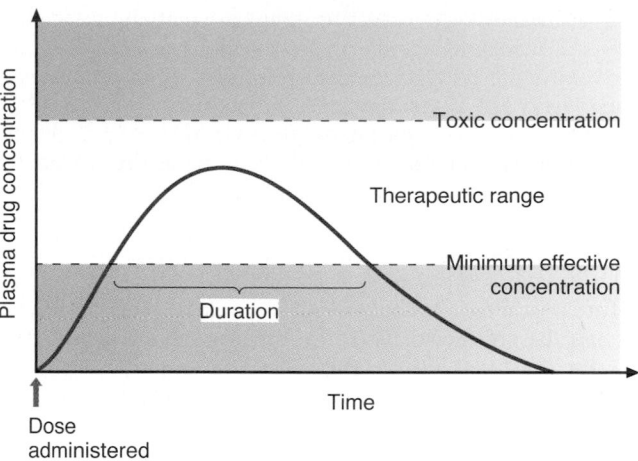

Figure 4–13 ■ Single-dose time course.

of this wide therapeutic range, dosage does not need to be highly precise; a broad range of doses can be employed to produce plasma levels that will be above the MEC but will not reach the toxic concentration. In contrast, lithium (used for bipolar disorder [manic-depressive illness]) has a very narrow therapeutic range: The toxic concentration is only 3 times greater than the MEC. Since toxicity can result from lithium levels that are not much greater than those needed to produce therapeutic effects, lithium dosing must be done carefully if therapeutic effects are to be achieved without causing toxicity. If lithium had a wider therapeutic range, the drug would be much easier to use.

Understanding the concept of therapeutic range can facilitate patient care. Because drugs with a narrow therapeutic range are more dangerous than drugs with a wide therapeutic range, patients taking drugs with a narrow therapeutic range are the most likely to require intervention for drug-related complications. The nurse who is aware of this fact can focus attention on these patients. In contrast, the nurse who has no basis for predicting which drugs are most likely to produce toxicity has no basis for allocating attention, and therefore is obliged to monitor all patients with equal diligence—a process that is both stressful and inefficient.

However, lest you get the wrong impression, the above advice should not be construed as a license to be lax about patients taking drugs that have a wide therapeutic range. Even these drugs can cause harm. Hence, although patients receiving drugs with a narrow therapeutic range should be monitored most closely, common sense dictates that patients receiving safer drugs must not be neglected.

Single-Dose Time Course

Figure 4–13 shows how plasma drug levels change over time after a single dose of an oral medication. The rise in drug levels occurs as the medicine undergoes absorption. Drug levels then decline as metabolism and excretion eliminate the drug from the body.

Because responses cannot occur until plasma drug levels have reached the MEC, there is a period of latency between drug administration and onset of effects. The extent of this delay is determined by the rate of absorption.

The duration of effects is determined largely by the combination of metabolism and excretion. As long as drug levels remain above the MEC, therapeutic responses will be maintained; when levels fall below the MEC, responses will cease. Since metabolism and excretion are the processes most responsible for causing plasma drug levels to fall, these processes are the primary determinants of how long drug effects will persist.

Drug Half-Life

Before proceeding to the topic of multiple dosing, we need to discuss the concept of half-life. When a patient ceases drug use, the combination of metabolism and excretion will cause the amount of drug in the body to decline. The half-life of a drug is an index of just how rapidly that decline occurs.

Drug half-life is defined as *the time required for the amount of drug in the body to decrease by 50%*. A few drugs have half-lives that are extremely short—on the order of minutes. In contrast, the half-lives of some drugs exceed 1 week. Drugs with short half-lives leave the body quickly. Drugs with long half-lives leave slowly.

Note that, in our definition of half-life, a *percentage*—not a specific *amount*—of drug is lost during one half-life. That is, the half-life does not specify, for example, that 2 gm or 18 mg will leave the body in a given time. Rather, the half-life tells us that, no matter what the amount of drug in the body may be, half (50%) will leave during a specified period of time (the half-life). The actual amount of drug that is lost during one half-life will depend upon just how much drug is present: The more drug that is in the body, the larger the amount lost during one half-life.

The concept of half-life is best understood through an example. Morphine provides a good illustration. The half-life of morphine is approximately 3 hours. By definition, this means that body stores of morphine will decrease by 50% every 3 hours—regardless of how much morphine is in the body. If there is 50 mg of morphine in the body, 25 mg (50%) will be lost in 3 hours; if there is only 2 mg of morphine in the body,

only 1 mg (50% of 2 mg) will be lost in 3 hours. Note that, in both cases, morphine levels drop by 50% during an interval of one half-life. However, the actual *amount* lost is larger when total body stores of the drug are higher.

The half-life of a drug determines the dosing interval (i.e., how much time separates each dose). For drugs with a short half-life, the dosing interval must be correspondingly short; if a long dosing interval were used, drug levels would fall below the MEC between doses, and therapeutic effects would be lost. Conversely, if a drug has a long half-life, a long time can separate doses without loss of effect.

Drug Levels Produced with Repeated Doses

Multiple dosing leads to drug accumulation. When a patient takes a single dose of a drug, plasma levels simply go up and then come down. In contrast, when a patient takes repeated doses of a drug, the process is more complex and results in drug accumulation. The factors that determine the rate and extent of accumulation are considered below.

The Process by Which Plateau Drug Levels Are Achieved

Administering repeated doses of a drug will cause that drug to build up in the body until a *plateau* (steady level) has been achieved. What causes drug levels to reach plateau? To begin with, common sense tells us that, if a second dose of a drug is administered before all of the prior dose has been eliminated, total body stores of that drug will be higher after the second dose than after the initial dose. As succeeding doses are administered, drug levels will climb even higher. The drug will continue to accumulate until a state has been achieved in which the amount of drug eliminated between doses equals the amount administered. *When the amount of drug eliminated between doses equals the dose administered, average drug levels will remain constant and plateau will have been reached.*

The process by which multiple dosing produces a plateau is illustrated in Figure 4–14. The drug in this figure is a hypothetical agent with a half-life of exactly 1 day. The regimen consists of a 2-gm dose administered once daily. For the purpose of illustration, we will assume that absorption takes place instantly. Upon administration of the first 2-gm dose (day 1 in the figure), total body stores go from zero to 2 gm. Within one half-life (1 day), body stores drop by 50%—from 2 gm down to 1 gm. At the beginning of day 2, the second 2-gm dose is given, causing body stores to rise from 1 gm up to 3 gm. Over the next day (one half-life), body stores again drop by 50%, this time from 3 gm down to 1.5 gm. When the third dose is given, body stores go from 1.5 gm up to 3.5 gm. Over the next half-life, stores drop by 50% down to 1.75 gm. When the fourth dose is given, drug levels climb to 3.75 gm and, between doses, levels again drop by 50%, this time to approximately 1.9 gm. When the fifth dose is given (at the beginning of day 5), drug levels go up to about 3.9 gm. This process of accumulation continues until body stores reach 4 gm. When total body stores of this drug are 4 gm, 2 gm will be lost each day (i.e., over one half-life). Since a 2-gm dose is being administered each day, when body stores reach 4 gm, the amount lost between doses will equal the dose administered. At this point, body stores will

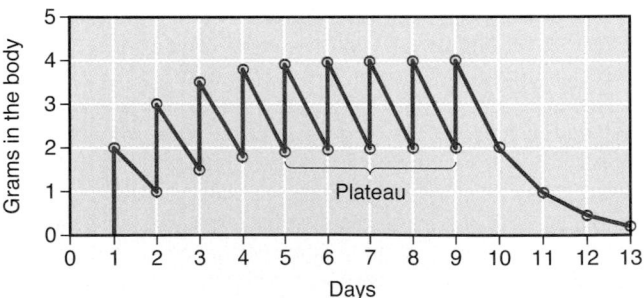

Figure 4–14 ■ Drug accumulation with repeated administration.
This figure illustrates the accumulation of a hypothetical drug during repeated administration. The drug has a half-life of 1 day. The dosing schedule is 2 gm given once a day on days 1 through 9. Note that plateau is reached at about the beginning of day 5 (i.e., after four half-lives). Note also that, when administration is discontinued, it takes about 4 days (four half-lives) for most (94%) of the drug to leave the body.

simply alternate between 4 gm and 2 gm; average body stores will be stable, and plateau will have been reached. Note that the reason that plateau is finally reached is that the actual amount of drug lost between doses gets larger each day. That is, although 50% of total body stores is lost each day, the *amount* in grams grows progressively larger because total body stores are getting larger day by day. Plateau is reached when the amount lost between doses grows to be as large as the amount administered.

Time to Plateau

When a drug is administered repeatedly in the same dose, *plateau will be reached in approximately four half-lives.* For the hypothetical agent illustrated in Figure 4–14, total body stores approached their peak near the beginning of day 5, or approximately 4 full days after treatment began. Since the half-life of this drug is 1 day, reaching plateau in 4 days is equivalent to reaching plateau in four half-lives.

As long as dosage remains constant, the time required to reach plateau is independent of dosage size. Put another way, the time required to reach plateau when giving repeated large doses of a particular drug is identical to the time required to reach plateau when giving repeated small doses of that drug. Referring to the drug in Figure 4–14, just as it took four half-lives (4 days) to reach plateau when a dose of 2 gm was administered daily, it would also take four half-lives to reach plateau if a dose of 4 gm were administered each day. It is true that the *height* of the plateau would be greater if a 4-gm dose were given, but the time required to reach plateau would not be altered by the increase in dosage. To confirm this statement, substitute a dose of 4 gm in the exercise we just went through and see when plateau is reached.

Techniques for Reducing Fluctuations in Drug Levels

As we can see in Figure 4–14, when a drug is administered repeatedly, its level will fluctuate between doses. The highest level is referred to as the *peak concentration,* and the lowest level is referred to as the *trough concentration.* How high the peaks and how low the troughs can be will depend upon the drug's therapeutic range: The peaks must be kept below the toxic concentration, and the troughs must be kept above the MEC. If there is not much difference between the toxic concentration and the MEC, then fluctuations must be kept to a minimum.

Two procedures can be employed to reduce fluctuations in drug levels. One technique is to *administer drugs by continuous infusion.* With this procedure, plasma levels can be kept nearly constant. The second procedure is to *reduce both the dosage size and dosing interval* (keeping the total daily dose constant). For example, rather than giving the drug from Figure 4–14 in 2-gm doses once every 24 hours, we could give this drug in 1-gm doses every 12 hours. With this altered dosing schedule, the total daily dose would remain unchanged, as would total body stores at plateau. However, instead of fluctuating over a range of 2 gm between doses, levels would fluctuate over a range of 1 gm.

Loading Doses Versus Maintenance Doses

As discussed above, if we administer a drug in repeated doses of equal size, an interval equivalent to about four half-lives is required to achieve plateau. For drugs whose half-lives are long, achieving plateau could take days or even weeks. When plateau must be achieved more quickly, a large initial dose can be administered. This large initial dose is called a *loading dose.* After high drug levels have been established with a loading dose, plateau can be maintained by giving smaller doses. These smaller doses are referred to as *maintenance doses.*

The claim that use of a loading dose will shorten the time to plateau may appear to contradict an earlier statement, which said that the time to plateau is not affected by dosage size. However, there is no contradiction. For any *specified* dosage, it will always take about four half-lives to reach plateau. When a loading dose is administered followed by maintenance doses, we have not reached plateau *for the loading dose.* Rather, we have simply used the loading dose to rapidly produce a drug level equivalent to the plateau level for a smaller dose. If we wished to achieve plateau level for the loading dose, we would be obliged to either administer repeated doses equivalent to the loading dose for a period of four half-lives or administer a dose even larger than the original loading dose. Think about it.

Decline From Plateau

When drug administration is discontinued, most (94%) of the drug in the body will be eliminated over an interval equal to about four half-lives. This statement can be validated with simple arithmetic. Let's consider a patient who has been taking morphine. In addition, let's assume that, at the time dosing ceased, the total body store of morphine was 40 mg. Within one half-life after drug withdrawal, morphine stores will decline by 50%—down to 20 mg. During the second half-life, stores will again decline by 50%, dropping from 20 mg to 10 mg. During the third half-life, the level will decline once more by 50%—from 10 mg down to 5 mg. During the fourth half-life, the level will again decline by 50%—from 5 mg down to 2.5 mg. Hence, over a period of four half-lives, total body stores of morphine will drop from an initial level of 40 mg down to 2.5 mg, an overall decline of 94%. Most of the drug in the body will be cleared within four half-lives.

The time required for drugs to leave the body is important when toxicity develops. Let's consider the elimination of digitoxin (a drug once used for heart failure). Digitoxin, true to its name, is a potentially dangerous drug with a narrow therapeutic range. In addition, the half-life of digitoxin is very long—about 7 days. What will be the consequence of digitoxin overdose? Toxic levels of the drug will remain in the body for a long time: Since digitoxin has a half-life of 7 days, and since four half-lives are required for most of the drug to be cleared from the body, it could take weeks for digitoxin stores to fall to a safe level. During the time that excess drug remains in the body, significant effort will be required to keep the patient alive. If digitoxin had a shorter half-life, body stores would decline more rapidly, thereby making management of overdose less difficult. (Because of its long half-life and potential for toxicity, digitoxin has been replaced by digoxin, a drug with identical actions but a much shorter half-life.)

It is important to note that the concept of half-life does not apply to the elimination of all drugs. A few agents, most notably ethanol (alcohol), leave the body at a *constant rate,* regardless of how much is present. The implications of this kind of decline for ethanol are discussed in ■ Chapter 37.

⁙ KEY POINTS

- Pharmacokinetics consists of four basic processes: absorption, distribution, metabolism, and excretion.
- Pharmacokinetic processes determine the concentration of a drug at its sites of action, and thereby determine the intensity and time course of responses.
- To cross membranes, most drugs must dissolve directly into the lipid bilayer of the membrane. Accordingly, lipid-soluble drugs can cross membranes easily, whereas drugs that are polar or ionized cannot.
- Acidic drugs ionize in basic (alkaline) media, whereas basic drugs ionize in acidic media.
- Absorption is defined as the movement of a drug from its site of administration into the blood.
- Absorption is enhanced by rapid drug dissolution, high lipid solubility of the drug, a large surface area for absorption, and high blood flow to the site of administration.
- Intravenous administration has several advantages: rapid onset, precise control over the amount of drug entering the blood, suitability for use with large volumes of fluid, and suitability for irritant drugs.
- Intravenous administration has several disadvantages: high cost; difficulty; inconvenience; danger because of irreversibility; and the potential for fluid overload, infection, and embolism.
- Intramuscular administration has two advantages: suitability for insoluble drugs and suitability for depot preparations.
- Intramuscular administration has two disadvantages: inconvenience and the potential for discomfort.
- Subcutaneous administration has the same advantages and disadvantages as IM administration.
- Oral administration has the advantages of ease, convenience, economy, and safety.
- The principal disadvantage of oral administration is high variability.
- Enteric-coated oral formulations are designed to release their contents in the small intestine—not in the stomach.
- Sustained-release oral formulations are designed to release their contents slowly, thereby permitting a longer interval between doses.
- Distribution is defined as the movement of drugs throughout the body.
- In most tissues, drugs can easily leave the vasculature through spaces between the cells that compose the capillary wall.
- The term *blood-brain barrier* refers to the presence of tight junctions between the cells that compose capillary walls in the CNS. Because of this barrier, drugs must pass through the cells of the capillary wall (rather than between them) in order to reach the CNS.
- The membranes of the placenta do not constitute an absolute barrier to the passage of drugs. The same factors that determine drug movements across all other membranes determine the movement of drugs across the placenta.
- Many drugs bind reversibly to plasma albumin. While bound to albumin, drug molecules cannot leave the vascular system.
- Drug metabolism (biotransformation) is defined as the enzymatic alteration of drug structure.
- Most drug metabolism takes place in the liver and is catalyzed by the cytochrome P450 system of enzymes.
- The most important consequence of drug metabolism is promotion of renal drug excretion (by converting lipid-soluble drugs into more polar [less lipid-soluble] forms).
- Other consequences of drug metabolism are conversion of drugs to less active (or inactive) forms, conversion of drugs to more active forms, conversion of prodrugs to their active forms, and conversion of drugs to more toxic or less toxic forms.
- Some drugs can induce (stimulate) synthesis of hepatic drug-metabolizing enzymes, and can thereby accelerate their own metabolism and the metabolism of other drugs.
- The term *first-pass effect* refers to the rapid inactivation of some oral drugs on their first pass through the liver.
- Most drugs are excreted by the kidneys.
- Renal drug excretion has three steps: glomerular filtration, passive tubular reabsorption, and active tubular secretion.
- Drugs that are highly lipid soluble undergo extensive passive reabsorption back into the blood, and therefore cannot be excreted by the kidney (until they are converted to more polar forms by the liver).
- Drugs can be excreted into breast milk, thereby posing a threat to the nursing infant.
- For most drugs, there is a direct correlation between the level of drug in plasma and the intensity of therapeutic and toxic effects.
- The minimum effective concentration (MEC) of a drug is defined as the plasma drug level below which therapeutic effects will not occur.
- The therapeutic range of a drug lies between the MEC and the toxic concentration.
- Drugs with a wide therapeutic range are relatively easy to use safely, whereas drugs with a narrow therapeutic range are difficult to use safely.
- The half-life of a drug is defined as the time required for the amount of drug in the body to decline by 50%.
- Drugs that have a short half-life must be administered more frequently than drugs that have a long half-life.
- When drugs are administered repeatedly, drug levels will gradually rise and then reach a steady plateau.
- The time required to reach plateau is equivalent to about four half-lives.

■ The time required to reach plateau is independent of dosage size, although the height of the plateau will be higher with larger doses.

■ If plasma drug levels fluctuate too much between doses, the fluctuations could be reduced by (1) giving smaller doses at shorter intervals (keeping the total daily dose the same) or (2) using a continuous infusion.

■ For a drug with a long half-life, it may be necessary to use a loading dose to achieve plateau quickly.

■ When drug administration is discontinued, most (94%) of the drug in the body will be eliminated over four half-lives.

CHAPTER

5

Pharmacodynamics

Pharmacodynamics is defined as the study of the biochemical and physiologic effects of drugs and the molecular mechanisms by which those effects are produced. In short, pharmacodynamics is the study of what drugs do to the body and how they do it.

In order to participate rationally in achieving the therapeutic objective, nurses need a basic understanding of pharmacodynamics. You must know about drug actions in order to educate patients about their medication, make PRN decisions, and evaluate patients for drug responses, both beneficial and harmful. You will also need to understand drug actions when conferring with physicians about drug therapy; if you believe that a patient is receiving inappropriate medication or is being denied a required drug, you will need to support that conviction with arguments based at least in part on knowledge of pharmacodynamics.

DOSE-RESPONSE RELATIONSHIPS

The dose-response relationship (i.e., the relationship between the size of an administered dose and the intensity of the response produced) is a fundamental concern in therapeutics. Dose-response relationships determine the minimum amount of drug we can use, the maximum response a drug can elicit, and how much we need to increase the dosage to produce the desired increase in response.

Basic Features of the Dose-Response Relationship

The basic characteristics of dose-response relationships are illustrated in Figure 5–1. Part A of the figure shows dose-

response data plotted on *linear* coordinates. Part B shows the same data plotted on *semilogarithmic* coordinates (i.e., the scale on which dosage is plotted is logarithmic rather than linear). The most obvious and important characteristic revealed by these curves is that the dose-response relationship is *graded*. That is, as dosage is increased, the response becomes progressively larger. Because drug responses are graded, therapeutic effects can be adjusted to fit the needs of each patient. To tailor treatment to a particular patient, all we need do is raise or lower the dosage until a response of the desired intensity is achieved. If drug responses were *all-or-nothing* instead of graded, drugs could produce only one intensity of response. If that response were too strong or too weak for a particular patient, there would be nothing we could do to adjust its intensity to better suit the patient. Clearly, the graded nature of the dose-response relationship is essential for successful drug therapy.

As indicated in Figure 5–1, the dose-response relationship can be viewed as having three phases. Phase 1 (see Fig. 5–1B) occurs at low doses; the curve is flat during this phase because doses are too low to elicit a measurable response. During phase 2, an increase in dose elicits a corresponding increase in the response; it is during this phase that the dose-response relationship is graded. As the dose is raised higher, we eventually reach a point where an increase in dose is unable to elicit a further increase in response; at this point, the curve flattens out into phase 3.

Maximal Efficacy and Relative Potency

Dose-response curves reveal two characteristic properties of drugs: *maximal efficacy* and *relative potency*. Curves that reflect these properties are shown in Figure 5–2.

Maximal Efficacy

Maximal efficacy is defined as *the largest effect that a drug can produce.* Maximal efficacy is indicated by the *height* of the dose-response curve.

The concept of maximal efficacy is illustrated by the dose-response curves for meperidine [Demerol] and pentazocine [Talwin], two morphine-like pain relievers (Fig. 5–2A). As we can see, the curve for pentazocine levels off at a maximum height below that of the curve for meperidine. This tells us that the maximum degree of pain relief we can achieve with pentazocine is less than the maximum degree of pain relief we can achieve with meperidine. Put another way, no matter how much pentazocine we administer, we can never produce the degree of pain relief that we can with meperidine. Accordingly, we would say that meperidine has greater maximal efficacy than pentazocine.

Despite what intuition might tell us, a drug with very high maximal efficacy is not always more desirable than a drug

44

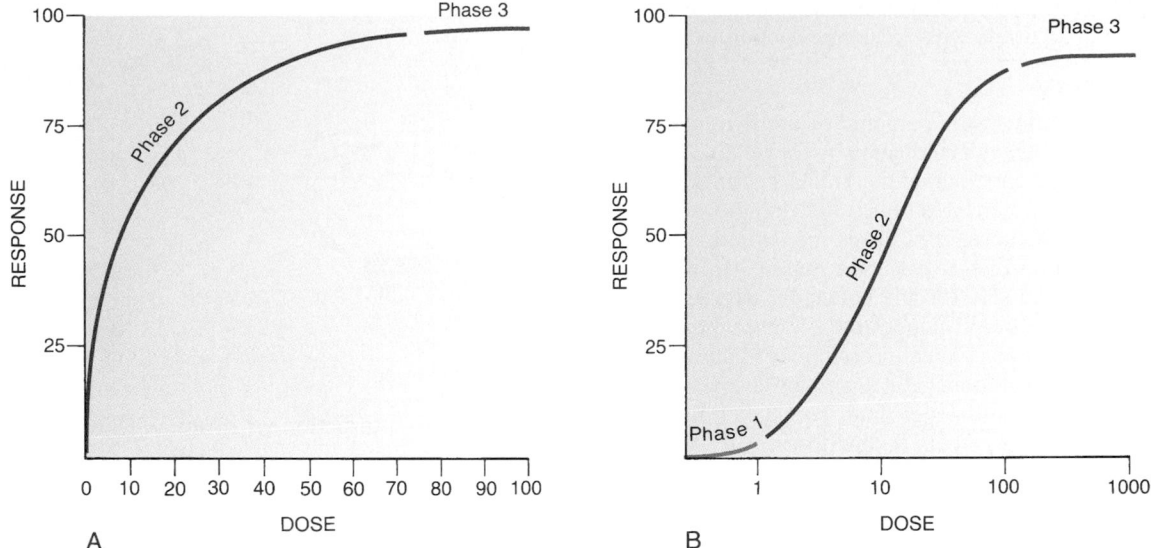

Figure 5–1 ■ Basic components of the dose-response curve.
A, A dose-response curve with dose plotted on a linear scale. *B,* The same dose-response relationship shown in *A* but with the dose plotted on a logarithmic scale. Note the three phases of the dose-response curve: *Phase 1,* The curve is relatively flat; doses are too low to elicit a significant response. *Phase 2,* The curve climbs upward as bigger doses elicit a corresponding increase in response. *Phase 3,* The curve levels off; bigger doses are unable to elicit a further increase in response. (Phase 1 is not indicated in *A* because very low doses cannot be shown on a linear scale.)

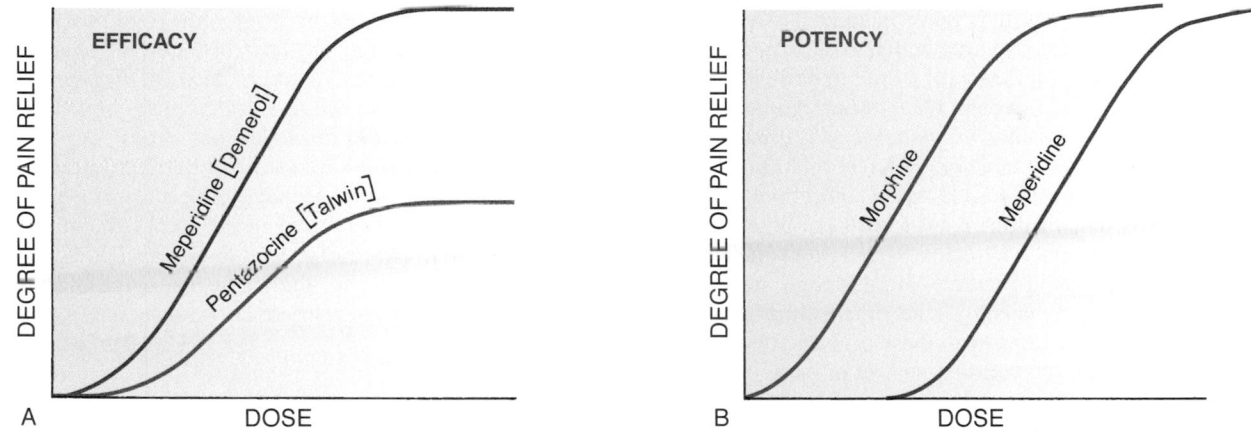

Figure 5–2 ■ Dose-response curves demonstrating efficacy and potency.
A, Efficacy, or "maximal efficacy," is an index of the maximal response that a drug can produce. The efficacy of a drug is indicated by the height of its dose-response curve. In this example, meperidine has greater efficacy than pentazocine. Efficacy is an important quality in a drug. *B,* Potency is an index of how much drug must be administered to elicit a desired response. In this example, achieving pain relief with meperidine requires higher doses than with morphine. We would say that morphine is more potent than meperidine. Note that, if administered in sufficiently high doses, meperidine can produce just as much pain relief as morphine. Potency is usually not an important quality in a drug.

with lower efficacy. Recall that we want to match the intensity of the response to the patient's needs. This may be difficult to do with a drug that produces extremely intense responses. For example, certain diuretics (e.g., furosemide) have such high maximal efficacy that they can cause dehydration. If we only

want to mobilize a modest volume of water, a diuretic with lower maximal efficacy (e.g., hydrochlorothiazide) would be preferred. Similarly, if a patient has a headache, we would not select a powerful analgesic (e.g., morphine) for relief; rather, we would select an analgesic with lower maximal efficacy, such as aspirin. Put another way, it is neither appropriate nor desirable to hunt squirrels with an atomic cannon.

Relative Potency

The term *potency* refers to the amount of drug we must give to elicit an effect. Potency is indicated by the relative position of the dose-response curve along the *x* (dosage) axis.

The concept of potency is illustrated by the curves in Figure 5–2*B*. These curves plot doses for two analgesics—morphine and meperidine—versus the degree of pain relief achieved. As you can see, for any particular degree of pain relief, the required dose of meperidine is larger than the required dose of morphine. Since morphine produces pain relief at lower doses than meperidine, we would say that morphine is more potent than meperidine. That is, a potent drug is one that produces its effects at low doses.

Potency is rarely an important characteristic of a drug. The fact that morphine is more potent than meperidine does not mean that morphine is a superior medicine. In fact, the only consequence of morphine's greater potency is that morphine can be given in smaller doses. The difference between providing pain relief with morphine versus meperidine is much like the difference between purchasing candy with a dime instead of two nickels; although the dime is smaller (more potent) than the two nickels, the purchasing power of the dime and the two nickels is identical.

Although potency is usually of no clinical concern, it can be important if a drug is so lacking in potency that doses become inconveniently large. For example, if a drug were of extremely low potency, we might need to administer that drug in huge doses multiple times a day to achieve beneficial effects. In a case such as this, an alternative drug with higher potency would be desirable. Fortunately, it is rare for a drug to be so lacking in potency that doses of inconvenient magnitude need be given.

It is important to note that the potency of a drug implies nothing about its maximal efficacy! Potency and efficacy are completely independent qualities. Drug A can be more effective than drug B even though drug B may be more potent. Also, drugs A and B can be equally effective even though one may be more potent. As we saw in Figure 5–2*B*, although meperidine happens to be less potent than morphine, the maximal degree of pain relief that we can achieve with these drugs is identical.

A final comment on the word *potency* is in order. In everyday parlance, we tend to use the word *potent* to express the pharmacologic concept of effectiveness. That is, when most people say, "This drug is very potent," what they mean is, "This drug produces powerful effects." They do not mean, "This drug produces its effects at low doses." In pharmacology, we use the words *potent* and *potency* with the specific meanings given above. Accordingly, whenever you see those words in this book, they will refer only to the dosage needed to produce effects—never to the maximal effects a drug can produce.

DRUG-RECEPTOR INTERACTIONS

Introduction to Drug Receptors

Drugs are not "magic bullets"; they are simply chemicals. Being chemicals, the only way drugs can produce their effects is by interacting with other chemicals. Receptors are the special "chemicals" in the body that drugs interact with to produce effects.

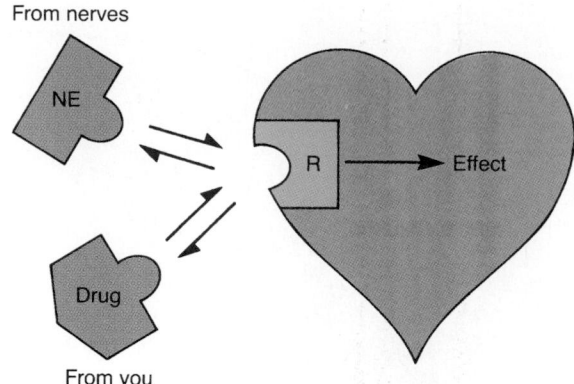

Figure 5–3 ■ Interaction of drugs with receptors for norepinephrine.
Under physiologic conditions, cardiac output can be increased by the binding of norepinephrine (NE) to receptors (R) on the heart. Norepinephrine is supplied to these receptors by nerves. These same receptors can be acted on by drugs. Drugs can act at these receptors to mimic endogenous NE (and thereby increase cardiac output), or they can block the actions of endogenous NE (and thereby reduce cardiac output).

We can define a receptor as *any functional macromolecule in a cell to which a drug binds to produce its effects.* Under this broad definition, many cellular components could be considered drug receptors, since drugs bind to many cellular components (e.g., enzymes, ribosomes, tubulin) to produce their effects. However, although the formal definition of a receptor encompasses all functional macromolecules, *the term* receptor *is generally reserved for what is arguably the most important group of macromolecules through which drugs act: the body's own receptors for hormones, neurotransmitters, and other regulatory molecules.* The other macromolecules to which drugs bind, such as enzymes and ribosomes, can be thought of simply as target molecules, rather than as true receptors.

The general equation for the interaction between drugs and their receptors is as follows (where D = drug and R = receptor):

$$D + R \rightleftharpoons D\text{-}R \text{ COMPLEX} \rightarrow RESPONSE$$

As suggested by the equation, binding of a drug to its receptor is usually *reversible.*

A receptor is analogous to a light switch, in that it has two configurations: "ON" and "OFF." Like the switch, a receptor must be in the "ON" configuration to influence cellular function. Receptors are activated ("turned on") by interaction with other molecules. Under physiologic conditions, receptor activity is regulated by endogenous compounds (neurotransmitters, hormones, other regulatory molecules). When a drug binds to a receptor, all that it can do is mimic or block the actions of endogenous regulatory molecules. By doing so, the drug will either increase or decrease the rate of the physiologic activity normally controlled by that receptor.

An illustration will help clarify the receptor concept. Let's consider receptors for norepinephrine (NE) in the heart. Cardiac output is controlled in part by NE acting at specific receptors in the heart. Norepinephrine is supplied to those receptors by neurons of the autonomic nervous system (Fig. 5–3). When the need

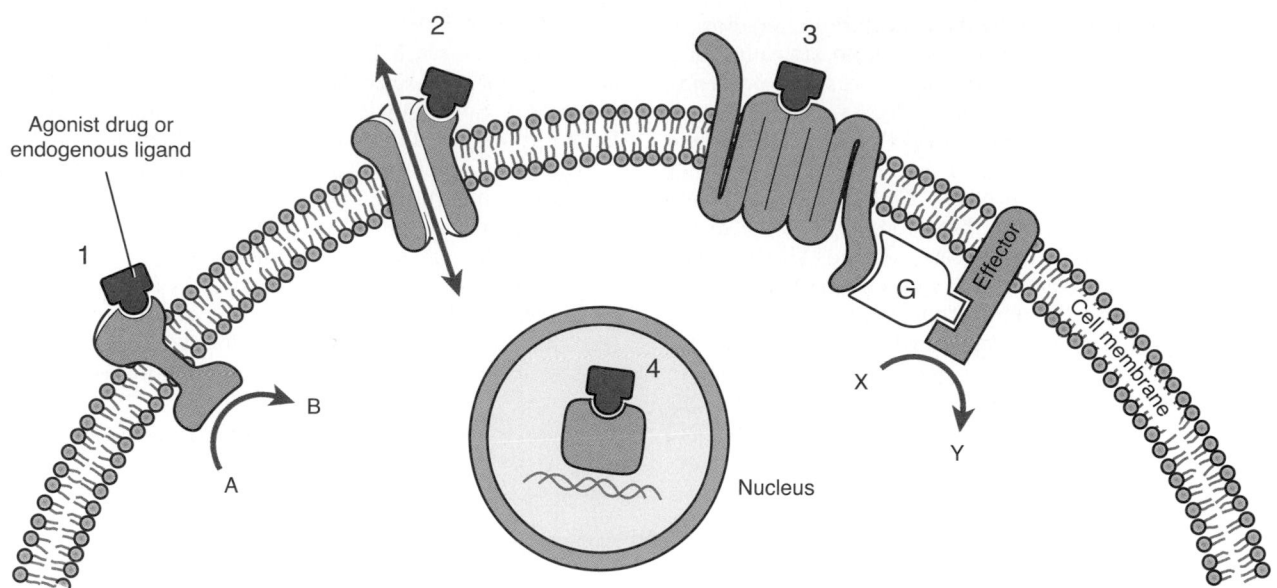

Figure 5–4 ■ The four primary receptor families.
1, Cell membrane–embedded enzyme. *2,* Ligand-gated ion channel. *3,* G protein–coupled receptor system (G = G protein). *4,* Transcription factor.

to increase cardiac output arises, the following events take place: (1) the firing rate of autonomic neurons to the heart is increased, causing increased release of NE; (2) NE then binds to receptors on the heart; and (3) as a consequence of the interaction between NE and its receptors, both the rate and force of cardiac contractions are increased, thereby increasing cardiac output. When the demand for cardiac output subsides, the autonomic neurons reduce their firing rate, binding of NE to its receptors diminishes, and cardiac output returns to resting levels.

The same cardiac receptors whose function is regulated by endogenous NE can also serve as receptors for drugs. That is, just as endogenous molecules can bind to these receptors, so can compounds that enter the body as drugs. The binding of drugs to these receptors can have one of two effects· (1) drugs can *mimic* the action of endogenous NE (and thereby increase cardiac output), or (2) drugs can *block* the action of endogenous NE (and thereby prevent stimulation of the heart by autonomic neurons).

Several important properties of receptors and drug-receptor interactions are illustrated by this example:

- The receptors through which drugs act are normal points of control of physiologic processes.
- Under physiologic conditions, receptor function is regulated by molecules supplied by the body.
- All that drugs can do at receptors is mimic or block the action of the body's own regulatory molecules.
- Because drug action is limited to mimicking or blocking the body's own regulatory molecules, drugs cannot give cells new functions. Rather, drugs can only alter the rate of pre-existing processes. In other words, drugs cannot make the body do anything that it is not already capable of doing.*

---

*The only exception to this rule is gene therapy. By inserting genes into cells, we actually *can* make them do something they were previously incapable of doing.

- Drugs produce their therapeutic effects by helping the body use its pre-existing capacities to the patient's best advantage. Put another way, medications simply help the body help itself.
- In theory, it should be possible to synthesize drugs that can alter the rate of any biologic process for which receptors exist.

The Four Primary Receptor Families

Although the body has many different receptors, they comprise only four primary families: cell membrane–embedded enzymes, ligand-gated ion channels, G protein–coupled receptor systems, and transcription factors. These families are depicted in Figure 5–4. In the discussion below, the term *ligand-binding domain* refers to the specific region of the receptor where binding of drugs and endogenous regulatory molecules takes place.

Cell Membrane–Embedded Enzymes. As shown in Figure 5–4, receptors of this type span the cell membrane. The ligand-binding domain is located on the cell surface, and the enzyme's catalytic site is inside. Binding of an endogenous regulatory molecule or agonist drug (one that mimics the action of the endogenous regulatory molecule) activates the enzyme, thereby increasing its catalytic activity. Responses to activation of these receptors occur in seconds. Insulin is representative of the endogenous ligands that act through this type of receptor.

Ligand-Gated Ion Channels. Like membrane-embedded enzymes, ligand-gated ion channels span the cell membrane. The function of these receptors is to regulate flow of ions into and out of cells. Each ligand-gated channel is specific for a particular ion (e.g., Na^+, Ca^{++}). As shown in Figure 5–4, the ligand-binding domain is on the cell surface. When an endogenous ligand or agonist drug binds the receptor, the channel opens, allowing ions to flow inward or outward. (The direction of flow is determined by the concentration gradient of the ion across the membrane.) Responses to activation of a ligand-gated ion channel are extremely fast, usually occurring in milliseconds. Several neurotransmitters, including acetylcholine and gamma-aminobutyric acid (GABA), act through this type of receptor.

G Protein–Coupled Receptor Systems. G protein–coupled receptor systems have three components: the receptor itself, G protein (so named because it binds GTP), and an effector (typically an ion channel or an enzyme). These systems work as follows: binding of an endogenous ligand or agonist drug activates the receptor, which in turn activates G protein, which in turn activates the effector. Responses to activation of this type of system develop rapidly. Numerous endogenous ligands, including NE, serotonin, histamine, and many peptide hormones, act through G protein–coupled receptor systems.

As shown in Figure 5–4, the receptors that couple to G proteins are serpentine structures that traverse the cell membrane seven times. For some of these receptors, the ligand-binding domain is found on the cell surface. For others, the ligand-binding domain is located in a pocket accessible from the cell surface.

Transcription Factors. Transcription factors differ from other receptors in two ways: (1) transcription factors are found *within* the cell rather than on the surface, and (2) responses to activation of these receptors are *delayed.* Transcription factors are situated on DNA in the cell nucleus. Their function is to regulate protein synthesis. Activation of these receptors by endogenous ligands or by agonist drugs stimulates transcription of messenger RNA molecules, which then act as templates for synthesis of specific proteins. The entire process—from activation of the transcription factor through completion of protein synthesis—may take hours or even days. Because transcription factors are intracellular, they can be activated only by ligands that are sufficiently lipid soluble to cross the cell membrane. Endogenous ligands that act through transcription factors include thyroid hormone and all of the steroid hormones (e.g., progesterone, testosterone, cortisol).

Receptors and Selectivity of Drug Action

In Chapter 1 we noted that selectivity is a highly desirable characteristic of a drug, since the more selective a drug is, the fewer side effects it will produce. Selective drug action is possible, in large part, because drugs act through specific receptors.

The body employs many different kinds of receptors to regulate its sundry physiologic activities. There are receptors for each neurotransmitter (e.g., NE, acetylcholine, dopamine); there are receptors for each hormone (e.g., progesterone, insulin, thyrotropin); and there are receptors for all of the other molecules the body uses to regulate physiologic processes (e.g., histamine, prostaglandins, leukotrienes). As a rule, each type of receptor participates in the regulation of just a few processes.

Selective drug action is made possible by the existence of many types of receptors, each regulating just a few processes. Common sense tells us that, if a drug interacts with only one type of receptor, and if that receptor type regulates just a few processes, then the effects of the drug will be limited. Conversely, intuition also tells us that, if a drug interacts with several different receptor types, then that drug is likely to elicit a wide variety of responses.

How can a drug interact with one receptor type and not with others? In some important ways, a receptor is analogous to a lock and a drug is analogous to a key for that lock: Just as only those keys with the proper profile can fit a particular lock, only those drugs with the proper size, shape, and physical properties can bind to a particular receptor.

The binding of acetylcholine (a neurotransmitter) to its receptor illustrates the lock-and-key analogy (Fig. 5–5). To bind with its receptor, acetylcholine must have a shape that is complementary to the shape of the receptor; in addition, acetylcholine must possess positive charges that are positioned so as to permit their interaction with corresponding negative sites on the receptor. If acetylcholine lacked these properties, it would be unable to interact with the receptor.

Like the acetylcholine receptor, all other receptors impose specific requirements on the molecules with which they will interact. Because receptors have such specific requirements, it is possible to synthesize drugs that interact

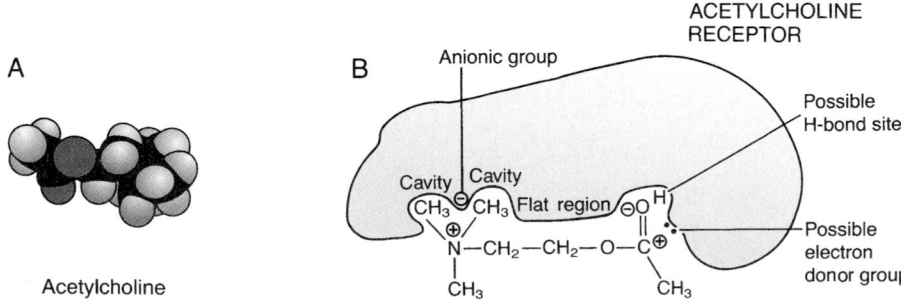

Figure 5–5 ■ Interaction of acetylcholine with its receptor.
A, Three-dimensional model of the acetylcholine molecule. *B,* Binding of acetylcholine to its receptor. Note how the shape of acetylcholine closely matches the shape of the receptor. Note also how the positive charges on acetylcholine align with the negative sites on the receptor. (Modified from Goldstein A, Aronow L, Sumner MK. Principles of Drug Action: The Basis of Pharmacology, 2nd ed. New York, John Wiley & Sons, 1974.)

with just one receptor type to the exclusion of all others. Such medications tend to elicit selective responses.

Even though a drug is selective for only one type of receptor, is it possible for that drug to produce nonselective effects? Yes: If a single receptor type is responsible for regulating several physiologic processes, then drugs that interact with that receptor will also influence a variety of processes. For example, in addition to modulating perception of pain, morphine receptors help regulate other processes, including respiration and motility of the bowel. Consequently, although morphine is selective for one class of receptor, the drug can still produce a variety of effects. In clinical practice, it is common for morphine to cause respiratory depression and constipation along with reduction of pain. Note that morphine produces these varied effects not because it lacks receptor selectivity, but because the receptor for which morphine is selective helps regulate a variety of physiologic processes.

One final comment on selectivity: *Selectivity does not guarantee safety.* A compound can be highly selective for a particular receptor and yet still be dangerous. For example, although botulinum toxin is highly selective for one type of receptor, the compound is anything but safe: Botulinum toxin can cause paralysis of the muscles of respiration, resulting in death from respiratory arrest.

Theories of Drug-Receptor Interaction

In the discussion below, we consider two theories of drug-receptor interaction: (1) the simple occupancy theory and (2) the modified occupancy theory. These theories help explain dose-response relationships and the ability of drugs to mimic or block the actions of endogenous regulatory molecules.

Simple Occupancy Theory

The simple occupancy theory of drug-receptor interaction states that (1) the intensity of the response to a drug is proportional to the number of receptors occupied by that drug and that (2) a maximal response will occur when *all* available receptors have been occupied. This relationship between receptor occupancy and the intensity of the response is depicted in Figure 5–6.

Although certain aspects of dose-response relationships can be explained by the simple occupancy theory, other important phenomena cannot. Specifically, there is nothing in this theory to explain why one drug should be more potent than another. In addition, this theory cannot explain how one drug can have higher maximal efficacy than another. That is, according to this theory, two drugs acting at the same receptor should produce the same maximal effect, providing that their dosages were high enough to produce 100% receptor occupancy. However, we have already seen this is not true. As illustrated in Figure 5–2A, there is a dose of pentazocine above which no further increase in response can be elicited. Presumably, all receptors are occupied when the dose-response curve levels off. However, at 100% receptor occupancy, the response elicited by pentazocine is less than that elicited by morphine. Simple occupancy theory cannot account for this difference.

Modified Occupancy Theory

The modified occupancy theory of drug-receptor interaction explains certain observations that cannot be accounted for with the simple occupancy theory. The simple occupancy

theory assumes that all drugs acting at a particular receptor are identical with respect to (1) the ability to bind to the receptor and (2) the ability to influence receptor function once binding has taken place. The modified occupancy theory is based on different assumptions.

The modified theory ascribes two qualities to drugs: *affinity* and *intrinsic activity*. The term *affinity* refers to the strength of the attraction between a drug and its receptor. *Intrinsic activity* refers to the ability of a drug to activate the receptor following binding. *Affinity and intrinsic activity are independent properties.*

Affinity. As noted, the term *affinity* refers to the strength of the attraction between a drug and its receptor. Drugs with high affinity are strongly attracted to their receptors. Conversely, drugs with low affinity are weakly attracted.

The affinity of a drug for its receptors is reflected in its *potency*. Because they are strongly attracted to their receptors, drugs with high affinity can bind to their receptors when present in low concentrations. Because they bind to receptors at low concentrations, drugs with high affinity are effective in low doses. That is, *drugs with high affinity are very potent.* Conversely, drugs with low affinity must be present in high concentrations to bind to their receptors. Accordingly, these drugs are not very potent.

Intrinsic Activity. The term *intrinsic activity* refers to the ability of a drug to activate a receptor upon binding. Drugs with high intrinsic activity cause intense receptor activation. Conversely, drugs with low intrinsic activity cause only slight activation.

The intrinsic activity of a drug is reflected in its *maximal efficacy*. Drugs with high intrinsic activity have high maximal efficacy. That is, by causing intense receptor activation, they

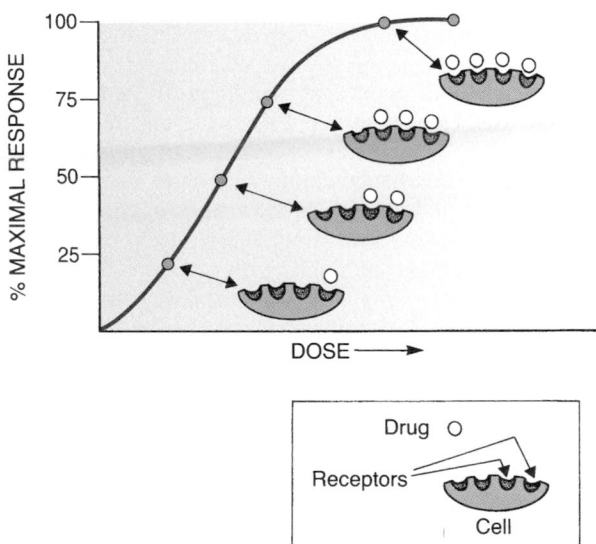

Figure 5–6 ■ Model of simple occupancy theory.
The simple occupancy theory states that the intensity of response to a drug is proportional to the number of receptors occupied; maximal response is reached with 100% receptor occupancy. Since the hypothetical cell in this figure has only four receptors, maximal response is achieved when all four receptors are occupied. (Please note: Real cells have thousands of receptors.)

are able to cause intense responses. Conversely, if intrinsic activity is low, maximal efficacy will be low as well.

It should be noted that, under the modified occupancy theory, the intensity of the response to a drug is still related to the number of receptors occupied. The wrinkle added by the modified theory is that intensity is also related to the ability of the drug to activate receptors once binding has occurred. Under the modified theory, two drugs can occupy the same number of receptors but produce effects of different intensity; the drug with greater intrinsic activity will produce the more intense response.

Agonists, Antagonists, and Partial Agonists

As noted above, when drugs bind to receptors they can do one of two things: they can either *mimic* the action of endogenous regulatory molecules or they can *block* the action of endogenous regulators. Drugs that mimic the body's own regulatory molecules are called *agonists*. Drugs that block the actions of endogenous regulators are called *antagonists*. Like agonists, *partial agonists* also mimic the actions of endogenous regulatory molecules, but they produce responses of intermediate intensity.

Agonists

Agonists are molecules that activate receptors. Since neurotransmitters, hormones, and all other endogenous regulators of receptor function activate the receptors to which they bind, all of these compounds are considered agonists. When drugs act as agonists, they simply bind to receptors and mimic the actions of the body's own regulatory molecules.

In terms of the modified occupancy theory, an agonist is a drug that has both *affinity* and *high intrinsic activity*. Affinity allows the agonist to bind to receptors, while intrinsic activity allows the bound agonist to "activate" or "turn on" receptor function.

Many therapeutic agents produce their effects by functioning as agonists. Dobutamine, for example, is a drug that mimics the action of NE at receptors on the heart, thereby causing heart rate and force of contraction to increase. The insulin that we administer as a drug mimics the actions of endogenous insulin at receptors. Norethindrone, a component of many oral contraceptives, acts by "turning on" receptors for progesterone.

It is important to note that agonists do not necessarily make physiologic processes go faster; receptor activation can also slow down a particular process. For example, there are receptors on the heart that, when activated by acetylcholine (the body's own agonist for these receptors), will cause heart rate to decrease. Drugs that mimic the action of acetylcholine at these receptors will also decrease heart rate. Since such drugs produce their effects by causing receptor activation, they would be called agonists—even though they cause heart rate to decline.

Antagonists

Antagonists produce their effects by preventing receptor activation by endogenous regulatory molecules and drugs. Antagonists have virtually no effects of their own on receptor function.

In terms of the modified occupancy theory, an antagonist is a drug with affinity for a receptor but with no intrinsic activity. Affinity allows the antagonist to bind to receptors, but lack of intrinsic activity prevents the bound antagonist from causing receptor activation.

Although antagonists do not cause receptor activation, they most certainly *do* produce pharmacologic effects. Antagonists produce their effects by *preventing the activation of receptors by agonists*. Antagonists can produce beneficial effects by blocking the actions of endogenous regulatory molecules or by blocking the actions of drugs. (The ability of antagonists to block the actions of drugs is employed most commonly in the treatment of overdose.)

It is important to note that the response to an antagonist is determined by how much *agonist* is present. Since antagonists act by preventing receptor activation, *if there is no agonist present, administration of an antagonist will have no observable effect;* the drug will bind to its receptors but nothing will happen. On the other hand, if receptors are undergoing activation by agonists, administration of an antagonist will shut the process down, resulting in an observable response. This is an important concept; please think about it.

Many therapeutic agents produce their effects by acting as receptor antagonists. Antihistamines, for example, suppress allergy symptoms by binding to receptors for histamine, thereby preventing activation of these receptors by histamine released in response to allergens. The use of antagonists to treat drug toxicity is illustrated by naloxone, an agent that blocks receptors for morphine and related opioids; by preventing activation of opioid receptors, naloxone can completely reverse all symptoms of opioid overdose.

Noncompetitive Versus Competitive Antagonists. Antagonists can be subdivided into two major classes: (1) noncompetitive antagonists and (2) competitive antagonists. Most antagonists are competitive.

Noncompetitive (Insurmountable) Antagonists. Noncompetitive antagonists bind *irreversibly* to receptors. The effect of irreversible binding is equivalent to reducing the total number of receptors available for activation by an agonist. Since the intensity of the response to an agonist is proportional to the total number of receptors occupied, and since noncompetitive antagonists decrease the number of receptors available for activation, noncompetitive antagonists *reduce the maximal response* that an agonist can elicit. If sufficient antagonist is present, agonist effects will be blocked completely. Dose-response curves illustrating inhibition by a noncompetitive antagonist are shown in Figure 5–7A.

Since the binding of noncompetitive antagonists is irreversible, inhibition by these agents cannot be overcome—no matter how much agonist may be available. Because inhibition by noncompetitive antagonists cannot be reversed, these agents are rarely used therapeutically. (Recall from Chapter 1 that reversibility is one of the properties of an ideal drug.)

Although noncompetitive antagonists bind irreversibly, this does not mean that their effects last forever. Cells are constantly breaking down "old" receptors and synthesizing new ones. Consequently, the effects of noncompetitive antagonists wear off as the receptors to which they are bound are replaced. Since the life cycle of a receptor can be relatively short, the effects of noncompetitive antagonists may subside in a few days.

Competitive (Surmountable) Antagonists. Competitive antagonists bind *reversibly* to receptors. As their name implies, competitive antagonists produce receptor blockade by competing with agonists for receptor binding. If an agonist and a competitive antagonist have equal affinity for a particular receptor, then the receptor will be occupied by whichever agent—agonist or antagonist—is present in the highest concentration. If there are more antagonist molecules present than agonist molecules, antagonist molecules will occupy the receptors and receptor activation will be blocked. Conversely, if agonist molecules outnumber the antagonists, receptors will be occupied mainly by the agonist and little inhibition will occur.

Because competitive antagonists bind reversibly to receptors, the inhibition they cause is *surmountable*. In the presence of sufficiently high amounts

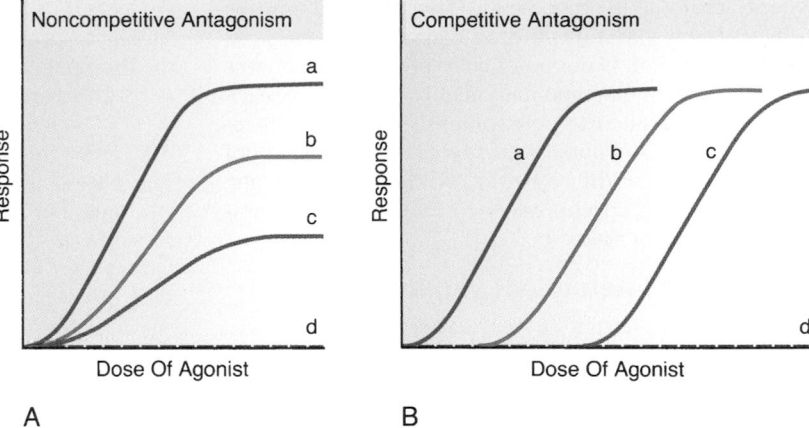

Figure 5–7 ■ Dose-response curves in the presence of competitive and noncompetitive antagonists.
A, Effect of a noncompetitive antagonist on the dose-response curve of an agonist. Note that noncompetitive antagonists decrease the maximal response achievable with an agonist. *B,* Effect of a competitive antagonist on the dose-response curve of an agonist. Note that the maximal response achievable with the agonist is not reduced. Competitive antagonists simply increase the amount of agonist required to produce any given intensity of response.

of agonist, agonist molecules will occupy all receptors and inhibition will be completely overcome. The dose-response curves shown in Figure 5–7*B* illustrate the process of overcoming the effects of a competitive antagonist with large doses of an agonist.

Partial Agonists

A partial agonist is an agonist that has only moderate intrinsic activity. As a result, *the maximal effect that a partial agonist can produce is lower than that of a full agonist.* Pentazocine is an example of a partial agonist. As the curves in Figure 5–2*A* indicate, the degree of pain relief that can be achieved with pentazocine is much lower than the relief that can be achieved with meperidine (a full agonist).

Partial agonists are interesting in that they can act as *antagonists* as well as *agonists.* For example, when pentazocine is administered by itself, it occupies opioid receptors and produces moderate relief of pain. In this situation, the drug is acting as an agonist. However, if a patient is already taking meperidine (a full agonist at opioid receptors) and is then given a large dose of pentazocine, pentazocine will occupy the opioid receptors and prevent their activation by meperidine. As a result, rather than experiencing the high degree of pain relief that meperidine can produce, the patient will experience only the limited relief that pentazocine can produce. In this situation, pentazocine is acting as both an agonist (producing moderate pain relief) and an antagonist (blocking the higher degree of relief that could have been achieved with meperidine by itself).

Regulation of Receptor Sensitivity

Receptors are dynamic components of the cell. In response to continuous activation or continuous inhibition, the number of receptors on the cell surface can change, as can their sensitivity to agonist molecules (drugs and endogenous ligands). For example, when the receptors of a cell are continually exposed to an *agonist,* the cell usually becomes less responsive. When this occurs, the cell is said to be *desensitized* or *refractory,* or

to have undergone *down-regulation.* Several mechanisms may be responsible, including destruction of receptors by the cell and modification of receptors such that they respond less fully. Continuous exposure to antagonists has the opposite effect, causing the cell to become *hypersensitive* (also referred to as *supersensitive*). One mechanism that can cause hypersensitivity is synthesis of more receptors.

DRUG RESPONSES THAT DO NOT INVOLVE RECEPTORS

Although the effects of most drugs result from drug-receptor interactions, some drugs do not act through receptors. Rather, they act through simple physical or chemical interactions with other small molecules.

Common examples of "receptorless drugs" include antacids, antiseptics, saline laxatives, and chelating agents. Antacids reduce gastric acidity by direct chemical interaction with stomach acid. The antiseptic action of ethyl alcohol results from precipitating bacterial proteins. Magnesium hydroxide, a powerful laxative, acts by retaining water in the intestinal lumen through an osmotic effect. Dimercaprol, a chelating agent, prevents toxicity from heavy metals (e.g., arsenic, mercury) by forming complexes with these compounds. All of these pharmacologic effects are the result of simple physical or chemical interactions, and not interactions with cellular receptors.

INTERPATIENT VARIABILITY IN DRUG RESPONSES

The dose required to produce a therapeutic response can vary substantially among patients. Why? Because people differ from one another. In this section we consider interpatient variation as a general issue. The specific kinds of differences that underlie variability in drug responses are discussed in Chapter 8.

In order to promote the therapeutic objective, you must be alert to interpatient variation in drug responses. Because of interpatient variation, it is not possible to predict exactly how an individual patient will respond to medication. Hence, each patient must be evaluated to determine his or her actual response to treatment. The nurse who appreciates the reality of interpatient variability will be better prepared to anticipate, evaluate, and respond appropriately to each patient's therapeutic needs.

Measurement of Interpatient Variability

An example of how interpatient variability is measured will facilitate our discussion. Let's assume we've just developed a drug that suppresses production of stomach acid, and now want to evaluate variability in patient responses. To make this evaluation, we must first define a specific *therapeutic objective* or *endpoint*. Since our drug reduces gastric acidity, an appropriate endpoint is elevation of gastric pH to a value of 5.

Having defined a therapeutic endpoint, we can now perform our study. Subjects for this study are 100 people with gastric ulcers. We begin our experiment by giving each subject a low initial dose (100 mg) of our drug. We then measure gastric pH to determine how many individuals achieved the therapeutic goal of pH 5. Let's assume that only two people responded to the initial dose. To the remaining 98 subjects, we give an additional 20-mg dose and again determine whose gastric pH rose to 5. Let's assume that six more subjects responded to this dose (120 mg total). We continue the experiment, administering doses in 20-mg increments, until all 100 subjects have responded with the desired elevation in gastric pH.

The data from our hypothetical experiment are plotted in Figure 5–8. The plot is called a *frequency distribution curve*. We can see from the curve that a wide range of doses was required to produce the desired response in all subjects. For some subjects, a dose of only 100 mg was sufficient to produce the target response. For other subjects, the therapeutic endpoint was not achieved until the dose totaled 240 mg.

The ED₅₀

The dose at the middle of the frequency distribution curve is termed the ED_{50} (see Fig. 5–8B). (ED_{50} is an abbreviation for *average effective dose.*) The ED_{50} is defined as *the dose that is required to produce a defined therapeutic response in 50% of the population.* In the case of our new drug, the ED_{50} was 170 mg—the dose needed to elevate gastric pH to a value of 5 in 50 of the 100 people tested.

The ED_{50} can be considered a "standard" dose and, as such, is frequently the dose selected for initial treatment. After evaluating a patient's response to this "standard" dose, we can then adjust subsequent doses up or down in accordance with the patient's need.

Clinical Implications of Interpatient Variability

Interpatient variation has four important clinical consequences. As a nurse you should be aware of these implications:

■ *The initial dose of a drug is necessarily an approximation. Subsequent doses must be "fine tuned" based on the patient's response.* Because initial doses are approximations, it would be wise not to challenge the physician if the prescribed initial dose differs by a small amount (e.g., 10% to 20%) from recommended doses in a published drug reference. Rather, you should administer the medication as prescribed and evaluate the response; dosage adjustments can then be made as needed. Of course, if the physician's order calls for a dose that differs from the recommended dose by a large amount, that order should be challenged.

■ *When given an average effective dose (ED_{50}), some patients will be undertreated, whereas others will have received more*

Dose of Drug (mg)	Number of Subjects Responding at Each Dose
100	2
120	6
140	17
160	25
180	25
200	17
220	6
240	2

A

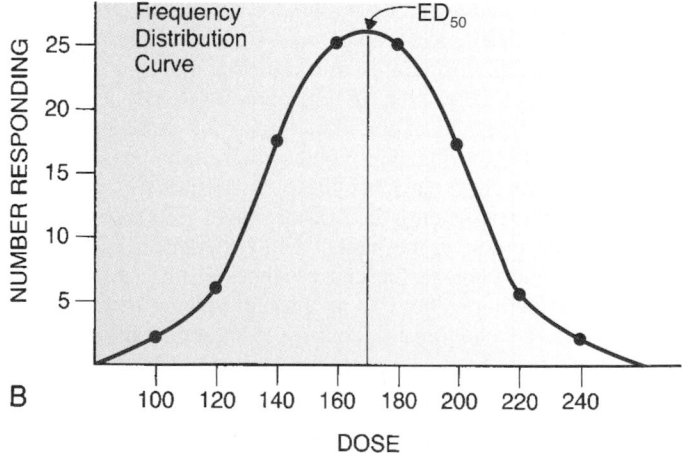

B

Figure 5–8 ■ **Interpatient variation in drug responses.**
A, Data from tests of a hypothetical acid-suppressing drug in 100 patients. The goal of the study was to determine the dosage required by each patient to elevate gastric pH to 5. Note the wide variability in doses needed to produce the target response for the 100 subjects. *B,* Frequency distribution curve for the data in *A.* The dose at the middle of the curve is termed the ED_{50}—the dose that will produce a predefined intensity of response in 50% of the population.

drug than they need. Accordingly, when therapy is initiated with a dose equivalent to the ED_{50}, it is especially important to evaluate the patient's response. Patients who fail to respond may need an increase in dosage. Conversely, patients who show signs of toxicity will need a dosage reduction.

- *Since drug responses are not completely predictable, you must look at the patient (and not the* Physicians' Desk Reference*) to determine if too much or too little medication has been administered.* In other words, doses should be adjusted on the basis of the patient's response and not just on the basis of what some reference says is supposed to work. For example, although many postoperative patients receive adequate pain relief with an "average" dose of morphine, this dose is not appropriate for everyone: An average dose may be effective for some patients, ineffective for others, and toxic for still others. Clearly, dosage must be adjusted on the basis of the patient's response, and must not be given in blind compliance with the dosage recommended in a book.

- *Because of variability in responses, nurses, patients, and other concerned individuals must evaluate actual responses and be prepared to inform the prescribing physician about these responses so that proper adjustments in dosage can be made.*

THE THERAPEUTIC INDEX

The therapeutic index is a measure of a drug's safety. The therapeutic index, determined using laboratory animals, is defined as *the ratio of a drug's LD_{50} to its ED_{50}.* (The LD_{50}, or average lethal dose, is the dose that is lethal to 50% of the animals treated.) A large therapeutic index indicates that a drug is relatively safe. Conversely, a small therapeutic index indicates that a drug is relatively unsafe.

The concept of therapeutic index is illustrated by the frequency distribution curves in Figure 5–9. Part *A* of the figure shows curves for therapeutic and lethal responses to drug "X." Part *B* shows equivalent curves for drug "Y." We can see in Figure 5–9*A* that the average lethal dose (100 mg) for drug X is much larger than the average therapeutic dose (10 mg). Since this drug's lethal dose is much larger than its therapeutic dose, common sense tells us that the drug should be relatively safe. The safety of this drug is reflected in its large therapeutic index, which is 10. In contrast, drug Y is unsafe. As shown in Figure 5–9*B*, the average lethal dose for drug Y (20 mg) is only twice the average therapeutic dose (10 mg). Hence, for drug Y, a dose only twice the ED_{50} could be lethal to 50% of those treated. Clearly, drug Y is not safe. This lack of safety is reflected in its small therapeutic index.

The curves for drug Y illustrate a phenomenon that is even more important than the therapeutic index. As we can see, there is *overlap* between the curve for therapeutic effects and the curve for lethal effects. This overlap tells us that the high doses needed to produce therapeutic effects in some people may be large enough to cause death. The message here is that, if a drug is to be truly safe, the highest dose required to produce therapeutic effects must be substantially lower than the lowest dose capable of causing death.

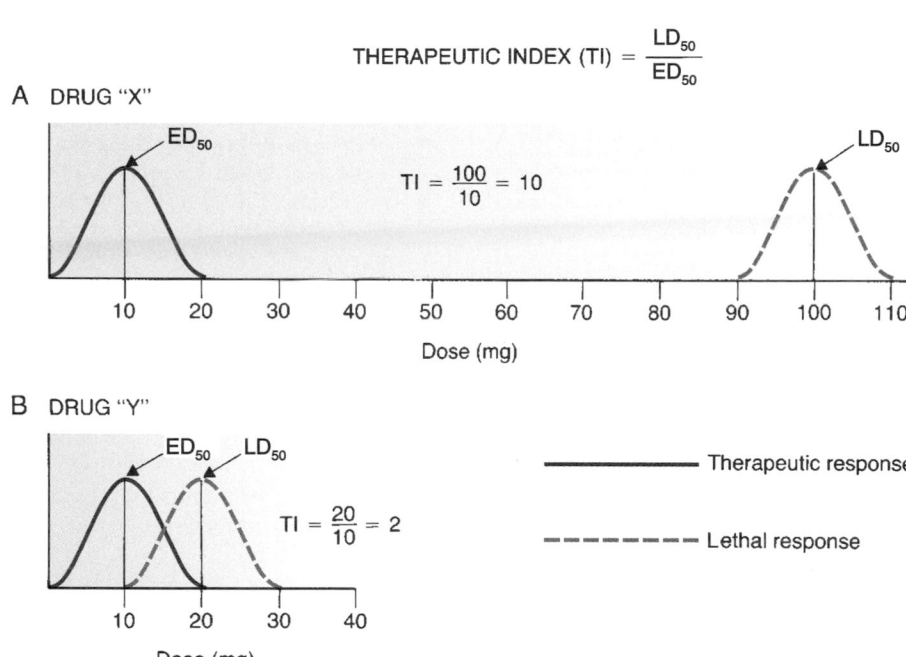

$$\text{THERAPEUTIC INDEX (TI)} = \frac{LD_{50}}{ED_{50}}$$

A   DRUG "X"

ED_{50} $\text{TI} = \dfrac{100}{10} = 10$ LD_{50}

Dose (mg)

B   DRUG "Y"

ED_{50} LD_{50} $\text{TI} = \dfrac{20}{10} = 2$

Dose (mg)

————— Therapeutic response

- - - - - - - Lethal response

Figure 5–9 ■ The therapeutic index.
A, Frequency distribution curves indicating the ED_{50} and LD_{50} for drug "X." Because its LD_{50} is much greater than its ED_{50}, drug X is relatively safe. *B,* Frequency distribution curves indicating the ED_{50} and LD_{50} for drug "Y." Because its LD_{50} is very close to its ED_{50}, drug Y is not very safe. Also note the overlap between the effective-dose curve and the lethal-dose curve.

⁙ KEY POINTS

- Pharmacodynamics is the study of the biochemical and physiologic effects of drugs and the molecular mechanisms by which those effects are produced.
- For most drugs, the dose-response relationship is graded. That is, the response gets more intense with increasing dosage.
- Maximal efficacy is defined as the biggest effect a drug can produce.
- Although efficacy is important, there are many situations in which a drug with relatively low efficacy is preferable to a drug with very high efficacy.
- A potent drug is simply a drug that produces its effects at low doses. As a rule, potency is not important.
- Potency and efficacy are independent qualities. Drug A can be more effective than drug B even though drug B may be more potent. Also, drugs A and B can be equally effective, although one may be more potent than the other.
- A receptor can be defined as any functional macromolecule in a cell to which a drug binds to produce its effects.
- Binding of drugs to their receptors is almost always reversible.
- The receptors through which drugs act are normal points of control for physiologic processes.
- Under physiologic conditions, receptor function is regulated by molecules supplied by the body.
- All that drugs can do at receptors is mimic or block the action of the body's own regulatory molecules.
- Because drug action is limited to mimicking or blocking the body's own regulatory molecules, drugs cannot give cells new functions. Rather, drugs can only alter the rate of pre-existing processes.
- Receptors make selective drug action possible.
- There are four primary families of receptors: cell membrane–embedded enzymes, ligand-gated ion channels, G protein–coupled receptor systems, and transcription factors.
- If a drug interacts with only one type of receptor, and if that receptor type regulates just a few processes, then the effects of the drug will be relatively selective.
- If a drug interacts with only one type of receptor, but that receptor type regulates multiple processes, then the effects of the drug will be nonselective.
- If a drug interacts with multiple receptors, its effects will be nonselective.
- Selectivity does not guarantee safety.
- The term *affinity* refers to the strength of the attraction between a drug and its receptor.
- Drugs with high affinity have high relative potency.
- The term *intrinsic activity* refers to the ability of a drug to activate receptors.
- Drugs with high intrinsic activity have high maximal efficacy.
- Agonists are molecules that activate receptors.
- In terms of the modified occupancy theory, agonists have both affinity and high intrinsic activity. Affinity allows them to bind to receptors, while intrinsic activity allows them to "activate" the receptor after binding.
- Antagonists are drugs that prevent receptor activation by endogenous regulatory molecules and by other drugs.
- In terms of the modified occupancy theory, antagonists have affinity for receptors but no intrinsic activity. Affinity allows the antagonist to bind to receptors, but lack of intrinsic activity prevents the bound antagonist from causing receptor activation.
- Antagonists have no observable effects in the absence of agonists.
- Partial agonists have only moderate intrinsic activity. Hence their maximal efficacy is lower than that of full agonists.
- Partial agonists can act as agonists (if there is no full agonist present) and as antagonists (if a full agonist is present).
- Continuous exposure of cells to agonists can result in receptor desensitization (aka refractoriness or down-regulation), whereas continuous exposure to antagonists can result in hypersensitivity (aka supersensitivity).
- Some drugs act through simple physical or chemical interactions with other small molecules rather than through receptors.
- The ED_{50} is defined as the dose required to produce a defined therapeutic response in 50% of the population.
- The initial dose of a drug is necessarily an approximation. Subsequent doses must be "fine tuned" based on the patient's response.
- An average effective dose (ED_{50}) is perfect for some people, insufficient for others, and excessive for still others.
- Since drug responses are not completely predictable, you must look at the patient (and not some drug reference book) to determine if dosage is appropriate.
- The therapeutic index—defined as the $LD_{50}:ED_{50}$ ratio—is a measure of a drug's safety. Drugs with a high therapeutic index are safe; drugs with a low therapeutic index are not.

Drug Interactions

In this chapter we consider the interactions of drugs with other drugs, with foods, and with herbal medicines. Our principal focus is on the mechanisms and clinical consequences of drug-drug interactions and drug-food interactions. Drug-herb interactions are discussed briefly here and at greater length in Chapter 104.

DRUG-DRUG INTERACTIONS

Drug-drug interactions can occur whenever a patient takes two or more drugs. Some interactions are both intended and desired, as when we combine drugs to treat hypertension. In contrast, some interactions are both unintended and undesired, as when we precipitate malignant hyperthermia in a patient receiving halothane and succinylcholine. Some adverse interactions are well known, and hence generally avoidable. Many others are yet to be documented.

Drug interactions occur because patients frequently take more than one drug. They may take multiple drugs to treat a single disorder. They may have multiple disorders that require treatment with different drugs. They may take over-the-counter drugs in addition to their prescription medicines. And they may take caffeine, nicotine, alcohol, and other drugs that have nothing to do with their illness.

Our objective in this chapter is to establish an overview of drug interactions, emphasizing the basic mechanisms by which drugs can interact. We will not attempt to catalog the huge number of specific interactions that are known. For information on interactions of specific drugs, you can refer to the chapters in which those drugs are discussed.

Consequences of Drug-Drug Interactions

When drug A interacts with drug B, there are three possible outcomes: (1) drug A may intensify the effects of drug B; (2) drug A may reduce the effects of drug B; or (3) the combination may produce a new response not seen with either drug alone.

Intensification of Effects

When a patient is taking two medications, one drug may intensify the effects of the other. This type of interaction is often termed *potentiative*. Potentiative interactions may be beneficial or detrimental. A potentiative interaction that enhances therapeutic effects is clearly beneficial. Conversely, a potentiative interaction that intensifies adverse effects is clearly detrimental. Examples of beneficial and detrimental potentiative interactions follow.

Increased Therapeutic Effects. The interaction between sulbactam and ampicillin represents a beneficial potentiative interaction. When administered alone, ampicillin undergoes rapid inactivation by bacterial enzymes. Sulbactam inhibits those enzymes, and thereby prolongs and intensifies ampicillin's therapeutic effects.

Increased Adverse Effects. The interaction between aspirin and warfarin represents a detrimental potentiative interaction. Warfarin is an anticoagulant used to suppress formation of blood clots. Unfortunately, if the dosage of warfarin is too high, the patient is at risk of spontaneous bleeding. Accordingly, for therapy to be safe and effective, the dosage must be high enough to suppress clot formation but not so high that spontaneous bleeding occurs. Like warfarin, aspirin also suppresses clotting. As a result, if aspirin and warfarin are taken concurrently, the risk of spontaneous bleeding is significantly increased. Clearly, potentiative interactions such as this are undesirable.

Reduction of Effects

Interactions that result in reduced drug effects are often termed *inhibitory*. As with potentiative interactions, inhibitory interactions can be beneficial or detrimental. Inhibitory interactions that reduce toxicity are beneficial. Conversely, inhibitory interactions that reduce therapeutic effects are detrimental. Examples of these interactions follow.

Reduced Therapeutic Effects. The interaction between propranolol and terbutaline represents a detrimental inhibitory interaction. Terbutaline is taken by people with asthma to dilate the bronchi. Propranolol, a drug for cardiovascular disorders, can act in the lung to block the effects of terbutaline. Hence, if propranolol and terbutaline are taken together, propranolol can reduce terbutaline's therapeutic effects. Inhibitory actions such as this, which can result in therapeutic failure, are clearly detrimental.

Reduced Adverse Effects. The use of naloxone to treat morphine overdose is an excellent example of a beneficial inhibitory interaction. When administered in excessive dosage, morphine can produce coma and profound respiratory depression; death can result. Naloxone, a drug that blocks morphine's actions, can completely reverse all symptoms of toxicity. The benefits of such an inhibitory interaction are obvious.

Creation of a Unique Response

Rarely, the combination of two drugs produces a new response not seen with either agent alone. To illustrate, let's consider the combination of alcohol with disulfiram [Antabuse], a drug used to treat alcoholism. When alcohol and disulfiram are combined, a host of unpleasant and dangerous responses can result. These effects do not occur when disulfiram or alcohol is used alone.

Basic Mechanisms of Drug-Drug Interactions

Drugs can interact through four basic mechanisms: (1) direct chemical or physical interaction, (2) pharmacokinetic interaction, (3) pharmacodynamic interaction, and (4) combined toxicity.

Direct Chemical or Physical Interaction

Some drugs, because of their physical or chemical properties, can undergo direct interaction with other drugs. Direct physical and chemical interactions usually render both drugs inactive.

Direct interactions occur most commonly when drugs are combined in IV solutions. Frequently, but not always, the interaction produces a precipitate. If a precipitate appears when drugs are mixed together, that solution should be discarded. Keep in mind, however, that direct drug interactions may not always leave visible evidence. Hence you cannot rely on simple inspection to reveal all direct interactions. Because drugs can interact in solution, *never combine two or more drugs in the same container unless it has been established that a direct interaction will not occur.*

The same kinds of interactions that can take place when drugs are mixed together in a bottle can also occur when drugs are mixed together in the patient. However, since drugs are diluted in body water following administration, and since dilution decreases chemical interactions, significant interactions within the patient are much less likely than in a bottle.

Pharmacokinetic Interactions

Drug interactions can affect all four of the basic pharmacokinetic processes. That is, when two drugs are taken together, one may alter the absorption, distribution, metabolism, or excretion of the other.

Altered Absorption. Drug absorption may be enhanced or reduced by drug interactions. In some cases, these interactions have great clinical significance. There are several mechanisms by which one drug can alter the absorption of another:

■ By elevating gastric pH, antacids can decrease the ionization of basic drugs in the stomach, thereby increasing the ability of basic drugs to cross membranes and be absorbed. Antacids have the opposite effect on acidic drugs.

■ Laxatives can reduce absorption of other drugs by accelerating their passage through the intestine.

■ Drugs that depress peristalsis (e.g., morphine, atropine) prolong drug transit time in the intestine, thereby increasing the time for absorption.

■ Drugs that induce vomiting can decrease absorption of oral drugs.

■ Cholestyramine and certain other adsorbent drugs, which are administered orally but do not undergo absorption, can adsorb other drugs onto themselves, thereby preventing absorption of the other drug into the blood.

■ Drugs that reduce regional blood flow can reduce absorption of other drugs from that region. For example, when epinephrine is injected together with a local anesthetic (as is often done), the epinephrine causes local vasoconstriction, thereby reducing regional blood flow and delaying absorption of the anesthetic.

Altered Distribution. There are two principal mechanisms by which one drug can alter the distribution of another: (1) competition for protein binding and (2) alteration of extracellular pH.

Competition for Protein Binding. When two drugs bind to the same site on plasma albumin, coadministration of those drugs produces competition for binding. As a result, binding of one or both agents is reduced, causing plasma levels of free drug to rise. In theory, the increase in free drug can intensify effects. However, since the newly freed drug usually undergoes rapid elimination, the increase in plasma levels of free drug is rarely sustained or significant.

Alteration of Extracellular pH. Because of the pH partitioning effect (see Chapter 4), a drug with the ability to change extracellular pH can alter the distribution of other drugs. For example, if a drug were to increase extracellular pH, that drug would increase the ionization of acidic drugs present in extracellular fluids (i.e., plasma and interstitial fluid). As a result, acidic drugs would be drawn from within cells (where the pH was below that of the extracellular fluid) into the extracellular space. Hence, the alteration in pH would change drug distribution.

The ability of drugs to alter pH and thereby alter the distribution of other drugs can be put to practical use in the management of poisoning. For example, symptoms of aspirin toxicity can be reduced with sodium bicarbonate, a drug that elevates extracellular pH. By increasing the pH outside cells, bicarbonate causes aspirin to move from intracellular sites into the interstitial fluid and plasma, thereby minimizing injury to cells.

Altered Metabolism. Altered metabolism is one of the most important—and most complex—mechanisms by which drugs interact. Some drugs *increase* the metabolism of other drugs; some drugs *decrease* the metabolism of other drugs. Drugs that increase the metabolism of other drugs do so by inducing synthesis of hepatic drug-metabolizing enzymes. Drugs that decrease the metabolism of other drugs do so by inhibiting those enzymes.

As we discussed in Chapter 4, the majority of drug metabolism is catalyzed by the cytochrome P450 (CYP) group of enzymes, which is composed of a large number of isozymes (closely related enzymes). Of all the isozymes in the P450 group, five are responsible for the metabolism of most drugs. These five isozymes of CYP are designated CYP1A2, CYP2C9, CYP2C19, CYP2D6, and CYP3A4. Table 6–1 lists the drugs that are metabolized by each isozyme, and indicates the drugs that can inhibit or induce them.

Induction of CYP Isozymes. Drugs that stimulate the synthesis of CYP isozymes are referred to as *inducing agents.* The classic example of an inducing agent is phenobarbital, a member of the barbiturate family. By increasing the synthesis of specific CYP isozymes, phenobarbital and other inducing agents can stimulate their own metabolism as well as that of other drugs.

Inducing agents can increase the rate of drug metabolism by as much as two- to threefold. This increase develops over 7 to 10 days. Rates of metabolism return to normal 7 to 10 days after the inducing agent has been withdrawn.

TABLE 6–1 ■ Drugs That Are Important Substrates, Inhibitors, or Inducers of Specific CYP Isozymes

CYP	Substrates	Inhibitors	Inducers
CYP1A2	Caffeine, clomipramine, theophylline	Cimetidine Fluvoxamine Ticlopidine Fluoroquinolones	Omeprazole Tobacco
CYP2C9	Diclofenac, ibuprofen, piroxicam, losartan, tolbutamide, warfarin	Azole antifungals Fluvastatin Zafirlukast	Rifampin
CYP2C19	Omeprazole, lansoprazole, diazepam, nelfinavir	Cimetidine Fluvoxamine	Rifampin
CYP2D6	*CNS Drugs:* amitriptyline, desipramine, imipramine, paroxetine, haloperidol, thioridazine *Antidysrhythmic Drugs:* mexiletine, propafenone *Beta Blockers:* propranolol, metoprolol, timolol *Opioids:* codeine, hydrocodone	Cimetidine Fluoxetine Paroxetine Quinidine Amiodarone Ritonavir	
CYP3A4	*Calcium Channel Blockers:* felodipine, nimodipine, nifedipine, nisoldipine, nitrendipine, verapamil *Immunosuppressants:* cyclosporine, tacrolimus *Steroids:* budesonide, cortisol, progesterone, 17-beta-estradiol, testosterone *Macrolide Antibiotics:* clarithromycin, erythromycin, troleandomycin *Anticancer Drugs:* cyclophosphamide, tamoxifen, vincristine, vinblastine, ifosfamide *Nonsedating Antihistamines:* astemizole,* terfenadine* *Benzodiazepines:* alprazolam, midazolam, triazolam *Opioids:* alfentanil, fentanyl, sufentanil *HMG-CoA Reductase Inhibitors:* lovastatin, simvastatin, atorvastatin, cerivastatin* *HIV Protease Inhibitors:* indinavir, nelfinavir, ritonavir, saquinavir, amprenavir *Others:* cisapride,* quinidine, sildenafil	Azole antifungals Amiodarone Clarithromycin Erythromycin Grapefruit juice Mibefradil Indinavir Ritonavir Troleandomycin	Rifampin Carbamazepine Phenobarbital Phenytoin Troglitazone

CNS = central nervous system, HIV = human immunodeficiency virus, HMG-CoA = 3-hydroxy-3methylglutaryl coenzyme A.
*No longer available in the United States.
Adapted from *The Medical Letter,* 41(1056):62, July 2, 1999.

When an inducing agent is taken concurrently with another medicine, dosage of the other medicine may need adjustment. For example, if a woman taking oral contraceptives were to begin taking phenobarbital, induction of drug metabolism by phenobarbital would accelerate metabolism of the contraceptive, thereby lowering its level. If drug metabolism is increased enough, protection against pregnancy would be lost. To maintain contraceptive efficacy, dosage of the contraceptive should be increased. Conversely, when a patient *discontinues* an inducing agent, dosages of other drugs may need to be *lowered.* If dosage is not reduced, drug levels may climb dangerously high as rates of hepatic metabolism decline to their baseline (noninduced) values.

Inhibition of CYP Isozymes. If drug A inhibits the metabolism of drug B, then levels of drug B will rise. The result may be beneficial or harmful. The interaction of ketoconazole (an antifungal drug) with cisapride* (a GI stimulant) and cyclosporine (an expensive immunosuppressant) provides an interesting case in point. Ketoconazole inhibits CYP3A4, the CYP isozyme that metabolizes cisapride and cyclosporine. If ketoconazole is combined with either drug, that drug's level will rise. In the case of cisapride, the result can be a fatal cardiac dysrhythmia—a clearly undesirable outcome. However, in the case of cyclosporine, inhibition of CYP3A4 allows us to achieve therapeutic drug levels at lower doses, thereby greatly reducing the cost of treatment—a clearly beneficial result.

Although inhibition of drug metabolism can be beneficial, as a rule inhibition has undesirable results. That is, in most cases, when an inhibitor increases the level of another drug, the outcome is toxicity. Accordingly, when a patient is taking an inhibitor along with his or her other medicines, you should be alert for possible adverse effects. Unfortunately, since the number of possible interactions of this type is large, keeping track of them is a challenge.

Altered Renal Excretion. Drugs can alter all three phases of renal excretion (filtration, reabsorption, and active secretion). By doing so, one drug can alter the renal excretion of another. Glomerular filtration can be decreased by drugs that reduce cardiac output: A reduction in cardiac output decreases renal blood flow, which decreases drug filtration at the glomerulus, which in turn decreases the rate of drug excretion. By altering urinary pH, one drug can alter the ionization of another, thereby increasing or decreasing the extent to which that drug undergoes passive tubular reabsorption. Lastly, competition between two drugs for active tubular secretion can decrease the renal excretion of both agents.

Pharmacodynamic Interactions

By influencing pharmacodynamic processes, one drug can alter the effects of another. Pharmacodynamic interactions are of two basic types: (1) interactions in which the interacting drugs act at the *same* site and (2) interactions in which the in-

*Cisapride [Propulsid] is no longer available in the United States.

teracting drugs act at *separate* sites. Pharmacodynamic interactions may be potentiative or inhibitory, and are of great clinical significance.

Interactions at the Same Receptor. Interactions that occur at the same receptor are almost always *inhibitory*. Inhibition occurs when an antagonist drug blocks access of an agonist drug to its receptor. These agonist-antagonist interactions are described in Chapter 5. There are many agonist-antagonist interactions of clinical importance. Some reduce therapeutic effects and are therefore undesirable. Others reduce toxicity and are of obvious benefit. The interaction between naloxone and morphine noted above is an example of a beneficial inhibitory interaction: By blocking access of morphine to its receptors, naloxone can reverse all symptoms of morphine overdose.

Interactions Resulting from Actions at Separate Sites. Even though two drugs have different mechanisms of action and act at separate sites, if both drugs influence the same physiologic process, then one drug can alter responses produced by the other. Interactions resulting from effects produced at different sites may be potentiative or inhibitory.

The interaction between morphine and diazepam [Valium] illustrates a potentiative interaction resulting from concurrent use of drugs that act at separate sites. Morphine and diazepam are central nervous system (CNS) depressants, but these drugs do not share the same mechanism of action. Hence, when these agents are administered together, the ability of each to depress CNS function reinforces the depressant effects of the other. This potentiative interaction can result in profound CNS depression.

The interaction between two diuretics—hydrochlorothiazide and spironolactone—illustrates how the effects of a drug acting at one site can *counteract* the effects of a second drug acting at a different site. Hydrochlorothiazide acts on the distal convoluted tubule of the nephron to *increase* excretion of potassium. Acting at a different site in the kidney, spironolactone works to *decrease* renal excretion of potassium. Consequently, when these two drugs are administered together, the potassium-sparing effects of spironolactone tend to balance the potassium-wasting effects of hydrochlorothiazide, leaving renal excretion of potassium at about the same level it would have been had no drugs been given at all.

Combined Toxicity

Common sense tells us that if drug A and drug B are both toxic to the same organ, then taking them together will cause more injury than if they were not combined. For example, when we treat tuberculosis with isoniazid and rifampin, both of which are hepatotoxic, we cause more liver injury than we would using just one of the drugs. As a rule, drugs with overlapping toxicity are not used together. Unfortunately, when treating tuberculosis, the combination is essential, and hence can't be avoided.

Clinical Significance of Drug-Drug Interactions

From the foregoing it should be clear that drug interactions have the potential to affect the outcome of therapy. As a result of drug-drug interactions, the intensity of responses may be increased or reduced. Interactions that increase therapeutic effects or reduce toxicity are desirable. Conversely, interactions that reduce therapeutic effects or increase toxicity are detrimental.

Common sense tells us that the risk of a serious drug interaction is proportional to the number of drugs that a patient is taking. That is, the more drugs the patient receives, the greater the risk of a detrimental interaction. Since the average hospitalized patient receives 6 to 10 drugs, interactions are common. Accordingly, you should always be alert for them.

Interactions are especially important for drugs that have a low therapeutic index. For these agents, an interaction that produces a modest increase in drug levels can cause toxicity. Conversely, an interaction that produces a modest decrease in drug levels can cause therapeutic failure.

Although a large number of important interactions have been documented, many more are yet to be identified. Therefore, if a patient develops unusual symptoms, it is wise to suspect that a drug interaction may be the cause—especially since yet another drug might be given to control the new symptoms.

We can minimize adverse interactions in several ways. The most obvious is to minimize the number of drugs a patient receives. Indiscriminate use of multiple-drug therapy does not constitute good treatment—and increases the risk of undesired interactions. A second and equally important way to avoid detrimental interactions is to take a thorough drug history. A history that identifies all drugs the patient is taking allows the prescriber to adjust the regimen accordingly. Please note, however, that patients taking illicit drugs or over-the-counter preparations may fail to report such drug use. You should be aware of this possibility and make a special effort to ensure that the patient's drug use profile is complete. Additional measures for reducing adverse interactions include adjusting the dosage when an inducer of metabolism is added to or deleted from the regimen, adjusting the timing of administration to minimize interference with absorption, and monitoring for early signs of toxicity when combinations of toxic agents cannot be avoided.

DRUG-FOOD INTERACTIONS

Drug-food interactions are both important and poorly understood. They are important because they can result in toxicity or therapeutic failure. They are poorly understood because research has been sorely lacking.

Impact of Food on Drug Absorption

Decreased Absorption. Food frequently decreases the *rate* of drug absorption, and occasionally decreases the *extent* of absorption. Reducing the rate of absorption merely delays the onset of effects; peak effects are not lowered. In contrast, reducing the extent of absorption reduces the intensity of peak responses.

The interaction between calcium-containing foods and tetracycline antibiotics is perhaps the classic example of food reducing drug absorption. Tetracyclines bind with calcium to form an insoluble and nonabsorbable complex. Hence, if tetracyclines are administered with milk products or calcium supplements, absorption is reduced and antibacterial effects may be lost.

High-fiber foods can reduce absorption of some drugs. For example, absorption of digoxin [Lanoxin], a drug used for cardiac disorders, is reduced significantly by wheat bran, rolled oats, and sunflower seeds. Since digoxin has a low therapeutic index, reduced absorption can result in therapeutic failure.

Increased Absorption. With some drugs, food increases the extent of drug absorption. When this occurs, peak effects are heightened. For example, a high-calorie meal more than doubles the absorption of saquinavir [Invirase], a drug for HIV infection. If saquinavir is taken without food, absorption may be insufficient for antiviral activity.

Impact of Food on Drug Metabolism: The Grapefruit Juice Effect

Grapefruit juice can inhibit the metabolism of certain drugs, thereby raising their blood levels. The effect is quite remarkable. In one study, coadministration of grapefruit juice produced a 406% increase in blood levels of felodipine [Plendil], a calcium channel blocker used for hypertension. In addition to felodipine and other calcium channel blockers, grapefruit juice can increase blood levels of lovastatin [Mevacor], cyclosporine [Sandimmune], midazolam [Versed], and several other drugs (Table 6–2). This effect is *not* seen with other citrus juices, including orange juice.

Grapefruit juice raises drug levels by inhibiting metabolism. Specifically, grapefruit juice inhibits CYP3A4, an isozyme of cytochrome P450 found in the liver and the intestinal wall. Grapefruit juice inhibits the intestinal isozyme much more than the liver isozyme. By inhibiting CYP3A4, grapefruit juice decreases the intestinal metabolism of certain drugs (see Table 6–2), and thereby increases the amount available for absorption. As a result, blood levels of these drugs rise, causing peak effects to be more intense. Since inhibition of CYP3A4 in the liver is minimal, grapefruit juice does not affect metabolism of drugs after they have been absorbed. Accordingly, their half-lives are not prolonged. Inhibition of CYP3A4 is dose dependent: The more grapefruit juice the patient drinks, the greater the inhibition.

Inhibition of CYP3A4 persists for some time after grapefruit juice is consumed. Therefore, a drug needn't be administered concurrently with grapefruit juice for an interaction to occur. Put another way, metabolism can still be inhibited even if a patient drinks grapefruit juice in the morning but waits until later in the day to take his or her medicine. Recent evidence indicates that, if grapefruit juice is consumed on a regular basis, inhibition can persist up to 3 days after the last glass.

The compound in grapefruit juice that inhibits CYP3A4 has not been established. Candidates include *flavonoids* and *psoralen derivatives*. Early studies had implicated *naringenin*, a compound that can inhibit CYP3A4 *in vitro*. However, when commercial naringenin was given to human subjects, no effect on drug metabolism was observed.

The effects of grapefruit juice vary considerably among patients. This is because levels of CYP3A4 show great individual variation. In patients with very little CYP3A4, inhibition by grapefruit juice may be sufficient to stop metabolism completely. As a result, large increases in drug levels may occur. Conversely, in patients with lots of CYP3A4, metabolism may continue more or less normally, despite inhibition by grapefruit juice. Hence, drug levels will be largely unaffected.

The clinical consequences of inhibition may be good or bad. As indicated in Table 6–2, by elevating levels of certain drugs, grapefruit juice can increase the risk of serious toxicity, an outcome that is obviously bad. On the other hand, by increasing levels of two other drugs—saquinavir and cyclosporine—grapefruit juice can intensify therapeutic effects, an outcome that is clearly good.

What should patients do if the drugs they are taking can be affected by grapefruit juice? Until more is known, prudence dictates avoiding grapefruit juice entirely.

TABLE 6–2 ■ Drugs Whose Levels Can Be Increased By Grapefruit Juice

Drug	Indications	Potential Consequences of Increased Drug Levels
Dihydropyridine calcium channel blockers: Amlodipine Felodipine Nifedipine Nicardipine Nimodipine Nisoldipine	Hypertension; angina pectoris	Toxicity: flushing, headache, tachycardia, hypotension
Verapamil	Hypertension; angina pectoris	Toxicity: bradycardia, AV heart block, hypotension, constipation
Caffeine	Prevents sleepiness	Toxicity: restlessness, insomnia, convulsions, tachycardia
Carbamazepine	Seizures; bipolar disorder	Toxicity: ataxia, drowsiness, nausea, vomiting, tremor
Estrogens	Replacement therapy	Clinical consequences are not yet known
Buspirone	Anxiety	Drowsiness, dysphoria
Triazolam	Anxiety; insomnia	Increased sedation
Midazolam	Induction of anesthesia; production of conscious sedation	Increased sedation
Lovastatin	Lowers cholesterol	Toxicity: headache, GI disturbances, liver and muscle toxicity
Terfenadine*	Allergy symptoms	Toxicity: prolonged QT interval leading to potentially fatal dysrhythmias
Saquinavir	HIV infection	Increased therapeutic effect
Cyclosporine	Prevents rejection of organ transplants	Increased therapeutic effects. If levels rise too high, toxicity (nephrotoxicity, hepatotoxicity) will occur
Cisapride*	Gastroesophageal reflux	Toxicity: prolonged QT interval leading to potentially fatal dysrhythmias

AV = atrioventricular, GI = gastrointestinal, HIV = human immunodeficiency virus.
*No longer available in the United States

Impact of Food on Drug Toxicity

Drug-food interactions sometimes increase toxicity. The most dramatic example is the interaction between monoamine oxidase (MAO) inhibitors (a family of antidepressants) and foods rich in tyramine (e.g., aged cheeses, yeast extracts, Chianti wine): Combining an MAO inhibitor with these foods can raise blood pressure to a life-threatening level. To avoid disaster, patients taking MAO inhibitors must be warned about the consequences of consuming tyramine-rich foods, and must be given a list of foods to strictly avoid (see Chapter 31). Other drug-food combinations that can increase toxicity include the following:

- Theophylline (an asthma medicine) plus caffeine, which can result in excessive CNS excitation
- Potassium-sparing diuretics (e.g., spironolactone) plus salt substitutes, which can result in dangerously high potassium levels
- Aluminum-containing antacids (e.g., Maalox) plus citrus beverages (e.g., orange juice), which can result in excessive absorption of aluminum

Impact of Food on Drug Action

Although most drug-food interactions concern drug absorption or drug metabolism, food may also (rarely) have a direct impact on drug action. For example, foods rich in vitamin K (e.g., broccoli, Brussels sprouts, cabbage) can reduce the effects of warfarin, an anticoagulant. How? As discussed in Chapter 50, warfarin acts by inhibiting vitamin K–dependent clotting factors; when vitamin K is more abundant, warfarin is less able to inhibit the clotting factors, and therapeutic effects are reduced.

Timing of Drug Administration with Respect to Meals

Administration of drugs at the appropriate time with respect to meals is an important facet of drug therapy. As discussed, the absorption of some drugs can be significantly decreased by food; hence, these drugs should be administered on an empty stomach. Conversely, the absorption of other drugs can be increased by food, and hence these drugs should be administered with meals.

Many drugs cause stomach upset when taken without food. If food does not reduce their absorption, then these drugs should definitely be administered with meals. However, if food does reduce their absorption, then we have a difficult choice: we can administer them with food and thereby reduce stomach upset (good news), but reduce absorption (bad news)—or, we can administer them without food and thereby improve absorption (good news), but increase stomach upset (bad news). Unfortunately, the correct choice is not obvious. The best solution may be to select an alternative drug that doesn't upset the stomach.

When the medication order says to administer a drug "with food" or "on an empty stomach," just what does this mean? To administer a drug with food means to administer it with or shortly after a meal. To administer a drug on an empty stomach means to administer it either 1 hour before a meal or 2 hours after.

Medication orders frequently fail to indicate when a drug should be administered with respect to meals. As a result, inappropriate administration may occur. If you are uncertain about when to give a drug, ask the prescriber if it should be taken on an empty stomach or with food, and if there are any foods or beverages to avoid.

DRUG-HERB INTERACTIONS

Herbal supplements (herbal medicines) are used widely in the United States, creating the potential for frequent and significant interactions with conventional drugs. Of greatest concern are interactions that reduce beneficial responses to conventional drugs and interactions that increase toxicity. How do these interactions occur? Through the same pharmacokinetic and pharmacodynamic mechanisms by which conventional drugs interact with each other. Unfortunately, reliable information about herbal supplements is largely lacking—including information on interactions with conventional agents. Interactions that *have* been well documented are discussed as appropriate throughout this text. In Chapter 31, for example, we discuss the well-known ability of St. John's wort to induce drug-metabolizing enzymes, and thereby reduce blood levels of many drugs. Herbal medicines and their interactions are discussed further in Chapter 104 (Herbal Supplements).

⁞▪ KEY POINTS

- Some drug-drug interactions are intended and beneficial; others are unintended and detrimental.
- Drug-drug interactions may result in intensified effects, diminished effects, or an entirely new effect.
- Potentiative interactions are beneficial when they increase therapeutic effects and detrimental when they increase adverse effects.
- Inhibitory interactions are beneficial when they decrease adverse effects and detrimental when they decrease beneficial effects.
- Because drugs can interact in solution, you should never combine two or more drugs in the same container unless you are certain that a direct interaction will not occur.
- Drug interactions can result in increased or decreased absorption.
- Competition for protein binding rarely results in a sustained or significant increase in plasma levels of free drug.
- Drugs that induce hepatic drug-metabolizing enzymes can accelerate the metabolism of other drugs.
- When an inducing agent is added to the regimen, it may be necessary to increase the dosages of other drugs. Conversely, when an inducing agent is discontinued, dosages of other drugs may need to be reduced.
- A drug that inhibits the metabolism of other drugs will increase their levels. Sometimes the result is beneficial, but usually it's detrimental.
- Drugs that act as antagonists at a particular receptor will diminish the effects of drugs that act as agonists at that receptor. The result may be beneficial (if the

antagonist prevents toxic effects of the agonist), or it may be detrimental (if the antagonist prevents therapeutic effects of the agonist).

▪ Drugs that are toxic to the same organ should not be combined (if at all possible).

▪ We can help reduce the risk of adverse interactions by minimizing the number of drugs the patient is given and by taking a thorough drug history.

▪ Food may reduce the rate or extent of drug absorption. Reducing the extent of absorption reduces peak therapeutic responses; reducing the rate of absorption merely delays the onset of effects.

▪ For some drugs, food may increase the extent of absorption.

▪ Grapefruit juice can inhibit the intestinal metabolism of certain drugs, thereby increasing their absorption, which in turn increases their blood levels.

▪ Foods may increase drug toxicity. The combination of an MAO inhibitor with tyramine-rich food is the classic example.

▪ When the medication order says to administer a drug on an empty stomach, this means administer it either 1 hour before a meal or 2 hours after.

▪ Conventional drugs can interact with herbal preparations. The biggest concerns are increased toxicity and reduced therapeutic effects of the conventional agent.

Adverse Drug Reactions and Medication Errors

ADVERSE DRUG REACTIONS

An adverse drug reaction (ADR), as defined by the World Health Organization, is any noxious, unintended, and undesired effect that occurs at normal drug doses. Note that this definition excludes undesired effects that occur when dosage is excessive (e.g., because of accidental poisoning or medication error). Adverse reactions can range in intensity from annoying to life threatening. Fortunately, when drugs are used properly, many ADRs can be avoided, or at least kept to a minimum.

Scope of the Problem

Drugs can adversely affect all body systems in varying degrees of intensity. Among the more mild reactions are drowsiness, nausea, itching, and rash. Severe reactions include respiratory depression, neutropenia, hepatocellular injury, anaphylaxis, and hemorrhage—all of which can result in death.

Although ADRs can occur in all patients, some patients are more vulnerable than others. Adverse events are most common in the elderly and the very young. (Patients over 60 account for nearly 50% of all ADR cases.) Severe illness also increases the risk of an ADR. Likewise, adverse events are more common in patients receiving multiple drugs than in patients taking just one.

Some data on ADRs will underscore their significance. Among hospitalized patients, the overall incidence of *serious* ADRs is 6.7%. Of these, about 5% result in death. One esti-

mate indicates that, in 1994, about 2.2 million hospitalized patients experienced serious ADRs, of which 106,000 proved fatal. If these numbers are correct, ADRs would be the fourth leading cause of death, exceeded only by heart disease, cancer, and stroke.

Definitions
Side Effect

A side effect is formally defined as *a nearly unavoidable secondary drug effect produced at therapeutic doses.* Common examples include drowsiness caused by antihistamines and gastric irritation caused by aspirin. Side effects are generally predictable and their intensity is dose dependent. Some side effects develop soon after the onset of drug use, whereas others may not appear until a drug has been taken for weeks or months.

Toxicity

The formal definition of toxicity is *an adverse drug reaction caused by excessive dosing.* Examples include coma from an overdose of morphine and severe hypoglycemia from an overdose of insulin. Although the formal definition of toxicity includes only those severe reactions that occur when dosage is excessive, in everyday parlance the term *toxicity* has come to mean any severe ADR, regardless of the dose that caused it. For example, when administered in therapeutic doses, many anticancer drugs cause neutropenia (profound loss of neutrophilic white blood cells), thereby putting the patient at high risk of infection. This neutropenia would be called a toxicity even though it was produced when dosage was therapeutic.

Allergic Reaction

An allergic reaction is an immune response. For an allergic reaction to occur there must be prior sensitization of the immune system. Once the immune system has been sensitized to a drug, re-exposure to that drug can trigger an allergic response. The intensity of allergic reactions can range from mild itching to severe rash to anaphylaxis. (Anaphylaxis is a life-threatening response characterized by bronchospasm, laryngeal edema, and a precipitous drop in blood pressure.) Estimates suggest that less than 10% of ADRs are of the allergic type.

The intensity of an allergic reaction is determined primarily by the degree of sensitization of the immune system—not by drug dosage. That is, *the intensity of allergic reactions is largely independent of dosage.* As a result, a dose that elicits a very strong reaction in one allergic patient may elicit a very mild reaction in another. Furthermore, since a patient's sensitivity to a drug can change over time, a dose that elicits a mild reaction early in treatment may produce an intense reaction later on.

Very few medications cause severe allergic reactions. In fact, most serious reactions are caused by just one drug family—the *penicillins*. Other drugs noted for causing allergic reactions include the nonsteroidal anti-inflammatory drugs (e.g., aspirin) and the sulfonamide group of compounds, which includes certain diuretics, antibiotics, and oral hypoglycemic agents.

Idiosyncratic Effect

An idiosyncratic effect is defined as *an uncommon drug response resulting from a genetic predisposition.* To illustrate this concept, let's consider responses to succinylcholine, a drug used to produce flaccid paralysis of skeletal muscle. In most patients, succinylcholine-induced paralysis is brief, lasting only a few minutes. In contrast, genetically predisposed patients may become paralyzed for hours. Why the difference? Because in all patients the effects of succinylcholine are terminated through enzymatic inactivation of the drug. Since most people have very high levels of the inactivating enzyme, paralysis is short lived. However, in a small percentage of patients, the genes that code for succinylcholine-metabolizing enzymes are abnormal, producing enzymes that inactivate the drug very slowly. As a result, paralysis is greatly prolonged.

Iatrogenic Disease

The word *iatrogenic* is derived from two words: *iatros,* the Greek word for physician and *-genic,* a combining form meaning *to produce.* Hence, an iatrogenic disease is *a disease produced by a physician.* The term *iatrogenic disease* is also used to denote *a disease produced by drugs.*

Iatrogenic diseases are nearly identical to idiopathic (naturally occurring) diseases. For example, patients taking certain antipsychotic drugs may develop a syndrome whose symptoms closely resemble those of Parkinson's disease. Because this syndrome is (1) drug induced and (2) essentially identical to a naturally occurring pathology, we would call the syndrome an iatrogenic disease.

Physical Dependence

Physical dependence develops during long-term use of certain drugs, such as opioids, alcohol, barbiturates, and amphetamines. We can define physical dependence as a state in which the body has adapted to prolonged drug exposure in such a way that an abstinence syndrome will result if drug use is discontinued. The precise nature of the abstinence syndrome is determined by the drug involved.

Although physical dependence is usually associated with "narcotics" (heroin, morphine, and other opioids), these are not the only dependence-inducing drugs. In addition to the opioids, a variety of other centrally acting drugs (e.g., ethanol, barbiturates, amphetamines) can promote dependence. Furthermore, some drugs that work outside the central nervous system can cause physical dependence of a sort. Because a variety of drugs can cause physical dependence of one type or another, and because withdrawal reactions have the potential for harm, *patients should be warned against abrupt discontinuation of any medication without first consulting a knowledgeable health professional.*

Carcinogenic Effect

The term *carcinogenic effect* refers to the ability of certain medications and environmental chemicals to cause cancers. Fortunately, only a few therapeutic agents are carcinogenic. Ironically, several of the drugs used to *treat* cancer are among the drugs with the greatest carcinogenic potential.

Evaluating drugs for the ability to cause cancer is extremely difficult. Evidence of neoplastic disease may not appear until 20 or more years after initial exposure to a cancer-causing compound. Consequently, it is unlikely that carcinogenic potential will be detected during preclinical and clinical drug trials. Accordingly, when a new drug is released for general marketing, we cannot know with certainty that the drug will not eventually prove carcinogenic.

Diethylstilbestrol (DES) illustrates the problem posed by the delayed appearance of cancer following exposure to a carcinogenic drug. DES is a synthetic hormone with actions similar to those of estrogen. At one time DES was used to prevent spontaneous abortion during high-risk pregnancies. It was not until years later, when vaginal and uterine cancers developed in females who had been exposed to this drug *in utero,* that the carcinogenic actions of DES became known.

Teratogenic Effect

A *teratogenic effect* can be defined as a drug-induced birth defect. Medicines and other chemicals capable of causing birth defects are called teratogens. Teratogenesis is discussed at length in Chapter 9.

Organ-Specific Toxicity

Many drugs are toxic to specific organs. Common examples include injury to the kidneys caused by amphotericin B (an antifungal drug), injury to the heart caused by doxorubicin (an anticancer drug), injury to the lungs caused by amiodarone (an antidysrhythmic drug), and injury to the inner ear caused by aminoglycoside antibiotics (e.g., gentamicin). Patients using such drugs should be monitored for signs of developing injury. In addition, patients should be educated about these signs and advised to seek medical attention if they appear.

Two types of organ-specific toxicity deserve special comment. These are (1) injury to the liver and (2) altered cardiac function, as evidenced by a prolonged QT interval on the electrocardiogram. Both are discussed below.

Hepatotoxic Drugs

Drugs are the leading cause of acute liver failure, a rare condition that can rapidly prove fatal. Most cases end with a liver transplant or in death. The ability to cause severe liver damage is the most common reason for withdrawing drugs from the market.

Fortunately, liver failure from using known hepatotoxic drugs is rare. The incidence is less than 1 in 50,000. (Drugs that cause liver failure more often than this are removed from the market—unless they are indicated for a life-threatening illness.) Some drugs known to cause liver injury are listed in Table 7–1.

How do drugs damage the liver? Recall that the liver is the primary site of drug metabolism. As some drugs undergo metabolism, they are converted to toxic products that can injure liver cells.

TABLE 7–1 ■ Some Hepatotoxic Drugs

Statins and Other Lipid-Lowering Drugs	*Antiseizure Drugs*	*Antiretroviral Drugs*
Atorvastatin [Lipitor]	Carbamazepine [Tegretol]	Ritonavir [Norvir]
Cerivastatin [Baycol]*	Felbamate [Felbatol]	Nevirapine [Viramune]
Fluvastatin [Lescol]	Valproic acid [Depakene, others]	*Other Drugs*
Lovastatin [Mevacor]	*Antifungal Drugs*	Acetaminophen [Tylenol, others], but
Pravastatin [Pravachol]	Itraconazole [Sporanox]	only when combined with alcohol
Simvastatin [Zocor]	Ketoconazole [Nizoral]	Amiodarone [Cordarone]
Fenofibrate [Tricor]	Terbinafine [Lamisil]	Diclofenac [Voltaren]
Gemfibrozil [Lopid]	*Drugs for Tuberculosis*	Halothane [Fluothane]
Niacin [Niaspan, others]	Isoniazid	Leflunomide [Arava]
Oral Hypoglycemics	Pyrazinamide	Methyldopa [Aldomet]
Acarbose [Precose]	Rifampin [Rifadin]	Nefazodone [Serzone]
Pioglitazone [Actos]	*Immunosuppressants*	Tacrine [Cognex]
Rosiglitazone [Avandia]	Azathioprine [Imuran]	Tamoxifen [Nolvadex]
Troglitazone [Rezulin]*	Methotrexate [Rheumatrex]	Zileuton [Zyflo]
		Nitrofurantoin [Macrodantin]

*Withdrawn from the market.

Combining a hepatotoxic drug with certain other drugs may increase the risk of liver damage. Perhaps the best example is the combination of acetaminophen [Tylenol, others] with alcohol. When taken in therapeutic doses in the absence of alcohol, acetaminophen cannot harm the liver. However, if the drug is taken with just two or three drinks, severe liver injury can result.

Patients taking hepatotoxic drugs should undergo liver function tests (LFTs) at baseline and periodically thereafter. How do we assess liver function? By testing a blood sample for the presence of two liver enzymes: *aspartate aminotransferase* (AST, formerly known as SGOT) and *alanine aminotransferase* (ALT, formerly known as SGPT). Under normal conditions blood levels of AST and ALT are low. However, when liver cells are injured, blood levels of these enzymes rise. LFTs are performed on a regular schedule (e.g., every 3 months) in hopes of detecting injury early. Unfortunately, since drug-induced liver injury can develop very quickly, it may progress from being undetectable to advanced between scheduled tests.

All patients receiving hepatotoxic drugs should be informed about signs of liver injury—jaundice (yellow skin and eyes), dark urine, light-colored stools, nausea, vomiting, malaise, abdominal discomfort, loss of appetite—and should be advised to seek medical attention if these develop.

QT Interval Drugs

The term *QT interval drugs*—or simply *QT drugs*—refers to the ability of some medications to prolong the QT interval on the electrocardiogram, thereby creating a risk of serious dysrhythmias. As discussed in Chapter 47 (Antidysrhythmic Drugs), the QT interval is a measure of the time required for the ventricles to repolarize after each contraction. When the QT interval is prolonged, patients can develop a dysrhythmia known as *torsades de pointes,* which can progress to potentially fatal ventricular fibrillation.

More than 50 drugs are known to cause QT prolongation, torsades de pointes, or both (Table 7–2). As shown in Table 7–2, QT drugs can be found in many drug families, ranging from antihistamines to antibiotics to antipsychotics. Recently, four QT drugs—astemizole [Hismanal], terfenadine [Seldane], cisapride [Propulsid], and grepafloxacin [Raxar]—were removed from the market because of deaths associated with their use. In re-sponse to heightened awareness of the risks posed by QT drugs, the Food and Drug Administration (FDA) now requires that all new drugs be tested to see if they cause QT prolongation.

When QT drugs are used, care should be taken to minimize the risk of dysrhythmias. These agents should be used with caution in patients predisposed to dysrhythmias. Among these are the elderly and patients with bradycardia, heart failure, congenital QT prolongation, and low levels of potassium or magnesium. Women are also at risk. Why? Because their normal QT interval is longer than the QT interval in men. Concurrent use of two or more QT drugs should be avoided—as should the concurrent use of a QT drug with another drug that can raise its blood level (e.g., by inhibiting its metabolism). Obviously, excessive dosing should be avoided. Additional information on QT drugs, including a current list of these agents, is available online at *www.QTdrugs.org.*

Identifying Adverse Drug Reactions

It can be very difficult to determine whether a specific drug is responsible for an observed adverse event. Why? Because other factors—especially the underlying illness and other drugs being taken—could be the actual cause. To help determine if a particular drug is responsible, the following questions should be asked:

- Did symptoms appear shortly after the drug was first used?
- Did symptoms abate when the drug was discontinued?
- Did symptoms reappear when the drug was reinstituted?
- Is the illness itself sufficient to explain the event?
- Are other drugs in the regimen sufficient to explain the event?

If the answers reveal a temporal relationship between the presence of the drug and the adverse event, and if the event cannot be explained by the illness itself or by other drugs in the regimen, then there is a high probability that the drug under suspicion is indeed the culprit. Unfortunately, this process is limited: It can only identify adverse effects that occur while the drug is being used; it cannot identify adverse events that develop years after a drug has been discontinued. Nor can it identify effects that develop slowly, that is, over the course of prolonged drug use.

TABLE 7–2 ▪ **Drugs That Prolong the QT Interval, Induce Torsades de Pointes, or Both**		
Antidysrhythmics	*Antibiotics*	*Antihistamines*
Amiodarone [Cordarone]	Clarithromycin [Biaxin]	Astemizole [Hismanal]*
Bretylium [Bretylol]	Erythromycin	Terfenadine [Seldane]*
Disopyramide [Norpace]	Gatifloxacin [Tequin]	*ACE Inhibitors/Calcium Channel Blockers*
Dofetilide [Tikosyn]	Grepafloxacin [Raxar]*	Bepridil [Vascor]
Flecainide [Tambocor]	Levofloxacin [Levaquin]	Isradipine [DynaCirc]
Ibutilide [Corvert]	Moxifloxacin [Avelox]	Nicardipine [Cardene]
Procainamide [Procan, Pronestyl]	Sparfloxacin [Zagam]	*Others*
Propafenone [Rhythmol]	*Triptans*	Cisapride [Propulsid]*
Quinidine	Naratriptan [Amerge]	Droperidol [Inapsine]
Sotalol [Betapace]	Sumatriptan [Imitrex]	Felbamate [Felbatol]
Antidepressants	Zolmitriptan [Zomig]	Foscarnet [Foscavir]
Amitriptyline [Elavil, Endep]	*Anticancer Drugs*	Fosphenytoin [Cerebyx]
Citalopram [Celexa]	Arsenic trioxide [Trisenox]	Halofantrine [Halfan]
Desipramine [Norpramin]	Tamoxifen [Nolvadex]	Indapamide [Lozol]
Doxepin [Sinequan]	*Antipsychotics*	Levomethadyl [Orlaam]
Fluoxetine [Prozac]	Chlorpromazine [Thorazine]	Octreotide [Sandostatin]
Imipramine [Tofranil]	Haloperidol [Haldol]	Pentamidine [Pentam, Nebupent]
Paroxetine [Paxil]	Mesoridazine [Serentil]	Probucol [Lorelco]
Sertraline [Zoloft]	Pimozide [Orap]	Salmeterol [Serevent]
Venlafaxine [Effexor]	Quetiapine [Seroquel]	Tacrolimus [Prograf]
	Risperidone [Risperdal]	Tizanidine [Zanaflex]
	Thioridazine [Mellaril]	
	Ziprasidone [Geodon]	

ACE = angiotensin-converting enzyme.
*Withdrawn from the market.

Adverse Reactions to New Drugs

As we discussed in Chapter 3, preclinical and clinical trials of new drugs cannot detect all of the ADRs that a drug may be able to cause. Accordingly, when a new drug is released for general marketing, information regarding ADRs is incomplete.

Because newly released drugs may have as-yet unreported adverse effects, you should be alert for unusual responses when giving new drugs. If the patient develops new symptoms, it is wise to suspect that the drug may be responsible—even if the symptoms are not described in the literature. If the drug is especially new, you may be the first clinician to have observed this particular effect.

If you suspect a drug of causing a previously unknown adverse effect, you should report the effect to MEDWATCH, the FDA Medical Products Reporting Program. You can file your report electronically via the MEDWATCH Internet site (*www.fda.gov/medwatch*). The form used for reporting is shown in Figure 7–1. Since voluntary reporting by healthcare professionals is an important mechanism for bringing ADRs to light, you should report all suspected ADRs, even if absolute proof of the drug's complicity has not been established.

Ways to Minimize Adverse Drug Reactions

The responsibility for reducing ADRs lies with everyone associated with drug manufacture and use. The pharmaceutical industry must strive to produce the safest possible medicines; the prescriber must select the least harmful medicine for a particular patient; the nurse must evaluate patients for ADRs and must educate patients in ways to avoid or minimize harm; and patients and their families must watch for signs that an ADR may be developing, and should seek medical attention if they appear.

Anticipation of ADRs can help minimize them. Both the nurse and the patient should know the major ADRs that a drug can produce. This knowledge will allow early identification of adverse effects, thereby permitting timely implementation of measures to minimize harm.

As noted, certain drugs are toxic to specific organs. When patients are using these drugs, function of the target organ should be monitored. The liver, kidneys, and bone marrow are important sites of drug toxicity. For drugs that are toxic to the liver, the patient should be monitored for signs and symptoms of liver damage (jaundice, dark urine, light-colored stools, nausea, vomiting, malaise, abdominal discomfort, loss of appetite); also, periodic LFTs should be performed. For drugs that are toxic to the kidneys, the patient should undergo routine urinalysis and measurement of serum creatinine; in addition, periodic tests of creatinine clearance should be performed. For drugs that are toxic to bone marrow, periodic blood cell counts are required.

Adverse effects can be reduced by individualizing therapy. When prescribing a drug for a particular patient, the physician must balance potential risks of that drug versus its probable benefits. Drugs that are likely to harm a specific patient should be avoided. For example, if a patient has a history of penicillin allergy, we can avoid a potentially severe reaction by withholding penicillin and administering a suitable substitute. Similarly, when treating pregnant patients, we must withhold drugs that can injure the fetus (see Chapter 9).

Lastly, we must be aware that patients with chronic disorders are especially vulnerable to ADRs. In this group are patients with hypertension, epilepsy, heart disease, and psychoses. When drugs must be used long term, the patient should

U.S. Department of Health and Human Services

MEDWATCH

The FDA Safety Information and Adverse Event Reporting Program

For VOLUNTARY reporting of
adverse events and product problems

Page ___ of ___

Form Approved: OMB No. 0910-0291 Expires: 04/30/03
See OMB statement on reverse

FDA Use Only

Triage unit
sequence #

A. Patient information

1. Patient identifier	2. Age at time of event: ___ or Date of birth:	3. Sex ☐ female ☐ male	4. Weight ___ lbs or ___ kgs
In confidence			

B. Adverse event or product problem

1. ☐ **Adverse event** and/or ☐ **Product problem** (e.g., defects/malfunctions)

2. **Outcomes attributed to adverse event** (check all that apply)
☐ death ___ (mo/day/yr)
☐ life-threatening
☐ hospitalization - initial or prolonged
☐ disability
☐ congenital anomaly
☐ required intervention to prevent permanent impairment/damage
☐ other: ___

3. Date of event (mo/day/yr)	4. Date of this report (mo/day/yr)

5. **Describe event or problem**

6. **Relevant tests/laboratory date,** including dates

7. **Other relevant history, including preexisting medical conditions** (e.g., allergies, race, pregnancy, smoking and alcohol use, hepatic/renal dysfunction, etc.)

C. Suspect medication (s)

1. **Name** (give labeled strength & mfr/labeler, in known)
#1
#2

2. **Dose, frequency & route used** #1 #2	3. **Therapy dates** (if unknown, give duration) from/to (or best estimate) #1 #2

4. **Diagnosis for use** (indication)
#1
#2

5. **Event abated after use stopped or dose reduced**
#1 ☐ yes ☐ no ☐ doesn't apply
#2 ☐ yes ☐ no ☐ doesn't apply

6. **Lot #** (if known) #1 #2	7. **Exp. date** (if known) #1 #2

8. **Event reappeared after introduction**
#1 ☐ yes ☐ no ☐ doesn't apply
#2 ☐ yes ☐ no ☐ doesn't apply

9. **NDC #** (for product problems only)

10. **Concomitant medical products** and therapy dates (exclude treatment of event)

D. Suspect medical device

1. **Brand name**

2. **Type of device**

3. **Manufacturer name & address**	4. **Operator of device** ☐ health professional ☐ lay user/patient ☐ other: ___

6. model # ___ –
catalog # ___ –
serial # ___ –
lot # ___ –
other #

5. **Expiration date** (mo/day/yr)

7. **If implanted, give date** (mo/day/yr)

8. **If explanted, give date** (mo/day/yr)

9. **Device available for evaluation?** **(Do not send to FDA)**
☐ yes ☐ no ☐ returned to manufacturer on ___ (mo/day/yr)

10. **Concomitant medical products** and therapy dates (exclude treatment of event)

E. Reporter (see confidentiality section on back)

1. **Name & address** | phone #

2. **Health professional?** ☐ yes ☐ no	3. **Occupation**	4. **Also reported to** ☐ manufacturer ☐ user facility ☐ distributor

5. If you do NOT want your identity disclosed to the manufacturer, place an "X" in this box. ☐

Mail to: **MEDWATCH**
5600 Fishers Lane
Rockville, MD 20852-9787

or FAX to:
1-800-FDA-0178

FDA Form 3500

Submission of a report does not constitute an admission that medical personnel or the product caused or contributed to the event.

Figure 7–1 ■ **FDA form for reporting adverse drug events.**

be informed about the adverse effects that may develop over time and should be monitored periodically for their appearance.

MEDICATION ERRORS

Medication errors are a major cause of morbidity and mortality. In 1999, the problem rose to national prominence with the publication of *To Err is Human,* a report on medical errors issued by the Institute of Medicine (IOM), a branch of the National Academy of Sciences. According to the IOM report, 7000 people die in U.S. hospitals each year because of medication errors—and tens of thousands more die outside of hospitals. In addition, the IOM estimates that fully half of all ADRs result from medication mistakes. Some authorities argue that the IOM estimates exaggerate the problem; others argue that the estimates are far too low. However, all agree that medication errors are a very real problem—even if the IOM estimates *are* in dispute. In response to the IOM report, healthcare organizations throughout the country have intensified efforts to reduce medical errors and thereby improve patient safety. The full text of the IOM report is available as pdf files online at *bob.nap.edu/html/to_err_is_human.*

What's a Medication Error and Who Makes Them?

The National Coordinating Council for Medication Error Reporting and Prevention (NCC MERP) defines a medication error as "any preventable event that may cause or lead to inappropriate medication use or patient harm, while the medication is in the control of the healthcare professional, patient, or consumer. Such events may be related to professional practice, healthcare products, procedures, and systems, including prescribing; order communication; product labeling, packaging and nomenclature; compounding; dispensing; distribution; administration; education; monitoring; and use." Note that, by this definition, medication errors can be made by many people—beginning with workers in the pharmaceutical industry, followed by people in the healthcare delivery system, and ending with patients and their family members.

In the hospital setting, a medication order must be processed by several people before it reaches the patient. All of these people can make a mistake. Fortunately, most are also in a position to catch mistakes made by others. The process typically begins with a physician writing a prescription; then someone transcribes the order; in the pharmacy, someone enters the order into a computer; then a pharmacy technician prepares the order, after which a pharmacist checks it; and finally a nurse checks the order again and then administers the drug. Each of these people is in a position to make an error. Except for the prescriber, each is also in a position to catch errors made by others as the order moves down the line. Because the nurse is the last person in the sequence, the nurse is the patient's last line of defense against mistakes—and also the last person with the opportunity to make one. Note also that the nurse is the only person whose actions are not routinely checked by anyone else. Because the nurse is the last person who can catch mistakes made by others, and because no one is there to catch mistakes the nurse might make, the nurse bears a heavy responsibility for ensuring patient safety. Can you think of a better reason to learn all you can about drugs?

Types of Medication Errors

Medication errors fall into 13 major categories (Table 7–3). Some types of errors cause harm directly, and some cause harm indirectly. For example, giving an excessive dose can cause direct harm (adverse effects or even death) from having too much drug in the body. Conversely, giving too little medication can lead to harm, not through direct effects of the drug, but through failure to adequately treat the patient's illness. According to the 1999 IOM report, among *fatal* medication errors, the most common types are giving an overdose (36.4%), giving the wrong drug (16.2%), and using the wrong route (9.5%).

Causes of Medication Errors

Medication errors can result from many causes (Table 7–4). Among fatal medication errors, the 1999 IOM report identified three categories—human factors, communication mistakes, and name confusion—that account for 90% of all errors. Of the human factors that can cause errors, performance deficits (e.g., administering a drug IV instead of IM) are the most common (29.8%), followed by knowledge deficits (14.2%) and miscalculation of dosage (13%).

Miscommunication involving oral and written orders underlies 15.8% of fatal errors. Poor handwriting is an infamous cause of mistakes. In one example, an order for 2 mg of warfarin (an anticoagulant) was misread as 5 mg, and resulted in death from hemorrhage. In another case, a woman with arthritis died because her prescription to take 10 mg of methotrexate (an immunosuppressant) once a week was misread as 10 mg once a day. Because of illegible handwriting by prescribers, pharmacists make an estimated 150 million phone calls a year for clarification. When patients are admitted to the hospital, errors can result from poor communication regarding medications they were taking at home. For example, a child who was taking cisapride at home died because his prescription for one-fourth of a 10-mg tablet 4 times a day was incorrectly transcribed to read one 10-mg tablet 4 times a day.

TABLE 7–3 ■ Types of Medication Errors
Wrong patient
Wrong drug
Wrong route
Wrong time
Wrong dose
Overdose
Underdose
Extra dose
Omitted dose
Wrong dosage form
Wrong diluent
Wrong strength/concentration
Wrong infusion rate
Wrong technique (includes inappropriate crushing of tablets)
Deteriorated drug error (dispensing a drug after its expiration date)
Wrong duration of treatment (continuing too long or stopping too soon)

TABLE 7–4 ■ Causes of Medication Errors	
Cause	**Examples**
Human Factors	
Performance deficit	Administration by IV infusion when IM injection was intended
Knowledge deficit	Failure to know and follow reasonable practice standards
Miscalculation of dosage	
Drug preparation	Using the wrong diluent; using the wrong amount of diluent; adding the wrong drug; adding the wrong amount of drug
Computer error	Incorrect selection from a list by computer operator; incorrect programming into the database; inadequate screening for allergies, interactions, etc.
Stocking error	Error in stocking or restocking; error in cart filling
Transcription error	Original to paper/carbon paper; original to computer; original to FAX
Stress	High-volume workload, etc.
Fatigue or lack of sleep	
Communication	
Written miscommunication	Illegible handwriting; misreading or failure to read; confusion regarding decimal point placement in dosage
Oral miscommunication	
Name Confusion	
Trade name confusion	Name sounds or looks like another drug name
Generic name confusion	Name sounds or looks like another drug name
Packaging, Formulations, and Delivery Devices	
Inappropriate packaging	Topical product packaged in sterile IV multidose vial
Tablet or capsule confusion	Confusion because the tablet or capsule is similar in color, shape, or size to tablets or capsules that contain a different drug or a different strength of the same drug
Delivery device problems	Malfunction; infusion pump problems; selection of wrong device
Labeling and Reference Materials	
Manufacturer's carton	Carton looks similar to other cartons from the same manufacturer or cartons from another manufacturer
Manufacturer's container label	Label looks similar to other labels from the same manufacturer or to labels from another manufacturer
Label of dispensed product	Wrong patient name; wrong drug name; wrong strength; wrong or incomplete directions
Reference materials (package insert and other printed material, electronic material)	Inaccurate, incomplete, misleading, or outdated information

Other causes of communication errors include careless use of zeros and decimal points, and confusion between metric and apothecary units.

Confusion over drug names leads to 8.9% of fatal errors. Why is there confusion? Because many drugs have names that sound like or look like the names of other drugs. Table 7–5 lists some good examples, such as *Anaspaz/Antispas, Celebrex/Cerebyx,* and *Renagel/Remegel.* Note that most of the examples in Table 7–5 are trade names, not generic names. The potential for lethal confusion among trade names is a powerful reason for abandoning them in favor of universal use of generic names. (In case you skipped the discussion on trade names in Chapter 3, your author feels very strongly that trade names should be outlawed.)

Ways to Reduce Medication Errors

Healthcare organizations throughout the country are working to design and implement measures to reduce medication errors. Much of this effort was triggered by the 1999 IOM report, and much was already in progress before the report was released. A central theme in these efforts is to change institutional culture—from one that focuses on "naming, shaming, and blaming" those who make mistakes to one focused on designing institution-wide processes and systems that can prevent errors from happening.

In southeastern Pennsylvania, a consortium of hospitals has developed a unique system for reducing medication errors. This system, known as the Regional Medication Safety Program for Hospitals (RMSPH), can be considered a model for other hospitals to follow. The RMSPH has a total of 16 action goals divided into four major categories: institutional culture, infrastructure, clinical practice, and technology (Table 7–6). Note that creating an institutional culture dedicated to safety tops the list, and that the institutional environment should be nonpunitive so as to encourage both the identification of errors and the development of new safety systems. This is a radical departure from the past, in which organizations focused largely on identifying and punishing caregivers who made mistakes. As you read through Table 7–6, the potential benefits of all 16 objectives should be apparent. To aid practitioners in achieving these 16 goals, the RMSPH contains a "tool kit" with detailed supporting information on how to meet each objective. For example, the kit includes safety checklists to follow when using high-alert drugs, such as anticoagulants, thrombolyt-

TABLE 7–5 ■ Examples of Drugs with Names That Sound Alike or Look Alike*

Amicar	*Amikin*
Anaspaz	*Antispas*
Carbastat	*Carbatrol*
Celebrex	*Cerebyx*
Clinoril	*Clozaril*
Clomiphene	Clomipramine
Cycloserine	Cyclosporine
Depo-Estradiol	*Depo-Testadiol*
Dioval	*Diovan*
Estratab	*Estratest*
Etidronate	Etretinate
Flomax	*Volmax*
Inderal	*Adderall*
Lamictal	*Lamisil*
Levoxine	*Levoxyl*
Lithobid	*Lithostat*
Lodine	Iodine
Lomotil	*Lamictal*
Naprelan	*Naprosyn*
Nasarel	*Nizoral*
Neoral	*Neosar*
Nephron	*Nephrox*
Nicoderm	*Nitroderm*
Plendil	*Pletal*
Preven	*Preveon*
Renagel	*Remegel*
Sarafem	*Serophene*
Serentil	*Seroquel*
Tamiflu	*Theraflu*
Zyvox	*Vioxx*

*Trade names are italicized; generic names are not.

TABLE 7–6 ■ Sixteen Ways to Cut Medication Errors*

Institutional Culture
- Establish an organizational commitment to a culture of safety.
- Provide medication safety education for all new and existing professional employees.
- Maintain ongoing recognition of safety innovation.
- Create a nonpunitive environment that encourages identification of errors and the development of new patient safety systems.

Infrastructure
- Designate a medication safety coordinator/officer and identify physician champions.
- Promote greater use of clinical pharmacists in high-risk areas.
- Establish area-specific guidelines for unit-stocked medications.
- Establish a mechanism to ensure availability of critical medication information to all members of the patient's care team.

Clinical Practice
- Eliminate dangerous abbreviations and dose designations.
- Implement safety checklists for high-alert medications.
- Implement safety checklists for infusion pumps.
- Develop limitations and safeguards regarding verbal orders.
- Perform failure-mode analysis during procurement process.
- Implement triggers and markers to indicate potential adverse medication events.

Technology
- Eliminate the use of infusion pumps that lack free-flow protection.
- Prepare for implementation of computerized prescriber order entry systems.

*These strategies are recommended in the Regional Medication Safety Program for Hospitals (RMSPH), developed by a consortium of hospitals in southeastern Pennsylvania.

ics, and neuromuscular blocking agents. (About 20 such drugs cause 80% of medication error-related deaths.)

Some measures to reduce errors have had remarkable success. For example,

- Replacing handwritten medication orders with a computerized order entry system has reduced medications errors by 50%.
- In ICUs, medication errors have been reduced by 66% by having a senior clinical pharmacist accompany physicians on rounds.
- Hospitals in the Veterans Administration system have reduced medication errors by up to 70% with a bar-code system. In this system, all nurses and patients wear bar-coded ID strips, and all medications have bar codes too. Before giving a medication, the nurse scans all three codes into a computer, which then either (1) verifies that the patient-drug match is correct and adverse interactions are unlikely or (2) flashes a warning if there is a potential problem.

There is a wealth of information available on reducing medication errors. If you would like more, a good place to start is *www.nccmerp.org,* the web site of the National Coordinating Council for Medication Error Reporting and Prevention. The NCC MERP was established to facilitate the reporting, understanding, and prevention of medication errors. Member organizations include the American Nurses Association, American Medical Association, American Hospital Association, Food and Drug Administration (FDA), and U.S. Pharmacopeia (USP). The NCC MERP web site has extensive recommendations for reducing medication errors related to drug administration, medication dispensing, and verbal medication orders and prescriptions. In addition, the site presents recommendations for promoting and standardizing bar coding on medication packaging. Even more information is available from the Institute for Safe Medical Practices (at *www.ismp. org/MSAarticles/AHA-ISMP.html*) and from the FDA (at *www. fda.gov/cder/drug/mederrors*).

How to Report a Medication Error

You can report a medication error via the *Medication Errors Reporting (MER) Program,* a nationwide program set up by the USP in cooperation with the Institute for Safe Medical Practices (ISMP). All reporting is confidential and can be done by phone or fax, or through the Internet. Details on submitting a report are available online at *www.usp.org/reporting/mer.htm.* The MER Program encourages participation by all healthcare providers, including pharmacists, nurses, physicians, and students. The objective is not to establish blame, but to improve patient safety by increasing our knowledge of medication errors. All information gathered by the MER Program is forwarded to the FDA, the ISMP, and the product manufacturer. The form for submitting a report is shown in Figure 7–2.

USP MEDICATION ERRORS REPORTING PROGRAM

MEDI-CATION ERRORS REPORTING PROGRAM

Presented in cooperation with the Institute for Safe Medication Practices

The USP Practitioners' Reporting Network^{SM} is an FDA MEDWATCH partner

☐ ACTUAL ERROR   ☐ POTENTIAL ERROR

Please describe the error. Include sequence of events, personnel involved, and work environment (e.g., code situation, change of shift, short staffing, no 24-hr. pharmacy, floor stock). If more space is needed, please attach separate page.

Was the medication administered to or used by the patient? ☐ No ☐ Yes   Date and time of event: _____

What type of staff or health care practitioner made the initial error? _____

Describe outcome (e.g., death, type of injury, adverse reaction). _____

If the medication did not reach the patient, describe the intervention. _____

Who discovered the error? _____

When and how was error discovered? _____

Where did the error occur (e.g., hospital, outpatient or retail pharmacy, nursing home, patient's home)? _____

Was another practitioner involved in the error? ☐ No ☐ Yes   If yes, what type of practitioner? _____

Was patient counseling provided? ☐ No ☐ Yes   If yes, before or after error was discovered? _____

If a product was involved, please complete the following:

	Product #1	Product #2
Brand name of product involved		
Generic name		
Manufacturer		
Labeler (if different from mfr.)		
Dosage form		
Strength/concentration		
Type and size of container		
NDC number		

If available, please provide relevant patient information (age, gender, diagnosis, etc.). Patient identification not required.

Reports are most useful when relevant materials such as product label, copy of prescription/order, etc. can be reviewed.

Can these materials be provided?   ☐ No ☐ Yes If yes, please specify. _____

Suggest any recommendations you have to prevent recurrence of this error or describe policies or procedures you have instituted to prevent future similar errors.

A copy of this report is routinely sent to the Institute for Safe Medication Practices (ISMP), to the manufacturer/labeler, and to the Food and Drug Administration (FDA). **USP may release my identity to: (check boxes that apply)**

☐ ISMP ☐ The manufacturer and/or labeler as listed above ☐ FDA ☐ Other persons requesting a copy of this report   ☐ Anonymous to all

Your name and title

Your facility name, address, and ZIP

Telephone number (include area code)

Signature

Date

Return to the attention of:
Diane D. Cousins, R.Ph.
USP PRN
12601 Twinbrook Parkway
Rockville, MD 20852-1790

Call Toll Free: 800-23-ERROR (800-233-7767)
or FAX 301-816-8532
USP home page: http://www.usp.org/prn

Date Received by USP:

File Access Number:

C-194
WEB pdf
10/14/97

Additional forms can be found in the *USP DI Vol. I* and *Vol. III* and in all monthly *Updates.*

Figure 7–2 ■ **Form for reporting medication errors to the USP Medication Errors Reporting Program.**

⁘ KEY POINTS

- An adverse drug reaction can be defined as any noxious, unintended, and undesired effect that occurs at normal drug doses.
- Patients at increased risk of adverse drug events include the very young, the elderly, the very ill, and those taking multiple drugs.
- An iatrogenic disease is defined as a drug- or physician-induced disease.
- An idiosyncratic effect is defined as an adverse drug reaction based on a genetic predisposition.
- A carcinogenic effect is defined as a drug-induced cancer.
- A teratogenic effect is defined as a drug-induced birth defect.
- The intensity of an allergic drug reaction is based on the degree of immune system sensitization—not on drug dosage.
- Drugs are the most common cause of acute liver failure, and hepatotoxicity is the most common reason for removing drugs from the market.
- Drugs that prolong the QT interval pose a risk of torsades de pointes, a dysrhythmia that can progress to fatal ventricular fibrillation.
- At the time a new drug is released, it well may have the ability to cause adverse effects that are as yet unknown.
- Measures to minimize adverse drug events include avoiding drugs that are likely to harm a particular patient, monitoring the patient for signs and symptoms of likely adverse effects, educating the patient about possible adverse effects, and monitoring organs that are vulnerable to a particular drug.
- Medication errors are a major cause of morbidity and mortality.
- Medication errors can be made by many people, including pharmaceutical workers, pharmacists, physicians, transcriptionists, nurses, and patients and their families.
- In a hospital, a medication order is processed by several people. Each is in a position to introduce errors, and, except for the prescribing physician, each is in a position to catch errors made by others.
- The nurse is the patient's last line of defense against medication errors made by others—and the last person with the opportunity to introduce an error.
- Because the nurse is the last person who can catch mistakes made by others, and because no one is there to catch mistakes the nurse might make, the nurse bears a unique responsibility for ensuring patient safety.
- The three most common *types* of fatal medication errors are giving an overdose, giving the wrong drug, and using the wrong route.
- The three most common *causes* of fatal medication errors are human factors (e.g., performance or knowledge deficits), miscommunication (e.g., because of illegible prescriber handwriting), and confusion caused by similarities in drug names.
- At the heart of efforts to reduce medication errors is a change in institutional culture—from a punitive system focused on "naming, blaming, and shaming" to a nonpunitive system in which medication errors can be discussed openly, thereby facilitating the identification of errors and the development of new safety procedures.
- Effective measures for reducing medication errors include (1) using a safety checklist for high-alert drugs, (2) replacing handwritten medication orders with a computerized order entry system, (3) having a clinical pharmacist accompany ICU physicians on rounds, and (4) using a computerized bar-code system that (a) identifies the administering nurse and (b) ensures that the drug is going to the right patient and that adverse interactions are unlikely.

Individual Variation in Drug Responses

Individual variation in drug responses has been a recurrent theme throughout the early chapters of this text. We noted that, because of individual variation, we must tailor drug therapy to each patient. In this chapter we discuss the major factors that can cause one patient to respond to drugs differently than another. With this information you will be better prepared to reduce individual variation in drug responses, thereby maximizing the benefits of treatment and reducing the potential for harm. As we discuss sources of individual variation, we will review and integrate much of the information presented in previous chapters.

BODY WEIGHT AND COMPOSITION

In the absence of adjustments in dosage, body size can be a significant determinant of drug effects. Recall that the intensity of the response to a drug is determined in large part by the concentration of the drug at its sites of action—the higher the concentration, the more intense the response. Common sense tells us that, if a small person and a large person are given the same amount of the same drug, the drug will achieve a higher concentration in the small person, and therefore will produce more intense effects. To

compensate for this potential source of individual variation, dosages must be adapted to the size of the patient.

When adjusting dosage to account for body weight, the clinician may base the adjustment on *body surface area* rather than on weight per se. Why? Because surface area determinations account not only for the patient's weight but also for how fat or lean the patient may be. Since percentage body fat can change drug distribution, and since altered distribution can change the concentration of a drug at its sites of action, dosage adjustments based on body surface area provide a more precise means of controlling drug responses than do adjustments based on weight alone.

AGE

Drug sensitivity varies with age. Infants are especially sensitive to drugs, as are the elderly. In the very young, heightened drug sensitivity is the result of organ immaturity. In the elderly, heightened sensitivity results largely from organ degeneration. Other factors that affect sensitivity in the elderly are increased severity of illness, the presence of multiple pathologies, and treatment with multiple drugs. The clinical challenge created by heightened drug sensitivity in the very young and the elderly is discussed at length in Chapters 10 and 11, respectively.

GENDER

Men and women can respond differently to the same drug. A drug may be more effective in men than in women, or vice versa. Likewise, adverse effects may be more intense in men than in women, or vice versa. Unfortunately, for most drugs, we don't know much about gender-related differences. Why? Because, until recently, essentially all drug research was done in men. Nonetheless, enough research has been done to indicate that gender-related differences really do exist. For example, we know that alcohol is metabolized more slowly by women than by men. As a result, a woman who drinks the same amount as a man (on a weight-adjusted basis) will become more intoxicated. Similarly, women are more sensitive to the cardiotoxic effects of terfenadine* [Seldane] than are men. As a result, women taking this drug are at higher risk of developing fatal dysrhythmias. In 1997, the Food and Drug Administration put pressure on drug companies to include women in trials of new drugs, especially drugs directed at serious or life-threatening illnesses. The information generated by these trials will permit drug therapy to be more rational in women than is possible today. In the mean-

---

*Terfenadine is a nonsedating antihistamine that was withdrawn from the U.S. market in 1998.

time, clinicians must keep in mind that the information currently available may fail to accurately predict responses in female patients. Accordingly, clinicians should remain alert for treatment failures and unexpected adverse effects.

PATHOPHYSIOLOGY

Abnormal physiology can alter responses to drugs. In this section we examine the impact on drug responses produced by four pathologic conditions: (1) kidney disease, (2) liver disease, (3) acid-base imbalance, and (4) altered electrolyte status.

Kidney Disease

Kidney disease can reduce drug excretion, causing drugs to accumulate in the body. If dosage is not lowered, drugs may accumulate to toxic levels. Consequently, if a patient is taking a drug whose elimination is dependent upon renal function, and if renal failure develops, dosage must be decreased.

The impact of renal disease on plasma drug levels is illustrated in Figure 8–1. The figure shows the decline in plasma levels of kanamycin (an antibiotic) following injection into two patients, one with healthy kidneys and one with renal failure. (Elimination of kanamycin is exclusively renal.) As shown in the figure, kanamycin levels fall off rapidly in the patient with good kidney function. In this patient, the drug's half-life is brief—only 1.5 hours. In contrast, drug levels decline very slowly in the patient with renal failure. Because of kidney disease, the half-life of kanamycin has increased by nearly 17-fold—from 1.5 hours to 25 hours. Under these conditions, if dosage is not reduced, kanamycin will quickly accumulate to toxic levels.

Liver Disease

Like kidney disease, liver disease can cause drugs to accumulate. Recall that the liver is the major site of drug metabolism. Hence, if the liver ceases to function, rates of metabolism will

fall and drug levels will climb. To prevent accumulation to toxic levels, patients with liver disease should have their dosages reduced. Of course, this guideline applies only to those drugs that are eliminated primarily by the liver; liver dysfunction will not affect plasma levels of drugs that are eliminated largely by nonhepatic mechanisms (e.g., renal excretion).

Acid-Base Imbalance

By altering pH partitioning (see Chapter 4), changes in acid-base status can alter the absorption, distribution, metabolism, and excretion of drugs.

Figure 8–2 illustrates the impact of altered acid-base status on drug distribution. Specifically, it shows the results of altered acid-base status on the distribution of phenobarbital (a weak acid) in a dog. The upper curve shows plasma levels of phenobarbital. The lower curve shows plasma pH. Acid-base status was altered by having the dog inhale a mixture of gas rich in carbon dioxide (CO_2), thereby causing respiratory acidosis. In the figure, acidosis is indicated by the drop in plasma pH. Note that the decline in pH is associated with a parallel drop in levels of phenobarbital. Upon discontinuation of CO_2 administration, plasma pH returned to normal and phenobarbital levels moved upward.

Why did acidosis alter plasma levels of phenobarbital? Recall that, because of pH partitioning, if there is a difference in pH on two sides of a membrane, a drug will accumulate on the side where the pH most favors its ionization. Hence, because acidic drugs ionize in alkaline media, acidic drugs will accumulate on the alkaline side of the membrane. Conversely, basic drugs will accumulate on the acidic side. Since phenobarbital is a weak acid, it tends to accumulate in alkaline environments. Accordingly, when the dog inhaled CO_2, causing extracellular pH to decline, phenobarbital left the plasma and entered cells, where the environment was less acidic (more alkaline) than in plasma. When CO_2 administration ceased and plasma pH returned to normal, the pH partitioning effect caused phenobarbital to leave cells and re-enter the blood, causing blood levels to rise.

Altered Electrolyte Status

Electrolytes (e.g., potassium, sodium, calcium, magnesium) have important roles in cell physiology. Consequently, when electrolyte levels become disturbed, multiple cellular processes can be disrupted. Excitable tissues (nerves and muscles) are especially sensitive to alterations in electrolyte status. Given that disturbances in electrolyte balance can have widespread effects on cell physiology, we might expect that electrolyte imbalances would cause profound and widespread effects on responses to drugs. However, this does not seem to be the case; examples in which electrolyte changes have a significant impact on drug responses are rare.

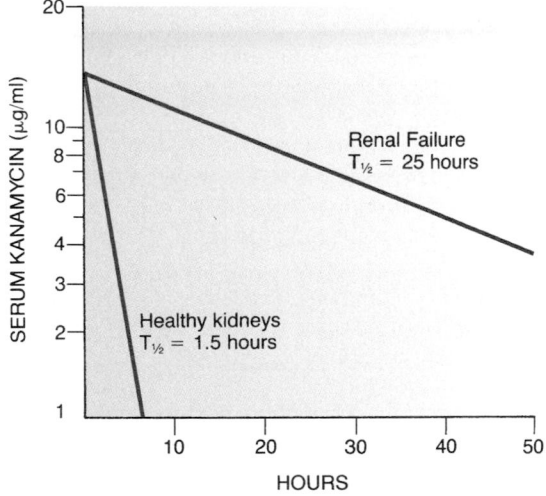

Figure 8–1 ■ Effect of renal failure on kanamycin half-life. Kanamycin was administered at time "0" to two patients, one with healthy kidneys and one with renal failure. Note that drug levels declined very rapidly in the patient with healthy kidneys and extremely slowly in the patient with renal failure, indicating that renal failure greatly reduced the capacity to remove this drug from the body.

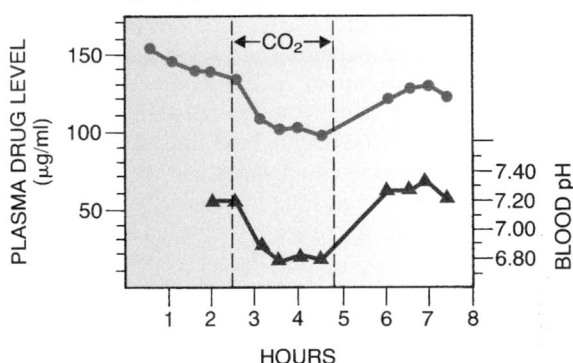

Figure 8–2 ■ Altered drug distribution in response to altered plasma pH.
Lower curve, Plasma (extracellular) pH. Note the decline in pH in response to inhalation of CO_2. *Upper curve,* Plasma levels of phenobarbital. Note the decline in plasma drug levels during the period of extracellular acidosis. This decline results from the redistribution of phenobarbital into cells. (See text for details.) (Redrawn from Waddell WJ, Butler TC. The distribution and excretion of phenobarbital. J Clin Invest 1957;36:1217.)

Perhaps the most important example of an altered drug effect occurring in response to electrolyte imbalance involves digoxin, a drug used to treat heart disease. The most serious toxicity of digoxin is production of potentially fatal cardiac dysrhythmias. The tendency of digoxin to disturb cardiac rhythm is related to levels of potassium: When potassium levels are depressed, the ability of digoxin to induce dysrhythmias is greatly increased. Accordingly, all patients receiving digoxin must undergo regular measurement of serum potassium to ensure that levels remain within a safe range. Digoxin toxicity and its relationship to potassium levels are discussed at length in Chapter 46.

TOLERANCE

Tolerance can be defined as *decreased responsiveness to a drug as a result of repeated drug administration*. Patients who are tolerant to a drug require higher doses to produce the same effects that were achievable with lower doses before tolerance had developed. There are three categories of drug tolerance: (1) pharmacodynamic tolerance, (2) metabolic tolerance, and (3) tachyphylaxis.

Pharmacodynamic Tolerance

The term *pharmacodynamic tolerance* refers to the familiar type of tolerance associated with long-term administration of drugs such as morphine and heroin. The person who is pharmacodynamically tolerant requires increased drug levels to produce effects that could formerly be elicited at lower drug levels. Put another way, in the presence of pharmacodynamic tolerance, the minimum effective concentration (MEC) of a drug is abnormally high. Pharmacodynamic tolerance is thought to result from adaptive processes that occur in response to chronic receptor occupation.

Metabolic Tolerance

Metabolic tolerance is defined as tolerance resulting from accelerated drug metabolism. This form of tolerance is brought about by the ability of certain drugs (e.g., barbiturates) to induce synthesis of hepatic drug-metabolizing enzymes, thereby causing rates of drug metabolism to increase. Because of increased metabolism, dosage must be increased to maintain therapeutic drug levels. Unlike pharmacodynamic tolerance, which causes the MEC to increase, metabolic tolerance does not affect the MEC.

The experiment summarized in Table 8–1 demonstrates the development of metabolic tolerance in response to repeated administration of pentobarbital, a central nervous system depressant. The study employed two groups of rabbits, a control group and an experimental group. Rabbits in the experimental group were pretreated with pentobarbital for 3 days (60 mg/kg/day SC) and then given an IV challenging dose (30 mg/kg) of the same drug. Drug effect (sleeping time) and plasma drug levels were then measured. The control rabbits received the challenging dose of pentobarbital but did not receive any pretreatment. As indicated in Table 8–1, the challenging dose of pentobarbital had less effect on the pretreated rabbits than on the control animals. Specifically, whereas the control rabbits slept an average of 67 minutes, the average sleeping time for the pretreated animals was only 30 minutes—less than half the effect seen in controls.

Why was pentobarbital less effective in the pretreated animals? The data on half-life suggest an answer. As shown in the table, the half-life of pentobarbital was much shorter in the experimental group than in the control group. Since pentobarbital is eliminated primarily by hepatic metabolism, the reduced half-life indicates accelerated metabolism. This increase in metabolism, which was brought on by pentobarbital pretreatment, explains why the experimental rabbits were more tolerant than the controls.

You might ask, "How do we know that the experimental rabbits had not developed *pharmacodynamic* tolerance?" The absence of pharmacodynamic tolerance is indicated by the plasma drug levels measured at the time the rabbits awoke. In the pretreated rabbits, the waking drug levels were slightly below the waking drug levels in the control group. Had the experimental animals developed pharmacodynamic tolerance, they would have required an *increase* in drug concentration to maintain sleep. Hence, if pharmacodynamic tolerance were present, drug levels would have been abnormally high at the time of awakening, rather than reduced.

Tachyphylaxis

Tachyphylaxis is a form of tolerance that can be defined as a reduction in drug responsiveness brought on by repeated dosing *over a short time*. Hence, unlike pharmacodynamic and metabolic tolerance, which take days or longer to develop, tachyphylaxis occurs quickly. Tachyphylaxis is not a common mechanism of drug tolerance.

Transdermal nitroglycerin provides a good example of tachyphylaxis. When nitroglycerin is administered using a transdermal patch, effects are lost in less than 24 hours (if the patch is left in place around the clock). As discussed in Chapter 49, the loss of effect results from depletion of a co-factor required for nitroglycerin to act. When nitroglycerin is administered on an intermittent schedule, rather than continuously, the co-factor can be replenished and no loss of effect occurs.

PLACEBO EFFECT

A *placebo* is a preparation that is devoid of intrinsic pharmacologic activity. Hence, any response that a patient may have to a placebo is based solely on his or her psychologic reaction to the idea of taking a medication and not to any direct physiologic or biochemical action of the placebo itself. The primary use of the placebo is as a control preparation during clinical trials.

In pharmacology, the *placebo effect* is defined as that component of a drug response that is caused by psychologic factors and not by the biochemical or physiologic properties of the drug. Although it is impossible to assess with precision the contribution that psychologic factors make to the overall response to any particular drug, it is widely believed that, with practically all medications, some fraction of the total response results from a placebo effect. Although placebo effects are determined by psychologic factors and not physiologic ones, the presence of a placebo response does not imply that a patient's original pathology was "all in the head."

Not all placebo responses are beneficial; placebo responses can also be negative. If a patient believes that a medication is going to be effective, then placebo responses are likely to help pro-

TABLE 8–1 ▪▪ Development of Metabolic Tolerance as a Result of Repeated Pentobarbital Administration		
	Type of Pretreatment	
Results	**None**	**Pentobarbital**
Sleeping time (minutes)	67 ± 4	30 ± 7
Pentobarbital half-life in plasma (minutes)	79 ± 3	26 ± 2
Plasma level of pentobarbital upon awakening (μg/ml)	9.9 ± 1.4	7.9 ± 0.6

Data from Remmer H. Drugs as activators of drug enzymes. In Brodie BB, Erdos EG (eds). Metabolic Factors Controlling Duration of Drug Action (Proceedings of First International Pharmacological Meeting, Vol 6). New York, Macmillan, 1962:235. (See text for details.)

Special Interest Topic

BOX 8-1 ■ HAS THE PLACEBO LOST ITS EFFECT?

In 1955, H. K. Beecher wrote his famous paper—"The Powerful Placebo"[1]—which was heralded as solid proof for the long-held (but largely unsubstantiated) belief that placebos can effectively relieve symptoms in many patients. This widely cited paper had gone unchallenged until 2001, when two Danish scientists—Hróbjartsson and Gøtzsche—wrote their own paper on the subject, titled "Is the Placebo Powerless?"[2] From their research, the Danes concluded that, at least in the context of clinical trials, placebo treatment has little or no measurable effect. Who's right? Let's consider both papers and see if we can decide.

Beecher analyzed the data from 15 placebo-controlled clinical trials. In all of these trials, patients in the placebo groups were evaluated at baseline, treated with placebo for a prescribed time, and then re-evaluated. Beecher then looked to see if improvement took place between baseline and the end of the treatment period. Based on his analysis, he concluded "It is evident that placebos have a high degree of effectiveness, decided improvement...being produced in 35.2% of cases." Pretty impressive. Unfortunately, there's a flaw: How do we know the placebos produced the benefits? Perhaps 35.2% of the patients would have improved with no treatment, owing simply to the natural course of their disease or to other factors. After all, many people *do* get better on their own—without doctors, drugs, placebos, or anything else. Furthermore, although Beecher claims to have selected the 15 papers at random, this seems improbable in that 7 of them were his own.

To address questions left open by Beecher, Hróbjartsson and Gøtzsche took a different approach. First, they analyzed data from 114 published trials—not just 15. More than 8500 patients were involved. More importantly, in all of these trials, placebo treatment was compared with *no treatment*. That is, in each trial, some subjects received placebo treatment and some received no treatment. (Of course, in most [112] of the trials, there was a third group of subjects who received an active treatment.) The trials involved 40 clinical conditions, including anemia, asthma, hypertension, hyperglycemia, epilepsy, Parkinson's disease, schizophrenia, depression, smoking, and pain. In 38 of the trials, the measured outcomes were *objective* (e.g., reduction in blood pressure, increase in red blood cell count), and in 76 the outcomes were *subjective* (e.g., improvement in mood, reduction of pain). Of the 114 trials, 45 evaluated pharmacologic interventions, 26 evaluated physical interventions, and 43 evaluated psychologic interventions. The type of placebo employed was matched to the active treatment: for the pharmacologic studies, typical placebo treatment consisted of giving a lactose pill; for the physical studies (e.g., evaluating the effect of transcutaneous electrical nerve stimulation on pain), typical placebo treatment consisted of performing the procedure but with the equipment turned off; and for the psychologic studies (e.g., evaluating the effect of psychotherapy on depression), typical placebo treatment

consisted of nondirectional, neutral discussion between the patient and the treatment provider.

What did the analysis reveal? In trials with *objective* outcomes, placebo treatment had *virtually no measurable effect:* outcomes in patients receiving placebo treatment were identical to those in patients receiving no treatment at all. However, in some trials with *subjective* outcomes, placebo treatment *did* have a convincing effect—but it was small, and limited primarily to studies of *pain.* In their conclusion, the authors stated, "We found little evidence that placebos in general have powerful clinical effects," although they go on to say they did find "significant effects of placebo...for the treatment of pain." In addition, they concede that their analysis does "leave open the question of whether placebo effects in clinical practice might differ from placebo effects among research subjects."

Is this the end of the story? Is the placebo effect really just a myth? Well, we really can't say. Yes, the Danish study (which was far superior to Beecher's) failed to reveal a powerful effect of placebo treatment. However, this does not prove there is no placebo effect. Rather, it may simply indicate that we can't readily measure a placebo effect in clinical trials. There are some good arguments supporting this possibility:

- If the placebo response is based primarily on the clinician-patient relationship, then, even if there is a placebo response, it would be invisible in clinical trials—because subjects who receive placebo treatment and those who receive no treatment all share the same relationship with the clinician.
- Placebo responses (assuming they exist) are based on the patient's strong belief that he or she is getting an effective treatment. However, in clinical trials, there is always *doubt*—because all participants are aware that they may be getting a placebo, rather than the real deal. In the presence of significant doubt, the placebo effect may be greatly diminished. If this is true, then placebo effects would not be expected in clinical trials.
- If placebo effects exist only in real practice—and not in clinical trials—then proving their existence may well be impossible. Why? Because we'd have to do a clinical trial to prove they exist—and we already know we can't see them in clinical trials.

What's the bottom line? First, owing to a major weakness in design, Beecher's study does not constitute proof that placebos have beneficial effects. Second, by using a more appropriate design, Hróbjartsson and Gøtzsche have shown clearly that, in the context of clinical trials, placebo interventions are largely devoid of measurable effects—with the exception of producing modest reductions in pain. Third, although Hróbjartsson and Gøtzsche failed to see a placebo effect, their study does not rule out the possibility that, in the real world, placebo treatments can indeed be beneficial. However, this is yet to be proved—and possibly never will be.

[1] Beecher HK. The powerful placebo. JAMA 1955;159;1602–1606.

[2] Hróbjartsson A, Gøtzsche PC. Is the placebo powerless? An analysis of clinical trials comparing placebo with no treatment. N Engl J Med 2001; 344:1594–1602.

mote recovery. Conversely, if a patient is convinced that a particular medication is ineffective or perhaps even harmful, then placebo effects are likely to detract from his or her progress.

Because the placebo effect depends on the patient's attitude toward medicine, fostering a positive attitude may help promote beneficial effects. In this regard, it is desirable that all members of the healthcare team present the patient with an optimistic (but realistic) assessment of the effects that therapy is likely to produce. It is also important that members of the team be consistent with one another; the beneficial placebo responses may well be decreased if, for example, nurses on the day shift repeatedly reassure a patient about the likely benefits of his or her regimen, while nurses on the night shift express pessimism about those same drugs.

Until recently, the power of the placebo effect was unquestioned by most clinicians and researchers. However, new evidence suggests that responses to placebos may be much smaller than previously believed (see Box 8–1).

GENETICS

A patient's unique genetic makeup can lead to drug responses that are qualitatively and quantitatively different from those of the population at large. Unique drug responses based on genetic heritage are often referred to as *idiosyncratic effects* (see Chapter 7).

The most common mechanism by which genetic differences modify drug responses is through altered drug metabolism. Gene-based variations can increase or decrease metabolism of certain drugs. Some people, for example, have a genetically determined insufficiency in the ability to metabolize succinylcholine (a muscle relaxant). Hence, if succinylcholine is administered to these people, muscle relaxation is prolonged. Other drugs whose rate of metabolism is genetically determined include isoniazid (a drug for tuberculosis) and tolbutamide (a drug for diabetes). If genetically determined abnormalities in rates of drug metabolism are not too great, they can be compensated for by adjustments in dosage. However, when the alteration in metabolic rate is extremely large, as it is with succinylcholine, then the drug should not be administered.

Some genetically determined drug responses are based on factors other than altered metabolism. For example, some individuals have red blood cells that are deficient in an enzyme called glucose-6-phosphate dehydrogenase. This deficiency puts them at risk of hemolysis (red blood cell destruction) if given certain drugs, including aspirin, sulfanilamide (an antibiotic), and primaquine (an antimalarial agent). About 10% of African American males and many Near Eastern and Mediterranean males are subject to this idiosyncratic reaction. Additional examples of genetically based drug responses include the following:

- Approximately 1 in 14 Caucasians lacks the enzyme needed to convert codeine into morphine, its active form. As a result, codeine cannot relieve pain in these people.
- Trastuzumab [Herceptin], a drug for breast cancer, only works against tumors that overexpress the HER2 protein.
- Tamoxifen [Nolvadex] can reduce the risk of breast cancer in women at high risk—but only in women with mutations in the BRCA2 gene, not in the BRCA1 gene.

VARIABILITY IN ABSORPTION

Both the rate and extent of drug absorption can vary among patients. As a result, both the timing and intensity of responses can be changed. Differences in manufacturing are a major cause of variability in drug absorption. Other causes include the presence or absence of food, diarrhea or constipation, and differences in gastric emptying time. Several causes of variable absorption are discussed in previous chapters, primarily Chapter 4 (Pharmacokinetics) and Chapter 6 (Drug Interactions), and hence their discussion here is brief.

Bioavailability

The term *bioavailability* refers to the ability of a drug to reach the systemic circulation from its site of administration. Different preparations of the same drug can vary in bioavailability. As discussed in Chapter 4, such factors as tablet disintegration time, enteric coatings, and sustained-release formulations can alter bioavailability, and can thereby make drug responses variable.

Differences in bioavailability occur primarily with oral preparations and not with parenteral preparations. Fortunately, even with oral agents, when differences in bioavailability do exist between preparations, those differences are usually so small as to lack clinical significance.

Differences in bioavailability are of greatest concern for drugs with a narrow therapeutic range. When the therapeutic range is narrow, a relatively small change in drug level can produce a significant change in response: A small decline in drug level may cause therapeutic failure, whereas a small increase in drug level may cause toxicity. Under these conditions, differences in bioavailability could have a significant impact.

Other Causes of Variable Absorption

Several factors in addition to bioavailability can alter drug absorption, and thereby lead to variations in drug responses. Alterations in gastric pH can affect absorption through the pH partitioning effect. For drugs that undergo absorption in the intestine, absorption will be delayed when gastric emptying time is prolonged. Diarrhea can reduce absorption by accelerating transport of drugs through the intestine. Conversely, constipation can enhance absorption by prolonging the time available for absorption. The presence of food in the stomach tends to *delay* absorption of most drugs; in some cases, food can decrease the *extent* of absorption as well. For example, absorption of tetracycline will be reduced substantially if this drug is ingested together with milk (and other dairy products that contain calcium). Lastly, there are multiple mechanisms by which drug interactions can decrease or increase absorption (see Chapter 6).

FAILURE TO TAKE MEDICINE AS PRESCRIBED

Medications are not always administered as prescribed: dosage size and timing may be altered, doses may be omitted, and extra doses may be taken. Failure to administer medication as prescribed is a common explanation for variability in the response to a prescribed dose. As a rule, such failure results from either poor patient compliance or medication errors made by hospital staff.

Patient compliance (adherence) can be defined as cooperative and accurate participation in one's own drug therapy. Multiple factors can influence compliance. These include manual dexterity, visual acuity, intellectual capacity, psychologic state, attitude toward drugs, and the ability to pay for medication.

Patient education is an important means of promoting compliance. Instruction must be convincing and clear. In most cases, it is the responsibility of the nurse to provide instruction. By promoting compliance, you can contribute greatly to reducing variability.

Medication errors are an obvious source of individual variation. Medication errors can originate with physicians, nurses, technicians, and pharmacists. However, since the nurse is usually the last member of the healthcare team to check medications prior to administration, it is ultimately the nurse's responsibility to ensure that medication errors are avoided.

DRUG INTERACTIONS

A drug interaction is a process in which one drug alters the effects of another. Drug interactions can be an important source of variability in responses. The mechanisms by which one drug can alter the effects of another and the clinical consequences of drug interactions are discussed at length in Chapter 6.

DIET

Diet can affect responses to drugs, primarily by affecting the patient's general health status. A diet that promotes good health can enable drugs to elicit therapeutic responses and increase the patient's capacity to tolerate adverse effects. Poor nutrition can have the opposite effect.

Starvation can affect responses by reducing protein binding. Starvation causes plasma levels of albumin to fall. As a result, binding of drugs to albumin declines, causing levels of free drug to rise, which in turn causes drug responses to become more intense. For certain drugs (e.g., warfarin, an anticoagulant), the resultant increase in effects could be disastrous.

Although nutrition can affect drug responses by the general mechanisms noted, there are only a few examples of a specific nutritional factor affecting the response to a specific drug. Perhaps the best illustration of the impact of diet on drug responses involves the monoamine oxidase (MAO) inhibitors—drugs used for depression. The most serious adverse effect of these drugs is malignant hypertension, a reaction that can be triggered by foods that contain tyramine, a breakdown product of the amino acid tyrosine. Accordingly, patients taking MAO inhibitors must rigidly avoid all tyramine-rich foods (e.g., beef liver, ripe cheeses, yeast products, Chianti wine). The interaction of tyramine-containing foods with MAO inhibitors is discussed at length in Chapter 31.

⸫ KEY POINTS

- In order to maximize beneficial drug responses and minimize harm, we must adjust therapy to account for sources of individual variation.
- As a rule, small patients need smaller doses than large patients.
- Dosage adjustments made to account for size are often based on body surface area, rather than simply on body weight.
- Infants and the elderly are more sensitive to drugs than are older children and younger adults.
- Therapeutic and adverse effects of drugs may differ between males and females. Unfortunately, for most drugs, there are insufficient data to predict what the differences might be.
- Kidney disease can decrease drug excretion, thereby causing drug levels to rise. To prevent toxicity, drugs that are eliminated by the kidneys should be given in reduced dosage.
- Liver disease can decrease drug metabolism, thereby causing levels to rise. To prevent toxicity, drugs that are eliminated by the liver should be given in reduced dosage.
- When a patient becomes tolerant to a drug, the dosage must be increased to maintain beneficial effects.
- Pharmacodynamic tolerance results from adaptive changes that occur in response to prolonged drug exposure. Pharmacodynamic tolerance increases the MEC of a drug.
- Pharmacokinetic tolerance results from accelerated drug metabolism. Pharmacokinetic tolerance does not change the MEC.
- A placebo effect is defined as the component of a drug response that can be attributed to psychologic factors, rather than to direct physiologic or biochemical actions of the drug. Solid proof that placebo effects are real is lacking.
- Genetic factors—especially genetically determined rates of drug metabolism—can be a source of individual variation.
- Bioavailability refers to the ability of a drug to reach the systemic circulation from its site of administration.
- Differences in bioavailability matter most for drugs that have a narrow therapeutic range.
- Poor patient compliance is a major source of individual variation.

Drug Therapy During Pregnancy and Breast-Feeding

Our topic for this chapter is drug therapy in women who are pregnant or breast-feeding. The clinical challenge is to provide effective treatment for the mother while avoiding harm to the fetus or nursing infant. Unfortunately, meeting this challenge is confounded by a shortage of reliable data on toxicity from drug use during pregnancy or breast-feeding.

DRUG THERAPY DURING PREGNANCY: BASIC CONSIDERATIONS

Drug use during pregnancy is common: Between one-half and two-thirds of pregnant women take at least one medication, and the majority take more. Some drugs are used to treat pregnancy-related conditions, such as nausea, constipation, and pre-eclampsia. Some are used to treat chronic disorders, such as hypertension, diabetes, and epilepsy. And some are used for infectious diseases or cancer. In addition to taking these therapeutic agents, pregnant women frequently take drugs of abuse, such as alcohol, cocaine, and heroin.

Drug therapy in pregnancy presents a vexing dilemma. In pregnant patients, as in all other patients, the benefits of treatment must balance the risks. Of course, when drugs are used during pregnancy, risks apply to the fetus as well as the mother. Unfortunately, the risks for most drugs used in pregnancy have not been determined—hence the dilemma: The clinician is obliged to balance risks versus benefits, without knowing what the risks really are. The reasons that underlie our lack of knowledge are discussed below under *Identification of Teratogens*.

Despite the imposing challenge of balancing risks versus benefits, drug therapy during pregnancy cannot and should not be avoided. The health of the fetus depends on the health of the mother. Hence, conditions that threaten the mother's health must be addressed—for the sake of the baby as well as the mother. Chronic asthma provides a good example. Uncontrolled maternal asthma is far more dangerous to the fetus than the drugs used to treat it. Among asthmatic women who fail to take medication, the incidence of stillbirth is doubled. If all women with asthma took medication, an estimated 2000 babies would be saved each year.

Physiologic Changes During Pregnancy and Their Impact on Drug Disposition and Dosing

Pregnancy brings on physiologic changes that can alter drug disposition. Changes in the kidney, liver, and GI tract are of particular interest. Because of these changes, a compensatory change in dosage may be needed.

By the third trimester, renal blood flow is doubled, causing a large increase in glomerular filtration rate. As a result, there is accelerated clearance of drugs that are eliminated by glomerular filtration. Elimination of lithium, for example, is increased by 100%. To compensate for accelerated excretion, dosage must be increased.

For some drugs, hepatic metabolism increases during pregnancy. Three anticonvulsants—phenytoin, carbamazepine, and valproic acid—provide examples.

Tone and motility of the bowel decrease in pregnancy, causing intestinal transit time to increase. Because of prolonged transit, there is more time for drugs to be absorbed. In theory, this could increase levels of drugs whose absorption is normally poor. Similarly, there is more time for reabsorption of drugs that undergo enterohepatic recirculation; hence, effects of these drugs could be prolonged. In both cases, a reduction in dosage might be needed.

Placental Drug Transfer

Essentially all drugs can cross the placenta, although some cross more readily than others. The factors that determine drug passage across the membranes of the placenta are the same factors that determine drug passage across all other membranes. Accordingly, drugs that are lipid soluble cross the placenta easily, whereas drugs that are ionized, highly polar, or protein bound cross with difficulty. Nonetheless, for practical purposes, the clinician should assume that *any drug taken during pregnancy will reach the fetus.*

Adverse Reactions During Pregnancy

Drugs taken during pregnancy can adversely affect both the mother and fetus. The effect of greatest concern is *teratogenesis* (production of birth defects). This issue is discussed separately below. Not only are pregnant women subject to the same adverse effects as everyone else, they may also suffer effects unique to pregnancy. For example, when heparin (an anticoagulant) is taken by pregnant women, it can cause osteoporosis, which in turn can cause compression fractures of the spine. Use of prostaglandins (e.g., misoprostol), which stimulate uterine contraction, can cause abortion. Conversely, use of aspirin near term can suppress contractions in labor. In addition, aspirin increases the risk of serious bleeding.

Regular use of dependence-producing drugs (e.g., heroin, barbiturates, alcohol) during pregnancy can result in the birth of a drug-dependent infant. If the infant is not supplied with a drug that can support its dependence, a withdrawal syndrome will ensue. Symptoms include shrill crying, vomiting, and extreme irritability. The neonate should be weaned from dependence by giving progressively smaller doses of the drug on which he or she is dependent.

Certain pain relievers used during delivery can depress respiration in the neonate. The infant should be closely monitored until respiration becomes normal.

DRUG THERAPY DURING PREGNANCY: TERATOGENESIS

The term *teratogenesis* is derived from *teras,* the Greek word for monster. Translated literally, teratogenesis means *to produce a monster.* Consistent with this derivation, we usually think of birth defects in terms of gross malformations, such as cleft palate, clubfoot, and hydrocephalus. However, birth defects are not limited to distortions of gross anatomy; they also include behavioral and biochemical anomalies.

Incidence and Causes of Congenital Anomalies

The incidence of *major* structural abnormalities (e.g., abnormalities that are life threatening or require surgical correction) is about 6%. Half of these are obvious and are reported at birth. The other half involve internal organs (e.g., heart, liver, GI tract) and are not discovered until later in life or at autopsy. The incidence of minor structural abnormalities is unknown, as is the incidence of functional abnormalities (e.g., growth retardation, mental retardation).

Congenital anomalies have multiple causes, including genetic heritage, environmental chemicals, and drugs. Genetic factors account for about 25% of all birth defects. Of the genetically based anomalies, Down's syndrome is the most common. Only 3% of all birth defects are caused by drugs. For the majority of congenital anomalies, the cause is unknown.

Teratogenesis and Stage of Development

Fetal sensitivity to teratogens changes during development; hence, the effect of a teratogen is highly dependent upon when the drug is given. As shown in Figure 9–1, development occurs in three major stages: the *preimplantation/presomite period* (conception through week 2), the *embryonic period* (weeks 3 through 8), and the *fetal period* (week 9 through term). During the preimplantation/presomite period, teratogens act in an "all or nothing" fashion. That is, if the dose is sufficiently high, the result is death of the conceptus. Conversely, if the dose is sublethal, the conceptus is likely to recover fully.

Gross malformations are produced by exposure to teratogens during the *embryonic period* (roughly the first trimester). This is the time when the basic shape of internal organs and other structures is being established. Hence, it is not surprising that interference at this stage results in conspicuous anatomic distortions. Because the fetus is especially vulnerable during the embryonic period, expectant mothers must take special care to avoid exposure to teratogens during this time.

Teratogen exposure during the *fetal period* (i.e., the second and third trimesters) usually disrupts *function* rather than gross anatomy. Of the developmental processes that occur in the fetal period, growth and development of the brain are especially important. Disruption of brain development can result in learning deficits and behavioral abnormalities.

Identification of Teratogens

For the following reasons, human teratogens are extremely difficult to identify:

- The incidence of congenital anomalies is generally low.
- Animal tests may not be applicable.
- Prolonged exposure may be required.
- Teratogenic effects may be delayed.
- Behavioral effects are difficult to document.
- Controlled experiments can't be done in humans.

As a result, only a few drugs are considered *proven* teratogens. Drugs whose teratogenicity has been documented (or at least highly suspected) are listed in Table 9–1. It is important to note, however, that *lack of proof of teratogenicity does not mean that a drug is safe;* it only means that the available information is insufficient to make a definitive judgment. Conversely, *proof of teratogenicity does not mean that every exposure will result in a birth defect.* In fact, with most teratogens, the risk of malformation following exposure is only about 10%.

To prove that a drug is a teratogen, three criteria must be met:

- The drug must cause a characteristic set of malformations.
- It must act only during a specific window of vulnerability (e.g., weeks 4 through 7 of gestation).
- The incidence of malformations should increase with increasing dosage and duration of exposure.

Obviously, we can't do experiments in humans to see if a drug meets these criteria. The best we can do is systematically collect and analyze data on drugs taken dur-

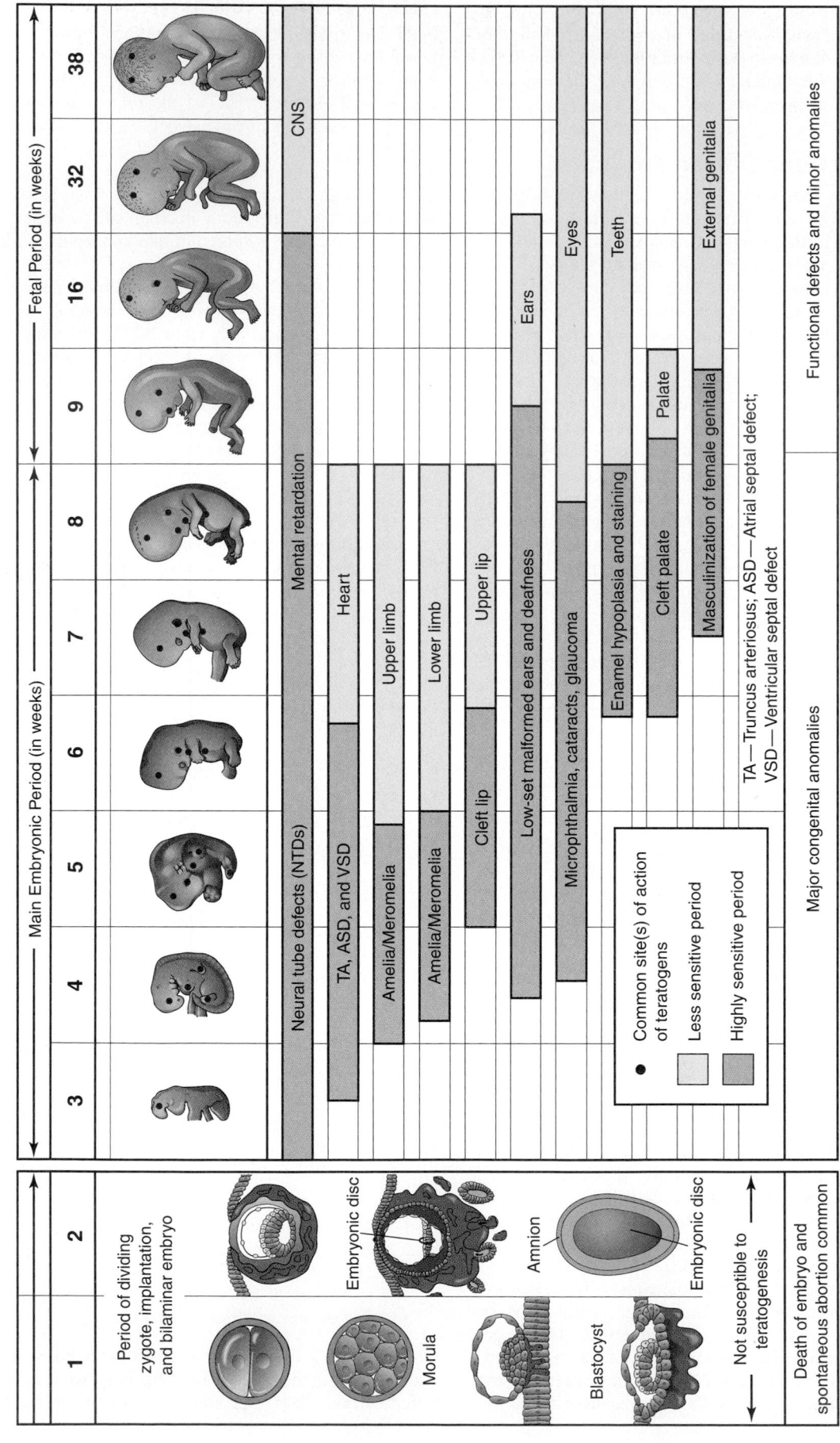

Figure 9–1 ■ Effects of teratogens at various stages of development of the fetus. (From Moore KL. The Developing Human: Clinically Oriented Embryology, 5th ed. Philadelphia, WB Saunders Company, 1993, with permission.)

TABLE 9–1 ■ Drugs That Should Be Avoided During Pregnancy Because of Proven or Strongly Suspected Teratogenicity*	
Drug	**Teratogenic Effect**
Anticancer/Immunosuppressant Drugs	
Cyclophosphamide	CNS malformation, secondary cancer
Methotrexate	CNS and limb malformations
Antiseizure Drugs	
Carbamazepine	Neural tube defects
Valproic acid	Neural tube defects
Phenytoin	Growth retardation, CNS defects
Sex Hormones	
Androgens (e.g., danazol)	Masculinization of the female fetus
Diethylstilbestrol	Vaginal carcinoma in female offspring
Other Drugs	
	Fetal alcohol syndrome, stillbirth, spontaneous abortion, low birth weight, mental retardation
Angiotensin-converting enzyme inhibitors	Renal failure, renal tubular dysgenesis, skull hypoplasia (from exposure during the second and third trimesters)
Antithyroid drugs (propylthiouracil, methimazole)	Goiter and hypothyroidism
Nonsteroidal anti-inflammatory drugs	Premature closure of the ductus arteriosus
Lithium	Ebstein's anomaly (cardiac defects)
Sulfonylurea or oral hypoglycemic drugs (e.g., tolbutamide)	Neonatal hypoglycemia
Vitamin A derivatives (isotretinoin, etretinate, megadoses of vitamin A)	Multiple defects (CNS, craniofacial, cardiovascular, others)
Tetracycline	Tooth and bone anomalies
Thalidomide	Shortened limbs, internal organ defects
Warfarin	Skeletal and CNS defects

CNS = central nervous system.
*The absence of a drug from this table does not mean that the drug is not a teratogen; it only means that teratogenicity has not been proved. For most proven teratogens, the risk of a congenital anomaly is only 10%.

ing pregnancy in the hope that useful information on teratogenicity will be revealed.

Studies in animals may be of limited value, in part because teratogenicity may depend on species. That is, drugs that are teratogens in laboratory animals may nonetheless be safe in humans. Conversely, and more importantly, drugs that fail to cause anomalies in animals may later prove teratogenic in humans. The most notorious example is thalidomide. In studies with pregnant animals, thalidomide was harmless. However, when thalidomide was taken by pregnant women, about 30% had babies with severe malformations. The take-home message is this: *Lack of teratogenicity in animals is not proof of safety in humans.* Accordingly, we cannot assume that a new drug is safe for use in human pregnancy just because it has met Food and Drug Administration (FDA) requirements, which are based on tests done in pregnant animals.

Some teratogens act quickly, whereas others require prolonged exposure. Thalidomide represents a fast-acting teratogen; a single dose can cause malformation. In contrast, alcohol (ethanol) must be taken repeatedly in high doses if gross malformation is to result. (Lower doses of alcohol may produce subtle anomalies.) Because a single exposure to a rapid-acting teratogen can produce obvious malformation, rapid-acting teratogens are easier to identify than slow-acting teratogens.

Teratogens that produce delayed effects are among the hardest to identify. The best example is diethylstilbestrol, an estrogenic substance that causes vaginal cancer in female offspring 18 or so years after birth.

Teratogens that affect behavior may be nearly impossible to identify. Behavioral changes are often delayed, and therefore may not become apparent until the child goes to school. By this time, it may be difficult to establish a correlation between drug use during pregnancy and the behavioral deficit. Furthermore, if the deficit is subtle, it may not even be recognized.

FDA Pregnancy Risk Categories

In 1983, the FDA established a system for classifying drugs according to their probable risks to the fetus. According to this system, drugs can be put into one of five categories: A, B, C, D, and X (Table 9–2). Drugs in Risk Category A are the least dangerous; controlled studies have been done in pregnant women and have failed to demonstrate a risk of fetal harm. In contrast, drugs in Category X are the most dangerous; these drugs are known to cause human fetal harm, and their risk to the fetus outweighs any possible therapeutic benefit. Drugs in Categories B, C, and D are progressively more dangerous than drugs in Category A and less dangerous than drugs in Category X. The law does not

TABLE 9–2 ■ FDA Pregnancy Risk Categories

Category	Category Description
A	*Remote Risk of Fetal Harm:* Controlled studies in women have been done and have failed to demonstrate a risk of fetal harm during the first trimester, and there is no evidence of risk in later trimesters.
B	*Slightly More Risk Than A:* Animal studies show no fetal risk, but controlled studies have not been done in women *or* animal studies do show a risk of fetal harm, but controlled studies in women have failed to demonstrate a risk during the first trimester, and there is no evidence of risk in later trimesters.
C	*Greater Risk Than B:* Animal studies show a risk of fetal harm, but no controlled studies have been done in women *or* no studies have been done in women or animals.
D	*Proven Risk of Fetal Harm:* Studies in women show proof of fetal damage, but the potential benefits of use during pregnancy may be acceptable despite the risks (e.g., treatment of life-threatening disease for which safer drugs are ineffective). A statement on risk will appear in the "WARNINGS" section of drug labeling.
X	*Proven Risk of Fetal Harm:* Studies in women or animals show definite risk of fetal abnormality *or* adverse reaction reports indicate evidence of fetal risk. The risks clearly outweigh any possible benefit. A statement on risk will appear in the "CONTRAINDICATIONS" section of drug labeling.

TABLE 9–3 ■ Drugs That Are Contraindicated During Breast-Feeding

Controlled Substances
Amphetamine
Cocaine
Heroin
Marijuana
Phencyclidine

Anticancer Agents/Immunosuppressants
Cyclophosphamide
Cyclosporine
Doxorubicin
Methotrexate

Others
Bromocriptine
Ergotamine
Lithium
Nicotine

require classification of drugs that were in use before 1983; hence many drugs are not classified.

Minimizing the Risk of Teratogenesis

Common sense tells us that the best way to minimize teratogenesis is to minimize use of drugs. If possible, pregnant women should avoid drugs entirely. At the least, all *unnecessary* drug use should be eliminated. Alcohol and cocaine, for example, which are known to harm the developing fetus, have no valid indications and their use cannot be justified. Nurses and other health professionals should warn pregnant women against use of all nonessential drugs.

As noted above, some disease states (e.g., epilepsy, asthma, diabetes) pose a greater risk to fetal health than do the drugs used for treatment. However, even with these disorders, in which drug therapy reduces the risk of disease-induced fetal harm, we must still take steps to minimize harm from drugs. Accordingly, drugs that pose a high risk of teratogenesis should be discontinued and safer alternatives substituted.

Rarely, a pregnant woman has a disease that requires use of drugs that have a high probability of causing teratogenesis. Some anticancer drugs, for example, are highly toxic to the developing fetus, yet cannot be ethically withheld from the pregnant patient. If a woman elects to use such drugs, termination of pregnancy should be considered.

Reducing the risk of teratogenesis also applies to female patients who are *not* pregnant but are taking teratogenic drugs. If they are of reproductive age, they should be educated about the teratogenic risk as well as the necessity of using at least one reliable form of birth control.

Responding to Teratogen Exposure

When a pregnant woman has been exposed to a known teratogen, the first step is to determine exactly when the drug was taken, and exactly when the pregnancy began. If drug exposure was not during the period of organogenesis (i.e., weeks 3 through 8), the patient should be reassured that the risk of drug-induced malformation is minimal. In addition, she should be reminded that 3% of all babies have some kind of conspicuous malformation, independent of teratogen exposure. This is important because otherwise the drug is sure to be blamed if the baby is abnormal.

What should be done if the exposure *did* occur during organogenesis? First, a reference (e.g., Briggs GG, Freeman RK, Yaffe SJ. *Drugs in Pregnancy and Lactation.* Philadelphia, JB Lippincott, 2002) should be consulted to determine the type of malformation expected. Next, at least two ultrasound scans should be done to assess the extent of injury. If the malformation is severe, termination of pregnancy should be considered. If the malformation is minor (e.g., cleft palate), it may be correctable by surgery, either shortly after birth or later in childhood.

DRUG THERAPY DURING BREAST-FEEDING

Drugs taken by lactating women can be excreted in breast milk. If drug concentrations in milk are high enough, a pharmacologic effect can occur in the infant, raising the question of possible harm. Unfortunately, there has been very little systematic research done on this issue. As a result, although a few drugs are known to be hazardous (Table 9–3), the possible danger posed by many others remains undetermined.

TABLE 9–4 ■ Drugs of Choice for Breast-Feeding Women*

Drug Category	Drugs and Drug Groups of Choice	Comments
Analgesic drugs	Acetaminophen, ibuprofen, flurbiprofen, ketorolac, mefenamic acid, sumatriptan, morphine	Sumatriptan may be given for migraine. Morphine may be given for severe pain.
Anticoagulant drugs	Warfarin, acenocoumarol, heparin (unfractionated and low molecular weight)	Among breast-fed infants whose mothers were taking warfarin, the drug was undetectable in plasma and bleeding time was not affected.
Antidepressant drugs	Sertraline, tricyclic antidepressants	Other antidepressants, such as fluoxetine [Prozac], may be given with caution.
Antiepileptic drugs	Carbamazepine, phenytoin, valproic acid	The estimated level of exposure to these drugs in infants is less than 10% of the therapeutic dose standardized by weight.
Antihistamines (histamine₁ blockers)	Loratadine	Other antihistamines may be given, but data on the concentrations of these drugs in breast milk are lacking.
Antimicrobial drugs	Penicillins, cephalosporins, aminoglycosides, macrolides	Avoid chloramphenicol and tetracycline.
Beta-adrenergic antagonists	Labetalol, propranolol	Angiotensin-converting enzyme inhibitors and calcium channel–blocking agents are also considered safe.
Endocrine drugs	Propylthiouracil, insulin, levothyroxine	The estimated level of exposure to propylthiouracil in breast-feeding infants is less than 1% of the therapeutic dose standardized by weight; thyroid function of the infants is not affected.
Glucocorticoids	Prednisolone and prednisone	The amount of prednisolone the infant would ingest in breast milk is less than 0.1% of the therapeutic dose standardized by weight.

*This list is not exhaustive. Cases of overdoses of these drugs must be assessed on an individual basis.
Adapted from Shinya I. Drug therapy for breast-feeding women. N Engl J Med 2000;343:118–126.

Although nearly all drugs can enter breast milk, the extent of entry varies greatly. The factors that determine entry into breast milk are the same factors that determine passage of drugs across membranes. Accordingly, drugs that are lipid soluble enter breast milk readily, whereas drugs that are ionized, highly polar, or protein bound tend to be excluded.

Most drugs can be detected in milk, but concentrations are generally too low to be harmful. Hence, breast-feeding is usually safe, even though drugs are being taken. Nonetheless, prudence is always in order: If the nursing mother can avoid drugs, she certainly should. Moreover, when drugs *must* be used, steps should taken to minimize risk. These include

- Dosing immediately *after* breast-feeding (to minimize drug concentrations in milk at the next feeding)
- Avoiding drugs that have a long half-life
- Choosing drugs that tend to be excluded from milk
- Choosing drugs that are least likely to affect the infant (Table 9–4).
- Avoiding drugs that are known to be hazardous (see Table 9–3).

⁙ KEY POINTS

- Because hepatic metabolism and glomerular filtration increase during pregnancy, dosages of some drugs may need to be increased.
- Lipid-soluble drugs cross the placenta readily, whereas drugs that are ionized, polar, or protein bound cross with difficulty. Nonetheless, all drugs cross to some extent.
- When prescribing drugs during pregnancy, the clinician must try to balance the benefits of treatment versus the risks—often without knowing what the risks really are.
- About 6% of all babies are born with gross structural malformations.
- Only 3% of birth defects are caused by drugs.
- Teratogen-induced gross malformations result from exposure early in pregnancy (weeks 3 through 8 of gestation)—the time of organogenesis.
- Functional impairments (e.g., mental retardation) result from exposure to teratogens later in pregnancy.
- For most drugs, we lack reliable data on the risks of use during pregnancy.
- Lack of teratogenicity in animals is not proof of safety in humans.
- Some drugs (e.g., thalidomide) cause birth defects with just one dose, whereas others (e.g., alcohol) require prolonged exposure.
- FDA Pregnancy Risk Categories indicate the relative risks of drug use. Drugs in Category X pose the highest risk of fetal harm and are contraindicated during pregnancy.

■ Any woman of reproductive age who is taking a known teratogen must be counseled about the teratogenic risk and the necessity of using at least one reliable form of birth control.

■ Drugs that are lipid soluble readily enter breast milk, whereas drugs that are ionized, polar, or protein bound tend to be excluded. Nonetheless, all drugs enter to some extent.

■ Although most drugs can be detected in breast milk, concentrations are usually too low to harm the nursing infant.

■ If possible, drugs should be avoided during breast-feeding.

■ If drugs cannot be avoided during breast-feeding, common sense dictates choosing drugs known to be safe (Table 9–4) and avoiding drugs known to be dangerous (Table 9–3).

Drug Therapy in Pediatric Patients

Patients who are very young or very old respond differently to drugs than does the rest of the population. Most differences are *quantitative*. That is, patients in both age groups are more sensitive to drugs than other patients, and they show greater individual variation. Drug sensitivity in the very young results largely from *organ system immaturity*. Drug sensitivity in the elderly results largely from *organ system degeneration*. Because of heightened drug sensitivity, patients in both age groups are at increased risk of adverse drug reactions. In this chapter we discuss the physiologic factors that underlie heightened drug sensitivity in pediatric patients, as well as ways to promote safe and effective drug use. Drug therapy in geriatric patients is the topic of Chapter 11.

Pediatrics covers all patients under the age of 16. Because of ongoing growth and development, pediatric patients in different age groups present different therapeutic challenges. Traditionally, the pediatric population is subdivided into six groups:

- Premature infants (less than 36 weeks' gestational age)
- Full-term infants (36 to 40 weeks' gestational age)
- Neonates (first 4 postnatal weeks)
- Infants (weeks 5 to 52 postnatal)
- Children (1 to 12 years)
- Adolescents (12 to 16 years)

Not surprisingly, as young patients grow older, they become more like adults physiologically, and hence more like adults with regard to drug therapy. Conversely, the very young—those less than 1 year old, and especially those less than 1 month old—are very different from adults. If drug therapy in these patients is to be safe and effective, we must account for these differences.

Pediatric drug therapy is made even more difficult by insufficient drug information. Until recently, the Food and Drug Administration (FDA) did not require drug trials in children.* As a result, for many drugs given to young patients, we lack good information on dosing, pharmacokinetics, and effects, both therapeutic and adverse. Despite lack of good information, the clinician must nonetheless use drugs to treat pediatric patients. Hence, similar to drug therapy during pregnancy, the clinician must try to balance benefits versus risks, without knowing with precision what the benefits and risks really are.

PHARMACOKINETICS: NEONATES AND INFANTS

As discussed in Chapter 4, pharmacokinetic factors determine the concentration of a drug at its sites of action, and hence determine the intensity and duration of responses. If drug levels are elevated, responses will be more intense. If drug elimination is delayed, responses will be prolonged. Because the organ systems that regulate drug levels are not fully developed in the very young, these patients are at risk of both possibilities: drug effects that are unusually intense *and* prolonged. By accounting for pharmacokinetic differences in the very young, we can increase the chances that drug therapy will be both effective and safe.

Figure 10–1 illustrates how drug levels differ between infants and adults following administration of equivalent doses (i.e., doses adjusted for body weight). When a drug is administered *intravenously* (Fig. 10–1A), levels decline more slowly in the infant than in the adult. As a result, drug levels in the infant remain above the minimum effective concentration (MEC) longer than in the adult, thereby causing effects to be prolonged. When a drug is administered *subcutaneously* (Fig. 10–1B), not only do levels in the infant remain above the MEC *longer* than in the adult, but these levels also rise *higher,* causing effects to be more intense as well as more prolonged. From these illustrations, it is clear that adjustment of dosage for infants on the basis of body size alone is not sufficient to achieve safe results.

If small body size is not the major reason for heightened drug sensitivity in infants, what is? The increased sensitivity of infants is due largely to the immature state of five pharmacokinetic processes: (1) drug absorption, (2) protein binding of drugs, (3) exclusion of drugs from the central nervous system (CNS) by the blood-brain barrier, (4) hepatic drug metabolism, and (5) renal drug excretion.

---

*On November 27, 1998, the FDA announced regulations requiring that, for all new drugs with potential pediatric applications, pharmaceutical companies must provide information on effects and dosages in children. In certain compelling circumstances, drug companies may also be required to develop pediatric dosing information on drugs already in use. As a result of these new regulations, safe and effective drug therapy in children will be greatly facilitated.

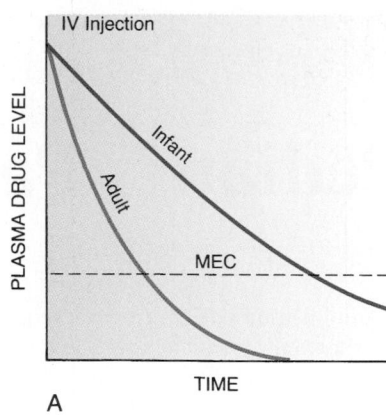
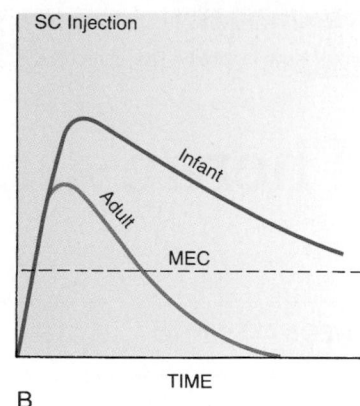

Figure 10–1 ■ Comparison of plasma drug levels in adults and infants. *A,* Plasma drug levels following IV injection. Dosage was adjusted for body weight. Note that plasma levels remain above the minimum effective concentration (MEC) much longer in the infant. *B,* Plasma drug levels following SC injection. Dosage was adjusted for body weight. Note that both the maximum drug level and the duration of action are greater in the infant. (Redrawn from Levine RR. Pharmacology: Drug Actions and Reactions. Boston, Little, Brown, 1973:238.)

Absorption

Oral Administration. Gastrointestinal physiology in the infant is very different from that in the adult. As a result, drug absorption may be enhanced or impeded, depending on the physicochemical properties of the drug involved.

Gastric emptying time is both prolonged and irregular in early infancy, and then gradually reaches adult values by 6 to 8 months. For drugs that are absorbed primarily from the stomach, delayed gastric emptying enhances absorption. On the other hand, for drugs that are absorbed primarily from the intestine, absorption is delayed. Because gastric emptying time is irregular, the precise impact on absorption is not predictable.

Gastric acidity is very low 24 hours after birth and does not reach adult values for 2 years. Because of low acidity, absorption of acid-labile drugs is increased.

Intramuscular Administration. Drug absorption following IM injection in the *neonate* is *slow* and *erratic.* Delayed absorption is due in part to low blood flow through muscle during the first days of postnatal life. By early *infancy,* absorption of IM drugs becomes more rapid than in neonates and adults.

Percutaneous Absorption. Because the skin of the very young is thin, percutaneous drug absorption is significantly greater than in older children and adults. This increases the risk of toxicity from topical drugs.

Distribution

Protein Binding. Binding of drugs to albumin and other plasma proteins is limited in the infant. This is because (1) the amount of albumin is relatively low and (2) endogenous compounds (e.g., fatty acids, bilirubin) compete with drugs for available binding sites. Consequently, drugs that ordinarily undergo extensive protein binding in adults undergo much less binding in infants. As a result, the concentration of *free* levels of such drugs is relatively high in the infant, thereby intensifying effects. To ensure that effects are not too intense,

		Duration of Drug-Induced Sleep	
Age	Percentage of Hexobarbital Metabolized (in 1 hr)	10-mg/kg Dose	50-mg/kg Dose
Newborn	"0"	6 hr	Eternal*
Adult	28–39	<5 min	12–22 min

TABLE 10–1 ■ Comparison of the Metabolism and Effects of Hexobarbital in Adult Versus Newborn Animals

*The 50-mg/kg dose was lethal to newborn animals.
Data from Jondorf WR, Maickel RP, Brodie BB. Inability of newborn mice and guinea pigs to metabolize drugs. Biochem Pharmacol 1958;1:352.

dosages in infants should be reduced. Protein-binding capacity reaches adult values within 10 to 12 months.

Blood-Brain Barrier. The blood-brain barrier is not fully developed at birth. As a result, drugs and other chemicals have relatively easy access to the CNS, making the infant especially sensitive to drugs that affect CNS function. Accordingly, all medicines employed for their CNS effects (e.g., morphine, phenobarbital) should be given in reduced dosage. Dosage should also be reduced for drugs used for actions *outside* the CNS if those drugs are capable of producing CNS toxicity as a side effect.

Hepatic Metabolism

The drug-metabolizing capacity of newborns is low. As a result, neonates are especially sensitive to drugs that are eliminated primarily by hepatic metabolism. When these drugs are used, dosages must be reduced. The capacity of the liver to metabolize many drugs increases rapidly about 1 month after birth, and approaches adult levels a few months later. Complete maturation of the liver develops by 1 year.

TABLE 10–2 ▪ Renal Function in Adults Versus Infants		
	Average Infant	Average Adult
Body Weight (kg)	3.5	70
Inulin Clearance		
Rate (ml/min)	3 (approximate)	130
Half-time (min)	630	120
Para-aminohippuric Acid (PAH) Clearance		
Rate (ml/min)	12 (approximate)	650
Half-time (min)	160	43

Adapted from Goldstein A, Aronow L, Kalman SM. Principles of Drug Action: The Basis of Pharmacology, 2nd ed. New York, Churchill Livingstone, 1974:215.

The minimal drug-metabolizing capacity of newborns is illustrated by the data in Table 10–1. These data are from experiments on the metabolism and effects of hexobarbital (a CNS depressant) in newborn and adult animals. *Metabolism* was measured in microsomal enzyme preparations made from the livers of *guinea pigs*. The *effect* of hexobarbital—CNS depression—was assessed in *mice*. Duration of sleeping time following hexobarbital injection was used as the index of CNS depression.

As indicated in Table 10–1, the drug-metabolizing capacity of the adult liver is much greater than the drug-metabolizing capacity of the newborn liver. Whereas the adult liver preparation metabolized an average of 33% of the hexobarbital presented to it, there was virtually no measurable metabolism by the newborn preparation.

The physiologic impact of limited drug-metabolizing capacity is indicated by observing sleeping time in newborns versus sleeping time in adults following injection of hexobarbital. As shown in Table 10–1, a low dose (10 mg/kg) of hexobarbital caused adult mice to sleep less than 5 minutes. In contrast, the same dose caused newborns to sleep 6 hours. The differential effects on adults and newborns are much more dramatic at a higher dose (50 mg/kg): Whereas the adults merely slept for 20 minutes, this dose was *lethal* to newborns.

Renal Excretion

Renal drug excretion is significantly reduced at birth. Renal blood flow, glomerular filtration, and active tubular secretion are all low during infancy. Because the drug-excreting capacity of infants is limited, drugs that are eliminated primarily by renal excretion must be given in reduced dosage. Adult levels of renal function are achieved by 1 year.

The relative inability of the infant kidney to excrete foreign compounds is illustrated by the data in Table 10–2. These data show rates of renal excretion for two compounds: inulin and *para*-aminohippuric acid (PAH). Inulin is excreted entirely by glomerular filtration. PAH is excreted by a combination of glomerular filtration and active tubular secretion. Note that the half-life for inulin is 630 minutes in infants but only 120 minutes in adults. Since inulin is eliminated by glomerular filtration alone, these data tell us that the glomerular filtration rate in the infant is much slower than in the adult. From the data for clearance of PAH, taken together with the data for clearance of inulin, we can conclude that tubular secretion in infants is also much slower than in adults.

PHARMACOKINETICS: CHILDREN 1 YEAR AND OLDER

By the age of 1 year, most pharmacokinetic parameters in children are similar to those in adults. Hence, drug sensitivity in children over the age of 1 is more like that of adults than that of the very young. Although pharmacokinetically similar to adults, children do differ in one important way: They metabolize drugs

TABLE 10–3 ▪ Adverse Drug Reactions Unique to Pediatric Patients	
Drug	Adverse Effect
Androgens	Premature puberty in males; reduced adult height from premature epiphyseal closure
Aspirin and other salicylates	Severe intoxication from acute overdose (acidosis, hyperthermia respiratory depression); Reye's syndrome in children with chickenpox or influenza
Chloramphenicol	Gray syndrome (neonates and infants)
Glucocorticoids	Growth suppression with prolonged use
Fluoroquinolones	Tendon rupture
Hexachlorophene	CNS toxicity (infants)
Nalidixic acid	Cartilage erosion
Phenothiazines	Sudden infant death syndrome
Sulfonamides	Kernicterus (neonates)
Tetracyclines	Staining of developing teeth

faster than adults. Drug-metabolizing capacity is markedly elevated until the age of 2 years, and then gradually declines. A further sharp decline takes place at puberty, when adult values are reached. Because of enhanced drug metabolism in children, an increase in dosage or a reduction in dosing interval may be needed for drugs that are eliminated by hepatic metabolism.

ADVERSE DRUG REACTIONS

Like adults, pediatric patients are subject to adverse reactions when drug levels rise too high. In addition to these dose-related reactions, pediatric patients are vulnerable to unique adverse effects related to the immature state of organ systems and to ongoing growth and development. Among these age-related effects are growth suppression (caused by glucocorticoids), discoloration of developing teeth (caused by tetracyclines), and kernicterus (caused by sulfonamides). Table 10–3 presents a list of drugs that can cause unique adverse effects in pediatric patients of various ages. Care should be taken to avoid these drugs in patients whose age renders them vulnerable.

DOSAGE DETERMINATION

Because of the pharmacokinetic factors discussed above, dosage selection for pediatric patients is difficult. Selecting a dosage is especially difficult in the very young, since pharmacokinetic factors are undergoing rapid change.

Pediatric doses have been established for some drugs but not others. For drugs that do not have an established pediatric dose, dosage can be extrapolated from adult doses. The method of conversion employed most commonly is based on body surface area:

$$\text{Approximate child's dose} = \frac{\text{Body surface area of the child} \times \text{Adult dose}}{1.73 \text{ m}^2}$$

Please note that initial pediatric doses—whether based on established pediatric doses or extrapolated from adult doses—are at best an *approximation*. Subsequent doses must be adjusted on the basis of clinical outcome and plasma drug concentrations. These adjustments are especially important in neonates and younger infants. Clearly, if dosage adjustments are to be optimal, it is essential that we monitor the patient for therapeutic and adverse responses.

PROMOTING COMPLIANCE

Achieving accurate and timely dosing requires informed participation of the child's parents or guardian and, to the extent possible, active involvement of the child too. Effective education is critical. The following issues should be addressed:

- Dosage size and timing
- Route and technique of administration
- Duration of treatment
- Drug storage
- The nature and time course of desired responses
- The nature and time course of adverse responses

Written instructions should be provided. For techniques of administration that are difficult, a demonstration should be made, after which the parents should repeat the procedure to ensure they understand. With young children, spills and spitting out are common causes of inaccurate dosing; parents should be taught to estimate the amount of drug lost and to re-administer that amount, being careful not to overcompensate. When more than one person is helping medicate a child, all participants should be warned against multiple dosing. Multiple dosing can be avoided by maintaining a drug administration chart. With some disorders—especially infections—symptoms may resolve before the prescribed course of treatment has been completed. Parents should be instructed to complete the full treatment nonetheless. Additional ways to promote compliance include (1) selecting the most convenient dosage form and dosing

schedule, (2) suggesting mixing oral drugs with food or juice (when allowed) to improve palatability, (3) providing a calibrated medicine spoon or syringe for measuring liquid formulations, and (4) taking extra time with young or disadvantaged parents to help ensure conscientious and skilled participation.

⁂ KEY POINTS

- Because of organ system immaturity, very young patients are highly sensitive to drugs.
- In neonates and young infants, drug responses may be unusually intense and prolonged.
- Absorption of IM drugs in *neonates* is slower than in adults. In contrast, absorption of IM drugs in *infants* is more rapid than in adults.
- Protein-binding capacity is limited early in life. Hence, free concentrations of some drugs may be especially high.
- The blood-brain barrier is not fully developed at birth. Hence, neonates are especially sensitive to drugs that affect the CNS.
- The drug-metabolizing capacity of neonates is low. Hence, neonates are especially sensitive to drugs that are eliminated primarily by hepatic metabolism.
- Renal excretion of drugs is low in neonates. Hence, drugs that are eliminated primarily by the kidney must be given in reduced dosage.
- In children 1 year and older, most pharmacokinetic parameters are similar to those in adults. Hence, drug sensitivity is more like that of adults than of the very young.
- Children (1 to 12 years) differ pharmacokinetically from adults in that children metabolize drugs faster.
- Initial pediatric doses are at best an approximation. Hence, subsequent doses must be adjusted on the basis of clinical outcome and plasma drug levels.

Drug Therapy in Geriatric Patients

Drug use among the elderly is disproportionately high. Whereas the elderly (those 65 years and older) constitute only 12% of the U.S. population, they consume 31% of the nation's prescribed drugs. Reasons for this intensive use of drugs include increased severity of illness, the presence of multiple pathologies, and excessive prescribing.

Drug therapy in the elderly represents a special therapeutic challenge. As a rule, older patients are more sensitive to drugs than are younger adults, and they show wider individual variation. In addition, the elderly experience more adverse drug reactions and drug-drug interactions. The principal factors underlying these complications of therapy are (1) altered pharmacokinetics (secondary to organ system degeneration), (2) multiple and severe illnesses, (3) multiple-drug therapy, and (4) poor compliance. To help ensure that drug therapy is as safe and effective as possible, *individualization of treatment is essential: each patient must be monitored for desired responses and adverse responses, and the regimen must be adjusted accordingly.* Since the elderly typically suffer from chronic illnesses, the usual objective is to reduce symptoms and improve quality of life, since cure is generally impossible.

PHARMACOKINETIC CHANGES IN THE ELDERLY

The aging process can affect all phases of pharmacokinetics. From early adulthood on, there is a gradual, progressive decline in organ function. This decline can alter the absorption, distribution, metabolism, and excretion of drugs. As a rule, these pharmacokinetic changes increase drug sensitivity (largely from reduced hepatic and renal drug elimination). It should be noted, however, that the extent of change varies greatly among patients: Pharmacokinetic changes may be minimal in patients who have remained physically fit, whereas they may be dramatic in patients who have aged less gracefully. Accordingly, you should keep in mind that age-related changes in pharmacokinetics are not only a potential source of increased sensitivity to drugs, they are also a potential source of increased variability. The physiologic changes that underlie alterations in pharmacokinetics are summarized in Table 11-1.

Absorption

Altered GI absorption is not a major factor in drug sensitivity in the elderly. As a rule, the *percentage* of an oral dose that becomes absorbed does not change with age. However, the *rate* of absorption may be slowed (because of delayed gastric emptying and reduced splanchnic blood flow). As a result, drug responses may be somewhat delayed. Gastric acidity is reduced in the elderly and may alter the absorption of certain drugs. For example, some drug formulations require high acidity to dissolve. Absorption of these formulations may be reduced.

Distribution

Four major factors can alter drug distribution in the elderly: (1) increased percent body fat, (2) decreased percent lean body mass, (3) decreased total body water, and (4) reduced concentration of serum albumin. The increase in body fat seen in the elderly provides a storage depot for *lipid-soluble* drugs (e.g., thiopental). As a result, plasma levels of these drugs are reduced, causing a reduction in responses. Because of the decline in lean body mass and total body water, *water-soluble* drugs (e.g., ethanol) become distributed in a smaller volume

TABLE 11–1 ■ Physiologic Changes That Can Affect Pharmacokinetics in the Elderly
Absorption of Drugs
Increased gastric pH
Decreased absorptive surface area
Decreased splanchnic blood flow
Decreased GI motility
Delayed gastric emptying
Distribution of Drugs
Increased body fat
Decreased lean body mass
Decreased total body water
Decreased serum albumin
Decreased cardiac output
Metabolism of Drugs
Decreased hepatic blood flow
Decreased hepatic mass
Decreased activity of hepatic enzymes
Excretion of Drugs
Decreased renal blood flow
Decreased glomerular filtration rate
Decreased tubular secretion
Decreased number of nephrons

than in younger adults. As a result, the concentration of these drugs is increased, causing their effects to be more intense. Although albumin levels are only slightly reduced in healthy adults, these levels can be significantly reduced in adults who are malnourished. Because of reduced albumin levels, protein binding of drugs decreases, causing levels of free drug to rise. As a result, drug effects may be more intense.

Metabolism

Rates of hepatic drug metabolism tend to decline with age. Principal factors underlying the decline are reduced hepatic blood flow, reduced liver mass, and decreased activity of some hepatic enzymes. Because liver function is diminished, the half-lives of certain drugs may be increased, thereby prolonging responses. Responses to oral drugs that ordinarily undergo extensive first-pass metabolism may be enhanced. It must be noted, however, that the degree of decline in drug metabolism varies greatly among individuals. As a result, we cannot predict whether drug responses will be significantly reduced in any particular patient.

Excretion

Renal drug function, and hence drug excretion, undergoes progressive decline beginning in early adulthood. *Drug accumulation secondary to reduced renal excretion is the most important cause of adverse drug reactions in the elderly.* The decline in renal function is the result of reductions in renal blood flow, glomerular filtration rate, active tubular secretion, and number of nephrons. Co-existence of renal pathology can further compromise kidney function. The degree of decline in renal function varies greatly among individuals. Accordingly, when patients are taking drugs that are eliminated primarily by the kidneys, renal function should be assessed. In the elderly, the proper index of renal function is *creatinine clearance*—not serum *creatinine levels*. Creatinine levels do not reflect kidney function in the elderly because the source of serum creatinine—lean muscle mass—declines in parallel with the decline in kidney function. As a result, creatinine levels may be normal even though renal function is greatly reduced.

PHARMACODYNAMIC CHANGES IN THE ELDERLY

Alterations in receptor properties may underlie altered sensitivity to some drugs. However, information on such pharmacodynamic changes is limited. In support of the possibility of altered pharmacodynamics is the observation that beta-adrenergic blocking agents (drugs used for cardiac disorders) are *less* effective in the elderly than in younger adults when present in the same concentrations. Possible explanations for this observation include (1) a reduction in the number of available beta receptors and (2) a reduction in the affinity of beta receptors for beta-receptor blocking agents. Other drugs (certain central nervous system depressants, warfarin) produce effects that are more intense in the elderly than in younger adults when present at the same concentrations, suggesting a possible increase in receptor number, receptor affinity, or both. Unfortunately, our knowledge of pharmacodynamic changes in the elderly is restricted to a few families of drugs.

ADVERSE DRUG REACTIONS AND DRUG INTERACTIONS

Adverse drug reactions (ADRs) are seven times more common in the elderly than in younger adults, accounting for about 16% of hospital admissions among older individuals and 50% of all medication-related deaths. The vast majority of these reactions are dose related—not idiosyncratic. Symptoms in the elderly are often nonspecific (e.g., dizziness, cognitive impairment), making identification of ADRs difficult.

Perhaps surprisingly, the increase in ADRs seen in the elderly is not the direct result of aging per se; rather, multiple factors predispose older patients to ADRs. The most important factors are

- Drug accumulation secondary to reduced renal function
- Polypharmacy (treatment with multiple drugs)
- Greater severity of illness
- The presence of multiple pathologies
- Greater use of drugs that have a low therapeutic index (e.g., digoxin, a drug for heart failure)
- Increased individual variation secondary to altered pharmacokinetics
- Inadequate supervision of long-term therapy
- Poor patient compliance

The majority of ADRs in the elderly are avoidable. Measures that can reduce the incidence of ADRs include

- Taking a thorough drug history, including over-the-counter medications
- Accounting for the pharmacokinetic and pharmacodynamic changes that occur with aging
- Initiating therapy with low doses
- Monitoring clinical responses and plasma drug levels to provide a rational basis for dosage adjustment
- Employing the simplest regimen possible
- Monitoring for drug-drug interactions and iatrogenic illness
- Periodically reviewing the need for continued drug therapy, and discontinuing medications as appropriate
- Encouraging the patient to dispose of old medications
- Taking steps to promote compliance (see below)

PROMOTING COMPLIANCE

As many as 40% or more of elderly patients fail to take their medicines as prescribed. Some patients never fill their prescriptions, some fail to refill their prescriptions, and some don't follow the prescribed dosing schedule. Noncompliance can result in therapeutic failure (from underdosing or erratic dosing) or toxicity (from overdosing). Of the two possibilities, underdosing with resulting therapeutic failure is by far (90%) the more common.

Multiple factors underlie nonadherence to the prescribed regimen (Table 11–2). Among these are forgetfulness; failure to comprehend instructions (because of intellectual, visual, or auditory impairment); inability to pay for medications; and use of complex regimens (several drugs taken several times a day). All of these factors can contribute to *unintentional* noncompliance. However, in the majority of cases (about 75%), noncompliance among the elderly is *intentional*. The principal reason given for intentional noncompli-

TABLE 11–2 ■ Factors That Contribute To Poor Compliance in the Elderly
Multiple chronic disorders
Multiple prescription medications
Multiple doses/day for each medication
Multiple prescribers
Changes in the regimen (addition of drugs, changes in dosage size or timing)
Cognitive or physical impairment (reduction in memory, hearing, visual acuity, color discrimination, or manual dexterity)
Living alone
Recent discharge from hospital
Low literacy
Inability to pay for drugs
Personal conviction that a drug is unnecessary or the dosage is too high
Presence of side effects

ance is the patient's conviction that the drug was simply not needed in the dosage prescribed. Unpleasant side effects and expense also contribute to intentional noncompliance.

Several steps can be taken to promote adherence to the prescribed regimen. These include

- Simplifying the regimen so that the number of drugs and doses per day is the smallest possible
- Explaining the treatment plan using clear, concise verbal and written instructions
- Choosing an appropriate dosage form (e.g., a liquid formulation if the patient has difficulty swallowing)
- Labeling drug containers clearly, and avoiding containers that are difficult to open by patients with impaired dexterity (e.g., those with arthritis)
- Suggesting the use of a calendar, diary, or pill counter to record drug administration
- Asking the patient if he or she has access to a pharmacy and can afford the medication
- Enlisting the aid of a friend, relative, or visiting healthcare professional
- Monitoring for therapeutic responses, adverse reactions, and plasma drug levels

It must be noted, however, that the benefits of these measures will be restricted primarily to patients whose nonadherence is *unintentional*. Unfortunately, these measures are generally inapplicable to the patient whose nonadherence is *intentional*. For these patients, intensive education may help.

■ KEY POINTS

- Older patients are generally more sensitive to drugs than are younger adults, and they show wider individual variation.
- Individualization of therapy for the elderly is essential: Each patient must be monitored for desired and adverse responses, and the regimen must be adjusted accordingly.
- Aging-related organ system decline can change drug absorption, distribution, metabolism, and (especially) excretion.
- The *rate* of drug absorption may be slowed in the elderly, although the *extent* of absorption is usually unchanged.
- Plasma concentrations of lipid-soluble drugs may be low in the elderly, and concentrations of water-soluble drugs may be high.
- Reduced liver function may prolong drug effects.
- Reduced renal function, with resultant drug accumulation, is the most important cause of adverse drug reactions in the elderly.
- Because the degree of renal impairment among the elderly varies, creatinine clearance (a test of renal function) should be determined for all patients taking drugs that are eliminated primarily by the kidneys.
- Adverse drug reactions are much more common in the elderly than in younger adults.
- Factors underlying the increase in adverse reactions include polypharmacy, severe illness, multiple pathologies, and treatment with dangerous drugs.
- Noncompliance is common among the elderly.
- Reasons for *unintentional* noncompliance include forgetfulness, side effects, low income, complex regimens, and failure to comprehend instructions.
- Most (90%) cases of noncompliance among the elderly are *intentional*. Reasons include expense, side effects, and the patient's conviction that the drug is unnecessary or the dosage too high.

Basic Principles of Neuropharmacology

Neuropharmacology can be defined as *the study of drugs that alter processes controlled by the nervous system.* Neuropharmacologic drugs produce effects equivalent to those produced by excitation or suppression of neuronal activity. Neuropharmacologic agents can be divided into two broad categories: (1) peripheral nervous system drugs and (2) central nervous system (CNS) drugs.

The neuropharmacologic drugs constitute a large and important family of therapeutic agents. These drugs are used to treat conditions that range from depression to epilepsy to hypertension to asthma. The clinical significance of neuropharmacologic agents is reflected in the fact that over 25% of the chapters in this text are dedicated to them.

Why do we have so many neuropharmacologic drugs? The answer can be found in a concept discussed in Chapter 5: Most therapeutic agents act by helping the body help itself. That is, most drugs produce their therapeutic effects by coaxing the body to perform normal processes in a fashion that benefits the patient. Since the nervous system participates in the regulation of practically all bodily processes, practically all bodily processes can be influenced by drugs that alter neuronal regulation. By mimicking or blocking neuronal regulation, neuropharmacologic drugs can modify such diverse processes as skeletal muscle contraction, cardiac output, vascular tone, respiration, GI function, uterine motility, glandular secretion, and functions unique to the CNS, such as pain perception, ideation, and mood. Given the broad spectrum of processes that neuropharmacologic drugs can alter, and given the potential benefits to be gained by manipulating those processes, it should be no surprise that neuropharmacologic drugs have widespread clinical applications.

We begin our study of neuropharmacology by discussing peripheral nervous system drugs (Chapters 14 through 19), after which we discuss CNS drugs (Chapters 20 through 38). The principal rationale for this order of presentation is that our understanding of peripheral nervous system pharmacology is much clearer than our understanding of CNS pharmacology. Why? Because the peripheral nervous system is much less complex than the CNS, and also more accessible to experimentation. By placing our initial focus on the peripheral nervous system, we can establish a firm knowledge base in neuropharmacology before proceeding to the less definitive and vastly more complex realm of CNS pharmacology.

HOW NEURONS REGULATE PHYSIOLOGIC PROCESSES

As a rule, if we want to understand the effects of a drug on a particular physiologic process, we must first understand the process itself. Accordingly, if we wish to understand the impact of drugs on neuronal regulation of bodily function, we must first understand how neurons regulate bodily function when drugs are absent.

The primary steps by which a neuron elicits a response from another cell are illustrated in Figure 12–1. This figure depicts two cells: a neuron and a postsynaptic cell. The postsynaptic cell might be another neuron, a muscle cell, or a cell within a secretory gland. There are three major steps in the process by which the neuron influences the behavior of the postsynaptic cell: (1) conduction of an action potential along the axon of the neuron, (2) release of neurotransmitter molecules from the axon terminal, and (3) binding of transmitter molecules (T) to receptors on the postsynaptic cell. As a result of transmitter-receptor binding, a series of events is initiated in the postsynaptic cell, leading to a change in its behavior. The precise nature of the change depends on the identity of the neurotransmitter and the type of cell involved. If the postsynaptic cell is another neuron, it may increase or decrease its firing rate; if the cell is part of a muscle, it may contract or relax; and if the cell is glandular, it may increase or decrease its rate of secretion.

The three steps discussed above can be viewed as constituting two primary processes: *(1) axonal conduction* and *(2) synaptic transmission.* Axonal conduction is simply the process of conducting an action potential down the axon of the neuron; synaptic transmission is the process by which information is carried across the gap between the neuron and the postsynaptic cell.

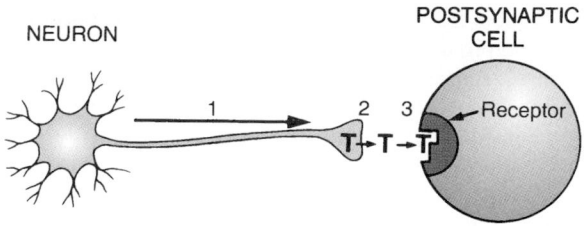

Figure 12–1 ■ How neurons regulate other cells.
The basic steps in the process by which neurons elicit responses from other cells are (1) axonal conduction, (2) transmitter (T) release, and (3) binding of transmitter to its receptor on the postsynaptic cell. Steps 2 and 3 are components of the process known as *synaptic transmission.*

BASIC MECHANISMS BY WHICH NEUROPHARMACOLOGIC AGENTS ACT

Sites of Action: Axons Versus Synapses

In order to influence a process under neuronal control, a drug can alter one of two basic neuronal activities: axonal conduction or synaptic transmission. *Most neuropharmacologic agents act by altering synaptic transmission*—only a few alter axonal conduction. Why do drugs usually target synaptic transmission? Because drugs that alter synaptic transmission can produce effects that are much more *selective* than those produced by drugs that alter axonal conduction.

Axonal Conduction

Drugs that act by altering axonal conduction are not very selective. Recall that the process of conducting an impulse along an axon is essentially the same in all neurons. As a consequence, a drug that alters axonal conduction will affect conduction in all nerves to which it has access. Such a drug cannot produce selective effects.

Local anesthetics are the only drugs proved to work by altering (decreasing) axonal conduction. Since these agents produce nonselective inhibition of axonal conduction, they will suppress transmission in any nerve they reach. Hence, although local anesthetics are certainly valuable, their indications are limited.

Synaptic Transmission

In contrast to drugs that alter axonal conduction, drugs that alter synaptic transmission can produce effects that are highly selective. These drugs can elicit selective responses because synapses, unlike axons, are not all the same. Synapses at different sites employ different transmitters. In addition, for many transmitters, the body employs more than one type of receptor. Hence, by using a drug that selectively influences a specific type of neurotransmitter or receptor, we can alter one neuronally regulated process while leaving most others unaffected. Because of this capacity for selectivity, drugs that alter synaptic transmission have numerous uses.

Receptors

The ability of a neuron to influence the behavior of another cell depends, ultimately, upon the ability of that neuron to alter receptor activity on the target cell. As discussed, neurons alter receptor activity by releasing transmitter molecules,

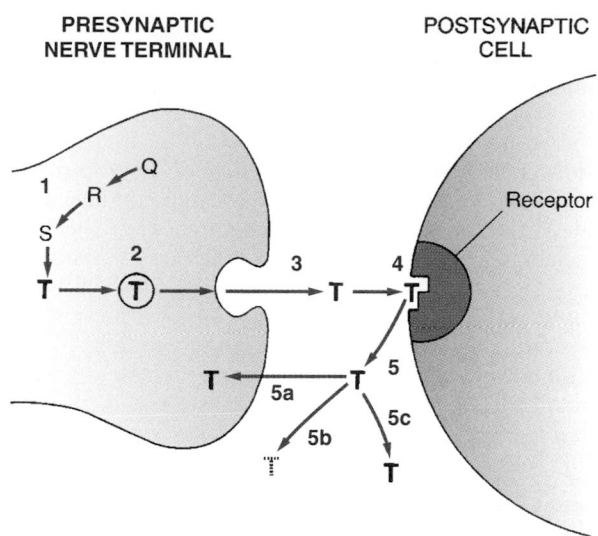

Figure 12–2 ■ Steps in synaptic transmission.
Step 1, Synthesis of transmitter (T) from precursor molecules (Q, R, and S). *Step 2,* Storage of transmitter in vesicles. *Step 3,* Release of transmitter: In response to an action potential, vesicles fuse with the terminal membrane and discharge their contents into the synaptic gap. *Step 4,* Action at receptor: Transmitter binds (reversibly) to its receptor on the postsynaptic cell, causing a response in that cell. *Step 5,* Termination of transmission: Transmitter dissociates from its receptor and is then removed from the synaptic gap by (a) reuptake into the nerve terminal, (b) enzymatic degradation, or (c) diffusion away from the gap.

which diffuse across the synaptic gap and bind to receptors on the postsynaptic cell. If the target cell lacked receptors for the transmitter that a particular neuron released, that neuron would be unable to affect the target cell.

The effects of neuropharmacologic drugs, like those of neurons, are dependent upon altering receptor activity. That is, no matter what its precise mechanism of action, a neuropharmacologic drug ultimately produces its effects through influencing receptor activity on target cells. This common-sense concept is central to understanding the actions of neuropharmacologic drugs. In fact, this concept is so critical to our understanding of neuropharmacologic agents that I will repeat it: *The impact of a drug on a neuronally regulated process is dependent upon the ability of that drug to directly or indirectly influence receptor activity on target cells.*

Steps in Synaptic Transmission

To understand how drugs alter receptor activity, we must first understand the steps by which synaptic transmission takes place, since it is by modifying these steps that neuropharmacologic drugs influence receptor function. The steps in synaptic transmission are summarized in Figure 12–2.

Step 1: Transmitter Synthesis. For synaptic transmission to take place, molecules of transmitter must be present in the nerve terminal. Hence, we can look upon transmitter synthesis as the first step in transmission. In the figure, the letters Q, R, and S represent the precursor molecules from which the transmitter (T) is made.

Step 2: Transmitter Storage. Once transmitter is synthesized, it must be stored until the time of its release. Transmitter storage takes place within vesicles—tiny packets present in the axon terminal. Each nerve terminal contains a large number of transmitter-filled vesicles.

Step 3: Transmitter Release. Release of transmitter is triggered by the arrival of an action potential at the axon terminal. The action potential initiates a process in which vesicles undergo fusion with the terminal membrane, causing release of their contents into the synaptic gap. With each action potential, only a small fraction of all vesicles present in the axon terminal are caused to discharge their contents.

Step 4: Receptor Binding. Following release, transmitter molecules diffuse across the synaptic gap and then undergo *reversible* binding to receptors on the postsynaptic cell. This binding initiates a cascade of events that result in altered behavior of the postsynaptic cell.

Step 5: Termination of Transmission. Transmission is terminated by dissociation of transmitter from its receptors, followed by removal of free transmitter from the synaptic gap. Transmitter can be removed from the synaptic gap by three processes: (1) reuptake, (2) enzymatic degradation, and (3) diffusion. In those synapses where transmission is terminated by reuptake, axon terminals contain "pumps" that transport transmitter molecules back into the neuron from which they were released (step 5a in Fig. 12–2). Following reuptake, molecules of transmitter may be degraded, or they may be packaged in vesicles for reuse. In synapses where transmitter is cleared by enzymatic degradation (step 5b), the synapse contains large quantities of transmitter-inactivating enzymes. Although simple diffusion away from the synaptic gap (step 5c) is a potential means of terminating transmitter action, this process is very slow and generally of little significance.

Effects of Drugs on the Steps of Synaptic Transmission

As noted, all neuropharmacologic agents (except anesthetics) produce their effects by directly or indirectly altering receptor activity. We also noted that the way in which drugs alter receptor activity is by interfering with synaptic transmission. Because synaptic transmission has multiple steps, the process offers a number of potential targets for drugs. In this section, we examine the specific ways in which drugs can alter the steps of synaptic transmission. By way of encouragement, although this information may appear complex, it isn't. In fact, it's largely self-evident.

Before discussing specific mechanisms by which drugs can alter receptor activity, we need to understand what drugs are capable of doing to receptors in general terms. From the broadest perspective, when a drug influences receptor function, that drug can do just one of two things: it can enhance receptor activation or it can reduce receptor activation. What do we mean by receptor activation? For our purposes, we can define *activation* as *an effect on receptor function equivalent to that produced by the natural neurotransmitter at a particular synapse.* Hence, a drug whose effects mimic the effects of a natural transmitter would be said to *increase* receptor activation. Conversely, a drug whose effects were equivalent to reducing the amount of natural transmitter available for receptor binding would be said to *decrease* receptor activation.

Please note that activation of a receptor does not necessarily mean that a physiologic process will go faster; receptor activation can also make a process go slower. For example, a drug that mimicked acetylcholine at receptors on the heart would cause the heart to beat more slowly. Since the effect of this drug on receptor function mimicked the effect of the natural neurotransmitter, we would say that the drug activated acetylcholine receptors, even though activation caused heart rate to decline.

Having defined receptor activation, we are ready to discuss the mechanisms by which drugs, acting on specific steps of synaptic transmission, can increase or decrease the receptor activity. These mechanisms are summarized in Table 12–1. As we consider these mechanisms one by one, their common-sense nature should become apparent.

Transmitter Synthesis. There are three different effects that drugs are known to have on transmitter synthesis. They can (1) increase transmitter synthesis, (2) decrease transmitter synthesis, or (3) cause the synthesis of transmitter molecules that are more effective than the natural transmitter itself.

The impact of increased or decreased transmitter synthesis on receptor activity should be obvious. A drug that increases transmitter synthesis will cause receptor activation to increase. The process is this: As a result of increased transmitter synthesis, storage vesicles will contain transmitter in abnormally high amounts; hence, when an action potential reaches the axon terminal, more transmitter will be released, and therefore more transmitter will be available to receptors on the postsynaptic cell, causing activation of those receptors to increase. Conversely, a drug that decreases transmitter synthesis will cause the transmitter content of vesicles to decline, resulting in reduced transmitter release and decreased receptor activation.

Some drugs can cause neurons to synthesize transmitter molecules whose structure is different from that of normal transmitter molecules. For example, by acting as substrates for enzymes in the axon terminal, drugs can be converted into "super" transmitters (molecules whose ability to activate receptors is greater than that of the naturally occurring transmitter at a particular

TABLE 12–1 ▐▪ Effects of Drugs on Synaptic Transmission and the Resulting Impact on Receptor Activation		
Step of Synaptic Transmission	**Drug Action**	**Impact on Receptor Activation***
1: Synthesis of transmitter	Increased synthesis of T Decreased synthesis of T Synthesis of "super" T	Increase Decrease Increase
2: Storage of transmitter	Reduced storage of T	Decrease
3: Release of transmitter	Promotion of T release Inhibition of T release	Increase Decrease
4: Binding to receptor	Direct receptor stimulation Enhanced response to T Blockade of T binding	Increase Increase Decrease
5: Termination of transmission	Blockade of T reuptake Prevention of T breakdown	Increase Increase

T = transmitter

*Receptor activation is defined as production of an effect equivalent to that produced by the natural transmitter that acts on a particular receptor.

site). Release of these supertransmitters will cause receptor activation to increase. In theory, it should be possible to cause the synthesis of *faulty* transmitter molecules (i.e., molecules with a reduced ability to activate a particular receptor). However, we have no medicines that are known to act this way.

Transmitter Storage. Drugs that interfere with transmitter storage will cause receptor activation to decrease. Why? Because disruption of storage depletes vesicles of their transmitter content, thereby decreasing the amount of transmitter available for release.

Transmitter Release. Drugs can either *promote* release or *inhibit* release. Drugs that promote release will increase receptor activation; drugs that inhibit release will reduce receptor activation. The amphetamines (CNS stimulants) represent drugs that act by promoting transmitter release. Botulinum toxin, in contrast, acts by inhibiting transmitter release.*

Receptor Binding. Many drugs act directly at receptors. These agents can either (1) bind to receptors and cause activation, (2) bind to receptors and thereby block receptor activation by other agents, or (3) bind to receptor components and thereby enhance receptor activation by the natural transmitter at the site.

In the terminology introduced in Chapter 5, drugs that directly activate receptors are called *agonists,* whereas drugs that prevent receptor activation are called *antagonists.* We have no special name for drugs that bind to receptors and thereby enhance the effects of the natural transmitter. The direct-acting receptor agonists and antagonists constitute the largest and most important groups of neuropharmacologic drugs.

Examples of drugs that act directly at receptors are numerous. Drugs that bind to receptors and cause *activation* include

---

*Botulinum toxin blocks release of acetylcholine from the neurons that control skeletal muscles, including the muscles of respiration. The potential for disaster is obvious.

morphine (used for its effects on the CNS), epinephrine (used mainly for its effects on the cardiovascular system), and insulin (used for its effects in diabetes). Drugs that bind to receptors and *prevent* their activation include naloxone (used to treat overdose with morphine-like drugs), antihistamines (used to treat allergic disorders), and propranolol (used to treat hypertension, angina pectoris, and dysrhythmias). The principal examples of drugs that bind to receptors and thereby enhance the actions of a natural transmitter are the benzodiazepines. Drugs in this family—which includes diazepam [Valium] and related agents—are used to treat anxiety, seizure disorders, and muscle spasm.

Termination of Transmitter Action. Drugs can interfere with the termination of transmitter action by two mechanisms: (1) blockade of transmitter reuptake and (2) inhibition of transmitter degradation. Drugs that act by either mechanism will cause the concentration of transmitter in the synaptic gap to rise, thereby causing receptor activation to increase.

MULTIPLE RECEPTOR TYPES AND SELECTIVITY OF DRUG ACTION

As we discussed in Chapter 1, selectivity is one of the most desirable qualities a drug can have, since a selective drug is able to alter a disease process while leaving other physiologic processes largely unaffected.

Many neuropharmacologic agents display a high degree of selectivity. This selectivity is possible because the nervous system works through multiple types of receptors to regulate the organs under its control. If neurons had only one or two types of receptors through which to act, selective effects by neuropharmacologic drugs could not be achieved.

The relationship between multiple receptor types and selective drug action is illustrated by Mort and Merv, whose

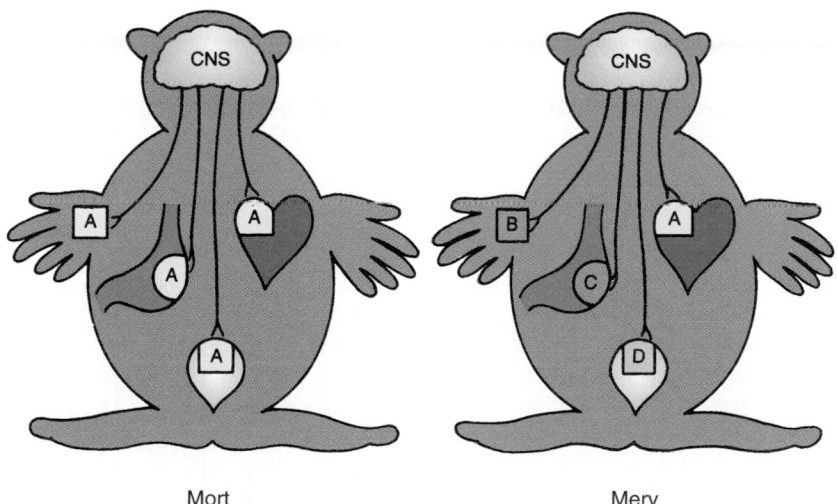

Figure 12–3 ■ Multiple drug receptors and selective drug action.
Mort, All organs are regulated through stimulation of type A receptors. Drugs that affect type A receptors on one organ will affect type A receptors on all other organs. Hence, selective drug action is impossible. *Merv,* Merv has four types of receptors (A, B, C, and D) to regulate his four organs. A drug that acts at one type of receptor will not affect the others. Hence, selective drug action is possible.

unique physiologies are depicted in Figure 12–3. Let's begin by considering Mort. Mort can perform four functions: he can pump blood, digest food, shake hands, and empty his bladder. As indicated in the figure, all four functions are under neuronal control, and, in all cases, that control is exerted by activation of the same type of receptor (designated A).

As long as Mort remains healthy, having only one type of receptor to regulate his various functions presents no problem. Selective *physiologic* regulation can be achieved simply by sending impulses down the appropriate nerves. When there is a need to increase cardiac output, impulses are sent down the nerve to his heart; when digestion is needed, impulses are sent down the nerve to his stomach; and so forth.

Although having only one receptor type is no disadvantage when all is well, if Mort gets sick, having only one receptor type creates a therapeutic problem. Let's assume he develops heart disease and we need to give a drug that will help increase cardiac output. To stimulate cardiac function, we need to administer a drug that will activate receptors on his heart. Unfortunately, since the receptors on his heart are the same as the receptors on his other organs, a drug that stimulates cardiac function will stimulate his other organs too. Consequently, any attempt to improve cardiac output with drugs will necessarily be accompanied by side effects. These will range from silly (compulsive handshaking) to embarrassing (enuresis) to hazardous (gastric ulcers). Such side effects are not likely to elicit either gratitude or compliance. Please note that all of these undesirable effects are the direct result of Mort having a nervous system that works through just one type of receptor to regulate all organs. That is, the presence of only one receptor type has made selective drug action impossible.

Now let's consider Merv. Although Merv appears to be Mort's twin, Merv differs in one important way: Whereas all functions in Mort are regulated through just one type of receptor, Merv employs different receptors to control each of his four functions. Because of this simple but important difference, the selective drug action that was impossible with Mort can be achieved easily with Merv. We can, for example, selectively enhance cardiac function in Merv without risking the side effects to which Mort was predisposed. This can be done simply by administering an agonist agent that binds selectively to receptors on the heart (type A receptors). If this medication is sufficiently selective for type A receptors, it will not interact with receptor types B, C, or D. Hence, function in structures regulated by those receptors will be unaffected. Note that our ability to produce selective drug action in Merv is made possible because his nervous system works through different types of receptors to regulate function in his various organs. The message from this example is clear: *The more types of receptors we have to work with, the greater our chances of producing selective drug effects.*

AN APPROACH TO LEARNING ABOUT PERIPHERAL NERVOUS SYSTEM DRUGS

As discussed, to understand the ways in which drugs can alter a process under neuronal control, you must first understand how the nervous system itself regulates that process. Accordingly, when preparing to study peripheral nervous system pharmacology, you must first establish a working knowledge of the peripheral nervous system itself. In particular, you need to know two basic types of information about peripheral nervous system function. First, you need to know the types of receptors through which the peripheral nervous system works when influencing the function of a specific organ. Second, you need to know what the normal response to activation of those receptors is. All of the information you need about peripheral nervous system function is reviewed in Chapter 13.

Once you understand the peripheral nervous system itself, you can go on to learn about peripheral nervous system drugs. Although learning about these drugs will require significant effort, the learning process itself is straightforward. To understand any particular peripheral nervous system drug, you need three types of information: (1) the type (or types) of receptor through which the drug acts, (2) the normal response to activation of those receptors, and (3) what the drug in question does to receptor function (i.e., does the drug increase or decrease receptor activation?). Armed with these three types of information, you can readily predict the major effects of any peripheral nervous system drug.

An example will illustrate this process. Let's consider a drug named *isoproterenol* as our example. The first information we need is the identity of the receptors at which isoproterenol acts. Isoproterenol acts at two types of receptors, named beta$_1$ and beta$_2$. Next, we need to know the normal responses to activation of these receptors. The most prominent responses to activation of beta$_1$ receptors are *increased heart rate* and *increased force of cardiac contraction*. The primary responses to activation of beta$_2$ receptors are *bronchial dilation* and *elevation of glucose levels in blood*. Lastly, we need to know whether isoproterenol increases or decreases the activation of beta$_1$ and beta$_2$ receptors. At both types of receptor, isoproterenol causes *activation*. Armed with these three primary pieces of information about isoproterenol, we can now predict the principal effects of this drug. By *activating* beta$_1$ and beta$_2$ receptors, isoproterenol can elicit three major responses: (1) increased cardiac output (by increasing heart rate and force of contraction), (2) dilation of the bronchi, and (3) elevation of blood glucose levels. Depending on the patient to whom this drug is given, these responses may be beneficial or detrimental.

From this example, you can see how easy it is to predict the effects of a peripheral nervous system drug. Accordingly, I strongly encourage you to take the approach suggested when studying these agents. That is, for each peripheral nervous system drug, you should learn (1) the identity of the receptors at which that drug acts, (2) the normal responses to activation of those receptors, and (3) whether the drug increases or decreases receptor activation.

⁙ KEY POINTS

- Except for local anesthetics, which suppress axonal conduction, all neuropharmacologic drugs act by altering synaptic transmission.
- Synaptic transmission consists of five basic steps: transmitter synthesis, transmitter storage, transmitter release, binding of transmitter to its receptors, and termination of transmitter action by dissociation of transmitter from the receptor followed by transmitter reuptake or degradation.

- Ultimately, the impact of a drug on a neuronally regulated process is dependent on the drug's ability to directly or indirectly alter receptor activity on target cells.
- Drugs can do one of two things to receptor function: they can increase receptor activation or they can decrease receptor activation.
- Drugs that increase transmitter synthesis increase receptor activation.
- Drugs that decrease transmitter synthesis decrease receptor activation.
- Drugs that promote synthesis of "super" transmitters increase receptor activation.
- Drugs that impede transmitter storage decrease receptor activation.
- Drugs that promote transmitter release increase receptor activation.
- Drugs that suppress transmitter release decrease receptor activation.

- Agonist drugs increase receptor activation.
- Antagonist drugs decrease receptor activation.
- Drugs that bind to receptors and enhance the actions of the natural transmitter at the receptor increase receptor activation.
- Drugs that block transmitter reuptake increase receptor activation.
- Drugs that inhibit transmitter degradation increase receptor activation.
- The presence of multiple receptor types increases our ability to produce selective drug effects.
- For each peripheral nervous system drug that you study, you should learn the identity of the receptors at which the drug acts, the normal responses to activation of those receptors, and whether the drug increases or decreases receptor activation.

Physiology of the Peripheral Nervous System

To understand peripheral nervous system drugs, we must first understand the peripheral nervous system itself. The purpose of this chapter is to help you develop that understanding.

It is not uncommon for students to be at least slightly apprehensive about studying the peripheral nervous system—especially the autonomic component. In fact, it is not uncommon for students who have studied this subject before to be thoroughly convinced that they will never, ever really understand it. This reaction is unfortunate in that, although there is a lot to know about the peripheral nervous system, the information is not terribly difficult. In this chapter, I take a nontraditional approach to teaching this material. Hopefully, this approach will facilitate your learning.

Since our ultimate goal concerns pharmacology—and not physiology—we do not address everything there is to know about the peripheral nervous system. Rather, discussion is limited to those aspects of peripheral nervous system physiology that have a direct bearing on your ability to understand drugs.

DIVISIONS OF THE NERVOUS SYSTEM

The nervous system has two main divisions, the *central nervous system* and the *peripheral nervous system.* The central nervous system is subdivided into the brain and the spinal cord.

The peripheral nervous system has two major subdivisions: (1) the *somatic motor system* and (2) the *autonomic nervous system.* The autonomic nervous system is further subdivided into the *parasympathetic nervous system* and the *sympathetic nervous system.* The somatic motor system controls movement of voluntary muscles, whereas the two subdivisions of the autonomic nervous system regulate many "involuntary" processes.

The autonomic nervous system is the principal focus of this chapter. The somatic motor system is also considered, but discussion is limited.

OVERVIEW OF AUTONOMIC NERVOUS SYSTEM FUNCTIONS

The autonomic nervous system has three principal functions: (1) regulation of the *heart,* (2) regulation of *secretory glands* (salivary, gastric, sweat, and bronchial glands), and (3) regulation of *smooth muscles* (muscles of the bronchi, blood vessels, urogenital system, and GI tract). These regulatory activities are shared between the sympathetic and parasympathetic divisions of the autonomic nervous system.

Functions of the Parasympathetic Nervous System

The parasympathetic nervous system performs seven regulatory functions that have particular relevance to drugs. Specifically, stimulation of appropriate parasympathetic nerves causes

- Slowing of heart rate
- Increased gastric secretion
- Emptying of the bladder
- Emptying of the bowel
- Focusing of the eye for near vision
- Constriction of the pupil
- Contraction of bronchial smooth muscle

Just how the parasympathetic nervous system elicits these responses is discussed later under *Functions of Cholinergic Receptor Subtypes.*

From the above we can see that the parasympathetic nervous system is concerned primarily with what might be called the "housekeeping" chores of the body (digestion of food and excretion of wastes). In addition, the system helps control vision and conserve energy (by reducing cardiac work).

As you might guess, therapeutic agents that work by altering parasympathetic nervous system function are used primarily for their effects on the GI tract, the bladder, and the eye. Occasionally, these drugs are also used for their effects on the heart and lungs.

A variety of poisons act by mimicking or blocking effects of parasympathetic stimulation. Among these are insecticides, nerve gases, and toxic compounds found in certain mushrooms and plants.

Functions of the Sympathetic Nervous System

The sympathetic nervous system has three main functions:

- Regulation of the cardiovascular system
- Regulation of body temperature
- Implementation of the "fight-or-flight" reaction

The sympathetic nervous system exerts multiple influences on the heart and blood vessels. Stimulation of sympathetic nerves to the heart increases cardiac output. Stimulation of sympathetic nerves to arterioles and veins causes vasoconstriction. Release of epinephrine from the adrenal medulla results in vasoconstriction in most vascular beds and vasodilation in certain others. By influencing the heart and blood vessels, the sympathetic nervous system can achieve three homeostatic objectives: (1) maintenance of blood flow to the brain, (2) redistribution of blood flow during exercise, and (3) compensation for loss of blood, primarily by causing vasoconstriction.

The sympathetic nervous system helps regulate body temperature in three ways: (1) By regulating blood flow to the skin, sympathetic nerves can increase or decrease heat loss. By *dilating* surface vessels, sympathetic nerves increase blood flow to the skin and thereby accelerate heat loss. Conversely, *constriction* of cutaneous vessels conserves heat. (2) Sympathetic nerves to sweat glands promote secretion of sweat, thereby helping the body cool. (3) By inducing piloerection (erection of hair), sympathetic nerves can promote heat conservation.

When we are faced with adversity, the sympathetic nervous system orchestrates the fight-or-flight response, which consists of

- Increased heart rate and blood pressure
- Shunting of blood away from the skin and viscera and into skeletal muscles
- Dilation of the bronchi to improve oxygenation
- Dilation of the pupils (perhaps to enhance visual acuity)
- Mobilization of stored energy, which provides glucose for the brain and fatty acids for muscles

The sensation of being "cold with fear" is brought on by the shunting of blood away from the skin. The phrase "wide-eyed with fear" may be based on pupillary dilation.

Many therapeutic agents produce their effects by altering functions under sympathetic control. Such drugs are used primarily for effects on the heart, blood vessels, and lungs. Agents that alter cardiovascular function are used to treat hy-

pertension, heart failure, angina pectoris, and other disorders. Drugs affecting the lungs are used primarily for asthma.

BASIC MECHANISMS BY WHICH THE AUTONOMIC NERVOUS SYSTEM REGULATES PHYSIOLOGIC PROCESSES

To understand how drugs influence processes under autonomic control, we must first understand how the autonomic nervous system itself regulates those activities. The basic mechanisms by which the autonomic nervous system regulates physiologic processes are discussed below.

Patterns of Innervation and Control

Most structures under autonomic control are innervated by sympathetic nerves *and* parasympathetic nerves. The relative influence of the sympathetic and parasympathetic nerves depends on the organ under consideration.

In many of the organs that receive dual innervation, the influence of sympathetic nerves *opposes* that of parasympathetic nerves. For example, in the heart, *sympathetic* nerves *increase* heart rate, whereas *parasympathetic* nerves *slow* heart rate (Fig. 13–1).

In some organs that receive nerves from both divisions of the autonomic nervous system, the effects of sympathetic and parasympathetic nerves are *complementary,* rather than opposite. For example, in the male reproductive system, erection is regulated by parasympathetic nerves while ejaculation is controlled by sympathetic nerves; if attempts at reproduction are to succeed, cooperative interaction of both systems is needed.

A few structures under autonomic control receive innervation from only one division. The principal example is blood vessels, which are innervated exclusively by sympathetic nerves.

In summary, there are three basic patterns of autonomic innervation and regulation:

- Innervation by *both* divisions of the autonomic nervous system in which the effects of the two divisions are *opposed*
- Innervation by *both* divisions of the autonomic nervous system in which the effects of the two divisions are *complementary*
- Innervation and regulation by *only one* division of the autonomic nervous system.

Feedback Regulation

Feedback regulation is a process that allows a system to adjust itself by responding to incoming information. Practically all physiologic processes are regulated at least in part by feedback control.

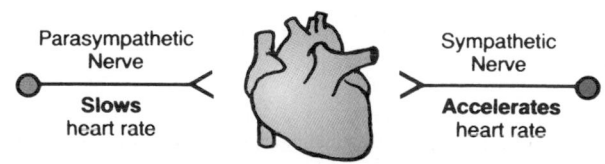

Figure 13–1 ■ Opposing effects of parasympathetic and sympathetic nerves.

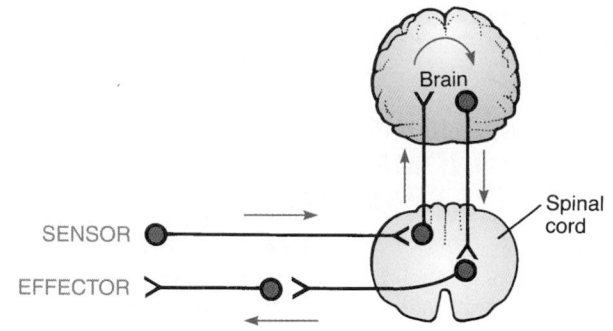

Figure 13–2 ■ Feedback loop of the autonomic nervous system.

Figure 13–2 depicts a feedback loop typical of those used by the autonomic nervous system. The main elements of this loop are (1) a *sensor*, (2) an *effector*, and (3) neurons connecting the sensor to the effector. The purpose of the sensor is to monitor the status of a physiologic process. Information picked up by the sensor is sent to the central nervous system (spinal cord and brain), where it is integrated with other relevant information. Signals (instructions for change) are then sent from the central nervous system along nerves of the autonomic system to the effector. In response to these instructions, the effector makes appropriate adjustments in the process. The entire procedure is termed a *reflex*.

Baroreceptor Reflex. From a pharmacologic perspective, the most important feedback loop of the autonomic nervous system is one that helps regulate blood pressure. This system is referred to as the *baroreceptor reflex*. (Baroreceptors are receptors that sense blood pressure.) This reflex is important to us because it frequently opposes our attempts to modify blood pressure with drugs.

Feedback (reflex) control of blood pressure is achieved as follows: (1) Baroreceptors located in the carotid sinus and aortic arch monitor changes in blood pressure and send this information to the brain. (2) In response to alterations in blood pressure, the brain sends impulses along nerves of the autonomic nervous system, instructing the heart and blood vessels to behave in such a way as to restore blood pressure to normalcy. Accordingly, when blood pressure *falls*, the baroreceptor reflex causes vasoconstriction and elevation of cardiac output so as to bring blood pressure back up. Conversely, when blood pressure *rises* too high, the baroreceptor reflex causes vasodilation and a reduction in cardiac output, thereby causing blood pressure to decline. The baroreceptor reflex is discussed in greater detail in Chapter 41 (Review of Hemodynamics).

Autonomic Tone

The term *autonomic tone* refers to the steady, day-to-day influence exerted by the autonomic nervous system on a particular organ or organ system. Autonomic tone provides a basal level of control over which reflex regulation is superimposed.

When an organ is innervated by both divisions of the autonomic nervous system, one division—either sympathetic or parasympathetic—provides most of the basal control, thereby obviating conflicting instruction. Recall that, when an organ receives nerves from both divisions of the autonomic nervous system, those nerves frequently exert opposing influences. If

both divisions were to send impulses simultaneously, the resultant conflicting instructions would be counterproductive. By having only one division of the autonomic nervous system provide the basal control to an organ, this possible source of conflict is avoided.

The branch of the autonomic nervous system that controls organ function most of the time is said to provide the *predominant tone* to that organ. *In most organs, the parasympathetic nervous system provides the predominant tone.* The vascular system, which is regulated almost exclusively by the *sympathetic* nervous system, is the principal exception to this general rule.

ANATOMIC CONSIDERATIONS

Although a great deal is known about the anatomy of the peripheral nervous system, very little of this information helps us understand peripheral nervous system drugs. The few details of peripheral nervous system anatomy that *do* pertain to pharmacology are summarized in Figure 13–3.

Parasympathetic Nervous System

Pharmacologically relevant aspects of parasympathetic anatomy are shown in Figure 13–3. Note that there are *two* neurons in the pathway leading from the spinal cord to organs innervated by parasympathetic nerves. The junction (synapse) between these two neurons occurs within a structure called a *ganglion*. (A ganglion is simply a lump created by a group of nerve cell bodies.) Not surprisingly, the neurons that go from the spinal cord to the parasympathetic ganglia are called *preganglionic neurons*, whereas the neurons that go from the ganglia to effector organs are called *postganglionic neurons*.

The anatomy of the parasympathetic nervous system offers two general sites at which drugs can act. These are (1) the synapses between preganglionic neurons and postganglionic neurons and (2) the junctions between postganglionic neurons and their effector organs.

Sympathetic Nervous System

Pharmacologically relevant aspects of sympathetic nervous system anatomy are illustrated in Figure 13–3. As you can see, these features are nearly identical to those of the parasympathetic nervous system. Like the parasympathetic nervous system, the sympathetic nervous system employs two neurons in the pathways leading from the spinal cord to organs under its control. As with the parasympathetic nervous system, the junctions between those neurons are located in *ganglia*. Neurons leading from the spinal cord to the sympathetic ganglia are termed *preganglionic neurons*, and neurons leading from ganglia to effector organs are termed *postganglionic neurons*.

The *medulla of the adrenal gland* is a feature of the sympathetic nervous system that requires comment. Although not a neuron per se, the adrenal medulla can be looked on as the functional equivalent of a postganglionic neuron of the sympathetic nervous system. (The adrenal medulla influences the body by releasing epinephrine into the bloodstream, which then produces effects much like those that occur in response to stimulation of postganglionic sympathetic nerves.) Since the adrenal medulla is similar in function to a postganglionic neuron, it is appropriate to refer to the nerve

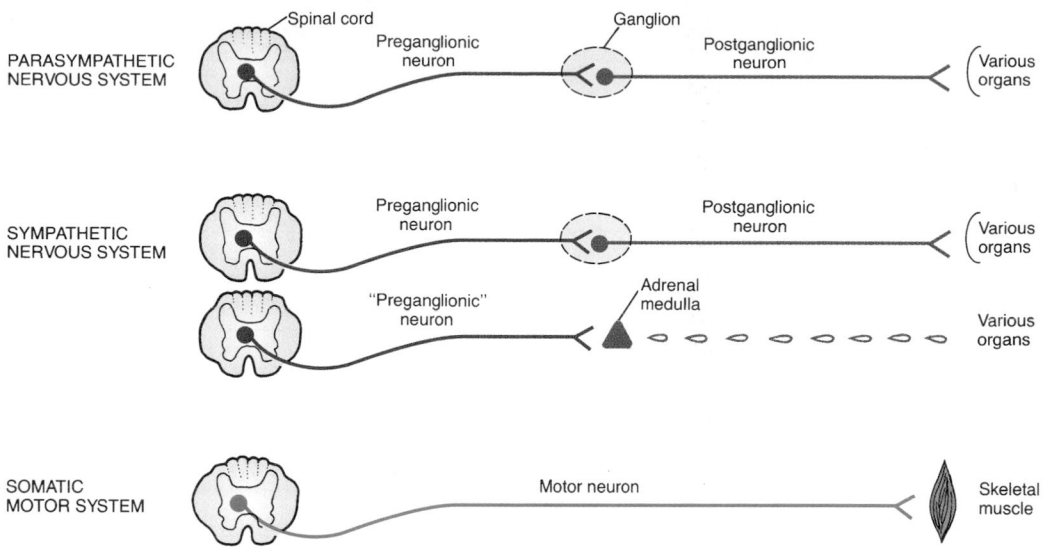

Figure 13–3 ■ **The basic anatomy of the parasympathetic and sympathetic nervous systems and the somatic motor system.**

leading from the spinal cord to the adrenal as preganglionic, even though there is no ganglion, as such, in this pathway.

As with the parasympathetic nervous system, drugs that affect the sympathetic nervous system have two general sites of action: (1) the synapses between preganglionic and postganglionic neurons (including the adrenal medulla), and (2) the junctions between postganglionic neurons and their effector organs.

Somatic Motor System

Pharmacologically relevant anatomy of the somatic motor system is depicted in Figure 13–3. Note that there is *only one* neuron in the pathway from the spinal cord to the muscles innervated by somatic motor nerves. Because this pathway contains only one neuron, peripherally acting drugs that affect somatic motor system function have only one site of action: the *neuromuscular junction* (i.e., the junction between the somatic motor nerve and the muscle).

INTRODUCTION TO TRANSMITTERS OF THE PERIPHERAL NERVOUS SYSTEM

The peripheral nervous system employs three neurotransmitters: *acetylcholine, norepinephrine,* and *epinephrine.* Any given junction in the peripheral nervous system uses only one of these transmitter substances. A fourth compound—*dopamine*—may also serve as a peripheral nervous system transmitter, but this role has not been demonstrated conclusively.

To understand peripheral nervous system pharmacology, it is necessary to know the identity of the transmitter employed at each of the junctions of the peripheral nervous system. This information is summarized in Figure 13–4.

As the figure indicates, *acetylcholine* is the transmitter employed at most junctions of the peripheral nervous system. Acetylcholine is the transmitter released by (1) all preganglionic neurons of the parasympathetic nervous system, (2) all preganglionic neurons of the sympathetic nervous sys-

tem, (3) all postganglionic neurons of the parasympathetic nervous system, (4) all motor neurons to skeletal muscles, and (5) most postganglionic neurons of the sympathetic nervous system that go to sweat glands.

Norepinephrine is the transmitter released by practically all postganglionic neurons of the sympathetic nervous system. The only exceptions are the postganglionic sympathetic neurons that go to sweat glands, which employ acetylcholine as their transmitter.

Epinephrine is the major transmitter released by the adrenal medulla. (The adrenal medulla also releases some norepinephrine.)

Much of what follows in this chapter is based on the information summarized in Figure 13–4. Accordingly, I strongly urge you to learn (memorize) this information now.

INTRODUCTION TO RECEPTORS OF THE PERIPHERAL NERVOUS SYSTEM

The peripheral nervous system works through several different types of receptors. Understanding of these receptors is central to understanding of peripheral nervous system pharmacology. All effort that you invest in learning about these receptors now will be richly rewarded as we discuss peripheral nervous system drugs in the chapters that follow.

Primary Receptor Types: Cholinergic Receptors and Adrenergic Receptors

There are two basic categories of receptors associated with the peripheral nervous system: *cholinergic receptors* and *adrenergic receptors.* Cholinergic receptors are defined as receptors that mediate responses to acetylcholine. These receptors mediate responses at all junctions where acetylcholine is the transmitter. Adrenergic receptors are defined as receptors that mediate responses to epinephrine (adrenaline) and norepinephrine. These receptors mediate responses at all junctions where norepinephrine or epinephrine is the transmitter.

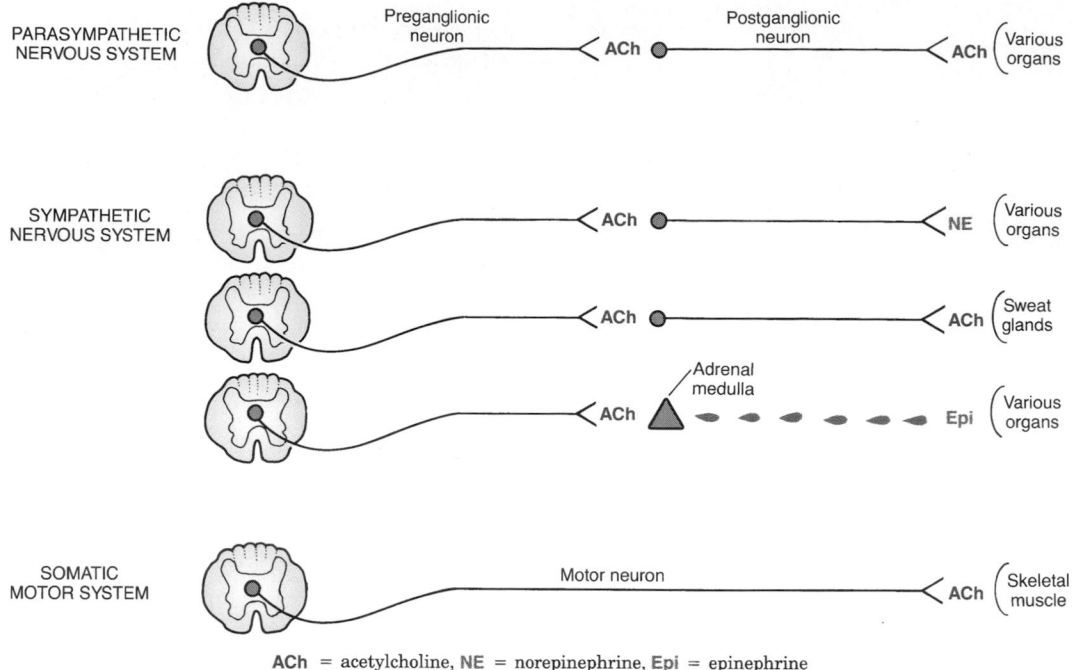

ACh = acetylcholine, **NE** = norepinephrine, **Epi** = epinephrine

Figure 13–4 ■ **Transmitters employed at specific junctions of the peripheral nervous system.** Summary:
1. *All preganglionic* neurons of the *parasympathetic* and *sympathetic* nervous systems release *acetylcholine* as their transmitter.
2. *All postganglionic* neurons of the *parasympathetic* nervous system release *acetylcholine* as their transmitter.
3. *Most postganglionic* neurons of the *sympathetic* nervous system release *norepinephrine* as their transmitter.
4. *Postganglionic* neurons of the sympathetic nervous system that innervate *sweat glands* release *acetylcholine* as their transmitter.
5. *Epinephrine* is the principal transmitter released by the *adrenal medulla*.
6. *All motor neurons* to *skeletal muscles* release *acetylcholine* as their transmitter.

Subtypes of Cholinergic and Adrenergic Receptors

Not all cholinergic receptors are the same; likewise, not all adrenergic receptors are the same. For each of these two major receptor classes there are receptor subtypes. There are three major subtypes of cholinergic receptors, referred to as nicotinic$_N$, nicotinic$_M$, and muscarinic.* There are four major subtypes of adrenergic receptors, referred to as alpha$_1$, alpha$_2$, beta$_1$, and beta$_2$.

In addition to the four major subtypes of adrenergic receptors, there is another adrenergic receptor type, referred to as the *dopamine* receptor. Although dopamine receptors are classified as adrenergic, these receptors do not respond to epinephrine or norepinephrine. Rather, they respond only to dopamine, a neurotransmitter found primarily in the central nervous system.

---

*Evidence gathered in recent years indicates that not all muscarinic receptors are the same. That is, like nicotinic receptors, muscarinic receptors come in subtypes. Five subtypes have been identified. However, since our understanding of these receptors is relatively new, and since drugs that can selectively alter their function are few, we will defer discussion of muscarinic subtypes to a future edition of this text.

EXPLORING THE CONCEPT OF RECEPTOR SUBTYPES

The concept of receptor subtypes is important and potentially confusing. In this section we discuss what a receptor subtype is and why receptor subtypes matter to us.

What Do We Mean by the Term *Receptor Subtype?*

Receptors that respond to the same transmitter but nonetheless are different from one another would be called receptor subtypes. For example, peripheral receptors that respond to acetylcholine can be found (1) in ganglia of the autonomic nervous system, (2) at neuromuscular junctions, and (3) on organs regulated by the parasympathetic nervous system. However, even though all of these receptors can be activated by acetylcholine, there is clear evidence that the receptors at these three sites are, in fact, different from one another. Hence, although all of these receptors belong to the same major receptor category (cholinergic), they are sufficiently different as to constitute distinct receptor subtypes.

How Do We Know That Receptor Subtypes Exist?

Historically, our knowledge of receptor subtypes came from observing responses to drugs. In fact, were it not for drugs, receptor subtypes might never have been discovered.

The data in Table 13–1 illustrate the types of drug responses that led to the realization that receptor subtypes exist. These data summarize the results of an experiment designed to study the effects of a natural transmitter (acetylcholine) and a series of drugs (nicotine, muscarine, *d*-tubocurarine, and atropine) on two tissues: skeletal muscle and ciliary muscle. (The ciliary muscle is the muscle responsible for focusing the eye for near vision.) As these data indicate, although skeletal muscle and ciliary muscle both contract in response to acetylcholine, these tissues differ in their responses to drugs. In the discussion below, we examine the selective responses of these tissues to drugs and see how those responses reveal the existence of receptor subtypes.

At synapses on skeletal muscle and ciliary muscle, acetylcholine is the transmitter employed by neurons to elicit contraction. Since both types of muscle respond to acetylcholine, it is safe to conclude that both muscles have receptors for this substance. Since acetylcholine is the natural transmitter for these receptors, we would classify these receptors as *cholinergic*.

What do the effects of nicotine on skeletal muscle and ciliary muscle suggest? The effects of nicotine on these muscles suggest four possible conclusions: (1) Since skeletal muscle contracts when nicotine is applied, we can conclude that skeletal muscle has receptors at which nicotine can act. (2) Since ciliary muscle does *not* respond to nicotine, we can tentatively conclude that ciliary muscle does not have receptors for nicotine. (3) Since nicotine mimics the effects of acetylcholine on skeletal muscle, we can conclude that nicotine may act at the same receptors on skeletal muscle as does acetylcholine. (4) Since both types of muscle have receptors for acetylcholine, and since nicotine appears to act only at the acetylcholine receptors on skeletal muscle, we can tentatively conclude that the acetylcholine receptors on skeletal muscle are different from the acetylcholine receptors on ciliary muscle.

What do the responses to muscarine suggest? The conclusions that can be drawn regarding responses to muscarine are exactly parallel to those drawn for nicotine. These conclusions are: (1) ciliary muscle has receptors that respond to muscarine, (2) skeletal muscle may not have receptors for muscarine, (3) muscarine may be acting at the same receptors on ciliary muscle as does acetylcholine, and (4) the receptors for acetylcholine on ciliary muscle may be different from the receptors for acetylcholine on skeletal muscle.

The responses of skeletal muscle and ciliary muscle to nicotine and muscarine suggest, but do not prove, that the cholinergic receptors on these two tissues are different; the responses of these two tissues to d-*tubocurarine* and *atropine*, both of which are receptor *blocking agents*, eliminate any doubts as to the presence of cholinergic receptor subtypes. When both types of muscle are pretreated with *d*-tubocurarine and then exposed to acetylcholine, the response to acetylcholine is blocked—but only in skeletal muscle. Tubocurarine pretreatment does not reduce the ability of acetylcholine to stimulate ciliary muscle. Conversely, pretreatment with atropine selectively blocks the response to acetylcholine in ciliary muscle; however, atropine does nothing to prevent acetyl-

TABLE 13–1 ▪ Responses of Skeletal Muscle and Ciliary Muscle to a Series of Drugs

Drug	Response	
	Skeletal Muscle	Ciliary Muscle
Acetylcholine	Contraction	Contraction
Nicotine	Contraction	No response
Muscarine	No response	Contraction
Acetylcholine		
After *d*-tubocurarine	No response	Contraction
After atropine	Contraction	No response

choline from stimulating receptors on skeletal muscle. Since tubocurarine can selectively block cholinergic receptors in skeletal muscle, whereas atropine can selectively block cholinergic receptors in ciliary muscle, we can conclude with certainty that the receptors for acetylcholine in these two types of muscle must be different from each other.

The data just discussed illustrate the essential role of drugs in revealing the presence of receptor subtypes. If acetylcholine were the only probe that we had, all that we would have been able to observe is that both skeletal muscle and ciliary muscle can respond to this agent. This simple observation would provide no basis for suspecting that the receptors for acetylcholine in these two tissues were different. It is only through the use of selectively acting drugs that the presence of receptor subtypes was initially revealed.

Today, the technology for identifying receptors and their subtypes is extremely sophisticated—not that studies like the one just discussed are no longer of value. In addition to performing traditional drug-based studies, scientists are now cloning receptors using DNA hybridization technology. As you can imagine, this allows us to understand receptors in ways that were unthinkable in the past.*

How Can Drugs Be More Selective Than Natural Transmitters at Receptor Subtypes?

Drugs achieve their selectivity for receptor subtypes by having structures that are different from those of natural transmitters. The relationship between structure and receptor selectivity is illustrated in Figure 13–5. In this figure, cartoon drawings are used to represent drugs (nicotine and muscarine), receptor subtypes (nicotinic and muscarinic), and acetylcholine (the natural transmitter at nicotinic and muscarinic receptors). From the structures shown, we can easily imagine how acetylcholine is able to interact with both kinds of receptor subtypes, whereas nicotine and muscarine can interact only with the receptor subtypes whose structure is complementary to their own. By synthesizing chemicals that are structurally related to natural transmitters, pharmaceutical scientists have been able

---

*In addition to revealing exciting new information about receptors previously identified, this spiffy technology is so powerful that new receptors and receptor subtypes are being discovered at a dizzying rate. Which means, of course, that students in the future will have many more receptors to contend with than you do. So, when it seems like you're working awfully hard to master the information on receptors in this chapter and the ones that follow, look on the bright side—you could be studying pharmacology 10 years from now.

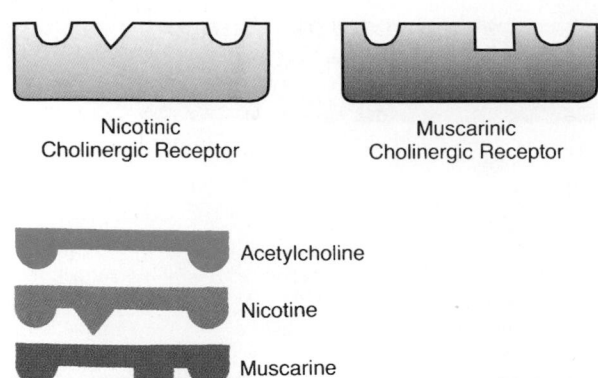

Figure 13–5 ■ Drug structure and receptor selectivity. These cartoon figures illustrate the relationship between structure and receptor selectivity. The structure of acetylcholine allows this transmitter to interact with both receptor subtypes. In contrast, because of their unique configurations, nicotine and muscarine are selective for the cholinergic receptor subtypes whose structure complements their own.

to produce drugs that are more selective for specific receptor subtypes than are the natural transmitters that act at those sites.

Why Do Receptor Subtypes Exist?

It is not unreasonable for us to wonder why Mother Nature bothered to create more than one type of receptor for any given transmitter. Unfortunately, a definitive answer to that question will have to come from Mother Nature herself. That is, the physiologic benefits of having multiple receptor subtypes for the same transmitter are not immediately obvious. In fact, as noted earlier, were it not for drugs, we probably wouldn't know that receptor subtypes existed at all.

Do Receptor Subtypes Matter to Us? You Bet!

Although receptor subtypes are of uncertain physiologic relevance, from the viewpoint of therapeutics, receptor subtypes are invaluable. The presence of receptor subtypes makes possible a dramatic increase in drug selectivity. For example, thanks to the existence of subtypes of cholinergic receptors (and the development of drugs selective for those receptor subtypes), it is possible to influence the activity of certain cholinergic receptors (e.g., receptors of the neuromuscular junction) without altering the activity of all other cholinergic receptors (e.g., the cholinergic receptors found in all autonomic ganglia and all target organs of the parasympathetic nervous system). Were it not for the existence of receptor subtypes, a drug that acted on cholinergic receptors at one site would alter the activity of cholinergic receptors at all other sites. Clearly, the existence of receptor subtypes for a particular transmitter makes possible drug actions that are much more selective than could be achieved if all of the receptors for that transmitter were the same.

LOCATIONS OF RECEPTOR SUBTYPES

Since many of the drugs discussed in the following chapters are selective for specific receptor subtypes, knowledge of the sites at which specific receptor subtypes are located will help

us predict which organs a drug will affect. Accordingly, in laying our foundation for studying peripheral nervous system drugs, it is important to learn the sites at which the subtypes of adrenergic and cholinergic receptors are located. This information is summarized in Figure 13–6. You will find it very helpful to master the contents of this figure before proceeding much further. (In the interest of minimizing confusion, subtypes of adrenergic receptors in Figure 13–6 are listed simply as alpha and beta rather than as $alpha_1$, $alpha_2$, $beta_1$, and $beta_2$. The locations of all four subtypes of adrenergic receptors are discussed in the section that follows.)

FUNCTIONS OF CHOLINERGIC AND ADRENERGIC RECEPTOR SUBTYPES

Knowledge of receptor function is an absolute requirement for understanding peripheral nervous system drugs. By knowing the receptors at which a drug acts, and by knowing what those receptors do, we can predict the major effects of any peripheral nervous system drug.

Tables 13–2 and 13–3 summarize the pharmacologically relevant functions of peripheral nervous system receptors. Table 13–2 summarizes responses elicited by activation of cholinergic receptor subtypes. Table 13–3 summarizes responses to activation of adrenergic receptor subtypes. Before attempting to study specific peripheral nervous system drugs, you should master (memorize) the contents of the appropriate table. Table 13–2 should be mastered before studying cholinergic drugs (Chapters 14, 15, and 16). Table 13–3 should be mastered before studying adrenergic drugs (Chapters 17, 18, and 19). If you study these tables in preparation for learning about peripheral nervous system drugs, you will find the process of learning the pharmacology relatively simple (and perhaps even enjoyable). Conversely, if you attempt to study the pharmacology without first mastering the appropriate table, you are likely to meet with frustration.

Functions of Cholinergic Receptor Subtypes

Table 13–2 summarizes the pharmacologically relevant responses to activation of the three major subtypes of cholinergic receptors: nicotinic$_N$, nicotinic$_M$, and muscarinic. Please commit the information in this table to memory.

We can group responses to cholinergic receptor activation into three major categories based on the subtype of receptor involved:

■ Activation of *nicotinic$_N$* (neuronal) receptors promotes *ganglionic transmission* at all ganglia of the sympathetic and parasympathetic nervous systems. In addition, activation of nicotinic$_N$ receptors promotes *release of epinephrine from the adrenal medulla.*

■ Activation of *nicotinic$_M$* (muscle) receptors causes *contraction of skeletal muscle.*

■ Activation of *muscarinic* receptors, which are located on target organs of the parasympathetic nervous system, elicits an appropriate response from the organ involved. Specifically, muscarinic activation causes (1) increased glandular secretions (from pulmonary, gastric, intestinal, and sweat glands);

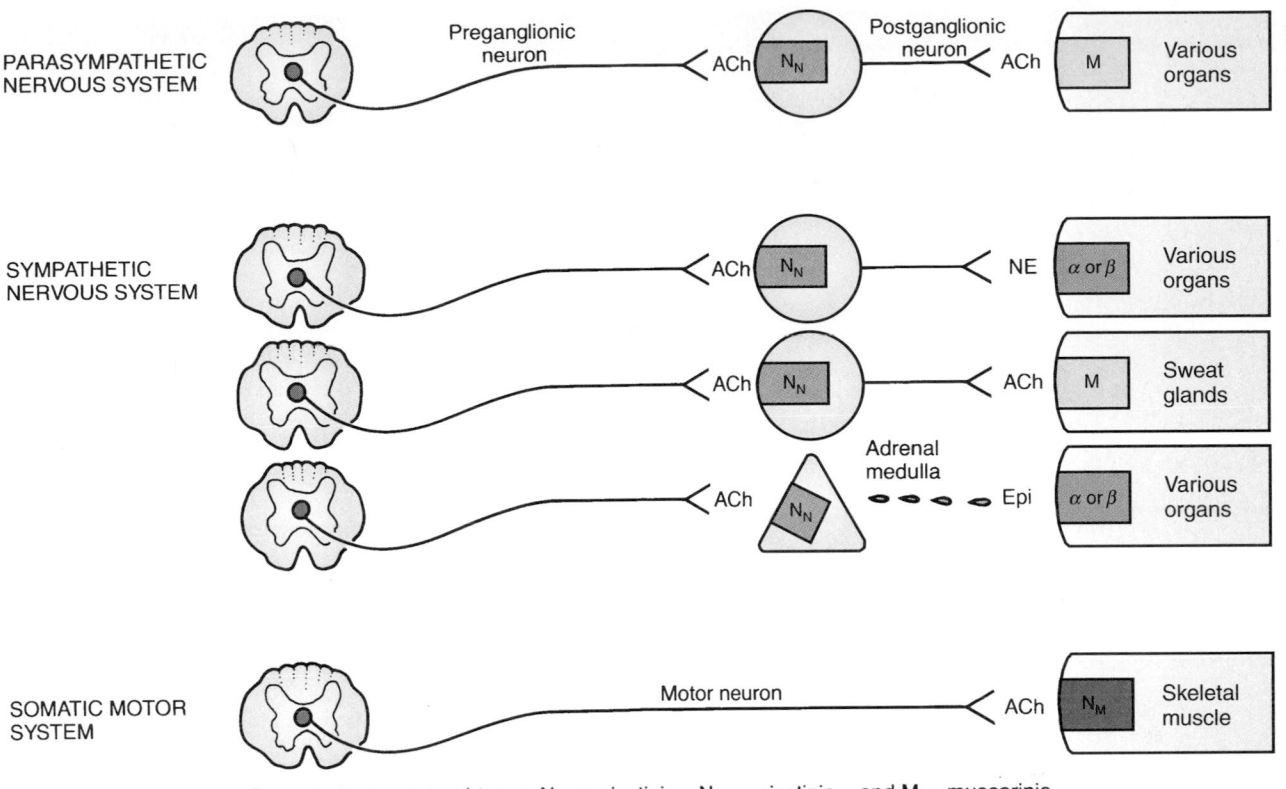

Cholinergic receptor subtypes: N_N = nicotinic$_N$, N_M = nicotinic$_M$, and M = muscarinic.
Adrenergic receptor subtypes: α = alpha and β = beta.

Figure 13–6 ■ Locations of cholinergic and adrenergic receptor subtypes.
Summary:
1. *Nicotinic$_N$* receptors are located on the *cell bodies of all postganglionic neurons* of the *parasympathetic* and *sympathetic* nervous systems. *Nicotinic$_N$* receptors are also located on cells of the *adrenal medulla*.
2. *Nicotinic$_M$* receptors are located on *skeletal muscle*.
3. *Muscarinic* receptors are located on *all organs* regulated by the *parasympathetic* nervous system (i.e., organs innervated by postganglionic parasympathetic nerves). *Muscarinic* receptors are also located on *sweat glands*.
4. *Adrenergic receptors*—alpha, beta, or both—are located on *all organs* (except sweat glands) regulated by the *sympathetic* nervous system (i.e., organs innervated by postganglionic sympathetic nerves). *Adrenergic* receptors are also located on organs regulated by epinephrine released from the *adrenal medulla*.

(2) contraction of smooth muscle in the bronchi, bladder, and GI tract; (3) slowing of heart rate; (4) contraction of the sphincter muscle of the iris, resulting in miosis (reduction in pupillary diameter); and (5) contraction of the ciliary muscle of the eye, causing the lens to focus for near vision.

Muscarinic cholinergic receptors on blood vessels require additional comment. These receptors are not associated with the nervous system in any way. That is, no nerves terminate at vascular muscarinic receptors. It is not at all clear as to how, or even if, these receptors are activated physiologically. However, regardless of their physiologic relevance, the cholinergic receptors on blood vessels do have *pharmacologic* significance, in that drugs that are able to activate these receptors will cause vasodilation, which in turn will cause blood pressure to fall.

Functions of Adrenergic Receptor Subtypes

Adrenergic receptor subtypes and their functions are summarized in Table 13–3. You should commit this information to memory.

Alpha₁ Receptors

Alpha₁ receptors are located in the eyes, blood vessels, male sex organs, bladder, and prostatic capsule.

Ocular alpha₁ receptors are present on the *radial muscle* of the iris. Activation of these receptors leads to mydriasis (dilation of the pupil). As depicted in Table 13–3, the fibers of the radial muscle are arranged like the spokes of a wheel. Because of this configuration, contraction of the radial muscle causes the pupil to enlarge. (If you have difficulty remembering that *mydriasis* means pupillary enlargement, whereas

TABLE 13–2 ■ Functions of Peripheral Cholinergic Receptor Subtypes

Receptor Subtype	Location	Response to Receptor Activation
Nicotinic$_N$	All autonomic nervous system ganglia and the adrenal medulla	Stimulation of parasympathetic and sympathetic postganglionic nerves and release of epinephrine from the adrenal medulla
Nicotinic$_M$	Neuromuscular junction	Contraction of skeletal muscle
Muscarinic	All parasympathetic target organs:	
	Eye	Contraction of the ciliary muscle focuses the lens for near vision Contraction of the iris sphincter muscle causes miosis (decreased pupil diameter)
	Heart	Decreased rate
	Lung	Constriction of bronchi Promotion of secretions
	Bladder	Voiding
	GI tract	Salivation Increased gastric secretions Increased intestinal tone and motility Defecation
	Sweat glands*	Generalized sweating
	Sex organs	Erection
	Blood vessels†	Vasodilation

*Although sweating is due primarily to stimulation of muscarinic receptors by acetylcholine, the nerves that supply acetylcholine to sweat glands belong to the sympathetic nervous system rather than the parasympathetic nervous system.
†Cholinergic receptors on blood vessels are not associated with the nervous system.

miosis means pupillary constriction, just remember that mydriasis [enlargement] is a bigger word than miosis.)

Activation of alpha$_1$ receptors in *blood vessels* produces *vasoconstriction.* Alpha$_1$ receptors are present on veins and on arterioles in many capillary beds.

Activation of alpha$_1$ receptors in the sexual apparatus of males causes *ejaculation.*

Activation of alpha$_1$ receptors in smooth muscle of the *bladder neck* and *prostatic capsule* causes *contraction.*

Alpha$_2$ Receptors

Alpha$_2$ receptors of the peripheral nervous system are located on *nerve terminals* (see Table 13–3) and not on the organs innervated by the autonomic nervous system. Because alpha$_2$ receptors are located on nerve terminals, these receptors are referred to as *presynaptic* or *prejunctional.* The function of these receptors is to regulate transmitter release. As depicted in Table 13–3, norepinephrine can bind to alpha$_2$ receptors located on the same neuron from which it was released. The consequence of this norepinephrine-receptor interaction is suppression of further norepinephrine release. Hence, presynaptic alpha$_2$ receptors can help reduce transmitter release when too much transmitter has accumulated in the synaptic gap. Drug effects resulting from activation of *peripheral* alpha$_2$ receptors are of minimal clinical significance.

Alpha$_2$ receptors are also present in the central nervous system. In contrast to peripheral alpha$_2$ receptors, central alpha$_2$ receptors are therapeutically relevant. We will consider these receptors in later chapters.

Beta$_1$ Receptors

Beta$_1$ receptors are located in the heart and the kidney. *Cardiac* beta$_1$ receptors have great therapeutic significance. Activation of these receptors increases *heart rate, force of contraction,* and *velocity of impulse conduction through the atrioventricular (AV) node.*

Activation of beta$_1$ receptors in the *kidney* causes release of *renin* into the blood. Since renin promotes synthesis of angiotensin, a powerful vasoconstrictor, activation of renal beta$_1$ receptors is a means by which the nervous system helps elevate blood pressure. (The role of renin in the regulation of blood pressure is discussed in depth in Chapter 42.)

Beta$_2$ Receptors

Beta$_2$ receptors mediate several important processes. Activation of beta$_2$ receptors in the lung leads to *bronchial dilation.* Activation of beta$_2$ receptors in the uterus causes *relaxation of uterine smooth muscle.* Activation of beta$_2$ receptors in arterioles of the heart, lungs, and skeletal muscles causes *va-*

TABLE 13–3 ⊞■ Functions of Peripheral Adrenergic Receptor Subtypes

Receptor Subtype	Location	Response to Receptor Activation
Alpha₁	Eye	Contraction of the radial muscle of the iris causes mydriasis (increased pupil size)
	Arterioles Skin Viscera Mucous membranes	Constriction
	Veins	Constriction
	Sex organs, male	Ejaculation
	Bladder neck and prostatic capsule	Contraction
Alpha₂	Presynaptic nerve terminals*	Inhibition of transmitter release
Beta₁	Heart	Increased rate Increased force of contraction Increased AV conduction velocity
	Kidney	Renin release
Beta₂	Arterioles Heart Lung Skeletal muscle	Dilation
	Bronchi	Dilation
	Uterus	Relaxation
	Liver	Glycogenolysis
	Skeletal muscle	Enhanced contraction, glycogenolysis
Dopamine	Kidney	Dilation of kidney vasculature

AV = atrioventricular, NE = norepinephrine, R = receptor.
*Alpha₂ receptors in the central nervous system are postsynaptic.

sodilation (an effect opposite to that of alpha₁ activation). Activation of beta₂ receptors in the liver and skeletal muscle promotes *glycogenolysis* (breakdown of glycogen into glucose), thereby increasing blood levels of glucose. In addition, activation of beta₂ receptors in skeletal muscle enhances contraction.

Dopamine Receptors

In the periphery, the only dopamine receptors of clinical significance are located in the vasculature of the kidney. Activation of these receptors *dilates renal blood vessels,* thereby enhancing renal perfusion.

In the central nervous system, receptors for dopamine are of great therapeutic significance. The functions of these receptors are discussed in Chapter 21 (Drugs for Parkinson's Disease) and Chapter 30 (Antipsychotic Agents).

RECEPTOR SPECIFICITY OF THE ADRENERGIC TRANSMITTERS

The receptor specificity of adrenergic transmitters is more complex than the receptor specificity of acetylcholine. Whereas acetylcholine can activate all three subtypes of cholinergic receptors, not every adrenergic transmitter (epinephrine, norepinephrine, dopamine) can interact with each of the five subtypes of adrenergic receptors.

Receptor specificity of adrenergic transmitters is as follows: (1) *epinephrine* can activate all alpha and beta receptors, but not dopamine receptors; (2) *norepinephrine* can activate alpha₁, alpha₂, and beta₁ receptors, but not beta₂ or dopamine receptors; and (3) *dopamine* can activate alpha₁, beta₁, and dopamine receptors. (Note that dopamine itself is the only transmitter capable of activating dopamine receptors.) Receptor specificity of the adrenergic transmitters is summarized in Table 13–4.

TABLE 13–4 ■ Receptor Specificity of Adrenergic Transmitters*					
	Adrenergic Receptor Subtype				
Transmitter	**Alpha₁**	**Alpha₂**	**Beta₁**	**Beta₂**	**Dopamine**
Epinephrine	←			→	
Norepinephrine	←			→	
Dopamine	←	→	←	→	← →

*Arrows indicate the range of receptors that the transmitters can activate.

Knowing that epinephrine is the only transmitter that acts at beta₂ receptors can serve as an aid to remembering the functions of this receptor subtype. Recall that epinephrine is released from the adrenal medulla (and not from neurons) and that the function of epinephrine is to prepare the body for fight or flight. Accordingly, since epinephrine is the only transmitter that activates beta₂ receptors, and since epinephrine is released only in preparation for fight or flight, times of fight or flight will be the only occasions on which beta₂ receptors will undergo significant physiologic activation. As it turns out, the physiologic changes elicited by beta₂ activation are precisely those needed for success in the fight-or-flight response. Specifically, activation of beta₂ receptors will cause (1) dilation of blood vessels in the heart, lungs, and skeletal muscles, thereby increasing blood flow to these organs; (2) dilation of the bronchi, thereby increasing oxygenation; (3) increased glycogenolysis, thereby increasing available energy; and (4) relaxation of uterine muscle, thereby preventing delivery (a process that would be inconvenient for a pregnant woman preparing to fight or flee). Hence, if you think of the physiologic requirements for success during fight or flight, you will have a good picture of the responses that beta₂ activation can cause.

TRANSMITTER LIFE CYCLES

In this section we consider the life cycles of acetylcholine, norepinephrine, and epinephrine. Since a number of drugs produce their effects by interfering with specific phases of the transmitters' life cycles, knowledge of these cycles helps us understand drug actions.

Life Cycle of Acetylcholine

The life cycle of acetylcholine (ACh) is depicted in Figure 13–7. The cycle begins with the synthesis of ACh from two precursors: choline and acetylcoenzyme A. Following synthesis, ACh is stored in vesicles and is later released in response to an action potential. Following release, ACh binds to receptors (nicotinic_N, nicotinic_M, or muscarinic) located on the postjunctional cell. Upon dissociating from its receptors, ACh is destroyed almost instantaneously by *acetylcholinesterase* (AChE), an enzyme present in abundance on the surface of the postjunctional cell. AChE degrades ACh into two inactive products: acetate and choline. Uptake of choline into the cholinergic nerve terminal completes the life cycle of ACh. Note that an inactive substance (choline), and not the active transmitter (acetylcholine), is taken back up for reuse.

Therapeutic and toxic agents can interfere with the ACh life cycle at several points. Botulinum toxin inhibits ACh release. A number of medicines and poisons act at cholinergic receptors to mimic or block the actions of ACh. Several therapeutic and toxic agents act by inhibiting AChE, thereby causing ACh to accumulate in the junctional gap.

Life Cycle of Norepinephrine

The life cycle of norepinephrine is depicted in Figure 13–8. As indicated, the cycle begins with synthesis of norepinephrine from a series of precursors. The final step of synthesis takes place within vesicles, where norepinephrine is then stored prior to release. Following release, norepinephrine binds to

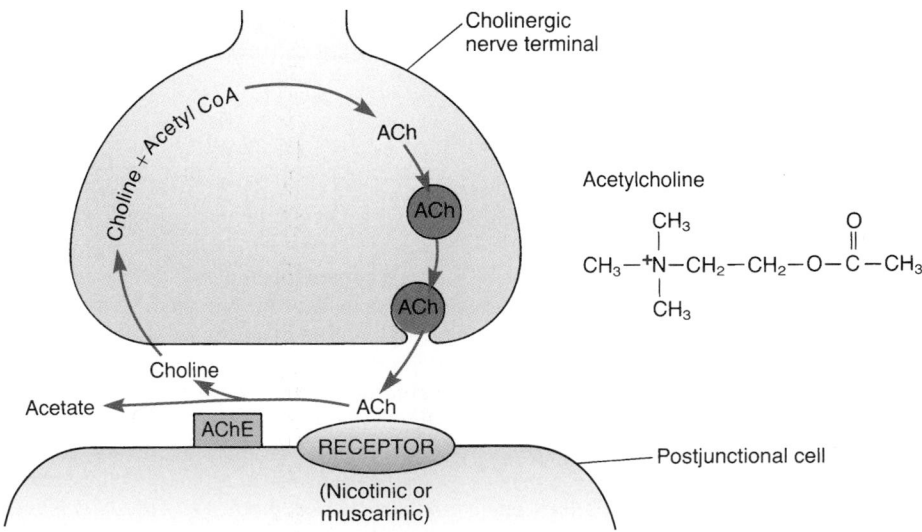

Figure 13–7 ■ Life cycle of acetylcholine.
Note that transmission is terminated by enzymatic degradation of ACh and not by uptake of intact ACh back into the nerve terminal. (ACh = acetylcholine, AChE = acetylcholinesterase, Acetyl CoA = acetyl coenzyme A)

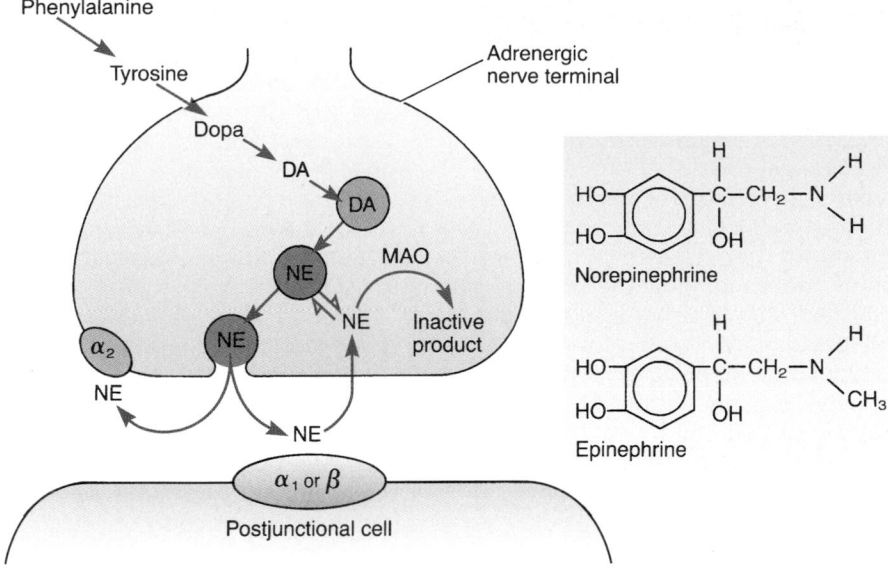

Figure 13–8 ▪ **Life cycle of norepinephrine.**
Note that transmission is terminated by reuptake of NE into the nerve terminal and not by enzymatic degradation. Note also the structural similarity between epinephrine and norepinephrine. (DA = dopamine, NE = norepinephrine, MAO = monoamine oxidase)

adrenergic receptors. As shown in the figure, norepinephrine can interact with *postsynaptic* alpha$_1$ and beta receptors and with *presynaptic* alpha$_2$ receptors. Transmission is terminated by *reuptake* of norepinephrine back into the nerve terminal. (Note that the termination process for norepinephrine differs from that for acetylcholine, whose effects are terminated by enzymatic degradation rather than reuptake.) Following reuptake, norepinephrine can undergo one of two fates: (1) uptake into vesicles for reuse or (2) inactivation by monoamine oxidase (MAO), an enzyme found in the nerve terminal.

Practically every step in the life cycle of norepinephrine can be altered by therapeutic agents. We have drugs that alter the synthesis, storage, and release of norepinephrine; we have drugs that act at adrenergic receptors to mimic or block the effects of norepinephrine; we have drugs, such as cocaine and tricyclic antidepressants, that inhibit the reuptake of norepinephrine (and thereby intensify transmission); and we have drugs that inhibit the breakdown of norepinephrine by MAO, causing an increase in the amount of transmitter available for release.

Life Cycle of Epinephrine

The life cycle of epinephrine is much like that of norepinephrine—although there are significant differences. The cycle begins with synthesis of epinephrine within chromaffin cells of the adrenal medulla. These cells produce epinephrine by first making norepinephrine, which is then converted enzymatically to epinephrine. (Since sympathetic neurons lack the enzyme needed to convert norepinephrine to epinephrine, epinephrine is not produced in sympathetic nerves.) Following synthesis, epinephrine is stored in vesicles to await release. Once released, epinephrine travels via the bloodstream to target organs throughout the body. Termination of epinephrine's actions is accomplished primarily by hepatic metabolism, and not by uptake into nerves.

▪▪ KEY POINTS

- The peripheral nervous system has two major divisions: the autonomic nervous system and the somatic motor system.
- The autonomic nervous system has two major divisions: the sympathetic nervous system and the parasympathetic nervous system.
- The parasympathetic nervous system has several functions relevant to pharmacology: it slows heart rate, increases gastric secretion, empties the bladder and bowel, focuses the eye for near vision, constricts the pupil, and contracts bronchial smooth muscle.
- Principal functions of the sympathetic nervous system are regulation of the cardiovascular system, regulation of body temperature, and implementation of the fight-or-flight response.
- In some organs (e.g., the heart), sympathetic and parasympathetic nerves have opposing effects; in other organs (e.g., male sex organs), the sympathetic and parasympathetic systems have complementary effects; and in still other organs (most notably the blood vessels), function is regulated by only one branch of the autonomic nervous system.
- The baroreceptor reflex helps regulate blood pressure.
- In most organs regulated by the autonomic nervous system, the parasympathetic nervous system provides the dominant tone.
- In blood vessels, the sympathetic nervous system provides the dominant tone.
- Pathways from the spinal cord to organs under sympathetic and parasympathetic control consist of two

neurons: a preganglionic neuron and a postganglionic neuron.

■ The adrenal medulla is the functional equivalent of a postganglionic sympathetic neuron.

■ Somatic motor pathways from the spinal cord to skeletal muscles have only one neuron.

■ The peripheral nervous system employs three transmitters: acetylcholine, norepinephrine, and epinephrine.

■ Acetylcholine is the transmitter released by all preganglionic neurons of the sympathetic nervous system, all preganglionic neurons of the parasympathetic nervous system, all postganglionic neurons of the parasympathetic nervous system, postganglionic neurons of the sympathetic nervous system that go to sweat glands, and all motor neurons.

■ Norepinephrine is the transmitter released by all postganglionic neurons of the sympathetic nervous system, except those that go to sweat glands.

■ Epinephrine is the major transmitter released by the adrenal medulla.

■ There are three major subtypes of cholinergic receptors: nicotinic$_N$, nicotinic$_M$, and muscarinic.

■ There are four major subtypes of adrenergic receptors: alpha$_1$, alpha$_2$, beta$_1$, and beta$_2$.

■ Although receptor subtypes are of uncertain physiologic significance, they are of great pharmacologic significance.

■ Activation of nicotinic$_N$ receptors promotes transmission at all autonomic ganglia, and promotes release of epinephrine from the adrenal medulla.

■ Activation of nicotinic$_M$ receptors causes contraction of skeletal muscle.

■ Activation of muscarinic receptors increases glandular secretion (from pulmonary, gastric, intestinal, and sweat glands); contracts smooth muscle in the bronchi, bladder, and GI tract; slows heart rate; contracts the iris sphincter; contracts the ciliary muscle (thereby focusing the lens for near vision); and dilates blood vessels.

■ Activation of alpha$_1$ receptors contracts the radial muscle of the eye (causing mydriasis), constricts veins and arterioles, promotes ejaculation, and contracts smooth muscle in the bladder neck and prostatic capsule.

■ Activation of *peripheral* alpha$_2$ receptors is of minimal pharmacologic significance.

■ Activation of beta$_1$ receptors increases heart rate, force of myocardial contraction, and conduction through the AV node, and promotes release of renin by the kidney.

■ Activation of beta$_2$ receptors dilates the bronchi, relaxes uterine smooth muscle, increases glycogenolysis, enhances contraction of skeletal muscle, and dilates arterioles (in the heart, lungs, and skeletal muscle).

■ Activation of dopamine receptors dilates blood vessels in the kidney.

■ Neurotransmission at cholinergic junctions is terminated by degradation of acetylcholine by acetylcholinesterase.

■ Neurotransmission at adrenergic junctions is terminated by reuptake of intact norepinephrine into nerve terminals.

■ Following reuptake, norepinephrine may be stored in vesicles for reuse or destroyed by monoamine oxidase.

I know it's a lot of work, but there's really no way around it: You've got to incorporate this information into your personal database (i.e., ya gotta memorize it).

Introduction to Cholinergic Drugs

The cholinergic drugs are agents that influence the activity of cholinergic receptors. Most of these drugs act directly at cholinergic receptors, where they mimic or block the actions of acetylcholine. Some of these drugs—the cholinesterase inhibitors—influence cholinergic receptors indirectly by preventing the breakdown of acetylcholine.

The cholinergic drugs have both therapeutic and toxicologic significance. Therapeutic applications of cholinergic drugs are limited but valuable. The toxicology of cholinergic drugs is extensive, encompassing such agents as nicotine, insecticides, and compounds designed for chemical warfare.

There are six categories of cholinergic drugs. These categories, along with representative agents, are summarized in Table 1. The *muscarinic agonists,* represented by bethanechol, selectively mimic the effects of acetylcholine at muscarinic receptors. The *muscarinic antagonists,* represented by atropine, selectively block the effects of acetylcholine (and other agonists) at muscarinic receptors. *Ganglionic stimulating agents,* represented by nicotine itself, selectively mimic the effects of acetylcholine at nicotinic$_N$ receptors of autonomic ganglia. *Ganglionic blocking agents,* represented by trimethaphan, selectively block ganglionic nicotinic$_N$ receptors. *Neuromuscular blocking agents,* represented by *d*-tubocurarine and succinylcholine, selectively block the effects of acetylcholine at nicotinic$_M$ receptors of the neuromuscular junction. The *cholinesterase inhibitors,* represented by neostigmine and physostigmine, prevent the breakdown of acetylcholine by acetylcholinesterase, and thereby increase the stimulation of all cholinergic receptors in the body.

Table 2 is your master key to understanding the cholinergic drugs. This table lists the three subtypes of cholinergic receptors (muscarinic, nicotinic$_N$, and nicotinic$_M$) and indicates for each receptor type: (1) location, (2) responses to activation, (3) drugs that produce activation (agonists), and (4) drugs that prevent activation (antagonists). This information, along with the detailed information on cholinergic receptor function summarized in Table 13–2, is just about all you need to predict the actions of cholinergic drugs.

An example will demonstrate the combined value of Tables 2 and 13-2. Let's consider *bethanechol.* As indicated in Table 2, bethanechol is a selective *agonist at muscarinic* cholinergic receptors. Referring to Table 13–2, we see that activation of muscarinic receptors can produce the following: ocular effects (miosis and ciliary muscle contraction), slowing of heart rate, bronchial constriction, urination, glandular secretion, stimulation of the GI tract, penile erection,

TABLE 1 ■ Categories of Cholinergic Drugs

Category	Representative Drugs
Muscarinic agonists	Bethanechol
Muscarinic antagonists	Atropine
Ganglionic stimulating agents	Nicotine
Ganglionic blocking agents	Trimethaphan
Neuromuscular blocking agents	*d*-Tubocurarine, succinylcholine
Cholinesterase inhibitors	Neostigmine, physostigmine

TABLE 2 ■ Summary of Cholinergic Drugs and Their Receptors

	Receptor Subtype		
	Muscarinic	*Nicotinic$_N$*	*Nicotinic$_M$*
Receptor Location	Sweat glands Blood vessels All organs regulated by the parasympathetic nervous system	All ganglia of the autonomic nervous system	Neuromuscular junctions (NMJ)
Effects of Receptor Activation	Many, including: ↓ Heart rate ↑ Gland secretion Smooth muscle contraction	Promotes ganglionic transmission	Skeletal muscle contraction
Receptor Agonists	Bethanechol	Nicotine	(Nicotine*)
	Cholinesterase inhibitors: physostigmine, neostigmine (these drugs indirectly activate all cholinergic receptors)		
Receptor Antagonists	Atropine	Trimethaphan	*d*-Tubocurarine, succinylcholine

*The doses of nicotine needed to activate nicotinic$_M$ receptors of the NMJ are much higher than the doses needed to activate nicotinic$_N$ receptors in autonomic ganglia.

and vasodilation. Since bethanechol *activates* muscarinic receptors, the drug is capable of eliciting all of these responses. Hence, by knowing which receptors bethanechol stimulates (from Table 2), and by knowing what those receptors do (from Table 13–2), you can predict the kinds of responses you might expect bethanechol to produce.

In the chapters that follow, we will employ the approach just described. That is, for each drug discussed, you will want to know (1) the receptors that the drug affects, (2) the normal responses to activation of those receptors, and (3) whether the drug in question increases or decreases receptor activation. All of this information is contained in Tables 2 and Table 13–2. Accordingly, if you master the information in these tables now, you will be prepared to follow discussions in succeeding chapters with relative ease—and perhaps even with pleasure. In contrast, if you postpone mastery of these tables, you are likely to find it both difficult and dissatisfying to proceed.

Muscarinic Agonists and Antagonists

The muscarinic agonists and antagonists produce their effects through direct interaction with muscarinic receptors. The muscarinic agonists cause receptor activation; the antagonists produce receptor blockade.

MUSCARINIC AGONISTS

The muscarinic agonists bind to muscarinic receptors and thereby cause receptor activation. Since nearly all muscarinic receptors are associated with the parasympathetic nervous system, responses to muscarinic agonists closely resemble those produced by stimulation of parasympathetic nerves. Accordingly, muscarinic agonists are also known as *parasympathomimetic agents*.

Bethanechol

Bethanechol embodies the characteristics that typify all muscarinic agonists, and hence will serve as our prototype for the group.

Mechanism of Action

Bethanechol is a direct-acting muscarinic agonist. The drug binds reversibly to muscarinic cholinergic receptors and causes activation. At therapeutic doses, bethanechol acts selectively at muscarinic receptors, having little or no effect on nicotinic receptors, either in ganglia or in skeletal muscle.

Pharmacologic Effects

Bethanechol can elicit all of the responses typical of muscarinic receptor activation. Accordingly, we can readily predict the effects of bethanechol by knowing the information on muscarinic responses summarized in Table 13–2.

The principal structures affected by muscarinic activation are the *heart, exocrine glands, smooth muscles, and eye*. Muscarinic agonists act on the heart to cause bradycardia (decreased heart rate) and on exocrine glands to increase sweating, salivation, bronchial secretions, and secretion of gastric acid. In smooth muscles of the lung, GI tract, and bladder, muscarinic agonists promote contraction. The result is constriction of the bronchi, increased tone and motility of GI smooth muscle, and contraction of the detrusor muscle of the bladder. In vascular smooth muscle, these drugs cause relaxation; the resultant vasodilation can produce hypotension. Activation of muscarinic receptors in the eye has two effects: (1) miosis (pupillary constriction); and (2) contraction of the ciliary muscle, resulting in accommodation for near vision. (The ciliary muscle, which is attached to the lens, focuses the eye for near vision by altering lens curvature.)

Pharmacokinetics

Bethanechol may be administered orally or by SC injection. Following oral administration, effects begin in 30 to 60 minutes and persist for about 1 hour. With SC injection, effects begin more rapidly (in 5 to 15 minutes).

To produce an equivalent therapeutic response, oral doses must be about 40 times larger than SC doses. As indicated in Figure 14–1, bethanechol is a *quaternary ammonium compound,* and hence always carries a positive charge. This charge greatly impedes passage across membranes of the GI tract. As a result, only a small fraction of oral bethanechol is absorbed. In contrast, since barriers to absorption are minimal with SC administration, SC bethanechol is completely absorbed. These differences underlie the differences in dosage for the two routes (see below).

Therapeutic Uses

Although bethanechol can produce a broad spectrum of pharmacologic effects, its clinical applications are limited. The principal indication is urinary retention.

Urinary Retention. Bethanechol relieves urinary retention by activating muscarinic receptors of the urinary tract. Muscarinic activation relaxes the urinary sphincters and increases voiding pressure (by contracting the detrusor muscle of the bladder). Bethanechol is used to treat urinary retention in postoperative and postpartum patients. The drug should not be used to treat urinary retention caused by physical obstruction of the urinary tract. Why? Because increased pressure in the tract in the presence of blockage could cause injury. When patients are treated with bethanechol, a bedpan or urinal should be readily available.

Gastrointestinal Uses. Bethanechol has been used on an investigational basis to treat *gastroesophageal reflux.* Benefits may result from increased esophageal motility and increased pressure in the lower esophageal sphincter.

Bethanechol can help treat disorders associated with GI paralysis. Benefits derive from increased tone and motility of GI smooth muscle. Specific

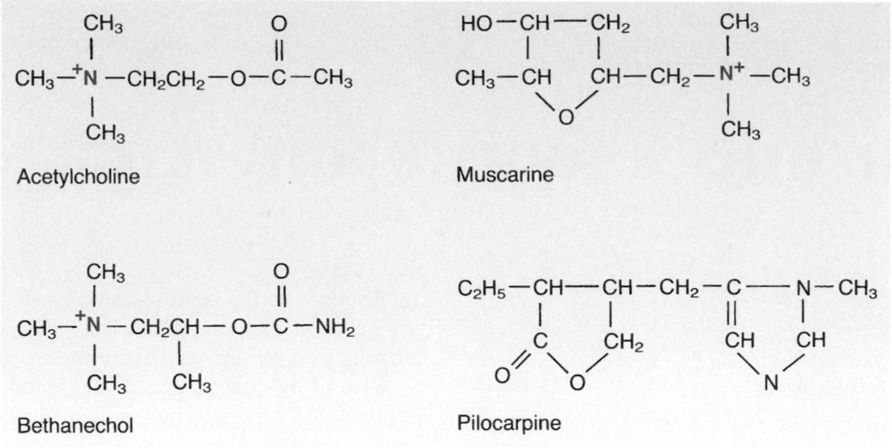

Figure 14–1 ■ **Structures of muscarinic agonists.**
Note that, with the exception of pilocarpine, all of these agents are quaternary ammonium compounds, and therefore always carry a positive charge. Because of this charge, these compounds cross membranes poorly.

applications are *adynamic ileus, gastric atony,* and *postoperative abdominal distention.* Bethanechol should not be given if physical obstruction of the GI tract is present, because, in the presence of blockage, increased propulsive contractions might result in damage to the intestinal wall.

Adverse Effects

In theory, bethanechol can produce the full range of muscarinic responses as side effects. However, in actual practice, side effects are relatively rare, and their incidence depends on the route of administration. With oral administration, side effects are uncommon. In contrast, when bethanechol is given SC, the incidence of side effects is relatively high.

Cardiovascular System. Bethanechol can cause *hypotension* (secondary to vasodilation) and *bradycardia.* Accordingly, the drug is contraindicated for patients with low blood pressure or low cardiac output.

Alimentary System. At usual therapeutic doses, bethanechol can cause *excessive salivation, increased secretion of gastric acid, abdominal cramps,* and *diarrhea.* Higher doses can cause *involuntary defecation.* Bethanechol is contraindicated in patients with gastric ulcers, since stimulation of acid secretion could intensify gastric erosion, causing bleeding and possibly perforation. The drug is also contraindicated for patients with *intestinal obstruction* and for those recovering from *recent surgery of the bowel.* In both cases, the ability of bethanechol to increase the tone and motility of intestinal smooth muscle could result in rupture of the bowel wall.

Urinary Tract. Because of its ability to contract the bladder, and thereby increase pressure within the urinary tract, bethanechol can be hazardous to patients with urinary tract obstruction or weakness of the bladder wall. In both groups of patients, elevation of pressure within the urinary tract could rupture the bladder. Accordingly, bethanechol is contraindicated for patients with either disorder.

Exacerbation of Asthma. By stimulating muscarinic receptors in the lungs, bethanechol can cause bronchoconstriction. Accordingly, the drug is contraindicated for patients with latent or active asthma.

Dysrhythmias in Hyperthyroid Patients. Bethanechol can cause *dysrhythmias* in hyperthyroid patients. Accordingly, the drug is contraindicated for these people. The mechanism of dysrhythmia induction is explained below.

If given to hyperthyroid patients, bethanechol may increase heart rate to the point of initiating a dysrhythmia. (Note that increased heart rate is opposite to the effect that muscarinic agonists have in most patients.) When hyperthyroid patients are given bethanechol, their initial cardiovascular responses are like those of anyone else: bradycardia and hypotension. In reaction to hypotension, the baroreceptor reflex attempts to return blood pressure to normal. Part of this reflex involves the release of norepinephrine from sympathetic nerves that regulate heart rate. In patients who are not hyperthyroid, norepinephrine release serves to increase cardiac output, and thereby helps restore blood pressure. However, in hyperthyroid patients, norepinephrine release can induce cardiac dysrhythmias. The reason for this unusual response is that in hyperthyroid patients the heart is exquisitely sensitive to the effects of norepinephrine; hence, relatively small amounts of norepinephrine can cause stimulation sufficient to elicit a dysrhythmia.

Preparations, Dosage, and Administration

Preparations. Bethanechol is available in tablets (5, 10, 25, and 50 mg) for oral therapy and in solution (5 mg/ml) for SC therapy.

Dosage and Administration. Oral. Adult dosages range from 10 to 50 mg 3 to 4 times a day. Administration with meals can cause nausea and vomiting. Accordingly, dosing should be done 1 hour before meals or 2 hours after.

Subcutaneous. The usual adult dosage is 5 mg administered up to 4 times a day. (Note that this dosage is significantly lower than the oral dosage.) The injectable form of bethanechol is intended for *subcutaneous* administration only. *Bethanechol must never be injected IM or IV.* Why? Because doing so could produce dangerously high blood levels, posing a risk of bloody diarrhea, bradycardia, profound hypotension, and cardiovascular collapse.

Other Muscarinic Agonists
Cevimeline

Actions and Uses. Cevimeline [Evoxac] is a muscarinic agonist with actions like those of bethanechol. This new drug, a derivative of acetylcholine, is indicated for relief of *xerostomia* (dry mouth) in patients with Sjögren's syndrome, an autoimmune disorder characterized by xerostomia, keratoconjunctivitis sicca (inflammation of the cornea and conjunctiva), and connective tissue disease (typically rheumatoid arthritis). Dry mouth results from extensive damage to salivary glands. Left untreated, it can lead to multiple complications, including periodontal disease, dental caries, altered taste, oral ulcers and candidiasis, and difficulty eating and speaking. Cevimeline relieves dry mouth by activating muscarinic receptors on residual healthy tissue in salivary glands, thereby promoting salivation. The drug also increases tear production, which can help relieve keratoconjunctivitis. Because it stimulates salivation, cevimeline may also benefit patients with xerostomia induced by radiation therapy for head and neck cancer, although the drug is not approved for this use.

Adverse Effects. Adverse effects result from activating muscarinic receptors, and hence are similar to those of bethanechol. The most common effects are excessive sweating (18.9%), nausea (13.8%), rhinitis (11.2%), and diarrhea (10.3%). To compensate for fluid loss caused by sweating and diarrhea, patients should increase fluid intake. Like bethanechol, cevimeline promotes miosis (constriction of the pupil) and may also blur vision. Both actions can make driving dangerous, especially at night.

Activation of cardiac muscarinic receptors can reduce heart rate and slow cardiac conduction. Accordingly, cevimeline should be used with caution in patients with a history of heart disease.

Because muscarinic activation increases airway resistance, cevimeline is contraindicated for patients with uncontrolled asthma and should be used with caution in patients with controlled asthma, chronic bronchitis, or chronic obstructive pulmonary disease.

Because miosis can exacerbate symptoms of both narrow-angle glaucoma and iritis (inflammation of the iris), cevimeline is contraindicated for people with these disorders.

Drug Interactions. Cevimeline can intensify cardiac depression caused by beta blockers (because both drugs decrease heart rate and cardiac conduction).

Beneficial effects of cevimeline can be antagonized by drugs that block muscarinic receptors. Among these are atropine, tricyclic antidepressants (e.g., imipramine), antihistamines (e.g., diphenhydramine), and phenothiazine antipsychotics (e.g., chlorpromazine).

Preparations, Dosage, and Administration. Cevimeline [Evoxac] is dispensed in 30-mg capsules. The dosage is 30 mg 3 times a day. The drug can be administered with food to reduce gastric upset.

Pilocarpine

Pilocarpine is a muscarinic agonist used mainly for topical therapy of glaucoma, an ophthalmic disorder characterized by elevated intraocular pressure with subsequent injury to the optic nerve. The basic pharmacology of pilocarpine and its use in glaucoma are discussed in Chapter 100 (Drugs for the Eye).

In addition to its use in glaucoma, pilocarpine is approved for oral therapy of dry mouth resulting from salivary gland damage caused by radiation therapy for head and neck cancer. For this application, pilocarpine is available in 5-mg tablets under the trade name *Salagen*. The recommended dosage is 5 mg 3 times a day. At this dosage, the principal adverse effect is sweating, which occurs in 29% of patients. However, if dosage is excessive, pilocarpine can produce the full spectrum of muscarinic effects.

Acetylcholine

Clinical use of acetylcholine [Miochol] is limited primarily to producing rapid miosis following lens delivery in cataract surgery. Two factors explain the limited utility of this drug. First, acetylcholine lacks selectivity (in addition to stimulating muscarinic cholinergic receptors, acetylcholine can also stimulate all nicotinic cholinergic receptors). Second, because of rapid destruction by cholinesterases, acetylcholine has a half-life that is extremely short—too short for most clinical applications.

Muscarine

Although muscarine is not used clinically, this agent has historic and toxicologic significance. Muscarine is of historic interest because of its role in the discovery of cholinergic receptor subtypes. The drug has toxicologic significance because of its presence in certain poisonous mushrooms.

Toxicology of Muscarinic Agonists

Sources of Muscarinic Poisoning. Muscarinic poisoning can result from ingestion of certain mushrooms and from overdose with two kinds of medications: (1) direct-acting muscarinic agonists (e.g., bethanechol, pilocarpine), and (2) cholinesterase inhibitors.

Of the mushrooms that cause poisoning, only a few do so through muscarinic stimulation. Mushrooms of the *Inocybe*

and *Clitocybe* species have lots of muscarine, hence their ingestion can produce typical signs of muscarinic toxicity. Interestingly, *Amanita muscaria,* the mushroom from which muscarine was originally extracted, actually contains very little muscarine; poisoning by this mushroom is due to toxins other than muscarinic agonists.

Symptoms. Manifestations of muscarinic poisoning result from excessive stimulation of muscarinic receptors. Prominent symptoms are profuse salivation, lacrimation (tearing), visual disturbances, bronchospasm, diarrhea, bradycardia, and hypotension. Severe poisoning can produce cardiovascular collapse.

Treatment. Management is direct and specific: administer *atropine* (a selective muscarinic blocking agent) and provide supportive therapy. By blocking access of muscarinic agonists to their receptors, atropine can reverse most signs of toxicity.

MUSCARINIC ANTAGONISTS

Muscarinic antagonists competitively block the actions of acetylcholine at muscarinic receptors. Because the majority of muscarinic receptors are located on structures innervated by parasympathetic nerves, the muscarinic antagonists are also known as *parasympatholytic drugs*. Additional names for these agents are *antimuscarinic drugs, muscarinic blockers,* and *anticholinergic drugs*.

The term *anticholinergic* can be a source of confusion and requires comment. This term is unfortunate in that it implies blockade at *all* cholinergic receptors. However, as normally used, the term *anticholinergic* only indicates blockade of *muscarinic* receptors. Therefore, when a drug is described as being anticholinergic, you can take this to mean that the drug produces selective *muscarinic* blockade—and not blockade of all cholinergic receptors.

Atropine

Atropine is the best known muscarinic antagonist and will serve as our prototype for the group. The actions of all other muscarinic antagonists are much like those of this drug.

Atropine is found naturally in a variety of plants, including *Atropa belladonna* (deadly nightshade) and *Datura stramonium* (also known as Jimson weed, stinkweed, and devil's apple). Because of its presence in *Atropa belladonna*, atropine is referred to as a *belladonna alkaloid*.

Mechanism of Action

Atropine produces its effects through competitive blockade at muscarinic receptors. Like all other receptor antagonists, atropine has no direct effects of its own. Rather, all responses to atropine result from *preventing receptor activation* by endogenous acetylcholine (or by drugs that act as muscarinic agonists).

At therapeutic doses, atropine produces selective blockade of muscarinic cholinergic receptors. However, if the dosage is sufficiently high, the drug will produce some blockade of nicotinic receptors too.

Pharmacologic Effects

Since atropine acts by causing muscarinic receptor blockade, its effects are opposite to those caused by muscarinic activation. Accordingly, we can readily predict the effects of atropine by knowing the normal responses to muscarinic receptor activation (see Table 13–2) and by knowing that atropine will reverse those responses. Like the muscarinic agonists, the muscarinic antagonists exert their influence primarily on the *heart, exocrine glands, smooth muscles,* and *eye.*

Heart. Atropine *increases heart rate.* Since stimulation of cardiac muscarinic receptors decreases heart rate, blockade of these receptors with atropine will cause heart rate to rise.

Exocrine Glands. Atropine *decreases secretion* from salivary glands, bronchial glands, sweat glands, and the acid-secreting cells of the stomach. Note that these effects are opposite to those of muscarinic agonists, which increase secretion from exocrine glands.

Smooth Muscle. By preventing activation of muscarinic receptors on smooth muscle, atropine causes *relaxation of the bronchi, decreased tone of the urinary bladder,* and *decreased tone and motility of the GI tract.* In the absence of an exogenous muscarinic agonist (e.g., bethanechol), muscarinic blockade has no effect on vascular smooth muscle tone. Why? Because there is no parasympathetic innervation to muscarinic receptors in blood vessels.

Eye. Blockade of muscarinic receptors on the iris sphincter causes *mydriasis* (dilation of the pupil). Blockade of muscarinic receptors on the ciliary muscle produces *cycloplegia* (relaxation of the ciliary muscle), thereby focusing the lens for far vision.

Central Nervous System (CNS). At therapeutic doses, atropine can cause mild CNS *excitation.* Toxic doses can cause *hallucinations* and *delirium,* which can resemble psychosis. Extremely high doses can result in coma, respiratory arrest, and death.

Dose Dependency of Muscarinic Blockade. It is important to note that not all muscarinic receptors are equally sensitive to blockade by atropine and most other muscarinic antagonists: At some sites, muscarinic receptors can be blocked with relatively low doses, whereas at other sites much higher doses are needed. Table 14–1 indicates the sequence in which specific muscarinic receptors are blocked as the dose of atropine is increased.

Differences in receptor sensitivity to muscarinic blockers are of clinical significance. As indicated in Table 14–1, the

TABLE 14–1 ■ Relationship Between Dosage and Responses to Atropine	
Dosage of Atropine	**Response Produced**
Low Doses	Salivary glands—decreased secretion
	Sweat glands—decreased secretion
	Bronchial glands—decreased secretion
	Heart—increased rate
	Eye—mydriasis, blurred vision
	Urinary tract—interference with voiding
	Intestine—decreased tone and motility
	Lung—dilation of bronchi
High Doses	Stomach—decreased acid secretion

Note that doses of atropine that are high enough to decrease gastric acid secretion or dilate the bronchi will also affect all other structures under muscarinic control. As a result, atropine and most other muscarinic antagonists are not very desirable for treating peptic ulcer disease or asthma.

doses needed to block muscarinic receptors in the stomach and bronchial smooth muscle are higher than the doses needed to block muscarinic receptors at all other locations. Accordingly, if we want to use atropine to treat peptic ulcer disease (by suppressing gastric acid secretion) or asthma (by dilating the bronchi), we cannot do so without also affecting the heart, exocrine glands, many smooth muscles, and the eye. Because of these obligatory side effects, atropine and most other muscarinic antagonists are not preferred drugs for treating peptic ulcers or asthma.

Pharmacokinetics

Atropine may be administered orally, topically (to the eye), and by injection (IM, SC, and IV). The drug is rapidly absorbed following oral administration and distributes to all tissues, including the CNS. Elimination is by a combination of hepatic metabolism and urinary excretion. Atropine has a half-life of approximately 3 hours.

Therapeutic Uses

Preanesthetic Medication. The cardiac effects of atropine can be helpful during surgery. Procedures that stimulate baroreceptors of the carotid body can initiate reflex slowing of the heart, resulting in profound bradycardia. Since this reflex is mediated by muscarinic receptors on the heart, pretreatment with atropine can prevent dangerous reductions in heart rate.

Certain anesthetics—especially ether, which is obsolete—irritate the respiratory tract, and thereby stimulate secretion from salivary, nasal, pharyngeal, and bronchial glands. If these secretions are sufficiently profuse, they can interfere with respiration. By blocking muscarinic receptors on secretory glands, atropine can help prevent excessive secretions. Fortunately, modern anesthetics are much less irritating than ether. The availability of these new anesthetics has greatly reduced the use of atropine as an antisecretagogue during anesthesia.

Disorders of the Eye. By blocking muscarinic receptors in the eye, atropine can cause mydriasis and paralysis of the ciliary muscle. Both actions can be of help during eye examinations and ocular surgery. The ophthalmic uses of atropine and other muscarinic antagonists are discussed in Chapter 100.

Bradycardia. Atropine can accelerate heart rate in certain patients with bradycardia. Heart rate is increased because blockade of cardiac muscarinic receptors prevents the parasympathetic nervous system from slowing the heart.

Intestinal Hypertonicity and Hypermotility. By blocking muscarinic receptors in the intestine, atropine can decrease both the tone and motility of intestinal smooth muscle. This can be beneficial in conditions characterized by excessive intestinal motility, such as mild dysentery and diverticulitis. When taken for these disorders, atropine can reduce both the frequency of bowel movements and associated abdominal cramps.

Muscarinic Agonist Poisoning. Atropine is a specific antidote to poisoning by agents that activate muscarinic receptors. By blocking muscarinic receptors, atropine can reverse all signs of muscarinic poisoning. As discussed above, muscarinic poisoning can result from an overdose with medications that promote muscarinic activation (e.g., bethanechol, cholinesterase inhibitors) or from ingestion of certain mushrooms.

Peptic Ulcer Disease. Because it can suppress secretion of gastric acid, atropine has been used to treat peptic ulcer disease. Unfortunately, when administered in doses that are strong enough to block the muscarinic receptors that regulate secretion of gastric acid, atropine also blocks most other muscarinic receptors. Hence, treatment of ulcers is necessarily associated with a broad range of antimuscarinic side effects (dry mouth, blurred vision, urinary retention, constipation, and so on). Because of these side effects, atropine is not a first-choice drug for ulcer therapy. Rather, atropine is reserved for cases in which symptoms cannot be relieved with preferred medications (e.g., antibiotics, histamine$_2$ receptor antagonists, proton pump inhibitors).

Asthma. By blocking bronchial muscarinic receptors, atropine can promote bronchial dilation, thereby improving respiration in patients with asthma. Unfortunately, in addition to dilating the bronchi, atropine also causes drying and thickening of bronchial secretions, effects that can be harmful to patients with asthma. Furthermore, when given in the doses needed to dilate the bronchi, atropine causes a variety of antimuscarinic side effects. Because of the potential for harm, and because superior medicines are available, atropine has a very limited role in asthma therapy.

Biliary Colic. Biliary colic is characterized by intense abdominal pain brought on by passage of a gallstone through the bile duct. This pain is usually treated with morphine. In some cases, atropine may be combined with morphine to relax biliary tract smooth muscle, thereby helping alleviate discomfort.

Adverse Effects

Most adverse effects of atropine and other muscarinic antagonists are the direct result of muscarinic receptor blockade. Accordingly, they can be predicted from your knowledge of muscarinic receptor function.

Xerostomia (Dry Mouth). Blockade of muscarinic receptors on salivary glands can inhibit salivation, thereby causing dry mouth. Not only is this uncomfortable, it can impede swallowing. Patients should be informed that dryness can be alleviated by chewing gum, sucking on hard candy, and sipping fluids.

Blurred Vision and Photophobia. Blockade of muscarinic receptors on the ciliary muscle and the sphincter of the iris can paralyze these muscles. Paralysis of the ciliary muscle focuses the eye for far vision, causing nearby objects to appear blurred. Patients should be forewarned about this effect and advised to avoid hazardous activities if vision is impaired.

Paralysis of the iris sphincter prevents constriction of the pupil, thereby rendering the eye unable to adapt to bright light. Patients should be advised to wear dark glasses if photophobia (intolerance to light) is a problem. Room lighting for hospitalized patients should be kept low.

Elevation of Intraocular Pressure. Paralysis of the iris sphincter can cause intraocular pressure (IOP) to rise. The mechanism of this effect is discussed in Chapter 100 (Drugs for the Eye). Because they can raise IOP, muscarinic blockers are contraindicated for patients with glaucoma, a disease characterized by abnormally high IOP. In addition, antimuscarinic drugs should be used with caution in patients who may not have glaucoma per se but for whom a predisposition to glaucoma may be present; included in this group are all people older than 40.

Urinary Retention. Blockade of muscarinic receptors in the urinary tract reduces pressure within the bladder and increases the tone of the urinary sphincter. These effects can produce urinary hesitancy or urinary retention. In the event of severe urinary retention, catheterization or treatment with a muscarinic agonist (e.g., bethanechol) may be required. Patients should be advised that urinary retention can be minimized by voiding just prior to taking their medication.

Constipation. Muscarinic blockade decreases the tone and motility of intestinal smooth muscle. The resultant delay in transit through the intestine can produce constipation. Patients should be informed that constipation can be minimized by increasing dietary fiber and fluids. A laxative may be needed if constipation is severe. Because of their ability to decrease smooth muscle tone, muscarinic antagonists are contraindicated for patients with intestinal atony, a condition in which intestinal tone is low already.

Anhidrosis. Blockade of muscarinic receptors on sweat glands can produce anhidrosis (a deficiency or absence of sweat). Since sweating is necessary for cooling, people who cannot sweat are at risk of hyperthermia. Patients should be warned of this possibility and advised to avoid activities that might lead to overheating (e.g., exercising on a hot day).

Tachycardia. Blockade of cardiac muscarinic receptors eliminates parasympathetic influence on the heart. By removing the "braking" influence of parasympathetic nerves, muscarinic antagonists can cause tachycardia (excessive heart rate). Caution must be exercised in patients with pre-existing tachycardia.

Asthma. In patients with asthma, antimuscarinic drugs can cause thickening and drying of bronchial secretions, which can lead to bronchial plugging. Consequently, although muscarinic antagonists can be used to treat asthma, they can also be harmful.

Drug Interactions

A number of drugs that are not classified as muscarinic antagonists can nonetheless produce significant muscarinic blockade. These include *antihistamines, phenothiazine antipsychotics,* and *tricyclic antidepressants.* Because of their prominent antimuscarinic actions, these drugs can greatly enhance the antimuscarinic effects of atropine and related agents. Accordingly, it is wise to avoid combined use of atropine with other drugs capable of causing muscarinic blockade.

Preparations, Dosage, and Administration

Atropine sulfate is dispensed in 0.4-mg tablets; as an ointment or solution for ophthalmic use; and in solution for SC, IM, and IV injection. The average systemic dose for adults is 0.5 mg.

Drugs for Urge Incontinence (Overactive Bladder)

Urinary incontinence, defined as *frequent involuntary urination,* is extremely common. About 12 to 15 million American adults are affected (although only 10% of cases get diagnosed). Among the elderly, incontinence affects between 15% and 30% of those living in the community, and up to 60% of those living in nursing homes. Incontinence has several forms, the most common being *urge incontinence,* defined as involuntary urination occurring in association with a strong urge to void. Episodes occur often throughout the day and night. With any episode, the volume of urine lost can range from just a few drops to the entire contents of the bladder. In almost all cases, urge incontinence results from *involuntary contraction of the bladder detrusor muscle,* which is under parasympathetic (muscarinic) control.

Urge incontinence can be treated with behavioral techniques (e.g., bladder training exercises, biofeedback) and with drugs. Behavioral therapy can be highly effective (even more effective than drugs), and hence should be tried first. As a rule, drugs should be reserved for patients who don't respond. In some cases, a combination of both approaches may be needed.

The two drugs used most for urge incontinence are *oxybutynin* [Ditropan, Ditropan XL] and *tolterodine* [Detrol, Detrol LA]. Both are muscarinic antagonists. By blocking muscarinic receptors on the detrusor muscle, these drugs prevent involuntary bladder contraction and subsequent voiding. Both appear equally effective: With both, treatment can greatly reduce the number of episodes each day, and some patients may experience complete remission. Formulations and dosages for these drugs are summarized in Table 14–2.

Oxybutynin and tolterodine can cause typical *anticholinergic side effects.* However, *dry mouth* is by far the biggest concern, occurring in up to 60% of patients. Other side effects include constipation, dyspepsia, and dry eyes. Since therapeutic effects and side effects are both the result of muscarinic blockade, it would seem that these antimuscarinic side effects are unavoidable. With both drugs, side effects can be intensified by concurrent use of other drugs that have anticholinergic properties (e.g., antihistamines, tricyclic antidepressants, phenothiazine antipsychotic agents).

Both oxybutynin and tolterodine are available in *immediate-release* (IR) and *extended-release* (ER) formulations. With the ER formulations, blood levels are more steady and peak levels are lower than with the IR formulations. Dry mouth is less intense and less frequent with the ER formulations, presumably because peak blood levels are lower. Although the ER formulations have not been compared directly, it seems likely that both are equally effective.

Other Muscarinic Antagonists

Scopolamine. Scopolamine is a muscarinic antagonist with actions much like those of atropine, but with two exceptions: (1) whereas therapeutic doses of atropine produce mild CNS *excitation,* therapeutic doses of scopolamine produce *sedation;* and (2) scopolamine *suppresses emesis and motion sickness,* whereas atropine does not. Principal uses for scopolamine are motion sickness (see Chapter 75), production of cycloplegia and mydriasis for ophthalmic procedures (see Chapter 100), and production of preanesthetic sedation and obstetric amnesia.

Ipratropium Bromide. Ipratropium [Atrovent] is an antimuscarinic drug used to treat asthma, chronic obstructive pulmonary disease, and rhinitis caused by allergies or the common cold. The drug is administered by inhalation and systemic absorption is minimal. As a result, therapy is not associated with typical antimuscarinic side effects (dry mouth, blurred vision, urinary hesitancy, constipation, and so forth). Ipratropium is discussed at length in Chapter 71.

Antisecretory Anticholinergics. Muscarinic blockers can be used to suppress gastric acid secretion in patients with peptic ulcer disease. However, since superior antiulcer drugs are available, and since anticholinergic agents produce significant side effects (dry mouth, blurred vision, urinary retention, and so forth), most of these drugs have been withdrawn. Today, only four—*glycopyrrolate* [Robinul], *mepenzolate* [Cantil], *methscopolamine* [Pamine], and *propantheline* [Pro-Banthine]—remain on the market. All four are administered orally, and one—glycopyrrolate—may also be given IM and IV.

Dicyclomine. This drug is indicated for irritable bowel syndrome (spastic colon, mucous colitis) and functional bowel disorders (diarrhea, hypermotility). Administration may be oral (40 mg 4 times a day) or by IM injection (20 mg 4 times a day). Trade names include *Antispas, Bentyl,* and *Dibent.*

Pirenzepine and Telenzepine. These drugs produce selective blockade of M_1-muscarinic receptors—the subtype of muscarinic receptor involved in regulating the secretion of gastric acid. Both drugs can effectively suppress acid secretion in patients with peptic ulcer disease, but neither is currently available in the United States. Because these drugs are selective blockers of M_1-muscarinic receptors, the incidence of dry mouth, blurred vision, and other typical antimuscarinic side effects is minimal.

Mydriatic Cycloplegics. Five muscarinic antagonists—*atropine, homatropine, scopolamine, cyclopentolate,* and *tropicamide*—are employed to produce mydriasis and cycloplegia in ophthalmic procedures. These applications are discussed in Chapter 100.

Centrally Acting Anticholinergics. Several anticholinergic drugs, including *trihexyphenidyl* [Artane] and *benztropine* [Cogentin], are used to treat Parkinson's disease and drug-induced parkinsonism. Benefits derive from blockade of muscarinic receptors in the CNS. The centrally acting anticholinergics and their use in Parkinson's disease are discussed in Chapter 21.

Toxicology of Muscarinic Antagonists

Sources of Antimuscarinic Poisoning. Sources of poisoning include natural products (e.g., *Atropa belladonna, Datura stramonium*); selective antimuscarinic drugs (e.g., atropine, scopolamine); and other drugs with pronounced antimuscarinic properties (e.g., antihistamines, phenothiazines, tricyclic antidepressants).

Symptoms. Symptoms of antimuscarinic poisoning, which are the direct result of excessive muscarinic blockade, include dry mouth, blurred vision, photophobia, hyperthermia, CNS effects (hallucinations, delirium), and skin that is hot, dry, and flushed. Death results from respiratory depression secondary to blockade of cholinergic receptors in the brain.

Treatment. Treatment consists of (1) minimizing absorption of the antimuscarinic agent and (2) administering an antidote. Absorption can be reduced by giving syrup of ipecac followed by activated charcoal. Ipecac induces vomiting, thereby removing unabsorbed poison from the stomach. Charcoal adsorbs poison within the intestine, thereby preventing its absorption into the blood.

The most effective antidote to antimuscarinic poisoning is *physostigmine,* an inhibitor of acetylcholinesterase. By inhibiting cholinesterase, physostigmine causes acetylcholine to accumulate at all cholinergic junctions. As acetylcholine builds up, it competes with the antimuscarinic agent for receptor binding, thereby reversing excessive muscarinic blockade. The pharmacology of physostigmine is discussed in Chapter 15.

Warning. It is important to differentiate between antimuscarinic poisoning, which often resembles psychosis (hallucinations, delirium), and an actual psychotic episode. We need to make the differential diagnosis because antipsychotic drugs, which have antimuscarinic properties of their own, will intensify symptoms if given to a victim of antimuscarinic poisoning. Fortunately, since a true psychotic episode is not ordinarily associated with signs of excessive muscarinic blockade (dry mouth, hyperthermia, dry skin, and so forth), differentiation is not usually difficult.

TABLE 14–2 ■ Drugs for Urge Incontinence		
Generic Name [Trade Names]	**Formulation***	**Adult Dosage**
Oxybutynin		
[Ditropan]	Syrup (1 mg/ml)	5 mg 2 or 3 times/day†
[Ditropan]	IR tablets (5 mg)	5 mg 2 or 3 times/day†
[Ditropan XL]	ER tablets (5, 10, 15 mg)	5–30 mg once a day†
Tolterodine		
[Detrol]	IR tablets (1, 2 mg)	1–2 mg 2 times a day
[Detrol LA]	ER capsules (2, 4 mg)	2–4 mg once a day

*IR = immediate release, ER = extended release.
†Begin at lowest dose and titrate upward as needed and tolerated.

∴ KEY POINTS

■ Muscarinic agonists work through direct activation of muscarinic cholinergic receptors, thereby causing bradycardia; increased secretion from sweat, salivary, bronchial, and gastric glands; contraction of intestinal, bronchial, and urinary tract smooth muscle; and, in the eye, miosis and accommodation for near vision.

■ Bethanechol, the prototype of the muscarinic agonists, is used primarily to relieve urinary retention.

■ Subcutaneous doses of bethanechol are 40 times smaller than oral doses.

■ Muscarinic agonist poisoning is characterized by profuse salivation, tearing, visual disturbances, bronchospasm, diarrhea, bradycardia, and hypotension.

■ Muscarinic agonist poisoning is treated with atropine.

■ Atropine, the prototype of the muscarinic antagonists, blocks the actions of acetylcholine (and all other muscarinic agonists) at muscarinic cholinergic receptors, and thereby (1) increases heart rate; (2) reduces secretion from sweat, salivary, bronchial, and gastric glands; (3) relaxes intestinal, bronchial, and urinary tract smooth muscle; (4) acts in the eye to cause mydriasis and cycloplegia; and (5) acts in the CNS to produce excitation (at low doses) and delirium and hallucinations (at toxic doses).

■ Important uses of muscarinic antagonists include preanesthetic medication, ophthalmic examinations, reversal of bradycardia, and treatment of muscarinic agonist poisoning.

■ Classic adverse effects of muscarinic antagonists are dry mouth, blurred vision, photophobia, tachycardia, urinary retention, constipation, and anhidrosis (suppression of sweating).

■ Certain drugs—especially antihistamines, tricyclic antidepressants, and phenothiazine antipsychotics—have prominent antimuscarinic actions. These should be used cautiously, if at all, in patients receiving atropine or other muscarinic antagonists.

■ Muscarinic antagonist poisoning is characterized by dry mouth, blurred vision, photophobia, hyperthermia, hallucinations and delirium, and skin that is hot, dry, and flushed.

■ The best antidote for muscarinic antagonist poisoning is physostigmine, an inhibitor of acetylcholinesterase.

Summary of Major Nursing Implications*

BETHANECHOL

Preadministration Assessment

Therapeutic Goal

Treatment of nonobstructive urinary retention.

Baseline Data

Record fluid intake and output.

Identifying High-Risk Patients

Bethanechol is *contraindicated* for patients with peptic ulcer disease, urinary tract obstruction, intestinal obstruction, coronary insufficiency, hypotension, asthma, and hyperthyroidism.

Implementation: Administration

Routes

Oral, SC
Never administer IM or IV!

Administration

Oral. Advise patients to take bethanechol 1 hour before meals or 2 hours after to reduce gastric upset.

Subcutaneous. Subcutaneous doses are much smaller than oral doses. Check SC doses carefully.

Both Routes. Since effects on the intestine and urinary tract can be rapid and dramatic, ensure that a bedpan or bathroom is readily accessible.

Ongoing Evaluation and Interventions

Evaluating Therapeutic Effects

Monitor fluid intake and output to evaluate treatment of urinary retention.

Minimizing Adverse Effects

Excessive muscarinic stimulation can cause salivation, sweating, urinary urgency, bradycardia, and hypotension. Monitor blood pressure and pulse rate. Observe for signs of muscarinic excess and report these to the physician. Inform patients about manifestations of muscarinic excess and advise them to notify the nurse or physician if they occur.

Management of Acute Toxicity

Overdose produces manifestations of excessive muscarinic stimulation (salivation, sweating, involuntary urination and defecation, bradycardia, severe hypotension). Treat with atropine (SC or IV) and supportive measures.

ATROPINE AND OTHER MUSCARINIC ANTAGONISTS

Preadministration Assessment

Therapeutic Goal

Atropine has many applications, including preanesthetic medication and treatment of bradycardia, biliary colic, intestinal hypertonicity and hypermotility, and muscarinic agonist poisoning.

*Patient education information is highlighted as blue text.

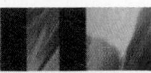

Summary of Major Nursing Implications*—cont'd

Identifying High-Risk Patients

Atropine and other muscarinic antagonists are *contraindicated* for patients with glaucoma, intestinal atony, urinary tract obstruction, and tachycardia. Use with *caution* in patients with asthma.

Implementation: Administration

Routes

Atropine is administered PO, IV, IM, and SC.

Administration

Dry mouth from muscarinic blockade may interfere with swallowing. **Advise patients to moisten the mouth by sipping water prior to oral administration.**

Ongoing Evaluation and Interventions

Minimizing Adverse Effects

Xerostomia (Dry Mouth). Decreased salivation can dry the mouth. **Teach patients that xerostomia can be relieved by chewing gum, sucking on hard candy, and sipping fluids.**

Blurred Vision. Paralysis of the ciliary muscle may reduce visual acuity. **Warn patients to avoid hazardous activities if vision is impaired.**

Photophobia. Muscarinic blockade prevents the pupil from constricting in response to bright light. Keep hospital room lighting low to reduce visual discomfort. **Advise patients to wear sunglasses outdoors.**

Urinary Retention. Muscarinic blockade in the bladder and urinary sphincter can cause urinary hesitancy or retention. **Advise patients that urinary retention can be mini-**mized by voiding just prior to taking anticholinergic medication. If urinary retention is severe, catheterization or treatment with bethanechol (a muscarinic agonist) may be required.

Constipation. Reduced tone and motility of the gut may cause constipation. **Advise patients that constipation can be reduced by increasing dietary fiber and fluids.** A laxative may be needed if constipation is severe.

Hyperthermia. Suppression of sweating may result in hyperthermia. **Advise patients to avoid vigorous exercise in warm environments.**

Tachycardia. Blockade of cardiac muscarinic receptors can accelerate heart rate. Monitor pulse rate and report significant increases.

Minimizing Adverse Interactions

Antihistamines, tricyclic antidepressants, and *phenothiazines* have prominent antimuscarinic actions. Combining these agents with atropine and other muscarinic antagonists can cause excessive muscarinic blockade.

Management of Acute Toxicity

Symptoms. Overdose produces dry mouth, blurred vision, photophobia, hyperthermia, hallucinations, and delirium; the skin becomes hot, dry, and flushed. Differentiate muscarinic antagonist poisoning from psychosis!

Treatment. Treatment centers on removing ingested poison (with syrup of ipecac); adsorbing ingested poison onto activated charcoal; and administering *physostigmine,* an inhibitor of acetylcholinesterase.

*Patient education information is highlighted as blue text.

CHAPTER 15

Cholinesterase Inhibitors and Their Use in Myasthenia Gravis

REVERSIBLE CHOLINESTERASE INHIBITORS
- **Neostigmine**
- **Other Reversible Cholinesterase Inhibitors**

"IRREVERSIBLE" CHOLINESTERASE INHIBITORS
- **Basic Pharmacology**
- **Toxicology**

MYASTHENIA GRAVIS
- **Pathophysiology**
- **Treatment with Cholinesterase Inhibitors**

Cholinesterase inhibitors are drugs that prevent the degradation of acetylcholine (ACh) by acetylcholinesterase (also known simply as cholinesterase [ChE]). By preventing the inactivation of ACh, the cholinesterase inhibitors enhance the actions of ACh released from cholinergic neurons. Hence, the cholinesterase inhibitors can be viewed as indirect-acting cholinergic agonists. Since cholinesterase inhibitors can intensify transmission at all cholinergic junctions (muscarinic, ganglionic, and neuromuscular), these drugs can elicit a broad spectrum of responses. Because they lack selectivity, cholinesterase inhibitors have limited therapeutic applications. An alternative name for the cholinesterase inhibitors is *anticholinesterase agents.*

There are two basic categories of cholinesterase inhibitors: (1) *reversible inhibitors* and (2) *"irreversible" inhibitors.* The reversible inhibitors produce effects of moderate duration. In contrast, the irreversible inhibitors produce effects that are long lasting.

REVERSIBLE CHOLINESTERASE INHIBITORS

Neostigmine

Neostigmine [Prostigmin] typifies the reversible cholinesterase inhibitors and will serve as our prototype for the group. The drug's only indication is *myasthenia gravis.*

Chemistry

As indicated in Figure 15–1, neostigmine contains a quaternary nitrogen atom, and hence always carries a positive charge. Because of this charge, neostigmine cannot readily cross membranes, including those of the GI tract, the blood-brain barrier, and the placenta. Consequently, neostigmine is absorbed poorly following oral administration and has minimal effects on the brain and fetus.

Mechanism of Action

Neostigmine and the other reversible cholinesterase inhibitors can be envisioned as poor substrates for ChE. As indicated in Figure 15–2, the normal function of ChE is to break down acetylcholine into choline and acetic acid. This process is termed a *hydrolysis* reaction because of the water molecule involved. As depicted in Figure 15–3*A*, hydrolysis of ACh takes place in two steps: (1) binding of ACh to the active center of ChE, followed by (2) splitting of ACh, which regenerates free ChE. The overall reaction between ACh and ChE is extremely fast. As a result, one molecule of ChE can break down a huge amount of ACh in a very short time.

As depicted in Figure 15–3*B*, the reaction between neostigmine and ChE is very similar to the reaction between ACh and ChE. The difference between the two reactions is simply that ChE splits neostigmine more slowly than it splits ACh. Hence, once neostigmine becomes bound to the active center

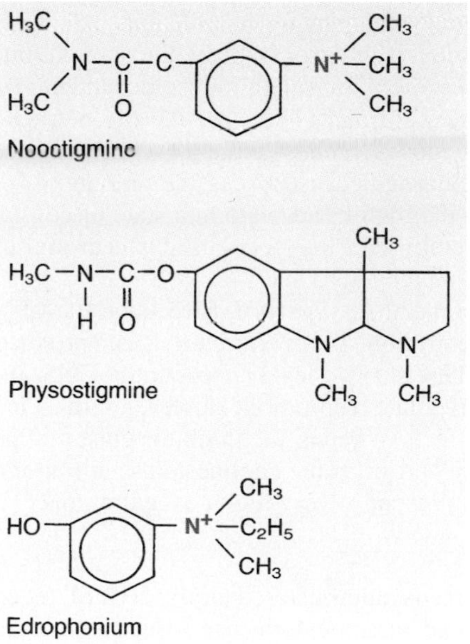

Figure 15–1 ■ Structural formulas of reversible cholinesterase inhibitors.
Note that neostigmine and edrophonium are quaternary ammonium compounds, but physostigmine is not. What does this difference imply about the relative abilities of these drugs to cross membranes, including the blood-brain barrier?

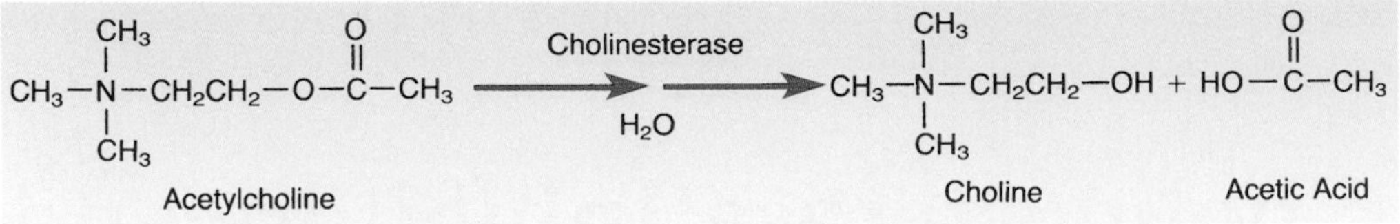

Figure 15–2 ■ **Hydrolysis of acetylcholine by cholinesterase.**

of ChE, the drug remains in place for a relatively long time, thereby preventing ChE from catalyzing the breakdown of ACh. ChE remains inhibited until it finally succeeds in splitting neostigmine off.

Pharmacologic Effects

By preventing inactivation of ACh, neostigmine and the other cholinesterase inhibitors can intensify transmission at virtually all junctions where ACh is the transmitter. In sufficient doses, cholinesterase inhibitors can produce skeletal muscle stimulation, activation of muscarinic receptors, ganglionic stimulation, and activation of cholinergic receptors in the central nervous system (CNS). However, when used *therapeutically,* cholinesterase inhibitors usually affect only muscarinic receptors and nicotinic receptors of the neuromuscular junction (NMJ). Ganglionic transmission and CNS function are usually unaltered.

Muscarinic Responses. Muscarinic effects of the cholinesterase inhibitors are identical to those of the direct-acting muscarinic agonists. By preventing breakdown of ACh, cholinesterase inhibitors can cause increased glandular secretions, increased tone and motility of GI smooth muscle, bradycardia, urinary urgency, bronchial constriction, miosis, and focusing of the lens for near vision.

Neuromuscular Effects. The effects of cholinesterase inhibitors on skeletal muscle are dose dependent. At *therapeutic* doses, these drugs *increase* force of contraction. In contrast, *toxic* doses *reduce* force of contraction. Contractile force is reduced because excessive amounts of ACh at the NMJ keep the motor end-plate in a state of constant depolarization, thereby causing depolarizing neuromuscular blockade (see Chapter 16).

Central Nervous System. Effects on the CNS vary with drug concentration. *Therapeutic* levels can produce mild *stimulation,* whereas *toxic* levels *depress* the CNS, including the areas that regulate respiration. However, it must be noted that, for CNS effects to occur, the inhibitor must first penetrate the blood-brain barrier; some cholinesterase inhibitors can do this only when present in very high concentrations.

Pharmacokinetics

Neostigmine is administered orally. (Until recently, it was also available for parenteral use.) Because neostigmine carries a positive charge, the drug is poorly absorbed following oral administration. Once absorbed, neostigmine can reach sites of action at the NMJ and peripheral muscarinic receptors, but cannot cross the blood-brain barrier to affect the CNS. Duration of action is 2 to 4 hours. Neostigmine is eliminated by enzymatic degradation: Cholinesterase, the enzyme that neostigmine inhibits, eventually converts neostigmine itself to an inactive product.

Therapeutic Uses

Currently, neostigmine is used only for oral therapy of myasthenia gravis. In the past, the drug was also used parenterally to reverse the effects of nondepolarizing neuromuscular blocking agents. Treatment of myasthenia is discussed later.

Adverse Effects

Excessive Muscarinic Stimulation. Accumulation of ACh at muscarinic receptors can result in excessive salivation, increased gastric secretions, increased tone and motility of the GI tract, urinary urgency, bradycardia, sweating, miosis, and spasm of accommodation (focusing of the lens for near vision). If necessary, these responses can be suppressed with atropine.

Neuromuscular Blockade. If administered in toxic doses, cholinesterase inhibitors can cause accumulation of ACh in amounts sufficient to produce depolarizing neuromuscular blockade. Paralysis of respiratory muscles can be fatal.

Precautions and Contraindications

Most of the precautions and contraindications regarding the cholinesterase inhibitors are the same as those for the direct-acting muscarinic agonists. These include (1) obstruction of the GI tract, (2) obstruction of the urinary tract, (3) peptic ulcer disease, (4) asthma, (5) coronary insufficiency, and (6) hyperthyroidism. The rationales underlying these precautions are discussed in Chapter 14. In addition to precautions related to muscarinic stimulation, cholinesterase inhibitors are contraindicated for patients receiving succinylcholine.

Drug Interactions

Muscarinic Antagonists. The effects of cholinesterase inhibitors at muscarinic receptors are opposite to those of atropine (and other muscarinic antagonists). Consequently, cholinesterase inhibitors can be used to overcome excessive muscarinic blockade caused by atropine. Conversely, atropine can be used to reduce excessive muscarinic stimulation caused by cholinesterase inhibitors.

Nondepolarizing Neuromuscular Blockers. By causing accumulation of ACh at the NMJ, cholinesterase inhibitors can reverse muscle relaxation induced with tubocurarine and other nondepolarizing neuromuscular blocking agents.

Depolarizing Neuromuscular Blockers. Cholinesterase inhibitors do not reverse the muscle-relaxant effects of succinylcholine, a depolarizing neuromuscular blocker. In fact, since cholinesterase inhibitors will decrease the breakdown of succinylcholine by cholinesterase, cholinesterase inhibitors will actually *intensify* neuromuscular blockade caused by succinylcholine.

A REACTION BETWEEN ACh and ChE

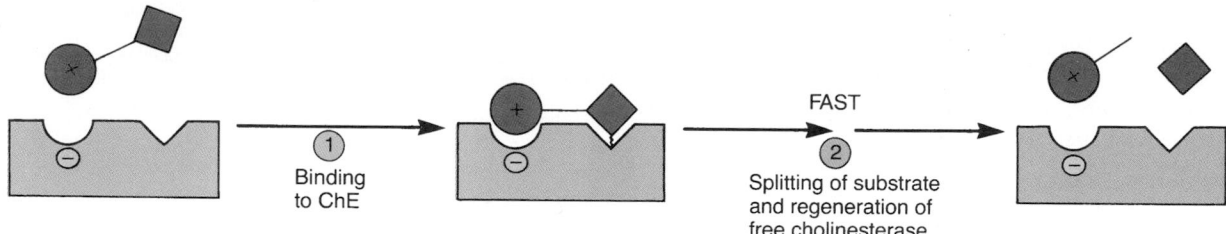

B REVERSIBLE INHIBITION OF ChE (BY NEOSTIGMINE)

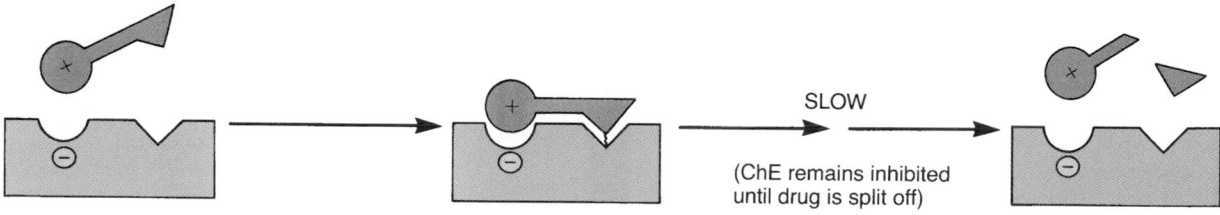

C "IRREVERSIBLE" INHIBITION OF ChE (BY ECHOTHIOPHATE)

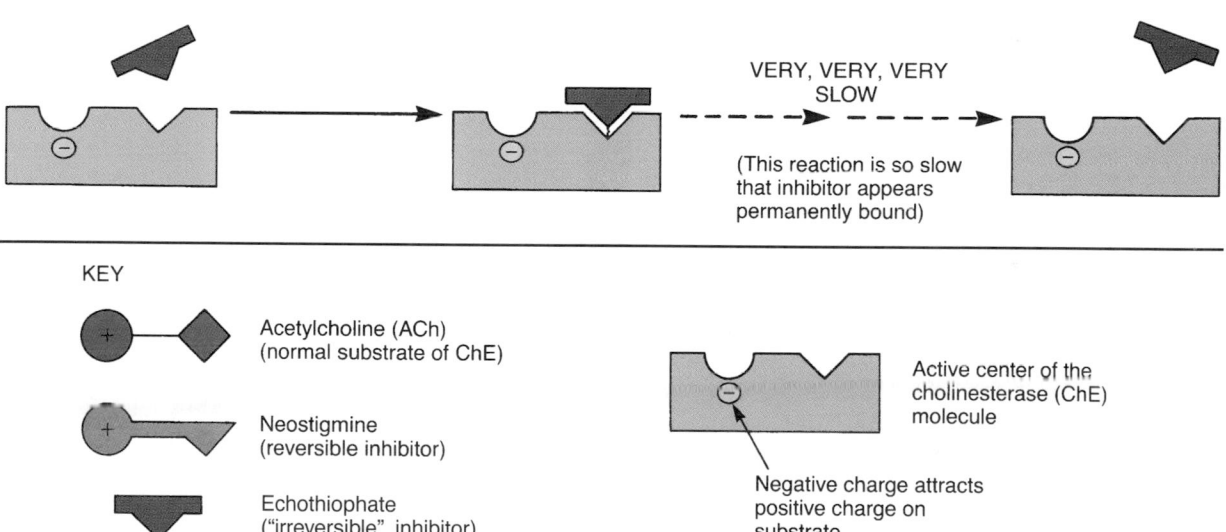

Figure 15–3 ■ **Inhibition of cholinesterase by reversible and "irreversible" inhibitors. (See text for details.)**

Acute Toxicity

Symptoms. Overdose with cholinesterase inhibitors causes *excessive muscarinic stimulation* and *respiratory depression*. (Respiratory depression results from a combination of depolarizing neuromuscular blockade and CNS depression.) The state produced by cholinesterase inhibitor poisoning is sometimes referred to as *cholinergic crisis*.

Treatment. Intravenous *atropine* will alleviate the muscarinic effects of cholinesterase inhibition. Respiratory depression from cholinesterase inhibitors cannot be managed with drugs. Hence, treatment consists of mechanical ventilation with oxygen. Suctioning may be necessary if atropine fails to suppress bronchial secretions.

Preparations, Dosage, and Administration

Neostigmine [Prostigmin] is available in 15-mg tablets for oral use. Dosages for *myasthenia gravis* are highly individualized, ranging from 15 to 375 mg/day administered in divided doses every 3 to 4 hours.

Other Reversible Cholinesterase Inhibitors
Physostigmine

The basic pharmacology of physostigmine is identical to that of neostigmine—except that physostigmine readily crosses membranes whereas neostigmine does not. Why? Because, in contrast to neostigmine, physostigmine is *not* a quaternary ammonium compound and hence does *not* carry a charge. Because physostigmine is uncharged, the drug crosses membranes with ease.

Physostigmine is the drug of choice for treating *poisoning by atropine and other drugs that cause muscarinic blockade* (e.g., antihistamines, tricyclic antidepressants, phenothiazine antipsychotics). Physostigmine counteracts antimuscarinic poisoning by causing ACh to build up at muscarinic junctions. The accumulated ACh competes with the muscarinic blocker for receptor binding, and thereby reverses receptor blockade. Physostigmine is preferred to neostigmine for antimuscarinic poisoning because, lacking a charge, physostigmine is able to cross the blood-brain barrier to reverse muscarinic blockade in the CNS. The usual dosage to treat antimuscarinic poisoning is 2 mg given by IM or slow IV injection.

Ambenonium, Demecarium, Edrophonium, and Pyridostigmine

These four drugs have pharmacologic effects much like those of neostigmine, our prototype cholinesterase inhibitor. One of these drugs—edrophonium—is noteworthy for its very brief duration of action. All four drugs are used for *myasthenia gravis*. Routes of administration for these drugs are summarized in Table 15–1.

In addition to treating myasthenia gravis, edrophonium and pyridostigmine are used to *reverse the effects of nondepolarizing neuromuscular blocking agents* (e.g., tubocurarine). These drugs reverse blockade by causing accumulation of ACh at the NMJ. This ability has two clinical applica-tions: (1) reversal of neuromuscular blockade in postoperative patients and (2) treatment of overdose with nondepolarizing neuromuscular blockers. In patients being treated for neuromuscular blocker overdose, artificial respiration must be maintained until muscle function has fully recovered. At the doses employed to reverse neuromuscular blockade, these drugs are likely to elicit substantial muscarinic responses; if needed, these can be reduced with atropine. It is important to note that cholinesterase inhibitors cannot be employed to counteract the effects of succinylcholine, a *depolarizing* neuromuscular blocker.

Demecarium and Echothiophate

These two drugs are used to lower intraocular pressure in patients with glaucoma. One of them—echothiophate—is the only *irreversible* cholinesterase inhibitor employed clinically. Glaucoma and its treatment are discussed in Chapter 100 (Drugs for the Eye).

Drugs for Alzheimer's Disease

Four cholinesterase inhibitors—*donepezil* [Aricept], *galantamine* [Reminyl], *rivastigmine* [Exelon], and *tacrine* [Cognex]—are used for Alzheimer's disease. Benefits derive from inhibiting cholinesterase in the CNS. These drugs are discussed in Chapter 22.

"IRREVERSIBLE" CHOLINESTERASE INHIBITORS

The "irreversible" cholinesterase inhibitors are highly toxic. These agents are employed primarily as *insecticides*. During World War II, huge quantities of irreversible cholinesterase inhibitors were produced for possible use as *nerve agents,* but were never deployed. Today, there is concern that these agents might be employed as weapons of terrorism. The only clinical indication for the irreversible inhibitors is *glaucoma*.

TABLE 15–1 ■ Clinical Applications of Cholinesterase Inhibitors

Generic Name [Trade Name]	Routes	Myasthenia Gravis Diagnosis	Myasthenia Gravis Treatment	Glaucoma	Reversal of Nondepolarizing Neuromuscular Blockade	Antidote to Poisoning by Muscarinic Antagonists	Alzheimer's Disease
Reversible Inhibitors							
Neostigmine [Prostigmin]	PO		✔				
Ambenonium [Mytelase]	PO		✔				
Pyridostigmine [Mestinon, Regonol]	PO, IM, IV		✔		✔		
Edrophonium [Tensilon, Enlon, Reversol]	IM, IV	✔			✔		
Physostigmine [Antilirium]	IM, IV					✔	
Demecarium [Humorsol]	Topical			✔			
Donepezil [Aricept]	PO						✔
Galantamine [Reminyl]	PO						✔
Rivastigmine [Exelon]	PO						✔
Tacrine [Cognex]	PO						✔
Irreversible Inhibitor							
Echothiophate [Phospholine Iodide]	Topical			✔			

Basic Pharmacology

Chemistry

All irreversible cholinesterase inhibitors contain an atom of *phosphorus* (Fig. 15–4). Because of this phosphorus atom, the irreversible inhibitors are known as *organophosphate* cholinesterase inhibitors.

Almost all irreversible cholinesterase inhibitors are *highly lipid soluble*. As a result, these drugs are readily absorbed from all routes of administration. They can even be absorbed directly through the skin. It is because of their easy absorption and high toxicity that these drugs are useful insecticides and have potential as agents of chemical warfare. Once absorbed, the organophosphate inhibitors have ready access to all tissues and organs, including the CNS.

Mechanism of Action

The irreversible cholinesterase inhibitors bind to the active center of cholinesterase, thereby preventing the enzyme from hydrolyzing ACh. Although these drugs can be split from ChE, the splitting reaction takes place *extremely* slowly (see Fig. 15–3C). Hence, under normal conditions, their binding to ChE can be considered irreversible. Because binding is permanent, effects persist until new molecules of cholinesterase can be synthesized.

Although we normally consider the bond between irreversible inhibitors and cholinesterase to be permanent, this bond can, in fact, be broken. To break the bond, and thereby reverse the inhibition of cholinesterase, we must administer *pralidoxime* (see below).

Pharmacologic Effects

The irreversible cholinesterase inhibitors produce essentially the same spectrum of effects as the reversible inhibitors. The principal difference is that responses to the irreversible inhibitors last a long time, whereas responses to the reversible inhibitors are short lived.

Therapeutic Uses

The irreversible cholinesterase inhibitors have only one indication: treatment of *glaucoma*—and for that indication, only one drug (echothiophate) is available. The limited indications for these drugs should be no surprise given their potential for toxicity. The use of echothiophate for glaucoma is discussed in Chapter 100 (Drugs for the Eye).

Toxicology

Sources of Poisoning. Poisoning by organophosphate cholinesterase inhibitors is not uncommon. Agricultural workers have been poisoned by accidental ingestion of organophosphate insecticides and by absorption of these lipid-soluble compounds through the skin. In addition, because organophosphate insecticides are readily available to the general public, poisoning may occur accidentally or from attempted homicide or suicide. Exposure could also occur if these drugs were used as instruments of warfare or terrorism.

Symptoms. Toxic doses of irreversible cholinesterase inhibitors produce a state of *cholinergic crisis,* a condition characterized by *excessive muscarinic stimulation and depolarizing neuromuscular blockade.* Overstimulation of muscarinic receptors results in profuse secretions from salivary and bronchial glands, involuntary urination and defecation, laryngospasm, and bronchoconstriction. Neuromuscular blockade can result in paralysis, followed by death from apnea. Convulsions of CNS origin precede paralysis and apnea.

Treatment. Treatment involves the following: (1) mechanical ventilation using oxygen, (2) giving *atropine* to reduce muscarinic stimulation, (3) giving *pralidoxime* to reverse inhibition of cholinesterase (primarily at the NMJ), and (4) giving *diazepam* to suppress convulsions.

Pralidoxime. Pralidoxime [Protopam] is a specific antidote to poisoning by the irreversible (organophosphate) cholinesterase inhibitors. This drug is *not* effective against poisoning by reversible cholinesterase inhibitors. Pralidoxime reverses poisoning by causing organophosphate inhibitors to dissociate from the active center of cholinesterase. Reversal is most effective at the NMJ; the drug is much less effective at reversing cholinesterase inhibition at muscarinic and ganglionic sites. Furthermore, since pralidoxime is a quaternary ammonium compound, it cannot cross the blood-brain barrier, and therefore cannot reverse cholinesterase inhibition in the CNS.

To be effective, pralidoxime must be administered soon after organophosphate poisoning has occurred. If too much time is allowed to elapse, a process called *aging* takes place. In this process, the bond between the organophosphate inhibitor and cholinesterase increases in strength. Once aging has occurred, pralidoxime is unable to cause the inhibitor to dissociate from the enzyme. The time required for aging depends on the agent involved. For example, with a nerve agent called *soman,*

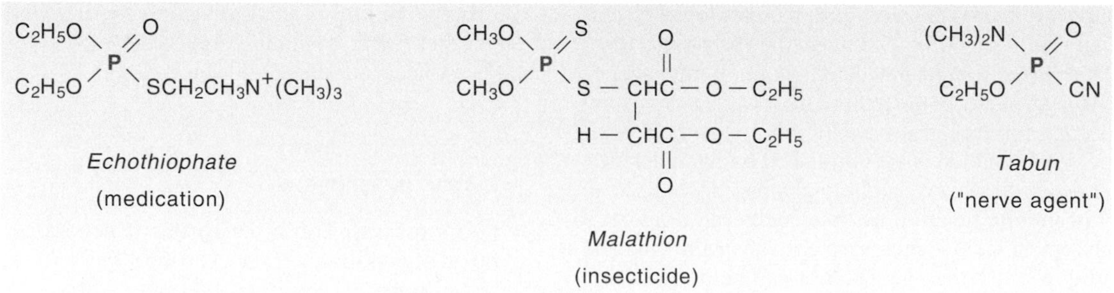

Figure 15–4 ▪ Structural formulas of "irreversible" cholinesterase inhibitors.
Note that irreversible cholinesterase inhibitors contain an atom of phosphorus. Because of this atom, these drugs are known as organophosphate cholinesterase inhibitors. With the exception of echothiophate, all of these drugs are highly lipid soluble, and therefore move throughout the body with ease.

aging occurs in just 2 minutes; however, with a nerve agent called *tabun* (see Fig. 15–4), aging requires 13 hours.

The usual dosage for pralidoxime is 1 to 2 gm administered IV or IM. Intravenous doses should be infused slowly (over 20 to 30 minutes) to avoid hypertension. For prolonged treatment, dosing can be repeated every hour, or the drug can be given by continuous infusion (500 mg/hr).

MYASTHENIA GRAVIS

Pathophysiology

Myasthenia gravis (MG) is a neuromuscular disorder characterized by fluctuating muscle weakness and a predisposition to rapid fatigue. Common symptoms include ptosis (drooping eyelids), difficulty swallowing, and weakness of skeletal muscles. Patients with severe MG may have difficulty breathing owing to weakness of the muscles of respiration.

Symptoms of MG result from an autoimmune process in which the patient's immune system produces antibodies directed against nicotinic$_M$ receptors on skeletal muscle. As a result of attack by these antibodies, the number of functional receptors at the neuromuscular junction is reduced by 70% to 90%, resulting in the muscle weakness that characterizes myasthenia.

Treatment with Cholinesterase Inhibitors

Beneficial Effects. Reversible cholinesterase inhibitors (e.g., neostigmine) are the mainstay of therapy. By preventing ACh inactivation, anticholinesterase agents can intensify the effects of ACh released from motor neurons, and can thereby increase muscle strength. Cholinesterase inhibitors do not cure myasthenia; they only produce symptomatic relief. Consequently, patients are likely to need therapy lifelong.

When working with a hospitalized patient, keep in mind that muscle strength may be insufficient to permit swallowing. Accordingly, you should assess the ability to swallow before giving oral medications. Assessment is accomplished by giving the patient a few sips of water. If the patient is unable to swallow the water, parenteral medication must be substituted for oral medication.

Side Effects. Since cholinesterase inhibitors can inhibit acetylcholinesterase at any location, these drugs will cause ACh to accumulate at muscarinic junctions as well as at neuromuscular junctions. If muscarinic responses are excessive, atropine may be given to suppress them. However, atropine should not be employed *routinely* since this drug can mask the early signs (e.g., excessive salivation) of overdose with anticholinesterase agents.

Dosage Adjustment. In the treatment of MG, establishing an optimal dosage for cholinesterase inhibitors can be a challenge. Dosage determination is accomplished by administering a small initial dose followed by additional small doses until an optimal level of muscle function has been achieved. Important signs of improvement include increased ease of swallowing and increased ability to raise the eyelids. You can help establish a correct dosage by keeping records of (1) times of drug administration, (2) times at which fatigue occurs, (3) the state of muscle strength before and after drug administration, and (4) signs of excessive muscarinic stimulation.

To maintain optimal responses, patients must occasionally modify dosage themselves. To do this, they must be taught to recognize signs of undermedication (difficulty in swallowing, ptosis) and signs of overmedication (excessive salivation and other muscarinic responses). Patients may also need to modify dosage in anticipation of exertion. For example, they may find it necessary to take supplementary medication 30 to 60 minutes prior to such activities as eating and shopping.

Usual adult dosages for the three agents used to treat myasthenia gravis are as follows:

- *Ambenonium*—15 to 100 mg/day in divided doses
- *Neostigmine*—15 to 375 mg/day in divided doses
- *Pyridostigmine*—60 to 1500 mg/day in divided doses

Myasthenic Crisis and Cholinergic Crisis. *Myasthenic Crisis.* Patients who are inadequately medicated may experience myasthenic crisis, a state characterized by extreme muscle weakness (caused by insufficient ACh at the neuromuscular junction). Left untreated, myasthenic crisis can result in death from paralysis of the muscles of respiration. A cholinesterase inhibitor (e.g., neostigmine) is used to relieve the crisis.

Cholinergic Crisis. As noted, overdose with a cholinesterase inhibitor can produce cholinergic crisis. Like myasthenic crisis, cholinergic crisis is characterized by extreme muscle weakness or frank paralysis. In addition, cholinergic crisis is accompanied by signs of excessive muscarinic stimulation. Treatment consists of respiratory support plus atropine. The offending cholinesterase inhibitor should be withheld until muscle strength has returned.

Distinguishing Myasthenic Crisis from Cholinergic Crisis. Since myasthenic crisis and cholinergic crisis share similar symptoms (muscle weakness or paralysis), but are treated very differently, it is essential to distinguish between them. A history of medication use or signs of excessive muscarinic stimulation are usually sufficient to permit a differential diagnosis. If these clues are inadequate, the differential diagnosis can be made by administering a challenging dose of *edrophonium,* an ultrashort-acting cholinesterase inhibitor. If edrophonium-induced elevation of ACh levels alleviates symptoms, the crisis is myasthenic. Conversely, if edrophonium intensifies symptoms, the crisis is cholinergic. Since the symptoms of cholinergic crisis will be made even worse by edrophonium, atropine and oxygen should be immediately available whenever edrophonium is used for this test.

Use of Identification by the Patient. Because of the possibility of experiencing either myasthenic crisis or cholinergic crisis, and because both crises can be fatal, patients with MG should be encouraged to wear a Medic Alert bracelet or some other form of identification to inform emergency medical personnel of their condition.

⁘ KEY POINTS

- Cholinesterase inhibitors prevent breakdown of ACh by acetylcholinesterase, causing ACh to accumulate in synapses, which in turn causes stimulation of muscarinic receptors, nicotinic receptors in ganglia and the NMJ, and cholinergic receptors in the CNS.
- The major use of reversible cholinesterase inhibitors is treatment of myasthenia gravis. Benefits derive from accumulation of ACh at the NMJ.

■ Secondary uses for reversible cholinesterase inhibitors are reversal of nondepolarizing neuromuscular blockade and treatment of glaucoma, Alzheimer's disease, and poisoning by muscarinic antagonists.

■ Because physostigmine crosses membranes easily, this drug is preferred for treating poisoning by muscarinic antagonists.

■ Irreversible cholinesterase inhibitors, also known as organophosphate cholinesterase inhibitors, are used primarily as insecticides. The only indication for these potentially toxic drugs is glaucoma.

■ Most organophosphate cholinesterase inhibitors are highly lipid soluble and therefore can be absorbed directly through the skin and can distribute easily to all tissues and organs.

■ Overdose with cholinesterase inhibitors produces cholinergic crisis, a state characterized by depolarizing neuromuscular blockade plus signs of excessive muscarinic stimulation (hypersalivation, tearing, sweating, bradycardia, involuntary urination and defecation, miosis, and spasm of accommodation). Death results from respiratory depression.

■ Poisoning by *reversible* cholinesterase inhibitors is treated with atropine (to reverse muscarinic stimulation) plus mechanical ventilation.

■ Poisoning by *organophosphate* cholinesterase inhibitors is treated with atropine, mechanical ventilation, pralidoxime (to reverse inhibition of cholinesterase, primarily at the NMJ), and diazepam (to suppress seizures).

Summary of Major Nursing Implications*

REVERSIBLE CHOLINESTERASE INHIBITORS

Ambenonium
Demecarium
Donepezil
Edrophonium
Galantamine
Neostigmine
Physostigmine
Pyridostigmine
Rivastigmine
Tacrine

Preadministration Assessment

Therapeutic Goal

Applications are treatment of myasthenia gravis, glaucoma, Alzheimer's disease, and poisoning by muscarinic antagonists and reversal of nondepolarizing neuromuscular blockade. Applications of individual agents are summarized in Table 15–1.

Baseline Data

Myasthenia Gravis. Determine the extent of neuromuscular dysfunction by assessing muscle strength, fatigue, ptosis, and ability to swallow.

Identifying High-Risk Patients

Cholinesterase inhibitors are *contraindicated* for patients with mechanical obstruction of the intestine or urinary tract. Exercise *caution* in patients with peptic ulcer disease, bradycardia, asthma, or hyperthyroidism.

Implementation: Administration

Routes

These drugs are given orally, topically, and parenterally (IM or IV). Routes for individual agents are summarized in Table 15–1.

Administration and Dosage in Myasthenia Gravis

Administration. Assess the patient's ability to swallow before giving oral medication. If swallowing is impaired, substitute a parenteral medication.

Optimizing Dosage. Monitor for therapeutic responses (see below) and adjust the dosage accordingly. **Teach patients to distinguish between insufficient and excessive dosing so they can participate effectively in dosage adjustment.**

Reversing Nondepolarizing Neuromuscular Blockade

To reverse toxicity from overdose with a nondepolarizing neuromuscular blocking agent (e.g., tubocurarine), administer pyridostigmine or edrophonium IV. Support respiration until muscle strength has recovered fully.

Treating Muscarinic Antagonist Poisoning

Physostigmine is the drug of choice for this indication. The usual dose is 2 mg administered by IM or slow IV injection.

Implementation: Measures to Enhance Therapeutic Effects

Myasthenia Gravis

Promoting Compliance. **Inform patients that MG is not usually curable, and hence treatment may be lifelong. Encourage patients to take their medication as prescribed.**

Using Identification. **Since patients with MG are at risk of fatal complications (cholinergic crisis, myasthenic crisis), encourage them to wear a Medic Alert bracelet or similar identification to inform emergency medical personnel of their condition.**

Ongoing Evaluation and Interventions

Evaluating Therapeutic Effects

Myasthenia Gravis. Monitor and record (1) times of drug administration; (2) times at which fatigue occurs; (3) state of muscle strength, ptosis, and ability to

*Patient education information is highlighted as blue text.

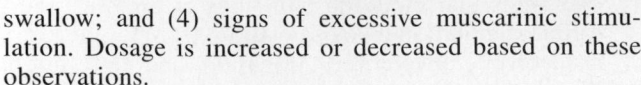

Summary of Major Nursing Implications*—cont'd

swallow; and (4) signs of excessive muscarinic stimulation. Dosage is increased or decreased based on these observations.

Monitor for *myasthenic crisis* (extreme muscle weakness, paralysis of respiratory muscles), which can occur when cholinesterase inhibitor dosage is insufficient. Manage with respiratory support and increased dosage.

Be certain to distinguish myasthenic crisis from cholinergic crisis. How? By observing for signs of excessive muscarinic stimulation, which will accompany cholinergic crisis but not myasthenic crisis. If necessary, these crises can be differentiated by giving *edrophonium,* which will reduce symptoms of myasthenic crisis and intensify symptoms of cholinergic crisis.

Minimizing Adverse Effects

Excessive Muscarinic Stimulation. Accumulation of ACh at muscarinic receptors can cause profuse salivation, increased tone and motility of the gut, urinary urgency, sweating, miosis, spasm of accommodation, bronchoconstriction, and bradycardia. **Inform patients about signs of excessive muscarinic stimulation and advise them to notify the physician if these occur.** Excessive muscarinic responses can be reduced with *atropine.*

Cholinergic Crisis. This condition results from cholinesterase inhibitor overdose. Manifestations are skeletal muscle paralysis (from depolarizing neuromuscular blockade) and signs of excessive muscarinic stimulation (e.g., salivation, sweating, miosis, bradycardia).

Manage with mechanical ventilation and atropine. Cholinergic crisis must be distinguished from myasthenic crisis.

*Patient education information is highlighted as blue text.

Neuromuscular Blocking Agents and Ganglionic Blocking Agents

The drugs discussed in this chapter act through blockade of nicotinic cholinergic receptors. The *neuromuscular* blocking agents block nicotinic$_M$ receptors at the neuromuscular junction. The *ganglionic* blocking agents block nicotinic$_N$ receptors in autonomic ganglia. The neuromuscular blockers have important clinical applications. In contrast, the ganglionic blockers, once used widely for hypertension, have been largely replaced by newer drugs.

NEUROMUSCULAR BLOCKING AGENTS

Neuromuscular blocking agents prevent acetylcholine from activating nicotinic$_M$ receptors on skeletal muscles, and thereby cause muscle relaxation. These drugs are given to produce muscle relaxation during surgery, endotracheal intubation, mechanical ventilation, and other procedures.

Control of Muscle Contraction

Before we discuss the neuromuscular blockers themselves, it will help to review physiologic control of muscle contraction. In particular, we need to understand *excitation-contraction coupling,* the process by which an action potential in a motor neuron leads to contraction of a muscle.

Basic Concepts: Polarization, Depolarization, and Repolarization

The concepts of *polarization, depolarization,* and *repolarization* are important to understanding both muscle contraction and neuromuscular blocking drugs. In *resting* muscle there is uneven distribution of electrical charge across the inner and outer surfaces of the cell membrane. As shown in Figure 16–1, positive charges cover the outer surface of the membrane and negative charges cover the inner surface. Because of this uneven charge distribution, the resting membrane is said to be *polarized.*

When the membrane *depolarizes,* positive charges move from outside to inside. So many positive charges move inward that the inside of the membrane becomes more positive than the outside (see Fig. 16–1).

Under physiologic conditions, depolarization of the muscle membrane is followed almost instantaneously by *repolarization.* Repolarization is accomplished by pumping positively charged ions out of the cell. Repolarization restores the original resting membrane state, with positive charges on the outer surface and negative charges on the inner surface.

Steps in Muscle Contraction

The steps leading to muscle contraction are summarized in Figure 16–2. The process begins with the arrival of an action potential at the terminal of a motor neuron, causing release of acetylcholine (ACh) into the subneural space. Acetylcholine then binds reversibly to nicotinic$_M$ receptors on the motor end-plate (a specialized region of the muscle membrane that contains the receptors for ACh) and causes the end-plate to *depolarize.* This depolarization initiates a muscle action potential (i.e., a wave of depolarization that spreads rapidly over the entire muscle membrane), which in turn triggers the release of calcium from the sarcoplasmic reticulum (SR) of the muscle. This calcium permits the interaction of actin and myosin, thereby causing contraction. Very rapidly, ACh dissociates from the motor end-plate, the motor end-plate repolarizes, the muscle membrane repolarizes, and calcium is taken back up into the SR. Because there is no longer any calcium available to support the interaction of actin and myosin, the muscle relaxes.

Sustained muscle contraction requires a continuous series of motor neuron action potentials. These action potentials cause repeated release of ACh, which causes repeated activation of nicotinic receptors on the motor end-plate. As a result, the end-plate goes through repeating cycles of depolarization and repolarization, which results in sufficient release of calcium to sustain contraction. If for some reason the motor end-plate fails to repolarize—that is, if the end-plate remains in a *depolarized* state—the signal for calcium release will stop, calcium will undergo immediate reuptake into the SR, and contraction will cease.

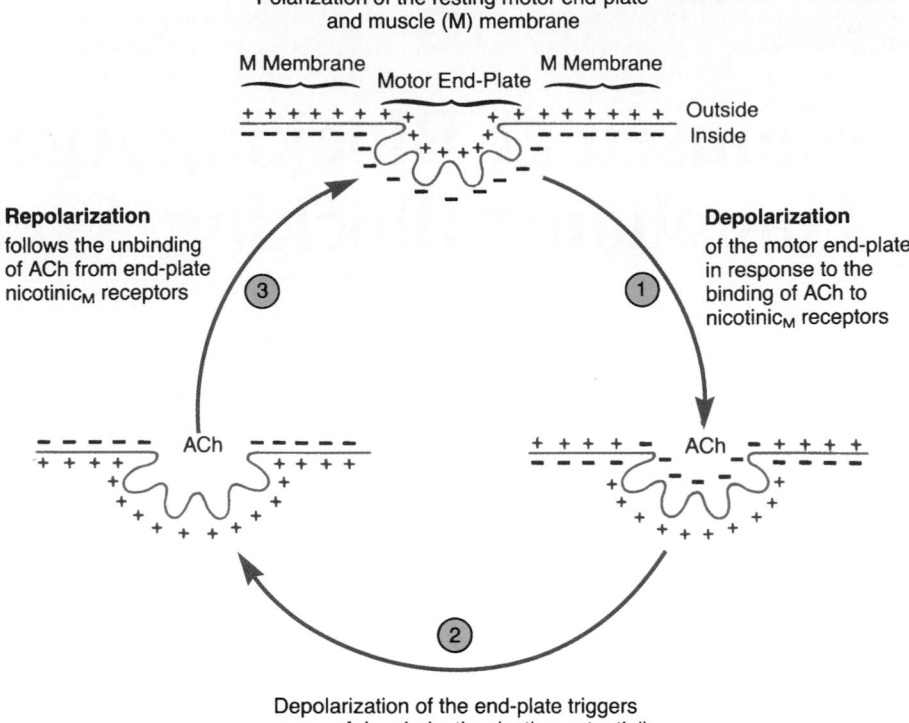

Figure 16–1 ■ The depolarization-repolarization cycle of the motor end-plate and muscle membrane.

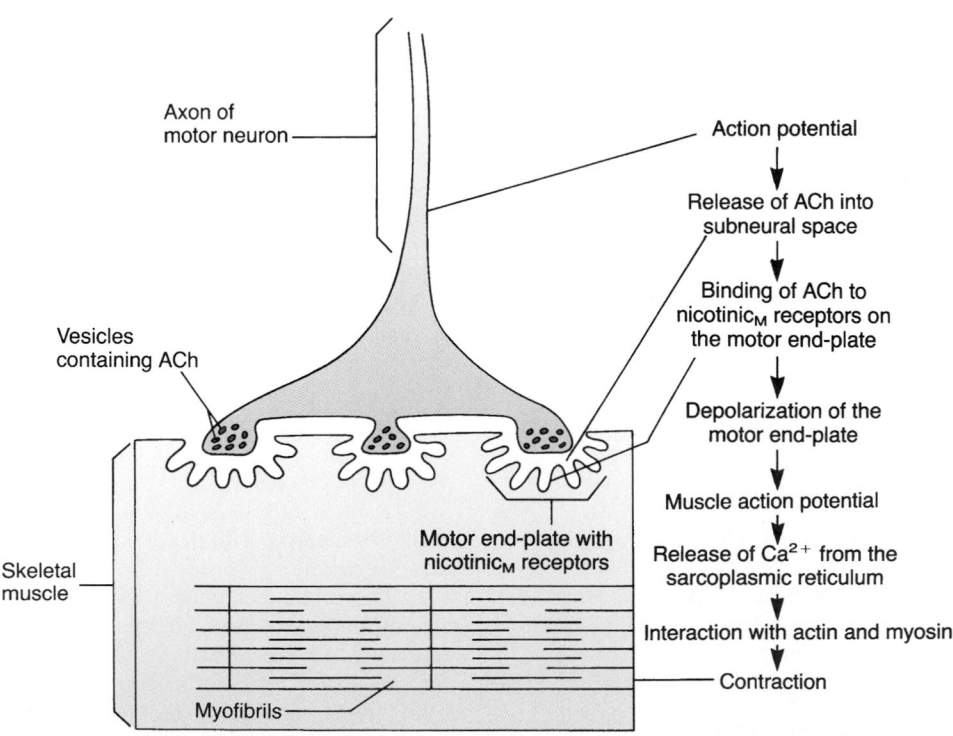

Figure 16–2 ■ Steps in excitation-contraction coupling.

Classification of Neuromuscular Blockers

The neuromuscular blockers can be classified according to *mechanism of action* and *time course of action*. When classified by mechanism of action, these drugs fall into two categories: nondepolarizing agents and depolarizing agents. When classified by time course, these drugs fall into four categories: long acting, intermediate acting, short acting, and ultrashort acting.

Nondepolarizing Neuromuscular Blockers I: Tubocurarine

Tubocurarine is the oldest nondepolarizing neuromuscular blocker and will serve as our prototype for the group.

The pharmacologic powers of tubocurarine were known to primitive hunters long before coming to the attention of modern scientists. Tubocurarine is one of several active principles found in *curare,* an arrow poison used for hunting by South American Indians. When shot into a monkey or other small animal, curare-tipped arrows cause relaxation (paralysis) of skeletal muscles. Death results from paralyzing the muscles of respiration.

The clinical utility of tubocurarine is based on the same action that is useful in hunting: production of skeletal muscle relaxation. Relaxation of skeletal muscles is helpful in patients undergoing surgery, endotracheal intubation, mechanical ventilation, and other procedures.

Chemistry

Tubocurarine and all other neuromuscular blocking agents contain a *quaternary nitrogen* atom (Fig. 16–3). As a result, these drugs always carry a positive charge, and therefore cannot readily cross membranes.

The inability to cross membranes has three clinical consequences. First, neuromuscular blockers cannot be administered orally. Instead, they must all be administered parenterally (almost always IV). Second, these drugs cannot cross the blood-brain barrier, and hence have no effect on the central nervous system (CNS). Third, neuromuscular blockers cannot readily cross the placenta. Thus, effects on the fetus are minimal.

Mechanism of Action

Tubocurarine acts by competing with ACh for binding to nicotinic$_M$ receptors on the motor end-plate (Fig. 16–4). Since tubocurarine does not activate these receptors, binding does not result in contraction. Muscle relaxation persists as long as the amount of tubocurarine at the neuromuscular junction (NMJ) is sufficient to prevent receptor occupation by ACh. Muscle function can be restored by eliminating tubocurarine from the body or by increasing the amount of ACh at the NMJ.

Pharmacologic Effects

Muscle Relaxation. The primary effect of tubocurarine is relaxation of skeletal muscles. Muscle relaxation produces a state of *flaccid paralysis.*

Although tubocurarine can paralyze all skeletal muscles, not all muscles are affected at once. The first to become paralyzed are the levator muscle of the eyelid and the muscles of mastication. Paralysis occurs next in muscles of the limbs, abdomen, and glottis. The last muscles affected are the muscles of respiration—the intercostals and diaphragm.

Hypotension. Tubocurarine can lower blood pressure by two mechanisms: (1) release of histamine and (2) partial ganglionic blockade. Histamine lowers blood pressure by pro-

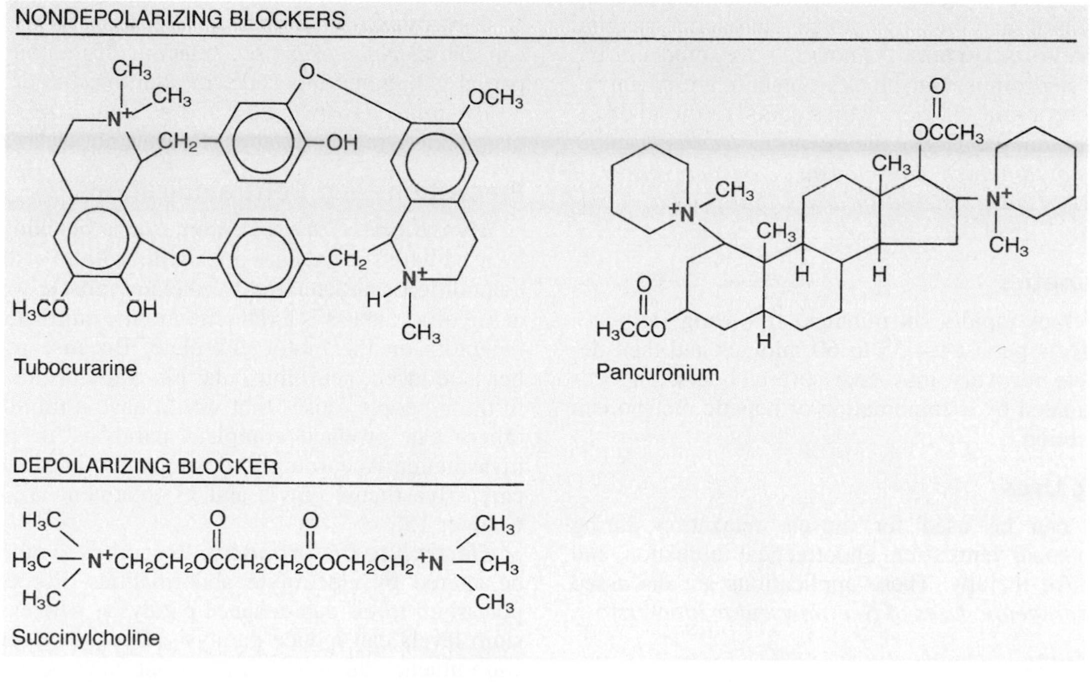

NONDEPOLARIZING BLOCKERS

Tubocurarine

Pancuronium

DEPOLARIZING BLOCKER

Succinylcholine

Figure 16–3 ■ **Structural formulas of representative neuromuscular blocking agents.** Note that all of these agents contain quaternary nitrogen atoms and therefore cross membranes poorly. Consequently, these drugs must be administered parenterally and have little effect on the central nervous system or the developing fetus.

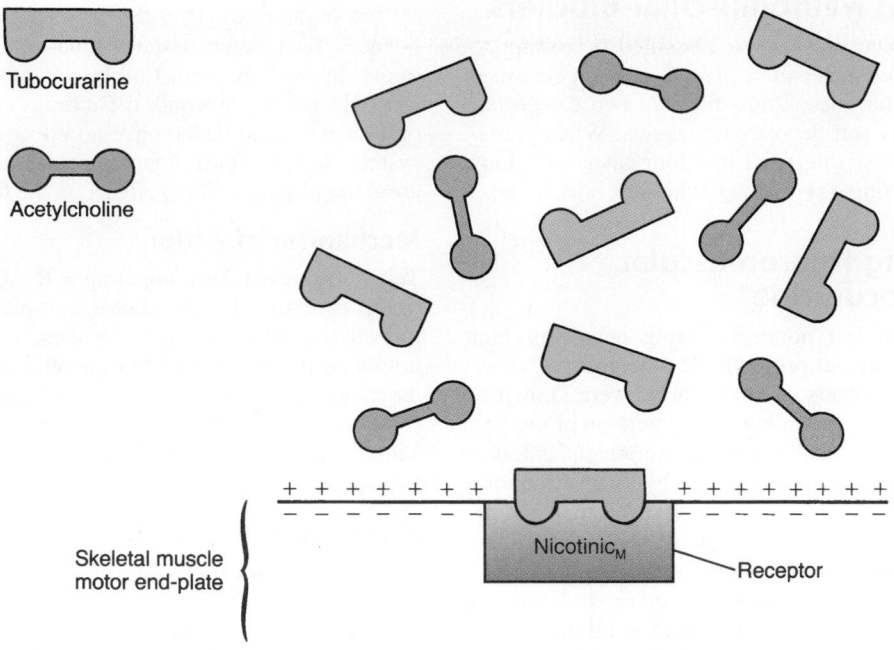

Figure 16–4 ■ Mechanism of nondepolarizing neuromuscular blockade. Tubocurarine competes with ACh for binding to nicotinic$_M$ receptors on the motor end-plate. Binding of tubocurarine does not depolarize the end-plate, and therefore does not cause contraction. At the same time, the presence of tubocurarine prevents ACh from binding to the receptor, hence contraction is prevented.

moting vasodilation. Ganglionic blockade lowers blood pressure by decreasing sympathetic tone to arterioles and veins. Tubocurarine suppresses ganglionic transmission by causing partial blockade of nicotinic$_N$ receptors in autonomic ganglia.

Central Nervous System. As noted above, tubocurarine and the other neuromuscular blocking agents are unable to cross the blood-brain barrier. Consequently, these drugs have no effect on the CNS. Please note: *Neuromuscular blockers do not diminish consciousness or perception of pain—even when administered in doses that produce complete paralysis.*

Pharmacokinetics

Paralysis develops rapidly (in minutes) following IV injection. Peak effects persist for 35 to 60 minutes and then decline. Complete recovery may take several hours. Tubocurarine is eliminated by a combination of hepatic metabolism and renal excretion.

Therapeutic Uses

Tubocurarine can be used for muscle relaxation during surgery, mechanical ventilation, endotracheal intubation, and electroconvulsive therapy. These applications are discussed later under *Therapeutic Uses of Neuromuscular Blockers.*

Adverse Effects

The principal adverse effects of tubocurarine concern the respiratory and cardiovascular systems.

Respiratory Arrest. Paralysis of respiratory muscles can produce respiratory arrest. Because of this risk, facilities for artificial ventilation must be immediately available. Patients

must be monitored closely and continuously. When tubocurarine is withdrawn, vital signs must be monitored until muscle function has fully recovered.

Cardiovascular Effects. As noted above, tubocurarine can cause *hypotension* secondary to histamine release and partial ganglionic blockade. In addition, the drug can cause *bradycardia, dysrhythmias,* and *cardiac arrest.* The mechanism underlying these latter effects is not clear.

Precautions and Contraindications

Myasthenia Gravis. Neuromuscular blocking agents must be used with special care in patients with myasthenia gravis, a condition characterized by skeletal muscle weakness. The cause of weakness is a reduction in the number of nicotinic$_M$ receptors on the motor end-plate. Because receptor number is reduced, neuromuscular blockade occurs very readily in these people; doses that would have a minimal effect on others can produce complete paralysis in patients with myasthenia. Accordingly, dosing must be done with great care. Myasthenia gravis and its treatment are discussed in Chapter 15.

Electrolyte Disturbances. Responses to tubocurarine can be altered by electrolyte abnormalities. For example, low potassium levels can enhance paralysis, whereas high potassium levels can reduce paralysis. Because electrolyte status can influence the depth of neuromuscular blockade, it is important to maintain normal electrolyte levels.

Drug Interactions

Tubocurarine can interact with many other drugs. Interactions of primary interest are discussed below.

TABLE 16–1 ▪ Neuromuscular Blockers: Time Course of Action*

Generic Name	Route	Time to Maximum Paralysis (min)	Duration of Effective Paralysis (min)	Time to Nearly Full Spontaneous Recovery†
Long Acting				
Doxacurium [Nuromax]	IV	4–10	100	Hours
Metocurine [Metubine]	IV	3–5	25–90	Hours
Pipecuronium [Arduan]	IV	3–5	90–120	Hours
Tubocurarine	IV, IM‡	2–5	60–90	Hours
Intermediate Acting				
Atracurium [Tracrium]	IV	2–5	20–35	60–70 min
Cisatracurium [Nimbex]	IV	2–5	20–35	—
Pancuronium [Pavulon]	IV	3–4	35–45	60–70 min
Rocuronium [Zemuron]	IV	1–3	20–40	—
Vecuronium [Norcuron]	IV	3–5	25–30	45–60 min
Short Acting				
Mivacurium [Mivacron]	IV	2–5	10–15	21–34 min
Ultrashort Acting				
Succinylcholine [Anectine, Quelicin]	IV, IM‡	1	4–6	—

*Time course of action can vary widely with dosage and route of administration. The values presented are for an average adult dose administered as a single IV injection.
†Because spontaneous recovery can take a long time, recovery from the *nondepolarizing* agents (all of the drugs listed except succinylcholine) is often accelerated by giving a cholinesterase inhibitor.
‡Intramuscular administration is rare.

General Anesthetics. All inhalation anesthetics produce some degree of skeletal muscle relaxation, and can thereby enhance the actions of tubocurarine and other neuromuscular blockers. Consequently, when general anesthetics and neuromuscular blockers are combined (as they often are), the dosage of the neuromuscular blocker should be reduced so as to avoid excessive neuromuscular blockade.

Antibiotics. Several antibiotics can intensify responses to neuromuscular blockers. Among them are *aminoglycosides* (e.g., gentamicin), *tetracyclines,* and certain other nonpenicillin antibiotics.

Cholinesterase Inhibitors. Cholinesterase inhibitors can *decrease* the effects of tubocurarine and other *nondepolarizing* neuromuscular blockers. (As discussed later in the chapter, cholinesterase inhibitors have the opposite effect on responses to succinylcholine, a *depolarizing* neuromuscular blocker.)

How do cholinesterase inhibitors decrease the effects of tubocurarine? Recall that nondepolarizing blockers compete with ACh for binding to nicotinic$_M$ receptors. By decreasing the degradation of ACh, cholinesterase inhibitors increase the amount of ACh available to compete with tubocurarine for receptor binding. As more ACh (and less tubocurarine) occupies nicotinic$_M$ receptors, the degree of neuromuscular blockade declines.

The ability of cholinesterase inhibitors to decrease responses to nondepolarizing neuromuscular blockers has two clinical applications: (1) management of overdose with a nondepolarizing neuromuscular blocker and (2) reversal of neuromuscular blockade following surgery and other procedures.

Toxicology

Overdose with tubocurarine has three major effects: (1) prolonged apnea, (2) massive histamine release, and (3) cardiovascular collapse. Apnea is managed with respiratory support plus a cholinesterase inhibitor (e.g., neostigmine) to reverse neuromuscular blockade. Antihistamines are given to counteract released histamine. Cardiovascular toxicity must be assessed and treated as indicated.

Preparations, Dosage, and Administration

Tubocurarine is always administered parenterally. The usual route is IV. Intramuscular injections are employed rarely.

Because of their potential for harm, tubocurarine and other neuromuscular blockers are administered only by clinicians specially trained in their use. Whenever these drugs are given, facilities for artificial respiration and management of cardiovascular complications must be at hand.

Tubocurarine is dispensed in solution (20 units/ml) for IM and IV injection. The dosage depends on the indication. A typical dosage for adult surgical patients is 40 to 60 units IV at the time of the initial incision, followed by 20 to 30 units a few minutes later. During long operations, additional doses of 20 to 30 units may be administered as needed.

Nondepolarizing Neuromuscular Blockers II: Others

In addition to tubocurarine, nine other nondepolarizing blockers are approved for use in the United States. Like tubocurarine, they all act by competing with acetylcholine at nicotinic$_M$ receptors on the motor end-plate. Differences among the drugs relate primarily to time course of action (Table 16–1) and cardiovascular effects. With all of these agents, respiratory depression secondary to neuromuscular blockade is the major concern. Respiratory depression can be reversed by giving a cholinesterase inhibitor.

Long-Acting Agents

Doxacurium. Doxacurium [Nuromax] is a long-acting neuromuscular blocker used for muscle relaxation during general anesthesia and intubation. The drug is eliminated by the kidneys, and hence muscle relaxation is prolonged in patients with renal failure. Doxacurium is devoid of adverse cardiovascular effects.

Metocurine. Metocurine [Metubine] is a semisynthetic derivative of tubocurarine and has a similar time course. The drug is used primarily for muscle relaxation during surgery. Metocurine causes less histamine release than tubocurarine and less ganglionic blockade. As a result, the risk of hypotension is low.

Pipecuronium. Pipecuronium [Arduan] is indicated for muscle relaxation during surgery and intubation. Because its effects are long lasting, the drug is not recommended for procedures that last less than 90 minutes. Pipecuronium does not release histamine, does not cause vagal block, and is generally free of adverse cardiovascular effects. Duration of paralysis may be prolonged and unpredictable in obese patients and patients with renal failure.

Intermediate-Acting Agents

Atracurium. Atracurium [Tracrium] is approved for muscle relaxation during surgery, intubation, and mechanical ventilation. The drug can cause hypotension secondary to histamine release. Like succinylcholine, atracurium is eliminated by *plasma cholinesterases,* not by the liver or kidneys. Hence, atracurium may be desirable for patients with renal or hepatic dysfunction since these disorders will not prolong the drug's effects.

Cisatracurium. Cisatracurium [Nimbex], a close relative of atracurium, is approved for muscle relaxation during surgery, intubation, and mechanical ventilation. Elimination is by spontaneous degradation, not by hepatic metabolism or renal excretion. Hence, like atracurium, cisatracurium would seem desirable for patients with kidney or liver dysfunction. Histamine release is minimal.

Pancuronium. Pancuronium [Pavulon] is approved for muscle relaxation during general anesthesia, intubation, and mechanical ventilation. The drug does not cause histamine release, ganglionic blockade, or hypotension. Vagolytic effects may produce tachycardia. Elimination is primarily renal.

Rocuronium. Rocuronium [Zemuron] has a rapid onset and intermediate duration of action. The only neuromuscular blockers with a faster onset are rapacuronium and succinylcholine. In contrast to succinylcholine and rapacuronium, whose effects fade relatively quickly, rocuronium has effects that persist for 20 to 40 minutes. Rocuronium does not cause histamine release. Elimination is by hepatic metabolism. The drug is approved for muscle relaxation during intubation, surgery, and mechanical ventilation.

Vecuronium. Vecuronium [Norcuron], an analog of pancuronium, is used for muscle relaxation during intubation and general anesthesia. The drug does not produce ganglionic or vagal block and does not release histamine. Consequently, cardiovascular effects are minimal. Vecuronium is excreted primarily in the bile; hence paralysis may be prolonged in patients with liver dysfunction. Paralysis may also be prolonged in obese patients.

Short-Acting Agents

Mivacurium. Mivacurium [Mivacron] is the shortest acting *nondepolarizing* neuromuscular blocker. The only neuromuscular blocker with a shorter duration is succinylcholine, a *depolarizing* neuromuscular blocker. Paralysis is maximal 2 to 5 minutes after IV injection and persists only 10 to 15 minutes. Like succinylcholine, mivacurium is metabolized by plasma cholinesterase. As a result, effects are prolonged in patients with low cholinesterase levels. Mivacurium can cause facial flushing secondary to histamine release. Other cardiovascular effects are minimal.

Depolarizing Neuromuscular Blockers: Succinylcholine

Succinylcholine, an ultrashort-acting drug, is the only depolarizing neuromuscular blocker in clinical use. This drug differs from the nondepolarizing blockers with regard to mechanism of action, mode of elimination, interaction with cholinesterase inhibitors, and management of toxicity.

Mechanism of Action

Succinylcholine produces a state known as *depolarizing neuromuscular blockade.* Like acetylcholine, succinylcholine binds to nicotinic$_M$ receptors on the motor end-plate and thereby causes depolarization. This depolarization produces transient muscle contractions (fasciculations). Then, instead of dissociating rapidly from the receptor, succinylcholine remains bound. By remaining bound, the drug prevents the end-plate from repolarizing. That is, succinylcholine maintains the end-plate in a state of *constant depolarization.* Since the end-plate must repeatedly depolarize and repolarize to maintain muscle contraction, succinylcholine's ability to keep the end-plate depolarized causes paralysis (following the brief initial period of contraction). Paralysis persists until plasma levels of succinylcholine decline, thereby allowing the drug to dissociate from its receptors.

Pharmacologic Effects

Muscle Relaxation. The muscle-relaxant effects of succinylcholine are much like those of tubocurarine: both drugs produce a state of flaccid paralysis. However, despite this similarity, there are two important differences: (1) paralysis from succinylcholine is preceded by transient contractions and (2) paralysis from succinylcholine abates much more rapidly.

Central Nervous System. Like tubocurarine, succinylcholine has no effect on the CNS. The drug can produce complete paralysis without decreasing consciousness or the ability to feel pain.

Pharmacokinetics

Succinylcholine has an extremely short duration of action. Paralysis peaks about 1 minute after IV injection and fades completely 4 to 10 minutes later.

Paralysis is brief because succinylcholine is rapidly degraded by *pseudocholinesterase,* an enzyme present in plasma. (This enzyme is called pseudocholinesterase to distinguish it from "true" cholinesterase, the enzyme found at synapses where ACh is the transmitter.) Because of its presence in plasma, pseudocholinesterase is also known as *plasma cholinesterase.* In most individuals, pseudocholinesterase is highly active and can eliminate succinylcholine in minutes.

Therapeutic Uses

Succinylcholine is used primarily for muscle relaxation during endotracheal intubation, electroconvulsive therapy, endoscopy, and other short procedures. Because of its brief duration, succinylcholine is less desirable than tubocurarine and other nondepolarizing blockers for use in prolonged procedures (i.e., surgery and mechanical ventilation). Clinical applications are discussed further under *Therapeutic Uses of Neuromuscular Blockers.*

Adverse Effects

Prolonged Apnea in Patients with Low Pseudocholinesterase Activity. A few people, because of their genetic heritage, produce a form of pseudocholinesterase that has extremely low activity. As a result, they are unable to degrade succinylcholine rapidly. If succinylcholine is given to these people, paralysis can persist for hours, instead of just a few minutes. Not surprisingly, succinylcholine is contraindicated for these individuals.

Patients suspected of having low pseudocholinesterase activity should be tested for this possibility before receiving full succinylcholine doses. Pseudocholinesterase activity can be assessed by direct measurement of a blood sample or by administering a tiny test dose of succinylcholine. If the test dose produces muscle relaxation that is unexpectedly intense and prolonged, pseudocholinesterase activity is probably low.

Malignant Hyperthermia. Malignant hyperthermia is a rare and potentially fatal condition that can be triggered by succinylcholine, and by all inhalation anesthetics as well. The condition is characterized by muscle rigidity associated with a profound elevation of temperature—sometimes to as high as 43°C. Temperature becomes elevated because of excessive and uncontrolled metabolic activity in muscle. Left untreated, the condition can rapidly prove fatal. Malignant hyperthermia is a genetically determined reaction that has an incidence of about 1 in 25,000. Individuals with a family history of the reaction should not receive succinylcholine.

Treatment of malignant hyperthermia includes (1) immediate discontinuation of succinylcholine and the accompanying anesthetic, (2) cooling patient with ice or with an infusion of iced saline, and (3) administering *dantrolene,* a drug that stops heat generation by acting directly on skeletal muscle to reduce its metabolic activity. The pharmacology of dantrolene is discussed in Chapter 24 (Drugs for Muscle Spasm and Spasticity).

Postoperative Muscle Pain. Between 10% and 70% of patients receiving succinylcholine experience postoperative muscle pain, most commonly in the neck, shoulders, and back. Pain develops 12 to 24 hours after surgery and may persist several hours or even days. The cause of pain may be the muscle contractions that occur during the initial phase of succinylcholine action.

Hyperkalemia. Succinylcholine promotes release of potassium from tissues. Rarely, potassium release is sufficient to cause severe hyperkalemia. Death from cardiac arrest has resulted. Significant hyperkalemia is most likely in patients with major burns, multiple trauma, denervation of skeletal muscle, or upper motor neuron injury. Accordingly, the drug is contraindicated for these patients.

Drug Interactions

Cholinesterase Inhibitors. These drugs *potentiate* (intensify) the effects of succinylcholine. Potentiation occurs because cholinesterase inhibitors decrease the activity of pseudocholinesterase, the enzyme that inactivates succinylcholine. Note that the effect of cholinesterase inhibitors on succinylcholine is opposite to their effect on *nondepolarizing* neuromuscular blockers.

Antibiotics. The effects of succinylcholine, like those of tubocurarine, can be intensified by certain antibiotics. Among these are aminoglycosides, tetracyclines, and certain other nonpenicillin antibiotics.

Toxicology

Overdose can produce prolonged apnea. Since there is no specific antidote to succinylcholine poisoning, management is purely supportive. Recall that, with tubocurarine overdose, paralysis can be reversed with a cholinesterase inhibitor. Since cholinesterase inhibitors *delay* the degradation of succinylcholine, use of these agents would prolong—not reverse—succinylcholine toxicity.

Preparations, Dosage, and Administration

Succinylcholine chloride [Anectine, Quelicin] is available in solution and as a powder. The drug is usually administered IV but can also be given IM. Solutions of succinylcholine are unstable and should be used within 24 hours. Multidose vials are stable for up to 2 weeks.

Dosage must be individualized and depends on the specific application. A typical adult dose for a brief procedure is 25 to 75 mg administered as a single IV injection. For prolonged procedures, succinylcholine may be administered by infusion at a rate of 2.5 to 4.3 mg/min.

Therapeutic Uses of Neuromuscular Blockers

The primary applications of the neuromuscular blocking agents are discussed below. No one agent is used for every application.

Muscle Relaxation During Surgery

Production of muscle relaxation during surgery offers two benefits. First, relaxation of skeletal muscles, especially those of the abdominal wall, makes the surgeon's work easier. Second, muscle relaxants allow us to decrease the dosage of the general anesthetic, thereby decreasing the risks associated with anesthesia. Before neuromuscular blockers became available, surgical muscle relaxation had to be achieved with the general anesthetic alone, often requiring high levels of anesthetic. (As noted earlier, inhalation anesthetics have muscle relaxant properties of their own.) By combining a neuromuscular blocker with the general anesthetic, we can achieve adequate surgical muscle relaxation with less anesthetic than was possible when paralysis had to be achieved with an anesthetic by itself. By allowing a reduction in anesthetic levels, neuromuscular blockers have decreased the risk of respiratory depression from anesthesia. In addition, since less anesthetic is administered, recovery from anesthesia occurs faster.

Whenever neuromuscular blockers are employed during surgery, it is very, very important that anesthesia be maintained at a level sufficient to produce unconsciousness. Recall that neuromuscular blockers do not enter the CNS, and therefore have no effect on hearing, thinking, or the ability to feel pain; all these drugs do is produce paralysis. Neuromuscular blockers are obviously and definitely not a substitute for anesthesia. It does not require much imagination to appreciate the horror of the surgical patient who is completely paralyzed from neuromuscular blockade yet fully awake because of inadequate anesthesia. Does this really happen? Yes. In fact, it happens in between 0.1% and 0.2% of surgeries in which neuromuscular blockers are used. Clearly, full anesthesia must be provided whenever surgery is performed on a patient who is under neuromuscular blockade.

Full recovery from neuromuscular blockade may take from one to several hours. During the recovery period, patients must be monitored closely to ensure adequate ventilation. A patent airway should be maintained until the patient can swallow or speak. Recovery from the effects of *nondepolarizing* neuromuscular blockers (e.g., tubocurarine) can be accelerated with a cholinesterase inhibitor.

Facilitation of Mechanical Ventilation

Some patients who require mechanical ventilation still have some spontaneous respiratory movements—movements that can fight the rhythm of the respirator. By suppressing these movements, neuromuscular blocking agents can reduce resistance to ventilation.

When neuromuscular blockers are used to facilitate mechanical ventilation, patients should be treated as if they were awake—even though they will appear to be asleep. (Remember that the patient is paralyzed, and hence there is no way to assess state of consciousness.) Because the patient may be fully awake, steps should be taken to ensure comfort at all times. Furthermore, since neuromuscular blockade does not affect hearing, nothing should be said in the patient's presence that might be inappropriate for him or her to hear.

Being fully awake but completely paralyzed can be a stressful and generally horrific experience. (Think about it.) Accordingly, many clinicians do not recommend routine use of neuromuscular blockers during prolonged mechanical ventilation in intensive care units.

Adjunct to Electroconvulsive Therapy

Electroconvulsive therapy is an effective treatment for severe depression (see Chapter 31). Benefits derive strictly from the effects of electroshock on the brain; the convulsive movements that can accompany electroshock don't help relieve depression. Since convulsions per se serve no useful purpose, and since electroshock-induced convulsions can be harmful, neuromuscular blockers are now used to prevent convulsive movements during electroshock therapy. Because of its short duration of action, *succinylcholine* is the preferred neuromuscular blocker for this application.

Endotracheal Intubation

An endotracheal tube is a large catheter that is inserted past the glottis and into the trachea to facilitate ventilation. Gag reflexes can fight tube insertion. By suppressing these reflexes, neuromuscular blockers can make intubation easier. Because of its short duration of action, succinylcholine is the preferred agent for this use.

Diagnosis of Myasthenia Gravis

Tubocurarine can be used to diagnose myasthenia gravis when safer diagnostic procedures have been inconclusive. To diagnose myasthenia, a small test dose of tubocurarine is administered. Since the dose is too small to affect individuals who do not have myasthenia, a significant reduction in muscle strength would be diagnostic of myasthenia. If the test dose does decrease strength, neostigmine (a cholinesterase inhibitor) should be administered immediately; the resultant elevation in ACh at the NMJ will reverse neuromuscular blockade. It must be stressed that use of tubocurarine to diagnose myasthenia gravis is not without risk: If the patient does have myasthenia, the challenging dose may be

sufficient to cause pronounced respiratory depression. Consequently, facilities for artificial ventilation must be immediately available.

GANGLIONIC BLOCKING AGENTS

Ganglionic blocking agents produce a broad spectrum of pharmacologic effects. Because they lack selectivity, ganglionic blockers have limited applications. These drugs are used only to lower blood pressure—and then only under special circumstances. In the United States, two ganglionic blockers are available: *trimethaphan* and *mecamylamine*. Trimethaphan will serve as our prototype.

Trimethaphan
Mechanism of Action

Trimethaphan [Arfonad] interrupts impulse transmission through ganglia of the autonomic nervous system. The drug blocks transmission by competing with ACh for binding to nicotinic$_N$ receptors in autonomic ganglia. Since the nicotinic$_N$ receptors of sympathetic and parasympathetic ganglia are the same, trimethaphan blocks transmission at *all* autonomic ganglia. By blocking all ganglionic transmission, the drug can, in effect, shut down the entire autonomic nervous system, thereby depriving organs of autonomic regulation.

In addition to blocking ganglionic transmission, trimethaphan has two other actions: (1) vasodilation (from a direct effect on blood vessels) and (2) release of histamine. Both actions can reduce blood pressure.

Pharmacologic Effects

Since trimethaphan acts by depriving organs of autonomic regulation, to predict the drug's effects, we need to know how the autonomic nervous system is affecting specific organs at the time of drug administration. That is, we need to know which branch of the autonomic nervous system is providing the predominant tone to specific organs. By knowing the source of predominant tone to an organ, and by knowing that ganglionic blockade will remove that tone, we can predict the effects that ganglionic blockade will produce.

Table 16–2 indicates (1) the major structures innervated by autonomic nerves, (2) the branch of the autonomic nervous system that provides the predominant tone to those structures, and (3) the responses to ganglionic blockade. As the table shows, *the predominant autonomic tone to most organs is provided by the parasympathetic nervous system*. The sympathetic branch provides the predominant tone only to *sweat glands, arterioles,* and *veins*.

Since the parasympathetic nervous system provides the predominant tone to most organs, and since the parasympathetic nervous system works through muscarinic receptors to influence organ function, *most responses to ganglionic blockade resemble those produced by muscarinic antagonists*. These responses include dry mouth, blurred vision, photophobia, urinary retention, constipation, tachycardia, and anhidrosis.

In addition to their parasympatholytic effects, ganglionic blockers produce *hypotension*. These drugs lower blood pressure by causing dilation of arterioles and veins. Vasodilation results primarily from blocking sympathetic nerve traffic to vascular smooth muscle.

TABLE 16–2 ■ Predominant Autonomic Tone and Responses to Ganglionic Blockade		
Location	**Predominant Tone**	**Response to Ganglionic Blockade**
Salivary glands	Parasympathetic	Dry mouth
Ciliary muscle	Parasympathetic	Blurred vision
Iris sphincter	Parasympathetic	Photophobia (from mydriasis)
Urinary bladder	Parasympathetic	Urinary retention
Gastrointestinal tract	Parasympathetic	Constipation
Heart	Parasympathetic	Tachycardia
Sweat glands	Sympathetic*	Anhidrosis
Arterioles	Sympathetic	Hypotension (from vasodilation)
Veins	Sympathetic	Orthostatic hypotension (from pooling of blood in veins secondary to venous dilation)

*Sympathetic nerves to sweat glands release acetylcholine as their transmitter, which acts at muscarinic receptors on the sweat glands.

Pharmacokinetics

Trimethaphan is a quaternary ammonium compound and therefore always carries a positive charge. As a result, the drug cannot readily cross membranes. Accordingly, trimethaphan must be administered parenterally. The drug has a brief duration of action and is eliminated by renal excretion.

Therapeutic Use

Controlled Hypotension in Surgery. Trimethaphan can produce controlled hypotension during surgery. Controlled reductions in blood pressure can (1) reduce blood loss and (2) facilitate surgery by decreasing the amount of blood in the surgical field.

Hypertensive Crisis. A hypertensive crisis is a condition in which blood pressure has risen so high as to constitute an immediate danger. Trimethaphan is one of several drugs that can be used to reduce blood pressure in patients with acute, severe hypertension.

Adverse Effects

Trimethaphan produces a broad spectrum of undesired effects, all of which are the predictable consequence of generalized inhibition of the autonomic nervous system. Side effects fall into two major groups: (1) antimuscarinic effects (caused by parasympathetic blockade) and (2) hypotension (caused largely by sympathetic blockade).

Antimuscarinic Effects. Blockade of parasympathetic ganglia produces typical antimuscarinic responses: dry mouth, blurred vision, photophobia, urinary retention, constipation, tachycardia, and anhidrosis. Antimuscarinic responses are discussed in detail in Chapter 14.

Hypotension. By causing arteriolar dilation, ganglionic blockers can produce a profound reduction in blood pressure. Excessive hypotension can be the most serious adverse effect of ganglionic blockade. If blood pressure drops too low, it may be necessary to administer a vasoconstrictor (e.g., norepinephrine) to restore pressure to a safe level.

Orthostatic Hypotension. Orthostatic hypotension is defined as a drop in blood pressure that occurs upon assuming an upright posture. Ganglionic blockers promote orthostatic hypotension by dilating veins, which causes blood to "pool" in veins when the patient moves from a recumbent position to an upright position. As a result of venous pooling, return of blood to the heart is significantly reduced, causing a reduction in cardiac output and a subsequent fall in blood pressure.

Since much of the hypotension that results from ganglionic blockade is dependent upon posture, patients who are supine or in Trendelenburg's position (head down) experience less hypotension than patients in reverse Trendelenburg's position (head up). Consequently, the blood pressure of patients receiving trimethaphan can be raised or lowered by the simple expedient of changing body position: if blood pressure is too low, lower the head and raise the feet; if blood pressure is too high, raise the head and lower the feet.

Preparations, Dosage, and Administration

Trimethaphan camsylate [Arfonad] is available in solution (50 mg/ml) for IV infusion. The drug must be diluted to 1 mg/ml with 5% dextrose prior to use. The average infusion rate is 3 to 4 ml/min (3 to 4 mg/min). The rate is adjusted to achieve the desired reduction in blood pressure. No other drugs should be added to the infusion fluid.

Mecamylamine

Mecamylamine is a ganglionic blocking agent with pharmacologic properties much like those of trimethaphan. The principal difference between the two drugs is pharmacokinetic: mecamylamine can cross membranes with ease, whereas trimethaphan can't. As a result, mecamylamine can be administered orally. In addition, the drug can cross the blood-brain barrier to produce CNS effects.

Therapeutic Use. Mecamylamine is indicated for essential hypertension in selected patients. The drug is reserved for those rare cases in which blood pressure cannot be reduced with more desirable medications.

Adverse Effects. The principal concern is *orthostatic hypotension.* Inform patients that hypotension can be minimized by moving slowly when assuming an upright posture. Also, warn them that hypotension can cause fainting and, consequently, they should sit or lie down if they become dizzy or lightheaded. In addition to hypotension, mecamylamine can cause typical antimuscarinic effects (dry mouth, blurred vision, photophobia, urinary retention, tachycardia, constipation, anhidrosis). Because it readily crosses the blood-brain barrier, trimethaphan can cause CNS effects, including tremor, convulsions, and mental aberrations. However, these reactions are rare.

Preparations, Dosage, and Administration. Trimethaphan hydrochloride [Inversine] is available in 2.5-mg tablets for oral use. The dosage is 2.5 mg twice daily initially and then is gradually increased until the target blood pressure is achieved. The average daily maintenance dose is 25 mg.

■▪ KEY POINTS

All of these key points apply to the *neuromuscular blocking* agents—not to ganglionic blocking agents.

■ Sustained contraction of skeletal muscle results from repetitive stimulation of nicotinic$_M$ receptors on the motor end-plate, causing the end-plate to go through repeating cycles of depolarization and repolarization.

■ Neuromuscular blockers interfere with nicotinic$_M$ receptor activation, and thereby cause muscle relaxation.

■ Nondepolarizing neuromuscular blockers act by competing with ACh for binding to nicotinic$_M$ receptors.

■ Succinylcholine, the only depolarizing neuromuscular blocker in use, binds to nicotinic$_M$ receptors, causing the end-plate to depolarize; the drug then remains bound, which keeps the end-plate from repolarizing.

■ The neuromuscular blockers are used to produce muscle relaxation during surgery, endotracheal intubation, mechanical ventilation, and electroshock therapy.

■ Neuromuscular blockers do not reduce consciousness or pain.

■ The major adverse effect of neuromuscular blockers is respiratory depression.

■ Cholinesterase inhibitors can reverse the effects of nondepolarizing neuromuscular blockers but will intensify the effects of succinylcholine.

■ Succinylcholine can cause malignant hyperthermia, a life-threatening condition.

■ Succinylcholine is eliminated by plasma cholinesterases. Accordingly, effects are greatly prolonged in patients with low plasma cholinesterase activity.

■ All of the neuromuscular blockers are quaternary ammonium compounds, and therefore must be administered parenterally (almost always IV).

Summary of Major Nursing Implications*

NEUROMUSCULAR BLOCKING AGENTS

Atracurium
Cisatracurium
Doxacurium
Metocurine
Mivacurium
Pancuronium
Pipecuronium
Rocuronium
Succinylcholine
Tubocurarine
Vecuronium

Except where noted otherwise, the implications summarized below apply to all of the neuromuscular blocking agents.

Preadministration Assessment

Therapeutic Goal

Provision of muscle relaxation during surgery, endotracheal intubation, mechanical ventilation, electroconvulsive therapy, and other procedures.

Identifying High-Risk Patients

Use all neuromuscular blockers with caution in patients with myasthenia gravis.

Succinylcholine is contraindicated for patients with low pseudocholinesterase activity, a personal or familial history of malignant hyperthermia, or conditions that predispose them to hyperkalemia (major burns, multiple trauma, denervation of skeletal muscle, upper motor neuron injury).

Implementation: Administration

Routes

Intravenous. *All* neuromuscular blockers.
Intramuscular. *Tubocurarine* and *succinylcholine.*

Administration

Neuromuscular blockers are dangerous drugs that should be administered only by clinicians skilled in their use.

Implementation: Measures to Enhance Therapeutic Effects

Neuromuscular blockers do not affect consciousness or perception of pain. When used during surgery, these drugs must be accompanied by adequate anesthesia. When neuromuscular blockers are used for prolonged paralysis during mechanical ventilation, care should be taken to ensure comfort (e.g., positioning the patient comfortably, moistening the mouth periodically). Since patients may be awake (but won't appear to be), conversations held in their presence should convey only information that is appropriate for them to hear.

Ongoing Evaluation and Interventions

Minimizing Adverse Effects

Apnea. All neuromuscular blockers can cause respiratory arrest. Facilities for intubation and mechanical ventilation should be immediately available.

Monitor respiration constantly during the period of peak drug action. When drug administration is discontinued, take vital signs at least every 17 minutes until recovery is complete.

A cholinesterase inhibitor can be used to reverse respiratory depression caused by *nondepolarizing* neuromuscular blockers—but not by succinylcholine, a *depolarizing* blocker.

Hypotension. Some neuromuscular blockers can cause hypotension secondary to ganglionic blockade or release of histamine. Antihistamines may help counteract this effect.

Malignant Hyperthermia. *Succinylcholine* can trigger malignant hyperthermia. Predisposition to this reaction is genetic. Assess for a family history of the reaction.

Hyperkalemia with Cardiac Arrest. *Succinylcholine* can cause severe hyperkalemia resulting in cardiac arrest if given to patients with major burns, multiple trauma, denervation of skeletal muscle, or upper motor neuron injury. Accordingly, the drug is contraindicated for these people.

Muscle Pain. *Succinylcholine* may cause muscle pain. Reassure the patient that this response, although unpleasant, is not unusual.

Minimizing Adverse Interactions

Antibiotics. Certain antibiotics, including *aminoglycosides* and *tetracyclines,* can intensify neuromuscular blockade. Use them with caution.

Cholinesterase Inhibitors. These drugs delay inactivation of *succinylcholine,* thereby greatly prolonging paralysis. Accordingly, cholinesterase inhibitors are contraindicated for patients receiving succinylcholine.

---

*Patient education information is highlighted as blue text.

Adrenergic Agonists

Adrenergic agonists produce their effects by activating adrenergic receptors. Since the sympathetic nervous system acts through these same receptors, responses to adrenergic agonists and responses to stimulation by the sympathetic nervous system are very similar. Because of this similarity, adrenergic agonists are often referred to as *sympathomimetics*. Adrenergic agonists have a broad spectrum of clinical applications, ranging from treatment of heart failure to relief of asthma to delay of preterm labor.

Learning about adrenergic agonists can be a challenge. To facilitate learning, we will approach these drugs in four stages. First we will discuss the general mechanisms by which drugs can activate adrenergic receptors. Next we will establish an overview of the major adrenergic agonists, focusing on their receptor specificity and chemical classifica-

tion. After that, we will address the adrenergic receptors themselves; for each receptor type—alpha₁, alpha₂, beta₁, beta₂, and dopamine—we will discuss the beneficial and harmful effects that can result from receptor activation. To finish, we will integrate all of this information by discussing the characteristic properties of representative individual sympathomimetic drugs.

Please note that this chapter is intended only as an *introduction* to the adrenergic agonists. Our objective here is to discuss the basic properties of the sympathomimetic drugs and establish an overview of their applications and adverse effects. In later chapters, the clinical applications of these agents are presented in greater depth.

MECHANISMS OF ADRENERGIC RECEPTOR ACTIVATION

Drugs can activate adrenergic receptors by four basic mechanisms: (1) direct receptor binding, (2) promotion of norepinephrine (NE) release, (3) blockade of NE reuptake, and (4) inhibition of NE inactivation. Note that only the first mechanism is *direct*. With the other three mechanisms, receptor activation occurs by an *indirect* process. Examples of drugs that act by these four mechanisms are presented in Table 17–1.

Direct Receptor Binding. Direct interaction with receptors is the most common mechanism by which drugs activate peripheral adrenergic receptors. The direct-acting receptor stimulants produce their effects by binding to adrenergic receptors and mimicking the actions of natural transmitters (NE, epinephrine, dopamine). In this chapter, all of the drugs discussed activate adrenergic receptors directly.

Promotion of NE Release. By acting on terminals of sympathetic nerves to cause NE release, drugs can bring about activation of adrenergic receptors. Agents that promote receptor activation by this indirect mechanism include the amphetamines and ephedrine. (Ephedrine can also stimulate adrenergic receptors directly.)

Inhibition of NE Reuptake. Recall that reuptake of NE into terminals of sympathetic nerves is the major mechanism by which adrenergic transmission is terminated. By blocking NE reuptake, drugs can cause NE to accumulate within the synaptic gap, and can thereby increase receptor activation. Agents that act by this mechanism include cocaine and the tricyclic antidepressants (e.g., imipramine).

Inhibition of NE Inactivation. As discussed in Chapter 13, some of the NE in terminals of adrenergic neurons is subject to inactivation by monoamine oxidase (MAO). Hence, drugs that inhibit MAO can increase the amount of NE available for release, and can thereby enhance receptor

TABLE 17-1 ▪■ Mechanisms of Adrenergic Receptor Activation

Mechanism of Stimulation	Examples
Direct Mechanism	
Binding to receptor to cause activation	Epinephrine
	Isoproterenol
	Ephedrine*
Indirect Mechanisms	
Promotion of NE release	Ephedrine*
	Amphetamines
Inhibition of NE reuptake	Cocaine
	Tricyclic antidepressants
Inhibition of MAO	MAO inhibitors

MAO = monoamine oxidase, NE = norepinephrine.
*Ephedrine is a mixed-acting drug that activates receptors directly and also promotes release of norepinephrine.

activation. (It should be noted that, in addition to being present in sympathetic nerves, MAO is present in the liver and the intestinal wall. The significance of MAO at these other sites is considered later in the chapter.)

In this chapter, which is dedicated to *peripherally* acting sympathomimetics, practically all of the drugs discussed act exclusively by *direct* receptor activation. The only exception is *ephedrine,* an agent that works by a combination of direct receptor activation and promotion of NE release.

Most of the indirect-acting adrenergic agonists are used for their ability to activate adrenergic receptors in the central nervous system (CNS)—not for their effects in the periphery. The indirect-acting sympathomimetics (e.g., amphetamine, cocaine) are mentioned here to emphasize that, although these agents are employed for effects on the brain, they can and will cause activation of adrenergic receptors in the periphery. Peripheral activation is responsible for certain toxicities of these drugs (e.g., cardiac dysrhythmias, hypertension).

OVERVIEW OF THE ADRENERGIC AGONISTS

Chemical Classification: Catecholamines Versus Noncatecholamines

The adrenergic agonists fall into two major chemical classes: catecholamines and noncatecholamines. As we shall see, the catecholamines and noncatecholamines differ in three important respects: (1) oral usability, (2) duration of action, and (3) the ability to act in the CNS. Accordingly, if we know which category a particular adrenergic agonist belongs to, we will know three of that drug's prominent features.

Catecholamines

The catecholamines are so named because they contain a *catechol* group and an *amine* group. A catechol group is simply a benzene ring that has hydroxyl groups on two adjacent carbons (Fig. 17–1). The amine component of the catecholamines is *ethylamine.* Structural formulas for each of the

major catecholamines—epinephrine, norepinephrine, isoproterenol, dopamine, and dobutamine—are presented in Figure 17–1. Because of their chemistry, all of the catecholamines have three properties in common: (1) they cannot be used orally, (2) they have a brief duration of action, and (3) they cannot cross the blood-brain barrier.

The actions of two enzymes—*monoamine oxidase* and *catechol-O-methyltransferase* (COMT)—explain why the catecholamines have short half-lives and cannot be used orally. MAO and COMT are located in the liver and the intestinal wall. Both enzymes are very active and quickly destroy catecholamines administered by any route. Because these enzymes are located in the liver and intestinal wall, catecholamines that are administered orally become inactivated before they can reach the systemic circulation. Hence, catecholamines are ineffective if given by mouth. Because of rapid inactivation by MAO and COMT, three catecholamines—norepinephrine, dopamine, and dobutamine—are effective only if administered by continuous infusion. Administration by other parenteral routes (e.g., SC, IM) will not permit adequate blood levels to be achieved.

The catecholamines cannot cross the blood-brain barrier because they are polar. (Recall from Chapter 4 that polar compounds penetrate membranes poorly.) The polar nature of the catecholamines is due to the hydroxyl groups on the catechol portion of the molecule. Because they cannot cross the blood-brain barrier, catecholamines have minimal effects on the CNS.

Be aware that catecholamine-containing solutions, which are colorless when first prepared, turn pink or brown over time. This pigmentation is caused by oxidation of the catecholamine molecule. As a rule, *catecholamine solutions should be discarded as soon as discoloration appears.* The only exception to this rule is dobutamine, which can be used up to 24 hours after the solution was made, even if discoloration has developed.

Noncatecholamines

The noncatecholamines have ethylamine in their structure (see Fig. 17–1) but do not contain the catechol portion that characterizes the catecholamines. In this chapter, we discuss three noncatecholamines: ephedrine, phenylephrine, and terbutaline.

The noncatecholamines differ from the catecholamines in three important respects. First, because they lack a catechol group, noncatecholamines are not substrates for COMT and are metabolized slowly by MAO. As a result, noncatecholamines have half-lives that are much longer than those of catecholamines. Second, since they do not undergo rapid degradation by MAO and COMT, noncatecholamines can be given orally, whereas catecholamines cannot. Third, noncatecholamines are considerably less polar than catecholamines. As a result, noncatecholamines are more able to penetrate the blood-brain barrier and influence the CNS.

Receptor Specificity

To understand the actions of individual adrenergic agonists, we need to know their receptor specificity. Since the sympathomimetic drugs differ widely with respect to the receptors they can activate, learning the receptor specificity of these drugs will take some effort.

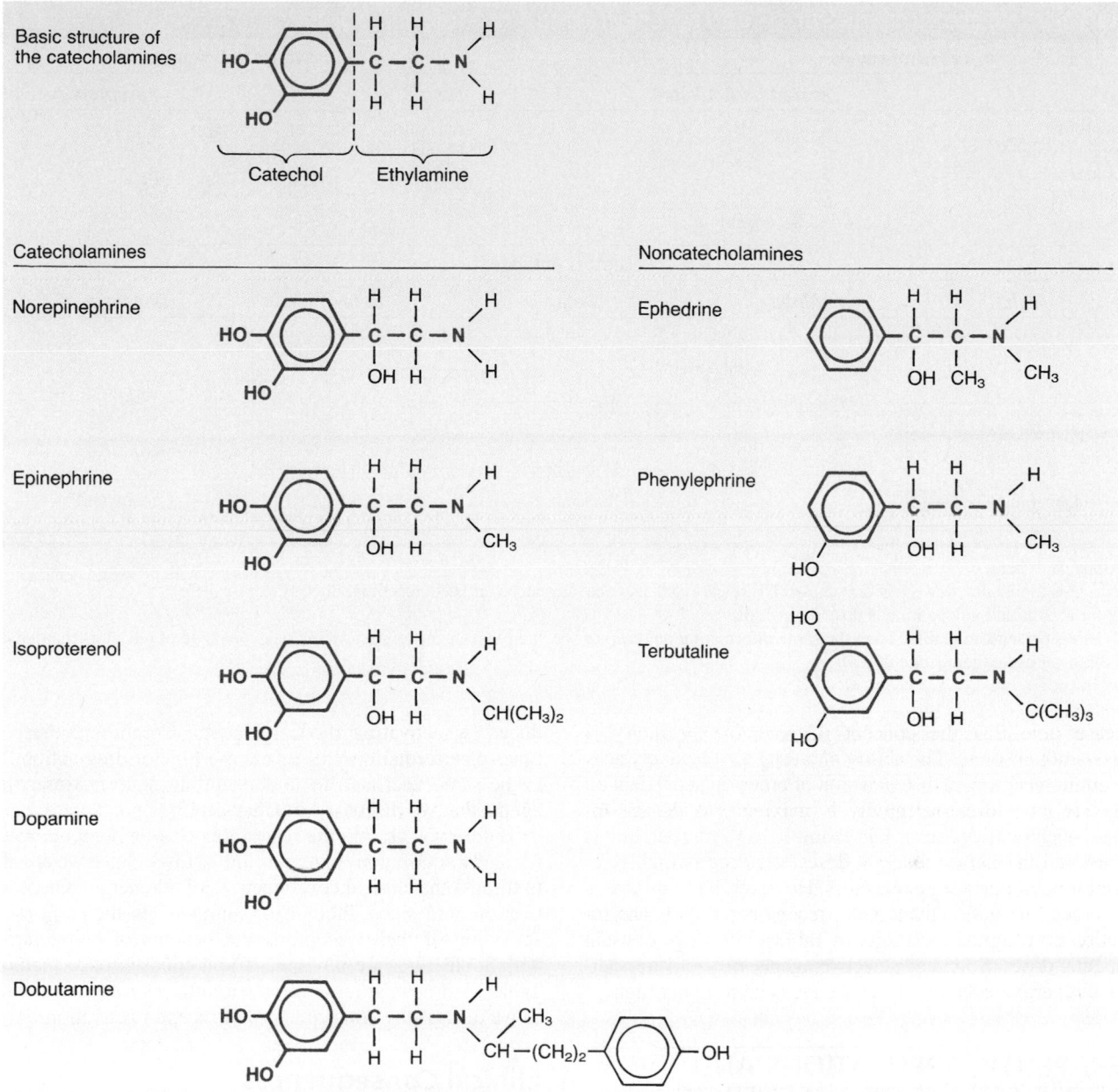

Figure 17–1 ■ Structures of catecholamines and noncatecholamines.
Catecholamines: Note that all of the catecholamines share the same basic chemical formula. Because of their biochemical properties, the catecholamines cannot be used orally, cannot cross the blood-brain barrier, and have short half-lives (owing to rapid inactivation by MAO and COMT).
Noncatecholamines: Although structurally similar to catecholamines, noncatecholamines differ from catecholamines in three important ways: (1) noncatecholamines are usable orally; (2) they can cross the blood-brain barrier; and (3) since they are not rapidly metabolized by MAO or COMT, they have much longer half-lives than the catecholamines.

Variability in receptor specificity among the adrenergic agonists can be illustrated with three drugs: terbutaline, isoproterenol, and epinephrine. Terbutaline is highly selective, acting at beta$_2$ receptors only. Isoproterenol is less selective, acting at beta$_1$ receptors as well as beta$_2$ receptors. Epinephrine is less selective yet, acting at all four subtypes (alpha$_1$, alpha$_2$, beta$_1$, and beta$_2$) of adrenergic receptors.

The receptor specificities of the major adrenergic agonists are summarized in Table 17–2. In the upper part of the table, receptor specificity is presented in tabular form. In the lower part, the same information is presented schematically. By learning (memorizing) the content of Table 17–2, you will have taken a major step toward understanding the pharmacology of the sympathomimetic drugs.

TABLE 17–2 ■ Receptor Specificity of Representative Adrenergic Agonists

Catecholamines		Noncatecholamines	
Drug	**Receptors Activated**	**Drug**	**Receptors Activated**
Epinephrine	$\alpha_1, \alpha_2, \beta_1, \beta_2$	Ephedrine*	$\alpha_1, \alpha_2, \beta_1, \beta_2$
Norepinephrine	$\alpha_1, \alpha_2, \beta_1$	Phenylephrine	α_1
Isoproterenol	β_1, β_2	Terbutaline	β_2
Dobutamine	β_1		
Dopamine†	$\alpha_1, \beta_1,$ dopamine		

Receptors Activated‡				
Alpha₁	**Alpha₂**	**Beta₁**	**Beta₂**	**Dopamine**
←———————————————— Epinephrine ———————————————→				
←———————————————— Ephedrine* ———————————————→				
←———————— Norepinephrine ————————→				
←—— Phenylephrine ——→		←———————— Isoproterenol ————————→		
		←—— Dobutamine ——→	←—— Terbutaline ——→	
←—— Dopamine† ——→		←—— Dopamine† ——→		←———— Dopamine† ————→

α = Alpha, β = beta.
*Ephedrine is a mixed-acting agent that causes NE release and also activates alpha and beta receptors directly.
†Receptor activation by dopamine is dose dependent.
‡This chart represents in graphic form the same information on receptor specificity given above. Arrows indicate the range of receptors that the drugs can activate (at usual therapeutic doses).

Please note that the concept of receptor specificity is *relative*—not absolute. The ability of a drug to selectively activate certain receptors to the exclusion of others is dependent on dosage: at low doses, selectivity is maximal; as dosage increases, selectivity declines. For example, when terbutaline is administered in low to moderate doses, the drug is highly selective for beta₂-adrenergic receptors. However, if the dosage is high, terbutaline will activate beta₁ receptors as well. The information on receptor specificity in Table 17–2 refers to usual therapeutic doses. So-called selective agents will activate additional adrenergic receptors if the dosage is abnormally high.

THERAPEUTIC APPLICATIONS AND ADVERSE EFFECTS OF ADRENERGIC RECEPTOR ACTIVATION

In this section we discuss the responses—both therapeutic and adverse—that can be elicited with sympathomimetic drugs. Since many adrenergic agonists activate more than one type of receptor (see Table 17–2), it could be quite confusing if we were to talk about the effects of the sympathomimetics while employing specific drugs as examples. Consequently, rather than attempting to structure this presentation around representative drugs, we will discuss the actions of the adrenergic agonists one receptor at a time. Our discussion begins with alpha₁ receptors, and then moves to alpha₂ receptors, beta₁ receptors, beta₂ receptors, and dopamine receptors. For each receptor type, we discuss both the therapeutic and the adverse responses that can result from receptor activation.

To understand the effects of any specific adrenergic agonist, all you need is two types of information: (1) the identity of the receptors at which the drug acts and (2) the effects produced by activating those receptors. Combining these two types of information will reveal a profile of drug action. This is the same approach to understanding neuropharmacologic agents that we discussed in Chapter 12.

Before you go into the rest of this chapter, I encourage you (strongly advise you) to review Table 13–3. Since we are about to discuss the clinical consequences of adrenergic receptor activation, and since Table 13–3 summarizes the responses to activation of these receptors, the benefits of being familiar with Table 13–3 are obvious. If you choose not to memorize Table 13–3 now, at least be prepared to refer back to the table as we discuss the consequences of receptor activation.

Clinical Consequences of Alpha₁ Activation

In this section we discuss the therapeutic and adverse effects that can result from activation of alpha₁-adrenergic receptors. As shown in Table 17–2, drugs capable of activating alpha₁ receptors include epinephrine, norepinephrine, phenylephrine, ephedrine, and dopamine.

Therapeutic Applications of Alpha₁ Activation

Activation of alpha₁ receptors elicits two responses that can be of therapeutic use: (1) *vasoconstriction* (in blood vessels of the skin, viscera, and mucous membranes), and (2) *mydriasis.* Of the two, vasoconstriction is the one for which alpha₁ agonists are most often employed. Use of alpha₁-activating agents to produce mydriasis is relatively rare.

Hemostasis. Hemostasis is defined as the arrest of bleeding. Drugs capable of alpha₁ activation produce hemostasis by causing vasoconstriction. Alpha₁ stimulants are given to stop bleeding primarily in the skin and mucous membranes. Epinephrine, applied topically, is the alpha₁-activating agent used most for this purpose.

Nasal Decongestion. Nasal congestion results from dilation and engorgement of blood vessels in the nasal mucosa. Drugs can relieve congestion by causing alpha₁-mediated vasoconstriction. Specific alpha₁-activating agents employed as nasal decongestants include phenylephrine (applied topically) and ephedrine (taken orally).

Adjunct to Local Anesthesia. Alpha₁ agonists are frequently combined with local anesthetics to delay anesthetic absorption. Absorption is delayed because alpha₁-mediated vasoconstriction reduces blood flow to the site of anesthetic administration. Delay of anesthetic absorption has three benefits: (1) it prolongs anesthesia, (2) it allows a reduction in anesthetic dosage, and (3) it reduces the systemic effects that a local anesthetic might produce. The drug used most frequently to delay anesthetic absorption is epinephrine.

Elevation of Blood Pressure. Because of their ability to cause vasoconstriction, alpha₁ agonists can be used to elevate blood pressure in hypotensive states. Please note, however, that alpha₁ agonists are not the primary therapy for hypotension; rather, these drugs are reserved for situations in which other measures, including fluid replacement, have failed to restore blood pressure to a satisfactory level.

Mydriasis. Activation of alpha₁ receptors on the radial muscle of the iris causes mydriasis (dilation of the pupil). Production of mydriasis can facilitate eye examinations and ocular surgery. Note that the ophthalmic applications of alpha₁ activation are the only applications that are not based on vasoconstriction.

Adverse Effects of Alpha₁ Activation

All of the adverse effects caused by alpha₁ activation result directly or indirectly from vasoconstriction.

Hypertension. Alpha₁ agonists can produce hypertension by causing widespread vasoconstriction. Severe hypertension is most likely with parenteral administration. Accordingly, when alpha₁ agonists are given parenterally, cardiovascular status must be monitored continuously; never leave the patient unattended.

Necrosis. If the IV line employed to administer an alpha₁ agonist becomes extravasated, local seepage of the drug may result in necrosis (tissue death). The cause of necrosis is lack of blood flow secondary to intense local vasoconstriction. If extravasation occurs, the area should be infiltrated with an alpha₁-blocking agent (e.g., phentolamine). By counteracting alpha₁-mediated vasoconstriction, the antagonist will help minimize injury.

Bradycardia. Alpha₁ agonists can cause reflex slowing of the heart. The mechanism is this: Alpha₁-mediated vasoconstriction elevates blood pressure, which triggers the baroreceptor reflex, causing heart rate to decline. In patients with marginal cardiac reserve, the decrease in cardiac output may compromise tissue perfusion.

Clinical Consequences of Alpha₂ Activation

As discussed in Chapter 13, alpha₂ receptors in the periphery are located *presynaptically,* and their activation inhibits NE release. Several adrenergic agonists (e.g., epinephrine, NE,

ephedrine) are capable of causing alpha₂ activation. However, the ability of drugs to activate alpha₂ receptors in the periphery has little clinical significance. There are no therapeutic applications related to activation of peripheral alpha₂ receptors. Furthermore, activation of these receptors rarely causes significant adverse effects.

In contrast to alpha₂ receptors in the *periphery,* alpha₂ receptors in the *CNS* are of great clinical significance. The principal response to stimulation of central alpha₂ receptors is a reduction of sympathetic outflow to the heart and blood vessels. By decreasing sympathetic outflow, drugs that stimulate central alpha₂ receptors act to *reduce* stimulation of adrenergic receptors in the periphery. The drugs that stimulate alpha₂ receptors in the CNS are discussed in Chapter 19 (Indirect-Acting Antiadrenergic Agents).

Clinical Consequences of Beta₁ Activation

All of the clinically relevant responses to activation of beta₁ receptors result from activating beta₁ receptors in the *heart;* activation of renal beta₁ receptors is not associated with either beneficial or adverse effects. As indicated in Table 17–2, beta₁ receptors can be activated by epinephrine, NE, isoproterenol, dopamine, dobutamine, and ephedrine.

Therapeutic Applications of Beta₁ Activation

Cardiac Arrest. By activating cardiac beta₁ receptors, drugs can initiate contraction in a heart that has stopped beating. It should be noted, however, that drugs are not the preferred treatment for cardiac arrest; rather, drugs should be used only after more desirable procedures (mechanical thumping, direct-current cardioversion) have failed to restart the heart. When a beta₁ agonist is indicated, epinephrine—injected directly into the heart—is the preferred drug.

Heart Failure. Heart failure is characterized by a reduction in the force of myocardial contraction, resulting in insufficient cardiac output. Since activation of beta₁ receptors in the heart has a positive inotropic effect (i.e., increases the force of contraction), drugs that activate these receptors can improve cardiac performance.

Shock. This condition is characterized by profound hypotension and greatly reduced tissue perfusion. The primary goal of treatment is to maintain blood flow to vital organs. By increasing heart rate and force of contraction, beta₁ stimulants can increase cardiac output and can thereby improve tissue perfusion.

Atrioventricular Heart Block. Atrioventricular (AV) heart block is a condition in which impulse conduction from the atria to the ventricles is impeded—or blocked entirely. As a consequence, the ventricles are no longer driven at an appropriate rate. Since activation of cardiac beta₁ receptors can enhance impulse conduction through the AV node, beta₁ stimulants can help overcome AV block. It should be noted, however, that drugs are only a temporary form of treatment; for long-term management, a pacemaker is implanted.

Adverse Effects of Beta₁ Activation

All of the adverse effects of beta₁ activation result from activating beta₁ receptors in the heart; activating renal beta₁ receptors is not associated with untoward effects.

Altered Heart Rate or Rhythm. Overstimulation of cardiac beta$_1$ receptors can produce *tachycardia* (excessive heart rate) and *dysrhythmias* (irregular heart beat).

Angina Pectoris. In some patients, drugs that activate beta$_1$ receptors can precipitate an attack of angina pectoris, a condition characterized by substernal pain in the region of the heart. Anginal pain occurs when oxygen supply (blood flow) to the heart is insufficient to meet the heart's oxygen needs. The most common cause of angina is coronary atherosclerosis (accumulation of lipids and other substances in coronary arteries). Since beta$_1$ agonists increase cardiac oxygen demand (by increasing heart rate and force of contraction), patients with compromised coronary blood flow are at risk of an anginal attack.

Clinical Consequences of Beta$_2$ Activation
Therapeutic Applications of Beta$_2$ Activation

Therapeutic applications of beta$_2$ activation are limited to the *lung* and *uterus*. Drugs used for their beta$_2$-activating ability include epinephrine, isoproterenol, and terbutaline.

Asthma. Asthma is a chronic condition characterized by inflammation and bronchoconstriction occurring in response to a variety of stimuli. During a severe attack, airflow can be reduced so much as to threaten life. Since drugs that activate beta$_2$ receptors in the lung promote *bronchodilation,* these agents can help relieve or prevent asthma attacks.

For therapy of asthma, adrenergic agonists that are *selective for beta$_2$ receptors* (e.g., terbutaline) are preferred to less selective agents (e.g., epinephrine, isoproterenol). This is especially true for patients who suffer from *angina pectoris* or *tachycardia.* Why? Because drugs that can activate beta$_1$ receptors would aggravate their cardiac disorder.

Several of the beta$_2$ agonists used to treat asthma are administered by *inhalation.* This route is desirable in that it helps minimize adverse systemic effects. It should be noted, however, that inhalation does not guarantee safety: Serious systemic toxicity can result from overdosing with inhaled sympathomimetics. Accordingly, patients must be warned against inhaling too much medication.

Delay of Preterm Labor. Activation of beta$_2$ receptors in the uterus relaxes uterine smooth muscle. This action can be exploited to delay preterm labor.

Adverse Effects of Beta$_2$ Activation

Hyperglycemia. The most important adverse response to beta$_2$ activation is *hyperglycemia* (elevation of blood glucose). Beta$_2$ agonists can cause hyperglycemia by acting on the liver and skeletal muscles to promote breakdown of glycogen into glucose. As a rule, these drugs produce hyperglycemia only in patients with *diabetes;* in patients with normal pancreatic function, insulin will be released in response to glucose elevation, thereby maintaining blood glucose at an appropriate level. If hyperglycemia develops in the diabetic patient, insulin dosage should be increased.

Tremor. Tremor is the most common side effect of beta$_2$ agonists. It occurs because activation of beta$_2$ receptors in skeletal muscle enhances contraction. Tremor generally fades over time and can be minimized by initiating therapy with low doses.

Clinical Consequences of Dopamine Receptor Activation

Activation of peripheral dopamine receptors causes dilation of the vasculature of the kidneys. This effect is exploited in the treatment of *shock:* by dilating renal blood vessels, we can improve renal perfusion and can thereby reduce the risk of renal failure. *Dopamine* itself is the only drug available that can activate dopamine receptors. It should be noted that, when dopamine is given to treat shock, the drug also enhances cardiac performance (because it activates beta$_1$ receptors in the heart).

Multiple Receptor Activation: Treatment of Anaphylactic Shock

Pathophysiology of Anaphylaxis. Anaphylactic shock is a manifestation of severe allergy. The reaction is characterized by *hypotension* (from widespread vasodilation), *bronchoconstriction,* and *edema of the glottis.* Although histamine contributes to these responses, symptoms are due largely to release of other mediators (e.g., leukotrienes). Anaphylaxis can be triggered by a variety of substances, including bee venom, wasp venom, and certain drugs (e.g., penicillins).

Treatment. Epinephrine, injected subcutaneously, is the treatment of choice for anaphylactic shock. Beneficial responses derive from the ability of epinephrine to activate three types of adrenergic receptors: alpha$_1$, beta$_1$, and beta$_2$. By activating these receptors, epinephrine can reverse the most severe manifestations of the anaphylactic reaction. Activation of beta$_1$ receptors increases cardiac output, thereby helping to elevate blood pressure. Blood pressure is also increased because epinephrine can promote alpha$_1$-mediated vasoconstriction. In addition to increasing blood pressure, vasoconstriction helps suppress glottal edema. By activating beta$_2$ receptors, epinephrine can counteract bronchoconstriction. Individuals who are prone to severe allergic responses should carry a syringe of epinephrine at all times. (Antihistamines are not especially useful against anaphylaxis because histamine is only a minor contributor to the reaction.)

PROPERTIES OF REPRESENTATIVE ADRENERGIC AGONISTS

Our aim in this section is to establish an overview of the adrenergic agonists. This overview is presented in the form of "drug digests" that highlight characteristic features of representative sympathomimetic agents.

As noted above, there are two major keys to understanding individual adrenergic agonists: (1) knowledge of the receptors that the drug can activate and (2) knowledge of the therapeutic and adverse effects that receptor activation can elicit. Integrating these two types of information will reveal the spectrum of effects that a particular drug can produce.

Unfortunately, knowing the effects that a drug is capable of producing does not always allow us to predict the *actual clinical applications* of that drug. Why? Because some adrenergic agonists are not used for all of the effects that they are able to produce. Norepinephrine, for example, can activate alpha$_1$ receptors and can therefore produce mydriasis; however, although NE can produce mydriasis, the drug is not actually used for this purpose. Similarly, although isoproterenol is capable of producing uterine relaxation (through beta$_2$ activation), isoproterenol is not employed clinically for this effect. Because receptor specificity is not always a predictor of the therapeutic applications of a particular adrenergic agonist, for each of the drugs discussed below, approved clinical applications are indicated.

Epinephrine

- *Receptor specificity:* alpha$_1$, alpha$_2$, beta$_1$, beta$_2$
- *Chemical classification:* catecholamine

Epinephrine [Adrenalin, others] was among the first adrenergic agonists employed clinically and can be considered the prototype of the sympathomimetic drugs. Because of its prototypic status, epinephrine is discussed in detail.

Therapeutic Uses

Epinephrine can activate all four subtypes of adrenergic receptors. As a consequence, the drug can produce a broad spectrum of beneficial sympathomimetic effects:

- Because of its ability to cause alpha$_1$-mediated vasoconstriction, epinephrine is used to (1) delay absorption of local anesthetics, (2) control superficial bleeding, (3) reduce nasal congestion, and (4) elevate blood pressure.
- Activation of alpha$_1$ receptors on the iris is employed to produce mydriasis during ophthalmologic procedures.
- Because of its ability to activate beta$_1$ receptors, epinephrine is used to (1) overcome AV heart block and (2) restore cardiac function in patients undergoing cardiac arrest.
- Activation of beta$_2$ receptors in the lung promotes bronchodilation in patients with asthma.
- Because of its ability to activate a combination of alpha and beta receptors, epinephrine is the treatment of choice for anaphylactic shock.

Pharmacokinetics

Absorption. Epinephrine may be administered topically, by injection, and by inhalation. The drug cannot be given orally because, as discussed, epinephrine and other catecholamines undergo destruction by MAO and COMT before reaching the systemic circulation. Following SC injection, absorption is slow owing to epinephrine-induced local vasoconstriction. Absorption is more rapid following IM injection. When epinephrine is inhaled (to treat asthma), systemic absorption is usually minimal; however, if dosing is excessive, systemic absorption can be sufficient to cause toxicity.

Inactivation. Epinephrine has a short half-life because of two processes: enzymatic inactivation and uptake into adrenergic nerves. The enzymes that inactivate epinephrine and other catecholamines are MAO and COMT.

Adverse Effects

Because of its ability to activate the four major adrenergic receptor subtypes, epinephrine can produce multiple adverse effects.

Hypertensive Crisis. Vasoconstriction secondary to excessive alpha$_1$ activation can produce a dramatic increase in blood pressure. Cerebral hemorrhage can occur. Because of the potential for severe hypertension, patients receiving *parenteral* epinephrine must undergo continuous cardiovascular monitoring.

Dysrhythmias. Excessive activation of beta$_1$ receptors in the heart can produce dysrhythmias. Because of their sensitivity to catecholamines, hyperthyroid patients are at high risk for epinephrine-induced dysrhythmias.

Angina Pectoris. By activating beta$_1$ receptors in the heart, epinephrine can increase cardiac work and oxygen demand. If the increase in oxygen demand is big enough, an anginal attack may ensue. Precipitation of angina is especially likely in patients with coronary atherosclerosis.

Necrosis Following Extravasation. If an IV line containing epinephrine becomes extravasated, the resultant localized vasoconstriction may cause necrosis. Because of this possibility, patients receiving IV epinephrine should be monitored closely. If extravasation occurs, injury can be minimized by local injection of phentolamine, an alpha-adrenergic antagonist.

Hyperglycemia. In diabetic patients, epinephrine can cause hyperglycemia. This results from breakdown of glycogen in response to activation of beta$_2$ receptors in liver and skeletal muscle. If hyperglycemia develops, insulin dosage should be increased.

Drug Interactions

MAO Inhibitors. MAO inhibitors suppress the activity of MAO. These drugs are used primarily to treat depression (see Chapter 31). Since MAO is one of the enzymes that inactivate epinephrine and other catecholamines, inhibition of MAO will prolong and intensify epinephrine's effects. As a rule, patients receiving an MAO inhibitor should not receive epinephrine.

Tricyclic Antidepressants. Tricyclic antidepressants block the uptake of catecholamines into adrenergic neurons. Since neuronal uptake is one mechanism by which the actions of norepinephrine and other catecholamines are terminated, blockade of uptake can intensify and prolong epinephrine's effects. Accordingly, patients receiving a tricyclic antidepressant may require a reduction in epinephrine dosage.

General Anesthetics. Several inhalation anesthetics render the myocardium hypersensitive to activation by beta$_1$ agonists. When the heart is in this hypersensitive state, exposure to epinephrine and other beta$_1$ agonists can cause dysrhythmias.

Alpha-Adrenergic Blocking Agents. Drugs that block alpha-adrenergic receptors can prevent receptor activation by epinephrine. Alpha blockers (e.g., phentolamine) can be used to treat toxicity (e.g., hypertension, local vasoconstriction) caused by excessive epinephrine-induced alpha activation.

Beta-Adrenergic Blocking Agents. Drugs that block beta-adrenergic receptors can prevent receptor activation by epinephrine. Beta-blocking agents (e.g., propranolol) can reduce adverse effects (e.g., dysrhythmias, anginal pain) caused by epinephrine and other beta$_1$ agonists.

Preparations, Dosage, and Administration

Epinephrine [Adrenalin, EpiPen] is dispensed in solution for administration by several routes: IV, SC, IM, intracardiac, intraspinal, inhalation, and topical. As indicated in Table 17–3, the strength of the epinephrine solution employed depends on the route of administration. Note that solutions intended for *intravenous* administration are *less concentrated* than solutions intended for administration by most other routes. The reason that epinephrine must be diluted for IV use is that *intravenous administration of a concentrated epinephrine*

TABLE 17–3 ■■ Epinephrine Solutions: Concentrations for Different Routes of Administration	
Concentration of Epinephrine Solution	**Route of Administration**
1% (1:100)	Oral inhalation
0.1% (1:1,000)	Subcutaneous Intramuscular Intraspinal
0.01% (1:10,000)	Intravenous Intracardiac
0.001% (1;100,000)	In combination with local anesthetics

solution can produce potentially fatal reactions (severe dysrhythmias and hypertension). Therefore, *before epinephrine is administered intravenously, the solution should be carefully checked to ensure that its concentration is appropriate!* Aspirate prior to IM or SC injection to avoid inadvertent injection into a vein.

Patients receiving IV epinephrine should be monitored constantly. They should be observed for signs of excessive cardiovascular activation (e.g., dysrhythmias, hypertension) and for possible extravasation of the IV line. If systemic toxicity develops, epinephrine should be discontinued; if indicated, an alpha-adrenergic blocker, a beta-adrenergic blocker, or both should be given to suppress symptoms. If an epinephrine-containing IV line becomes extravasated, administration should be discontinued and the region of extravasation infiltrated with an alpha-adrenergic blocker.

Norepinephrine

■ *Receptor specificity:* alpha$_1$, alpha$_2$, beta$_1$
■ *Chemical classification:* catecholamine

Norepinephrine is similar to epinephrine in many respects. With regard to receptor specificity, NE differs from epinephrine only in that NE does not activate beta$_2$ receptors. Accordingly, NE can elicit all of the responses that epinephrine can, except those that are beta$_2$ mediated. Because NE is a catecholamine, the drug is subject to rapid inactivation by MAO and COMT and cannot be given orally. Adverse effects are nearly identical to those of epinephrine: dysrhythmias, angina, hypertension, and local necrosis upon extravasation. In contrast to epinephrine, NE does not promote hyperglycemia, a response that is mediated by beta$_2$ receptors. As with epinephrine, responses to NE can be modified by MAO inhibitors, tricyclic antidepressants, general anesthetics, and adrenergic blocking agents.

Despite its similarity to epinephrine, NE has limited clinical applications. The only recognized indications are *hypotensive states* and *cardiac arrest.*

Norepinephrine [Levophed] is dispensed in solution (1 mg/ml) for administration by IV infusion only. Never leave patients unattended. Monitor cardiovascular status continuously. Take care to avoid extravasation.

Isoproterenol

■ *Receptor specificity:* beta$_1$ and beta$_2$
■ *Chemical classification:* catecholamine

Isoproterenol [Isuprel, others] differs significantly from NE and epinephrine in that isoproterenol acts only at beta-adrenergic receptors. Isoproterenol was the first beta-selective agent employed clinically and will serve as our prototype of the beta-selective adrenergic agonists.

Therapeutic Uses

Cardiovascular. By activating beta$_1$ receptors on the heart, isoproterenol can benefit patients with cardiovascular disorders. Specifically, it can help overcome AV heart block, restart the heart following cardiac arrest, and increase cardiac output during shock.

Asthma. By activating beta$_2$ receptors in the lung, isoproterenol can cause bronchodilation, thereby decreasing airway resistance. Following its introduction, isoproterenol became a mainstay of asthma therapy. However, because of the development of even more selective beta-adrenergic agonists (i.e., drugs that activate beta$_2$ receptors only), use of isoproterenol for asthma has been abandoned.

Bronchospasm. Although isoproterenol is no longer used for asthma, it *is* used to treat bronchospasm during anesthesia. Benefits derive from activating beta$_2$ receptors in the lung.

Adverse Effects

Since isoproterenol does not activate alpha-adrenergic receptors, the drug produces fewer adverse effects than NE or epinephrine. The major undesired responses are cardiac. Excessive activation of beta$_1$ receptors in the heart can cause *dysrhythmias* and *angina pectoris.* In diabetic patients, isoproterenol can cause *hyperglycemia* by promoting beta$_2$-mediated glycogenolysis.

Drug Interactions

The major drug interactions of isoproterenol are nearly identical to those of epinephrine. Effects are enhanced by MAO inhibitors and tricyclic antidepressants and reduced by beta-adrenergic blocking agents. Like epinephrine, isoproterenol can cause dysrhythmias in patients receiving certain inhalation anesthetics.

Preparations and Administration

Isoproterenol hydrochloride [Isuprel] is available in solution (0.2 and 0.02 mg/ml) for parenteral administration.

When used to *stimulate the heart,* isoproterenol can be administered IV and IM and by intracardiac injection. The dosage for IM administration is about 10 times greater than the dosage employed by the other two routes.

When used to relieve *bronchospasm,* isoproterenol is administered IV.

Dopamine

■ *Receptor specificity:* dopamine, beta$_1$, and, at high doses, alpha$_1$
■ *Chemical classification:* catecholamine

Receptor Specificity

The degree of receptor specificity displayed by dopamine is dose dependent. When administered in low therapeutic doses, dopamine acts on dopamine receptors only. At moderate therapeutic doses, dopamine activates beta$_1$ receptors in addition to dopamine receptors. At very high doses, dopamine activates alpha$_1$ receptors along with beta$_1$ and dopamine receptors.

Therapeutic Uses

Shock. The major indication for dopamine is shock. Benefits derive from effects on the heart and renal blood vessels. By activating beta$_1$ receptors in the heart, dopamine can increase cardiac output, thereby improving tissue perfusion. By activating dopamine receptors in the kidney, dopamine can dilate renal blood vessels, thereby improving renal perfusion. Success can be evaluated by monitoring output of urine.

Heart Failure. Heart failure is characterized by reduced tissue perfusion secondary to reduced cardiac output. Dopamine can help alleviate symptoms by activating beta$_1$ receptors on the heart, which increases myocardial contractility, and thereby increases cardiac output.

Acute Renal Failure. Because of its ability to increase renal blood flow and urine output, low-dose dopamine has long been used in efforts to preserve renal function in patients with evolving acute renal failure (ARF). However, recent evidence indicates that the drug is not effective: in patients with early ARF, dopamine failed to protect renal function, shorten hospital stays, or reduce the number of patients needing a kidney transplant. Accordingly, it would appear to be time to abandon low-dose dopamine as a treatment for ARF.

Adverse Effects

The most common adverse effects of dopamine—*tachycardia, dysrhythmias,* and *anginal pain*—result from activation of beta$_1$ receptors in the heart. Because of its cardiac actions, dopamine is contraindicated for patients with tachydysrhythmias or ventricular fibrillation. Since high concentrations of dopamine cause alpha$_1$ activation, extravasation may result in *necrosis* from localized vasoconstriction; tissue injury can be minimized by local infiltration of phentolamine, an alpha-adrenergic blocking agent.

Drug Interactions

MAO inhibitors can intensify the effects of dopamine on the heart and blood vessels. If a patient is receiving an MAO inhibitor, the dosage of dopamine must be reduced by at least 90%. *Tricyclic antidepressants* can also intensify dopamine's actions, but not to the extent seen with MAO inhibitors. Certain *general anesthetics* can sensitize the myocardium to stimulation by dopamine and other catecholamines, thereby creating a risk of dysrhythmias. *Diuretics* can complement the beneficial effects of dopamine on the kidney.

Preparations, Dosage, and Administration

Preparations. Dopamine hydrochloride [Intropin] is dispensed in aqueous solutions that range in concentration from 40 to 160 mg/ml.

Dosage. Dopamine must be diluted prior to infusion. For treatment of *shock,* a dilution of 400 µg/ml can be used. The recommended initial rate of infusion is 2 to 5 µg/kg/min. If needed, the infusion rate can be gradually increased to a maximum of 20 to 50 µg/kg/min.

Administration. Dopamine is administered IV. Because of extremely rapid inactivation by MAO and COMT, the drug must be given by *continuous infusion.* A metering device is needed to control flow rate. Cardiovascular status must be closely monitored. If extravasation occurs, the infusion should be stopped and the affected area infiltrated with an alpha-adrenergic antagonist.

Dobutamine

■ *Receptor specificity:* beta$_1$
■ *Chemical classification:* catecholamine

Actions and Uses. At therapeutic doses, dobutamine causes selective activation of beta$_1$-adrenergic receptors. The only indication for the drug is *heart failure.*

Adverse Effects. The major adverse effect is tachycardia. Blood pressure and the electrocardiogram (EKG) should be monitored closely.

Drug Interactions. Effects of dobutamine on the heart and blood vessels are intensified greatly by *MAO inhibitors.* In patients receiving an MAO inhibitor, the dosage of dobutamine must be reduced by at least 90%. Concurrent use of *tricyclic antidepressants* may cause a moderate increase in the cardiovascular effects. Certain *general anesthetics* can sensitize the myocardium to the stimulant actions of dobutamine, thereby increasing the risk of dysrhythmias.

Preparations, Dosage, and Administration. Dobutamine hydrochloride [Dobutrex] is dispensed in solution (12.5 mg/ml) in 20-ml vials. This concentrated solution must be diluted to at least 50 ml prior to use. Because of rapid inactivation by MAO and COMT, dobutamine is administered by IV infusion only. Rates of infusion usually range from 2.5 to 10 µg/kg/min.

Phenylephrine

■ *Receptor specificity:* alpha$_1$
■ *Chemical classification:* noncatecholamine

Phenylephrine is a selective alpha$_1$ agonist. The drug can be administered locally to reduce nasal congestion and parenterally to elevate blood pressure. In addition, phenylephrine eye drops can be used to dilate the pupil. Also, phenylephrine can be coadministered with local anesthetics to retard absorption of the anesthetic.

Terbutaline

■ *Receptor specificity:* beta$_2$
■ *Chemical classification:* noncatecholamine

Therapeutic Uses

Asthma. Terbutaline can reduce airway resistance in asthma by causing beta$_2$-mediated bronchodilation. Since terbutaline is "selective" for beta$_2$ receptors, it produces much less activation of cardiac beta$_1$ receptors than does isoproterenol. Accordingly, terbutaline and other beta$_2$-selective agents have replaced isoproterenol for therapy of asthma. It must be remembered, however, that receptor selectivity is only relative: If administered in large doses, terbutaline will lose selectivity and activate beta$_1$ receptors as well as beta$_2$ receptors. Accordingly, patients should be warned not to exceed recommended doses, since doing so may cause undesired cardiac stimulation.

Delay of Preterm Labor. By activating beta$_2$ receptors in the uterus, terbutaline can relax uterine smooth muscle, thereby delaying labor. However, although terbutaline can be employed to delay labor, a different beta$_2$ agonist—ritodrine—is the drug of choice for this indication.

Adverse Effects

Adverse effects are minimal at therapeutic doses. *Tremor* is most common. If the dosage is excessive, terbutaline can cause *tachycardia* by activating beta$_1$ receptors in the heart.

Ephedrine

■ *Receptor specificity:* alpha$_1$, alpha$_2$, beta$_1$, beta$_2$
■ *Chemical classification:* noncatecholamine

Ephedrine is referred to as a *mixed-acting drug* because it activates adrenergic receptors by direct *and* indirect mechanisms. *Direct* activation results from binding of the drug to alpha and beta receptors. *Indirect* activation results from release of NE from adrenergic neurons.

Therapeutic Uses

Nasal Congestion. Ephedrine can reduce nasal congestion by causing alpha$_1$-mediated vasoconstriction. When used for this indication, the drug can be administered topically or by mouth. As a rule, topical administration is preferred. This is because systemic reactions to topical administration are minimal, whereas oral administration results in activation of adrenergic receptors throughout the body.

Narcolepsy. Narcolepsy is a CNS disorder characterized by sudden and irresistible "attacks" of sleep. Ephedrine is one of several medications

TABLE 17–4 ■ Discussion of Adrenergic Agonists In Other Chapters

Drug Class	Indication/Type	Chapter
Alpha₁ Agonists	Nasal congestion	72
	Ophthalmology	100
Alpha₂ Agonists	Basic pharmacology	19
	Hypertension	45
Beta₁ Agonists	Heart failure	46
Beta₂ Agonists	Asthma	71
	Preterm labor	62
Amphetamines	Basic pharmacology	35
	Attention-deficit/hyperactivity disorder	35
	Appetite suppression	78

employed for treatment. Benefits are thought to result from activation of adrenergic receptors in the brain. Ephedrine has access to CNS receptors because, being a noncatecholamine, the drug is able to cross the blood-brain barrier.

Adverse Effects

Since ephedrine activates the same receptors as epinephrine, both drugs share the same adverse effects: *hypertension, dysrhythmias, angina,* and *hyperglycemia.* In addition to these shared effects, ephedrine can act in the CNS to cause *insomnia.*

DISCUSSION OF ADRENERGIC AGONISTS IN OTHER CHAPTERS

All of the drugs presented in this chapter are discussed again in chapters that address specific applications. For example, the use of alpha₁ agonists to relieve nasal congestion is discussed in Chapter 72. Table 17–4 summarizes the chapters in which adrenergic agonists are discussed again.

⸪ KEY POINTS

- Adrenergic agonists are also known as sympathomimetics because their effects mimic those caused by the sympathetic nervous system.
- Most adrenergic agonists act by direct stimulation of adrenergic receptors. A few act by indirect mechanisms: promotion of norepinephrine release, blockade of norepinephrine uptake, and inhibition of norepinephrine degradation.
- Adrenergic agonists in the catecholamine family cannot be taken orally (because of destruction by MAO and COMT), have a brief duration of action (because of destruction by MAO and COMT), and cannot cross the blood-brain barrier (because they are polar molecules).
- Adrenergic agonists that are not catecholamines can be taken orally, have a longer duration than the catecholamines, and cross the blood-brain barrier.
- Activation of alpha₁ receptors causes vasoconstriction and mydriasis.

- Alpha₁ agonists are used for hemostasis, nasal decongestion, and elevation of blood pressure, and as adjuncts to local anesthetics.
- Major adverse effects that can result from alpha₁ activation are hypertension and local necrosis (if extravasation occurs).
- Activation of alpha₂ receptors in the periphery is of minimal clinical significance. In contrast, drugs that activate alpha₂ receptors in the CNS produce useful effects (see Chapter 19).
- All of the clinically relevant responses to activation of beta₁ receptors result from activating beta₁ receptors in the heart.
- Activation of cardiac beta₁ receptors increases heart rate, force of contraction, and conduction through the AV node.
- Drugs that activate beta₁ receptors can be used to treat heart failure, AV block, and cardiac arrest.
- Potential adverse effects from beta₁ activation are tachycardia, dysrhythmias, and angina.
- Drugs that activate beta₂ receptors are used to treat asthma and delay preterm labor.
- Principal adverse effects from beta₂ activation are hyperglycemia (in diabetic patients) and tremor.
- Activation of dopamine receptors dilates renal blood vessels, which helps maintain renal perfusion in shock.
- Epinephrine is a catecholamine that activates alpha₁, alpha₂, beta₁, and beta₂ receptors.
- Epinephrine is the drug of choice for treating anaphylactic shock: By activating alpha₁, beta₁, and beta₂ receptors, epinephrine can elevate blood pressure, suppress glottal edema, and counteract bronchoconstriction.
- Epinephrine can also be used to control superficial bleeding, restart the heart after cardiac arrest, and delay absorption of local anesthetics.
- Epinephrine should not be combined with MAO inhibitors, and should be used cautiously in patients taking tricyclic antidepressants.
- Isoproterenol is a catecholamine that activates beta₁ and beta₂ receptors.
- Isoproterenol can be used to enhance cardiac performance (by activating beta₁ receptors) and to treat bronchospasm (by activating beta₂ receptors).
- Dopamine is a catecholamine whose receptor specificity is highly dose dependent: at low therapeutic doses, dopamine acts on dopamine receptors only; at moderate doses, dopamine activates beta₁ receptors in addition to dopamine receptors; and at high doses, dopamine activates alpha₁ receptors along with beta₁ receptors and dopamine receptors.
- Terbutaline is a noncatecholamine that produces selective activation of beta₂ receptors.
- Terbutaline can be used to treat asthma and to delay preterm labor.
- Because terbutaline is "selective" for beta₂ receptors, it produces much less stimulation of the heart than does isoproterenol. Accordingly, terbutaline (and related drugs) has replaced isoproterenol for therapy of asthma.

Summary of Major Nursing Implications*

EPINEPHRINE

Preadministration Assessment

Therapeutic Goal

Epinephrine has multiple uses. Major applications include *treatment of anaphylaxis* and *cardiac arrest.* Other uses include *control of superficial bleeding, delay of local anesthetic absorption,* and *nasal decongestion.*

Identifying High-Risk Patients

Epinephrine must be used with *great caution* in patients with hyperthyroidism, cardiac dysrhythmias, organic heart disease, or hypertension. *Caution* is also needed in patients with angina pectoris or diabetes and in those receiving MAO inhibitors, tricyclic antidepressants, or general anesthetics.

Implementation: Administration

Routes

Topical, oral inhalation, and parenteral (IV, IM, SC, intracardiac, intraspinal). Rapid inactivation by MAO and COMT prohibits oral (enteral) use.

Administration

The concentration of epinephrine solutions varies according to the route of administration (see Table 17–3). To avoid serious injury, check solution strength to ensure that the concentration is appropriate for the intended route. Aspirate prior to SC and IM administration to avoid inadvertent injection into a vein.

Epinephrine solutions oxidize over time, causing them to turn pink or brown. Discard discolored solutions.

Ongoing Evaluation and Interventions

Evaluating Therapeutic Effects

In patients receiving IV epinephrine, monitor cardiovascular status continuously.

Minimizing Adverse Effects

Cardiovascular Effects. By stimulating the heart, epinephrine can cause *anginal pain, tachycardia,* and *dysrhythmias.* These responses can be reduced with a beta-adrenergic blocking agent (e.g., propranolol).

By stimulating alpha$_1$ receptors on blood vessels, epinephrine can cause intense vasoconstriction, which can result in *severe hypertension.* Blood pressure can be lowered with an alpha-adrenergic blocking agent (e.g., phentolamine).

Necrosis. If an IV line delivering epinephrine becomes extravasated, necrosis may result. Exercise care to avoid extravasation. If extravasation occurs, infiltrate the region with phentolamine to minimize injury.

Hyperglycemia. Epinephrine may cause hyperglycemia in diabetic patients. If hyperglycemia develops, insulin dosage should be increased.

Minimizing Adverse Interactions

MAO Inhibitors and Tricyclic Antidepressants. These drugs prolong and intensify the actions of epinephrine. Patients taking these antidepressants require a reduction in epinephrine dosage.

General Anesthetics. When combined with certain general anesthetics, epinephrine can induce cardiac dysrhythmias. Dysrhythmias may respond to a beta$_1$-adrenergic blocker.

DOPAMINE

Preadministration Assessment

Therapeutic Goal

Improvement of hemodynamic status in patients with *shock* or *heart failure.* Benefits derive from enhanced cardiac performance and increased renal perfusion.

Baseline Data

Full assessment of cardiac, hemodynamic, and renal status is needed.

Identifying High-Risk Patients

Dopamine is *contraindicated* for patients with tachydysrhythmias or ventricular fibrillation. Use with *extreme caution* in patients with organic heart disease, hyperthyroidism, or hypertension and in patients receiving MAO inhibitors. *Caution* is also needed in patients with angina pectoris and in those receiving tricyclic antidepressants or general anesthetics.

Implementation: Administration

Route

Intravenous.

Administration

Administer by continuous infusion, employing a metering device to control flow rate.

If extravasation occurs, stop the infusion immediately and infiltrate the region with an alpha-adrenergic antagonist.

Ongoing Evaluation and Interventions

Evaluating Therapeutic Effects

Monitor cardiovascular status continuously. Increased urine output is one index of success. Diuretics may complement the beneficial effects of dopamine on the kidney.

Minimizing Adverse Effects

Cardiovascular Effects. By stimulating the heart, dopamine may cause *anginal pain, tachycardia,* or *dysrhythmias.* These reactions can be decreased with a beta-adrenergic blocking agent (e.g., propranolol).

Necrosis. If the IV line delivering dopamine becomes extravasated, necrosis may result. Exercise care to avoid extravasation. If extravasation occurs, infiltrate the region with phentolamine.

Minimizing Adverse Interactions

MAO Inhibitors. Concurrent use of MAO inhibitors and dopamine can result in severe cardiovascular toxicity. If a patient is taking an MAO inhibitor, dopamine dosage must be reduced by at least 90%.

Tricyclic Antidepressants. These drugs prolong and intensify the actions of dopamine. Patients receiving them may require a reduction in dopamine dosage.

*Patient education information is highlighted as blue text.

Summary of Major Nursing Implications*—cont'd
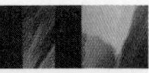

General Anesthetics. When combined with certain general anesthetics, dopamine can induce dysrhythmias. These may respond to a beta$_1$-adrenergic blocker.

DOBUTAMINE

Preadministration Assessment

Therapeutic Goal

Improvement of hemodynamic status in patients with heart failure.

Baseline Data

Full assessment of cardiac, renal, and hemodynamic status is needed.

Identifying High-Risk Patients

Use with *great caution* in patients with organic heart disease, hyperthyroidism, tachydysrhythmias, or hypertension and in those taking an MAO inhibitor. *Caution* is also needed in patients with angina pectoris and in those receiving tricyclic antidepressants or general anesthetics.

Implementation: Administration

Route

Intravenous.

Administration

Administer by continuous infusion. Dilute concentrated solutions prior to use. Infusion rates usually range from 2.5 to 10 μg/kg/min. Adjust the infusion rate on the basis of the cardiovascular response.

*Patient education information is highlighted as blue text.

Ongoing Evaluation and Interventions

Evaluating Therapeutic Effects

Monitor cardiac function (heart rate, EKG), blood pressure, and urine output. When possible, monitor central venous pressure and pulmonary wedge pressure.

Minimizing Adverse Effects

Major adverse effects are *tachycardia* and *dysrhythmias.* Monitor the EKG and blood pressure closely. Adverse cardiac effects can be reduced with a beta-adrenergic antagonist.

Minimizing Adverse Interactions

MAO Inhibitors. Concurrent use of an MAO inhibitor with dobutamine can cause severe cardiovascular toxicity. If a patient is taking an MAO inhibitor, dobutamine dosage must be reduced by at least 90%.

Tricyclic Antidepressants. These drugs can prolong and intensify the actions of dobutamine. Patients receiving them may require a reduction in dobutamine dosage.

General Anesthetics. When combined with certain general anesthetics, dobutamine can cause cardiac dysrhythmias. These may respond to a beta$_1$-adrenergic antagonist.

Adrenergic Antagonists

TABLE 18–1 ▪ Receptor Specificity of Adrenergic Antagonists

Category	Drugs	Receptors Blocked
Alpha-Adrenergic Blocking Agents	Phentolamine	$alpha_1$, $alpha_2$
	Phenoxybenzamine*	$alpha_1$, $alpha_2$
	Doxazosin	$alpha_1$
	Prazosin	$alpha_1$
	Terazosin	$alpha_1$
	Tamsulosin	$alpha_1$
Beta-Adrenergic Blocking Agents	Carteolol	$beta_1$, $beta_2$
	Carvedilol†	$beta_1$, $beta_2$
	Labetalol†	$beta_1$, $beta_2$
	Nadolol	$beta_1$, $beta_2$
	Penbutolol	$beta_1$, $beta_2$
	Pindolol	$beta_1$, $beta_2$
	Propranolol	$beta_1$, $beta_2$
	Sotalol	$beta_1$, $beta_2$
	Timolol	$beta_1$, $beta_2$
	Acebutolol	$beta_1$
	Atenolol	$beta_1$
	Betaxolol	$beta_1$
	Bisoprolol	$beta_1$
	Esmolol	$beta_1$
	Metoprolol	$beta_1$

*No longer available in the United States.
†Also blocks $alpha_1$-adrenergic receptors.

The adrenergic antagonists cause direct blockade of adrenergic receptors. With one exception, all of the adrenergic antagonists produce *reversible* (competitive) receptor blockade.

In contrast to some adrenergic *agonists* (e.g., epinephrine), the adrenergic *antagonists* display a high degree of receptor specificity. Because of this specificity, the adrenergic antagonists can be neatly divided into two major groups: (1) *alpha-adrenergic blocking agents* (drugs that produce selective blockade of alpha-adrenergic receptors) and (2) *beta-adrenergic blocking agents* (drugs that produce selective blockade of beta receptors). The drugs that belong to these two groups are listed in Table 18–1.

Our approach to the adrenergic antagonists mirrors the approach we took with the adrenergic agonists. That is, we begin by discussing the therapeutic and adverse effects that can result from blocking alpha- and beta-adrenergic receptors, after which we discuss the individual drugs that produce receptor blockade.

Remember that it is much easier to understand responses to the adrenergic drugs if you first understand the responses to activation of adrenergic receptors. Accordingly, if you have not yet mastered (memorized) Table 13–3, you should do so now (or at least be prepared to consult the table as we proceed).

ALPHA-ADRENERGIC ANTAGONISTS I: THERAPEUTIC AND ADVERSE RESPONSES TO ALPHA BLOCKADE

In this section we discuss the beneficial and adverse responses that can result from blockade of alpha-adrenergic receptors. Properties of individual alpha blocking agents are discussed later.

Therapeutic Applications of Alpha Blockade

Most clinically useful responses to alpha-adrenergic antagonists result from blockade of $alpha_1$ receptors on blood vessels. Blockade of $alpha_1$ receptors in the bladder and prostate can help men with benign prostatic hyperplasia (BPH). Blockade of $alpha_1$ receptors in the eye and blockade of $alpha_2$ receptors have no recognized therapeutic applications.

Essential Hypertension. Hypertension (high blood pressure) can be treated with a variety of drugs, including the alpha-adrenergic antagonists. Alpha antagonists lower blood pressure by blocking $alpha_1$ receptors on arterioles and veins, causing vasodilation. Dilation of arterioles reduces arterial pressure directly. Dilation of veins lowers arterial pressure by an indirect process: In response to venous dilation, return of blood to the heart decreases, thereby decreasing cardiac output, which in turn reduces arterial pressure. The role of alpha-adrenergic blockers in essential hypertension is discussed further in Chapter 45 (Drugs for Hypertension).

Reversal of Toxicity from Alpha₁ Agonists. Overdose with an alpha-adrenergic agonist (e.g., epinephrine) can produce *hypertension* secondary to excessive stimulation of alpha₁ receptors on blood vessels. When this occurs, blood pressure can be lowered by reversing the vasoconstriction with an alpha-adrenergic antagonist.

If an IV line containing an alpha agonist becomes extravasated, necrosis can occur secondary to intense local vasoconstriction. By infiltrating the region with phentolamine (an alpha-adrenergic antagonist), we can block the vasoconstriction and thereby prevent injury.

Benign Prostatic Hyperplasia. BPH results from proliferation of cells in the prostate gland. Symptoms include dysuria, increased frequency of daytime urination, nocturia, urinary hesitance and intermittence, urinary urgency, a sensation of incomplete voiding, and a reduction in the size and force of the urinary stream. All of these symptoms can be improved with drugs that block alpha₁ receptors; benefits result from reduced contraction of smooth muscle in the bladder neck and prostatic capsule. BPH is discussed further in Chapter 103.

Pheochromocytoma. A pheochromocytoma is a catecholamine-secreting tumor derived from cells of the sympathetic nervous system. These tumors are usually located in the adrenal medulla. If secretion of catecholamines (epinephrine, norepinephrine) is sufficiently great, persistent hypertension can result. The principal cause of hypertension is activation of alpha₁ receptors on blood vessels, although activation of beta₁ receptors on the heart can also contribute. The preferred treatment is surgical removal of the tumor, but alpha-adrenergic blockers may also be employed.

Alpha-blocking agents have two roles in managing pheochromocytoma. First, in patients with inoperable tumors, alpha blockers are given chronically to suppress hypertension. Second, when surgery is indicated, alpha blockers are administered preoperatively to reduce the risk of acute hypertension during the procedure. (The surgical patient is at risk of acute hypertension because manipulation of the tumor can cause massive catecholamine release.)

Raynaud's Disease. Raynaud's disease is a peripheral vascular disorder characterized by vasospasm in the toes and fingers. Prominent symptoms are local sensations of pain and cold. Alpha-adrenergic blocking agents can suppress symptoms by preventing alpha-mediated vasoconstriction. It should be noted, however, that although alpha blockers can relieve symptoms of Raynaud's disease, they are generally ineffective against other peripheral vascular disorders that involve inappropriate vasoconstriction.

Adverse Effects of Alpha Blockade

The most significant adverse effects of the alpha-adrenergic antagonists result from blockade of alpha₁ receptors. Detrimental effects associated with alpha₂ blockade are minor.

Adverse Effects of Alpha₁ Blockade

Orthostatic Hypotension. This is the most serious adverse response to alpha-adrenergic blockade. Orthostatic hypotension can reduce blood flow to the brain, thereby causing dizziness, lightheadedness, and even syncope (fainting).

The cause of orthostatic hypotension is blockade of alpha receptors on *veins*, which reduces muscle tone in the venous wall. Because of reduced venous tone, blood tends to pool (accumulate) in veins when the patient assumes an erect posture. As a result, return of blood to the heart is reduced, which decreases cardiac output, which in turn causes blood pressure to fall.

Patients should be informed about symptoms of hypotension (lightheadedness, dizziness) and advised to sit or lie down if these occur. In addition, patients should be informed that orthostatic hypotension can be minimized by avoiding abrupt transitions from a supine or sitting position to an erect posture.

Reflex Tachycardia. Alpha-adrenergic antagonists can increase heart rate by triggering the baroreceptor reflex. Activation of the reflex occurs as follows: (1) blockade of vascular alpha₁ receptors causes vasodilation; (2) vasodilation reduces blood pressure; (3) baroreceptors sense the reduction in blood pressure and, in an attempt to restore normal pressure, initiate a reflex increase in heart rate via the autonomic nervous system. If necessary, reflex tachycardia can be suppressed with a beta-adrenergic blocking agent.

Nasal Congestion. Alpha blockade can dilate the blood vessels of the nasal mucosa, producing nasal congestion.

Inhibition of Ejaculation. Since activation of alpha₁ receptors is required for ejaculation (see Table 13–3), blockade of these receptors can cause impotence. This form of drug-induced impotence is reversible and resolves when the alpha blocker is withdrawn.

The ability of alpha blockers to inhibit ejaculation can be a major reason for noncompliance. If a patient deems the adverse sexual effects of alpha blockade unacceptable, a change in medication will be required. Since males may be reluctant to discuss such concerns, a tactful interview will be needed to discern if drug-induced impotence is discouraging drug use.

Sodium Retention and Increased Blood Volume. By reducing blood pressure, alpha blockers can promote renal retention of sodium and water, thereby causing blood volume to increase. The steps in this process are as follows: (1) by reducing blood pressure, alpha₁ blockers decrease renal blood flow; (2) in response to reduced perfusion, the kidney excretes less sodium and water; and (3) the resultant retention of sodium and water increases blood volume. As a result, blood pressure is elevated, blood flow to the kidney is increased, and, as far as the kidney is concerned, all is well. Unfortunately, when alpha blockers are used to treat hypertension (which they often are), this compensatory elevation in blood pressure can negate beneficial effects. In order to prevent the kidney from "neutralizing" hypotensive actions, alpha-blocking agents are usually combined with a diuretic when used in patients with hypertension.

Adverse Effects of Alpha₂ Blockade

The most significant adverse effect associated with alpha₂ blockade is *potentiation of the reflex tachycardia that can occur in response to blockade of alpha₁ receptors.* Why does alpha₂ blockade intensify reflex tachycardia? Recall that peripheral alpha₂ receptors are located presynaptically and that activation of these receptors inhibits norepinephrine release. Hence, if alpha₂ receptors are blocked, release of norepinephrine will increase. Since the reflex tachycardia caused by alpha₁ blockade is ultimately the result of increased firing of the sympathetic nerves to the heart, and since alpha₂ blockade will cause each nerve impulse to release a greater amount of norepinephrine, alpha₂ blockade will potentiate reflex tachycardia initiated by blockade of alpha₁ receptors. Accordingly, drugs such as phentolamine, which block alpha₂ as well as alpha₁ receptors, cause greater reflex tachycardia than do drugs that block alpha₁ receptors only.

ALPHA-ADRENERGIC ANTAGONISTS II: PROPERTIES OF INDIVIDUAL ALPHA BLOCKERS

Only five alpha-adrenergic antagonists are employed clinically. Because the alpha blockers often cause postural hypotension, therapeutic uses are limited.

As indicated in Table 18–1, the alpha-adrenergic blocking agents can be subdivided into two groups. One group—the *nonselective* alpha-blocking agents—contains drugs that block alpha₁ *and* alpha₂ receptors. Phentolamine is the prototype for this group. The second group, represented by *prazosin*, contains drugs that produce *selective alpha₁ blockade*.

Prazosin

Actions and Uses. Prazosin [Minipress] is a competitive antagonist that produces selective blockade of alpha₁-adrenergic receptors. By blocking alpha₁ receptors, prazosin can cause dilation of arterioles and veins, and relaxation of smooth muscle in the bladder neck and prostatic capsule. The drug is approved only for hypertension. However, it can also benefit men with BPH.

Pharmacokinetics. Prazosin is administered orally. Antihypertensive effects peak in 1 to 3 hours and persist for 10 hours. The drug undergoes extensive hepatic metabolism followed by excretion in the bile. Only about 10% is eliminated in the urine. The half-life is 2 to 3 hours.

Adverse Effects. Blockade of alpha₁ receptors can cause *orthostatic hypotension, reflex tachycardia, inhibition of ejaculation,* and *nasal congestion.* The most serious of these is hypotension. Patients should be educated about the symptoms of hypotension (dizziness, lightheadedness) and advised to sit or lie down if they occur. Patients should also be informed that orthostatic hypotension can be minimized by moving slowly when making the transition from a supine or sitting position to an upright position.

About 1% of patients lose consciousness 30 to 60 minutes after receiving their first prazosin dose. This "first-dose" effect is the result of severe postural hypotension. To minimize the first-dose effect, the initial dose should be small (1 mg or less). After this low initial dose, doses can be gradually increased with little risk of fainting. Patients who are beginning treatment should be forewarned about the first-dose effect and advised to avoid driving and other hazardous activities for 12 to 24 hours. Administering the initial dose at bedtime eliminates the risk of a first-dose effect.

Preparations, Dosage, and Administration. Prazosin hydrochloride [Minipress] is available in capsules (1, 2, and 5 mg) for oral use. The initial adult dosage for essential hypertension is 1 mg taken 2 or 3 times a day. For maintenance therapy, the dosage is 6 to 15 mg/day administered in divided doses.

Terazosin

Actions and Uses. Like prazosin, terazosin [Hytrin] is a selective, competitive antagonist at alpha₁-adrenergic receptors. The drug is approved for hypertension and BPH.

Pharmacokinetics. Terazosin is administered orally, and peak effects develop in 1 to 2 hours. The drug's half-life is prolonged (9 to 12 hours), allowing benefits to be maintained with just one dose a day. Terazosin undergoes hepatic metabolism followed by excretion in the bile and urine.

Adverse Effects. Like other alpha-blocking agents, terazosin can cause *orthostatic hypotension, reflex tachycardia, nasal congestion,* and *inhibition of ejaculation.* In addition, terazosin is associated with a high incidence (16%) of *headache.* As with prazosin, the first dose can cause profound hypotension. To minimize this first-dose effect, the initial dose should be administered at bedtime.

Preparations, Dosage, and Administration. Terazosin [Hytrin] is available in capsules (1, 2, 5, and 10 mg) for oral use. *Antihypertensive* therapy is initiated with a 1-mg dose, administered at bedtime to minimize the first-dose effect. Dosage can be gradually increased as needed and tolerated. The recommended dosage range for maintenance therapy is 1 to 5 mg once daily. Dosing for *benign prostatic hyperplasia* is similar to that for hypertension, except that a maintenance dosage of 10 mg/day is needed for most men.

Doxazosin

Actions and Uses. Doxazosin [Cardura] is a selective, competitive inhibitor of alpha₁-adrenergic receptors. The drug is indicated for hypertension and BPH.

Pharmacokinetics. Doxazosin is administered orally, and peak effects develop in 2 to 3 hours. The drug has a prolonged half-life (22 hours), and once-a-day dosing is adequate. Most (98%) of the drug in blood is protein bound. Doxazosin undergoes extensive hepatic metabolism followed by biliary excretion.

Adverse Effects. Like prazosin and terazosin, doxazosin can cause *orthostatic hypotension, reflex tachycardia, nasal congestion,* and *inhibition of ejaculation.* As with prazosin, the first dose can cause profound hypotension. First-dose hypotension can be minimized by giving the initial dose at bedtime.

Preparations, Dosage, and Administration. Doxazosin [Cardura] is dispensed in tablets (1, 2, 4, and 8 mg) for oral administration. The initial dosage for hypertension or BPH is 1 mg once a day. The dosage may be gradually increased as needed, up to a maximum of 16 mg once daily for hypertension or 8 mg once daily for BPH.

Tamsulosin

Actions and Uses. Tamsulosin [Flomax] is a selective alpha₁-adrenergic antagonist. The drug is approved only for BPH. It is not indicated for hypertension. In men with BPH, tamsulosin increases urine flow rate and decreases residual urine volume. Maximum benefits develop within 2 weeks.

Pharmacokinetics. Tamsulosin is administered orally, and absorption is slow. Food further decreases the rate and extent of absorption. The drug is metabolized in the liver and excreted in the urine.

Adverse Effects and Interactions. Like other alpha₁ blockers, tamsulosin can cause *orthostatic hypotension, nasal congestion,* and *abnormal ejaculation* (ejaculation failure, ejaculation decrease, retrograde ejaculation). In addition, the drug is associated with increased *infection.* Combined use with *cimetidine* increases levels of tamsulosin, and may thereby cause toxicity.

Preparations, Dosage, and Administration. Tamsulosin [Flomax] is available in 0.4-mg capsules for oral administration. The usual dosage is 0.4 mg, administered 30 minutes after the same meal each day. Dosage may be increased to 0.8 mg/day if needed.

Phentolamine

Actions and Uses. Like prazosin, phentolamine [Regitine] is a competitive adrenergic antagonist. However, in contrast to prazosin, phentolamine blocks alpha₂ receptors as well as alpha₁ receptors. Phentolamine has two applications: (1) treatment of pheochromocytoma and (2) prevention of tissue necrosis following extravasation of drugs that produce alpha₁-mediated vasoconstriction (e.g., norepinephrine).

Adverse Effects. Like prazosin, phentolamine can produce the typical adverse effects associated with alpha-adrenergic blockade: *orthostatic hypotension, reflex tachycardia, nasal congestion,* and *inhibition of ejaculation.* Because of its ability to block alpha₂ receptors, *phentolamine produces greater reflex tachycardia than prazosin.* If reflex tachycardia is especially severe, heart rate can be reduced with a beta-adrenergic blocker. Since tachycardia can aggravate angina pectoris and myocardial infarction (MI), phentolamine is contraindicated for patients with either disorder.

Overdose can produce profound hypotension. If necessary, blood pressure can be elevated with *norepinephrine. Epinephrine* should *not* be used, because the drug can cause blood pressure to drop even further! Why? Because in the presence of alpha₁ blockade, the ability of epinephrine to promote vasodilation (via activation of vascular beta₂ receptors) may outweigh the ability of epinephrine to cause vasoconstriction (via activation of vascular alpha₁ receptors). Further lowering of blood pressure is not a problem with norepinephrine because norepinephrine does not activate beta₂ receptors.

Preparations, Dosage, and Administration. Phentolamine [Regitine] is dispensed in solution (5 mg/25 ml) for IM and IV administration. The dosage for preventing hypertension during surgical excision of a *pheochromocytoma* is 5 mg (IM or IV). To prevent *necrosis following extravasation* of IV norepinephrine, the region should be infiltrated with 5 to 10 mg of phentolamine diluted in 10 ml of saline.

Phenoxybenzamine

Phenoxybenzamine [Dibenzyline] is an old drug that, like phentolamine, blocks alpha₁ and alpha₂ receptors. However, unlike all of the other alpha-adrenergic antagonists, phenoxybenzamine is a *noncompetitive* receptor antagonist. Hence, receptor blockade is *not reversible.* As a result, the effects of phenoxybenzamine are long lasting. (Responses to a single dose can persist for several days.) Effects subside as newly synthesized receptors replace the ones that have been irreversibly blocked. Because irreversibility makes phenoxybenzamine difficult to work with, and because superior (reversible) drugs are available, phenoxybenzamine has been withdrawn from the United States market. Prior to being withdrawn, phenoxybenzamine was used for patients with pheochromocytoma.

Like the other alpha-adrenergic antagonists, phenoxybenzamine can produce *orthostatic hypotension, reflex tachycardia, nasal congestion,* and *inhibition of ejaculation.* Reflex tachycardia is greater than that caused by prazosin and about equal to that caused by phentolamine.

If administered in excessive amounts, phenoxybenzamine, like phentolamine, will cause profound hypotension. Furthermore, since hypotension is the result of *irreversible* alpha₁ blockade, phenoxybenzamine-induced hypotension cannot be corrected with an alpha₁ agonist. To restore blood pressure, patients must be given IV fluids, which elevate blood pressure by increasing blood volume.

BETA-ADRENERGIC ANTAGONISTS I: THERAPEUTIC AND ADVERSE RESPONSES TO BETA BLOCKADE

In this section we consider the beneficial and adverse responses that can result from blockade of beta-adrenergic receptors. Properties of individual beta-blocking agents are discussed later.

Therapeutic Applications of Beta Blockade

Practically all of the therapeutic effects of the beta-adrenergic antagonists result from blockade of beta₁ receptors in the heart. The major consequences of blocking these receptors are (1) reduced heart rate, (2) reduced force of contraction, and (3) reduced velocity of impulse conduction through the atrioventricular (AV) node. Because of these effects, beta blockers are useful in a variety of pathologic states.

Angina Pectoris. Angina pectoris (paroxysmal pain in the region of the heart) occurs when oxygen supply (blood flow) to the heart is insufficient to meet cardiac oxygen demand. Anginal attacks can be precipitated by exertion, intense emotion, and other factors. Beta-adrenergic blockers are a mainstay of antianginal therapy. By blocking beta₁ receptors in the heart, these drugs decrease cardiac work. This brings oxygen demand back into balance with oxygen supply, and thereby prevents pain. Angina pectoris and its treatment are the subject of Chapter 49.

Hypertension. Beta-adrenergic blocking agents are drugs of choice for hypertension. Because of their use in this common disorder, beta blockers are one of our most widely prescribed families of drugs.

The exact mechanism by which beta blockers reduce blood pressure is not known. Older proposed mechanisms include reduction of cardiac output through blockade of beta₁ receptors in the heart and suppression of renin release through blockade of beta₁ receptors in the kidney (see Chapter 42 for a discussion of the role of renin in blood pressure control). More recently, we have learned that, with long-term use, beta blockers reduce peripheral vascular resistance, which could account for much of their antihypertensive effects. The role of beta-adrenergic blocking agents in hypertension is discussed further in Chapter 45.

Cardiac Dysrhythmias. Beta-adrenergic blocking agents are especially useful for treating dysrhythmias that involve excessive electrical activity in the sinus node and atria. By blocking cardiac beta₁ receptors, these drugs can (1) decrease the rate of sinus nodal discharge and (2) suppress conduction of atrial impulses through the AV node, thereby preventing the ventricles from being driven at an excessive rate. The use of beta-adrenergic blockers to treat dysrhythmias is discussed at length in Chapter 47.

Myocardial Infarction. An MI is a region of myocardial necrosis caused by localized interruption of blood flow to the heart wall. Treatment with a beta blocker can reduce pain, infarct size, mortality, and the risk of reinfarction. To be effective, therapy with a beta-blocker must commence soon after an MI has occurred, and should be continued for several years. The role of beta blockers in treating MI is discussed further in Chapter 51.

Heart Failure. Beta blockers are now considered standard therapy for heart failure. This application is relatively new and may come as a surprise to some readers. Why? Because, until recently, heart failure was considered an absolute *contraindication* to beta blockers. At this time, only two beta blockers—carvedilol and metoprolol—are approved for treatment of heart failure. Use of beta blockers for heart failure is discussed at length in Chapter 46.

Hyperthyroidism. Hyperthyroidism (excessive production of thyroid hormone) is associated with an increase in the sensitivity of the heart to catecholamines (e.g., norepinephrine, epinephrine). As a result, normal levels of sympathetic activity to the heart can generate tachydysrhythmias and angina pectoris. Blockade of cardiac beta₁ receptors suppresses these responses.

Migraine. When taken prophylactically, beta-adrenergic blocking agents can reduce the frequency of migraine attacks. However, although beta blockers are effective as prophylaxis, these drugs are not able to abort a migraine headache once it has begun. The mechanism by which beta blockers prevent migraine is not known. Treatment of migraine and other headaches is the subject of Chapter 29.

Stage Fright. Public speakers and other performers sometimes experience "stage fright." Prominent symptoms are tachycardia and sweating brought on by generalized discharge of the sympathetic nervous system. Beta blockers help by preventing beta₁-mediated tachycardia.

Pheochromocytoma. As discussed above, a pheochromocytoma secretes large amounts of catecholamines, which can cause excessive stimulation of the heart. Cardiac stimulation can be counteracted by beta₁ blockade.

Glaucoma. Beta blockers are important drugs for treating glaucoma, a condition characterized by elevated intraocular pressure with subsequent injury to the optic nerve. The group of beta blockers used in glaucoma (see Table 100–2) is different from the group of beta blockers discussed in this chapter. Glaucoma and its treatment are addressed in Chapter 100 (Drugs for the Eye).

Adverse Effects of Beta Blockade

Although therapeutic responses to beta blockers are due almost entirely to blockade of beta$_1$ receptors, adverse effects involve both beta$_1$ and beta$_2$ blockade. Consequently, the nonselective beta-adrenergic blocking agents (drugs that block beta$_1$ *and* beta$_2$ receptors) produce a broader spectrum of adverse effects than do the "cardioselective" beta-adrenergic antagonists (drugs that selectively block beta$_1$ receptors at usual therapeutic doses).

Adverse Effects of Beta$_1$ Blockade

All of the adverse effects of beta$_1$ blockade are the result of blocking beta$_1$ receptors in the heart. Blockade of renal beta$_1$ receptors does not produce significant adverse effects.

Bradycardia. Blockade of cardiac beta$_1$ receptors can produce bradycardia (excessively slow heart rate). If necessary, heart rate can be increased using a combination of isoproterenol (a beta-adrenergic agonist) and atropine (a muscarinic antagonist). Isoproterenol competes with the beta blocker for cardiac beta$_1$ receptors, thereby promoting cardiac stimulation. By blocking muscarinic receptors on the heart, atropine prevents slowing of the heart by the parasympathetic nervous system.

Reduced Cardiac Output. Beta$_1$ blockade can reduce cardiac output by decreasing heart rate and the force of myocardial contraction. Because they can decrease cardiac output, *beta blockers must be used with great caution in patients with heart failure or reduced cardiac reserve.* In both cases, any further decrease in cardiac output could result in insufficient tissue perfusion.

Precipitation of Heart Failure. In some patients, suppression of cardiac function with a beta blocker can be so great as to cause heart failure. Patients should be informed about the early signs of heart failure (shortness of breath, night coughs, swelling of the extremities) and instructed to notify the physician if these occur. It is important to appreciate that, although beta blockers can precipitate heart failure, they are also used to *treat* heart failure.

AV Heart Block. Atrioventricular heart block is defined as suppression of impulse conduction through the AV node. In its most severe form, AV block prevents *all* atrial impulses from reaching the ventricles. Since blockade of cardiac beta$_1$ receptors can suppress AV conduction, production of AV block is a potential complication of beta-blocker therapy. These drugs are contraindicated for patients with pre-existing AV block.

Rebound Cardiac Excitation. Long-term use of beta blockers can sensitize the heart to catecholamines. As a result, if a beta blocker is withdrawn *abruptly,* anginal pain or ventricular dysrhythmias may develop. This phenomenon of increased cardiac activity in response to abrupt cessation of beta-blocker therapy is referred to as *rebound excitation.* The risk of rebound excitation can be minimized by withdrawing these drugs gradually (e.g., by tapering the dosage over a period of 1 to 2 weeks). If rebound excitation occurs, dosing should be temporarily resumed. Patients should be warned against abrupt cessation of treatment. Also, they should be advised to carry an adequate supply of their beta blocker when traveling.

Adverse Effects of Beta$_2$ Blockade

Bronchoconstriction. Blockade of beta$_2$ receptors in the lung can cause constriction of the bronchi. (Recall that activation of these receptors promotes bronchodilation.) For most people, the degree of bronchoconstriction is insignificant. However, when bronchial beta$_2$ receptors are blocked in patients with asthma, the resulting increase in airway resistance can be life threatening. Accordingly, *drugs that block beta$_2$ receptors are contraindicated for people with asthma.* If these individuals must use a beta blocker, they should use an agent that is beta$_1$ selective (e.g., metoprolol).

Inhibition of Glycogenolysis. As noted in Chapter 13, epinephrine, acting at beta$_2$ receptors in skeletal muscle and the liver, can stimulate glycogenolysis (breakdown of glycogen into glucose). Beta$_2$ blockade will inhibit this process. Although suppression of beta$_2$-mediated glycogenolysis is inconsequential for most people, interference with this process can be detrimental to patients with *diabetes.* Why? Because these people are especially dependent on beta$_2$-mediated glycogenolysis as a way to overcome severe reductions in blood glucose levels (caused by overdosing with insulin). If the diabetic patient requires a beta blocker, a beta$_1$-selective agent should be chosen.

BETA-ADRENERGIC ANTAGONISTS II: PROPERTIES OF INDIVIDUAL BETA BLOCKERS

The beta-adrenergic antagonists can be subdivided into two groups: *nonselective* beta blockers and *cardioselective* beta blockers. The nonselective agents, represented by propranolol, block beta$_1$ *and* beta$_2$ receptors. The cardioselective agents, represented by metoprolol, produce selective blockade of beta$_1$ receptors (at usual therapeutic doses). Our discussion of the individual beta blockers focuses on the two prototypes: propranolol and metoprolol.

Propranolol

Propranolol [Inderal] was the first beta-adrenergic blocker to receive widespread clinical use and remains one of our most important beta-blocking agents. Propranolol blocks beta$_1$ *and* beta$_2$ receptors, and is the prototype of the nonselective beta-adrenergic antagonists.

Pharmacologic Effects

By blocking cardiac beta$_1$ receptors, propranolol can *reduce heart rate, decrease the force of ventricular contraction,* and *suppress impulse conduction through the AV node.* The net response to these effects is a reduction in cardiac output.

By blocking beta$_1$ receptors in the kidney, propranolol can *suppress secretion of renin.*

Blockade of beta$_2$ receptors has three major effects: (1) blockade of beta$_2$ receptors in the lung can cause *bronchoconstriction,* (2) blockade of beta$_2$ receptors on certain blood vessels can produce *vasoconstriction,* and (3) blockade of beta$_2$ receptors in skeletal muscle and the liver can cause *inhibition of glycogenolysis.*

Pharmacokinetics

Propranolol is *highly lipid soluble* and therefore can readily cross membranes. The drug is well absorbed following oral administration, but, because of extensive metabolism on its first pass through the liver, less than 30% of each dose reaches the systemic circulation. Because of its ability to cross membranes, propranolol is widely distributed to all tissues and organs, including the central nervous system (CNS). Propranolol is inactivated by hepatic metabolism, and the metabolites are excreted in the urine.

Therapeutic Uses

Practically all of the applications of propranolol are based on blockade of beta$_1$ receptors in the heart. The drug's most important indications are *hypertension, angina pectoris, cardiac dysrhythmias,* and *myocardial infarction.* The role of propranolol and other beta blockers in these disorders is discussed in Chapter 45 (Drugs for Hypertension), Chapter 49 (Drugs for Angina Pectoris), Chapter 47 (Antidysrhythmic Drugs), and Chapter 51 (Management of Myocardial Infarction). Additional indications include *migraine headache* and *"stage fright."*

Adverse Effects

The most serious adverse effects of propranolol result from blockade of beta$_1$ receptors in the heart and blockade of beta$_2$ receptors in the lung.

Bradycardia. Beta$_1$ blockade in the heart can cause bradycardia. Heart rate should be assessed before each dose. If necessary, heart rate can be increased by administering atropine and isoproterenol.

AV Heart Block. By slowing conduction of impulses through the AV node, propranolol can cause AV heart block. The drug is contraindicated for patients with pre-existing AV block (if the block is greater than first degree).

Heart Failure. In patients with cardiac disease, suppression of myocardial contractility by propranolol can result in heart failure. Patients should be informed about the early signs of heart failure (shortness of breath, night coughs, swelling of the extremities) and instructed to notify the physician if these occur. Propranolol is generally contraindicated for patients with pre-existing heart failure.

Rebound Cardiac Excitation. Abrupt withdrawal of propranolol can cause rebound excitation of the heart, resulting in tachycardia and ventricular dysrhythmias. To avoid rebound excitation, propranolol should be withdrawn slowly (i.e., by giving progressively smaller doses over 1 to 2 weeks). Patients should be warned against abrupt cessation of treatment. In addition, they should be advised to carry an adequate supply of propranolol when traveling.

Bronchoconstriction. Blockade of beta$_2$ receptors in the lung can cause bronchoconstriction. As a rule, increased airway resistance is hazardous only to patients with asthma and other obstructive pulmonary disorders.

Inhibition of Glycogenolysis. Blockade of beta$_2$ receptors in skeletal muscle and the liver can inhibit glycogenolysis. This effect can be dangerous for people with diabetes (see below).

CNS Effects. Because of its lipid solubility, propranolol can readily cross the blood-brain barrier to reach sites in the CNS. Primary neuropsychiatric responses are *depression* and *insomnia.* The drug may also cause *nightmares* and *hallucinations.* Propranolol should be used with caution in patients with a history of major depression.

Precautions, Warnings, and Contraindications

Severe Allergy. Propranolol should be avoided in patients with a history of severe allergic reactions (anaphylaxis). Recall that epinephrine, the drug of choice for anaphylaxis, relieves symptoms in large part by activating beta$_1$ receptors in the heart and beta$_2$ receptors in the lung. If these receptors are blocked by propranolol, the ability of epinephrine to act will be dangerously impaired.

Diabetes. Propranolol can be detrimental to diabetic patients in two ways. First, by blocking beta$_2$ receptors in muscle and liver, propranolol can suppress glycogenolysis, thereby eliminating an important mechanism for correcting hypoglycemia (which can occur when insulin dosage is excessive). Second, by blocking beta$_1$ receptors, propranolol can suppress tachycardia, which normally serves as an early warning signal that blood glucose levels are falling too low. (When glucose drops below a safe level, the sympathetic nervous system is activated, causing an increase in heart rate.) By "masking" tachycardia, propranolol can delay awareness of hypoglycemia, thereby compromising the patient's ability to correct the problem in a timely fashion. Diabetic patients who are taking propranolol should be warned that tachycardia may no longer be a reliable indicator of hypoglycemia. In addition, they should be taught to recognize alternative signs (sweating, hunger, fatigue, poor concentration) that blood glucose is falling perilously low. Because of its ability to suppress glycogenolysis and mask tachycardia, propranolol must be used with caution by diabetic patients. Also, patients may need to reduce their dosage of insulin.

Cardiac, Respiratory, and Psychiatric Disorders. Propranolol can exacerbate *heart failure, AV heart block, sinus bradycardia, asthma,* and *bronchospasm.* The drug is contraindicated for patients with these disorders. In addition, propranolol should be used with caution in patients with a history of *depression.*

Drug Interactions

Calcium Channel Blockers. The cardiac effects of certain calcium channel blockers (e.g., verapamil) are identical to those of propranolol: reduction of heart rate, suppression of AV conduction, and suppression of myocardial contractility. When propranolol and these calcium channel blockers are used concurrently, there is a risk of excessive cardiac suppression.

Insulin. As discussed above, propranolol can impede early recognition of insulin-induced hypoglycemia. In addition, propranolol can block glycogenolysis, the body's mechanism for correcting hypoglycemia.

Preparations, Dosage, and Administration

General Dosing Considerations. Establishing an effective propranolol dosage is difficult for two reasons: (1) patients vary widely in their requirements for propranolol and (2) there is a poor correlation between blood levels of propranolol and the response. The explanation for these observations is that responses to propranolol are dependent on the activity of the sympathetic nervous system. If sympathetic activity is high, then the dose needed to reduce receptor activation will be high as well. Conversely, if sympathetic activity is low, then low doses will be sufficient to produce receptor blockade. Since sympathetic activity varies among patients, propranolol requirements vary also. Accordingly, the dosage must be adjusted by monitoring the patient's response, and not by relying on dosing information in a drug reference.

TABLE 18–2 ■ Clinical Pharmacology of the Beta-Adrenergic Blocking Agents

Generic Name	Trade Name	Receptors Blocked	ISA	Lipid Solubility	Half-Life (hr)	Route*	Maintenance Dosage in Hypertension†
Acebutolol	Sectral		+	Low	3–4	PO	400 mg once/day
Atenolol	Tenormin		0	Low	6–9	PO, IV	50 mg once/day
Betaxolol	Kerlone		0	Low	14–22	PO	10 mg once/day
Bisoprolol	Zebeta, Monocor	Beta₁	0	Low	9–12	PO	5 mg once/day
Esmolol	Brevibloc		0	Low	0.15	IV	Not for hypertension
Metoprolol	Lopressor		0	Moderate	3–7	PO, IV	100 mg once/day
slow release	Toprol XL					PO	100 mg once/day
Carteolol	Cartrol		++	Low	6	PO	2.5 mg once/day
Carvedilol‡	Coreg		0	High	5–11	PO	12.5 mg twice/day
Labetalol‡	Normodyne, Trandate		0	Moderate	6–8	PO, IV	300 mg twice/day
Nadolol	Corgard	Beta₁	0	Low	20–24	PO	40 mg once/day
Penbutolol	Levatol	and	+	High	5	PO	20 mg once/day
Pindolol	Visken	Beta₂	+++	Moderate	3–4	PO	10 mg twice/day
Propranolol	Inderal		0	High	3–5	PO, IV	60 mg twice/day
slow release	Inderal LA					PO	120 mg once/day
Sotalol	Betapace		0	Low	12	PO	Not for hypertension
Timolol	Blocadren		0	Low	4	PO	20 mg twice/day

ISA = intrinsic sympathomimetic activity (partial agonist activity).

*Oral administration is used for essential hypertension. Intravenous administration is reserved for acute myocardial infarction (atenolol, metoprolol), cardiac dysrhythmias (esmolol, propranolol), and severe hypertension (labetalol).

†These are the lowest doses normally used for maintenance in hypertension.

‡Blocks alpha₁-adrenergic receptors in addition to beta receptors.

Preparations. Propranolol hydrochloride [Inderal] is available in three oral formulations: (1) tablets (10 to 90 mg), (2) sustained-release capsules (60 to 160 mg), and (3) solution (4 and 8 mg/ml). The drug is also available in solution (1 mg/ml) for IV administration.

Dosage. For treatment of *hypertension*, the initial dosage is 40 mg twice a day. Daily maintenance dosages usually range from 120 to 240 mg (in divided doses), although some patients may need as much as 640 mg/day. The usual adult dosage for *angina pectoris* is 160 mg/day.

Metoprolol

Metoprolol [Lopressor, Toprol XL] is the prototype of the cardioselective beta-adrenergic antagonists. At usual therapeutic doses, metoprolol blocks beta₁ receptors only. Please note, however, that selectivity for beta₁ receptors is not absolute: At higher doses, metoprolol and the other "cardioselective" agents will block beta₂ receptors as well. Because their effects on beta₂ receptors are normally minimal, the cardioselective agents are not likely to cause bronchoconstriction or suppression of glycogenolysis. Accordingly, these drugs are preferred to the nonselective beta blockers for patients with asthma or diabetes.

Pharmacologic Effects. By blocking cardiac beta₁ receptors, metoprolol has the same impact on the heart as propranolol: the drug reduces heart rate, force of contraction, and conduction velocity through the AV node. Also like propranolol, metoprolol reduces secretion of renin by the kidney. In contrast to propranolol, metoprolol does not block bronchial beta₂ receptors (at usual therapeutic doses), and therefore does not increase airway resistance.

Pharmacokinetics. Metoprolol is moderately lipid soluble and well absorbed following oral administration. Like propranolol, metoprolol under-

goes extensive metabolism on its first pass through the liver. As a result, only about 40% of an oral dose reaches the systemic circulation. Elimination is by hepatic metabolism and renal excretion.

Therapeutic Uses. The primary indication for metoprolol is *hypertension*. The drug is also approved for *angina pectoris, heart failure,* and *myocardial infarction.*

Adverse Effects. The major adverse effects of metoprolol involve the heart. Like propranolol, metoprolol can cause *bradycardia, reduction of cardiac output, AV heart block,* and *rebound cardiac excitation following abrupt withdrawal.* Also, even though metoprolol is approved for *treating* heart failure, it can *cause* heart failure if used incautiously. In contrast to propranolol, metoprolol causes minimal bronchoconstriction and does not interfere with beta₂-mediated glycogenolysis.

Precautions, Warnings, and Contraindications. Like propranolol, metoprolol is contraindicated for patients with *sinus bradycardia* and *AV heart block that is greater than first degree.* In addition, it should be used with great care in patients with *heart failure.* Because metoprolol produces only minimal blockade of beta₂ receptors, the drug is safer than propranolol for patients with asthma or a history of severe allergic reactions. In addition, since metoprolol does not suppress beta₂-mediated glycogenolysis, it can be used more safely than propranolol by patients with diabetes. Please note, however, that metoprolol, like propranolol, will "mask" tachycardia, thereby depriving the diabetic patient of an early indication that hypoglycemia is developing.

Preparations, Dosage, and Administration. Metoprolol is available in standard oral tablets (50 and 100 mg) under the trade name Lopressor and in sustained-release oral tablets (25, 50, 100, and 200 mg) under the trade name Toprol XL. The drug is also available in solution (1 mg/ml) for IV

TABLE 18–3 ■ Beta-Adrenergic Blocking Agents: Summary of Therapeutic Uses*

	Hypertension	Angina Pectoris	Cardiac Dysrhythmias	Myocardial Infarction	Migraine Prophylaxis	Stage Fright	Heart Failure
Acebutolol	A	I	A				
Atenolol	A	A	I	A	I	I	
Betaxolol	A						
Bisoprolol	A	I	I				I
Carteolol	A	I					
Carvedilol	A	I					A
Esmolol		I	A				
Labetalol	A						
Metoprolol	A	A	I	A	I		A
Nadolol	A	A	I		I	I	
Penbutolol	A						
Pindolol	A		I			I	
Propranolol	A	A	A	A	A	I	
Sotalol			A				
Timolol	A		I	A	A	I	

A = FDA-approved use, I = investigational use.
*A group of beta blockers not discussed in this chapter is used to treat glaucoma. These beta blockers are discussed in Chapter 100 (Drugs for the Eye).

administration. The initial dosage for *hypertension* is 100 mg/day in single or divided doses. The dosage for maintenance therapy ranges from 100 to 400 mg/day in divided doses. Intravenous administration is reserved for *myocardial infarction*.

Other Beta-Adrenergic Blockers

In the United States, 15 beta blockers are approved for treatment of cardiovascular disorders (hypertension, angina pectoris, cardiac dysrhythmias, MI). Principal differences among these drugs concern receptor specificity, pharmacokinetics, indications, and side effects.

In addition to the agents used for cardiovascular disorders, there is a group of beta blockers used to treat glaucoma. These drugs are discussed in Chapter 100 (Drugs for the Eye).

Properties of the beta blockers employed for cardiovascular disorders are discussed below.

Receptor Specificity. As noted above, the beta blockers fall into two major groups: nonselective agents and cardioselective agents. The nonselective agents block beta₁ *and* beta₂ receptors, whereas the cardioselective agents block beta₁ receptors only (at usual therapeutic doses). Because of their limited side effects, the cardioselective agents are preferred for patients with asthma or diabetes. Two beta blockers—*labetalol* and *carvedilol*—differ from all the others in that they block *alpha* adrenergic receptors in addition to beta receptors. The receptor specificity of individual beta blockers is indicated in Tables 18–1 and 18–2.

Pharmacokinetics. Pharmacokinetic properties of the beta blockers are summarized in Table 18–2. The relative lipid solubility of these agents is of particular importance. The drugs with the highest lipid solubility—carvedilol, propranolol, and penbutolol—have two prominent features: (1) they penetrate the blood-brain barrier with ease and (2) they are eliminated primarily by hepatic metabolism. The drugs with

low lipid solubility (e.g., acebutolol, atenolol) penetrate the blood-brain barrier poorly and are eliminated primarily by renal excretion. The drugs with moderate lipid solubility—metoprolol, labetalol, and pindolol—are able to penetrate the blood-brain barrier and are eliminated by a combination of hepatic metabolism and renal excretion.

Therapeutic Uses. Principal indications for the beta-adrenergic blockers are *hypertension, angina pectoris,* and *cardiac dysrhythmias.* Other uses include prophylaxis of *migraine headache,* treatment of *myocardial infarction,* suppression of symptoms in individuals with *situational anxiety* (e.g., stage fright), and, surprisingly, treatment of *heart failure* (see Chapter 46). Approved and investigational uses of the beta blockers are summarized in Table 18–3.

Esmolol and *sotalol* differ from the other beta blockers in that they are not used for hypertension. Because of its very short half-life (15 minutes), *esmolol* is clearly unsuited for treating hypertension, which requires that blood levels be maintained throughout the day, every day, for an indefinite time. The only approved indication for esmolol is emergency IV therapy of *supraventricular tachycardia. Sotalol* is approved only for *ventricular dysrhythmias.* Esmolol and sotalol are discussed further in Chapter 47 (Antidysrhythmic Drugs).

Adverse Effects. By blocking beta₁ receptors in the heart, all of the beta blockers can cause *bradycardia, AV heart block,* and, rarely, *heart failure.* By blocking beta₂ receptors in the lung, the nonselective agents can cause significant *bronchoconstriction* in patients with asthma or chronic obstructive pulmonary disease. In addition, by blocking beta₂ receptors in the liver and skeletal muscle, the *nonselective* agents can *inhibit glycogenolysis,* thereby compromising the ability of diabetic patients to compensate for insulin-induced hypoglycemia. Because of their ability to block alpha-adrenergic receptors, *carvedilol* and *labetalol* can cause *postural hypoten-*

sion. Although *CNS effects* (insomnia, depression) can occur with all beta blockers, these effects may be more prominent with the highly lipid-soluble agents. Abrupt discontinuation of any beta blocker can produce *rebound cardiac excitation.* Accordingly, all beta blockers should be withdrawn slowly (by tapering the dosage over 1 to 2 weeks).

Intrinsic Sympathomimetic Activity (Partial Agonist Activity). The term *intrinsic sympathomimetic activity* (ISA) refers to the ability of certain beta blockers—especially *pindolol*—to act as *partial agonists* at beta-adrenergic receptors. (As discussed in Chapter 5, a partial agonist is a drug whose binding to a receptor produces a limited degree of receptor activation while preventing strong agonists from binding to the receptor to cause full activation.)

In contrast to other beta blockers, agents with ISA have very little effect on resting heart rate and cardiac output. When patients are at rest, stimulation of the heart by the sympathetic nervous system is low. If an ordinary beta blocker is given, it will block sympathetic stimulation, causing heart rate and cardiac output to decline. However, if a beta blocker has ISA, its own ability to cause limited receptor activation will compensate for blocking receptor activation by the sympathetic nervous system; consequently, resting heart rate and cardiac output are not reduced.

Because of their ability to provide a low level of cardiac stimulation, beta blockers with ISA are preferred to other beta blockers for use in patients with bradycardia. Conversely, these agents should not be given to patients with myocardial infarction, since their ability to cause even limited cardiac stimulation can be detrimental.

Dosage and Administration. With the exception of esmolol, all of the beta blockers discussed in this chapter can be administered *orally.* Three drugs—*atenolol, labetalol,* and *propranolol*—may be given *intravenously* as well. *Esmolol* is administered only by IV injection.

Maintenance dosages for hypertension are summarized in Table 18–2. For most beta blockers, dosing can be done just once a day. For the drugs with especially short half-lives, twice-a-day dosing is required (unless an extended-release formulation is available).

.ː. KEY POINTS

- Most beneficial responses to alpha blockers, including reduction of blood pressure in patients with hypertension, result from blockade of alpha₁ receptors on blood vessels.
- Alpha blockers reduce symptoms of BPH by blocking alpha₁ receptors in the bladder neck and prostatic capsule, which causes smooth muscle at those sites to relax.
- The major adverse effects of alpha blockers are *orthostatic hypotension* (caused by blocking alpha₁

receptors on veins); *reflex tachycardia* (caused by blocking alpha₁ receptors on arterioles); *nasal congestion* (caused by blocking alpha₁ receptors in blood vessels of the nasal mucosa); and *inhibition of ejaculation* (caused by blocking alpha₁ receptors in male sex organs).
- The first dose of an alpha blocker can cause fainting from profound orthostatic hypotension, the so-called first-dose effect.
- The alpha blockers used most frequently—prazosin, doxazosin, and terazosin—produce selective blockade of alpha₁ receptors.
- Beta blockers produce most of their beneficial effects by blocking beta₁ receptors in the heart, thereby reducing heart rate, force of contraction, and AV conduction.
- Principal indications for beta blockers are hypertension, angina pectoris, heart failure, and supraventricular tachydysrhythmias.
- Potential adverse effects from beta₁ blockade are bradycardia, reduced cardiac output, AV block, and precipitation of heart failure (even though some beta blockers are used to *treat* heart failure).
- Potential adverse effects from beta₂ blockade are bronchoconstriction (a concern for people with asthma) and reduced glycogenolysis (a concern for people with diabetes).
- In addition to adverse effects caused by blockade of receptors in the periphery, beta blockers can cause depression and insomnia from actions in the CNS.
- Beta blockers can be divided into two groups: (1) nonselective beta blockers (e.g., propranolol), which block beta₁ *and* beta₂ receptors; and (2) cardioselective beta blockers (e.g., metoprolol), which block beta₁ receptors only (at usual therapeutic doses).
- Beta blockers can be hazardous to patients with severe allergies because they can block beneficial actions of epinephrine, the drug of choice for treating anaphylactic shock.
- Beta blockers can be detrimental to diabetic patients because they suppress glycogenolysis (an important mechanism for correcting insulin-induced hypoglycemia), and they suppress tachycardia (an early warning signal that glucose levels are falling too low).
- Combining a beta blocker with a calcium channel blocker can produce excessive cardiosuppression.
- Cardioselective beta blockers are preferred to nonselective beta blockers for patients with asthma or diabetes.

Summary of Major Nursing Implications*

ALPHA₁-ADRENERGIC ANTAGONISTS

Doxazosin
Prazosin
Tamsulosin
Terazosin

Preadministration Assessment

Therapeutic Goal

Doxazosin, Prazosin, Terazosin. Reduction of blood pressure in patients with *essential hypertension*.
All Four Drugs. Reduction of symptoms in patients with *benign prostatic hyperplasia*.

Baseline Data

Essential Hypertension. Determine blood pressure.
Benign Prostatic Hyperplasia. Determine the degree of nocturia, daytime frequency, hesitance, intermittency, terminal dribbling (at the end of voiding), urgency, impairment of size and force of urinary stream, dysuria, and sensation of incomplete voiding.

Identifying High-Risk Patients

The only contraindication is hypersensitivity to these drugs.

Implementation: Administration

Route

Oral.

Administration

Instruct patients to take the initial dose at bedtime to minimize the "first-dose" effect. Except for *tamsulosin*, which is administered *after* eating, these drugs may be taken with food.

Ongoing Evaluation and Interventions

Evaluating Therapeutic Effects

Essential Hypertension. Evaluate by monitoring blood pressure.
Benign Prostatic Hyperplasia. Evaluate for improvement in the symptoms listed above under *Baseline Data*.

Minimizing Adverse Effects

Orthostatic Hypotension. Alpha₁ blockade can cause postural hypotension. Inform patients about the symptoms of hypotension (dizziness, lightheadedness) and advise them to sit or lie down if these occur. Advise patients to move slowly when changing from a supine or sitting position to an upright posture.
First-Dose Effect. The first dose may cause fainting from severe orthostatic hypotension. Forewarn patients about this effect and advise them to avoid driving and other hazardous activities for 12 to 24 hours after the initial dose. To minimize risk, advise patients to take the first dose at bedtime.

*Patient education information is highlighted as blue text.

BETA-ADRENERGIC ANTAGONISTS

Acebutolol
Atenolol
Betaxolol
Bisoprolol
Carteolol
Carvedilol
Labetalol
Metoprolol
Nadolol
Penbutolol
Pindolol
Propranolol
Timolol

Except where noted, the implications summarized here apply to all beta-adrenergic blocking agents.

Preadministration Assessment

Therapeutic Goal

Principal indications are *hypertension, angina pectoris, heart failure,* and *cardiac dysrhythmias.* Indications for individual agents are summarized in Table 18–3.

Baseline Data

Hypertension. Determine standing and supine blood pressure.
Angina Pectoris. Determine the incidence, severity, and circumstances of anginal attacks.
Cardiac Dysrhythmias. Obtain a baseline electrocardiogram (EKG).

Identifying High-Risk Patients

All beta blockers are *contraindicated* for patients with sinus bradycardia or AV heart block (greater than first degree), and must be used with *great caution* in patients with heart failure. Use with *caution* (especially the nonselective agents) in patients with asthma, bronchospasm, diabetes, or a history of severe allergic reactions. Use all beta blockers with *caution* in patients with a history of depression and in those taking calcium channel blockers.

Implementation: Administration

Routes

Oral. All beta blockers.
Intravenous. Atenolol, labetalol, metoprolol, and propranolol.

Administration

For maintenance therapy of hypertension, administer once or twice daily (see Table 18–2).
Warn patients against abrupt discontinuation of treatment.

Summary of Major Nursing Implications*—cont'd

Ongoing Evaluation and Interventions

Evaluating Therapeutic Effects

Hypertension. Monitor blood pressure and heart rate prior to each dose. **Advise outpatients to monitor blood pressure and heart rate daily.**

Angina Pectoris. **Advise patients to record the incidence, circumstances, and severity of anginal attacks.**

Cardiac Dysrhythmias. Monitor for improvement in the EKG.

Minimizing Adverse Effects

Bradycardia. Beta$_1$ blockade can reduce heart rate. If bradycardia is severe, withhold medication and notify the physician. If necessary, administer atropine and isoproterenol to restore heart rate.

AV Heart Block. Beta$_1$ blockade can decrease AV conduction. Do not give beta blockers to patients with AV block greater than first degree.

Heart Failure. Suppression of myocardial contractility can cause heart failure. **Inform patients about early signs of heart failure (shortness of breath, night coughs, swelling of the extremities), and instruct them to notify the physician if these occur.**

Rebound Cardiac Excitation. Abrupt withdrawal of beta blockers can cause tachycardia and ventricular dysrhythmias. **Warn patients against abrupt discontinuation of drug use. Advise patients to carry an adequate supply of medication when traveling.**

Postural Hypotension. By blocking alpha-adrenergic receptors, *carvedilol* and *labetalol* can cause postural hypotension. **Inform patients about signs of hypotension (lightheadedness, dizziness) and advise them to sit or lie**

down **if these develop. Advise patients to move slowly when changing from a supine or sitting position to an upright posture.**

Bronchoconstriction. Beta$_2$ blockade can cause substantial airway constriction in patients with asthma. The risk of bronchoconstriction is much lower with the cardioselective agents than with the nonselective agents.

Effects in Diabetic Patients. Beta$_1$ blockade can "mask" tachycardia, an early sign of hypoglycemia. **Warn patients that tachycardia cannot be relied on as an indicator of impending hypoglycemia, and teach them to recognize other indicators (sweating, hunger, fatigue, poor concentration) that blood glucose is falling dangerously low.** Beta$_2$ blockade can prevent glycogenolysis, an emergency means of increasing blood glucose. Patients may need to reduce their insulin dosage. Cardioselective beta blockers are preferred to nonselective agents in patients with diabetes.

CNS Effects. Beta blockers can cause depression, insomnia, and nightmares. If these occur, it may be helpful to switch to a beta blocker with low lipid solubility (see Table 18–2).

Minimizing Adverse Interactions

Calcium Channel Blockers. Two calcium channel blockers—verapamil and diltiazem—can intensify the cardiosuppressant effects of the beta blockers. Use the combination with caution.

Insulin. Beta blockers can prevent the compensatory glycogenolysis that normally occurs in response to insulin-induced hypoglycemia. Diabetic patients may need to reduce their insulin dosage.

*Patient education information is highlighted as blue text.

Indirect-Acting Antiadrenergic Agents

ADRENERGIC NEURON-BLOCKING AGENTS
  Reserpine
  Guanethidine
  Guanadrel
CENTRALLY ACTING ALPHA$_2$ AGONISTS
  Clonidine
  Guanabenz and Guanfacine
  Methyldopa and Methyldopate

The indirect-acting antiadrenergic agents are drugs that prevent stimulation of peripheral adrenergic receptors, but they do so by mechanisms that do not involve direct interaction with peripheral receptors. There are two categories of indirect-acting antiadrenergic drugs. The first group—*adrenergic neuron-blocking agents*—consists of drugs that act within the terminals of sympathetic neurons to decrease norepinephrine release. The second group—*centrally acting alpha$_2$ agonists*—consists of drugs that act within the central nervous system (CNS) to reduce the outflow of impulses along sympathetic neurons. With both groups, the net result is reduced stimulation of peripheral adrenergic receptors. Hence, the pharmacologic effects of the indirect-acting adrenergic blocking agents are similar to those of drugs that block adrenergic receptors directly.

ADRENERGIC NEURON-BLOCKING AGENTS

The adrenergic neuron-blocking agents are drugs that act presynaptically to reduce the release of norepinephrine (NE) from sympathetic neurons. (These drugs have very little effect on the release of epinephrine from the adrenal medulla.) Our discussion of the adrenergic neuron blockers focuses on two agents: reserpine and guanethidine.

Reserpine

Reserpine is a naturally occurring compound prepared from the root of *Rauwolfia serpentina,* a shrub indigenous to India. Because of its source, reserpine is classified as a *Rauwolfia alkaloid.* The primary indication for reserpine is hypertension. The side effect of greatest concern is severe depression.

Mechanism of Action

Reserpine causes *depletion of NE from postganglionic sympathetic neurons.* By doing so, the drug can decrease stimulation of practically all adrenergic receptors. Hence, the effects

of reserpine closely resemble those produced by a combination of alpha- and beta-adrenergic blockade.

Reserpine depletes NE in two ways. First, the drug acts on vesicles within the nerve terminal to cause displacement of stored NE, thereby exposing the transmitter to destruction by monoamine oxidase. Second, reserpine suppresses NE synthesis. As depicted in Figure 19–1, reserpine decreases NE synthesis by blocking the uptake of dopamine (the immediate precursor of NE) into presynaptic vesicles, which contain the enzymes needed to convert dopamine into NE. A week or two may be required for maximal transmitter depletion to develop.

In addition to its peripheral effects, reserpine can cause depletion of transmitters (serotonin, catecholamines) from neurons in the CNS. Depletion of these CNS transmitters underlies the most serious side effect of reserpine—deep emotional depression—and also explains the occasional use of reserpine in psychiatry.

Pharmacologic Effects

Peripheral Effects. By depleting sympathetic neurons of NE, reserpine decreases the activation of alpha- and beta-adrenergic receptors. Decreased activation of beta receptors slows heart rate and reduces cardiac output. Decreased alpha activation promotes vasodilation. All three effects cause a *decrease in blood pressure.*

Effects on the CNS. Reserpine produces sedation and a state of indifference to the environment. In addition, the drug can cause severe depression. These effects are thought to result from depletion of certain neurotransmitters (catecholamines, serotonin) from neurons in the brain.

Therapeutic Uses

Hypertension. The principal indication for reserpine is hypertension. Antihypertensive effects result from vasodilation and reduced cardiac output. Since these effects occur secondary to depletion of NE, and since transmitter depletion occurs slowly, full antihypertensive responses can take a week or more to develop. Conversely, when reserpine is discontinued, effects may persist for several weeks as the NE content of sympathetic neurons becomes replenished. Because its side effects can be severe, and because more desirable drugs are available (see Chapter 45), reserpine is not a preferred drug for hypertension.

Psychotic States. Reserpine can be used to treat agitated psychotic patients, such as those suffering from certain forms of schizophrenia. However, since superior drugs are available (e.g., phenothiazine antipsychotics), reserpine is rarely employed in psychotherapy.

Adverse Effects

Depression. Reserpine can produce severe depression that may persist for months after the drug is withdrawn. Suicide has occurred. All patients should be informed about the

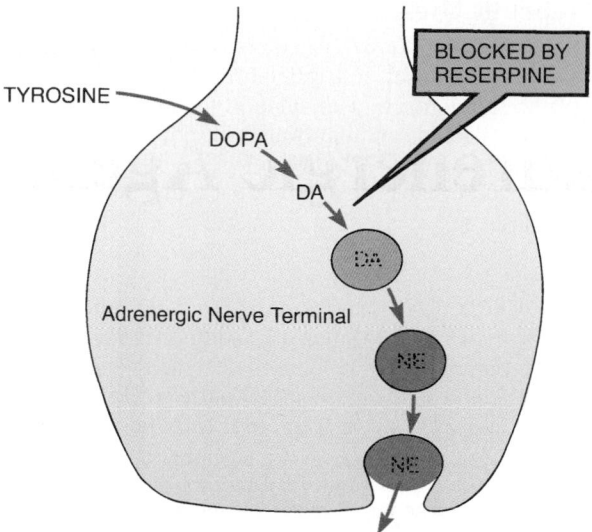

Figure 19–1 ■ Mechanism of reserpine action.
Reserpine depletes neurons of norepinephrine (NE) by two mechanisms. (1) As indicated in this figure, reserpine blocks the uptake of dopamine (DA) into vesicles, thereby preventing NE synthesis. (2) Reserpine displaces NE from vesicles, thereby allowing degradation of NE by monoamine oxidase present in the nerve terminal (not shown).

risk of depression. Also, they should be educated about signs of depression (e.g., early morning insomnia, loss of appetite, change in mood) and instructed to notify the physician immediately if these develop. Because of the risk of suicide, patients who develop depression may require hospitalization. *Reserpine is contraindicated for patients with a history of depressive disorders.* The risk of depression can be minimized by keeping the dosage low (0.25 mg/day or less).

Cardiovascular Effects. Depletion of NE from sympathetic neurons can result in *bradycardia, orthostatic hypotension,* and *nasal congestion.* Bradycardia is caused by decreased activation of beta₁ receptors in the heart. Hypotension and nasal congestion result from decreased activation of alpha receptors on blood vessels. Patients should be informed that orthostatic hypotension, the most serious cardiovascular effect, can be minimized by moving slowly when changing from a seated or supine posture to an upright posture. In addition, patients should be advised to sit or lie down if lightheadedness or dizziness occurs.

GI Effects. By mechanisms that are not understood, reserpine can stimulate several aspects of GI function. The drug can increase secretion of gastric acid, which may result in ulcer formation. In addition, reserpine can increase the tone and motility of intestinal smooth muscle, thereby causing cramps and diarrhea.

Preparations, Dosage, and Administration

Reserpine is available in tablets (0.1 and 0.25 mg) for oral use. The drug may be administered with food if GI upset occurs. The usual initial dosage for hypertension in adults is 0.5 mg/day for 1 to 2 weeks. The usual maintenance dosage is 0.1 to 0.25 mg/day.

Guanethidine

Guanethidine [Ismelin] is an adrenergic neuron-blocking agent with hypotensive actions similar to those of reserpine. However, in contrast to reserpine, guanethidine cannot cross the blood-brain barrier, and hence does cause

adverse CNS effects. The most prominent adverse effects are diarrhea and profound orthostatic hypotension. Because of these effects, guanethidine is rarely used.

Mechanism of Action

Primary Action: Inhibition of NE Release. Guanethidine acts presynaptically to inhibit release of NE from sympathetic neurons. In order to inhibit NE release, guanethidine must first be taken up into nerve terminals. Uptake takes place via the same transport system employed for reuptake of NE. Once inside the sympathetic nerve terminal, guanethidine prevents NE release. The precise mechanism by which the drug inhibits release is unknown.

Secondary Actions. In addition to blocking NE release, guanethidine has two other actions. First, during *initial* use, guanethidine can *promote NE release.* As a result, the early phase of therapy may be associated with transient *sympathomimetic effects,* rather than sympathetic blockade. Second, with chronic use, guanethidine, like reserpine, *depletes NE from sympathetic nerves.*

Pharmacologic Effects

The pharmacologic effects of guanethidine, like those of reserpine, result from decreased activation of alpha- and beta-adrenergic receptors. The most pronounced cardiovascular effects are *bradycardia, decreased cardiac output,* and *a great reduction in venous smooth muscle tone.* As a result, systolic blood pressure falls, especially when the patient is standing.

Therapeutic Use

The only indication for guanethidine is *hypertension.* Because of its tendency to cause diarrhea and severe orthostatic hypotension, guanethidine is not used routinely. Rather, the drug is reserved for patients whose blood pressure cannot be controlled with more desirable drugs.

Adverse Effects

Diarrhea. Like reserpine, guanethidine stimulates the GI system; diarrhea is the most common result. Usually, diarrhea can be managed with drugs (e.g., diphenoxylate, loperamide, anticholinergic agents). The mechanism underlying diarrhea is in dispute.

Orthostatic Hypotension. Guanethidine-induced orthostatic hypotension can be severe. Blood pressure may fall so low that perfusion of the heart and brain is seriously compromised. Supine and standing blood pressure should be monitored. If standing blood pressure drops too low, guanethidine should be withheld and the physician notified. Patients should be warned about orthostatic hypotension and informed that it can be minimized by moving slowly when changing from a supine or seated position to an upright position. Also, patients should be informed that factors that promote vasodilation (e.g., alcohol consumption, warm environments, strenuous exercise) can intensify orthostatic hypotension and hence should be avoided.

Hypertension. Although guanethidine is used to *treat* hypertension, the drug can *cause* hypertension in patients with a pheochromocytoma (a catecholamine-secreting tumor). Recall that guanethidine stimulates NE release during the initial phase of treatment. Since pheochromocytomas contain massive amounts of NE, guanethidine-induced NE release can result in a dramatic rise in blood pressure.

Drug Interactions

Tricyclic antidepressants and other drugs that block the uptake of NE into adrenergic neurons will also block the uptake of guanethidine, thereby keeping the drug from its site action. Hence, reuptake blockers will reduce guanethidine's effects.

Preparations, Dosage, and Administration

Guanethidine monosulfate [Ismelin] is available in 10- and 25-mg tablets for oral use. The initial dosage for hypertension in adults is 10 mg once a day. The dosage can be increased every 5 to 7 days to a maintenance level of 25 to 50 mg once daily. Dosage should be reduced in patients who develop orthostatic hypotension or severe diarrhea.

Guanadrel

Guanadrel [Hylorel] is a close relative of guanethidine. Both drugs share the same mechanism of action, therapeutic use, drug interactions, and adverse effects (although diarrhea is less troubling with guanadrel). Guanadrel has a shorter half-life than guanethidine, and hence must be administered twice daily rather than once daily. The usual initial dosage for adults is 10 mg/day. Maintenance dosages range from 20 to 75 mg/day.

CENTRALLY ACTING ALPHA₂ AGONISTS

The drugs discussed in this section act within the CNS to reduce the firing of sympathetic neurons. These drugs are used primarily for hypertension.

Why are we discussing centrally acting drugs in a unit on peripheral nervous system pharmacology? Because the effects of these drugs are ultimately the result of decreased activation of alpha- and beta-adrenergic receptors in the periphery. That is, by inhibiting the firing of sympathetic neurons, the centrally acting agents decrease the release of NE from sympathetic nerves, and thereby decrease activation of peripheral adrenergic receptors. Hence, although these drugs act within the CNS, their effects are like those of the direct-acting adrenergic receptor blockers. Accordingly, it seems appropriate to discuss these agents in the context of peripheral nervous system pharmacology—rather than presenting them in the context of CNS drugs.

Clonidine

Clonidine [Catapres] is an *antihypertensive drug* that acts within the CNS. Except for rare instances of rebound hypertension, the drug is generally free of serious adverse effects. Because it is both effective and safe, clonidine is widely used. To treat hypertension, the drug is administered by mouth or by transdermal patch.

In addition to its use in hypertension, clonidine is used to relieve *severe pain of cancer.* To provide pain relief, the drug must be administered by epidural infusion. The preparation employed for this purpose is marketed under the trade name *Duraclon.* Because clonidine's analgesic pharmacology differs substantially from its antihypertensive pharmacology, the analgesic pharmacology is discussed separately in Chapter 28.

Mechanism of Antihypertensive Action

Clonidine is an alpha₂-adrenergic agonist that causes "selective" stimulation of alpha₂ receptors in the CNS—specifically, in brainstem areas associated with autonomic regulation of the cardiovascular system. By stimulating central alpha₂ receptors, clonidine reduces sympathetic outflow to blood vessels and the heart.

Pharmacologic Effects

The most significant effects of clonidine occur in the heart and vascular system. By suppressing the firing of sympathetic nerves to the heart, clonidine can cause *bradycardia* and *a decrease in cardiac output.* By suppressing sympathetic regulation of blood vessels, the drug promotes *vasodilation.* The net result of cardiac suppression and vasodilation is *decreased blood pressure.* Blood pressure is reduced in both supine and standing subjects. (Note that the effect of clonidine on blood pressure is unlike that of the peripheral alpha-adrenergic blockers, which tend to decrease blood pressure only when the patient is standing.) Since the hypotensive effects of clonidine are not posture dependent, orthostatic hypotension with this drug is minimal.

Pharmacokinetics

Clonidine is very lipid soluble. As a result, the drug is readily absorbed following oral administration and is widely distributed throughout the body, including the CNS. Hypotensive responses begin 30 to 60 minutes after administration and peak in 4 hours. Effects of a single dose may persist for as long as 1 day. Clonidine is eliminated by a combination of hepatic metabolism and renal excretion.

Therapeutic Uses

Clonidine has two *approved* applications: treatment of hypertension (its main use) and relief of severe pain (see Chapter 28). *Investigational* uses include treatment of migraine; menopausal flushing; withdrawal from opioids, alcohol, and tobacco; and Tourette's syndrome (a CNS disease characterized by uncontrollable tics and verbal outbursts that are frequently obscene).

Adverse Effects

Drowsiness. CNS depression is common. About 35% of patients experience drowsiness; an additional 8% experience outright sedation. These responses become less intense with continued drug use. Patients in their early weeks of treatment should be advised to avoid hazardous activities if alertness is impaired.

Xerostomia. Xerostomia (dry mouth) is common, occurring in about 40% of patients. The reaction usually diminishes over the first 2 to 4 weeks of therapy. Although not dangerous, xerostomia can be annoying enough to discourage drug use. Patients should be advised that discomfort can be reduced by chewing gum, sucking on hard candy, and taking frequent sips of fluids.

Rebound Hypertension. Rebound hypertension is characterized by a large increase in blood pressure occurring in response to abrupt clonidine withdrawal. This rare but serious reaction is caused by overactivity of the sympathetic nervous system, and can be accompanied by nervousness, tachycardia, and sweating. Left untreated, the reaction may persist for a week or more. If blood pressure climbs dangerously high, it should be lowered with a combination of alpha- and beta-adrenergic blocking agents. Rebound effects can be avoided by withdrawing clonidine slowly (over 2 to 4 days). Patients should be informed about rebound hypertension and warned not to discontinue clonidine without consulting the physician.

Use in Pregnancy. Clonidine is embryotoxic in animals. Because of the possibility of fetal harm, clonidine is not recommended for use by pregnant women. Pregnancy should be ruled out before clonidine is given.

Other Adverse Effects. Clonidine can cause a variety of adverse effects, including *constipation, impotence, gynecomastia,* and *adverse CNS effects* (e.g., vivid dreams, nightmares, anxiety, depression). *Localized skin reactions* are common with transdermal clonidine patches.

Preparations, Dosage, and Administration

Preparations. Clonidine hydrochloride is available in oral and transdermal formulations. Oral clonidine [Catapres] is available in 0.1-, 0.2-, and 0.3-mg tablets. Transdermal clonidine [Catapres-TTS] is available in 2.5-, 5-, or 7.5-mg patches that deliver 0.1, 0.2, and 0.3 mg/24 hours respectively.

Dosage and Administration. Oral. For treatment of hypertension, the initial adult dosage is 0.1 mg twice a day. The usual maintenance dosage is 0.2 to 0.6 mg/day administered in divided doses. By taking the majority of the daily dose at bedtime, daytime sedation can be minimized.

Transdermal. Transdermal patches are applied to a region of hairless, intact skin on the upper arm or torso. A new patch is applied every 7 days.

Guanabenz and Guanfacine

The pharmacology of guanabenz [Wytensin] and guanfacine [Tenex] is very similar to that of clonidine. Like clonidine, both drugs stimulate brainstem alpha₂-adrenergic receptors, and thereby reduce sympathetic outflow to the heart and blood vessels. The result is a reduction in cardiac output and blood pressure. Both drugs also share the major adverse effects of clonidine: sedation and dry mouth. In addition, both can cause rebound hypertension following abrupt withdrawal. Guanabenz is available in 4- and 8-mg tablets.

Dosing is begun at 4 mg twice daily and can be increased to 32 mg twice daily. Guanfacine is available in 1- and 2-mg tablets. The usual dosage is 1 mg/day, taken at bedtime to minimize daytime sedation.

Methyldopa and Methyldopate

Methyldopa [Aldomet] is an oral antihypertensive agent that lowers blood pressure by acting at sites within the CNS. Two side effects—hemolytic anemia and hepatic necrosis—can be severe. Methyldopate [Aldomet], an intravenous agent, is nearly identical to methyldopa in structure and pharmacologic effects.

Mechanism of Action

Methyldopa has a mechanism of action similar to that of clonidine. Like clonidine, methyldopa inhibits sympathetic outflow from the CNS by causing alpha$_2$ stimulation in the brain. However, methyldopa differs from clonidine in that methyldopa itself is not an alpha$_2$ agonist. Hence, before it can act, methyldopa must first be taken up into brainstem neurons, where it is then converted to methylnorepinephrine, a compound that is an effective alpha$_2$ agonist. Release of methylnorepinephrine results in alpha$_2$ stimulation.

Pharmacologic Effects

The most prominent response to methyldopa is a drop in blood pressure. The drug reduces blood pressure primarily by causing vasodilation—and not by suppressing the heart. Vasodilation occurs because of reduced sympathetic traffic to blood vessels. At usual therapeutic doses, methyldopa does not decrease heart rate or cardiac output. Hence, hypotensive actions cannot be ascribed to cardiac depression. The hemodynamic effects of methyldopa are very much like those of clonidine: Both drugs lower blood pressure in supine and standing subjects, and both produce relatively little orthostatic hypotension.

Therapeutic Use

The only indication for methyldopa is *hypertension*. Methyldopa was one of the earliest antihypertensive agents available and remains in wide use.

Adverse Effects

Positive Coombs' Test and Hemolytic Anemia. A positive Coombs' test* develops in 10% to 20% of patients who take methyldopa chronically. The test usually turns positive between the 6th and 12th month of treatment. Of the patients who have a positive Coombs' test, only a few (about 5%) develop hemolytic anemia. Coombs-positive patients who do not develop hemolytic anemia may continue methyldopa treatment. However, if hemolytic anemia does develop, methyldopa should be withdrawn immediately. For most patients, hemolytic anemia resolves shortly after drug withdrawal—

---

*The Coombs' test detects the presence of antibodies directed against the patient's own red blood cells. These antibodies can cause hemolysis (i.e., red blood cell lysis).

although the Coombs' test may remain positive for months. A Coombs' test should be performed prior to treatment and 6 to 12 months later. Blood counts (hematocrit, hemoglobin, or red cell count) should be obtained prior to treatment and periodically thereafter.

Hepatotoxicity. Methyldopa has been associated with hepatitis, jaundice, and, rarely, fatal hepatic necrosis. All patients should undergo periodic assessment of liver function. If signs of hepatotoxicity appear, methyldopa should be discontinued immediately. Liver function usually normalizes after drug withdrawal.

Other Adverse Effects. Methyldopa can cause *xerostomia, sexual dysfunction, orthostatic hypotension,* and a variety of *CNS effects,* including drowsiness, reduced mental acuity, nightmares, and depression. These responses are not usually dangerous, but they can detract from compliance.

Preparations, Dosage, and Administration

Preparations. *Methyldopa* [Aldomet] is available in tablets (125, 250, and 500 mg) and in a suspension (50 mg/ml) for oral use. *Methyldopate* [Aldomet] is available as an injection (50 mg/ml in 5- and 10-ml vials) for IV use.

Oral Therapy. For treatment of hypertension, the initial adult dosage is 250 mg 2 to 3 times a day. Daily maintenance dosages usually range from 0.5 to 2 gm administered in two to four divided doses.

Intravenous Therapy. Methyldopate, administered by slow IV infusion, is indicated for hypertensive emergencies. However, since faster-acting drugs are available, use of methyldopate is rare. Methyldopate for infusion should be diluted in 5% dextrose to a concentration of 10 mg/ml. The usual adult dose is 250 to 500 mg infused over 30 to 60 minutes. Dosing may be repeated every 6 hours as required.

⋰ KEY POINTS

- All of the drugs discussed in this chapter reduce stimulation of peripheral alpha- and beta-adrenergic receptors, but they do so by mechanisms other than direct receptor blockade.
- The principal indication for these drugs is hypertension.
- Reserpine acts by depleting NE from adrenergic neurons.
- Guanethidine is taken up by adrenergic neurons, where it blocks NE release and, eventually, depletes NE from storage vesicles.
- Clonidine and methyldopa reduce sympathetic outflow to the heart and blood vessels by causing stimulation of alpha$_2$-adrenergic receptors in the brainstem.
- The principal adverse effect of reserpine is depression.
- The principal adverse effects of guanethidine are orthostatic hypotension and diarrhea.
- The principal adverse effects of clonidine are drowsiness and dry mouth. Rebound hypertension can occur if the drug is abruptly withdrawn.
- The principal adverse effects of methyldopa are hemolytic anemia and liver damage.

Summary of Major Nursing Implications*

RESERPINE

Preadministration Assessment

Therapeutic Goal

Reduction of blood pressure in hypertensive patients.

Baseline Data

Determine blood pressure.

Identifying High-Risk Patients

Reserpine is *contraindicated* for patients with active peptic ulcer disease or a history of depression.

Implementation: Administration

Route

Oral.

Administration

Administer with food to reduce gastric upset.

Ongoing Evaluation and Interventions

Evaluating Therapeutic Effects

Full antihypertensive effects may take a week or more to develop. Monitor blood pressure to evaluate treatment.

Minimizing Adverse Effects

Depression. Reserpine can cause profound depression. **Inform patients about signs of depression (e.g., early morning insomnia, loss of appetite, change in mood) and instruct them to notify the physician if these develop.** Hospitalization may be required. Avoid reserpine in patients with a history of depression. To minimize the risk of depression, keep the dosage low (0.25 mg/day or less).

Orthostatic Hypotension. **Inform patients that orthostatic hypotension can be minimized by moving slowly when changing from a seated or supine position to an upright position. Advise patients to sit or lie down if dizziness or lightheadedness occurs.**

GUANETHIDINE

Preadministration Assessment

Therapeutic Goal

Reduction of blood pressure in hypertensive patients.

Baseline Data

Determine blood pressure in supine and standing positions, and, if possible, immediately after exercise.

Identifying High-Risk Patients

Guanethidine is *contraindicated* for patients with pheochromocytoma.

Implementation: Administration

Route

Oral.

Administration

For ambulatory patients, the entire daily dose is usually taken at one time.

Ongoing Evaluation and Interventions

Evaluating Therapeutic Effects

Monitor supine and standing blood pressure. Dosage is adjusted on the basis of the response.

Minimizing Adverse Effects

Orthostatic Hypotension. Orthostatic hypotension can be severe. Monitor supine and standing blood pressure. If standing blood pressure falls too low, withhold medication and notify the physician. **Educate patients about the signs of hypotension (dizziness, lightheadedness) and advise them to sit or lie down if these occur. Advise patients to move slowly when changing from a supine or sitting position to an upright position. Warn patients to avoid factors that can promote hypotension (e.g., alcohol, warm environments, strenuous exercise).**

Diarrhea. Diarrhea is common. If necessary, manage with antidiarrheal drugs.

Hypertension. Guanethidine can cause severe hypertension in patients with pheochromocytoma. The drug is contraindicated for these patients.

Minimizing Adverse Interactions

Tricyclic antidepressants and other drugs that block the NE uptake pump can decrease the effects of guanethidine, and hence should be avoided.

CLONIDINE

Preadministration Assessment

Therapeutic Goal

Reduction of blood pressure in hypertensive patients.

Baseline Data

Determine blood pressure.

Identifying High-Risk Patients

Clonidine is embryotoxic to animals and should not be used during pregnancy. Rule out pregnancy before initiating treatment.

Implementation: Administration

Routes

Oral, transdermal.

Administration

Oral. **Advise the patient to take the major portion of the daily dose at bedtime to minimize daytime sedation.**

Transdermal. **Instruct the patient to apply transdermal patches to hairless, intact skin on the upper arm or torso. A new patch is applied every 7 days.**

*Patient education information is highlighted as blue text.

Summary of Major Nursing Implications*—cont'd

Ongoing Evaluation and Interventions

Evaluating Therapeutic Effects

Monitor blood pressure.

Minimizing Adverse Effects

Drowsiness and Sedation. Inform patients about possible CNS depression and warn them to avoid hazardous activities if alertness is impaired.

Xerostomia. Dry mouth is common. Inform patients that discomfort can be reduced by chewing gum, sucking on hard candy, and taking frequent sips of fluids.

Rebound Hypertension. Severe hypertension occurs rarely following abrupt clonidine withdrawal. Treat with a combination of alpha- and beta-adrenergic blockers. To avoid rebound hypertension, withdraw clonidine slowly (over 2 to 4 days). **Inform patients about rebound hypertension and warn them against abrupt discontinuation of treatment.**

METHYLDOPA

Preadministration Assessment

Therapeutic Goal

Reduction of blood pressure in hypertensive patients.

Baseline Data

Obtain baseline values for blood pressure, blood counts (hematocrit, hemoglobin, or red cell count), Coombs' test, and liver function tests.

*Patient education information is highlighted as blue text.

Identifying High-Risk Patients

Methyldopa is *contraindicated* for patients with active liver disease or a history of methyldopa-induced liver dysfunction.

Implementation: Administration

Routes

Oral. For routine management of hypertension.
Intravenous. For hypertensive emergencies.

Administration

Most patients on oral therapy require divided (two to four) daily doses. For some patients, blood pressure can be controlled with a single daily dose at bedtime.

Ongoing Evaluation and Interventions

Evaluating Therapeutic Effects

Monitor blood pressure.

Minimizing Adverse Effects

Hemolytic Anemia. If hemolysis occurs, withdraw methyldopa immediately; hemolytic anemia usually resolves soon. Obtain a Coombs' test prior to treatment and 6 to 12 months later. Obtain blood counts (hematocrit, hemoglobin, or red cell count) prior to treatment and periodically thereafter.

Hepatotoxicity. Methyldopa can cause hepatitis, jaundice, and fatal hepatic necrosis. Assess liver function prior to treatment and periodically thereafter. If liver dysfunction develops, discontinue methyldopa immediately. In most cases, liver function returns to normal soon.

Introduction to Central Nervous System Pharmacology

TABLE 20–1 ▪ Neurotransmitters of the CNS

Monoamines	Peptides
Norepinephrine	Dynorphins
Epinephrine	Endorphins
Dopamine	Enkephalins
Serotonin	Neurotensin
Amino Acids	Somatostatin
Aspartate	Substance P
Glutamate	Oxytocin
GABA	Vasopressin
Glycine	Others
	Acetylcholine
	Histamine

GABA = gamma-aminobutyric acid.

The central nervous system (CNS) drugs—agents that act on the brain and spinal cord—are used widely for medical and nonmedical purposes. Medical applications include treatment of psychiatric disorders, suppression of seizures, relief of pain, and production of anesthesia. CNS drugs are used nonmedically for their stimulant, depressant, euphoriant, and other "mind-altering" abilities.

Despite the widespread use of CNS drugs, knowledge of these agents is limited. Much of our ignorance stems from the anatomic and neurochemical complexity of the brain and spinal cord. (There are more than 50 billion neurons in the cerebral hemispheres alone.) Because of this complexity, we are a long way from fully understanding both the CNS itself and the drugs used to influence its function.

TRANSMITTERS OF THE CNS

In contrast to the peripheral nervous system, in which only three compounds—acetylcholine, norepinephrine, and epinephrine—serve as neurotransmitters, the CNS contains more than a dozen compounds that appear to serve as neurotransmitters (Table 20–1). Furthermore, since there are numerous sites within the CNS for which no transmitter has been identified, it is clear that additional compounds, yet to be discovered, also mediate neurotransmission in the brain and spinal cord.

It is important to note that none of the compounds that are thought to be CNS neurotransmitters has actually been proved to serve this function. The reason for uncertainty lies with the technical difficulties involved in CNS research. However, although absolute proof may be lacking, the evidence supporting a neurotransmitter role for several compounds (e.g., dopamine, norepinephrine, serotonin, enkephalins) is completely convincing.

Although much is known about the actions of CNS transmitters at various sites in the brain and spinal cord, it is not usually possible to relate these known actions in a precise way to behavioral or psychologic processes. For example, although we know the locations of specific CNS sites at which norepinephrine appears to act as a transmitter, and although we know the effect of norepinephrine at most of these sites (suppression of neuronal excitability), we do not know the precise relationship between suppression of neuronal excitability at each of these sites and the impact of that suppression on the overt function of the organism. This example illustrates the general state of our knowledge of CNS transmitter function: We have a great deal of detailed information about the biochemistry and electrophysiology of CNS transmitters, but we are as yet unable to assemble those details into a completely meaningful picture.

THE BLOOD-BRAIN BARRIER

As discussed in Chapter 4, the blood-brain barrier impedes the entry of drugs into the brain. Passage across the barrier is limited to lipid-soluble agents and to drugs that are able to cross by way of specific transport systems. Drugs that are protein bound and drugs that are highly ionized cannot cross.

From a therapeutic perspective, the blood-brain barrier is a mixed blessing. On the positive side, the barrier protects the brain from injury by potentially toxic substances. On the negative side, the barrier can be a significant obstacle to entry of therapeutic agents.

The blood-brain barrier is not fully developed at birth. Accordingly, infants are much more sensitive to CNS drugs than are older children and adults.

HOW DO CNS DRUGS PRODUCE THERAPEUTIC EFFECTS?

Although much is known about the biochemical and electrophysiologic effects of CNS drugs, in most cases we cannot state with certainty the relationship between these effects and production of beneficial responses. Why? In order to fully understand how a drug alters symptoms, we need to understand, at a biochemical and physiologic level, the pathophysiology of the disorder being treated. In the case of most CNS disorders, our knowledge is limited. That is, we do not fully understand the brain in either health or disease. Given our incomplete understanding of the CNS itself, we must exercise caution when attempting to assign a precise mechanism for a drug's therapeutic effects.

Although we can't state with certainty how CNS drugs act, we do have sufficient data to permit formulation of plausible hypotheses. Consequently, as we study CNS drugs in the chapters that follow, proposed mechanisms of action are presented. Keep in mind, however, that these mechanisms are tentative, representing our best guesses based on data available today. As we learn more, it is almost certain that these concepts will be modified, if not discarded entirely.

ADAPTATION OF THE CNS TO PROLONGED DRUG EXPOSURE

When CNS drugs are taken chronically, their effects may differ from those produced during initial use. These altered effects are the result of adaptive changes that occur in the brain in response to prolonged drug exposure. The brain's ability to adapt to drugs can produce alterations in therapeutic effects and side effects. Adaptive changes are often beneficial, although they can also be detrimental.

Increased Therapeutic Effects. Certain drugs used in psychiatry—antipsychotics and antidepressants—must be taken for several weeks before full therapeutic effects develop. It would appear that beneficial responses are delayed because they result from adaptive changes—and not from the direct effects of drugs on synaptic function. Hence, full therapeutic effects are not seen until the CNS has had time to modify itself in response to prolonged drug exposure.

Decreased Side Effects. When CNS drugs are taken chronically, the intensity of side effects may decrease (while therapeutic effects remain undiminished). For example, phenobarbital (an anticonvulsant) produces sedation during the initial phase of therapy; however, with continued treatment, sedation declines while full protection from seizures is retained. Similarly, when morphine is given to control pain, nausea is a common side effect early on; however, as treatment continues, nausea diminishes while analgesic effects persist. Adaptations within the brain are believed to underlie these phenomena.

Tolerance and Physical Dependence. Tolerance and physical dependence are special manifestations of CNS adaptation. (*Tolerance* is defined as a decreased response occurring in the course of prolonged drug use. *Physical dependence* is defined as a state in which abrupt discontinuation of drug use will precipitate a withdrawal syndrome.) Research indicates that the kinds of adaptive changes that underlie tolerance and dependence are such that, once they have taken place, continued drug use is required for the brain to function "normally." If drug use is stopped, the drug-adapted brain can no longer function properly and a withdrawal syndrome ensues. The withdrawal reaction continues until the adaptive changes have had time to revert, thereby restoring the CNS to its pretreatment state.

DEVELOPMENT OF NEW PSYCHOTHERAPEUTIC DRUGS

Because of deficiencies in our knowledge of the neurochemical and physiologic changes that underlie mental disease, it is impossible to take a rational approach to the development of truly new (nonderivative) psychotherapeutic agents. History bears this out: Virtually all of the major advances in psychopharmacology have been happy accidents.

In addition to our relative ignorance about the neurochemical and physiologic correlates of mental illness, two other factors contribute to the difficulty in generating truly new psychotherapeutic agents. (1) In contrast to many other diseases, we lack adequate animal models of mental illness. Accordingly, animal research is not likely to reveal new types of psychotherapeutic agents. (2) Mentally healthy individuals cannot be used as subjects to assess potential psychotherapeutic agents. Why? Because most psychotherapeutic drugs either have no effect on healthy individuals or produce paradoxical effects.

Once a new drug has been stumbled upon, variations on that agent can be developed systematically. The following process is employed: (1) structural analogs of the new agent are synthesized, (2) these analogs are run through biochemical and physiologic screening tests to determine whether or not they possess activity similar to that of the parent compound, and (3) after serious toxicity has been ruled out, promising agents are tested in humans for possible psychotherapeutic activity. By following this procedure, it is possible to develop drugs that have fewer side effects than the original drug and perhaps even superior therapeutic effects. However, although this procedure may produce small advances, it is not likely to yield a major therapeutic breakthrough.

APPROACHING THE STUDY OF CNS DRUGS

Because our understanding of the CNS is less complete than our understanding of the peripheral nervous system, our approach to studying CNS drugs differs from the approach we took with peripheral nervous system agents. When we studied the pharmacology of the peripheral nervous system, we emphasized the importance of understanding transmitters and their receptors prior to embarking on a study of drugs. Since our knowledge of CNS transmitters is insufficient to allow this approach, rather than making a detailed examination of CNS transmitters before we study CNS drugs, we will discuss drugs and transmitters concurrently. Hence, for now, all that you need to know about CNS transmitters is that (1) there are a lot of them, (2) their precise functional roles are not clear, and (3) their complexity makes it difficult for us to know with certainty just how CNS drugs produce their effects.

⁂ KEY POINTS

- In the CNS, many compounds appear to act as neurotransmitters, whereas in the periphery, only three compounds act as neurotransmitters.
- As a rule, we do not understand with precision how CNS drugs produce their effects.
- The blood-brain barrier can protect the CNS from toxic substances—but can also block entry of medicines into the CNS.
- The CNS often undergoes adaptive changes during prolonged drug exposure. The result can be increased therapeutic effects, decreased side effects, tolerance, and physical dependence.

Drugs for Parkinson's Disease

Parkinson's disease (PD) is a neurodegenerative disorder first described in 1817 by Dr. James Parkinson, a London physician. The disease afflicts over 1 million Americans, making it second only to Alzheimer's disease as the most common degenerative disease of neurons. Primary symptoms are tremor, rigidity, postural instability, and slowed movement. The underlying cause is loss of dopaminergic neurons in the substantia nigra. Although there is no cure for PD, drug therapy can maintain functional mobility for years, and can thereby substantially prolong quality of life and life expectancy. The most effective drug for PD is levodopa, almost always given in combination with carbidopa. Unfortunately, as neurodegeneration progresses, levodopa eventually becomes ineffective.

PATHOPHYSIOLOGY OF PARKINSON'S DISEASE

Parkinson's disease is a disorder of the *extrapyramidal system,* a complex neuronal network that helps regulate movement. When extrapyramidal function is disrupted, dyskinesias (disorders of movement) result. The *dyskinesias* that characterize PD are tremor at rest, rigidity, postural instability, and bradykinesia (slowed movement); in severe disease, bradykinesia may progress to *akinesia* (complete absence of movement). In addition to movement disorders, patients frequently experience psychologic disturbances, including dementia, depression, and impaired memory. As a rule, symptoms first appear in middle age and progress relentlessly.

Symptoms of PD result from disruption of neurotransmission within the *striatum,* an important component of the extrapyramidal system. A simplified model of striatal neurotransmission is depicted in Figure 21-1A. As indicated, proper function of the striatum requires a balance between two neurotransmitters: *dopamine* and *acetylcholine* (ACh). Dopamine is an *inhibitory* transmitter; ACh is *excitatory.* According to the model, the neurons that release dopamine inhibit neurons that release gamma-aminobutyric acid (GABA, another inhibitory transmitter). In contrast, the neurons that release ACh excite the neurons that release GABA. Movement is normal when the inhibitory influence of dopamine and the excitatory influence of ACh are in balance. Note that the neurons that supply dopamine to the striatum originate in the *substantia nigra.* Between 70% and 80% of these neurons must be lost before PD becomes clinically recognizable. This loss takes place over 5 to 20 years. Put another way, neuronal degeneration begins long before overt symptoms of PD appear.

In PD, there is an imbalance between dopamine and ACh in the striatum (Fig. 21-1B). As noted, the imbalance results from *degeneration of the neurons that supply dopamine to the striatum.* In the absence of dopamine, the excitatory influence of ACh goes unopposed, causing excessive stimulation of the neurons that release GABA. Overactivity of these GABAergic neurons contributes to the movement disorders seen in PD.

What causes degeneration of dopaminergic neurons? No one knows for sure. However, recent evidence strongly implicates *alpha-synuclein*—a potentially toxic protein synthesized by dopaminergic neurons. Under normal conditions, alpha-synuclein is rapidly degraded. As a result, it does not accumulate and no harm occurs. Degradation of alpha-synuclein requires two other proteins: *parkin* and *ubiquitin.* (Parkin is an enzyme that catalyzes the binding of alpha-synuclein to ubiquitin. Once bound to ubiquitin, alpha-synuclein can be degraded.) If any of these proteins—alpha-synuclein, parkin, or ubiquitin—is defective, degradation of alpha-synuclein cannot take place. When this occurs, alpha-synuclein accumulates inside the cell, forming neurotoxic fibrils. At autopsy, these fibrils are visible as so-called Lewy bodies, which are characteristic of PD pathology. Failure to degrade alpha-synuclein appears to result from two causes: genetic vulnerability and toxins in the environment. Defective genes coding for all three proteins have been found in families with inherited forms of PD. In people with PD that is not inherited, environmental toxins may explain the inability to degrade alpha-synuclein.

As discussed in Chapter 30, movement disorders similar to those of PD can occur as side effects of therapy with antipsychotic agents. These dyskinesias, which are referred to as *extrapyramidal side effects,* result from blockade of dopamine receptors in the striatum. This drug-induced parkinsonism can be managed with some of the drugs used to treat PD.

A Normal

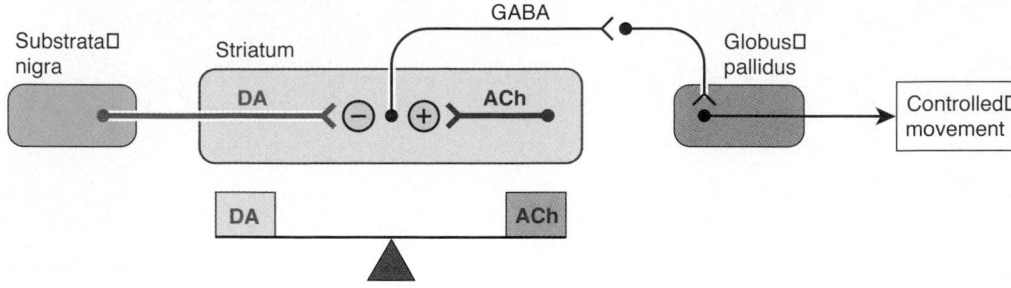

B Parkinson's Disease

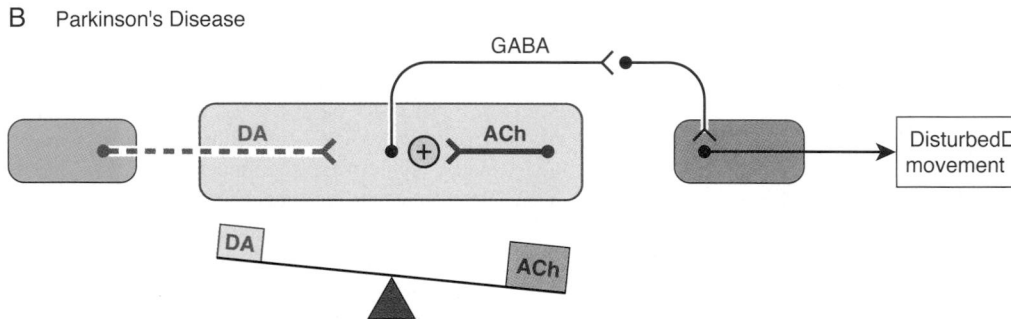

Figure 21–1 ■ A model of neurotransmission in the healthy striatum and parkinsonian striatum.
A, In the healthy striatum, dopamine (DA) released from neurons originating in the substantia nigra *inhibits* the firing of neurons in the striatum that release gamma-aminobutyric acid (GABA) as their transmitter. Conversely, neurons located within the striatum, which release acetylcholine (ACh) as their transmitter, *excite* the GABAergic neurons. Hence, under normal conditions, the inhibitory actions of DA are balanced by the excitatory actions of ACh, and controlled movement results.
B, In Parkinson's disease, the neurons that supply DA to the striatum degenerate. In the absence of sufficient DA, the excitatory effects of ACh go unopposed, and disturbed movement results.

OVERVIEW OF DRUG THERAPY

Therapeutic Goal

Ideally, treatment would reverse neuronal degeneration, or at least prevent further degeneration, and control symptoms. Unfortunately, the ideal treatment doesn't exist. Hence, the goal with currently available drugs is simply to improve the patient's ability to carry out activities of daily life. Drug selection and dosage are determined by the extent to which PD interferes with work, walking, dressing, eating, bathing, and other activities. Drugs benefit the patient most by improving bradykinesia, gait disturbance, and postural instability. Tremor and rigidity, although disturbing, are less disabling. It is important to note that drugs only provide symptomatic relief; they do not cure PD. Furthermore, with the possible exception of selegiline, these drugs do not alter disease progression.

Drugs Employed

Given the neurochemical basis of parkinsonism—too little striatal dopamine and too much ACh—the approach to treatment is obvious: Give drugs that can restore the functional balance between dopamine and ACh. To accomplish this, two types of drugs are used: (1) *dopaminergic agents* (i.e., drugs that directly or indirectly activate dopamine receptors), and (2) *anticholinergic agents* (i.e., drugs that block receptors for ACh). Of the two, dopaminergic agents are by far the more widely employed.

As shown in Table 21–1, the dopaminergic drugs act by several mechanisms: levodopa promotes dopamine synthesis; the dopamine agonists stimulate dopamine receptors directly; selegiline inhibits dopamine breakdown; amantadine promotes dopamine release (and may also block dopamine reuptake); and the inhibitors of catecholamine-*O*-methyl transferase (COMT) enhance the effects of levodopa (by blocking its degradation).

In contrast to the dopaminergic drugs, which act by multiple mechanisms, all of the anticholinergic agents share the same mechanism: blockade of muscarinic receptors in the striatum.

Drug Selection

Treatment of PD has two mainstays: levodopa (combined with carbidopa) and the dopamine agonists. Levodopa is the most effective treatment for PD. However, long-term use carries a high risk of disabling dyskinesias, and beneficial effects diminish over time. The dopamine agonists are less effective than levodopa, but also are less likely to cause dyskinesias.

TABLE 21-1 ■ Dopaminergic Agents for Parkinson's Disease

Drug	Mechanism of Action	Therapeutic Role
Dopamine Replacement		
Levodopa Levodopa/carbidopa	Levodopa undergoes conversion to DA in the brain and then activates DA receptors (carbidopa just blocks destruction of levodopa in the periphery)	First-line drug, or supplement to a dopamine agonist
Dopamine Agonists		
Bromocriptine Pergolide Pramipexole Ropinirole	Direct activation of DA receptors	First-line drug, or supplement to levodopa (The nonergot agents—pramipexole and ropinirole—are preferred)
COMT Inhibitors		
Entacapone Tolcapone	Inhibit breakdown of levodopa by COMT	Adjunct to levodopa (to increase "on time" and decrease "wearing off"); entacapone is preferred to tolcapone
Dopamine Releaser		
Amantadine	Promotes release of DA from remaining DA neurons; may also block DA reuptake	Second-line therapy for motor fluctuations
MAO-B Inhibitor		
Selegiline	Inhibits breakdown of DA by MAO-B	Used in newly diagnosed patients for possible neuroprotection; second- or third-line agent as adjunct to levodopa

COMT = catechol-*o*-methyltransferase, DA = dopamine, MAO-B = type B monoamine oxidase.

However, the dopamine agonists frequently cause troubling side effects, especially hallucinations, confusion, hypotension, nausea, vomiting, and daytime sedation.

Which option—levodopa or a dopamine agonist—should be used for *initial* therapy? Until recently, levodopa was the preferred choice. However, according to a new clinical guideline—"An Algorithm (Decision Tree) for the Management of Parkinson's Disease," published in a June 2001 supplement to the journal *Neurology*—dopamine agonists are now recommended as initial therapy for most patients. If a dopamine agonist alone is insufficient, it can be supplemented with levodopa. For patients in their 70s and older, levodopa may the better choice. Why? Because the elderly are less able to tolerate the side effects of dopamine agonists. If needed, levodopa can be supplemented with a dopamine agonist.

For patients with *advanced* disease, levodopa is the treatment of choice. If levodopa by itself is inadequate, it can be combined with a dopamine agonist, amantadine, or a COMT inhibitor. Levodopa may also be combined with an anticholinergic agent, except in elderly patients and those with a history of psychosis, since the risk of adverse psychologic reactions is high.

PHARMACOLOGY OF THE DRUGS USED FOR PARKINSON'S DISEASE

Levodopa

Levodopa was introduced over 30 years ago, and has been a cornerstone of PD treatment ever since. Unfortunately, although the drug is highly effective, beneficial effects diminish over time. The most troubling adverse effects are dyskinesias.

Use in Parkinson's Disease

Beneficial Effects. Levodopa [Dopar, Larodopa] is the most effective drug for PD. At the beginning of treatment, about 75% of patients experience a 50% reduction in symptom severity. Levodopa is so effective, in fact, that a diagnosis of PD should be questioned if the patient fails to respond.

Full therapeutic responses may take several months to develop. Consequently, although the effects of levodopa can be significant, patients should not expect improvement immediately. Rather, they should be informed that beneficial effects are likely to increase steadily over the first few months.

In contrast to the dramatic improvements seen during initial therapy, long-term therapy with levodopa has been disappointing. Although symptoms may be well controlled during the first 2 years of treatment, by the end of 5 years the patient's ability to function may deteriorate to pretreatment levels. This probably reflects progression of the disease and not development of tolerance to levodopa.

Acute Loss of Effect. Acute loss of effect occurs in two patterns: gradual loss and abrupt loss. Gradual loss ("wearing off") develops near the end of the dosing interval, and simply indicates that plasma drug levels have declined to a subtherapeutic value. Wearing off can be minimized in three ways: (1) shortening the dosing interval, (2) giving a drug that prolongs levodopa's plasma half-life (e.g., entacapone), and (3) giving a direct-acting dopamine agonist. Wearing off can also be reduced by using Sinemet CR, a controlled-release formulation of levodopa.

Abrupt loss of effect, often referred to as the "on-off" phenomenon, can occur at any time during the dosing interval—even while drug levels are high. "Off" times may last from minutes to hours. Over the course of treatment, "off" periods are likely to increase in both intensity and frequency. The "on-off" phenomenon is difficult to correct. As discussed below, avoidance of high-protein meals may help.

Mechanism of Action

Levodopa reduces symptoms by promoting synthesis of dopamine in the striatum (Fig. 21–2). Levodopa enters the brain via an active transport system that carries it across the blood-brain barrier. Once in the brain, the drug undergoes uptake into the few dopaminergic nerve terminals that remain in the striatum. Following uptake, levodopa, which has no direct effects of its own, is converted to dopamine, its active form. By undergoing conversion to dopamine, levodopa helps restore a proper balance between dopamine and ACh.

Conversion of levodopa to dopamine is depicted in Figure 21–3. As indicated, the enzyme that catalyzes the reaction is called a *decarboxylase* (because it removes a carboxyl group from levodopa). The activity of decarboxylases is enhanced by *pyridoxine* (vitamin B_6).

Why is PD treated with levodopa and not with dopamine itself? There are two reasons. First, dopamine cannot cross the blood-brain barrier (see Fig. 21–2). As noted, levodopa crosses the barrier by means of an active transport system; this system will not transport dopamine. Second, dopamine has such a short half-life in the blood that it would be impractical to use even if it could cross the blood-brain barrier.

Pharmacokinetics

Levodopa is administered orally and undergoes rapid absorption from the small intestine. Food delays absorption by slowing gastric emptying. Furthermore, since neutral amino acids compete with levodopa for intestinal absorption (and for transport across the blood-brain barrier as well), high-protein foods will reduce therapeutic effects.

Only a small fraction of each dose of levodopa reaches the brain. The majority is metabolized in the periphery, primarily by *decarboxylase enzymes,* and, to a lesser extent, by COMT. Peripheral decarboxylases convert levodopa into dopamine, an active metabolite. In contrast, COMT converts levodopa into an inactive metabolite. Like the enzymes that decarboxylate levodopa within the brain, peripheral decarboxylases work faster in the presence of pyridoxine. Because of peripheral metabolism, less than 2% of each dose enters the brain.

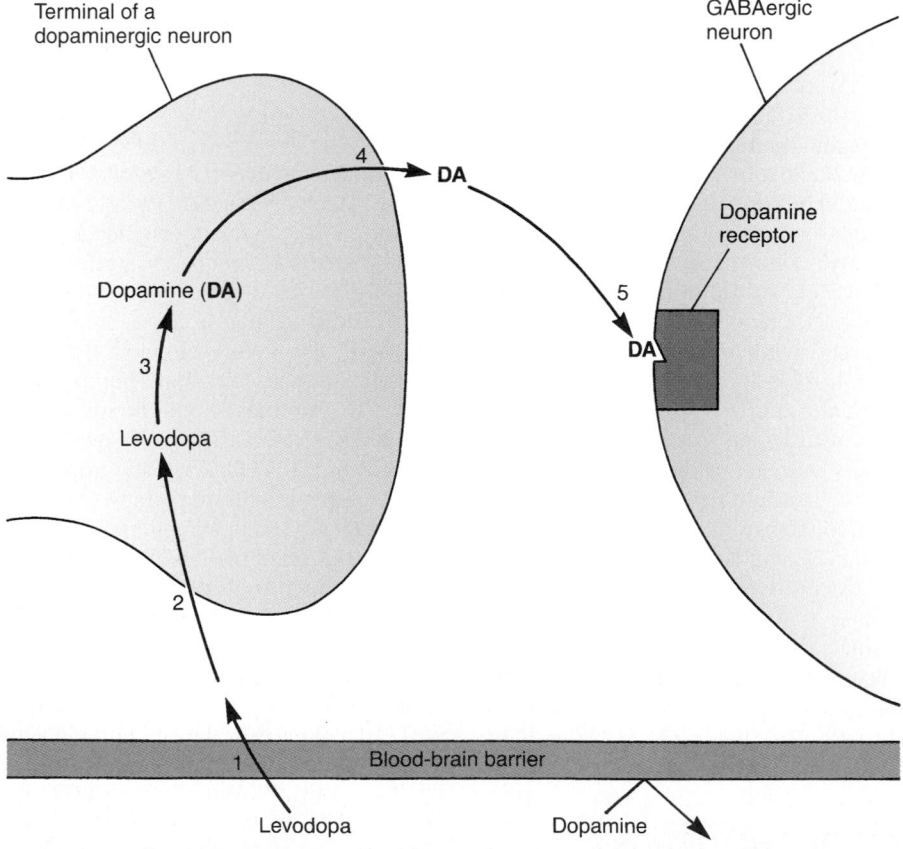

Figure 21–2 ■ Steps leading to alteration of CNS function by levodopa.
To produce its beneficial effects in PD, levodopa must be (1) transported across the blood-brain barrier; (2) taken up by dopaminergic nerve terminals in the striatum; (3) converted into dopamine; (4) released into the synaptic space; and (5) bound to dopamine receptors on striatal GABAergic neurons, causing them to fire at a slower rate. Note that dopamine itself is unable to cross the blood-brain barrier, and hence cannot be used to treat PD.

Adverse Effects

Most side effects of levodopa are dose dependent. The elderly, who are the primary users of levodopa, are especially sensitive to adverse effects.

Nausea and Vomiting. Most patients experience nausea and vomiting early in treatment. These effects result from activation of dopamine receptors in the chemoreceptor trigger zone (CTZ) of the medulla. Nausea and vomiting can be reduced by administering levodopa in low initial doses and with meals. (The presence of food retards levodopa absorption, causing a decrease in peak plasma drug levels and a corresponding decrease in stimulation of the CTZ.) However, since administration with food can reduce therapeutic effects (by decreasing levodopa absorption), administration with meals should be avoided if possible.

Dyskinesias. Ironically, levodopa, which is given to *alleviate* movement disorders, actually *causes* movement disorders in many patients. About 80% develop involuntary movements within the first year of treatment. Some dyskinesias are just annoying (e.g., head bobbing, tics, grimacing), whereas others can be disabling (e.g., ballismus, choreoathetosis). These dyskinesias develop just before or soon after optimal levodopa dosage has been achieved. With the exception of surgery (see discussion of pallidotomy in Box 21–1), the only treatment for dyskinesias is to reduce levodopa dosage. Unfortunately, dosage reduction is likely to permit re-emergence of PD symptoms.

Cardiovascular Effects. *Postural hypotension* is common early in treatment. The mechanism of this paradoxical effect is unknown. Hypotension can be reduced by increasing intake of salt and water. An alpha-adrenergic agonist can also help.

Conversion of levodopa to dopamine in the periphery can produce excessive activation of beta$_1$ receptors in the heart. *Dysrhythmias* can result, especially in patients with cardiac disease.

Psychosis. Psychosis develops in about 20% of levodopa-treated patients. Prominent symptoms are visual hallucinations, vivid dreams or nightmares, and paranoid ideation (fears of personal endangerment, sense of persecution, feelings of being followed or spied on). Stimulation of dopamine receptors is in some way involved. Symptoms can be reduced by lowering levodopa dosage, but this will reduce beneficial effects as well.

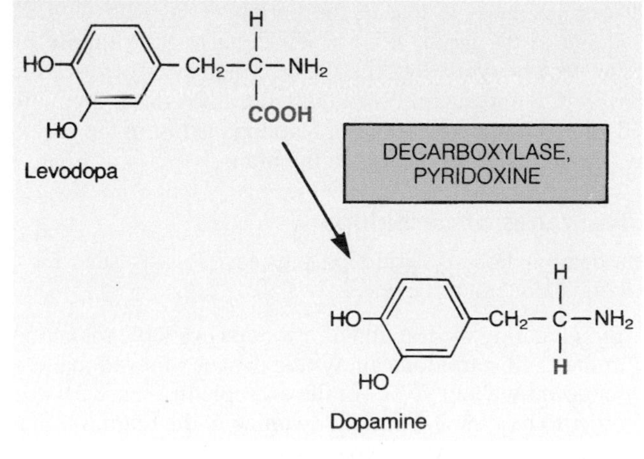

Treatment of levodopa-induced psychosis with traditional antipsychotic drugs is problematic. Yes, these agents can decrease psychologic symptoms. However, they will also *intensify* symptoms of PD. Why? Because they block receptors for dopamine in the striatum. In fact, when traditional antipsychotic agents are used for schizophrenia, the biggest problem is parkinsonian side effects, referred to as extrapyramidal symptoms (EPS).

Clozapine (an atypical antipsychotic agent) has been used successfully to manage levodopa-induced psychosis. Unlike traditional antipsychotic drugs, clozapine does not block dopamine receptors in the striatum, and hence does not cause EPS. In patients taking levodopa, clozapine can reduce psychotic symptoms without intensifying symptoms of PD. Interestingly, the dosage employed is only 25 mg/day, about 20 times lower than the dosage for schizophrenia. The pharmacology of clozapine is discussed at length in Chapter 30.

Neurotoxicity. There is concern that long-term use of levodopa may accelerate loss of dopaminergic neurons. The proposed mechanism is conversion of levodopa into dopamine, which in turn becomes converted to reactive metabolites (e.g., hydrogen peroxide). These reactive products could harm mitochondria and other cell components. However, although cellular injury is a theoretical possibility, there is no proof that it actually occurs.

Other Adverse Effects. Levodopa may *darken sweat and urine;* patients should be forewarned of this harmless effect. The drug can *activate malignant melanoma* and consequently should be avoided in patients with undiagnosed skin lesions.

Drug Holidays

With long-term use of levodopa, adverse effects tend to increase and therapeutic effects tend to diminish. For some patients, the situation may improve following a "drug holiday," defined as a brief (e.g., 10-day) interruption of treatment. When the holiday is successful, beneficial effects are achieved with lower doses. Because doses are lower, the incidence of dyskinesias and psychosis is lowered as well. Unfortunately, drug holidays do not correct the "on-off" phenomenon.

Drug holidays are dangerous. Since drug withdrawal will immobilize the patient, the holiday must take place in a hospital. In addition to severe psychologic distress, immobilization presents a risk of deep vein thrombosis, aspiration pneumonitis, and decubitus ulcers.

Drug Interactions

Interactions between levodopa and other drugs can (1) increase beneficial effects of levodopa, (2) decrease beneficial effects of levodopa, and (3) increase toxicity from levodopa. Major interactions are summarized in Table 21–2. Several interactions are discussed immediately below; others are discussed later.

Conventional Antipsychotic Drugs. All of the conventional antipsychotic drugs (e.g., chlorpromazine, haloperidol) block receptors for dopamine in the striatum. As a result, they can decrease therapeutic effects of levodopa. Accordingly, concurrent use of levodopa and these drugs should be avoided. As discussed above, clozapine, an atypical antipsy-

Figure 21–3 ■ Conversion of levodopa to dopamine. Decarboxylases present in the brain, liver, and intestine convert levodopa into dopamine. Pyridoxine (vitamin B$_6$) accelerates the reaction.

TABLE 21–2 ■ Major Drug Interactions of Levodopa

Drug Category	Drug	Mechanism of Interaction
Drugs that *increase* beneficial effects of levodopa	Carbidopa	Inhibits peripheral decarboxylation of levodopa
	Tolcapone, entacapone	Inhibit destruction of levodopa by COMT in the intestine and peripheral tissues
	Bromocriptine, pergolide, pramipexole, ropinirole	Stimulate dopamine receptors directly, and thereby add to the effects of dopamine derived from levodopa
	Amantadine	Promotes release of dopamine
	Anticholinergic drugs	Block cholinergic receptors in the CNS, and thereby help restore the balance between dopamine and ACh
Drugs that *decrease* beneficial effects of levodopa	Pyridoxine (vitamin B$_6$)	Enhances destruction of levodopa by decarboxylases
	Antipsychotic drugs*	Block dopamine receptors in the striatum
Drugs that increase levodopa toxicity	MAO inhibitors	Inhibition of MAO increases the risk of severe levodopa-induced hypertension

ACh = acetylcholine, CNS = central nervous system, COMT = catechol-*o*-methyltransferase, MAO = monoamine oxidase.
*Conventional antipsychotic agents block dopamine receptors in the striatum and thereby nullify the therapeutic effects of levodopa. Clozapine, an atypical antipsychotic drug, does not block dopamine receptors in the striatum, and hence does not nullify the therapeutic effects of levodopa.

chotic agent, does not block dopamine receptors in the striatum, and hence can be used safely in patients with PD.

Monoamine Oxidase Inhibitors. Levodopa can cause a hypertensive crisis if administered to an individual taking a nonselective inhibitor of monoamine oxidase (MAO). The mechanism of this interaction is as follows: (1) Levodopa elevates neuronal stores of dopamine and norepinephrine (NE) by promoting synthesis of both compounds. (2) Since intraneuronal MAO serves to inactivate dopamine and NE, inhibition of MAO allows elevated neuronal stores of these transmitters to grow even larger. (3) Since both dopamine and NE promote vasoconstriction, release of these agents in supranormal amounts can lead to massive vasoconstriction, thereby causing blood pressure to rise dangerously high. To avoid hypertensive crisis, MAO inhibitors should be withdrawn at least 2 weeks prior to initiating levodopa.

Anticholinergic Drugs. As discussed above, excessive stimulation of cholinergic receptors contributes to the dyskinesias of PD. Therefore, by blocking these receptors, anticholinergic agents can enhance responses to levodopa.

Pyridoxine. Pyridoxine (vitamin B$_6$) stimulates decarboxylase activity. By accelerating decarboxylation of levodopa in the periphery, pyridoxine can decrease the amount of levodopa that reaches the central nervous system (CNS). As a result, therapeutic effects of levodopa are reduced. Patients should be informed about this interaction and instructed to avoid multivitamin preparations that contain pyridoxine.

Food Interactions

Meals with a high protein content can reduce therapeutic responses to levodopa. Why? Because neutral amino acids compete with levodopa for absorption from the intestine and for transport across the blood-brain barrier. Hence, a high-protein meal can significantly reduce both the amount of levodopa that gets absorbed and the amount that gets transported into the brain. It has been suggested that a high-protein meal could trigger an abrupt loss of effect (i.e., an "off" episode). Accordingly, patients should be advised to spread their protein consumption evenly throughout the day's meals.

Preparations, Dosage, and Administration

Levodopa [Dopar, Larodopa] is dispensed in tablets and capsules (100, 250, and 500 mg) for oral administration. To minimize adverse effects, especially drug-induced dyskinesias, dosage must be individualized. The usual initial dosage is 0.5 to 1.0 gm/day administered in two or more divided doses. The total daily dosage can be increased gradually to a maximum of 8 gm. Full therapeutic responses may take 6 months to develop.

Levodopa Plus Carbidopa

The combination of levodopa plus carbidopa, marketed as Sinemet, is our most effective therapy for PD. The combination is much more effective than levodopa alone.

Mechanism of Action

Carbidopa is used to enhance the effects of levodopa. Carbidopa has no therapeutic effects of its own, and therefore is always used in conjunction with levodopa. Carbidopa inhibits decarboxylation of levodopa in the intestine and peripheral tissues, thereby making more levodopa available to the CNS. Carbidopa does not prevent the conversion of levodopa to dopamine by decarboxylases within the brain. Why? Because carbidopa is unable to cross the blood-brain barrier.

The impact of carbidopa is shown schematically in Figure 21–4, which compares the fate of levodopa in the presence and absence of carbidopa. In the absence of carbidopa, about 98% of levodopa is lost in the periphery, leaving only 2% available to the brain. Why is levodopa lost? Primarily because decarboxylases in the GI tract and peripheral tissues convert it to dopamine. When these decarboxylases are inhibited by carbidopa, only 90% of levodopa is lost in the periphery, leaving 10% for actions in the brain.

Advantages of Carbidopa

The combination of carbidopa plus levodopa is superior to levodopa alone in three ways:

■ By increasing the fraction of levodopa available for actions in the CNS, carbidopa allows the dosage of levodopa to be reduced by about 75%. (In the example in Figure 21–4, in order to provide 2.5 mg of dopamine to the brain, we must administer 125 mg of levodopa if carbidopa is absent, but only 25 mg if carbidopa is present.)

■ By reducing production of dopamine in the periphery, carbidopa reduces cardiovascular responses to levodopa and also reduces nausea and vomiting.

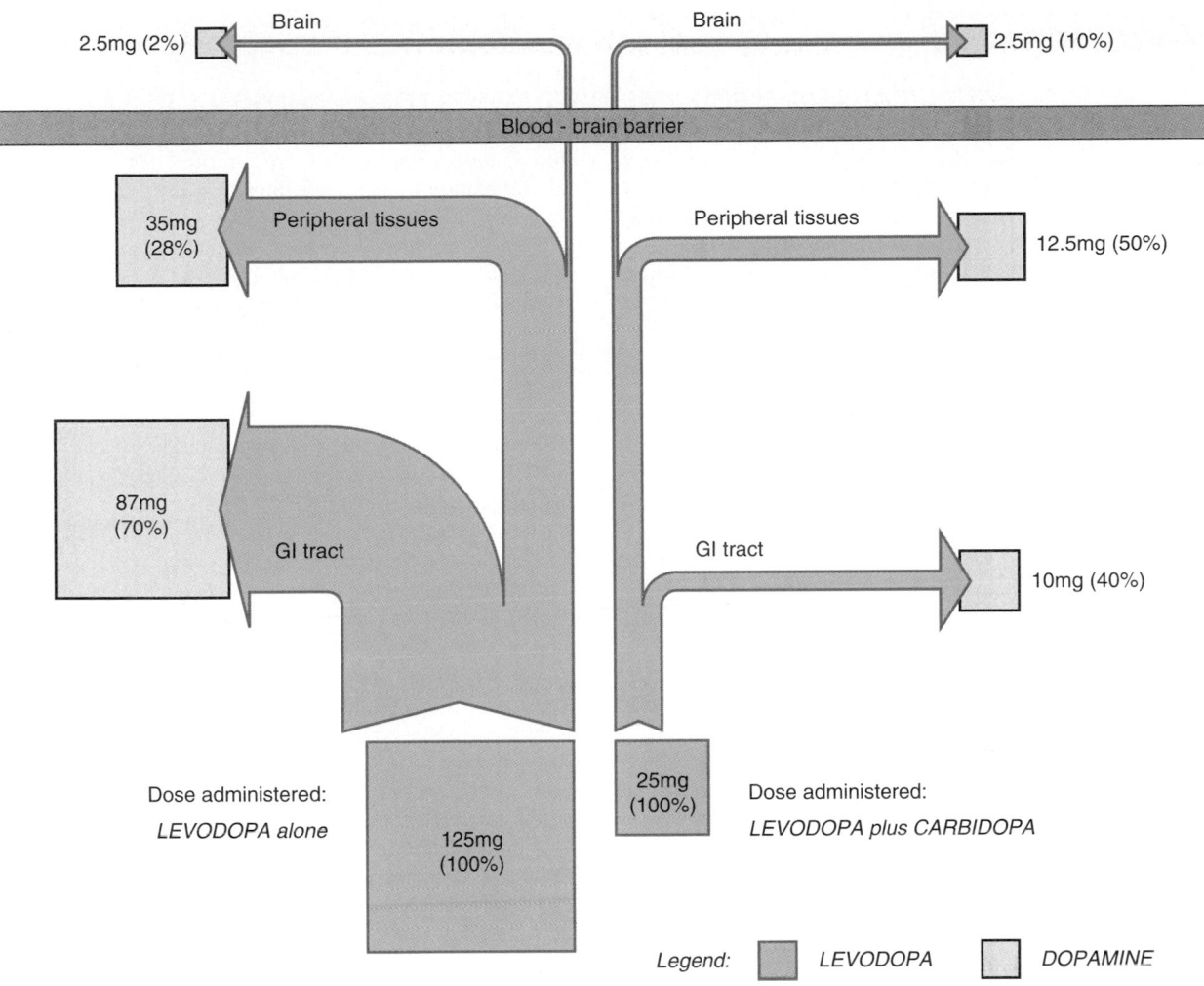

Figure 21–4 ■ Fate of levodopa in the presence and absence of carbidopa.
In the absence of carbidopa, 98% of an administered dose of levodopa is metabolized in GI tract and peripheral tissues—either by decarboxylases or COMT—leaving only 2% for actions in the brain. Hence, in order to deliver 2.5 mg of levodopa to the brain, the dose of levodopa must be large (125 mg). By inhibiting intestinal and peripheral decarboxylases, carbidopa increases the percentage of levodopa available to the brain. Hence, the dose needed to deliver 2.5 mg is greatly reduced (to 25 mg in this example). Since carbidopa cannot cross the blood-brain barrier, it does not suppress conversion of levodopa to dopamine in the brain. Furthermore, since carbidopa reduces peripheral production of dopamine (from 35 mg to 12.5 mg in this example), peripheral toxicity (nausea, cardiovascular effects) is greatly reduced. (Data in the figure are extrapolated from Nutt JG, Fellman JH. Pharmacokinetics of levodopa. Clin Neuropharmacol 1984;7:35.)

■ By causing direct inhibition of decarboxylase, carbidopa obviates stimulation of decarboxylase by pyridoxine. As a result, carbidopa eliminates concern about decreasing the effects of levodopa through inadvertent use of vitamin preparations that contain pyridoxine.

Disadvantages of Carbidopa

Carbidopa has no adverse effects of its own, and hence any adverse responses that may occur are due to potentiation of levodopa. When levodopa is combined with carbidopa, abnormal movements and psychiatric disturbances may occur sooner and may be more intense than when levodopa is employed alone.

Preparations, Dosage, and Administration

Carbidopa is almost always administered with levodopa in a formulation that contains both drugs. These combination products (standard and sustained-release tablets) are marketed under the trade name *Sinemet*. Standard Sinemet tablets are available in three strengths: (1) 10 mg carbidopa/100 mg levodopa, (2) 25 mg carbidopa/100 mg levodopa, and (3) 25 mg carbidopa/250 mg levodopa. The sustained-release tablets [Sinemet CR] are available in two strengths: 25 mg carbidopa/100 mg levodopa, and 50 mg carbidopa/200 mg levodopa.

Carbidopa without levodopa, dispensed under the trade name *Lodosyn*, is available by special request for investiga-

Special Interest Topic

BOX 21–1 ▐▪ SURGICAL AND ELECTRICAL TREATMENTS FOR PARKINSON'S DISEASE

For patients with advanced Parkinson's disease (PD), levodopa therapy is far from ideal. Over time, the drug becomes less and less effective. Patients typically experience "off" times as well as drug-induced dyskinesias. For these patients, nondrug therapies may help. Potential options include pallidotomy, deep brain stimulation, and cell implants. Pallidotomy and brain stimulation have been very successful; cell implants have not.

Pallidotomy

Posteroventral medial pallidotomy, or simply pallidotomy, is a neurosurgical procedure for destroying a region of the globus pallidus. As indicated in Figure 21–1, the globus pallidus, which helps regulate movement, receives input from the striatum. In patients with PD, striatal input to the globus pallidus is disrupted, causing the globus pallidus itself to malfunction. It has been argued that altered output from the globus pallidus underlies many of the symptoms of PD, including tremor, rigidity, and bradykinesia. The results of pallidotomy support this argument: For many patients with PD, *unilateral* destruction of the posteroventral medial region of the globus pallidus produces a substantial improvement in symptoms. The most consistent benefit is a reduction in levodopa-induced dyskinesias. Motor control during levodopa "off" times also improves. In contrast, very little improvement is seen during levodopa "on" times. Following pallidotomy, about 50% of patients who previously needed help with activities of daily living are able to live independently. Pallidotomy may also permit a temporary reduction in levodopa dosage. Although complications of the procedure are generally mild, intracerebral hemorrhage is a potential and serious risk.

Because pallidotomy is irreversible, and because complications can be serious, the procedure should be limited to patients with intractable levodopa-induced dyskinesias and to patients who are disabled by levodopa "off" times. Furthermore, because brain tissue is permanently destroyed, pallidotomy is usually performed unilaterally; this leaves the other side of the brain intact, just in case something goes wrong.

Deep Brain Stimulation

Electrical stimulation of specific brain areas can improve symptoms in patients with PD. Three areas have been targeted: the subthalamic nucleus (STN), the globus pallidus internus, and the ventralis intermedius nucleus of the thalamus. Stimulation of the STN has produced the best results. Compared with pallidotomy, electrical stimulation has several advantages: it's reversible and adjustable, and, because brain tissue is not permanently damaged, it can be done bilaterally with low risk. On the other hand, electrical stimulation is very expensive. Several studies on STN stimulation have been conducted. One is described below.

In 1998, researchers reported that continuous, long-term electrical stimulation of the STN can improve symptoms in patients with advanced PD. This work was based on animal models of PD in which (1) motor symptoms were associated with abnormal neuronal activity in the STN and (2) electrical stimulation of the STN improved the symptoms. In patients with PD, electrodes were implanted *bilaterally* in the STN and then connected by a subcutaneous lead to a pulse generator implanted in the subclavicular region (much like a cardiac pacemaker). The pulse generator was then programmed by telemetry to adjust stimulation parameters (e.g., voltage, frequency). All patients in the study had advanced PD and all were experiencing "on-off" phenomena with levodopa.

Electrical stimulation produced substantial benefits during "off" times but only modest benefits during "on" times. During "off" times, there was a 60% improvement in motor function; bradykinesia, rigidity, tremor, and gait all improved. During "on" times, improvement was only 10%. Stimulation allowed all patients to become independent in most activities of daily living. On average, stimulation permitted a 50% reduction in levodopa dosage.

Adverse effects were generally mild, but serious sequelae of the neurosurgery are possible. Of the 20 patients in this study, 8 experienced transient CNS effects, including confusion, hallucinations, temporospatial disorientation, and abulia (lack of will; inability to make decisions). All symptoms resolved within 2 weeks of the surgery. Of much greater concern, the procedure carries a 2% to 8% risk of intracerebral hematoma. Because of this risk, the procedure should be reserved for patients with advanced PD who are otherwise good candidates for surgery.

How does STN stimulation improve PD symptoms? The answer is unclear. One theory, based on animal studies, suggests that electrical stimulation may *inhibit* overactivity of neurons in the STN. The net result would be to *increase* excitatory input to the cerebral cortex.

Electrical stimulation is expensive. The surgery costs about $25,000. The pulse generator costs another $10,000. And every 3 to 5 years, additional costs arise when the batteries in the pulse generator must be replaced.

Cell Implants

The objective with cell implants is to replace degenerated dopaminergic neurons. Implants have been tried with human adrenal cells and with fetal brain cells from humans and pigs. Human brain cells work best, and even then benefits are modest.

In 1995, researchers finally obtained definitive proof that transplanting fetal dopaminergic neurons into the brain can benefit a patient with PD. In this case study, the patient had severe parkinsonism that would no longer respond to drug therapy. Following the transplant, symptoms steadily improved over 3 months, eventually allowing the patient to perform all activities of daily living without assistance. The improvements were sustained for 15 months, at which time the patient died of a massive pulmonary embolism unrelated to the transplant. Autopsy revealed that the grafts not only took but had become seamlessly integrated into the surrounding tissue. This was the

tional use. This preparation is employed when dosages of levodopa and carbidopa must be titrated separately.

When patients who have been taking levodopa alone are switched over to the combination of carbidopa plus levodopa, at least 8 hours should elapse between the last dose of levodopa and the first dose of the combination. This delay is needed to prevent excessive potentiation of residual levodopa by carbidopa. Also, when switching from levodopa alone to the combination, the total daily dose of levodopa must be reduced substantially: The dose of levodopa within the combination should be only 25% of the former dose. For patients who are not currently receiving levodopa, therapy can be initiated with either 10 mg carbidopa/100 mg levodopa or 25 mg carbidopa/100 mg levodopa, each taken 3 times a day.

Dopamine Agonists

Dopamine agonists are first-line drugs for PD. Beneficial effects result from direct activation of dopamine receptors in the striatum. For patients with mild or moderate symptoms, dopamine agonists are now considered drugs of first choice. Although dopamine agonists are less effective than levodopa, they still have advantages. Specifically, in contrast to levodopa, they aren't dependent on enzymatic conversion to become active, aren't converted to potentially toxic metabolites, and don't compete with dietary proteins for uptake from the intestine or transport across the blood-brain barrier. In addition, when used long-term, dopamine agonists have a lower incidence of response failures and are less likely to cause disabling dyskinesias. However, these drugs do cause more serious side effects—especially hallucinations, daytime sleepiness, and postural hypotension. As a result, these drugs are usually reserved for younger patients, who tolerate these side effects better than do the elderly.

At this time, four dopamine agonists are available. Two are derivatives of ergot (an alkaloid found in plants) and two are not. The nonergot derivatives (pramipexole and ropinirole), which are relatively new, cause fewer side effects than the ergot derivatives (bromocriptine and pergolide). Why? Because the nonergot drugs are selective for dopamine receptors, whereas the ergot derivatives interact with alpha-adrenergic and serotonergic receptors, in addition to dopamine receptors. Because the newer (nonergot) drugs are better tolerated than the ergot derivatives, the newer drugs are preferred.

Pramipexole

Actions and Uses. Pramipexole [Mirapex] is a nonergot dopamine-receptor agonist. The drug is used alone in early-stage PD, and combined with levodopa in advanced-stage PD. Pramipexole binds selectively to dopamine D_2 and D_3 receptor subtypes. Binding to D_2 receptors underlies therapeutic effects. The significance of D_3 binding is unknown. When used as monotherapy in early PD, pramipexole can produce significant improvement in motor performance. When combined with levodopa in advanced PD, the drug can reduce fluctuations in motor control and may permit a reduction in levodopa dosage. In both cases, maximal benefits take several weeks to develop.

Pharmacokinetics. Pramipexole is rapidly absorbed and reaches peak plasma levels in 1 to 2 hours. Food reduces the speed of absorption but not the extent. Pramipexole undergoes wide distribution, and achieves a high concentration red blood cells. The drug is eliminated unchanged in the urine.

Adverse Effects and Interactions. Pramipexole can produce a variety of adverse effects. Most are the direct result of activating dopamine receptors. The most common effects seen when pramipexole is used *alone* are nausea (28%), dizziness (25%), daytime somnolence (22%), insomnia (17%), constipation (14%), weakness (14%), and hallucinations (9%). When the drug is *combined with levodopa,* many patients experience orthostatic hypotension (54%) and dyskinesias (47%), which are not seen when the drug is used by itself. In addition, the incidence of hallucinations nearly doubles—to 17%.

A few patients have experienced *sleep attacks* (overwhelming and irresistible sleepiness that comes on without warning). Sleep attacks can be a real danger for people who are driving (and a potential blessing for those in faculty meetings). Sleep attacks should not be equated with the normal sleepiness that occurs with dopaminergic agents. Patients who experience a sleep attack should inform their physician.

Cimetidine (a drug for peptic ulcer disease) can inhibit renal excretion of pramipexole, thereby increasing its blood level.

Preparations, Dosage, and Administration. Pramipexole [Mirapex] is available in tablets (0.125, 0.25, 1.0, and 1.5 mg) for oral administration. The drug may be taken with food to reduce nausea. To minimize other adverse effects, dosage should be low initially and then gradually increased. The recommended starting dosage is 0.125 mg 3 times a day. This can be increased over 7 weeks to a maximum of 1.5 mg 3 times a day. In patients with significant renal impairment, dosage should be reduced.

Ropinirole

Actions, Uses, and Adverse Effects. Ropinirole [Requip], a nonergot dopamine agonist, is similar to pramipexole with respect to receptor specificity, mechanism of action, and therapeutic and adverse effects. Like pramipexole, ropinirole is highly selective for D_2 and D_3 receptors. The drug can be used as monotherapy in early PD and as an adjunct to levodopa in advanced PD. In contrast to pramipexole, which is eliminated entirely by renal excretion, ropinirole is eliminated by hepatic metabolism. Some adverse effects are more common than with pramipexole. When ropinirole is used *alone,* the most common effects are nausea (60%), dizziness (40%), somnolence (40%), and hallucinations (5%). Rarely, sleep attacks occur. When ropinirole is *combined with levodopa,* the most important side effects are dyskinesias (34%), hallucinations (10%), and postural hypotension (2%). Note that these occur less frequently than when pramipexole is combined with levodopa. Animal tests indicate that ropinirole can harm the developing fetus. Accordingly, the drug should not be used during pregnancy.

Preparations, Dosage, and Administration. Ropinirole [Requip] is available in film-coated tablets (0.25, 0.5, 1, 2, and 5 mg) for oral administration. The drug may be taken with food to decrease nausea. Dosage should be low initially and then gradually increased. The recommended starting dosage is 0.25 mg 3 times a day. Dosage can be increased over several weeks to a maximum of 8 mg 3 times a day.

Bromocriptine

Actions and Uses. Bromocriptine [Parlodel], a derivative of ergot, is a direct-acting dopamine agonist. Beneficial effects result from activating dopamine receptors in the striatum. Responses are equivalent to those seen with pramipexole and ropinirole. Bromocriptine is used alone in early PD and in combination with levodopa in advanced PD. When combined with levodopa, bromocriptine can prolong therapeutic responses and reduce motor fluctuations. In addition, since bromocriptine allows the dosage of levodopa to be reduced, the incidence of levodopa-induced dyskinesias may be reduced too.

Adverse Effects. Adverse effects are dose dependent and seen in 30% to 50% of patients. Nausea is most common, occurring in over 50% of those treated. The most common dose-limiting effects are psychologic reactions (confusion, nightmares, agitation, hallucinations, paranoid delusions). These occur in about 30% of patients and are most likely when the dosage is high. Like levodopa, bromocriptine can cause dyskinesias and postural hypotension. Rarely, bromocriptine causes retroperitoneal fibrosis, pulmonary infiltrates, a Raynaud-like phenomenon, and erythromelalgia (vasodilation in the feet, and sometimes hands, resulting in swelling, redness, warmth, and burning pain).

Preparations, Dosage, and Administration. Bromocriptine is available in 5-mg capsules [Parlodel] and 2.5-mg tablets [Parlodel Snap Tabs]. The initial dosage is 1.25 mg twice daily, administered with meals. Dosage is gradually increased until the desired response has been achieved, or until side effects become intolerable. Maintenance dosages range from 30 to 100 mg/day.

Pergolide

Actions, Uses, and Adverse Effects. Pergolide [Permax], an ergot derivative, is similar to bromocriptine with respect to chemistry, actions, uses, and adverse effects. Like other dopamine agonists, pergolide reduces symptoms of PD through direct activation of dopamine receptors in the striatum. When used as an adjunct to levodopa, pergolide can prolong symptomatic control, reduce fluctuations in motor responses, and reduce the incidence of levodopa-induced dyskinesias. Like bromocriptine, pergolide can cause nausea, dyskinesias, postural hypotension, and adverse psychologic reactions (hallucinations, confusion, sedation, paranoid delusions)—as well as rare cases of retroperitoneal fibrosis, pulmonary infiltrates, erythromelalgia, and a Raynaud-like phenomenon.

Preparations, Dosage, and Administration. Pergolide mesylate [Permax] is dispensed in tablets (0.05, 0.25, and 1 mg) for oral use. The recommended initial dosage is 0.05 mg once daily. Dosage is gradually increased to a maximum of 5 mg/day (in three divided doses).

COMT Inhibitors

Two COMT inhibitors are available: entacapone and tolcapone. Benefits of both derive from inhibiting metabolism of levodopa in the periphery; these drugs have no direct therapeutic effects of their own. Rarely, tolcapone has caused fatal liver damage. Accordingly, entacapone is preferred.

Entacapone

Actions and Therapeutic Use. Entacapone [Comtan] is a selective, reversible inhibitor of COMT indicated only for use with levodopa. Like carbidopa, entacapone inhibits metabolism of levodopa in the intestine and peripheral tissues. However, the drugs inhibit different enzymes: carbidopa inhibits decarboxylases, whereas entacapone inhibits COMT. By inhibiting COMT, entacapone prolongs the half-life of levodopa in blood, and thereby prolongs the time that levodopa is available to the brain. In addition, entacapone increases levodopa availability by a second mechanism: By inhibiting COMT, entacapone decreases production of levodopa metabolites that compete with levodopa for transport across the blood-brain barrier. In clinical trials, entacapone increased the half-life of levodopa by 50% to 75%, and thereby caused levodopa blood levels to be smoother and more sustained. As a result, "wearing off" was delayed and "on" times were extended. Entacapone may also permit a reduction in levodopa dosage.

Pharmacokinetics. Entacapone is rapidly absorbed and reaches peak levels in 2 hours. Elimination is by hepatic metabolism followed by excretion in the feces and urine. The plasma half-life is 1.5 to 3.5 hours.

Adverse Effects. Most adverse effects result from increasing levodopa levels, and some are caused by entacapone itself. By increasing levodopa levels, entacapone can cause dyskinesias, orthostatic hypotension, nausea, hallucinations, and sleep disturbances. These can be managed by decreasing levodopa dosage. Entacapone itself can cause vomiting, diarrhea, constipation, and yellow-orange discoloration of the urine.

Drug Interactions. Because it inhibits COMT, entacapone can, in theory, increase levels of drugs that COMT metabolizes. In addition to levodopa, these include methyldopa (an antihypertensive agent), dobutamine (an adrenergic agonist), and isoproterenol (a beta-adrenergic blocker). If entacapone is combined with these drugs, a reduction in their dosages may be needed.

Preparations, Dosage, and Administration. Entacapone [Comtan] is available in 200-mg tablets. The recommended dosage is 200 mg taken with each dose of carbidopa/levodopa—to a maximum of 8 doses (1600 mg) a day.

Tolcapone

Actions and Therapeutic Use. Tolcapone [Tasmar] is a COMT inhibitor used only in conjunction with levodopa—and only if safer agents are ineffective or inappropriate. As with entacapone, benefits derive from inhibiting levodopa metabolism in the periphery, which prolongs levodopa availability. When given to patients taking levodopa, tolcapone improves motor function and may allow a reduction in levodopa dosage. For many patients, the drug reduces the "wearing off" effect that can occur with levodopa, thereby extending levodopa "on" time by as much as 2.9 hours a day. Unfortunately, although tolcapone is effective, it is also dangerous: Deaths from liver failure have occurred. Because it carries a serious risk, tolcapone should be reserved for patients who cannot be treated with safer drugs. Also, when tolcapone *is* used, treatment should be limited to 3 weeks in the absence of a beneficial response.

Pharmacokinetics. Tolcapone is well absorbed following oral administration. Plasma levels peak 2 hours after dosing. In the blood, tolcapone is highly bound (>99.9%) to plasma proteins, primarily albumin. The drug undergoes extensive hepatic metabolism followed by renal excretion. The plasma half-life is 2 to 3 hours.

Adverse Effects. *Liver Failure.* Tolcapone can cause severe hepatocellular injury. At least three patients have died from acute, fulminant liver failure. Prior to treatment, patients should be fully apprised of the risks. Patients with pre-existing liver dysfunction should not take the drug. Patients taking tolcapone should be informed about signs of emergent liver dysfunction (persistent nausea, fatigue, lethargy, anorexia, jaundice, dark urine) and instructed to report these immediately. If liver injury is diagnosed, tolcapone should be discontinued and never used again.

Laboratory monitoring of liver enzymes is required. Tests for serum alanine aminotransferase (ALT) and aspartate aminotransferase (AST) should be conducted prior to treatment and then throughout treatment as follows: every 2 weeks for the first year, every 4 weeks for the next 6 months, and every 8 weeks thereafter. If ALT or AST levels exceed the upper limit of normal, tolcapone should be discontinued. Monitoring may not prevent liver injury, but early detection and immediate drug withdrawal can minimize harm.

Other Adverse Effects. By increasing the availability of levodopa, tolcapone can intensify levodopa-related effects, especially dyskinesias, orthostatic hypotension, nausea, hallucinations, and sleep disturbances; a reduction in levodopa dosage may be required. Tolcapone itself can cause diarrhea, hematuria, and yellow-orange discoloration of the urine. Abrupt withdrawal of tolcapone can produce symptoms that resemble neuroleptic malignant syndrome (fever, muscular rigidity, altered consciousness). In rats, large doses have caused renal tubular necrosis and tumors of the kidneys and uterus.

Preparations, Dosage, and Administration. Tolcapone [Tasmar] is available in 100- and 200-mg tablets, and may be taken with or without food. The usual dosage is 100 mg 3 times a day. The first dose should be administered in the morning along with levodopa. The next two doses are taken 6 and 12 hours later. If necessary, the dosage can be increased to 200 mg 3 times a day. However, elevations in ALT are more likely at the higher dosage.

Selegiline: An MAO-B Inhibitor

Selegiline [Eldepryl, Carbex]—also known as deprenyl—is considered a second- or third-line drug for PD. When combined with levodopa, it can reduce the "wearing-off" effect, but benefits are modest. There is great interest in the possibility that selegiline may be neuroprotective, and hence may delay disease progression. Unfortunately, research has yet to provide any conclusive evidence that selegiline prevents neuronal degeneration. Nonetheless, current guidelines suggest that physicians consider giving selegiline to newly diagnosed patients, just in case the drug *does* confer protection.

Actions and Uses

Selegiline causes *selective, irreversible inhibition of type B monoamine oxidase* (MAO-B), the enzyme that inactivates dopamine in the striatum. Another form of MAO, known as MAO-A, inactivates NE and serotonin. As discussed in Chapter 31, nonselective inhibitors of MAO (i.e., drugs that inhibit MAO-A *and* MAO-B) are used to treat depression—and pose a risk of hypertensive crisis as a side effect. Since selegiline is a selective inhibitor of MAO-B, the drug is not an antidepressant and, at recommended doses, does not present a risk of hypertensive crisis.

Selegiline appears to benefit patients with PD in two ways. First, when used as an adjunct to levodopa, selegiline can suppress destruction of dopamine derived from levodopa. The mechanism is inhibition of MAO-B. By helping preserve dopamine, selegiline can prolong the effects of levodopa, and can thereby decrease fluctuations in motor control. Unfortunately, these benefits decline dramatically within 12 to 24 months.

In addition to preserving dopamine, there is some hope that selegiline may delay the progression of PD. When used early in the disease, selegiline can delay the need for levodopa. This may reflect a delay in the progression of the disease, or it may simply reflect direct symptomatic relief from selegiline itself.

If selegiline does slow the progression of PD, what might be the mechanism? In experimental animals, selegiline can prevent development of parkinsonism following exposure to 1-methyl-4-phenyl-1,2,3,6-tetrahydropyridine (MPTP), a neurotoxin that causes selective degeneration of dopaminergic neurons. (Humans accidentally exposed to MPTP develop severe parkinsonism.) Neuronal degeneration is caused not by MPTP itself but rather by a *toxic metabolite.* Formation of this metabolite is catalyzed by MAO-B. By inhibiting MAO-B, selegiline prevents formation of the toxic metabolite, and thereby protects against neuronal injury. If selegiline does retard progression of PD, this mechanism could explain the effect. That is, just as selegiline protects animals by suppressing formation of a neurotoxic metabolite of MPTP, the drug may retard progression of PD by suppressing formation of a neurotoxic metabolite of an as-yet unidentified compound.

One study raises serious doubts about the benefits of selegiline—and indicates the drug may actually be harmful. In the study, patients were treated either with levodopa alone or with levodopa plus selegiline. After 5 years, the degree of disability in both groups was the same, indicating that selegiline had no long-term effect on disease progression. Even more striking, however, were the data on mortality: The death rate for the group receiving levodopa plus selegiline was nearly double the death rate for the group receiving levodopa alone. Most of the difference could be accounted for by deaths directly due to PD.

Pharmacokinetics

Selegiline is rapidly absorbed following oral administration and readily penetrates the blood-brain barrier. Irreversible inhibition of MAO-B follows. Selegiline undergoes hepatic metabolism followed by renal excretion. Two metabolites—L-amphetamine and L-methamphetamine—are CNS stimulants. These metabolites do not appear to have any beneficial effects, and they can be harmful.

Adverse Effects

When selegiline is used alone, the principal adverse effect is *insomnia,* presumably because of CNS excitation by amphetamine and methamphetamine. Insomnia can be minimized by administering the last daily dose at noon.

Drug Interactions

Levodopa. When used with *levodopa,* selegiline can intensify adverse responses to levodopa-derived dopamine. These reactions—orthostatic hypotension, dyskinesias, and psychologic disturbances (hallucinations, confusion)—can be reduced by decreasing the dosage of levodopa.

Meperidine. Like the nonselective MAO inhibitors, selegiline can cause a dangerous interaction with meperidine [Demerol]. Symptoms include stupor, rigidity, agitation, and hyperthermia. The combination should be avoided.

Fluoxetine. Selegiline should not be combined with fluoxetine [Prozac]. The combination of a nonselective MAO inhibitor plus fluoxetine has been fatal. Although this interaction has not been reported with selegiline, prudence dictates caution. Accordingly, fluoxetine should be withdrawn at least 14 days before giving selegiline.

Preparations, Dosage, and Administration

Selegiline [Eldepryl, Carbex] is available in 5-mg tablets and capsules. The usual dosage is 5 mg taken with breakfast and lunch. Since a total daily dose of 10 mg is sufficient to produce complete inhibition of MAO-B, larger doses are unnecessary.

Amantadine

Actions and Uses. Amantadine [Symmetrel] was developed as an antiviral agent (see Chapter 89), and later found to be effective in PD. Benefits derive primarily from promoting the release of dopamine from surviving dopaminergic terminals in the striatum. The drug may also block dopamine reuptake. Responses develop rapidly—often within 2 to 3 days—but are less profound than with levodopa. Furthermore, responses may begin to diminish within 3 to 6 months. Amantadine is considered a second-line drug for PD.

Adverse Effects. Amantadine can cause adverse *CNS effects* (confusion, lightheadedness, anxiety) and peripheral effects that are thought to result from *muscarinic blockade* (blurred vision, urinary retention, dry mouth, constipation). All of these are generally mild when amantadine is used alone. However, if amantadine is combined with an anticholinergic agent, both the CNS and peripheral responses will be intensified.

Patients taking amantadine for 1 month or longer often develop *livedo reticularis,* a condition characterized by mottled discoloration of the skin. Livedo reticularis is a benign condition that gradually subsides following amantadine withdrawal.

Preparations, Dosage, and Administration. Amantadine [Symmetrel] is dispensed in 100-mg capsules and in a syrup (10 mg/ml). The usual dosage is 100 mg twice daily. Because amantadine is eliminated primarily by the kidneys, dosage must be reduced in patients with renal impairment.

Amantadine often loses effectiveness after several months. If effects diminish, they can be restored by increasing the dosage or by interrupting treatment for several weeks.

Amantadine can enhance responses to levodopa and anticholinergic agents. When combined with these drugs, amantadine is administered in the same doses employed when taken alone.

Centrally Acting Anticholinergic Drugs

Anticholinergic drugs have been used in PD since 1867, making them the oldest medicines for this disease. These drugs alleviate symptoms by blocking muscarinic receptors in the striatum, thereby restoring the functional balance between dopamine and ACh. Anticholinergic drugs can reduce tremor and possibly rigidity, but not bradykinesia. These agents are less effective than levodopa, but better tolerated. Today, anticholinergics are used as second-line therapy for tremor. They are most appropriate for younger patients with mild symptoms. Anticholinergics are generally avoided in the elderly, who are intolerant of CNS side effects (sedation, confusion, delusions, and hallucinations).

Although the anticholinergic drugs used today are somewhat selective for cholinergic receptors in the CNS, they can also block cholinergic receptors in the periphery. As a result, they can cause *dry mouth, blurred vision, photophobia, urinary retention, constipation,* and *tachycardia.* These effects are usually dose limiting. Blockade of cholinergic receptors in the eye may precipitate or aggravate *glaucoma.* Accordingly, intraocular pressure should be measured periodically. Peripheral anticholinergic effects are discussed fully in Chapter 14.

The anticholinergic agents used most often are *trihexyphenidyl* [Artane] and *benztropine* [Cogentin]. Doses are low initially and then gradually increased—until the desired response is achieved or until side effects become intolerable. For trihexyphenidyl, the initial dosage is 1.0 mg once a day, and the maximum dosage is 2 mg 3 times a day. For benztropine, the initial dosage is 0.5 mg twice a day, and the maximum dosage is 2 mg twice a day. If anticholinergic drugs are discontinued abruptly, symptoms of parkinsonism may be intensified. Accordingly, they should be withdrawn gradually.

⁙ KEY POINTS

- Parkinson's disease is a neurodegenerative disorder characterized by tremor at rest, rigidity, postural instability, and bradykinesia.
- The primary pathology in PD is degeneration of neurons in the substantia nigra that supply dopamine to the striatum. The result is an imbalance between dopamine and ACh.
- Parkinson's disease is treated primarily with drugs that directly or indirectly activate dopamine receptors. Drugs that block cholinergic receptors can also be used.
- Levodopa (combined with carbidopa) is the most effective treatment for PD.

- Levodopa relieves symptoms by undergoing conversion to dopamine in surviving nerve terminals in the striatum.
- The enzyme that converts levodopa to dopamine is called a decarboxylase.
- Acute loss of response to levodopa occurs in two patterns: gradual "wearing off," which develops at the end of the dosing interval, and abrupt loss of effect ("on-off" phenomenon), which can occur at any time during the dosing interval.
- The principal adverse effects of levodopa are nausea, dyskinesias, hypotension, and psychosis.
- Conventional antipsychotic drugs block dopamine receptors in the striatum, and can thereby negate the effects of levodopa. Clozapine, an atypical antipsychotic agent, does not block dopamine receptors in the striatum, and hence can be used safely to treat levodopa-induced psychosis.
- Combining levodopa with a nonselective MAO inhibitor can result in hypertensive crisis.
- Because amino acids compete with levodopa for absorption from the intestine and for transport across the blood-brain barrier, high-protein meals can reduce therapeutic effects.
- Carbidopa enhances the effects of levodopa by preventing decarboxylation of levodopa in the GI tract and peripheral tissues. Since carbidopa cannot cross the blood-brain barrier, it does not prevent conversion of levodopa to dopamine in the brain.
- Pramipexole, a dopamine agonist, is a first-line drug for PD. It can be used alone in early PD and combined with levodopa in advanced PD.
- Pramipexole and other dopamine agonists relieve symptoms of PD by causing direct activation of dopamine receptors in the striatum.
- The major adverse effects of pramipexole—nausea, dyskinesia, postural hypotension, and hallucinations—result from excessive activation of dopamine receptors.
- Entacapone, a COMT inhibitor, is combined with levodopa to enhance levodopa effects. The drug inhibits metabolism of levodopa by COMT in the intestine and peripheral tissues, thereby making more levodopa available to the brain.
- Selegiline enhances responses to levodopa by inhibiting MAO-B, the brain enzyme that inactivates dopamine.
- Amantadine relieves symptoms of early PD primarily by promoting release of dopamine from remaining dopaminergic neurons in the striatum.
- Anticholinergic drugs relieve symptoms of PD by blocking cholinergic receptors in the striatum.

Summary of Major Nursing Implications*

LEVODOPA/CARBIDOPA [SINEMET]

Preadministration Assessment

Therapeutic Goal

The goal of treatment is to improve the patient's ability to carry out activities of daily living. Levodopa does not cure PD or delay its progression.

Baseline Data

Assess overt manifestations of PD (bradykinesia, akinesia, postural instability, tremor, rigidity) and the extent to which these interfere with activities of daily living (ability to work, dress, bathe, walk, etc.).

Identifying High-Risk Patients

Levodopa is *contraindicated* for patients with malignant melanoma (it can activate this neoplasm) and for patients taking MAO inhibitors. Exercise *caution* in patients with cardiac disease and psychiatric disorders.

Implementation: Administration

Route

Oral.

Administration

Parkinsonism may render self-medication impossible. Assist the patient with dosing when needed. If appropriate, involve family members in medicating outpatients.

Inform patients that levodopa may be taken with food to reduce nausea and vomiting. However, high-protein meals should be avoided.

If the patient has been taking levodopa alone, allow at least 8 hours between the last dose of levodopa and the first dose of levodopa/carbidopa. The dosage of levodopa in the combination should be reduced to no more than 25% of the dosage employed when levodopa was taken alone.

So that expectations may be realistic, inform patients that effects of levodopa may be delayed for weeks to months. This knowledge will facilitate compliance.

Ongoing Evaluation and Interventions

Evaluating Therapeutic Effects

Evaluate for improvements in activities of daily living and for reductions in bradykinesia, postural instability, tremor, and rigidity.

Managing Acute Loss of Effect

Gradual "wearing off" at the end of the dosing interval can be reduced by using a controlled-release formulation of levodopa/carbidopa, or by adding entacapone or a dopamine agonist to the regimen. **Forewarn patients about possible abrupt loss of therapeutic effects ("on-off" phenomenon) and instruct them to notify the physician if this occurs. Avoiding high-protein meals may help.**

*Patient education information is highlighted as blue text.

Minimizing Adverse Effects

Nausea and Vomiting. Inform patients that nausea and vomiting can be reduced by taking levodopa with food. Instruct patients to notify the physician if nausea and vomiting persist or become severe.

Dyskinesias. Inform patients about possible levodopa-induced movement disorders (tremor, dystonic movements, twitching) and instruct them to notify the physician if these develop.

If the hospitalized patient develops dyskinesias, withhold levodopa and consult the physician about a possible reduction in dosage.

Dysrhythmias. Inform patients about signs of excessive cardiac stimulation (palpitations, tachycardia, irregular heartbeat) and instruct them to notify the physician if these occur.

Orthostatic Hypotension. Inform patients about symptoms of hypotension (dizziness, lightheadedness) and advise them to sit or lie down if these occur. Advise patients to move slowly when assuming an erect posture.

Psychosis. Inform patients about possible levodopa-induced psychosis (visual hallucinations, vivid dreams, paranoia) and instruct them to notify the physician if these develop. Clozapine (an atypical antipsychotic agent) can help.

Minimizing Adverse Interactions

Conventional Antipsychotic Drugs. These can block responses to levodopa and should be avoided. Clozapine, an atypical antipsychotic agent, can be used safely.

MAO Inhibitors. Concurrent use of levodopa and an MAO inhibitor can produce severe hypertension. Withdraw MAO inhibitors at least 2 weeks before initiating levodopa.

Anticholinergic Drugs. These can enhance therapeutic responses to levodopa, but they also increase the risk of adverse psychiatric effects.

High-Protein Meals. Amino acids compete with levodopa for absorption from the intestine and for transport across the blood-brain barrier. **Instruct patients to avoid high-protein meals.**

DOPAMINE AGONISTS

Bromocriptine
Pergolide
Pramipexole
Ropinirole

Preadministration Assessment

Therapeutic Goal

The goal of treatment is to improve the patient's ability to carry out activities of daily living. Dopamine agonists do not cure PD or delay its progression.

Summary of Major Nursing Implications*—cont'd

Baseline Data

Assess overt manifestations of PD (bradykinesia, akinesia, postural instability, tremor, rigidity) and the extent to which these interfere with activities of daily living (ability to work, dress, bathe, walk, etc.).

Identifying High-Risk Patients

Use *all dopamine agonists* with *caution* in elderly patients and in patients with psychiatric disorders. Use *pramipexole* with caution in patients with kidney dysfunction. Avoid *ropinirole* during pregnancy.

Implementation: Administration

Route

Oral.

Administration

Parkinsonism may render self-medication impossible. Assist the patient with dosing when needed. If appropriate, involve family members in medicating outpatients.

Inform patients that dopamine agonists may be taken with food to reduce nausea and vomiting.

To minimize adverse effects, dosage should be low initially and then gradually increased.

Reduce dosage of pramipexole in patients with significant renal dysfunction.

*Patient education information is highlighted as blue text.

Ongoing Evaluation and Interventions

Evaluating Therapeutic Effects

Evaluate for improvements in activities of daily living and for reductions in bradykinesia, postural instability, tremor, and rigidity.

Minimizing Adverse Effects

Nausea and Vomiting. Inform patients that nausea and vomiting can be reduced by taking dopamine agonists with food. Instruct patients to notify the physician if nausea and vomiting persist or become severe.

Orthostatic Hypotension. Inform patients about symptoms of hypotension (dizziness, lightheadedness) and advise them to sit or lie down if these occur. Advise patients to move slowly when assuming an erect posture.

Dyskinesias. Inform patients about possible movement disorders (tremor, dystonic movements, twitching) and instruct them to notify the physician if these develop.

Hallucinations. Forewarn patients that dopamine agonists can cause hallucinations, especially in the elderly, and instruct them to notify the physician if these develop.

Sleep Attacks. Warn patients that *pramipexole* and *ropinirole* may cause sleep attacks. Instruct patients that, if a sleep attack occurs, they should inform the physician and avoid potentially hazardous activities (e.g., driving).

Fetal Injury. Inform women of child-bearing age that *ropinirole* may harm the developing fetus, and advise them to use effective birth control. If pregnancy occurs, switching to a different dopamine agonist is advised.

Alzheimer's Disease

Alzheimer's disease (AD) is a devastating illness characterized by progressive memory loss, impaired thinking, personality change, and inability to perform routine tasks of daily living. AD affects about 2.3 million Americans and kills about 100,000 each year, making it the fourth leading cause of death among adults. The annual cost of AD—over $70 billion—is exceeded only by the costs of heart disease and cancer. Major pathologic findings in AD are degeneration of cholinergic neurons and the presence of neuritic plaques and neurofibrillary tangles. The neuronal damage in AD is irreversible, and hence the disease cannot be cured. Furthermore, we have no highly effective drugs for relieving symptoms, and no prospect of one in the near future.

PATHOPHYSIOLOGY

The underlying cause of AD is unknown. Scientists have discovered important pieces of the AD puzzle, but still don't know how they fit together. It may well be that AD results from a combination of factors, rather than from a single cause.

Degeneration of Neurons

Neuronal degeneration occurs in the hippocampus early in AD, followed later by degeneration of neurons in the cerebral cortex. The hippocampus serves an important role in memory. The cerebral cortex is central to speech, perception, reasoning, and other higher functions. As hippocampal neurons degenerate, short-term memory begins to fail. As cortical neurons degenerate, patients begin having difficulty with language. With advancing cortical degeneration, more severe symptoms appear. These include complete loss of speech, loss of bladder and bowel control, and complete inability for self-care. AD eventually destroys enough brain function to cause death.

Reduced Cholinergic Transmission

In patients with advanced AD, levels of acetylcholine (ACh) are 90% below normal. This dramatic loss contrasts with the small loss that occurs normally with age. Loss of ACh is significant for two reasons. First, ACh is an important transmitter in the hippocampus and cerebral cortex, the regions where neuronal degeneration occurs. Second, ACh is critical to forming memories, and its decline has been linked to memory loss in AD. However, although loss of cholinergic function is clearly important, it cannot be the whole story. Why? Because in 1999, researchers reported that, in patients with *mild* AD, markers for cholinergic transmission are essentially normal. Hence, loss of cholinergic function cannot explain the cognitive deficits that occur early in the disease process.

Neuritic Plaques and Beta-Amyloid

Neuritic plaques, which form outside of neurons, are a hallmark of AD. These spherical bodies are composed of a central core of beta-amyloid (a protein fragment) surrounded by remnants of axons and dendrites. Neuritic plaques are seen mainly in the hippocampus and cerebral cortex. The relationship of neuritic plaques to the disease process is unknown.

In patients with AD, beta-amyloid is present in high levels and may contribute to neuronal injury. Several lines of evidence support this possibility: beta-amyloid can kill hippocampal cells grown in culture; it can release free radicals, which injure cells; it can disrupt potassium channels; and it may form channels in the cell membrane that permit excessive entry of calcium. Also, low doses of beta-amyloid cause vasoconstriction, and high doses cause permanent blood vessel injury (secondary to release of oxygen free radicals). By disrupting blood vessels, beta-amyloid could slowly starve neurons to death. Perhaps the strongest evidence linking beta-amyloid to AD is the observation that injection of the compound directly into the brains of rhesus monkeys produces pathology essentially identical to that of AD. Interestingly, beta-amyloid was harmful only to old monkeys; young monkeys were not affected. This may indicate that, as the brain ages, it produces substances that act in concert with beta-amyloid to permit neurotoxic effects.

Neurofibrillary Tangles and Tau

Like neuritic plaques, neurofibrillary tangles are a prominent feature of AD. These tangles, which form inside neurons, result when the orderly arrangement of microtubules becomes disrupted (Fig. 22–1). The underlying cause is production of an abnormal form of tau, a protein that, in healthy neurons, forms cross-bridges between microtubules, and thereby keeps them in a stable configuration. In patients with AD, tau twists into paired helical filaments. As a result, the orderly arrangement of microtubules transforms into neurofibrillary tangles.

Apolipoprotein E4

Apolipoprotein E (apoE), long known for its role in cholesterol transport, may also contribute to AD. Like some other proteins, apoE has more than one form. In fact, it has three forms, named apoE2, apoE3, and apoE4. (Don't ask what happened to apoE1.) Only one form—apoE4—is associated with AD. Genetics research has shown that individuals with one or two copies of the gene that codes for apoE4 are at increased risk for AD. In contrast, apoE2 seems to protect in some way.

What does apoE4 do? One possibility is that it promotes formation of neuritic plaques. ApoE4 binds quickly and tightly to beta-amyloid, causing this normally soluble substance to become insoluble, which could promote deposition of beta-amyloid in plaque.

It is important to note that apoE4 is neither necessary nor sufficient to cause AD. There are many people with AD who do not have the gene for apoE4. Conversely, in one study involving people who were 90 years old and homozygous for apoE4, 50% had not developed AD.

Endoplasmic Reticulum–Associated Binding Protein

The recent discovery of endoplasmic reticulum–associated binding protein (ERAB) adds another piece to the AD puzzle. Involvement of ERAB in AD is supported by several observations: ERAB is present in high concentration in the brains of patients with AD; ERAB is found in association with beta-amyloid, a compound with neurotoxic effects; high concentrations of ERAB enhance the neurotoxic effects of beta-amyloid; and the neurotoxic effects of beta-amyloid can be blocked by blocking the actions of ERAB.

Homocysteine

Elevated plasma levels of homocysteine are associated with an increased risk of AD. (Homocysteine is an amino acid formed from dietary methionine.) An elevation of 5 mmol/L appears to increase the risk by 40%; an elevation of 14 mmol/L appears to double the risk. How might homocysteine promote AD? One possibility is reduced blood flow secondary to blockage of cerebral blood vessels. (As discussed in Box 48–1, homocysteine is thought to accelerate atherosclerosis.) Another possibility is direct injury to nerve cells. Fortunately, even if homocysteine really does promote AD, the risk can be easily reduced: Levels of homocysteine can be lowered by eating foods rich in folic acid and vitamins B_6 and B_{12}—or by taking dietary supplements that contain these compounds.

RISK FACTORS, SYMPTOMS, AND DIAGNOSIS

Risk Factors

The major known risk factor for AD is advancing age. In 90% of patients, the age of onset is 65 years or older. After age 65, the risk of AD increases exponentially, doubling every 10 years. The only other known risk factor is a family history of AD. Being female *may* be a risk factor. However, the higher incidence of AD in women may occur simply because women live longer than men. *Possible* risk factors include head injury, low educational level, production of apoE4, high levels of homocysteine, and nicotine in cigarette smoke.

Symptoms

Alzheimer's is a disease in which symptoms progress relentlessly from mild to moderate to severe (Table 22–1). Symptoms typically begin after age 65, but may appear in people as young as 40. Early in the disease, patients begin to experience memory loss and confusion. They may be disoriented and get lost in familiar surroundings. Judgment becomes impaired and personality may change. As the disease progresses, patients have increasing difficulty with self-care. Between 70% and 90% eventually develop behavior problems (wandering,

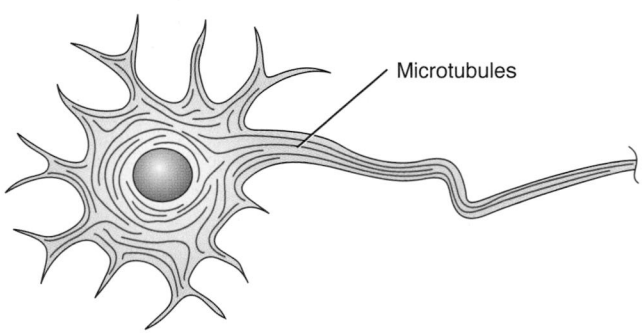

A Normal

Microtubules

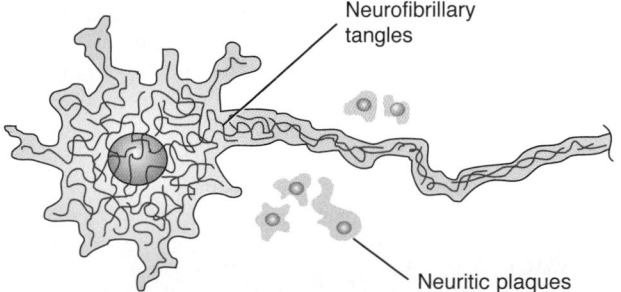

B Alzheimer's Disease

Neurofibrillary tangles

Neuritic plaques

FIGURE 22–1 ■ Histologic changes in Alzheimer's disease. *A*, Healthy neuron. *B*, Neuron affected by Alzheimer's disease, showing characteristic intracellular neurofibrillary tangles. Note also extracellular neuritic plaques.

TABLE 22–1 ■ Symptoms of Alzheimer's Disease
Mild Symptoms
Confusion and memory loss
Disorientation; getting lost in familiar surroundings
Problems with routine tasks
Changes in personality and judgment
Moderate Symptoms
Difficulty with activities of daily living, such as feeding and bathing
Anxiety, suspiciousness, agitation
Sleep disturbances
Wandering, pacing
Difficulty recognizing family and friends
Severe Symptoms
Loss of speech
Loss of appetite; weight loss
Loss of bladder and bowel control
Total dependence on caregiver

pacing, agitation, screaming). Symptoms may intensify in the evening, a phenomenon known as "sundowning." In the final stages of AD, the patient is unable to recognize close family members or communicate in any way. All sense of identity is lost and the patient is completely dependent on others for survival. The time from onset of symptoms to death may be 20 years or longer, but is usually 4 to 8 years. Although there is no clearly effective therapy for *core* symptoms, other symptoms (e.g., incontinence, depression) can be treated. In addition, resources are available to help families cope with AD and prepare for future caregiving needs.

Diagnosis

There is no specific test for AD. Hence, a definitive diagnosis is possible only at autopsy, when the brain can be examined for characteristic neuritic plaques and neurofibrillary tangles. Prior to autopsy, diagnosis is done largely by exclusion. That is, when all other possible causes of dementia have been ruled out, a probable diagnosis of AD can be made. Criteria for a probable diagnosis are summarized in Table 22–2.

DRUG THERAPY

In 2001, the American Academy of Neurology issued evidence-based guidelines that urge early diagnosis and treatment of AD. The guidelines were published as a four-article series in *Neurology* (Vol. 56, 2001) and are available free on the Internet at *www.aan.com/professionals/practice/guidelines.cfm*. Ideally, the goal of treatment is to improve symptoms and reverse decline. However, a more realistic goal is to slow loss of memory and cognition, and to preserve independent function as long as possible. To achieve these goals, the guidelines recommend using a cholinesterase inhibitor (e.g., donepezil [Aricept]) for all patients with mild to moderate disease. Cholinesterase inhibitors modestly improve cognition, behavior, and function, and slightly delay disease progression. The guidelines also recommend considering high-dose vitamin E to slow progression of AD, although the recommendation is not as strong as for cholinesterase inhibitors. Estrogen is specifically excluded as a *treatment* for AD, although it may help *prevent* AD in postmenopausal women. Other recommendations include use of antipsychotics to help manage agitation or psychosis, and antidepressants (especially selective serotonin reuptake inhibitors [SSRIs]) to help manage depression.

TABLE 22–2 ▪ Diagnostic Criteria for Probable Alzheimer's Disease*

- Dementia established by clinical examination, documented by mental status testing, and confirmed by neuropsychological testing
- Deficits in two or more cognitive areas (e.g., memory, attention, language, personality, visuospatial functions)
- Cognitive deterioration is progressive
- Cognitive deterioration occurs in the presence of a clear sensorium (i.e., in the absence of delirium)
- Age of onset is between 40 and 90 years
- The individual has no systemic or other illnesses that affect the brain and that can produce dementia

*Established by the National Institute of Neurological and Communicative Disorders and Stroke (NINCDS) and by the Alzheimer's Disease and Related Disorders Association (ADRDA).

Cholinesterase Inhibitors

Cholinesterase inhibitors are the only drugs approved by the Food and Drug Administration for treatment of AD. These drugs are the best treatment we have for AD, and should be tried in all patients with mild to moderate disease.

Group Properties

Mechanism of Action. Cholinesterase inhibitors prevent the breakdown of ACh by acetylcholinesterase (AChE), and thereby increase the availability of ACh at cholinergic synapses. In patients with AD, the result is enhanced transmission by cholinergic neurons that have not yet been destroyed. Cholinesterase inhibitors do not cure AD, and they do not stop disease progression—although they may *slow* progression by a few months.

Therapeutic Effect. Cholinesterase inhibitors are currently approved for patients with mild to moderate symptoms, and are being studied in patients with more severe symptoms. Among patients with mild to moderate symptoms, only 25% and 30% respond. Among those who do respond, improvements are seen in quality of life and cognitive functions (e.g., memory, thought, reasoning). However, these improvements are modest and short lasting. There is no convincing evidence of marked improvement or significant delay of disease progression. Nonetheless, although improvements are neither universal, dramatic, nor long lasting, and although side effects are common (see below), the benefits still seem well worth the risks—given the devastating effects of AD and the need for any drug that offers some hope of relief.

Adverse Effects. By elevating ACh in the periphery, all cholinesterase inhibitors can cause typical cholinergic effects. Gastrointestinal effects—nausea, vomiting, dyspepsia, diarrhea—occur often. Dizziness and headache are also common. Elevation of ACh at synapses in the lungs can cause bronchoconstriction. Accordingly, cholinesterase inhibitors should be used with caution in patients with asthma or chronic obstructive pulmonary disease (COPD). One drug—tacrine—carries a high risk of liver injury.

Drug Interactions. Drugs that block cholinergic receptors (e.g., first-generation antihistamines, tricyclic antidepressants, conventional antipsychotics) can reduce therapeutic effects, and hence should be avoided.

Dosage and Duration of Treatment. Dosage should be carefully titrated, and treatment should continue as long as clinically indicated. The highest doses produce the greatest benefits—but also the most intense side effects. Accordingly, dosage should be low initially and then gradually increased to the highest tolerable amount. Treatment can continue indefinitely—or until side effects become intolerable or benefits are lost. Abrupt cessation of treatment can lead to rapid progression of symptoms, and hence should be avoided unless cessation is merited owing to severe side effects.

Properties of Individual Cholinesterase Inhibitors

Four cholinesterase inhibitors are available (Table 22–3). Of these, only three are recommended: donepezil, galantamine, and rivastigmine. The fourth—tacrine—carries a significant risk of liver damage, and hence should be avoided. Although the cho-linesterase inhibitors have not been directly compared with one another in clinical trials, they all appear equally effective. Nonetheless, these drugs are not identical. Accordingly, if a patient fails to respond to one, a trial with a another

TABLE 22–3 ▪■ Cholinesterase Inhibitors Used in Alzheimer's Disease

Drug	Year Approved	Dosing Schedule	Mode of Metabolism	Comments
Tacrine [Cognex]	1993	qid, apart from food	Hepatic P450	Rarely used owing to hepatotoxicity and qid dosing
Donepezil [Aricept]	1996	Once daily at bedtime	Hepatic P450	Well tolerated with convenient dosing, hence drug of choice
Rivastigmine [Exelon]	2000	bid, with AM and PM meal	Cholinesterase	Causes "irreversible" inhibition of cholinesterase; no drug interactions
Galantamine [Reminyl]	2001	bid, with AM and PM meal	Hepatic P450	

may be warranted. Because the cholinesterase inhibitors have similar clinical efficacy, selection among them is based on side effects and ease of dosing. Donepezil [Aricept] is better tolerated than the rest and has the simplest dosing schedule (once a day). Accordingly, donepezil is usually preferred.

Tacrine. Tacrine [Cognex], introduced in 1993, was the first cholinesterase inhibitor approved for AD. The drug causes reversible inhibition of AChE. Benefits derive from increasing ACh concentrations at cholinergic synapses in the brain. Tacrine has two major drawbacks: (1) it can cause liver injury, and (2) has a short half-life, and hence must be administered 4 times a day.

Tacrine is administered orally, and food decreases absorption. Bioavailability is low because of substantial first-pass metabolism. Blood levels peak in 2 hours, and decline with an elimination half-life of 3 hours. Tacrine crosses the blood-brain barrier with ease, and is retained in the central nervous system.

Tacrine carries a high risk of serious liver injury. Damage is monitored by assessing serum for elevations in alanine aminotransferase (ALT), an enzyme released from liver cells when they are injured. In 50% of patients taking tacrine, ALT levels are greater than 3 times the amount considered normal. Depending on the degree of ALT elevation and other indices of liver damage (e.g., jaundice, elevation of serum bilirubin), tacrine must be given in reduced dosage or discontinued. In most patients, liver damage reverses after tacrine is withdrawn. The recommended schedule for ALT measurement is every 2 weeks during weeks 4 through 16 of treatment, and every 3 months thereafter. If ALT levels exceed twice normal, more frequent monitoring is required. If ALT levels exceed 5 times normal, tacrine should be discontinued. Treatment can resume when ALT levels return to normal. If the patient develops clinical jaundice (defined here as bilirubin levels above 3 mg/ml), or if there are signs and symptoms of hypersensitivity (e.g., rash, fever) in association with elevated ALT, tacrine should be immediately and permanently discontinued.

Tacrine is dispensed in capsules (10, 20, 30, and 40 mg) for oral administration. Administration is 4 times a day—preferably between meals to enhance absorption. However, tacrine can be given with meals if stomach upset occurs. Dosing is begun at 10 mg 4 times a day, and then gradually increased to a maximum of 40 mg 4 times a day, as tolerated. When treatment is resumed after temporary discontinuation, the original titration sequence should be repeated.

Donepezil. Donepezil [Aricept], approved in 1996, was the second cholinesterase inhibitor approved for AD. The drug is better tolerated and easier to use than other cholinesterase inhibitors, and hence is the current agent of choice. Like tacrine, donepezil causes reversible inhibition of AChE—but is more selective for the form of AChE found in the brain than in the periphery. Therapeutic responses appear equal to those of tacrine. Like tacrine, donepezil does not affect the underlying disease process.

Donepezil is well absorbed following oral administration and undergoes metabolism by hepatic P450 enzymes. Elimination is mainly in the urine and partly in the bile. Donepezil has a prolonged plasma half-life (about 60 hours), and hence can be administered just once a day.

Although donepezil is somewhat selective for brain cholinesterase, it can still cause peripheral cholinergic effects; nausea (11%) and diarrhea (10%) are most common. Bradycardia may also develop, especially in patients with predisposing heart disorders. Unlike tacrine, donepezil is not hepatotoxic.

Donepezil is available in 5- and 10-mg tablets. Dosing is begun at 5 mg once a day, and can be increased to 10 mg once a day.

Rivastigmine. Rivastigmine [Exelon] was approved in 2000, thereby becoming the third cholinesterase inhibitor indicated for AD. Unlike tacrine and donepezil, which cause *reversible* inhibition of AChE, rivastigmine causes *irreversible* inhibition. As with tacrine and donepezil, clinical benefits are modest.

Rivastigmine is well absorbed from the GI tract, especially in the presence of food. In contrast to other cholinesterase inhibitors, rivastigmine is converted to inactive metabolites by AChE, and not by P450 enzymes in the liver.

Like other cholinesterase inhibitors, rivastigmine can cause peripheral cholinergic side effects. The most common are nausea (47%), vomiting (31%), diarrhea (19%), abdominal pain (13%), and anorexia (17%). Significant weight loss (7% of initial weight) occurs in 18% to 26% of patients. By enhancing cholinergic transmission, rivastigmine can intensify symptoms in patients with peptic ulcer disease, bradycardia, sick sinus syndrome, urinary obstruction, and lung disease; caution is advised. In contrast to tacrine, rivastigmine is not hepatotoxic. Rivastigmine has no significant drug interactions—probably because it does not interact with drug-metabolizing enzymes in the liver.

Rivastigmine is available in tablets (1.5, 3, 4.5, and 6 mg) for oral use. The initial dosage is 1.5 mg twice daily. The maximum dosage is 6 mg twice daily. All doses should be administered with food to enhance absorption.

Galantamine. Galantamine [Reminyl], approved in 2001, is a reversible cholinesterase inhibitor indicated for mild to moderate AD. The drug is prepared by extraction from daffodil bulbs. In clinical trials, galantamine improved cognitive function, behavioral symptoms, quality of life, and ability to perform activities of daily living. However, as with other cholinesterase inhibitors, benefits were modest and short lasting.

Galantamine is rapidly and completely absorbed following oral administration. Protein binding in plasma is low. Elimination is by hepatic metabolism and renal excretion. Moderate to severe hepatic or renal impairment delays elimination and increases blood levels. In healthy adults, the half-life is about 7 hours.

The most common adverse effects are nausea (13% to 17%), vomiting (6% to 10%), diarrhea (6% to 12%), anorexia (7% to 9%), and weight loss (5%). Nausea and other GI complaints are greater than with donepezil, but less than with rivastigmine. Like other cholinesterase inhibitors, galantamine can cause bronchoconstriction, and hence must be used with caution in patients with asthma or COPD. Unlike tacrine, galantamine is not hepatotoxic. Drugs that block cholinergic receptors (e.g., first-generation antihistamines, tricyclic antidepressants, typical antipsychotics) can reduce therapeutic effects, and hence should be avoided.

Galantamine is available in tablets (4, 8, and 12 mg) and in solution (4 mg/ml). Dosing is begun at 4 mg twice daily (taken with the morning and evening meals). After a minimum of 4 weeks, dosage may be increased to 8 mg twice daily. Four weeks later, dosage may be increased again to 12 mg twice daily. For patients with moderate hepatic or renal impairment, the maximum dosage is 8 mg twice daily (16 mg/day). For patients with severe hepatic or renal impairment, galantamine should be avoided. For all patients, dosage should be titrated carefully to minimize GI complaints. An antiemetic may be used if needed.

Other Drugs for Alzheimer's Disease
Vitamin E and Selegiline

The treatment guidelines issued by the American Academy of Neurology recommend vitamin E and selegiline as optional treatments for AD. This recommendation is based on a 1997 paper that reported that vitamin E (1000 IU twice daily) and selegiline (5 mg twice daily) can slow disease progression in patients with moderately severe AD. Both drugs have antioxidant properties. The authors hypothesized that benefits derived from decreasing neuronal injury that can be caused by oxidative processes.

Unfortunately, the study had significant problems, and hence the authors' conclusions may not be valid. Most importantly, neither drug was able to slow cognitive decline—the hallmark of AD. Rather, the drugs slightly delayed the time to (1) institutionalization, (2) death, (3) progression to severe dementia, or (4) loss of the ability to perform certain activities of daily living (e.g., eating, using the toilet). Since cognitive decline is a core characteristic of AD, and since the drugs did not retard cognitive decline, it is questionable that they altered the natural course of the disease. The authors' conclusions are further undermined by the observation that giving the drugs together did not yield additive benefits. In fact, benefits were somewhat lower when the drugs were combined. Although the results of this study are encouraging, we need more research to determine if vitamin E and/or selegiline can truly slow the progression of AD.

Nonsteroidal Anti-inflammatory Drugs

There is mounting evidence that long-term use of nonsteroidal anti-inflammatory drugs (NSAIDs) such as ibuprofen, naproxen, and aspirin may protect against development of AD. The most convincing study to date, published in 2001, followed nearly 7000 patients over a 7-year period. All were over the age of 54 and all were taking prescription NSAIDs (e.g., ibuprofen, naproxen)—but not aspirin, which is available without prescription. The results? Taking NSAIDs for 2 years or more—regardless of dosage—decreased the risk of developing AD by 80%. Taking NSAIDs for less than 2 years conferred little or no protection. Furthermore, NSAIDs were of no help if they were taken after symptoms of AD developed, or if they were taken during the 2 year interval prior to symptom onset. This suggests that there is a critical period—which ends 2 years before symptoms begin—during which NSAIDs can be of benefit. Accordingly, for NSAIDs to help, dosing must begin at least 4 years before symptoms would have started. Because protection is conferred at low doses as well as high doses, and because low doses are not anti-inflammatory, it would seem that protection against AD is not due to suppression of inflammation. Instead, there is evidence that NSAIDs may actually help by inhibiting production of Ab_{42}, a specific form of beta-amyloid. Does *aspirin* protect against AD? Yes: Two recent studies suggest that long-term, low-dose aspirin protects against AD, although the degree of protection is not as great as with nonaspirin NSAIDs.

Estrogens

Estrogens may help *prevent* AD, but they are no good for treating existing AD. In a study of postmenopausal women, those who used hormone replacement therapy (HRT) had a 30% to 40% reduction in the risk of AD after 10 years. In those who developed AD despite using HRT, the onset of symptoms was delayed. However, in women who already have AD, estrogens do not reduce symptoms. Accordingly, these drugs are not recommended as treatment.

Ginkgo Biloba

In a 1997 study, an extract made from the leaves of the maidenhair tree (*Ginkgo biloba*) was able to stabilize or improve cognitive performance and social behavior for 6 to 12 months in patients with uncomplicated AD. These benefits are about equal to those seen with tacrine. Patients in the study were given 120 mg/day of a standardized *Gingko biloba* extract containing 24% ginkgo flavonoids and 6% terpenoids, both of which have biologic activity. An equivalent extract—marketed as *Ginkgold*—is available commercially. *Ginkgo biloba* extracts have antioxidant, antiplatelet, and anti-inflammatory actions. The role of these actions in AD is unknown. Significant adverse effects with *Ginkgo biloba* are uncommon. However, because the extract can inhibit platelet aggregation, it may pose a risk of bleeding. Accordingly, combined use with antiplatelet drugs (e.g., aspirin) or anticoagulants (e.g., warfarin, heparin) should be done with caution. *Ginkgo biloba* is discussed further in Chapter 104.

Drugs for Delusions, Agitation, Anxiety, and Depression

Patients with AD may need medication for delusions, agitation, depression, or anxiety. Delusions and agitation may respond to antipsychotics. Conventional agents, such as haloperidol [Haldol], have been used a lot, and their benefits are well established. The newer, atypical agents, such as risperidone [Risperdal] and olanzapine [Zyprexa], also appear effective, and are better tolerated than the older antipsychotics. Anxiety can be lowered with lorazepam [Ativan] or buspirone [BuSpar]. SSRIs, such as fluoxetine [Prozac], can help relieve depression. Tricyclic antidepressants, which have significant anticholinergic actions, should be used with caution, since they may intensify symptoms of AD.

⠢ KEY POINTS

- Alzheimer's disease (AD) is a relentless illness characterized by progressive memory loss, impaired thinking, personality changes, and inability to perform routine tasks of daily living.
- The histopathology of AD is characterized by neuritic plaques, neurofibrillary tangles, and degeneration of cholinergic neurons in the hippocampus and cerebral cortex.
- Neuritic plaques are spherical, extracellular bodies that consist of a beta-amyloid core surrounded by remnants of axons and dendrites.
- In patients with AD, beta-amyloid is present in high levels and may contribute to neuronal injury.
- Neurofibrillary tangles result from production of a faulty form of tau, a protein that in healthy neurons serves to maintain the orderly arrangement of neurotubules.
- The major known risk factor for AD is advancing age.
- Cholinesterase inhibitors (e.g., donepezil) increase the availability of acetylcholine at cholinergic synapses, and thereby enhance transmission by cholinergic neurons that have not yet been destroyed by AD.
- Cholinesterase inhibitors produce modest improvements in cognition, behavior, and function in 30% to 60% of AD patients.
- Cholinesterase inhibitors do not cure AD, and they do not stop disease progression—although they may delay it for a short time.
- The efficacy of all cholinesterase inhibitors appears equal.
- By elevating ACh in the periphery, all cholinesterase inhibitors can cause typical cholinergic effects. Gastrointestinal effects—nausea, vomiting, dyspepsia, diarrhea—are most common.
- Drugs that block cholinergic receptors (e.g., first-generation antihistamines, tricyclic antidepressants, conventional antipsychotics) can reduce responses to cholinesterase inhibitors.
- Donepezil is better tolerated than other cholinesterase inhibitors and more convenient to administer, and hence is the current drug of choice.
- High doses of vitamin E may slow progression of AD.
- Long-term use of NSAIDs may protect against developing AD.

CHAPTER 23

Drugs for Epilepsy

The term *epilepsy* refers to a group of disorders characterized by excessive excitability of neurons within the central nervous system (CNS). This abnormal neuronal activity can produce a variety of symptoms, ranging from brief periods of unconsciousness to violent convulsions. In the United States, 2.3 million people have epilepsy. Every year, 100,000 new cases are diagnosed. The incidence is highest among the elderly. Nonetheless, epilepsy affects about 300,000 children under 14 years old. Between 60% and 70% of patients can be rendered seizure free with drugs. Unfortunately, this means that 30% to 40% cannot.

The terms *seizure* and *convulsion* are not synonymous. *Seizure* is a general term that applies to all types of epileptic events. In contrast, *convulsion* has a more limited meaning, applying only to abnormal motor phenomena, for example, the jerking movements that occur during a tonic-clonic (grand mal) attack. Accordingly, although all convulsions may be called seizures, it is not correct to call all seizures convulsions. Absence seizures, for example, manifest as brief periods of un-consciousness, that may or may not be accompanied by involuntary movements. Since not all epileptic seizures involve convulsions, we will refer to the agents used to treat epilepsy as *antiepileptic drugs* (AEDs), rather than anticonvulsants.

SEIZURE GENERATION

Seizures are initiated by synchronous, high-frequency discharge from a group of hyperexcitable neurons, called a *focus*. A focus may result from several causes, including congenital defects, hypoxia at birth, head trauma, and cancer. Seizures result when discharge from a focus spreads to other brain areas, thereby recruiting normal neurons to discharge abnormally along with the focus.

The overt manifestations of any particular seizure disorder depend on the location of the seizure focus and the neuronal connections to that focus. (The connections to the focus determine the brain areas to which seizure activity can spread.) If seizure activity invades a very limited part of the brain, a partial or local seizure occurs. In contrast, if seizure activity spreads to a large portion of the brain, a generalized seizure develops.

An experimental procedure referred to as *kindling* may explain how a focal discharge is eventually able to generate a seizure. Experimental kindling is performed by implanting a small electrode into the brain of an animal. The electrode is used to deliver localized stimuli for a brief interval once a day. When stimuli are first administered, no seizures result. However, after repeated once-a-day delivery, these stimuli eventually elicit a seizure. If brief, daily stimulations are continued long enough, spontaneous seizures will begin to occur.

The process of kindling may tell us something about seizure development in humans. For example, kindling may account for the delay that can take place between injury to the head and eventual development of seizures. Furthermore, kindling may explain why the seizures associated with some forms of epilepsy become more frequent as time passes. Also, the progressive nature of kindling suggests that early treatment might prevent seizure disorders from becoming more severe over time.

TYPES OF SEIZURES

Seizure can be divided into two broad categories: *partial (focal) seizures* and *generalized seizures*. In partial seizures, seizure activity begins focally in the cerebral cortex and usually undergoes limited spread to adjacent cortical areas. In generalized seizures, focal seizure activity is conducted widely throughout both hemispheres. As a rule, partial seizures and generalized seizures are treated with different drugs (Table 23–1).

TABLE 23–1 ■ Drugs for Specific Types of Seizures

Seizure Type	Drugs Used for Treatment		
	Effective and Well Tolerated	Effective but Less Well Tolerated	Newer Alternatives*
Partial Seizures			
Simple partial	Carbamazepine Oxcarbazepine Phenytoin Valproic acid	Clorazepate Phenobarbital Primidone	Gabapentin Lamotrigine Levetiracetam Topiramate Tiagabine Zonisamide Felbamate†
Complex partial	*Same as simple partial*	*Same as simple partial*	*Same as simple partial*
Secondarily generalized	*Same as simple partial*	Phenobarbital Primidone	Gabapentin Lamotrigine Topiramate Tiagabine Zonisamide Felbamate†
Primary Generalized Seizures			
Tonic-clonic (grand mal)	Carbamazepine Oxcarbazepine Phenytoin Valproic acid	Phenobarbital Primidone	Lamotrigine Topiramate Zonisamide Felbamate†
Absence (petit mal)	Ethosuximide Valproic acid	Clonazepam Trimethadione	Lamotrigine
Myoclonic	Clonazepam Valproic acid		Lamotrigine Topiramate Felbamate†
Atonic	*Same as myoclonic*		*Same as myoclonic*

*These drugs appear effective for the seizures indicated. However, because experience with them is limited, their clinical role has not been firmly established.

†Felbamate can cause aplastic anemia and liver failure, both of which can be fatal. Accordingly, the drug is reserved for patients who have not responded to safer alternatives.

Partial Seizures

Partial seizures fall into three groups: simple partial seizures, complex partial seizures, and partial seizures that evolve into secondarily generalized seizures.

Simple Partial Seizures. These seizures manifest with discrete symptoms that are determined by the brain region involved. Hence, the patient may experience discrete motor symptoms (e.g., twitching thumb), sensory symptoms (e.g., local numbness; auditory, visual, or olfactory hallucinations), autonomic symptoms (e.g., nausea, flushing, salivation, urinary incontinence), or psychoillusory symptoms (e.g., feelings of unreality, fear, or depression). Simple partial seizures are distinguished from complex partial seizures in that there is *no loss of consciousness.* These seizures persist for 20 to 60 seconds.

Complex Partial Seizures. These seizures are characterized by *impaired consciousness* and lack of responsiveness. At seizure onset, the patient becomes motionless and stares with a fixed gaze. This state is followed by a period of *automatism,* in which the patient performs repetitive, purposeless movements, such as lip smacking or hand wringing. Seizures last for 45 to 90 seconds.

Secondarily Generalized Seizures. These seizures begin as simple or complex partial seizures, and then evolve into generalized tonic-clonic seizures. Consciousness is lost. These seizures last for 1 to 2 minutes.

Generalized Seizures

Generalized seizures may be convulsive or nonconvulsive. As a rule, they produce immediate loss of consciousness. The major generalized seizures are discussed briefly below.

Tonic-Clonic Seizures (Grand Mal). In tonic-clonic seizures, neuronal discharge spreads throughout the entire cerebral cortex. These seizures manifest as major convulsions, characterized by a period of muscle rigidity (tonic phase) followed by synchronous muscle jerks (clonic phase). These seizures often cause urination, but not defecation. Convulsions may be preceded by a loud cry, caused by forceful expiration of air across the vocal cords. Tonic-clonic seizures are accompanied by marked impairment of consciousness and are followed by a period of CNS depression, referred to as the *postictal state.* The seizure itself is over in 90 seconds or less.

Absence Seizures (Petit Mal). Absence seizures are characterized by loss of consciousness for a brief time (10 to 30 seconds). Seizures usually involve mild, symmetric motor activity (e.g., eye blinking) but may occur with no motor activity at all. The patient may experience hundreds of absence attacks a day. Absence seizures occur primarily in children and usually cease during the early teens.

Atonic Seizures. These seizures are characterized by sudden loss of muscle tone. If seizure activity is limited to the muscles of the neck, "head drop" occurs. However, if the muscles of the limbs and trunk are involved, a "drop attack" can occur, causing the patient to suddenly collapse. Atonic seizures occur mainly in children.

Myoclonic Seizures. These seizures consist of sudden muscle contractions that last for just 1 second. Seizure activity may be limited to one limb (focal myoclonus) or it may involve the entire body (massive myoclonus).

Status Epilepticus. Status epilepticus (SE) is defined as a seizure that persists for 30 minutes or more. There are several types of SE, including generalized convulsive SE, absence SE, and myoclonic SE. Generalized convulsive SE, which can be life threatening, is discussed later.

Febrile Seizures. Fever-associated seizures are common among children ages 6 months to 5 years. Febrile seizures typically manifest as generalized tonic-clonic convulsions of short duration. Children who experience these seizures are *not* at high risk of developing epilepsy later in life.

HOW ANTIEPILEPTIC DRUGS WORK

We have long known that AEDs can (1) suppress discharge of neurons within a seizure focus and (2) suppress propagation of seizure activity from the focus to other areas of the brain. However, until recently we did not know how these effects were achieved. It now appears that AEDs act through three basic mechanisms: suppression of sodium influx, suppression of calcium influx, and potentiation of gamma-aminobutyric acid (GABA).

Suppression of Sodium Influx. Before discussing AED actions, we need to review sodium channel physiology. Neuronal action potentials are propagated by influx of sodium through sodium channels, which are gated pores in the cell membrane that control sodium entry. For sodium influx to occur, the channel must be in an *activated state.* Immediately following sodium entry, the channel goes into an *inactivated state,* during which further sodium entry is prevented. Under normal circumstances, the inactive channel very quickly returns to the activated state, thereby permitting more sodium entry and propagation of another action potential.

Several AEDs, including phenytoin, carbamazepine, valproic acid, and lamotrigine, reversibly bind to sodium channels while they are in the inactivated state, and thereby prolong channel inactivation. By delaying return to the active state, these drugs decrease the ability of neurons to fire at high frequency. As a result, seizures that depend on high-frequency discharge are suppressed.

Suppression of Calcium Influx. Valproic acid and ethosuximide, which are used to treat absence seizures, act by inhibiting influx of calcium ions through a special class of calcium channels, known as *T-type calcium channels.* In most neurons, T currents (the electric currents generated by influx of calcium ions through T-type channels) play a minimal role in action potential generation. However, in certain neurons of the hypothalamus, T currents are large enough to cause an action potential. This is significant because these same hypothalamic neurons are responsible for generating absence seizures. Hence, by blocking calcium inflow through T-type channels, valproic acid and ethosuximide are able to suppress generation of absence seizures.

Potentiation of GABA. Several AEDs potentiate the actions of GABA, an inhibitory neurotransmitter that is widely distributed throughout the brain. By augmenting the inhibitory influence of GABA, these drugs decrease neuronal excitability and thereby suppress seizure activity. Drugs increase the influence of GABA by several mechanisms. Benzodiazepines and barbiturates enhance the effects of GABA by mechanisms that involve direct binding to GABA receptors. Gabapentin acts by promoting GABA release. Vigabatrin inhibits the enzyme that degrades GABA, and thereby increases GABA availability. Tiagabine inhibits GABA reuptake.

GENERAL THERAPEUTIC CONSIDERATIONS

Therapeutic Goal and Treatment Options

The goal in treating epilepsy is to reduce seizures to an extent that enables the patient to live a normal or near-normal life. Ideally, treatment should eliminate seizures entirely. However, this may not be possible without causing intolerable side effects. Hence, we must balance the desire for complete seizure control against the acceptability of undesired side effects.

Epilepsy may be treated with drugs or with nondrug therapies. As noted, drugs can benefit 60% to 70% of patients. This means that, of the 2.3 million Americans with epilepsy, between 690,000 and 920,000 *cannot* be treated successfully with drugs. For these people, nondrug therapy may well help. Three options exist: surgery, vagal nerve stimulation, and the ketogenic diet. Of the three, surgery has the best success rate. All three nondrug therapies are discussed in Box 23–1.

Diagnosis and Drug Selection

Control of seizures requires proper drug selection. As indicated in Table 23–1, many AEDs are selective for specific seizure disorders. Phenytoin, for example, is useful for treating tonic-clonic and partial seizures but not absence seizures. Conversely, ethosuximide is active against absence seizures but does not work against tonic-clonic or partial seizures. Only one drug—valproic acid—appears effective against practically all forms of epilepsy. Since most AEDs are selective for specific seizure disorders, effective treatment requires a proper match between the drug and the seizure. To make this match, the seizure type must be accurately diagnosed.

Making a diagnosis requires physical, neurologic, and laboratory evaluations along with a thorough history. The history should determine the age at which seizures began, the frequency and duration of seizure events, precipitating factors, and times when seizures occur. Physical and neurologic evaluations may reveal signs of head injury or other disorders that could underlie seizure activity, although in many patients the physical and neurologic evaluations may be normal. An elec-

Special Interest Topic

BOX 23–1 ■■ NONDRUG THERAPIES FOR EPILEPSY: SURGERY, VAGUS NERVE STIMULATION, AND THE KETOGENIC DIET

Surgery: The Cure That's Rarely Used

Surgical treatment of epilepsy is highly effective, yet used only rarely. For more than 100 years, surgical intervention has been the only *cure* for epilepsy. (Although drugs can control symptoms, they don't offer a cure.) The safety and efficacy of surgery have been documented in literally thousands of papers. Among patients with forms of epilepsy that can be treated surgically, the procedure can render between 70% and 90% seizure free—and, even when seizures do continue, their frequency is often decreased. This degree of success is all the more remarkable when we consider that, in order to qualify for surgery, candidates must first be proved refractory to drugs. Put another way, surgery is only performed on patients who have epilepsy that is especially hard to treat. Yet, despite its proven efficacy, surgery remains grossly underutilized: Each year, only 1500 surgeries are performed, although more than 100,000 patients are eligible. This is especially unfortunate because, among people who are refractory to drugs, surgery can greatly improve seizure control, thereby improving quality of life, along with attendance at work and at school.

Vagus Nerve Stimulation: Fighting Impulses with Impulses

The vagus nerve stimulator (VNS) is the first medical device for reducing seizures. The only commercial VNS, known as the NeuroCybernetic Prosthesis System, received FDA approval in 1997. This system is intended for use in conjunction with drugs by patients with severe, uncontrolled seizures. Responses to vagal stimulation develop slowly: Initial responses usually occur in 3 months, but full responses take longer to develop.

The heart of the VNS is a small, programmable pulse generator that is implanted under the collarbone, much like a cardiac pacemaker. Subcutaneous leads connect the generator to the left branch of the vagus nerve in the neck. Stimulation is typically applied for 30 seconds every 5 minutes around the clock. When needed, stimulation parameters (voltage, frequency, duration) can be adjusted externally by the physician. By holding a small magnet over the generator, patients can activate the device manually if they feel a seizure coming on. In addition, patients can use the magnet to turn the generator off. VNS batteries last 3 to 5 years. Replacement is done in an outpatient procedure that takes 30 to 60 minutes.

In clinical trials, some patients responded dramatically and most showed at least some improvement. However, with a few patients, seizures *increased.* Specific results were as follows:

- In 26% of patients, seizure frequency decreased by 25% to 50%.
- In 11% of patients, seizure frequency decreased by more than 75%.
- In one patient, seizures stopped entirely.
- In 6% of patients, seizure frequency increased.

Vagal stimulation does not eliminate the need for drugs—but it can permit a simpler regimen. Up to 50% of patients can decrease the number of drugs they are taking (e.g., two instead of three; one instead of two). Please note, however, that stimulation does *not* permit a reduction in dosage of the drugs that remain.

Vagal stimulation is well tolerated by most patients, although side effects are very common. During stimulation, patients experience hoarseness (100%), coughing (50%), voice alteration (73%), and shortness of breath (25%). In addition, there is a 2% to 3% risk of infection at the implant site. Stimulation does not cause cognitive effects and, perhaps surprisingly, does not cause autonomic effects (e.g., bradycardia, GI disturbances, hypotension).

How does vagal stimulation decrease seizure frequency? No one knows. What we do know is that vagal fibers project to the brainstem, and from there to areas of the brain involved in seizure generation. When we stimulate the vagus, the resultant impulses in some way interrupt or prevent abnormal neuronal firing.

The Ketogenic Diet: It's Tough but It Works

The ketogenic diet for epilepsy can decrease seizure frequency, but it's hard to implement and potentially dangerous. The diet was introduced in the 1920s, but fell out of use when AEDs became available. Today, the diet is under renewed study as a way to control seizures when drug therapy fails. Because the diet is both difficult and hazardous, close medical supervision is essential.

The ketogenic diet has two cornerstones: high intake of fat and very low intake of carbohydrates. Fats—usually butter or heavy cream—comprise 80% of daily calories. In contrast, the carbohydrate allowance very low—so low, in fact, that the sugar in a dose of valproic acid [Depakene] syrup would exceed the daily limit. With strict adherence to the diet, ketosis develops in a few days. However, with just a minor deviation from the diet (e.g., ingestion of two cookies), ketosis will be lost in hours.

How does a high-fat, low-carbohydrate diet reduce seizures? By causing ketoacidosis. Because carbohydrate availability is low, the body burns fat to meet its needs. Burning fat produces large amounts of ketone bodies (beta-hydroxybutyric acid, acetoacetic acid, acetone), whose presence creates a state of ketoacidosis. For reasons that are unclear, ketoacidosis can decrease seizures in some patients.

The principal candidates for dietary therapy are children under the age of 10 who have not responded to AEDs. Depending on the child, the ketogenic diet may be very effective, moderately effective, or ineffective. In clinical trials, about one-third of children became seizure free and were able to discontinue AEDs; one-third showed some improvement but still required AEDs; and one-third failed to benefit at all.

Continued.

troencephalogram (EEG) is essential for diagnosis. Other diagnostic tests that may be employed include computerized tomography (CT), positron emission tomography (PET), and magnetic resonance imaging (MRI).

Very often, patients must try several AEDs before a regimen that is both effective and well tolerated can be established. Initial treatment should be done with just one AED. If this drug fails, it should be discontinued and a different AED should be tried. If this second drug fails, two options are open: (1) treatment with a third AED alone, or (2) treatment with a combination of two AEDs.

Drug Evaluation

Once an AED has been selected, a trial period is needed to determine its effectiveness. During this time there is no guarantee that seizures will be controlled. Accordingly, until seizure control is certain, the patient should be warned not to participate in activities that could be hazardous if a seizure were to occur (e.g., driving, operating dangerous machinery).

During the process of drug evaluation, adjustments in dosage are often needed. No drug should be considered ineffective until it has been tested in sufficiently high dosage and for a reasonable time. Knowledge of plasma drug levels can be a valuable tool for establishing dosage and evaluating the effectiveness of a specific drug.

Maintenance of a seizure frequency chart is essential for evaluating treatment. The chart should be maintained by the patient or a family member and should contain a complete record of all seizure events. This record will enable the physician to determine if treatment has been effective. The nurse should teach the patient how to create and use a seizure frequency chart.

Monitoring Plasma Drug Levels

Monitoring plasma levels of AEDs is common. Safe and effective plasma levels have been firmly established for older AEDs (see Table 23-2), although they have not been established for newer AEDs. For those drugs whose therapeutic level has been established, knowledge of the plasma level can help guide dosage adjustments.

Monitoring plasma drug levels is especially helpful when treating major convulsive disorders (e.g., tonic-clonic seizures). Since these seizures can be dangerous, and since delay of therapy may allow the condition to worsen, rapid control of seizures is desirable. However, since these seizures occur infrequently, a long time may be needed to establish control if clinical outcome is relied on as the only means of determining an effective dosage. By adjusting initial doses on the basis of plasma drug levels (rather than on the basis of seizure control), we can readily achieve drug levels that are likely to be effective, thereby increasing our chances of establishing control quickly.

Measurements of plasma drug levels are not especially important for determining effective dosages for absence seizures. Because absence seizures occur very frequently (up to several hundred a day), observation of the patient is the best means for establishing an effective dosage: if seizures stop, dosage is sufficient; if seizures continue, more drug is needed.

In addition to serving as a guide for dosage adjustment, knowledge of plasma drug levels can serve as an aid to (1) monitoring compliance, (2) determining the cause of lost seizure control, and (3) identifying causes of toxicity, especially in patients taking more than one drug.

Promoting Compliance

Epilepsy is a chronic condition that requires regular and continuous therapy. As a result, seizure control is highly dependent on patient compliance. In fact, it is estimated that noncompliance accounts for about 50% of all treatment failures. Accordingly, promoting compliance should be a priority for all members of the healthcare team. Measures that can help compliance include

- Educating patients and families about the chronic nature of epilepsy and the importance of adhering to the prescribed regimen
- Monitoring plasma drug levels so as to encourage and evaluate compliance
- Deepening patient and family involvement by having them maintain a seizure frequency chart.

Withdrawing Antiepileptic Drugs

Some forms of epilepsy undergo spontaneous remission; hence discontinuing treatment may at some time be appropriate. Unfortunately, there are no firm guidelines to indicate the most appropriate time to withdraw AEDs. However, once the decision to discontinue treatment has been made, agreement does exist on how drug withdrawal should be accomplished. *The most important rule is that AEDs be withdrawn slowly (over a period of 6 weeks to several months).* Failure to gradually reduce dosage is a frequent cause of SE. If the patient is taking two drugs to control seizures, they should be withdrawn sequentially, not simultaneously.

BASIC PHARMACOLOGY OF THE ANTIEPILEPTIC DRUGS

The AEDs can be grouped into two major categories: *older (conventional)* AEDs and *newer* AEDs. The drugs that we classify as older were introduced before 1990, and the ones

TABLE 23–2 ▌■ Clinical Pharmacology of the Antiepileptic Drugs

Drug	Product Name	Dosing Schedule	Daily Maintenance Dosage		Target Serum Level* (μg/ml)	Induces Hepatic Drug Metabolism
			Adults (mg)	Children (mg/kg)		
Conventional Antiepileptic Drugs						
Carbamazepine	Tegretol	tid–qid	600–1800	10–35	6–12	Yes
	Tegretol-XR	bid				
	Carbatrol	bid				
Ethosuximide	Zarontin	qd–bid	750	15–40	40–100	No
Phenobarbital	(generic)	qd–bid	60–100	3–6	15–40	Yes
Phenytoin	Phenytoin, prompt	bid–tid	200–300	4–8	10–20	Yes
	Dilantin Infatab	bid–tid				
	Dilantin suspension	bid–tid				
	Phenytoin, extended	qd				
	Dilantin Kapseals	qd				
Primidone	Mysoline	tid–qid	500–750	10–25	5–15†	Yes
Valproic acid	Depakene	tid–qid	750–3000	15–45	50–150	No
	Depakote					
	Depakote ER	bid				
Newer Antiepileptic Drugs						
Felbamate	Felbatol	tid	2400–3600	15–45	ND	No
Gabapentin	Neurontin	tid	1200–3600	25–50	ND	No
Lamotrigine	Lamictal	bid	400‡§	5‡§	ND	No
Levetiracetam	Keppra	bid	2000–3000	40–60	ND	No
Oxcarbazepine	Trileptal	bid	900–2400	30–46	ND	No‖
Tiagabine	Gabitril	bid–qid	16–32	0.4§	ND	No
Topiramate	Topamax	bid	200–400	3–9	ND	No
Zonisamide	Zonegran	qd–bid	200–400	4–12	ND	No

*ND = not determined.

†Target serum level is 5–15 μg/ml for primidone itself, and 15–40 μg/ml for phenobarbital derived from primidone.

‡Dosage must be decreased in patients taking valproic acid.

§Dosage must be increased in patients taking drugs that induce hepatic drug-metabolizing enzymes.

‖Oxcarbazepine does not induce enzymes that metabolize AEDs, but does induce enzymes that metabolize other kinds of drugs.

we classify as newer were introduced after 1990. Because we have much more clinical experience with the older agents, these drugs are generally preferred to the newer ones. Drugs that belong to each category are indicated in Table 23–2.

The AEDs used most frequently are phenytoin, carbamazepine, valproic acid, and ethosuximide—all of which are in the conventional category. Most of our discussion focuses on these drugs.

Applications of the AEDs are summarized in Table 23–1. Dosages and therapeutic levels are summarized in Table 23–2.

Phenytoin

Phenytoin [Dilantin] is probably our most widely used AED—despite having tricky kinetics and troublesome adverse effects. The drug is active against partial seizures as well as primary generalized tonic-clonic seizures. Phenytoin is of historic importance in that it was the first drug to suppress seizures without producing generalized depression of the CNS. Hence, phenytoin heralded the development of selective medications that could treat epilepsy while leaving most CNS functions undiminished.

Mechanism of Action

At the concentrations achieved clinically, phenytoin causes selective inhibition of sodium channels. Specifically, the drug slows recovery of sodium channels from their inactive state back to their active state. As a result, entry of sodium into neurons is inhibited, and hence action potentials are suppressed. Blockade of sodium entry is limited to neurons that are hyperactive. Therefore, the drug suppresses activity of seizure-generating neurons while leaving healthy neurons unaffected.

Pharmacokinetics

Phenytoin has unusual pharmacokinetics that must be accounted for in therapy. Absorption of the drug varies substantially among patients. In addition, because of saturable kinetics, small changes in dosage can produce disproportionately large changes in serum drug levels. As a result, a dosage that is both effective and safe is difficult to establish.

Absorption. Absorption varies between the different oral formulations of phenytoin. With some—Dilantin Infatab, Dilantin suspension, phenytoin (prompt)—absorption is relatively fast, whereas with others—Dilantin Kapseals, phenytoin (extended)—absorption is delayed and prolonged.

In the past, there was concern that absorption also varied between preparations of phenytoin made by different manufacturers. However, it is now clear that all Food and Drug Administration (FDA)–approved equivalent products have equivalent bioavailability. As a result, switching from one brand of phenytoin to another produces no more variability than switching between lots of phenytoin produced by the same manufacturer.

Metabolism. The capacity of the liver to metabolize phenytoin is very limited. As a result, the relationship between dosage and plasma levels of phenytoin is unusual. Doses of phenytoin needed to produce therapeutic effects are only slightly smaller than the doses needed to saturate the hepatic enzymes that metabolize phenytoin. Consequently, if phenytoin is administered in doses only slightly greater than those needed for therapeutic effects, the liver's capacity to metabolize the drug will be overwhelmed, causing plasma levels of phenytoin to rise dramatically. This unusual relationship between dosage and plasma levels is illustrated in Figure 23–1*A*. As we can see, once plasma levels have reached the therapeutic range, small changes in dosage produce large changes in drug levels. As a result, small increases in dosage can cause toxicity, and small decreases can cause therapeutic failure. This relationship makes it difficult to establish and maintain a dosage that is both safe and effective.

Figure 23–1*B* indicates the relationship between dosage and plasma drug levels that exists for most drugs. As we can see here, this relationship is *linear,* in contrast to the nonlinear relationship that exists for phenytoin. Accordingly, for most drugs, if the patient is taking doses that produce plasma levels that are within the therapeutic range, small deviations from that dosage produce only small deviations in plasma drug levels. Because of this relationship, for most drugs it is relatively easy to maintain plasma levels that are safe and effective.

Because of saturation kinetics, the half-life of phenytoin varies with dosage. At low doses, the half-life is relatively short—about 8 hours. However, at higher doses, the half-life becomes prolonged—in some cases up to 60 hours. Why? Because, at higher doses, there is more drug present than the liver can process. As a result, metabolism is delayed, causing the half-life to increase.

Therapeutic Uses

Epilepsy. Phenytoin can be used to treat all major forms of epilepsy except absence seizures. The drug is especially effective against tonic-clonic seizures, and is a drug of choice for treating these in adults and older children. (Carbamazepine is preferred to phenytoin for treating tonic-clonic seizures in young children.) Although phenytoin can be used to treat simple and complex partial seizures, the drug is less effective against these seizures than against tonic-clonic seizures. Phenytoin can be administered IV to treat generalized convulsive SE. However, other drugs are preferred.

Cardiac Dysrhythmias. Phenytoin is active against certain types of dysrhythmias. Antidysrhythmic applications are discussed in Chapter 47.

Adverse Effects

Effects on the CNS. Although phenytoin acts on the CNS in a relatively selective fashion to suppress seizures, the drug is not completely devoid of CNS side effects—especially when dosage is excessive. At therapeutic levels (10 to 20 μg/ml), sedation and other CNS effects are mild. At plasma levels above 20 μg/ml, toxic effects can occur. Nystagmus (continuous back-and-forth movements of the eyes) is relatively common. Other manifestations of excessive dosage include sedation, ataxia (staggering gait), diplopia (double vision), and cognitive impairment.

Gingival Hyperplasia. Gingival hyperplasia (excessive growth of gum tissue) is characterized by swelling, tenderness, and bleeding of the gums. This effect occurs in about 20% of patients. Gingival hyperplasia can be minimized by good oral hygiene, including dental flossing and gum massage. Patients should be given instruction in these techniques and encouraged to practice them. In some cases, gingival hyperplasia is so great as to require gingivectomy (surgical removal of excess gum tissue).

Skin Rash. Between 2% and 5% of patients develop a morbilliform (measles-like) rash. Rarely, morbilliform rash

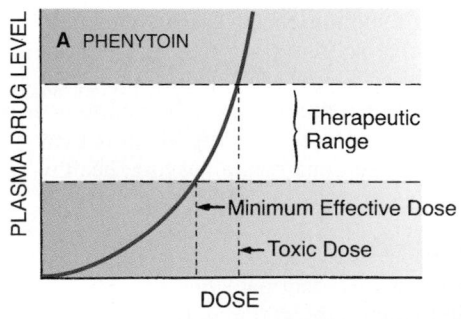
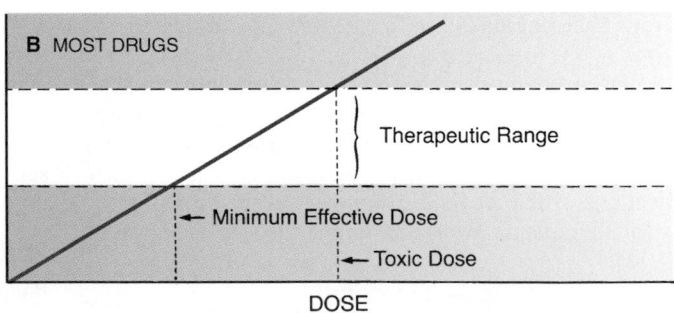

Figure 23–1 ■ Relationship between dose and plasma level for phenytoin compared with most other drugs.
A, Within the therapeutic range, small increments in phenytoin dosage produce sharp increases in plasma drug levels. This relationship makes it difficult to maintain plasma phenytoin levels within the therapeutic range.
B, Within the therapeutic range, small increments in dosage produce small increases in drug levels. With this relationship, moderate fluctuations in dosage are unlikely to result in either toxicity or loss of therapeutic effects.

progresses to exfoliative dermatitis or Stevens-Johnson syndrome (an inflammatory skin disease characterized by red macules, papules, and tubercles). If a rash develops, phenytoin should be discontinued.

Effects in Pregnancy. Phenytoin is a teratogen in animals and humans. In animals, the drug can cause cleft palate, hydrocephalus, renal defects, and micromelia (small or shortened limbs). In humans, phenytoin can cause cleft palate, heart malformations, and *fetal hydantoin syndrome,* characterized by growth deficiency, motor or mental deficiency, microcephaly, craniofacial distortion, positional deformities of the limbs, hypoplasia of the nails and fingers, and impaired neurodevelopment. Accordingly, phenytoin should be used during pregnancy only if the benefits of seizure control outweigh the risk to the fetus.

Phenytoin can decrease synthesis of vitamin K–dependent clotting factors, and can thereby cause *bleeding tendencies in newborns.* The risk of neonatal bleeding can be decreased by giving the mother prophylactic vitamin K for 1 month prior to delivery and during delivery and to the infant immediately after delivery.

Cardiovascular Effects. When phenytoin is administered by IV injection (to treat SE), cardiac dysrhythmias and hypotension may result. These dangerous responses can be minimized by injecting phenytoin slowly and in dilute solution.

Other Adverse Effects. *Hirsutism* (overgrowth of hair in unusual places) can be a disturbing response, especially in young women. Interference with vitamin D metabolism may cause *rickets* and *osteomalacia* (softening of the bones). Interference with vitamin K metabolism can lower prothrombin levels, thereby causing *bleeding tendencies in newborns.*

Drug Interactions

Phenytoin interacts with a large number of drugs. The more important interactions are discussed below.

Interactions Resulting from Induction of Hepatic Drug-Metabolizing Enzymes. Phenytoin stimulates synthesis of hepatic drug-metabolizing enzymes. As a result, phenytoin can decrease the effects of other drugs, including *oral contraceptives, warfarin* (an anticoagulant), and *glucocorticoids* (anti-inflammatory/immunosuppressive drugs). Because avoiding pregnancy is desirable while taking antiseizure medications, and because phenytoin can decrease the effectiveness of oral contraceptives, women should increase the dosage of the contraceptive.

Drugs That Increase Plasma Levels of Phenytoin. Since the therapeutic range of phenytoin is narrow, slight increases in phenytoin levels can cause toxicity. Consequently, caution must be exercised when phenytoin is used with drugs that can increase its level. Drugs known to elevate phenytoin levels include *diazepam* (an antianxiety agent and AED), *isoniazid* (a drug for tuberculosis), *cimetidine* (a drug for gastric ulcers), and *alcohol* (when taken acutely). These agents increase phenytoin levels by reducing the rate at which phenytoin is metabolized. *Valproic acid* (an AED) elevates levels of free phenytoin by displacing phenytoin from binding sites on plasma proteins.

Drugs That Decrease Plasma Levels of Phenytoin. *Carbamazepine* and *phenobarbital,* and *alcohol* when used chronically, can accelerate the metabolism of phenytoin, thereby decreasing its level. Breakthrough seizures can result.

CNS Depressants. The depressant effects of *alcohol, barbiturates,* and *other CNS depressants* will add to those of phenytoin. Advise patients to avoid alcohol and all other drugs with CNS-depressant properties.

Preparations, Dosage, and Administration

Preparations. Phenytoin [Dilantin] is available in solution for injection and in four oral formulations: chewable tablets [Dilantin Infatab], oral suspension [Dilantin-125], prompt-acting capsules, and extended-release capsules [Dilantin Kapseals]. Phenytoin products made by different manufacturers have equivalent bioavailability. Hence, although switching between products from different manufacturers was a concern in the past, it is not a concern today.

Dosage. *Dosing is highly individualized.* Initial doses are usually given twice daily. Once a maintenance dosage has been established, once-a-day dosing is often possible (using extended-release capsules). For *adults,* a typical initial dosage is 150 mg twice a day; maintenance dosages usually range between 200 and 300 mg/day. For *children,* a typical initial dosage is 2.5 mg/kg twice a day; maintenance dosages usually range between 4 and 8 mg/kg/day.

Plasma drug levels are often monitored as an aid to dosage determination. *The dosing objective is to produce levels between 10 and 20 μg/ml.* Levels below 10 μg/ml are too low to control seizures; at levels above 20 μg/ml, signs of toxicity begin to appear. Because phenytoin has a relatively narrow therapeutic range (between 10 and 20 μg/ml), and because of the nonlinear relationship between phenytoin dosage and phenytoin plasma levels, *once a safe and effective dosage has been established, the patient should adhere to it rigidly, because small deviations from the established dosage can cause toxicity or therapeutic failure.*

When treatment with phenytoin is discontinued, dosage should be reduced gradually. Abrupt withdrawal may precipitate seizures.

Administration. *Oral* preparations may cause gastric discomfort. Patients should be informed that gastric upset can be reduced by administering phenytoin with or immediately after a meal. Patients using the oral suspension should shake it well before dispensing, since failure to do so can result in uneven dosing.

Intravenous administration is used to treat generalized convulsive SE. *It is imperative that infusions be performed slowly* (no faster than 50 mg/min). Why? Because rapid administration can cause cardiovascular collapse. Phenytoin should not be added to an existing IV infusion, since mixing phenytoin with other solutions is likely to produce a precipitate. Solutions of phenytoin are highly alkaline and can cause local venous irritation. Irritation can be reduced by flushing the IV needle or catheter with sterile saline immediately after completing the infusion.

Fosphenytoin

Fosphenytoin [Cerebyx] is a prodrug form of phenytoin used to treat convulsive SE. The drug is administered IV and undergoes immediate conversion to phenytoin in the blood. Fosphenytoin differs from phenytoin in two important ways: (1) solutions are prepared in 0.5% dextrose or 0.9% saline (compared with ethylene glycol for phenytoin), and (2) solutions have a neutral pH (compared with pH 12 for phenytoin). As a result, solutions of fosphenytoin do not irritate veins. In addition, fosphenytoin can be infused faster than phenytoin (150 mg/min versus 50 mg/min) without risking cardiovascular collapse. Obviously, rapid administration is a benefit when treating convulsive SE.

Carbamazepine

Carbamazepine [Tegretol, Carbatrol, others] is a mainstay of epilepsy therapy. The drug is active against partial seizures and tonic-clonic seizures but not absence seizures.

Mechanism of Action

Carbamazepine suppresses high-frequency neuronal discharge in and around seizure foci. The mechanism appears to be the same as that of phenytoin: delayed recovery of sodium channels from their inactivated state.

Pharmacokinetics

Absorption of carbamazepine is delayed and variable. Peak levels are achieved in 4 to 12 hours. Overall bioavailability is about 80%. The drug distributes well to tissues.

Elimination is by hepatic metabolism. Carbamazepine is unusual in that its half-life decreases as therapy progresses. During the initial phase of treatment, the half-life is about 40 hours. The half-life decreases to about 15 hours with continued treatment. Why? Because carbamazepine, like phenytoin and phenobarbital, induces hepatic drug-metabolizing enzymes; by increasing its own metabolism, carbamazepine causes its own half-life to decline.

Therapeutic Uses

Epilepsy. Carbamazepine is effective against tonic-clonic, simple partial, and complex partial seizures. Because the drug causes fewer adverse effects than phenytoin and phenobarbital, it is often preferred to these agents. Many clinicians consider carbamazepine the drug of first choice for partial seizures. Carbamazepine is not effective against absence, myoclonic, or atonic seizures.

Bipolar Disorder. Carbamazepine can provide symptomatic control in patients with bipolar disorder (manic-depressive illness), and is often effective in patients who are refractory to lithium. The role of carbamazepine in bipolar disorder is discussed in Chapter 32.

Trigeminal and Glossopharyngeal Neuralgias. A neuralgia is a severe, stabbing pain that occurs along the course of a nerve. Carbamazepine can reduce neuralgia associated with the trigeminal and glossopharyngeal nerves. The mechanism of this analgesic effect is unknown. It should be noted that, although carbamazepine can reduce pain in these specific neuralgias, it is not generally effective as an analgesic, and is not indicated for other kinds of pain.

Adverse Effects

CNS Effects. In contrast to phenytoin and phenobarbital, carbamazepine has minimal effects on cognitive function. This is a primary reason for selecting carbamazepine over these other drugs.

Carbamazepine can cause a variety of *neurologic effects,* including visual disturbances (nystagmus, blurred vision, diplopia), ataxia, vertigo, unsteadiness, and headache. These reactions are common during the first weeks of treatment, affecting 35% to 50% of patients. Fortunately, tolerance usually develops with continued use. These effects can be minimized by initiating therapy at low doses and giving the largest portion of the daily dose at bedtime.

Hematologic Effects. Carbamazepine-induced bone marrow suppression can cause *leukopenia, anemia,* and *thrombocytopenia.* However, serious reactions are rare. Thrombocytopenia and anemia, which have an incidence of 5%, respond to drug discontinuation. Leukopenia, which has an incidence of 10%, is usually transient and subsides even with continued drug use; accordingly, carbamazepine should not be withdrawn unless the white blood cell count drops below 3000/mm³.

Fatal *aplastic anemia* has occurred during carbamazepine therapy. This reaction is extremely rare, having an incidence of 1 in 200,000. Very few cases have been reported since 1964, and in many of these cases a direct cause-and-effect relationship could not be established.

To reduce the risk of serious hematologic effects, complete blood counts should be performed before treatment and periodically thereafter. Patients with pre-existing hematologic abnormalities should not be given the drug. Patients should be informed about manifestations of hematologic abnormalities (fever, sore throat, pallor, weakness, infection, easy bruising, petechiae) and instructed to notify the physician if these occur.

Birth Defects. Carbamazepine may be teratogenic. In humans, the drug is associated with an increased risk of neural tube defects. In mice, it has caused cleft palate, dilated cerebral ventricles, and growth retardation. Because it can harm the fetus, carbamazepine is classified in FDA Pregnancy Risk Category D, and hence should be used only if the benefits of seizure control are deemed to outweigh risks to the fetus.

Hypo-osmolarity. Carbamazepine can inhibit renal excretion of water, apparently by promoting secretion of antidiuretic hormone. Water retention can reduce the osmolarity of blood and other body fluids, thereby posing a threat to patients with heart failure. Periodic monitoring of serum sodium content is recommended.

Dermatologic Effects. Carbamazepine has been associated with a number of dermatologic effects, including morbilliform rash (10% incidence), photosensitivity reactions, Stevens-Johnson syndrome, and exfoliative dermatitis. Mild reactions can often be treated with prednisone (an anti-inflammatory agent) or an antihistamine. Severe reactions necessitate drug withdrawal.

Drug-Drug and Drug-Food Interactions

Induction of Drug-Metabolizing Enzymes. Carbamazepine is an effective inducer of hepatic drug-metabolizing enzymes. By promoting synthesis of these enzymes, carbamazepine can increase the rate at which it and other drugs are inactivated. Accelerated inactivation of *oral contraceptives* and *warfarin* is of particular concern.

Phenytoin and Phenobarbital. Both phenytoin and phenobarbital are effective inducers of hepatic drug metabolism. Hence, if either drug is taken with carbamazepine, induction of metabolism is likely to be greater than with carbamazepine alone. Accordingly, phenytoin and phenobarbital can further accelerate the metabolism of carbamazepine, thereby decreasing its effects.

Grapefruit Juice. As discussed in Chapter 6, grapefruit juice can inhibit the metabolism of many drugs, thereby causing their plasma levels to rise. Grapefruit juice can increase peak and trough levels of carbamazepine by 40%. Accordingly, patients taking the drug should be advised to avoid grapefruit juice.

Preparations, Dosage, and Administration

Carbamazepine [Tegretol, Tegretol-XR, Carbatrol, others] is available in standard tablets (200 mg); chewable tablets (100 mg); extended-release tablets (100, 200, and 400 mg), sold as Tegretol-XR; extended-release capsules (200 and 300 mg), sold as Carbatrol; and an oral suspension (20 mg/ml). The drug should be administered with meals to reduce gastric upset. Administering the largest portion of the daily dose at bedtime can help reduce adverse CNS effects. Carbamazepine suspension should not be administered with other liquid-formulation medicines.

Therapy is initiated with small doses (100 to 200 mg twice a day) to minimize side effects. Dosage is then increased gradually (every 1 to 3 weeks) until seizure control is achieved. Maintenance dosages for *adults* range from 600 to 1800 mg/day, administered in divided doses. Maintenance dosages for *children* range from 10 to 35 mg/kg/day, administered in divided doses.

Valproic Acid

Valproic acid [Depakene, Depakote, Depacon] is an important AED used widely to treat all major seizure types. Serious adverse effects are limited to rare cases of severe hepatotoxicity and pancreatitis, both of which can be fatal. In addition to its use in epilepsy, valproic acid is used to treat bipolar disorder and to prevent migraine headache.

Nomenclature

Valproic acid is available in three closely related chemical forms: (1) valproic acid itself, (2) the sodium salt of valproic acid, known as *valproate,* and (3) *divalproex sodium,* a combination of valproic acid plus its sodium salt. All three forms have identical antiseizure actions. In this chapter, the term *valproic acid* is used in reference to all three forms.

Mechanism of Action

Valproic acid appears to act by three mechanisms. First, it shares the same mechanism as phenytoin and carbamazepine: suppression of high-frequency neuronal firing through blockade of sodium channels. Second, it suppresses calcium influx through T-type calcium channels. Third, it may augment the inhibitory influence of GABA.

Pharmacokinetics

Valproic acid is readily absorbed from the GI tract and is widely distributed throughout the body. The drug undergoes extensive hepatic metabolism followed by renal excretion.

Therapeutic responses are often seen at plasma levels of 50 to 150 mg/ml. However, the correlation between plasma levels and therapeutic effects is not very tight.

Therapeutic Uses

Seizure Disorders. As shown in Table 23–1, valproic acid is considered a first-line drug for all partial and generalized seizures.

Bipolar Disorder. Like carbamazepine, valproic acid can provide symptomatic control in patients with bipolar disorder (manic-depressive illness). This application is discussed in Chapter 32.

Migraine. Valproic acid is approved for prophylaxis of migraine. This use is discussed in Chapter 29.

Adverse Effects

Valproic acid is generally well tolerated and causes minimal sedation and cognitive impairment. Gastrointestinal effects are most common. Hepatotoxicity and pancreatitis are rare but serious.

Gastrointestinal Effects. Nausea, vomiting, and indigestion are common—but transient. These effects are most intense with formulations that are not enteric coated. Gastrointestinal reactions can be minimized by administering valproic acid with food and by using an enteric-coated formulation (see Table 23–3).

Hepatotoxicity. Rarely, valproic acid has been associated with fatal liver failure. Most deaths have occurred within the first few months of therapy. The overall incidence of fatal hepatotoxicity is about 1 in 40,000. However, in high-risk patients—children under the age of 2 years who are receiving multidrug therapy—the incidence is much higher: 1 in 500. To minimize the risk of fatal liver injury, the following guidelines have been established:

- Don't use valproic acid in conjunction with other drugs in children less than 3 years old.
- Don't use valproic acid in patients with pre-existing liver dysfunction.
- Evaluate liver function before initiating treatment and periodically thereafter. (Unfortunately, monitoring liver func-

tion may fail to provide advance warning of severe hepatotoxicity: Fatal liver failure can develop so rapidly that it is not preceded by an abnormal test result.)

- Inform patients about signs and symptoms of liver injury (reduced appetite, malaise, nausea, abdominal pain, jaundice) and instruct them to notify the physician if these develop.
- Use valproic acid in the lowest effective dosage.

Pancreatitis. Life-threatening pancreatitis has developed in children and adults taking valproic acid. Some cases have been hemorrhagic, progressing rapidly from initial symptoms to death. Pancreatitis can develop soon after starting therapy or after years of drug use. Patients should be informed about signs of pancreatitis (abdominal pain, nausea, vomiting, anorexia) and instructed to obtain immediate evaluation if these develop. If pancreatitis is diagnosed, valproic acid should be withdrawn. Alternative medication should be substituted as indicated.

Teratogenic Effects. Like most other AEDs, valproic acid can harm the developing fetus. Neural tube defects (e.g., spina bifida) are the greatest concern. Women of child-bearing age should use an effective form of contraception, and should take folic acid supplements (5 mg/day), which can help protect against neural tube damage in case pregnancy occurs. Valproic acid is classified in FDA Pregnancy Risk Category D: There is evidence of human fetal risk, but the drug may be used during pregnancy if the potential benefits are considered to outweigh the risks to the fetus.

Other Adverse Effects. Valproic acid may cause *rash, weight gain, hair loss, tremor,* and *blood dyscrasias* (leukopenia, thrombocytopenia, red blood cell aplasia). Significant CNS effects are uncommon.

Drug Interactions

Phenobarbital. Valproic acid decreases the rate at which phenobarbital is metabolized. Blood levels of phenobarbital may rise by 40%, resulting in significant CNS depression. When the combination is used, levels of phenobarbital should be monitored and, if they rise too high, phenobarbital dosage should be reduced.

Phenytoin. Valproic acid can displace phenytoin from binding sites on plasma proteins. The resultant increase in free phenytoin may lead to toxicity. Phenytoin levels and clinical status should be monitored.

Preparations, Dosage, and Administration

Preparations. Valproic acid is available in several oral formulations (Table 23–3) and in a 100-mg/ml solution [Depacon] for IV use.

Oral Dosage and Administration. Daily doses are small initially and then gradually increased. For *adults and older children,* the initial dosage is 5 to 15 mg/kg/day, usually administered in two divided doses. The usual maintenance dosage is 0.75 to 3 gm/day. For *children ages 1 to 12 years,* the initial dosage is 10 to 30 mg/kg/day, usually administered in divided doses. The usual maintenance dosage is 15 to 45 mg/kg/day. For both adults and children, the dosage should be increased if phenobarbital or another inducer of hepatic drug metabolism is taken concurrently.

Patients should be instructed to swallow the tablets and capsules intact, without chewing or crushing. Gastric discomfort can be decreased by administering valproic acid with meals and by using an enteric-coated formulation.

Ethosuximide

Therapeutic Use. Ethosuximide [Zarontin] is a drug of choice for absence seizures, the only seizures for which it is indicated. Absence seizures are abolished in 60% of patients, and, in newly diagnosed patients, practical control is achieved in 80% to 90%. Ethosuximide is inactive against tonic-clonic, simple partial, and complex partial seizures.

TABLE 23–3 ■ Oral Preparations of Valproic Acid and Its Derivatives

Chemical Form	Trade Name	Product Description	Comments
Valproic acid	Depakene	Capsules (250 mg)	Immediate release; GI upset is common.
Valproate sodium	Depakene	Syrup (250 mg/5 ml)	Immediate release; GI upset is common.
Divalproex sodium	Depakote	Delayed-release, enteric-coated tablets (125, 250, 500 mg)	Released over 8–12 hours, and hence *not* for once daily administration. *Not interchangeable with Depakote ER* (extended-release tablets) because rate of drug release is different. Less GI upset than Depakene.
	Depakote ER	Extended-release, enteric-coated tablets (500 mg)	Released over 18 to 24 hours, and hence *can* be administered once daily. *Not interchangeable with regular Depakote* (delayed-release tablets) because rate of drug release is different. Not approved for epilepsy (but is used anyway). Less GI upset than Depakene.
	Depakote	"Sprinkle" capsules containing enteric-coated granules (125 mg)	Immediate release. Less GI upset than Depakene. May swallow capsule whole or open and sprinkle granules on a small amount (1 teaspoon) of soft food.

Mechanism of Action. Ethosuximide suppresses neurons in the thalamus that are responsible for generating absence seizures. The specific mechanism is inhibition of low-threshold calcium currents, known as T currents. Ethosuximide does not block sodium channels, and does not enhance GABA-mediated neuronal inhibition.

Pharmacokinetics. Ethosuximide is well absorbed following oral administration. Therapeutic plasma levels range between 40 and 100 mg/ml. The drug is eliminated by a combination of hepatic metabolism and renal excretion. Its half-life is 60 hours in adults and 30 hours in children. Ethosuximide does not induce hepatic drug-metabolizing enzymes.

Adverse Effects and Drug Interactions. Ethosuximide is generally devoid of significant adverse effects and interactions. During initial treatment, it may cause *drowsiness, dizziness,* and *lethargy.* These diminish with continued use. *Nausea* and *vomiting* may occur and can be reduced by administering the drug with food. Rare but serious reactions include *systemic lupus erythematosus, leukopenia,* and *aplastic anemia.*

Preparations, Dosage, and Administration. Ethosuximide [Zarontin] is available in capsules (250 mg) and in a syrup (250 mg/5 ml). For *children ages 3 to 6 years,* the initial dosage is 250 mg/day. For *older children and adults,* the initial dosage is 500 mg/day. Dosage should be gradually increased until control of seizures is obtained. The usual maintenance dosage is 750 mg/day for adults, and between 15 and 40 mg/kg/day for children. Because ethosuximide has a long half-life, dosing can be done just once a day. However, dosing twice a day is better tolerated.

Since absence seizures occur many times each day, monitoring the clinical response rather than plasma drug levels is the preferred method for dosage determination. Dosage should be increased until seizures have been controlled or until adverse effects become too great.

When withdrawing ethosuximide, dosage should be reduced gradually.

Phenobarbital

Phenobarbital is one of our oldest AEDs. The drug is effective, inexpensive, and can be administered just once a day. Unfortunately, certain side effects—lethargy, depression, learning impairment—can be significant. Hence, although phenobarbital was used widely in the past, it has largely been replaced by newer drugs that are equally effective but better tolerated.

Phenobarbital belongs to the barbiturate family. However, in contrast to most barbiturates, which produce generalized depression of the CNS, phenobarbital is able to suppress seizures at doses that produce only moderate disruption of CNS function. Because it can reduce seizures without causing sedation, phenobarbital is classified as an *anticonvulsant barbiturate* (to distinguish it from most other barbiturates, which are employed as daytime sedatives or "sleeping pills").

The basic pharmacology of the barbiturates is discussed in Chapter 33. Discussion here is limited to the use of phenobarbital for seizures.

Mechanism of Antiseizure Action

Phenobarbital suppresses seizures by potentiating the effects of GABA. Specifically, the drug binds to GABA receptors, causing the receptor to respond more intensely to GABA itself.

Pharmacokinetics

Phenobarbital is administered orally and absorption is complete. Elimination occurs through hepatic metabolism and renal excretion. Phenobarbital has a *long half-life*—about 4 days. As a result, once-daily dosing is adequate for most patients. In addition to permitting once-daily dosing, the long half-life has another consequence: 2 to 3 weeks are required for plasma levels to reach plateau. (Recall that, in the absence of a loading dose, an interval equivalent to four half-lives is required to reach plateau.)

Therapeutic Uses

Epilepsy. Phenobarbital is effective against partial seizures and generalized tonic-clonic seizures but not against absence seizures. Until recently, phenobarbital had been a drug of choice for tonic-clonic seizures and partial seizures in older children and adults. However, most clinicians now prefer to treat these epilepsies with carbamazepine, phenytoin, or valproic acid—drugs that cause fewer neuropsychologic effects than phenobarbital. Intravenous phenobarbital can be used for generalized convulsive SE, but lorazepam and phenytoin are preferred.

Sedation and Induction of Sleep. Like other barbiturates, phenobarbital can be used for daytime sedation and promotion of sleep at night. These applications are discussed in Chapter 33.

Adverse Effects

Neuropsychologic Effects. Drowsiness is the most common CNS effect. During the initial phase of therapy, sedation develops in practically all patients. With continued treatment, tolerance to sedation develops. Some children experience paradoxical responses: Instead of becoming sedated, they may become irritable and hyperactive. Depression may occur in adults. Elderly patients may experience agitation and confusion.

Physical Dependence. Like all other barbiturates, phenobarbital can cause physical dependence. However, at the doses employed to treat epilepsy, significant dependence is unlikely.

Exacerbation of Intermittent Porphyria. Phenobarbital and other barbiturates can increase the risk of acute intermittent porphyria. Accordingly, barbiturates are absolutely contraindicated for patients with a history of this disorder. The relationship of barbiturates to intermittent porphyria is discussed further in Chapter 33.

Use in Pregnancy. Use of barbiturates during pregnancy has been associated with congenital abnormalities. Women who take phenobarbital during pregnancy or become pregnant while taking the drug should be informed of the potential risk to the fetus.

Like phenytoin, phenobarbital can decrease synthesis of vitamin K–dependent clotting factors, and can thereby cause *bleeding tendencies in newborns.* The risk of neonatal bleeding can be decreased by administering vitamin K to the mother for 1 month prior to delivery and during delivery, and to the infant immediately after delivery.

Other Adverse Effects. Like phenytoin, phenobarbital can interfere with the metabolism of vitamins D and K. Disruption of vitamin D metabolism can cause *rickets* and *osteomalacia.*

Toxicity

When taken in moderately excessive doses, phenobarbital causes nystagmus and ataxia. Severe overdose produces generalized CNS depression; death results from depression of respiration. Barbiturate toxicity and its treatment are discussed at length in Chapter 33.

Drug Interactions

Induction of Drug-Metabolizing Enzymes. Phenobarbital induces hepatic drug-metabolizing enzymes, and can thereby accelerate the metabolism of other drugs, causing a loss of therapeutic effects. This is particular concern with oral contraceptives and warfarin.

CNS Depressants. Being a CNS depressant itself, phenobarbital can intensify CNS depression caused by other drugs (e.g., alcohol, benzodiazepines, opioids). Severe respiratory depression and coma could result. Patients should be warned against combining phenobarbital with other drugs that have CNS-depressant actions.

Valproic Acid. Valproic acid is an AED that has been used in combination with phenobarbital. By competing with phenobarbital for drug-metabolizing enzymes, valproic acid can increase plasma levels of phenobarbital by approximately 40%. Hence, when this combination is used, the dosage of phenobarbital must be reduced.

Drug Withdrawal

When phenobarbital is withdrawn, *dosage should be reduced gradually,* since abrupt withdrawal can precipitate SE. Patients should be warned of this danger and instructed not to discontinue phenobarbital too quickly.

Preparations, Dosage, and Administration

Preparations. Phenobarbital is dispensed in three oral formulations: tablets, capsules, and elixir. The drug is also available in solution for IM and IV administration.

Dosage. *Adult* maintenance dosages range from 60 to 100 mg/day administered as a single dose or two divided doses. *Pediatric* maintenance dosages range from 3 to 6 mg/kg/day. When dosage is being established, plasma drug levels may be used as a guide; target levels are 15 to 40 mg/ml.

Loading doses may be needed. Because phenobarbital has a long half-life, several weeks are required for drug levels to reach plateau. If plateau must be reached sooner, a loading schedule can be employed. For example, doses that are twice normal can be given for 4 days. Unfortunately, these large doses are likely to produce substantial CNS depression.

Administration. Phenobarbital may be administered orally, IV, or IM. Oral administration is employed for routine therapy. Intravenous administration is needed for SE.

Intravenous injection must be done slowly. If done too fast, excessive CNS depression may result. Phenobarbital is highly alkaline and may cause local tissue injury if extravasation occurs.

Primidone

Primidone [Mysoline] is active against all major seizure disorders except absence seizures. The drug is nearly identical in structure to phenobarbital. As a result, the pharmacology of both agents is very similar.

Pharmacokinetics. Primidone is readily absorbed following oral administration. In the liver, much of the drug undergoes conversion to two active metabolites: phenobarbital and phenylethylmalonamide. Seizure control is produced by primidone itself and by its metabolites. Therapeutic plasma levels range from 5 to 15 mg/ml.

Therapeutic Uses. Primidone is effective against tonic-clonic, simple partial, and complex partial seizures. The drug is not active against absence seizures.

As a rule, primidone is employed in combination with another AED, usually phenytoin or carbamazepine. Primidone is never taken together with phenobarbital. Why? Because phenobarbital is an active metabolite of primidone, and hence concurrent use would be irrational.

Adverse Effects. Sedation, ataxia, and dizziness are common during initial treatment but diminish with continued drug use. Like phenobarbital, primidone can cause confusion in the elderly and paradoxical hyperexcitability in children. A sense of acute intoxication can occur shortly after administration. As with phenobarbital, primidone is absolutely contraindicated for patients with acute intermittent porphyria. Serious adverse reactions (acute psychosis, leukopenia, thrombocytopenia, systemic lupus erythematosus) can occur but are rare.

Drug Interactions. Drug interactions for primidone are similar to those for phenobarbital. Primidone can induce hepatic drug-metabolizing enzymes and can thereby reduce the effects of oral contraceptives, warfarin, and other drugs. In addition, primidone can intensify responses to other CNS depressants.

Preparations, Dosage, and Administration. Primidone [Mysoline] is available in tablets (50 and 250 mg) and an oral suspension (250 mg/5 ml). Therapy in *adults* is initiated with 100 to 125 mg at bedtime. Dosage is gradually increased over the next 10 days to a maintenance level of 250 mg 3 or 4 times a day. The maximum dosage is 500 mg 4 times a day.

Newer Antiepileptic Drugs

All of the newer AEDs were introduced after 1990. Because clinical experience with these drugs is limited, they are generally reserved for patients who have not responded to older (conventional) agents. Oxcarbazepine is the principal exception to this rule.

Oxcarbazepine

Actions and Uses. Oxcarbazepine [Trileptal], a derivative of carbamazepine, is indicated for oral therapy of partial seizures in adults and children. The drug is as effective as carbamazepine and better tolerated. Unfortunately, it's also much more expensive. Antiseizure effects are thought to result from blockade of voltage-sensitive sodium channels in neuronal membranes, an action that stabilizes hyperexcitable neurons and thereby suppresses seizure spread. The drug does not affect neuronal GABA receptors. Oxcarbazepine was approved for use in the United States on January 17, 2000, but has been available in Mexico and other countries for years.

Pharmacokinetics. Oxcarbazepine is well absorbed both in the presence and absence of food. In the liver, the drug undergoes rapid conversion to a 10-monohydroxy metabolite (MHD), its active form. MHD has a half-life of 9 hours and undergoes excretion in the urine.

Adverse Effects. The most common adverse effects are dizziness (22% to 49%), drowsiness (19% to 36%), double vision (14% to 40%), nystagmus (7% to 26%), headache (13% to 32%), nausea (15% to 29%), vomiting (7% to 36%), and ataxia (5% to 31%). Individuals should avoid driving and other hazardous activities, unless the degree of drowsiness is low.

Clinically significant *hyponatremia* (sodium concentration less than 125 mmol/L) develops in 2.5% of patients. Signs include nausea, drowsiness, headache, and confusion. If carbamazepine is combined with other drugs that can decrease sodium levels (especially diuretics), monitoring of sodium levels may be needed.

Oxcarbazepine has not caused the severe hematologic abnormalities seen with carbamazepine. Accordingly, routine monitoring of blood counts is not required.

Oxcarbazepine has not been associated with the severe skin reactions that have occurred (rarely) with carbamazepine. However, because of possible cross sensitivity, oxcarbazepine should be used with caution—if at all—by patients who have experienced a severe reaction (e.g., Stevens-Johnson syndrome) with carbamazepine.

Use in Pregnancy and Breast-Feeding. Like carbamazepine (FDA Pregnancy Risk Category D), oxcarbazepine (FDA Pregnancy Risk Category C) may pose a risk of birth defects. Accordingly, women of child-bearing potential should use effective contraception. Clearly, the drug should be avoided by women who are already pregnant. In addition, since both oxcarbazepine and its metabolite are excreted in breast milk, the drug should be avoided by women who are breast-feeding.

Drug Interactions. Oxcarbazepine induces some drug-metabolizing enzymes and inhibits others. The drug does not induce enzymes that metabolize other AEDs. However, it does induce enzymes that metabolize *oral contraceptives,* and can thereby render them less effective. Accordingly, women should employ an alternative birth control method.

Oxcarbazepine inhibits the enzymes that metabolize phenytoin, and can thereby raise phenytoin levels. Toxicity can result. Phenytoin levels should be monitored and dosage adjusted accordingly.

Drugs that induce drug-metabolizing enzymes (e.g., phenytoin, phenobarbital, carbamazepine) can reduce levels of MHD, the active form of oxcarbazepine. Accordingly, dosage of oxcarbazepine may need to be increased.

Alcohol can intensify CNS depression caused by oxcarbazepine, and hence should be avoided.

As noted, oxcarbazepine should be used with caution in patients taking *diuretics* and other drugs that can lower sodium levels.

Preparations, Dosage, and Administration. Oxcarbazepine [Trileptal] is available in 150-, 300-, and 600-mg film-coated oral tablets.

For *monotherapy in adults,* the initial dosage is 300 mg twice daily. The maximum dosage is 1200 mg twice daily.

For *adjunctive therapy in adults,* the initial dosage is 300 mg twice daily. The maximum dosage is 600 mg twice daily.

For *adjunctive therapy in children* (ages 4 to 16), the initial dosage is 8 to 10 mg/kg/day in two divided doses. Maintenance dosages are related to body weight: For children weighing 20 to 29 kg, the dosage is 900 mg/day; for children 29.1 to 30 kg, the dosage is 1200 mg/day; and for children above 39 kg, the dosage is 1800 mg/day.

Lamotrigine

Actions and Uses. Lamotrigine [Lamictal] has a broad spectrum of antiseizure activity, but approved uses are limited. Currently, the drug is indicated only for (1) adjunctive or monotherapy of partial seizures and (2) adjunctive therapy of Lennox-Gastaut syndrome. Investigational uses include absence, myoclonic, and generalized tonic-clonic seizures. Benefits appear to derive from suppressing release of excitatory neurotransmitters secondary to blockade of sodium channels. Because serious toxicity (life-threatening rash) occurs often in younger patients, *lamotrigine should not be used by patients under the age of 16.* In addition to its use in epilepsy, lamotrigine is under study for use in bipolar disorder (manic-depressive illness).

Pharmacokinetics. Administration is oral and absorption is nearly complete, both in the presence and absence of food. Blood levels peak in 1.5 to 5 hours and decline with a half-life of 24 hours. The drug undergoes hepatic metabolism followed by renal excretion.

Drug Interactions. The half-life is dramatically affected by drugs that induce or inhibit hepatic drug-metabolizing enzymes. Enzyme inducers (e.g., carbamazepine, phenytoin, phenobarbital) decrease the half-life of lamotrigine to 10 hours, whereas valproate (an enzyme inhibitor) increases the half-life to about 60 hours.

Adverse Effects. Lamotrigine can cause *life-threatening rashes,* including Stevens-Johnson syndrome and toxic epidermal necrolysis. Deaths have occurred. The incidence of severe rash is about 1% in pediatric patients (<16 years old) and 0.3% in adults. If a rash develops, lamotrigine should be withdrawn immediately. Patients younger than 16 should not use the drug.

In addition to severe rash, lamotrigine commonly causes dizziness, diplopia (double vision), blurred vision, nausea, vomiting, and headache. Safety in pregnancy and breast-feeding has not been established.

Preparations, Dosage, and Administration. Lamotrigine [Lamictal] is dispensed in standard tablets (25, 100, 150, and 200 mg) and chewable tablets (5 and 25 mg). The dosage depends on what other drugs are being taken. For patients taking an *inducer* of drug metabolism (e.g., carbamazepine, phenytoin, phenobarbital), dosing is begun at 50 mg/day, and then gradually increased to between 150 and 500 mg twice a day for maintenance. For patients taking *valproate* (an enzyme inhibitor), dosing is begun at 25 mg every other day, and then gradually increased to between 50 and 75 mg twice daily for maintenance.

Gabapentin

Actions and Uses. Gabapentin [Neurontin] has a broad spectrum of anticonvulsant activity, but use in epilepsy is limited to adjunctive therapy of partial seizures (with or without secondary generalization). Gabapentin is an analog of GABA, but does not directly affect GABA receptors. Rather, it appears to act by enhancing GABA release, thereby increasing GABA-mediated inhibition of neuronal firing. In 2002, gabapentin was aproved for relief of postherpetic neuralgia. Investigational uses include bipolar disorder, neuropathic pain, prophylaxis of migraine, and leg cramps.

Pharmacokinetics. Gabapentin is rapidly absorbed following oral administration and reaches peak plasma levels in 2 to 3 hours. Absorption is not affected by food. However, as the dosage gets larger, the percent absorbed gets smaller. Why? Because, at high doses, the intestinal transport system for uptake of the drug becomes saturated. Gabapentin is not metabolized and is excreted intact in the urine. The half-life is 5 to 7 hours.

Drug Interactions. Unlike most AEDs, gabapentin is devoid of significant interactions. Gabapentin neither induces nor inhibits hepatic drug-metabolizing enzymes, and does not affect the metabolism of other drugs. As a result, gabapentin is well suited for combined therapy with other AEDs.

Adverse Reactions. Gabapentin is very well tolerated. The most common side effects are somnolence, dizziness, ataxia, fatigue, and nystagmus. These are usually mild to moderate and often diminish with continued drug use. Patients should avoid driving and other hazardous activities until they are confident they are not impaired. Safety in pregnancy and breast-feeding has not been established.

Preparations, Dosage, and Administration. Gabapentin [Neurontin] is dispensed in capsules (100, 300, and 400 mg), tablets (600 and 800 mg), and an oral solution (50 mg/ml). Dosing for adults is begun with a 300-mg dose at bedtime, followed the next day by 600 mg (in two divided doses), and the next day by 900 mg (in three divided doses). Thereafter, the dosage can be raised rapidly to maintenance levels, typically 1200 to 3600 mg/day in three divided doses. Dosage should be reduced in patients with renal impairment.

Levetiracetam

Levetiracetam [Keppra] is a unique agent approved for adjunctive therapy of partial seizures in adults. The drug is chemically and pharmacologically different for all other AEDs. How levetiracetam acts is unknown. All we do know is that it does not bind to receptors for GABA or any other known neurotransmitter.

Levetiracetam is administered PO and undergoes rapid and complete GI absorption, both in the presence and absence of food. Metabolism is minimal and not mediated by hepatic P450 enzymes. Levetiracetam is excreted in the urine, largely (66%) unchanged.

Adverse effects are generally mild to moderate. The most common are drowsiness (14.8%) and asthenia (14.7%). Neuropsychiatric symptoms (agitation, anxiety, depression, psychosis, hallucinations, depersonalization) occur in less than 1% of patients. In contrast to other AEDs, levetiracetam does not impair speech, concentration, or other cognitive functions. Safety for use during pregnancy or breast feeding has not been determined.

Unlike other AEDs, levetiracetam does not interact with other drugs. It does not alter plasma concentrations of oral contraceptives, warfarin, digoxin, or other AEDs. Given that levetiracetam is not metabolized by P450 enzymes, its lack of interactions is no surprise.

Levetiracetam is available in tablets (250, 500, and 750 mg) for oral administration. The initial adult dosage is 500 mg twice daily. The maximum dosage is 3000 mg/day. Because levetiracetam is eliminated by the kidneys, dosage should be reduced in patients with significant renal impairment.

Topiramate

Actions and Uses. Topiramate [Topamax] is approved for adjunctive therapy of partial seizures and primary tonic-clonic seizures in adults and children, and for seizures associated with Lennox-Gastaut syndrome. Three possible mechanisms are involved: (1) potentiation of inhibition by GABA,

(2) inhibition of voltage-dependent sodium channels, and (3) blockade of receptors for glutamate, an excitatory neurotransmitter. Unlabeled uses include bipolar disorder, cluster headaches, and infantile spasm.

Pharmacokinetics. Topiramate is rapidly absorbed following oral administration. Bioavailability is not affected by food. Plasma levels peak 2 hours after dosing. Most of the drug is eliminated unchanged in the urine.

Adverse Effects. Although topiramate is generally well tolerated, it can cause multiple adverse effects. Common effects include somnolence (30%), dizziness (28%), ataxia (21%), nervousness (20%), diplopia (15%), nausea (13%), anorexia (12%), and weight loss (12%). Cognitive effects (confusion, memory difficulties, altered thinking, reduced concentration, difficulty finding words) can occur, but the incidence appears low at recommended dosages. Kidney stones and paresthesias occur rarely.

Recent case reports indicate that topiramate can cause *angle-closure glaucoma.* Left untreated, this rapidly leads to blindness. Patients should be informed about symptoms of glaucoma (ocular pain, unusual redness, sudden worsening or blurring of vision) and instructed to seek immediate attention if these develop. Fortunately, topiramate-induced glaucoma is rare: Although 825,000 patients have used the drug, as of August 2001, only 23 cases had been reported.

Drug Interactions. Phenytoin and carbamazepine can decrease levels of topiramate by about 45%. Topiramate may increase levels of phenytoin.

Preparations, Dosage, and Administration. Topiramate [Topamax] is available in tablets (50, 100, and 200 mg) and "sprinkle" capsules (15 and 25 mg). *Adult* dosing is begun at 50 mg/day and then gradually increased to 200 mg twice daily for maintenance. *Pediatric* dosing is begun at 25 mg (or less) per day and gradually increased to 3 to 9 mg/kg/day administered in two divided doses. Advise patients not to break the tablets because of bitter taste. The capsules can be swallowed whole or opened and sprinkled onto a small amount (1 teaspoon) of soft food.

Tiagabine

Actions and Uses. Tiagabine [Gabitril] is approved for adjunctive therapy of partial seizures in patients over the age of 12. The drug blocks reuptake of GABA by neurons and glia. As a result, the inhibitory influence of GABA is intensified, and seizures are suppressed.

Pharmacokinetics. Tiagabine has uncomplicated kinetics. Administration is oral. Absorption is rapid and nearly complete. Food reduces the rate of absorption but not the extent. Plasma levels peak about 45 minutes after administration. In the blood, tiagabine is highly (96%) bound to plasma proteins. Elimination is by hepatic metabolism followed by excretion in the bile and, to a lesser extent, the urine. The serum half-life is 7 to 9 hours.

Adverse Effects. Tiagabine is generally well tolerated. Common adverse effects are dizziness (27%), somnolence (18%), asthenia (20%), nausea (11%), nervousness (10%), and tremor (9%). Like most other AEDs, tiagabine can cause dose-related cognitive effects (e.g., confusion, abnormal thinking, trouble concentrating).

Drug Interactions. Tiagabine does not alter the metabolism or serum concentrations of other AEDs. However, levels of tiagabine can be decreased by phenytoin, phenobarbital, and carbamazepine—all of which induce drug-metabolizing enzymes.

Preparations, Dosage, and Administration. Tiagabine [Gabitril] is available in tablets (4, 12, 16, and 20 mg) for oral administration. Dosing should be done with food. The initial dosage for adults and children is 4 mg once a day. Dosage can be increased by 4 to 8 mg/day at weekly intervals. The maximum daily dose, administered in two to four divided doses, is 56 mg for adults and 32 mg for children under 18. Dosage should be increased in patients taking drugs that can accelerate tiagabine metabolism.

Zonisamide

Actions and Uses. Zonisamide [Zonegran] is an oral drug indicated for adjunctive therapy of partial seizures in patients at least 16 years old. The drug belongs to the same chemical family as the sulfonamide antibiotics, although it lacks antimicrobial activity. In animal models, zonisamide suppresses both seizure spread and focal seizure activity. However, the mechanism underlying these effects is unknown. What we do know is that zonisamide can impair ion flow through neuronal sodium channels and calcium channels. In addition, we know that the drug can facilitate transmission at dopaminergic and serotonergic synapses, but not at GABAergic synapses. What we don't know is how these actions relate to seizure control.

Pharmacokinetics. Zonisamide undergoes rapid absorption from the GI tract. Bioavailability is nearly 100%, both in the presence and absence of food. In the blood, zonisamide is extensively bound to erythrocytes. As a result, its concentration in erythrocytes is 8 times higher than in plasma. Zon-

isamide is metabolized in the liver by the 3A4 isozyme of cytochrome P450 (CYP3A4). Excretion occurs in the urine, in the form of zonisamide itself (30%) and metabolites. The drug's plasma half-life is 63 hours.

Adverse Effects. The most common adverse effects are drowsiness (17%), dizziness (13%), anorexia (13%), headache (10%), and nausea (9%). Like most AEDs, zonisamide can impair speech, concentration, and other cognitive processes. Because the drug can reduce alertness and impair cognition, patients should avoid driving and other hazardous activities until they know how the drug affects them.

Zonisamide can have severe *psychiatric effects.* During clinical trials, 2.2% of patients either discontinued treatment or were hospitalized because of severe depression; 1.1% attempted suicide. Psychosis caused another 2.2% to discontinue treatment.

Like all other sulfonamides, zonisamide can trigger *hypersensitivity reactions,* including some that are potentially fatal (e.g., Stevens-Johnson syndrome, toxic epidermal necrolysis, fulminant hepatic necrosis). Accordingly, zonisamide is contraindicated for patients with a history of sulfonamide hypersensitivity. Patients who develop a rash should be followed closely, because rash can evolve into a more serious event. If severe hypersensitivity develops, zonisamide should be withdrawn immediately. Fortunately, serious reactions and fatalities are rare.

Zonisamide has adverse effects on the kidney. In clinical trials, about 4% of patients developed *nephrolithiasis* (kidney stones). The risk can be reduced by drinking 6 to 8 glasses of water a day, which will maintain hydration and urine flow. Patients should be informed about signs of kidney stones (sudden back pain, abdominal pain, painful urination, bloody or dark urine) and instructed to report them to the physician. In addition to nephrolithiasis, zonisamide can *impair glomerular filtration.* Because of its effects on the kidney, zonisamide should be used with caution in patients with kidney disease.

Rarely, zonisamide causes *oligohidrosis* (decreased sweating) and *hyperthermia* (elevation of body temperature). Pediatric patients may be at special risk for these effects. In warm weather, oligohidrosis may lead to heat stroke and subsequent hospitalization. Patients should be monitored closely for reduced sweating and increased body temperature.

Use in Pregnancy and Breast-Feeding. Zonisamide is teratogenic and embryolethal in laboratory animals. Cardiovascular abnormalities are common. Women of child-bearing potential should use effective contraception. Zonisamide is classified in FDA Pregnancy Risk Category C, and hence should be avoided during pregnancy unless the benefits to the mother are deemed to outweigh the potential risks to the fetus. We do not know if zonisamide enters breast milk. Until more is known, prudence dictates that women who are breast-feeding should not take the drug.

Drug and Food Interactions. Levels of zonisamide can be affected by agents that induce or inhibit CYP3A4. Inducers of CYP3A4—including St. John's wort (an herbal supplement used for depression) and several AEDs (e.g., phenytoin, phenobarbital, carbamazepine)—can accelerate the metabolism of zonisamide, and thereby reduce the drug's half-life to as little as 27 hours. Conversely, inhibitors of CYP3A4—including grapefruit juice, azole antifungal agents (e.g., ketoconazole), and several protease inhibitors (e.g., amprenavir)—can slow the metabolism of zonisamide, and thereby prolong and intensify its effects.

Preparations, Dosage, and Administration. Zonisamide is available in 100-mg tablets for oral use. The initial adult dosage is 100 mg once daily. The maximum dosage is 600 mg/day in one or two divided doses.

Vigabatrin

Vigabatrin [Sabril] can suppress partial and secondarily generalized seizures, but may exacerbate absence and myoclonic seizures. The drug acts by inhibiting GABA transaminase, the enzyme that degrades GABA. By preventing GABA degradation, vigabatrin increases GABA availability in the CNS, and thereby enhances GABA-mediated inhibition of neuronal activity. Adverse effects include nausea, sedation, depression, psychosis, weight gain, and visual field constriction. The maintenance dosage is 2 to 4 gm once a day. Vigabatrin is available in Europe but not the United States.

Felbamate

Felbamate [Felbatol] is an effective AED with a broad spectrum of antiseizure activity. Unfortunately, the drug has potentially fatal adverse effects: aplastic anemia and liver failure. Accordingly, use is restricted to patients with severe epilepsy refractory to other therapy.

Mechanism of Action. Felbamate increases seizure threshold and suppresses seizure spread. The underlying mechanism is unknown. Unlike some AEDs (e.g., phenobarbital, benzodiazepines), felbamate does not interact with GABA receptors and does enhance the inhibitory actions of GABA.

Pharmacokinetics. Felbamate is well absorbed following oral administration, even in the presence of food. Peak plasma levels are achieved in 1 to 4 hours. The drug readily penetrates to the CNS. Although therapeutic plasma levels have not been established, levels of 20 to 120 mg/ml have been measured during clinical trials. Felbamate is eliminated in the urine, primarily unchanged. Its half-life is 14 to 23 hours.

Therapeutic Uses. Felbamate is approved for (1) adjunctive or monotherapy in adults with partial seizures (with or without generalization), and (2) adjunctive therapy in children with Lennox-Gastaut syndrome. However, because of toxicity, use of the drug is very limited.

Adverse Effects. Felbamate can cause *aplastic anemia* and *liver damage.* Aplastic anemia has occurred in at least 21 patients, 3 of whom died. Acute liver failure occurred in eight patients, four of whom died. Because of the risk of liver failure, felbamate should not be used by patients with pre-existing liver dysfunction. In addition, patients taking the drug should be monitored for indications of liver injury.

The most common adverse effects are GI disturbances (anorexia, nausea, vomiting) and CNS effects (insomnia, somnolence, dizziness, headache, diplopia). These occur more frequently when felbamate is combined with other drugs.

Drug Interactions. Felbamate can alter plasma levels of other AEDs and vice versa. Felbamate increases levels of phenytoin and valproic acid. Levels of felbamate are increased by valproic acid and reduced by phenytoin and carbamazepine. Increased levels of phenytoin and valproic acid (and possibly felbamate) could lead to toxicity; reduced levels of felbamate could lead to therapeutic failure. Therefore, to keep levels of these drugs within the therapeutic range, their levels should be monitored and dosages adjusted accordingly.

Preparations, Dosage, and Administration. Felbamate [Felbatol] is available in tablets (400 and 600 mg) and an oral suspension (120 mg/ml). For *older children* (over 14 years old) and *adults,* the initial dosage is 1200 mg/day in three divided doses; the maximum dosage is 3600 mg/day in three divided doses. For *younger children* (2 to 14 years old), the initial dosage is 15 mg/kg/day in three divided doses; the maximum dosage is 45 mg/kg/day or 3600 mg/day, whichever is less, administered in three divided doses.

MANAGEMENT OF EPILEPSY DURING PREGNANCY

Managing epilepsy during pregnancy is a challenge. Why? Because AEDs can harm the fetus, but so can uncontrolled seizures. There is solid evidence that all of the conventional AEDs increase the risk of minor malformations, major malformations, and growth retardation. At this time, the teratogenic potential of the newer AEDs is unclear. The most common malformations associated with AEDs are oral-facial clefts and midline heart defects. Valproic acid poses an especially high risk of spina bifida and other neural tube defects. The risk of malformation is proportional to AED dosage and to the number of AEDs used. As with other teratogens, the risk of birth defects is greatest from exposure during the first trimester. How do AEDs cause birth defects? One likely mechanism is conversion to reactive epoxide metabolites. In addition to causing birth defects, certain AEDs can cause neonatal hemorrhage.

Uncontrolled seizures carry their own risks—although they don't cause fetal malformation. Generalized tonic-clonic seizures can induce labor and, very rarely, miscarriage. Major seizures during the last month of pregnancy can injure the baby. Seizures of all types can delay development and promote epilepsy in the child. Of course, seizures also pose a risk of falls and injury to the mother.

Given that seizures and AEDs both carry risks, what should be done? Should the drugs be withdrawn, thereby increasing the risk of injury from seizures? Or should the drugs be continued, thereby posing a risk of drug-induced injury? Most authorities agree that the risk to the fetus from uncontrolled seizures is greater than the risk from AEDs. Hence, as a general rule, women with major seizure disorders should continue to take AEDs throughout pregnancy. To minimize fetal risk, the lowest effective dosage should be determined and maintained. In addition, since the risk of malformation is proportional to the number of drugs taken, just one drug should be used whenever possible.

As discussed in Chapter 9, drug disposition changes during pregnancy. In particular, renal excretion of drugs increases, as do hepatic metabolism and protein binding. As a result, the level of free (active) drug falls, posing a risk of breakthrough seizures. Accordingly, dosage should be increased. To determine dosing requirements, drug levels should be measured at least once a month.

To reduce the risk of neural tube defects, women should take supplemental folic acid prior to conception and throughout pregnancy. A dose of 2 mg/day has been recommended. (This is 5 times the dosage recommended for women not taking AEDs.) Although supplemental folic acid can prevent neural tube defects in the absence of AEDs, it may not prevent AED-induced defects.

Four drugs—*phenobarbital, phenytoin, carbamazepine,* and *primidone*—reduce levels of vitamin K–dependent clotting factors (by inducing hepatic enzymes). As a result, these drugs increase the risk of bleeding. To reduce this risk, women should be given 20 mg of vitamin K daily during the last few weeks of pregnancy, and the baby should be given a 1-mg IM injection of vitamin K at birth.

In addition to their influence on clotting, inducers of hepatic metabolism can decrease blood levels of oral contraceptives, thereby rendering them ineffective. All women of child-bearing age should be informed of this drug interaction, and dosages of oral contraceptives should be increased as required.

MANAGEMENT OF GENERALIZED CONVULSIVE STATUS EPILEPTICUS

Convulsive SE is defined as a continuous series of tonic-clonic seizures that lasts for at least 20 to 30 minutes. Consciousness is lost during the entire attack. Tachycardia, elevation of blood pressure, and hyperthermia are typical. Metabolic sequelae include hypoglycemia and acidosis. If SE persists for more than 20 minutes, it can cause permanent neurologic injury (cognitive impairment, memory loss, worsening of the underlying seizure disorder) and even death. About 125,000 Americans suffer SE each year. About 20% of these die.

Generalized convulsive SE is a medical emergency that requires immediate treatment. Ideally, treatment should commence within 5 minutes of seizure onset. Experience has shown that, as time passes, SE becomes more and more resistant to therapy.

The goal of treatment is to maintain ventilation, correct hypoglycemia, and terminate the seizure. An IV line is established to draw blood for analysis of glucose levels, electrolyte levels, and drug levels. The line is also used to administer glucose and AEDs.

An IV benzodiazepine—either *lorazepam* [Ativan] or *diazepam* [Valium]—is used initially. Both drugs can terminate seizures quickly. Diazepam has a short duration of action, and hence must be administered repeatedly. In contrast, effects of lorazepam last up to 72 hours. Because of its prolonged effects, lorazepam is generally preferred to diazepam. The dosage for lorazepam is 0.1 mg/kg administered at a rate of 2 mg/min. The initial dose for diazepam is 0.2 mg/kg administered at a rate of 5 mg/min.

Once seizures have been stopped with a benzodiazepine, either *phenytoin* [Dilantin] or *fosphenytoin* [Cerebyx] is given for long-term suppression. Because the effects of diazepam are short lived, follow-up treatment with a long-acting drug is essential when diazepam is used for initial control. However, when lorazepam is used for initial control, follow-up therapy may be unnecessary.

⸬ KEY POINTS

- Seizures are initiated by discharge from a group of hyperexcitable neurons, called a focus.
- In partial seizures, excitation undergoes limited spread from the focus to adjacent cortical areas.
- In generalized seizure, excitation spreads widely throughout both hemispheres of the brain.
- AEDs act through three basic mechanisms: suppression of sodium influx, suppression of calcium influx, and potentiation of the inhibitory effects of GABA.
- The goal in treating epilepsy is to reduce seizures to an extent that enables the patient to live a normal or near-normal life. Complete elimination of seizures may not be possible without causing intolerable side effects.
- Many AEDs are selective for particular seizures, and hence successful treatment depends on choosing the correct drug.
- Monitoring plasma drug levels can be valuable for adjusting dosage, monitoring compliance, determining the cause of lost seizure control, and identifying the cause of toxicity, especially in patients taking more than one drug.
- Noncompliance accounts for nearly half of all treatment failures. Hence, promoting compliance is a treatment priority.
- Withdrawal of AEDs must be done very gradually, since abrupt withdrawal can trigger SE.
- Most AEDs cause CNS depression, which can be deepened by concurrent use of other CNS depressants (e.g., alcohol, antihistamines, opioids, other AEDs).
- Phenytoin is active against partial seizures and tonic-clonic seizures but not absence seizures.
- The capacity of the liver to metabolize phenytoin is limited. As a result, doses only slightly greater than those needed for therapeutic effects can push phenytoin levels into the toxic range.
- The therapeutic range for phenytoin is 10 to 20 μg/ml.
- When phenytoin levels rise above 20 μg/ml, CNS toxicity develops. Signs include nystagmus, sedation, ataxia, diplopia, and cognitive impairment.
- Phenytoin causes gingival hyperplasia in 20% of patients.
- Like phenytoin, carbamazepine is active against partial seizures and tonic-clonic seizures.
- Because carbamazepine is better tolerated than phenytoin, it is often preferred.
- Carbamazepine can cause leukopenia, anemia, and thrombocytopenia—and, very rarely, fatal aplastic anemia. To reduce the risk of serious hematologic toxicity, complete blood counts should be obtained prior to treatment and periodically thereafter.
- Valproic acid is a very-broad-spectrum AED, having activity against partial seizures and most generalized seizures, including tonic-clonic, absence, atonic, and myoclonic seizures.
- Valproic acid can cause potentially fatal liver injury, especially in children under 2 years old who are taking other AEDs.
- Valproic acid can cause potentially fatal pancreatitis.
- In contrast to other barbiturates, phenobarbital is able to suppress seizures without causing generalized CNS depression.
- Phenytoin, carbamazepine, and phenobarbital induce the synthesis of hepatic drug-metabolizing enzymes, and can thereby accelerate inactivation of other drugs. Inactivation of oral contraceptives and warfarin is of particular concern.
- AEDs can interact with one another in complex ways, causing their blood levels to change. Dosages must be adjusted to compensate for these interactions.
- All conventional AEDs (and possibly the newer AEDs) can harm the developing fetus, especially during the first trimester. However, the fetus and mother are at greater risk from uncontrolled seizures than from AEDs. Accordingly, women with major seizure disorders should continue taking AEDs throughout pregnancy.
- Fetal risk can be minimized by using just one AED (if possible) and in the lowest effective dosage.
- Initial control of generalized convulsive status epilepticus is accomplished with an IV benzodiazepine—either diazepam or lorazepam. When diazepam is used, follow-up treatment with phenytoin or fosphenytoin is essential for prolonged suppression.

Summary of Major Nursing Implications*

NURSING IMPLICATIONS THAT APPLY TO ALL ANTIEPILEPTIC DRUGS

Preadministration Assessment

Therapeutic Goal

The goal of treatment is to minimize or eliminate seizure events, thereby allowing the patient to live a normal or near-normal life.

Baseline Data

Before initiating treatment, it is essential to know the type of seizure involved (e.g., absence, generalized tonic-clonic) and the frequency of seizure events.

Implementation: Administration

Dosage Determination

Dosages are often highly individualized and difficult to establish. Clinical evaluation of therapeutic and adverse effects is essential to establish a dosage that is both safe and effective. For several AEDs (especially those used to treat tonic-clonic seizures), knowledge of plasma AED levels can be a significant aid to dosage determination.

Promoting Compliance

Seizure control requires rigid adherence to the prescribed regimen; noncompliance is a major cause of therapeutic failure. **To promote compliance, educate patients about the importance of taking AEDs exactly as prescribed.** Monitoring plasma AED levels can motivate compliance and facilitate assessment of noncompliance.

Ongoing Evaluation and Interventions

Evaluating Therapeutic Effects

Teach the patient (or a family member) to maintain a seizure frequency chart, indicating the date, time, and nature of all seizure events. The physician can use this record to evaluate treatment, make dosage adjustments, and alter drug selections.

Minimizing Danger from Uncontrolled Seizures

Advise patients to avoid potentially hazardous activities (e.g., driving, operating dangerous machinery) until seizure control has been achieved. Also, because seizures may recur after they are largely under control, advise patients to carry some form of identification (e.g., Medic Alert bracelet) to aid in diagnosis and treatment if a seizure occurs.

Minimizing Adverse Effects

CNS Depression. Practically all AEDs depress the CNS. Signs of CNS depression (sedation, drowsiness, lethargy) are most prominent during the initial phase of treatment and decline with continued drug use. **Forewarn patients about CNS depression, and advise them to avoid driving and other hazardous activities if CNS depression is significant.**

Withdrawal Seizures. Abrupt discontinuation of AEDs can lead to status epilepticus (SE). Consequently, withdrawal of medication should be done slowly (over 6 weeks to several months). **Forewarn patients about the dangers of abrupt drug withdrawal, and instruct them never to discontinue drug use without consulting the physician. Advise patients who are planning to travel to carry extra medication to ensure an uninterrupted supply in the event they become stranded where medication is unavailable.**

Usage in Pregnancy. In most cases, the risk from uncontrolled seizures exceeds the risk from medication, hence women with major seizure disorders should continue to take AEDs during pregnancy. However, the lowest effective dosage should be employed and, if possible, only one drug should be used. To reduce the risk of neural tube defects, women should take folic acid supplements prior to and throughout pregnancy.

Minimizing Adverse Interactions

CNS Depressants. Drugs with CNS-depressant actions (e.g., alcohol, antihistamines, barbiturates, opioids) will intensify the depressant effects of AEDs, thereby posing a risk of excessive CNS depression. **Warn patients against using alcohol and other CNS depressants.**

PHENYTOIN

Nursing implications for phenytoin include those presented below as well as those presented above for all AEDs.

Preadministration Assessment

Therapeutic Goal

Oral phenytoin is used to treat partial seizures (simple and complex) and tonic-clonic seizures. Intravenous phenytoin is used to treat convulsive SE.

Identifying High-Risk Patients

Intravenous phenytoin is *contraindicated* for patients with sinus bradycardia, sinoatrial block, second- or third-degree atrioventricular block, or Stokes-Adams syndrome.

Implementation: Administration

Routes

Oral, IV, and (rarely) IM.

Administration

Oral. **Instruct patients to take phenytoin exactly as prescribed. Inform them that, once a safe and effective dosage has been established, small deviations in dosage can lead to toxicity or to loss of seizure control.**

Advise patients to take phenytoin with meals to reduce gastric discomfort.

Instruct patients to shake the phenytoin oral suspension before dispensing in order to provide consistent dosing.

Intravenous. To minimize the risk of severe reactions (e.g., cardiovascular collapse), infuse phenytoin slowly (no faster than 50 mg/min).

Do not mix phenytoin solutions with other drugs.

To minimize venous inflammation at the site of injection, flush the needle or catheter with saline immediately after completing the phenytoin infusion.

*Patient education information is highlighted as blue text.

Summary of Major Nursing Implications*—cont'd

Ongoing Evaluation and Interventions

Minimizing Adverse Effects

CNS Effects. Inform patients that excessive doses can produce sedation, ataxia, diplopia, and interference with cognitive function. Instruct them to notify the physician if these occur.

Gingival Hyperplasia. Inform patients that phenytoin often promotes overgrowth of gum tissue. To minimize harm and discomfort, instruct them in proper techniques of brushing, flossing, and gum massage.

Use in Pregnancy. Phenytoin can cause fetal hydantoin syndrome and bleeding tendencies in the neonate. The risk of bleeding can be decreased by giving the mother vitamin K for 1 month prior to delivery and during delivery and to the infant immediately after delivery. The risk of fetal hydantoin syndrome can be decreased by using the lowest effective phenytoin dosage.

Skin Rash. Inform patients that phenytoin can cause a morbilliform (measles-like) rash that may progress to a more serious reaction. Instruct them to notify the physician immediately if a rash develops. Use of phenytoin should stop.

Withdrawal Seizures. Abrupt discontinuation of phenytoin can trigger convulsive SE. **Warn patients against abrupt cessation of treatment.**

Minimizing Adverse Interactions

Phenytoin is subject to a large number of significant interactions with other drugs; a few arc noted below. **Warn patients against use of any drugs not specifically approved by the physician.**

CNS Depressants. Warn patients against use of alcohol and all other drugs with CNS-depressant properties, including opioids, barbiturates, and antihistamines.

Warfarin and Oral Contraceptives. Phenytoin can decrease the effects of these agents (as well as other drugs) by inducing hepatic drug-metabolizing enzymes. Dosages of warfarin and oral contraceptives may need to be increased.

CARBAMAZEPINE

Nursing implications for carbamazepine include those presented below as well as those presented above for all AEDs.

Preadministration Assessment

Therapeutic Goal

Carbamazepine is used to treat partial seizures (simple and complex) and tonic-clonic seizures.

Baseline Data

Obtain complete blood counts prior to treatment.

Identifying High-Risk Patients

Carbamazepine is *contraindicated* for patients with a history of bone marrow depression or adverse hematologic reactions to other drugs.

Implementation: Administration

Route

Oral.

Administration

Advise patients to administer carbamazepine with meals to decrease gastric upset.

To minimize adverse CNS effects, use low initial doses and give the largest portion of the daily dose at bedtime.

Ongoing Evaluation and Interventions

Minimizing Adverse Effects

CNS Effects. Carbamazepine can cause headache, visual disturbances (nystagmus, blurred vision, diplopia), ataxia, vertigo, and unsteadiness. To minimize these effects, initiate therapy with low doses and have the patient take the largest portion of the daily dose at bedtime.

Hematologic Effects. Carbamazepine can cause leukopenia, anemia, thrombocytopenia, and, very rarely, fatal aplastic anemia. To reduce the risk of serious hematologic effects, (1) obtain complete blood counts prior to treatment and periodically thereafter, (2) avoid carbamazepine in patients with pre-existing hematologic abnormalities, and (3) **inform patients about manifestations of hematologic abnormalities (fever, sore throat, pallor, weakness, infection, easy bruising, petechiae), and instruct them to notify the physician if these occur.**

Birth Defects. Carbamazepine can cause neural-tube defects. Use in pregnancy only if the benefits of seizure suppression outweigh the risks to the fetus.

Minimizing Adverse Interactions

Interactions Due to Induction of Drug Metabolism. Carbamazepine can decrease responses to other drugs by inducing hepatic drug-metabolizing enzymes. Effects on oral contraceptives and oral anticoagulants are of particular concern. Patients using these drugs will require increased dosages to maintain therapeutic responses.

Phenytoin and Phenobarbital. These drugs can decrease responses to carbamazepine by inducing drug-metabolizing enzymes (beyond the degree of induction caused by carbamazepine itself). Dosage of carbamazepine may need to be increased.

Grapefruit Juice. Grapefruit juice can increase levels of carbamazepine. **Instruct patients not to drink grapefruit juice.**

VALPROIC ACID

Nursing implications for valproic acid include those presented below as well as those presented above for all AEDs.

Preadministration Assessment

Therapeutic Goal

Valproic acid is used to treat all major seizure disorders: tonic-clonic, absence, myoclonic, atonic, and partial (simple, complex, and secondarily generalized).

*Patient education information is highlighted as blue text.

Summary of Major Nursing Implications*—cont'd

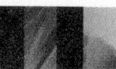

Baseline Data

Obtain baseline tests of liver function.

Identifying High-Risk Patients

Valproic acid is *contraindicated* for patients with significant hepatic dysfunction and for children under the age of 3 years who are taking other AEDs.

Implementation: Administration

Routes

Oral, IV.

Administration

Advise patients to take valproic acid with meals.

Instruct patients to ingest tablets and capsules intact, without crushing or chewing.

Ongoing Evaluation and Interventions

Minimizing Adverse Effects

Gastrointestinal Effects. Nausea, vomiting, and indigestion are common. These can be reduced by using an enteric-coated formulation (see Table 23–3) and by taking valproic acid with meals.

Hepatotoxicity. Rarely, valproic acid has caused fatal liver injury. To minimize risk, (1) don't use valproic acid in conjunction with other drugs in children under the age of 3 years; (2) don't use valproic acid in patients with pre-existing liver dysfunction; (3) evaluate liver function before initiating treatment and periodically thereafter; (4) **inform patients about signs and symptoms of liver injury (reduced appetite, malaise, nausea, abdominal pain, jaundice), and instruct them to notify the physician if these develop;** and (5) use valproic acid in the lowest effective dosage.

Pancreatitis. Valproic acid can cause life-threatening pancreatitis. **Inform patients about signs of pancreatitis (abdominal pain, nausea, vomiting, anorexia) and instruct them to get immediate evaluation if these develop.** If pancreatitis is diagnosed, valproic acid should be withdrawn.

Teratogenesis. Valproic acid may cause neural tube defects and other birth defects. **Advise women of child-bearing age to use an effective form of birth control and to take 5 mg of folic acid daily (to reduce the risk of neural tube defects.)**

Minimizing Adverse Interactions

Anticonvulsants. Valproic acid can elevate plasma levels of phenytoin and phenobarbital. Levels of phenobarbital and phenytoin should be monitored and their dosages adjusted accordingly.

PHENOBARBITAL

Nursing implications that apply to the antiseizure applications of phenobarbital include those presented below and those presented above for all AEDs. Nursing implications that apply to the barbiturates as a group are summarized in Chapter 33.

Preadministration Assessment

Therapeutic Goal

Oral phenobarbital is used to treat partial seizures (simple and complex) and tonic-clonic seizures. Intravenous therapy is used for convulsive SE.

Identifying High-Risk Patients

Phenobarbital is *contraindicated* for patients with a history of acute intermittent porphyria. The drug should be used with *caution* during pregnancy.

Implementation: Administration

Routes

Oral and IV.

Administration

Oral. A loading schedule may be employed to initiate treatment. Monitor for excessive CNS depression when these large doses are used.

Intravenous. Rapid IV infusion can cause severe adverse effects. Perform infusions slowly.

Ongoing Evaluation and Interventions

Minimizing Adverse Effects

Neuropsychologic Effects. **Warn patients that sedation may occur during the initial phase of treatment. Advise them to avoid hazardous activities if sedation is significant.**

Inform parents that children may become irritable and hyperactive, and instruct them to notify the physician if these behaviors occur.

Exacerbation of Intermittent Porphyria. Phenobarbital can exacerbate acute intermittent porphyria, and hence is absolutely contraindicated for patients with a history of this disorder.

Use in Pregnancy. **Warn women of child-bearing age that barbiturates may cause birth defects.**

Withdrawal Seizures. Abrupt withdrawal of phenobarbital can trigger seizures. **Warn patients against abrupt cessation of treatment.**

Minimizing Adverse Interactions

Interactions Caused by Induction of Drug Metabolism. Phenobarbital induces hepatic drug-metabolizing enzymes, and can thereby can decrease responses to other drugs. Effects on *oral contraceptives* and *warfarin* are a particular concern; their dosages should be increased.

CNS Depressants. **Warn patients against use of alcohol and all other drugs with CNS-depressant properties (e.g., opioids, benzodiazepines).**

Valproic Acid. Valproic acid increases blood levels of phenobarbital. To avoid toxicity, phenobarbital dosage should be reduced.

*Patient education information is highlighted as blue text.

Drugs for Muscle Spasm and Spasticity

DRUG THERAPY OF MUSCLE SPASM:
CENTRALLY ACTING MUSCLE RELAXANTS
DRUGS FOR SPASTICITY
 Baclofen
 Diazepam
 Dantrolene

In this chapter we consider two groups of drugs that cause skeletal muscle relaxation. One group is used to treat localized muscle spasm. The other is used to treat spasticity. With only one exception (dantrolene), these drugs produce their effects through actions in the central nervous system (CNS). As a rule, the drugs used to treat spasticity do not relieve acute muscle spasm and vice versa. Hence, the two groups are not interchangeable.

DRUG THERAPY OF MUSCLE SPASM: CENTRALLY ACTING MUSCLE RELAXANTS

Muscle spasm is defined as involuntary contraction of a muscle or muscle group. Muscle spasm is often painful and decreases the patient's level of functioning. Spasm can result from a variety of causes, including epilepsy, hypocalcemia, acute and chronic pain syndromes, and trauma (localized skeletal muscle injury). Discussion here is limited to spasm resulting from muscle injury.

Treatment of spasm involves physical measures as well as drug therapy. Physical measures include immobilization of the affected muscle, application of cold compresses,

whirlpool baths, and physical therapy. For drug therapy, two groups of medicines are used: (1) analgesic anti-inflammatory agents (e.g., aspirin), and (2) centrally acting muscle relaxants. The analgesic anti-inflammatory agents are discussed in Chapter 67. The centrally acting muscle relaxants are discussed below.

The family of centrally acting muscle relaxants consists of 10 drugs (Table 24–1). All have similar pharmacologic properties. Hence, we will consider them as a group.

Mechanism of Action

For most centrally acting muscle relaxants, the mechanism of spasm relief is unclear. In laboratory animals, high doses can depress spinal motor reflexes. However, these doses are much higher than those used in humans. Hence, many investigators believe that relaxation of spasm results primarily from the *sedative properties* of these drugs, and not from specific actions exerted on CNS pathways that control muscle tone.

Two drugs—diazepam and tizanidine—are thought to relieve spasm by enhancing presynaptic inhibition of motor neurons in the CNS. Diazepam promotes presynaptic inhibition by enhancing the effects of gamma-aminobutyric acid (GABA), an inhibitory neurotransmitter. Tizanidine promotes inhibition by acting as an agonist at presynaptic alpha$_2$ receptors.

Therapeutic Use

The centrally acting muscle relaxants are used to treat localized spasm resulting from muscle injury. These agents can decrease local pain and tenderness and can increase range of motion. Treatment is almost always associated with sedation. The ability of central muscle relaxants to relieve discomfort

TABLE 24–1 ▪ Drugs for Muscle Spasm: Centrally Acting Muscle Relaxants		
Generic Name	Trade Names	Usual Adult Oral Maintenance Dosage
Baclofen	Lioresal	15–20 mg 3 or 4 times/day
Carisoprodol	Soma	350 mg 3 or 4 times/day
Chlorphenesin	Maolate	400–800 mg 4 times/day
Chlorzoxazone	Paraflex, Parafon Forte, Remular-S	250 mg 3 or 4 times/day
Cyclobenzaprine	Flexeril	10 mg 3 times/day
Diazepam	Valium	2–10 mg 3 or 4 times/day
Metaxalone	Skelaxin	800 mg 3 or 4 times/day
Methocarbamol	Robaxin	1000 mg 4 times/day
Orphenadrine	Norflex	100 mg morning and evening
Tizanidine	Zanaflex	4 mg 3 or 4 times/day

of muscle spasm appears about equal to that of aspirin and the other analgesic anti-inflammatory drugs. Since there are no studies to indicate the superiority of one centrally acting muscle relaxant over another, drug selection is based largely on the prescriber's preference and the patient's response. With the exception of diazepam, the central muscle relaxants are not useful for treating spasticity or other muscle disorders resulting from CNS pathology.

Adverse Effects

CNS Depression. All of the centrally acting muscle relaxants can produce generalized depression of the CNS. Drowsiness, dizziness, and lightheadedness are common. Patients should be warned not to participate in hazardous activities (e.g., driving) if CNS depression is significant. In addition, they should be advised to avoid alcohol and all other CNS depressants.

Hepatic Toxicity. *Tizanidine* [Zanaflex] and *metaxalone* [Skelaxin] can cause liver damage. Liver function should be assessed before starting treatment and periodically thereafter. If liver injury develops, these drugs should be discontinued. If the patient has pre-existing liver disease, these drugs should be avoided.

Chlorzoxazone [Paraflex, others] can cause hepatitis and potentially fatal hepatic necrosis. Because of this potential for harm, and because the benefits of chlorzoxazone are questionable, the drug should not be used.

Physical Dependence. Chronic, high-dose therapy can cause physical dependence, manifesting as a potentially life-threatening abstinence syndrome if these drugs are abruptly withdrawn. Accordingly, withdrawal should be done slowly.

Other Adverse Effects. *Cyclobenzaprine* and *orphenadrine* have significant anticholinergic (atropine-like) properties, and hence may cause dry mouth, blurred vision, photophobia, urinary retention, and constipation. *Methocarbamol* may turn urine brown, black, or dark green; patients should be forewarned of this harmless effect. *Tizanidine* can cause dry mouth, hypotension, hallucinations, and psychotic symptoms. *Carisoprodol* can be hazardous to patients predisposed to intermittent porphyria, and hence is contraindicated for these people.

Dosage and Administration

All centrally acting skeletal muscle relaxants can be administered orally. In addition, two agents—methocarbamol and diazepam—can be administered by injection (IM and IV). Average oral maintenance dosages for adults are listed in Table 24–1.

DRUGS FOR SPASTICITY

The term *spasticity* refers to a group of movement disorders of CNS origin. These disorders are characterized by heightened muscle tone, spasm, and loss of dexterity. The most common causes are multiple sclerosis and cerebral palsy. Other causes include traumatic spinal cord lesions and stroke. Spasticity is managed with a combination of drugs and physical therapy.

Three drugs—baclofen, diazepam, and dantrolene—can relieve spasticity. Two of these agents—baclofen and diazepam—act in the CNS. The third drug—dantrolene—acts directly on skeletal muscle. With the exception of diazepam, the drugs employed to treat muscle spasm (i.e., the centrally acting muscle relaxants) are not effective against spasticity.

Baclofen
Mechanism of Action

Baclofen [Lioresal] acts within the spinal cord to suppress hyperactive reflexes involved in regulation of muscle movement. The precise mechanism of reflex attenuation is unknown. Since baclofen is a structural analog of the inhibitory neurotransmitter GABA (Fig. 24–1), it may act by mimicking the actions of GABA on spinal neurons. Baclofen has no direct effects on skeletal muscle.

Therapeutic Use

Baclofen can reduce spasticity associated with multiple sclerosis, spinal cord injury, and cerebral palsy—but not with stroke. The drug decreases flexor and extensor spasms and suppresses resistance to passive movement. These actions reduce the discomfort of spasticity and allow increased performance. Since baclofen has no direct muscle-relaxant action, and hence does not decrease muscle strength, baclofen is preferred to dantrolene in patients whose spasticity is associated with significant muscle weakness. Baclofen does not relieve the spasticity of Parkinson's disease or Huntington's chorea.

Adverse Effects

The most common side effects involve the CNS and GI tract. Serious adverse effects are rare.

CNS Effects. Baclofen is a CNS depressant and hence frequently causes drowsiness, dizziness, weakness, and fatigue. These responses are most intense during the early phase of therapy and diminish with continued drug use. CNS depression can be minimized with doses that are small initially and then gradually increased. Patients should be cautioned to avoid alcohol and other CNS depressants, since baclofen potentiates the depressant actions of these drugs.

Overdose with baclofen can produce coma and respiratory depression. Since there is no antidote to baclofen poisoning, treatment is supportive.

Although baclofen does not appear to cause physical dependence, abrupt discontinuation has been associated with adverse reactions, including visual hallucinations, paranoid ideation, and seizures. Accordingly, drug withdrawal should be done slowly (over 1 to 2 weeks).

Other Adverse Effects. Baclofen frequently causes *nausea, constipation,* and *urinary retention.* Patients should be warned about these possible reactions.

Preparations, Dosage, and Administration

Oral. Baclofen [Lioresal] is dispensed in tablets (10 and 20 mg) for oral use. Dosages are low initially (e.g., 5 mg 3 times a day) and then gradually increased. Maintenance dosages range from 15 to 20 mg administered 3 to 4 times a day.

Intrathecal. Baclofen can be administered by intrathecal infusion using an implantable pump. The average maintenance dosage is 300 to 800 mg/day. Intrathecal administration is reserved for patients who are unresponsive to or intolerant of oral baclofen.

Diazepam

Diazepam [Valium] is a member of the benzodiazepine family. Although diazepam is the only benzodiazepine labeled for treating spasticity, other benzodiazepines would probably be effective. The basic pharmacology of the benzodiazepines is discussed in Chapter 33.

Actions. Like baclofen, diazepam acts within the CNS to suppress spasticity. Beneficial effects appear to result from mimicking the actions of GABA at receptors in the spinal cord and brain. Diazepam does not affect skeletal muscle directly. Since diazepam has no direct effects on muscle strength, the drug is preferred to dantrolene in patients whose strength is marginal.

Adverse Effects. *Sedation* is common when treating spasticity. To minimize sedation, initiate therapy with low doses. Other adverse effects are discussed in Chapter 33.

Preparations, Dosage, and Administration. For oral use, diazepam [Valium] is dispensed in tablets (2, 5, and 10 mg), sustained-release capsules (15 mg), and solution (1 and 5 mg/ml). The drug is also available as an injection (5 mg/ml) for IM and IV administration. The usual oral dosage for adults is 2 to 10 mg 3 or 4 times a day.

Dantrolene

Mechanism of Action

Unlike baclofen and diazepam, which act within the CNS, dantrolene [Dantrium] acts directly on skeletal muscle. The drug relieves spasm by suppressing release of calcium from the sarcoplasmic reticulum (SR), and hence the muscle is less able to contract. Fortunately, therapeutic doses have only minimal effects on contraction of smooth muscle and cardiac muscle.

Therapeutic Uses

Spasticity. Dantrolene can relieve spasticity associated with multiple sclerosis, cerebral palsy, and spinal cord injury. Unfortunately, since dantrolene suppresses spasticity by causing a generalized reduction in the ability of skeletal muscle to contract, treatment may be associated with a significant decrease in strength. As a result, for some patients, overall function may be reduced rather than improved. Accordingly, care must be taken to ensure that the benefits of therapy (reduced spasticity) outweigh the harm (reduced strength).

Malignant Hyperthermia. Malignant hyperthermia is a rare, life-threatening syndrome that can be triggered by any general anesthetic and by succinylcholine, a neuromuscular blocking agent. Onset of symptoms is most abrupt with succinylcholine (when used alone or in combination with an anesthetic). Prominent symptoms are muscle rigidity and profound elevation of temperature. The heat of malignant hyperthermia is generated by muscle contraction occurring secondary to massive release of calcium from the SR. Dantrolene relieves symptoms by acting on the SR to block calcium release. Malignant hyperthermia is discussed further in Chapter 16.

Adverse Effects

Hepatic Toxicity. Dose-related liver damage is dantrolene's most serious adverse effect. The incidence is 1 in 1000. Deaths have occurred. Hepatotoxicity is most common in women over age 35. By contrast, liver injury is rare in children under 10 years. To reduce the risk of liver damage, tests of liver function should be performed before initiating treatment and periodically thereafter. Because of the potential for liver damage, dantrolene should be administered in the lowest effective dosage and for the shortest time necessary.

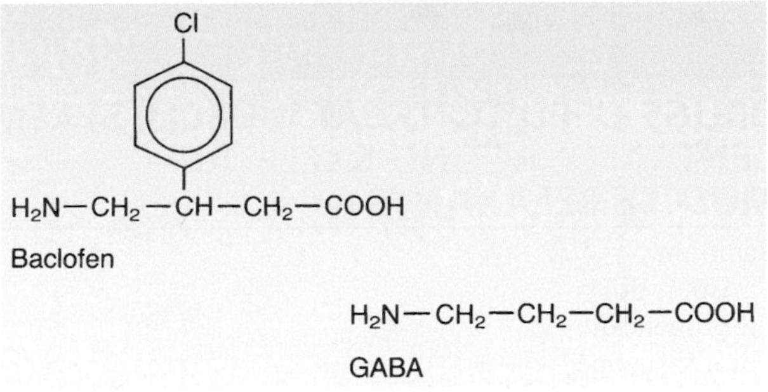

Figure 24–1 ■ **Structural similarity between baclofen and gamma-aminobutyric acid (GABA).**

Other Adverse Effects. *Muscle weakness, drowsiness,* and *diarrhea* are the most common side effects. Muscle weakness is a direct extension of dantrolene's pharmacologic action. Other disturbing reactions include *anorexia, nausea, vomiting,* and *acne-like rash.*

Preparations, Dosage, and Administration

Preparations. Dantrolene sodium [Dantrium] is dispensed in capsules (25, 50, and 100 mg) for oral use and as a powder to be reconstituted for IV injection.

Use in Spasticity. For treatment of spasticity, administration is oral. The initial adult dosage is 25 mg once daily. The usual maintenance dosage is 100 mg 2 to 4 times a day. If beneficial effects do not develop within 45 days, dantrolene should be stopped.

Use in Malignant Hyperthermia. *Preoperative Prophylaxis.* Patients with a history of malignant hyperthermia can be given dantrolene for prophylaxis prior to elective surgery. The dosage is 4 to 8 mg/kg/day in four divided doses for 1 to 2 days preceding surgery.

Treatment of an Ongoing Crisis. For treatment of malignant hyperthermia, dantrolene is administered by IV push. The initial dose is 2 mg/kg. Administration is repeated until symptoms are controlled or until a total dose of 10 mg/kg has been given. Other management measures are discussed in Chapter 16.

⸫ KEY POINTS

- Localized muscle spasm is treated with centrally acting muscle relaxants and aspirin-like drugs.
- Spasticity is treated with three drugs: baclofen, diazepam, and dantrolene.
- All centrally acting muscle relaxants produce generalized CNS depression.
- Chlorzoxazone, a central muscle relaxant, is marginally effective and can cause fatal hepatic necrosis. Accordingly, the drug should not be used.
- Baclofen and diazepam relieve spasticity by mimicking the inhibitory actions of GABA in the CNS.
- Like the centrally acting muscle relaxants, baclofen and diazepam cause generalized CNS depression.
- In contrast to all other drugs discussed in this chapter, dantrolene acts directly on muscle to promote relaxation.
- With prolonged use, dantrolene can cause potentially fatal liver damage. Monitor liver function and minimize dosage and duration of treatment.
- In addition to relief of spasticity, dantrolene is used to treat malignant hyperthermia, a potentially fatal condition caused by succinylcholine and general anesthetics.

Summary of Major Nursing Implications*

DRUGS USED TO TREAT MUSCLE SPASM: CENTRALLY ACTING SKELETAL MUSCLE RELAXANTS

Baclofen
Carisoprodol
Chlorphenesin
Chlorzoxazone
Cyclobenzaprine
Diazepam
Metaxalone
Methocarbamol
Orphenadrine
Tizanidine

Except where noted otherwise, the nursing implications summarized below apply to all centrally acting muscle relaxants used to treat muscle spasm.

Preadministration Assessment

Therapeutic Goal

Relief of signs and symptoms of muscle spasm.

Identifying High-Risk Patients

Avoid *chlorzoxazone, metaxalone,* and *tizanidine* in patients with liver disease.

Implementation: Administration

Routes

Oral. All central skeletal muscle relaxants.
Parenteral. Methocarbamol and *diazepam* may be given IM and IV as well as PO.

Dosage

See Table 24–1.

Implementation: Measures to Enhance Therapeutic Effects

The treatment plan should include appropriate physical measures (e.g., immobilization of the affected muscle, application of cold compresses, whirlpool baths, and physical therapy).

Ongoing Evaluation and Interventions

Minimizing Adverse Effects

CNS Depression. All central muscle relaxants cause CNS depression. **Inform patients about possible effects (drowsiness, dizziness, lightheadedness, fatigue) and advise them to avoid hazardous activities (e.g., driving) if significant impairment occurs.**
Hepatic Toxicity. Metaxalone and *tizanidine* can cause liver damage. Determine liver function before treatment and periodically thereafter. If liver damage develops, discontinue treatment. Avoid these drugs in patients with pre-existing liver disease.
Chlorzoxazone can cause hepatitis and potentially fatal hepatic necrosis. This drug should not be used.

Minimizing Adverse Interactions

CNS Depressants. **Caution patients to avoid CNS depressants (e.g., alcohol, benzodiazepines, opioids, antihistamines)** since these drugs will intensify the depressant effects of muscle relaxants.

Avoiding Withdrawal Reactions

Central muscle relaxants can cause physical dependence. To avoid an abstinence syndrome, withdraw gradually. **Warn the patient against abrupt discontinuation of treatment.**

BACLOFEN

Preadministration Assessment

Therapeutic Goal

Relief of signs and symptoms of spasticity.

Baseline Data

Assess for spasm, rigidity, pain, range of motion, and dexterity.

Implementation: Administration

Route

Oral.

Administration

Patients with muscle spasm may be unable to self-medicate. Provide assistance if needed.

Ongoing Evaluation and Interventions

Evaluating Therapeutic Effects

Monitor for reductions in rigidity, muscle spasm, and pain and for improvements in dexterity and range of motion.

Minimizing Adverse Effects

CNS Depression. Baclofen is a CNS depressant. **Inform patients about possible depressant effects (drowsiness, dizziness, lightheadedness, fatigue) and advise them to avoid hazardous activities (e.g., driving) if significant impairment occurs.**

Minimizing Adverse Interactions

CNS Depressants. **Caution patients to avoid CNS depressants (e.g., alcohol, benzodiazepines, opioids, antihistamines)** since these drugs will intensify the depressant effects of baclofen.

Avoiding Withdrawal Reactions

Abrupt withdrawal can cause visual hallucinations, paranoid ideation, and seizures. **Caution the patient against abrupt discontinuation of treatment.**

DANTROLENE

The nursing implications summarized here apply only to the use of dantrolene for spasticity.

*Patient education information is highlighted as blue text.

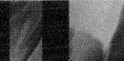

Summary of Major Nursing Implications*—cont'd

Preadministration Assessment

Therapeutic Goal

Relief of signs and symptoms of spasticity.

Baseline Data

Assess for spasm, rigidity, pain, range of motion, and dexterity. Obtain laboratory tests of liver function.

Identifying High-Risk Patients

Dantrolene is *contraindicated* for patients with active hepatic disease (e.g., cirrhosis, hepatitis).

Implementation: Administration

Route

Oral.

Administration

Patients with muscle spasm may be unable to self-medicate. Provide assistance if needed.

Ongoing Evaluation and Interventions

Summary of Monitoring

Therapeutic Effects. Monitor for reductions in rigidity, spasm, and pain and for improvements in dexterity and range of motion.

Adverse Effects. Monitor liver function tests and for reductions in muscle strength.

*Patient education information is highlighted as blue text.

Minimizing Adverse Effects

CNS Depression. Dantrolene is a CNS depressant. Inform patients about possible depressant effects (drowsiness, dizziness, lightheadedness, fatigue) and advise them to avoid hazardous activities (e.g., driving) if significant impairment occurs.

Hepatic Toxicity. Dantrolene is hepatotoxic. Assess liver function at baseline and periodically thereafter. If signs of liver dysfunction develop, withdraw dantrolene. Inform patients about signs of liver dysfunction (e.g., jaundice, abdominal pain, malaise) and instruct them to seek medical attention if these develop.

Muscle Weakness. Dantrolene can decrease muscle strength. Evaluate muscle function to ensure that benefits of therapy (decreased spasticity) are not outweighed by reductions in strength.

Minimizing Adverse Interactions

CNS Depressants. Warn patients to avoid CNS depressants (e.g., alcohol, benzodiazepines, opioids, antihistamines), since these drugs will intensify depressant effects of dantrolene.

DIAZEPAM

Nursing implications for diazepam and the other benzodiazepines are summarized in Chapter 33.

CHAPTER

25

Local Anesthetics

Local anesthetics are drugs that suppress pain by blocking impulse conduction along axons. Conduction is blocked only in neurons located near the site of anesthetic administration. The great advantage of local anesthesia, as compared with inhalational anesthesia, is that pain can be suppressed without causing generalized depression of the entire nervous system. Hence, local anesthetics allow performance of medical and surgical procedures with much less risk than is associated with general anesthetics.

We begin the chapter by considering the pharmacology of the local anesthetics as a group. After that, we discuss three prototypic agents: procaine, lidocaine, and cocaine. We conclude by discussing specific routes of anesthetic administration.

BASIC PHARMACOLOGY OF THE LOCAL ANESTHETICS

Classification

There are two major groups of local anesthetics: *esters* and *amides*. As shown in Figure 25–1, the ester-type anesthetics, represented by *procaine* [Novocain], contain an ester linkage in their structure. In contrast, the amide-type agents, represented by *lidocaine* [Xylocaine], contain an amide linkage. The ester-type agents and amide-type agents differ in two important ways: method of inactivation and ability to promote allergic responses. Contrasts between the esters and amides are summarized in Table 25–1.

Mechanism of Action

Local anesthetics stop axonal conduction by *blocking sodium channels* in the axonal membrane. Recall that propagation of an action potential requires movement of sodium ions from outside the axon to the inside. This influx takes place through specialized sodium channels. By blocking axonal sodium channels, local anesthetics prevent sodium entry, and thereby bring conduction to a halt.

Selectivity of Anesthetic Effects

Local anesthetics are nonselective modifiers of neuronal function. That is, these drugs will block action potentials in all neurons to which they have access. The only way we can achieve selectivity is by delivering anesthetic to a limited area.

Although local anesthetics can block traffic in all neurons, blockade develops more rapidly in some neurons than in others. Specifically, small, nonmyelinated neurons are blocked more rapidly than large, myelinated neurons. Because of this differential sensitivity, some sensations are blocked sooner than others: perception of pain is lost first, followed in order by perception of cold, warmth, touch, and deep pressure.

It should be noted that the effects of local anesthetics are not limited to sensory neurons; these drugs also block conduction in motor neurons.

Time Course of Local Anesthesia

Ideally, local anesthesia would begin promptly and would persist no longer (or shorter) than needed. Unfortunately, although onset of anesthesia is usually rapid (see Tables 25–2 and 25–3), duration of anesthesia is often less than ideal. In some cases, anesthesia persists longer than needed; in others, repeated administration is required to maintain anesthesia of sufficient duration.

Onset of local anesthesia is determined largely by the molecular properties of the anesthetic. Before anesthesia can occur, the anesthetic must diffuse from its site of administration to its sites of action within the axon membrane; anesthesia is delayed until this movement has occurred. The ability of an anesthetic to penetrate the axon membrane is determined by three properties: *molecular size, lipid solubility,* and *degree of ionization at tissue pH*. Anesthetics of small size, high lipid solubility, and low ionization cross the axon membrane rapidly. In contrast, anesthetics of large size, low lipid solubility, and high ionization cross slowly. Obviously, anesthetics that penetrate the axon most rapidly have the fastest onset.

Termination of local anesthesia occurs as molecules of anesthetic diffuse out of neurons and are carried away in the blood. The same factors that determine onset of anesthesia

214

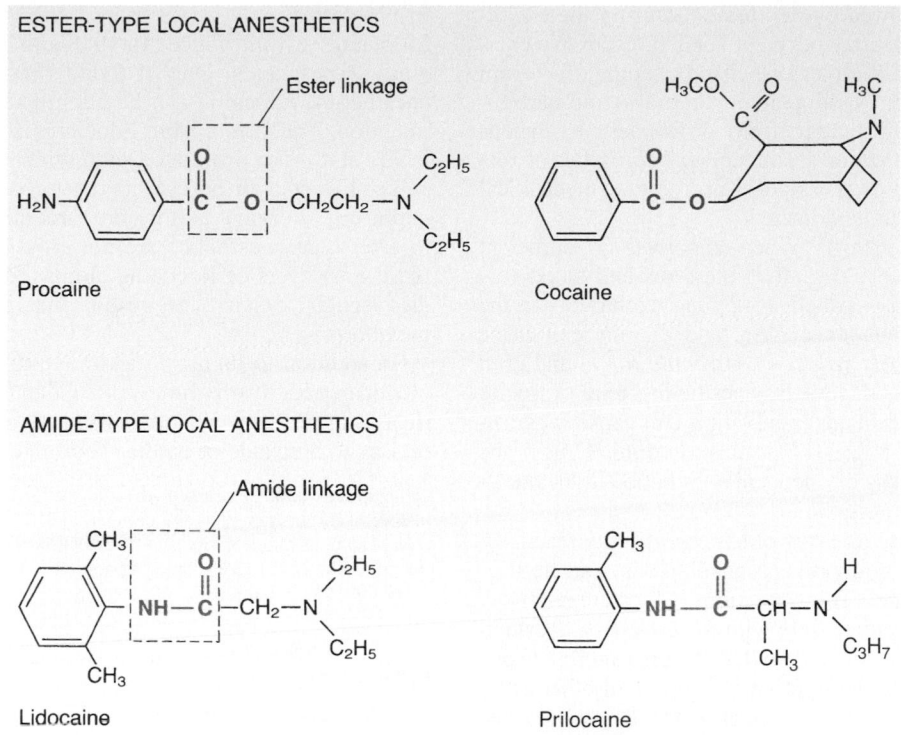

Figure 25–1 ■ **Structural formulas of representative local anesthetics.**

(molecular size, lipid solubility, degree of ionization) also help determine duration. In addition, *regional blood flow* is an important determinant of how long anesthesia will last. In areas where blood flow is high, anesthetic is carried away quickly, and hence effects terminate with relative haste. In regions where blood flow is low, anesthesia is more prolonged.

Use with Vasoconstrictors

Local anesthetics are frequently administered in combination with a vasoconstrictor—usually *epinephrine*. The vasoconstrictor decreases local blood flow and thereby delays systemic absorption of the anesthetic. Delaying absorption has two benefits: It *prolongs anesthesia* and *reduces the risk of toxicity*. Why is toxicity reduced? First, because absorption is slowed, we can use less anesthetic. Second, by slowing absorption, we can establish a more favorable balance between the rate of entry of anesthetic into circulation and the capacity of the body to convert the anesthetic into inactive metabolites.

It should be noted that absorption of the vasoconstrictor itself can result in systemic toxicity (e.g., palpitations, tachycardia, nervousness, hypertension). If adrenergic stimulation from absorption of epinephrine is excessive, symptoms can be controlled with alpha- and beta-adrenergic antagonists.

Fate in the Body

Absorption and Distribution. Although administered for local effects, local anesthetics do get absorbed into the blood and become distributed to all parts of the body. The rate of absorption is determined largely by blood flow to the site of administration.

TABLE 25–1 ■ Contrasts Between Ester and Amide Local Anesthetics		
	Ester-type Anesthetics	Amide-type Anesthetics
Characteristic Chemistry	Ester bond	Amide bond
Representative Agents	Procaine	Lidocaine
Incidence of Allergic Reactions	Low	Very low
Method of Metabolism	Plasma esterases	Hepatic enzymes

Metabolism. The process by which a local anesthetic is metabolized depends on the class—ester or amide—to which it belongs. *Ester-type* local anesthetics are metabolized in the blood by enzymes known as *esterases*. In contrast, *amide-type* anesthetics are metabolized by enzymes in the *liver*. For both types of anesthetic, metabolism results in inactivation.

The balance between rate of absorption and rate of metabolism is clinically significant. If a local anesthetic is absorbed more slowly than it is metabolized, its level in blood will remain low, and hence systemic reactions will be minimal. Conversely, if absorption outpaces metabolism, plasma drug levels will rise, and the risk of systemic toxicity will increase.

Adverse Effects

Adverse effects can occur locally or distant from the site of administration. Local effects are less common.

Central Nervous System. When absorbed in sufficient amounts, local anesthetics cause central nervous system

(CNS) excitation followed by depression. During the excitation phase, convulsions may occur. If needed, excessive excitation can be managed with an IV benzodiazepine (diazepam or midazolam) or with IV thiopental (a rapid-acting barbiturate). Depressant effects range from drowsiness to unconsciousness. Death can occur secondary to depression of respiration. If respiratory depression is prominent, mechanical ventilation with oxygen is indicated.

Cardiovascular System. When absorbed in sufficient amounts, local anesthetics can affect the heart and blood vessels. In the heart, local anesthetics suppress excitability in the myocardium and conducting system, and thereby can cause *bradycardia, heart block, reduced contractile force,* and *even cardiac arrest.* In blood vessels, anesthetics relax vascular smooth muscle; the resultant vasodilation can cause *hypotension.* As discussed in Chapter 47 (Antidysrhythmic Drugs), the cardiosuppressant actions of one local anesthetic—lidocaine— are exploited to treat dysrhythmias.

Allergic Reactions. An array of hypersensitivity reactions, ranging from allergic dermatitis to anaphylaxis, can be triggered by local anesthetics. These reactions, which are relatively uncommon, are much more likely with the *ester-type* anesthetics (e.g., procaine) than with the amides. Patients allergic to one ester-type anesthetic are likely to be allergic to all other ester-type agents. Fortunately, cross-hypersensitivity between the esters and amides has not been observed. Hence, the amides can be used when allergies contraindicate use of ester-type anesthetics. Because they are unlikely to cause hypersensitivity reactions, the amide-type anesthetics have largely replaced the ester-type agents when administration by injection is required.

Use in Labor and Delivery. Local anesthetics can depress uterine contractility and maternal expulsion effort. Both actions can prolong labor. Also, local anesthetics can cross the placenta, causing bradycardia and CNS depression in the neonate.

PROPERTIES OF INDIVIDUAL LOCAL ANESTHETICS

Procaine

Procaine [Novocain] was synthesized in 1905 and is the prototype of the ester-type local anesthetics. The drug is not effective topically, and hence must be given by injection. Administration in combination with epinephrine delays absorption. Although procaine is readily absorbed, systemic toxicity is rare. Why? Because plasma esterases rapidly convert the drug to inactive, nontoxic products. Being an ester-type anesthetic, procaine poses a greater risk of allergic reactions than do the amide-type anesthetics. Individuals allergic to procaine should be considered allergic to all other ester-type anesthetics—but not to the amides.

For many years, procaine was the local anesthetic most preferred for use by injection. However, with the development of newer agents, use of procaine has sharply declined. Once popular in dentistry, procaine is rarely employed in that setting today.

Preparations. Procaine hydrochloride [Novocain] is available in solution (1%, 2%, and 10%) for administration by injection. Dilution is required for use by some routes. Epinephrine (at a final concentration of 1:100,000 or 1:200,000) may be combined with procaine to delay absorption.

Lidocaine

Lidocaine was introduced in 1948 and is the prototype of the amide-type agents. One of today's most widely used local anesthetics, lidocaine can be administered topically and by injection. Anesthesia from lidocaine is more rapid, more intense, and more prolonged than with an equal dose of procaine. Effects can be extended by coadministration of epinephrine. Allergic reactions are rare, and individuals allergic to ester-type anesthetics are not cross-allergic to lidocaine. If plasma levels of lidocaine climb too high, CNS and cardiovascular toxicity can result. Inactivation is by hepatic metabolism.

In addition to its use in local anesthesia, lidocaine is employed to treat dysrhythmias (see Chapter 47). Control of dysrhythmias results from suppression of cardiac excitability secondary to blockade of cardiac sodium channels.

Preparations. Lidocaine hydrochloride [Xylocaine, others] is dispensed in several formulations (cream, ointment, jelly, solution, aerosol, patch) for topical administration. Lidocaine for injection is available in concentrations ranging from 0.5% to 5%; some preparations contain epinephrine (1:50,000, 1:100,000, or 1:200,000).

Cocaine

Cocaine was our first local anesthetic. Clinical use was initiated in 1884 by Sigmund Freud and Karl Koller. Freud described the physiologic effects of cocaine while Koller focused on the drug's anesthetic actions. As you can see from its structure (Fig. 25–1), cocaine is an ester-type anesthetic. In addition to causing local anesthesia, cocaine has pronounced effects on the sympathetic and central nervous systems. Sympathetic and CNS effects are due in large part to the drug's ability to block uptake of norepinephrine by adrenergic neurons.

Anesthetic Use. Cocaine is an excellent local anesthetic. Administration is topical. The drug is employed for anesthesia of the ear, nose, and throat. Anesthesia develops rapidly and persists for about an hour. Unlike other local anesthetics, cocaine causes intense vasoconstriction (by blocking norepinephrine uptake at sympathetic nerve terminals on blood vessels). Accordingly, the drug should not be given in combination with epinephrine or other vasoconstrictors. Despite its ability to constrict blood vessels, cocaine is readily absorbed following application to mucous membranes; significant effects on the brain and heart can result. The drug is inactivated by plasma esterases and by enzymes in the liver.

CNS Effects. Cocaine produces generalized CNS stimulation. Moderate doses cause euphoria, loquaciousness, reduced fatigue, and increased sociability and alertness. Excessive doses can cause seizures. Excitation is followed by CNS depression; respiratory arrest and death can result.

Although cocaine does not seem to cause substantial physical dependence, psychologic dependence can be profound. The drug is subject to widespread abuse and is classified under Schedule II of the Controlled Substances Act. Cocaine abuse is discussed in Chapter 38.

Cardiovascular Effects. Cocaine stimulates the heart and causes vasoconstriction. These effects result from (1) central stimulation of the sympathetic nervous system and (2) blockade

TABLE 25–2 ■ Topical Local Anesthetics: Trade Names, Indications, and Time Course of Action

	Generic Name	Trade Name	Indications Skin	Indications Mucous Membranes	Time Course of Action* Peak Effect (min)	Time Course of Action* Duration (min)
Amides	Dibucaine†	Nupercainal	✔		<5	15–45
	Lidocaine†	Xylocaine, others	✔	✔	2–5	15–45
Esters	Benzocaine	Many names	✔	✔	<5	15–45
	Butamben	Butesin	✔		—	—
	Cocaine			✔	1–5	30–60
	Tetracaine†	Pontocaine, Viractin	✔	✔	3–8	30–60
Others	Dyclonine	Dyclone		✔	<10	<60
	Pramoxine	Tronothane, others	✔		3–5	—

*Based primarily on application to mucous membranes.
†Also administered by injection.

of norepinephrine uptake in the periphery. Stimulation of the heart can produce tachycardia and potentially fatal dysrhythmias. Vasoconstriction can cause hypertension. Cocaine presents an especially serious risk to individuals with cardiovascular disease (e.g., hypertension, dysrhythmias, angina pectoris).

When used for local anesthesia, cocaine should not be combined with epinephrine, since the combination would increase the risk of cardiovascular toxicity. Furthermore, since a vasoconstrictor would not significantly retard cocaine absorption, the combination would be irrational in addition to dangerous.

Preparations and Administration. Cocaine hydrochloride is available as a powder (5 and 25 gm) and in solution (4% and 10%). Administration is topical. For application to the ear, nose, or throat, a 4% solution is usually employed. The drug must be dispensed in accord with the Controlled Substances Act.

Other Local Anesthetics

In addition to the drugs discussed above, several other local anesthetics are available. These agents differ with respect to indications, route of administration, mode of elimination, duration of action, and toxicity.

The local anesthetics can be grouped according to route of administration: topical versus injection. (Very few agents are administered by both routes, largely because the drugs that are suitable for topical application are usually too toxic for parenteral use.) Table 25–2 lists the topically administered local anesthetics along with trade names and time course of action. Table 25–3 presents equivalent information for the injectable agents.

CLINICAL USE OF LOCAL ANESTHETICS

Local anesthetics may be administered *topically* (for surface anesthesia) and *by injection* (for infiltration anesthesia, nerve block anesthesia, intravenous regional anesthesia, epidural anesthesia, and spinal anesthesia). The uses and hazards of these anesthesia techniques are discussed below.

Topical Administration

Surface anesthesia is accomplished by applying the anesthetic directly to the skin or a mucous membrane. The agents employed most commonly are *lidocaine, tetracaine,* and *cocaine.*

Therapeutic Uses. Local anesthetics are applied to the *skin* to relieve pain, itching, and soreness of various causes, including infection, thermal burns, sunburn, diaper rash, wounds, bruises, abrasions, plant poisoning, and insect bites. Application may be made to *mucous membranes* of the nose, mouth, pharynx, larynx, trachea, bronchi, vagina, and urethra. In addition, local anesthetics may be used to relieve discomfort associated with hemorrhoids, anal fissures, and pruritus ani.

Systemic Toxicity. Topical anesthetics can be absorbed in amounts sufficient to produce systemic toxicity. Cardiovascular reactions and CNS reactions are the principal concerns. Because the extent of absorption is proportional to the surface area covered, the risk of toxicity is greatest when the surface area is large. Also, because absorption occurs more readily through mucous membranes than through the skin, application to mucous membranes poses the greater risk. If the skin is abraded or otherwise injured, absorption will be increased, thereby increasing risk.

Administration by Injection

Injection of local anesthetics carries significant risk and requires special skills. Accordingly, injections are usually performed by an anesthesiologist. Because severe systemic reactions may occur, equipment for resuscitation should be immediately available. Also, an IV line should be in place to permit rapid treatment of toxicity. Inadvertent injection into an artery or vein can cause severe toxicity. To ensure the needle is not in a blood vessel, it should be aspirated prior to injection. Following administration, the patient should be monitored for cardiovascular status, respiratory function, and state of consciousness. To reduce the risk of toxicity, local anesthetics should be administered in the lowest effective dose.

TABLE 25–3 ▪■ Injectable Local Anesthetics: Trade Names and Time Course of Action

	Generic Name	Trade Name	Time Course of Action*	
			Onset (min)	Duration (hr)
Amides	Lidocaine†	Xylocaine, Octocaine	<2	0.5–1
	Articaine	Septocaine	1–6‡	1‡
	Bupivacaine	Marcaine, Sensorcaine	5	2–4
	Levobupivacaine	Chirocaine	10§	8§
	Mepivacaine	Carbocaine, Polocaine	3–5	0.75–1.5
	Prilocaine	Citanest	<2	≥1
	Ropivacaine	Naropin	10–30§	0.5–6§
Esters‖	Procaine	Novocain	2–5	0.25–1.0
	Chloroprocaine	Nesacaine	6–12	0.5
	Tetracaine†	Pontocaine	≤15	2–3

*Values are for *infiltration* anesthesia in the absence of epinephrine (epinephrine prolongs duration two- to threefold).
†Also administered topically.
‡Values are for *infiltration* anesthesia *with* epinephrine.
§Values are for *epidural* administration (without epinephrine).
‖Because of the risk of allergic reactions, the ester anesthetics are rarely administered by injection.

Infiltration Anesthesia

Infiltration anesthesia is achieved by injecting a local anesthetic directly into the immediate area of surgery or manipulation. Anesthesia can be prolonged by combining the anesthetic with epinephrine. However, epinephrine should not be used in areas supplied by end arteries (toes, fingers, nose, ears, penis), since restriction of blood flow at these sites may result in gangrene. The agents employed most frequently for infiltration anesthesia are *lidocaine* and *bupivacaine*.

Nerve Block Anesthesia

Nerve block anesthesia is achieved by injecting a local anesthetic into or near nerves that supply the surgical field, but at a site *distant* from the field itself. This technique has the advantage of producing anesthesia with doses that are smaller than those needed for infiltration anesthesia.

Drug selection is based on required duration of anesthesia. For shorter procedures, *lidocaine* or *mepivacaine* might be used. For longer procedures, *bupivacaine* would be appropriate.

Intravenous Regional Anesthesia

Intravenous regional anesthesia is employed to anesthetize the extremities—hands, feet, arms, and lower legs, but not the entire leg (because too much anesthetic would be needed). Anesthesia is produced by injection into a distal vein of an arm or leg. Prior to giving the anesthetic, blood is removed from the limb (by gravity or by application of an Esmarch bandage), and a tourniquet is applied to the limb (proximal to the site of anesthetic injection) to prevent anesthetic from entering the systemic circulation. To ensure complete blockade of arterial flow throughout the procedure, a double tourniquet is used. Following injection, the anesthetic diffuses out of the vasculature and becomes evenly distributed to all areas of the occluded limb. When the tourniquet is loosened at the end of surgery, about 15% to 30% of administered anesthetic is released into the systemic circulation. *Lidocaine—without epinephrine—*is the preferred agent for intravenous regional anesthesia.

Epidural Anesthesia

Epidural anesthesia is achieved by injecting a local anesthetic into the epidural space (i.e., within the spinal column but outside the dura mater). A catheter placed in the epidural space allows administration by bolus or by continuous infusion. Following administration, diffusion of anesthetic across the dura into the subarachnoid space blocks conduction in nerve roots and in the spinal cord itself. Diffusion through intervertebral foramina blocks nerves located in the paravertebral region. With epidural administration, anesthetic can reach the systemic circulation in significant amounts. As a result, when the technique is used during delivery, neonatal depression may result. *Lidocaine* and *bupivacaine* are popular drugs for epidural anesthesia. Because of the risk of death from cardiac arrest, the concentrated (0.75%) solution of bupivacaine should not be used in obstetric patients.

Spinal (Subarachnoid) Anesthesia

Technique. Spinal anesthesia is produced by injecting local anesthetic into the subarachnoid space. Injection is made in the lumbar region below the termination of the cord. Spread of anesthetic within the subarachnoid space determines the level of anesthesia achieved. Movement of anesthetic within the subarachnoid space is determined by two factors: (1) the density of the anesthetic solution and (2) the position in which the patient is lying. Anesthetics employed most commonly are *bupivacaine, lidocaine,* and *tetracaine*. All must be free of preservatives.

Adverse Effects. The most significant adverse effect of spinal anesthesia is *hypotension*. Blood pressure is reduced by venous dilation secondary to blockade of sympathetic nerves. (Loss of venous tone decreases the return of blood to the heart, causing a reduction in cardiac output and a corresponding fall in blood pressure.) Loss of venous tone can be compensated for by placing the patient in a 10- to 15-degree head-down position, which promotes venous return to the heart. If blood pressure cannot be restored through head-down positioning, drugs may be indicated; ephedrine and phenylephrine have been employed to promote vasoconstriction and enhance cardiac performance.

Autonomic blockade may disrupt function of the intestinal and urinary tracts, causing fecal incontinence and either urinary incontinence or urinary retention. The physician should be notified if the patient fails to void within 8 hours of the end of surgery.

Spinal anesthesia frequently causes headache. These "spinal" headaches are posture dependent and can be relieved by having the patient assume a supine position.

▪▪ KEY POINTS

- Local anesthetics stop nerve conduction by blocking sodium channels in the axon membrane.
- Small, unmyelinated neurons are blocked more rapidly than large, myelinated neurons.
- There are two classes of local anesthetics: ester-type anesthetics and amide-type anesthetics.
- Ester-type anesthetics (e.g., procaine) occasionally cause allergic reactions and are inactivated by esterases in the blood.
- Amide-type anesthetics (e.g., lidocaine) rarely cause allergic reactions and are inactivated by enzymes in the liver.

- Onset of anesthesia occurs most rapidly with anesthetics that are small, lipid soluble, and un-ionized at physiologic pH.
- Termination of local anesthesia is determined in large part by regional blood flow. Hence, coadministration of epinephrine, a vasoconstrictor, will prolong anesthesia.
- Local anesthetics can be absorbed in amounts sufficient to cause systemic toxicity. Principal concerns are

cardiac depression, vasodilation, and CNS excitation followed by depression.
- Because of the risk of systemic toxicity, an IV line should be in place prior to anesthetic administration (to permit administration of required emergency drugs), and facilities for resuscitation should be immediately available.

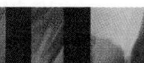

Summary of Major Nursing Implications*

INJECTED LOCAL ANESTHETICS

Articaine
Bupivacaine
Chloroprocaine
Levobupivacaine
Lidocaine
Mepivacaine
Prilocaine
Procaine
Ropivacaine
Tetracaine

Preadministration Assessment

Therapeutic Goal

Production of local anesthesia for surgical, dental, and obstetric procedures.

Identifying High-Risk Patients

Ester-type local anesthetics are *contraindicated* for patients with a history of serious allergic reactions to these drugs.

Implementation: Administration

Preparation of the Patient

The nurse may be responsible for preparing the patient to receive an injectable local anesthetic. Preparation includes cleansing the injection site, shaving the site when indicated, and placing the patient in a position appropriate to receive the injection. Children, elderly patients, and uncooperative patients may require restraint prior to injection by some routes.

Administration

Injection of local anesthetics is performed by clinicians with special training in their use (physicians, dentists, nurse anesthetists).

Ongoing Evaluation and Interventions

Minimizing Adverse Effects

Systemic Reactions. Absorption into the general circulation can cause systemic toxicity. Effects on the CNS and heart are of greatest concern. CNS toxicity manifests as a brief period of excitement, possibly including convulsions, followed by CNS depression, which can result in respiratory depression. Cardiotoxicity can manifest as bradycardia, atri-

oventricular (AV) heart block, and cardiac arrest. Monitor blood pressure, pulse rate, respiratory rate, and state of consciousness. Have facilities for cardiopulmonary resuscitation available. Manage CNS excitation with IV diazepam or IV thiopental.

Allergic Reactions. Severe allergic reactions are rare but can occur. These are most likely with ester-type anesthetics. Avoid ester-type agents in patients with a history of allergy to these drugs.

Labor and Delivery. Use of local anesthetics during delivery can cause bradycardia and CNS depression in the newborn. Monitor cardiac status.

Self-Inflicted Injury. Since anesthetics eliminate pain, and since pain warns us about injury, patients recovering from anesthesia must be protected from inadvertent harm until anesthesia wears off. **Caution the patient against activities that might result in unintentional harm.** Position the patient comfortably.

Spinal Headache and Urinary Retention. Patients recovering from spinal anesthesia may experience headache and urinary retention. Headache is posture dependent and can be minimized by having the patient remain supine for about 12 hours. Notify the physician if the patient fails to void within 8 hours.

TOPICAL LOCAL ANESTHETICS

Benzocaine
Butamben
Cocaine
Dibucaine
Dyclonine
Lidocaine
Pramoxine
Tetracaine

Preadministration Assessment

Therapeutic Goal

Reduction of discomfort associated with local disorders of the skin and mucous membranes.

Identifying High-Risk Patients

Ester-type local anesthetics are *contraindicated* for patients with a history of serious allergic reactions to these drugs.

*Patient education information is highlighted as blue text.

Summary of Major Nursing Implications*—cont'd

Implementation: Administration

Routes

Topical application to skin and mucous membranes.

Administration

Apply in the lowest effective dosage to the smallest area required. If possible, avoid application to skin that is abraded or otherwise injured.

Ongoing Evaluation and Interventions

Minimizing Adverse Effects

Systemic Toxicity. Absorption into the general circulation can cause systemic toxicity. Effects on the heart (brady-cardia, AV heart block, cardiac arrest) and CNS (excitation, possibly including convulsions, followed by depression) are of greatest concern. Monitor blood pressure, pulse rate, respiratory rate, and state of consciousness. Have facilities for cardiopulmonary resuscitation available.

The risk of systemic toxicity is determined by the extent of absorption. To minimize absorption, apply topical anesthetics to the smallest surface area needed and, when possible, avoid application to injured skin.

Allergic Reactions. Severe allergic reactions are rare but can occur. Allergic reactions are most likely with ester-type anesthetics. Avoid ester-type agents in patients with a history of allergy to these drugs.

*Patient education information is highlighted as blue text.

General Anesthetics

General anesthetics are drugs that produce unconsciousness and a lack of responsiveness to all painful stimuli. In contrast, *local anesthetics* do not reduce consciousness and they blunt sensation only in a limited area (see Chapter 25).

General anesthetics can be divided into two groups: (1) inhalation anesthetics and (2) intravenous anesthetics. The inhalation anesthetics are the main focus of the chapter.

When considering the anesthetics, we need to distinguish between the terms *analgesia* and *anesthesia*. Analgesia refers specifically to loss of sensibility to pain. In contrast, anesthesia refers not only to loss of pain but to loss of all other sensations as well (e.g., touch, temperature, taste). Hence, while analgesics (e.g., aspirin, morphine) can selectively reduce pain without affecting other sensory modalities and without reducing consciousness, the general anesthetics have no such selectivity: During general anesthesia, all sensation is lost, and consciousness is lost as well.

The development of general anesthetics has had an incalculable impact on the surgeon's art. The first general anesthetic—ether—was introduced by Dr. William T. Morton in 1846. Prior to this, surgery was a brutal and exquisitely painful ordeal, undertaken only under the most desperate circumstances. Immobilization of the surgical field was accomplished with the aid of strong men and straps. Survival of the patient was determined by the surgeon's speed—not his finesse. With the advent of general anesthesia, all of this changed. General anesthesia produced a patient who slept through surgery and experienced no pain. These changes allowed surgeons to develop the lengthy and intricate procedures that are routine today. Such procedures were unthinkable before general anesthetics became available.

BASIC PHARMACOLOGY OF THE INHALATION ANESTHETICS

In this section, we consider the inhalation anesthetics as a group. Our focus is on (1) properties of an ideal anesthetic, (2) pharmacokinetic aspects of inhalation anesthesia, (3) adverse effects of the inhalation anesthetics, and (4) drugs employed as adjuncts to anesthesia.

Properties of an Ideal Inhalation Anesthetic

An ideal inhalation anesthetic would produce unconsciousness, analgesia, muscle relaxation, and amnesia. Furthermore, induction of anesthesia would be brief and pleasant, as would the process of emergence. Depth of anesthesia could be raised or lowered with ease. Adverse effects would be minimal, and the margin of safety would be large. As you might guess, the ideal inhalation anesthetic does not exist: No single agent has all of these properties.

Balanced Anesthesia

The term *balanced anesthesia* refers to the use of a combination of drugs to accomplish what we cannot achieve with an inhalation anesthetic alone. Put another way, balanced anesthesia is a technique employed to compensate for the lack of an ideal anesthetic. Drugs are combined in balanced anesthesia to ensure that induction is smooth and rapid, and that analgesia and muscle relaxation are adequate. The agents used most commonly to achieve these goals are (1) short-acting barbiturates (for induction of anesthesia), (2) neuromuscular blocking

221

agents (for muscle relaxation), and (3) opioids and nitrous oxide (for analgesia). The primary benefit of combining drugs to achieve surgical anesthesia is that doing so permits full general anesthesia at doses of the inhalation anesthetic that are lower (safer) than those that would be required if surgical anesthesia were attempted using an inhalation anesthetic alone.

Stages of Anesthesia

The state of anesthesia has four stages of increasing depth. These stages were first described for patients undergoing anesthesia with ether, an agent whose effects develop slowly. Because modern anesthetics act much more rapidly than ether, the early stages of anesthesia usually pass so quickly as to be indiscernible. Hence, the stages of anesthesia described below, which are conspicuous during anesthesia with ether, are rarely seen in modern practice.

I: Stage of Analgesia. The initial stage of anesthesia begins with the onset of anesthetic administration and extends until consciousness is lost. Stage I is characterized by analgesia and moderate muscle relaxation. Some major surgeries can be performed at this stage.

II: Stage of Delirium. Stage II begins with loss of consciousness and extends to the onset of the stage of surgical anesthesia. Stage II is characterized by delirious excitement and reflex muscle activity. Respiration is typically irregular. Vomiting and urinary or fecal incontinence may occur. Stage II can be troublesome, hence anesthesiologists try to hasten passage through it.

III: Stage of Surgical Anesthesia. Stage III extends from the end of stage II to the point where spontaneous respiration ceases. Stage III is characterized by deep unconsciousness, varying degrees of respiratory depression, and suppression of certain reflexes. Muscle relaxation is greater than in stages I and II. Stage III can be subdivided into four planes of increasing depth. As the patient passes through these planes, respiration becomes progressively weaker.

IV: Stage of Medullary Paralysis. Stage IV begins when all spontaneous respiration is lost. Passage into stage IV results from anesthetic overdose. During this stage, vital signs are dangerously depressed; death results from circulatory collapse.

Molecular Mechanism of Action

Our understanding of how inhalation anesthetics act has changed dramatically in recent years. Attention has shifted from nonspecific effects on neuronal membranes to selective alteration of synaptic transmission. However, despite recent advances, we still don't know with certainty just how these drugs work.

For many years it was postulated that inhalation anesthetics acted by disrupting the lipid bilayer of the neuronal membrane. This long-standing theory was based on the observation that there is a direct correlation between the potency of an anesthetic and its lipid solubility. That is, the more readily an anesthetic could dissolve in the lipid matrix of the neuronal membrane, the more readily that agent could produce anesthesia. Hence the theory that anesthetics dissolve into neuronal membranes, disrupt their structure, and thereby suppress axonal conduction and possibly synaptic transmission.

More recent data suggest that inhalation anesthetics work primarily by activating receptors for gamma-aminobutyric acid (GABA), the principal inhibitory transmitter in the central nervous system (CNS). By activating GABA receptors, these drugs can cause generalized inhibition of CNS function. Inhalation anesthetics appear to activate GABA receptors in two ways: (1) at *high* concentrations, they bind to GABA receptors and thereby cause *direct* receptor activation, and (2) at *low* concentrations, they bind to GABA receptors and thereby *enhance the effects of GABA* (rather than activating receptors directly).

Minimum Alveolar Concentration

The minimum alveolar concentration (MAC) is an index of inhalation anesthetic potency. The MAC is defined as *the minimum concentration of drug in the alveolar air that will produce immobility in 50% of patients exposed to a painful stimulus.* Please note that, by this definition, a *low* MAC indicates *high* anesthetic potency.

From a clinical perspective, knowledge of the MAC of an anesthetic is of great practical value: The MAC tells us approximately how much anesthetic the inspired air must contain to produce anesthesia. A low MAC indicates that the inspired air need contain only low concentrations of drug to produce anesthesia. Conversely, when a drug has a high MAC, anesthesia can be achieved only when drug concentration in the inspired air is high. Fortunately, most inhalation anesthetics have very low MACs (Table 26–1), and therefore can act at low concentrations. However, one important agent—nitrous oxide—has a very high MAC. The MAC is so high, in fact, that surgical anesthesia cannot be achieved using nitrous oxide alone.

Pharmacokinetics
Uptake and Distribution

To produce therapeutic effects, an inhalation anesthetic must reach a concentration in the CNS that is sufficient to suppress neuronal excitability. The principal determinants of anesthetic

---

TABLE 26–1 ■ Properties of the Major Inhalation Anesthetics

Drug	MAC* (%)	Analgesic Effect	Effect on Blood Pressure	Effect on Respiration	Muscle Relaxant Effect	Extent of Metabolism	Compatible with Epinephrine
Nitrous oxide	105	++++	→	→	0	0	Yes
Halothane	0.75	++	↓	↓↓	+	15%	No
Desflurane	4.58	++	↓	↓↓	++	2–3%	Yes
Enflurane	1.68	++	↓	↓↓	++	2–5%	Yes†
Isoflurane	1.15	++	↓	↓↓	++	1–2%	Yes
Sevoflurane	1.71	++	↓	↓↓	++	<1%	Yes

0	=	No effect	→ =	Little or no change
+	=	Small effect		
++	=	Moderate effect	↓ =	Moderate decrease
+++	=	Large effect		
++++	=	Very large effect	↓↓ =	Large decrease

*Minimal alveolar concentration.

†Enflurane sensitizes the myocardium to catecholamines, but less so than halothane.

concentration are (1) uptake from the lungs and (2) distribution to the CNS and other tissues. The kinetics of anesthetic uptake and distribution are complex and hence are considered only briefly.

Uptake. A major determinant of anesthetic uptake is the concentration of anesthetic in the inspired air: The greater the anesthetic concentration, the more rapid uptake will be. Other factors that contribute to anesthetic uptake are pulmonary ventilation, solubility of the anesthetic in blood, and blood flow through the lungs. An increase in any of these factors increases the rate of uptake.

Distribution. Distribution to specific tissues is determined largely by regional blood flow. Anesthetic levels rise rapidly in the brain, kidney, heart, and liver—tissues that receive the largest fraction of the cardiac output. Anesthetic levels in these tissues equilibrate with those in blood 5 to 15 minutes after the onset of drug administration. In skin and skeletal muscle—tissues with an intermediate blood flow—equilibration occurs more slowly. The most poorly perfused tissues—fat, bone, ligaments, and cartilage—are the last to equilibrate with anesthetic levels in the blood.

Elimination

Export in the Expired Breath. Inhalation anesthetics are eliminated almost entirely via the lungs; hepatic metabolism is only a minor determinant of elimination. The same factors that determine anesthetic uptake (pulmonary ventilation, blood flow to the lungs, anesthetic solubility in blood and tissues) also determine the rate of elimination. Since blood flow to the brain is high, anesthetic levels in the brain drop rapidly once administration has stopped. Anesthetic levels in tissues that have a lower blood flow decline more slowly. Because anesthetic levels in the CNS decline more rapidly than levels in other tissues, patients can awaken from anesthesia long before all of the anesthetic has left the body.

Metabolism. Most inhalation anesthetics undergo very little metabolism. Hence, metabolism does not influence the time course of anesthesia. However, since some metabolites can be toxic, metabolism is nonetheless clinically significant.

Adverse Effects

The adverse effects discussed here apply to the inhalation anesthetics as a group. Not all of these effects are seen with every anesthetic.

Respiratory and Cardiac Depression. Depression of respiratory and cardiac function is a concern with virtually all inhalation anesthetics. Doses only 2 to 4 times greater than those needed for surgical anesthesia are sufficient to cause potentially lethal depression of pulmonary and cardiac function. To compensate for respiratory depression, almost all patients require mechanical support of ventilation.

Sensitization of the Heart to Catecholamines. Some anesthetics—most notably *halothane*—can increase the sensitivity of the heart to stimulation by catecholamines (e.g., norepinephrine, epinephrine). While in this sensitized state, the heart may develop dysrhythmias in response to catecholamines. Exposure to catecholamines may result from two causes: (1) release of endogenous catecholamines (in response to pain or other stimuli of the sympathetic nervous system), and (2) topical application of catecholamines to control bleeding in the surgical field.

Malignant Hyperthermia. Malignant hyperthermia is a rare but potentially fatal reaction that can be triggered by all inhalation anesthetics. Predisposition to the reaction is genetic. Malignant hyperthermia is characterized by muscle rigidity and a profound elevation of temperature—sometimes to as high as 43°C. Left untreated, the reaction can rapidly prove fatal. The risk of malignant hyperthermia is greatest when an inhalation anesthetic is used in combination with *succinylcholine,* a neuromuscular blocker that also can trigger the reaction. Diagnosis and management of malignant hyperthermia are discussed in Chapter 16.

Aspiration of Gastric Contents. During the state of anesthesia, reflexes that normally prevent aspiration of gastric contents into the lungs are abolished. Aspiration of gastric fluids can cause bronchospasm and pneumonia. Use of an endotracheal tube isolates the trachea and can thereby help prevent these complications.

Toxicity to Operating Room Personnel. Chronic exposure to low levels of anesthetics may harm operating room personnel. Suspected reactions include headache, reduced alertness, and spontaneous abortion. Risk can be reduced simply by venting anesthetic gases from the operating room.

Hepatotoxicity. Rarely, patients receiving inhalation anesthesia develop serious liver dysfunction. In the past, we thought that halothane was more hepatotoxic than other anesthetics. However, it now appears that the risk is about equal with all anesthetics.

Drug Interactions

Several classes of drugs—analgesics, CNS depressants, CNS stimulants—can influence the amount of anesthetic required to produce anesthesia. Opioid analgesics allow a reduction in anesthetic dosage. Why? Because, when opioids are present, analgesia needn't be produced by the anesthetic alone. Similarly, because CNS depressants (barbiturates, benzodiazepines, alcohol) add to the depressant effects of anesthetics, concurrent use of CNS depressants lowers the required dose of anesthetic. Conversely, concurrent use of CNS stimulants (amphetamines, cocaine) increases the required dose of anesthetic.

Adjuncts to Inhalation Anesthesia

Adjuncts to anesthesia are drugs employed to complement the beneficial effects of inhalation anesthetics and to counteract their adverse effects. Some adjunctive agents are administered before surgery, some during surgery, and some after surgery.

Preanesthetic Medications

Preanesthetic medications are administered for three main purposes: (1) reduction of anxiety, (2) production of perioperative amnesia, and (3) relief of preoperative and postoperative pain. In addition, preanesthetic medications may be used to suppress certain adverse responses: excessive salivation, excessive bronchial secretion, coughing, bradycardia, and vomiting.

Benzodiazepines. Benzodiazepines (e.g., diazepam) are given preoperatively to reduce anxiety and promote amnesia. The doses employed produce mild sedation with little or no respiratory depression.

Barbiturates. Like the benzodiazepines, barbiturates can relieve anxiety and induce sedation. Respiratory and cardiovascular effects are minimal. Barbiturates with an intermediate duration of action are employed (e.g., pentobarbital, secobarbital).

Opioids. Opioids (e.g., morphine) are administered to relieve preoperative and postoperative pain. These drugs may also help by suppressing cough.

Opioids can have adverse effects. Because they depress the CNS, opioids can delay awakening after surgery. Effects on the bowel and urinary tract may result in postoperative constipation and urinary retention. Stimulation of the chemoreceptor trigger zone promotes vomiting. Opioid-induced respiratory depression adds with anesthetic-induced respiratory depression, thereby increasing the risk of postoperative respiratory distress.

Clonidine, an Alpha₂-Adrenergic Agonist. Clonidine is a centrally acting alpha₂ agonist used for both hypertension and pain reduction. When administered prior to surgery, the drug reduces anxiety and causes sedation. In addition, it permits a reduction in anesthetic and analgesic dosages. Analgesic properties of clonidine are discussed further in Chapter 27; antihypertensive properties are discussed in Chapters 19 and 45. The formulation used for analgesia is marketed under the trade name *Duraclon;* the antihypertensive formulation is marketed as *Catapres.*

Anticholinergic Drugs. Anticholinergic drugs (e.g., atropine) may be given to decrease the risk of bradycardia during surgery. Surgical manipulations can trigger parasympathetic reflexes, which in turn can produce profound vagal slowing of the heart. Pretreatment with a cholinergic antagonist prevents bradycardia from this cause.

At one time, anticholinergic drugs were needed to prevent excessive bronchial secretions associated with anesthesia. Older anesthetic agents (e.g., ether) irritate the respiratory tract, and thereby cause profuse bronchial secretions. Cholinergic blockers were given to suppress this response. Since the inhalation anesthetics used today are much less irritating, bronchial secretions are minimal. Consequently, although anticholinergic agents are still employed as adjuncts to anesthesia, their purpose is no longer to suppress secretions.

Neuromuscular Blocking Agents

Performance of most surgical procedures requires that skeletal muscles be relaxed; neuromuscular blocking agents (e.g., succinylcholine, pancuronium) are given to induce relaxation. By using neuromuscular blockers, we can reduce the dose of general anesthetic. That is, although it is possible to produce

surgical muscle relaxation with an anesthetic alone, the required degree of muscle relaxation can be achieved only with deep anesthesia. When skeletal muscles have been relaxed with a neuromuscular blocker, anesthesia need not be so deep.

Muscle relaxants can have adverse effects. Neuromuscular blocking agents prevent contraction of all skeletal muscles, including the diaphragm and other muscles of respiration. Accordingly, patients require mechanical support of ventilation during surgery. Patients recovering from anesthesia may have reduced respiratory capacity owing to residual neuromuscular blockade. Accordingly, respiration must be monitored until recovery is complete.

It is important to appreciate that neuromuscular blockers produce a state of total flaccid paralysis. In this condition, a patient could be fully awake while seeming to be asleep. Incidents in which paralyzed patients have been awake during surgery, but unable to communicate their agony, have been reported. Because neuromuscular blockade can obscure depth of anesthesia, and because failure to maintain adequate anesthesia can result in true horror, the anesthesiologist must be especially watchful to ensure that patients receiving neuromuscular blocking agents also receive adequate amounts of anesthetic.

Postanesthetic Medications

Analgesics. Analgesics are needed to control postoperative pain. If pain is severe, opioids are indicated. For mild pain, aspirin-like drugs may suffice.

Antiemetics. Patients recovering from anesthesia often experience nausea and vomiting. This can be suppressed with antiemetics. Among the most effective is *ondansetron* [Zofran], a drug developed to suppress nausea and vomiting in patients undergoing cancer chemotherapy. Other commonly used antiemetics are *promethazine* and *droperidol.*

Muscarinic Agonists. Abdominal distention (from atony of the bowel) and urinary retention are potential postoperative complications. Both conditions can be relieved through stimulation of muscarinic receptors. The muscarinic agonist employed most often is *bethanechol.*

Dosage and Administration

Administration of inhalation anesthetics is performed only by anesthesiologists (physicians) and anesthetists (nurses). Clinicians who lack the training of these specialists have no authority to administer anesthesia. Since knowledge of anesthetic dosage and administration is the responsibility of specialists, and since this text is designed for beginning students, details on dosage and administration are not presented. If you need this information, consult a textbook of anesthesiology.

Classification of Inhalation Anesthetics

Inhalation anesthetics fall into two basic categories: *gases* and *volatile liquids*. The gases, as their name implies, exist in a gaseous state at atmospheric pressure. The volatile liquids exist in a liquid state at atmospheric pressure, but can be easily volatilized for administration by inhalation. The inhalation anesthetics in current use are listed in Table 26–2. The volatile liquids—halothane, enflurane, isoflurane, desflurane, and sevoflurane—are similar to one another in structure and function. The only gas in current use is nitrous oxide.

TABLE 26–2 ■ Classification of the Inhalation Anesthetics		
	Anesthetic	
Class	**Generic Name**	**Trade Name**
Volatile Liquids	Halothane	Fluothane
	Enflurane	Ethrane
	Isoflurane	Forane
	Desflurane	Suprane
	Sevoflurane	Ultane
Gases	Nitrous oxide	

PROPERTIES OF INDIVIDUAL INHALATION ANESTHETICS

Halothane

Halothane [Fluothane] is the prototype of the volatile inhalation anesthetics. Halothane was introduced in 1956 and remains the standard against which the newer volatile liquids are compared. The drug is widely used in children. However, because of concerns about liver failure (see below), use of halothane in adults has sharply declined.

Anesthetic Properties

Halothane is an effective anesthetic. For some procedures, anesthesia may be produced with halothane alone. Other procedures require addition of other drugs.

Potency. Halothane is a high-potency anesthetic. This high potency is reflected in halothane's low MAC (0.75%), which tells us that unconsciousness can be produced when the concentration of halothane in alveolar air is only 0.75%.

Time Course. Induction of anesthesia is smooth and relatively rapid. However, although halothane can act quickly, in actual practice, induction is usually produced with thiopental, a rapid-acting barbiturate. Once the patient is unconscious, depth of anesthesia can be raised or lowered with ease. Patients awaken about 1 hour after ceasing halothane inhalation.

Analgesia. Halothane is a weak analgesic. Consequently, when this agent is used for surgical anesthesia, coadministration of a strong analgesic is usually required. The analgesics most commonly employed are opioids (e.g., morphine) and nitrous oxide.

Muscle Relaxation. Although halothane has muscle-relaxant actions, the degree of relaxation produced is generally inadequate for surgery. Accordingly, concurrent use of a neuromuscular blocking agent (e.g., pancuronium) is usually required. Although relaxation of skeletal muscle is only moderate, halothane does promote significant relaxation of uterine smooth muscle. Consequently, when used in obstetrics, halothane may inhibit uterine contractions, thereby delaying delivery and possibly increasing postpartum bleeding.

Adverse Effects

Hypotension. Halothane causes a dose-dependent reduction in blood pressure. Doses only twice those needed for surgical anesthesia can produce complete circulatory failure and death.

Halothane promotes hypotension by two mechanisms. First, the drug has a direct depressant effect on the myocardium; the resultant decrease in contractility can reduce cardiac output by 20% to 50%. Second, halothane increases vagal tone, thereby slowing heart rate and reducing cardiac output even further.

Respiratory Depression. Halothane produces significant depression of respiration. To ensure adequate oxygenation, two measures are implemented: (1) mechanical or manual ventilatory support and (2) enrichment of the inspired gas mixture with additional oxygen.

Promotion of Dysrhythmias. Halothane promotes dysrhythmias in two ways. First, the drug sensitizes the myocardium to catecholamines. Second, it prolongs the QT interval (see discussion of QT interval drugs in Chapter 7). To

reduce the risk of dysrhythmias, epinephrine and other catecholamines should be used with caution. Also, caution is required in patients with existing QT prolongation and in those taking other drugs known to prolong the QT interval.

Malignant Hyperthermia. Genetically predisposed patients may experience malignant hyperthermia. Accordingly, patients with a personal or familial history of malignant hyperthermia should receive halothane only if there is no option. Also, if halothane *is* employed, it must not be combined with succinylcholine (which would further increase the risk of malignant hyperthermia).

Hepatotoxicity. Rarely, halothane produces hepatitis, sometimes progressing to massive hepatic necrosis and death. The incidence of fulminant hepatic failure is 1 in 30,000. Hepatotoxicity is thought to result from an autoimmune process triggered by metabolites of halothane that have formed complexes with liver proteins. Halothane-induced liver failure has occurred in adults only—never in children. Because of concerns about liver damage, halothane is rarely given to adults in the United States. However, the drug enjoys continued widespread use in children.

Other Adverse Effects. Postoperative *nausea* and *vomiting* may occur, but these reactions are less common with halothane than with older anesthetics (e.g., ether). By decreasing blood flow to the kidney, halothane can cause a substantial *decrease in urine output.*

Elimination

The majority (60% to 80%) of an administered dose is eliminated intact in the exhaled breath. Hepatic metabolism accounts for only 15% of elimination.

Isoflurane

Isoflurane [Forane] is our most widely used inhalation anesthetic. The drug is potent (MAC = 1.15%) and has properties much like those of halothane. Induction of anesthesia is smooth and rapid, depth of anesthesia can be adjusted with speed and ease, and patients emerge from anesthesia rapidly. Like other volatile liquids, isoflurane causes respiratory depression and hypotension. With isoflurane, hypotension results from vasodilation rather than from reduced cardiac output. Isoflurane is a more effective muscle relaxant than halothane, but nonetheless is usually employed with a neuromuscular blocker. Like halothane, isoflurane suppresses uterine contraction. In contrast to halothane, isoflurane is not associated with renal or hepatic toxicity. Isoflurane is eliminated almost entirely in the expired breath; only 0.2% undergoes metabolism.

The cardiac actions of isoflurane differ significantly from those of halothane. Unlike halothane, isoflurane does not cause myocardial depression. Hence, cardiac output is not decreased. Furthermore, isoflurane does not sensitize the myocardium to catecholamines. Hence, patients can be given epinephrine and other catecholamines with little fear of precipitating a dysrhythmia. Finally, isoflurane is not associated with QT prolongation.

Enflurane

Enflurane [Ethrane] has pharmacologic properties very similar to those of halothane. Enflurane was introduced in 1973 and still enjoys widespread use.

Comparison of enflurane with halothane reveals important similarities and a few significant differences. Both anesthetics are very potent: the MAC of enflurane is 1.68%, compared with 0.75% for halothane. As with halothane, induction of anesthesia is smooth and rapid, and depth of anesthesia can be changed quickly and easily. Like halothane, enflurane produces substantial depression of respiration. Accordingly, patients are likely to need ventilatory support; the concentration of inspired oxygen should be at least 35%. Muscle relaxation induced by enflurane is greater than with halothane. However, despite this action, a neuromuscular blocker is usually employed (to permit a reduction of enflurane dosage). Like halothane, enflurane can suppress uterine contraction, thereby impeding labor. Significantly, sensitization of the myocardium to catecholamines is less than with halothane. As a result, patients can be given catecholamines with relative safety. High doses of enflurane can induce seizures, a response not seen with halothane. Obviously, enflurane should be avoided in patients with a history of seizure disorders. Like halothane, enflurane is eliminated primarily in the exhaled breath as the intact parent compound. Only 2% to 5% is eliminated by hepatic metabolism.

Desflurane

Desflurane [Suprane] is nearly identical in structure to isoflurane. Induction occurs more rapidly than with any other volatile anesthetic, depth of anesthesia can be changed quickly, and recovery occurs only minutes after ceasing administration. Desflurane is indicated for *maintenance* of anesthesia in adults and children and for *induction* of anesthesia in adults. The drug is not approved for induction in children and infants because of a high incidence of respiratory difficulties (laryngospasm, apnea, increased secretions), which are due to the drug's pungency. Like isoflurane, desflurane can cause respiratory depression and hypotension secondary to vasodilation. During induction, or in response to an abrupt increase in desflurane blood levels, heart rate and blood pressure may increase, causing tachycardia and hypertension. Postoperative nausea and vomiting are possible. Malignant hypertension has occurred in experimental animals. Desflurane undergoes even less metabolism than isoflurane. Hence, the risk of postoperative organ injury is probably low.

Sevoflurane

Sevoflurane [Ultane] is a relatively new anesthetic similar to desflurane. The drug is approved for induction and maintenance of anesthesia in adults and children. As with desflurane, induction is rapid, depth of anesthesia can be adjusted easily, and recovery occurs minutes after ceasing inhalation. In contrast to desflurane, sevoflurane has a pleasant odor and is not a respiratory irritant. Accordingly, the drug is suitable for mask induction in children. Sevoflurane has a MAC of 1.7% and is eliminated primarily in the exhaled breath. Adverse effects are minimal. The most common problem is postoperative nausea and vomiting. In contrast to desflurane, sevoflurane does not cause tachycardia or hypertension.

Nitrous Oxide

Nitrous oxide (aka "laughing gas") differs from the volatile liquid anesthetics with respect to pharmacologic properties and uses. The pharmacologic properties of nitrous oxide differ from those of the inhalation anesthetics in two important ways: (1) whereas other inhalation agents have high *anesthetic* potency, the anesthetic potency of nitrous oxide is very low, and (2) whereas other inhalation agents lack *analgesic* potency, the analgesic potency of nitrous oxide is very *high*. Because of these properties, nitrous oxide has a unique pattern of use: Because of its low anesthetic potency, nitrous oxide is never employed as a primary anesthetic agent; however, because of its high analgesic potency, nitrous oxide is frequently employed as an adjuvant to other inhalation agents to provide supplemental analgesia.

Because nitrous oxide has such low anesthetic potency, *it is virtually impossible to produce surgical anesthesia employing nitrous oxide alone.* The low anesthetic potency of nitrous oxide is reflected in the drug's extremely high MAC, which is greater than 100%. A MAC of this value tells us that, even if it were possible to administer 100% nitrous oxide (i.e., inspired gas that contains only nitrous oxide and no oxygen), this concentration of nitrous oxide would still be insufficient to produce surgical anesthesia. Since practical considerations (i.e., the need to administer at least 30% oxygen) limit the maximum usable concentration of nitrous oxide to 70%, and since much higher concentrations are needed to approach production of surgical anesthesia, it is clear that full anesthesia cannot be achieved with nitrous oxide by itself.

Despite its low anesthetic potency, nitrous oxide may well be our most widely used inhalation agent: *Almost all patients undergoing general anesthesia receive nitrous oxide to supplement the analgesic effects of the primary anesthetic.* As indicated in Table 26–1, the analgesic effects of nitrous oxide are substantially greater than those of the other inhalation agents. In fact, nitrous oxide is such a potent analgesic that inhaling 20% nitrous oxide can produce pain relief equivalent to that of morphine. The advantage of providing analgesia with nitrous oxide, rather than relying entirely on the primary anesthetic for pain relief, is that nitrous oxide allows the dosage of the primary anesthetic to be significantly decreased—usually by 50% or more. This reduction in dosage results in decreased respiratory and cardiovascular depression and permits faster emergence. When employed in combination with other inhalation anesthetics, nitrous oxide is administered at a concentration of 70%.

When administered at therapeutic concentrations, nitrous oxide has no serious adverse effects. The drug is not toxic to the CNS, and does not cause cardiovascular or respiratory depression. Furthermore, it is not likely to precipitate malignant hyperthermia. The major concern with nitrous oxide is postoperative *nausea* and *vomiting,* which occurs more often with this agent than with any other inhalation anesthetic.

In certain settings, nitrous oxide can be used alone. When administered by itself, nitrous oxide is employed for *analgesia*—not anesthesia. Nitrous oxide alone is used for analgesia in dentistry and during delivery.

Obsolete Inhalation Anesthetics

Several once-popular anesthetics are now obsolete. Five of these agents—*ethylene, cyclopropane, diethyl ether (ether), vinyl ether,* and *ethyl chloride*—are *gases.* They were abandoned because they are *explosive* and because they offer no advantages over newer, less hazardous anesthetics. Only one volatile liquid—*methoxyflurane*—has become obsolete. The reason is concern about kidney damage.

INTRAVENOUS ANESTHETICS

Intravenous anesthetics may be used alone or to supplement the effects of inhalation agents. When combined with inhalation anesthetics, IV agents offer two potential benefits: (1) they permit dosage of the inhalation agent to be reduced and (2) they produce effects that cannot be achieved with an inhalation agent alone. Three of the drug families discussed in this section—opioids, barbiturates, and benzodiazepines—are considered at length in other chapters. Discussion here is limited to their use in anesthesia.

Short-Acting Barbiturates (Thiobarbiturates)

Short-acting barbiturates, administered intravenously, are employed for *induction of anesthesia*. Two agents are available: *thiopental sodium* [Pentothal] and *methohexital sodium* [Brevital]. Almost every time an inhalation anesthetic is used, a short-acting barbiturate is administered first for induction.

Thiopental. Thiopental [Pentothal] was the first short-acting barbiturate and is the prototype for the group. This drug acts rapidly to produce unconsciousness. Analgesic and muscle-relaxant effects are weak.

Thiopental has a rapid onset and short duration. Unconsciousness occurs 10 to 20 seconds after IV injection. If thiopental is not followed by inhalation anesthesia, the patient will wake up in about 10 minutes.

The time course of thiopental-induced anesthesia is determined by the drug's pattern of distribution. Thiopental is highly lipid soluble, and therefore enters the brain rapidly to begin its effects. Anesthesia is terminated as thiopental undergoes redistribution from the brain and blood to other tissues. Practically no metabolism of the drug takes place between the time of administration and the time of awakening.

Like most of the inhalation anesthetics, thiopental causes cardiovascular and respiratory depression. If administered too rapidly, the drug may cause apnea.

Benzodiazepines

When administered in large doses, benzodiazepines produce unconsciousness and amnesia. Because of this ability, IV benzodiazepines are occasionally given to induce anesthesia. However, short-acting barbiturates are generally preferred. Three benzodiazepines—diazepam, lorazepam, and midazolam—are administered IV for induction. Diazepam is the prototype for the group. The basic pharmacology of the benzodiazepines is discussed in Chapter 33.

Diazepam. Induction with IV diazepam [Valium] is slower than with barbiturates; unconsciousness develops in about 1 minute. Diazepam causes very little muscle relaxation and no analgesia. Cardiovascular and respiratory depression are usually only moderate. However, on occasion respiratory depression is severe. Therefore, whenever diazepam is administered IV, facilities for respiratory support must be immediately available.

Midazolam. Intravenous midazolam [Versed] may be used for *induction of anesthesia* and to produce *conscious sedation*. When used for induction, midazolam is usually combined with a short-acting barbiturate. Unconsciousness develops in 80 seconds.

Conscious sedation can be produced by combining midazolam with an opioid analgesic (e.g., morphine). The state is characterized by sedation, analgesia, amnesia, and lack of anxiety. The patient is unperturbed and passive, but responsive to commands, such as "open your eyes." Conscious sedation persists for an hour or so and is suitable for minor surgeries and endoscopic procedures.

Midazolam can cause dangerous cardiorespiratory effects, including respiratory depression and respiratory and cardiac arrest. Accordingly, the drug should be used only in settings that permit constant monitoring of cardiac and respiratory status. Facilities for resuscitation must be immediately available. The risk of adverse effects can be minimized by injecting midazolam slowly (over 2 or more minutes) and by waiting another 2 or more minutes for full effects to develop before giving additional doses.

Propofol

Actions and Uses. Propofol [Diprivan] is an IV sedative-hypnotic used for induction and maintenance of anesthesia. In addition, propofol can be used to sedate patients undergoing mechanical ventilation and certain noninvasive procedures (e.g., radiation therapy, endoscopy, magnetic resonance imaging). Like thiopental, propofol has a rapid onset and short duration of action. Unconsciousness develops within 60 seconds and lasts for 3 to 5 minutes following a single injection. As with thiopental, redistribution from the brain to other tissues explains the speed of awakening. For extended effects, a continuous, low-dose infusion is used.

Adverse Effects. Propofol can cause profound *respiratory depression* (including apnea) and *hypotension*. Accordingly, the drug should be used with caution in elderly patients, hypovolemic patients, and patients with compromised cardiac function. Whenever the drug is used, facilities for respiratory support should be immediately available.

Propofol poses a high risk of *bacterial infection.* Why? Because the drug is supplied in a mixture of soybean oil, glycerol, and egg lecithin—an excellent medium for bacteria to grow in. In surgical patients, use of preparations that have become contaminated after opening has caused sepsis and death. To minimize the risk of infection, propofol solutions and opened vials should be discarded within 6 hours. Unopened vials should be stored at 22°C.

Propofol can cause transient pain at the site of IV injection. This can be minimized by using a large vein and by injecting IV lidocaine (a local anesthetic) at the site just prior to injecting propofol.

Etomidate

Etomidate [Amidate] is a potent hypnotic agent used for induction of surgical anesthesia. Unconsciousness develops rapidly and lasts about 5 minutes. The drug has no analgesic actions. Adverse effects associated with single injections include transient apnea, venous pain at the injection site, and suppression of plasma cortisol levels for 6 to 8 hours. Repeated administration can cause hypotension, oliguria, electrolyte disturbances, and a high incidence (50%) of postoperative nausea and vomiting. Cardiovascular effects are less than with barbiturates; hence, the drug is preferred to barbiturates for patients with cardiovascular disorders.

Ketamine

Anesthetic Effects. Ketamine [Ketalar] produces a state known as *dissociative anesthesia* in which the patient feels dissociated from his or her environment. In addition, the drug causes sedation, immobility, analgesia, and amnesia; responsiveness to pain is lost. Induction is rapid and emergence begins within 10 to 15 minutes. Full recovery, however, may take several hours.

Adverse Psychologic Reactions. During recovery from ketamine, unpleasant psychologic reactions may occur. Possible reactions include hallucinations, disturbing dreams, and delirium. In some cases, these reactions recur days or even weeks after ketamine has been used. To minimize adverse psychologic effects, the patient should be kept in a soothing, stimulus-free environment until recovery is complete. Premedication with diazepam or midazolam reduces the risk of adverse reactions. Psychologic reactions are least likely in children under the age of 15 and in adults over the age of 65.

Therapeutic Uses. Ketamine is especially valuable for anesthesia in young children undergoing minor surgical and diagnostic procedures; the drug is frequently used to facilitate changing of burn dressings. Because of its potential for adverse psychologic effects, ketamine should be avoided in patients with a history of psychiatric illness.

Neuroleptic-Opioid Combination: Droperidol Plus Fentanyl

A unique state, known as *neurolept analgesia,* can be produced with a combination of fentanyl, a potent opioid, plus droperidol, a neuroleptic (antipsychotic) agent. The combination of fentanyl plus droperidol is available premixed under the trade name *Innovar.*

Neurolept analgesia is characterized by quiescence, indifference to surroundings, and insensitivity to pain. The patient appears to be asleep but is not (i.e., complete loss of consciousness does not occur). In large part, neurolept analgesia is similar to the dissociative anesthesia produced by ketamine. Neurolept analgesia is employed for diagnostic and minor surgical procedures (e.g., bronchoscopy, repeated changing of burn dressings).

Recent data show that droperidol prolongs the QT interval on the electrocardiogram, indicating that it can cause potentially fatal dysrhythmias. Accordingly, droperidol should be used only when safer drugs are ineffective or intolerable. Droperidol is contraindicated for patients with existing QT prolongation, and should be used with great caution in those at risk of developing QT prolongation. The issue of drug-induced QT prolongation is discussed at length in Chapter 6 (Adverse Drug Reactions and Medication Errors).

Other adverse effects include hypotension and respiratory depression. Respiratory depression can be severe and may persist for hours. Respiratory assistance is likely to be required. Like other neuroleptics, droperidol blocks receptors for dopamine, and hence should not be given to patients with Parkinson's disease.

For some procedures, the combination of fentanyl plus droperidol is supplemented with nitrous oxide. The state produced by this three-drug regimen is called *neurolept anesthesia.* Neurolept anesthesia produces more analgesia and a greater reduction of consciousness than seen with *neurolept analgesia.* Neurolept anesthesia can be used for major surgical procedures.

⁝▪ KEY POINTS

- General anesthetics produce unconsciousness and insensitivity to painful stimuli. In contrast, analgesics reduce sensitivity to pain but need not reduce consciousness.
- The term *balanced anesthesia* refers to the use of several drugs to ensure that induction of anesthesia is smooth and rapid and that analgesia and muscle relaxation are adequate.
- The minimum alveolar concentration (MAC) of an inhalation anesthetic is defined as the minimum concentration of drug in alveolar air that will produce immobility in 50% of patients exposed to a painful stimulus. A *low* MAC indicates *high* anesthetic potency!
- Inhalation anesthetics are eliminated almost entirely in the expired air. As a rule, they undergo minimal hepatic metabolism.
- The principal adverse effects of general anesthetics are depression of respiration and cardiac performance.
- Malignant hyperthermia is a rare, genetically determined, life-threatening reaction to general anesthetics. Coadministration of succinylcholine, a neuromuscular blocker, increases the risk of the reaction.
- By enhancing analgesia, opioids reduce the required dosage of general anesthetic.
- By enhancing muscle relaxation, neuromuscular blockers reduce the required dosage of general anesthetic.
- Nitrous oxide differs from other general anesthetics in two important ways: (1) it has a very high MAC, and therefore cannot be used alone to produce general anesthesia; and (2) it has high analgesic potency, and therefore is frequently combined with other general anesthetics to supplement their analgesic effects.
- Induction of anesthesia is usually accomplished with a short-acting barbiturate, such as thiopental.
- Ketamine is an IV anesthetic that produces a state known as dissociative anesthesia. Patients recovering from ketamine may experience adverse psychologic reactions.

Summary of Major Nursing Implications*

ALL GENERAL ANESTHETICS

Nursing management of the patient receiving general anesthesia is almost exclusively preoperative and postoperative; intraoperative management is the responsibility of anesthesiologists and anesthetists. Accordingly, our summary of anesthesia-related nursing implications is divided into two sections: (1) implications that pertain to the preoperative patient and (2) implications that pertain to the postoperative patient. Intraoperative implications are not considered.

The nursing implications summarized here are limited to ones that are directly related to anesthesia. Nursing implications regarding the overall management of the surgical patient (i.e., implications unrelated to anesthesia) are not presented. (Overall nursing management of the surgical patient is discussed fully—and appropriately—in medical-surgical texts.)

Nursing implications for drugs employed as adjuncts to anesthesia (barbiturates, benzodiazepines, anticholinergic agents, opioids, neuromuscular blocking agents) are summarized in other chapters. Only those implications that apply specifically to the adjunctive use of these agents are addressed here.

Preoperative Patients: Counseling, Assessment, and Medicating

Counseling

Anxiety is common among patients anticipating surgery: the patient may fear the surgery itself, or may be concerned about the possibility of waking up or experiencing pain during the procedure. Since excessive anxiety can disrupt the smoothness of the surgical course (in addition to being distressing to the patient), you should attempt to dispel preop-

*Patient education information is highlighted as blue text.

Summary of Major Nursing Implications*—cont'd

erative fears. To some extent, fear can be allayed by reassuring the patient that anesthesia will keep him or her asleep for the entire procedure, will prevent pain, and will create amnesia about the experience.

Assessment

Medication History. The patient may be taking drugs that can affect responses to anesthetics. Drugs that act on the respiratory and cardiovascular systems are of particular concern. To decrease the risk of adverse interactions, obtain a thorough history of drug use. *All* drugs—prescription medications, over-the-counter preparations, and illicit agents—should be considered. With illicit drugs (e.g., heroin, barbiturates) and with alcohol, it is important to determine both the duration of use and the amount used per day.

Respiratory and Cardiovascular Function. Most general anesthetics produce cardiovascular and respiratory depression. In order to evaluate the effects of anesthesia, baseline values for blood pressure, heart rate, and respiration are required. Also, any disease of the cardiovascular and respiratory systems should be noted.

Preoperative Medication

Preoperative medications (e.g., benzodiazepines, opioids, anticholinergic agents) are employed to (1) calm the patient, (2) provide analgesia, and (3) counteract adverse effects of general anesthetics. As a rule, the nurse is responsible for administering these drugs. Since preoperative medication can have a significant impact on the overall response to anesthesia, it is important that these drugs be administered at an appropriate time—typically 30 to 60 minutes before surgery. Because preoperative medication may produce drowsiness or reduce blood pressure, the patient should remain in bed. A calm environment will complement the effect of sedatives.

Postoperative Patients: Ongoing Evaluation and Interventions

When receiving a patient for postoperative care, you should know all of the drugs the patient has received in the hospital (anesthetics and adjunctive medications). In addition, you should know what medications the patient was taking at home (especially drugs for hypertension). With this information, you will be able to anticipate the time course of emergence from anesthesia as well as potential drug-related postoperative complications.

Evaluations and Interventions That Pertain to Specific Organ Systems

Cardiovascular and Respiratory Systems. Anesthetics depress cardiovascular and respiratory function. Mon-

itor vital signs until they return to baseline. Determine blood pressure, pulse rate, and respiration immediately upon receipt of the patient, and repeat monitoring at brief intervals until recovery is complete. During the recovery period, observe the patient for respiratory and cardiovascular distress. Be alert for (1) reductions in blood pressure, (2) altered cardiac rhythm, and (3) shallow, slow, or noisy breathing. Have facilities for respiratory support available.

Central Nervous System. Return of CNS function is gradual, and precautions must be taken until recovery is complete. When appropriate, employ side rails or straps to avoid accidental falls. Assist ambulation until the patient is able to stand steadily. During the early stage of emergence, the patient may be able to hear, even though he or she may appear unconscious. Accordingly, exercise discretion in conversation.

Gastrointestinal Tract. Bowel function may be compromised by the surgery itself or by the drugs employed as adjuncts to anesthesia (e.g., opioids, anticholinergics). Constipation or atony of the bowel may occur. Monitor bowel function. A muscarinic agonist (e.g., bethanechol) may be needed to restore peristalsis. Determine bowel sounds before giving oral medications.

Nausea and vomiting are potential postanesthetic reactions. To reduce the risk of aspiration, position the patient with his or her head to the side. Have equipment for suctioning available. Antiemetic medication may be needed.

Urinary Tract. Anesthetics and their adjuncts can disrupt urinary tract function. Anesthetics can decrease urine production by reducing renal blood flow. Opioids and anticholinergic drugs can cause urinary retention. Monitor urine output. If the patient fails to void, follow hospital protocol. Catheterization or medication (e.g., bethanechol) may be required.

Management of Postoperative Pain

As anesthesia wears off, the patient may experience postoperative pain. An opioid may be required. Since respiratory depression from opioids will add to residual respiratory depression from anesthesia, use opioids with caution; balance the need to relieve pain against the need to maintain ventilation.

Implications for Ketamine

Adverse psychologic reactions can develop as the patient emerges from ketamine-induced anesthesia. To minimize these reactions, provide a calm and stimulus-free environment until recovery is complete.

*Patient education information is highlighted as blue text.

Opioid (Narcotic) Analgesics, Opioid Antagonists, and Nonopioid Centrally Acting Analgesics

Analgesics are drugs that relieve pain without causing loss of consciousness. In this chapter, our principal focus is on the opioid analgesics—the most effective pain relievers available. The opioid family, whose name derives from *opium*, includes such widely used agents as morphine, codeine, oxycodone [OxyContin], and propoxyphene [Darvon].

INTRODUCTION TO THE OPIOIDS

Terminology

Opioid is a general term defined as any drug, natural or synthetic, that has actions similar to those of morphine. The term *opiate* is more specific and applies only to compounds present in opium (e.g., morphine, codeine).

The term *narcotic* has had so many definitions that it can no longer be used with precision. *Narcotic* has been used to mean an analgesic, a central nervous system (CNS) depressant, and any drug capable of causing physical dependence. *Narcotic* has also been employed in a legal context to designate not only the opioids but also such diverse drugs as cocaine, marijuana, and lysergic acid diethylamide (LSD). Because of its more precise definition, *opioid* is clearly preferable to *narcotic* as a label for a discrete family of pharmacologic agents.

Endogenous Opioid Peptides

The body has three families of peptides that have opioid-like properties. These families are named *enkephalins, endorphins,* and *dynorphins.* Although we know that endogenous opioid peptides serve as neurotransmitters, neurohormones, and neuromodulators, their precise physiologic role is not fully understood. Endogenous opioid peptides are found in the CNS and in peripheral tissues.

Opioid Receptors

There are three main classes of opioid receptors, designated *mu, kappa,* and *delta.* From a pharmacologic perspective, mu receptors are the most important. Why? Because opioid analgesics act primarily through activation of mu receptors, although they also produce weak activation of kappa receptors. As a rule, opioid analgesics do not interact with delta receptors. In contrast to opioid analgesics, endogenous opioid peptides act through all three types of opioid receptors, including delta receptors. Important responses to activation of mu and kappa receptors are summarized in Table 27–1.

Mu Receptors. Responses to activation of mu receptors include analgesia, respiratory depression, euphoria, and sedation. In addition, mu activation is related to development of physical dependence.

A study in genetically engineered mice underscores the importance of mu receptors in drug action. In this study, researchers employed mice from which the gene for mu receptors had been deleted. When these mice were given morphine, the drug had no effect. It did not produce analgesia, it did not produce physical dependence, and it did not reinforce social behaviors that are thought to indicate subjective effects.

TABLE 27–1 ▮▪ Important Responses to Activation of Mu and Kappa Receptors

Response	Receptor Type	
	Mu	Kappa
Analgesia	✓	✓
Respiratory depression	✓	
Sedation	✓	✓
Euphoria	✓	
Physical dependence	✓	
Decreased GI motility	✓	✓

TABLE 27–2 ▮▪ Drug Actions At Mu and Kappa Receptors

Drugs	Receptor Type	
	Mu	Kappa
Pure Opioid Agonists		
Morphine, codeine, meperidine, and other morphine-like drugs	Agonist	Agonist
Agonist-Antagonist Opioids		
Pentazocine, nalbuphine, and butorphanol	Antagonist	Agonist
Buprenorphine	Partial agonist	Antagonist
Pure Opioid Antagonists		
Naloxone, naltrexone, and nalmefene	Antagonist	Antagonist

Hence, at least in mice, mu receptors appear both necessary and sufficient to mediate the major actions of opioid drugs.

Kappa Receptors. As with mu receptors, activation of kappa receptors can produce analgesia and sedation. In addition, kappa activation may underlie psychotomimetic effects seen with certain opioids.

Classification of Drugs That Act at Opioid Receptors

Drugs that act at opioid receptors are classified on the basis of how they affect receptor function. At each type of receptor, a drug can act in one of three ways: as an *agonist, partial agonist,* or *antagonist.* (Recall from Chapter 5 that a partial agonist is a drug that produces low to moderate receptor activation when administered alone, but will block the actions of a full agonist if the two drugs are given together.) Based on these actions, drugs that bind opioid receptors fall into three major groups: (1) pure opioid agonists, (2) agonist-antagonist opioids, and (3) pure opioid antagonists. The actions of drugs in these groups at mu and kappa receptors are summarized in Table 27–2.

Pure Opioid Agonists. The pure opioid agonists activate mu and kappa receptors. By activating these receptors, the pure agonists can produce analgesia, euphoria, sedation, respiratory depression, physical dependence, constipation, and other effects. As indicated in Table 27–3, the pure agonists can be subdivided into two groups: *strong opioid agonists* and *moderate to strong opioid agonists.* Morphine is the prototype of the strong agonists. Codeine is the prototype of the moderate to strong agonists.

Agonist-Antagonist Opioids. Five agonist-antagonist opioids are available: pentazocine, nalbuphine, butorphanol, dezocine, and buprenorphine. The actions of these drugs at mu and kappa receptors are summarized in Table 27–2. When administered alone, the agonist-antagonist opioids produce analgesia. However, if given to a patient who is taking a pure opioid agonist, these drugs can *antagonize* analgesia caused by the pure agonist. Pentazocine [Talwin] is the prototype of the agonist-antagonists.

Pure Opioid Antagonists. The pure opioid antagonists act as antagonists at mu and kappa receptors. These drugs do not produce analgesia or any of the other effects caused by opioid agonists. The principal use for these agents is reversal of respiratory and CNS depression caused by overdose with opioid agonists. Naloxone [Narcan] is the prototype of the pure antagonists.

BASIC PHARMACOLOGY OF THE OPIOIDS

Morphine

Morphine is the prototype of the strong opioid analgesics and remains the standard by which newer opioids are measured. Morphine has multiple pharmacologic effects, including analgesia, sedation, euphoria, respiratory depression, cough suppression, and suppression of bowel motility. The drug is named after Morpheus, the Greek god of dreams.

Source

Morphine is found in the seedpod of the poppy plant, *Papaver somniferum.* The drug is prepared by extraction from opium, which is the dried juice of the poppy seedpod. In addition to morphine, opium contains two other medicinal compounds: codeine (an analgesic) and papaverine (a smooth muscle relaxant).

Overview of Pharmacologic Actions

Morphine has multiple pharmacologic actions. In addition to relieving pain, the drug causes drowsiness, mental clouding, reduction of anxiety, and a sense of well-being. Through actions in the CNS and periphery, morphine can cause respiratory depression, constipation, urinary retention, orthostatic hypotension, emesis, miosis, cough suppression, and biliary colic. With prolonged use, the drug produces tolerance and physical dependence.

Individual effects of morphine may be beneficial, detrimental, or both. For example, analgesia is clearly beneficial, whereas respiratory depression and urinary retention are clearly detrimental. Certain other effects, such as sedation and reduced bowel motility, may be beneficial or detrimental, depending on the circumstances of drug use.

Therapeutic Use: Relief of Pain

The principal indication for morphine is relief of moderate to severe pain. The drug can relieve postoperative pain, chronic pain of cancer, and pain associated with labor and delivery. In addition, morphine can be used to relieve pain of myocardial infarction and dyspnea associated with left ventricular failure and pulmonary edema—although it is no longer the drug of choice for such patients. Morphine may also be administered preoperatively for sedation and reduction of anxiety.

TABLE 27–3 ■ Opioid Analgesics: Abuse Liability and Maximal Pain Relief

Drug and Category	CSA* Schedule	Abuse Liability	Maximal Pain Relief
Strong Opioid Agonists			
Alfentanil	II	High	High
Fentanyl	II	High	High
Hydromorphone	II	High	High
Levorphanol	II	High	High
Meperidine	II	High	High
Methadone	II	High	High
Morphine	II	High	High
Oxymorphone	II	High	High
Remifentanil	II	—	High
Sufentanil	II	High	High
Moderate to Strong Opioid Agonists			
Codeine	II	Moderate	Low
Hydrocodone	III†	Moderate	Moderate
Oxycodone	II	Moderate	Moderate
Propoxyphene	IV	Low	Low
Agonist-Antagonist Opioids			
Buprenorphine	V	Low	Moderate to high
Dezocine	NR‡	Low	Moderate
Butorphanol	IV	Low	Moderate to high
Nalbuphine	NR‡	Low	Moderate to high
Pentazocine	IV	Low	Moderate

*CSA = Controlled Substances Act.

†In the United States, hydrocodone is available only in combination with aspirin or acetaminophen. These combination products are classified under Schedule III.

‡NR = not regulated under the Controlled Substances Act.

Morphine relieves pain without affecting other senses (e.g., sight, touch, smell, hearing) and without causing loss of consciousness. The drug is more effective against constant, dull pain than against sharp, intermittent pain. However, even sharp pain can be relieved by large doses. The ability of morphine to cause mental clouding, sedation, euphoria, and anxiety reduction can contribute to relief of pain.

The use of morphine and other opioids to relieve pain is discussed further under *Clinical Use of Opioids* and in Chapter 28.

Mechanism of Analgesic Action. Morphine and other opioid agonists are thought to relieve pain by mimicking the actions of endogenous opioid peptides, primarily at mu receptors. This hypothesis is based on the following observations:

■ Opioid peptides and morphine-like drugs both produce analgesia when administered to experimental subjects.
■ Opioid peptides and morphine-like drugs share structural similarities (Fig. 27–1).
■ Opioid peptides and morphine-like drugs bind to the same receptors in the CNS.
■ The receptors to which opioid peptides and morphine-like drugs bind are located in regions of the brain and spinal cord that are associated with perception of pain.

■ Subjects rendered tolerant to analgesia from morphine-like drugs show cross-tolerance to analgesia from opioid peptides.
■ The analgesic effects of opioid peptides and morphine-like drugs can both be blocked by the same antagonist (naloxone).

From these data it is postulated that (1) opioid peptides serve a physiologic role as modulators of pain perception, and (2) morphine-like drugs produce analgesia by mimicking the actions of endogenous opioid peptides.

Adverse Effects

Respiratory Depression. Respiratory depression is the most serious adverse effect of the opioids. At equianalgesic doses, all of the pure opioid agonists depress respiration to the same extent. Death following overdose is almost always from respiratory arrest. Opioids depress respiration primarily through activation of mu receptors, although activation of kappa receptors also contributes.

The time course of respiratory depression varies with route of administration. Depressant effects begin about 7 minutes after IV injection, 30 minutes after IM injection, and up to 90 minutes after SC injection. With all three routes, significant depression may persist for 4 to 5 hours. When morphine

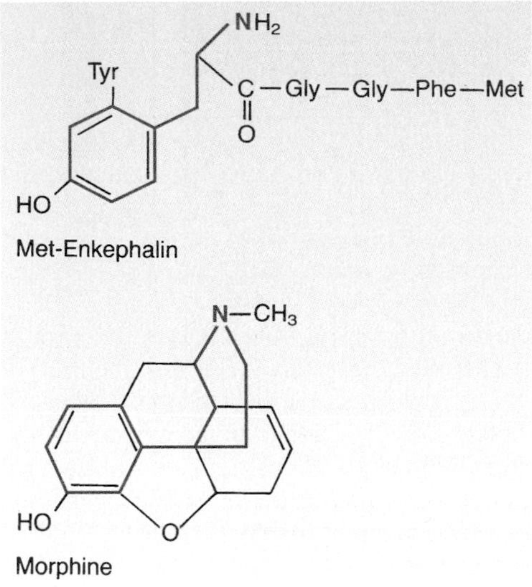

Figure 27–1 ■ Structural similarity between morphine and metenkephalin.
In the morphine structural formula, color highlighting indicates the part of the molecule thought responsible for interaction with opioid receptors. In the metenkephalin structural formula, color highlighting indicates the region of structural similarity with morphine.

is administered by spinal injection, onset of respiratory depression may be delayed for hours; you should be alert to this possibility.

With prolonged use of opioids, tolerance develops to respiratory depression. Huge doses that would be lethal to nontolerant individuals have been taken by opioid addicts without noticeable effect. Similarly, tolerance to respiratory depression develops during long-term clinical use of opioids (e.g., in patients with cancer).

When administered at usual therapeutic doses, opioids rarely cause significant respiratory depression. However, although uncommon, substantial respiratory depression can occur. Accordingly, respiratory rate should be determined prior to opioid administration. If the rate is 12 breaths per minute or less, the opioid should be withheld and the physician notified. Certain patients, including the very young, the elderly, and those with respiratory disease (e.g., asthma, emphysema) are especially sensitive to respiratory depression and must be monitored closely. Outpatients should be informed about the risk of respiratory depression and instructed to notify the physician if respiratory distress occurs.

Respiratory depression is increased by concurrent use of other drugs with CNS-depressant actions (e.g., alcohol, barbiturates, benzodiazepines). Accordingly, these drugs should be avoided. Outpatients should be warned against use of alcohol and all other CNS depressants.

Constipation. Opioids promote constipation through a combination of effects on the GI tract. Through actions exerted in the CNS and locally, these drugs suppress propulsive intestinal contractions, intensify nonpropulsive contractions, increase the tone of the anal sphincter, and inhibit secretion of fluids into the intestinal lumen. As a result, constipation can develop within a few days of starting opioid therapy.

The risk of opioid-induced constipation can be reduced with a combination of pharmacologic and nonpharmacologic measures. The goal is to produce a soft, formed stool every 1 to 2 days. Principal nondrug measures are physical activity and increased fluid intake. Most patients also require prophylactic drugs. A stimulant laxative, such as senna [Senokot], is given to counteract reduced bowel motility. A stool softener, such as docusate [Colace, others], provides additional benefit. If the stimulant laxative and stool softener fail to prevent constipation, bisacodyl [Dulcolax, others] may be added to the regimen. Severe constipation can be managed with an osmotic laxative (e.g., magnesium citrate, milk of magnesia).

Recent studies indicate that an opioid antagonist can be used to treat opioid-induced constipation. In one study, patients who were taking large doses of opioids were given oral *methylnaltrexone,* an opioid antagonist that cannot be absorbed from the GI tract. By blocking opioid receptors in the intestine, the drug induced laxation and reversed slowing of intestinal transit time. Because the drug cannot be absorbed into the systemic circulation, it was able to reverse constipation without blocking opioid receptors in the brain and spinal cord, and hence did not reduce analgesia.

Because of their effects on the intestine, opioids are highly effective for managing diarrhea. In fact, antidiarrheal use of these drugs preceded their analgesic use by centuries. The effect of opioids on intestinal function is an interesting example of how a drug response can be viewed as detrimental (constipation) or beneficial (relief of diarrhea) depending on who is taking the medication. Opioids employed specifically to treat diarrhea are discussed in Chapter 75.

Orthostatic Hypotension. Morphine-like drugs lower blood pressure by blunting the baroreceptor reflex and by dilating peripheral arterioles and veins. Peripheral vasodilation results primarily from morphine-induced release of histamine. Hypotension is mild in the recumbent patient but can be substantial when the patient stands up. Patients should be informed about symptoms of hypotension (lightheadedness, dizziness) and instructed to sit or lie down if these occur. Also, patients should be informed that hypotension can be minimized by moving slowly when changing from a supine or seated position to an upright position. Patients should be warned against ambulation if hypotension is significant. Hospitalized patients may require ambulatory assistance. Hypotensive drugs can exacerbate opioid-induced hypotension.

Urinary Retention. Morphine can cause urinary hesitancy and urinary retention by increasing tone in the sphincter of the bladder. Also, by increasing tone in the detrusor muscle, the drug can elevate pressure within the bladder, causing urinary urgency. In addition to its direct effects on the urinary tract, morphine may interfere with voiding by suppressing awareness of bladder stimuli. Accordingly, patients should be encouraged to void every 4 hours. Urinary hesitancy or retention is especially likely in patients with prostatic hypertrophy. Drugs with anticholinergic properties (e.g., tricyclic antidepressants, antihistamines) can exacerbate urinary retention.

Urinary retention should be assessed by monitoring intake and output and by palpating the lower abdomen every 4 to 6 hours for bladder distention. If a change in intake-output ratio develops, or if bladder distention is detected, or if the patient reports difficulty voiding, the physician should be notified. Catheterization may be required.

In addition to causing urinary retention, morphine may decrease urine production. The drug reduces urine formation largely by decreasing renal blood flow, and partly by promoting release of antidiuretic hormone.

Cough Suppression. Morphine-like drugs act at opioid receptors in the medulla to suppress cough. Suppression of spontaneous cough may lead to accumulation of secretions in the airway. Accordingly, patients should be instructed to actively cough at regular intervals. Lung status should be assessed by auscultation for rales. The ability of opioids to suppress cough is put to clinical use in the form of codeine- and hydrocodone-based cough remedies.

Biliary Colic. Morphine can induce spasm of the common bile duct, causing pressure within the biliary tract to rise dramatically. Symptoms range from epigastric distress to biliary colic. In patients with pre-existing biliary colic, morphine may intensify pain rather than relieve it. Certain opioids (e.g., meperidine) cause less smooth muscle spasm than morphine, and hence are less likely to exacerbate biliary colic.

Emesis. Morphine promotes nausea and vomiting through direct stimulation of the chemoreceptor trigger zone of the medulla. Emetic reactions are greatest with the initial dose and diminish with subsequent doses. Nausea and vomiting are uncommon in recumbent patients, but occur in 15% to 40% of ambulatory patients, suggesting a vestibular component. Nausea and vomiting can be reduced by pretreatment with an antiemetic (e.g., prochlorperazine) and by having the patient remain still.

Elevation of Intracranial Pressure. Morphine can elevate intracranial pressure (ICP). The mechanism is indirect: By suppressing respiration, morphine increases the CO_2 content of blood, which dilates the cerebral vasculature, causing ICP to rise. Accordingly, if respiration is maintained at a normal rate, ICP will remain normal too.

Euphoria/Dysphoria. *Euphoria* is defined as an exaggerated sense of well-being. Morphine often produces euphoria when given to patients in pain. Although euphoria can enhance pain relief, it also contributes to the drug's potential for abuse. Euphoria is caused by activation of mu receptors.

In some individuals, morphine causes *dysphoria* (a sense of anxiety and being ill at ease). Dysphoria is uncommon among patients in pain, but may occur when morphine is taken in the absence of pain.

Sedation. When administered to relieve pain, morphine is likely to cause drowsiness and some mental clouding. Although these effects can complement the drug's analgesic actions, they can also be detrimental. Outpatients should be warned about CNS depression and advised to avoid hazardous activities (e.g., driving) if sedation is significant. Sedation can be minimized by (1) taking smaller doses more often, (2) using opioids that have short half-lives, and (3) giving small doses of a CNS stimulant (methylphenidate or dextroamphetamine) in the morning and early afternoon.

Miosis. Morphine and other opioids cause pupillary constriction (miosis). In response to toxic doses, the pupils may constrict to "pinpoint" size. Since miosis can impair vision in dim light, room light should be kept bright during waking hours.

Pharmacokinetics

Morphine is administered by several routes: oral, IM, IV, SC, epidural, and intrathecal. Onset of effects is slower with oral administration than with parenteral administration. With three routes—IM, IV, and SC—analgesia lasts 4 to 5 hours. With two routes—epidural and intrathecal—analgesia may persist up to 24 hours. With oral therapy, duration of action depends on the formulation. For example, with standard tablets, effects last 4 to 5 hours, whereas with extended-release capsules, effects last 24 hours.

In order to relieve pain, morphine must cross the blood-brain barrier and enter the CNS. Because the drug is not very lipid soluble, it does not cross the barrier easily. Consequently, only a small fraction of an administered dose reaches sites of analgesic action. Since the blood-brain barrier is not well developed in infants, these patients generally require lower doses than older children and adults.

Morphine is inactivated by hepatic metabolism. When taken by mouth, the drug must pass through the liver on its way to the systemic circulation. Much of an oral dose is inactivated during this first pass through the liver. Consequently, oral doses need to be substantially larger than parenteral doses to produce equivalent analgesic effects. Analgesia and other effects may be intensified and prolonged in patients with liver disease; hence, it may be necessary to reduce the dosage or lengthen the dosing interval.

Tolerance and Physical Dependence

With continuous use, morphine can cause tolerance and physical dependence. These phenomena, which are generally inseparable, reflect cellular adaptations that occur in response to prolonged opioid exposure.

Tolerance. Tolerance can be defined as a state in which a larger dose is required to produce the same response that could formerly be elicited by a smaller dose. Alternatively, tolerance can be defined as a condition in which a particular dose now produces a smaller response than it did when treatment began. Because of tolerance, dosage must be increased to maintain analgesic effects.

Tolerance develops to many—but not all—of morphine's actions. With prolonged treatment, tolerance develops to *analgesia, euphoria,* and *sedation.* As a result, with long-term therapy, an increase in dosage may be required to maintain these desirable effects. Fortunately, as tolerance develops to these therapeutic effects, tolerance also develops to *respiratory depression.* As a result, the high doses needed to control pain in the tolerant individual are not associated with increased respiratory depression.

Very little tolerance develops to *constipation* and *miosis.* Even in highly tolerant addicts, constipation remains a chronic problem, and constricted pupils are characteristic.

Cross-tolerance exists among the opioid agonists (e.g., oxycodone, methadone, codeine, heroin). Accordingly, individuals tolerant to one of these agents will be tolerant to the others. No cross-tolerance exists between opioids and general CNS depressants (e.g., barbiturates, ethanol, benzodiazepines, general anesthetics).

Physical Dependence. Physical dependence is defined as a state in which an abstinence syndrome will occur if drug use is abruptly discontinued. Opioid dependence results from adaptive cellular changes that occur in response to the continuous presence of these drugs. Although the exact nature of these changes is unknown, it is clear that, once these compensatory changes have taken place, the body requires the continued presence of opioids to function normally. If opioids are withdrawn, an abstinence syndrome will result.

The intensity and duration of the opioid abstinence syndrome depends on two factors: the half-life of the drug being used and the degree of physical dependence. With opioids that have relatively short half-lives (e.g., morphine), symptoms of abstinence are intense but brief. In contrast, with opioids that have long half-lives (e.g., methadone), symptoms are less intense but more prolonged. With any opioid, the intensity of withdrawal symptoms parallels the degree of physical dependence.

For individuals who are highly dependent, the abstinence syndrome can be extremely unpleasant. Initial reactions include yawning, rhinorrhea, and sweating. Onset occurs about 10 hours after the last dose. These early responses are followed by anorexia, irritability, tremor, and "gooseflesh"—hence the term *cold turkey*. At its peak, the syndrome manifests as violent sneezing, weakness, nausea, vomiting, diarrhea, abdominal cramps, bone and muscle pain, muscle spasm, and kicking movements—hence, "kicking the habit." Giving an opioid at any time during withdrawal rapidly reverses all signs and symptoms. Left untreated, the morphine withdrawal syndrome runs its course in 7 to 10 days. It should be emphasized that, although withdrawal from opioids is unpleasant, the syndrome is rarely dangerous. In contrast, withdrawal from general CNS depressants (e.g., barbiturates, alcohol) can be lethal (see Chapter 33).

To minimize the abstinence syndrome, opioids should be withdrawn gradually. When the degree of dependence is moderate, symptoms can be avoided by administering progressively smaller doses over 3 days. When the patient is highly dependent, dosage should be tapered more slowly—over 7 to 10 days. With a proper withdrawal procedure, symptoms of abstinence will resemble those of a mild case of flu—even when the degree of dependence is high.

It is important to note that physical dependence is rarely a complication when opioids are taken *acutely* to treat pain. Hospitalized patients receiving morphine 2 to 3 times a day for up to 2 weeks show no significant signs of dependence. If morphine is withheld from these patients, no significant signs of withdrawal can be detected. The issue of physical dependence as a clinical concern is discussed further later in the chapter.

Infants exposed to opioids *in utero* may be born drug dependent. If the infant is not provided with opioids, an abstinence syndrome will occur. Signs of withdrawal include excessive crying, sneezing, tremor, hyperreflexia, fever, and diarrhea. The infant can be weaned from drug dependence by administering dilute opium tincture in progressively smaller doses.

Cross-dependence exists among pure opioid agonists. As a result, any pure agonist will prevent withdrawal in a patient who is physically dependent on any other pure agonist.

Abuse Liability

Morphine and the other opioids are subject to abuse, largely because of their ability to cause pleasurable experiences (e.g., euphoria, sedation, a sensation in the lower abdomen resembling orgasm). Physical dependence contributes to abuse: Once dependence exists, the ability of opioids to ward off withdrawal serves to reinforce their desirability in the mind of the abuser.

The abuse liability of the opioids is reflected in their classification under the Controlled Substances Act. (The provisions of this act are discussed in Chapter 36.) As shown in Table 27–3, morphine and all other strong opioid agonists are classified under Schedule II of the act. This classification reflects a moderate to high abuse liability. The agonist-antagonist opioids have a lower abuse liability and hence are classified under Schedule IV (butorphanol, pentazocine) or Schedule V (buprenorphine), or have no classification at all (dezocine, nalbuphine). Members of the healthcare team who prescribe, dispense, and administer opioids must adhere to the procedures set forth in the Controlled Substances Act.

Fortunately, abuse is rare when opioids are employed to treat pain. The issue of abuse as a clinical concern is discussed further later in the chapter.

Precautions

Some patients are more likely than others to experience adverse reactions to opioids. Common sense dictates that opioids be used with special caution in these people. Conditions that can predispose patients to adverse reactions are discussed immediately below.

Decreased Respiratory Reserve. Because of its respiratory depressant action, morphine can further compromise respiration in patients with impaired pulmonary function. Accordingly, the drug should be used with caution in patients with asthma, emphysema, kyphoscoliosis, chronic cor pulmonale, and extreme obesity. Caution is also needed in patients taking other drugs that can depress respiration (e.g., barbiturates, benzodiazepines, general anesthetics).

Pregnancy. Morphine does not cause birth defects in humans. However, regular use of opioids during pregnancy *can* cause physical dependence in the fetus. Accordingly, prolonged use by pregnant women should be avoided if possible.

Labor and Delivery. Use of morphine during delivery can suppress uterine contractions and cause respiratory depression in the neonate. Following delivery, respiration in the neonate should be monitored closely. Respiratory depression can be reversed with naloxone. The use of opioids in obstetrics is discussed further later in the chapter.

Head Injury. Morphine and other opioids must be used with caution in patients with head injury. Head injury can cause respiratory depression accompanied by elevation of ICP. Morphine can exacerbate these symptoms. In addition, since miosis, mental clouding, and vomiting can be valuable diagnostic signs following head injury, and since morphine can cause these same effects, use of opioids can confound diagnosis.

Other Precautions. *Infants* and *elderly patients* are especially sensitive to the respiratory-depressant action of morphine. In patients with *inflammatory bowel disease,* morphine may cause toxic megacolon or paralytic ileus. Since morphine and all other opioids are inactivated by the liver, effects of these agents may be intensified and prolonged in patients with *liver impairment.* Severe hypotension may occur in patients with pre-existing *hypotension* or *reduced blood volume.* In patients with *prostatic hypertrophy,* opioids may cause acute urinary retention; repeated catheterization may be required.

Drug Interactions

The major interactions between morphine and other drugs are summarized in Table 27–4. Some of these interactions are adverse; others are beneficial.

CNS Depressants. All drugs with CNS-depressant actions (e.g., barbiturates, benzodiazepines, alcohol) can intensify sedation and respiratory depression caused by morphine and other opioids. Outpatients should be warned against use of alcohol and all other CNS depressants.

Anticholinergic Drugs. These agents (e.g., antihistamines, tricyclic antidepressants, atropine-like drugs) can exacerbate morphine-induced constipation and urinary retention.

Hypotensive Drugs. Antihypertensive drugs and other drugs that lower blood pressure can exacerbate morphine-induced hypotension.

Monoamine Oxidase Inhibitors. The combination of meperidine (a morphine-like drug) with a monoamine oxidase (MAO) inhibitor has produced a syndrome characterized by excitation, delirium, hyperpyrexia, convulsions, and severe respiratory depression. Death has occurred. Although this reaction has not been reported with combined use of an MAO inhibitor and morphine, prudence suggests that the combination nonetheless be avoided.

Agonist-Antagonist Opioids. These drugs (e.g., pentazocine, buprenorphine) can precipitate a withdrawal syndrome if administered to an individual who is physically dependent on a pure opioid agonist. The basis of this reaction is considered later in the chapter. Patients taking pure opioid agonists should be weaned from these drugs before beginning treatment with an agonist-antagonist.

Opioid Antagonists. Opioid antagonists (e.g., naloxone) can counteract most actions of morphine and other pure opioid agonists. Opioid antagonists are employed primarily to treat opioid overdose. The actions and uses of the opioid antagonists are discussed in detail later in the chapter.

Other Interactions. *Antiemetics* of the phenothiazine type (e.g., promethazine [Phenergan]) may be combined with opioids to reduce nausea and vomiting. *Amphetamines, clonidine,* and *dextromethorphan* can enhance opioid-induced analgesia. *Amphetamines* can also offset sedation.

Toxicity

Clinical Manifestations. Opioid overdose produces a classic triad of signs: *coma, respiratory depression,* and *pinpoint pupils.* Coma is profound, and the patient cannot be aroused. Respiratory rate may be as low as 2 to 4 breaths per minute. Although the pupils are constricted initially, they may dilate as hypoxia sets in (secondary to respiratory depression). Hypoxia may cause blood pressure to fall. Prolonged hypoxia may result in shock. When death occurs, respiratory arrest is almost always the immediate cause.

Treatment. Treatment consists primarily of *ventilatory support* and giving an *opioid antagonist.* Traditionally, naloxone [Narcan] has been the antagonist of choice. However, nalmefene [Revex], a newer and longer acting antagonist, may be preferred for many patients. The pharmacology of the opioid antagonists is discussed later in the chapter.

Preparations, Dosage, and Administration

General Guidelines on Dosage and Administration. Dosage must be individualized. High doses are required for patients with a low tolerance to pain or with extremely painful disorders. Patients with sharp, stabbing pain need higher doses than patients with dull pain. Elderly adults generally require lower doses than younger adults. Neonates require relatively low doses because the blood-brain barrier is not fully

---

TABLE 27–4 ■ Interactions of Morphine-Like Drugs with Other Drugs	
Interacting Drugs	**Outcome of the Interaction**
Adverse Interactions	

CNS depressants
   Barbiturates
   Benzodiazepines
   Alcohol
   General anesthetics
   Antihistamines
   Phenothiazines
	Increased respiratory depression and sedation

Agonist-antagonist opioids	Precipitation of a withdrawal reaction

Anticholinergic drugs
   Atropine-like drugs
   Antihistamines
   Phenothiazines
   Tricyclic antidepressants
	Increased constipation and urinary retention

Hypotensive agents	Increased hypotension
Monoamine oxidase inhibitors	Hyperpyrexic coma
Beneficial Interactions	
Amphetamines	Increased analgesia and decreased sedation
Antiemetics	Suppression of nausea and vomiting
Naloxone	Suppression of symptoms of opioid overdose
Dextromethorphan	Increased analgesia; possible reduction in tolerance

developed. For all patients, dosage should be reduced as pain subsides. Outpatients should be warned not to increase dosage without consulting the physician.

Before an opioid is administered, respiratory rate, blood pressure, and pulse rate should be determined. The drug should be withheld and the physician notified if respiratory rate is at or below 12 breaths per minute, if blood pressure is significantly below the pretreatment value, or if pulse rate is significantly above or below the pretreatment value.

As a rule, *opioids should be administered on a fixed schedule—not PRN*. With a fixed schedule, medication is given before intense pain returns. As a result, the patient is spared needless discomfort. Furthermore, anxiety about recurrence of pain is reduced. If breakthrough pain occurs, supplemental doses of a short-acting preparation should be given.

Morphine and practically all other opioid agonists are classified under Schedule II of the Controlled Substances Act and must be dispensed accordingly.

Preparations. Morphine sulfate is available in 10 formulations: *standard tablets* [MSIR] (15 and 30 mg); *soluble tablets* (10, 15, and 30 mg); *controlled-release tablets* [MS Contin, Oramorph SR] (15, 30, 60, 100, and 200 mg); *extended-release tablets* (15, 30, 60, and 100 mg); *standard capsules* [MSIR] (15 and 30 mg), *sustained-release capsules* [Kadian] (20, 50, and 100 mg); *extended-release capsules* [Avinza] (30, 60, 90, and 120 mg); *oral solution* [MSIR, Roxanol] (4 and 20 mg/ml); *rectal suppositories* [RMS] (5, 10, 20, and 30 mg); and *solution for injection* [Astramorph PF, Duramorph, Infumorph] (0.5, 1, 2, 4, 5, 8, 10, 15, 25, and 50 mg/ml).

Dosage and Routes of Administration. Oral. Oral administration is generally reserved for patients with chronic, severe pain, such as that associated with cancer. Because oral morphine undergoes extensive metabolism on its first pass through the liver, oral doses are usually higher than parenteral doses. A typical dosage is 10 to 30 mg repeated every 4 hours as needed. However, oral dosing is highly individualized; hence, some patients may require 75 mg or more. Controlled-release formulations may be administered every 8 to 12 hours, and the extended-release formulation [Avinza] is given every 24 hours. Patients should be instructed to swallow these products intact, without crushing or chewing.

Intramuscular and Subcutaneous. Both routes are painful and unreliable, and hence should generally be avoided. For adults, dosing is initiated at 5 to 10 mg every 4 hours, and then adjusted up or down as needed. The usual dosage for children is 0.1 to 0.2 mg/kg repeated every 4 hours as needed.

Intravenous. Intravenous morphine should be injected slowly (over 4 to 5 minutes). Rapid IV injection can cause severe adverse effects (profound hypotension, cardiac arrest, respiratory arrest) and should be avoided. When IV injections are made, an opioid antagonist (e.g., naloxone) and facilities for respiratory support should be available. Injections should be given with the patient lying down to minimize hypotension. The usual dose for adults is 4 to 10 mg (diluted in 4 to 5 ml of water for injection). The usual pediatric dose is 0.05 to 0.1 mg/kg.

Epidural and Intrathecal. When morphine is employed for spinal analgesia, epidural injection is preferred to intrathecal. With either route, onset of analgesia is rapid and the duration prolonged (up to 24 hours). The most troubling side effects are delayed respiratory depression and delayed cardiac depression. Be alert for possible late reactions. The usual adult epidural dose is 5 mg. Intrathecal doses are much smaller—about one-tenth the epidural dose.

Other Strong Opioid Agonists

In an effort to produce a strong analgesic with a low potential for respiratory depression and abuse, pharmaceutical scientists have created many new opioid analgesics. However, none of the newer pure opioid agonists can be considered truly superior to morphine: The newer pure opioids are essentially equal to morphine with respect to analgesic action, abuse liability, and the ability to cause respiratory depression. Also, to

varying degrees, all of these drugs cause sedation, euphoria, constipation, urinary retention, cough suppression, hypotension, and miosis. However, despite similarities to morphine, the newer drugs do have unique qualities. These special characteristics may render one agent more desirable than another in a particular clinical situation. With all of the newer pure opioid agonists, toxicity can be reversed with an opioid antagonist (e.g., naloxone). Important differences between morphine and the newer strong opioid analgesics are discussed below. Table 27–5 summarizes dosages, routes, and time courses for morphine and the newer opioid agonists.

Fentanyl

Fentanyl [Sublimaze, Duragesic, Fentanyl Oralet, Actiq] is a strong opioid analgesic with a high milligram potency (about 100 times that of morphine). The drug is available for parenteral, transdermal, and transmucosal administration. All preparations are regulated under Schedule II of the Controlled Substances Act.

Parenteral. Parenteral fentanyl [Sublimaze] is employed primarily for induction and maintenance of surgical anesthesia. The drug is well suited for these applications because it has a rapid onset and short duration. Most effects are like those of morphine. In addition, fentanyl can cause muscle rigidity, which can interfere with induction of anesthesia. As discussed in Chapter 26 (General Anesthetics), the combination of fentanyl plus droperidol, available commercially as Innovar, is used to produce a state known as "neurolept analgesia."

Transdermal. The fentanyl transdermal system [Duragesic] consists of a fentanyl-containing "patch" that is applied to the skin of the upper torso. The drug is slowly released from the patch and absorbed through the skin, reaching effective levels in 24 hours. Levels remain steady for another 48 hours, after which the patch should be replaced. If a new patch is not applied, effects will nonetheless persist for several hours (owing to continued absorption of residual fentanyl remaining in the skin after the old patch was removed).

Transdermal fentanyl is indicated for chronic severe pain, such as that associated with cancer. Because analgesia is delayed, fentanyl patches are not suited for acute or postoperative pain. The patches should not be used in children under 12 years old, or in anyone under 18 who weighs less than 110 pounds. Also, patches should not be used for mild pain that responds to a less powerful analgesic.

Transdermal fentanyl has the same adverse effects as other opioids: respiratory depression, sedation, constipation, urinary retention, nausea, and so forth. Adverse effects may persist for hours following patch removal because of continued absorption from the skin. Signs of toxicity can be reversed with an opioid antagonist (e.g., naloxone). Used patches should be flushed down the toilet. Unused patches should be stored out of reach of children.

Fentanyl patches are available in four sizes, which deliver fentanyl to the systemic circulation at rates of 25, 50, 75, and 100 μg/hr. If the patient is not already tolerant to opioids, therapy should begin with the smallest patch. If a dosage greater than 100 μg/hr is required, a combination of patches can be applied. Because full analgesic effects can take up to 24 hours to develop, PRN therapy with a short-acting opioid may be required until the patch takes effect. For the majority of patients, patches can be replaced every 72 hours, although

TABLE 27–5 ■ Clinical Pharmacology of Pure Opioid Agonists

Drug and Route*	Equianalgesic Dose (mg)†	Time Course of Analgesic Effects		
		Onset (min)	Peak (min)	Duration (hr)
Codeine				
PO	200	30–45	60–120	4–6
IM	120	10–30	30–60	4–6
SC	120	10–30	30–60	4–6
Hydrocodone				
PO	10	10–30	30–60	4–6
Hydromorphone				
PO	7.5	30	90–120	4
IM	1.5	15	30–60	4–5
IV	1.5	10–15	15–30	2–3
SC	1.5	15	30–90	4
Levorphanol				
PO	4	10–60	90–120	6–8
IM	2	—	60	6–8
IV	2	—	Within 20	6–8
SC	2	—	60–90	6–8
Meperidine				
PO	300	15	60–90	2–4
IM	75	10–15	30–50	2–4
IV	75	1	5–7	2–4
SC	75	10–15	30–50	2–4
Methadone				
PO	20	30–60	90–120	4–6‡
IM	10	10–20	60–120	4–5‡
IV	10	—	15–30	3–4‡
Morphine				
PO	60	—	60–120	4–5§
IM	10	10–30	30–60	4–5
IV	10	—	20	4–5
SC	10	10–30	50–90	4–5
Epidural	10	15–60	—	Up to 24
Intrathecal	10	15–60	—	Up to 24
Oxycodone				
PO	30	15–30	60	3–4
Oxymorphone				
IM	1	10–15	30–90	3–6
IV	1	5–10	15–30	3–4
SC	1	10–20	—	3–6
Rectal	10	15–30	120	3–6
Propoxyphene				
PO	—‖	15–60	120	4–6

*IM administration should be avoided whenever possible.
†Dose in milligrams that produces a degree of analgesia equivalent to that produced by a 10-mg IM dose of morphine.
‡With repeated doses, methadone's duration of action may increase up to 48 hours.
§Effects of extended-release tablets may persist for 8 to 12 hours.
‖A dose of propoxyphene equivalent to 10 mg of morphine would be too toxic to administer.

some patients may require a new patch every 48 hours. As with other long-acting opioids, if breakthrough pain occurs, supplemental dosing with a short-acting opioid is indicated.

Transmucosal. Fentanyl is available in two transmucosal systems: a lozenge [Fentanyl Oralet] and a lozenge on a stick [Actiq]. The two formulations differ with respect to indications and strength.

Fentanyl Lozenges. Fentanyl Oralets are raspberry-flavored lozenges that come in four sizes: 100, 200, 300, and 400 μg. Oralets are approved *for preanesthetic medication before surgery* and for *inducing conscious sedation prior to painful diagnostic or therapeutic procedures.*

Despite their benign appearance, fentanyl lozenges are powerful and dangerous analgesics approved for use only in a hospital setting. Administration should be done by someone trained in the use of anesthetic drugs. Because of the risk of hypoventilation, continuous direct monitoring is required. Facilities for respiratory and cardiac resuscitation must be immediately available. The drug is contraindicated for children who weigh less than 10 kg (22 lb) and for treatment of acute or chronic pain in any patient.

When patients suck on a Fentanyl Oralet, some of the drug is absorbed directly and rapidly through the oral mucosa, and some is swallowed and absorbed slowly from the GI tract. Total bioavailability is about 50%. Analgesia begins in 10 to 15 minutes, peaks in 20 minutes, and persists for 1 to 2 hours.

Adverse effects are like those of other opioids. Preoperative itching of the nose and eyes is common, as are postoperative nausea and vomiting. However, the biggest danger is profound respiratory depression.

The recommended dosage for adults is 5 μg/kg, up to a maximum of 400 μg. Pediatric dosages range from 5 to 15 μg/kg. Patients should be instructed to suck the lozenge, not chew it. Consumption of the entire lozenge takes 10 to 20 minutes. Because onset of analgesia is delayed, dosing should begin 20 to 40 minutes prior to anticipated need. If the desired effect is achieved before the entire lozenge is consumed, the remainder should be flushed down a toilet.

Fentanyl Lozenge on a Stick. The Actiq system looks like a lollipop, consisting of a raspberry-flavored lozenge on a plastic handle. Six strengths are available: 200, 400, 600, 800, 1200, and 1600 μg. The *Actiq system* is approved only for *breakthrough cancer pain* in patients who are already taking opioids and have developed some degree of tolerance. (Tolerance is defined as needing more than 60 mg of morphine/day, more than 50 μg of fentanyl/hr, or an equianalgesic dose of another opioid for a week or more.) It is essential to appreciate that the dose of fentanyl in each Actiq unit is sufficient to kill nontolerant individuals—especially children. Accordingly, the drug must be stored in a secure, child-resistant location.

To administer the unit, patients place it between the cheek and the lower gum and actively suck it. Periodically, the unit should be moved from one side of the mouth to the other. Consumption of the entire lozenge should take 15 minutes. As the patient sucks, some of the drug is absorbed directly and rapidly through the oral mucosa, and some is swallowed and absorbed slowly from the GI tract. Analgesia begins in 10 to 15 minutes, peaks in 20 minutes, and persists for 1 to 2 hours.

Dosing should begin with a 200-μg unit. If breakthrough pain persists, the patient can take another 200-μg unit 15 minutes after finishing the first one (i.e., 30 minutes after starting the first). Unit size should be gradually increased until an effective dose is determined. If the patient needs more than 4 units a day, it may be time to give the patient a higher dose of his or her long-acting opioid.

Adverse effects of the Actiq system are like those of other opioids. The most common are dizziness, anxiety, confusion, nausea, vomiting, constipation, dyspnea, weakness, and headache. The biggest concerns are respiratory depression and shock. If dizziness, nausea, or signs of overdose develop during administration, the unit should be removed from the patient's mouth and disposed of immediately.

To promote safe and effective use of the Actiq system, the manufacturer provides an Actiq Welcome Kit with the initial drug supply. The kit contains educational materials and safe storage containers for unused, partially used, and completely used units.

Meperidine

Meperidine [Demerol] shares the major pharmacologic properties of morphine. Administration is oral and analgesia is strong. Until recently, meperidine was considered a first-line drug for relief of moderate to severe pain. Now, however, use of meperidine is in decline. Why? First, the drug has a short half-life, and hence dosing must be repeated at short intervals. Second, meperidine interacts adversely with a number of drugs. Third, with continuous use, there is a risk of harm owing to accumulation of a toxic metabolite. Accordingly, routine use of the drug should be avoided. However, meperidine may still be appropriate for patients who can't take other opioids, and for patients with drug-induced rigors or post-anesthesia shivering.

Meperidine can interact with MAO inhibitors to cause excitation, delirium, hyperpyrexia, and convulsions. Coma and death can follow. The underlying mechanism appears to be excessive activation of serotonin receptors owing to meperidine-induced blockade of serotonin reuptake. Clearly, the combination of meperidine with an MAO inhibitor should be avoided. Other drugs that increase serotonin availability (e.g., tricyclic antidepressants, selective serotonin reuptake inhibitors) may also pose a risk.

Repeated dosing results in accumulation of normeperidine, a toxic metabolite that can cause dysphoria, irritability, tremors, and seizures. To avoid toxicity, *treatment should not exceed 48 hours, and the dosage should not exceed 600 mg/24 hours.*

Meperidine is available in tablets (50 and 100 mg) and a syrup (10 mg/ml) for oral use, and in solution (50 and 100 mg/ml) for injection (IV, IM, or SC). In addition, the drug is available in single-dose vials, ampules, and syringes. The usual adult dosage is 50 to 150 mg (IM, SC, or PO) repeated every 3 to 4 hours as needed—up to a maximum of 600 mg/day. The usual dosage for children is 1 to 1.8 mg/kg (IM, SC, or PO) repeated every 3 to 4 hours as needed. As noted, prolonged use must be avoided.

Methadone

Methadone [Dolophine, Methadose] has pharmacologic properties very similar to those of morphine. The drug is effective orally and has a long duration of action. Repeated dosing can result in accumulation. Methadone is used to relieve pain and to treat opioid addicts. The use of methadone in drug-abuse treatment programs is discussed in Chapter 38.

Methadone is dispensed in standard tablets (5 and 10 mg) and solution (1, 2, and 10 mg/ml) for oral use, and in solution (10 mg/ml) for IM and SC administration. In addition, the drug is available in dispensable 40-mg tablets and bulk containers (50, 100, 500, and 1000 g) for detoxification and maintenance of opioid addicts. Usual oral analgesic doses for adults range from 2.5 to 20 mg repeated every 3 to 4 hours as needed.

Heroin

Heroin is a strong opioid agonist that is very similar to morphine in structure and actions. Heroin is an effective analgesic and is employed legally in Europe to relieve pain. In the United States, federal legislation prohibits the medical use of this drug. Heroin has been banned from American medicine because of its high abuse liability and because it does not appear to offer any benefits over opioids with a lower abuse potential.

Why is heroin preferred to other opioids as a drug of abuse? Because of its pharmacokinetic properties. Heroin has greater lipid solubility than morphine, and therefore crosses the blood-brain barrier more readily. As a result, when heroin is injected IV, the drug accumulates in the brain more rapidly and to a higher level than would an equivalent dose of IV morphine. Once in the brain, heroin (diacetylmorphine) is rapidly converted into active metabolites: monoacetylmorphine and morphine (Fig. 27–2). It is these metabolites, and not heroin itself, that produce the subjective effects that follow heroin injection. In this regard, heroin can be viewed as a vehicle for facilitating transport of morphine into the brain.

Alfentanil and Sufentanil

Alfentanil [Alfenta] and sufentanil [Sufenta] are intravenous opioids related to fentanyl. Both drugs are used for induction of anesthesia, for maintenance of anesthesia (in combination with other agents), and as sole anesthetic agents. Pharmacologic effects are like those of morphine. Sufentanil has an especially high milligram potency (about 1000 times that of morphine); alfentanil is about 10 times more potent than morphine. Both alfentanil and sufentanil have a rapid onset of action. Both drugs are Schedule II agents.

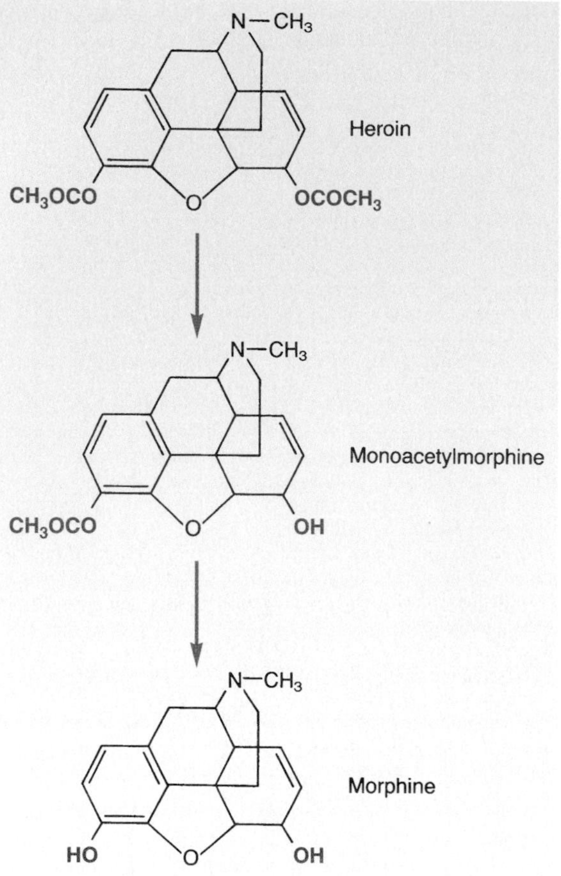

Figure 27–2 ■ **Biotransformation of heroin into morphine.** Heroin, as such, is biologically inactive. After crossing the blood-brain barrier, heroin is converted to monoacetylmorphine (MAM) and then into morphine itself. MAM and morphine are responsible for the effects elicited by injection of heroin.

Remifentanil

Remifentanil [Ultiva] is an intravenous opioid with a rapid onset and brief duration. The brief duration results from rapid metabolism by plasma and tissue esterases, and not from hepatic metabolism or renal excretion. Like fentanyl, remifentanil is about 100 times more potent than morphine. Remifentanil is approved for analgesia during surgery and during the immediate postoperative period. Administration is by continuous IV infusion. Effects begin in minutes, and terminate 5 to 10 minutes after the infusion is stopped. For surgical analgesia, the infusion rate is 0.05 to 2 μg/min. For postoperative analgesia, the infusion rate is 0.025 to 0.2 μg/min. Adverse effects during the infusion include respiratory depression, hypotension, bradycardia, and muscle rigidity sufficient to compromise breathing. Postinfusion effects include nausea (44%), vomiting (22%), and headache (18%). Remifentanil is regulated under Schedule II of the Controlled Substances Act.

Hydromorphone, Oxymorphone, and Levorphanol

Basic Pharmacology. All three drugs are strong opioid agonists with pharmacologic actions like those of morphine. All three are indicated for relief of moderate to severe pain. Dosages and time courses are summarized in Table 27–5. Adverse effects include respiratory depression, sedation, cough suppression, constipation, urinary retention, nausea, and vomiting. Toxicity can be reversed with an opioid antagonist (e.g., naloxone). All three drugs are Schedule II substances.

Preparations, Dosage, and Administration. Hydromorphone. Hydromorphone [Dilaudid] is available in tablets (1, 2, 3, 4, and 8 mg), oral liquid (1 mg/ml), rectal suppositories (3 mg), and solution (1, 2, 4, and 10 mg/ml) for IM and SC injection. The usual adult oral dosage is 2 mg

every 4 to 6 hours. The adult rectal dosage is 3 mg every 6 to 8 hours. Usual SC and IM dosages are 1 to 4 mg every 4 to 6 hours.

Oxymorphone. Oxymorphone [Numorphan] is available in solution (1 and 1.5 mg/ml) for parenteral administration and in 5-mg rectal suppositories. The initial IV dose is 0.5 mg. Usual SC and IM dosages are 1 to 1.5 mg every 4 to 6 hours as needed. The rectal dosage is 5 mg every 4 to 6 hours.

Levorphanol. Levorphanol [Levo-Dromoran] is available in 2-mg oral tablets. The usual adult dosage is 2 to 3 mg.

Moderate to Strong Opioid Agonists

The moderate to strong opioid agonists are similar to morphine in most respects. Like morphine, these drugs produce analgesia, sedation, and euphoria. In addition, they can cause respiratory depression, constipation, urinary retention, cough suppression, and miosis. Differences between the moderate to strong opioids and morphine are primarily quantitative: The moderate to strong opioids produce less analgesia and respiratory depression than morphine and have a somewhat lower potential for abuse. As with morphine, toxicity from the moderate to strong agonists can be reversed with naloxone.

Codeine

Actions and Uses. Codeine is indicated for relief of mild to moderate pain. The drug is usually administered by mouth. Side effects are dose limiting. As a result, although codeine is a strong analgesic, the degree of pain relief that can be achieved *safely* is quite low—much lower than can be achieved safely with morphine. When taken in its usual analgesic dose (30 mg), codeine produces about as much pain relief as 325 mg of aspirin or 325 mg of acetaminophen.

For analgesic use, codeine is dispensed alone and in combination with a nonopioid analgesic (either aspirin or acetaminophen). Since codeine and nonopioid analgesics relieve pain by different mechanisms, the combination of codeine with a nonopioid can produce greater pain relief than either agent alone. Codeine alone is classified under Schedule II of the Controlled Substances Act. The combination preparations are classified under Schedule III. Although codeine is classified along with morphine in Schedule II, the abuse liability of codeine appears to be significantly lower.

Codeine is an extremely effective cough suppressant and is widely used for this action. The antitussive dose (10 mg) is lower than analgesic doses. Codeine is dispensed in combination with various agents for suppression of cough. These mixtures are classified under Schedule V.

Preparations, Dosage, and Administration. Codeine is administered orally and parenterally (IV, IM, and SC). For oral therapy, the drug is available in tablets (15, 30, and 60 mg) and in solution (3 mg/ml). For parenteral therapy, the drug is dispensed in solution (30 and 60 mg/ml).

The usual analgesic dosage for adults is 15 to 60 mg (PO, IV, IM, or SC) every 3 to 6 hours (to a maximum of 120 mg/24 hours). The usual analgesic dosage for children 1 year and older is 0.5 mg/kg (PO, IM, or SC) every 4 to 6 hours (to a maximum of 60 mg/24 hours).

Oxycodone

Oxycodone [OxyContin, Percodan, Percocet, Roxicodone, others] has analgesic actions equivalent to those of codeine. Administration is oral. Oxycodone is available by itself in 5-mg immediate-release tablets and capsules, controlled-release tablets (10, 20, 40, 80, and 160 mg), and oral solution (1 and 20 mg/ml). In addition, the drug is available in combination with aspirin (marketed as Percodan) or acetaminophen (marketed as Percocet). All formulations are classified under Schedule II.

Controlled-release oxycodone [OxyContin] is a long-acting analgesic designed to relieve moderate to severe pain around-the-clock for an extended time. Dosing is done every 12 hours—not PRN. If breakthrough pain occurs, supplemental dosing with a short-acting analgesic is indicated.

Recently, there have been increasing reports of OxyContin abuse. As a result, safety warnings have been strengthened. When prescribed and used properly, controlled-release oxycodone tablets are safe and effective. However, abusers do not take them properly. Rather, they crush the tablets and then "snort" the resulting powder, or dissolve the powder in water and inject it IV. Both practices allow *immediate* absorption of the entire dose, and thereby produce drug blood levels that are much higher than those produced when the tablets are ingested whole and absorbed gradually. The result can be an intense "high" coupled with a risk of fatal respiratory depression. At least 39 deaths have been reported. To prevent the immediate release of a potentially fatal dose, the controlled-release tablets must be swallowed whole, without breaking, crushing, or chewing. Furthermore, the 80- and 160-mg formulations must be reserved for patients who are already opioid tolerant. OxyContin tablets should never be dissolved and injected. Why? Because the tablets contain insoluble particulate matter (especially talc) that can cause local tissue necrosis, pulmonary granulomas, endocarditis, and valvular heart injury. As with all other opioids, concerns about abuse and addiction should not interfere with using OxyContin to manage pain. Rather, the drug must simply be prescribed appropriately and then used as prescribed.

Hydrocodone

Hydrocodone [Vicodin, Vicoprofen, others] has analgesic actions equivalent to those of codeine. The drug is taken orally to relieve pain and to suppress cough. The usual dosage is 5 mg. Hydrocodone is available only in combination with other drugs. For analgesic use, hydrocodone is combined with aspirin, acetaminophen, or ibuprofen. For cough suppression, the drug is combined with antihistamines and nasal decongestants. All of these combination products are classified under Schedule III.

Propoxyphene

Propoxyphene [Darvon] has analgesic effects about equal to those of aspirin. The drug is frequently prescribed in combination with a nonopioid analgesic, either aspirin or acetaminophen. These combinations can produce greater pain relief than either propoxyphene or the nonopioid alone. Propoxyphene has a low potential for abuse, primarily because large doses cause toxic psychosis. Furthermore, excessive doses often prove fatal. Accordingly, the drug should not be dispensed to patients with suicidal tendencies. Physical dependence is minimal. Propoxyphene—alone or in combination with a nonopioid analgesic—is classified under Schedule IV.

Propoxyphene is available as two salts: propoxyphene hydrochloride and propoxyphene napsylate. Both are administered orally. Propoxyphene hydrochloride is dispensed in 65-mg capsules, and the usual adult dosage is 65 mg repeated every 4 hours as needed. Propoxyphene napsylate is dispensed in 100-mg tablets, and the usual adult dosage is 100 mg repeated every 4 hours as needed.

Agonist-Antagonist Opioids

Five agonist-antagonist opioids are available: pentazocine, nalbuphine, butorphanol, dezocine, and buprenorphine. With the exception of buprenorphine, all of these drugs act as antagonists at mu receptors and as agonists at kappa receptors (see Table 27–2). Compared with pure opioid agonists, the agonist-antagonists have a low potential for abuse, produce

less respiratory depression, and generally have less powerful analgesic effects. If given to a patient who is physically dependent on a pure opioid agonist, these drugs can precipitate a withdrawal reaction. The clinical pharmacology of the agonist-antagonists is summarized in Table 27–6.

Pentazocine

Actions and Uses. Pentazocine [Talwin] was the first agonist-antagonist opioid available and can be considered the prototype for the group. The drug is indicated for mild to moderate pain. Pentazocine is much less effective than morphine against severe pain.

Pentazocine acts as an *agonist* at kappa receptors and as an *antagonist* at mu receptors. By activating kappa receptors, the drug produces analgesia, sedation, and respiratory depression. However, unlike the respiratory depression caused by morphine, *respiratory depression caused by pentazocine is limited:* Beyond a certain dose, no further depression occurs. Because it lacks agonist actions at mu receptors, pentazocine produces little or no euphoria. In fact, at supratherapeutic doses, pentazocine produces unpleasant reactions (anxiety, strange thoughts, nightmares, hallucinations). These psychotomimetic effects may result from stimulation of kappa receptors. Because of its subjective effects, pentazocine has a low potential for abuse and is classified under Schedule IV.

Adverse effects are generally like those of morphine. However, in contrast to the pure opioid agonists, pentazocine increases cardiac work. Accordingly, a pure agonist (e.g., morphine) is preferred to pentazocine for relieving pain in patients with myocardial infarction.

If administered to a patient who is physically dependent on a pure opioid agonist, pentazocine can precipitate an abstinence syndrome. Recall that mu receptors mediate physical dependence on pure opioid agonists and that pentazocine acts as an antagonist at these receptors. By blocking access of the pure agonist to mu receptors, pentazocine will prevent receptor activation, thereby triggering withdrawal. Accordingly, *pentazocine and other drugs that block mu receptors should never be administered to a person who is physically dependent on a pure opioid agonist.* If a pentazocine-like agent is to be used, the pure opioid agonist must first be withdrawn.

Physical dependence can occur with pentazocine, but symptoms of withdrawal are generally mild (e.g., cramps, fever, anxiety, restlessness). Treatment is rarely required. As with pure opioid agonists, toxicity from pentazocine can be reversed with naloxone.

Preparations, Dosage, and Administration. *Oral.* For oral therapy, pentazocine [Talwin NX] is dispensed in 50-mg tablets that also contain 0.5 mg of naloxone (to prevent abuse). The usual adult dosage is 50 mg every 3 to 4 hours as needed. The drug is also available in combination with aspirin [Talwin Compound] and in combination with acetaminophen [Talacen].

Parenteral. For parenteral therapy, pentazocine [Talwin] is available in solution (30 mg/ml as the lactate salt). Administration is IV, IM, and SC. The usual adult dosage is 30 mg every 3 to 4 hours as needed.

Nalbuphine

Nalbuphine [Nubain] has pharmacologic actions similar to those of pentazocine. The drug is an agonist at kappa receptors and an antagonist at mu receptors. At low doses, nalbuphine has analgesic actions equal to those of morphine. However, as dosage increases, a ceiling to analgesia is reached. As a result, the maximal pain relief that can be produced with nalbuphine is much lower than the maximal pain relief that can be produced with morphine. As with pain relief, there is also a ceiling to respiratory depression. Like pen-

TABLE 27–6 ■ Clinical Pharmacology of Opioid Agonists-Antagonists

Drug and Route*	Equianalgesic Dose (mg)†	Time Course of Analgesic Effects		
		Onset (min)	Peak (min)	Duration (hr)
Buprenorphine				
IM	0.3	15	60	Up to 6
IV	0.3	<15	<60	Up to 6
Butorphanol				
IM	2–3	10	30–60	3–4
IV	2–3	2–3	30	2–4
Intranasal	2–3	Within 15	60–120	4–5
Dezocine				
IM	10	30	30–150	2–4
IV	10	15	30–150	2–4
Nalbuphine				
IM	10	Within 15	60	3–6
IV	10	2–3	30	3–4
SC	10	Within 15	—	3–6
Pentazocine				
PO	180	15–30	60–90	3‡
IM	60	15–20	30–60	2–3‡
IV	60	2–3	15–30	2–3‡
SC	60	15–20	30–60	2–3‡

*IM administration should be avoided whenever possible.
†Dose in milligrams that produces a degree of analgesia equivalent to that produced by a 10-mg IM dose of morphine.
‡Duration may increase greatly in patients with liver disease.

tazocine, nalbuphine can cause psychotomimetic reactions. With prolonged treatment, physical dependence can develop. Symptoms of abstinence are less intense than with morphine but more intense than with pentazocine. Nalbuphine has a low abuse potential and is not regulated under the Controlled Substances Act. As with the pure opioid agonists, toxicity can be reversed with naloxone. Like pentazocine, nalbuphine will precipitate a withdrawal reaction if administered to an individual who is physically dependent on a pure opioid agonist. Nalbuphine is dispensed in solution (10 and 20 mg/ml) for IV, IM, and SC injection. The usual adult dosage is 10 mg repeated every 3 to 6 hours as needed.

Butorphanol

Butorphanol [Stadol] has actions similar to those of pentazocine. The drug is an agonist at kappa receptors and an antagonist at mu receptors. Analgesic effects are less than those of morphine. As with pentazocine, there is a "ceiling" to respiratory depression. The drug can cause psychotomimetic reactions, but these are rare. Butorphanol increases cardiac work and should not be given to patients with myocardial infarction. Physical dependence can occur, but symptoms of withdrawal are relatively mild. The drug may induce a withdrawal reaction in patients physically dependent on a pure opioid agonist. Butorphanol has a low potential for abuse and is regulated under Schedule IV of the Controlled Substances Act. Toxicity can be reversed with naloxone.

Butorphanol is administered parenterally (IM and IV) and by nasal spray (primarily to treat migraine headache). The usual adult IV dosage is 1 mg every 3 to 4 hours as needed. The usual IM dosage is 2 mg every 3 to 4 hours as needed. The usual intranasal dosage is 1 mg (one spray from the metered-dose spray device) repeated in 60 to 90 minutes if needed. The two-dose sequence may then be repeated every 3 to 4 hours as needed.

Dezocine

Dezocine [Dalgan] has analgesic effects equivalent to those of morphine. The drug's adverse effects are like those of the pure opioid agonists, except there is a ceiling to respiratory depression. Fatal respiratory depression has not been reported. Effects on cardiac performance are modest, but caution should be exercised in patients with coronary artery disease. Dezocine appears to have a low potential for abuse and is not regulated under the Controlled Sub-

stances Act. The drug is dispensed in solution (5, 10, and 15 mg/ml) for IM and IV administration. The usual IM dosage is 5 to 20 mg every 3 to 6 hours as needed. The usual IV dosage is 2.5 to 10 mg every 2 to 4 hours.

Buprenorphine

Buprenorphine [Buprenex] differs significantly from other opioid agonist-antagonists. The drug is a partial agonist at mu receptors and an antagonist at kappa receptors. Analgesic effects are like those of morphine, but significant tolerance has not been observed. Although buprenorphine can depress respiration, severe respiratory depression has not been reported. Like pentazocine, buprenorphine can precipitate a withdrawal reaction in persons physically dependent on pure opioid agonists. Psychotomimetic reactions can occur but are rare. Physical dependence develops but symptoms of abstinence are delayed; peak responses may not occur until 2 weeks after the last dose was taken. Buprenorphine is currently classified as a Schedule III substance. In addition to its use for analgesia, buprenorphine is used to treat opioid addiction (see Chapter 38).

Although pretreatment with naloxone can prevent toxicity from buprenorphine, naloxone cannot readily reverse toxicity that has already developed. It appears that buprenorphine binds very tightly to its receptors, and hence cannot be readily displaced by naloxone.

Buprenorphine is dispensed in solution (0.3 mg/ml) for administration by IM or slow IV injection. The usual dosage for patients age 13 and older is 0.3 mg repeated every 6 hours as needed.

CLINICAL USE OF OPIOIDS

Dosing Guidelines
Assessment of Pain

Assessment is an essential component of pain management. Pain status should be evaluated prior to opioid administration and about 1 hour after. Unfortunately, because pain is a subjective experience, affected by multiple factors (e.g., cultural

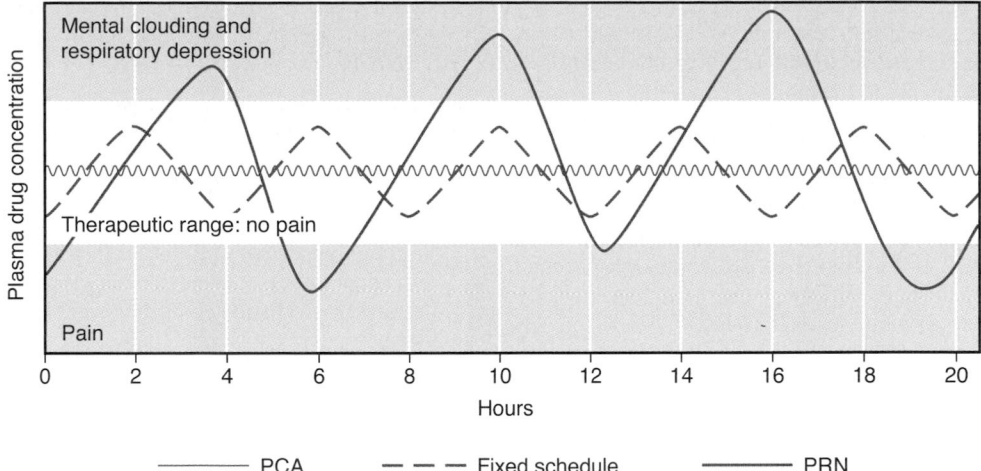

Figure 27–3 ■ Fluctuations in opioid blood levels seen with three dosing procedures.
Note that, with PRN dosing, opioid levels can fluctuate widely, going from subtherapeutic to excessive and back again. In contrast, when opioids are administered with a PCA device or on a fixed schedule, levels stay within the therapeutic range, allowing continuous pain relief with minimal adverse effects.

influences, patient expectations, associated disease), there is no reliable objective method for determining just how much discomfort the patient is feeling. That is, we cannot measure pain with instruments equivalent to those employed to monitor blood pressure, cardiac performance, and other physiologic parameters. As a result, assessment must ultimately be based on the patient's description of his or her experience. Accordingly, you should ask the patient where the pain is located, what type of pain is present (e.g., dull, sharp, stabbing), how the pain changes with time, what makes the pain better, and what makes it worse. In addition, you should assess for psychologic factors that can reduce pain threshold (anxiety, depression, fear, anger).

When attempting to assess pain, keep in mind that, on occasion, what the patient says may not accurately reflect his or her experience. For example, a few patients who are pain free may claim to feel pain so as to receive medication for its euphoriant effects. Conversely, some patients may claim to feel fine even though they are experiencing considerable discomfort. Reasons for under-reporting pain include fear of addiction, fear of needles, and a need to be stoic and bear the pain. Patients suspected of under-reporting pain must be listened to with care if their true pain status is to be evaluated.

Pain assessment is discussed at length in Chapter 28 (Pain Management in Patients with Cancer).

Dosage Determination

Dosage of opioid analgesics must be adjusted to accommodate individual variation. "Standard" doses cannot be relied upon as appropriate for all patients. For example, if a "standard" 10-mg dose of morphine were employed for all adults, only 70% would receive adequate relief; the other 30% would be undertreated. Not all patients have the same tolerance for pain, and hence some will need larger doses than others for the same disorder. Some conditions hurt more than others. For example, patients recovering from open chest surgery are likely to experience greater pain and need larger doses than

patients recovering from an appendectomy. Elderly patients metabolize opioids slowly, and therefore require lower doses than younger adults. Because the blood-brain barrier of newborns is poorly developed, these patients are especially sensitive to opioids; therefore, they generally require smaller doses than older infants and young children.

Dosing Schedule

As a rule, *opioids should be administered on a fixed schedule* (e.g., every 4 hours) rather than PRN. With a fixed schedule, each dose is given before pain returns, thereby sparing the patient needless discomfort. In contrast, when PRN dosing is employed, there can be a long delay between onset of pain and production of relief: Each time pain returns, the patient must call the nurse, wait for the nurse to respond, wait for the nurse to evaluate the pain, wait for the nurse to sign out medication, wait for the nurse to prepare and administer the injection, and then wait for the drug to undergo absorption and finally produce analgesia. This delay causes unnecessary discomfort and creates anxiety about pain recurrence. Use of a fixed dosing schedule reduces these problems. As discussed below, allowing the patient to self-administer opioids with a patient-controlled analgesia (PCA) device can provide even greater protection against pain recurrence than can be achieved by having the nurse administer opioids on a fixed schedule. The differences between PRN dosing, fixed-schedule dosing, and use of a PCA device are shown graphically in Figure 27–3.

Avoiding Withdrawal

When opioids are administered in high doses for 20 days or more, clinically significant physical dependence may develop. Under these conditions, abrupt withdrawal will precipitate an abstinence syndrome. To minimize symptoms of abstinence, opioids should be withdrawn slowly, tapering the dosage over 3 days. If the degree of dependence is especially high, as can occur in opioid addicts, dosage should be tapered over 7 to 10 days.

Physical Dependence, Abuse, and Addiction as Clinical Concerns

Most people in our society, including many health professionals, harbor strong fears about the ability of "narcotics" to cause "addiction." In a clinical setting, such excessive concern is both unwarranted and counterproductive. Because of inappropriate fears, physicians frequently prescribe less pain medication than patients need, and nurses frequently administer less medication than was prescribed. The result, according to one estimate, is that only 25% of patients receive doses of opioids that are sufficient to relieve suffering. One pain specialist described this unacceptable situation as follows: "The excessive and unrealistic concern about the dangers of addiction in the hospitalized medical patient is a significant and potent force for the undertreatment with narcotics [opioids]."

When treating a patient for pain, you may have to decide how much opioid to give and when to give it. If you are excessively concerned about the ability of opioids to cause physical dependence and addiction, you will be unable to make a rational decision. Furthermore, in your role as patient advocate, it is your responsibility to intervene and request an increase in dosage if the prescribed dosage has proved inadequate. If you fear that dosage escalation may cause "addiction," you are less likely to make the request.

The object of the following discussion is to dispel excessive concerns about dependence, abuse, and addiction in the medical patient so these concerns do not result in undermedication and needless suffering.

Definitions

Before we can discuss the clinical implications of physical dependence, abuse, and addiction, we need to define these three terms.

Physical Dependence. As noted, physical dependence is a state in which an abstinence syndrome will occur if the dependence-producing drug is abruptly withdrawn. *Physical dependence should NOT be equated with addiction.*

Abuse. Abuse can be broadly defined as *drug use that is inconsistent with medical or social norms.* By this definition, abuse is determined primarily by the reason for drug use and by the setting in which that use occurs—and not by the pharmacologic properties of the drug itself. For example, whereas it is *not* considered abuse to administer 20 mg of morphine in a hospital to relieve pain, it *is* considered abuse to administer the same dose of the same drug on the street to produce euphoria. The concept of abuse is discussed at length in Chapter 36.

Addiction. Addiction can be defined as a behavior pattern characterized by continued use of a psychoactive substance despite physical, psychologic, or social harm. Note that nowhere in this definition is addiction equated with physical dependence. In fact, physical dependence is not even part of the definition. The concept of addiction is discussed further in Chapter 36.

Although physical dependence is not required for addiction to occur, physical dependence *can* contribute to addictive behavior. If an individual has already established a pattern of compulsive drug use, physical dependence can reinforce that pattern. For the individual with a marginal resolve to discontinue opioid use, the desire to avoid symptoms of withdrawal may be sufficient to promote continued drug use. However, in the presence of a strong desire to become drug free, physical dependence, by itself, is insufficient to motivate continued addictive behavior.

Minimizing Fears About Physical Dependence

For two important reasons, there is little to fear regarding physical dependence on opioids in the hospitalized patient:

▪ Development of significant physical dependence is extremely rare when opioids are given acutely to relieve pain. For most patients, the doses employed and the duration of treatment are insufficient to cause significant dependence.

▪ Even when physical dependence *does* occur, patients rarely develop addictive behavior and continue opioid administration after their pain has subsided. The vast majority of patients who become physically dependent in a clinical setting simply go through gradual withdrawal and never take opioids again. This observation emphasizes the point that physical dependence per se is insufficient to cause addiction.

From the preceding, we can see there is little to fear regarding physical dependence during the therapeutic use of opioids. We can conclude, therefore, that there is no justification for withholding opioids from patients in pain on the basis of concerns about physical dependence.

Minimizing Fears About Addiction

The principal reason for abandoning fears about opioid addiction in patients is simple: *Development of addiction to opioids as a result of clinical exposure to these drugs is extremely rare.* Results of the Boston Collaborative Drug Study showed that, of 12,000 patients taking opioids, only 4 became drug abusers. Furthermore, as discussed below, if abuse or addiction *does* occur, it is probable that these behaviors reflect tendencies that existed before the patient entered the hospital, and hence are not the result of inappropriate medical use of opioids during the hospital stay.

For the purpose of this discussion, the population can be divided into two groups: individuals who are prone to drug abuse and individuals who are not. One source estimates that about 8% of the population is prone to drug abuse, whereas the other 92% is not. Individuals who are prone to drug abuse have a tendency to abuse drugs inside the hospital and out. Nonabusers, on the other hand, will not abuse drugs in a clinical setting or anywhere else. Withholding analgesics from abuse-prone individuals is not going to reverse their tendency to abuse drugs. Conversely, administering opioids to non–abuse-prone persons will not change their personalities and convert them into "drug fiends."

If a patient who did not formerly abuse opioids does abuse these drugs following therapeutic exposure, you should not feel responsible for having created an addict. That is, if a patient tries to continue opioid use after leaving the hospital, it is probable that the patient is of the abuse-prone personality type. Therefore, the pattern of abuse that emerged during clinical exposure to opioids was the result of tendencies that were established before the patient ever entered the hospital—and not the consequence of therapy. The only action that might have prevented opioid abuse by such a patient would have been to withhold opioids entirely—an action that would not have been feasible.

Balancing the Need to Provide Pain Relief with the Desire to Minimize Abuse

Although concerns about opioid abuse in the clinical setting are small, they cannot be dismissed entirely. You are still obliged to administer opioids with discretion in an effort to minimize abuse. Some reasonable attempt must be made to determine who is likely to abuse drugs and who is not. As a rule, distinguishing abusers from nonabusers can be done with some confidence. When nonabusers say they need more pain relief, believe them and provide it. In contrast, when an obvious abuser requests more analgesic, some healthy skepticism is in order. When there is doubt as to whether a patient is abuse prone or not, logic dictates giving the patient the benefit of the doubt and providing the medication. If the patient is an abuser, little harm will result from giving unneeded medication. However, if the patient is a nonabuser, failure to provide medication would intensify suffering for no justifiable reason.

In order to minimize physical dependence and abuse, opioid analgesics should be administered in the lowest effective dosages for the shortest time needed. Be aware, however, that larger doses are needed for patients who have more intense pain and for those who have developed tolerance. As pain diminishes, opioid dosage should be reduced. As soon as possible, the patient should be switched to a nonopioid analgesic, such as aspirin or acetaminophen.

In summary, when working with opioids, as with any other drugs, you must balance the risks of therapy against the benefits. The risk of addiction from therapeutic use of opioids is real but very small. Consequently, concerns about addiction should play a real but secondary role in making decisions about giving these drugs. Dosages should be sufficient to relieve pain. Suffering because of insufficient dosage is unacceptable. However, it is also unacceptable to promote possible abuse through failure to exercise good judgment.

Patient-Controlled Analgesia

Patient-controlled analgesia (PCA) is a method of drug delivery that permits the patient to self-administer parenteral (IV, SC, epidural) opioids on an "as-needed" basis. PCA has been employed primarily for relief of pain in postoperative patients. Other candidates include patients experiencing pain caused by cancer, trauma, myocardial infarction, vaso-occlusive sickle cell crisis, and labor. As discussed below, PCA offers several advantages over opioids administered by the nurse.

PCA Devices. PCA has been made possible by the development of reliable PCA devices. A PCA device consists of an electronically controlled infusion pump that can be activated by the patient to deliver a preset bolus dose of an opioid. The opioid is delivered through an indwelling catheter. In addition to providing bolus doses on demand, some PCA devices can deliver a basal infusion of opioid.

An essential feature of all PCA devices is a timing control. This control limits the total dose that can be administered each hour, thereby minimizing the risk of overdose. In addition, the timing control regulates the minimum interval (e.g., 10 minutes) between doses. This interval, referred to as the "lock-out" or "delay" interval, prevents the patient from administering a second dose before the first has had time to produce its full effect.

Drug Selection and Dosage Regulation. The opioid used most extensively for PCA is morphine. Other pure opioid agonists (e.g., methadone, hydromorphone, fentanyl) have also been employed, as have agonist-antagonist opioids (e.g., nalbuphine, buprenorphine).

Prior to starting PCA, the postoperative patient should be given an opioid loading dose (e.g., 2 to 10 mg of morphine). Once effective opioid levels have been established with the loading dose, PCA can be initiated, provided the patient has recovered sufficiently from anesthesia. For PCA with morphine, initial bolus doses of 1 mg are typical. The size of the bolus should be increased if analgesia is inadequate, and decreased if excessive sedation occurs. The size of the bolus dose is usually increased during sleeping hours, thereby promoting rest by prolonging the interval between doses.

Comparison of PCA with Traditional Intramuscular Therapy. The objective of therapy with analgesics is to provide comfort while minimizing sedation and other side effects, especially respiratory depression. This objective is best achieved by maintaining plasma levels of opioids that are steady (i.e., that have minimal fluctuations). In this manner, side effects from excessively high levels can be avoided, as can the return of severe pain when levels dip too low.

In the traditional management of postoperative pain, patients are given an IM injection of an opioid every 3 to 4 hours. With this dosing schedule, plasma levels of the opioid can vary widely. Shortly after the injection, plasma levels may rise very high, causing excessive sedation and possibly respiratory depression. Late in the dosing interval, pain may return as plasma levels drop to their lowest point.

In contrast to traditional therapy, PCA is ideally suited to maintain steady levels of opioids. Why? Because PCA relies on small doses given frequently (e.g., 1 mg of morphine every 10 minutes) rather than on large doses given infrequently (e.g., 20 mg of morphine every 3 hours). Maintenance of steady drug levels can be facilitated further if the PCA device is capable of delivering a basal opioid infusion. Because plasma drug levels remain relatively steady, PCA can provide continuous control of pain while avoiding the adverse effects associated with excessive drug levels.

An additional advantage of PCA is rapid relief of pain. Because the patient can self-administer an IV dose of opioid as soon as pain begins to return, there is minimal delay between detection of pain and restoration of an adequate drug level. With traditional therapy, the patient must wait for the nurse to respond to a request for more drug; this delay allows pain to grow more intense.

Studies indicate that PCA is associated with accelerated recovery. When compared with patients receiving traditional IM analgesia, postoperative patients receiving PCA show improved early mobilization, greater cooperation during physical therapy, and a shorter hospital stay.

Patient Education. Patient education is essential for successful PCA. Surgical patients should be educated preoperatively. Education should include an explanation of what PCA is along with instruction on how to activate the PCA device.

Patients should be told not to fear overdose; the PCA device will not permit self-administration of excessive doses. Patients should be informed that there is a time lag (about 10 minutes) between activation of the device and production of maximal analgesia. To reduce discomfort associated with physical therapy, changing of dressings, ambulation, and other potentially painful activities, patients should be taught to activate the pump prophylactically (e.g., 10 minutes prior to the anticipated activity). Patients should be informed that, at night, the PCA device will be adjusted to deliver larger doses than during waking hours; the purpose of this adjustment is to prolong the interval between doses and thereby facilitate sleep.

Use of Opioids in Specific Settings

Postoperative Pain. Opioid analgesics offer several benefits to the postoperative patient. The most obvious is increased comfort through reduction of pain. In addition, by reducing painful sensation, opioids can facilitate early movement and intentional cough. In patients who have undergone thoracic surgery, opioids permit chest movement that would otherwise be too uncomfortable to allow adequate ventilation. By promoting ventilation, opioids can reduce the risk of hypoxia and pneumonitis.

Opioids are not without drawbacks for the postoperative patient. These agents can cause constipation and urinary retention. Suppression of reflex cough can result in respiratory tract complications. In addition, analgesia may delay diagnosis of postoperative complications—because pain will not be present to signal their development.

Obstetric Analgesia. When administered to relieve pain during delivery, opioids may depress fetal respiration and uterine contractions. Since these effects are less likely with meperidine than with other strong opioids, *meperidine* is often the preferred opioid for obstetric use. Dosage should be high enough to reduce maternal discomfort to a tolerable level, but not so high as to cause pronounced respiratory depression in the neonate. Because opioids cross the blood-brain barrier of the infant more readily than that of the mother, doses that have little effect on maternal respiration may nonetheless cause profound respiratory depression in the infant. For meperidine, the usual dosage is 50 to 100 mg every 2 to 3 hours. Administration should be parenteral (IV or IM). Timing of administration is important: if the drug is given too early, it can inhibit or delay the progress of uterine contractions; if given too late, it can cause excessive neonatal sedation and respiratory depression. Following delivery, respiration in the neonate should be monitored closely. Naloxone can reverse respiratory depression and should be on hand.

Myocardial Infarction. Morphine is the opioid of choice for decreasing pain of myocardial infarction. With careful control of dosage, morphine can reduce discomfort without causing excessive respiratory depression and adverse cardiovascular effects. In addition, by lowering blood pressure, morphine can decrease cardiac work. If excessive hypotension or respiratory depression occurs, it can be reversed with naloxone. Because *pentazocine* and *butorphanol* increase cardiac work and oxygen demand, these agonist-antagonist opioids should generally be avoided.

Head Injury. Opioids must be employed with caution in patients with head injury. Head injury can cause respiratory depression accompanied by elevation of ICP; opioids can exacerbate these symptoms. In addition, since miosis, mental clouding, and vomiting can be valuable diagnostic signs following had injury, and since opioids can cause these same effects, us of opioids can complicate diagnosis.

Cancer. Treating chronic pain of cancer differs substantially from treating acute pain of other disorders. When treating cancer pain, the objective is to maximize comfort. Psychologic and physical dependence are minimal concerns. Patients should be given as much medication as needed to relieve pain. In the words of one pain specialist, "No patient should wish for death because of the physician's reluctance to use adequate amounts of opioids." With proper therapy, cancer pain can be effectively managed in about 90% of patients. Cancer pain is discussed fully in Chapter 28.

OPIOID ANTAGONISTS

Opioid antagonists are drugs that block the effects of opioid agonists. Principal uses are treatment of opioid overdose, reversal of postoperative opioid effects (e.g., respiratory depression), and management of opioid addiction. Three pure antagonists are available: naloxone [Narcan], nalmefene [Revex], and naltrexone [ReVia, Depade].

Naloxone

Mechanism of Action

Naloxone [Narcan] is a structural analog of morphine that acts as a competitive antagonist at opioid receptors. By blocking access of opioid agonists to these receptors, naloxone prevents the agonists from producing effects. Naloxone can reverse most actions of the opioid agonists, including respiratory depression, coma, and analgesia.

Pharmacologic Effects

When administered in the absence of opioids, naloxone has no significant effects. If administered prior to giving an opioid, naloxone will block opioid actions. If administered to a patient who is already receiving opioids, naloxone will reverse analgesia, sedation, euphoria, and respiratory depression. If administered to an individual who is physically dependent on opioids, naloxone will precipitate an immediate withdrawal reaction.

Pharmacokinetics

Naloxone may be administered IV, IM, or SC. Following IV injection, effects begin almost immediately and persist for about 1 hour. Following IM or SC injection, effects begin within 2 to 5 minutes and persist for several hours. Elimination is by hepatic metabolism. The half-life is approximately 2 hours. Naloxone cannot be used orally because of rapid first-pass inactivation.

Therapeutic Uses

Reversal of Opioid Overdose. Naloxone is the drug of choice for treating overdose with pure opioid agonists. The drug reverses respiratory depression, coma, and other signs of opioid toxicity. Naloxone can also reverse toxicity from agonist-antagonist opioids (e.g., pentazocine, nalbuphine). However, the doses required may be higher than those needed to reverse poisoning by pure agonists.

Dosage must be carefully titrated when treating toxicity in opioid addicts. Because the degree of physical dependence in these individuals is likely to be high, if dosage is excessive, naloxone can transport the patient from a state of poisoning to one of acute withdrawal. Accordingly, treatment should be initiated with a series of small doses rather than a single large dose. Because the half-life of naloxone is shorter than that of most opioids, repeated doses are required until the crisis has passed.

In some cases of accidental poisoning, there may be uncertainty as to whether unconsciousness is due to opioid overdose or to overdose with a general CNS depressant (e.g., barbiturate, alcohol, benzodiazepine). When uncertainty exists, naloxone is nonetheless indicated. If the cause of poisoning is a barbiturate or another general CNS depressant, naloxone will be of no benefit—but neither will it cause any harm. If a cumulative dose of 10 mg fails to elicit a response, it is unlikely that opioids are involved, and hence other intoxicants should be suspected.

Reversal of Postoperative Opioid Effects. Following surgery, naloxone may be employed to reverse excessive respiratory and CNS depression caused by opioids given preoperatively or intraoperatively. Dosage should be titrated with care; the objective is to achieve adequate ventilation and alertness without reversing opioid actions to the point of unmasking pain.

Reversal of Neonatal Respiratory Depression. When opioids are given for analgesia during labor and delivery, respiratory depression may occur in the neonate. If respiratory depression is substantial, naloxone should be administered to restore ventilation.

Preparations, Dosage, and Administration

Preparations and Routes. Naloxone [Narcan] is available in solution (0.4 and 1 mg/ml) for IV, IM, and SC injection. A dilute solution (0.02 mg/ml) is available for treating neonates.

Opioid Overdose. The initial dosage is 0.4 mg for adults and 10 μg/kg for children. The preferred route is IV. However, IM or SC injection may be employed if IV administration is not possible. Dosing is repeated at 2- to 3-minute intervals until a satisfactory response has been achieved. Additional doses may be needed at 1- to 2-hour intervals for up to 72 hours, depending on the duration of action of the offending opioid.

Postoperative Opioid Effects. Initial therapy for adults consists of 0.1 to 0.2 mg IV repeated every 2 to 3 minutes until an adequate response has been achieved. Additional doses may be required at 1- to 2-hour intervals.

Neonatal Respiratory Depression. The initial dose is 10 μg/kg (IV, IM, or SC). This dose is repeated every 2 to 3 minutes until respiration is satisfactory.

Other Opioid Antagonists

Naltrexone

Naltrexone [ReVia, Depade] is a pure opioid antagonist approved for treating opioid abuse and alcohol abuse. In opioid abuse, the objective is to prevent euphoria if the abuser should take an opioid. Since naltrexone can precipitate a withdrawal reaction in persons who are physically dependent on opioids, candidates for treatment must be rendered opioid-free before naltrexone is given. Although naltrexone can block opioid-induced euphoria, the drug does not prevent craving for opioids. As a result, many addicts fail to comply with treatment. Therapy with naltrexone has been considerably less successful than therapy with methadone, a drug that eliminates craving for opioids while blocking euphoria. Naltrexone is dispensed in 50-mg tablets. A typical dosing schedule consists of 100 mg on Monday and Wednesday and 150 mg on Friday. Alternatively, the drug can be administered daily in 50-mg doses. Use of naltrexone in alcoholism is discussed in Chapter 37.

Nalmefene

Uses. Nalmefene [Revex] is a *long-acting* analog of naltrexone. The drug is approved for reversing postoperative opioid effects and treating opioid overdose. Nalmefene must be used with caution when treating overdose in patients suspected of being opioid dependent, because too much nalmefene could precipitate prolonged withdrawal.

Pharmacokinetics. Effects begin 2 minutes after IV injection (the usual route) and peak within 5 minutes. Duration of action depends on dosage: Effects may fade within 30 to 60 minutes after a small dose, and may last many hours after a large dose. Most importantly, when nalmefene dosage is adequate, effects persist longer than those of most opioids. Nalmefene undergoes complete but slow hepatic metabolism, followed by renal excretion. The half-life is 11 hours—considerably longer than that of naloxone.

Preparations, Dosage, and Administration. Nalmefene [Revex] is available in two concentrations. The low concentration (100 μg/ml), dispensed in blue-labeled ampules, is used to reverse postoperative opioid effects. The high concentration (1 mg/ml), dispensed in green-labeled ampules, is used for opioid overdose.

The usual route is IV. However, if IV access is impossible, nalmefene may be given IM or SC. Dosages are the same for all routes. However, with IM or SC administration, onset is delayed.

For postoperative use, the initial dose is 0.25 μg/kg. This dose is repeated at 2- to 5-minute intervals (for a maximum of four total doses) until the desired degree of opioid reversal has been achieved.

Treatment of opioid overdose depends on whether the victim is opioid dependent. If the victim is not dependent, treatment consists of two doses: 0.5 mg/70 kg initially, followed by 1 mg/70 kg 2 to 5 minutes later. If opioid dependency is suspected, a small (0.1 mg/70 kg) challenge dose is given. If the challenge dose does not precipitate withdrawal, then treatment continues as for patients who are not dependent.

NONOPIOID CENTRALLY ACTING ANALGESICS

Two centrally acting analgesics—tramadol [Ultram] and clonidine [Duraclon]—relieve pain by mechanisms largely unrelated to opioid receptors. These agents do not cause respiratory depression, dependence, or abuse, and are not regulated under the Controlled Substances Act.

Tramadol

Tramadol [Ultram, Ultracet] is a moderately strong analgesic with minimal potential for dependence, abuse, or respiratory depression. The drug relieves pain through a combination of opioid and nonopioid mechanisms.

Mechanism of Action. Tramadol is an analog of codeine that relieves pain in part through weak agonist activity at mu opioid receptors. However, it seems to work primarily by blocking uptake of norepinephrine and serotonin, thereby activating monoaminergic spinal inhibition of pain. Naloxone, an opioid antagonist, only partially blocks tramadol's effects.

Therapeutic Use. Tramadol is approved for moderate to moderately severe pain. The drug is less effective than morphine and no more effective than codeine combined with aspirin or acetaminophen. Analgesia begins 1 hour after oral administration, is maximal at 2 hours, and continues for 6 hours.

Pharmacokinetics. Tramadol is administered by mouth and reaches peak plasma levels in 2 hours. Elimination is by hepatic metabolism and renal excretion. The half-life is 5 to 6 hours.

Adverse Effects and Interactions. Tramadol has been used by millions of patients, and serious adverse effects have been rare. The most common side effects are sedation, dizziness, headache, dry mouth, and constipation. Respiratory depression is minimal. *Seizures* have been reported in over 280 patients, and hence the drug should be avoided in patients with epilepsy and other neurologic disorders. Severe allergic reactions have developed rarely.

Drug Interactions. Tramadol can intensify responses to *CNS depressants* (e.g., alcohol, benzodiazepines), and therefore should not be combined with these drugs. By inhibiting uptake of norepinephrine, tramadol can precipitate a hypertensive crisis if combined with an *MAO inhibitor.* Accordingly, the combination is absolutely contraindicated. By inhibiting uptake of serotonin, tramadol can cause serotonin syndrome in patients taking *drugs that enhance serotonergic transmission* (e.g., tricyclic antidepressants, selective serotonin reuptake inhibitors).

Abuse Liability. The abuse liability of tramadol is very low and the drug is not regulated under the Controlled Substances Act. Nonetheless, there have been a few reports of abuse, dependence, withdrawal, and intentional overdose, presumably for subjective effects. Consequently, tramadol should not be given to patients with a history of drug abuse, and the recommended dosage should not be exceeded.

Preparations, Dosage, and Administration. Tramadol is available alone (under the trade name Ultram) and in combination with acetaminophen (under the trade name Ultracet).

Tramadol alone [Ultram] is dispensed in 50-mg oral tablets. The recommended adult dosage is 50 to 100 mg every 4 to 6 hours as needed, up to a *maximum of 400 mg/day.* The dosing interval should be increased for patients with hepatic or renal dysfunction.

Tramadol combined with acetaminophen [Ultracet] is indicated for short-term therapy of acute pain. Each tablet contains 37.5 mg tramadol and 325 mg acetaminophen. The recommended dosage is 2 tablets every 4 to 6 hours (but should not exceed 8 tablets/day). Treatment duration should not exceed 5 days.

Clonidine

Clonidine [Duraclon] has two approved applications: treatment of hypertension and relief of severe pain. To relieve pain, clonidine is administered by continuous epidural infusion. To treat hypertension, the drug is given by mouth or by transdermal patch. Because the antihypertensive pharmacology of clonidine differs dramatically from its analgesic pharmacology, antihypertensive pharmacology is discussed separately (in Chapters 19 and 45). To avoid errors, you should know that the trade name employed for clonidine depends on the application: When used for pain relief, clonidine is marketed as *Duraclon;* when used for hypertension, the drug is marketed as *Catapres.* Clonidine has no abuse potential and is not regulated under the Controlled Substances Act.

Mechanism of Pain Relief. As discussed in Chapter 19, clonidine is an alpha$_2$-adrenergic agonist. The drug appears to relieve pain by binding to presynaptic and postsynaptic alpha$_2$ receptors in the spinal cord. The result is blockade of nerve traffic in pathways that transmit pain signals from the periphery to the brain. Pain relief is not blocked by opioid antagonists.

Analgesic Use. Clonidine is employed in combination with an opioid analgesic to relieve severe cancer pain that cannot be relieved by an opioid alone. Administration is by continuous infusion through an implanted epidural catheter. The drug is more effective against neuropathic pain (electrical, burning, or shooting in nature) than diffuse (unlocalized) visceral pain. Pain relief occurs only in regions innervated by sensory nerves that come from the part of the spinal cord where clonidine is present in high concentration.

Pharmacokinetics. Clonidine is a highly lipid soluble, and hence readily moves from the spinal cord to the blood. About half of each dose undergoes hepatic metabolism. The rest is excreted unchanged in the urine. Because urinary excretion is substantial, dosage should be reduced in patients with significant renal impairment.

Adverse Effects. Hypotension. The greatest concern is *severe hypotension* secondary to massive vasodilation. The cause of vasodilation is stimulation of alpha$_2$ receptors in the CNS. Hypotension is most likely during the first 4 days of treatment—and is most intense following infusion into the upper thoracic region of the spinal cord. Because of the risk of hypotension, vital signs should be monitored closely, especially during the first few days of treatment. Hypotension can be managed by infusing IV fluids. If necessary, IV ephedrine can be used to promote vasoconstriction.

Bradycardia. Clonidine can slow heart rate. The underlying mechanism is stimulation of alpha$_2$ receptors in the CNS. Severe bradycardia can be managed with atropine.

Rebound Hypertension. As discussed in Chapter 19, abrupt discontinuation of clonidine can cause rebound hypertension. Accordingly, when the drug is withdrawn, dosage should be tapered over 2 to 4 days. Rebound hypertension can be managed with IV clonidine or phentolamine.

Catheter-Related Infection. Infection is common with implanted epidural catheters. If the patient develops a fever of unknown origin, infection should be suspected.

Other Adverse Effects. As with oral clonidine, epidural clonidine can cause dry mouth, dizziness, sedation, anxiety, and depression.

Contraindications. Because of the risk of severe hypotension and bradycardia, epidural clonidine is contraindicated for patients who are hemodynamically unstable, and for obstetric, postpartum, or surgical patients. Additional contraindications are infection at the site of infusion, administration above the C4 dermatome, and use by patients receiving anticoagulants.

Preparations, Dosage, and Administration. Clonidine [Duraclon] is dispensed in 10-ml vials containing 100 or 500 μg/ml. The drug is administered through an implanted epidural catheter using a continuous infusion device. The initial infusion rate is 30 μg/hr.

:·: KEY POINTS

- Analgesics are drugs that relieve pain without causing loss of consciousness.
- Opioids are the most effective analgesics available.
- There are three major classes of opioid receptors, designated mu, kappa, and delta.
- Morphine and other pure opioid agonists relieve pain by mimicking the actions of endogenous opioid peptides—primarily at mu receptors (and partly at kappa receptors).
- Opioid-induced sedation and euphoria can complement pain relief.
- Because opioids produce desirable subjective effects (e.g., euphoria), they have a high liability for abuse.
- Respiratory depression is the most serious adverse effect of the opioids.
- Other important adverse effects are constipation, urinary retention, orthostatic hypotension, emesis, and elevation of ICP.
- Because of first-pass metabolism, oral doses of morphine must be larger than parenteral doses to produce equivalent effects.
- Because the blood-brain barrier is poorly developed in infants, these patients need smaller doses of opioids (adjusted for body weight) than do older children and adults.
- With prolonged opioid use, tolerance develops to analgesia, euphoria, sedation, and respiratory depression, but not to constipation and miosis.
- Cross-tolerance exists among the various opioid agonists, but not between opioid agonists and general CNS depressants.
- With prolonged opioid use, physical dependence develops. An abstinence syndrome will occur if the opioid is abruptly withdrawn.
- In contrast to the withdrawal syndrome associated with general CNS depressants, the withdrawal syndrome associated with opioids, although unpleasant, is not dangerous.
- To minimize symptoms of abstinence, opioids should be withdrawn gradually.
- Precautions to opioid use include pregnancy, labor and delivery, head injury, and decreased respiratory reserve.
- Patients taking opioids should avoid alcohol and other CNS depressants—because these drugs can intensify opioid-induced sedation and respiratory depression.
- Patients taking opioids should avoid anticholinergic drugs (e.g., antihistamines, tricyclic antidepressants, atropine-like drugs)—because these drugs can exacerbate opioid-induced constipation and urinary retention.
- Opioid overdose produces a classic triad of signs: coma, respiratory depression, and pinpoint pupils.
- All strong opioid agonists are essentially equal to morphine with regard to analgesia, abuse liability, and respiratory depression.
- Use of meperidine [Demerol] should not exceed 48 hours—so as to avoid accumulation of normeperidine, a toxic metabolite.

- Like morphine, codeine and other moderate to strong opioid agonists produce analgesia, sedation, euphoria, respiratory depression, constipation, urinary retention, cough suppression, and miosis. These drugs differ from morphine in that they produce less analgesia and respiratory depression and have a lower potential for abuse.
- The combination of codeine with a nonopioid analgesic (e.g., aspirin, acetaminophen) produces greater pain relief than can be achieved with either agent alone.
- Most agonist-antagonist opioids act as agonists at kappa receptors and antagonists at mu receptors.
- Pentazocine and other agonist-antagonist opioids produce less analgesia than morphine and have a lower potential for abuse.
- With agonist-antagonist opioids, there is a ceiling to respiratory depression.
- If given to a patient who is physically dependent on pure opioid agonists, an agonist-antagonist will precipitate withdrawal.
- Pure opioid antagonists act as antagonists at mu receptors and at kappa receptors.
- Naloxone and other pure opioid antagonists can reverse respiratory depression, coma, analgesia, and most other effects of pure opioid agonists.
- Pure opioid antagonists are used primarily to treat opioid overdose.
- If administered in excessive dosage to an individual who is physically dependent on opioid agonists, naloxone will precipitate an immediate withdrawal reaction.

- Opioid dosage must be individualized. Patients with a low tolerance to pain or with extremely painful conditions need high doses. Patients with sharp, stabbing pain need higher doses than patients with dull pain. Elderly adults generally require lower doses than younger adults. Neonates require relatively low doses.
- As a rule, opioids should be administered on a fixed schedule (with supplemental doses for breakthrough pain) rather than PRN.
- A PCA device is an electronically controlled pump that can be activated by the patient to deliver a preset dose of opioid through an indwelling catheter. Some PCA devices also deliver a basal opioid infusion.
- PCA devices provide steady plasma drug levels, thereby maintaining continuous pain control while avoiding unnecessary sedation and respiratory depression.
- Use of parenteral opioids during delivery can suppress uterine contractions and cause respiratory depression in the neonate.
- Addiction is a behavior pattern characterized by continued use of a psychoactive substance despite physical, psychologic, or social harm. Physical dependence and addiction are not the same.
- Abuse is defined as drug use that is inconsistent with medical or social norms.
- Because of excessive and inappropriate fears about addiction and abuse, physicians frequently prescribe less pain medication than patients need, and nurses frequently administer less medication than was prescribed.
- Please! Dispel your concerns about abuse and addiction and give your patients the medication they need to relieve suffering. That's what opioids are for, after all.

Summary of Major Nursing Implications*

PURE OPIOID AGONISTS

Alfentanil
Codeine
Fentanyl
Hydrocodone
Hydromorphone
Levorphanol
Meperidine
Methadone
Morphine
Oxycodone
Oxymorphone
Propoxyphene
Remifentanil
Sufentanil

Preadministration Assessment

Therapeutic Goal

Relief or prevention of moderate to severe pain while causing minimal respiratory depression, constipation, urinary retention, and other adverse effects.

*Patient education information is highlighted as blue text.

Baseline Data

Pain Assessment. Assess pain before administration and 1 hour later. Determine the location, time of onset, and quality of pain (e.g., sharp, stabbing, dull). Also, assess for psychologic factors that can lower pain threshold (anxiety, depression, fear, anger). Because pain is subjective and determined by multiple factors (e.g., cultural influences, patient expectations, associated disease), there is no reliable objective method for determining how much discomfort the patient is experiencing. Ultimately, you must rely on your ability to interpret what patients have to say about their pain. When listening to patients, be aware that a few may claim discomfort when their pain is under control, whereas others may claim to feel fine when they actually hurt.

Vital Signs. Prior to administration, determine respiratory rate, blood pressure, and pulse rate.

Identifying High-Risk Patients

All opioids are *contraindicated* for premature infants (both during and after delivery). *Morphine* is *contraindicated* fol-

Summary of Major Nursing Implications*—cont'd

lowing biliary tract surgery. *Meperidine* is *contraindicated* for patients taking MAO inhibitors.

Use opioids with *caution* in patients with head injury, profound CNS depression, coma, respiratory depression, pulmonary disease (e.g., emphysema, asthma), cardiovascular disease, hypotension, reduced blood volume, prostatic hypertrophy, urethral stricture, and liver impairment. *Caution* is also required when treating infants, elderly or debilitated patients, and patients receiving MAO inhibitors, CNS depressants, anticholinergic drugs, and hypotensive agents.

Implementation: Administration

Routes

Oral, IM, IV, SC, rectal, epidural, intrathecal, transdermal (fentanyl), and transmucosal (fentanyl). Routes for specific opioids are summarized in Tables 27–5 and 27–6.

Dosage

General Guidelines. Adjust dosage to meet individual needs. Higher doses are required for patients with low pain tolerance or with especially painful conditions. Patients with sharp, stabbing pain need higher doses than patients with dull, constant pain. Elderly patients generally require lower doses than younger adults. Neonates require relatively low doses because of their poorly developed blood-brain barriers. For all patients, dosage should be reduced as pain subsides.

Oral doses are larger than parenteral doses. Check to ensure that the dose is appropriate for the intended route.

Tolerance may develop with prolonged treatment, necessitating dosage escalation.

Warn outpatients not to increase dosage without consulting the physician.

Dosage in Patients with Cancer. Cancer is the principal disease for which opioids are used chronically. The objective is to maximize comfort. Physical dependence is a minor concern. Cancer patients should receive opioids on a fixed schedule around the clock—not PRN. If breakthrough pain occurs, fixed dosing should be supplemented PRN with a short-acting opioid. Because of tolerance to opioids or intensification of pain, dosage escalation may be required. Hence, patients should be re-evaluated on a regular basis to determine if pain control is adequate.

Discontinuing Opioids. Although significant dependence in hospitalized patients is rare, it can occur. To minimize symptoms of abstinence, withdraw opioids slowly, tapering the dosage over 3 days. **Warn outpatients against abrupt discontinuation of treatment.**

Administration

Prior to administration, determine respiratory rate, blood pressure, and pulse rate. Withhold medication and notify the physician if respiratory rate is at or below 12 breaths per minute, if blood pressure is significantly below the pretreatment value, or if pulse rate is significantly above or below the pretreatment value.

As a rule, opioids should be administered on a fixed schedule, with supplemental doses as needed.

Perform IV injections slowly (over 4 to 5 minutes). Rapid injection may produce severe adverse effects (profound hypotension, respiratory arrest, cardiac arrest) and should be avoided. When making an IV injection, have an opioid antagonist (e.g., naloxone) and facilities for respiratory support available.

Perform injections (especially IV) with the patient lying down to minimize hypotension.

Opioid agonists are regulated under the Controlled Substances Act and must be dispensed accordingly. All of the pure agonists are Schedule II substances, except propoxyphene (Schedule IV) and hydrocodone (Schedule III).

Concern for Opioid Abuse as a Factor in Dosage and Administration

Although opioids have a high potential for abuse, abuse is rare in the clinical setting. Consequently, when balancing the risk of abuse against the need to relieve pain, do not give excessive weight to concerns about abuse. The patient must not be allowed to suffer because of your unwarranted fears about abuse and dependence.

Although abuse is rare in the clinical setting, it can occur. To keep abuse to a minimum: (1) exercise clinical judgment when interpreting requests for opioid doses that seem excessive, (2) use opioids in the lowest effective doses for the shortest time required, (3) reserve opioid analgesics for patients with moderate to severe pain, and (4) switch to a nonopioid analgesic when the intensity of pain no longer justifies an opioid.

Responses to analgesics can be reinforced by nondrug measures, such as positioning the patient comfortably, showing concern and interest, and reassuring the patient that the medication will provide relief. Rest, mood elevation, and diversion can raise pain threshold and should be promoted. Conversely, anxiety, depression, fatigue, fear, and anger can lower pain threshold and should be minimized.

Ongoing Evaluation and Interventions

Evaluating Therapeutic Effects

Evaluate for pain control 1 hour after opioid administration. If analgesia is insufficient, consult the physician about an increase in dosage. Patients taking opioids chronically for suppression of cancer pain should be re-evaluated on a regular basis to determine if dosage is adequate.

Minimizing Adverse Effects

Respiratory Depression. Monitor respiration in all patients. If respiratory rate is 12 breaths per minute or less, withhold medication and notify the physician. **Warn outpatients about respiratory depression and instruct them to notify the physician if respiratory distress occurs.**

Certain patients, including the very young, the elderly, and those with respiratory disease (e.g., asthma, emphysema), are especially sensitive to respiratory depression and must be monitored closely.

*Patient education information is highlighted as blue text.

Summary of Major Nursing Implications*—cont'd

Delayed respiratory depression may develop following spinal administration of morphine. Be alert to this possibility.

When employed during labor and delivery, opioids may cause respiratory depression in the neonate. Monitor the infant closely. Have naloxone available to reverse opioid toxicity.

Sedation. **Inform patients that opioids may cause drowsiness. Warn them against doing hazardous activities (e.g., driving) if sedation is significant.** Sedation can be minimized by (1) using smaller doses given more frequently, (2) using opioids with short half-lives, and (3) giving small doses of a CNS stimulant (methylphenidate or dextroamphetamine) in the morning and early afternoon.

Orthostatic Hypotension. Monitor blood pressure and pulse rate. **Inform patients about symptoms of hypotension (dizziness, lightheadedness), and advise them to sit or lie down if these occur. Inform patients that hypotension can be minimized by moving slowly when assuming an erect posture. Warn patients against ambulation if hypotension is significant.** If appropriate, assist hospitalized patients with ambulation.

Constipation. The risk of constipation can be reduced by maintaining physical activity, increasing fluid intake, and prophylactic treatment with a stimulant laxative (e.g., senna) plus a stool softener (e.g., docusate). Severe constipation can be managed with an osmotic laxative (e.g., magnesium citrate, milk of magnesia).

Urinary Retention. To evaluate urinary retention, monitor intake and output, and palpate the lower abdomen for bladder distention every 4 to 6 hours. If there is a change in intake-output ratio, if bladder distention is detected, or if the patient reports difficulty voiding, notify the physician. Catheterization may be required. Difficulty with voiding is especially likely in patients with prostatic hypertrophy.

Because opioids may suppress awareness of bladder stimuli, encourage patients to void every 4 hours.

Biliary Colic. By constricting the common bile duct, morphine can increase pressure within the biliary tract, thereby causing severe pain. Biliary colic may be less pronounced with meperidine.

Emesis. Initial doses of opioids may cause nausea and vomiting. These reactions can be minimized by pretreatment with an antiemetic (e.g., promethazine) and by having the patient remain still. Tolerance to emesis develops quickly.

Cough Suppression. Cough suppression may result in accumulation of secretions in the airway. **Instruct patients to cough at regular intervals.** Auscultate the lungs for rales.

Miosis. Miosis can impair vision in dim light. Keep hospital room lighting bright during waking hours.

Opioid Dependence in the Neonate. The infant whose mother abused opioids during pregnancy may be born drug dependent. Observe the infant for signs of withdrawal (e.g., excessive crying, sneezing, tremor, hyperreflexia, fever, diarrhea) and notify the physician if these develop (usually within a few days after birth). The infant can be weaned from drug dependence by administering dilute opium tincture in progressively smaller doses.

Minimizing Adverse Interactions

CNS Depressants. Opioids can intensify responses to other CNS depressants (e.g., barbiturates, benzodiazepines, alcohol, antihistamines), thereby presenting a risk of profound sedation and respiratory depression. **Warn patients against use of alcohol and other CNS depressants.**

Agonist-Antagonist Opioids. These drugs (e.g., pentazocine, nalbuphine) can precipitate an abstinence syndrome if administered to a patient who is physically dependent on a pure opioid agonist. Before administering an agonist-antagonist, make certain the patient has been withdrawn from opioid agonists.

Anticholinergic Drugs. These agents (e.g., atropine-like drugs, tricyclic antidepressants, phenothiazines, antihistamines) can exacerbate opioid-induced constipation and urinary retention.

Hypotensive Drugs. Antihypertensive agents and other drugs that lower blood pressure can exacerbate opioid-induced orthostatic hypotension.

Opioid Antagonists. Opioid antagonists (e.g., naloxone) can precipitate an abstinence syndrome if administered in excessive dosage to a patient who is physically dependent on opioids. To avoid this reaction, carefully titrate the dosage of the antagonist.

MAO Inhibitors. Combining *meperidine* with an MAO inhibitor can cause delirium, hyperthemia, rigidity, convulsion, coma, and death. Obviously, the combination must be avoided.

AGONIST-ANTAGONIST OPIOIDS

Buprenorphine
Butorphanol
Dezocine
Nalbuphine
Pentazocine

Except for the differences presented below, the nursing implications for these drugs are much like those for the pure opioid agonists.

Therapeutic Goal

Relief of moderate to severe pain.

Routes

Oral, IV, IM, SC, and intranasal (butorphanol). Routes for individual agents are summarized in Table 27–6.

Differences from Pure Opioid Agonists

Maximal pain relief with the agonist-antagonists is generally lower than with pure opioid agonists.

Most agonist-antagonists have a ceiling to respiratory depression, thereby minimizing concerns about insufficient oxygenation.

*Patient education information is highlighted as blue text.

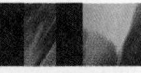

Summary of Major Nursing Implications*—cont'd

Agonist-antagonists cause little euphoria. Hence, abuse liability is low.

Agonist-antagonists increase cardiac work and should not be given to patients with acute myocardial infarction.

Because of their antagonist properties, agonist-antagonists can precipitate an abstinence syndrome in patients physically dependent on opioid agonists. Accordingly, patients must be withdrawn from pure opioid agonists before receiving an agonist-antagonist.

NALOXONE

Therapeutic Goal

Reversal of (1) postoperative opioid effects, (2) opioid-induced neonatal respiratory depression, and (3) overdose with pure opioid agonists.

*Patient education information is highlighted as blue text.

Routes

Intravenous, IM, and SC. For initial treatment, administer IV. Once opioid-induced CNS depression and respiratory depression have been reversed, IM or SC administration may be employed.

Dosage

Titrate dosage carefully. In opioid addicts, excessive doses can precipitate withdrawal. In postoperative patients, excessive doses can unmask pain by reversing opioid-mediated analgesia.

Pain Management in Patients with Cancer

TABLE 28–1 ■ Barriers to Cancer Pain Management

Barriers Related to Healthcare Professionals

Inadequate knowledge of pain management
Poor assessment of pain
Concerns stemming from regulations on controlled substances
Fear of patient addiction
Concern about side effects of analgesics
Concern about tolerance to analgesics

Barriers Related to Patients

Reluctance to report pain
   Fear of distracting physicians from treating the cancer
   Fear that pain means the cancer is worse
   Concern about not being a "good" patient
Reluctance to take pain medication
   Fear of addiction or being thought of as an addict
   Worries about unmanageable side effects
   Concern about becoming tolerant to pain medications
Inability to pay for treatment

Barriers Related to the Healthcare System

Low priority given to cancer pain management
Inadequate reimbursement: The most appropriate treatment may
   not be reimbursed
Restrictive regulation of controlled substances
Treatment is unavailable or access is limited

Adapted from Jacox A, Carr DB, Payne R, et al. *Management of Cancer Pain* (Clinical Practice Guideline No. 9; AHCPR Publication No. 94-0592). Rockville, MD, Agency for Health Care Policy and Research, 1994.

Our topic for this chapter—cancer pain management—is of note both for its good news and bad news. The good news is that pain can be relieved with simple interventions in 90% of cancer patients. The bad news is that, despite the availability of effective treatments, pain goes unrelieved far too often. Multiple factors contribute to undertreatment (Table 28–1). Important among these are inadequate physician training in pain management; unfounded fears of addiction (shared by physicians, patients, and families); and a healthcare system that focuses more on treating disease than relieving suffering.

Pain has a profound impact on both the patient and the family. Pain undermines quality of life for the patient and puts a heavy burden on the family. Unrelieved pain compromises that patient's ability to work, enjoy leisure activities, and fulfill his or her role in the family and in society at large. Furthermore, pain can impede recovery, hasten death from cancer, and possibly even create a risk of suicide.

Every patient has the right to expect that pain management will be an integral part of treatment throughout the course of his or her disease. The goal is to minimize pain and thereby maintain a reasonable quality of life, including the ability to function at work and at play, and within the family and society. In addi-

tion, if the cancer is incurable, treatment should permit the patient a relatively painless death when the time comes.

Much of this chapter is based on information in *Management of Cancer Pain* (Clinical Practice Guideline No. 9), sponsored by the Agency for Healthcare Research and Quality, formerly named the Agency for Health Care Policy and Research (AHCPR). You can order a copy by calling 1-800-4-CANCER.

PATHOPHYSIOLOGY OF PAIN

What Is Pain?

The International Association for the Study of Pain defines pain as "an unpleasant sensory and emotional experience associated with actual or potential tissue damage, or described in terms of such damage." Note that, by this definition, pain is not simply a sensory experience resulting from activation of pain receptors. Rather, it also includes the patient's emotional and cognitive responses to both the sensation of pain and the underlying cause (e.g., tissue damage caused by cancer). Most importantly, we must appreciate that pain is inherently *personal and subjective*. Hence, when assessing pain, the most reliable method is to have the patient describe his or her experience.

Neurophysiologic Basis of Painful Sensations

The discussion that follows is a gross oversimplification of how we perceive pain. Nonetheless, it should be adequate as a basis for understanding the interventions used for pain relief.

Sensation of pain is the net result of activity in two opposing neuronal pathways. The first pathway carries pain impulses from their site of origin to the brain, and thereby generates pain sensation. The second pathway, which originates in the brain, suppresses impulse conduction along the first pathway, and thereby diminishes pain sensation.

Pain impulses are initiated by activation of pain receptors, which are simply free nerve endings. These receptors can be activated by three types of stimuli: mechanical (e.g., pressure), thermal, and chemical (e.g., bradykinin, serotonin, histamine). In addition, *prostaglandins* and *substance P* can enhance the sensitivity of pain receptors to activation, although these compounds do not activate pain receptors directly.

Conduction of pain impulses from the periphery to the brain occurs by way of a multineuron pathway. The first neuron carries impulses from the periphery to a synapse in the spinal cord, where it releases either *glutamate* or *substance P* as a transmitter. The next neuron carries the impulse up the cord to a synapse in the thalamus. And the next neuron carries impulses from the thalamus to the cerebral cortex.

The brain is able to suppress pain conduction using endogenous opioid compounds, especially *enkephalins* and *beta-endorphin*. These compounds are released at synapses in both the brain and the spinal cord. Release within the spinal cord is controlled by a descending neuronal pathway that originates in the brain. The opioids that we give as drugs (e.g., morphine) produce analgesia by activating the same receptors that are activated by this endogenous pain-suppressing system.

Nociceptive Pain Versus Neuropathic Pain

In patients with cancer, pain has two major forms, referred to as *nociceptive* and *neuropathic*. Nociceptive pain results from injury to *tissues*, whereas neuropathic pain results from injury to *peripheral nerves*. These two forms of pain respond differently to analgesic drugs. Accordingly, it is important to differentiate between them. Among cancer patients, nociceptive pain is more common than neuropathic pain.

Nociceptive pain has two forms, known as *somatic and visceral*. Somatic pain results from injury to somatic tissues (bones, joints, muscles), whereas visceral pain results from injury to visceral organs (e.g., small intestine). Patients generally describe somatic pain as localized and sharp in quality. In contrast, they describe visceral pain as vaguely localized with a diffuse, aching quality. Both forms of nociceptive pain respond well to *opioid analgesics* (e.g., morphine). In addition, they may respond to *nonopioids* (e.g., ibuprofen).

Neuropathic pain produces different sensations than nociceptive pain and responds to different drugs. Patients describe neuropathic pain with such words as "burning," "shooting," "jabbing," "tearing," "numb," "dead," and "cold." Unlike nociceptive pain, neuropathic pain responds poorly to opioid analgesics. However, it does respond to drugs known as *adjuvant analgesics*. Among these are certain antidepressants (e.g., imipramine), anticonvulsants (e.g., carbamazepine), and local anesthetic/antidysrhythmics (e.g., lidocaine).

Pain in Cancer Patients

Among patients with cancer, pain can be caused by the cancer itself and by therapeutic interventions. Cancer can cause pain through direct invasion of surrounding tissues (e.g., nerves, muscles, visceral organs) and through metastatic invasion at distant sites. Metastases to bone are very common, causing pain in up to 50% of patients. Cancer can cause neuropathic pain through infiltration of nerves, and visceral pain through infiltration, obstruction, and compression of visceral structures.

The incidence and intensity of cancer-induced pain is a function of cancer type and stage of disease progression. Among patients with advanced disease, about 75% experience significant pain. Of these, 40% to 50% report moderate to severe pain, and 25% to 30% report very severe pain.

Therapeutic interventions—especially chemotherapy, radiation, and surgery—cause significant pain in at least 25% of patients, and probably more. Chemotherapy can cause painful mucositis, diffuse neuropathies, and aseptic necrosis of joints. Radiation can cause osteonecrosis, chronic visceral pain, and peripheral neuropathy (secondary to causing fibrosis of nerves). Surgery can cause a variety of pain syndromes, including phantom limb syndrome and postmastectomy syndrome.

MANAGEMENT STRATEGY

Management of cancer pain is an ongoing process that involves repeating cycles of assessment, intervention, and reassessment. The goal is to create and implement a flexible treatment plan that can meet the changing needs of the individual patient. The flow chart in Figure 28–1 summarizes the steps involved. Management begins with a comprehensive assessment. Once the nature of the pain has been determined, a treatment modality is selected. Analgesic drugs are preferred, and hence are usually tried first. If drugs are ineffective, other modalities can be implemented. Among these are radiation, surgery, and nerve blocks. After each intervention, pain is reassessed. Once relief has been achieved, the effective intervention is continued, accompanied by frequent reassessments. If severe pain returns or new pain develops, a new comprehensive assessment should be performed—followed by appropriate interventions and reassessment. Throughout this process, the healthcare team should make every effort to ensure active involvement of the patient and his or her family. Without their involvement, maximal benefits cannot be achieved. The importance of patient and family involvement is reflected in the clinical approach to pain management recommended by the AHCPR:

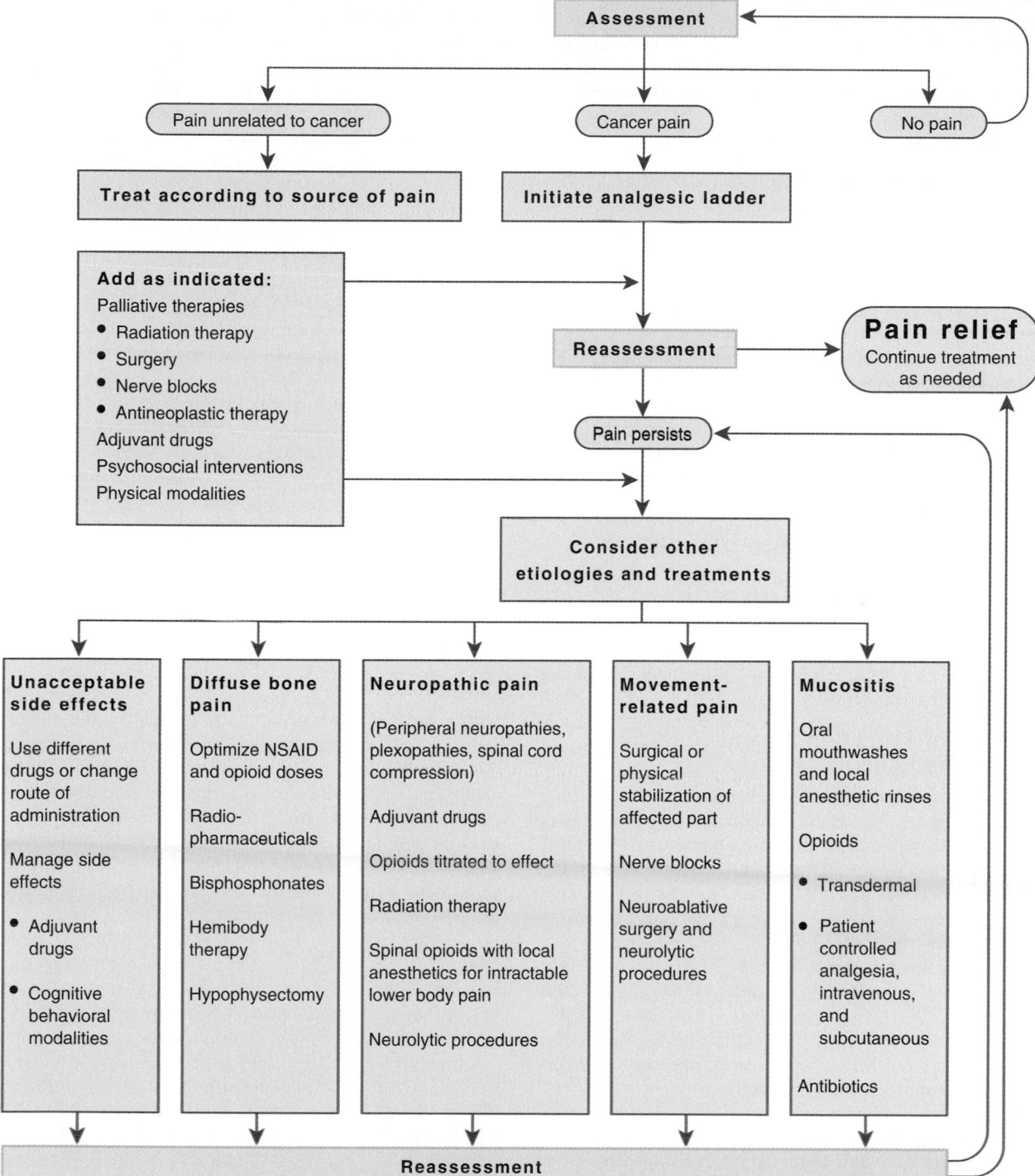

Figure 28–1 ■ **Flowchart for pain management in patients with cancer.**
NSAIDs = nonsteroidal anti-inflammatory drugs. (Adapted from Jacox A, Carr DB, Payne R, et al. Management of Cancer Pain [Clinical Practice Guideline No. 9; AHCPR Publication No. 94-0592]. Rockville, MD, Agency for Health Care Policy and Research, 1994.)

A Ask about pain regularly.
   Assess pain systematically.
B Believe the patient and family in their reports of pain and what relieves it.
C Choose pain control options appropriate for the patient, family, and setting.
D Deliver interventions in a timely, logical, coordinated fashion.
E Empower patients and their families.
   Enable patients to control their treatment to the greatest extent possible.

ASSESSMENT AND ONGOING EVALUATION

Assessment is the foundation of treatment. In the absence of thorough assessment, effective pain management is impossible. Assessment begins with a comprehensive evaluation and then continues with regular follow-up evaluations. The initial assessment provides the basis for designing the treatment program. The follow-ups let us know how well treatment is working.

Comprehensive Initial Assessment

The initial assessment employs an extensive array of tests. The primary objective is to characterize the pain and identify its cause. This information provides the basis for designing a pain management plan. In addition, by documenting the patient's baseline pain status, the initial assessment provides a basis for evaluating the efficacy of treatment.

Assessment of Pain Intensity and Character: The Patient Self-Report

The patient's description of his or her pain is the cornerstone of pain assessment. No other component of assessment is more important! Remember, pain is a personal experience. Accordingly, if we want to assess pain, we must rely on the patient to tell us about it. Furthermore, we must act on what the patient says—even if we personally believe the patient may not be telling the truth.

The best way to ensure an accurate report is to ask the right questions and listen carefully to the answers. We cannot elicit comprehensive information by asking, "How do you feel?" Rather, we must ask a series of specific questions. The answers should be recorded on a pain inventory form. The following information should be obtained:

- *Onset and temporal pattern*—When did your pain begin? How often does it occur? Has the intensity increased, decreased, or remained constant?
- *Location*—Where is your pain? Do you feel pain in more than one place? Ask patients to point to the exact location of the pain, either on themselves, on yourself, or on a full-body drawing.
- *Quality*—What does your pain feel like? Is it sharp or dull? Does it ache? Is it shooting or stabbing pain? Burning or tingling pain? These questions can help distinguish neuropathic pain from nociceptive pain.
- *Intensity*—On a scale of 0 to 10, with 0 being no pain and 10 the most intense pain you can imagine, how would you rank your pain now? How would you rank your pain at its worst? And at its best? A pain intensity scale (see below) can be very helpful for this assessment.
- *Modulating factors*—What makes your pain worse? What makes it better?
- *Previous treatment*—What treatments have you tried to relieve your pain (e.g., analgesics, acupuncture, relaxation techniques)? Are they effective now? If not, were they ever effective in the past?
- *Impact*—How does the pain affect your ability to function, both physically and socially? For example, does the pain interfere with your general mobility, work, eating, sleeping, socializing, or sex life?

Physical and Neurologic Examinations

The physical and neurologic examinations help to further characterize the pain, identify its source, and identify any complications related to the underlying pathology. The physician should examine the site of pain and determine if palpation or manipulation makes it worse. Nonverbal cues (e.g., protecting the painful area, limited movement in an arm or leg) that may indicate pain should be noted. Common patterns of referred pain should be assessed. For example, if the patient has hip pain, the physician should determine if the pain actually originates in the hip or if it is referred pain caused by pathology in the lumbar spine. Potential neurologic complications should be considered. For example, patients with back pain should be evaluated for impaired motor and sensory function in the limbs, and for impaired rectal and urinary sphincter function.

Diagnostic Tests

Diagnostic tests are performed to identify the underlying cause of pain (e.g., progression of cancer, tissue injury caused by cancer treatments). The repertoire of diagnostic tests includes imaging studies (e.g., computerized tomography scan, magnetic resonance imaging), neurophysiologic tests, and tests for tumor markers in blood. To ensure that abnormalities identified in the diagnostic tests really do explain the patient's pain, these findings should be correlated with findings from the physical and neurologic examinations.

Psychosocial Assessment

Psychosocial assessment is directed at both the patient and his or her family. The information is used in making pain management decisions. Some important issues to address include

- The impact of significant pain on the patient in the past
- The patient's usual coping responses to pain and stress
- The patient's preferences regarding pain management methods
- The patient's concerns about using opioids and other controlled substances (anxiolytics, stimulants)
- Changes in the patient's mood (anxiety, depression) brought on by cancer and pain
- The impact of cancer and its treatment on the family
- The level of care the family can provide and the potential need for outside help (e.g., hospice)

Pain Intensity Scales

Pain intensity scales are useful tools for assessing pain intensity. Representative scales are shown in Figures 28–2 and 28–3. The *descriptive scale* and *numeric scale* (Fig. 28–2) are used for adults and older children. The *pain affect FACES scale* (Fig. 28–3) is used for young children and for patients with cognitive impairment, who may have difficulty understanding the descriptive and numeric scales.

Pain intensity scales are valuable not only for assessing pain intensity, but also for *setting pain relief goals and evaluating treatment.* When setting goals, the patient and physician should agree on a target pain intensity rating that will permit the patient to participate in recovery activities, perform activities of daily living, and enjoy activities that contribute to quality of life. The objective of treatment is to reduce pain to the agreed-upon level—and lower, if possible.

Ongoing Evaluation

Once a treatment plan has been implemented, pain should be reassessed frequently. The objective is to determine the efficacy of treatment and to allow early diagnosis and treatment of new pain. Each time an analgesic drug is administered, pain should be evaluated after sufficient time has elapsed for the drug to take effect. Because most patients are treated at home, patients and caregivers should be taught how to conduct and document pain evaluations. The physician will use the documented record to make adjustments to the pain management plan.

Physicians, patients, and caregivers should be alert for development of new pain. In the majority of cases, new pain results from a new cause (e.g., metastasis, infection, fracture). Accordingly, whenever new pain occurs, a rigorous diagnostic work-up should be conducted.

Barriers to Assessment

As stressed above, pain assessment relies heavily on a report from the patient. Unfortunately, the report is not always accurate: Some patients report more pain than they have, some report less, and some are unable to report at all. With other patients, cultural and language differences impede assessment. In all cases, reliance on behavioral cues and facial expression is a poor substitute for an accurate report by the patient.

Many patients under-report pain, frequently because of misconceptions. Some fear addiction to opioids, and hence want to minimize opioid use. Some believe they are expected to be stoic and "tough it out." Some deny their pain because they fear pain signifies disease progression. When under-reporting of pain is suspected, the patient should be interviewed in an effort to discover the reason. If a misconception is responsible for under-reporting, educating the patient can help fix the problem.

Some patients fear they may be denied sufficient pain medication, and hence, to ensure adequate dosing, report more pain than they actually have. When exaggeration is suspected, the patient should be reassured that adequate pain relief will be provided, and should be taught that inaccurate reporting serves only to make appropriate treatment more difficult.

Language barriers and cultural barriers can impede pain assessment. For patients who do not speak English, a translator should be provided. Obtaining a pain rating scale in the patient's own language would obviously help. A *pain affect FACES scale* can be useful, since facial expressions representing discomfort are the same in all cultures. Cultural beliefs may cause some patients to hide overt expression of pain and report less pain than is present. The interviewer should be alert to this possibility.

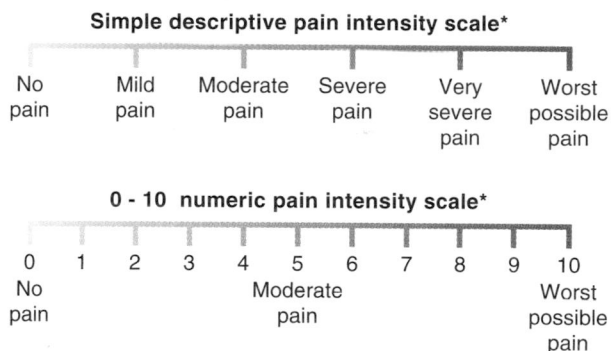

Figure 28–2 ■ Linear pain intensity scales.
*If used as a graphic rating scale, a 10-cm baseline is recommended. (From Acute Pain Management Guideline Panel. Acute Pain Management: Operative or Medical Procedures and Trauma [Clinical Practice Guideline No. 1; AHCPR Publication No. 92-0032]. Rockville, MD, Agency for Health Care Policy and Research, 1992, with permission.)

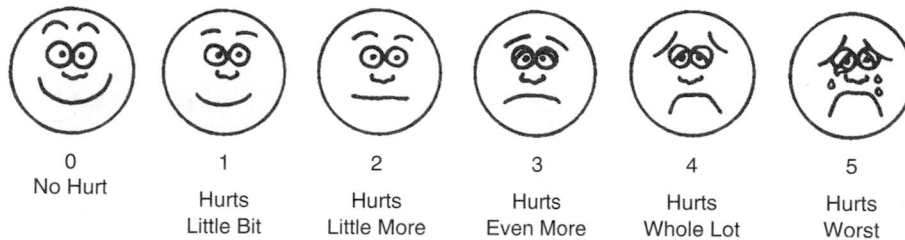

Figure 28–3 ■ Wong-Baker FACES Pain Rating Scale.
Explain to the patient that the first face represents a person who feels happy because he or she has no pain, and that the other faces represent people who feel sad because they have pain, ranging from a little to a lot. Explain that face 5 represents a person who hurts as much as you can imagine, but that you don't have to be crying to feel this bad. Ask the patient to choose the face that best reflects how he or she is feeling. The numbers below the faces correspond to the values in the numeric pain scale shown in Figure 28-2. (From Wong DL. Wong's Essentials of Pediatric Nursing, 6th ed. St. Louis, CV Mosby, 2003, with permission.)

When assessing pain, we must keep in mind that behavior and facial expression may be poor indicators of pain status. For example, in patients approaching the end of life, behavioral cues of pain (e.g., vocalizing, grimacing) are often absent. Other patients may simply have good coping skills, and hence may smile and move around in apparent comfort, even though they are in considerable pain. Because appearances can be deceiving, we must not rely on them to assess pain.

Assessment in young children and other nonverbal patients is a special challenge. By definition, nonverbal patients are unable to self-report pain. Accordingly, we must use less reliable methods of assessment, including observing the patient for cues. Assessment in children is discussed further under *Pain Management in Special Populations.*

DRUG THERAPY

Analgesic drugs are the most powerful weapons we have for conquering cancer pain. With proper use, these agents can relieve pain in 90% of patients. Because analgesics are so effective, drug therapy is the principal modality for pain treatment. Three types of analgesics are employed:

- Nonopioid analgesics (nonsteroidal anti-inflammatory drugs [NSAIDs] and acetaminophen)
- Opioid analgesics (e.g., oxycodone, morphine)
- Adjuvant analgesics (e.g., amitriptyline, carbamazepine, dextroamphetamine)

These classes differ in their abilities to relieve pain. With the nonopioid and adjuvant analgesics, there is a ceiling to how much pain relief we can achieve. In contrast, there is no ceiling to the relief that opioids can provide.

Selection among the analgesics is based on pain intensity and pain type. To guide drug selection, the World Health Organization (WHO) has devised a drug selection ladder (Fig. 28–4). The first step of the ladder—for mild to moderate pain—consists of nonopioid analgesics: NSAIDs and acetaminophen. The second step—for more severe pain—*adds* opioid analgesics of moderate strength (e.g., oxycodone, hydrocodone). The top step—for severe pain—substitutes powerful opioids (e.g., morphine, fentanyl) for the weaker ones. Adjuvant analgesics, which are especially effective against neuropathic pain, can be used on any step of the ladder. Specific drugs to *avoid* are listed in Table 28–2.

It is common practice to combine an opioid with a nonopioid. Why? Because the combination can be more effective than either drug alone. When pain is only moderate, opioids and nonopioids can be given in a fixed-dose combination formulation, thereby simplifying dosing. However, when pain is severe, these drugs must be given separately. Why? Because, with a fixed-dose combination, side effects of the nonopioid would become intolerable as the dosage grew large, and hence would limit how much opioid could be given.

Drug therapy of cancer pain should adhere to the following principles:

- Perform a comprehensive pretreatment assessment to identify pain intensity and the underlying cause.
- Individualize the treatment plan.
- Use the WHO ladder to guide drug selection.
- Use oral therapy whenever possible.

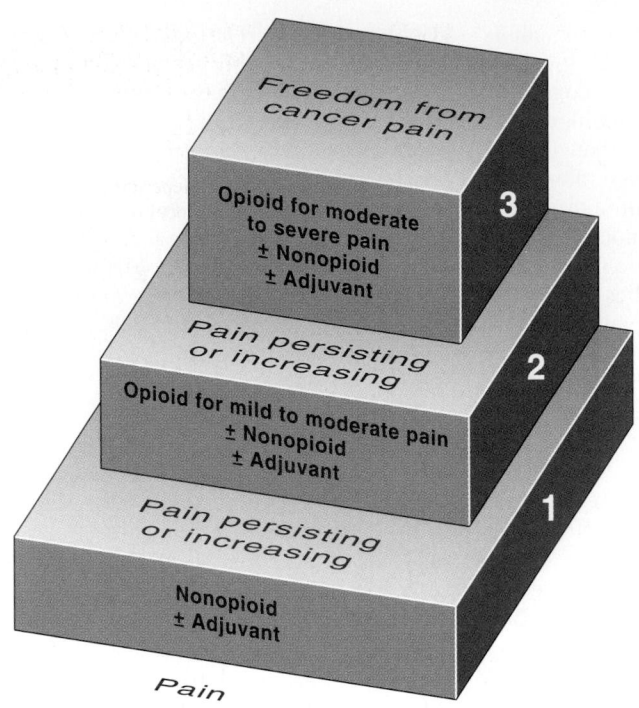

Figure 28–4 ■ The WHO analgesic ladder for cancer pain management. (Adapted from Cancer Pain Relief, 2nd ed. Geneva, World Health Organization, 1996.)

- Avoid IM injections whenever possible.
- For persistent pain, administer analgesics on a fixed-schedule around the clock (ATC), and provide additional rescue doses of a short-acting agent if breakthrough pain occurs.
- Evaluate the patient frequently for pain relief and drug side effects.

Nonopioid Analgesics

The nonopioid analgesics—NSAIDs and acetaminophen—constitute the first rung of the WHO analgesic ladder. These agents are the initial drugs of choice for patients with mild to moderate pain. There is a ceiling to how much pain relief nonopioid drugs can provide. Hence, there is no benefit to exceeding recommended dosages (Table 28–3). Acetaminophen is about equal to the NSAIDs in *analgesic* efficacy but lacks *anti-inflammatory* actions. Because of this difference and others, acetaminophen is considered separately. The NSAIDs and acetaminophen are discussed at length in Chapter 67. Accordingly, discussion here is brief.

Nonsteroidal Anti-inflammatory Drugs

NSAIDs (e.g., aspirin, ibuprofen) can produce a variety of effects. Primary beneficial effects are pain relief, suppression of inflammation, and reduction of fever. Primary adverse effects are gastric ulceration, acute renal failure, and bleeding. In contrast to opioids, NSAIDs do not cause tolerance, physical dependence, or psychologic dependence.

NSAIDs are effective analgesics that can relieve mild to moderate pain. All of the NSAIDs have essentially equal analgesic efficacy, although individual patients may respond better to one NSAID than to another. NSAIDs relieve pain by a mechanism different from that of the opioids. As a result,

TABLE 28–2 ■ Drugs That Are Not Recommended for Treating Cancer Pain

Class	Drug	Why the Drug Is Not Recommended
Opioids		
Pure agonists	Meperidine Codeine	A toxic metabolite accumulates with prolonged use Maximal pain relief is limited owing to dose-limiting side effects
Agonist-antagonists	Buprenorphine Butorphanol Dezocine Nalbuphine Pentazocine	Ceiling to analgesic effects; can precipitate withdrawal in opioid-dependent patients; cause psychotomimetic reactions
Opioid Antagonists	Naloxone Naltrexone	Can precipitate withdrawal in opioid-dependent patients; limit use to reversing life-threatening respiratory depression caused by opioid overdose
Benzodiazepines	Diazepam Lorazepam others	Sedation from benzodiazepines limits opioid dosage; no demonstrated analgesic action
Barbiturates	Amobarbital Secobarbital others	Sedation from barbiturates limits opioid dosage; no demonstrated analgesic action
Miscellaneous	Cocaine	No analgesic efficacy, either alone or in combination with an opioid
	Marijuana	Side effects (dysphoria, drowsiness, hypotension, bradycardia) preclude routine use as an analgesic
	Brompton's cocktail	Analgesic efficacy is no better than that of a single opioid

combined use of an NSAID with an opioid can produce greater pain relief than either agent alone.

NSAIDs produce their effects—both good and bad—by inhibiting cyclooxygenase (COX), an enzyme that has two forms: cyclooxygenase-1 (COX-1) and cyclooxygenase-2 (COX-2). COX-1 is present in the stomach, kidneys, platelets, and practically all other tissues. In contrast, COX-2 is produced mainly at sites of tissue injury. Both COX isoforms participate in the synthesis of prostaglandins and related compounds, chemicals that have both harmful and beneficial effects:

- At sites of tissue injury, these compounds promote inflammation and sensitize receptors to painful stimuli.
- In the brain, they modulate perception of pain and promote fever.
- In the stomach, they protect the gastric mucosa from self-digestion.
- In platelets, they promote aggregation.
- In the kidney, they promote vasodilation, and thereby help maintain renal blood flow.

Because COX-1 and COX-2 are found at different sites and have different functions, inhibition of these enzymes has different effects. Specifically, inhibition of *COX-1* promotes *adverse* effects: gastric ulceration, acute renal failure, and bleeding (by inhibiting platelet aggregation). In contrast, inhibition of *COX-2* promotes *beneficial* effects: reduction of pain, inflammation, and fever.

Individual NSAIDs differ in their abilities to inhibit COX-1 and COX-2. Conventional NSAIDs (e.g., aspirin, ibuprofen) inhibit both forms of the enzyme. As a result, conventional NSAIDs cannot reduce pain and inflammation (through COX-2 inhibition) without also posing a risk of gastric ulceration, kidney damage, and bleeding (through COX-1 inhibition). Recently, selective COX-2 inhibitors (e.g., celecoxib, rofecoxib) were introduced. Because of their selectivity, these drugs can reduce pain and inflammation while posing a relatively small risk of adverse effects. Unfortunately, COX-2 inhibitors are much more expensive than conventional NSAIDs. Accordingly, COX-2 inhibitors are generally reserved for patients who cannot tolerate the conventional agents.

For patients undergoing chemotherapy, inhibition of platelet aggregation by NSAIDs is a serious concern. Many anticancer drugs suppress bone marrow function, and thereby decrease platelet production. The resultant thrombocytopenia puts patients at risk of bruising and bleeding. Obviously, this risk will be increased by drugs that inhibit platelet function. Among the conventional NSAIDs, only one subclass—the nonacetylated salicylates (e.g., choline salicylate)—does not inhibit platelet aggregation, and hence is safe for patients with thrombocytopenia. All other conventional NSAIDs should be avoided. *Aspirin* is especially dangerous because it causes *irreversible* inhibition of platelet aggregation. Hence, its effects persist for the life of the platelet (about 8 days). Because COX-2 inhibitors do not affect platelets, these drugs are safe for patients with thrombocytopenia.

Acetaminophen

Acetaminophen [Tylenol, others] is similar to the NSAIDs in some respects and different in others. Like the NSAIDs, acetaminophen is an effective analgesic, and hence can relieve mild to moderate pain in patients with cancer. The drug relieves pain

TABLE 28–3 ▪■ Dosages for Nonopioid Analgesics: Acetaminophen and Selected NSAIDS

Drug	Usual Adult Dosage*	
	Body Weight ≥50 kg	**Body Weight <50 kg**
Acetaminophen	650 mg q 4 h *or* 975 mg q 6 h	10–15 mg/kg q 4 h *or* 15–20 mg/kg q 4 h (rectal)
NSAIDs: Salicylates		
Aspirin	650 mg q 4 h *or* 975 mg q 6 h	10–15 mg/kg q 4 h *or* 15–20 mg/kg q 4 h (rectal)
Choline salicylate [Arthropan]	870 mg q 3–4 h	—
Magnesium salicylate [Magan]	650 mg q 4 h	—
Sodium salicylate	325–650 mg q 3–4 h	—
NSAIDs: Propionic Acid Derivatives		
Fenoprofen [Nalfon]	300–600 mg q 6 h	—
Ibuprofen [Motrin, Advil, others]	400–600 mg q 6 h	10 mg/kg q 6–8 h
Ketoprofen [Orudis]	25–60 mg q 6–8 h	—
Naproxen [Naprosyn]	250–275 mg q 6–8 h	5 mg/kg q 8 h
Naproxen sodium [Anaprox, Aleve, Naprelan, others]	275 mg q 6–8 h	—
NSAIDs: Miscellaneous		
Diflunisal [Dolobid]	500 mg q 12 h	—
Etodolac [Lodine]	200–400 mg q 6–8 h	—
Meclofenamate sodium	50–100 mg q 6 h	—
Mefenamic acid [Ponstel]	250 mg q 6 h	—
NSAIDs: Selective COX-2 Inhibitors		
Celecoxib [Celebrex]	200 mg q 12 h	—
Rofecoxib [Vioxx]	25–50 mg q 12 h	—

*All dosages are oral except where indicated.

by inhibiting COX in the central nervous system (CNS)—but not in the periphery. Combining acetaminophen with an opioid can produce greater analgesia than either drug used alone (because acetaminophen and opioids relieve pain by different mechanisms).

Acetaminophen differs from the NSAIDs in several important ways. Because it does not inhibit COX in the periphery, acetaminophen lacks anti-inflammatory actions, does not promote gastric ulceration or renal failure, and does not inhibit platelet aggregation. Because acetaminophen does not affect platelets, the drug is safe for patients with thrombocytopenia.

Acetaminophen has important interactions with two other drugs: alcohol and warfarin (an anticoagulant). Combining acetaminophen with alcohol, even in moderate amounts, can result in potentially fatal liver damage. Accordingly, patients taking acetaminophen should minimize alcohol consumption. Acetaminophen also can increase the risk of bleeding in patients taking warfarin. The mechanism appears to be inhibition of warfarin metabolism, which causes warfarin to accumulate to dangerous levels.

Opioid Analgesics

Opioids are the most effective analgesics available, and hence are the primary drugs for treating moderate to severe cancer pain. With proper dosing, opioids can safely relieve pain in over 90% of cancer patients. Unfortunately, many patients are denied adequate doses, owing primarily to unfounded fears of addiction. In the past, opioids were known as *narcotics,* a term that is now obsolete.

Opioids produce a variety of pharmacologic effects. In addition to analgesia, they can cause sedation, euphoria, constipation, respiratory depression, urinary retention, and miosis. With continuous use, tolerance develops to most of these effects, with the notable exception of constipation. Continuous use also results in physical dependence, which must not be equated with addiction.

The opioids are discussed at length in Chapter 27. Discussion here focuses on their use in patients with cancer.

Mechanism of Action and Classification

Opioid analgesics relieve pain by mimicking the actions of endogenous opioid peptides (enkephalins, dynorphins, endorphins), primarily at mu receptors and partly at kappa receptors.

Based on their actions at mu and kappa receptors, the opioids fall into two major groups: (1) *pure (full) agonists* (e.g., morphine) and (2) *agonist-antagonists* (e.g., butorphanol). The pure agonists can be subdivided into (1) agents for mild to moderate pain and (2) agents for moderate to severe pain. The pure agonists act as agonists at mu receptors *and* kappa receptors. In contrast, the agonist-antagonists act as agonists only at kappa receptors; at mu receptors, these drugs act as *antagonists.* Because their agonist actions are limited to kappa receptors, the agonist-antagonists have a ceiling to their analgesic effects. Furthermore, because of their antagonist actions, the agonist-antagonists can block access of the pure agonists to mu receptors, and can thereby prevent the pure agonists from relieving pain. Accordingly, agonist-antagonists are not recommended for managing cancer pain.

Tolerance and Physical Dependence

Over time, opioids cause tolerance and physical dependence. These phenomena, which are generally inseparable, reflect neuronal adaptations to prolonged opioid exposure. Some degree of tolerance and physical dependence will develop after 1 to 2 weeks of opioid use.

Tolerance. Tolerance can be defined as a state in which a specific dose (e.g., 5 mg of morphine) produces a smaller effect than it could when treatment began. Put another way, tolerance is a state in which dosage must be increased to maintain the desired response. In patients with cancer, however, a need for larger doses isn't always a sign of tolerance. In fact, it's usually a sign that pain is getting worse (owing to disease progression).

Tolerance develops to some opioid effects but not to others. Tolerance does develop to analgesia, euphoria, respiratory depression, and sedation. In contrast, little or no tolerance develops to constipation.

There is cross-tolerance among opioids. Accordingly, significant tolerance to one opioid confers a similar degree of tolerance to all others.

Physical Dependence. Physical dependence is a state in which an abstinence syndrome will occur if a drug is abruptly withdrawn. With opioids, the abstinence syndrome can be very unpleasant—but not dangerous. The intensity and duration of the abstinence syndrome are determined in part by the duration of drug use and in part by the half-life of the drug taken. Because drugs with a short half-life leave the body rapidly, the abstinence syndrome is brief but intense. Conversely, for drugs with long half-lives, the syndrome is prolonged but relatively mild. The abstinence syndrome can be minimized by withdrawing opioids slowly (i.e., by giving progressively smaller doses over several days). Please note that *physical dependence is not the same as addiction!*

Addiction

Opioid addiction is an important issue in pain management—not because addiction occurs (it rarely does), but because *inappropriate fears of addiction* are a major cause for undertreatment.

The American Society of Addiction Medicine defines addiction as *a disease process characterized by continued use of a psychoactive substance despite physical, psychologic, or social harm.* According to this definition, addiction is primarily a *behavior pattern*—and is *not* equated with physical dependence. Although it is true that physical dependence can contribute to addictive behavior, other factors—especially *psychologic dependence*—are the primary underlying cause. All cancer patients who take opioids chronically develop substantial physical dependence, but only a few (much less than 1%) develop addictive behavior. Most patients, if their cancer were cured, would simply go through gradual withdrawal, and never think about or use opioids again. Clearly, these patients cannot be considered addicted, despite their physical dependence.

Because of misconceptions about opioid addiction, physicians often prescribe lower doses than patients need, nurses administer lower doses than were prescribed, patients report less pain than they actually have, and family members dis-

TABLE 28–4 ■ Equianalgesic Doses of Pure Opioid Agonists

Drug	Equianalgesic Dose* Parenteral	Equianalgesic Dose* Oral
Agents for Mild to Moderate Pain		
Codeine†	130 mg q 3–4 h	200 mg q 3–4 h
Hydrocodone	NA	30 mg q 3–4 h
Oxycodone	NA	15 mg q 3–4 h
Oxycodone SR	NA	45–60 mg q 12 h
Agents for Moderate to Severe Pain		
Morphine	10 mg q 3–4 h	30 mg q 3–4 h
Morphine SR	NA	90–120 mg q 12 h
Morphine ER	NA	180–240 mg q 24 h
Hydromorphone	1.5 mg q 3–4 h	7.5 mg q 3–4 h
Levorphanol	2 mg q 6–8 h	4 mg q 6–8 h
Methadone	1 mg q 6–8 h	20 mg q 6–8h
Oxymorphone	1 mg q 3–4 h	NA
Fentanyl	100 μg/hr (SC, IV, or transdermal) equals 4 mg/hr IV morphine	

SR = sustained release, ER = extended release, NA = not available.
*Equianalgesic dose = dose that will produce the same degree of analgesia as 10 mg of parenteral morphine given every 3 to 4 hours.
†Codeine is not generally recommended for chronic therapy because the doses required to produce significant analgesia also produce significant side effects.

courage opioid use. The end result? The majority of cancer patients receive lower doses of opioids than they need. How can we improve this unacceptable situation? We must educate physicians, nurses, patients, and family members. Specifically, we must teach them about the nature of addiction and inform them that development of addiction in the therapeutic setting is very rare. Hopefully, this information will dispel unfounded fears of addiction, and will thereby help ensure delivery of opioids in doses that are sufficient to relieve suffering. After all, that *is* what opioids are for.

Drug Selection

Preferred Opioids. For all cancer patients, *pure opioid agonists* are preferred to the agonist-antagonists. If pain is not too intense, a moderately strong opioid (e.g., oxycodone) is appropriate. If pain is moderate to severe, a strong opioid (e.g., morphine) should be used. Since morphine is inexpensive, available in multiple dosage forms, and clinically well understood, this opioid is used more than any other. Preferred opioids are listed in Table 28–4.

Opioids to Use with Special Caution. Methadone [Dolophine, Methadose] and *levorphanol* [Levo-Dromoran] must be used with caution. Both drugs have prolonged half-lives, which makes dosage titration difficult. If dosing is not done skillfully, these drugs can accumulate to dangerous levels, causing excessive sedation and respiratory depression.

Codeine deserves special comment. Although codeine is capable of producing significant analgesia, side effects limit the dose that can be given. As a result, the degree of pain relief that can be achieved safely is quite low.

Opioids to Avoid. Meperidine [Demerol], a pure opioid agonist, may be used for a few days, but no longer. When the drug is taken chronically, a toxic metabolite (normeperidine) can accumulate, thereby posing a risk of adverse CNS effects (dysphoria, agitation, seizures).

The *agonist-antagonists*—buprenorphine, butorphanol, dezocine, nalbuphine, and pentazocine—should be avoided. Why? First, these drugs are much less effective than pure opioid agonists; hence, there is little reason to choose them. Second, if given to a patient who is physically dependent on a pure opioid agonist, these drugs can prevent the pure agonist from working, and can thereby block analgesia and precipitate withdrawal. Third, the agonist-antagonists can cause adverse psychologic reactions (nightmares, hallucinations, dysphoria).

Dosage

Dosage must be individualized. The objective is to find a dosage that can relieve pain without causing intolerable side effects. For patients with moderate pain and low opioid tolerance, very low doses (e.g., 2 mg of parenteral morphine every 4 hours) can be sufficient. In contrast, when pain is severe or tolerance is high, much larger doses (e.g., 600 mg of parenteral morphine every few hours) may be required. The upper limit to dosage is determined only by the intensity of side effects. Accordingly, as pain and/or tolerance increase, dosage should be increased until pain is relieved—unless intolerable side effects (e.g., excessive respiratory depression) occur first.

The dosing schedule is determined by the temporal pattern of the pain. If pain is intermittent and infrequent, PRN dosing can suffice. However, since most patients have persistent pain, PRN dosing is inappropriate. Instead, dosing should be done *on a fixed schedule around the clock* (ATC). Why? Because a fixed schedule can prevent opioid levels from becoming subtherapeutic, and can thereby prevent pain recurrence. As a result, the patient is spared needless suffering, both from the pain itself and from anxiety about its return.

What dose should be used when switching from one opioid to another, or from one route of administration to another? To help make this decision, an *equianalgesia table* (Table 28–4) should be consulted. Equianalgesia tables indicate equivalent analgesic doses for different opioids, and for the same opioid administered by different routes. Let's assume, for example, that our patient has been getting 10 mg of IV morphine every 4 hours, and we want to switch to oral hydromorphone. By consulting Table 28–4, we can see that 7.5 mg of oral hydromorphone is about equivalent to 10 mg of parenteral morphine, with both drugs being given every 4 hours. Hence, we might begin oral hydromorphone at 7.5 mg. However, there is a caveat: Because cross-tolerance among opioids is incomplete, the listed equianalgesic dose may actually produce a *stronger* effect than advertised. Accordingly, when switching drugs, it is safer to use a dose that is somewhat *lower* than the equianalgesic dose, and then titrate up.

Routes of Administration

Since most patients with cancer pain must take analgesics continuously, the chosen route should be as convenient, affordable, and noninvasive as possible. Oral administration meets these criteria best, and hence is the preferred route for most patients. If oral medication cannot be used, the preferred alternatives are rectal and transdermal: Both are relatively convenient, affordable, and noninvasive. If these routes are ineffective or inappropriate, then parenteral administration (IV or SC) is indicated (IM injections should be avoided). For patients who cannot be managed with IV or SC therapy, more invasive routes—intraspinal or intraventricular—can be tried.

Oral. Oral administration is the preferred method for chronic therapy. Why? Because oral dosing is cheap, convenient, and noninvasive. Accordingly, in the absence of contraindications (e.g., vomiting, inability to swallow), the oral route should be considered for all patients. Opioids are available in several formulations (e.g., tablets, capsules, solution) for oral use. To reduce the number of daily doses, a long-acting formulation (e.g., controlled-release morphine) can be used. Because oral opioids undergo substantial first-pass metabolism, oral doses must be larger than parenteral doses to achieve equivalent analgesic effects.

Rectal. Rectal administration is a preferred alternative for patients who cannot take drugs by mouth. Three opioids—morphine, hydromorphone, and oxymorphone—are available in rectal formulations (suppositories). When switching from oral to rectal administration, dosing is begun with the same dose that was used orally, and then adjusted as needed. Rectal administration is inappropriate for patients with diarrhea or lesions of the rectum or anus. Also, children frequently object to this route.

Transdermal. Transdermal administration is a preferred alternative to oral therapy. Only one opioid—fentanyl [Sublimaze]—is available for transdermal use. Fentanyl "patches" provide steady analgesia for 72 hours, and hence are appropriate for patients with pain that is continuous and does not fluctuate much in intensity. Absorption from the patch is very slow. As a result, when the first patch is applied, effective analgesia may take 12 to 24 hours to develop. During this time, PRN therapy with a short-acting opioid may be required. Fentanyl patches are available in four strengths, and hence allow dosage to be matched with pain intensity. As with other long-acting opioids, rescue doses with a short-acting opioid are needed when breakthrough pain occurs.

Intravenous and Subcutaneous. Intravenous and SC administration are acceptable alternatives when less invasive routes (oral, transdermal, rectal) cannot be used. The IV and SC routes have two advantages: (1) onset of analgesia is quick and (2) these routes permit rapid escalation of dosage. Obvious disadvantages are inconvenience and increased cost. In addition, frequent SC dosing is uncomfortable. Conditions that might justify IV or SC administration include

- Persistent nausea and vomiting (which preclude oral dosing)
- Inability to swallow (which precludes oral dosing)
- Delirium or stupor (which preclude oral dosing)
- Pain that requires a large number of pills (which makes oral dosing inconvenient)
- Unstable pain that requires rapid dosage escalation (which precludes oral, rectal, and transdermal administration)

Dosages for IV and SC administration are the same.

Intramuscular. Intramuscular administration should be avoided. Intramuscular injections are painful, and hence unacceptable for repeated dosing. In addition, absorption from IM sites is inconsistent, hence pain relief is unpredictable.

Intraspinal. Intraspinal administration is reserved for patients with intractable pain that cannot be controlled with less invasive routes (e.g., IV, SC). In this technique, opioids are delivered to the epidural or subarachnoid space via a percutaneous catheter connected to an infusion pump or injection port. By using this route, we can achieve high opioid concentrations at receptors on pain pathways in the spinal cord. It is important to note, however, that effects will not be limited to the spinal cord: Intraspinal opioids undergo absorption into the blood in amounts sufficient to cause systemic effects. In fact, blood levels may be equivalent to those achieved with conventional routes (e.g., SC). Intraspinal administration is especially useful for patients with severe pain in the lower body: Pain is relieved in up to 90% of appropriate candidates. Patients who are tolerant to opioids delivered by other routes will also be tolerant to opioids given intraspinally; dosage should be adjusted accordingly. Patients should have access to rescue medication in case breakthrough pain occurs—because of either system malfunction or inadequate dosing. Side effects with intraspinal administration are the same as with other routes. In addition, there is a risk of *delayed* respiratory depression as well as infection associated with the catheter.

Intraventricular. Like intraspinal administration, intraventricular administration is reserved for patients whose pain cannot be controlled with less invasive routes. In this procedure, morphine is delivered to the cerebral ventricles via a catheter connected to an external infusion pump (for continuous administration) or a subcutaneous reservoir (for intermittent administration). Because morphine is delivered directly to the brain, bypassing the blood-brain barrier, analgesia can be achieved with extremely low doses (e.g., 5 mg daily). Pain is relieved in 90% of patients. Intraventricular administration is especially helpful for patients with intractable pain caused by head and neck malignancies or tumors that affect the brachial plexus.

Patient-Controlled Analgesia. Patient-controlled analgesia (PCA) is a method of drug delivery that permits patients to control the amount of opioid they receive. PCA is accomplished using a PCA device to deliver opioids through an indwelling IV or SC catheter. The PCA device is an electronically controlled infusion pump that (1) delivers a continuous basal infusion of opioid and (2) can be activated manually by the patient to deliver additional bolus doses for breakthrough pain. To prevent an overdose, the device (1) limits the total dose of opioid that can be delivered per hour and (2) sets a minimum interval (e.g., 10 minutes) between bolus doses, thereby preventing the patient from giving a second dose before the prior one can take full effect. PCA devices are safe for use in the hospital and at home, but should not be used by patients who are sedated or confused. PCA administration is discussed at length in Chapter 27.

Managing Breakthrough Pain

Many patients whose pain is well controlled most of the day experience transient episodes of moderate to severe pain, known as breakthrough pain. Breakthrough pain develops quickly, reaches peak intensity in minutes, and may persist from minutes to hours (the median duration is 30 minutes). At least 50% of cancer patients experience these episodes, typically 1 to 4 times a day. Breakthrough pain may occur spontaneously, or it may be precipitated by coughing or other movements. In contrast to end-of-dose pain, which occurs because analgesic levels are lowest at that time, breakthrough pain can occur at any time in the dosing interval.

All patients receiving ATC opioids for persistent pain should have access to a rescue medication to manage breakthrough pain. Because breakthrough pain is both severe and self-limited, the best medication is a strong opioid with a rapid onset and short duration. The rapid onset permits speedy relief, and the short duration facilitates dosage titration. For ease of administration, oral and transmucosal formulations are preferred; examples include immediate-release oral morphine and transmucosal fentanyl [Actiq]. The dosage, as recommended by the American Pain Society, should be equivalent to one-sixth of the total daily opioid dose, repeated in 2 hours if needed.

Managing Side Effects

Side effects of the opioids include respiratory depression, sedation, constipation, orthostatic hypotension, nausea, and vomiting. All can be effectively managed. In many patients, side effects can be reduced simply by decreasing the dosage (typically by 25%). If dosage reduction causes pain to return, adding a nonopioid analgesic may take care of the problem. Over time, tolerance develops to sedation, respiratory depression, nausea, and vomiting—but not to constipation.

Respiratory Depression. Respiratory depression is the most serious side effect of the opioids; death can result. Fortunately, when dosage and monitoring are appropriate, significant respiratory depression is rare. Pain counteracts the depressant actions of opioids. Hence, as pain decreases, respiratory depression may deepen.

Respiratory depression is greatest at the outset of treatment and then decreases as tolerance develops. As a result, small initial doses of opioids (e.g., 5 mg of IV morphine every hour) can pose a greater risk than much larger doses (e.g., 1000 mg of IV morphine every hour) given later on.

Significant respiratory depression is most likely when dosage is being titrated up. The best way to assess the risk of impending respiratory depression is to monitor opioid-induced sedation. Why? Because an increase in sedation generally precedes an increase in respiratory depression. Hence, if excessive sedation is observed, further dosing should be delayed.

Respiratory depression is increased by other drugs with CNS-depressant actions (e.g., alcohol, barbiturates, benzodiazepines). Accordingly, these agents should be avoided.

Severe respiratory depression can be reversed with *naloxone* [Narcan], a pure opioid antagonist. However, caution is required: Excessive dosing will reverse analgesia, thereby putting the patient in great pain. Accordingly, naloxone dosage must be titrated carefully.

When death is near, should opioids be withheld out of fear that respiratory depression may bring death sooner? For several reasons, the answer is "No." First, significant respiratory depression is rare in the tolerant patient. Hence, concerns about hastening death are largely unfounded. Second, unrelieved pain can itself hasten death. Third, when death is imminent, it is more important to provide comfort than prolong life. Accordingly, adequate opioids should be provided, even if doing so means life may be shortened a little.

Constipation. Constipation occurs in most patients. Opioids promote constipation by decreasing propulsive intestinal contractions, increasing nonpropulsive contractions, increasing the tone of the anal sphincter, and reducing fluid secretion into the intestinal lumen. No tolerance to these effects develops. To reduce constipation, all patients should increase dietary fiber and fluid. However, most patients also need pharmacologic help. Options include stool softeners (e.g., docusate), stimulant laxatives (e.g., senna), and osmotic laxatives (e.g., milk of magnesia). For prophylaxis of constipation, current guidelines recommend daily therapy with a combination product, such as Senokot-S, which contains both senna and docusate. Drugs with anticholinergic properties (e.g., tricyclic antidepressants, antihistamines) can exacerbate opioid-induced constipation (by further depressing bowel function), and hence should be avoided.

Sedation. Sedation is common early in therapy, but tolerance develops quickly. If sedation persists, it can be reduced by giving smaller doses of the opioid more frequently, while keeping the total dose the same. This dosing schedule will decrease peak opioid levels, and hence reduce excessive CNS depression. If necessary, sedation can be opposed with a CNS stimulant (e.g., caffeine, methylphenidate, dextroamphetamine).

Other Side Effects. Initial doses of opioids may cause *nausea* and *vomiting*. Fortunately, tolerance develops rapidly. Nausea and vomiting can be minimized by pretreatment with an antiemetic (e.g., prochlorperazine, metoclopramide).

Opioids promote histamine release, and can thereby cause *itching*. Itching can be relieved with an antihistamine (e.g., diphenhydramine).

Opioids increase the tone in the urinary bladder sphincter, and can thereby cause *urinary retention*. Prostatic hypertrophy and use of anticholinergic drugs will exacerbate the problem. Patients should be monitored for urinary retention and encouraged to void every 4 hours.

Opioids can cause *orthostatic hypotension*. Patients should be informed about symptoms of hypotension (lightheadedness, dizziness) and instructed to sit or lie down if they occur. Orthostatic hypotension can be minimized by moving slowly when changing from a supine or seated position to an upright posture.

Adjuvant Analgesics

Adjuvant analgesics are used to *complement* the effects of opioids. Accordingly, these drugs are employed in *combination* with opioids—not as substitutes. Adjuvant analgesics can (1) enhance analgesia from opioids, (2) help manage concurrent symptoms that exacerbate pain, and (3) treat side effects caused by opioids. Several of the adjuvants are especially useful for *neuropathic pain*. The adjuvant analgesics differ from opioids in that pain relief is limited and less predictable, and often develops slowly. Adjuvant agents may be employed at any step on the analgesic ladder. The adjuvants are interesting in that, although they can relieve pain, they were developed to treat other conditions (e.g., depression, seizures, dysrhythmias). Accordingly, it is important to reassure patients that the adjuvant is being used to alleviate pain, and not for its original purpose. Dosages for the adjuvant analgesics are summarized in Table 28–5.

TABLE 28–5 ■ **Adjuvant Drugs for Cancer Pain**

Drug	Usual Adult Dosage	Beneficial Actions
Tricyclic Antidepressants		
Amitriptyline [Elavil]	25–150 mg/day PO	Reduce neuropathic pain
Desipramine [Norpramin]	25–150 mg/day PO	
Doxepin [Sinequan]	25–150 mg/day PO	
Imipramine [Tofranil]	20–100 mg/day PO	
Nortriptyline [Aventyl, Pamelor]	25–150 mg/day PO	
Anticonvulsants		
Carbamazepine [Tegretol]	200–1600 mg/day PO	Reduce neuropathic pain
Gabapentin [Neurontin]	300–3600 mg/day PO	
Phenytoin [Dilantin]	300–500 mg/day PO	
Local Anesthetics/Antidysrhythmics		
Lidocaine	5 mg/kg/day IV or SC	Reduce neuropathic pain
Mexiletine [Mexitil]	450–600 mg/day PO	
CNS Stimulants		
Dextroamphetamine [Dexedrine]	5–10 mg/day PO	Enhance analgesia and reduce
Methylphenidate [Ritalin]	10–15 mg/day PO	sedation from opioids
Antihistamine		
Hydroxyzine [Vistaril]	300–450 mg/day IM	Enhances analgesia and reduces anxiety, insomnia, and nausea
Glucocorticoids		
Dexamethasone [Decadron, others]	16–96 mg/day PO or IV	Reduce pain associated with brain
Prednisone [Deltasone, Orasone]	40–100 mg/day PO	metastases and epidural spinal cord compression
Bisphosphonates		
Etidronate [Didronel]	7.5 mg/kg IV for 3 days	Reduce hypercalcemia and
Pamidronate [Aredia]	60–90 mg IV once	possibly bone pain

Tricyclic Antidepressants

Amitriptyline [Elavil] and other tricyclic antidepressants (TCAs) can reduce pain of *neuropathic* origin. TCAs have analgesic effects of their own and they enhance the effects of opioids, and may thereby allow a reduction in opioid dosage. As a side benefit, TCAs can elevate mood. Important adverse effects are orthostatic hypotension, sedation, anticholinergic effects (dry mouth, urinary retention, constipation), and weight gain (secondary to improved appetite). Dosing at bedtime takes advantage of sedative effects, and minimizes hypotension during the day. Effects begin in 1 to 2 weeks and reach their maximum in 4 to 6 weeks. The TCAs are discussed at length in Chapter 31.

Anticonvulsants

Certain antiseizure drugs can help relieve *neuropathic pain.* Lancinating pain (sharp, darting pain) is especially responsive, although other forms of neuropathic pain (cramping pain, aching pain, burning pain) also respond. Analgesia is thought to result from suppressing spontaneous neuronal firing. Of the available anticonvulsants, *carbamazepine* [Tegretol] has been used most widely. Because carbamazepine is myelosuppressive, it must be used with caution in patients receiving anticancer drugs that suppress bone marrow function. Recent experience indicates that *gabapentin* [Neurontin] can be very effective, while causing fewer side effects than carbamazepine. Dosage should be low initially (100 mg once a day) and then gradually increased; dosages as high as 1200 mg 3 times a day have been employed. The anticonvulsants are discussed at length in Chapter 23.

Local Anesthetics/Antidysrhythmics

Lidocaine (a local anesthetic and antidysrhythmic) and *mexiletine* (an antidysrhythmic related to lidocaine) are considered second-line agents for *neuropathic pain.* Intravenous infusion of lidocaine produces analgesia in 10 to 15 minutes. The drug may be most appropriate for rapidly escalating neuropathic pain. Both lidocaine and mexiletine are discussed in Chapter 47 (Antidysrhythmic Drugs). Lidocaine is also discussed in Chapter 25 (Local Anesthetics).

CNS Stimulants

The CNS stimulants, such as dextroamphetamine [Dexedrine] and methylphenidate [Ritalin] have two beneficial effects: they can enhance opioid-induced analgesia and they can counteract opioid-induced sedation. In addition, they can be used for rapid elevation of mood. Principal adverse effects are weight loss (because of appetite suppression) and insomnia (because of CNS stimulation). To minimize interference with sleep, dosing late in the day should be avoided. The CNS stimulants are discussed fully in Chapter 35.

Antihistamines

Hydroxyzine [Vistaril], an antihistamine, has several useful properties. It can reduce pain, anxiety, and nausea, and it also has sedative actions. Hydroxyzine may be especially useful for promoting analgesia in patients with anxiety. The antihistamines are discussed fully in Chapter 66.

Glucocorticoids

Although glucocorticoids lack direct analgesic actions, they can help manage painful cancer-related conditions. Because glucocorticoids can reduce cerebral and spinal edema, these drugs are essential for the emergency management of elevated intracranial pressure and epidural spinal cord compression. Similarly, glucocorticoids are part of the standard therapy for tumor-induced spinal cord compression. In addition to these benefits, glucocorticoids can improve appetite and impart a general sense of well-being; both actions help in managing anorexia (loss of appetite) and cachexia (weakness and emaciation) associated with terminal illness.

Glucocorticoids are very safe when used short term (even in high doses) and very dangerous when used long term (even in low doses). In particular, long-term therapy can cause adrenal insufficiency, osteoporosis, glucose intolerance (hyperglycemia), increased vulnerability to infection, thinning of the skin, and, possibly, peptic ulcer disease (PUD). Concurrent therapy with NSAIDs augments the risk of PUD. The risk of osteoporosis can be reduced by giving calcium supplements and vitamin D along with calcitonin or a bisphosphonate (e.g., etidronate). The glucocorticoids are discussed fully in Chapter 68.

Bisphosphonates

Bisphosphonates, such as etidronate [Didronel] and pamidronate [Aredia], can reduce cancer-related bone pain in some patients. Bone pain is common when cancers metastasize to bone. The cause of pain may be tumor-induced bone resorption, which can also cause hypercalcemia, osteoporosis, and related fractures. Bisphosphonates inhibit bone resorption and are approved for treating hypercalcemia of malignancy—but not bone pain. However, when these drugs were given to treat hypercalcemia, many patients reported a reduction in bone pain, although others did not. Hence, although these drugs appear promising, their use for management of bone pain is still considered investigational. The bisphosphonates are discussed further in Chapter 70.

NONDRUG THERAPY

Invasive Procedures

Invasive therapies are the last resort for relieving intractable pain. Hence, for most patients, all other options should be exhausted before these are tried.

Neurolytic Nerve Block

The goal of this procedure is to destroy neurons that transmit pain from a limited area, thereby providing permanent pain relief. Nerve destruction is accomplished through local injection of a neurolytic (neurotoxic) substance, typically alcohol or phenol. To ensure that the right nerves are destroyed, reversible nerve block is done first, using a local anesthetic. If the local anesthetic relieves the pain, a neurolytic agent is then applied to the same site. Neurolytic nerve block can eliminate pain in up to 80% of patients. However, even if pain relief is only partial, the procedure can still permit some reduction in opioid dosage, and can thereby decrease side effects (e.g., sedation, constipation). When nerve block is successful and opioids are discontinued, opioid dosage should be tapered gradually to avoid withdrawal. Nerve block is not without risk. Potential complications include hypotension, paresis (slight paralysis), paralysis, and disruption of bowel and bladder function (e.g., diarrhea, incontinence). The incidence of complications ranges between 0.5% and 2%.

Neurosurgery

Neurosurgeons relieve cancer pain in several ways. They can destroy neurons that transmit pain signals; they can implant opioid infusion systems; and, in a procedure known as neuroaugmentation, they can implant electrodes to stimulate neurons that release endogenous opioid peptides (e.g., endorphins). Nerve damage incurred during these surgeries can result in neurologic deficits and new pain. Less than 10% of cancer patients undergo neurosurgery for pain relief.

Tumor Surgery

When curative excision of a tumor is not feasible, it may still be appropriate to surgically debulk the tumor with the goal of relieving pain. Unfortunately, palliative debulking only provides temporary relief: Growth of residual cancer cells eventually causes pain to return. Radiation therapy following the surgery may extend pain relief.

Radiation Therapy

Radiation therapy relieves pain by causing tumor regression. Palliative treatment can be directed at primary tumors and at metastases anywhere in the body.

Radiation can be delivered in three forms: *brachytherapy* (implanted radioactive pellets), *teletherapy* (external beam radiation), and *intravenous radiopharmaceuticals*. With brachytherapy, cell kill is limited to the immediate area of the implanted pellets; hence, the technique is suited only for localized tumors. With teletherapy, cell kill can be localized or widespread, depending on the size of the beam employed; hence, the technique can be used for both local tumors as well as metastases. Intravenous radiopharmaceuticals travel throughout the body, and hence are best suited for widespread metastases.

With radiation therapy, as with chemotherapy, damage to normal tissue is dose limiting. Therefore, the challenge is to deliver a dose of radiation that is large enough to kill cancer cells, but not so large that it causes intolerable damage to healthy tissue.

Some side effects of radiation occur early and some occur late. Early effects develop during or immediately after radiation exposure. Late reactions develop months or years later. The most common early effects are skin inflammation and lesions of the GI mucosa. Fortunately, in the regimens employed for palliation, these acute effects are generally mild. The most common late reaction is fibrosis, which occurs mainly in tissues that have a limited ability to regenerate (e.g., brain, peripheral neurons, lung). Late reactions are of limited concern, however, because most patients die from their cancer before late reactions have time to develop.

Physical and Psychosocial Interventions

Physical and psychosocial interventions can help reduce pain, but the degree of relief is limited. Accordingly, these interventions should be used only in conjunction with drug therapy—not as substitutes.

Physical Interventions

Physical interventions (e.g., heat, massage, vibration) can help relieve aches and pains associated with cancer.

Heat. Application of heat can benefit the patient in at least two ways: (1) heat promotes vasodilation, and can thereby increase delivery of oxygen and nutrients to damaged tissue, and (2) heat increases elasticity in muscle, and can thereby reduce stiffness. Heat may be applied in several ways, including use of hot compresses, hot water bottles, and electric heating pads. Heat may be harmful to tissue exposed to radiation, and hence these areas should be avoided. There is some concern that heat may actually stimulate tumor growth and metastatic spread, although convincing data are lacking.

Cold. Application of cold can reduce inflammation and muscle spasm. Cold can be applied using ice packs, chemical gel packs, and towels soaked in ice water. Application should last no longer than 15 minutes. Cold should not be applied to areas damaged by radiation. In addition, because cold promotes vasoconstriction, it should be avoided in patients with peripheral vascular disease, Raynaud's syndrome, and all other disorders that can be exacerbated by vasoconstriction.

Massage. Massage is primarily a comfort measure that provides relief through distraction and relaxation. In addition, massage may help ease discomfort at specific sites by increasing local circulation.

Exercise. Exercise can reduce subacute and chronic pain by increasing muscle strength and joint mobility. Additional benefits include improved cardiovascular conditioning and restoration of coordination and balance. Range-of-motion exercises can preserve strength and joint function. When patients cannot perform these exercises on their own, family members should be taught to assist them. Although weight-bearing exercise is desirable, it should be avoided in patients at risk of fractures because of tumor invasion or osteoporosis.

Acupuncture and Transcutaneous Electrical Nerve Stimulation. In theory, these techniques reduce pain by stimulating peripheral nerves, which in turn activate central pain-modulating pathways. However, the efficacy of both techniques in cancer patients is uncertain. Acupuncture is performed by inserting solid needles through the skin into the underlying muscle. Transcutaneous electrical nerve stimulation (TENS) is performed using low-voltage cutaneous electrodes. Because the efficacy of these techniques is questionable, pain status must be closely monitored.

Psychosocial Interventions

Psychosocial interventions can help patients cope by (1) increasing the sense of control over pain, (2) reversing negative thoughts and feelings, and (3) offering social support. Interventions that require learning and practice should be introduced early so that they can be perfected while the patient still has sufficient energy and strength to learn them.

Relaxation and Imagery. The aim of these techniques is to reduce pain by inducing both mental relaxation (alleviation of anxiety) and physical relaxation (release of tension in skeletal muscles). These techniques are easy to learn and require little or no special equipment. Examples include (1) meditation, (2) slow rhythmic breathing, (3) imagining a peaceful scene (e.g., gentle waves breaking on a secluded, sunny beach), and (4) active listening to recorded music (e.g., tapping a finger in time to an enjoyable tune).

Cognitive Distraction. The goal of cognitive distraction is to divert attention away from pain and associated negative emotions. Distractions may be internal or external. Examples of internal distractions include praying, counting or singing in one's head, and repeating positive thoughts, such as "I can cope." External distractions include watching TV, listening to music, and conversing with friends.

Peer Support Groups. Support groups composed of other cancer patients can help members cope with pain and all other sequelae of the disease. These groups can provide emotional support, cancer-related information, and a sense of social belonging. Talking with other cancer survivors can be especially helpful for patients with newly diagnosed disease. Some support groups welcome patients who have any form of cancer; others are dedicated to just one form of the disease (e.g., breast cancer). Resources for locating a support group in your community include (1) the National Coalition for Cancer Survivorship, at 1-877-622-7937; (2) the National Cancer Information Service, at 1-800-4-CANCER; and (3) your local chapter of the American Cancer Society, whose number should be in your phone book.

PAIN MANAGEMENT IN SPECIAL POPULATIONS

The Elderly

In elderly patients, two issues are of special concern: (1) undertreatment of pain and (2) increased risk of adverse effects. Paradoxically, a third issue—heightened drug sensitivity—contributes to both problems.

Heightened Drug Sensitivity. The elderly are more sensitive to drugs than are younger adults, owing largely to a decline in organ function. In particular, rates of hepatic metabolism and renal excretion decline with age. As a result, drugs tend to accumulate in the body, causing responses to be more intense and prolonged.

Undertreatment of Pain. Undertreatment is common in the elderly. In addition to the usual reasons (fears about tolerance, addiction, and adverse effects), the elderly are denied adequate medication for two more: difficulties with assessment and erroneous ideas about old age.

Assessment is made difficult by cognitive impairment (e.g., delirium, dementia) and by impairment of vision and hearing. As a result, self-reporting of pain may be inaccurate or even impossible. Because of these obstacles, special effort must be made to help ensure that assessment is accurate. However, because accuracy cannot be guaranteed, frequent reassessment is recommended.

Misconceptions about the elderly contribute to undertreatment. Specifically, providers may believe (incorrectly) that dosage should be low because (1) the elderly are relatively insensitive to pain; (2) if pain occurs, the elderly can tolerate it well; and (3) the elderly are highly sensitive to opioid side effects. The first two concepts have no basis in fact, and therefore must not be allowed to influence treatment. Although there is some truth to the third concept, concern about side effects is no excuse for inadequate dosing.

Increased Risk of Side Effects and Adverse Interactions. For several reasons, elderly patients may experience more side effects than younger adults. As noted, drug elimination in the elderly is impaired, posing a risk that drug levels may rise dangerously high. However, with careful dosing, drug levels can be kept within a range that is both safe and effective. Drugs with prolonged half-lives (e.g., methadone) pose an increased risk of excessive accumulation, and hence should be avoided.

The risk of gastric ulceration and renal toxicity from NSAIDs is increased in older patients. Gastric erosion can be reduced by concurrent therapy with misoprostol. There is no specific way to prevent renal toxicity. Hence, the best we can do is monitor closely for evolving kidney damage.

Older patients are at increased risk of adverse drug-drug interactions. Why? Because, in addition to the disorder that's causing pain, the elderly are likely to have other disorders, and hence require more drugs than younger adults. The risk of serious injury from drug-drug interactions can be reduced by careful drug selection and by monitoring for potential reactions.

Young Children

Management of cancer pain in children is much like management in adults. The principal difference is that assessment in children is more difficult. In addition, children frequently experience more pain from chemotherapy and other interventions than from the cancer itself.

Assessment

Assessment must be tailored to the child's developmental level and personality. Selection of an appropriate assessment method is especially important for children with developmental delays, learning disabilities, and emotional disturbances. Assessment can be greatly facilitated by open communication about pain between the child, family, and healthcare team.

Assessment methods include self-reporting, behavioral observation, and measurement of physiologic parameters (e.g., heart rate, blood pressure, respiratory rate, sweating). As stressed earlier, self-reporting is preferred and should be employed whenever appropriate. Behavioral observation is a distant second choice. Because many factors other than pain can alter physiologic parameters, measuring these is the least reliable way to assess pain.

Verbal Children. For children who can verbalize and are over the age of 4, self-reporting is the most reliable way to assess pain. Since children rarely claim to have pain that isn't there, there is little risk of error from over-reporting. However, there *is* a significant risk of error from under-reporting. Children may report less pain than they have for several reasons. These include (1) fear that revealing their pain will lead to additional injections and other painful procedures, (2) lack of awareness that we can help their pain go away, (3) a desire to protect their parents from the knowledge that their cancer is getting worse, and (4) a desire to please. Because the self-report may conceal pain, it can be helpful to supplement the self-report with behavioral observation (see below).

Preverbal and Nonverbal Children. Since preverbal and nonverbal children cannot self-report pain, a less reliable method must be used for assessment. The principal alternative is *behavioral observation.* Behavioral cues suggesting pain include vocalization (crying, whining, groaning), facial expression (grimacing, frowning, reduced affect), muscle tension, inability to be consoled, protection of body areas, and reduced activity. The biggest drawback to behavioral observation is the risk of a false-negative conclusion. That is, a child may be in pain although his or her behavior may lead the observer to conclude otherwise. For example, sleeping, watching television, or laughing may suggest that a child is comfortable; however, these behaviors can actually represent an attempt to control pain. Similarly, although sitting quietly might indicate comfort, it could also mean that moving and talking are painful. When behavioral observation leaves doubt about whether the child is in pain, a trial with an analgesic can help confirm the assessment.

Treatment

Therapy of cancer pain in children is essentially the same as in adults. As in adults, drugs are the cornerstone of treatment; nondrug therapies are used only as supplements. Drug selection is guided by the WHO analgesic ladder. Because of the risk of Reye's syndrome, children with influenza or chickenpox should not receive NSAIDs; acetaminophen is a safe alternative. As in adults, oral administration is preferred; more invasive routes should be reserved for patients who cannot take drugs by mouth. Children generally object to rectal administration, and may refuse treatment by this route. Administration with a PCA device is an option for children over the age of 7.

Neonates and infants are highly sensitive to drugs, and hence must be treated with special caution. Drug sensitivity occurs for two reasons: (1) the blood-brain barrier is incompletely formed, giving drugs ready access to the CNS; and (2) the kidneys and liver are poorly developed, causing drug elimination to be slow. Because of heightened drug sensitivity, neonates and infants are at increased risk of respiratory depression from opioids. Accordingly, when opioids are given to nonventilated infants, the initial dosage should be very low (about one-third the dosage employed for older children). Furthermore, use of opioids should be accompanied by intensive monitoring of respiration.

Opioid Abusers

When treating cancer pain in opioid abusers, we have two primary obligations: we must (1) try to relieve the pain and (2) try to avoid giving opioids simply because the patient wants to get high. Both obligations are difficult to meet. Because of the challenge, treatment should be directed by a clinician trained in substance abuse as well as pain management.

Concerns about abuse can result in undertreatment of pain. This must be avoided. Remember, abusers feel pain like everyone else, and therefore need opioids like everyone else. Clinicians must take special care not to withhold opioids because they have confused relief-seeking behavior with drug-seeking behavior. In the end, we have little choice but to base treatment on the patient's self-report of pain. Hence, if the patient tells us that pain is persisting, adequate doses of opioids should be provided.

Because of opioid tolerance, initial doses in abusers must be higher than in nonabusers. To estimate how high the initial dosage should be, we must try to estimate the existing degree of tolerance by interviewing the patient about the extent of opioid use.

As with all other patients, drug selection is guided by the WHO ladder. If pain is sufficient to justify opioids, then opioids should be used; nonopioids (NSAIDs and acetaminophen) should not be substituted for opioids out of concern for addiction. If the patient is on methadone maintenance, methadone can be used for the pain. However, because regulations limit the dosage of methadone that drug-abuse clinics can dispense,

the increased dosage needed to manage pain will have to come from another source. One group of opioids—the agonist-antagonists—will precipitate withdrawal in opioid abusers, and hence must never be prescribed for these patients.

Paradoxically, drug delivery with a PCA device can be helpful. By using a PCA device, we can avoid potential conflicts between the patient and the clinician, who would otherwise have to administer each dose. Excessive dosing can be prevented by setting the PCA device to limit how much opioid the patient can self-administer.

PATIENT EDUCATION

Patient education is an integral part of cancer pain management. When education is successful, it can help reduce anxiety, dispel hopelessness, facilitate assessment, enhance compliance, decrease complications, provide a sense of control, and enable patients to take an active role in their care. All of these, of course, will promote pain relief.

General Issues

Common sense tells us that patient education should be accurate, comprehensive, and understandable. To reinforce communication, information should be presented at least twice and in more than one way. Major topics to discuss are (1) the nature and causes of pain, (2) assessment and the importance of honest self-reporting, and (3) plans for drug and nondrug therapy. Patients should be encouraged to express their fears and concerns about cancer, cancer pain, and pain treatment—and they should be reassured that pain can be effectively controlled in most cases. All patients should receive a written pain management plan. To facilitate ongoing education, patients should be invited to contact care providers whenever they feel the need—be it to discuss specific concerns with treatment or simply to acquire new information. Finally, patients should know when and how to contact the physician to report new pain, treatment failure, or serious side effects.

Drug Therapy

The goal in teaching patients about analgesic drugs is to maximize pain relief and minimize harm. To help achieve this goal, patients should know the following about each drug they take:

- Drug name and therapeutic category
- Dosage size and dosing schedule
- Route and technique of administration
- Expected therapeutic response and when it should develop
- Duration of treatment
- Method of drug storage
- Symptoms of major adverse effects and measures to minimize discomfort and harm
- Major adverse drug-drug and drug-food interactions
- Whom to contact in the event of therapeutic failure, severe adverse effects, or severe adverse interactions

The dosing schedule should be discussed. Patients should understand that PRN dosing is appropriate only if pain is intermittent. When pain is persistent (as it is for most patients), the objective is to *prevent* pain from returning. Hence, dosing should be done on a fixed schedule ATC, not PRN. However, even with

ATC dosing, breakthrough pain can occur. Hence, patients should be taught what dosage to use for rescue treatment.

Fears based on misconceptions about opioids can impair compliance, and can thereby impair pain control. The misconceptions that influence compliance most relate to tolerance, physical dependence, addiction, and side effects. To correct these misconceptions, and thereby dispel fears and improve compliance, the following topics should be discussed:

- *Tolerance*—Some patients fear that, because of tolerance, taking opioids now will decrease their effectiveness later on. Hence, to help ensure pain relief in the future, they limit current opioid use—and thus suffer needless pain. These patients should be reassured that, if tolerance does develop, efficacy can be restored by simply increasing the dosage; tolerance does not mean that efficacy is lost.
- *Physical Dependence and Addiction*—Many patients fear opioid addiction, and hence are reluctant to take these drugs. This fear is based largely on the misconception that physical dependence (which eventually develops in all patients) is equivalent to addiction. Patients should be taught that physical dependence is not the same as addiction, and that physical dependence itself is nothing to fear. In addition, they should be taught that the behavior pattern that constitutes addiction rarely develops in people who take opioids in a therapeutic setting.
- *Fear of Severe Side Effects*—Some patients fear that opioids cannot relieve pain without causing severe side effects. These patients should be reassured that, when used correctly, opioids are both safe and effective. The most dangerous side effect—respiratory depression—is uncommon.

The rationale for using an adjuvant analgesic should be discussed. With all of the adjuvants, the objective is to *complement* the effects of opioid and nonopioid analgesics. Adjuvants are not intended as substitutes for these drugs. Furthermore, because the drugs we use as adjuvants were originally developed to treat disorders other than pain, the rationale for prescribing specific adjuvants should be explained. For example, when imipramine is prescribed, the patients should understand that the objective is to relieve neuropathic pain—not depression, the disorder for which this drug was originally developed.

Basic issues related to patient education in drug therapy are discussed at length in Chapter 2.

Nondrug Therapy

Education regarding nondrug therapy focuses on psychosocial interventions. Patients should understand that these interventions are intended as complements to analgesics—not as alternatives. Techniques for imaging, relaxation, and distraction should be introduced early in treatment. Family caregivers should be taught how to apply heat and cold and how to give a therapeutic massage. Patients should be informed about the benefits of peer support groups and given assistance in locating one.

JCAHO PAIN MANAGEMENT STANDARDS

There's a new sheriff in town and she's laid down the law: Undertreatment of pain will no longer be tolerated! This is no idle threat. The "sheriff" is the *Joint Commission on*

Accreditation of Healthcare Organizations (JCAHO), an organization charged with accrediting hospitals and other healthcare institutions in the United States. The "law" is a new set of pain management standards, established by JCAHO, that took effect on January 1, 2001. The purpose of the standards is to make assessment and management of pain a priority in the nation's healthcare system. Under the standards, *accountability for pain management is shifted from individual practitioners to the institution as a whole.* Compliance is mandatory: Healthcare organizations that fail to meet the standards will lose accreditation. This is serious. Why? Because loss of accreditation would mean loss of insurance reimbursement, and would disqualify teaching hospitals from offering training programs. Hence, thanks to the enforcement power wielded by JCAHO, healthcare institutions in the United States now have a very real incentive to correct the persistent problem of pain undertreatment. It should be noted that the JCAHO standards are *not* a guideline on how to treat specific kinds of pain. Rather, the standards focus on (1) the rights of patients to receive appropriate assessment and management of pain and (2) ways for institutions to establish a formalized, systematic approach to pain management that involves interdisciplinary teams whose members have clearly identified responsibilities. Specific provisions include the following:

- Institutions must recognize assessment and management of pain as a right of all patients.
- Institutions must assess all patients for pain and, if pain is present, identify its nature and intensity.
- Pain must be regarded as a "fifth vital sign," and pain intensity must be quantified and recorded along with blood pressure, heart rate, respiration, and temperature.
- Institutions must educate patients and their families about pain management, and must provide ready access to educational materials.
- Institutions must educate clinical staff about assessment and management of pain and must document the education provided.
- Institutions must establish a system to monitor pain management, including a system of checks and balances in which individuals who assess and manage pain are monitored for compliance with standards set by the institution.
- Institutions must monitor patient satisfaction with pain management.
- Discharge planning must provide for continuing reassessment and management of pain.

Where can you find the new standards? Unfortunately, they don't exist as a separate document. Rather, JCAHO has inserted content related to pain management throughout existing manuals, including the *Comprehensive Accreditation Manual for Hospitals: The Official Handbook*. If you don't want to search through the manuals, a summary of the standards is available. You can purchase this document—*Pain Assessment and Management: An Organizational Approach* (published by Joint Commission Resources, Inc. [a subsidiary of JCAHO])—through the JCAHO web site (*www.jcaho.org*) or by calling 1-630-792-5800.

⁛ KEY POINTS

- Cancer pain can be relieved in 90% of patients.
- Despite the availability of effective treatments, cancer pain goes unrelieved in a large number of patients.
- Barriers to pain relief include inadequate physician training, fears of addiction, and a healthcare system that, until recently, has put a low priority on pain management.
- Pain is a personal, subjective experience that encompasses not only the sensory perception of pain but also the patient's emotional and cognitive responses to both the painful sensation and the underlying disease.
- Pain has two major forms: nociceptive pain, which results from injury to tissues, and neuropathic pain, which results from injury to peripheral nerves.
- Management of cancer pain is an ongoing process that involves repeated cycles of assessment, intervention, and reassessment. The goal is to create an individualized treatment plan that can meet the changing needs of the patient.
- The patient self-report is the cornerstone of assessment.
- Behavioral observation is a poor substitute for the patient self-report as a method of assessment.
- Analgesic drugs are the principal modality for treating cancer pain.
- Three groups of analgesics are employed: nonopioid analgesics (NSAIDs and acetaminophen), opioid analgesics, and adjuvant analgesics.
- Drug selection is guided by the WHO analgesic ladder: As pain intensity increases, treatment progresses from nonopioid analgesics to opioids of moderate strength (e.g., oxycodone), and then to powerful opioids (e.g., morphine). Adjuvant analgesics can be used at any time.
- Because nonopioids and opioids relieve pain by different mechanisms, combining an opioid with a nonopioid can be more effective than either drug alone.
- NSAIDs produce their effects by inhibiting COX-1 and COX-2. Inhibition of COX-1 promotes adverse effects: gastric ulceration, acute renal failure, and bleeding (by inhibiting platelet aggregation). Inhibition of COX-2 promotes beneficial effects: reduction of pain, inflammation, and fever.
- By inhibiting platelet aggregation, NSAIDs increase the risk of bruising and bleeding in patients with thrombocytopenia, a common side effect of cancer chemotherapy.
- In contrast to opioids, NSAIDs do not cause tolerance, physical dependence, or psychologic dependence.
- Acetaminophen relieves pain but does not suppress inflammation, inhibit platelet aggregation, or promote gastric ulceration or renal failure.
- Because acetaminophen does not affect platelets, the drug is safe for patients with thrombocytopenia.
- Combining acetaminophen with alcohol, even in moderate amounts, can result in potentially fatal liver damage.
- Opioids are the most effective analgesics available, and hence are the primary drugs for treating moderate to severe cancer pain.
- Opioids are especially effective against nociceptive pain; efficacy against neuropathic pain is limited.
- Opioid analgesics relieve pain by mimicking the actions of endogenous opioid peptides (enkephalins, dynorphins, endorphins), primarily at mu receptors in the CNS.
- The opioids fall into two major groups: pure (full) agonists (e.g., morphine) and agonist-antagonists (e.g., butorphanol).
- There is a ceiling to pain relief with the agonist-antagonists, but not with the pure agonists. Hence, pure agonists are generally preferred for patients with cancer pain.
- For most patients, opioids should be given on a fixed schedule ATC, with additional doses provided for breakthrough pain. PRN dosing should be limited to patients with intermittent pain.
- Oral administration is preferred for most patients; transdermal administration is a good alternative.
- Intramuscular opioids are painful and should be avoided.
- PCA is a desirable method of opioid delivery because it gives patients more control over their treatment.
- An equianalgesia table can facilitate dosage selection when switching from one opioid to another or from one route to another.
- Over time, opioids cause tolerance, a state in which a specific dose produces a smaller effect than it could when treatment began.
- Tolerance develops to analgesia, euphoria, respiratory depression, and sedation, but not to constipation.
- Over time, opioids produce physical dependence, a state in which an abstinence syndrome will occur if the drug is abruptly withdrawn. *Note:* Physical dependence is NOT the same as addiction!
- Addiction is a behavior pattern characterized by continued use of a psychoactive substance despite physical, psychologic, or social harm. *Note:* Addiction is NOT the same as physical dependence!
- Addiction to opioids is very rare in people taking opioids to relieve pain.
- Misconceptions about opioid addiction are a major cause for undertreatment of cancer pain. Accordingly, we must correct these misconceptions by teaching physicians, nurses, patients, and family members that (1) addiction is not the same as physical dependence and (2) addiction is very rare in therapeutic settings.
- Respiratory depression is the most dangerous side effect of the opioids. Fortunately, significant respiratory depression is rare.
- Respiratory depression is increased by other drugs with CNS-depressant actions (e.g., alcohol, barbiturates, benzodiazepines). Accordingly, combining these agents with opioids should be avoided.
- Severe respiratory depression can be reversed with naloxone [Narcan], an opioid antagonist. However, because excessive naloxone will reverse opioid analgesia and precipitate withdrawal, dosage must be titrated carefully.

- Opioids cause constipation in most patients. No tolerance develops. Constipation can be minimized by increasing dietary fiber and fluid, and by taking one or more appropriate drugs (stool softener, stimulant laxative, osmotic laxative).
- Use of meperidine (a pure opioid agonist) should be limited to a few days because, with longer use, a toxic metabolite can accumulate.
- Agonist-antagonist opioids must not be given to patients taking pure opioid agonists because doing so could reduce analgesia and precipitate withdrawal.
- Adjuvant analgesics can enhance analgesia from opioids, help manage concurrent symptoms that exacerbate pain, and treat side effects caused by opioids. In addition, several adjuvants are effective against neuropathic pain.
- Adjuvant analgesics are given to complement the effects of opioids. Accordingly, these drugs are employed in combination with opioids—not as substitutes.
- Invasive therapies (nerve blocks, neurosurgical procedures, radiation) are the last resort for relieving intractable pain. All other options should be exhausted before these are tried.
- Physical interventions (e.g., heat, cold, massage, acupuncture, TENS) and psychosocial interventions (e.g., relaxation, imaging, cognitive distraction, peer support groups) can help reduce pain, but the degree of relief is limited. Accordingly, these interventions should be used only in conjunction with drug therapy—not as substitutes.

- Elderly patients are more sensitive to drugs than are younger adults. The principal reason is drug accumulation secondary to a decline in hepatic metabolism and renal excretion.
- Undertreatment of pain is especially common in the elderly. Undertreatment is inexcusable and must not be allowed.
- The elderly are at risk of increased side effects and adverse drug interactions. Careful drug selection and monitoring can minimize risk.
- Management of cancer pain in children is much like management in adults, except that assessment is more difficult.
- For children who can verbalize and are older than 4 years, self-reporting is the most reliable way to assess pain. The self-report can be supplemented with behavioral observation to enhance accuracy.
- Preverbal and nonverbal children cannot self-report pain, and hence a less reliable assessment method must be used. The principal option is behavioral observation, a method that carries a significant risk of underassessment.
- When opioid abusers get cancer, they feel pain and need relief like everyone else. If pain is sufficient to justify opioids, then opioids should be used; nonopioids should not be substituted for opioids out of concern for addiction.
- New pain management standards from JCAHO are designed to make pain relief an institutional priority, and hence should greatly reduce the incidence of pain undertreatment.

Drugs for Headache

Headache is a common symptom that can be triggered by a variety of stimuli, including stress, fatigue, acute illness, and sensitivity to alcohol. Many people experience mild, episodic headaches that can be relieved with over-the-counter medications, such as aspirin, acetaminophen [Tylenol], and ibuprofen [Motrin, Advil]. For these individuals, medical intervention is unnecessary. In contrast, some people experience severe, recurrent, debilitating headaches that are frequently unresponsive to aspirin-like drugs. For these individuals, medical attention is merited. In this chapter, our focus is on severe forms of headache—specifically, migraine, cluster, and tension-type headaches. Characteristics of these headache types are summarized in Table 29–1.

When attempting to treat headache, we must differentiate between headaches that have an identifiable underlying cause (e.g., severe hypertension; hyperthyroidism; tumors; infection; disorders of the eye, ear, nose, sinuses, and throat) and headaches that have no identifiable cause (e.g., migraine and cluster headaches). Obviously, if there is a clear cause, it should be treated directly.

As we consider drugs for headache, keep three basic principles in mind. First, antiheadache drugs may be used in two ways: to abort an ongoing attack and to prevent attacks from occurring. Second, not all patients with a particular type of headache respond to the same drugs; hence, therapy must be individualized. Third, several of the drugs employed to treat severe headaches (e.g., ergotamine, butalbital, opioids) can cause physical dependence. Accordingly, every effort should be made to keep dependence from developing. If dependence does develop, a withdrawal procedure is needed.

TABLE 29–1 ▪ Characteristics of Major Headache Syndromes

	Migraine	Cluster Headache	Tension Headache
Pain Location	Unilateral (60%) Bilateral (40%)	Unilateral, behind the right or left eye	Bilateral, in "head band" configuration
Pain Quality	Throbbing	Throbbing, sometimes piercing	Nonthrobbing
Pain Severity	Moderate to severe	Severe	Mild to moderate
Duration	4 hr to 3 days	15 min to 2 hr*	30 min to 7 days†
Impact of Activity	Worsens pain	None	None
Associated Symptoms	Nausea, vomiting, photophobia, phonophobia	Conjunctival redness, lacrimation, nasal congestion, rhinorrhea, ptosis, miosis—all on the same side as the headache	Uncommon
Usual Time of Onset	Early morning	Nighttime	Daytime
Preceded by Aura	Yes, in 30%	No	No
Triggers	Many (see Table 29–2)	Usually unidentified	Tension, anxiety
Gender Prevalence	More common in females (3:1)	More common in males (5:1)	Slightly (10%) more common in females
Family History	Likely	Unlikely	Unlikely
Impact on Daily Life	Often substantial	Usually substantial	Minimal

*Headaches occur in clusters that typically consist of one or more headaches (lasting 15 minutes to 2 hours) every day for 2 to 3 months, with a headache-free interval (months to years) between each cluster.
†*Chronic* tension headaches occur at least 15 days/month for 6 months or longer.

MIGRAINE HEADACHE I: CHARACTERISTICS AND OVERVIEW OF TREATMENT

Characteristics

Migraine headache is characterized by unilateral, throbbing head pain of moderate to severe intensity. Most patients also experience nausea and vomiting, along with sensitivity to light and sound. Physical activity intensifies the pain. Migraines usually develop in the morning after arising. Pain increases gradually and lasts 4 to 72 hours (median duration 24 hours). On average, attacks occur 1.5 times a month. Precipitating factors include anxiety, fatigue, stress, menstruation, alcohol, and tyramine-containing foods (Table 29–2).

Migraine has two primary forms: migraine *with aura* (formerly called classic migraine) and migraine *without aura* (formerly called common migraine). In migraine with aura, the headache is preceded by visual symptoms (flashes of light, a blank area in the field of vision, zigzag patterns). Of the two forms, migraine without aura is more common, affecting about 70% of migraineurs.

In the United States, 28 million people suffer from migraine. The disorder affects nearly 1 in 5 women and 1 in 20 men. About 65% of migraineurs are women in their late teens, 20s, or 30s. With some women, migraine attacks are worse during menstruation but subside during pregnancy and cease after menopause, indicating a hormonal component to the attacks. A family history of the disease is typical.

Migraine is highly debilitating. An attack can prevent participation in social and leisure activities, and can result in lost productivity at home, at school, and on the job. According to the World Health Organization, disability caused by a severe migraine attack equals that caused by quadriplegia, psychosis, or dementia.

Pathophysiology

Migraine headache is a *neurovascular* disorder that involves *dilation* and *inflammation* of intracranial blood vessels. Headache generation begins with neural events that trigger vasodilation. Vasodilation then leads to pain, which leads to further neural activation, thereby amplifying pain-generating signals. Neurons of the trigeminal vascular system, which innervate intracranial blood vessels, are key components in the process.

The exact cause of migraine pain is not completely understood—although vasodilation and inflammation are clearly involved. Available data suggest that two compounds—*calcitonin gene–related peptide* (CGRP) and *serotonin* (5-hydroxytryptamine [5-HT])—play important roles. The role of CGRP is to *promote* migraine, whereas the role of 5-HT is to *suppress* migraine. Data that implicate CGRP as a cause of migraine include the following:

- Plasma levels of CGRP rise during a migraine attack.
- Stimulation of neurons of the trigeminal vascular system promotes release of CGRP, which in turn promotes vasodilation and release of inflammatory neuropeptides.
- Administration of sumatriptan, a drug that relieves migraine, lowers elevated levels of CGRP.
- Sumatriptan can suppress release of CGRP from cultured trigeminal neurons.

Data that support a suppressive role for 5-HT include the following:

- Plasma levels of 5-HT drop by 50% during a migraine attack.
- Depletion of 5-HT with reserpine can precipitate an attack in migraine-prone individuals.
- Administration of 5-HT or sumatriptan, both of which activate 5-HT receptors, can abort an ongoing attack.

Overview of Treatment

Drugs for migraine are employed in two ways: to abort an ongoing attack and to prevent attacks from occurring. Drugs used to abort an attack fall into two groups: nonspecific analgesics (aspirin-like drugs and opioid analgesics) and migraine-specific drugs (ergot alkaloids and serotonin$_{1B/1D}$ agonists [triptans]). Drugs employed for prophylaxis include beta-blockers (e.g., propranolol), tricyclic antidepressants (e.g., amitriptyline), and anticonvulsants (e.g., divalproex).

Nondrug measures can help. Patients should try to control or eliminate triggers (see Table 29–2) and should maintain a regular pattern of eating, sleeping, and exercise. Why? Because, in people with migraine, the brain seems to have a low tolerance for the ups and downs of life. Once an attack has begun, the migraineur should retire to a dark, quiet room. Placing an ice pack on the neck and scalp can help too.

TABLE 29–2 ■ Factors That Can Precipitate Migraine Headache

Emotions

Stress
Anticipation
Anxiety
Depression
Excitement
Frustration

Foods That Contain:

Tyramine (e.g., aged cheeses, Chianti wine)
Nitrates (e.g., cured meat products)
Phenylethylamine (e.g., chocolate)
Monosodium glutamate (e.g., Chinese food, canned soups)
Aspartame (e.g., diet sodas, artificial sweeteners)
Yellow food coloring

Drugs

Alcohol
Analgesics (excessive use or withdrawal)
Caffeine (excessive use or withdrawal)
Cimetidine
Cocaine
Estrogens (e.g., oral contraceptives)
Nitroglycerin

Others

Carbon monoxide
Hormonal changes in women
Flickering lights/glare
Loud noises
Hypoglycemia
Change in altitude or barometric pressure
Altered sleep pattern (excessive sleep or sleep deprivation)

MIGRAINE HEADACHE II: ABORTIVE THERAPY

The objective of abortive therapy is to eliminate headache pain and suppress associated nausea and vomiting. Treatment should commence at the earliest sign of an attack. Because migraine causes nausea, vomiting, and gastric stasis, oral therapy may be ineffective once an attack has begun. Hence, for treatment of an established attack, a drug that can be administered rectally, by injection, or by inhalation may be best. As noted, two types of drugs are used for abortive therapy: nonspecific analgesics and migraine-specific drugs. Representative agents are listed in Table 29–3.

Drug selection depends on the intensity of the attack. For mild to moderate symptoms, an *aspirin-like drug* (e.g., aspirin, ibuprofen, acetaminophen) may be sufficient. For moderate to severe symptoms, patients should take a migraine-specific drug—either an *ergot alkaloid* (ergotamine or dihydroergotamine) or a *serotonin$_{1B/1D}$ agonist*. If these agents fail to relieve pain, an *opioid analgesic* (e.g., butorphanol, meperidine) may be needed.

Use of abortive medications (both nonspecific and migraine specific) should be limited to 1 or 2 days a week. Why? Because more frequent use can lead to *medication overuse headache* (MOH), also known as drug-induced headache or drug-rebound headache (see Box 29–1).

Antiemetics are important adjuncts to migraine therapy. By reducing nausea and vomiting, these drugs can (1) make the patient more comfortable, and (2) permit therapy with oral antimigraine drugs. Two antiemetics—*metoclopramide* [Reglan] and *prochlorperazine* [Compazine]—are used most often. Of the two, metoclopramide is preferred. Why? Because, in addition to suppressing nausea and vomiting, metoclopramide can reverse gastric stasis caused by the attack, and can thereby facilitate absorption of oral antimigraine drugs. Like metoclopramide, prochlorperazine suppresses nausea and vomiting. However, because of its anticholinergic actions, prochlorperazine can make gastric stasis even worse.

Analgesics
Aspirin-like Drugs

Aspirin, acetaminophen, ibuprofen, and other aspirin-like analgesics can provide adequate relief of mild to moderate migraine attacks. In fact, when combined with metoclopramide (to enhance absorption), aspirin may work as well as sumatriptan, a highly effective antimigraine drug. Moreover, the combination of aspirin plus metoclopramide costs less than sumatriptan and causes fewer adverse effects.

Acetaminophen should be used in combination with other drugs. Use of acetaminophen alone is not recommended. One effective combination, marketed as *Excedrin Migraine,* consists of acetaminophen, aspirin, and caffeine. An older and less effective product, marketed as *Midrin,* consists of acetaminophen, isometheptene (a sympathomimetic drug), and dichloralphenazone (a sedative).

Opioid Analgesics

Opioid analgesics are reserved for severe migraine that has not responded to first-line medications. The agents used most often are *meperidine* [Demerol] and *butorphanol*

TABLE 29–3 ■ Migraine Headache: Drugs for Abortive Therapy

Nonspecific Analgesics

Aspirin-like Drugs
Nonsteroidal anti-inflammatory drugs (e.g., aspirin, ibuprofen)
Acetaminophen + Aspirin + Caffeine [Excedrin Migraine]

Opioid Analgesics
Butorphanol [Stadol NS]
Meperidine [Demerol]

Migraine-Specific Drugs

Ergot Alkaloids
Dihydroergotamine [D.H.E. 45, Migranal Nasal Spray]
Ergotamine [Ergomar, Ergostat]
Ergotamine + Caffeine [Cafergot, Ercaf, Wigraine]

Selective Serotonin$_{1B/1D}$-Receptor Agonists (Triptans)
Almotriptan [Axert]
Frovatriptan [Frova]
Naratriptan [Amerge]
Rizatriptan [Maxalt]
Sumatriptan [Imitrex]
Zolmitriptan [Zomig]

nasal spray [Stadol NS]. Of the two, butorphanol is preferred. Why? Because meperidine can cause all of the adverse effects associated with other pure opioid agonists (e.g., respiratory depression, sedation) and also has significant abuse potential. These drawbacks are less of a problem with butorphanol.

Ergot Alkaloids
Ergotamine

Mechanism of Antimigraine Action. The actions of ergotamine are complex, and the precise mechanism by which the drug aborts migraine attacks is unknown. Ergotamine can alter transmission at serotonergic, dopaminergic, and alpha-adrenergic junctions. Recent evidence suggests that antimigraine effects are related to agonist activity at subtypes of serotonin receptors, specifically 5-HT$_{1B}$ and 5-HT$_{1D}$ receptors. Recent evidence indicates that ergotamine can block inflammation associated with the trigeminal vascular system, perhaps by suppressing release of CGRP. Relief may also be related to vascular effects. In cranial arteries, ergotamine acts directly to promote constriction and reduce the amplitude of pulsations. In addition, the drug can affect blood flow by depressing the vasomotor center.

Therapeutic Uses. Ergotamine is a drug of choice for stopping an ongoing migraine attack. It is also used to treat cluster headaches. Because of the risk of dependence (see below), ergotamine should not be taken daily on a long-term basis.

Pharmacokinetics. Administration may be oral, sublingual, rectal, or by inhalation. Bioavailability with oral and sublingual administration is low. Bioavailability with rectal and inhalational administration is higher. Although the half-life of ergotamine is only 2 hours, pharmacologic effects can still be observed 24 hours after administration. The drug is eliminated primarily by hepatic metabolism. Metabolites are excreted in the bile.

Special Interest Topic

BOX 29–1 ▪▪ MEDICATION-OVERUSE HEADACHE: TOO MUCH OF A GOOD THING

People who take headache medicine every day often develop medication overuse headaches (MOHs), also known as drug-rebound headaches or drug-induced headaches. What's an MOH? A chronic headache that develops in response to frequent use of headache medicines, and that resolves days to weeks after the overused drug is withdrawn. The stage for MOH is set when headache drugs are taken too often—especially if the dosage is high. Once the stage has been set, discontinuation of medication brings on the MOH, which causes the patient to resume taking medicine—thereby setting up a repeating cycle of MOH, followed by medication use and discontinuation, followed by MOH, followed by more medication, and so on. One reason the cycle gets established is that patients don't realize that the drugs they're taking to *treat* headache can, if taken too often, become the *cause* of headache. Failing to recognize MOH for what it is, patients take more and more medicine to make their headaches go away—but only succeed in making MOH worse.

Which drugs can cause MOH? Almost all of the medicines used for abortive headache therapy. Hence, MOH can be caused by overuse of analgesics (aspirin-like drugs, opioids), ergotamine (but not dihydroergotamine), triptans, and caffeine.

How can MOH be treated? The only hope is to stop taking headache medicine. Unfortunately, when medication is withdrawn, headaches will increase for a while. Their duration and intensity depends on the drug that was overused. With triptans, these withdrawal headaches are relatively mild and often resolve in a few days. In contrast, with analgesics or ergots, withdrawal headaches are more intense and may persist for 2 weeks or more.

Several measures can decrease the risk of MOH. The most important is to limit use of abortive medicines. If possible, patients should take these drugs no more than 2 or 3 times a week—and doses should be no higher than actually needed. Alternating headache medicines may help too, since this would limit exposure to any one drug. If headaches begin to occur more than 2 or 3 times a month, prophylactic therapy should be tried. Implementing nondrug measures—stress reduction, avoidance of triggers, getting sufficient sleep, relaxation techniques, and biofeedback—can reduce the need for headache medicines, and can thereby decrease exposure to the drugs that cause MOH.

Adverse Effects. Ergotamine is well tolerated at usual therapeutic doses. The drug can stimulate the chemoreceptor trigger zone, causing nausea and vomiting in about 10% of patients. This action can augment nausea and vomiting caused by the migraine itself. Concurrent treatment with metoclopramide or a phenothiazine antiemetic (e.g., prochlorperazine) can help suppress these responses. Other common side effects include weakness in the legs, myalgia, numbness and tingling in fingers and toes, angina-like pain, and tachycardia or bradycardia.

Overdose. Acute or chronic overdose can cause serious toxicity (ergotism). In addition to the adverse effects seen at therapeutic doses, overdose can cause ischemia secondary to constriction of peripheral arteries and arterioles: the extremities become cold, pale, and numb; muscle pain develops; and gangrene may eventually result. Patients should be informed about these responses and instructed to seek immediate medical attention. The risk of ergotism is highest in patients with sepsis, peripheral vascular disease, and renal or hepatic impairment. Management consists of discontinuing ergotamine, followed by measures to maintain circulation (treatment with anticoagulants, low-molecular-weight dextran, and/or intravenous nitroprusside as appropriate).

Physical Dependence. Regular daily use of ergotamine, even in moderate doses, can cause physical dependence. The withdrawal syndrome is characterized by headache, nausea, vomiting, and restlessness. That is, withdrawal resembles a migraine attack. Patients who begin to experience these symptoms are likely to resume taking the drug, thereby perpetuating the cycle of dependence. Hospitalization may be required to break the cycle. To avoid dependence, dosage and duration of treatment must be limited (see dosing guidelines below).

Drug Interactions. Ergotamine should not be combined with triptans (e.g., sumatriptan, zolmitriptan) because a prolonged vasospastic reaction can occur. To avoid this problem, administration of ergotamine and serotonin agonists should be separated by at least 24 hours.

Contraindications. Ergotamine is contraindicated for patients with hepatic or renal impairment, sepsis (gangrene has resulted), coronary artery disease (CAD), and peripheral vascular disease. In addition, the drug should not be taken during pregnancy. Why? Because its ability to promote uterine contractions can cause fetal harm or abortion. Because of its effects on the uterus, ergotamine is classified in the Food and Drug Administration's Pregnancy Risk Category X: The risk of use by pregnant women clearly outweighs any possible benefits. Warn women of child-bearing age to avoid pregnancy while using this drug.

Preparations, Dosage, and Administration. Ergotamine by itself is available in tablets for sublingual use. In addition, ergotamine is dispensed in combination with other drugs for oral and rectal administration.

Sublingual. Ergotamine tartrate [Ergomar] is dispensed in 2-mg tablets for sublingual use. One tablet should be placed under the tongue immediately after onset of aura or headache. If needed, additional tablets can be administered at 30-minute intervals—up to a maximum of 3 tablets/24 hours or 5 tablets/week.

Oral. Three oral formulations [Cafergot, Ercaf, Wigraine] contain 1 mg ergotamine tartrate and 100 mg caffeine; a fourth formulation [Cafatine-PB] contains 30 mg pentobarbital and 0.125 mg belladonna alkaloids in addition to the ergotamine and caffeine. The caffeine is present to enhance vasoconstriction and ergotamine absorption. The pentobarbital provides sedation. The belladonna alkaloids suppress emesis. With all four oral formulations, 2 tablets are taken immediately after onset of aura or headache. One additional tablet can be administered every 30 minutes—up to a maximum of 6 per attack or 10/week.

Rectal. Ergotamine is available in four rectal formulations [Cafatine Supps, Cafergot Supps, Cafetrate Supps, Wigraine Supps]. Each contains 2 mg ergotamine tartrate and 100 mg caffeine. No more than two suppositories should be administered per attack.

Dihydroergotamine

Therapeutic Uses. Parenteral dihydroergotamine [D.H.E. 45, Migranal] is a drug of choice for terminating migraine and cluster headaches. Administration is by injection (IM, IV) and nasal spray.

Pharmacologic Effects and Contraindications. The actions of dihydroergotamine are similar to those of ergotamine. Like ergotamine, dihydroergotamine alters transmission at serotonergic, dopaminergic, and alpha-adrenergic junctions. In contrast to ergotamine, dihydroergotamine causes minimal peripheral vasoconstriction, little nausea and vomiting, and no physical dependence. However, diarrhea is prominent. Contraindications are the same as for ergotamine: CAD, peripheral vascular disease, sepsis, pregnancy, and hepatic or renal impairment. As with ergotamine, dihydroergotamine should not be administered within 24 hours of a serotonin agonist (e.g., sumatriptan).

Pharmacokinetics. Dihydroergotamine may be administered parenterally (IM, IV) or by nasal spray. Because of extensive first-pass metabolism, the drug is not active orally. Elimination is by hepatic metabolism. An active metabolite (8'-hydroxydihydroergotamine) contributes to therapeutic effects. The half-life of dihydroergotamine plus its active metabolite is about 21 hours.

Parenteral Administration. Dihydroergotamine mesylate [D.H.E. 45] is dispensed in solution (1 mg/ml) for IM and IV administration.

Intramuscular. The initial dose is 1 mg immediately after onset of symptoms. Additional 1-mg doses may be given hourly up to a maximum of 3 mg per attack. Dosage should be adjusted early in therapy to determine a minimal effective dose. This dose should be used for subsequent attacks.

Intravenous. One milligram is given initially followed by another 1 mg in 1 hour if needed. Dosage should not exceed 6 mg/week.

Intranasal Administration. The nasal spray device [Migranal] delivers 0.5 mg of dihydroergotamine per spray. The dosage is 1 spray in each nostril repeated in 15 minutes, for a total of 2 mg. Pain is relieved in 60% of patients by 2 hours after administration. The 24-hour recurrence rate is 15%. Sumatriptan is more effective than intranasal dihydroergotamine, but has a higher recurrence rate.

Serotonin₁ᵦ/₁ᴅ-Receptor Agonists (Triptans)

The serotonin$_{1B/1D}$-receptor agonists, also known as triptans, are first-line drugs for terminating a migraine attack. These agents relieve pain by constricting intracranial blood vessels and suppressing release of inflammatory neuropeptides. All are well tolerated. Rarely, they cause symptomatic coronary vasospasm.

Sumatriptan

Sumatriptan [Imitrex] was the first triptan and will serve as our prototype for the group. The drug can be administered by mouth, nasal inhalation, and SC injection.

Mechanism of Action. Sumatriptan, an analog of 5-HT, causes selective stimulation of 5-HT$_{1B}$ and 5-HT$_{1D}$ receptors (5-HT$_{1B/1D}$ receptors). The drug has no affinity for 5-HT$_2$ or 5-HT$_3$ receptors, nor does it bind to adrenergic, dopaminergic, muscarinic, or histaminergic receptors. Binding to 5-HT$_{1B/1D}$ receptors on intracranial blood vessels causes vasoconstriction. Binding to 5-HT$_{1B/1D}$ receptors on sensory nerves of the trigeminal vascular system suppresses release of CGRT, a compound that promotes release of inflammatory neuropeptides. As a result, sumatriptan reduces release of inflammatory neuropeptides, and thereby diminishes perivascular inflammation. Both actions—vasoconstriction and decreased perivascular inflammation—help relieve migraine pain.

Therapeutic Use. Sumatriptan is used to abort an ongoing migraine attack. The drug relieves both headache and associated symptoms (nausea, photophobia, phonophobia). In clinical trials, sumatriptan gave complete relief to the majority of patients. Beneficial effects begin about 15 minutes after SC or intranasal administration, and 30 to 60 minutes after oral administration. Complete relief occurs in 70% to 80% of patients 2 hours after SC administration, in 60% of patients 2 hours after intranasal administration, and in 50% to 60% of patients 4 hours after oral administration. Unfortunately headache returns in about 40% of patients within 24 hours. In comparison, the 24-hour recurrence rate with dihydroergotamine is only 18%. In patients who respond to SC sumatriptan, subsequent administration of oral sumatriptan can delay recurrence but does not prevent it. In addition to migraine, sumatriptan is approved for cluster headaches.

Pharmacokinetics. As noted, sumatriptan is available for oral, SC, and intranasal administration. With oral or intranasal administration, bioavailability is low (about 15%), whereas SC bioavailability is high (97%). As a result, oral and intranasal doses are considerably higher than SC doses. Once in the blood, sumatriptan undergoes hepatic metabolism followed by excretion in the urine. Its half-life is short—about 2.5 hours.

Adverse Effects. Sumatriptan is generally well tolerated. Most side effects are transient and mild. Coronary vasospasm is the biggest concern.

Chest Symptoms. About 50% of patients experience unpleasant chest symptoms, usually described as "heavy arms" or "chest pressure" rather than pain. These symptoms are transient and *not* related to ischemic heart disease. Possible causes are pulmonary vasoconstriction, esophageal spasm, intercostal muscle spasm, and bronchoconstriction. Patients should be forewarned of these symptoms and told they are not dangerous.

Coronary Vasospasm. Rarely, sumatriptan causes angina secondary to coronary vasospasm. Electrocardiographic changes have been observed in patients with CAD or Prinzmetal's (vasospastic) angina. To reduce the risk of angina, do not give sumatriptan to patients who have risk factors for CAD until CAD has been ruled out. These patients include postmenopausal women, men over 40, smokers, and patients with hypertension, hypercholesterolemia, obesity, diabetes, or a family history of CAD. Because of the risk of coronary vasospasm, sumatriptan is contraindicated for patients with a history of ischemic heart disease, myocardial infarction (MI), uncontrolled hypertension, or other heart disease.

Teratogenesis. *Sumatriptan should be avoided during pregnancy.* When given daily to pregnant rabbits, the drug is embryolethal at blood levels only 3 times higher than those achieved with a 6-mg SC injection in humans (a typical dose). Accordingly, unless the physician directs otherwise, women should be instructed to avoid the drug if they are pregnant or think they might be, if they are trying to become pregnant, or if they are not using an adequate form of contraception.

Other Adverse Effects. Mild reactions include vertigo, malaise, fatigue, and tingling sensations. Transient pain and redness may occur at sites of SC injection. Intranasal administration may cause irritation in the nose and throat as well as an offensive or unusual taste.

Drug Interactions. Ergot Alkaloids and Other Triptans. Sumatriptan, other triptans, and ergot alkaloids (e.g., ergotamine, dihydroergotamine) all cause vasoconstriction. Accordingly, if one triptan is combined with another or with an ergot alkaloid, excessive and prolonged vasospasm could result. Accordingly, sumatriptan should not be used within 24 hours of an ergot derivative or another triptan.

Monoamine Oxidase Inhibitors. Monoamine oxidase inhibitors (MAOIs) can suppress degradation of sumatriptan, causing plasma levels to rise. Toxicity can result. Accordingly, sumatriptan and MAOIs should not be used together. Furthermore, sumatriptan should not be administered within 2 weeks of stopping an MAOI.

Preparations, Dosage, and Administration. Subcutaneous. Sumatriptan succinate [Imitrex] is available in single-dose vials and prefilled syringes for SC injection. A new Imitrex STATdose Pen is available for self-injection. The maximum single dose is 6 mg. The maximum that may be given in 24 hours is two 6-mg doses, separated by at least 1 hour.

Oral. Sumatriptan [Imitrex] is available in 25-, 50-, and 100-mg tablets for oral use. The usual dose is 25 mg, but doses as high as 100 mg may be tried. If, after 2 hours, the response to the first dose is unsatisfactory, a second dose may be given.

Nasal Spray. Sumatriptan [Imitrex] is available in 5- and 20-mg unit-dose spray devices. The initial dose is 5 or 20 mg. This can be repeated in 2 hours if needed. The maximum dose that may be given in 24 hours is 40 mg.

Other Serotonin$_{1B/1D}$-Receptor Agonists

In addition to sumatriptan, the triptan family includes five other drugs: naratriptan [Amerge], rizatriptan [Maxalt], zolmitriptan [Zomig], almotriptan [Axert], and frovatriptan [Frova]. All five are administered orally; all are essentially equal to sumatriptan with respect to efficacy and safety; and all have the same mechanism of action: activation of 5-HT$_{1B/1D}$ receptors with subse-quent intracranial vasoconstriction and decreased perivascular inflammation. Because the triptans are very similar, selection among them is based on relatively small differences in kinetics and side effects. Dosage and time course are summarized in Table 29–4.

Zolmitriptan. Zolmitriptan [Zomig, Zomig ZMT] is indicated for terminating an ongoing migraine attack. The drug is similar to sumatriptan with regard to mechanism, efficacy, time course, side effects, and interactions. Zolmitriptan is available in two oral formulations: standard tablets (2.5 and 5 mg), sold as Zomig, and melt-in-the-mouth tablets (2.5 mg), sold as Zomig ZMT. Zomig ZMT dissolves in saliva present on the tongue; no water is needed. Because water is unnecessary, the drug can be taken conveniently as soon as an aura is perceived. Be aware, however, that onset of effects is no faster than with standard Zomig tablets. With either formulation, a 2.5-mg dose produces the most favorable response/tolerability ratio. About 65% of patients respond within 2 hours. Dosing can be repeated in 2 hours if headache persists. The maximum dose per 24 hours is 10 mg. Headache recurs in 8% to 32% of patients. Adverse effects are generally mild and transient. Like sumatriptan, zolmitriptan causes harmless, transient chest discomfort. Of much greater concern, the drug can cause coronary vasospasm, and hence is contraindicated for patients with ischemic heart disease, prior MI, or uncontrolled hypertension. To avoid excessive vasospasm, zolmitriptan should not be administered within 24 hours of an ergot alkaloid or another triptan, or within 2 weeks of stopping an MAOI.

Naratriptan. Naratriptan [Amerge] is indicated for oral therapy of an ongoing migraine attack. The drug differs from most other triptans in two respects: (1) it has a relatively long half-life (6 hours versus 2 to 3 hours for most other triptans), and (2) it can be safely combined with an MAOI. Onset of effects is slower than with other triptans, but the duration of effects is longer. Because effects persist, the 24-hour migraine recurrence rate may be reduced. Naratriptan is available in 1- and 2.5-mg tablets. The 2.5-mg strength is more effective but causes more side effects. The initial dose is 1 or 2.5 mg. Dosing may be repeated in 4 hours if needed. The maximum daily dose is 5 mg. Like other triptans, naratriptan causes transient chest discomfort. Also like other triptans, the drug can cause coronary vasospasm, and hence is contraindicated for patients with ischemic heart disease, prior MI, or

TABLE 29–4 ■ Clinical Pharmacology of the Triptans

Drug	Route	Onset (min)	Duration	Half-Life (hr)	Dosage	Comments
Sumatriptan [Imitrex]	Oral	30–60	Short	2.5	25, 50, or 100 mg; may repeat in 2 hr (max. 200 mg/24 hr)	First triptan available. Most widely used and best understood. Only triptan available in nasal and SC formulations, which act faster than oral triptans.
	Nasal	15–20			5 or 20 mg; may repeat in 2 hr (max. 40 mg/24 hr)	
	SC	10–15			6 mg; may repeat in 1 hr (max. 12 mg/24 hr)	
Almotriptan [Axert]	Oral	30–120	Short	3.1	6.25 or 12.5 mg; may repeat in 2 hr (max. 25 mg/24 hr)	Incidence of chest discomfort (pain, tightness, pressure) is lower than with other triptans. Safe for use with MAOIs.
Frovatriptan [Frova]	Oral	120–180	Long	26	2.5 mg; may repeat in 2 hr	Longest half-life; slowest onset—but also lowest rate of headache recurrence. Decrease dose if combined with propranolol. Safe for use with MAOIs.
Naratriptan [Amerge]	Oral	60–180	Long	6	1 or 2.5 mg; may repeat in 4 hr (max. 5 mg/24 hr)	Available in melt-in-the-mouth tablets that can be taken without water. Safe for use with MAOIs.
Rizatriptan [Maxalt]	Oral	30–120	Short	2–3	5 or 10 mg; may repeat in 2 hours (max. 30 mg/24 hr)	May be the most consistently effective triptan. Decrease dose if combined with propranolol.
Zolmitriptan [Zomig]	Oral	45	Short	3	2.5 or 5 mg; may repeat in 2 hr (max. 10 mg/24 hr)	Available in melt-in-the-mouth tablets that can be taken without water.

MAOI = monoamine oxidase inhibitor.

uncontrolled hypertension. To avoid excessive vasospasm, naratriptan should not be administered within 24 hours of an ergot alkaloid or another triptan.

Rizatriptan. Rizatriptan [Maxalt, Maxalt MLT] is used to terminate an ongoing migraine attack. The drug is similar to sumatriptan with regard to mechanism, efficacy, time course, side effects, and interactions. Rizatriptan is available in two oral formulations: standard tablets [Maxalt] and melt-in-the-mouth tablets [Maxalt MLT] that can be taken without water. Both formulations come in 5- and 10-mg strengths. The initial dose is 5 or 10 mg. Dosing may be repeated in 2 hours if needed. No more than 30 mg should be taken per day. Adverse effects are generally mild and transient. Like other triptans, rizatriptan causes harmless, transient chest discomfort. Also like other triptans, the drug can cause coronary vasospasm, and hence is contraindicated for patients with ischemic heart disease, prior MI, or uncontrolled hypertension. To avoid excessive vasospasm, rizatriptan should not be administered within 24 hours of an ergot alkaloid or another triptan, or within 2 weeks of stopping an MAOI. Propranolol can raise levels of rizatriptan; a dosage reduction may be needed. Rizatriptan may harm the developing fetus: in rats, the drug increased perinatal mortality, reduced learning capacity, and decreased pre- and post-weaning weight. Use with caution in pregnant women.

Almotriptan. Almotriptan [Axert] is indicated for oral therapy of an ongoing migraine attack. The drug is similar to sumatriptan with regard to mechanism, efficacy, and time course—and is better tolerated. Almotriptan is available in 6.25- and 12.5-mg tablets for oral use. The initial dosage is 6.25 or 12.5 mg. Dosing can be repeated in 2 hours if headache persists. The maximum dose per 24 hours is 25 mg. Adverse effects are minimal. Like other triptans, almotriptan can cause harmless, transient chest discomfort—but the incidence is very low (only 0.3%). Also like other triptans, the drug can cause coronary vasospasm, and hence is contraindicated for patients with ischemic heart disease, prior MI, or uncontrolled hypertension. To avoid excessive vasospasm, zolmitriptan should not be administered within 24 hours of an ergot alkaloid or another triptan. In contrast to some triptans, almotriptan can be combined safely with an MAOI.

Frovatriptan. Frovatriptan [Frova] is indicated for oral therapy of an ongoing migraine attack. The drug is similar to other triptans with regard to mechanism and side effects—but is less effective and has very different kinetics. Effects begin slowly, but are sustained—thanks to the drug's long half-life (26 hours). Although the number of patients responding at 2 hours is low (37% to 46%), rates of headache recurrence are low too (7% to 23%)—lower than with any other triptan. Frovatriptan is available in 2.5-mg tablets. The initial dosage is 2.5 mg. If headache recurs after initial relief, dosing can be repeated—but no sooner than 2 hours after the first dose. If there was no response to the first dose, repeat dosing is unlikely to help. The maximum dosage per 24 hours is 7.5 mg. Adverse effects are mild and transient. Like sumatriptan, frovatriptan can cause harmless, transient chest discomfort. In addition, the drug can cause coronary vasospasm, and hence is contraindicated for patients with ischemic heart disease, prior MI, or uncontrolled hypertension. To avoid excessive vasospasm, frovatriptan should not be administered within 24 hours of an ergot alkaloid or another triptan. However, it can be used concurrently with an MAOI. Dosage should be reduced in patients receiving propranolol.

MIGRAINE HEADACHE III: PREVENTIVE THERAPY

Prophylactic therapy can reduce both the frequency and intensity of migraine attacks. Preventive treatment is indicated for patients who have frequent attacks (two or more a month), attacks that are especially severe, or attacks that do not respond adequately to abortive agents. Preferred drugs for prophylaxis include propranolol, divalproex, and amitriptyline. All three are effective and well tolerated. A fourth drug—methysergide—is also very effective, but its use is limited owing to a risk of fibrosis. Commonly used preventive agents are listed in Table 29–5.

Beta Blockers

Beta blockers are preferred drugs for migraine prevention. These drugs are as effective as methysergide (see below) and much safer. Of the available agents, *propranolol* [Inderal] is

used most often. Treatment can reduce the number and intensity of attacks in 70% of patients. Benefits take a few weeks to develop. The most common side effects are extreme tiredness and fatigue, which occur in about 10% of patients. In addition, the drug can cause depression and can exacerbate symptoms of asthma. The usual dosage is 40 to 120 mg twice daily. In addition to propranolol, four other beta blockers—*timolol, atenolol, metoprolol,* and *nadolol*—can help prevent migraine attacks. In contrast, beta blockers that possess intrinsic sympathomimetic activity (e.g., acebutolol, pindolol) are *not* effective. The basic pharmacology of the beta blockers is discussed in Chapter 18.

Anticonvulsants

Several drugs that were developed as anticonvulsants can reduce migraine attacks. Proof of efficacy is strongest for divalproex [Depakote] and gabapentin [Neurontin]. Topiramate [Topamax] and tiagabine [Gabitril] appear promising, although extensive proof of efficacy is lacking.

Divalproex. Divalproex [Depakote ER], employed first for epilepsy and more recently for bipolar disorder (manic-depressive illness), is now approved for prophylaxis of migraine. The drug is a form of valproic acid (see Chapter 23). Divalproex reduces the incidence of attacks by 60%. However, when attacks do occur, their intensity and duration are not diminished. In migraineurs, the most common side effect is nausea. Other side effects include fatigue, weight gain, tremor, and reversible hair loss. Potentially fatal pancreatitis and hepatitis occur rarely. Divalproex can cause neural tube defects in the developing fetus, and hence is contraindicated during pregnancy. The drug is available in standard and extended-release (ER) tablets. Only the ER tablets are approved for prevention of migraine. The recommended dosage is 500 or 1000 mg once a day.

Tricyclic Antidepressants

Tricyclic antidepressants can prevent migraine and tension-type headaches in some patients. The underlying mechanism is unknown. The tricyclic agent used most often is *amitriptyline*

TABLE 29–5 ■ Migraine Headache: Drugs for Preventive Therapy
Beta-Adrenergic Blocking Agents
Propranolol [Inderal]
Timolol [Blocadren]
Anticonvulsants
Divalproex [Depakote ER]
Tricyclic Antidepressants
Amitriptyline [Elavil]
Calcium Channel Blockers
Verapamil [Calan]
Flunarizine*
Estrogens (for menstrual migraine)
Estrogen gel
Estrogen patches [Alora, Climara, Esclim, Estraderm, Vivelle]

*Not available in the United States.

[Elavil, others]. Benefits equal those of propranolol and methysergide. The usual dosage is 25 to 75 mg once daily at bedtime. Since amitriptyline is effective in patients who are not depressed, it would seem that benefits do not depend on elevation of mood. Like other tricyclic antidepressants, amitriptyline can cause hypotension and anticholinergic effects (dry mouth, constipation, urinary retention, blurred vision, tachycardia). Excessive doses can cause dysrhythmias. The basic pharmacology of amitriptyline is discussed in Chapter 31.

Estrogens (for Menstrual Migraine)

Menstrual migraine is defined as migraine that routinely occurs within 2 days of the onset of menses. An important trigger is the decline in estrogen levels that precedes menstruation. For many women, we can prevent menstrual migraine by giving estrogen supplements, which compensate for the premenstrual estrogen drop. Topical preparations—estrogen gel and estrogen patches [Climara, Estraderm, Vivelle]—work well. Effective dosages are 1.5 mg/day for the gel and 100 mg/day for the patches. Dosing is done for 7 days each month, beginning 2 days before the expected attack.

Other Drugs for Prophylaxis
Methysergide

Methysergide [Sansert], an ergot alkaloid, was the first effective drug for preventing migraine attacks. It can produce complete or partial relief in 60% to 70% of patients. The drug is more effective than propranol, but also more dangerous. Because of its potential for severe adverse effects, methysergide is reserved for patients who are unresponsive to or intolerant of safer drugs. The mechanism by which methysergide prevents migraine is not clear.

Methysergide causes a variety of adverse effects. Fibrotic changes, although rare, are most serious. With long-term therapy, methysergide can cause retroperitoneal, pleuropulmonary, and cardiac fibrosis. Retroperitoneal fibrosis can result in urinary tract obstruction. Pleuropulmonary fibrosis can cause chest pain, dyspnea, and plural effusion. Fibrosis of the aortic and mitral valves can cause heart murmurs and dyspnea. Fibrotic changes may reverse spontaneously upon cessation of drug use; however, surgical correction may be required. To minimize the risk of fibrosis, treatment should be interrupted every 6 months. Other adverse effects include vascular insufficiency (caused by excessive vasoconstriction); central nervous system reactions (insomnia, altered mood, depersonalization, hallucinations, nightmares); and GI disturbances (nausea, vomiting, diarrhea).

Several drugs increase the risk of methysergide-induced arterial spasm. Among these are other ergot alkaloids (e.g., ergotamine, dihydroergotamine), serotonin receptor agonists (e.g., sumatriptan), beta-adrenergic blockers, dopamine, and drugs that inhibit the cytochrome P450 3A4 subclass of hepatic drug-metabolizing enzymes.

The usual adult dosage is 2 mg 2 to 4 times a day. Because of its potential for causing fibrosis, methysergide should not be taken continuously. Rather, the manufacturer recommends discontinuing the drug for 3 to 4 weeks every 6 months. When treatment is discontinued, dosage should be reduced gradually.

Calcium Channel Blockers

Of the calcium channel blockers evaluated for migraine prevention, only two appear useful: *verapamil* and *flunarizine* (a drug not yet available in the United States). These agents are less effective than propranolol or divalproex, and their effects develop slowly, reaching a maximum in 1 to 2 months. Although these drugs can relieve vasospasm, it is not clear that vasodilation explains antimigraine effects. A direct effect on neurons is also possible. When used for prophylaxis, these drugs cause side effects in 20% to 60% of patients. Constipation and orthostatic hypotension are most common. The basic pharmacology of the calcium channel blockers is discussed in Chapter 43.

Riboflavin

Riboflavin (vitamin B_2) can reduce the number and severity of migraine attacks, but benefits are modest and develop slowly. In one study, migraineurs with frequent attacks took 400 mg of riboflavin a day. After 3 months, the number of attacks had decreased by 37%. In addition, the average duration of each attack also declined. Side effects were minimal.

Coenzyme Q-10

In a preliminary study, daily therapy with coenzyme Q-10 (CoQ-10) produced a significant reduction in the occurrence of migraine attacks. Subjects took 150 mg of CoQ-10 each morning. After 3 months, the number of days on which headaches occurred declined by at least 50% in 61.3% of study participants. However, although headache frequency declined, headache intensity was not affected. CoQ-10 was well tolerated.

CLUSTER HEADACHES

Characteristics

Cluster headaches occur in a series or "cluster" of attacks. Each attack lasts 15 minutes to 2 hours and is characterized by severe, throbbing, unilateral pain in the orbital-temporal area (i.e., near the eye). A typical cluster consists of one or two such attacks every day for 2 to 3 months. An attack-free interval of months to years separates each cluster. Along with headache, patients usually experience lacrimation, conjunctival redness, nasal congestion, rhinorrhea, ptosis (drooping eyelid), and miosis (constriction of the pupil)—all on the same side as the headache. Although related to migraine, cluster headaches differ in several ways: (1) they are not preceded by an aura, (2) they do not cause nausea and vomiting, (3) they can be more debilitating, (4) they are less common and occur mostly in males (5:1), (5) they are not associated with a family history of attacks, and (6) management is different.

Treatment

Primary therapy is directed at prophylaxis. Effective agents include *prednisone, methysergide, lithium,* and *verapamil.* High-dose prednisone (40 to 80 mg/day) acts rapidly, producing benefits in 48 hours. However, because long-term use of glucocorticoids carries serious risks (see Chapter 68), treatment should stop in 1 to 2 months. Methysergide (2 to 8 mg/day) can suppress cluster headaches, but benefits take up to 2 weeks to develop. In addition, because long-term therapy can cause fibrotic complications, treatment should be limited to 3 months or less. Lithium is a drug of choice for prevention of chronic cluster headache. Benefits begin in 1 to 2 weeks. To ensure therapeutic effects and minimize toxicity, blood levels of lithium must be monitored; the target range is 0.6 to 1.2 mEq/L. Verapamil (160 to 480 mg/day) is less effective than lithium but safer and easier to use.

If an attack occurs despite preventive therapy, it can be aborted with *oxygen, sumatriptan,* or an *ergot preparation.* Inhalation of 100% oxygen for 10 minutes or less brings rapid relief to most patients. The mechanism is unknown. Speedy relief can also be achieved with *sublingual* ergotamine tartrate, *intranasal* dihydroergotamine, or *subcutaneous* sumatriptan. Slower relief can be achieved with an ergotamine-caffeine *suppository. Oral* ergotamine acts too slowly to be of much help.

TENSION-TYPE HEADACHE

Characteristics

Tension-type headaches (formerly called muscle-contraction headaches) are the most common form of headache. These headaches are characterized by moderate, nonthrobbing pain, usually located in a "head band" distribution. Headache is often associated with scalp formication and a sense of tightness or pressure in the head and neck. Precipitating factors include eye strain, aggravation, frustration, and life's daily stresses. Depressive symptoms (sleep disturbances, including early and frequent awakening) are often present. Tension headaches may be episodic or chronic. By definition, chronic tension-type headaches occur 15 or more days per month for at least 6 months.

Treatment

An acute attack of mild to moderate intensity can be relieved with a nonopioid analgesic: acetaminophen or a nonsteroidal anti-inflammatory drug (e.g., aspirin, ibuprofen, naproxen). An analgesic-sedative combination (e.g., aspirin-butalbital) may also be used. However, because of their potential for dependence and abuse, these combinations should be reserved for acute therapy of episodic attacks; they are inappropriate for patients with chronic headache syndrome.

For prophylaxis, *amitriptyline* [Elavil, others], a tricyclic antidepressant, is the drug of choice. Administering the drug at bedtime will help relieve any depression-related sleep disturbances in addition to protecting against headache. Amitriptyline can cause anticholinergic side effects (e.g., dry mouth, constipation) and poses a risk of cardiotoxicity at high doses (see Chapter 31).

In addition to receiving drugs, patients should be taught how to manage stress. Instruction should include cognitive coping skills and information on relaxation techniques (e.g., massage, hot baths, biofeedback, deep muscle relaxation).

∴ KEY POINTS

- Migraine is a neurovascular disorder involving dilation and inflammation of intracranial arteries.
- Antimigraine drugs are used in two ways: abortive therapy and prophylactic therapy.
- The goal of abortive therapy is to eliminate headache pain and associated nausea and vomiting.
- The goal of prophylactic therapy is to reduce the incidence and intensity of migraine attacks.
- There are two kinds of drugs for abortive therapy: nonspecific analgesics (aspirin-like drugs, opioids) and migraine-specific drugs (ergot alkaloids, triptans).
- Aspirin-like analgesics (e.g., acetaminophen, aspirin, ibuprofen) are effective for abortive therapy of mild to moderate migraine.
- Opioid analgesics (e.g., butorphanol) are reserved for severe migraine that has not responded to other drugs.
- Ergotamine is a first-line drug for abortive therapy of severe migraine.
- Overdose with ergotamine can cause ergotism, a serious condition characterized by severe tissue ischemia secondary to generalized constriction of peripheral arteries.
- Ergotamine must not be taken routinely because physical dependence will occur.
- Ergotamine can cause uterine contraction and must not be taken during pregnancy.
- Triptans (e.g., sumatriptan) are first-line drugs for abortive therapy of moderate to severe migraine.
- Triptans activate $5-HT_{1B/1D}$ receptors and thereby constrict intracranial blood vessels and suppress release of inflammatory neuropeptides.
- All triptans are available in oral formulations, and one agent—sumatriptan—is also available in SC and intranasal formulations, which act faster than oral triptans.
- Triptans can cause coronary vasospasm, and hence are contraindicated for patients with ischemic heart disease, prior MI, or uncontrolled hypertension.
- Triptans should not be combined with one another or with ergot derivatives because excessive vasoconstriction could occur.
- Prophylactic therapy is indicated for migraineurs who have frequent attacks (two or more a month), especially severe attacks, or attacks that do not respond adequately to abortive agents.
- Propranolol, divalproex, and amitriptyline are preferred drugs for migraine prophylaxis.
- Estrogen supplements can help prevent menstrual-associated migraine.

Summary of Major Nursing Implications*

ERGOTAMINE AND DIHYDROERGOTAMINE

Preadministration Assessment

Therapeutic Goal

Termination of migraine or cluster headache.

Baseline Data

Determine the age of onset, frequency, location, intensity, and quality (throbbing or nonthrobbing) of headaches as well as the presence or absence of a prodromal aura. Assess for trigger factors (e.g., stress, anxiety, fatigue) and for a family history of severe headache.

Assess for possible underlying causes of headache (e.g., severe hypertension; hyperthyroidism; infection; tumors; disorders of the eye, ear, nose, sinuses, or throat). If present, these should be treated directly.

Identifying High-Risk Patients

Ergot alkaloids are *contraindicated* in patients with hepatic or renal impairment, sepsis, CAD, or peripheral vascular disease, and for patients who are pregnant or taking triptans.

Implementation: Administration

Routes

Ergotamine Alone: Sublingual.
Ergotamine Plus Caffeine: Oral, rectal.
Dihydroergotamine: Nasal spray, IM, IV.

Dosage and Administration

Instruct the patient to commence dosing immediately after onset of symptoms.

Nausea and vomiting from the headache and from ergotamine itself may prevent complete absorption of oral ergotamine. Concurrent treatment with metoclopramide or another antiemetic can minimize these effects. (Nausea and vomiting are minimal with dihydroergotamine.)

Ergotamine (but not dihydroergotamine) can cause physical dependence and serious toxicity if dosage is excessive. **Inform the patient about the risks of dependence and toxicity and the importance of not exceeding the prescribed dosage.**

*Patient education information is highlighted as blue text.

Summary of Major Nursing Implications*—cont'd

Implementation: Measures to Enhance Therapeutic Effects

Educate the patient in ways to control, avoid, or eliminate trigger factors (e.g., stress, fatigue, anxiety, alcohol, tyramine-containing foods).

Teach the patient about relaxation techniques (e.g., biofeedback, deep muscle relaxation). Advise the patient to rest in a quiet, dark room for 2 to 3 hours after drug administration and to apply an ice pack to the neck and scalp.

Ongoing Evaluation and Interventions

Evaluating Therapeutic Effects

Determine the size and frequency of doses used and the extent to which therapy has reduced the intensity and duration of attacks.

Minimizing Adverse Effects

Nausea and Vomiting. *Ergotamine* promotes nausea and vomiting. Minimize these by concurrent therapy with metoclopramide or a phenothiazine-type antiemetic.

Ergotism. Toxicity (ergotism) can result from acute or chronic overdose. **Teach patients the early manifestations of ergotism (muscle pain; paresthesias in fingers and toes; extremities become cold, pale, and numb) and instruct them to seek immediate medical attention.** Treat by withdrawing ergotamine and administering drugs (anticoagulants, low-molecular-weight dextran, intravenous nitroprusside) as appropriate to maintain circulation.

Physical Dependence. *Ergotamine* can cause physical dependence. **Warn patients not to overuse the drug, since physical dependence can result. Teach patients the signs and symptoms of withdrawal (headache, nausea, vomiting, restlessness) and instruct them to inform the physician if these develop during a drug-free interval.** Patients who become dependent may require hospitalization to bring about withdrawal.

Abortion. Ergot alkaloids are uterine stimulants that can cause abortion in high doses. **Warn women of child-bearing age to avoid pregnancy while using this drug.**

SEROTONIN$_{1B/1D}$-RECEPTOR AGONISTS (TRIPTANS)

Almotriptan
Frovatriptan
Naratriptan
Rizatriptan
Sumatriptan
Zolmitriptan

Preadministration Assessment

Therapeutic Goal

Termination of migraine headache.

Baseline Data

See *Ergotamine and Dihydroergotamine.*

Identifying High-Risk Patients

All triptans are *contraindicated* for patients with ischemic heart disease, prior MI, or uncontrolled hypertension, and for patients taking ergot alkaloids, other triptans, or MAOIs. Sumatriptan, rizatriptan, and zolmitriptan are contraindicated for patients taking MAOIs.

Implementation: Administration

Routes

Oral. All triptans.
Subcutaneous and Intranasal. *Sumatriptan.*

Dosage and Administration

Instruct patients to administer triptans immediately after onset of symptoms.

Teach patients how to use the sumatriptan auto-injector.

Implementation: Measures to Enhance Therapeutic Effects

Educate the patient in ways to control, avoid, or eliminate trigger factors (e.g., stress, fatigue, anxiety, alcohol, tyramine-containing foods).

Teach the patient biofeedback or another relaxation technique. Advise the patient to rest in a quiet, dark room for 2 to 3 hours after drug administration and to apply an ice pack to the neck and scalp.

Ongoing Evaluation and Interventions

Evaluating Therapeutic Effect

Determine the size and frequency of doses used and the extent to which therapy has reduced the intensity and duration of attacks.

Minimizing Adverse Effects

Coronary Vasospasm. All triptans can cause coronary vasospasm with resultant anginal pain. Avoid these drugs in patients with ischemic heart disease, prior MI, or uncontrolled hypertension. In patients with risk factors for CAD, rule out CAD before giving triptans.

Teratogenesis. *Sumatriptan* can cause birth defects in laboratory animals. Avoid the drug during pregnancy.

Minimizing Adverse Interactions

Ergot Alkaloids and Other Triptans. Combining a triptan with an ergot alkaloid (e.g., ergotamine, dihydroergotamine) or another triptan can cause prolonged vasospasm. Do not administer a triptan within 24 hours of an ergot alkaloid or another triptan.

MAOIs. MAOIs can intensify the effects of *sumatriptan, rizatriptan,* and *zolmitriptan.* Do not give these triptans to patients who are taking MAOIs or who stopped taking MAOIs within the last 14 days.

Propranolol. Propranolol can raise levels of frovatriptan and rizatriptan. Dosage of the triptan should be reduced.

*Patient education information is highlighted as blue text.

Antipsychotic Agents and Their Use in Schizophrenia

The antipsychotic agents are a chemically diverse group of compounds employed to treat a broad spectrum of psychotic disorders. Specific indications include schizophrenia, delusional disorders, acute mania, depressive psychoses, and drug-induced psychoses. In addition to their psychiatric applications, the antipsychotics are used to suppress emesis and to treat Tourette's syndrome and Huntington's chorea.

Since their introduction in the early 1950s, the antipsychotic agents have catalyzed revolutionary change in the management of psychotic illnesses. Before these drugs became available, psychoses were largely untreatable and patients were fated to a life of institutionalization. With the advent of antipsychotic medications, many patients with schizophrenia and other severe psychotic disorders have been able to leave psychiatric hospitals and return to the community. Others have been spared hospitalization en-

tirely. For those who must remain institutionalized, antipsychotic drugs have at least reduced suffering.

The antipsychotic drugs fall into two major groups: *conventional antipsychotics* and *atypical antipsychotics.* All of the conventional agents block receptors for dopamine in the central nervous system (CNS). As a result, they all can cause serious movement disorders, known as *extrapyramidal symptoms.* The atypical agents produce only moderate blockade of receptors for dopamine and much stronger blockade of receptors for serotonin. Because dopamine receptor blockade is low, the risk of extrapyramidal reactions is low as well. In recent years, the atypical antipsychotics have replaced the conventional antipsychotics as first-choice drugs for schizophrenia.

SCHIZOPHRENIA: CLINICAL FEATURES AND ETIOLOGY

Clinical Features

Schizophrenia is a chronic psychotic illness characterized by disordered thinking and a reduced ability to comprehend reality. Symptoms usually emerge during adolescence or early adulthood. The incidence of the disease the United States is about 1%. Diagnostic criteria for schizophrenia are presented in Table 30–1.

Positive and Negative Symptoms. Symptoms of schizophrenia can be divided into two groups: positive symptoms and negative symptoms (Table 30–2). Positive symptoms can be viewed as an exaggeration or distortion of normal function, whereas negative symptoms can be viewed as a loss or diminution of normal function. Positive symptoms include hallucinations, delusions, agitation, tension, and paranoia. Negative symptoms include lack of motivation, poverty of speech, blunted affect, poor self-care, and social withdrawal. Conventional antipsychotics relieve positive symptoms more effectively than negative symptoms. In contrast, atypical antipsychotic agents relieve both types of symptoms.

Acute Episodes. During an acute schizophrenic episode, delusions (fixed false beliefs) and hallucinations are frequently prominent. Delusions are typically religious, grandiose, or persecutory. Auditory hallucinations, which are more common than visual hallucinations, may consist of voices arguing or commenting on one's behavior. The patient may feel controlled by external influences. Disordered

TABLE 30–1 ▪▪ DSM-IV-TR Diagnostic Criteria for Schizophrenia

A. Characteristic Symptoms

At least two of the following are present for a significant time during a 1-month period (or less if successfully treated):

- Delusions
- Hallucinations
- Disorganized speech (e.g., frequent derailment or incoherence)
- Grossly disorganized or catatonic behavior
- Negative symptoms (affective flattening, alogia, or avolition)

Note: Only one symptom is required if delusions are bizarre or if hallucinations consist of either (1) a voice making running comments on the person's behavior or thoughts or (2) voices conversing with each other.

B. Social/Occupational Dysfunction

For a significant time since the onset of the disturbance, at least one major area of functioning (e.g., work, interpersonal relations, self-care) is markedly below the preonset level *or,* if the onset occurred in childhood or adolescence, the individual failed to achieve the expected level of interpersonal, academic, or occupational functioning.

C. Duration

Continuous signs of the disturbance persist for at least 6 months. This 6-month period must include at least 1 month of symptoms (or less if successfully treated) that meet Criterion A (i.e., active-phase symptoms). It may also include periods of prodromal or residual symptoms; during these times the disturbance is manifested only by negative symptoms or by at least two symptoms from Criterion A that are present in attenuated form (e.g., odd beliefs, unusual perceptual experience).

D. Schizoaffective and Mood Disorder Exclusion

Schizoaffective Disorder and Mood Disorder With Psychotic Features have been ruled out because either (1) no Major Depressive, Manic, or Mixed Episodes have occurred concurrently with the active-phase symptoms; or (2) if mood episodes have occurred during active-phase symptoms, their total duration has been brief relative to the duration of the active and residual periods.

E. Substance/General Medical Condition Exclusion

The disturbance is not due to the direct physiologic effects of a substance (e.g., drug of abuse, medication) or a general medical condition.

F. Relationship to a Pervasive Developmental Disorder

If there is a history of Autistic Disorder or another Pervasive Developmental Disorder, the additional diagnosis of Schizophrenia is made only if prominent delusions or hallucinations are present for at least 1 month (or less if successfully treated).

Adapted from the Diagnostic and Statistical Manual of Mental Disorders, Fourth Edition, Text Revision. Washington, DC, American Psychiatric Press, 2000, with permission. Copyright © 2000 American Psychiatric Association.

thinking and loose association may render rational conversation impossible. Affect may be blunted or labile. Misperception of reality may result in hostility and lack of cooperation. Impaired self-care skills may leave the patient disheveled and dirty. Patterns of sleeping and eating are usually disrupted.

Residual Symptoms. After florid symptoms (e.g., hallucinations, delusions) of an acute episode remit, less vivid symptoms may remain. These include suspiciousness, poor anxiety management, and diminished judgment, insight, motivation, and capacity for self-care. As a result of these changes, patients frequently find it difficult to establish close relationships, maintain employment, and function independently in society. Suspiciousness and poor anxiety management contribute to social withdrawal. An inability to appreciate the need for continued drug therapy may cause noncompliance, resulting in relapse and perhaps hospital readmission.

TABLE 30–2 ▪▪ Positive and Negative Symptoms of Schizophrenia

Positive Symptoms	Negative Symptoms
Hallucinations	Social withdrawal
Delusions	Emotional withdrawal
Disordered thinking	Lack of motivation
Disorganized speech	Poverty of speech
Combativeness	Blunted affect
Agitation	Poor insight
Paranoia	Poor judgment
	Poor self-care

Long-Term Course. The long-term course of schizophrenia is characterized by episodic acute exacerbations separated by intervals of partial remission. As the years pass, some patients experience progressive decline in mental status and social functioning. However, many others stabilize, or even

TABLE 30–3 ▌■ Antipsychotic Drugs: Relative Potency and Incidence of Side Effects

Drug	Equivalent Oral Dose (mg)*	Incidence of Side Effects					
		Extrapyramidal Effects†	Sedation	Orthostatic Hypotension	Anticholinergic Effects	Weight Gain	Significant QT Prolongation
Conventional Agents							
Low Potency							
Chlorpromazine	100	Moderate	High	High	Moderate	Moderate	Yes
Thioridazine	100	Low	High	High	High	Moderate	Yes
Mesoridazine	50	Low	High	Moderate	High	Moderate	Yes
Medium Potency							
Triflupromazine	25	Moderate	High	Moderate	Moderate	—	—
Loxapine	10	Moderate	Moderate	Low	Low	Low	—
Molindone	10	Moderate	Moderate	Low	Low	Low	—
Perphenazine	10	Moderate	Moderate	Low	Low	—	—
High Potency							
Trifluoperazine	5	High	Low	Low	Low	—	—
Thiothixene	2	High	Low	Moderate	Low	Moderate	—
Fluphenazine	2	High	Low	Low	Low	—	—
Haloperidol	2	High	Low	Low	Low	Moderate	Yes
Pimozide	0.5	High	Moderate	Low	Moderate	—	Yes
Atypical Agents							
Clozapine	50	Very low	High	Moderate	High	High	—
Risperidone	4	Very low	Low	Low	None	Moderate	Yes
Olanzapine	5	Very low	High	Moderate	High	High	—
Quetiapine	150	Very low	Moderate	Moderate	None	Moderate	Yes
Ziprasidone	NA	Very low	Moderate	Moderate	None	Low	Yes
Aripiprazole	NA	Very low	Low	Low	None	Low	No

*Doses listed are the therapeutic equivalent of 100 mg of oral chlorpromazine. NA = not available.
†Incidence refers to *early* extrapyramidal reactions (acute dystonia, parkinsonism, akathisia). The incidence of *late* reactions (tardive dyskinesia) is the same for all traditional antipsychotics; tardive dyskinesia has not been reported with atypical antipsychotics.

improve. Maintenance therapy with antipsychotic drugs reduces the risk of acute relapse, but may fail to prevent long-term deterioration.

Etiology

Although there is strong evidence that schizophrenia has a biologic basis, the exact etiology is unknown. Genetic, perinatal, neurodevelopmental, and neuroanatomic factors may all be involved. Possible primary defects include excessive activation of CNS receptors for dopamine, and insufficient activation of CNS receptors for glutamate. Although psychosocial stressors can precipitate acute exacerbations in susceptible patients, these stressors are not considered causative.

CONVENTIONAL ANTIPSYCHOTIC AGENTS I: GROUP PROPERTIES

In this section we discuss pharmacologic properties shared by all of the conventional agents. Much of our attention focuses on adverse effects. Of these, the extrapyramidal side effects are of particular concern. Because of these neurologic side effects, the conventional antipsychotics are known alternatively as *neuroleptics*.

Classification

The conventional antipsychotics can be classified by potency or chemical structure. From a clinical viewpoint, classification by potency is more useful.

Classification by Potency

Conventional antipsychotic agents can be classified as *low potency, medium potency,* or *high potency* (Table 30–3). The low-potency drugs, represented by chlorpromazine [Thorazine], and the high-potency drugs, represented by haloperidol [Haldol], are of particular interest.

It is important to note that, although the conventional antipsychotics differ from one another in potency, they all have the same ability to relieve symptoms of psychosis. Recall that the term *potency* refers only to the size of the dose needed to elicit a given response; potency implies nothing about the maximal effect a drug can produce. Hence, when we say that haloperidol is more potent than chlorpromazine, we mean only that the dose of haloperidol required to relieve psychotic symptoms is smaller than the required dose of chlorpromazine; we do not mean that haloperidol can produce greater effects. When administered in therapeutically equivalent doses, both drugs elicit an equivalent antipsychotic response.

TABLE 30–4 ■ Antipsychotic Drugs: Routes and Dosages

Chemical Group and Generic Name	Trade Name	Route	Total Daily Dose (mg)	
			Short Term	Maintenance
Conventional Agents				
Phenothiazine: aliphatic				
Chlorpromazine	Thorazine	PO, IM, R*	200–1000	50–400
Triflupromazine	Vesprin	IM	30–150	20–200
Phenothiazine: piperidine				
Mesoridazine	Serentil	PO, IM	100–400	25–200
Thioridazine	Mellaril	PO	200–800	50–400
Phenothiazine: piperazine				
Fluphenazine	Prolixin, Permitil	PO, IM	5–50	1–15
Perphenazine	Trilafon	PO, IM	12–64	8–24
Trifluoperazine	Stelazine	PO, IM	10–60	4–30
Thioxanthene				
Thiothixene	Navane	PO, IM	10–60	6–30
Butyrophenone				
Haloperidol	Haldol	PO, IM	5–50	1–15
Dihydroindolone				
Molindone	Moban	PO	40–225	15–100
Dibenzoxazepine				
Loxapine	Loxitane	PO, IM	20–160	10–60
Diphenylbutylpiperadine				
Pimozide	Orap	PO	1–2†	10†
Atypical Agents				
Dibenzodiazepine				
Clozapine	Clozaril	PO	300–900	300–600
Benzisoxazole				
Risperidone	Risperdal	PO	2–4	4–6
Thiobenzodiazepine				
Olanzapine	Zyprexa	PO	5–10	10–20
Dibenzothiozepine				
Quetiapine	Seroquel	PO	50	300–400
Benzisothiazolyl piperazine				
Ziprasidone	Geodon	PO, IM	40	80–120
Quinolinone				
Aripiprazole	Abilify	PO	10–15	10–15

*R = rectal (suppository)
†Dosage for Tourette's syndrome.

If low-potency and high-potency neuroleptics are equally effective, why distinguish between them? The answer is that, although these agents produce identical *antipsychotic* effects, they differ significantly in *side effects*. Hence, by knowing the potency category to which a particular neuroleptic belongs, we can better predict that drug's undesired responses. This knowledge is useful in drug selection and providing patient care and education.

Chemical Classification

The conventional antipsychotic agents fall into six major chemical categories (Table 30–4). One of these categories, the phenothiazines, has three subgroups. Drugs in all groups are equivalent with respect to antipsychotic actions. Because of this equivalence, chemical classification is not emphasized in this chapter.

Two chemical categories—the *phenothiazines* and the *butyrophenones*—deserve special attention. The phenothiazines were the first of the modern antipsychotic agents. Chlorpromazine, our prototype of the low-potency neuroleptics, is a member of the phenothiazine family. The butyrophenones stand out because they are the family to which haloperidol belongs. Haloperidol is the prototype of the high-potency antipsychotics.

Mechanism of Action

The conventional antipsychotic drugs block a variety of receptors within and outside the CNS. To varying degrees, these drugs block receptors for dopamine, acetylcholine, histamine, and norepinephrine. There is little question that blockade at these receptors is responsible for the major *adverse effects* of the antipsychotics. However, since the etiology of psychotic illness is entirely unknown, the relationship of receptor blockade to *therapeutic effects* can only be guessed at. The current dominant theory suggests that conventional antipsychotic drugs suppress symptoms of psychosis by blocking dopamine$_2$ (D$_2$) receptors in the mesolimbic area of the brain. In support of this theory is the observation that all of the conventional antipsychotics produce D$_2$ receptor blockade. Furthermore, there is a close correlation between the clinical potency of these drugs and their potency as D$_2$ receptor antagonists.

TABLE 30–5 ■ Receptor Blockade and Side Effects of Antipsychotic Drugs

Receptor Type	Consequence of Blockade
D$_2$ dopaminergic	EPS; prolactin release
H$_1$ histaminergic	Sedation
Muscarinic cholinergic	Dry mouth, blurred vision, urinary retention, constipation, tachycardia
Alpha$_1$-adrenergic	Orthostatic hypotension; reflex tachycardia
5-HT$_2$ serotoninergic	Weight gain

EPS = extrapyramidal symptoms.

Therapeutic Uses

Schizophrenia. Schizophrenia is the primary indication for antipsychotic drugs. These agents effectively suppress symptoms during acute psychotic episodes and, when taken chronically, can greatly decrease the risk of relapse. Initial effects may be seen in 1 to 2 days, but substantial improvement usually takes 2 to 4 weeks, and full effects may not develop for several months. Positive symptoms (e.g., delusions, hallucinations) respond better than negative symptoms (e.g., social and emotional withdrawal, blunted affect, poverty of speech). All of the conventional antipsychotic agents are equally effective, although individual patients may respond better to one drug than to another. Consequently, selection among these drugs is based primarily on their side effect profiles, rather than on therapeutic effects. It must be noted that antipsychotic drugs do not alter the underlying pathology of schizophrenia. Hence, treatment is not curative—it offers only symptomatic relief. Management of schizophrenia is discussed in depth later in the chapter.

Bipolar Disorder (Manic-Depressive Illness). Most patients with bipolar disorder are managed with a mood-stabilizing agent, almost always lithium or valproic acid. Neuroleptics may be employed acutely (in combination with lithium or valproic acid) to help manage patients going through a severe manic phase. In addition, one neuroleptic drug—olanzapine—is approved for monotherapy of acute mania. Bipolar disorder and its treatment are the subject of Chapter 32.

Tourette's Syndrome. This rare inherited disorder is characterized by severe motor tics, barking cries, grunts, and outbursts of obscene language, all of which are spontaneous and beyond control of the patient. In addition to these core symptoms, patients frequently have symptoms resembling those of obsessive-compulsive disorder (OCD) or attention-deficit/hyperactivity disorder (ADHD). Neuroleptic drugs (e.g., pimozide, fluphenazine, haloperidol) are the most effective agents for managing core symptoms. When core symptoms are mild, clonidine is the drug of choice. Symptoms of OCD can be managed with a selective serotonin reuptake inhibitor (e.g., fluoxetine [Prozac]). Symptoms of ADHD can be controlled with a CNS stimulant (e.g., methylphenidate [Ritalin]).

Prevention of Emesis. Neuroleptics suppress emesis by blocking dopamine receptors in the chemoreceptor trigger zone of the medulla. These drugs can be employed to suppress vomiting associated with cancer chemotherapy, gastroenteritis, uremia, and other conditions.

Other Applications. Neuroleptics can be used for *delusional disorders, schizoaffective disorder,* and *dementia and other organic mental syndromes* (i.e., psychiatric syndromes resulting from organic causes, such as infection, metabolic disorders, poisoning, and structural injury to the brain). In addition, neuroleptics can relieve symptoms of *Huntington's chorea.*

Adverse Effects

The antipsychotic drugs block several kinds of receptors, and hence produce an array of side effects. Side effects associated with blockade of specific receptors are summarized in Table 30–5.

Although antipsychotic agents produce a variety of undesired effects, these drugs are, on the whole, very safe; death from overdose is practically unheard of. Of the many side effects these drugs can produce, the most troubling are the extrapyramidal reactions—especially tardive dyskinesia (TD).

Extrapyramidal Symptoms

Extrapyramidal symptoms (EPS) are movement disorders resulting from effects of antipsychotic drugs on the extrapyramidal motor system. The extrapyramidal system is the same neuronal network whose malfunction is responsible for the movement disorders of Parkinson's disease (PD). Although the exact cause of EPS is unclear, blockade of D$_2$ receptors is strongly suspected.

Four types of EPS occur. These differ with respect to time of onset and management. Three of these reactions—acute dystonia, parkinsonism, and akathisia—occur early in therapy and can be managed with a variety of drugs. The fourth reaction—tardive dyskinesia—occurs late in therapy and has no satisfactory treatment. Characteristics of EPS are summarized in Table 30–6.

The *early* reactions occur *less frequently* with *low-potency* agents (e.g., chlorpromazine) than with high-potency agents (e.g., haloperidol). In contrast, the risk of TD is *equal* with *all* antipsychotics.

Acute Dystonia. Acute dystonia can be both disturbing and dangerous. The reaction develops within the first few days of therapy, and frequently within hours of the first dose. Typically, the patient develops severe spasm of the muscles of the tongue, face, neck, or back. Oculogyric crisis (involuntary upward deviation of the eyes) and opisthotonus (tetanic spasm of the back muscles causing the trunk to arch forward, while the head and lower limbs are thrust backward) may also occur. Severe cramping can cause joint dislocation. Laryngeal dystonia can impair respiration.

Intense dystonia constitutes a crisis that requires rapid intervention. Initial treatment consists of anticholinergic medication (e.g., benztropine, diphenhydramine) administered IM

TABLE 30–6 ■ Extrapyramidal Side Effects of Antipsychotic Drugs

Type of Reaction	Time of Onset	Features	Management
Early Reactions			
Acute dystonia	A few hours to 5 days	Spasm of muscles of tongue, face, neck, and back; opisthotonus	Anticholinergic drugs (e.g., benztropine) IM or IV
Parkinsonism	5–30 days	Bradykinesia, mask-like facies, tremor, rigidity, shuffling gait, drooling, cogwheeling, stooped posture	Anticholinergics (e.g., benztropine, diphenhydramine), amantadine, or both. For severe symptoms, switch to an atypical antipsychotic.
Akathisia	5–60 days	Compulsive, restless movement; symptoms of anxiety, agitation	Reduce dosage or switch to a low-potency antipsychotic. Treat with a benzodiazepine, beta blocker, or anticholinergic drug
Late Reaction			
Tardive dyskinesia	Months to years	Oral-facial dyskinesias, choreoathetoid movements	Best approach is prevention; no reliable treatment. Discontinue all anticholinergic drugs. Give benzodiazepines. Reduce antipsychotic dosage. For severe TD, switch to an atypical antipsychotic.

or IV. As a rule, symptoms resolve within 5 minutes of IV administration and within 15 to 20 minutes of IM administration.

It is important to differentiate between acute dystonia and psychotic hysteria. Why? Because misdiagnosis of acute dystonia as hysteria could result in escalation of antipsychotic dosage, thereby causing the acute dystonia to become even worse.

Parkinsonism. Antipsychotic-induced parkinsonism is characterized by bradykinesia, mask-like facies, drooling, tremor, rigidity, shuffling gait, cogwheeling, and stooped posture. Symptoms develop within the first month of therapy and are indistinguishable from those of idiopathic PD.

Neuroleptics cause parkinsonism by blocking dopamine receptors in the striatum. Since idiopathic PD is also due to reduced activation of striatal dopamine receptors (see Chapter 21), it is no wonder that PD and neuroleptic-induced parkinsonism share the same symptoms.

Neuroleptic-induced parkinsonism is treated with some of the drugs used for PD. Specifically, centrally acting *anticholinergic drugs* (e.g., benztropine, diphenhydramine) and *amantadine* [Symmetrel] may be employed. Levodopa, however, should be avoided. Why? Because levodopa promotes activation of dopamine receptors, and might thereby counteract the beneficial effects of antipsychotic treatment.

Use of antiparkinsonism drugs should not continue indefinitely. Antipsychotic-induced parkinsonism tends to resolve spontaneously, usually within months of its appearance. Accordingly, antiparkinsonism drugs should be withdrawn after a few months to determine if they are still needed.

If parkinsonism is severe, switching to an atypical antipsychotic is likely to help. As discussed below, the risk of parkinsonism with the atypical antipsychotics is much lower than with the conventional agents.

Akathisia. Akathisia is characterized by pacing and squirming brought on by an uncontrollable need to be in motion. This profound sense of restlessness can be very disturbing. The syndrome usually develops within the first 2 months of treatment. Like other early EPS, akathisia occurs most frequently with high-potency antipsychotics.

Three types of drugs have been used to suppress symptoms: *beta blockers, benzodiazepines,* and *anticholinergic drugs.* Although these can be helpful, a reduction in antipsychotic dosage or switching to a low-potency agent may be more effective.

It is important to differentiate between akathisia and exacerbation of psychosis. If akathisia were to be confused with anxiety or psychotic agitation, it is likely that antipsychotic dosage would be increased, thereby making akathisia more intense.

Tardive Dyskinesia. Tardive dyskinesia (TD), the most troubling EPS, develops in 15% to 20% of patients during long-term therapy. The risk is related to duration of treatment and dosage size. For many patients, symptoms are irreversible.

TD is characterized by involuntary choreoathetoid (twisting, writhing, worm-like) movements of the tongue and face. Patients may also present with lip-smacking movements, and their tongues may flick out in a "fly-catching" motion. One of the earliest manifestations of TD is slow, worm-like movement of the tongue. Involuntary movements that involve the tongue and mouth can interfere with chewing, swallowing, and speaking. Eating difficulties can result in malnutrition and weight loss. Over time, TD produces involuntary movements of the limbs, toes, fingers, and trunk. For some patients, symptoms decline following a dosage reduction or drug withdrawal. For others, TD is irreversible.

The cause of TD is complex and incompletely understood. One theory suggests that symptoms result from excessive *activation* of dopamine receptors. It is postulated that, in response to chronic receptor blockade, dopamine receptors of the extrapyramidal system undergo a functional change such that their sensitivity to activation is increased. Stimulation of these "supersensitive" receptors produces an imbalance in favor of dopamine, and thereby produces abnormal movement. In support of this theory is the observation that symptoms of TD can be reduced (temporarily) by *increasing* antipsychotic dosage, which causes greater dopamine receptor blockade. (Since symptoms eventually return even though antipsychotic dosage is kept high, dosage elevation cannot be used to treat TD.)

There is no reliable management for TD. Measures that may be tried include gradual withdrawal of anticholinergic drugs, administration of benzodiazepines, and reducing the dosage of the offending antipsychotic agent. For patients with severe TD, switching to an atypical antipsychotic agent (e.g., clozapine) may be beneficial. These drugs do not seem to cause TD, and may actually suppress symptoms in patients who have developed the disorder.

Since TD has no reliable means of treatment, prevention is the best approach. Antipsychotic drugs should be used in the lowest effective dosage for the shortest time required. After 12 months, the need for continued therapy should be assessed. If drug use must continue, a neurologic evaluation should be done at least every 3 months to detect early signs of TD. For patients with chronic schizophrenia, dosage should be tapered periodically (at least annually) to determine the need for continued treatment.

Other Adverse Effects

Neuroleptic Malignant Syndrome. Neuroleptic malignant syndrome (NMS) is a rare but serious reaction that carries a 4% risk of mortality (down from 30% a decade ago, thanks to early diagnosis and intervention). Primary symptoms are "lead-pipe" rigidity, sudden high fever (temperature may exceed 41°C), sweating, and autonomic instability, manifested as dysrhythmias and fluctuations in blood pressure. Level of consciousness may rise and fall, the patient may appear confused or mute, and seizures or coma may develop. Death can result from respiratory failure, cardiovascular collapse, dysrhythmias, and other causes. NMS is more likely with high-potency agents than with low-potency agents.

Treatment consists of supportive measures, drug therapy, and immediate withdrawal of antipsychotic medication. Hyperthermia should be controlled with cooling blankets and antipyretics (e.g., aspirin, acetaminophen). Hydration should be maintained with fluids. Benzodiazepines may relieve anxiety and help reduce blood pressure and tachycardia. Two drugs—*dantrolene* and *bromocriptine*—may be especially helpful. Dantrolene is a direct-acting muscle relaxant (see Chapter 24). In patients with NMS, this drug reduces rigidity and hyperthermia. Bromocriptine is a dopamine receptor agonist (see Chapter 21) that may relieve CNS toxicity.

Resumption of antipsychotic therapy carries a small risk of NMS recurrence. The risk can be minimized by (1) waiting at least 2 weeks before resuming antipsychotic treatment, (2) using the lowest effective dosage, and (3) avoiding high-potency agents. Some clinicians believe that the atypical agent clozapine carries little or no risk of NMS. Hence, if NMS recurs during treatment with a conventional antipsychotic drug, a switch to clozapine may be appropriate.

Anticholinergic Effects. Antipsychotic drugs produce varying degrees of muscarinic cholinergic blockade (see Table 30–3). By blocking muscarinic receptors, these drugs can elicit the full spectrum of anticholinergic responses (dry mouth, blurred vision, photophobia, urinary hesitancy, constipation, tachycardia). Patients should be informed about these responses and taught how to minimize danger and discomfort. As indicated in Table 30–3, anticholinergic effects are more likely with low-potency agents than with high-potency agents. Anticholinergic effects and their management are discussed in detail in Chapter 14.

Orthostatic Hypotension. Antipsychotic drugs promote orthostatic hypotension by blocking alpha₁-adrenergic receptors on blood vessels. Alpha-adrenergic blockade prevents compensatory vasoconstriction when the patient stands, thereby causing blood pressure to fall. Patients should be informed about signs of hypotension (lightheadedness, dizziness) and advised to sit or lie down if these occur. In addition, patients should be informed that hypotension can be minimized by moving slowly when assuming an erect posture. With hospitalized patients, blood pressure and pulses should be checked before drug administration and 1 hour after. Measurements should be made while the patient is lying down and again after the patient has been sitting or standing for 1 to 2 minutes. If blood pressure is low, or if pulse rate is high, the drug should be withheld and the physician consulted. Hypotension is more likely with low-potency antipsychotics than with the high-potency drugs (see Table 30–3). Tolerance to hypotension develops in 2 to 3 months.

Sedation. Sedation is common during the early days of treatment but subsides within a week or so. Neuroleptic-induced sedation is thought to result from blockade of histamine₁ receptors in the CNS. Daytime sedation can be minimized by administering the entire daily dose at bedtime. Patients should be warned against participation in hazardous activities (e.g., driving) until sedative effects diminish.

Neuroendocrine Effects. Antipsychotics increase levels of circulating prolactin by blocking the inhibitory action of dopamine on prolactin release. Elevation of prolactin levels promotes *gynecomastia* (breast growth) and *galactorrhea* in up to 57% of women. Up to 97% experience menstrual irregularities. Gynecomastia and galactorrhea can also occur in males. Since prolactin can promote growth of prolactin-dependent carcinoma of the breast, neuroleptics should be avoided in patients with this form of cancer. (It should be noted that, although antipsychotic drugs can promote the growth of cancers that already exist, there is no evidence that antipsychotic drugs actually *cause* cancer.)

Seizures. Antipsychotic drugs can reduce seizure threshold, thereby increasing the risk of seizure activity. The risk of seizures is greatest in patients with epilepsy and other seizure disorders. These patients should be monitored, and, if loss of seizure control occurs, the dosage of their antiseizure medication must be increased.

Sexual Dysfunction. Antipsychotics can cause sexual dysfunction in women and men. In women, these drugs can suppress libido and impair the ability to achieve orgasm. In men, neuroleptics can suppress libido and cause erectile and ejaculatory dysfunction; the incidence of these effects is 25% to 60%. Drug-induced sexual dysfunction can make treatment unacceptable to sexually active patients, thereby leading to poor compliance. A reduction in dosage or switching to a high-potency antipsychotic may reduce effects on sexual function. Patients should be counseled about possible sexual dysfunction and encouraged to report problems.

Dermatologic Effects. Drugs in the *phenothiazine* class can sensitize the skin to ultraviolet light, thereby increasing the risk of severe sunburn. Patients should be warned against excessive exposure to sunlight and advised to apply a sunscreen and wear protective clothing. Phenothiazines can also produce pigmentary deposits in the skin, cornea, and lens of the eye.

Handling antipsychotics can cause contact dermatitis in patients and in health care personnel. Dermatitis can be prevented by avoiding direct contact with these drugs.

Agranulocytosis. Agranulocytosis is a rare but serious reaction. Among the conventional antipsychotics, the risk is highest with chlorpromazine and certain other phenothiazines. Since agranulocytosis severely compromises the ability to fight infection, white blood cell (WBC) counts should be done whenever signs of infection (e.g., fever, sore throat) appear. If agranulocytosis is diagnosed, the neuroleptic should be withdrawn. Agranulocytosis reverses upon discontinuation of treatment.

Severe Dysrhythmias. Five conventional antipsychotics— *chlorpromazine, thioridazine, mesoridazine, haloperidol,* and *pimozide*—pose a risk of fatal cardiac dysrhythmias. The mechanism is prolongation of the QT interval, an index of cardiac function that can be measured with an electrocardiogram (EKG). As discussed in Chapter 7 (Adverse Drug Reactions and Medication Errors), drugs that prolong the QT interval increase the risk of torsades de pointes, a type of dysrhythmia than can progress to fatal ventricular fibrillation. To reduce the risk of dysrhythmias, patients should undergo an EKG and serum potassium determination prior to treatment and periodically thereafter. In addition, they should avoid other drugs that cause QT prolongation (see Table 7–2), as well as drugs that can increase levels of the drugs under consideration.

Physical and Psychologic Dependence

Development of physical and psychologic dependence is rare. Patients should be reassured that addiction and dependence are not likely.

Although physical dependence is minimal, abrupt withdrawal of antipsychotics *can* precipitate a mild abstinence syndrome. Symptoms, which are related to chronic cholinergic blockade, include restlessness, insomnia, headache, gastric distress, and sweating. This syndrome can be avoided by withdrawing antipsychotic medication gradually.

Drug Interactions

Anticholinergic Drugs. Drugs with anticholinergic properties will intensify anticholinergic responses to neuroleptics. Patients should be advised to avoid all drugs with anticholinergic actions, including antihistamines and certain over-the-counter sleep aids.

CNS Depressants. Neuroleptics can intensify CNS depression caused by other drugs. Patients should be warned against using alcohol and all other drugs with CNS-depressant actions (e.g., antihistamines, benzodiazepines, barbiturates).

Levodopa. Levodopa (a drug used to treat PD) may counteract the antipsychotic effects of neuroleptics. Conversely, neuroleptics may counteract the therapeutic effects of levodopa. These interactions occur because levodopa and neuroleptics have opposing effects on receptors for dopamine: Levodopa activates these receptors, whereas neuroleptics cause blockade.

Toxicity

Conventional antipsychotic drugs are very safe; death by overdose is extremely rare. With chlorpromazine, for example, the therapeutic index is about 200. That is, the lethal dose is 200 times the therapeutic dose.

Overdose produces hypotension, CNS depression, and extrapyramidal reactions. Extrapyramidal reactions can be treated with antiparkinsonism drugs. Hypotension can be

treated with IV fluids plus an alpha-adrenergic agonist (e.g., phenylephrine). There is no specific antidote to CNS depression. Excess drug should be removed from the stomach by gastric lavage. Emetics cannot be used because their effects would be blocked by the antiemetic action of the neuroleptic.

CONVENTIONAL ANTIPSYCHOTIC AGENTS II: PROPERTIES OF INDIVIDUAL AGENTS

All of the conventional antipsychotic drugs are equally effective at alleviating symptoms of schizophrenia, although individual patients may respond better to one drug than to another. Differences among these agents relate primarily to their side effect profiles (see Table 30–3). Because high-potency agents produce fewer side effects than the low-potency agents, high-potency agents are generally preferred. In recent years, the atypical antipsychotics, which cause fewer EPS than the conventional agents, have replaced the conventional agents as first-choice drugs for schizophrenia.

Low-Potency Agents
Chlorpromazine

Chlorpromazine [Thorazine] was the first modern antipsychotic medication and is the prototype for all that followed. None of the newer conventional agents is superior at relieving symptoms of psychotic illnesses. Chlorpromazine is a low-potency neuroleptic and belongs to the phenothiazine family of compounds.

Therapeutic Uses. Principal indications are schizophrenia and other psychotic disorders. Additional psychiatric indications are schizoaffective disorder and the manic phase of bipolar disorder. Other uses include suppression of emesis and relief of intractable hiccups.

Pharmacokinetics. Chlorpromazine may be administered PO, IM, and by rectal suppository. Following oral administration, the drug is well absorbed but undergoes extensive first-pass metabolism. As a result, oral bioavailability is only 30%. When chlorpromazine is given IM, peak plasma levels are 10 times those achieved with an equal oral dose. Excretion is renal, almost entirely as metabolites.

Adverse Effects. The most common adverse effects are sedation, orthostatic hypotension, and anticholinergic effects (dry mouth, blurred vision, urinary retention, photophobia, constipation, tachycardia). Neuroendocrine effects—galactorrhea, gynecomastia, and menstrual irregularities—occur occasionally. Photosensitivity reactions are possible, and patients should be warned to minimize unprotected exposure to sunlight. Because chlorpromazine is a low-potency neuroleptic, the risk of early extrapyramidal reactions (dystonia, akathisia, parkinsonism) is relatively low. However, the risk of TD is the same as with all other conventional agents. Chlorpromazine lowers seizure threshold. Accordingly, patients with seizure disorders should be especially diligent about taking antiseizure medication. Agranulocytosis and NMS occur rarely.

Drug Interactions. Chlorpromazine can intensify responses to CNS depressants (e.g., antihistamines, benzodiazepines, barbiturates) and anticholinergic drugs (e.g., antihistamines, tricyclic antidepressants, atropine-like drugs).

Preparations, Dosage, and Administration. Chlorpromazine [Thorazine] is available in six formulations: *tablets* (10, 25, 50, 100, and 200 mg), *sustained-release capsules* (30, 75, and 150 mg), *syrup* (2 mg/ml), *liquid con-*

centrate (30 and 100 mg/ml), *rectal suppositories* (25 and 100 mg), and *solution for injection* (25 mg/ml).

Oral Therapy. The initial dosage for adults is 25 mg 3 times a day. Dosage should be gradually increased until symptoms are controlled. The usual maintenance dosage is 400 mg/day. Elderly patients require less drug than younger patients.

Parenteral Therapy. Parenteral therapy is indicated for acutely psychotic, hospitalized patients. Intramuscular administration is preferred to IV administration. (Intravenous chlorpromazine is highly irritating and generally avoided.) The initial dose is 25 to 50 mg. Dosage may be increased gradually to a maximum of 400 mg every 4 to 6 hours. Once symptoms are controlled, oral therapy should be substituted for parenteral therapy.

Thioridazine

Thioridazine [Mellaril] is a low-potency antipsychotic that prolongs the QT interval, and hence can cause fatal cardiac dysrhythmias. Because of this danger, the drug should be reserved for treating schizophrenia in patients who have not responded to safer agents. The most common adverse effects are sedation, orthostatic hypotension, anticholinergic effects, weight gain, and inhibition of ejaculation. Effects seen occasionally include extrapyramidal reactions (dystonia, parkinsonism, akathisia, TD), galactorrhea, gynecomastia, menstrual irregularities, and photosensitivity reactions. NMS, convulsions, agranulocytosis, and pigmentary retinopathy occur rarely. Principal interactions are with anticholinergic drugs and CNS depressants. Thioridazine is available in three oral formulations: tablets (10, 15, 25, 50, 100, 150, and 200 mg), liquid concentrate (30 and 100 mg/ml), and a suspension (5 and 20 mg/ml). The initial dosage is 50 to 100 mg 3 times a day. Dosage may be gradually increased until symptoms are controlled, but should not exceed 800 mg/day. The usual maintenance dosage is 200 to 800 mg/day in two to four divided doses.

Mesoridazine

Mesoridazine [Serentil], an active metabolite of thioridazine, has pharmacologic properties much like those of the parent drug. Like thioridazine, mesoridazine can cause fatal dysrhythmias, and hence should be reserved for treatment of schizophrenia in patients who have not responded to safer medicines. Mesoridazine is available in tablets (10, 25, 50, and 100 mg/ml), a concentrated oral solution (25 mg/ml), and in solution for IM injection (25 mg/ml). The initial oral dosage is 50 mg 3 times a day. The usual maintenance dosage is 100 to 400 mg/day in divided doses.

Medium-Potency Agents

Loxapine. Loxapine [Loxitane] is a medium-potency agent indicated for schizophrenia and other psychotic disorders. The drug's side effect profile is similar to that of fluphenazine. Administration is oral and IM. Three formulations are available: capsules (5, 10, 25, and 50 mg), liquid concentrate (25 mg/ml), and solution for injection (50 mg/ml). The initial *oral* dosage is 10 mg twice a day. Dosage is increased until symptoms are controlled, typically with 60 to 100 mg/day in divided doses. The dosage should be reduced for maintenance therapy; the usual range is 20 to 60 mg/day. The *intramuscular* dosage is 12.5 to 50 mg every 4 to 6 hours.

Molindone. Molindone [Moban] is a medium-potency agent used to treat schizophrenia and other psychotic disorders. The most common adverse effects are early extrapyramidal reactions (dystonia, parkinsonism, akathisia) and anticholinergic effects (dry mouth, blurred vision, photophobia, urinary retention, constipation, tachycardia). Effects seen occasionally include sedation, menstrual irregularities, weight loss, and TD. Orthostatic hypotension and NMS occur rarely. Molindone is available in tablets (5, 10, 25, 50, and 100 mg) and an oral concentrate (20 mg/ml). The initial dosage is 50 to 75 mg/day in divided doses. Dosage is then increased until symptoms are controlled. As much as 225 mg/day has been given. Dosage should be reduced to the lowest effective amount for maintenance.

Perphenazine. Perphenazine [Trilafon] is a medium-potency agent used to treat schizophrenia and other psychotic disorders. The drug's side effect profile is like that of fluphenazine. For therapy of psychotic disorders, perphenazine is given orally and by IM injection. The drug is available in tablets (2, 4, 8, and 16 mg), a liquid concentrate (16 mg/5 ml), and solution for injection (5 mg/ml). The initial oral dosage is 4 to 8 mg 3 times daily. Once symptoms have been controlled, the dosage should be reduced to the lowest effective amount.

High-Potency Agents

High-potency agents differ from low-potency agents primarily in that high-potency agents cause more early EPS but less sedation, orthostatic hypotension, and anticholinergic effects. Because they cause fewer side effects, high-potency agents are generally preferred for initial therapy.

Haloperidol

Actions and Uses. Haloperidol [Haldol], a member of the *butyrophenone* family, is the prototype of the high-potency neuroleptics. Antipsychotic actions are equivalent to those of chlorpromazine. Principal indications are schizophrenia and acute psychosis. In addition, haloperidol is a preferred drug for Tourette's syndrome.

Pharmacokinetics. Haloperidol may be administered PO and IM. Oral bioavailability is about 60%. Hepatic metabolism is extensive. Parent drug and metabolites are excreted in the urine.

Adverse Effects. As indicated in Table 30–3, early extrapyramidal reactions (acute dystonia, parkinsonism, akathisia) occur frequently, whereas sedation, hypotension, and anticholinergic effects are uncommon. Note that the incidence of these reactions is exactly opposite to that seen with chlorpromazine and other low-potency agents. The incidence of TD with haloperidol is the same as with the low-potency drugs. Like chlorpromazine, haloperidol occasionally causes gynecomastia, galactorrhea, and menstrual irregularities. NMS, photosensitivity, convulsions, and impotence are rare. Haloperidol can prolong the QT interval, and hence may pose of risk of serious dysrhythmias.

Preparations, Dosage, and Administration. Haloperidol [Haldol] is dispensed in tablets (0.5, 1, 2, 5, 10, and 20 mg) and a liquid concentrate (2 mg/ml) for oral use. Two injectable forms—*haloperidol lactate* and *haloperidol decanoate*—are available for parenteral (IM) administration. Haloperidol lactate is employed for acute therapy. Haloperidol decanoate is a depot preparation used for long-term treatment.

Oral. The initial dosage for adults is 0.5 to 2 mg taken 2 or 3 times a day. For severe illness, daily doses up to 100 mg have been employed. Once symptoms have been controlled, the dosage should be reduced to the lowest effective amount.

Intramuscular. For acute therapy of severe psychosis, haloperidol lactate is administered IM in doses of 2 to 5 mg. Dosing may be repeated at intervals of 30 minutes to 8 hours. Once symptoms are under control, the patient should be switched to oral therapy. Long-term therapy with haloperidol decanoate is discussed later under *Depot Preparations.*

Other High-Potency Agents

Fluphenazine. Fluphenazine [Prolixin, Permitil] is a high-potency agent indicated for schizophrenia and other psychotic disorders. The drug belongs to the piperazine subclass of phenothiazines. As with other high-potency agents, the most common adverse effects are early extrapyramidal reactions (acute dystonia, parkinsonism, akathisia). The risk of TD equals that of other conventional antipsychotics. Effects seen occasionally include sedation, orthostatic hypotension, anticholinergic effects, gynecomastia, galactorrhea, and menstrual irregularities. NMS, convulsions, and agranulocytosis are rare.

Fluphenazine is administered PO and IM. For oral use, the drug is available in tablets (1, 2.5, 5, and 10 mg), an elixir (0.5 mg/ml), and a liquid concentrate (5 mg/ml). The liquid concentrate should be diluted with water, fruit juice, or some other suitable fluid—but not with beverages that contain caffeine, tannins (tea), or pectinates (apple juice) because of physical incompatibilities. The initial *oral* dosage is 2.5 to 10 mg/day given in divided doses every 6 to 8 hours. Daily dosages greater than 3 mg are rarely needed, although some patients may require as much as 30 mg. Once symptoms have been controlled, the dosage should be reduced to the lowest effective amount, typically 1 to 5 mg/day taken as a single dose.

Three injectable preparations are available: *fluphenazine* (2.5 mg/ml), *fluphenazine decanoate* (25 mg/ml), and *fluphenazine enanthate* (25 mg/ml). Fluphenazine itself is used for acute therapy. Fluphenazine enanthate and fluphenazine decanoate are depot preparations used for long-term therapy (see below). Intramuscular dosages for acute therapy are usually one-third to one-half the oral dosage.

Trifluoperazine. Trifluoperazine [Stelazine] is a high-potency agent used for schizophrenia and other psychotic disorders. The drug belongs to the piperazine subclass of phenothiazines. The most common adverse effects are

TABLE 30–7 ■ Depot Antipsychotic Preparations		
Generic Name [Trade Name]	**Route**	**Typical Maintenance Dosage**
Haloperidol decanoate [Haldol Decanoate]	IM	50–200 mg every 4 wk
Fluphenazine decanoate [Prolixin Decanoate]	IM, SC	2.5–25 mg every 2 wk

early extrapyramidal reactions (acute dystonia, parkinsonism, akathisia). Effects seen occasionally include sedation, orthostatic hypotension, anticholinergic effects, gynecomastia, galactorrhea, menstrual irregularities, and TD. NMS, convulsions, and agranulocytosis are rare.

Trifluoperazine is administered orally and by deep IM injection. Three formulations are available: tablets (1, 2, 5, and 10 mg), liquid concentrate (10 mg/ml), and solution for injection (2 mg/ml). *Oral* dosing is begun at 2 to 5 mg twice daily. Dosage is then increased until an optimal response has been produced, usually with 15 to 20 mg/day. *Intramuscular* therapy is employed acutely. The usual dosage is 1 to 2 mg every 4 to 6 hours as needed.

Thiothixene. Thiothixene [Navane] is a high-potency agent approved for schizophrenia and other psychotic disorders. The most common adverse effects are early extrapyramidal reactions (acute dystonia, parkinsonism, akathisia) and anticholinergic responses. Side effects seen occasionally include galactorrhea, gynecomastia, menstrual irregularities, sedation, orthostatic hypotension, and TD. Agranulocytosis, NMS, and convulsions are rare.

Thiothixene is administered by mouth. Two formulations are available: capsules (1, 2, 5, 10, and 20 mg) and a liquid concentrate (5 mg/ml). The initial dosage is 2 mg 3 times daily. Dosage is increased until an optimal response has been achieved, usually with 20 to 30 mg/day.

Pimozide. Pimozide [Orap] is a high-potency neuroleptic approved only for suppressing symptoms of *Tourette's syndrome,* a rare disorder characterized by severe motor tics and uncontrollable grunts, barking cries, and outbursts of obscene language. Like other neuroleptics, pimozide can cause sedation, postural hypotension, and extrapyramidal reactions (acute dystonia, parkinsonism, akathisia, TD). Pimozide can prolong the QT interval, and hence poses a risk of fatal cardiac dysrhythmias. The drug is available in 2-mg tablets for oral therapy. The initial dosage is 1 to 2 mg/day in divided doses. Dosage should be slowly increased to a maintenance level of 10 mg/day or 0.2 mg/kg/day (whichever is less).

Depot Preparations

The depot antipsychotics are long-acting, injectable preparations used for long-term maintenance therapy of schizophrenia. The objective is to prevent relapse and maintain the highest possible level of functioning. The rate of relapse is lower with depot therapy than with oral therapy. Depot preparations are valuable for all patients who need long-term treatment—not just for patients who have difficulty with compliance. There is no evidence that depot preparations pose an increased risk of side effects, including NMS and TD. In fact, because depot therapy permits a reduction in the total drug burden (the dose per unit time is lower than with oral therapy), the risk of TD is actually reduced.

The depot preparations used most often are *haloperidol decanoate* and *fluphenazine decanoate*. Following IM or SC injection, active drug (fluphenazine or haloperidol) is slowly absorbed into the blood. Because of this slow, steady absorption, plasma levels remain relatively constant between injections. The dosing interval is 2 to 4 weeks. Typical maintenance dosages are presented in Table 30–7.

ATYPICAL ANTIPSYCHOTIC AGENTS

Atypical antipsychotic agents differ from conventional agents in two important ways. First, atypical agents cause few or no EPS, including TD. Second, atypical agents can relieve positive *and* negative symptoms of schizophrenia, whereas benefits of conventional agents are limited primarily to positive symptoms. Because the atypical agents are largely devoid of EPS, they are more acceptable to patients. As a result, compliance is enhanced—which further increases therapeutic responses.

Although the atypical agents are generally very attractive, they do have some drawbacks. Weight gain is common. In addition, case reports suggest they may be able to cause diabetes. Of greater concern, at least three atypical agents can prolong the QT interval, and hence may pose a risk of severe dysrhythmias. Nonetheless, because of their efficacy and acceptability to patients, and because marketing has been aggressive, atypical agents have replaced the conventional agents as first-choice drugs for most patients.

Clozapine

Clozapine [Clozaril] was the first atypical agent available and will serve as our prototype for the group—even though other atypical agents are now used more widely. Clozapine is indicated for schizophrenia. However, because it can cause agranulocytosis, the drug should be reserved for patients who have not responded to safer alternatives.

Mechanism of Action

Antipsychotic effects result from blockade of receptors for dopamine and serotonin (5-hydroxytryptamine [5-HT]). Like conventional antipsychotic agents, clozapine blocks D_2 dopamine receptors, but its affinity for these receptors is low. In contrast, the drug produces strong blockade of $5\text{-}HT_2$ serotonin receptors. Combined blockade of D_2 receptors and $5\text{-}HT_2$ receptors is thought to underlie therapeutic effects. Low affinity for D_2 receptors may explain why EPS are uncommon. In addition to blocking receptors for dopamine and serotonin, clozapine blocks receptors for norepinephrine (alpha$_1$), histamine, and acetylcholine.

Therapeutic Use

Schizophrenia. Because of the risk of fatal agranulocytosis, clozapine should be reserved for patients with severe schizophrenia who have not responded to safer alternatives. Like conventional agents, clozapine improves positive symptoms of schizophrenia. However, in contrast to conventional agents, clozapine improves negative symptoms as well. Patients become more animated, behavior is more socially acceptable, and rates of rehospitalization are reduced. Because the incidence of EPS with clozapine is low, the drug is well suited for patients who have experienced severe EPS with a conventional agent.

Levodopa-Induced Psychosis. Psychosis is a common side effect of levodopa, a drug used for Parkinson's disease (PD). Clozapine is preferred to conventional antipsychotics for treatment. As discussed in Chapter 21, the movement disorders of PD result from insufficient dopamine in the striatum, a component of the extrapyramidal system. Levodopa reduces symptoms of PD by increasing dopamine availability. Since conventional antipsychotic agents cause profound blockade of dopamine receptors in the striatum, they will intensify symptoms of PD. In contrast, clozapine causes little or no blockade of striatal dopamine receptors, and hence can alleviate levodopa-induced psychosis without making symptoms of PD worse. The dosage of clozapine required is only 25 mg a day—about 20 times less than the dosage for schizophrenia.

Pharmacokinetics

Clozapine is rapidly absorbed following oral administration. Peak plasma levels develop in 3.2 hours. About 95% of the drug is bound to plasma proteins. Clozapine undergoes extensive metabolism followed by fecal and urinary excretion. Its half-life is approximately 12 hours.

Adverse Effects and Interactions

Common adverse effects include sedation (from blockade of H_1 histamine receptors; orthostatic hypotension (from blockade of alpha-adrenergic receptors); weight gain (from blockade of 5-HT_2 receptors; and dry mouth, blurred vision, urinary retention, constipation, and tachycardia (from blockade of muscarinic cholinergic receptors). Neuroendocrine effects (galactorrhea, gynecomastia, amenorrhea) and interference with sexual function are minimal.

In contrast to conventional antipsychotics, clozapine carries a low risk of extrapyramidal effects. TD has not been reported. In fact, tardive dyskinesia may improve when patients switch to clozapine from a conventional agent.

Agranulocytosis. Clozapine produces agranulocytosis in 1% to 2% of patients. The overall risk of death is about 1 in 5000. The usual cause is gram-negative septicemia. Agranulocytosis typically occurs during the first 6 months of treatment, and the onset is usually gradual. Why agranulocytosis occurs is unknown.

Because of the risk of fatal agranulocytosis, weekly hematologic monitoring is mandatory. If the total WBC count falls below 3000/mm^3 or if the granulocyte count falls below 1500/mm^3, treatment should be interrupted. When subsequent *daily* monitoring indicates that counts have risen above these values, clozapine can be resumed. If the total WBC count falls below 2000/mm^3 or if the granulocyte count falls below 1000/mm^3, clozapine should be permanently discontinued. Blood counts should be monitored for 4 weeks after drug withdrawal.

Patients should be informed about the risk of agranulocytosis and told that clozapine will not be dispensed if the weekly blood test has not been made. Also, patients should be informed about early signs of infection (fever, sore throat, fatigue, mucous membrane ulceration) and instructed to report these immediately.

Seizures. Generalized tonic-clonic convulsions occur in 3% of patients. The risk of seizures is dose related. Patients should be warned not to drive or to participate in other potentially hazardous activities if a seizure has occurred. Patients with a history of seizure disorders should use the drug with great caution.

Diabetes. Case reports indicate that clozapine may cause new-onset diabetes. Patients taking the drug have developed typical symptoms of diabetes (hyperglycemia, increased appetite, dehydration) and some have experienced diabetic ketoacidosis. At this time, the number of reported cases is small, and a definitive link between clozapine and diabetes has not been established. Nonetheless, it may be wise to monitor blood glucose in patients with diabetes risk factors (obesity, glucose intolerance, family history of diabetes). If diabetes develops, it can be managed with insulin or an oral hypoglycemic agent. Discontinuing the clozapine is also an option. However, if the psychosis is controlled, continuing clozapine and treating the diabetes might be preferable.

Weight Gain. Clozapine can promote significant weight gain. Increases in excess of 30 pounds have been reported. Patients should be informed about the possibility of weight gain and encouraged to get regular exercise, monitor their weight, and reduce caloric intake if their weight increases. If signifi-

cant weight gain occurs, blood levels of cholesterol, triglycerides, and glucose should be monitored.

Myocarditis. Clozapine may cause myocarditis (inflammation of the heart muscle). As of August 2001, 82 cases had been reported, including 31 that were fatal. However, since more that 262,000 patients have used the drug, the risk is clearly very low. If a patient develops signs and symptoms (e.g., unexplained fatigue, dyspnea, tachypnea, chest pain, palpitations), clozapine should be withheld until myocarditis has been ruled out. If myocarditis is diagnosed, clozapine should not be used again.

Drug Interactions. Because of its ability to cause agranulocytosis, clozapine is contraindicated for patients taking other drugs that can suppress bone marrow function (e.g., many anticancer drugs).

Preparations, Dosage, and Administration

Clozapine [Clozaril] is dispensed in 25- and 100-mg tablets for oral administration. To minimize side effects, treatment should begin with a 12.5-mg dose, followed by 25 mg once or twice daily. Dosage is then increased by 25 mg/day until it reaches 300 to 450 mg/day. Further increases can be made once or twice weekly in increments no larger than 100 mg. The usual maintenance dosage is 300 to 600 mg/day in three divided doses. The maximum dosage is 900 mg/day. If therapy is interrupted, it should resume with a 12.5-mg dose and then follow the original escalation guidelines.

Other Atypical Antipsychotics
Risperidone

Risperidone [Risperdal] is a rapid-acting drug that improves positive and negative symptoms of schizophrenia. Like other atypical antipsychotics, risperidone causes fewer extrapyramidal reactions than conventional agents. Risperidone is structurally unrelated to clozapine.

Mechanism of Action. We know that risperidone binds to multiple receptors, but we do not know with certainty how clinical benefits are produced. Risperidone is a powerful antagonist at 5-HT_2 receptors and a less powerful antagonist at D_2 receptors. Antagonism at both sites probably underlies therapeutic effects. Risperidone does not block cholinergic receptors but does block H_1 receptors as well as alpha-adrenergic receptors.

Pharmacokinetics. Absorption of risperidone is rapid and not affected by food. Plasma levels peak about 1 hour after oral administration. Much of each dose is metabolized to 9-hydroxyrisperidone, which has activity equivalent to that of risperidone itself. Parent drug and metabolite are excreted primarily in the urine. The effective half-life is 24 hours. In patients with hepatic or renal dysfunction, the half-life is prolonged.

Therapeutic Effects. Risperidone relieves positive and negative symptoms of schizophrenia. Significant improvement may be seen in 1 week. By contrast, benefits of haloperidol develop more slowly and are limited primarily to positive symptoms. In patients with severe TD, risperidone may have an antidyskinetic effect.

Adverse Effects. Side effects are generally infrequent and mild, and only rarely require discontinuation of treatment. The incidence of EPS is very low at the recommended dosage. However, at dosages above 10 mg/day, there is a dose-related increase in EPS. TD has not been observed. Risperidone increases prolactin levels, but symptoms (gynecomastia, galactorrhea) are uncommon. Like other atypical antipsychotics, risperidone can promote weight gain. Adverse effects that have led to discontinuing the drug include agitation, dizziness, somnolence, and fatigue. Excessive doses have caused difficulty concentrating, sedation, and disruption of sleep. Risperidone can prolong the QT interval, and hence may pose a risk of serious dysrhythmias.

Preparations, Dosage, and Administration. Risperidone [Risperdal] is dispensed in tablets (0.25, 0.5, 1, 2, 3, and 4 mg) and solution (1 mg/ml) for oral administration. The recommended dosage is 1 mg twice daily the first day, 2 mg twice daily the second day, and 3 mg twice daily thereafter. Dosages above 2 or 3 mg twice daily do not increase therapeutic effects, but do increase the risk of EPS and other side effects. Dosage should be reduced in patients with renal or hepatic impairment.

Olanzapine

Olanzapine [Zyprexa] is an atypical antipsychotic agent approved for schizophrenia and other psychotic disorders. The drug is similar to clozapine in structure and actions, but does not cause agranulocytosis.

Mechanism of Action. Olanzapine blocks receptors for serotonin, dopamine, histamine, acetylcholine, and norepinephrine. We believe that therapeutic effects result from blocking 5-HT$_2$ receptors and D$_2$ receptors. Adverse effects result in part from blocking receptors for histamine, acetylcholine, and norepinephrine.

Pharmacokinetics. Olanzapine is well absorbed following oral administration. Food does not alter the rate or extent of absorption. Plasma levels peak 6 hours after dosing and decline with a half-life of 30 hours. Hepatic metabolism of the drug is extensive.

Therapeutic Uses. *Schizophrenia.* In patients with schizophrenia, olanzapine is at least as effective as haloperidol or risperidone and produces fewer EPS than either drug. Comparative trials with clozapine have not been done. Interestingly, olanzapine can relieve psychosis induced by drugs taken for Parkinson's disease without reversing antiparkinsonism effects.

Bipolar Disorder. Olanzapine is approved for monotherapy of acute mania in patients with bipolar disorder (manic-depressive illness). Benefits appear equal to those of lithium, a drug of choice for this disorder (see Chapter 32).

Adverse Effects. Olanzapine is generally well tolerated and appears largely devoid of serious adverse effects. Acute EPS are minimal when the drug is used at the recommended dosage. TD has not been reported. Like clozapine, olanzapine may cause new-onset diabetes. However, in contrast to clozapine, olanzapine does not cause agranulocytosis. Following overdose, the only signs are slurred speech and drowsiness.

Although serious side effects are rare, mild effects are common. Olanzapine causes somnolence in 26% of patients, presumably by blocking H$_1$ receptors. Blockade of muscarinic receptors causes constipation and other anticholinergic effects. Alpha$_1$-adrenergic blockade causes orthostatic hypotension. Blockade of 5-HT$_2$ receptors results in weight gain. In addition, case reports indicate that olanzapine can cause sleepwalking and writer's cramp.

Preparations, Dosage, and Administration. Olanzapine [Zyprexa, Zyprexa Zydis] is dispensed in standard tablets (2.5, 5, 7.5, 10, and 25 mg) under the trade name Zyprexa, and in tablets formulated to disintegrate in the mouth (5 and 10 mg) under the trade name Zyprexa Zydis. For treatment of schizophrenia, the recommended dosage is 5 to 10 mg once a day for the first few days, and 10 mg once a day thereafter. Dosages greater than 10 mg/day are no more effective, but do increase the risk of side effects.

Quetiapine

Actions and Uses. Quetiapine [Seroquel] is an atypical antipsychotic agent indicated only for schizophrenia. The drug can improve both positive and negative schizophrenic symptoms, although negative symptoms respond less consistently. Like other atypical agents, quetiapine produces strong blockade of 5-HT$_2$ receptors and weaker blockade of D$_2$ receptors. Blockade of both receptor types is believed responsible for beneficial effects. In addition to blocking receptors for serotonin and dopamine, quetiapine blocks H$_1$ receptors and alpha-adrenergic receptors, but does not block receptors for acetylcholine.

Pharmacokinetics. Quetiapine is well absorbed following oral administration. The drug undergoes hepatic metabolism followed by excretion in the urine and feces. Its half-life is 6 hours.

Adverse Effects. Common side effects include sedation (from H$_1$ blockade), orthostatic hypotension (from alpha blockade), and weight gain (from 5-HT$_2$ blockade). In clinical trials, quetiapine raised plasma levels of cholesterol and triglycerides by 11% and 17%, respectively. As with other atypical agents, the risk of EPS is low (at therapeutic doses). Tardive dyskinesia has not been reported. Despite structural similarity to clozapine, quetiapine does not pose a risk of agranulocytosis. However, quetiapine may share the ability of clozapine to promote diabetes. Quetiapine can prolong the QT interval, and hence may pose a risk of serious dysrhythmias.

Cataracts are a concern. Cataracts developed in dogs fed 4 times the maximum human dose for 6 or 12 months. Lens changes have also developed in patients; quetiapine may have been the cause. Because quetiapine may pose a risk of cataracts, the manufacturer recommends examination of the lens for cataracts prior to treatment and every 6 months thereafter.

Drug Interactions. Metabolism of quetiapine is accelerated by phenytoin, a drug that induces cytochrome P450 (CYP) 3A4, an isozyme of hepatic CYP drug-metabolizing enzymes. As a result, a larger dose of quetiapine may be needed to maintain antipsychotic effects. Other inducers of CYP3A4 (e.g., barbiturates, carbamazepine, rifampin) may have the same effect.

Although clinical data are not yet available, it seems likely that inhibitors of CYP3A4 (e.g., ketoconazole, itraconazole, fluconazole, erythromycin) will increase levels of quetiapine, thereby posing a risk of toxicity. Caution is advised.

Preparations, Dosage, and Administration. Quetiapine is available in tablets (25, 100, 200, and 300 mg) for oral administration. The initial dosage is low—25 mg twice a day—to minimize orthostatic hypotension. Dosage is gradually increased over the next 3 days to a maintenance level of 300 to 400 mg/day, given in two or three divided doses. For patients who may be especially sensitive to quetiapine (e.g., the elderly, those with hepatic impairment, those predisposed to hypotension), a slower titration rate and lower maintenance dosage may be advisable.

Ziprasidone

Ziprasidone [Geodon] is a new atypical antipsychotic agent indicated for oral therapy of schizophrenia. Like other atypical antipsychotics, ziprasidone can improve both positive and negative symptoms of schizophrenia, and causes fewer EPS than traditional antipsychotics. Ziprasidone stands out from other atypical agents in three significant ways: (1) it causes less weight gain; (2) it causes greater prolongation of the QT interval, and hence poses a greater risk of dysrhythmias; and (3) it is the only atypical antipsychotic available for IM administration.

Mechanism of Action. Ziprasidone blocks multiple receptor types, including D$_2$, 5-HT$_2$, H$_1$, and alpha-adrenergic receptors. In addition, it blocks reuptake of two transmitters: serotonin and norepinephrine. As with other atypical antipsychotics, therapeutic effects are believed to result from blockade of D$_2$ and 5-HT$_2$ receptors. Blockade of serotonin and norepinephrine uptake may provide antidepressant effects.

Pharmacokinetics. Oral ziprasidone is well absorbed, especially in the presence of food. Binding to plasma proteins is extensive. Ziprasidone undergoes hepatic metabolism (primarily by CYP3A4) followed by excretion in the urine and feces. The elimination half-life is about 7 hours.

Adverse Effects. Ziprasidone is generally well tolerated. The most common side effects are somnolence (perhaps from H$_1$ blockade), orthostatic hypotension (perhaps from alpha-adrenergic blockade), and rash (the side effect most responsible for discontinuing the drug). EPS develop in about 5% of patients. Like other atypical antipsychotics, ziprasidone causes weight gain. However, the degree of weight gain is less than with the other agents. In contrast to clozapine, ziprasidone does not cause agranulocytosis.

Ziprasidone prolongs the QT interval, and thereby poses a risk of torsades de pointes, a dysrhythmia that can progress to fatal ventricular fibrillation. QT prolongation is greater than with haloperidol or with other atypical antipsychotics, but less than with thioridazine [Mellaril]. Because of QT prolongation, ziprasidone should not be given to patients with risk factors for torsades de pointes, the most important being hypokalemia, hypomagnesemia, bradycardia, congenital QT prolongation, or a history of dysrhythmias, myocardial infarction, or severe heart failure.

Drug Interactions. Ziprasidone should not be combined with other drugs that prolong the QT interval. Among these are tricyclic antidepressants, thioridazine, several antidysrhythmic drugs (e.g., amiodarone, dofetilide, quinidine), and certain antibiotics (e.g., clarithromycin, erythromycin, moxifloxacin, gatifloxacin, sparfloxacin).

Drugs that induce CYP3A4 (e.g., carbamazepine, phenytoin) can accelerate the metabolism of ziprasidone, and may thereby decrease its levels. Conversely, drugs that inhibit CYP3A4 (e.g., ketoconazole) may increase ziprasidone levels.

Preparations, Dosage, and Administration. Ziprasidone [Geodon] is available in oral capsules (20, 40, 60, and 80 mg) and 20-mg single-use vials for IM administration.

Oral. The initial dosage is 20 mg twice daily taken with food. The maximum dosage is 80 mg twice daily.

Intramuscular. Two dosing schedules may be employed: (1) 10-mg doses given at least 2 hours apart up to a maximum of 40 mg/day or (2) 20-mg doses administered at least 4 hours apart up to a maximum of 40 mg/day. Intramuscular therapy for more than 3 days has not been studied. If long-term treatment is indicated, switch to oral ziprasidone.

Aripiprazole

Contrasts with Other Atypical Antipsychotic Agents. Aripiprazole [Abilify] is the first representative of a new class of antipsychotic drugs, referred to by some as *dopamine system stabilizers* (DDSs). The new drug is just as effective as older atypical agents, but causes fewer side effects. Like other atypical antipsychotics, aripiprazole reduces positive symptoms of schizophrenia and improves negative symptoms, while posing little or no risk of EPS or TD. However, in contrast to other atypical agents, aripiprazole is unlikely to cause significant weight gain, hypotension, or prolactin release, and poses no risk of anticholinergic effects or dysrhythmias.

Mechanism of Action. Like other antipsychotic drugs, aripiprazole can affect multiple receptor types. It blocks H_1, 5-HT_2, and alpha$_1$ receptors, and has mixed effects on 5-HT_1 and D_2 receptors. The drug does not block cholinergic receptors.

As with other atypical antipsychotic agents, therapeutic effects are believed to result from interaction with dopamine and serotonin receptors. However, the nature of the interaction differs: Whereas other atypical agents act as *pure antagonists* at dopamine and serotonin receptors, aripiprazole acts as a *partial agonist* at 5-HT_1 and D_2 receptors, and as a pure antagonist only at 5-HT_2 receptors. Because aripiprazole is a partial agonist at 5-HT_1 and D_2 receptors, net effects on receptor activity will depend on how much transmitter (dopamine or serotonin) is present. Specifically, at synapses where transmitter concentrations are *low,* aripiprazole will bind to receptors and thereby cause *moderate activation.* Conversely, at synapses where transmitter concentrations are *high,* aripiprazole will compete with transmitter for receptor binding, and hence will *reduce receptor activation.* It is because of this ability to modulate the activity of dopamine receptors—rather than simply cause receptor activation or blockade—that aripiprazole has been dubbed a DDS. Researchers suggest that dopamine system stabilization explains why aripiprazole can improve positive and negative symptoms of schizophrenia while having little or no effect on the extrapyramidal system or prolactin release.

Pharmacokinetics. Aripiprazole is well absorbed following oral administration, both in the presence and absence of food. Plasma levels peak 3 to 5 hours after dosing. Protein binding in blood is high—more than 99%. In the liver, aripiprazole undergoes metabolism by two isozymes of cytochrome P450, designated CYP3A4 and CYP2D6. Aripiprazole and its active metabolite—dehydro-aripiprazole—have prolonged half-lives: 75 hours and 94 hours, respectively. Because elimination is slow, (1) dosing can be done once a day and (2) about 14 days (four half-lives) are required to achieve steady-state (plateau) plasma drug levels.

Drug Interactions. Drugs that induce CYP3A4 (e.g., barbiturates, carbamazepine, phenytoin, rifampin) can accelerate metabolism of aripiprazole, and can thereby reduce its blood level. Conversely, drugs that inhibit CYP3A4 (e.g., ketoconazole, itraconazole, fluconazole, erythromycin) can increase aripiprazole levels, as can drugs that inhibit CYP2D6 (e.g., quinidine, fluoxetine, paroxetine).

Adverse Effects. In clinical trials, aripiprazole was well tolerated. The most common side effects were headache, agitation, nervousness, anxiety, insomnia, nausea, vomiting, dizziness, and somnolence. The incidence of EPS was the same as in patients taking placebo. Tardive dyskinesia has not been observed. To date, only two cases of NMS have been reported. Very few patients have gained significant weight (presumably because aripiprazole is a partial agonist at 5-HT_2 receptors, rather than a pure antagonist). Although aripiprazole can block alpha$_1$-adrenergic receptors, the incidence of orthostatic hypotension is low (1.9% vs. 1.0% in patients on placebo). Aripiprazole does not prolong the QT interval, and hence does not pose a risk of dysrhythmias. Also, the drug does not increase prolactin levels, and hence does not cause gynecomastia or galactorrhea.

Preparations, Dosage, and Administration. Aripiprazole [Abilify] is available in 10-, 15-, 20-, and 30-mg tablets. The recommended dosage—both initial and maintenance—is 10 or 15 mg once a day, administered with or without food. Dosages above 15 mg/day do not increase therapeutic effects, but *can* intensify side effects. Dosage should be increased in patients taking inducers of CYP3A4, and reduced in patients taking inhibitors of CYP3A4 or CYP2D6.

MANAGEMENT OF SCHIZOPHRENIA

Drug Therapy

Drug therapy of schizophrenia has three major objectives: (1) suppression of acute episodes, (2) prevention of acute exacerbations, and (3) maintenance of the highest possible level of functioning.

Drug Selection

Drug selection in schizophrenia has changed dramatically in recent years. Use of conventional antipsychotic agents has declined, and use of atypical agents has risen sharply. Today, authorities on schizophrenia consider the atypical antipsychotics drugs of first choice in most situations. These drugs are preferred for initial therapy of acute episodes in most patients, and for treating breakthrough episodes in patients who are taking conventional agents. Therapy with conventional agents is now limited to (1) patients who have used them with success and can tolerate their side effects, (2) patients who are especially aggressive or violent, and (3) patients who need short-acting or long-acting IM medication (atypicals are not yet available for IM administration). Because clozapine can cause agranulocytosis, this atypical agent is reserved for patients who have failed to respond to trials with other atypical agents and with conventional agents.

The switch to atypical agents is due in large part to a better understanding of the real costs of treatment. The clinical superiority of these drugs has been clear for some time: They are more effective and better tolerated than conventional agents, and are associated with fewer relapses and dramatically fewer days of hospitalization. However, they are also much more expensive. For example, whereas haloperidol costs only $50 a year, risperidone costs about $2000 a year, and olanzapine costs about $4000. Nonetheless, even though these drugs are expensive, using them results in significant savings. Why? Because their cost is more than offset by the money saved as a result of fewer days of hospitalization.

Dosing

Dosing with antipsychotics is highly individualized. Elderly patients require relatively small doses—typically 30% to 50% of those for younger patients. Poorly responsive patients may need larger doses that are higher than average. However, very large doses should generally be avoided. Why? Because huge doses are probably no more effective than moderate doses—and will increase the risk of side effects.

Dosage size and timing are likely to change over the course of therapy. During the initial phase of treatment, antipsychotics should be administered in divided daily doses. Once an effective dosage has been determined, the entire daily dose may be given at bedtime. Since antipsychotics cause sedation, bedtime dosing helps promote sleep while decreasing daytime drowsiness. Doses used early in therapy to gain rapid control of behavior are often very high. For long-term therapy, the dosage should be reduced to the lowest effective amount.

Routes

Oral. Oral administration is preferred for most patients. Antipsychotics are available in tablets, capsules, and liquids for oral use.

The liquid formulations require special handling. These preparations are concentrated and must be diluted prior to administration. Dilution may be performed with a variety of fluids, including milk, fruit juices, and carbonated beverages. Some oral liquids are light sensitive and must be stored in amber or opaque containers. Liquid formulations of *phenothiazines* can cause contact dermatitis; nurses and patients should take care to avoid skin contact with these preparations.

Intramuscular. Intramuscular injection is generally reserved for patients with severe, acute schizophrenia and for long-term maintenance. Depot preparations are given every 2 to 4 weeks (see Table 30–7).

Initial Therapy

With adequate dosing, symptoms begin to resolve within 1 to 2 days. However, significant improvement takes 1 to 2 weeks, and full response may not be seen for several months.

Some symptoms resolve sooner than others. During the first week, the goal is to reduce agitation, hostility, anxiety, and tension and to normalize patterns of sleeping and eating. Over the next 6 to 8 weeks, symptoms should continue to steadily improve. The goals over this interval are increased socialization and improved self-care, mood, and formal thought processes. Of the patients who have not responded within 6 weeks, 50% are likely to respond by the end of 12 weeks.

It is important to note that not all symptoms respond equally. With conventional antipsychotics, positive symptoms respond much better than negative symptoms. However, with the atypical agents, positive and negative symptoms may both respond well.

Maintenance Therapy

Schizophrenia is a chronic disorder that usually requires prolonged treatment. The purpose of long-term therapy is to reduce the recurrence of acute florid episodes and to maintain the highest possible level of functioning. Unfortunately, although long-term treatment can be very effective, it also carries a risk of adverse effects, especially TD.

Following control of an acute episode, antipsychotic therapy should continue for at least 12 months. Withdrawal of medication prior to this time is associated with a 55% incidence of relapse, compared with only 20% in patients who continue drug use. Accordingly, patients must be convinced to continue therapy for the entire 12-month course, even though they may be symptom free and consider themselves "cured."

After 12 months, an attempt should be made to discontinue drug use, provided symptoms are absent. About 25% of patients do not need drugs beyond this time. To avoid a withdrawal reaction, dosage should be tapered gradually. It is important that medication not be withdrawn at a time of stress (e.g., when the patient is being discharged following hospitalization). If relapse occurs in response to withdrawal, treatment should be reinstituted. For many patients, resumption of therapy controls symptoms and prevents further deterioration.

When long-term therapy is conducted, dosage should be adjusted with care. To reduce the risk of TD and other adverse effects, a minimum effective dosage should be established. Annual attempts should be made to lower the dosage or to discontinue treatment entirely.

Long-acting (depot) antipsychotics are especially well suited for prolonged treatment. Depot therapy has three major advantages compared with oral therapy: (1) the relapse rate is lower, (2) drug levels are more stable between doses, and (3) the total dose per unit time is lower, thereby reducing the risk of adverse effects, including TD. In the United States, only 10% of patients receive depot therapy. This low rate is based in large part on the widely held (but unfounded) perception that depot therapy is for "losers"—patients who suffer recurrent relapse because of persistent noncompliance with oral therapy.

Adjunctive Drugs

Benzodiazepines (e.g., lorazepam, alprazolam) can suppress anxiety and promote sleep. Whether these drugs also improve core symptoms of schizophrenia is uncertain. In patients experiencing an acute psychotic episode, benzodiazepines can help suppress anxiety, irritability, and agitation. In addition, the benzodiazepine may allow the dosage of antipsychotic medication to be reduced.

Antidepressants are appropriate when schizophrenia is associated with depressive symptoms. A tricyclic antidepressant (e.g., imipramine) is usually chosen. Antidepressant dosage is the same as for major depression. The ideal duration is unknown.

Promoting Compliance

Poor compliance is a common cause of therapeutic failure, and underlies a significant proportion of hospital readmissions. Compliance can be difficult to achieve because treatment is prolonged and because patients may fail to appreciate the need for therapy, or they may be unwilling or unable to take medicine as prescribed. In addition, side effects can discourage compliance. Compliance can be enhanced by

- Ensuring that the medication given to hospitalized patients is actually swallowed and not "cheeked"
- Encouraging family members to oversee medication for outpatients
- Providing patients with written and verbal instructions on dosage size and timing, and encouraging them to take their medicine exactly as prescribed
- Informing patients and their families that antipsychotics must be taken on a regular schedule to be effective, and hence cannot be used PRN
- Informing patients about side effects of treatment and teaching them how to minimize undesired responses
- Assuring patients that antipsychotic drugs do not cause addiction
- Establishing a good therapeutic relationship with the patient and family
- Using a depot preparation (fluphenazine decanoate, haloperidol decanoate) for long-term therapy

Nondrug Therapy

Although drugs can be of great benefit in schizophrenia, medication alone does not constitute optimal treatment. The acutely ill patient needs care, support, and protection; a period of hospitalization may be essential. Counseling can offer the patient and family insight into the nature of schizophrenia and can facilitate adjustment and rehabilitation. Although conventional psychotherapy is of little value in reducing symptoms of schizophrenia, establishing a good therapeutic relationship can help promote compliance and can help the physician evaluate the patient, which in turn can facilitate dosage adjustment and drug selection. Behavioral therapy can help reduce stress. Vocational training in a sheltered environment offers the hope of productivity and some measure of independence. Ideally, the patient will be provided with a comprehensive therapeutic program to complement the benefits of medication. Unfortunately, ideal situations don't always exist, leaving many patients to rely on drugs as their sole treatment modality.

⁘ KEY POINTS

- Schizophrenia is the principal indication for antipsychotic drugs.
- Schizophrenia is a chronic illness characterized by disordered thinking and reduced comprehension of reality. Positive symptoms include hallucinations, delusions, and agitation. Negative symptoms include blunted affect, poverty of speech, and social withdrawal.
- Antipsychotic drugs fall into two major groups: conventional agents and atypical agents.
- Conventional antipsychotics are thought to relieve symptoms of schizophrenia by blocking D_2 receptors.
- Conventional antipsychotics improve positive symptoms of schizophrenia more effectively than negative symptoms.
- Therapeutic responses to antipsychotic drugs develop slowly, often taking several months to become maximal.
- Low-potency conventional agents and high-potency conventional agents produce equal therapeutic effects.
- Conventional antipsychotic drugs produce three types of early EPS: acute dystonia, parkinsonism, and akathisia.
- Acute dystonia and parkinsonism respond to anticholinergic drugs (e.g., benztropine). Akathisia is harder to treat, but may respond to anticholinergic drugs, benzodiazepines, or beta blockers.
- Tardive dyskinesia (TD), a late EPS, has no reliable treatment. For patients with severe TD, switching to an atypical agent may help.
- The risk of early EPS is much greater with high-potency agents than with low-potency agents, whereas the risk of TD is equal with both groups.
- Neuroleptic malignant syndrome, which can be fatal, is characterized by muscular rigidity, high fever, and autonomic instability. Dantrolene and bromocriptine are used for treatment.
- Low-potency agents produce more sedation, orthostatic hypotension, and anticholinergic effects than high-potency agents.
- Antipsychotic drugs increase levels of circulating prolactin by blocking the inhibitory action of dopamine on prolactin release.
- Levodopa can counteract the beneficial effects of conventional antipsychotic drugs and vice versa. Why? Because levodopa activates dopamine receptors, whereas conventional antipsychotic drugs block dopamine receptors.
- Chlorpromazine [Thorazine] is the prototype of the low-potency agents.
- Haloperidol [Haldol] is the prototype of the high-potency agents.
- Antipsychotic depot preparations—haloperidol decanoate and fluphenazine decanoate—are used for long-term maintenance therapy of schizophrenia.
- Atypical antipsychotics differ from conventional antipsychotics in three important ways: (1) they block receptors for serotonin in addition to receptors for dopamine; (2) they cause few or no EPS, including TD; and (3) they relieve positive and negative symptoms of schizophrenia, whereas conventional agents relieve primarily positive symptoms.
- Clozapine can cause potentially fatal agranulocytosis. Hence, (1) weekly blood tests are mandatory and (2) this drug is reserved for patients who have not responded to other atypical agents or conventional agents.
- With the exception of clozapine, the atypical antipsychotic agents are preferred to conventional agents for most patients with schizophrenia.

Summary of Major Nursing Implications*

CONVENTIONAL ANTIPSYCHOTIC DRUGS

Chlorpromazine
Fluphenazine
Haloperidol
Loxapine
Mesoridazine
Molindone
Perphenazine
Pimozide
Thioridazine
Thiothixene
Trifluoperazine
Triflupromazine

Except where indicated otherwise, these nursing implications apply to all conventional antipsychotic drugs.

*Patient education information is highlighted as blue text.

Preadministration Assessment

Therapeutic Goal

Treatment of schizophrenia has three goals: suppression of acute episodes, prevention of acute exacerbations, and maintenance of the highest possible level of functioning.

Baseline Data

Patients should receive a thorough mental status examination and a physical examination.

Observe and record such factors as overt behavior (e.g., gait, pacing, restlessness, volatile outbursts), emotional state (e.g., depression, agitation, mania), intellectual function (e.g., stream of thought, coherence, hallucinations, delusions), and responsiveness to the environment.

Obtain a complete family and social history.

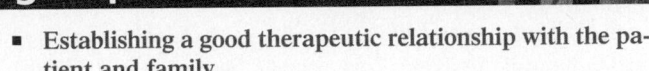

Summary of Major Nursing Implications*—cont'd

Determine vital signs and obtain complete blood counts, electrolytes, and evaluations of hepatic, renal, and cardiovascular function.

Identifying High-Risk Patients

Conventional antipsychotic agents are *contraindicated* for patients who are comatose or severely depressed and for patients with Parkinson's disease, prolactin-dependent carcinoma of the breast, bone marrow depression, and severe hypotension or hypertension. Use with *caution* in patients with glaucoma, adynamic ileus, prostatic hypertrophy, cardiovascular disease, hepatic or renal dysfunction, and seizure disorders.

Implementation: Administration

Routes

Oral, IM, SC, rectal (suppository). Routes for individual agents are summarized in Tables 30–4 and 30–7.

Administration

Dosing. Divided daily doses are employed initially. Once an effective dosage has been determined, the entire daily dose is usually administered at bedtime, thereby promoting sleep and minimizing daytime sedation. For long-term therapy, the smallest effective dosage should be employed.

Oral Liquids. Oral liquid formulations must be protected from light. Concentrated formulations should be diluted just prior to use. Dilution in fruit juice improves palatability.

Oral liquids can cause contact dermatitis. **Warn patients against making skin contact with these drugs, and instruct them to flush the affected area with water if a spill occurs.** Take care to avoid skin contact with these preparations yourself.

Intramuscular. Make injections into the deltoid or gluteal muscle. Rotate the injection site. Depot preparations are administered every 2 to 4 weeks (see Table 30–7).

Implementation: Measures to Enhance Therapeutic Effects

Promoting Compliance

Poor compliance is a common cause of therapeutic failure and rehospitalization. Compliance can be improved by

- Ensuring that medication is actually swallowed and not "cheeked"
- **Encouraging family members to oversee medication for outpatients**
- **Providing patients with written and verbal instructions on dosage size and timing, and encouraging them to take their medicine as prescribed**
- **Informing patients and their families that antipsychotic drugs must be taken on a regular schedule to be effective**
- **Informing patients about side effects and teaching them how to minimize undesired responses**
- **Assuring patients that antipsychotic drugs do not cause addiction**

- **Establishing a good therapeutic relationship with the patient and family**
- Using a depot preparation (e.g., fluphenazine decanoate, haloperidol decanoate) for long-term therapy.

Nondrug Therapy

Acutely ill patients need care, support, and protection; hospitalization may be essential. **Educate the patient and family about the nature of schizophrenia to facilitate adjustment and rehabilitation.** Behavioral therapy can help reduce stress. Vocational training in a sheltered environment offers the hope of productivity and some measure of independence.

Ongoing Evaluation and Interventions

Evaluating Therapeutic Effects

Success is indicated by improvement in psychotic symptoms. Evaluate for suppression of hallucinations, delusions, agitation, tension, and hostility, and for improvement in judgment, insight, motivation, affect, self-care, social skills, anxiety management, and patterns of sleeping and eating.

Minimizing Adverse Effects

Early EPS: Acute Dystonia, Parkinsonism, and Akathisia. These reactions develop within hours to months of the onset of treatment. The risk is greatest with high-potency agents. Take care to differentiate these reactions from worsening of psychotic symptoms. **Inform patients and their families about symptoms (e.g., muscle spasm of tongue, face, neck, or back; tremor; rigidity; restless movement), and instruct them to notify the physician if these appear.** Acute dystonia and parkinsonism respond to anticholinergic drugs (e.g., benztropine). Akathisia may respond to anticholinergic drugs, beta blockers, or benzodiazepines. For severe parkinsonism, switch to an atypical antipsychotic.

Late EPS: Tardive Dyskinesia. TD develops after months or years of continuous therapy. The risk is equal with all conventional antipsychotics. **Inform patients and their families about early signs (e.g., fine, worm-like movements of the tongue), and instruct them to notify the physician if these develop.** Although there is no reliable treatment, the following measures are recommended: discontinue all anticholinergic drugs; give a benzodiazepine; and discontinue the antipsychotic, or at least reduce the dosage. For severe TD, switch to an atypical antipsychotic.

Neuroleptic Malignant Syndrome. NMS is a rare reaction that carries a 4% risk of mortality. Symptoms include rigidity, fever, sweating, dysrhythmias, and fluctuations in blood pressure. NMS is most likely with high-potency agents.

Treatment consists of supportive measures (use of cooling blankets, rehydration), drug therapy (dantrolene, bromocriptine), and immediate withdrawal of the neuroleptic. If neuroleptic therapy is resumed after symptoms have subsided, the lowest effective dosage of a low-potency drug should be employed. If a second episode occurs, switching to an atypical agent may be helpful.

*Patient education information is highlighted as blue text.

Summary of Major Nursing Implications*—cont'd

Anticholinergic Effects. Inform patients about possible anticholinergic reactions (dry mouth, blurred vision, photophobia, urinary hesitancy, constipation, tachycardia, suppression of sweating), and teach them how to minimize discomfort. A complete summary of nursing implications for anticholinergic effects is given in Chapter 14. Anticholinergic effects are most likely with low-potency antipsychotics.

Orthostatic Hypotension. Inform patients about signs of hypotension (lightheadedness, dizziness) and advise them to sit or lie down if these occur. Inform patients that hypotension can be minimized by moving slowly when assuming an erect posture. Orthostatic hypotension is most likely with low-potency antipsychotics.

In hospitalized patients, measure blood pressure and pulses before dosing and 1 hour after. Make these measurements while the patient is lying down and again after he or she has been sitting or standing for 1 to 2 minutes. If blood pressure is low, withhold medication and consult the physician.

Sedation. Sedation is most intense during the first weeks of therapy and declines with continued drug use. Warn patients about sedative effects, and advise them to avoid hazardous activity until sedation subsides. Sedation is most likely with low-potency agents.

Seizures. Neuroleptics reduce seizure threshold, thereby increasing the risk of seizures, especially in patients with epilepsy and other seizure disorders. For patients with seizure disorders, adequate doses of antiseizure medication must be employed. Monitor the patient for seizure activity; if loss of seizure control occurs, dosage of antiseizure medication must be increased.

Sexual Dysfunction. In women, antipsychotics can suppress libido and impair the ability to achieve orgasm. In men, antipsychotics can suppress libido and cause erectile and ejaculatory dysfunction. Counsel patients about possible sexual dysfunction and encourage them to report problems. Dosage reduction or switching to a high-potency neuroleptic may be helpful.

Dermatologic Effects. Inform patients that phenothiazines can sensitize the skin to ultraviolet light, thereby increasing the risk of sunburn. Advise them to avoid excessive exposure to sunlight, apply a sunscreen, and wear protective clothing.

Oral liquid formulations of antipsychotics can cause contact dermatitis. Warn patients to avoid skin contact with these drugs.

Neuroendocrine Effects. Inform patients that antipsychotics can cause galactorrhea, gynecomastia, and menstrual irregularities.

Antipsychotics can promote growth of prolactin-dependent carcinoma of the breast and must not be used by patients with this cancer.

Agranulocytosis. Agranulocytosis greatly diminishes the ability to fight infection. Inform patients about early signs of infection (fever, sore throat), and instruct them to notify the physician if these develop. If blood tests indicate agranulocytosis, the antipsychotic should be withdrawn.

Severe Dysrhythmias. *Chlorpromazine, thioridazine, mesoridazine, haloperidol,* and *pimozide* prolong the QT interval, and can thereby induce torsades de pointes, a dysrhythmia that can progress to fatal ventricular fibrillation. The risk of dysrhythmias can be reduced by (1) ensuring that potassium and magnesium levels are normal, (2) avoiding other drugs that cause QT prolongation, and (3) avoiding drugs that can increase levels of the antipsychotic drug being used.

Minimizing Adverse Interactions

Anticholinergics. Drugs with anticholinergic properties will intensify anticholinergic responses to antipsychotics. Instruct patients to avoid all drugs with anticholinergic properties, including the antihistamines and certain over-the-counter sleep aids.

CNS Depressants. Antipsychotics will intensify CNS depression caused by other drugs. Warn patients against use of alcohol and all other drugs with CNS-depressant properties (e.g., barbiturates, opioids, antihistamines, benzodiazepines).

Levodopa. Levodopa promotes activation of dopamine receptors and may thereby diminish the therapeutic effects of antipsychotics. These drugs should not be used concurrently.

CLOZAPINE, AN ATYPICAL ANTIPSYCHOTIC AGENT

Preadministration Assessment

Therapeutic Goal and Baseline Data

See *Conventional Antipsychotic Agents.*

Identifying High-Risk Patients

Clozapine is *contraindicated* for patients with a history of clozapine-induced agranulocytosis, for patients with bone marrow depression, and for those taking myelosuppressive drugs (e.g., many anticancer drugs). Use with *caution* in patients with seizure disorders and diabetes risk factors.

Implementation: Administration

Route

Oral.

Dosing

To minimize side effects, dosage must be low initially and then gradually increased. If treatment is interrupted, it should resume at the original low dosage.

Ongoing Evaluation and Interventions

Evaluating Therapeutic Effects

See *Conventional Antipsychotic Agents.*

Minimizing Adverse Effects

In contrast to conventional antipsychotic drugs, clozapine carries a low risk of sexual dysfunction, neuroendocrine effects, and extrapyramidal reactions, including TD.

*Patient education information is highlighted as blue text.

Summary of Major Nursing Implications*—cont'd

Agranulocytosis. Clozapine produces agranulocytosis in 1% to 2% of patients, typically during the first 6 months of treatment. Deaths from gram-negative septicemia have occurred.

Weekly hematologic monitoring is mandatory. If the total WBC count falls below 3000/mm³ or if the granulocyte count falls below 1500/mm³, treatment should be interrupted. When subsequent daily monitoring indicates that cell counts have risen above these values, clozapine can be resumed. If the total WBC count falls below 2000/mm³ or if the granulocyte count falls below 1000/mm³, clozapine should be permanently discontinued. Continue monitoring blood counts for 4 weeks.

Warn patients about the risk of agranulocytosis, and inform them that clozapine will not be dispensed without weekly proof of blood counts. Inform patients about early signs of infection (fever, sore throat, fatigue, mucous membrane ulceration), and instruct them to report these immediately.

Seizures. Generalized tonic-clonic seizures occur in 3% of patients. **Warn patients against driving and other hazardous activities if seizures have occurred.**

Sedation. Sedation occurs in 40% of patients. **Warn patients against driving and participation in other hazardous activities if impairment is significant.**

*Patient education information is highlighted as blue text.

Weight Gain. Clozapine can promote significant weight gain. **Inform patients about this risk and encourage them to get regular exercise, monitor their weight, and reduce caloric intake if they gain weight.** In patients with significant weight gain, monitor blood levels of cholesterol, triglycerides, and glucose.

Diabetes. Clozapine may cause new-onset diabetes. To reduce the risk of harm, monitor blood glucose in patients with diabetes risk factors (obesity, glucose intolerance, family history of diabetes). If diabetes develops, it can be managed with insulin or an oral hypoglycemic agent, or by switching to a different antipsychotic.

Myocarditis. Very rarely, clozapine may cause myocarditis. **Inform patients about signs and symptoms (e.g., unexplained fatigue, dyspnea, tachypnea, chest pain, palpitations), and advise them to seek immediate medical attention if these develop.** Clozapine should be withheld until myocarditis has been ruled out. If myocarditis is diagnosed, clozapine should not be used again.

Orthostatic Hypotension and Anticholinergic Effects. See *Conventional Antipsychotic Agents.*

Minimizing Adverse Interactions

Myelosuppressive Drugs. Clozapine must not be given to patients taking other drugs that can suppress bone marrow function (e.g., many anticancer agents).

Antidepressants

MAJOR DEPRESSION: CLINICAL FEATURES,
PATHOGENESIS, AND TREATMENT MODALITIES

TRICYCLIC ANTIDEPRESSANTS

SELECTIVE SEROTONIN REUPTAKE INHIBITORS

Fluoxetine

Other SSRIs

MONOAMINE OXIDASE INHIBITORS

ATYPICAL ANTIDEPRESSANTS

Bupropion

Other Atypical Antidepressants

ELECTROCONVULSIVE THERAPY

TABLE 31–1 ▪ DSM-IV-TR Diagnostic Criteria for a Major Depressive Episode

A. For a diagnosis of major depression, at least five of the following symptoms must be present for 2 weeks or more, and must represent a change from previous functioning. Furthermore, at least one symptom must be (1) depressed mood or (2) loss of interest or pleasure. (*Note:* Do not include mood-incongruent delusions or hallucinations, or symptoms that are due to a general medical condition.)

- Depressed mood most of the day, nearly every day (*Note:* In children and adolescents, can be irritable mood.)
- Loss of interest or pleasure in all or almost all activities
- Significant weight loss or weight gain without dieting *or* decrease or increase in appetite (*Note:* In children, consider failure to make expected weight gains.)
- Insomnia or hypersomnia
- Psychomotor agitation or retardation
- Fatigue or loss of energy
- Feelings of worthlessness or excessive or inappropriate guilt
- Diminished ability to think or concentrate *or* indecisiveness
- Recurrent thoughts of death, recurrent suicidal ideation, a suicide attempt, or a specific suicide plan

B. The symptoms do not meet the criteria for a Mixed Episode (i.e., an episode in which criteria are met for a Major Depressive Episode *and* a Manic Episode)

C. The symptoms cause clinically significant distress or impairment in social, occupational, or other important areas of functioning.

D. The symptoms are not due to the direct physiologic effects of a substance (e.g., drug of abuse, medication) or a general condition (e.g., hypothyroidism).

E. Major depression should not be diagnosed in the context of bereavement (i.e., after the loss of a loved one), unless the symptoms persist for longer than 2 months, or are characterized by marked functional impairment, morbid preoccupation with worthlessness, suicidal ideation, psychotic symptoms, or psychomotor retardation.

Adapted from the Diagnostic and Statistical Manual of Mental Disorders, Fourth Edition, Text Revision. Washington, DC, American Psychiatric Press, 2000, with permission. Copyright © 2000 American Psychiatric Association.

As their name suggests, the antidepressants are used primarily to relieve symptoms of depression. In addition, these drugs can help patients with anxiety disorders. As a rule, antidepressants are not indicated for uncomplicated bereavement. The antidepressants fall into four major groups: tricyclic antidepressants, selective serotonin reuptake inhibitors, monoamine oxidase inhibitors, and atypical antidepressants.

MAJOR DEPRESSION: CLINICAL FEATURES, PATHOGENESIS, AND TREATMENT MODALITIES

Depression is the most common psychiatric disorder. In the United States, about 30% of the population will experience some form of depression during their lives. At any given time, about 5% of the adult population is depressed. The incidence in women is twice that in men. The risk of suicide among depressed people is about 25%. Unfortunately, depression is underdiagnosed and undertreated: Only 30% of depressed individuals receive treatment; the other 70% do not. This is especially sad in that treatment can help many people: about 40% of those given antidepressants achieve full remission; another 20% to 30% achieve at least a 50% reduction in symptom severity.

Clinical Features

Diagnostic criteria for a major depressive episode are summarized in Table 31–1. As indicated, the principal symptoms are *depressed mood* and *loss of pleasure or interest in all or nearly all of one's usual activities and pastimes.* Associated symptoms include insomnia (or sometimes hypersomnia); anorexia and weight loss (or sometimes hyperphagia and weight gain); mental slowing and loss of concentration; feelings of guilt, worthlessness, and helplessness; thoughts of

death and suicide; and overt suicidal behavior. For a diagnosis to be made, symptoms must be present most of the day, nearly every day, for at least 2 weeks.

It is important to distinguish between major depression and normal grief or sadness. Whereas major depression is an illness, grief or sadness is not. Rather, grief and sadness are appropriate reactions to a major life stressor (e.g., death of a loved one, loss of a job). In most cases, grief and sadness resolve spontaneously over several weeks and do not require

Special Interest Topic

BOX 31–1 ■ POSTPARTUM DEPRESSION

Remarkably, the vast majority (about 80%) of women experience depressive symptoms after giving birth. For most, the symptoms are mild and transient, reflecting a condition known as the "baby blues." For others, symptoms are severe and persistent, reflecting true postpartum depression, a condition that merits rapid medical attention.

An estimated 60% to 70% of women get the postpartum blues. Symptoms include tearfulness, sadness, nervousness, irritability, and anxiety, along with difficulty eating and sleeping. The new mom may feel overwhelmed, vulnerable, weak, and alone. She may cry for no clear reason. Her self-esteem and self-confidence may decline, and she may feel unqualified to care for her baby. Fortunately, all of these symptoms pass quickly: as a rule, they develop a few days after delivery and are gone by day 10. Because the baby blues are so common, they're considered a normal postpartum event. Treatment is neither necessary nor recommended.

True postpartum depression is a different matter. The condition is less common than the baby blues—but much more serious. Left untreated, postpartum depression typically lasts for months, and is likely to become worse as time passes. Not only is the condition detrimental to the mother, it can adversely affect the child, preventing secure attachment and impairing cognitive, emotional, and behavioral development. Accordingly, immediate intervention is indicated.

Just what is postpartum depression? Simply put, it's an episode of major depression that starts after giving birth. Otherwise, the diagnostic criteria are the same as for all other episodes of major depression (see Table 31–1). According to the *Diagnostic and Statistical Manual of Mental Disorders, Fourth Edition* (DSM-IV), for a depressive episode to qualify as having postpartum onset, symptoms must begin within *4 weeks* of delivery. However, most clinicians who study the disorder use a different criterion: To them, depression is considered postpartum if it begins within *3 months* of delivery—not just within 4 weeks.

Who is likely to suffer postpartum depression? Sometimes the condition occurs in first-time mothers, and sometimes it doesn't strike until a second, third, or fourth child is born. Among first-time mothers, the incidence is between 8% and 15% (about 1 in 8). For women with a history of the disorder, the risk increases to 33% (1 in 3). In addition to a prior history of the disorder, risk factors include a history of depression unrelated to childbirth, a history of premenstrual dysphoric disorder (i.e., severe premenstrual syndrome), and major stress related to family, work, or residence (e.g., death of a loved one, loss of a job, moving away from a familiar town or city).

The underlying cause of postpartum depression is unknown, but several factors are thought to contribute. Heading the list is the sharp drop in estrogen and progesterone levels that occurs after delivery. (Levels of these hormones increase 10-fold during pregnancy, and then return to baseline after the placenta is expelled.) However, since hormone levels fall in all women, but only some get postpartum depression, other factors—physical, emotional, and social—must be involved.

The birthing process leaves women feeling weak and fatigued. Caring for a baby, who needs round-the-clock attention and feeding, exacerbates tiredness and exhaustion. Emotional and social factors may also play a role. Feelings of loss are common: Women experience loss of freedom, loss of control, and even loss of identity. In addition, they may feel loss of attractiveness. Stress increases substantially, owing to increased workload and responsibilities, coupled with feelings of self-doubt and inadequacy, and compounded by a self-imposed (albeit highly unrealistic) expectation to be a "perfect" mom. Stress can be made even worse by financial insecurity and by inadequate support from one's partner, family, and friends. Thyroid insufficiency may also contribute: Levels of thyroid hormone often decline after delivery, thereby causing symptoms that can mimic depression. Accordingly, thyroid levels should be checked and, if indicated, replacement therapy should be implemented.

Screening for postpartum depression can be accomplished with a quick test: the Edinburgh Postnatal Depression Scale. The test is administered 6 to 8 weeks after delivery and contains the following short statements:

1. I have been able to laugh and see the funny side of things.
2. I have looked forward with enjoyment to things.
3. I have blamed myself unnecessarily when things went wrong.
4. I have been anxious or worried for no good reason.
5. I have felt scared or panicky for no very good reason.
6. Things have been getting on top of me.
7. I have been so unhappy that I have had difficulty sleeping.
8. I have felt sad or miserable.
9. I have been so unhappy that I have been crying.
10. The thought of harming myself has occurred to me.

Each statement has four possible responses, such as these for statement 10: (1) Yes, quite often, (2) sometimes, (3) hardly ever, and (4) never. When taking the test, the mother simply underlines the option that best reflects her feelings during the previous week. If her responses indicate she probably has postpartum depression, she should undergo clinical evaluation to establish a definitive diagnosis.

Treatment of postpartum depression is much like treatment of major depression unrelated to pregnancy. The goal is to normalize mood, and optimize maternal and social functioning. The principal treatment modalities are psychotherapy and antidepressant drugs, both of which can be effective. In addition, the woman should be encouraged to nurture herself as well as her baby: She should reduce isolation (by going out for at least a short time each day), she should ensure adequate rest (by doing only what's really needed and letting the rest go), and she should spend time alone with her partner. Other beneficial measures include joining a support group for new mothers and recruiting family members and friends to assist with household and baby-related chores.

Although antidepressants are clearly appropriate, there are few published data to guide selection. In one study of women

(Continued on next page)

Special Interest Topic—cont'd

with postpartum depression, fluoxetine [Prozac], a selective serotonin reuptake inhibitor (SSRI), was compared with psychotherapy. Both treatments were equally effective, and both were superior to placebo. Efficacy has also been demonstrated for sertraline [Zoloft], venlafaxine [Effexor], and certain tricyclic antidepressants (TCAs). For initial therapy, the SSRIs are an attractive choice. Why? Because they are effective and well tolerated, and present little risk of toxicity if taken in overdose. However, if a woman has responded to an antidepressant from a different class in the past, that drug should be tried first. To minimize side effects, dosage should be low initially (50% the usual starting dosage) and then gradually increased. To reduce the risk of relapse, treatment should continue for at least 6 months after symptoms have resolved. Unfortunately, even then the relapse rate is high: Between 50% and 85% of patients

experience at least one more depressive episode. With each succeeding episode, the risk of another recurrence increases. Accordingly, long-term prophylactic therapy should be considered.

Which antidepressants can be taken safely while breastfeeding? All of these drugs can be detected in breast milk—but the levels of some are much lower (safer) than the levels of others. Sertraline, for example, appears very safe. Studies show that drug activity in breast-fed infants is extremely low, and no adverse reactions have been observed. The TCAs (e.g., nortriptyline, desipramine) also appear safe: Levels are too low for detection in breast-fed infants, and follow-up studies have found no developmental deficits. In contrast to sertraline and the TCAs, fluoxetine appears unsafe: The drug and its metabolites reach therapeutic levels in breast-fed infants; potential consequences include colic and impaired weight gain.

medical intervention. However, if symptoms are unusually intense, and if they fail to abate within an appropriate time, a major depressive episode may have been superimposed. If this occurs, treatment is indicated.

Pathogenesis

The etiology of major depression is complex and incompletely understood. For some individuals, depression seems to descend "out of the blue"; otherwise healthy people—unexpectedly and without apparent cause—find themselves feeling profoundly depressed. For many others, depressive episodes are brought on by stressful life events, such a bereavement or loss of a job. Since depression does not occur in everyone, it would appear that some people are more vulnerable than others. Factors that may contribute to vulnerability include genetic heritage, a difficult childhood, and chronic low self-esteem.

Clinical observations made in the 1960s led to formulation of the *monoamine hypothesis of depression,* which asserts that depression is caused by a functional insufficiency of monoamine neurotransmitters (norepinephrine, serotonin, or both). This hypothesis is based in large part on two observations: (1) depression can be induced with reserpine, a drug that depletes monoamines from the brain, and (2) the drugs used to treat depression intensify monoamine-mediated neurotransmission. Although these observations lend support to the monoamine hypothesis, it is now clear that the hypothesis is too simplistic. However, despite its shortcomings, the monoamine hypothesis does provide a useful conceptual framework for understanding antidepressant drugs.

Treatment Modalities

Depression can be treated with three modalities: (1) pharmacotherapy, (2) depression-specific psychotherapy (e.g., cognitive behavioral therapy), and (3) electroconvulsive therapy (ECT). Each modality has a legitimate role. For patients with mild to moderate depression, drug therapy and psychotherapy can be equally effective. For those with more severe depression, a combination of drugs and psychotherapy is more effective than either intervention alone. ECT is used when a rapid response is needed, or when drugs and psychotherapy have not worked.

Drugs are the primary therapy for major depression. Available antidepressants are listed in Table 31–2. For many patients, the *tricyclic antidepressants* (TCAs) are drugs of first choice. These agents are inexpensive, effective, relatively safe, and easy to administer. *Selective serotonin reuptake inhibitors* (SSRIs) are just as effective as the tricyclics and better tolerated. Because of these qualities—and despite their high cost—the SSRIs have become our most widely prescribed antidepressants. *Monoamine oxidase inhibitors* (MAOIs) are generally reserved for patients who have not responded to TCAs or SSRIs. However, for patients with *atypical* depression, MAOIs are drugs of choice.

Electroconvulsive therapy is a valuable tool for treating depression. This procedure is safe and effective, and benefits develop more rapidly than with drugs or psychotherapy. Accordingly, ECT is especially appropriate when speed is critical. Candidates for ECT include (1) severely depressed, suicidal patients; (2) elderly patients at risk of starving to death because of depression-induced lack of appetite; and (3) patients who have not responded to antidepressant drugs.

TRICYCLIC ANTIDEPRESSANTS

The TCAs are drugs of first choice for many patients with major depression. The first tricyclic agent—imipramine—was introduced to psychiatry in the late 1950s. Since then, the ability of TCAs to relieve depressive symptoms has been firmly established. The most common adverse effects of TCAs are sedation, orthostatic hypotension, and anticholinergic effects. The most dangerous effect is cardiac toxicity. Because all of the TCAs have similar properties, we will discuss these drugs as a group, rather than focusing on a representative prototype.

Chemistry

The structure of imipramine, a representative TCA, is shown in Figure 31–1. As you can see, the nucleus of this drug has three rings—hence the classification *tricyclic antidepressant.*

As indicated in Figure 31–1, the three-ringed nucleus of the TCAs is very similar to the three-ringed nucleus of the

TABLE 31–2 ■ Antidepressants: Adverse Effects and Effects on Neurotransmitters

	Transmitter Reuptake Antagonism[a]		Anticho-linergic Activity	Sedation	Hypo-tension	Seizure Risk	Cardiac Toxicity	Weight Gain	Sexual Dysfunction	Other Side Effects
	NE	5-HT								
Tricyclic Antidepressants										
Amitriptyline	++	+++	++++	++++	++	+++	++++	++	++	
Clomipramine	+++	+++	+++	+++	++	++	++++	+	+++	
Desipramine	+++	0	+	c	+	++	+++	+	++	
Doxepin	+	++	++	+++	++	++	++	++	++	
Imipramine	++	+++	++	++	+++	++	++++	++	++	
Maprotiline	+++	0	++	++	+	+++	+++	+	++	
Nortriptyline	++	+++	++	++	+	++	+++	+	++	
Protriptyline	+++	0	+++	c	+	++	++++	+	++	
Trimipramine	+	+	++	+++	++	++	++++	++	++	
Monoamine Oxidase Inhibitors										
Isocarboxazid	b	b	+	+	+	0	0	+	++	Hypertensive crisis from tyramine in food
Phenelzine	b	b	+	+	+	0	0	+	+++	
Tranylcypromine	b	b	+	c	0	0	0	+	++	
Selective Serotonin Reuptake Inhibitors										
Citalopram	0	+++	0/+	0/+	0/+			+	+++	
Fluoxetine	0	+++	0	c	0/+	0/+	0	+	++++	
Fluvoxamine	0	+++		++		0		+	+++	
Paroxetine	0	+++	+	c	0/+	0	0	+	++++	
Sertraline	0	+++	0	c	0	0	0	+	+++	
Atypical Antidepressants										
Amoxapine	++d	+d	+++	++	+	+++	+	+	++	Parkinsonism Seizures
Bupropion	e	e	++	c	+	++++	+	0	g	
Mirtazapine	f	f	++	+++	++		0/+	+	0/+	
Nefazodone	0	+	+	++	+	0	0/+	0	0/+	
Trazodone	0	++	+	++++	+++	+	+	+	h	Priapism
Venlafaxine	++	+++	0	0	0	+	0/+	0	++	

[a]NE = norepinephrine; 5-HT = serotonin.
[b]MAOIs do not block transmitter reuptake. Rather, they increase intraneuronal stores of NE, 5-HT, and dopamine.
[c]Produces moderate *stimulation,* not sedation.
[d]In addition to blocking NE and 5-HT *reuptake,* amoxapine blocks *receptors* for dopamine.
[e]Bupropion primarily inhibits reuptake of dopamine rather than NE or 5-HT.
[f]Mirtazapine acts by promoting *release* of NE and 5-HT.
[g]Bupropion may actually increase sexual desire.
[h]Trazodone can cause priapism (persistent painful erection).

phenothiazine antipsychotics. Because of this structural similarity, TCAs and phenothiazines have several actions in common. Specifically, both groups produce varying degrees of *sedation, orthostatic hypotension,* and *anticholinergic effects.*

Mechanism of Action

The proposed mechanism of action of the TCAs is depicted in Figure 31–2. As shown, TCAs block neuronal reuptake of two monoamine transmitters: norepinephrine (NE) and serotonin. By blocking reuptake of these transmitters, TCAs intensify their effects. This mechanism is consistent with the monoamine hypothesis of depression, which asserts that depression stems from a *deficiency* in monoamine-mediated transmission—and hence should be relieved by drugs that can intensify monoamine effects. The relative ability of individual tricyclics to block reuptake of NE and serotonin is summarized in Table 31–2.

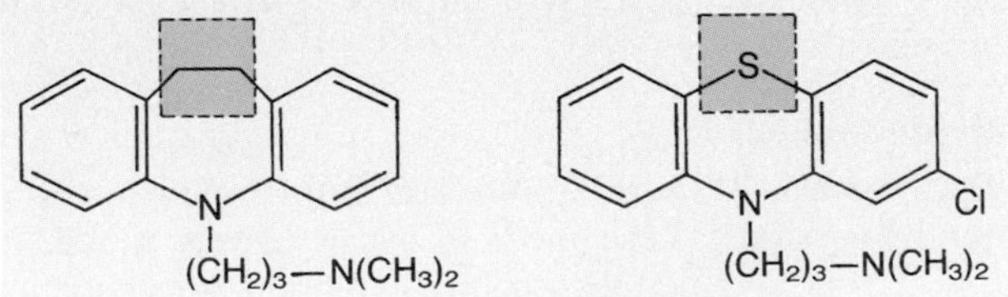

Imipramine
(a tricyclic antidepressant)

Chlorpromazine
(a phenothiazine antipsychotic)

Figure 31–1 ■ Structural similarities between tricyclic antidepressants and phenothiazine antipsychotics.
Except for the areas highlighted, the phenothiazine nucleus is nearly identical to that of TCAs. Because of their structural similarities, TCAs and phenothiazines have several pharmacologic properties in common.

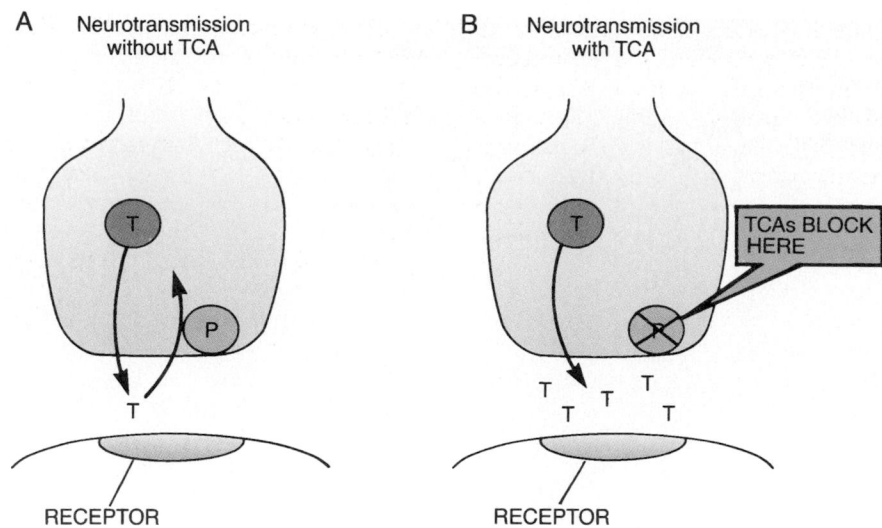

Figure 31–2 ■ Mechanism of action of tricyclic antidepressants.
A, Under drug-free conditions, the actions of norepinephrine and serotonin are terminated by active uptake of these transmitters back into the nerve terminals from which they were released.

B, By inhibiting the uptake pumps for norepinephrine and serotonin, tricyclic antidepressants cause these transmitters to accumulate in the synaptic space, thereby intensifying transmission.

(P = uptake pump, T = transmitter [norepinephrine or serotonin], TCA = tricyclic antidepressant.)

It is important to appreciate that blockade of reuptake, by itself, cannot fully account for therapeutic effects. Why? Because clinical responses to the TCAs (relief of depressive symptoms) and biochemical effects of the TCAs (blockade of transmitter reuptake) do not occur in the same time frame. That is, whereas TCAs block transmitter uptake within hours of their administration, relief of depression takes several weeks to develop. Hence, it would appear that, in the interval between the onset of uptake blockade and the onset of a therapeutic response, intermediary neurochemical events must be taking place. Just what these are is unknown.

Pharmacokinetics

TCAs have half-lives that are long and variable. Because their half-lives are long, TCAs can usually be administered in a single daily dose. Because their half-lives are variable, TCAs require individualization of dosage.

Therapeutic Uses

Depression. TCAs are preferred drugs for treatment of major depression. These medicines can elevate mood, increase activity and alertness, decrease morbid preoccupation, improve appetite, and normalize sleep patterns.

Like all other antidepressants, TCAs do not relieve symptoms immediately. *Initial* responses develop in 1 to 3 weeks. *Maximal* responses develop over 1 to 2 months. Because therapeutic effects are delayed, TCAs cannot be used PRN. Furthermore, a therapeutic trial should not be considered a failure until medication has been administered for at least 1 month without success.

Suicide is always a concern when treating depression. Why? Because the patient may be so despondent as to perceive death as the only means of relief. To reduce the chances of suicide, several precautions can be taken. First, since antidepressants take several weeks to alleviate symptoms, patients with suicidal tendencies should be hospitalized until treatment has had time to reduce suicide risk. In addition, since TCAs themselves can be vehicles for suicide, the patient should not be given access to a large supply. Accordingly, you should ensure that each dose is actually swallowed and not cheeked. This precaution will prevent the patient from accumulating multiple doses that might be taken with suicidal intent.

Bipolar Disorder. Bipolar disorder (manic-depressive illness) is characterized by alternating episodes of mania and depression (see Chapter 32). TCAs can help during depressive episodes.

Other Uses. TCAs can benefit patients with *pain* (see Chapter 28), *chronic insomnia* (see Chapter 33), *attention-deficit/hyperactivity disorder* (see Chapter 35), and *panic disorder* or *obsessive-compulsive disorder* (see Chapter 34).

Adverse Effects

The most common adverse effects are orthostatic hypotension, sedation, and anticholinergic effects. The most serious adverse effect is cardiotoxicity. These effects occur because, in addition to blocking uptake of monoamine transmitters, TCAs cause direct blockade of receptors for histamine, acetylcholine, and NE. Adverse effects of individual agents are summarized in Table 31–2.

Orthostatic Hypotension. Orthostatic hypotension is the most serious of the common adverse responses to TCAs. Hypotension is due in large part to blockade of alpha$_1$-adrenergic receptors on blood vessels. Patients should be informed that orthostatic hypotension can be minimized by moving slowly when assuming an upright posture. In addition, patients should be instructed to sit or lie down if symptoms (dizziness, lightheadedness) occur. For hospitalized patients, blood pressure and pulse rate should be monitored on a regular schedule (e.g., 4 times a day). These measurements should be taken while the patient is lying down and again after the patient has been sitting or standing for 1 to 2 minutes. If blood pressure is low or pulse rate is high, medication should be withheld and the physician notified.

Anticholinergic Effects. The TCAs block muscarinic cholinergic receptors, and can thereby cause an array of anticholinergic effects (dry mouth, blurred vision, photophobia, constipation, urinary hesitancy, and tachycardia). Patients should be informed about possible anticholinergic responses and instructed in ways to minimize discomfort. A detailed discussion of anticholinergic effects and their management is presented in Chapter 14.

Diaphoresis. Despite their anticholinergic properties, TCAs often cause diaphoresis (sweating). The mechanism of this paradoxical effect is unknown.

Sedation. Sedation is a common response to TCAs. The cause is blockade of histamine receptors in the central nervous system (CNS). Patients should be advised to avoid hazardous activities if sedation is prominent.

Cardiac Toxicity. Tricyclics can adversely affect cardiac function. However, in the absence of an overdose or pre-existing cardiac impairment, serious effects are rare. The TCAs affect the heart by (1) decreasing vagal influence on the heart (secondary to muscarinic blockade) and (2) acting directly on the bundle of His to slow conduction. Both effects increase the risk of dysrhythmias. To minimize risk, all patients—adults and children—should undergo electrocardiographic (EKG) evaluation prior to treatment and periodically thereafter.

Seizures. TCAs lower seizure threshold. Caution must be exercised in patients with epilepsy and other seizure disorders.

Hypomania. On occasion, TCAs produce too much of a good thing, elevating mood from depression all the way to hypomania (mild mania). If hypomania develops, the patient should be evaluated to determine whether elation is drug induced or symptomatic of bipolar disorder.

Yawngasm. Rarely, patients taking *clomipramine* [Anafranil] experience yawngasm. Experience what? A spontaneous orgasm while yawning. Honest. This unusual side effect, which affects both males and females, may be considered adverse or beneficial, depending on one's view of such things. In at least one documented case, yawngasms strongly influenced compliance, as evidenced by the patient asking how long she would be "allowed" to continue treatment. Although data are scarce, one might guess that the occasional yawngasm would help relieve depression.

Drug Interactions

Monoamine Oxidase Inhibitors. The combination of a TCA with an MAOI can lead to *severe hypertension* from excessive adrenergic stimulation of the heart and blood vessels. Excessive adrenergic stimulation occurs because (1) inhibition of monoamine oxidase (MAO) causes accumulation of NE in adrenergic neurons and (2) blockade of NE reuptake by the tricyclics decreases NE inactivation. Because of the potential for hypertensive crisis, combined therapy with TCAs and MAOIs is generally avoided.

Direct-Acting Sympathomimetic Drugs. Tricyclics *potentiate* responses to direct-acting sympathomimetics (i.e., drugs such as epinephrine and NE that produce their effects

by direct interaction with adrenergic receptors). Stimulation by these drugs is increased because TCAs block their uptake into adrenergic terminals, thereby prolonging their presence in the synaptic space.

Indirect-Acting Sympathomimetic Drugs. TCAs *decrease* responses to indirect-acting sympathomimetics (i.e., drugs such as ephedrine and amphetamine that promote release of transmitter from adrenergic nerves). Effects of indirect-acting sympathomimetics are reduced because TCAs block uptake of these agents into adrenergic nerves, thereby preventing them from reaching their site of action within the nerve terminal.

Anticholinergic Agents. Since TCAs have anticholinergic actions of their own, they will intensify the effects of other medications that have anticholinergic actions. Consequently, patients receiving TCAs should be advised to avoid all other drugs with anticholinergic properties, including antihistamines and certain over-the-counter sleep aids.

CNS Depressants. CNS depression caused by TCAs will add with CNS depression caused by other drugs. Accordingly, patients should be warned against taking all other CNS depressants, including alcohol, antihistamines, opioids, and barbiturates.

Toxicity

Overdose with a TCA can be life threatening. (The lethal dose is only 8 times the average daily dose.) To minimize the risk of death by suicide, acutely depressed patients should be given no more than a 1-week supply of TCAs at one time.

Clinical Manifestations. Symptoms result primarily from *anticholinergic* and *cardiotoxic* actions. The combination of cholinergic blockade and direct cardiotoxicity can produce *dysrhythmias,* including tachycardia, intraventricular blocks, complete atrioventricular block, ventricular tachycardia, and ventricular fibrillation. Responses to peripheral muscarinic blockade include hyperthermia, flushing, dry mouth, and dilation of the pupils.

CNS symptoms are prominent. Early responses are confusion, agitation, and hallucinations. Seizures and coma may follow.

Treatment. Absorption of ingested drug can be reduced with gastric lavage followed by ingestion of activated charcoal. Physostigmine (a cholinesterase inhibitor) is given to counteract anticholinergic actions. Propranolol, lidocaine, or phenytoin can be given to control dysrhythmias. Dysrhythmias should not be treated with procainamide or quinidine, because they will aggravate cardiac depression.

Dosage and Routes of Administration

Dosage. Dosages for individual TCAs are summarized in Table 31–3. General guidelines on dosing are discussed below.

Initial doses of TCAs should be low (e.g., 50 mg of imipramine a day for adult outpatients). Low initial doses minimize adverse reactions and thereby help promote compliance. High initial doses are both undesirable and unnecessary. High doses are undesirable in that they pose an increased risk of adverse reactions. They are unnecessary in that onset of therapeutic effects is delayed regardless of dosage; hence aggressive initial dosing offers no benefit.

Because of interpatient variability in TCA metabolism, dosing is highly individualized. As a rule, dosage is adjusted on the basis of clinical response. However, if there is no observable response, plasma drug levels can be used as a guide. For example, levels of imipramine must be above 225 ng/ml to be effective. If a patient has not responded to imipramine, measurements should be made to ensure that the plasma level is adequate. If the level is below 225 ng/ml, dosage should be increased.

Once an effective dosage has been established, most patients can take their entire daily dose at bedtime; the long half-lives of the TCAs make divided daily doses unnecessary. Once-a-day dosing at bedtime has three advantages: (1) it's easy, and hence facilitates compliance; (2) it promotes sleep by causing maximal sedation at night; and (3) it reduces the intensity of side effects during the day. If bedtime dosing causes residual sedation in the morning, dosing earlier in the evening can help. Although once-a-day dosing is generally desirable, not all patients can use this schedule. The elderly, for example, can be especially sensitive to the cardiotoxic actions of the tricyclics. As a result, if the entire daily dose were taken at one time, effects on the heart might be intolerable.

Once remission has been produced, therapy should continue for 6 months to a year. Failure to take medication for this period is likely to result in relapse. Patients should be encouraged to continue drug therapy even if they are symptom free and hence feel that further medication is unnecessary.

Routes of Administration. All TCAs can be administered by mouth, as they usually are. Two agents—*amitriptyline* and *imipramine*—may be given IM. Since effects take weeks to develop, there is no benefit to IV administration. Hence, this route is not used.

Preparations and Drug Selection

Preparations. In the United States, nine TCAs are available (see Tables 31–2 and 31–3). All nine are equally effective. Principal differences among these drugs concern side effects (see Table 31–2).

Drug Selection. Selection among TCAs is based on side effects. For example, if the patient is experiencing insomnia, a drug with prominent sedative properties (e.g., doxepin) might be selected. Conversely, if daytime sedation is undesirable, a less sedating agent (e.g., desipramine) might be preferred. Elderly patients with glaucoma or constipation and males with prostatic

TABLE 31–3 ■ Adult Dosage for Antidepressants

Generic Name	Trade Name	Initial Dose*† (mg/day)	Dose after 4–8 Wk* (mg/day)	Maximum Dose‡ (mg/day)
Tricyclic Antidepressants				
Amitriptyline	Elavil	50	100–200	300
Clomipramine	Anafranil	25	100–200	250
Desipramine	Norpramin	50	100–200	300
Doxepin	Sinequan	50	75–150	300
Imipramine	Tofranil	50	75–150	300
Maprotiline	generic only	50	100–150	225
Nortriptyline	Aventyl, Pamelor	20	75–100	125
Protriptyline	Vivactil	10	15–40	60
Trimipramine	Surmontil	50	100–200	300
Monoamine Oxidase Inhibitors				
Isocarboxazid	Marplan	20	20–60	80
Phenelzine	Nardil	15	45–60	90
Tranylcypromine	Parnate	10	30–40	60
Selective Serotonin Reuptake Inhibitors				
Citalopram	Celexa	20	20–60	60
Escitalopram	Lexapro	10	10	10
Fluoxetine	Prozac	20	20–80	80
Fluvoxamine	Luvox	50	50–300	300
Paroxetine	Paxil	10	20–50	50
Sertraline	Zoloft	50	50–150	200
Atypical Antidepressants				
Amoxapine	Asendin	50	200–300	400
Bupropion	Wellbutrin	150	50–300	450
Mirtazapine	Remeron	15	15–45	60
Nefazodone	Serzone	200	300–600	600
Reboxetine	Vestra	4–8	4–10	10
Trazodone	Desyrel	150	150–400	600
Venlafaxine	Effexor	37.5	75–225	375

*Doses listed are *total daily doses*. Depending on the drug and the patient, the total dose may be given in a single dose or in divided doses.
†Initial doses are employed for 4–8 weeks, the time required for most symptoms to respond. Dosage is gradually increased as required.
‡Doses higher than these may be needed for some patients with severe depression.

hypertrophy can be especially sensitive to anticholinergic effects. Hence, for these patients, a drug with weak anticholinergic properties (e.g., desipramine) would be appropriate.

SELECTIVE SEROTONIN REUPTAKE INHIBITORS

The SSRIs were introduced in 1987 and have since become our most commonly prescribed group of antidepressants, accounting for over $3 billion in annual sales. These drugs are as effective as the TCAs, but do not cause hypotension, sedation, or anticholinergic effects. Moreover, overdose does not cause cardiotoxicity. Death by overdose is extremely rare. Characteristic side effects of the SSRIs are nausea, insomnia, weight gain, and sexual dysfunction (especially anorgasmia). SSRIs can interact adversely with MAOIs, and hence the combination must be avoided. These drugs are used to treat major depression and a variety of other psychologic disorders (Table 31–4). Fluoxetine, the first SSRI available, will serve as our prototype for the group.

Fluoxetine

Fluoxetine [Prozac, Sarafem] is the most widely prescribed antidepressant in the United States. The drug is as effective as the TCAs, causes fewer side effects, and is less dangerous when taken in overdose. Combined use with MAOIs can cause serious adverse effects, and therefore must be avoided.

Mechanism of Action

Fluoxetine produces selective inhibition of serotonin reuptake, and thereby intensifies transmission at serotonergic synapses. As with TCAs, blockade of transmitter uptake occurs quickly, whereas therapeutic effects develop slowly. This delay suggests that therapeutic effects are the result of adaptive cellular changes that take place in response to prolonged uptake blockade. Fluoxetine does not block uptake of dopamine or NE. In contrast to the TCAs, fluoxetine does not block cholinergic, histaminergic, or alpha₁-adrenergic receptors. Furthermore, fluoxetine produces CNS excitation rather than sedation.

Therapeutic Uses

Fluoxetine is used primarily to treat major depression. Antidepressant effects begin in 1 to 3 weeks and are equivalent to those produced by TCAs. Fluoxetine is also approved for obsessive-compulsive disorder (Chapter 34), bulimia nervosa, and premenstrual dysphoric disorder (Chapter 59). Unlabeled uses include panic disorder, post-traumatic stress disorder, social phobia, alcoholism, attention-deficit/hyperactivity disorder, bipolar disorder, migraine, Tourette's syndrome, and obesity.

Pharmacokinetics

Fluoxetine is well absorbed following oral administration, even in the presence of food. The drug is widely distributed and highly bound (94%) to plasma proteins. Fluoxetine undergoes extensive hepatic conversion to norfluoxetine, an active metabolite. Norfluoxetine is eventually converted to inactive metabolites that are excreted in the urine. The half-life of fluoxetine is 2 days and the half-life of norfluoxetine is 7 days. Because the effective half-life is prolonged, about 4 weeks are required to produce steady-state plasma drug levels.

Adverse Effects

Fluoxetine is safer and better tolerated than TCAs and MAOIs. Death from overdose with fluoxetine alone has not been reported. In contrast to TCAs, fluoxetine does not block receptors for histamine, NE, or acetylcholine, and hence does not cause sedation, orthostatic hypotension, anticholinergic effects, or cardiotoxicity. The most common side effects are sexual dysfunction (70%), nausea (21%), headache (20%), and manifestations of CNS stimulation, including nervousness (15%), insomnia (14%), and anxiety (10%). Weight gain is also a problem. Fluoxetine and other SSRIs appear safe for use during pregnancy.

TABLE 31–4 ■ Therapeutic Uses of Selective Serotonin Reuptake Inhibitors

| Drug | Therapeutic Use*† | | | | | | | |
	Major Depression	OCD	Panic Disorder	Social Phobia	GAD	PTSD	PMDD	Bulimia Nervosa
Citalopram [Celexa]	A		U	U			U	
Escitalopram [Lexapro]	A							
Fluoxetine [Prozac]	A	A	U	U		U	A	A
Fluvoxamine [Luvox]	U	A	U	U	U	U	U	
Paroxetine [Paxil]	A	A	A	A	A	A	U	
Sertraline [Zoloft]	A	A	A		U	A	A	

*A = approved use, U = unlabeled use.
†GAD = generalized anxiety disorder, OCD = obsessive-compulsive disorder, PMDD = premenstrual dysphoric disorder, PTSD = post-traumatic stress disorder.

Sexual Dysfunction. Fluoxetine causes sexual problems (impotence, delayed or absent orgasm, delayed or absent ejaculation, decreased sexual interest) in nearly 70% of men and women. The underlying mechanism is unknown.

Sexual dysfunction can be managed in several ways. In some cases, reducing the dosage or taking "drug holidays" (e.g., discontinuing medication on Fridays and Saturdays) can help. Another solution is to add a drug that can overcome the problem. Among these are yohimbine, buspirone [BuSpar], and three atypical antidepressants: bupropion [Wellbutrin], nefazodone [Serzone], and mirtazapine [Remeron]. For men with erectile dysfunction, sildenafil [Viagra] can help. A third alternative is to switch antidepressants. Agents that cause the least sexual dysfunction are the same three atypical antidepressants named above.

Sexual problems often go unreported, either because patients are uncomfortable discussing them or because patients don't realize their medicine is the cause. Accordingly, patients should be informed about the high probability of sexual dysfunction and told to report any problems so they can be addressed.

Weight Gain. Like many other antidepressants, fluoxetine and other SSRIs cause weight gain. When these drugs were first introduced, we thought they caused weight *loss*. Why? Because during the first few weeks of therapy patients do lose weight, perhaps because of drug-induced nausea and vomiting. However, with long-term treatment, the lost weight is regained. Furthermore, about one-third of patients continue putting on weight—up to 20 pounds or more. Although the reason for weight gain is unknown, a good possibility is decreased sensitivity of serotonin receptors that regulate appetite.

Serotonin Syndrome. By increasing serotonergic transmission in the brainstem and spinal cord, fluoxetine and other SSRIs can cause *serotonin syndrome*. This syndrome usually begins 2 to 72 hours after initiation of treatment, and is most likely if an SSRI is combined with an MAOI. Signs and symptoms include altered mental status (agitation, confusion, disorientation, anxiety, hallucinations, poor concentration) as well as incoordination, myoclonus, hyperreflexia, excessive sweating, tremor, and fever. Deaths have occurred. The syndrome resolves spontaneously after discontinuing the drug. The risk of serotonin syndrome is increased by concurrent use of an MAOI, or by use of ritonavir [Norvir, Kaletra] and other drugs that can increase fluoxetine levels.

Withdrawal Syndrome. Abrupt discontinuation of SSRIs can cause a withdrawal syndrome. Symptoms include dizziness, headache, nausea, sensory disturbances, tremor, anxiety, and dysphoria. These begin within days to weeks of stopping dosing, and then persist for 1 to 3 weeks. Resumption of drug use will make symptoms subside. The withdrawal syndrome can be minimized by tapering the dosage slowly. Of the SSRIs in use today, fluoxetine is least likely to cause a withdrawal reaction. Why? Because fluoxetine has a prolonged half-life; hence, when dosing is stopped, plasma levels decline slowly. When SSRIs are discontinued, it is important to distinguish between symptoms of withdrawal and return of depression.

Extrapyramidal Side Effects. SSRIs cause extrapyramidal symptoms (EPS) in about 0.1% of patients. This is much less frequent than among patients taking antipsychotic medications (see Chapter 30). Among patients taking SSRIs, the most common EPS is akathisia, characterized by restlessness and agitation. However, parkinsonism, dystonic reactions, and tardive dyski-

nesia also occur. EPS typically develop during the first month of treatment. The risk is increased by concurrent use of an antipsychotic drug. The underlying cause of SSRI-induced EPS may be alteration of serotonergic transmission within the extrapyramidal system. For a detailed discussion of EPS, please refer to Chapter 30.

Bruxism. SSRIs may cause bruxism (clenching and grinding of teeth). However, since bruxism usually occurs during sleep, the condition often goes unrecognized. Sequelae of bruxism include headache, jaw pain, and dental problems (e.g., cracked fillings).

How do SSRIs cause bruxism? One theory is that SSRIs inhibit release of dopamine, a neurotransmitter that suppresses activity in certain muscles, including those of the jaw. By decreasing dopamine availability, SSRIs could release these muscles from inhibition, and excessive activity could result. This same mechanism may be responsible for SSRI-induced EPS.

How can bruxism can be managed? One option is to reduce the SSRI dosage. However, this may cause depression to return. Other options include switching to a different class of antidepressant, use of a mouth guard, and treatment with low-dose buspirone (5 to 10 mg 1 to 3 times a day).

Other Adverse Effects. Fluoxetine can cause *dizziness* and *fatigue;* patients should be warned against participation in hazardous activities (e.g., driving). *Skin rash,* which can be severe, has occurred in 4% of patients; in most cases, rashes readily respond to drug therapy (antihistamines, glucocorticoids) or to withdrawal of fluoxetine. Other common reactions include *diarrhea* (12%) and *excessive sweating* (8%).

Drug Interactions

Monoamine Oxidase Inhibitors. Fluoxetine should not be combined with MAOIs because serotonin syndrome can occur. (Like fluoxetine, MAOIs intensify serotonergic transmission.) MAOIs should be withdrawn at least 14 days before starting fluoxetine. When fluoxetine is discontinued, at least 5 weeks should elapse before giving an MAOI.

Warfarin. Because fluoxetine is highly bound to plasma proteins, it can displace other highly bound drugs. Displacement of warfarin (an anticoagulant) is of particular concern. Monitor responses to warfarin closely.

Tricyclic Antidepressants and Lithium. Fluoxetine can elevate plasma levels of TCAs and lithium. Exercise caution if fluoxetine is combined with these agents.

Preparations, Dosage, and Administration

Preparations. Fluoxetine is available in several oral formulations and is sold under three trade names: Prozac, Prozac Weekly, and Sarafem. Products available under each trade name are as follows:

- Prozac—tablets (10 mg), pulvules (10 and 20 mg), solution (20 mg/5 ml)
- Prozac Weekly—delayed-release, enteric-coated capsules (90 mg)
- Sarafem—pulvules (10 and 20 mg)

Dosage for Depression. Daily Dosing. The recommended initial dosage is 20 mg/day, taken with or without food. If needed, dosage may be increased gradually to a maximum of 80 mg/day. However, doses greater than 20 mg/day may just increase adverse effects without increasing benefits. If daily doses above 20 mg are used, they should be divided. For elderly patients and patients with impaired liver function, the dosage should be low initially and then cautiously increased if needed. Since fluoxetine often impairs sleep, evening dosing should generally be avoided.

Weekly Dosing. Patients who have been treated successfully with 20 mg of fluoxetine daily for at least 13 weeks can be switched to once-weekly dosing (using 90-mg delayed-release capsules) for maintenance. Weekly dosing is initiated 7 days after the last 20-mg dose of daily fluoxetine.

Other SSRIs

In addition to fluoxetine, four other SSRIs are available: citalopram [Celexa], fluvoxamine [Luvox], paroxetine [Paxil], and sertraline [Zoloft]. All four are similar to fluoxetine. Antidepressant effects equal those of TCAs. Like fluoxetine, the newer SSRIs do not cause hypotension or anticholinergic effects, and, with the exception of fluvoxamine, do not sedation. When taken in overdose, these drugs do not cause cardiotoxicity. All four can interact adversely with MAOIs; hence, the combination must be avoided. Characteristic side effects are nausea, insomnia, headache, nervousness, weight gain, and sexual dysfunction. Serotonin syndrome is a potential complication with all SSRIs. The principal differences among the SSRIs relate to duration of action. Patients who experience intolerable adverse effects with one SSRI may find a different SSRI more acceptable. Therapeutic uses for individual agents are summarized in Table 31–4.

Sertraline

Sertraline [Zoloft] is much like fluoxetine: both drugs block uptake of serotonin, both relieve symptoms of major depression, both cause CNS stimulation rather than sedation, and both have minimal effects on seizure threshold and the EKG. In contrast to fluoxetine, sertraline blocks uptake of dopamine (in addition to blocking uptake of serotonin). Sertraline is indicated for major depression, panic disorder, obsessive-compulsive disorder, post-traumatic stress disorder and premenstrual dysphoric disorder. The drug is being studied for use in generalized social phobia.

Common side effects include headache, tremor, insomnia, agitation, nervousness, nausea, diarrhea, weight gain, and sexual dysfunction. Because of the risk of serotonin syndrome, sertraline must not be combined with MAOIs. MAOIs should be withdrawn at least 14 days before starting sertraline, and sertraline should be withdrawn at least 14 days before starting an MAOI.

Sertraline is slowly absorbed following oral administration. Food increases the extent of absorption. In the blood, the drug is highly bound (99%) to plasma proteins. Sertraline undergoes extensive hepatic metabolism followed by elimination in the urine and feces. The plasma half-life is approximately 1 day.

Sertraline is available in tablets (25, 50, and 100 mg) and a concentrated oral solution (20 mg/ml). For treatment of depression, the initial adult daily dosage is 50 mg, administered in the morning or evening. After 4 to 8 weeks, the dosage may be increased by 50-mg increments to a maximum of 200 mg/day.

Fluvoxamine

Like other SSRIs, fluvoxamine [Luvox] produces powerful and selective inhibition of serotonin reuptake. At this time, the drug is approved only for obsessive-compulsive disorder. Unlabeled uses include major depression, panic disorder, social phobia, generalized anxiety disorder, post-traumatic stress disorder, premenstrual dysphoric disorder, and bulimia nervosa.

Fluvoxamine is rapidly absorbed from the GI tract, both in the presence and absence of food. The drug undergoes extensive hepatic metabolism followed by excretion in the urine. The half-life is about 15 hours.

Common side effects include nausea, vomiting, dry mouth, headache, constipation, weight gain, and sexual dysfunction. In contrast to other SSRIs, fluvoxamine has moderate sedative effects, although it nonetheless can cause insomnia. Some patients have developed abnormal liver function tests. Accordingly, liver function should be assessed prior to treatment and weekly during the first month of therapy. Like other SSRIs, fluvoxamine interacts adversely with MAOIs, and hence the combination must be avoided.

Fluvoxamine is available in 25-, 50-, and 100-mg tablets. The initial dosage for obsessive-compulsive disorder is 50 mg once a day. Dosage can be gradually increased to a maximum of 300 mg/day. Side effects are minimized by giving the daily dose at bedtime.

Paroxetine

Like other SSRIs, paroxetine [Paxil, Paxil CR] produces powerful and selective inhibition of serotonin uptake. The drug is indicated for major depression, obsessive-compulsive disorder, social phobia, panic disorder, generalized anxiety disorder, and post-traumatic stress disorder. Unlabeled uses include bipolar disorder and premenstrual dysphoric disorder.

Paroxetine is well absorbed following oral administration, even in the presence of food. The drug is widely distributed and highly bound (95%) to plasma proteins. Concentrations in breast milk equal those in plasma. The drug undergoes hepatic metabolism followed by renal excretion. The half-life is about 20 hours.

Side effects are dose dependent and generally mild. Early reactions include nausea, somnolence, sweating, tremor, and fatigue. These tend to diminish over time. After 5 to 6 weeks, the major complaints are headache, weight gain, and sexual dysfunction. Like fluoxetine, paroxetine causes signs of CNS stimulation (increased awakenings, reduced time in rapid-eye-movement sleep, insomnia). In contrast to TCAs, paroxetine has no effect on heart rate, blood pressure, or the EKG—but does have some antimuscarinic effects. Like other SSRIs, paroxetine interacts adversely with MAOIs, and hence the combination must be avoided.

Paroxetine is available in standard tablets (10, 20, 30, and 40 mg) and an oral suspension (2 mg/ml) as Paxil, and in controlled-release (CR) tablets (12.5, 25, and 37.5 mg) as Paxil CR. Please note that the CR tablets are *not* longer acting than the standard tablets. Rather, the CR tablets are designed to dissolve in the lower intestine, and hence may cause less GI disturbance than the standard tablets.

The initial dosage for depression is 20 mg/day. The entire daily dose is administered in the morning (to minimize sleep disturbance) and with food (to minimize GI upset). Dosage may be increased gradually (every 3 to 4 weeks) to a maximum of 50 mg/day.

Citalopram

Citalopram [Celexa] is very similar to fluoxetine and the other SSRIs. Benefits derive from selective blockade of serotonin uptake. The drug does not block receptors for serotonin, acetylcholine, NE, or histamine. At this time, citalopram is approved only for major depression. Unlabeled uses include panic disorder, social phobia, and premenstrual dysphoric disorder.

Citalopram is rapidly absorbed from the GI tract, both in the presence and absence of food. Plasma levels peak about 4 hours after administration. The drug undergoes hepatic metabolism followed by excretion in the urine and feces. The half-life is about 35 hours.

The most common adverse effects are nausea, somnolence, dry mouth, and sexual dysfunction. Additional side effects include weight gain, tachycardia, postural hypotension, headache, paresthesias, and inappropriate secretion of antidiuretic hormone. Large doses are teratogenic in animals. Citalopram enters breast milk in amounts sufficient to cause somnolence, reduced feeding, and weight loss in the infant.

Because of the risk of serotonin syndrome, citalopram should not be combined with an MAOI. Allow at least 14 days to pass between stopping an MAOI and starting citalopram, or vice versa.

Citalopram is available in tablets (10 and 20 mg) and an oral solution (2 mg/ml). The drug may be taken in the morning or evening, with or without food. The initial dosage for depression is 20 mg once a day. Dosage may be increased slowly to a maximum of 60 mg/day. Dosage should remain low in elderly patients and those with liver impairment.

Escitalopram

Escitalopram [Lexapro] is the S-isomer of citalopram [Celexa], which is a 50:50 mixture of S- and R-isomers. The S-isomer (escitalopram) is responsible for antidepressant effects. The R-isomer has no antidepressant actions, but does contribute to side effects. Accordingly, escitalopram retains the therapeutic benefits of citalopram, but may be better tolerated. Otherwise, the pharmacology of the two drugs is largely the same. Escitalopram is approved only for major depression.

Like citalopram and other SSRIs, escitalopram is generally well tolerated. In clinical trials, the most common side effects were nausea (15%), insomnia (9%), somnolence (6%), sweating (5%), and fatigue (5%). In addition, 9% of males reported ejaculatory disorders. However, the true incidence of sexual dysfunction may be higher. Why? Because, with other SSRIs, the incidence of sexual problems reported during clinical trials was considerably lower than the incidence seen in actual practice. As with other SSRIs, combined use with an MAOI can cause serotonin syndrome. Accordingly, at least 14 days should separate use of these drugs.

Escitalopram is available in 5-, 10-, and 20-mg tablets. The recommended initial dosage is 10 mg/day, taken in the morning or evening, with or without food. In clinical trials, dosages above 10 mg/day did not increase antidepressant effects, but did intensify side effects. There is no need to reduce the dosage in elderly patients or in patients with hepatic impairment or mild or moderate renal impairment; however, in patients with severe renal impairment, a dosage reduction may be required.

MONOAMINE OXIDASE INHIBITORS

The MAOIs are second- or third-choice antidepressants for most patients. Although these drugs are as effective as the tricyclics and SSRIs, they are more dangerous. Of particular concern is the risk of triggering hypertensive crisis by eating foods rich in tyramine. At this time, MAOIs are drugs of choice only for atypical depression. Three MAOIs are available: isocarboxazid [Marplan], phenelzine [Nardil], and tranylcypromine [Parnate].

Mechanism of Action

Before discussing the MAOIs, we need to discuss MAO itself. MAO is an enzyme found in the liver, the intestinal wall, and terminals of monoamine-containing neurons. The function of MAO in neurons is to convert monoamine neurotransmitters—NE, serotonin, and dopamine—into inactive products. In the liver and intestine, MAO serves to inactivate tyramine and other biogenic amines in food. In addition, these enzymes inactivate biogenic amines administered as drugs.

The body has two forms of MAO, named MAO-A and MAO-B. In the brain, MAO-A inactivates NE and serotonin, whereas MAO-B inactivates dopamine. In the liver, MAO-A acts on dietary tyramine and other compounds. Currently available antidepressant MAOIs are *nonselective*. That is, they inhibit both MAO-A and MAO-B. Antidepressant agents selective for MAO-A are in development. Selegiline, a selective inhibitor of MAO-B, is used to treat Parkinson's disease (see Chapter 21).

Antidepressant effects of the MAOIs result from inhibiting MAO-A in nerve terminals (Fig. 31–3). By inhibiting intraneuronal MAO-A, these drugs increase the amount of NE and serotonin available for release, and thereby intensify transmission at noradrenergic and serotonergic junctions.

It should be noted that antidepressant effects of the MAOIs cannot be fully explained by MAO inhibition alone. Why? Because the biochemical action of MAOIs (inhibition of MAO) takes place rapidly, whereas the clinical response to MAOIs (relief of depression) develops slowly. In the interval between initial inhibition of MAO and relief of depression, secondary neurochemical events must be taking place. It is these as-yet unknown events that are ultimately responsible for the beneficial response to treatment.

The MAOIs can act on MAO in two ways: reversibly and irreversibly. All of the MAOIs in current use cause *irreversible* inhibition. Since recovery from irreversible inhibition requires synthesis of new MAO molecules, effects of the irreversible inhibitors persist for about 2 weeks after drug withdrawal. In contrast, recovery from reversible inhibition is more rapid, occurring in 3 to 5 days.

Therapeutic Uses

Depression. MAOIs are as effective as TCAs and SSRIs for relieving depression. However, because they can be hazardous, MAOIs are generally reserved for patients who have not responded to TCAs, SSRIs, and other safer drugs. Nonetheless, there *is* one group of patients—those with *atypical depression*—for whom MAOIs are the treatment of choice. As with other antidepressants, beneficial effects do not reach their peak for several weeks.

Other Uses. MAOIs have been used with some success to treat *bulimia nervosa* and *obsessive-compulsive disorders*. Like TCAs and SSRIs, MAOIs can reduce *panic attacks* in patients with panic disorder.

Adverse Effects

CNS Stimulation. In contrast to TCAs, MAOIs cause direct CNS stimulation (in addition to exerting antidepressant effects). Excessive stimulation can produce anxiety, agitation, hypomania, and even mania.

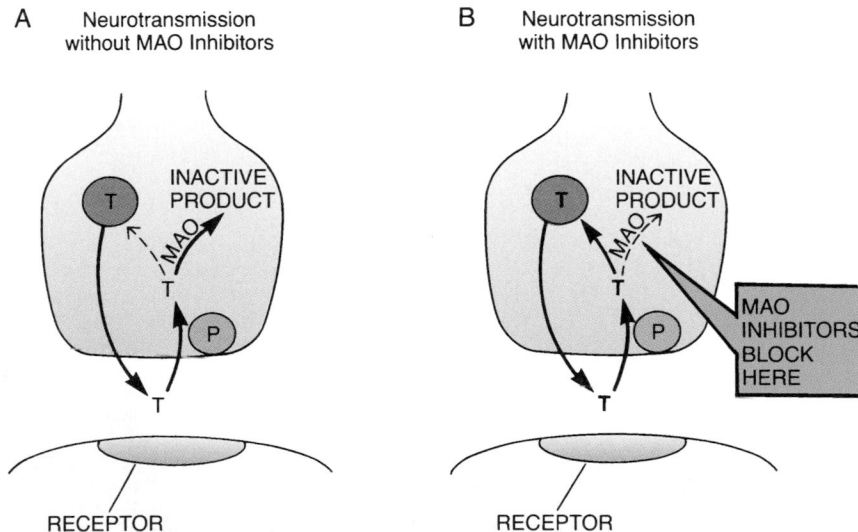

Figure 31–3 ■ Mechanism of action of monoamine oxidase inhibitors.
A, Under drug-free conditions, much of the norepinephrine or serotonin that undergoes reuptake into nerve terminals becomes inactivated by MAO. Inactivation helps maintain an appropriate concentration of transmitter within the terminal.
B, MAO inhibitors prevent inactivation of norepinephrine and serotonin, thereby increasing the amount of transmitter available for release. Release of supranormal amounts of transmitter intensifies transmission.
(P = uptake pump, MAO = monoamine oxidase, T = transmitter [norepinephrine or serotonin],.)

Orthostatic Hypotension. Despite their ability to increase the NE content of peripheral sympathetic neurons, the MAOIs *reduce blood pressure* when administered in usual therapeutic doses. Patients should be informed about signs of hypotension (dizziness, lightheadedness) and advised to sit or lie down if these occur. Also, they should be informed that hypotension can be minimized by moving slowly when assuming an erect posture. For the hospitalized patient, blood pressure and pulse rate should be monitored on a regular schedule (e.g., 4 times daily). These measurements should be taken while the patient is lying down and again after the patient has been sitting or standing for 1 to 2 minutes.

MAOIs lower blood pressure through actions in the CNS. The following sequence has been proposed: (1) inhibition of MAO increases the NE content of neurons within the vasomotor center; (2) when NE is released, it binds to postsynaptic alpha receptors on neurons within the vasomotor center, thereby decreasing the firing rate of sympathetic nerves that control vascular tone; (3) this reduction in sympathetic activity results in vasodilation, causing blood pressure to fall.

Hypertensive Crisis from Dietary Tyramine. Although the MAOIs normally produce *hypotension,* they can be the cause of severe *hypertension* if the patient eats food that is rich in *tyramine,* a substance that promotes the release of NE from sympathetic neurons. Hypertensive crisis is characterized by headache, tachycardia, hypertension, nausea, and vomiting.

Before considering the mechanism by which hypertensive crisis is produced, let's consider the effect of dietary tyramine under drug-free conditions. In the absence of MAO inhibition, dietary tyramine does not represent a threat. Much of the tyramine in food is metabolized by MAO in the intestinal wall. Furthermore, as shown in Figure 31–4*A,* any dietary tyramine

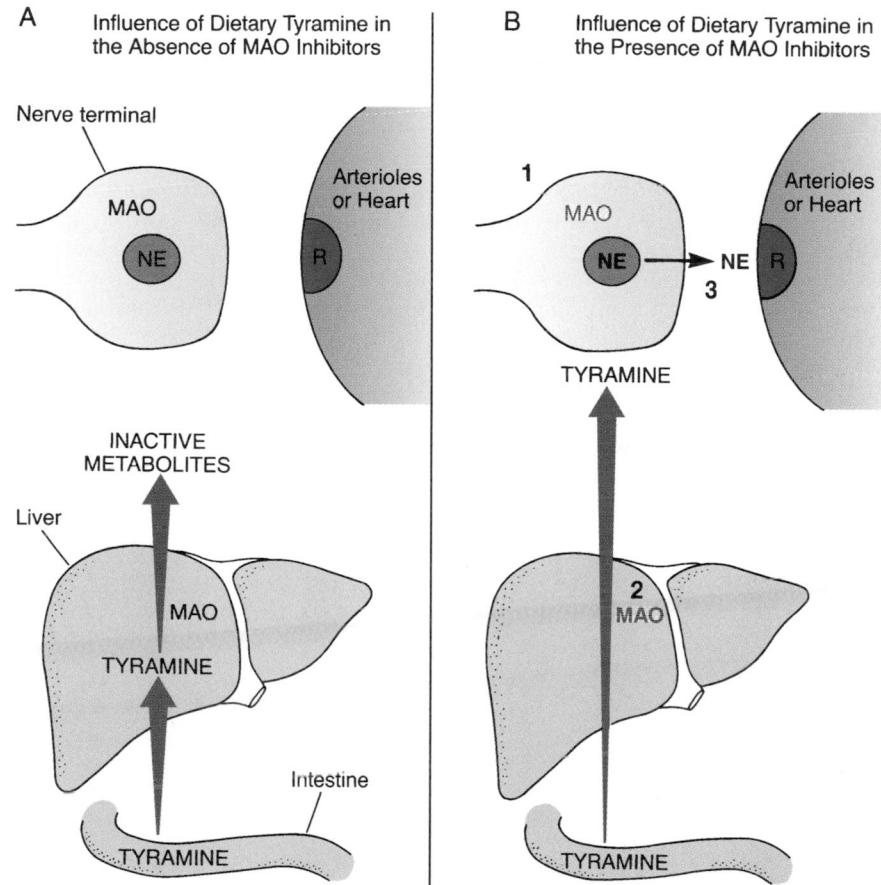

Figure 31–4 ■ Interaction between dietary tyramine and MAOIs.
A, In the absence of MAOIs, dietary tyramine is absorbed from the intestine, transported to the liver, and then immediately inactivated by hepatic MAO. No tyramine reaches the general circulation.

B, Three events occur in the presence of MAOIs: (1) Inhibition of neuronal MAO raises levels of norepinephrine in sympathetic nerve terminals. (2) Inhibition of hepatic MAO allows dietary tyramine to pass through the liver and enter the systemic circulation intact. (3) Upon reaching peripheral sympathetic nerve terminals, tyramine promotes the release of accumulate norepinephrine stores, thereby causing massive vasoconstriction and excessive stimulation of the heart.

(MAO = monoamine oxidase, NE = norepinephrine, R = receptor for norepinephrine.)

that does get absorbed passes directly to the liver via the hepatic portal circulation. Once in the liver, tyramine is immediately inactivated by MAO there. Hence, as long as hepatic MAO is functioning, dietary tyramine is prevented from reaching the general circulation, and therefore is devoid of adverse effects.

In the presence of MAOIs, the picture is very different: dietary tyramine can produce a life-threatening hypertensive crisis. The mechanism of this reaction has three components (Fig. 31–4B). First, inhibition of *neuronal* MAO augments NE levels within the terminals of sympathetic neurons that regulate cardiac function and vascular tone. Second, inhibition of *hepatic* MAO allows dietary tyramine to pass directly through the liver and enter the systemic circulation intact. Third, upon reaching peripheral sympathetic nerves, tyramine stimulates the release of the accumulated NE, thereby causing massive vasoconstriction and excessive stimulation of the heart. Hypertensive crisis results. To reduce the risk of tyramine-induced hypertensive crisis, the following precautions must be taken:

- MAOIs must not be dispensed to patients considered incapable of rigid adherence to dietary restrictions.
- Before an MAOI is dispensed, the patient must be fully informed about the hazard of ingesting tyramine-rich foods.
- The patient must be given a detailed list of foods and beverages to avoid. These foods—which include yeast extracts, most cheeses, fermented sausages (e.g., salami, pepperoni, bologna), and aged fish or meat—are listed in Table 31–5.
- The patient should be instructed to avoid all drugs not specifically approved by the physician.

The patient should be educated about the symptoms of hypertensive crisis (headache, tachycardia, palpitations, nausea, vomiting) and instructed to seek immediate medical attention if these develop. In the event of hypertensive crisis, blood pressure can be lowered with IV *phentolamine,* a short-acting alpha-adrenergic antagonist; blood pressure declines because of vasodilation secondary to blockade of alpha$_1$ receptors on blood vessels. Sublingual *nifedipine,* a calcium channel blocker, is an alternative; like IV phentolamine, sublingual nifedipine acts rapidly to promote vasodilation. Some physicians recommend that patients carry a 10-mg nifedipine capsule with them for use in emergencies.

In addition to tyramine, several other dietary constituents (e.g., caffeine, phenylethylamine) can precipitate hypertension in patients taking MAOIs. Foods that contain these compounds are listed in Table 31–5. The patient should be instructed to avoid them.

Drug Interactions

The MAOIs can interact with many drugs to cause potentially disastrous results. Accordingly, patients should be instructed to avoid all medications—prescription agents and over-the-counter drugs—that have not been specifically approved by the physician.

Indirect-Acting Sympathomimetic Agents. Indirect-acting sympathomimetics (e.g., ephedrine, amphetamine) are drugs that promote the release of NE from sympathetic nerves. In patients taking MAOIs, these drugs can produce *hypertensive crisis.* The mechanism is the same as that described for tyramine. Patients should be instructed to avoid all

---

TABLE 31–5 ■ Foods That Can Interact With MAO Inhibitors

Foods That Contain Tyramine

Category	Unsafe Foods (High Tyramine Content)	Safe Foods (Little or No Tyramine)
Vegetables	Avocados, especially if overripe; fermented bean curd; fermented soybean; soybean paste	Most vegetables
Fruits	Figs, especially if overripe; bananas, in large amounts	Most fruits
Meats	Meats that are fermented, smoked, or otherwise aged; spoiled meats; liver, unless *very* fresh	Meats that are known to be fresh (exercise caution in restaurants; meat may not be fresh)
Sausages	Fermented varieties: bologna, pepperoni, salami, others	Nonfermented varieties
Fish	Dried or cured fish; fish that is fermented, smoked, or otherwise aged; spoiled fish	Fish that is known to be fresh; vacuum-packed fish, if eaten promptly or refrigerated only briefly after opening
Milk, milk products	Practically all cheeses	Milk, yogurt, cottage cheese, cream cheese
Foods with yeast	Yeast extract (e.g., Marmite, Bovril)	Baked goods that contain yeast
Beer, wine	Some imported beers; Chianti wine	Major domestic brands of beer; most wines
Other foods	Protein dietary supplements; soups (may contain protein extract); shrimp paste; soy sauce	

Foods That Contain Other Vasopressors

Food	Comments
Chocolate	Contains phenylethylamine, a pressor agent; large amounts can cause a reaction.
Fava beans	Contain dopamine, a pressor agent; reactions are most likely with overripe beans.
Ginseng	Headache, tremulousness, and manic-like reactions have occurred.
Caffeinated beverages	Caffeine is a weak pressor agent; large amounts may cause a reaction.

sympathomimetic drugs, including ephedrine, methylphenidate, amphetamines, and cocaine. Sympathomimetic agents may be present in cold remedies, nasal decongestants, and asthma medications; all of these should be avoided unless approved by the physician.

Interactions Secondary to Inhibition of Hepatic MAO. Inhibition of MAO in the liver can decrease the metabolism of several drugs, including epinephrine, NE, and dopamine. These drugs must be used with caution because their effects will be intensified and prolonged.

Antidepressants: TCAs and SSRIs. The combination of a TCA with an MAOI may produce hypertensive episodes or hypertensive crisis. As a result, this combination of antidepressants is not employed routinely. However, although potentially dangerous, the combination can benefit certain patients. If this combination is employed, caution must be exercised.

Combining an MAOI with an SSRI can produce serotonin syndrome. Accordingly, the combination must be avoided.

Antihypertensive Drugs. Combined use of MAOIs and antihypertensive agents may result in excessive lowering of blood pressure. This response should be no surprise considering that MAOIs, by themselves, can cause hypotension.

Meperidine. Meperidine [Demerol] can cause hyperpyrexia (excessive elevation of temperature) in patients receiving MAOIs. Accordingly, if a strong analgesic is required, an agent other than meperidine should be chosen. Furthermore, the analgesic should be administered in its lowest effective dosage.

Preparations, Dosage, and Administration

All MAOIs are administered orally. Formulations are as follows: isocarboxazid [Marplan], 10-mg tablets; phenelzine [Nardil], 15-mg tablets; and tranylcypromine [Parnate], 10-mg tablets. Dosages are summarized in Table 31–3.

ATYPICAL ANTIDEPRESSANTS

Bupropion

Actions and Uses. Bupropion [Wellbutrin] is a unique antidepressant similar in structure to amphetamine. Like amphetamine, bupropion has stimulant actions and suppresses appetite. Antidepressant effects begin in 1 to 3 weeks and equal those of amitriptyline (a TCA). The mechanism by which depression is relieved is unclear, but may be related to blockade of dopamine uptake. The drug does not affect serotonergic, cholinergic, or histaminergic transmission. In contrast to SSRIs, bupropion does not cause weight gain or sexual dysfunction. In fact, it appears to *increase* sexual desire and pleasure—hence bupropion has been used to (1) counteract sexual dysfunction in patients taking SSRIs, and (2) heighten sexual interest in women with hypoactive sexual desire disorder. Because of its efficacy and side effect profile, bupropion is a good alternative to SSRIs for patients who cannot tolerate SSRI side effects. The most serious adverse effect is seizures, which can occur when dosage is too high. In addition to its use in depression, bupropion is indicated as an aid to quit smoking (see Chapter 38).

Adverse Effects. Bupropion is generally well tolerated, but can cause seizures. The most common adverse effects are agitation (31%), headache (27%), dry mouth (27%), constipation (26%), weight loss (23%), GI upset (22%), dizziness (21%), tremor (21%), insomnia (19%), blurred vision (15%), and tachycardia (11%).

At doses greater than 450 mg/day, bupropion produces seizures in about 0.4% of patients. The risk is greatly increased in patients with predisposing factors, such as head trauma, pre-existing seizure disorder, CNS tumor, and use of other drugs that lower seizure threshold. Careful dosing reduces seizure risk.

Drug Interactions. MAOIs can increase the risk of bupropion toxicity. Accordingly, patients should discontinue MAOIs at least 2 weeks before starting bupropion.

Preparations, Dosage, and Administration. For treatment of depression, bupropion [Wellbutrin] is available in standard tablets (75 and 100 mg) and sustained-release tablets (100 and 150 mg). Dosing must be done carefully to minimize the risk of seizures. Dosage escalation should be done slowly. The initial dosage is 75 mg twice a day. After 4 days, the dosage can be increased to 100 mg 3 times a day. If necessary, the dosage can be increased to a maximum of 150 mg 3 times a day.

The formulation used to help smokers quit is marketed under the trade name *Zyban* (see Chapter 38 for dosage).

Other Atypical Antidepressants
Nefazodone

Nefazodone [Serzone] is a novel drug indicated only for depression. Neuropharmacologic actions include blockade of serotonin₂ receptors and alpha₁-adrenergic receptors, and weak inhibition of NE and serotonin reuptake. The contribution of these actions to therapeutic effects is unknown. Life-threatening liver failure is the adverse effect of greatest concern.

Nefazodone is rapidly and completely absorbed following oral administration. Food delays absorption and decreases bioavailability by 20%. Plasma drug levels peak about 1 hour after an oral dose. In the liver, nefazodone undergoes conversion to three active metabolites. The effective half-life of the parent drug and metabolites is 11 to 24 hours.

Nefazodone is generally well tolerated. The most common side effects are headache, somnolence, dry mouth, nausea, dizziness, blurred vision, and other visual disturbances. Sexual dysfunction and weight gain are minimal.

Nefazodone can cause life-threatening liver failure. However, the incidence is extremely low: only 1 case leading to death or liver transplant for every 250,000 to 300,000 patient years. As a rule, nefazodone should not be given to patients with pre-existing liver disease. Patients who develop signs of liver injury (e.g., nausea, anorexia, abdominal pain, malaise, jaundice) should seek immediate medical attention. If laboratory tests confirm hepatocellular injury, nefazodone should be withdrawn.

Drugs that block uptake of serotonin, NE, or both can cause serious reactions if combined with an MAOI. Accordingly, nefazodone and MAOIs must not be combined. If the patient has been taking an MAOI, it should be discontinued at least 2 weeks before starting nefazodone. Conversely, when switching from nefazodone to an MAOI, nefazodone should be discontinued at least 7 days before starting the MAOI.

Nefazodone inhibits hepatic drug-metabolizing enzymes, and can thereby raise levels of other drugs. When present at high levels, terfenadine* or astemizole* (two nonsedating antihistamines) can cause fatal ventricular dysrhythmias. Accordingly, since nefazodone can raise levels of these drugs, it must not be combined with either one.

Nefazodone is dispensed in tablets (50, 100, 150, 200, and 250 mg) for oral use. Dosing is begun at 100 mg twice daily. If needed, the dose can be gradually increased to between 150 and 300 mg twice daily. For elderly patients, dosing is begun at 50 mg twice daily; the usual effective range is 50 to 200 mg twice daily.

Venlafaxine

Venlafaxine [Effexor] is indicated for major depression and generalized anxiety disorder. The drug produces powerful blockade of NE and serotonin uptake and weak blockade of dopamine uptake. The relationship of these actions to therapeutic effects is uncertain. Venlafaxine does not block cholinergic, histaminergic, or alpha₁-adrenergic receptors. For treatment of depression, the drug is more effective than SSRIs, and is more likely to produce complete remission. Venlafaxine is often effective in patients who were not helped by other antidepressant drugs.

---

*No longer available in the United States.

Special Interest Topic

BOX 31–2 ■ ST. JOHN'S WORT: MOTHER NATURE'S PROZAC?

St. John's wort is an herbal preparation used widely to treat depression. Limited clinical studies suggest that it can help people with mild to moderate depression—but not severe depression. Side effects are minimal. However the herb *can* interact adversely with many drugs.

St. John's wort is the common name for *Hypericum perforatum,* a perennial herb found in Europe, Asia, and North America. The plant has blue-green leaves and small yellow flowers that bloom in profusion around June 24, the date celebrated as the birthday of St. John the Divine.

In Germany, extract of St. John's wort is a prescription medicine licensed for treatment of depression, anxiety, and insomnia. About 3 million prescriptions are written each year. In the United States, St. John's wort can be purchased without prescription in health food stores, vitamin shops, and pharmacies. The preparation is considered a dietary supplement here, and hence has not been evaluated by the Food and Drug Administration.

St. John's wort has multiple active components. Among these are naphthodianthrones, flavonoids, and xanthones. The component generally believed responsible for antidepressant effects is *hypericin,* a naphthodianthrone. As one might expect, the hypericin content of St. John's wort can vary widely. In an effort to make all batches of the herb therapeutically equivalent, some manufacturers ensure that each batch has the same hypericin content—typically 0.3%. However, even among batches that have the same amount of hypericin, the amount of other active constituents varies.

Several mechanisms may explain antidepressant effects. St. John's wort can decrease uptake of three neurotransmitters: serotonin, NE, and dopamine. In addition, it binds strongly to GABA receptors and produces mild inhibition of MAO. Blockade of serotonin uptake and inhibition of MAO mimic the actions of conventional antidepressants. Although the hypericin in St. John's wort may be responsible for blockade of transmitter uptake, it is not responsible for inhibition of MAO. We know this because pure synthetic hypericin has practically no effect on the enzyme. In contrast, preparations of St. John's wort that have very high flavonoid concentrations produce the strongest MAO inhibition—suggesting that flavonoids are responsible for inhibiting the enzyme.

How effective is St. John's wort? At this time, it's hard to say. In 1996, researchers reviewed 23 randomized clinical trials in which St. John's wort was compared with placebo and standard antidepressant drugs for treating mild to moderate depression. The reviewers concluded that the herb is superior to placebo and about equal to the standard antidepressants. However, these conclusions are shaky because of design flaws in the trials. Specifically,

* Diagnosis of depression was not well established.
* Antidepressant dosages were low.
* Hypericin content of the herbal preparations varied sixfold.
* Placebo responses were unusually low, which would make the test compounds appear more effective.

Furthermore, duration of treatment was relatively short: one trial lasted 12 weeks; the rest lasted 8 weeks or less. Hence, information on long-term efficacy is lacking. Nonetheless, these trials do suggest that St. John's wort has real—albeit mild—antidepressant effects. This conclusion is supported by two recent, well-designed trials, which showed that, for patients with mild to moderate depression, St. John's wort works as well as imipramine and is better tolerated.

However, although the herb may be effective for *mild* depression, it does not seem to help in *severe* depression: Data from a randomized controlled trial, published in the April 18, 2001, issue of *JAMA,* indicate that, for patients with moderate to severe depression, St. John's wort is no more effective than placebo. Similarly, another major and eagerly anticipated paper—"Effect of *Hypericum perforatum* (St. John's Wort) in major depressive disorder"—published 1 year later in *JAMA,* came to the same conclusion. However, the conclusion doesn't seem justified by the data. Why? Because, in this study—which compared the effects of placebo, St. John's wort, and sertraline [Zoloft] in patients with moderately severe depression—not only was St. John's wort no better than placebo, neither was sertraline, an antidepressant whose efficacy has been clearly documented by many other studies. Hence, if the authors want to conclude that St. John's wort doesn't work, they must also conclude that sertraline doesn't work either—a conclusion that would be hard to defend. The bottom line? St. John's wort is probably effective against mild depression, and may (or may not) be effective against more severe depression.

In trials done to date, St. John's wort was devoid of serious adverse effects. Dry mouth, dizziness, confusion, and constipation and other GI complaints were reported. Only 2% of patients dropped out because of side effects. Because the trials were relatively short, long-term adverse effects are unknown. Recent data suggest the drug may increase the risk of cataracts.

Ingestion of St. John's wort by grazing sheep and cattle has caused photosensitivity reactions, manifesting as welts. Severe photosensitivity has been reported in one patient taking the herb. To reduce the risk of phototoxic reactions, patients should minimize exposure to sunlight, wear protective clothing, and apply a sunscreen to exposed skin.

St. John's wort is known to interact adversely with many drugs—and the list continues to grow. Three mechanisms are involved: induction of cytochrome P450 enzymes, induction of P-glycoprotein, and intensification of serotonin effects. Let's consider these one by one:

* *Induction of P450* can accelerate the metabolism of many drugs, thereby decreasing their effects. This mechanism appears responsible for breakthrough bleeding in women taking oral contraceptives, transplant rejection in patients taking cyclosporine (an immunosuppressant), reduced antiretroviral effects in patients taking indinavir (an HIV protease inhibitor), and reduced anticoagulation in patients taking warfarin. Other drugs whose effects are likely to be reduced by this mechanism include non-nucleoside reverse

(Continued on next page)

transcriptase inhibitors (delavirdine, efavirenz, nevirapine), all protease inhibitors (amprenavir, indinavir, nelfinavir, ritonavir, saquinavir), theophylline, and glucocorticoids.

- *P-glycoprotein* is a transport protein found in cells that line the intestine and renal tubules. In the intestine, P-glycoprotein transports drugs *out* of cells into the intestinal lumen; in renal tubules, P-glycoprotein transports drugs *out* of tubular cells into the urine. Hence, by increasing P-glycoprotein synthesis, St. John's wort can accelerate elimination of drugs, and can thereby reduce their effects. This is the mechanism by which St. John's wort greatly reduces levels of *digoxin,* a drug for heart failure. Other drugs whose levels can probably be reduced by this mechanism include calcium channel blockers, steroid hormones, protease inhibitors, and certain anticancer drugs (e.g., etoposide, paclitaxel, vinblastine, vincristine).

- Combining St. John's wort with certain drugs can intensify serotonergic transmission to a degree sufficient to cause potentially fatal *serotonin syndrome.* Although St. John's wort can enhance serotonergic transmission by itself, its effect is relatively weak. Hence, when used alone, the herb poses little risk of harm. However, if St. John's wort is combined with other serotonin-enhancing agents, the risk is greatly increased. Obviously, St. John's wort should not be combined with such drugs. Among these are amphetamine, cocaine, MAO inhibitors, two atypical antidepressants (nefazodone and venlafaxine), certain tricyclic antidepressants

(e.g., amitriptyline, clomipramine), and all SSRIs (e.g., fluoxetine, paroxetine).

Because St. John's wort has a variety of known adverse interactions—and is likely to have more that are as yet unknown—caution is clearly advised. Accordingly, prescribers should ask patients if they are using the herb. For patients who are, prescribers should either (1) limit prescriptions to drugs that are not likely to interact adversely, or (2) instruct patients to stop taking the herb if a medication known to interact adversely must be prescribed.

Because reliable information about St. John's Wort is very limited, rational use of the herb is difficult. Yes, the preparation seems safe and somewhat effective for people with mild depression, but is probably not effective for more severe depression. Furthermore, we don't know its long-term effects—either beneficial or harmful. Nor do we know how it works, or even which of its components is responsible for beneficial effects. These issues are compounded by variability in the potency and purity of herbal preparations. Hence, until more is known, patients with moderate to severe depression should be treated with conventional antidepressant drugs—drugs whose efficacy and risks are well documented. For people with mild depression, St. John's wort may be a reasonable alternative—provided its use doesn't dissuade them from seeking proper medical help as needed.

Venlafaxine is well absorbed following oral administration, both in the presence and absence of food. Much of each dose is converted to an active metabolite by the liver. The half-life is 5 hours for the parent drug and 11 hours for the major metabolite.

Venlafaxine can cause a variety of adverse effects. The most common is nausea (37%), followed by headache, anorexia, nervousness, sweating, somnolence, and insomnia. Dose-dependent weight loss may occur secondary to anorexia. Venlafaxine can also cause dose-related sustained diastolic hypertension; blood pressure should be monitored. Sexual dysfunction (e.g., impotence, anorgasmia) may occur too.

Abrupt discontinuation of venlafaxine can cause a withdrawal syndrome. Symptoms include anxiety, agitation, tremors, headache, vertigo, nausea, tachycardia, and tinnitus. Worsening of pretreatment symptoms may also occur. Withdrawal symptoms can be minimized by tapering the dosage over 2 to 4 weeks. Warn patients not to stop venlafaxine abruptly.

Venlafaxine and other drugs that block uptake of NE and serotonin can cause serious reactions if combined with an MAOI. Accordingly, MAOIs should be withdrawn at least 14 days before starting venlafaxine. When switching from venlafaxine to an MAOI, venlafaxine should be discontinued 7 days before starting the MAOI.

Venlafaxine is available in standard tablets (25, 37.5, 50, 75, and 100 mg) and extended-release capsules (37.5, 75, and 150 mg). The recommended initial dosage for depression is 75 mg/day (in two or three divided doses) taken with food. If needed, the dosage may be gradually increased. The usual maximum dosage is 225 mg/day. However, dosages as large as 375 mg/day have been used for severely depressed patients. A dosage reduction is needed for patients with liver disease, and possibly for those with kidney disease.

Mirtazapine

Mirtazapine [Remeron] is the first representative of a new class of antidepressants. Antidepressant effects equal those of SSRIs and may develop faster. Benefits appear to result from increased *release* of serotonin and NE. The mechanism is blockade of presynaptic alpha$_2$-adrenergic receptors that

serve to inhibit release. In addition to promoting transmitter release, mirtazapine is a powerful blocker of two serotonin receptor subtypes: 5-HT$_2$ and 5-HT$_3$. The contribution of this effect is unclear. Mirtazapine blocks histamine receptors, and thereby promotes sedation and weight gain.

Mirtazapine is well absorbed following oral administration and reaches peak plasma levels in 2 hours. The drug undergoes extensive hepatic metabolism followed by excretion in the urine (75%) and feces (25%). The elimination half-life is 20 to 40 hours.

Mirtazapine is generally well tolerated. Somnolence is the most prominent adverse effect, occurring in 54% of patients. Other side effects include increased appetite (17%), weight gain (8%), cholesterol elevation (15%), and dizziness (7%). Sexual dysfunction is less than with SSRIs. Reversible agranulocytosis and neutropenia occur rarely. Blockade of muscarinic receptors is moderate, and hence anticholinergic effects are mild. Mirtazapine-induced somnolence can be exacerbated by alcohol, benzodiazepines, and other CNS depressants. Accordingly, these agents should be avoided. Mirtazapine should not be combined with MAOIs.

Mirtazapine is available in standard tablets (15, 30, and 45 mg) under the trade name *Remeron,* and orally disintegrating tablets (15, 30, and 45 mg) under the trade name *Remeron SolTab.* The initial dosage is 15 mg once a day at bedtime. Dosage may be gradually increased to a maximum of 45 mg/day.

Amoxapine

Amoxapine [Asendin] is chemically related to the antipsychotic agent loxapine, and has both antidepressant and neuroleptic properties. Antidepressant effects are equivalent to those of the TCAs. Because it can cause serious side effects, amoxapine should be reserved for patients with psychotic depression.

Amoxapine is generally well tolerated. Anticholinergic and sedative effects are moderate. Following overdose, the risk of seizures is greater than with TCAs. Exercise caution in patients with epilepsy.

Like loxapine and the other antipsychotics, amoxapine can block receptors for dopamine. As a result, the drug can cause extrapyramidal side effects (e.g., parkinsonism, akathisia). Because of the risk of tardive dyskinesia (an extrapyramidal effect that develops with prolonged use of dopamine antagonists), long-term use of amoxapine should generally be avoided.

Amoxapine is available in tablets (25, 50, 100, and 200 mg) for oral use. The usual dosage for depression is 200 to 300 mg/day.

Reboxetine

Reboxetine [Vestra] is the first representative of a new class of antidepressants: the *selective norepinephrine reuptake inhibitors* (SNRIs). The drug is not related chemically to TCAs, MAOIs, or SSRIs. Biochemical effects are limited almost entirely to enhancing transmission at receptors for norepinephrine. The drug has little or no impact on receptors for serotonin, dopamine, acetylcholine, or histamine.

In clinical trials, antidepressant effects were comparable to those of TCAs and fluoxetine [Prozac], an SSRI. With short-term use, reboxetine induced remission and, with long-term use, it prevented relapse. Because reboxetine is a new drug, its therapeutic niche has not been established. However, available data suggest that it may be especially good for patients with severe depression and for those in whom social functioning is severely impaired.

Reboxetine is rapidly absorbed following oral administration. Plasma levels peak within 2 hours. High-fat meals delay absorption, but do not reduce the extent of absorption. Reboxetine undergoes extensive hepatic metabolism followed by excretion in the urine. The drug's half-life is 12 to 16 hours, but may be prolonged in patients with liver dysfunction.

Reboxetine is generally well tolerated. The most common side effects are dry mouth, hypotension, constipation, urinary hesitancy or retention, and decreased libido. Other effects include dizziness, headache, nausea, insomnia, tremor, diaphoresis, and tachycardia. Reboxetine does not cause sedation or weight gain, and has minimal effects on psychomotor or cognitive function.

Combining reboxetine with an MAOI may pose a risk of hypertensive crisis. Accordingly, MAOIs should be withdrawn at least 14 days before giving reboxetine.

The recommended starting dosage is 4 mg twice daily. In patients with liver dysfunction, the initial dosage should be reduced to 2 mg twice daily. In clinical trials, dosages ranged between 4 and 12 mg/day.

Trazodone

Trazodone [Desyrel] is a second-line agent for treatment of depression. The drug is not very effective when used alone, but, because of its pronounced sedative effects, it can be a helpful adjunct for patients with antidepressant-induced insomnia. Trazodone produces selective (but moderate) blockade of serotonin reuptake. Antidepressant effects take several weeks to develop.

Common side effects are sedation, orthostatic hypotension, dry mouth, and nausea. In contrast to the tricyclic agents, trazodone has minimal anticholinergic actions and is not cardiotoxic. Accordingly, trazodone may be useful for elderly patients and other individuals for whom the cardiac and anticholinergic effects of the tricyclics may be intolerable.

Trazodone can cause priapism (prolonged, painful erection of the penis). In some cases, surgical intervention has been required. Priapism itself or the procedures required for relief can result in permanent impotence. Patients should be instructed to notify the physician or to go to an emergency department if persistent erection occurs. Prolonged clitoral erection can also occur, but the incidence is extremely low (0.016%).

Overdose with trazodone is considered safer than with tricyclic agents or MAOIs. Death from overdose with trazodone alone has not been reported (although death has occurred following overdose with trazodone in combination with another CNS depressant).

Trazodone is dispensed in tablets (50, 100, 150, and 300 mg) for oral administration. The initial dosage is 150 mg/day in divided doses. Dosage may be gradually increased to a maximum of 400 mg/day (for outpatients) and 600 mg/day (for hospitalized patients).

ELECTROCONVULSIVE THERAPY

Although outside the realm of pharmacology, ECT is a valuable treatment for depression and deserves our consideration. Success requires a series of treatments, typically three per week for 2 to 4 weeks. Since ECT as practiced today does not cause convulsions, a more appropriate name might be elec-tro*shock* therapy.

ECT has two characteristics that are especially desirable: *effectiveness* and *rapid onset* (relative to antidepressant drugs). Because of these properties, ECT is indicated primarily for two types of patients: (1) those who have failed to respond to pharmacologic treatment for depression (50% to 60% will respond to ECT), and (2) severely depressed, suicidal patients who need rapid relief of symptoms.

Thanks to the adjunctive use of drugs, ECT is much less dramatic and traumatic than it was in the past. Prior to the delivery of electroshock, patients are treated with a combination of *thiopental* and *succinylcholine*. Thiopental is an injectable, ultra-short-acting anesthetic that prevents conscious awareness of the ECT procedure (without interfering with beneficial actions). Succinylcholine is a short-acting neuromuscular blocking agent that prevents shock-induced convulsive movements, which are both hazardous and unnecessary for a therapeutic response.

ECT can terminate an ongoing depression episode, but a single series of treatments cannot prevent recurrence. Accordingly, some patients are now given "maintenance" treatments, at weekly or monthly intervals. In one study, the relapse rate at 6 months in the absence of maintenance was 73%, compared with only 8% when maintenance ECT was used. Maintenance with antidepressant drugs (e.g., lithium plus amitriptyline) is another option, but appears significantly less effective than maintenance with ECT.

The principal adverse effect of ECT is some loss of memory for events immediately surrounding treatment. Patients do not lose other memories, and their intellectual function is not affected. Minor adverse effects, which occur immediately after treatment, include nausea, headache, confusion, and muscle discomfort.

⠿ KEY POINTS

- The principal symptoms of major depression are depressed mood and loss of pleasure or interest in one's usual activities and pastimes.
- Patients with mild depression can be treated equally well with antidepressant drugs or with psychotherapy. Patients with severe depression respond better to a combination of drugs plus psychotherapy than they do to either intervention alone.
- Therapeutic responses to antidepressants develop slowly. Initial responses develop in 1 to 3 weeks. Maximal responses develop in 1 to 2 months.
- Antidepressant therapy should continue for 6 months to 1 year after symptoms have abated.
- TCAs block reuptake of NE and serotonin, and thereby intensify transmission at noradrenergic and serotonergic synapses. Over time, this induces adaptive cellular responses that are ultimately responsible for relieving depression.
- The most common adverse effects of TCAs are sedation, orthostatic hypotension, and anticholinergic effects (e.g., dry mouth, constipation).
- The most serious adverse effect of TCAs is cardiotoxicity, which can be lethal if an overdose is taken.
- TCAs can cause a hypertensive crisis if combined with an MAOI. Accordingly, the combination is generally avoided.

- TCAs intensify responses to direct-acting sympathomimetics (e.g., epinephrine) and diminish responses to indirect-acting sympathomimetics (e.g., amphetamine).
- SSRIs block reuptake of serotonin, and thereby intensify transmission at serotonergic synapses. Over time, this induces adaptive cellular responses that are ultimately responsible for relieving depression.
- SSRIs have two major advantages over TCAs: they cause fewer side effects and are safer when taken in overdose.
- Most SSRIs have stimulant properties, and hence can cause insomnia and nervousness. This contrasts with TCAs, which cause sedation.
- Like most other antidepressants, SSRIs can cause weight gain.
- Sexual dysfunction (e.g., impotence, anorgasmia) is more common with SSRIs than with other antidepressants.
- SSRIs can cause serotonin syndrome, especially when combined with MAOIs. Symptoms include agitation, confusion, hallucinations, hyperreflexia, tremor, and fever.
- MAOIs increase neuronal stores of NE and serotonin, and thereby intensify transmission at noradrenergic and serotonergic synapses. Over time, this induces

adaptive cellular responses that are ultimately responsible for relieving depression.
- MAOIs are as effective as TCAs and SSRIs, but are much more dangerous.
- MAOIs are first-choice drugs only for patients with atypical depression.
- Like SSRIs (and unlike TCAs), MAOIs cause direct CNS stimulation.
- Like TCAs (and unlike SSRIs), MAOIs cause orthostatic hypotension.
- Patients taking MAOIs must not eat tyramine-rich foods because hypertensive crisis can result.
- MAOIs must not be combined with indirect-acting sympathomimetics (e.g., ephedrine, amphetamine) because hypertensive crisis can result.
- MAOIs must not be combined with SSRIs because serotonin syndrome could result.
- ECT relieves depression faster than antidepressant drugs, and often helps when antidepressants have failed.
- ECT is now safer and less traumatic than in the past owing to adjunctive use of thiopental (which produces unconsciousness) and succinylcholine (which prevents convulsions).

Summary of Major Nursing Implications*

IMPLICATIONS THAT APPLY TO ALL ANTIDEPRESSANTS

Psychologic Assessment

Observe and record the patient's behavior. Factors to assess include affect, thought content, interest in the environment, appetite, sleep patterns, and appearance.

Reducing the Risk of Suicide

Patients who are so depressed that they are a risk to themselves and others should be hospitalized until symptoms are under control. Suicide potential should be evaluated carefully. To prevent patients from accumulating a potentially lethal supply of medication, ensure that each dose is swallowed and not cheeked. Provide outpatients with no more than a 1-week supply of medication at a time. For patients considered at high risk of suicide, TCAs and MAOIs should be avoided; SSRIs are much safer.

Promoting Compliance

Inform the patient that antidepressant effects usually develop slowly, over 1 to 3 weeks. This knowledge will make expectations more realistic, which should help promote compliance.

Premature discontinuation of therapy can result in relapse. **Educate patients about the importance of taking their medication as prescribed, even though they may be symp-**

tom free and therefore feel "cured." In general, treatment should continue for 6 months to a year after symptoms have subsided.

Nondrug Therapy

For patients with severe depression, treatment with drugs alone is not optimal. Emotional support and psychotherapy can complement and reinforce responses to antidepressants. ECT may be indicated for suicidal patients and for patients who fail to respond to antidepressant drugs and psychotherapy.

Evaluating Therapeutic Effects

Assess patients for improvement in symptoms, especially depressed mood and loss of interest or pleasure in usual activities.

TRICYCLIC ANTIDEPRESSANTS

Amitriptyline
Clomipramine
Desipramine
Doxepin
Imipramine
Maprotiline
Nortriptyline
Protriptyline
Trimipramine

*Patient education information is highlighted as blue text.

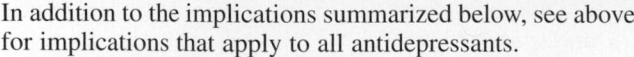

Summary of Major Nursing Implications*—cont'd

In addition to the implications summarized below, see above for implications that apply to all antidepressants.

Preadministration Assessment

Therapeutic Goal

Alleviation of symptoms of major depression.

Baseline Data

Assess psychologic status. Arrange for an EKG, especially for patients with cardiac disease and those over 40.

Identifying High-Risk Patients

TCAs are generally *contraindicated* for patients taking MAOIs.

Use TCAs with *caution* in patients with cardiac disorders (e.g., coronary heart disease, progressive heart failure, paroxysmal tachycardia), elevated intraocular pressure, urinary retention, hyperthyroidism, seizure disorders, and liver or kidney dysfunction.

Doxepin is *contraindicated* for patients with glaucoma or a tendency to urinary retention.

Maprotiline is *contraindicated* for patients with seizure disorders.

Implementation: Administration

Routes

Oral (usual); IM (occasional).

Administration

Instruct patients to take medication daily as prescribed and not PRN. Warn patients not to discontinue treatment once mood has improved, since doing so may result in relapse. Once an effective dosage has been established, the entire daily dose can usually be taken at bedtime.

Ongoing Evaluation and Interventions

Minimizing Adverse Effects

Orthostatic Hypotension. Inform patients about symptoms of hypotension (dizziness, lightheadedness), and advise them to sit or lie down if these occur. Inform patients that hypotension can be minimized by moving slowly when assuming an erect posture. For hospitalized patients, monitor blood pressure and pulse rate on a regular schedule; take measurements while the patient is lying down and again after the patient has been sitting or standing for 1 to 2 minutes. If blood pressure is low or pulse rate is high, withhold medication and inform the physician.

Anticholinergic Effects. Forewarn patients about possible anticholinergic effects (dry mouth, blurred vision, photophobia, urinary hesitancy, constipation, tachycardia), and advise them to notify the physician if these are troublesome. A detailed summary of nursing implications for anticholinergic drugs is presented in Chapter 14.

Diaphoresis. TCAs promote sweating (despite their anticholinergic properties). Excessive sweating may necessitate frequent changes of bedding and clothing.

Sedation. Sedation is most intense during the first weeks of therapy and declines with continued drug use. **Advise the patient to avoid hazardous activities (e.g., driving, operating dangerous machinery) if sedation is significant.** Giving TCAs at bedtime minimizes daytime sedation and promotes sleep.

Cardiotoxicity. TCAs can disrupt cardiac function, but usually only when taken in excessive doses or by patients with heart disease. All patients should receive an EKG prior to treatment and periodically thereafter.

Seizures. TCAs decrease seizure threshold. Exercise caution in patients with seizure disorders.

Hypomania. TCAs may shift mood from depression up to hypomania. If hypomania develops, the patient must be evaluated to determine if elation is drug induced or indicates bipolar disorder.

Minimizing Adverse Interactions

MAO Inhibitors. Rarely, the combination of a TCA and an MAOI has produced hypertensive episodes and hypertensive crisis. Exercise caution if this combination is employed.

Sympathomimetic Agents. TCAs decrease the effects of indirect-acting sympathomimetics (e.g., ephedrine, amphetamine), but potentiate the actions of direct-acting sympathomimetics (e.g., epinephrine, dopamine). If sympathomimetics are to be used, these effects must be accounted for.

Anticholinergic Agents. Drugs capable of blocking muscarinic receptors will enhance the anticholinergic effects of TCAs. **Warn patients against concurrent use of other anticholinergic drugs (e.g., scopolamine, antihistamines, phenothiazines).**

CNS Depressants. These will enhance the depressant effects of TCAs. **Warn patients against using alcohol and all other drugs with CNS-depressant properties (e.g., opioids, antihistamines, barbiturates, benzodiazepines).**

SELECTIVE SEROTONIN REUPTAKE INHIBITORS

Citalopram
Escitalopram
Fluoxetine
Fluvoxamine
Paroxetine
Sertraline

In addition to the implications summarized below, see above for implications that apply to all antidepressants.

Preadministration Assessment

Therapeutic Goal

Alleviation of Symptoms of Major Depression. All SSRIs except fluvoxamine are approved for treating depression.

Other Goals. SSRIs are used to relieve symptoms of many psychologic disorders, including obsessive-compulsive

*Patient education information is highlighted as blue text.

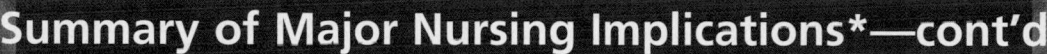

Summary of Major Nursing Implications*—cont'd

disorder, panic disorder, social phobia, generalized anxiety disorder, post-traumatic stress disorder, premenstrual dysphoric disorder, and bulimia nervosa (Table 31–4).

Identifying High-Risk Patients

SSRIs are *contraindicated* for patients taking MAOIs. Use with *caution* in patients with liver disease and in the elderly and women who are pregnant or breast-feeding.

Implementation: Administration
Route
Oral.

Administration

All SSRIs may be administered with food. Administration in the morning minimizes sleep disruption.

Warn patients not to discontinue treatment once mood has improved, since doing so could lead to relapse.

Ongoing Evaluation and Interventions
Minimizing Adverse Effects

CNS Stimulation. Citalopram, escitalopram, fluoxetine, paroxetine, and sertraline can cause nervousness, insomnia, and anxiety. These reactions may respond to a decrease in dosage. (Fluvoxamine causes mild sedation.)

Serotonin Syndrome. Symptoms of this potentially fatal syndrome include agitation, confusion, disorientation, anxiety, hallucinations, poor concentration, incoordination, myoclonus, hyperreflexia, excessive sweating, tremor, and fever. The risk is reduced by avoiding concurrent use of MAOIs. Serotonin syndrome resolves spontaneously after discontinuing the SSRI.

Sexual Dysfunction. **Forewarn patients about possible sexual dysfunction (anorgasmia, impotence, decreased libido), and encourage them to report problems.** Management strategies include dosage reduction, drug holidays, adding a drug to counteract sexual dysfunction (e.g., sildenafil, buspirone), and switching to an antidepressant that causes less sexual dysfunction (e.g., bupropion, nefazodone, mirtazapine).

Dizziness and Fatigue. **Inform patients about possible dizziness and fatigue, and advise them to exercise caution while performing hazardous tasks (e.g., driving).**

Rash. Fluoxetine may cause rash. **Inform patients about the risk of rash and instruct them to notify the physician if one develops.** Treatment consists of drug therapy (antihistamines, glucocorticoids) or withdrawal of fluoxetine.

Weight Gain. Long-term therapy can result in significant weight gain. **Advise patients to restrict caloric intake and to get appropriate exercise.**

Bruxism. SSRIs can cause bruxism (clenching and grinding of teeth), usually during sleep. **Alert patients to the sequelae of bruxism (headache, jaw pain, and dental problems, such as cracked fillings).** If these develop, investigate whether an SSRI is the cause. Bruxism can be managed by (1) a reduction in SSRI dosage (but then depression may re-

turn), (2) switching to a different class of antidepressants, (3) use of a mouth guard, and (4) treatment with low-dose buspirone.

Minimizing Adverse Interactions

MAO Inhibitors. MAOIs increase the risk of serotonin syndrome, and hence must not be combined with SSRIs. Withdraw MAOIs at least 14 days before starting an SSRI. Withdraw fluoxetine 5 weeks before starting an MAOI; withdraw other SSRIs at least 2 weeks before starting an MAOI.

TCAs and Lithium. Fluoxetine can increase levels of these drugs. Exercise caution.

MONOAMINE OXIDASE INHIBITORS

Isocarboxazid
Phenelzine
Tranylcypromine

Preadministration Assessment

In addition to the implications summarized below, see above for implications that apply to all antidepressants.

Therapeutic Goal

Alleviation of symptoms of major depression, especially atypical depression.

Identifying High-Risk Patients

MAOIs are *contraindicated* for patients taking SSRIs and for patients with pheochromocytoma, heart failure, liver disease, severe renal impairment, cerebrovascular defect (known or suspected), cardiovascular disease, and hypertension and for patients over the age of 60 (because of possible cerebral sclerosis associated with vessel damage).

Use with *caution* in patients taking TCAs.

Implementation: Administration
Route
Oral.

Administration

Instruct patients to take MAOIs every day as prescribed—not PRN. Warn patients not to discontinue treatment once mood has improved, since doing so may result in relapse.

Ongoing Evaluation and Interventions
Minimizing Adverse Effects

Hypertensive Crisis. Dietary tyramine, certain other dietary constituents (see Table 31–5), and indirect-acting sympathomimetics (e.g., amphetamine, methylphenidate, ephedrine, cocaine) can precipitate a hypertensive crisis in patients taking MAOIs.

Inform patients about symptoms of hypertensive crisis (headache, palpitations, tachycardia, nausea, vomiting), and instruct them to seek immediate medical attention if these develop.

*Patient education information is highlighted as blue text.

Summary of Major Nursing Implications*—cont'd

To reduce the risk of hypertensive crisis, the following precautions must be observed: (1) do not give MAOIs to patients who are suicidal or who are considered incapable of rigid adherence to dietary constraints; (2) forewarn patients about the hazard of hypertensive crisis and the need to avoid tyramine-rich foods and sympathomimetic drugs; (3) provide patients with a list of specific foods to avoid (see Table 31–5); and (4) instruct them to avoid all drugs not approved by the physician.

If hypertensive crisis develops, blood pressure can be lowered with IV phentolamine or sublingual nifedipine.

Orthostatic Hypotension. Inform patients about signs of hypotension (dizziness, lightheadedness), and advise them to sit or lie down if these occur. Inform patients that hypotension can be minimized by moving slowly when assuming an erect posture. For the hospitalized patient, monitor blood pressure and pulse rate on a regular schedule. Take these measurements while the patient is lying down and again after the patient has been sitting or standing for 1 to 2 minutes. If blood pressure is low, withhold medication and inform the physician.

*Patient education information is highlighted as blue text.

Minimizing Adverse Interactions

All Drugs. MAOIs can interact adversely with many other drugs. **Instruct the patient to avoid all medications—prescription and nonprescription—that have not been specifically approved by the physician.**

Indirect-Acting Sympathomimetics. Concurrent use with MAOIs can precipitate a hypertensive crisis. **Warn patients against use of any indirect-acting sympathomimetics (e.g., ephedrine, methylphenidate, amphetamines, cocaine).**

Tricyclic Antidepressants. Concurrent use with MAOIs can produce hypertensive episodes and hypertensive crisis. Use this combination with caution.

SSRIs. Concurrent use with MAOIs can cause serotonin syndrome. Avoid the combination.

Antihypertensive Drugs. These drugs will potentiate the hypotensive effects of MAOIs. If these agents are combined, monitor blood pressure periodically.

Meperidine. Meperidine can produce hyperthermia in patients taking MAOIs and hence should be avoided.

Drugs for Bipolar Disorder

Our topic for this chapter is drug therapy of bipolar disorder (BPD), formerly known as *manic-depressive illness.* The disease afflicts 1.2% of the adult population—or more than 2.2 million Americans. The mainstays of therapy are lithium and valproic acid, drugs with the ability to stabilize mood. Some patients may require an antidepressant or antipsychotic agent as well. Bipolar disorder is a chronic condition that usually requires treatment for life.

CHARACTERISTICS OF BIPOLAR DISORDER

Bipolar disorder is a severe biologic illness characterized by recurrent fluctuations in mood. Typically, patients experience alternating episodes in which mood is abnormally elevated or abnormally depressed—separated by periods in which mood is relatively normal. Onset of symptoms usually occurs in adolescence or early adulthood, but may also occur earlier in life or as late as the fourth or fifth decade. In the absence of treatment, episodes of mania or depression generally persist for several months. As time passes, manic and depressive episodes tend to recur more frequently. Although the precise etiology of BPD is unknown, it is clear that symptoms are caused by a change in brain chemistry—not by a character flaw or an unstable personality.

Types of Mood Episodes Seen in BPD

Patients with BPD may experience four types of mood episodes. These are described below.

Pure Manic Episode (Euphoric Mania). Manic episodes are characterized by persistently heightened, expansive, or irritable mood—typically associated with hyperactivity, excessive enthusiasm, and flight of ideas. Manic individuals display overactivity at work and at play and have a reduced need for sleep. Mania produces excessive sociability and talkativeness. Extreme self-confidence, grandiose ideas, and delusions of importance are common. Manic individuals often indulge in high-risk activities (e.g., questionable business deals, reckless driving, gambling, sexual indiscretions), giving no forethought to the consequences. In severe cases, symptoms may resemble those of paranoid schizophrenia (hallucinations, delusions, bizarre behavior). Specific diagnostic criteria for a manic episode, as described in the *Diagnostic and Statistical Manual of Mental Disorders, Fourth Edition,* are summarized in Table 32–1.

Hypomanic Episode (Hypomania). Hypomania can be viewed as a mild form of mania. As in mania, mood is persistently elevated, expansive, or irritable. However, symptoms are not severe enough to cause marked impairment in social or occupational functioning, or to require hospitalization. Psychotic symptoms are absent.

Major Depressive Episode (Depression). A major depressive episode is characterized by depressed mood and loss of pleasure or interest in all or nearly all of one's usual activities and pastimes. Associated symptoms include disruption of sleeping and eating patterns; difficulty concentrating; feelings of guilt, worthlessness, and helplessness; and thoughts of death and suicide. The characteristics of major depression are discussed further in Chapter 31.

Mixed Episode. In a true mixed episode, patients experience symptoms of mania and depression simultaneously. Patients may be agitated and irritable (as in mania), but may also feel worthless and depressed. The combination of high energy and depression puts them at significant risk of suicide.

Patterns of Mood Episodes

Among people with BPD, mood episodes can occur in a variety of patterns. Contrary to popular belief, not all patients alternate repeatedly between mania and depression. Some experience repeated episodes of mania, and some experience repeated episodes of depression (with an occasional episode of mania). Mood may be normal between episodes of mania and depression, or it may be slightly elevated (hypomania) or slightly depressed (dysphoria).

Mood episodes can vary greatly with respect to duration and how often they occur. A single episode may last for days, weeks, months, or more than a year. In the absence of treatment, episodes of mania or hypomania typically last a few months, whereas episodes of major depression typically last over 6 months. On average, people with BPD experience only 4 episodes during the first 10 years of their illness. However, some people cycle much more rapidly, experiencing many episodes every year.

TABLE 32–1 ■ DSM-IV-TR Criteria for a Manic Episode

A. A distinct period of abnormally and persistently elevated, expansive, or irritable mood, lasting at least 1 week (or any duration if hospitalization is necessary).

B. During the period of mood disturbance, three (or more) of the following symptoms have persisted (four if the mood is only irritable) and have been present to a significant degree:

- Inflated self-esteem or grandiosity
- Decreased need for sleep (e.g., feels rested after only 3 hours of sleep)
- More talkative than usual or pressure to keep talking
- Flight of ideas or subjective experience that thoughts are racing
- Distractibility (i.e., attention too easily drawn to unimportant or irrelevant external stimuli)
- Increase in goal-directed activity (either socially, at work or school, or sexually) or psychomotor agitation
- Excessive involvement in pleasurable activities that have a high potential for painful consequences (e.g., engaging in unrestrained buying sprees, sexual indiscretions, or foolish business investments)

C. The mood disturbance is sufficiently severe to cause marked impairment in occupational functioning or in usual social activities or relationships with others, or to necessitate hospitalization to prevent harm to self or others, or there are psychotic features.

D. The symptoms are not due to the direct physiologic effects of a substance (e.g., a drug of abuse, a medication, or other treatment) or a general medical condition (e.g., hyperthyroidism).*

*Manic-like episodes that are clearly caused by somatic antidepressant treatment (e.g., medication, electroconvulsive therapy, light therapy) should not count toward a diagnosis of bipolar disorder. Modified from the Diagnostic and Statistical Manual of Mental Disorders, Fourth Edition, Text Revision. Washington, DC, American Psychiatric Press, 2000, with permission. Copyright © 2000 American Psychiatric Association.

On the basis of mood episode type and frequency, BPD can be subdivided into three major categories:

- *Bipolar I Disorder*—Patients experience manic or mixed episodes, and usually depressive episodes too.
- *Bipolar II Disorder*—Patients experience hypomanic or depressive episodes, but not manic or mixed episodes.
- *Rapid-Cycling Bipolar Disorder*—Patients experience four or more episodes of any sort (manic, hypomanic, depressive, mixed) each year.

TREATMENT OF BIPOLAR DISORDER

Drug Therapy
Types of Drugs Employed

Bipolar disorder is treated with three major groups of drugs: mood stabilizers, antidepressants, and antipsychotics. In addition, benzodiazepines are frequently used for sedation.

Mood Stabilizers. Mood stabilizers are drugs that (1) relieve symptoms during manic and depressive episodes, (2) prevent recurrence of manic and depressive episodes, and (3) do not worsen symptoms of mania or depression, or accelerate the rate of cycling. The principal mood stabilizers in use are *lithium* and two drugs that were originally developed as anticonvulsants: *valproic acid* (and its derivatives), and *carbamazepine*. These drugs are the mainstays of treatment. The pharmacology of lithium and the anticonvulsants is discussed below.

Antidepressants. Antidepressants may be needed during a depressive episode. In patients with BPD, antidepressants are always combined with a mood stabilizer. Why? Because, when used alone, antidepressants can elevate mood so much that a hypomanic or manic episode can result. Although anti-depressants have been studied extensively in patients with major depression, very little research has been done in patients with BPD. As a result, reliable information on which to base antidepressant selection is lacking. Nonetheless, experts do have their preferences. Among clinicians with extensive experience in PBD, the following agents are considered antidepressants of choice: *bupropion* [Wellbutrin], *venlafaxine* [Effexor], and the *selective serotonin reuptake inhibitors* (SSRIs), such as fluoxetine [Prozac] and sertraline [Zoloft]. The pharmacology of the antidepressants is discussed in Chapter 31.

Antipsychotics. In patients with BPD, antipsychotic drugs are used to help control symptoms during severe manic episodes, even if psychotic symptoms are absent. Benefits include reduction of anxiety, insomnia, and agitation. Some antipsychotics also help stabilize mood. Although antipsychotics can be used alone, they are usually employed in combination with a mood stabilizer (e.g., lithium, valproic acid).

Which antipsychotics are preferred? As discussed in Chapter 30, the antipsychotics can be divided into two major groups: conventional agents (e.g., haloperidol) and atypical agents (e.g., olanzapine). Compared with the conventional agents, the atypical agents carry a much lower risk of extrapyramidal side effects, including tardive dyskinesia. Accordingly, the atypical agents are generally preferred. Of the four atypical agents available, three—*olanzapine* [Zyprexa], *quetiapine* [Seroquel], and *risperidone* [Risperdal]—are used most often. The fourth atypical agent—*clozapine* [Clozaril]—is highly effective in BPD, but can cause agranulocytosis, and hence is used only rarely.

Olanzapine deserves special mention. In 2000, olanzapine became the first antipsychotic agent to receive Food and Drug Administration (FDA) approval as monotherapy for acute mania in patients with BPD. The drug can reduce irritability, euphoria, and psychotic symptoms. In one study, benefits of

TABLE 32–2 ■ Initial Treatment of First Manic Episode

Clinical Presentation	Preferred Strategy	Preferred Drugs*	
		Mood Stabilizers	Antipsychotics
Euphoric mania	Mood stabilizer alone	Valproic acid or **lithium**	
Dysphoric mania or true mixed mania	Mood stabilizer alone	**Valproic acid** or lithium	
Mania with psychosis	Mood stabilizer plus an antipsychotic	**Valproic acid** or lithium	Olanzapine or risperidone
Rapid cycling (currently manic)	Mood stabilizer alone	**Valproic acid**	

*Drugs of choice, if established, are presented in **bold type.**

short-term olanzapine were equal to those of lithium—and olanzapine works faster. Although olanzapine appears to stabilize mood, we do not yet know if long-term use will prevent recurrence of mania or depression.

The pharmacology of the antipsychotics is presented in Chapter 30.

Drug Selection

Acute Therapy: Manic Episodes. Two mood stabilizers—lithium and valproic acid—are preferred drugs for acute management of manic episodes. The choice between them is based on clinical presentation (e.g., euphoric mania, mania with psychosis, rapid-cycling BPD). As shown in Table 32–2, valproic acid is preferred to lithium in most cases. In fact, the only exception is euphoric mania, for which lithium is the drug of choice. If the patient does not respond adequately to lithium or valproic acid alone, the two drugs may be used in combination. Responses to these mood stabilizers develop slowly, taking 2 or more weeks to become maximal.

If needed, an antipsychotic agent or a benzodiazepine may be added to the regimen. These adjuvants can help relieve symptoms (e.g., insomnia, anxiety, agitation) until the mood stabilizer takes full effect. For patients with mild mania, a benzodiazepine (e.g., lorazepam [Ativan]) may be adequate. For patients with severe mania or with symptoms of psychosis, an antipsychotic is preferred; olanzapine or risperidone would be a good choice.

Acute Therapy: Depressive Episodes. Depressive episodes may be treated with a mood stabilizer alone, or with a mood stabilizer *plus* an antidepressant—but *never* with an antidepressant alone (because hypomania or mania might result). If depression is mild, monotherapy with a mood stabilizer (lithium or valproic acid) may be sufficient. If the mood stabilizer alone is not adequate, an antidepressant should be added. Preferred agents are bupropion, venlafaxine, and the SSRIs.

Long-Term Preventive Treatment. The purpose of long-term therapy is to prevent recurrence of both mania and depression. One or more mood stabilizers is employed. Drug selection is based on what worked acutely. For example, if the patient responded to acute therapy with lithium alone, then lithium alone should be used long-term. Other long-term options include valproic acid alone, and valproic acid plus lithium. For patients with psychotic symptoms, long-term therapy with an antipsychotic agent (along with a mood stabilizer) may be needed.

Promoting Compliance

Poor patient compliance can frustrate attempts at treating manic episodes. Patients may resist treatment because they fail to see anything wrong with their thinking or behavior. Furthermore, the experience is not necessarily unpleasant. In fact, individuals going through a manic episode may well enjoy it. As a result, in order to ensure compliance, short-term hospitalization may be required. To achieve this, collaboration with the patient's family may be needed. Since hospitalization per se won't guarantee success, lithium administration should be observed to ensure that each dose is actually taken.

After an acute manic episode has been controlled, long-term prophylactic therapy is indicated, making compliance an ongoing issue. To promote compliance, the patient and family should be educated about the nature of BPD and the importance of taking medication as prescribed. Family members can help ensure compliance by overseeing medication use, and by urging the patient to visit a physician or psychiatric clinic if a pattern of noncompliance develops.

Nondrug Therapy
Education and Psychotherapy

Ideally, BPD should be treated with a combination of drugs and adjunctive psychotherapy (individual, group, or family); drug therapy alone is not optimal. Bipolar disorder is a chronic illness that requires supportive therapy and education for the patient and family. Counseling can help patients cope with the sequelae of manic episodes, such as strained relationships, reduced self-confidence, and a sense of shame regarding uncontrolled behavior. Certain life stresses (e.g., moving, job loss, bereavement, childbirth) can precipitate a mood change; therapy can help reduce the destabilizing impact of these events. Patients should be taught to recognize early symptoms of mood change, and encouraged to contact the physician immediately if these develop. Additional measures by which patients can help themselves include:

- Maintaining a stable sleep pattern
- Maintaining a regular pattern of activity
- Avoiding alcohol and psychoactive street drugs
- Enlisting the support of family and friends
- Taking steps to reduce stress at work
- Keeping a mood chart to monitor progress

Special Interest Topic

BOX 32–1 ■ OMEGA-3 FATTY ACIDS FOR BIPOLAR DISORDER: A FISH STORY WITH A HAPPY ENDING

In 1999, researchers from Harvard University made a very exciting discovery: Fish oil can stabilize mood in people with bipolar disorder. Their results were so striking, in fact, that the experiment was stopped after 4 months so that control patients could switch to the fish-oil regimen. All subjects in the study had diagnosed bipolar disorder. Some took 9.6 gm of fish oil daily, and some took olive oil as a control. All continued on their usual medications. Among the group that ate fish oil, 11 of 15 improved after 4 months—and only 2 suffered eventual relapse. Among the group that ate olive oil, only 6 of 20 improved after 4 months—and 11 experienced relapse. Patients taking the fish oil had longer periods of remission, and, when symptoms did appear, they were less severe. Several patients were able to discontinue their medications and remain symptom-free on fish oil alone. Side effects of the fish oil were minor—nausea, belching, fishy taste, loose stools—and easily controlled. At this time, the long-term benefits or detriments of fish oil are unknown. This study is of special interest in that it suggests that dietary therapy for a major illness can be as effective as drugs.

How does fish oil work? No one knows. Fish oil is composed of omega-3 fatty acids*—specifically, eicosapentaenoic acid and docosahexaenoic acid. The highest concentrations of omega-3s are found in the eyes and brain, where they are present in cell membranes. It may be that eating fish oil increases the concentration of omega-3s in neuronal membranes, and thereby slows nerve signaling, which in turn may stabilize mood. There is some evidence that omega-6 fatty acids—the kind found in vegetable oils, margarine, and mayonnaise—may negate the beneficial effects of omega-3s. Accordingly, patients taking fish oil for bipolar disorder should probably decrease intake of omega-6s.

*Omega-3 fatty acids are long-chain polyunsaturated fats that have a double bond located three carbons from the methyl terminus of the chain.

Electroconvulsive Therapy

Electroconvulsive therapy (ECT) is a very effective treatment that can be life-saving in patients with severe mania or depression. However, ECT is not a treatment of first choice. Rather, it should be reserved for patients who have not responded adequately to drugs. Candidates for ECT include patients with psychotic depression, severe nonpsychotic depression, severe mania, and rapid-cycling BPD. Details of ECT are discussed in Chapter 31.

PHARMACOLOGY OF THE MOOD-STABILIZING DRUGS

As noted above, a mood-stabilizing drug is one that can provide relief from an acute manic or depressive episode, and can prevent symptoms from recurring—all without aggravating mania or depression, and without accelerating cycling. At this time, the only drugs with a proven ability to stabilize mood are lithium and two anticonvulsants: valproic acid and carbamazepine.

Lithium

Lithium can stabilize mood in patients with BPD. Beneficial effects were first described in 1949 by John Cade, an Australian. However, because of concerns about toxicity, lithium was not approved for use in the United States until 1970. Lithium has a low therapeutic index. As a result, toxicity can occur at blood levels that are only slightly greater than therapeutic. Accordingly, monitoring of lithium levels is mandatory.

Chemistry

Lithium is a simple inorganic ion that carries a single positive charge. In the periodic table of elements, lithium is in the same group as potassium and sodium. Not surprisingly, lithium has properties in common with both elements. Lithium is found naturally in animal tissues but has no known physiologic function.

Therapeutic Uses

Bipolar Disorder. Lithium is a drug of choice for controlling acute manic episodes in patients with BPD and for long-term prophylaxis against recurrence of mania or depression. In manic patients, lithium reduces euphoria, hyperactivity, and other symptoms but does not cause sedation. Antimanic effects begin 5 to 7 days after the onset of treatment. However, full benefits may not develop for 2 to 3 weeks. In the past, lithium was considered the drug of choice for all patients experiencing an acute manic episode, regardless of clinical presentation. Today, however, lithium is preferred only for patients with classic (euphoric) mania; valproic acid is preferred to lithium for all others (see Table 32–2).

Other Uses. Although approved only for treatment of BPD, lithium has been used with varying degrees of success in other psychiatric disorders, including *alcoholism, bulimia, schizophrenia,* and *glucocorticoid-induced psychosis.* Nonpsychiatric uses include *hyperthyroidism, cluster headache, migraine,* and *syndrome of inappropriate secretion of antidiuretic hormone.* In addition, lithium can *raise neutrophil counts* in children with chronic neutropenia and in patients receiving anticancer drugs or zidovudine (AZT).

Mechanism of Action in Bipolar Disorder

Although lithium has been studied extensively, the precise mechanism by which it stabilizes mood is unknown. Research has focused on three areas: (1) altered distribution of certain ions (calcium, sodium, magnesium) that are critical to neuronal function; (2) effects on the synthesis and release of norepinephrine, serotonin, and dopamine; and (3) effects on second-messenger systems that mediate intracellular responses to neurotransmitters. At this time, effects on second messengers seem the most likely mechanism. (A second messenger is a compound that is formed inside a cell in response to the interaction of a first messenger [e.g., neurotransmitter] with its receptor on the cell surface. The second messenger then acts within the cell to mediate responses to the first messenger.) Lithium has the ability to suppress the synthesis of at least three second messengers: inositol-1,4,5-triphosphate, diacylglycerol, and cyclic AMP. It may be that, in patients with BPD, there is excessive activity in neuronal pathways that employ these second messengers. If so, the ability of lithium to suppress synthesis of these compounds could explain the drug's clinical benefits.

Pharmacokinetics

Absorption and Distribution. Lithium is well absorbed following oral administration. The drug distributes evenly to all tissues and body fluids.

Excretion. Lithium has a short half-life owing to rapid renal excretion. Because of its short half-life (and high toxicity), the drug must be administered in divided daily doses. Large, single daily doses cannot be used. Because lithium is excreted by the kidneys, it must be employed with great care in patients with renal impairment.

Renal excretion of lithium is affected by blood levels of sodium. Specifically, lithium excretion is *reduced* when blood levels of sodium are *low*. Why? Because the kidney processes lithium and sodium in the same way. Hence, when the kidney senses that sodium levels are inadequate, it retains lithium in an attempt to compensate. Because of this relationship, in the presence of low sodium, lithium can accumulate to toxic levels. Accordingly, it is important that sodium levels remain normal. Patients should be instructed to maintain normal sodium intake. Obviously, a sodium-free diet cannot be used. Since diuretics promote sodium loss, these agents must be employed with caution. Sodium loss secondary to diarrhea can be sufficient to cause lithium accumulation. The patient should be forewarned of this possibility.

Dehydration will cause lithium retention by the kidneys, posing the risk of accumulation to dangerous levels. Potential causes of dehydration include hot weather and diarrhea. Counsel patients to maintain adequate hydration.

Monitoring Plasma Lithium Levels. Measurement of plasma lithium levels is an essential component of treatment. *Lithium levels must be kept below 1.5 mEq/L; levels greater than this can produce significant toxicity.* For *initial* therapy of a manic episode, lithium levels should range from 0.8 to 1.4 mEq/L. Once the desired therapeutic effect has been achieved, the dosage should be reduced to produce *maintenance* levels of 0.4 to 1.0 mEq/L. Blood for lithium determinations should be drawn in the morning, 12 hours after the evening dose.

Adverse Effects

The adverse effects of lithium can be divided into two categories: (1) effects that occur at excessive drug levels and (2) effects that occur at therapeutic drug levels. In the discussion below, adverse effects produced at excessive lithium levels are considered as a group. Effects produced at therapeutic levels are considered individually.

Adverse Effects That Occur When Lithium Levels Are Excessive. Certain toxicities are closely correlated with the concentration of lithium in blood. As indicated in Table 32–3, mild responses (e.g., fine hand tremor, GI upset, thirst, muscle weakness) can develop at lithium levels that are still within the therapeutic range (i.e., below 1.5 mEq/L). When plasma levels exceed 1.5 mEq/L, more serious toxicities appear. At drug levels above 2.5 mEq/L, death has resulted. Patients should be informed about early signs of toxicity and instructed to interrupt lithium if these appear. In compliant patients, the most common cause of lithium accumulation is sodium depletion.

TABLE 32–3 ■ Toxicities Associated with Excessive Plasma Level of Lithium

Plasma Lithium Level (mEq/L)	Signs of Toxicity
<1.5	Nausea, vomiting, diarrhea, thirst, polyuria, lethargy, slurred speech, muscle weakness, fine hand tremor
1.5–2.0	Persistent GI upset, coarse hand tremor, confusion, hyperirritability of muscles, EKG changes, sedation, incoordination
2.0–2.5	Ataxia, giddiness, high output of dilute urine, serious EKG changes, fasciculations, tinnitus, blurred vision, clonic movements, seizures, stupor, severe hypotension, coma, death (usually secondary to pulmonary complications)
>2.5	Symptoms may progress rapidly to generalized convulsions, oliguria, and death

EKG = electrocardiogram.

To keep lithium levels within the therapeutic range, plasma drug levels should be monitored routinely. Levels should be measured every 2 to 3 days at the beginning of treatment and every 1 to 3 months during maintenance therapy.

Treatment of acute overdose is primarily supportive; there is no specific antidote. The severely intoxicated patient should be hospitalized. Hemodialysis is an effective means of lithium removal and should be considered whenever drug levels exceed 2.5 mEq/L.

Adverse Effects That Occur at Therapeutic Levels of Lithium. Early Adverse Effects. Several responses occur early in treatment and then usually subside. *Gastrointestinal effects* (e.g., nausea, diarrhea, abdominal bloating, anorexia) are common but transient. About 30% of patients experience transient *fatigue, muscle weakness, headache, confusion, and memory impairment. Polyuria* and *thirst* occur in 30% to 50% of those treated and may persist.

Tremor. Patients may develop a fine hand tremor, especially in the fingers, that can interfere with writing and other motor skills. Lithium-induced tremor can be augmented by stress, fatigue, and certain drugs (antidepressants, antipsychotics, caffeine). Tremor can be reduced with a beta-adrenergic blocking agent (e.g., propranolol) and by measures that reduce peak levels of lithium (i.e., dosage reduction, use of divided doses, or use of a sustained-release formulation).

Polyuria. Polyuria occurs in 50% to 70% of patients taking lithium chronically. In some patients, daily urine output may exceed 3 L. Lithium promotes polyuria by antagonizing the effects of antidiuretic hormone. To maintain adequate hydration, patients should be instructed to drink 8 to 12 glasses of fluids daily. Polyuria, nocturia, and excessive thirst can discourage patients from complying with the prescribed regimen.

Lithium-induced polyuria can be reduced with *amiloride* [Midamor], a potassium-sparing diuretic. Amiloride appears to help by reducing the entry of lithium into epithelial cells of the renal tubule. Polyuria can also be reduced with a thiazide diuretic. However, because thiazides can lower levels of sodium (see Chapter 39), and would thereby increase lithium retention, amiloride is preferred.

Renal Toxicity. Chronic lithium use has been associated with degenerative changes in the kidney. The risk of renal injury can be reduced by keeping the dosage low and, when possible, avoiding long-term lithium therapy. Kidney function should be assessed prior to treatment and once a year thereafter.

Goiter and Hypothyroidism. Lithium can reduce incorporation of iodine into thyroid hormone, and can inhibit thyroid hormone secretion. With long-term use, the drug can cause *goiter* (enlargement of the thyroid gland). Although usually benign, lithium-induced goiter is sometimes associated with *hypothyroidism*. Treatment with thyroid hormone (levothyroxine) or withdrawal of lithium will reverse both goiter and hypothyroidism. Levels of thyroid hormones—triiodothyronine (T_3) and thyroxine (T_4)—and levels of thyroid-stimulating hormone (TSH) should be measured prior to giving lithium and annually thereafter.

Teratogenesis. Lithium may—or may not—be a teratogen. In older studies, lithium appeared to have significant teratogenic effects: use of the drug during the first trimester of pregnancy was associated with an 11% incidence of birth defects (usually malformations of the heart). However, in newer studies, lithium showed little or no teratogenic potential. Nonetheless, lithium is still classified in FDA Pregnancy Risk Category D. To minimize any potential fetal risk, *lithium should be avoided during the first trimester of pregnancy* and, unless the benefits of therapy clearly outweigh the risks, the drug should be avoided during the remainder of pregnancy as well. Women of child-bearing age should be counseled to avoid pregnancy while taking lithium. Also, pregnancy should be ruled out before initiating lithium therapy.

Use in Lactation. Lithium readily enters breast milk and can achieve concentrations that are potentially harmful to the nursing infant. Consequently, breast-feeding during lithium therapy should be discouraged.

Other Effects. Lithium can cause mild, reversible *leukocytosis* (10,000 to 18,000 white blood cells/mm³); complete blood counts with a differential should be obtained prior to treatment and annually thereafter. Possible *dermatologic reactions* include psoriasis, acne, folliculitis, and alopecia.

Drug Interactions

Diuretics. Diuretics promote sodium loss, and can thereby increase the risk of lithium toxicity. Toxicity can occur because, in the presence of low sodium, renal excretion of lithium is reduced, causing lithium levels to rise.

Nonsteroidal Anti-inflammatory Drugs (NSAIDs). NSAIDs can increase lithium levels by as much as 60%. How? By suppressing synthesis of prostaglandins in the kidney, NSAIDs disrupt (increase) renal reabsorption of lithium (and also sodium), thereby causing lithium levels to rise. NSAIDs known to increase lithium levels include ibuprofen [Motrin, others], naproxen [Naprosyn], piroxicam [Feldene], indomethacin [Indocin], and celecoxib [Celebrex]. Interestingly, aspirin (the prototype of the NSAIDs) and sulindac [Clinoril] do *not* increase lithium levels. Accordingly, if a mild analgesic is needed, aspirin or sulindac would be a good choice.

Anticholinergic Drugs. Anticholinergics can cause urinary hesitancy. Coupled with lithium-induced polyuria, this can result in considerable discomfort. Accordingly, patients should avoid drugs with prominent anticholinergic properties (e.g., antihistamines, phenothiazine antipsychotics, tricyclic antidepressants).

Preparations, Dosage, and Administration

Preparations and Administration. Lithium is available as two salts: *lithium carbonate* and *lithium citrate*. With either salt, administration is oral. Lithium carbonate is dispensed in capsules, standard tablets, and slow-release tablets. Lithium citrate is dispensed in a syrup. Lithium formulations and trade names are summarized in Table 32–4.

Lithium can cause gastric upset. This can be reduced by administering lithium with meals or milk.

Dosing. Lithium dosing is highly individualized. Dosage adjustments are based on plasma drug levels and clinical response.

Plasma levels should be kept within the therapeutic range. Levels between 0.8 and 1.4 mEq/L are generally appropriate for *acute therapy* of manic episodes. For *maintenance therapy*, lithium levels should range from 0.4 to 1.0 mEq/L. (Levels of 0.6 to 0.8 mEq/L are effective for most patients.) To avoid serious toxicity, *lithium levels should not exceed 1.5 mEq/L.*

Knowledge of plasma drug levels is not the only guide to lithium dosing; the clinical response is at least as important. Accordingly, when evaluating the appropriateness of a lithium dosage, we must not forget to look at the patient. Laboratory tests are all well and good, but they are not a substitute for clinical assessment. If, for example, blood levels of lithium appear proper but clinical evaluation indicates toxicity, there is no question as to what should be done: The

TABLE 32–4 ■ Lithium Preparations			
Lithium Salt	**Formulation**	**Lithium Content***	**Trade Name**
Lithium carbonate (Li_2CO_3)	Capsules	4.06 mEq lithium (150 mg Li_2CO_3) 8.12 mEq lithium (300 mg Li_2CO_3) 16.24 mEq lithium (600 mg Li_2CO_3)	Eskalith, Lithonate
	Tablets	8.12 mEq lithium (300 mg Li_2CO_3)	Eskalith, Lithotabs
	Tablets: slow-release	8.12 mEq lithium (300 mg Li_2CO_3)	Lithobid
	Tablets: controlled release	12.18 mEq lithium (300 mg Li_2CO_3)	Eskalith CR
Lithium citrate	Syrup	8 mEq lithium/5 ml (equivalent to 300 mg Li_2CO_3)	

*Lithium content is expressed in two ways: (1) milliequivalents (mEq) of lithium ion and (2) milligrams (mg) of the particular lithium salt of which the preparation is composed.

dosage should be reduced—despite the apparent acceptability of the dosage as reflected by plasma lithium levels.

Because of its short half-life and low therapeutic index, *lithium cannot be administered in a single daily dose;* with once-a-day dosing, peak drug levels would be excessive. Hence, a typical dosage is 300 mg (of lithium carbonate) taken 3 or 4 times a day. A dosage of 600 mg twice a day is acceptable, provided an extended-release formulation is employed. However, even these preparations cannot be given on a once-daily basis.

Mood-Stabilizing Anticonvulsants

Certain anticonvulsants (e.g., valproic acid, carbamazepine) can suppress mania and stabilize mood in patients with BPD. The efficacy of these drugs is firmly established. In fact, one agent—valproic acid—is so effective that it has replaced lithium as the drug of choice for many patients. The basic pharmacology of the anticonvulsants and their use in seizure disorders is discussed in Chapter 23. Discussion here focuses on their use in BPD.

Valproic Acid

Valproic acid* [Depakene, Depakote, Depacon] is the only antiseizure agent that has been approved by the FDA for BPD. The drug can control symptoms in acute manic episodes and can provide prophylaxis against recurrent episodes of mania and depression. Valproic acid is as effective as lithium. Moreover, it works faster, and has a higher therapeutic index and more desirable side effect profile. Because of these properties, valproic acid has become a first-line treatment for BPD—and is preferred to lithium for initial therapy of patients with dysphoric mania, mixed mania, mania with psychosis, and rapid-cycling BPD. The starting dosage for acute mania in adults is 250 mg 3 times a day. Typical maintenance dosages range from 1000 to 2500 mg/day. The target trough plasma level is 50 to 125 mg/ml.

Although valproic acid has a higher therapeutic index than lithium and is generally better tolerated, it can cause serious toxicity. Of greatest concern are rare cases of thrombocytopenia, pancreatitis, and liver failure—all of which require immediate discontinuation of treatment. In addition, valproic acid is a teratogen, and hence should not be used during pregnancy. Gastrointestinal disturbances (nausea, vomiting, diarrhea, dyspepsia, indigestion) are common. These can be minimized by using Depakote, an enteric-coated formulation of divalproex sodium (a form of valproic acid). Despite causing GI distress, valproic acid frequently causes weight gain, a serious and chronic complication of treatment.

Carbamazepine

Carbamazepine [Tegretol, Carbatrol, others] was the first drug to be widely studied as an alternative to lithium for patients with BPD. Like lithium, carbamazepine reduces symptoms during manic and depressive episodes. In addition, when taken for maintenance, it can protect against recurrence of mania and depression. Like valproic acid, carbamazepine is preferred to lithium for patients with mixed mania or rapid-cycling BPD. For treatment of acute manic episodes, the dosage should be low initially (100 or 200 mg twice daily) and then gradually increased. The maximum dosage is 1600 to 2200 mg/day. The target trough plasma level is 6 to 12 mg/ml. Neurologic side effects (visual disturbances, ataxia, vertigo, unsteadiness, headache) are common early in treatment, but generally resolve despite continued drug use. Hematologic effects (leukopenia, anemia, thrombocytopenia, aplastic anemia) are relatively uncommon, but can be severe. Accordingly, complete blood counts including platelets should be obtained at baseline and periodically thereafter. Carbamazepine induces cytochrome P450 enzymes, and can thereby accelerate its own metabolism and the metabolism of other drugs (e.g., oral contraceptives, warfarin, valproic acid, tricyclic antidepressants). To maintain efficacy, dosages of carbamazepine and these other drugs should be increased as needed.

Lamotrigine, Gabapentin, and Topiramate

Lamotrigine [Lamictal], gabapentin [Neurontin], and topiramate [Topamax] are newer anticonvulsants that show some efficacy in BPD. Because experience with these drugs is limited, they should be reserved for patients who are unresponsive to or intolerant of standard therapies. Side effects of lamotrigine include headache, dizziness, double vision, and, rarely, life-threatening rashes (Stevens-Johnson syndrome, toxic epidermal necrolysis). To minimize the risk of serious rash, dosage must be titrated slowly. In contrast to lamotrigine, gabapentin is devoid of serious side effects. Topiramate is unique among the drugs used for BPD in that it promotes weight loss, rather than weight gain. Dosages for BPD are as follows:

- *Lamotrigine*—starting, 12.5 to 37.5 mg/day; maximum, 425 mg/day
- *Gabapentin*—starting, 400 to 1000 mg/day; maximum, 4000 mg/day
- *Topiramate*—starting, 25 to 75 mg/day; maximum, 600 mg/day

---

◾ KEY POINTS

- Mood stabilizers are drugs that (1) relieve symptoms during manic and depressive episodes, (2) prevent recurrence of manic and depressive episodes, and (3) do not worsen symptoms of mania or depression, and do not accelerate the rate of cycling.
- Lithium and valproic acid are the preferred mood stabilizers for BPD.
- To minimize the risk of toxicity, lithium levels must be monitored. The trough level, measured 12 hours after the evening dose, must be kept below 1.5 mEq/L.
- Common side effects that occur at therapeutic levels of lithium include tremor, goiter, and polyuria.
- Lithium may be teratogenic, and hence should be avoided during the first trimester of pregnancy. Also, unless the benefits outweigh the risks, lithium should be avoided during the second and third trimesters as well.
- A reduction in sodium levels will reduce lithium excretion, causing lithium levels to rise—possibly to toxic concentrations. Patients must maintain normal sodium intake and levels.
- Lithium levels can be increased by diuretics (especially thiazides) and by several nonsteroidal anti-inflammatory drugs.

---

*As discussed in Chapter 23, valproic acid is available in three closely related chemical forms: (1) valproic acid itself [Depakene, Depacon]; (2) the sodium salt of valproic acid [Depakene]; and (3) divalproex sodium [Depakote], a mixture of valproic acid and its sodium salt. All three forms have identical actions. In this chapter, the term *valproic acid* refers to all three forms.

Summary of Major Nursing Implications*

LITHIUM

Preadministration Assessment

Therapeutic Goal

Control of acute manic episodes in patients with BPD, and prophylaxis against recurrent mania and depression in these patients.

Baseline Data

Make baseline determinations of cardiac status (electrocardiogram, blood pressure, pulse), hematologic status (complete blood counts with differential), serum electrolytes, renal function (serum creatinine, creatinine clearance, urinalysis), and thyroid function (T_3, T_4, and TSH).

Identifying High-Risk Patients

Lithium should be *avoided* during the first trimester of pregnancy, and used with *caution* during the remainder of pregnancy and in the presence of renal disease, cardiovascular disease, dehydration, sodium depletion, and concurrent therapy with diuretics.

Implementation: Administration

Route

Oral.

Administration

Advise the patient to administer lithium with meals or milk to decrease gastric upset. Instruct the patient to swallow slow-release and controlled-release tablets intact, without crushing or chewing.

Promoting Compliance

Rigid adherence to the prescribed regimen is important. Deviations in dosage size and timing can cause toxicity. Inadequate dosing may cause relapse.

To promote compliance, educate the patient and his or her family about the nature of BPD and the importance of taking lithium as prescribed. Encourage family members to oversee lithium use, and advise them to urge the patient to visit the physician or a psychiatric clinic if a pattern of noncompliance develops.

When medicating inpatients, make certain that each lithium dose is ingested.

Ongoing Evaluation and Interventions

Monitoring Summary

Lithium Levels. Monitor lithium levels to ensure that they remain within the therapeutic range (0.8 to 1.4 mEq/L for initial therapy and 0.4 to 1.0 mEq/L for maintenance). Levels should be measured every 2 to 3 days during initial therapy, and every 1 to 3 months during maintenance. Blood for lithium determination should be drawn in the morning, 12 hours after the evening dose.

Other Parameters to Monitor. Evaluate the patient at least once a year for hematologic status (complete blood count with differential), serum electrolytes, renal function (serum creatinine, creatinine clearance, urinalysis), and thyroid function (T_3, T_4, and TSH).

Evaluating Therapeutic Effects

Evaluate the patient for abatement of manic symptoms (e.g., flight of ideas, pressure of speech, hyperactivity) and for mood stabilization.

Minimizing Adverse Effects

Effects Caused by Excessive Drug Levels. Excessive lithium levels can result in serious adverse effects (see Table 32–3). Lithium levels must be monitored (see *Monitoring Summary* above) and the dosage adjusted accordingly.

Teach patients about signs of toxicity, and instruct them to withhold medication and notify the physician if these develop.

Renal impairment can cause lithium accumulation. Kidney function should be assessed prior to treatment and once yearly thereafter.

Sodium deficiency can cause lithium to accumulate. Instruct the patient to maintain normal sodium intake. Forewarn the patient that diarrhea can cause significant sodium loss. Diuretics promote sodium excretion and must be used with caution.

In the event of severe toxicity, hospitalization may be required. If lithium levels exceed 2.5 mEq/L, hemodialysis should be considered.

Tremor. Lithium can cause fine hand tremor that can interfere with motor skills. Tremor can be reduced with a beta blocker (e.g., propranolol) and by measures that reduce peak lithium levels (dosage reduction; use of divided doses or a sustained-release formulation).

Hypothyroidism and Goiter. Lithium can promote goiter (thyroid enlargement) and frank hypothyroidism. Plasma levels of T_3, T_4, and TSH should be measured prior to treatment and yearly thereafter. Treat hypothyroidism with levothyroxine.

Renal Toxicity. Lithium can cause renal damage. Kidney function should be assessed prior to treatment and once a year thereafter. If renal impairment develops, lithium dosage must be reduced.

Polyuria. Lithium increases urine output. Polyuria can be suppressed with amiloride (a potassium-sparing diuretic). Instruct the patient to drink 8 to 12 glasses of fluid daily to maintain hydration.

Use in Pregnancy and Lactation. Lithium may cause birth defects. The drug should be avoided during pregnancy, especially in the first trimester. Counsel women of childbearing age about the importance of avoiding pregnancy. Rule out pregnancy before initiating therapy.

Lithium enters breast milk. Advise patients to avoid breast-feeding.

*Patient education information is highlighted as blue text.

Summary of Major Nursing Implications*—cont'd

Minimizing Adverse Interactions

Diuretics. By promoting sodium loss, diuretics can reduce lithium excretion, thereby causing lithium levels to rise. Monitor closely for signs of toxicity.

Anticholinergic Drugs. By causing urinary hesitancy, drugs with anticholinergic properties (e.g., antihistamines, phenothiazine antipsychotics, tricyclic antidepressants) can intensify discomfort associated with lithium-induced diuresis.

Nonsteroidal Anti-inflammatory Drugs (NSAIDs). Several NSAIDs (e.g., ibuprofen, naproxen, celecoxib), but *not* aspirin or sulindac, can increase renal absorption of lithium, thereby causing lithium levels to rise. If a mild analgesic is needed, aspirin or sulindac would be a good choice.

*Patient education information is highlighted as blue text.

Sedative-Hypnotic Drugs

The sedative-hypnotics are drugs that depress central nervous system (CNS) function. With some of these drugs, CNS depression is more generalized than with others. The sedative-hypnotics are used primarily to treat anxiety and insomnia. Because both disorders are common, the sedative-hypnotics are widely used. Agents given to relieve anxiety are known as *antianxiety agents* or *anxiolytics;* an older term is *tranquilizers.* Agents given to promote sleep are known as *hypnotics.* The distinction between antianxiety effects and hypnotic effects is often a matter of dosage: typically, sedative-hypnotics relieve anxiety in low doses and induce sleep in higher doses. Hence, a single drug may be considered both an antianxiety agent and a hypnotic agent, depending upon the reason for its use and the dosage employed.

Before the benzodiazepines became available, anxiety and insomnia were treated with barbiturates and other *general CNS depressants*—drugs with multiple undesirable qualities: (1) These drugs are powerful respiratory depressants that can readily prove fatal in overdose. As a result, they are "drugs of

choice" for suicide. (2) Because they produce subjective effects that many individuals find desirable, most general CNS depressants have a high potential for abuse. (3) With prolonged use, most of these drugs produce significant tolerance and physical dependence. (4) Barbiturates and some other CNS depressants induce synthesis of hepatic drug-metabolizing enzymes, and can thereby decrease responses to other drugs. Since the benzodiazepines are just as effective as the general CNS depressants, but do not share their undesirable properties, the benzodiazepines have largely replaced general CNS depressants in the management of anxiety and insomnia.

We begin the chapter by discussing the basic pharmacology of the sedative-hypnotics, and end by discussing their use in insomnia. Use of these drugs for anxiety is discussed in Chapter 34.

BENZODIAZEPINES

Benzodiazepines are drugs of first choice for treating anxiety and insomnia. In addition, these agents are used to induce general anesthesia and to manage seizure disorders, muscle spasm, panic disorder, and withdrawal from alcohol.

Benzodiazepines were introduced in the early 1960s and are among the most widely prescribed drugs in the United States. Perhaps the most familiar member of the family is diazepam [Valium]. The most frequently prescribed members are lorazepam [Ativan] and alprazolam [Xanax].

The popularity of the benzodiazepines as sedatives and hypnotics stems from their clear superiority over the alternatives—barbiturates and other general CNS depressants. The benzodiazepines are safer than the general CNS depressants and have a lower potential for abuse. In addition, benzodiazepines produce less tolerance and physical dependence and are sub-

TABLE 33–1 ▪ Contrasts Between Benzodiazepines and Barbiturates		
Area of Comparison	Benzodiazepines	Barbiturates
Relative safety	High	Low
Maximal ability to depress CNS function	Low	High
Respiratory depressant ability	Low	High
Suicide potential	Low	High
Ability to cause physical dependence	Low*	High
Ability to cause tolerance	Low	High
Abuse potential	Low	High
Ability to induce hepatic drug metabolism	Low	High

*Although dependence is low in most patients, significant dependence *can* develop with long-term high-dose use.

ject to fewer drug interactions. Contrasts between the benzodiazepines and barbiturates are summarized in Table 33–1.

Since all of the benzodiazepines produce nearly identical effects, we will consider the family as a group, rather than selecting a representative member as a prototype.

Overview of Pharmacologic Effects

Practically all responses to benzodiazepines result from actions in the CNS. Benzodiazepines have few direct actions outside the CNS. All of the benzodiazepines produce a similar spectrum of responses. However, because of pharmacokinetic differences, individual benzodiazepines may differ in clinical applications.

Central Nervous System. All beneficial effects of benzodiazepines and most adverse effects result from depressant actions in the CNS. With increasing dosage, effects progress from sedation to hypnosis to stupor.

Benzodiazepines depress neuronal function at multiple sites in the CNS. These drugs *reduce anxiety* through effects on the limbic system, a neuronal network associated with emotionality. They *promote sleep* through effects on cortical areas and on the sleep-wakefulness clock. They *induce muscle relaxation* through effects on supraspinal motor areas, including the cerebellum. Two important side effects—*confusion* and *anterograde amnesia*—result from effects on the hippocampus and cerebral cortex.

Cardiovascular System. When taken *orally,* benzodiazepines have almost no effect on the heart and blood vessels. In contrast, when administered *intravenously*—even in therapeutic doses—benzodiazepines can produce profound hypotension and cardiac arrest.

Respiratory System. In contrast to the barbiturates, the benzodiazepines are weak respiratory depressants. When taken alone in therapeutic doses, benzodiazepines produce little or no depression of respiration; with toxic doses, respiratory depression is moderate at most. With oral therapy, clinically significant respiratory depression occurs only when benzodiazepines are combined with other CNS depressants (e.g., opioids, barbiturates, alcohol).

Although benzodiazepines generally have minimal effects on respiration, they can be a problem for patients with respiratory disorders. In patients with chronic obstructive pulmonary disease, benzodiazepines may worsen hypoventilation and hypoxemia. In patients with obstructive sleep apnea (OSA), benzodiazepines may exacerbate apneic episodes. In patients who snore, benzodiazepines may convert partial airway obstruction into OSA.

Molecular Mechanism of Action

Benzodiazepines *potentiate the actions of gamma-aminobutyric acid* (GABA), an inhibitory neurotransmitter found throughout the CNS. These drugs enhance the actions of GABA by binding to specific receptors in a supramolecular structure known as the GABA receptor–chloride channel complex (Fig. 33–1). Please note that benzodiazepines act only by intensifying the effects of GABA; they do not act as direct GABA agonists.

Because benzodiazepines act by amplifying the actions of endogenous GABA, rather than by directly mimicking GABA, there is a limit to how much CNS depression they can produce. This explains why benzodiazepines are so much safer than the barbiturates—drugs that can directly mimic

GABA. Since benzodiazepines simply potentiate the inhibitory effects of endogenous GABA, and since the amount of GABA in the CNS is finite, there is a built-in limit to the depth of CNS depression the benzodiazepines can produce. In contrast, since the barbiturates are direct-acting CNS depressants, maximal effects are limited only by the amount of barbiturate administered.

Pharmacokinetics

Absorption and Distribution. Most benzodiazepines are well absorbed following oral administration. Because of their high lipid solubility, benzodiazepines readily cross the blood-brain barrier to reach sites in the CNS.

Metabolism. Most benzodiazepines undergo extensive metabolic alterations. With few exceptions, the *metabolites are pharmacologically active.* As a result, responses produced by administering a particular benzodiazepine often persist long after the parent drug has disappeared. Hence, there may be a poor correlation between the plasma half-life of the parent drug and duration of pharmacologic effects. Flurazepam, for example, whose plasma half-life is only 2 to 3 hours, is converted into an active metabolite whose half-life is 50 hours. Hence, administration of flurazepam produces long-lasting effects, even though flurazepam itself is gone from the plasma in 8 to 12 hours.

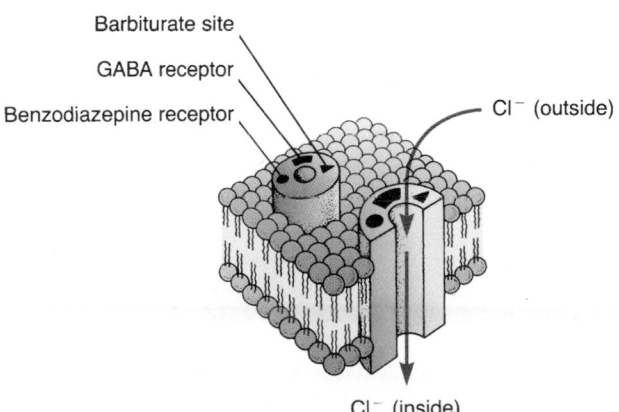

Figure 33–1 ■ **Schematic model of the GABA receptor–chloride channel complex showing binding sites for benzodiazepines and barbiturates.**
The GABA receptor–chloride channel complex, which spans the neuronal cell membrane, can exist in an open or closed configuration. Binding of GABA to its receptor causes the chloride channel to *open.* The resulting inward flow of chloride ions hyperpolarizes the neuron (makes the cell highly negative inside) and thereby decreases the cell's ability to fire. Hence GABA is an *inhibitory* neurotransmitter. Binding of a *benzodiazepine* to its receptor on the complex increases the frequency of channel opening, thereby increasing chloride influx. Hence, benzodiazepines enhance the inhibitory effects of GABA. In the absence of GABA, benzodiazepines have no effect on channel opening. Effects of *barbiturates* on the chloride channel are dose dependent: at low doses, barbiturates enhance the actions of GABA (by prolonging the duration of channel opening); at high doses, barbiturates directly mimic the actions of GABA.

In patients with liver disease, metabolism of benzodiazepines can decline, thereby prolonging and intensifying responses. Because certain benzodiazepines (oxazepam, temazepam, and lorazepam) undergo very little metabolic alteration, these agents may be preferred for patients with hepatic impairment.

Time Course of Action. Benzodiazepines differ significantly from one another with respect to time course. Specifically, they differ in onset and duration of action, and tendency to accumulate with repeated dosing.

Because all benzodiazepines have essentially equivalent pharmacologic actions, selection among them is based largely on differences in time course. For example, if a patient needs medication to accelerate falling asleep, a benzodiazepine with a rapid onset (e.g., triazolam) would be indicated. However, if medication is needed to prevent waking later in the night, a benzodiazepine with a slower onset (e.g., estazolam) would be preferred. For treatment of anxiety, a drug with an intermediate duration is desirable. For treatment of any benzodiazepine-responsive condition in the elderly, a drug such as lorazepam, which is not likely to accumulate with repeated dosing, is generally preferred.

Therapeutic Uses

The benzodiazepines have three principal indications: (1) anxiety, (2) insomnia, and (3) seizure disorders. In addition, they are employed as preoperative medication and to treat muscle spasm, panic disorder, and withdrawal from alcohol. Although all benzodiazepines share the same pharmacologic properties, and therefore might be equally effective for all applications, not every benzodiazepine is actually employed for all potential uses. The principal factors that determine the actual applications of a particular benzodiazepine are (1) the pharmacokinetic properties of the drug itself and (2) research and marketing decisions of pharmaceutical companies. Specific applications of individual benzodiazepines are summarized in Table 33–2.

Anxiety. Benzodiazepines are drugs of first choice for anxiety. Although all benzodiazepines have anxiolytic actions, only seven are marketed for this indication (see Table 33–2). Anxiolytic effects result from depressing neurotransmission in the limbic system and cortical areas. Use of benzodiazepines to treat anxiety is discussed in Chapter 34.

Insomnia. Benzodiazepines are drugs of first choice for insomnia. These drugs decrease latency time to falling asleep, reduce awakenings, and increase total sleeping time. The role of benzodiazepines in managing insomnia is discussed later.

Seizure Disorders. Four benzodiazepines—diazepam, clonazepam, lorazepam, and clorazepate—are employed for seizure disorders. Antiseizure applications are discussed in Chapter 23.

Muscle Spasm. One benzodiazepine—diazepam—is used to relieve muscle spasm and spasticity (see Chapter 24). Effects on muscle tone are secondary to actions in the CNS. Diazepam cannot relieve spasm without causing sedation.

Alcohol Withdrawal. Diazepam and other benzodiazepines may be administered to facilitate withdrawal from alcohol (see Chapter 37). These drugs are helpful because cross-dependence with alcohol enables them to suppress symptoms brought on by alcohol abstinence.

Panic Disorder. Alprazolam [Xanax], clonazepam [Klonopin], and lorazepam [Ativan] can provide effective treatment of panic disorder. These benzodiazepines and other drugs for panic disorder are discussed in Chapter 34.

Perioperative Applications. Three benzodiazepines—diazepam [Valium], lorazepam [Ativan], and midazolam [Versed]—are given IV for *induction of anesthesia*. In addition, midazolam (in combination with an opioid analgesic) can be used to produce *conscious sedation*—a semiconscious state suitable for endoscopic procedures and minor surgeries. Benzodiazepines are also used for *preoperative sedation*. All of these applications are discussed in Chapter 26.

TABLE 33–2 ■ Applications of the Benzodiazepines

Generic Name [Trade Name]	Approved Applications						
	Anxiety	Insomnia	Seizures	Muscle Spasm, Spasticity	Alcohol Withdrawal	Induction of Anesthesia	Panic Disorder
Alprazolam [Xanax]	✔						✔
Chlordiazepoxide [Librium, others]	✔				✔		
Clonazepam [Klonopin]			✔				
Clorazepate [Tranxene, Gen-Xene]	✔		✔		✔		
Diazepam [Valium, others]	✔		✔	✔	✔	✔	
Estazolam [ProSom]		✔					
Flurazepam [Dalmane]		✔					
Halazepam [Paxipam]	✔						
Lorazepam [Ativan]	✔		✔		✔	✔	
Midazolam [Versed]						✔*	
Oxazepam [Serax]	✔				✔		
Quazepam [Doral]		✔					
Temazepam [Restoril]		✔					
Triazolam [Halcion]		✔					

*Midazolam, in conjunction with an opioid analgesic, is also used to produce *conscious sedation,* a semiconscious state suitable for minor surgeries and endoscopic procedures.

Adverse Effects

Benzodiazepines are generally well tolerated, and serious adverse reactions are rare. In contrast to barbiturates and other general CNS depressants, benzodiazepines are remarkably safe.

CNS Depression. When taken in sleep-inducing doses, benzodiazepines cause drowsiness, lightheadedness, incoordination, and difficulty concentrating. When these effects occur at bedtime, they are generally inconsequential. However, if sedation and other manifestations of CNS depression persist beyond waking, interference with daytime activities can occur.

Anterograde Amnesia. Benzodiazepines can cause anterograde amnesia (impaired recall of events that take place after dosing). Anterograde amnesia has been especially troublesome with *triazolam* [Halcion]. If patients complain of forgetfulness, the possibility of drug-induced amnesia should be evaluated.

Paradoxical Effects. When employed to treat anxiety, benzodiazepines sometimes cause paradoxical responses, including insomnia, excitation, euphoria, heightened anxiety, and rage. If these occur, the benzodiazepine should be withdrawn.

Respiratory Depression. Benzodiazepines are weak respiratory depressants. Death from overdose with oral benzodiazepines alone has never been documented. Hence, in contrast to the barbiturates, benzodiazepines present little risk as vehicles for suicide. It must be emphasized, however, that although respiratory depression with *oral* therapy is rare, benzodiazepines can cause severe respiratory depression when administered *intravenously*. In addition, substantial respiratory depression can result from combining oral benzodiazepines with other CNS depressants (e.g., alcohol, barbiturates, opioids).

Abuse. Benzodiazepines have a lower abuse potential than barbiturates and most other general CNS depressants. The behavior pattern that constitutes "addiction" is uncommon among people who take benzodiazepines for therapeutic purposes. When asked about their drug use, individuals who regularly abuse drugs rarely express a preference for benzodiazepines over barbiturates. Because their potential for abuse is low, the benzodiazepines are classified under Schedule IV of the Controlled Substances Act. This contrasts with the barbiturates, most of which are classified under Schedule II or III.

Use in Pregnancy and Lactation. Benzodiazepines are highly lipid soluble and can readily cross the placental barrier. Use of benzodiazepines during the first trimester of pregnancy is associated with an increased risk of congenital malformations, such as cleft lip, inguinal hernia, and cardiac anomalies. Use near term can cause CNS depression in the neonate. Because they may represent a risk to the fetus, most benzodiazepines are classified in Food and Drug Administration (FDA) Pregnancy Risk Category D. Four of these drugs—estazolam, quazepam, temazepam, and triazolam—are classified in Category X. Women of child-bearing age should be warned about the potential for fetal harm and instructed to discontinue benzodiazepines if pregnancy occurs.

Benzodiazepines enter breast milk with ease and may accumulate to toxic levels in the breast-fed infant. Accordingly, these drugs should be avoided by nursing mothers.

Other Adverse Effects. Occasional reactions include weakness, headache, blurred vision, vertigo, nausea, vomiting, epigastric distress, and diarrhea. Neutropenia and jaundice occur rarely.

Drug Interactions

Benzodiazepines undergo very few important interactions with other drugs. Unlike barbiturates, benzodiazepines do not induce hepatic drug-metabolizing enzymes. Hence, benzodiazepines do not accelerate the metabolism of other drugs.

CNS Depressants. The CNS-depressant actions of benzodiazepines add with those of other CNS depressants (e.g., alcohol, barbiturates, opioids). Hence, although benzodiazepines are very safe when used alone, these drugs can be extremely hazardous in combination with other depressants. Combined overdose with a benzodiazepine plus another CNS depressant can cause profound respiratory depression, coma, and death. Patients should be warned against use of alcohol and all other CNS depressants.

Tolerance and Physical Dependence

Tolerance. With prolonged use of benzodiazepines, tolerance develops to some effects but not others. No tolerance develops to anxiolytic effects, and tolerance to hypnotic effects is generally low. In contrast, significant tolerance develops to antiseizure effects. Patients tolerant to barbiturates, alcohol, and other general CNS depressants show some cross-tolerance to benzodiazepines.

Physical Dependence. Benzodiazepines can cause physical dependence—but the incidence of *substantial* dependence is low. When benzodiazepines are discontinued following short-term use at therapeutic doses, the resulting withdrawal syndrome is generally mild and often goes unrecognized. Symptoms include anxiety, insomnia, sweating, tremors, and dizziness. Withdrawal from long-term, high-dose therapy can elicit more serious reactions, such as panic, paranoia, delirium, hypertension, muscle twitches, and outright convulsions. Symptoms of withdrawal are usually more intense with benzodiazepines that have a short duration of action. With one agent—*alprazolam* [Xanax]—dependence may be a greater problem than with other benzodiazepines. Because the benzodiazepine withdrawal syndrome can resemble an anxiety disorder, care must be taken to differentiate withdrawal symptoms from the return of original disease symptoms.

The intensity of withdrawal symptoms can be minimized by discontinuing treatment gradually. Doses should be slowly tapered over several weeks or months. Substituting a benzodiazepine with a long half-life for one with a short half-life is also helpful. Patients should be warned against abrupt cessation of treatment. Following discontinuation of treatment, patients should be monitored for 3 weeks for indications of withdrawal or recurrence of original symptoms.

Acute Toxicity

Oral Overdose. When administered in excessive dosage by mouth, benzodiazepines rarely cause serious toxicity. Symptoms include drowsiness, lethargy, and confusion. Significant cardiovascular and respiratory effects are uncommon. If an individual known to have taken an overdose of benzodiazepines does exhibit signs of serious toxicity, it is probable that another drug was taken too.

Intravenous Toxicity. When injected IV, even in therapeutic doses, benzodiazepines can cause severe adverse effects. Life-threatening reactions (e.g., profound hypotension, respiratory arrest, cardiac arrest) occur in about 2% of patients.

General Treatment Measures. Benzodiazepine-induced toxicity is managed the same as toxicity from barbiturates and other general CNS depressants. Oral benzodiazepines can be removed from the body with gastric lavage followed by ingestion of activated charcoal and a saline cathartic; dialysis may be helpful if symptoms are especially severe. Respiration should be monitored and the airway kept patent. Support of blood pressure with IV fluids and norepinephrine may be required.

Treatment with Flumazenil. Flumazenil [Romazicon] is a competitive benzodiazepine receptor antagonist. The drug can reverse the sedative effects of benzodiazepines but may not reverse respiratory depression. Flumazenil is approved for benzodiazepine overdose and for reversing the effects of benzodiazepines following general anesthesia. The principal adverse effect is precipitation of convulsions. This is most likely in patients taking benzodiazepines to treat epilepsy and in patients who are physically dependent on benzodiazepines. Flumazenil is administered IV. Doses are injected slowly (over 30 seconds) and may be repeated every minute as needed. The first dose is 0.2 mg, the second is 0.3 mg, and all subsequent doses are 0.5 mg. Effects of flumazenil fade in about 1 hour, hence additional dosing may be required.

Preparations, Dosage, and Administration

Preparations and Dosage. Preparations and dosages for *insomnia* are presented later in the chapter. Preparations and dosages of benzodiazepines used for other disorders are presented in Chapter 23 (Drugs for Epilepsy), Chapter 24 (Drugs for Muscle Spasm and Spasticity), Chapter 26 (General Anesthetics), and Chapter 34 (Management of Anxiety Disorders).

Routes. All benzodiazepines can be administered orally. In addition, three agents—diazepam, chlordiazepoxide, and lorazepam—may be administered parenterally (IM and IV). When used for sedation or induction of sleep, benzodiazepines are almost always administered by mouth. Parenteral administration is reserved for emergencies, including acute alcohol withdrawal, severe anxiety, and status epilepticus.

Oral. Patients should be advised to take oral benzodiazepines with food if gastric upset occurs. Also, they should be instructed to swallow sustained-release formulations intact, without crushing or chewing. Patients should be warned not to increase the dosage or discontinue therapy without consulting the physician.

For treatment of insomnia, benzodiazepines should be given on an intermittent schedule (e.g., 3 or 4 days a week) in the lowest effective dosage for the shortest duration required. This will minimize physical dependence and associated drug-dependency insomnia.

Intravenous. Intravenous administration is hazardous and must be performed with care. Life-threatening reactions (severe hypotension, respiratory arrest, cardiac arrest) have occurred. In addition, IV administration carries a risk of venous thrombosis, phlebitis, and vascular impairment.

To reduce complications, the following precautions should be taken: (1) inject the drug slowly; (2) take care to avoid intra-arterial injection and extravasation; (3) if direct venous injection is impossible, make the injection into infusion tubing as close to the vein as possible; (4) follow the manufacturer's instructions regarding suitable diluents for preparing solutions; and (5) have facilities for resuscitation available.

BENZODIAZEPINE-LIKE DRUGS

Zolpidem and zaleplon act much like the benzodiazepines—even though these drugs and benzodiazepines do not have similar structures. Like benzodiazepines, zolpidem and zaleplon produce their effects by acting as agonists at the benzo-

diazepine receptor site on the GABA receptor–chloride channel complex. Both agents, like the benzodiazepines, are drugs of first choice for short-term management of insomnia.

Zolpidem

Zolpidem [Ambien] is a sedative-hypnotic agent approved for short-term management of insomnia. Although structurally unrelated to the benzodiazepines, zolpidem binds to the benzodiazepine receptor site on the GABA receptor–chloride channel complex and shares some properties of the benzodiazepines. Like the benzodiazepines, zolpidem can reduce sleep latency and awakenings and can prolong sleep duration. The drug does not significantly reduce time in rapid-eye-movement (REM) sleep and causes little or no rebound insomnia when therapy is discontinued. In contrast to the benzodiazepines, zolpidem lacks anxiolytic, muscle relaxant, and anticonvulsant actions.

Zolpidem is rapidly absorbed following oral administration. Plasma levels peak in 2 hours. The drug is widely distributed, although levels in the brain remain low. Zolpidem is extensively metabolized to inactive compounds that are excreted in the bile, urine, and feces. The drug's half-life is 2.4 hours.

Zolpidem has a side effect profile like that of the benzodiazepines. *Daytime drowsiness* and *dizziness* are most common, and these occur in only 1% to 2% of patients. At therapeutic doses, zolpidem causes little or no respiratory depression. Safety in pregnancy has not been established.

Short-term treatment is not associated with significant tolerance or physical dependence. Withdrawal symptoms are minimal or absent. Similarly, the abuse liability of zolpidem is low. Accordingly, the drug is classified under Schedule IV of the Controlled Substances Act.

Like other sedative-hypnotics, zolpidem can intensify the effects of CNS depressants. Accordingly, patients should be warned against combining zolpidem with alcohol and all other drugs that depress CNS function.

Zolpidem [Ambien] is available in 5- and 10-mg tablets for oral use. The usual dosage is 10 mg. The initial dosage should be reduced to 5 mg for elderly and debilitated patients and for those with hepatic insufficiency. Zolpidem has a rapid onset, and hence should be taken just prior to bedtime. This timing will promote sleep while minimizing daytime sedation.

Zaleplon

Zaleplon [Sonata] is the first representative of a new class of hypnotics, the pyrazolopyrimidines. The drug has a very rapid onset and short duration of action. Although zaleplon is not chemically related to the benzodiazepines, these drugs share the same mechanism of action: they both bind to the benzodiazepine receptor site on the GABA receptor–chloride channel complex, and thereby enhance the depressant actions of endogenous GABA. Like the benzodiazepines, zaleplon has sedative, anxiolytic, muscle relaxant, and anticonvulsant effects.

Zaleplon is rapidly and completely absorbed from the GI tract. However, because of extensive first-pass metabolism, bioavailability is only 30%. A large or high-fat meal can delay absorption substantially. Plasma levels peak about 1 hour after administration and then rapidly decline, returning to baseline in 4 to 5 hours. Zaleplon is metabolized by hepatic aldehyde oxidase prior to excretion in the urine. Its half-life is only 1 hour.

Because of its kinetic profile, zaleplon is well suited for people who have trouble falling asleep, but not for people who can't maintain sleep. The drug can also help people who need a sedative in the middle of the night: because of its short duration, zaleplon can be taken at 3:00 AM without causing hangover when the alarm goes off at 7:00.

Zaleplon is well tolerated. The most common side effects are headache, nausea, drowsiness, dizziness, myalgia, and abdominal pain. Respiratory depression has not been observed. Physical dependence is minimal, the only sign being mild rebound insomnia the first night after drug withdrawal. Next-day sedation or hangover has not been reported. The abuse liability of zaleplon is like that of the benzodiazepines; hence, the drug is classified under Schedule IV of the Controlled Substances Act.

Cimetidine (a drug for peptic ulcer disease) inhibits hepatic aldehyde oxidase, and can thereby greatly increase levels of zaleplon. Accordingly, dosage of zaleplon must be reduced if these drugs are used concurrently.

Zaleplon is available in 5- and 10-mg capsules. The usual dose is 10 mg. The dose should be reduced to 5 mg for (1) the elderly, (2) small individuals, (3) patients with liver impairment, and (4) patients taking cimetidine. The maximum dose is 20 mg. Dosing is usually done just before retiring. However, dosing may also be done after going to bed on nights when sleep fails to come.

BARBITURATES

The barbiturates (pronounced bahr-bi-tewr′-ates or bahr-bitch′-oo-rates) have been available since the early 1900s. These drugs cause relatively nonselective depression of CNS function and are the prototypes of the general CNS depressants. Because they depress multiple aspects of CNS function, barbiturates can be used for daytime sedation, induction of sleep, suppression of seizures, and general anesthesia. Barbiturates cause tolerance and dependence, have a high abuse potential, and are subject to multiple drug interactions. Moreover, these drugs are powerful respiratory depressants that can readily prove fatal in overdose. Because of these undesirable properties, barbiturates are used much less than in the past, having been replaced by newer and safer drugs—primarily the benzodiazepines. However, although their use has declined greatly, barbiturates still have important applications in seizure control and anesthesia. Moreover, barbiturates are valuable from an instructional point of view: By understanding these prototypic agents, we gain an understanding of the general CNS depressants as a group, along with an appreciation of why these drugs are rarely used for anxiety and insomnia.

Classification

The barbiturates can be grouped into three classes based on duration of action: (1) ultrashort-acting agents, (2) short- to intermediate-acting agents, and (3) long-acting agents. As indicated in Table 33–3, the duration of action of these drugs is inversely related to their lipid solubility. Barbiturates with the highest lipid solubility have the shortest duration of action. Conversely, barbiturates with the lowest lipid solubility have the longest duration.

Duration of action influences the clinical applications of barbiturates. The ultrashort-acting agents (e.g., thiopental) are used for induction of anesthesia. The short- to intermediate-acting agents (e.g., secobarbital) are used as sedatives and hypnotics. The long-acting agents (e.g., phenobarbital) are used primarily as antiseizure drugs.

Mechanism of Action

Like benzodiazepines, barbiturates bind to the GABA receptor–chloride channel complex (see Fig. 33–1). By doing so, these drugs can (1) enhance the inhibitory actions of GABA and (2) directly mimic the actions of GABA.

Since barbiturates can directly mimic GABA, there is no ceiling to the degree of CNS depression they can produce. Hence, in contrast to the benzodiazepines, these drugs can readily cause death by overdose. Although barbiturates can cause general depression of the CNS, they show some selectivity for depressing the *reticular activating system* (RAS), a neuronal network that helps regulate the sleep-wakefulness cycle. By depressing the RAS, barbiturates produce sedation and sleep.

Pharmacologic Effects

CNS Depression. Most effects of barbiturates—both therapeutic and adverse—result from generalized depression of CNS function. With increasing dosage, responses progress from *sedation* to *sleep* to *general anesthesia*.

Most barbiturates can be considered *nonselective* CNS depressants. The main exception to this rule is phenobarbital, a drug used to control seizures. Seizure control is achieved at doses that have minimal effects on other aspects of CNS function.

Cardiovascular Effects. At hypnotic doses, barbiturates produce modest reductions in blood pressure and heart rate. In contrast, toxic doses can cause profound hypotension and shock. These reactions result from direct depressant effects on both the myocardium and vascular smooth muscle.

Induction of Hepatic Drug-Metabolizing Enzymes. Barbiturates stimulate synthesis of hepatic microsomal enzymes, the principal drug-metabolizing enzymes of the liver. As a result, barbiturates can accelerate their own metabolism as well as the metabolism of many other drugs.

Barbiturates stimulate drug metabolism by promoting the synthesis of porphyrin (Fig. 33–2). Porphyrin is then converted into heme, which in turn is converted into cytochrome P450, a key component of the hepatic drug-metabolizing enzyme system.

Tolerance and Physical Dependence

Tolerance. Tolerance is defined as reduced drug responsiveness that develops over the course of repeated drug use. When barbiturates are taken regularly, tolerance develops to many—but not all—of their CNS effects. Specifically, tolerance develops to sedative and hypnotic effects and to other effects that underlie barbiturate abuse. However, even with chronic use, *very little tolerance develops to toxic effects.*

In the tolerant user, doses must be increased to elicit the same intensity of response that could formerly be elicited with smaller doses. Hence, individuals who take barbiturates for prolonged periods—be it for therapy or abuse—require steadily increasing doses to achieve the effects they desire.

It is important to note that *very little tolerance develops to respiratory depression.* Because tolerance to respiratory depression is minimal, and because tolerance does develop to therapeutic effects, with continued treatment, the lethal (respiratory-depressant) dose remains relatively constant while the therapeutic dose climbs higher and higher (Fig. 33–3). As tolerance to therapeutic effects increases, the therapeutic dose grows steadily closer to the lethal dose—a situation that is clearly hazardous.

As a rule, tolerance to one general CNS depressant bestows tolerance to all other general CNS depressants. Hence, there is cross-tolerance among barbiturates, alcohol, benzodiazepines, general anesthetics, chloral hydrate, and a number of other agents. Tolerance to barbiturates and the other general CNS depressants does *not* produce significant cross-tolerance with opioids (e.g., morphine).

Physical Dependence. Prolonged administration of barbiturates results in physical dependence, a state in which continued drug use is required to avoid an abstinence syndrome. Physical dependence results from adaptive neurochemical changes that occur in response to chronic drug exposure.

Individuals who are physically dependent on barbiturates exhibit cross-dependence with other general CNS depressants. Because of cross-dependence,

			Time Course		
Barbiturate Subgroup	**Representative Drug**	**Lipid Solubility**	**Onset (min)**	**Duration (hr)**	**Applications**
Ultrashort-acting	Thiopental	High	0.5	0.2	Induction of anesthesia; treatment of seizures
Short- to intermediate-acting	Secobarbital	Moderate	10–15	3–4	Treatment of insomnia
Long-acting	Phenobarbital	Low	60 or less	10–12	Treatment of seizures

TABLE 33–3 ■ Characteristics of Barbiturate Subgroups

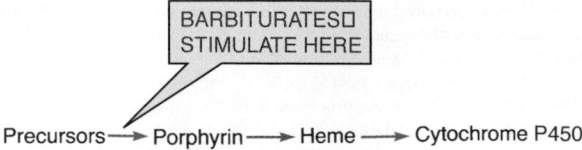

Figure 33–2 ■ **Induction of hepatic microsomal enzymes by barbiturates.**
By increasing synthesis of porphyrin, barbiturates increase production of cytochrome P450, a key component of the hepatic drug-metabolizing system.

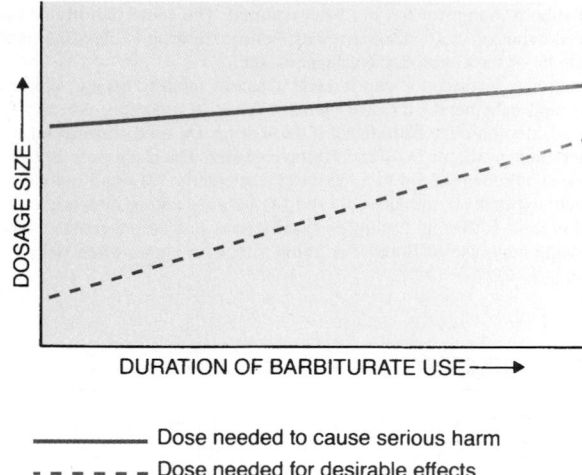

——— Dose needed to cause serious harm
- - - - - Dose needed for desirable effects

Figure 33–3 ■ **Development of tolerance to the toxic and subjective effects of barbiturates.**
With prolonged barbiturate use, tolerance develops. However, less tolerance develops to toxic effects than to desired effects. Consequently, as duration of use increases, the difference between the dose producing desirable effects and the dose producing toxicity becomes progressively smaller, thereby increasing the risk of serious harm.

a person physically dependent on barbiturates can prevent development of a withdrawal syndrome by taking any other general CNS depressant (e.g., alcohol, benzodiazepines). As a rule, cross-dependence exists among all of the general CNS depressants. However, there is no significant cross-dependence with opioids.

The general CNS depressant abstinence syndrome can be severe. Contrary to popular understanding, abrupt withdrawal from general CNS depressants is more dangerous than withdrawal from opioids. Although withdrawal from opioids is certainly unpleasant, the risk of serious injury is low. In contrast, the abstinence syndrome associated with general CNS depressants can be fatal.

The following description illustrates how dangerous withdrawal from general CNS depressants can be. Early reactions include weakness, restlessness, insomnia, hyperthermia, orthostatic hypotension, confusion, and disorientation. By the third day, major convulsive episodes may develop. Approximately 75% of patients experience psychotic delirium (a state similar to alcoholic delirium tremens). In extreme cases, these symptoms may be followed by exhaustion, cardiovascular collapse, and death. The entire abstinence syndrome evolves over approximately 8 days. The intensity of symptoms can be greatly reduced by withdrawing general CNS depressants slowly.

A long-acting barbiturate (e.g., phenobarbital) may be administered to facilitate the withdrawal process. Because of cross-dependence, phenobarbital can substitute for other CNS depressants, and can thereby suppress symptoms of withdrawal. Because of its long half-life, phenobarbital leaves the body slowly, thereby allowing a gradual transition from a drug-dependent state to a drug-free state. When phenobarbital is given to aid withdrawal, its dosage should be reduced gradually over 10 days to 3 weeks.

It is important to note that physical dependence should not be equated with addiction. Addiction is defined as a behavior pattern characterized by continued drug use despite physical, psychologic, or social harm. Although physical dependence can contribute to this behavior pattern, physical dependence, by itself, will neither cause nor sustain addictive behavior. The distinction between addiction and physical dependence is discussed further in Chapter 36 (Drug Abuse I: Basic Considerations).

Pharmacokinetics

Lipid solubility has a significant impact on the pharmacokinetic properties of individual barbiturates. As noted, barbiturates of high lipid solubility have a rapid onset and brief duration. Onset is rapid because lipid solubility allows these drugs to penetrate the blood-brain barrier with ease, thereby reaching sites of action quickly. As they undergo uptake by tissues other than the brain, levels in plasma fall, creating a concentration gradient favoring movement from the brain back into the blood. As a result, highly lipid-soluble barbiturates undergo rapid redistribution from the brain back into the blood and then into other tissues. This redistribution terminates CNS effects.

In comparison to the highly lipid-soluble agents, barbiturates of lower lipid solubility have effects of relatively slow onset but prolonged duration. Onset is delayed because low lipid solubility impedes passage across the blood-brain barrier. Effects are prolonged because termination is dependent on renal excretion and hepatic metabolism—processes that are slower than simple redistribution from the brain to other tissues.

With the exception of the highly lipid-soluble agents, all of the barbiturates have long plasma half-lives. These half-lives are so long, in fact, that significant amounts of barbiturate remain in plasma more than 24 hours after giving a single dose. This persistence has two clinical consequences: First, when barbiturates are taken at night to promote sleep, residual drug may cause sedation the following day. Second, since barbiturates are not eliminated entirely in 24 hours, daily administration causes

accumulation. As a result, the brain undergoes continuous exposure to progressively higher levels of drug—a phenomenon that promotes tolerance.

Therapeutic Uses

Insomnia. By depressing the CNS, barbiturates can promote sleep. However, because they can cause multiple undesired effects, barbiturates have long since been replaced by benzodiazepines as drugs of choice for insomnia.

Seizure Disorders. Two barbiturates—phenobarbital and mephobarbital—are employed to treat epilepsy and other seizure disorders (see Chapter 23). These anticonvulsant barbiturates suppress seizures at doses that are essentially nonsedative.

Induction of Anesthesia. Thiopental and other highly lipid-soluble barbiturates are given to induce general anesthesia (see Chapter 26). Unconsciousness develops within seconds of IV injection.

Other Uses. Barbiturates have been used to treat acute manic states and delirium. In children, they can decrease restlessness secondary to colic, pylorospasm, and whooping cough. In addition, they can help reduce anxiety in children prior to minor dental and medical procedures. Excessive excitation from overdose with CNS stimulants (e.g., amphetamine, theophylline, ephedrine) can be decreased with barbiturates. They can also be employed for emergency treatment of convulsions caused by tetanus, eclampsia, and epilepsy. When administered in anesthetic doses, barbiturates can help reduce mortality from head injury; deep anesthesia reduces the brain's requirements for oxygen and glucose and thereby helps preserve CNS function.

Adverse Effects

Respiratory Depression. Barbiturates reduce ventilation by two mechanisms: (1) depression of brainstem neurogenic respiratory drive and (2) depression of chemoreceptive mechanisms that control respiratory drive. Doses only 3 times greater than those needed to induce sleep can cause complete suppression of the neurogenic respiratory drive. With severe overdose, barbiturates can cause apnea and death.

For most patients, the degree of respiratory depression produced at therapeutic doses is not significant. However, in elderly patients and those with respiratory disease, therapeutic doses can compromise respiration substantially. Combining a barbiturate with another CNS depressant intensifies respiratory depression.

Suicide. Barbiturates have a low therapeutic index. Accordingly, overdose can readily cause death. Because of their toxicity, the barbiturates are frequently employed as vehicles for suicide. Accordingly, they should not be dispensed to patients with suicidal tendencies.

Abuse. Barbiturates produce subjective effects that many individuals find desirable. As a result, they are popular drugs of abuse. The barbiturates that are most prone to abuse are those in the short- to intermediate-acting group (e.g., secobarbital). Individual barbiturates within the group are classified under Schedule II or III of the Controlled Substances Act, reflecting their high potential for abuse. Although barbiturates are frequently abused in nonmedical settings, they are rarely abused during medical use.

Use in Pregnancy. Barbiturates readily cross the placenta and can injure the developing fetus. Women of child-bearing age should be informed about the potential for fetal harm and warned against becoming pregnant. Use of barbiturates during the third trimester may cause drug dependence in the infant.

Exacerbation of Intermittent Porphyria. Barbiturates can intensify attacks of acute intermittent porphyria, a condition brought on by excessive synthesis of porphyrin. Symptoms include nausea, vomiting, abdominal colic, neuromuscular disturbances, and disturbed behavior. Barbiturates exacerbate porphyria by stimulating porphyrin synthesis (see Fig. 33–2). Because of their ability to intensify porphyria, barbiturates are absolutely contraindicated for individuals with a history of the disorder.

Hangover. Barbiturates have long half-lives, and therefore can produce residual effects (hangover) when taken for insomnia. Hangover can manifest as sedation, impaired judgment, and reduced motor skills. Patients should be forewarned that their ability to perform complex tasks, both manual and intellectual, may be significantly decreased the day after taking a barbiturate to induce sleep.

Paradoxical Excitement. In some patients, especially the elderly and debilitated, barbiturates may cause excitation. The mechanism of this paradoxical response is unknown.

Hyperalgesia. Barbiturates can intensify sensitivity to pain. In addition, they may cause pain directly. These drugs have caused muscle pain, joint pain, and pain along nerves.

Drug Interactions

CNS Depressants. Drugs with CNS-depressant properties (e.g., barbiturates, benzodiazepines, alcohol, opioids, antihistamines) intensify each other's effects. If these agents are combined, the degree of CNS depression can be hazardous—perhaps even fatal. Accordingly, patients should be warned emphatically against combining barbiturates with alcohol and other drugs that can depress CNS function.

Interactions Resulting from Induction of Drug-Metabolizing Enzymes. As discussed above, barbiturates stimulate synthesis of hepatic drug-metabolizing enzymes, thereby accelerating metabolism of other drugs. Increased metabolism is of particular concern with *warfarin* (an anticoagulant), *oral contraceptives,* and *phenytoin* (an antiseizure agent). When these drugs are taken concurrently with a barbiturate, their dosages should be increased to account for accelerated degradation.

Following barbiturate withdrawal, rates of drug metabolism gradually decline to baseline values. Several weeks are required for this to occur. Drug dosages that had been increased to account for augmented metabolism must now be reduced to their prebarbiturate amount.

Acute Toxicity

Acute intoxication with barbiturates is a medical emergency; left untreated, overdose can be fatal. Poisoning is often the result of attempted suicide, although it can also occur by accident (usually in children and drug abusers). Since acute toxicity from barbiturates and other general CNS depressants is very similar, the discussion below applies to all of these drugs.

Symptoms. Acute overdose produces a classic triad of symptoms: *respiratory depression, coma,* and *pinpoint pupils.* (Pupils may later dilate as hypoxia caused by respiratory depression sets in.) The three classic symptoms are frequently accompanied by *hypotension* and *hypothermia.* Death is likely to be the result of pulmonary complications and renal failure.

Treatment. Proper management requires an intensive care unit. With vigorous treatment, most patients recover fully.

Treatment has two main objectives: (1) removal of barbiturate from the body and (2) maintenance of an adequate oxygen supply to the brain. Oxygenation can be maintained by keeping the airway patent and by administering oxygen.

Several measures can promote barbiturate removal. Unabsorbed drug can be removed from the stomach by gastric lavage and by induction of emesis (e.g., with apomorphine). A saline cathartic can reduce absorption by accelerating drug transit through the intestine. Drug that has already been absorbed can be removed rapidly with hemodialysis. (Peritoneal dialysis is significantly slower.) Forced diuresis and alkalinization of urine may facilitate drug removal via the kidneys.

Steps should be taken to prevent hypotension and loss of body heat. Blood pressure can be supported with fluid replacement and dopamine. Body heat can be maintained with blankets and warming devices.

Barbiturate poisoning has no specific antidote. CNS stimulants should definitely *not* be employed. Not only are stimulants ineffective, they are dangerous: Use of these drugs to treat barbiturate poisoning has been associated with a significant increase in mortality. Naloxone, a drug that can reverse poisoning by opioids, is not effective against poisoning by barbiturates.

Administration

Oral. Oral administration is employed for daytime sedation and to treat insomnia. Patients should be warned not to increase their dosage or discontinue treatment without consulting the physician. Dosages should be reduced for elderly patients. When terminating therapy, the dosage should be gradually tapered.

Intravenous. Intravenous administration is reserved for general anesthesia and emergency treatment of convulsions. Injections should be made slowly to minimize respiratory depression and hypotension. Blood pressure, pulses, and respiration should be monitored, and facilities for resuscitation should be available. The patient should be under continuous observation. Extravasation may result in local necrosis, hence care must be taken to ensure that extravasation does not occur. Solutions that are cloudy or contain a precipitate should not be used. Intra-arterial injection should be avoided, since using this route may cause arteriospasm of sufficient duration to cause gangrene.

Intramuscular. Barbiturate solutions are highly alkaline and can cause pain and necrosis when injected IM. Consequently, IM injection is generally avoided. Injection in the vicinity of peripheral nerves can cause irreversible neurologic injury.

MISCELLANEOUS SEDATIVE-HYPNOTICS

Basic Pharmacologic Profile

The drugs discussed in this section are nonselective CNS depressants, with actions much like those of the barbiturates. Their principal use is short-term management of insomnia.

At therapeutic doses, the nonselective CNS depressants can cause substantial drowsiness. Patients should be warned to avoid driving and other hazardous activities.

Taking these drugs with other CNS depressants (e.g., alcohol, barbiturates, benzodiazepines, opioids, antihistamines) can produce profound depression of CNS function. Accordingly, combined use with CNS depressants should be avoided.

Prolonged use can produce tolerance and physical dependence. Consequently, these agents should be reserved for short-term therapy. In patients who have been treated long term, termination should be done gradually to minimize the withdrawal reaction.

The nonselective CNS depressants can produce subjective effects that individuals prone to drug abuse consider desirable. Because of this abuse potential, agents in this group are classified under Schedule III or IV of the Controlled Substances Act.

In general, acute overdose resembles poisoning with barbiturates. Characteristic signs are respiratory depression, coma, miosis, and hypotension. Management is the same as with barbiturate poisoning. Because overdose can cause potentially fatal respiratory depression, these drugs should not be given to patients suspected of suicidal tendencies.

Nonselective CNS depressants should be avoided during pregnancy and lactation. Some of these agents may cause birth defects, especially if taken during the first trimester. In addition, if these drugs are taken late in pregnancy, the infant may be born drug dependent. These drugs can achieve concentrations in breast milk that are sufficient to cause lethargy in the infant. Accordingly, nursing mothers should not use them.

Chloral Hydrate

Chloral hydrate [Aquachloral Supprettes, generic] is a general CNS depressant with properties similar to those of the barbiturates. Chloral is a prodrug that undergoes rapid conversion to its active form in the liver. The drug's principal application is induction of sleep. However, tolerance to hypnotic effects develops quickly, and withdrawal is associated with sleep disruption and nightmares.

Chloral hydrate is dispensed in capsules (500 mg), a syrup (50 and 100 mg/ml), and suppositories (324, 500, and 648 mg). Patients should be instructed to swallow the capsules intact, without crushing or chewing. The syrup should be diluted with water, fruit juice, or ginger ale. With oral administration, epigastric distress, nausea, and flatulence are common.

The recommended dosage is 0.5 to 1 gm 30 minutes before bedtime. However, doses in this range are frequently too low to induce sleep. To elicit an adequate response, as much as 2 gm may be needed.

Chloral hydrate is subject to abuse and is classified as a Schedule IV drug. Abuse is similar to that seen in alcoholism. Prolonged consumption of chloral hydrate results in substantial tolerance and physical dependence. As a result, chloral hydrate addicts may ingest extremely large amounts of the drug. Abrupt withdrawal can cause delirium and seizures. Left untreated, the abstinence syndrome can be fatal.

Glutethimide

Glutethimide is a general CNS depressant similar to the barbiturates. In addition, the drug has prominent anticholinergic actions. Like the barbiturates, glutethimide can intensify episodes of intermittent porphyria and is contraindicated for patients with this disorder. Acute poisoning produces CNS depression together with anticholinergic responses (e.g., dry mouth, visual disturbance, decreased intestinal motility, atony of the urinary bladder, hyperpyrexia). Glutethimide has an abuse liability like that of the barbiturates, and hence is classified as a Schedule II substance.

Glutethimide is indicated only for short-term (3 to 7 days) management of insomnia. However, because superior agents are available, and because toxicity can be difficult to manage, the drug has little to recommend its use. Glutethimide is dispensed in 250-mg tablets. The usual adult dosage is 250 to 500 mg at bedtime.

Meprobamate

Meprobamate [Miltown, Equanil] has pharmacologic properties that lie midway between those of the barbiturates and the benzodiazepines. As a CNS depressant, meprobamate is more selective than barbiturates but less selective than benzodiazepines. Meprobamate induces hepatic drug-metabolizing enzymes and can exacerbate intermittent porphyria. The drug's only indication is short-term management of anxiety. However, it is rarely used today. Meprobamate is available in 200- and 400-mg tablets. The usual adult dosage is 1.2 to 1.6 gm/day in three or four divided doses. Meprobamate is classified as a Schedule IV drug.

Paraldehyde

Paraldehyde [Paral] is a general CNS depressant indicated for insomnia and management of alcoholic delirium tremens. The drug is employed almost exclusively in hospitals and institutions. Use by outpatients is rare.

Poisoning with paraldehyde is different from poisoning with other CNS depressants. In addition to causing respiratory depression and hypotension, paraldehyde causes prominent metabolic acidosis. Symptoms of toxicity include rapid, labored breathing; bleeding gastritis; toxic hepatitis; nephrosis; pulmonary hemorrhage; and edema. An oral dose of 25 ml can be fatal.

Solutions of paraldehyde decompose rapidly to acetic acid. Preparations that smell strongly of acetic acid (i.e., that smell like vinegar) should be discarded. Since decomposition occurs rapidly, containers that have been open for more than 24 hours should not be used.

Administration may be oral or rectal (as a retention enema). Oral paraldehyde has an unpleasant taste and irritates the throat and stomach. The usual oral dose for adults is 4 to 8 ml diluted in milk or iced fruit juice to improve palatability. Paraldehyde is a Schedule IV drug and must be dispensed accordingly.

Ethchlorvynol

Ethchlorvynol [Placidyl] is a CNS depressant with a rapid onset and short duration. Side effects include dizziness, hypotension, facial numbness, and a mint-like aftertaste. Like the barbiturates, ethchlorvynol can exacerbate acute intermittent porphyria. Ethchlorvynol is a Schedule IV drug approved only for short-term management of insomnia. The usual adult dosage is 500 to 1000 mg at bedtime.

MANAGEMENT OF TRANSIENT INSOMNIA

Insomnia can be defined as an inability to sleep well. Some people have difficulty falling asleep; some have difficulty maintaining sleep; and some are troubled by early morning awakening. For some insomnia is transient, and for others insomnia is chronic. As a result of sleep loss, insomniacs experience daytime drowsiness along with reductions in mood, memory, coordination, and the ability to concentrate and make decisions. Practically everyone has insomnia at some time in his or her life. In any given year, about 30% of Americans experience short-term insomnia, and about 10% experience chronic insomnia. In the United States, the direct costs of insomnia total $13.9 billion—a figure that includes the costs of testing, physician visits, and hypnotic drugs.

Loss of sleep is often the result of a medical disorder. Psychiatric disorders often disturb sleep, and pain can keep anyone awake. Sleep is frequently lost owing to concern regarding impending surgery and other procedures.

At one time or another, nearly everyone suffers from situational insomnia. Worry about exams may keep students awake. Job-related pressures may deprive workers of sleep. Unfamiliar surroundings may render sleeping difficult for travelers. Major life stressors (bereavement, divorce, loss of job) frequently disrupt sleep. Other factors, such as uncomfortable bedding, excessive noise, and bright light, can deprive us of sound sleep.

Sleep Physiology

Sleep is a complex state characterized by a reduced level of consciousness and minimal physical activity. The sleeping state has two primary divisions: *rapid-eye-movement* (REM) sleep and *non–rapid-eye-movement* (NREM) sleep. Sleeping begins with a period of NREM sleep, after which periods of REM sleep and NREM sleep alternate until waking takes place.

REM sleep is the phase during which most recallable dreams occur. A typical night's sleep has four to six REM periods, accounting for approximately 30% of total sleeping time. In males, penile erection is common during REM sleep. This curious phenomenon is independent of dream content. Except for the benzodiazepines, most of the drugs used to promote sleep cause significant reductions in total REM sleep time.

The precise physiologic benefits of sleep have not been established. Some studies suggest that deprivation of REM sleep can produce adverse psychologic reactions; other studies do not support this conclusion. One study indicated that REM sleep is important for consolidating perceptual learning. Regardless of the value that specific stages of sleep may or may not have, one thing is clear: When we don't get enough sleep, we tend to be drowsy the next day and hence less able to function. If fatigue or reduced alertness compromises daytime performance, some form of intervention may be needed.

Basic Management Principles
Cause-Specific Therapy

Treatment is highly dependent on the cause of insomnia. Accordingly, if therapy is to succeed, the underlying reason for sleep loss must be determined. To make this assessment, a thorough history is required.

When the cause of insomnia is a known medical disorder, primary therapy should be directed at the underlying illness; hypnotics should be employed only as adjuncts. For example, if pain is the reason for lack of sleep, analgesics should be prescribed. If insomnia is secondary to major depression, antidepressants are the appropriate treatment. If anxiety is the cause of insomnia, the patient should be given an anxiolytic.

Nondrug Therapy

Not everyone with insomnia should be treated with drugs. For some individuals, avoidance of naps and adherence to a regular sleep schedule is sufficient. For others, decreased consumption of caffeine-containing beverages (e.g., coffee, tea, cola drinks) may be all that is needed. Still others may benefit from restful activity as bedtime nears. If environmental factors are responsible for lack of sleep, the patient should be taught how to correct them or compensate for them. All patients should be counseled about sleep fitness (also known as sleep hygiene). Rules for sleep fitness are summarized in Table 33–4.

Therapy with Hypnotic Drugs

Hypnotics should be reserved for patients whose insomnia cannot be managed by other means. If nondrug measures can relieve insomnia, hypnotics should be avoided. Likewise, if insomnia is secondary to an identified and treatable pathology, specific therapies directed at that pathology are clearly preferred.

Drug therapy of transient insomnia should be short term (just 2 to 3 weeks). The patient should be reassessed on a regular basis to determine if drug therapy is still needed. If insomnia persists, an underlying pathology may well be the cause. Every effort should be made to diagnose this pathology rather than cover it up with continued use of drugs.

Escalation of dosage should be avoided. A need for increased dosage suggests development of tolerance. If hypnotic effects are lost in the course of treatment, it is preferable to interrupt therapy rather than elevate dosage. Interruption will allow tolerance to decline, thereby restoring responsiveness to treatment.

In certain patients, hypnotics must be employed with special caution. Patients who snore heavily and patients with respiratory disorders have reduced respiratory reserve, which can be further compromised by the respiratory-depressant actions of hypnotics. Hypnotic agents are generally contraindicated for use during pregnancy; these drugs have the potential to cause fetal harm, and their use is never an absolute necessity. Except for the benzodiazepines, most hypnotics can be lethal if taken in overdose. Accordingly, these drugs should not be given to individuals with suicidal tendencies.

Patients taking hypnotics should be forewarned that residual CNS depression may be present the next day. Although CNS depression may not be pronounced, it may still be sufficient to compromise intellectual or physical performance.

When hypnotics are employed, care must be taken to prevent *drug-dependency insomnia*, a condition that can lead to inappropriate prolongation of therapy. Drug-dependency insomnia is a particular problem with older hypnotics (e.g., barbiturates), and develops as follows: (1) Insomnia motivates treatment with hypnotics. (2) With continuous drug use, low-level physical dependence develops. (3) Upon cessation of treatment, a mild withdrawal syndrome occurs and disrupts sleep. (4) Failing to recognize that the inability to sleep is a manifestation of drug withdrawal, the patient becomes convinced that insomnia has

returned and resumes drug use. (5) Continued drug use leads to heightened physical dependence, making it even more difficult to withdraw medication without producing another episode of drug-dependency insomnia. To minimize drug-dependency insomnia, hypnotics should be employed judiciously. That is, they should be used in the lowest effective dosage for the shortest time required.

Drugs Used for Treatment

Transient insomnia can be treated with prescription drugs, nonprescription drugs, and alternative medicines. Among the prescription drugs, benzodiazepines and two benzodiazepine-like drugs—zolpidem and zaleplon—are agents of first choice. Older sedative-hypnotics, such as barbiturates and chloral hydrate, are rarely used today. Nonprescription drugs and alternative medicines are much less effective than the benzodiazepines, and hence should be reserved for people whose insomnia is mild.

As shown in Table 33–5, hypnotic drugs differ with respect to onset and duration of action, and, as a result, differ in their applications. Drugs with a rapid onset (e.g., zolpidem) are good for patients who have difficulty falling asleep, whereas drugs with a long duration (e.g., estazolam) are good for patients who have difficulty maintaining sleep. Drugs like flurazepam, which have both a rapid onset and long duration, are good for patients with both types of difficulties.

TABLE 33–4 ■ Rules for Sleep Fitness

- Establish a regular time to go to bed and a regular time to rise. This will help reset your biologic clock.
- Sleep only as long as needed to feel refreshed. Too much time in bed causes fragmented and shallow sleep. In contrast, restricting time in bed helps consolidate and deepen sleep.
- Insulate your bedroom against light and sounds that disturb your sleep (e.g., install carpeting and insulated curtains).
- Keep your bedroom temperature moderate. High temperature may disturb sleep.
- Exercise daily, but not later than 7:00 PM. Regular exercise helps deepen sleep.
- Avoid daytime naps. Staying awake during the day helps you sleep at night.
- Avoid caffeine, especially in the evening.
- Avoid consuming too much fluid in the evening so as to minimize nighttime trips to the bathroom.
- Avoid alcohol in the evening. Although alcohol can help you fall asleep, it causes sleep to be fragmented.
- Avoid tobacco; it disturbs sleep (and shortens your life, too).
- Try having a light snack near bedtime, since hunger can disturb sleep—but don't eat heavily.
- Relax before bedtime with soft music, mild stretching, yoga, or pleasurable reading.
- Leave your problems outside the bedroom. Reserve time earlier in the evening to work on problems and to plan tomorrow's activities.
- Reserve your bedroom for sleeping (and sex). This will help condition your brain to see the bedroom as a place where sleep happens. Don't eat, read, or watch TV in bed.
- If you don't fall asleep within 20 minutes or so, get up and do something relaxing (e.g., read, listen to music, watch TV), and then return to bed when you feel drowsy. Repeat as often as required.
- Don't look at the clock if you wake up during the night. If necessary, turn its face away from the bed.

Benzodiazepines

Benzodiazepines are drugs of first choice for short-term treatment of insomnia. These agents are safe and effective and lack the undesirable properties that typify barbiturates and other older hypnotics. Benzodiazepines have a low abuse potential, cause minimal tolerance and physical dependence, present a minimal risk of suicide, and undergo few interactions with other drugs. Only five benzodiazepines are marketed specifically for use as hypnotics (see Table 33–5). However, any benzodiazepine with a short to intermediate onset could be employed.

Benzodiazepines have multiple desirable effects on sleep: they decrease the latency to sleep onset, decrease the number of awakenings, and increase total sleeping time. In addition, they impart a sense of deep and refreshing sleep. With most benzodiazepines, tolerance to hypnotic actions develops slowly, allowing them to be used nightly for several weeks without a noticeable loss in hypnotic effects. Furthermore, with most benzodiazepines, treatment does not significantly reduce the amount of time spent in REM sleep, and withdrawal is not associated with significant rebound insomnia.

Two agents—*triazolam* [Halcion] and *flurazepam* [Dalmane]—can be considered prototypes of the benzodiazepines used to promote sleep. Triazolam has a rapid onset and short duration, making it a good choice for patients who have difficulty falling asleep (as compared with difficulty maintaining sleep). Flurazepam has a delayed onset and more prolonged duration, making it a good choice for patients who have difficulty maintaining sleep. However, because flurazepam has a relatively long half-life, the drug is likely to cause daytime drowsiness. Triazolam has a much shorter half-life than flurazepam, which is both good news and bad news. The good news is that, because it leaves the body rapidly, triazolam does not cause daytime sedation. The bad news is that, because triazolam is rapidly cleared, treatment is associated with two problems: (1) tolerance to hypnotic effects can develop quickly (in 11 to 18 days), which is much faster than with other benzodiazepines; and (2) triazolam causes more rebound insomnia than other benzodiazepines.

Benzodiazepine-like Drugs: Zolpidem and Zaleplon

Like the benzodiazepines, zolpidem [Ambien] and zaleplon [Sonata] are first-choice drugs for short-term therapy of insomnia. These drugs have the same mechanism of action as the benzodiazepines, and are just as safe and effective for insomnia. Both drugs have a rapid onset and short duration of action. As a result, both can help people with difficulty falling asleep (but not difficulty maintaining sleep), and neither causes daytime sedation. Despite their rapid clearance, they are not associated with rebound insomnia or tolerance to hypnotic effects. Because zaleplon has an ultrashort duration of action, it can be taken in the middle of the night and still not cause drowsiness the next day.

Trazodone

Trazodone [Desyrel] is an atypical antidepressant with strong sedative actions. The drug can decrease sleep latency and prolong sleep duration, and does not cause tolerance or physical dependence. Trazodone is especially useful for treating insomnia resulting from use of antidepressants that cause significant CNS stimulation (e.g., fluoxetine [Prozac], bupropion [Wellbutrin]). Principal adverse effects are daytime grogginess and postural hypotension. (Hypotension results from alpha-adrenergic blockade.) The basic pharmacology of trazodone is presented in Chapter 31.

TABLE 33–5 ■ Some Drugs Used for Insomnia

| Drug | Time course | | Use in Insomnia* | | Bedtime Dosage (mg) | |
	Onset (min)	Duration	DFA	DMS	Nonelderly	Elderly
Benzodiazepines						
Triazolam [Halcion]	15–30	Short	✔		0.125–0.25	0.13
Flurazepam [Dalmane]	30–60	Long	✔	✔	30	7.5
Quazepam [Doral]	20–45	Long	✔	✔	15	7.5
Estazolam [ProSom]	15–60	Long		✔	1–2	0.5–1
Temazepam [Restoril]	45–60	Intermediate		✔	15–30	7.5–15
Benzodiazepine-like Drugs						
Zolpidem [Sonata]	30	Short	✔		10	5
Zaleplon [Ambien]	15–30	Ultrashort	✔		10–20	5
Antidepressant						
Trazodone [Desyrel]	60–120	Long		✔	25–75	
Antihistamines						
Doxylamine [Unisom]	60–120	Long		✔	25	
Diphenhydramine [Nytol, Sominex, Sleep-Eze]	60–180	Long		✔	25–50	

*DFA = difficulty falling asleep, DMS = difficulty maintaining sleep.

Antihistamines

Two antihistamines—diphenhydramine [Nytol, Sominex, others] and doxylamine [Unisom]—are FDA-approved for use as "sleep aids," and can be purchased without a prescription. These drugs are less effective than benzodiazepines, and tolerance to hypnotic effects develops quickly (in 1 to 2 weeks). Daytime drowsiness and anticholinergic effects (e.g., dry mouth, blurred vision, urinary hesitancy, constipation) are common.

Older CNS Depressants

Barbiturates. The barbiturates are a distant second choice to the benzodiazepines, zolpidem, and zaleplon for short-term therapy of insomnia. Barbiturates are hazardous and have a high potential for abuse. Tolerance, dependence, and a host of drug interactions further decrease their desirability. Although several barbiturates are approved for insomnia, these agents have been largely abandoned in favor of benzodiazepines.

Several sleep-related effects of the barbiturates differ from those of the benzodiazepines. At the beginning of therapy, barbiturates tend to suppress REM sleep. However, with continued treatment, time spent in REM sleep returns to normal. "Hangover" and residual daytime sedation are relatively common. Tolerance develops rapidly to hypnotic effects, and withdrawal is associated with rebound insomnia and increased REM sleep.

Chloral Hydrate. Chloral hydrate is an effective hypnotic, but tolerance develops quickly (in 1 to 2 weeks). Prolonged use can cause physical dependence, resulting in disturbed sleep with intense nightmares when treatment stops.

Alternative Medicines

Of the alternative medicines employed to promote sleep, only two—valerian root (*Valeriana officinalis*) and melatonin—appear moderately effective. Several others—chamomile, passionflower, lemon balm, and lavender—have very mild sedative effects, and proof of benefits in insomnia is lacking. Valerian can help people fall asleep, but does not help them maintain sleep. Furthermore, hypnotic effects take a week or more to develop, and hence valerian is no good for acute therapy. Valerian root is discussed further in Chapter 104 (Herbal Supplements). Melatonin is discussed in Box 33–1.

Special Interest Topic

BOX 33–1 ■ MELATONIN: HYPNOTIC OR HYPE?

Melatonin has been the subject of at least four popular books and has received prominent coverage in the media. Proponents claim melatonin can treat insomnia and jet lag, protect against cancer and pregnancy, and prolong life and youthfulness. However, despite the publicity, very little is actually known about melatonin's efficacy or safety. Why? Because only a few clinical trials have been performed—and these were short, poorly designed, and involved just a few subjects. What follows is a summary of what we do know.

Melatonin is a hormone produced by the pineal gland, which is located at the base of the brain. Secretion is suppressed by environmental light and stimulated by darkness. Normally, secretion is low during the day, begins to rise around 9:00 PM, reaches a peak between 2:00 AM and 4:00 AM, and returns to baseline by morning. Signals that control secretion travel along a multineuron pathway that connects the retina to the pineal. Nocturnal secretion is greatest in children and declines with age. In blind people, melatonin secretion has no predictable pattern. Melatonin levels are low in insomniacs.

Although melatonin is a hormone, it is marketed as a dietary supplement—not as a drug. As a result, melatonin is not regulated by the FDA and has not been reviewed for safety and efficacy. Because melatonin is not regulated, commercial preparations may contain impurities and may not have the exact amount of melatonin advertised on the label (typically 0.3, 1.5, or 3 mg). Melatonin is the only hormone that can be purchased without a prescription. It is available in health food stores, vitamin shops, and even airport newsstands.

Several small, short-term trials suggest that melatonin can promote sleep. For example, doses of 0.3 to 1 mg taken at 1 to 2 hours before bedtime hastened onset of sleep and the time to REM sleep, without reducing total time in REM sleep. At a slightly higher dose (2 mg of a controlled-release formulation 2 hours before bedtime), melatonin hastened sleep onset by 14 minutes and decreased total time awake during the night

by 24 minutes. When taken in huge doses (80 to 100 mg) at noon, melatonin can cause daytime fatigue. In blind insomniacs, taking melatonin for 3 weeks normalized the melatonin production cycle and relieved insomnia. Because small doses may fail to elevate melatonin levels throughout the night, maintenance of sleep may be best with larger doses or with sustained-release formulations.

Benefits of melatonin in jet lag are in doubt. Two older studies suggest that melatonin can help. In one, the severity and duration of jet lag were reduced by taking 5 mg of melatonin once daily for 3 days before the flight and for 3 days after. In the other, subjective feelings of fatigue were reduced by taking 8 mg at 10:00 PM on the evening of the flight and for 3 days after. However, these results were not supported by a large, double-blind trial reported in 1999. This trial involved 257 Norwegian physicians flying home from New York. They were randomly assigned to one of four regimens: placebo, 0.5 mg of melatonin at bedtime, 5 mg at bedtime, or 0.5 mg taken at bedtime on the first night and then progressively earlier each day after. Dosing started on the day of their flight and continued for 5 days after. The result? Melatonin had no effect: Symptoms of jet lag in all three treatment groups were the same as those in the placebo group.

When used short term in low doses (e.g., under 2 mg), melatonin has not caused observable adverse effects. In contrast, short-term use of large doses has caused hangover, headache, nightmares, hypothermia, and transient depression. In one case, reversible psychosis occurred with a huge daytime dose. Possible adverse effects of long-term use are unknown.

In conclusion, melatonin is the miracle that awaits definitive proof. Although benefits in jet lag seem unlikely, small studies on insomnia *have* been encouraging. However, large-scale, long-term, carefully controlled trials are needed to prove that melatonin is truly safe and effective for insomnia, and to establish optimal dosages and dosing schedules.

⁘ KEY POINTS

- Drugs used to treat anxiety are called antianxiety agents, anxiolytics, or tranquilizers.
- Drugs that promote sleep are called hypnotics.
- Barbiturates and other general CNS depressants are very undesirable in that they can cause fatal respiratory depression, have a high potential for abuse, cause significant tolerance and physical dependence, and often induce hepatic drug-metabolizing enzymes.
- Benzodiazepines are preferred to barbiturates and other general CNS depressants because they are much safer, have a low abuse potential, cause less tolerance and dependence, and don't induce drug-metabolizing enzymes.
- Although benzodiazepines can cause physical dependence, the withdrawal syndrome is usually mild (except in patients who have undergone prolonged, high-dose therapy).
- To minimize withdrawal symptoms, benzodiazepines should be withdrawn gradually, over several weeks or even months.
- Benzodiazepines cause minimal respiratory depression when used alone, but can cause profound respiratory depression when combined with other CNS depressants (e.g., opioids, barbiturates, alcohol).
- Benzodiazepines produce their effects by enhancing the actions of GABA, the principal inhibitory neurotransmitter in the CNS.
- Although benzodiazepines undergo extensive metabolism, in most cases the metabolites are pharmacologically active. As a result, responses produced by administering a particular benzodiazepine often persist long after the parent drug has disappeared from the blood.
- All of the benzodiazepines have essentially equivalent pharmacologic actions; hence, selection among them is based in large part on differences in time course.
- The principal indications for benzodiazepines are anxiety, insomnia, and seizure disorders.
- The principal adverse effects of benzodiazepines are daytime sedation and anterograde amnesia.
- Flumazenil, a benzodiazepine receptor antagonist, can be used to treat benzodiazepine overdose.
- When insomnia has a treatable cause (e.g., pain, depression, schizophrenia), primary therapy should be directed at the underlying illness; hypnotics should be used only as adjuncts.
- Benzodiazepines are drugs of choice for transient insomnia.
- When benzodiazepines are used for transient insomnia, dosing should last only 2 to 3 weeks.

Summary of Major Nursing Implications*

BENZODIAZEPINES

Alprazolam
Chlordiazepoxide
Clorazepate
Diazepam
Estazolam
Flurazepam
Halazepam
Lorazepam
Oxazepam
Quazepam
Temazepam
Triazolam

The nursing implications summarized here apply to the benzodiazepines as a group and to their use in insomnia.

Preadministration Assessment

Therapeutic Goal

Benzodiazepines are used to promote sleep, relieve symptoms of anxiety (see Chapter 34), suppress seizure disorders (see Chapter 23), relax muscle spasm (see Chapter 24), and ease withdrawal from alcohol (see Chapter 37). They are also used for preanesthetic medication and to induce general anesthesia (see Chapter 26).

Baseline Data

Determine the nature of the sleep disturbance (prolonged latency, frequent awakenings, early morning awakening) and how long it has lasted. Assess for a possible underlying cause (e.g., medical illness, psychiatric illness, use of caffeine and other stimulants, poor sleep hygiene, major life stressor).

Identifying High-Risk Patients

Benzodiazepines are *contraindicated* during pregnancy and for patients who experience sleep apnea. Use with *caution* in patients with suicidal tendencies or a history of substance abuse.

Implementation: Administration

Routes

Oral. All benzodiazepines.
IM and IV. Diazepam, chlordiazepoxide, and lorazepam.
Rectal. Diazepam.

Administration

Oral. Advise patients to administer benzodiazepines with food if gastric upset occurs. Instruct patients to swallow sustained-release formulations intact, without crushing or chewing.

*Patient education information is highlighted as blue text.

Summary of Major Nursing Implications*—cont'd

Warn patients not to increase the dosage or discontinue treatment without consulting the physician.

To minimize physical dependence when treating insomnia, administer intermittently (three or four nights a week) and use the lowest effective dosage for the shortest duration required.

To minimize abstinence symptoms, taper the dosage gradually (over several weeks or even months).

Intravenous. Perform IV injections with care. Life-threatening reactions (severe hypotension, respiratory arrest, cardiac arrest) have occurred, along with less serious reactions (venous thrombosis, phlebitis, vascular impairment). To reduce complications, follow these guidelines: (1) make injections slowly; (2) take care to avoid intra-arterial injection and extravasation; (3) if direct venous injection is impossible, inject into infusion tubing as close to the vein as possible; (4) follow the manufacturer's instructions regarding suitable diluents for preparing solutions; and (5) have facilities for resuscitation available.

Implementation Measures to Enhance Therapeutic Effects

Educate patients about sleep fitness (see Table 33–4). Reassure patients with situational insomnia that sleep patterns will normalize once the precipitating stressor has been eliminated. Ensure that correctable underlying causes of insomnia (psychiatric or medical illness, use of stimulant drugs) are being managed.

Ongoing Evaluation and Interventions

Evaluating Therapeutic Effects

Insomnia is usually self-limiting. Consequently, drug therapy is usually short term. Benzodiazepines should be discontinued periodically to determine if they are still required. If insomnia is long term, make a special effort to identify possible underlying causes (e.g., psychiatric illness, medical illness, use of caffeine and other stimulants).

Minimizing Adverse Effects

CNS Depression. Drowsiness may be present the next day when benzodiazepines are used for insomnia. **Warn patients about possible residual CNS depression and advise them to avoid hazardous activities (e.g., driving) if daytime sedation is significant.**

Paradoxical Effects. **Inform patients about possible paradoxical reactions (rage, excitement, heightened anxiety), and instruct them to notify the physician if these occur.** If the reaction is verified, benzodiazepines should be withdrawn.

Physical Dependence. With most benzodiazepines, significant physical dependence is rare. However, with one agent—alprazolam [Xanax]—substantial dependence has been reported. With all benzodiazepines, development of dependence can be minimized by using the lowest effective

dosage for the shortest time necessary and by using intermittent dosing when treating insomnia.

When dependence is mild, withdrawal can elicit insomnia and other symptoms that resemble anxiety. These must be distinguished from a return of the patient's original sleep disorder. **Warn patients about possible drug-dependency insomnia during or after benzodiazepine withdrawal.**

When dependence is severe, withdrawal reactions may be serious (panic, paranoia, delirium, hypertension, convulsions). To minimize symptoms, withdraw benzodiazepines slowly (over several weeks or months). **Warn patients against abrupt discontinuation of treatment.** After drug cessation, patients should be monitored for 3 weeks for signs of withdrawal or recurrence of original symptoms.

Abuse. The abuse potential of the benzodiazepines is low. However, these drugs are abused by some individuals. Be alert to requests for increased dosage, since they may reflect an attempt at abuse. Benzodiazepines are classified under Schedule IV of the Controlled Substances Act and must be dispensed accordingly.

Use in Pregnancy and Lactation. Benzodiazepines may injure the developing fetus, especially during the first trimester. **Inform women of child-bearing age about the potential for fetal harm and warn them against becoming pregnant.** If pregnancy occurs, benzodiazepines should be withdrawn.

Benzodiazepines readily enter breast milk and may accumulate to toxic levels in the infant. **Warn mothers against breast-feeding.**

Minimizing Adverse Interactions

CNS Depressants. Combined overdose with a benzodiazepine plus another CNS depressant can cause profound respiratory depression, coma, and death. **Warn patients against use of alcohol and all other CNS depressants (e.g., opioids, barbiturates, antihistamines).**

BARBITURATES

Amobarbital
Aprobarbital
Butabarbital
Pentobarbital
Phenobarbital
Secobarbital

The nursing implications summarized below pertain to the barbiturates as a group. Implications specific to *phenobarbital* in the treatment of epilepsy are summarized in Chapter 23.

Preadministration Assessment

Therapeutic Goal

Barbiturates are used to promote sleep, suppress seizures (see Chapter 23), and induce general anesthesia (see Chapter 26).

*Patient education information is highlighted as blue text.

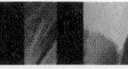

Summary of Major Nursing Implications*—cont'd

Baseline Data

For patients with *insomnia,* determine the nature of the sleep disturbance (prolonged latency, frequent awakenings, early morning awakening) and how long it has lasted. Assess for a possible underlying cause (e.g., medical illness, psychiatric illness, use of caffeine and other stimulants, poor sleep hygiene, major life stressor).

Identifying High-Risk Patients

Barbiturates are *contraindicated* for patients with severe respiratory disease and active or latent porphyria. Use with *caution* in elderly patients and those with respiratory disease. Do not dispense to individuals suspected of suicidal tendencies or to those with a history of sedative-hypnotic abuse.

Implementation: Administration

Routes

Oral, IV, and IM.

Administration

Oral. **Warn patients not to increase the dosage or discontinue treatment without consulting the physician.** Dosages should be reduced for elderly patients.

Intravenous. Make injections slowly to minimize respiratory depression and hypotension. Monitor blood pressure, pulses, and respiration. Have facilities for resuscitation immediately available. Observe the patient continuously. Do not inject solutions that are cloudy or contain a precipitate. Extravasation may cause local necrosis; take care to ensure that extravasation does not occur. Intra-arterial administration may cause gangrene (secondary to arteriospasm) and must be avoided.

Intramuscular. Barbiturate solutions are highly alkaline and can cause pain and necrosis when injected IM. Consequently, IM injection is generally avoided. Avoid injection in the vicinity of peripheral nerves since irreversible nerve damage may result.

Ongoing Evaluation and Interventions

Evaluating Therapeutic Effects

Since insomnia is usually self-limiting, drug therapy should be short term. If insomnia is long term, make a special effort to identify a possible underlying cause (e.g., psychiatric illness, medical illness, use of caffeine and other stimulants).

Minimizing Adverse Effects

CNS Depression. **Inform patients about symptoms of CNS depression (sedation, lethargy, incoordination) and warn them against participating in hazardous activities (e.g., driving, operating machinery).** Hospitalized patients may require ambulatory assistance.

Respiratory Depression. Barbiturates are strong respiratory depressants. Use with caution in elderly patients and those with respiratory disease.

Tolerance. Tolerance develops with prolonged treatment, and cross-tolerance exists with other general CNS depressants but not with opioids. If tolerance develops, temporary interruption of treatment is preferable to an increase in dosage. **Warn patients against escalation of dosage without consulting the physician.** To minimize tolerance, employ the lowest effective dosage for the shortest time necessary.

Physical Dependence. Physical dependence develops with prolonged treatment, and cross-dependence exists with other general CNS depressants, but not with opioids. The barbiturate abstinence syndrome can be severe, possibly life threatening. Manifestations can be minimized by withdrawing barbiturates slowly. **Warn patients against abrupt discontinuation of treatment.**

Drug-Dependency Insomnia. When used for insomnia, barbiturates may cause drug-dependency insomnia upon cessation of treatment. This must be distinguished from re-emergence of the original sleep disorder. To minimize drug-dependency insomnia, administer barbiturates in the lowest effective dosage for the shortest time necessary.

Abuse. Short- to intermediate-acting barbiturates (e.g., secobarbital) have a high potential for abuse. Be alert to escalating requests for medication, since these may reflect attempts at abuse. Barbiturates are regulated under the Controlled Substances Act and must be dispensed accordingly.

Suicide. Barbiturates are "drugs of choice" for suicide. Do not dispense to patients suspected of suicidal tendencies.

Use in Pregnancy. Barbiturates readily cross the placenta and can injure the developing fetus. **Inform women of child-bearing age about the potential for fetal harm and warn them against becoming pregnant.**

Infants exposed to barbiturates during the third trimester may be born drug dependent; an abstinence syndrome may develop several days after parturition.

Minimizing Adverse Interactions

CNS Depressants. Combined use of barbiturates and other CNS depressants (e.g., benzodiazepines, alcohol, opioids) can cause profound respiratory depression, coma, and death. **Warn patients against use of alcohol and all other CNS depressants.**

Interactions Secondary to Accelerated Drug Metabolism. Barbiturates induce hepatic drug-metabolizing enzymes, and thereby accelerate the degradation of other drugs. Increased metabolism is of particular concern with *warfarin, oral contraceptives,* and *phenytoin.* **Advise women taking oral contraceptives to consider an alternative form of birth control.**

Managing Toxicity

Overdose can be life threatening. Manifestations include respiratory depression, coma, pinpoint pupils, and hypotension. Death may result from pulmonary complications or renal failure. Treatment requires an intensive care unit. Principal management objectives are removal of the drug and maintenance of oxygenation. There is no specific antidote to barbiturate poisoning; CNS stimulants should not be used.

*Patient education information is highlighted as blue text.

Management of Anxiety Disorders

GENERALIZED ANXIETY DISORDER
PANIC DISORDER
OBSESSIVE-COMPULSIVE DISORDER
SOCIAL ANXIETY DISORDER (SOCIAL PHOBIA)
POST-TRAUMATIC STRESS DISORDER

Anxiety is an uncomfortable state that has both psychologic and physical components. The psychologic component can be characterized with terms such as *fear, apprehension, dread,* and *uneasiness.* The physical component manifests as tachycardia, palpitations, trembling, dry mouth, sweating, weakness, fatigue, and shortness of breath.

Anxiety is a nearly universal experience that often serves an adaptive function. When anxiety is moderate and situationally appropriate, therapy may not be needed or even desirable. In contrast, when anxiety is persistent and disabling, intervention is clearly indicated.

In the *Diagnostic and Statistical Manual of Mental Disorders, Fourth Edition* (DSM-IV), primary anxiety disorders are divided into six major classes: generalized anxiety disorder, panic disorder, obsessive-compulsive disorder, phobic disorders, post-traumatic stress disorder, and acute stress disorder. Although each class is distinct, they all have one element in common: an unhealthy level of anxiety. In addition, with all classes, depression is frequently comorbid.

Anxiety disorders are among the most common psychiatric illnesses. In the United States, about 25% of people develop pathologic anxiety at some time in their lives. As a rule, the incidence is higher in women than in men.

Fortunately, anxiety disorders respond well to treatment—either psychotherapy, drug therapy, or both. As indicated in Table 34–1, two classes of drugs are used most: *benzodiazepines* and *selective serotonin reuptake inhibitors* (SSRIs). Benzodiazepines are used primarily for one condition: generalized anxiety disorder (GAD). In contrast, the SSRIs are now used for *all* anxiety disorders. It should be noted that, although SSRIs were developed as antidepressants, they are highly effective against anxiety—whether or not depression is also present.

GENERALIZED ANXIETY DISORDER

Characteristics

Generalized anxiety disorder is a chronic condition characterized by uncontrollable worrying. Of all anxiety disorders, GAD is the least likely to remit. Most patients with GAD also have another psychiatric disorder, usually depression. GAD should not be confused with *situational anxiety,* which is a normal response to a stressful situation (e.g., family problems, exams, financial difficulties); symptoms may be intense, but they are temporary.

The hallmark of GAD is unrealistic or excessive anxiety about several events or activities (e.g., work or school per-

TABLE 34–1 ▪▪ First-Line Drugs for Anxiety Disorders			
Anxiety Disorder	**Benzodiazepines**	**SSRIs**	**Others**
Generalized Anxiety Disorder	Alprazolam Chlordiazepoxide Clorazepate Diazepam Halazepam Lorazepam Oxazepam	Paroxetine	Buspirone Venlafaxine
Panic Disorder		Paroxetine Sertraline	
Obsessive-Compulsive Disorder		Paroxetine Fluoxetine Fluvoxamine Sertraline	
Social Anxiety Disorder		Paroxetine	
Post-traumatic Stress Disorder		Paroxetine Sertraline	

SSRIs = selective serotonin reuptake inhibitors.

formance) that lasts 6 months or longer. Other psychologic manifestations include vigilance, tension, apprehension, poor concentration, and difficulty falling or staying asleep. Somatic manifestations include trembling, muscle tension, restlessness, and signs of autonomic hyperactivity, such as palpitations, tachycardia, sweating, and cold clammy hands. Diagnostic criteria for GAD, as described in DSM-IV, are shown in Table 34–2.

Treatment

GAD can be managed with nondrug therapy and with drugs. Nondrug approaches include supportive therapy, cognitive behavioral therapy, biofeedback, and relaxation training. These can help relieve symptoms and improve coping skills in anxiety-provoking situations. When symptoms are mild, nondrug therapy may be all that is needed. However, if symptoms are intensely uncomfortable or disabling, drugs are indicated. Current first-line choices are the benzodiazepines, buspirone, and two antidepressants: venlafaxine and paroxetine. With the benzodiazepines, onset of relief is rapid; in contrast, with buspirone and the antidepressants, onset is delayed. Accordingly, benzodiazepines are preferred drugs for immediate stabilization, especially when anxiety is severe. In contrast, buspirone and the antidepressants may be preferred for long-term management. Because GAD is a chronic disorder, initial drug therapy should be prolonged, lasting at least 2 to 6 months. Unfortunately, even after extended treatment, withdrawal frequently results in relapse. Hence, for many patients, drug therapy must continue indefinitely.

Benzodiazepines

Benzodiazepines are first-choice drugs for anxiety. As discussed in Chapter 33, benefits derive from enhancing responses to GABA, an inhibitory neurotransmitter. Onset of effects is immediate, and the margin of safety is high. Principal side effects are sedation and psychomotor slowing. Patients should be warned about these effects and informed they will subside within 7 to 10 days. Because of their abuse potential, benzodiazepines should be used with caution in patients known to abuse alcohol or other psychoactive substances.

Long-term use of benzodiazepines carries a risk of physical dependence. Withdrawal symptoms include panic, paranoia, and delirium. These can be especially troubling for patients with GAD. Furthermore, they can be confused with a return of pretreatment symptoms. Accordingly, care must be taken to differentiate between a withdrawal reaction and relapse. To minimize withdrawal symptoms, benzodiazepines should be tapered gradually—over a period of several months. If relapse occurs, treatment should resume.

Of the 14 benzodiazepines available, 7 are approved for anxiety. The agents prescribed most often are alprazolam [Xanax] and lorazepam [Ativan]. However, there is no proof that any one benzodiazepine is clearly superior to the others. Hence, selection among them is largely a matter of prescriber preference. Dosages for anxiety are summarized in Table 34–3.

TABLE 34–2 ■ DSM-IV-TR Diagnostic Criteria for GAD

A. Excessive anxiety and worry about several events or activities (such as work or school performance) that occur more days than not for at least 6 months.

B. The person finds the worry difficult to control.

C. The anxiety and worry are associated with three (or more) of the following six symptoms (with at least some symptoms present for more days than not for the past 6 months). *Note:* only one item is required in children.

- Restlessness or feeling keyed up or on edge
- Being easily fatigued
- Difficulty concentrating or mind going blank
- Irritability
- Muscle tension
- Sleep disturbance (difficulty falling asleep or staying asleep, or restlessness, unsatisfying sleep)

D. The focus of the anxiety and worry is not related to another psychiatric disorder.

E. The anxiety, worry, or physical symptoms cause clinically significant distress or impairment in social, occupational, or other important areas of functioning.

F. The disturbance is not due to the direct physiologic effects of a substance (e.g., drug of abuse, medication) or a general medical condition (e.g., hyperthyroidism) and does not occur exclusively during a mood disorder, psychotic disorder, or pervasive developmental disorder.

Modified from the Diagnostic and Statistical Manual of Mental Disorders, Fourth Edition, Text Revision. Washington, DC, American Psychiatric Press, 2000, with permission. Copyright © 2000 American Psychiatric Association.

The basic pharmacology of the benzodiazepines is discussed in Chapter 33.

Buspirone

Actions and Therapeutic Use. Buspirone [BuSpar] is an anxiolytic drug that differs significantly from the benzodiazepines. Most notably, buspirone is *not* a central nervous system (CNS) depressant. For treatment of anxiety, buspirone is as effective as the benzodiazepines and has three distinct advantages: It does not cause sedation, has no abuse potential, and does not intensify the effects of CNS depressants (benzodiazepines, alcohol, barbiturates, and related drugs). Its major disadvantage is that anxiolytic effects develop *slowly:* initial responses take a week to appear, and several more weeks must pass before responses peak. Because therapeutic effects are delayed, buspirone is not suitable for PRN use or for patients who need immediate relief. Since buspirone has no abuse potential, it may be especially appropriate for patients known to abuse alcohol and other drugs. Because it lacks depressant properties, buspirone is an attractive alternative to benzodiazepines in patients who require long-term therapy but cannot tolerate benzodiazepine-induced sedation and psychomotor slowing. Buspirone is labeled only for *short-term* treatment of anxiety. However, the drug has been taken for as long as a year with no reduction in beneficial effects. Buspirone does not display cross-dependence with benzodi-

TABLE 34–3 ■ Dosages of Benzodiazepines Approved for Anxiety

Generic Name	Trade Name	Dosage	
		Initial	Usual Range (mg/day)
Alprazolam	Xanax	0.25 mg tid	0.5–6
Chlordiazepoxide	Librium	—	15–100
Clorazepate	Tranxene, Gen-Xene	—	15–60
Diazepam	Valium	—	4–40
Halazepam	Paxipam	—	60–160
Lorazepam	Ativan	0.5 mg tid	2–6
Oxazepam	Serax	—	30–120

azepines. Hence, when patients are switched from a benzodiazepine to buspirone, the benzodiazepine must be tapered off slowly. Furthermore, since the effects of buspirone are delayed, buspirone should be initiated 2 to 4 weeks before beginning benzodiazepine withdrawal. In contrast to benzodiazepines, buspirone lacks sedative, muscle relaxant, and anticonvulsant actions—and hence cannot be used for insomnia, muscle spasm, or epilepsy.

The mechanism by which buspirone relieves anxiety has not been established. The drug binds with high affinity to receptors for serotonin and with lower affinity to receptors for dopamine. Buspirone does not bind to receptors for GABA or benzodiazepines.

Pharmacokinetics. Buspirone is well absorbed following oral administration but undergoes extensive metabolism on its first pass through the liver. Administration with food delays absorption but enhances bioavailability (by reducing first-pass metabolism). The drug is excreted in part by the kidneys, primarily as metabolites.

Adverse Effects. Buspirone is generally well tolerated. The most common reactions are *dizziness, nausea, headache, nervousness, lightheadedness,* and *excitement.* The drug is nonsedating and does not interfere with daytime activities. Furthermore, it poses little or no risk of suicide; huge doses (375 mg/day) have been given to healthy volunteers with only moderate adverse effects (nausea, vomiting, dizziness, drowsiness, miosis).

Drug and Food Interactions. Levels of buspirone can be greatly increased (5- to 13-fold) by *erythromycin* and *ketoconazole.* Levels can also be increased by *grapefruit juice.* Elevated levels may cause drowsiness and subjective effects (dysphoria, feeling "spacey"). Buspirone does not enhance the depressant effects of alcohol, barbiturates, and other general CNS depressants.

Tolerance, Dependence, and Abuse. Buspirone has been used for up to 1 year without evidence of tolerance, physical dependence, or psychologic dependence. No withdrawal symptoms have been observed upon termination. There is no cross-tolerance or cross-dependence between buspirone and the sedative-hypnotics (e.g., benzodiazepines, barbiturates). Buspirone appears to have no potential for abuse, and hence is not regulated under the Controlled Substances Act.

Preparations, Dosage, and Administration. Buspirone [BuSpar] is dispensed in 5- and 10-mg tablets. The initial dosage is 5 mg 3 times a day. Dosage may be increased to a maximum of 60 mg/day.

Antidepressants: Venlafaxine and Paroxetine

At this time, only two antidepressants—venlafaxine [Effexor XR] and paroxetine [Paxil]—are approved for treatment of GAD. Venlafaxine is an atypical antidepressant; paroxetine is an SSRI. Both drugs are especially well suited for patients who have depression in addition to GAD. However, both are effective even when depression is absent. As with buspirone, anxiolytic effects develop slowly: Initial responses can be seen a week, but optimal responses require several more weeks to develop. Because relief is delayed, the antidepressants cannot be used PRN. Compared with benzodiazepines, the antidepressants do a better job of decreasing cognitive and psychic symptoms of anxiety, but are not as good at decreasing somatic symptoms. In contrast to the benzodiazepines, antidepressants have no potential for abuse. However, abrupt discontinuation *can* produce withdrawal symptoms.

Venlafaxine was the first antidepressant approved for GAD. The drug has been proved effective for both short-term and long-term use. The most common side effect is nausea, which develops in 37% of patients. Fortunately, nausea subsides despite continued drug use. Other common reactions include headache, anorexia, nervousness, sweating, daytime somnolence, and insomnia. In addition, venlafaxine can cause hypertension, although this is unlikely at the doses used in GAD. Combing venlafaxine with a monoamine oxidase inhibitor can result in serious toxicity, and hence must be avoided. Venlafaxine is available in two formulations: standard tablets [Effexor] and extended-release capsules [Effexor XR]. Only the extended-release formulation is approved for GAD. The initial dosage is 37.5 mg once a day, and the maintenance range is 75 to 225 mg once a day.

Paroxetine is the only SSRI approved for GAD. The drug seems to be as effective as the benzodiazepines, but is less well tolerated. The initial dosage for GAD is 20 mg once a day in the morning. Dosage can be gradually increased to a maintenance range of 20 to 50 mg/day.

The basic pharmacology of venlafaxine and paroxetine is discussed in Chapter 31.

PANIC DISORDER

Characteristics

Panic disorder is characterized by recurrent, intensely uncomfortable episodes known as *panic attacks.* As defined in DSM-IV, panic attacks have a sudden onset, reach peak intensity within 10 minutes, and have four (or more) of the following symptoms:

- Palpitations, pounding heart, racing heartbeat
- Chest pain or discomfort
- Sensation of shortness of breath or smothering
- Feeling of choking
- Dizziness, lightheadedness
- Nausea or abdominal discomfort
- Derealization (feelings of unreality) or depersonalization (feeling detached from oneself)
- Fear of losing control or going crazy
- Fear of dying
- Tingling or numbness in the hands
- Flushes or chills

Symptoms typically dissipate within 30 minutes. Many patients go to emergency departments because they think they are having a heart attack. Some patients experience panic attacks daily, whereas others have only one or two a month. Panic disorder is a common condition that affects 1.6% of Americans at some time in their lives. The incidence in women is 2 to 3 times the incidence in men. Onset of panic disorder usually occurs in the late teens or early 20s.

Perhaps 50% of patients who get panic disorder also experience *agoraphobia,* a condition characterized by anxiety about being in places or situations from which escape might be difficult or embarrassing, or in which help might be unavailable in the event that a panic attack should occur. Agoraphobia leads to avoidance of certain places (e.g., elevators, bridges, tunnels, movie theaters) and situations (e.g., being outside the home alone; being in a crowd; standing on line; driving in traffic; traveling by bus, train, or plane). In extreme cases, agoraphobics may never set foot outside the home. Because of avoidance behavior, agoraphobia can severely limit occupational and social options.

What's the underlying cause of panic attacks? We don't know. However, malfunction of the brain's "alarm system" is suspected. This malfunction may result from abnormalities in noradrenergic systems, serotonergic systems, and/or benzodiazepine receptors. Genetic vulnerability also may play a role.

Treatment

Between 70% and 90% of patients with panic disorder respond well to treatment. Two modalities may be employed: drug therapy and cognitive behavioral therapy (CBT). Combining drug therapy with CBT is more effective than either modality alone. As a rule, patients experience rapid and significant improvement. Drug therapy helps suppress panic attacks, while CBT helps patients become more comfortable with situations and places they've been avoiding. Additional benefit can be derived from avoiding caffeine and sympathomimetics (which can trigger panic attacks), avoiding sleep deprivation (which can predispose to panic attacks), and doing regular aerobic exercise (which can reduce anxiety).

Drug therapy should continue for at least 6 to 9 months. Stopping sooner is associated with a high rate of relapse.

Antidepressants

Panic disorder responds well to all three major classes of antidepressants: SSRIs, tricyclic antidepressants (TCAs), and monoamine oxidase inhibitors (MAOIs). With all three, full benefits take 6 to 12 weeks to develop. Owing to better tolerability, SSRIs are preferred to TCAs and MAOIs. The basic pharmacology of the antidepressants is discussed in Chapter 31.

Selective Serotonin Reuptake Inhibitors. The SSRIs are first-line drugs for panic disorder. At this time, only two SSRIs—paroxetine [Paxil] and sertraline [Zoloft]—are approved for this disorder. However, the other SSRIs—citalopram [Celexa], fluoxetine [Prozac], and fluvoxamine [Luvox]—appear just as effective. The SSRIs decrease the frequency and intensity attacks, anticipatory anxiety, and avoidance behavior. Furthermore, they decrease panic attacks regardless of whether the patient is actually depressed. However, if the patient does have co-existing depression, antidepressants will benefit the depression and panic disorder simultaneously. Common side effects include nausea, headache, insomnia, and sexual dysfunction. Weight gain is also a problem. In addition, SSRIs can *increase* anxiety early in treatment. To minimize exacerbation of anxiety, dosage should be low initially and then gradually increased. For paroxetine, the initial dosage is 10 mg/day, and the target range is 20 to 40 mg/day. For sertraline, the initial dosage is 25 mg/day, and the target range is 50 to 200 mg/day.

Tricyclic Antidepressants. The TCAs (e.g., imipramine [Tofranil], clomipramine [Anafranil]) are second-line drugs for panic disorder. They should be used only after a trial with at least one SSRI has failed. Although TCAs are as effective as SSRIs, they are not as well tolerated. The most common side effects are sedation, orthostatic hypotension, and anticholinergic effects: dry mouth, blurred vision, urinary retention, constipation, and tachycardia. Of greater concern, TCAs can cause fatal dysrhythmias if taken in overdose. As with the SSRIs, dosage should be low initially and then gradually increased. For clomipramine, the initial dosage is 25 mg/day, and the target range is 50 to 200 mg/day. For imipramine, the initial dosage is 10 mg/day, and the target range is 100 to 300 mg/day.

Monoamine Oxidase Inhibitors. Although MAOIs (e.g., phenelzine) are very effective in panic disorder, they are difficult to use. MAOIs can cause significant side effects, including orthostatic hypotension, weight gain, and sexual dysfunction. In addition, they can cause hypertensive crisis if the patient takes certain drugs or consumes foods rich in tyramine. Because of these drawbacks, MAOIs are considered last-line drugs for panic disorder.

Benzodiazepines

Benzodiazepines are first-line drugs for panic disorder. The agents used most often are alprazolam [Xanax], clonazepam [Klonopin], and lorazepam [Ativan]. All three drugs provide rapid and effective protection against panic attacks. These drugs also reduce anticipatory anxiety and phobic avoidance. In contrast to antidepressants, which take weeks or even months to work, benzodiazepines often provide relief with the first few doses. Accordingly, benzodiazepines are especially useful as initial therapy while responses to antidepressants are developing. The principal side effect of the benzodiazepines is sedation, but some tolerance develops in 7 to 10 days. Benzodiazepines can cause physical dependence, which can make withdrawal extremely hard for some patients. The difficulty is that withdrawal produces intense anxiety, which people with panic disorder are often unable to tolerate. To minimize withdrawal symptoms, benzodiazepines should be withdrawn very slowly—over a period of several months. In addition, withdrawal symptoms can be reduced by concurrent treatment with an SSRI. The basic pharmacology of the benzodiazepines is discussed in Chapter 33.

OBSESSIVE-COMPULSIVE DISORDER
Characteristics

Obsessive-compulsive disorder (OCD) is a potentially disabling condition characterized by persistent obsessions and compulsions that cause marked distress, consume at least 1 hour a day, and significantly interfere with daily living. An *obsession* is defined as a recurrent, persistent thought, impulse, or mental image that is unwanted and distressing, and comes involuntarily to mind despite attempts to ignore or suppress it. Common obsessions include fear of contamination (e.g., acquiring a disease by touching another person), aggressive impulses (e.g., harming a family member), a need for orderliness or symmetry (e.g., personal bathroom items must be arranged in a precise way), and repeated doubts (e.g., did I unplug the iron?). A *compulsion* is a ritualized behavior or mental act that the patient is driven to perform in response to his or her obsessions. In the patient's mind, carrying out the compulsion is essential to prevent some horrible event from occurring (e.g., death of a parent). If performing the compulsion is suppressed or postponed, the patient experiences increased anxiety. Common compulsions include hand washing, mental counting, arranging objects symmetrically, and hoarding. Patients usually understand that their compulsive behavior is excessive and senseless, but nonetheless are unable to stop. Diagnostic criteria for OCD, as described in DSM-IV, are presented in Table 34–4.

Treatment

Patients with OCD respond to drugs and behavioral therapy. Optimal treatment consists of both.

Behavioral therapy is probably more important in OCD than in any other psychiatric disorder. In the technique employed, patients are exposed to sources of their fears, while being encouraged to refrain from acting out their compulsive rituals. When no dire consequences come to pass, despite the absence of "protective" rituals, patients are able to gradually give up their compulsive behavior. Although this form of therapy causes great anxiety, the success rate is high.

Five drugs are approved for OCD: four SSRIs and one TCA (clomipramine). All five enhance serotonergic transmission. The SSRIs are better tolerated than clomipramine, and hence are preferred.

Selective Serotonin Reuptake Inhibitors

The SSRIs are first-line drugs for OCD. Four agents are used: fluoxetine [Prozac], fluvoxamine [Luvox], sertraline [Zoloft], and paroxetine [Paxil]. All four reduce symptoms by enhancing serotonergic transmission. They all are equally effective, although individual patients may respond better to one than to another. With all four, beneficial effects develop slowly, taking several months to become maximal. Common side effects

---

TABLE 34–4 ▪ DSM-IV-TR Diagnostic Criteria for Obsessive-Compulsive Disorder

A. The presence of either obsessions or compulsions:

Obsessions

1. Recurrent and persistent thoughts, impulses, or images that are experienced, at some time during the disturbance, as intrusive and senseless and that cause marked anxiety and distress.

2. The thoughts, impulses, or images are not simply excessive worries about real-life problems.

3. The person attempts to ignore or suppress the thoughts, impulses, or images, or to neutralize them with some other thought or action.

4. The person recognizes that the obsessions are a product of his or her own mind.

Compulsions

1. Repetitive behaviors (e.g., hand washing, putting objects in order) or mental acts (e.g., praying, counting, repeating words silently) that the person feels driven to perform in response to an obsession or according to rigid rules.

2. The behaviors or mental acts are performed to prevent or reduce distress or to prevent some dreaded event; however, these behaviors or mental acts either have no realistic connection with what they are designed to neutralize or prevent, or are clearly excessive.

B. At some time during the disorder, the person recognizes that the obsessions or compulsions are excessive or unreasonable. (This does not apply to children.)

C. The obsessions or compulsions cause marked distress, are time consuming (take >1 hour a day), or significantly interfere with normal routines, occupational or academic functioning, or usual social activities or relationships.

D. The symptoms are not related to another psychiatric disorder, and are not caused by a substance, medication, or general medical illness.

Adapted from the Diagnostic and Statistical Manual of Mental Disorders, Fourth Edition, Text Revision. Washington, DC, American Psychiatric Press, 2000, with permission. Copyright © 2000 American Psychiatric Association.

include nausea, headache, insomnia, and sexual dysfunction. Weight gain can also occur. Despite this array of side effects, SSRIs are safer than clomipramine and better tolerated. Dosages are as follows:

- *Fluoxetine*—20 mg in the morning initially, increased to a maximum of 80 mg/day
- *Fluvoxamine*—50 mg at bedtime initially, increased to a maximum of 300 mg/day
- *Paroxetine*—20 mg in the morning initially, increased to a maximum of 60 mg/day
- *Sertraline*—25 to 50 mg once a day initially, increased to a maximum of 200 mg/day

How long should treatment last? Therapy of an initial episode should continue for at least 1 year, after which discontinuation can be tried. Withdrawal should be done slowly, reducing the dosage by 25% every 1 to 2 months. Unfortunately relapse is common; estimates range from 23% to as high as 90%. If relapse continues to occur after three or four attempts at withdrawal, lifelong treatment may be indicated.

Clomipramine

For patients with OCD, clomipramine [Anafranil] is as effective as SSRIs, but less well tolerated. Accordingly, clomipramine is considered a second-line drug for this disorder, and hence should be used only after treatment with one or more SSRIs has failed.

Clomipramine is the only TCA effective in OCD. About 70% of patients experience a significant improvement. Initial effects take 4 weeks to develop; maximal effects are seen in 12 weeks.

Clomipramine affects several neurotransmitter systems. As with the SSRIs, benefits in OCD derive from blocking uptake of serotonin. (Among the TCAs, clomipramine is the most effective inhibitor of serotonin uptake.) However, in contrast to SSRIs, which block reuptake of serotonin only, clomipramine blocks reuptake of norepinephrine as well as serotonin. Like other TCAs, clomipramine also blocks *receptors* for norepinephrine, acetylcholine, and histamine.

Clomipramine can cause a variety of side effects. Sedation, dry mouth, dizziness, and tremor occur in over 50% of patients. Other common effects include weight gain, constipation, blurred vision, insomnia, headache, and nausea. Of greatest concern, clomipramine can induce *seizures.* Because of seizure risk, the drug should be avoided in patients with a history of seizures or head injury. Clomipramine greatly increases the risk of hypertensive crisis from MAOIs, and therefore is contraindicated for patients taking these drugs.

Doses should be low initially (20 to 25 mg/day) and then gradually increased. Side effects can be minimized by dividing the early doses and taking them with meals. Maintenance doses of 150 to 250 mg/day are achieved in 2 to 4 weeks.

The basic pharmacology of clomipramine and other TCAs is discussed in Chapter 31.

SOCIAL ANXIETY DISORDER (SOCIAL PHOBIA)

Characteristics

Social anxiety disorder, formerly known as social phobia, is characterized by an intense, irrational fear of situations in which one might be scrutinized by others, or might do something that is embarrassing or humiliating. Exposure to the feared situation almost elicits anxiety. As a result, the person avoids the situation or, if it can't be avoided, endures it with intense anxiety (manifestations include blushing, stuttering, sweating, palpitations, dry throat, and muscle tension and twitches). Diagnostic criteria for social anxiety disorder, as defined in DSM-IV, are listed in Table 34–5.

Social anxiety disorder has two forms: generalized and nongeneralized. In the generalized form, the person fears nearly all social and performance situations. In the nongeneralized form, fear is limited to a specific type of situation, such as public speaking.

Not surprisingly, social anxiety disorder can be debilitating. In younger people, it can retard social development, inhibit participation in social activities, impair acquisition of friends, and make dating difficult or even impossible. It can also preclude pursuit of higher education. In older people, it can severely limit social and occupational options.

Social anxiety disorder is one of the most common psychiatric disorders, and *the* most common anxiety disorder. In the United States, 13% to 14% of the population is affected at some time in their lives. The disorder typically begins during the teenage years and, left untreated, is likely to continue lifelong.

Treatment

Social anxiety disorder can be treated with psychotherapy, drug therapy, or both. Studies indicate that psychotherapy—both cognitive and behavioral—can be as effective as drugs. A combination of psychotherapy and drugs may be more effective than either modality alone.

The SSRIs are considered first-line drugs for most patients. These drugs are especially well suited for patients who fear multiple situations and are obliged to face those situations on a regular basis. Currently, only one SSRI—paroxetine [Paxil]—is approved for social anxiety disorder. However, available data indicate that the other SSRIs are effective too. Initial effects take about 4 weeks to be seen; optimal effects develop in 8 to 12 weeks. Patients should be warned that benefits will be delayed. For paroxetine, the initial dosage is 20 mg once a day in the morning. The usual maintenance range is 20 to 40 mg/day. Treatment should continue for at least 1 year, after which gradual withdrawal can be tried. Unfortunately, withdrawal frequently results in relapse.

TABLE 34–5 ■ DSM-IV-TR Diagnostic Criteria for Social Anxiety Disorder (Social Phobia)

A. A marked and persistent fear of one or more social or performance situations in which the person is exposed to unfamiliar people or to possible scrutiny by others. The individual fears that he or she will act in a way that will be embarrassing or humiliating, or will show anxiety symptoms that will be embarrassing or humiliating.

B. Exposure to the feared situation almost always provokes anxiety.

C. The person recognizes that the fear is excessive or unreasonable (not required in children).

D. The feared situation is avoided, or endured with intense anxiety.

E. The avoidance or anxious anticipation causes marked distress or interferes significantly with the person's relationships, normal routine, social activities, or performance at work or at school.

F. For persons under age 18, the fear has lasted at least 6 months.

G. The fear or avoidance is not caused by a substance, medication, or general medical illness, and cannot be better accounted for by another psychiatric illness.

Adapted from the Diagnostic and Statistical Manual of Mental Disorders, Fourth Edition, Text Revision. Washington, DC, American Psychiatric Press, 2000, with permission. Copyright © 2000 American Psychiatric Association.

Benzodiazepines (e.g., clonazepam [Klonopin], alprazolam [Xanax]) are an option for some patients. These drugs are well tolerated and their benefits are immediate, unlike those of the SSRIs. As a result, benzodiazepines can (1) provide rapid relief and (2) be used PRN. Accordingly, these drugs are well suited for people whose fear is limited to specific situations, and who must face those situations only occasionally. The usual dosage is 1 to 3 mg/day for clonazepam, and 1 to 6 mg/day for alprazolam.

Propranolol [Inderal] and other beta blockers can benefit patients with performance anxiety, a form of nongeneralized social anxiety disorder. When taken 1 to 2 hours before a scheduled performance, these drugs can reduce symptoms caused by autonomic hyperactivity (e.g., tremors, sweating, tachycardia, palpitations). Doses are relatively small—only 10 to 80 mg for propranolol.

POST-TRAUMATIC STRESS DISORDER

Characteristics

As described in DSM-IV (see Table 34–6), post-traumatic stress disorder (PTSD) develops following a *traumatic event* that elicited an immediate reaction of *fear, helplessness,* or *horror.* PTSD has three core symptoms: *re-experiencing* the event, *avoidance of reminders* of the event (coupled with generalized emotional numbing), and a persistent state of *hyperarousal.* According to DSM-IV, a traumatic event is one that involves a threat of injury or death, or a threat to one's physical integrity. Many events meet this criterion. Among these are physical or sexual assault, rape, torture, combat, industrial explosions, serious accidents, natural disasters, being taken hostage, displacement as a refugee, and terrorist attacks, such as the ones that took place on September 11, 2001, against the World Trade Center and the Pentagon. It should be noted that PTSD can develop in persons who were only *witnesses* to a traumatic event—not just in those who were directly involved.

The epidemiology of PTSD is revealing. In the United States, PTSD develops in 5% to 6% of men at some time in their lives, and in 10% to 14% of women—making PTSD the fourth most common psychiatric disorder. Traumatic events that involve interpersonal violence (e.g., assault, rape, torture) are more likely to cause PTSD than are traumatic events that do not (e.g., car accidents, natural disasters). For example, among rape victims, the incidence of PTSD is 45.9% for women and 65% for men. In contrast, among natural disaster survivors, the incidence is only 5.4% for women and 3.7% for men. Combat carries a high risk of PTSD: the disorder develops in 2 of every 5 men who go to war.

Treatment

PTSD can be treated with psychotherapy and with drugs. For patients with mild symptoms, psychotherapy alone may be adequate. However, for patients with moderate or severe symptoms, a combination of psychotherapy and drugs is recommended.

Psychotherapy has several objectives. The initial goal is to provide education about PTSD, and establish a relationship that

---

TABLE 34–6 ■ DSM-IV-TR Diagnostic Criteria for Post-traumatic Stress Disorder

A. The person participated in (or witnessed) a *traumatic event,* and reacted with a sense of intense fear, helplessness, or horror. The event could involve serious physical injury, actual or threatened death, or a threat to physical integrity.

B. The traumatic event is *persistently re-experienced,* either through flashbacks, hallucinations, distressing dreams, or recurrent thoughts, or through intense psychologic or physiologic reactions triggered by exposure to cues associated with the event.

C. Persistent *avoidance* of reminders of the event stimuli along with *generalized emotional numbing,* as indicated by three or more of the following:

- Efforts to avoid thoughts, feelings, or conversations associated with the trauma
- Efforts to avoid activities, places, or people that arouse recollections of the trauma
- Inability to recall an important aspect of the trauma
- Markedly diminished interest or participation in significant activities
- Feeling detached or estranged from others
- Restricted range of affect (e.g., unable to have loving feelings)
- Sense of foreshortened future (e.g., does not expect to have a career, marriage, children, or a normal life span)

D. Persistent symptoms of increased arousal, as indicated by two or more of the following:

- Difficulty falling or staying asleep
- Irritability or outbursts of anger
- Difficulty concentrating
- Hypervigilance
- Exaggerated startle response

E. The symptoms (B, C, and D) have lasted more than 1 month.

F. The symptoms cause significant distress, or disrupt relationships, job performance, or some other important facet of life.

Adapted from the Diagnostic and Statistical Manual of Mental Disorders, Fourth Edition, Text Revision. Washington, DC, American Psychiatric Press, 2000, with permission. Copyright © 2000 American Psychiatric Association.

offers support and a sense of safety. Education can help the patient understand that his or her symptoms reflect psychologic and biologic responses to overwhelming trauma, and hence do not indicate a character flaw or personal weakness. Specific therapeutic techniques can help neutralize symptoms: Cognitive therapy can reduce guilt, shame, and demoralization; exposure therapy can reduce intrusive thoughts and avoidance behavior; and group therapy can reduce the sense of isolation and stigma.

Only two drugs—*paroxetine* [Paxil] and *sertraline* [Zoloft]—are approved by the Food and Drug Administration for PTSD. Both drugs are SSRIs, and both are safe and well tolerated. These drugs can reduce all three core symptoms of PTSD: re-experiencing, avoidance/emotional numbing, and hyperarousal. In addition, they can reduce associated anxiety and depression. Treatment is most effective when initiated within 3 months of the traumatic event. Initial responses can be seen in 2 weeks; responses become maximal in 2 to 3 months. Treatment should continue for 6 to 24 months after a full response is achieved. Withdrawal should be done slowly—over 1 to 3 months. The target dosage for paroxetine is 20 to 40 mg/day, and the target for sertraline is 50 to 150 mg/day.

KEY POINTS

- Anxiety is an uncomfortable state that has psychologic manifestations (fear, apprehension, dread, uneasiness) and physical manifestations (tachycardia, palpitations, trembling, dry mouth, sweating, weakness, fatigue, shortness of breath).
- When anxiety is persistent and disabling, intervention is indicated.
- As a rule, optimal therapy of anxiety disorders consists of psychotherapy combined with drug therapy.
- The drugs used most often for anxiety disorders are benzodiazepines and selective serotonin reuptake inhibitors (SSRIs).
- Benzodiazepines are used primarily for generalized anxiety disorder (GAD), whereas SSRIs are used for *all* anxiety disorders.
- GAD is a chronic condition characterized by uncontrollable worrying.
- First-line drugs for GAD are benzodiazepines, buspirone, and two antidepressants: venlafaxine and paroxetine.
- Benzodiazepines suppress symptoms of GAD immediately. Accordingly, these drugs are preferred agents for rapid stabilization, especially when anxiety is severe.
- With buspirone, venlafaxine, and paroxetine, anxiolytic effects are delayed. Accordingly, these drugs are best suited for long-term management—not rapid relief.
- Benzodiazepines are CNS depressants and hence can cause sedation and psychomotor slowing. In addition, they can intensify CNS depression caused by other drugs.
- Benzodiazepines have some potential for abuse, and hence should be used with caution in patients known to abuse alcohol or other psychoactive drugs.
- When taken long term, benzodiazepines can cause physical dependence. To minimize withdrawal symptoms, dosage should be tapered off gradually—over a period of several months.

- Buspirone has three advantages over benzodiazepines: It does not cause CNS depression, has no abuse potential, and does not intensify the effects of CNS depressants (e.g., benzodiazepines, alcohol, barbiturates).
- Buspirone levels can be increased by erythromycin, ketoconazole, and grapefruit juice.
- Venlafaxine and paroxetine are especially well suited for treating patients who have depression in addition to GAD. However, both drugs are effective even when depression is absent.
- Patients with panic disorder experience recurrent panic attacks, characterized by palpitations, pounding heart, chest pain, derealization or depersonalization, and fear of dying or going crazy.
- Many patients with panic disorder also experience agoraphobia, a condition characterized by anxiety about being in places or situations from which escape might be difficult or embarrassing, or in which help might be unavailable if a panic attack should occur.
- The principal drugs for panic disorder are SSRIs and benzodiazepines.
- SSRIs decrease the frequency and intensity of panic attacks, anticipatory anxiety, and avoidance behavior—and they work regardless of whether the patient has depression.
- Because benzodiazepines act much faster than SSRIs, benzodiazepines are especially useful as initial therapy while responses to SSRIs are developing.
- Weaning panic disorder patients from benzodiazepines must be done gradually, so as to minimize anxiety and other symptoms of withdrawal.
- Obsessive-compulsive disorder (OCD) is characterized by persistent obsessions and compulsions that cause marked distress, consume at least 1 hour a day, and significantly interfere with daily living.
- SSRIs are first-line drugs for OCD.
- Social anxiety disorder, formerly known as social phobia, is characterized by an intense, irrational fear of being scrutinized by others, or of doing something that is embarrassing or humiliating.
- The SSRIs are first-line drugs for most patients with social anxiety disorder.
- When social anxiety disorder is limited to fear of specific situations, and when those situations arise infrequently, PRN treatment with benzodiazepines may be preferred to long-term treatment with SSRIs.
- Post-traumatic stress disorder (PTSD) develops following a traumatic event that elicited an immediate reaction of fear, helplessness, or horror.
- PTSD has three core symptoms: re-experiencing, avoidance/emotional numbing, and hyperarousal.
- Events that can precipitate PTSD include physical or sexual assault, rape, torture, combat, industrial explosions, serious accidents, natural disasters, being taken hostage, displacement as a refugee, and terrorist attacks.
- Two SSRIs—paroxetine and sertraline—are the only drugs approved for PTSD. Both can reduce all three core symptoms of PTSD, and both can reduce associated anxiety and depression.

Central Nervous System Stimulants and Attention-Deficit/ Hyperactivity Disorder

Central nervous system (CNS) stimulants increase the activity of CNS neurons. Most stimulants act by enhancing neuronal excitation. A few act by suppressing neuronal inhibition. In sufficient doses, all CNS stimulants can cause convulsions.

Clinical applications of the CNS stimulants are limited. Currently these drugs have two principal indications: attention-deficit/hyperactivity disorder (ADHD) and narcolepsy. In the past, CNS stimulants were used to treat obesity and to counteract poisoning by CNS depressants, but these uses are no longer recommended.

Please note that CNS stimulants are not the same as antidepressants. The antidepressants act selectively to elevate mood, and hence can relieve depression without affecting other CNS functions. In contrast, CNS stimulants cannot elevate mood without producing generalized excitation. Accordingly, the role of CNS stimulants in treating depression is minor.

Our principal focus is on *amphetamines, methylphenidate* [Ritalin, others], and *methylxanthines* (e.g., caffeine). These agents are by far the most widely used CNS stimulants.

AMPHETAMINES

The amphetamine family consists of amphetamine, dextroamphetamine, and methamphetamine. All are powerful CNS stimulants. In addition to their CNS actions, amphetamines have significant actions in the periphery—actions that can cause cardiac stimulation and vasoconstriction. The amphetamines have a high potential for abuse.

Chemistry

Dextroamphetamine and Levamphetamine. The amphetamines are molecules that contain an asymmetric carbon atom. As a result, amphetamines can exist as mirror images of each other. Such compounds are termed *optical isomers* or *enantiomers*. Dextroamphetamine and levamphetamine, whose structures are shown in Figure 35–1, illustrate the mirror-image concept. As we can see, dextroamphetamine and levamphetamine both contain the same atomic components—but those components are arranged differently around the asymmetric carbon. Because of this structural difference, these compounds have somewhat different properties. For example, dextroamphetamine is more selective than levamphetamine for causing CNS stimulation, and hence produces fewer peripheral side effects.

Amphetamine. The term *amphetamine* refers not to a single compound but rather to a 50:50 mixture of dextroamphetamine and levamphetamine. (In chemistry, we refer to such equimolar mixtures of enantiomers as racemic.)

Methamphetamine. Methamphetamine is simply dextroamphetamine with an extra methyl group (see Fig. 35–1).

Mechanism of Action

The amphetamines act primarily by promoting release of norepinephrine (NE) and dopamine (DA), and partly by inhibiting reuptake of NE and DA. These actions take place in both the CNS and periphery. Most effects result from release of NE.

Pharmacologic Effects

Central Nervous System. The amphetamines have prominent effects on mood and arousal. At usual doses, these drugs increase wakefulness and alertness, reduce fatigue, elevate mood, and augment self-confidence and initiative. Eu-

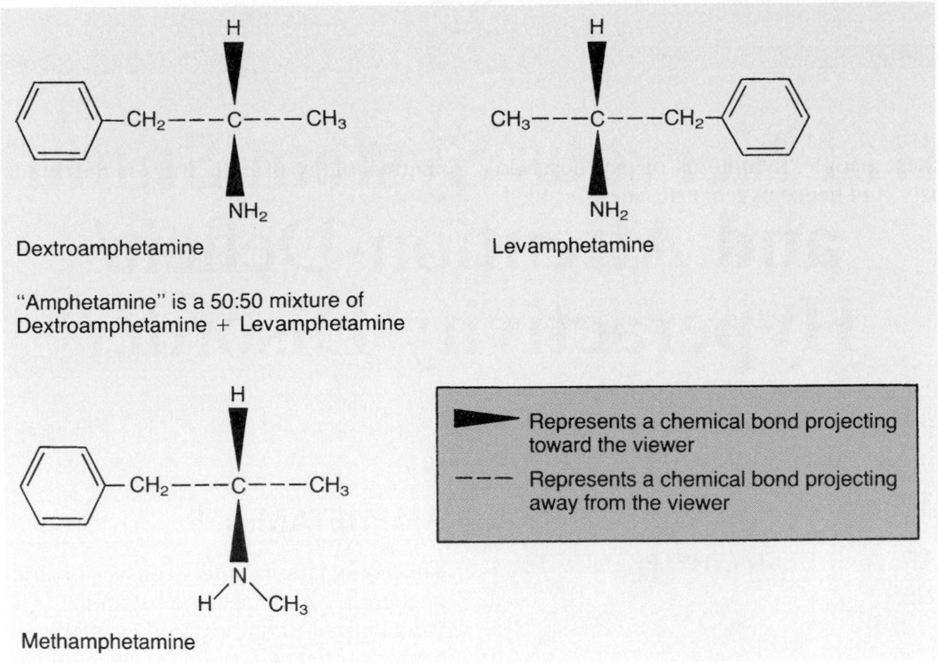

Figure 35–1 ■ **Structural formulas of the amphetamines.**
"Amphetamine" is a 50:50 mixture of dextroamphetamine and levamphetamine. Note that dextroamphetamine and levamphetamine are simply mirror images of each other. Both compounds contain the same atomic components.

phoria, talkativeness, and increased motor activity are likely. Task performance that had been reduced by fatigue or boredom improves.

In addition to their effects on mood and arousal, amphetamines can stimulate respiration and suppress appetite and perception of pain. Stimulation of the medullary respiratory center increases respiration. Effects on the hypothalamic feeding center depress appetite. By a mechanism that is not understood, amphetamines can enhance the analgesic effects of morphine and other opioids.

Cardiovascular System. Cardiovascular effects occur secondary to release of norepinephrine from sympathetic neurons. Norepinephrine acts in the heart to increase heart rate, atrioventricular (AV) conduction, and force of contraction. Excessive cardiac stimulation can produce dysrhythmias. In blood vessels, NE promotes constriction. Excessive vasoconstriction can produce hypertension.

Tolerance

With regular amphetamine use, tolerance develops to elevation of mood, suppression of appetite, and stimulation of the heart and blood vessels. In highly tolerant users, doses up to 1000 mg (IV) every few *hours* may be required to maintain *euphoric* effects. This compares with *daily* doses of 5 to 30 mg for nontolerant individuals.

Physical Dependence

Chronic use of amphetamines produces physical dependence. If amphetamines are abruptly withdrawn after prolonged use, an abstinence syndrome will result. Symptoms include exhaustion, depression, prolonged sleep, excessive eating, and a craving for more amphetamine. Sleep patterns may take months to normalize.

Abuse

Because amphetamines can produce euphoria (extreme mood elevation), these compounds have a high potential for abuse. Psychologic dependence can occur. (Users familiar with CNS stimulants find the psychologic effects of amphetamines nearly identical to those of cocaine.) Because of their abuse potential, amphetamines are classified under Schedule II of the Controlled Substances Act and must be dispensed accordingly. Whenever amphetamines are used therapeutically, their potential for abuse must be weighed against the potential benefits.

Adverse Effects

CNS Stimulation. Stimulation of the CNS can cause *insomnia, restlessness,* and *extreme loquaciousness.* These effects can occur at therapeutic doses.

Weight Loss. By suppressing appetite, amphetamines can cause weight loss. For people who are lean to start with, weight loss is considered an adverse effect. Conversely, for people who are obese, weight loss is desirable.

Cardiovascular Effects. Stimulation of the heart and blood vessels can result in *dysrhythmias, anginal pain,* and *hypertension.* Accordingly, amphetamines must be employed with extreme caution in patients with cardiovascular disease.

Psychosis. Excessive amphetamine use produces a state of paranoid psychosis, characterized by hallucinations and paranoid delusions (suspiciousness, feelings of being watched). Amphetamine-induced psychosis looks very much like schizophrenia. Symptoms are thought to result from release of DA. Consistent with this hypothesis is the observation that symptoms can be alleviated with a DA-receptor blocking agent (e.g., haloperidol). Following amphetamine withdrawal, psychosis usually resolves spontaneously within a week.

In some individuals, amphetamines can unmask latent schizophrenia. For these people, symptoms of psychosis do not clear spontaneously, and hence psychiatric care is needed.

Acute Toxicity

Symptoms. Overdose produces dizziness, confusion, hallucinations, paranoid delusions, palpitations, dysrhythmias, and hypertension. Death is rare. Fatal overdose is associated with convulsions, coma, and cerebral hemorrhage.

Treatment. Hallucinations can be controlled with chlorpromazine (an antipsychotic drug). An alpha-adrenergic blocker (e.g., phentolamine) can reduce hypertension (by promoting vasodilation). Because of its ability to block alpha receptors, chlorpromazine helps lower blood pressure. Seizures can be managed with diazepam. Acidification of the urine can accelerate amphetamine excretion.

Therapeutic Uses

Attention-Deficit/Hyperactivity Disorder. Amphetamines are useful in ADHD. This disorder and its treatment are discussed later.

Narcolepsy. Narcolepsy is a disorder characterized by daytime somnolence and uncontrollable attacks of sleep. By stimulating the CNS, amphetamines can promote arousal and thereby alleviate symptoms.

Obesity. Because they suppress appetite, amphetamines have been employed in programs for weight loss. However, because of their high potential for abuse, and because they offer no advantages over less dangerous drugs, amphetamines are not recommended for weight reduction.

Preparations, Dosage, and Administration

Three members of the amphetamine family are used clinically: dextroamphetamine sulfate, an amphetamine/dextroamphetamine mixture, and methamphetamine. A fourth agent—amphetamine sulfate (racemic amphetamine)—has been discontinued. In clinical practice, amphetamines are given *orally.* (These drugs are not approved for IV administration. Amphetamines for IV use are available only through illegal sources.) All amphetamines are regulated under Schedule II of the Controlled Substances Act and must be dispensed accordingly.

Dextroamphetamine Sulfate. Dextroamphetamine is available in short-duration (SD) and long-duration (LD) formulations. Both are indicated for ADHD.

Short-Duration. SD dextroamphetamine [Dexedrine, Dextrostat] is available in 5- and 10-mg tablets. Effects begin rapidly and last 4 to 6 hours. The usual dosage for ADHD is 5 mg at 8 AM, noon, and 4 PM.

Long-Duration. LD dextroamphetamine [Dexedrine Spansules] is available in 5-, 10-, and 15-mg capsules. Effects begin rapidly and last 6 to 8 hours. The usual dosage for ADHD is 10 mg once daily in the morning.

Amphetamine/Dextroamphetamine Mixture. Amphetamine mixture is available in SD and LD formulations. Both are used for ADHD.

Short-Duration. The SD formulation [Adderall] is available in 5-, 10-, 20-, and 30-mg tablets. Effects begin rapidly and last 4 to 6 hours. The usual dosage for ADHD is 5 mg twice daily, taken 5 hours apart.

Long-Duration. The LD formulation [Adderall-XR] is available in 5-, 10-, 15-, 20, 25-, and 30-mg capsules. Half of the dose is released immediately, and the remainder 4 hours later. As a result, effects begin rapidly and last 10 to 12 hours. The usual dosage is 20 mg once daily in the morning. This is equivalent to taking 10 mg of SD Adderall at 8 AM and again around noon.

Methamphetamine. Methamphetamine is indicated for ADHD and obesity, although it is not a preferred drug for either condition. The drug is available in SD and LD formulations. SD methamphetamine [Desoxyn] is available in 5-mg tablets. LD methamphetamine [Desoxyn Gradumet] is available in 5-, 10-, and 15-mg tablets. The usual daily dosage for ADHD is 20 to 25 mg, administered in two divided doses (if the SD tablets are used) or as one large dose (if the LD tablets are used).

METHYLPHENIDATE AND DEXMETHYLPHENIDATE

Methylphenidate and dexmethylphenidate are nearly identical in structure and pharmacologic actions. Furthermore, the pharmacology of both drugs is nearly identical to that of the amphetamines.

Methylphenidate

Although methylphenidate [Ritalin, others] is structurally dissimilar from the amphetamines, the pharmacologic actions of these drugs are essentially the same. Consequently, methylphenidate can be considered an amphetamine in all but structure and name. Methylphenidate and amphetamine share the same mechanism of action (promotion of NE and DA release, and inhibition of NE and DA reuptake), adverse effects (insomnia, reduced appetite, emotional lability), and abuse liability (Schedule II). Like amphetamine, methylphenidate is not a single compound, but rather a 50:50 mixture of dextro and levo isomers. The dextro isomer is highly active, whereas the levo isomer is not. Methylphenidate has two indications: ADHD and narcolepsy.

Preparations, Dosage, and Administration

Methylphenidate is available in three types of formulations: short duration (SD), intermediate duration (ID), and long duration (LD). All three are indicated for ADHD. As a rule, the SD and ID formulations must be taken bid or tid, whereas the LD formulations can be taken just once a day.

Short-Duration. SD methylphenidate [Ritalin, Methylin] is available in 5-, 10-, and 20-mg tablets. Effects begin rapidly and last 3 to 5 hours. Because effects are brief, dosing must be done 2 or 3 times a day. The usual dosage for ADHD is 10 mg at 8 AM and noon, and 5 mg at 4 PM.

Intermediate-Duration. ID methylphenidate [Ritalin SR, Metadate ER, Methylin ER] is available in 12- and 20-mg tablets. Effects are *delayed* and last 4 to 8 hours. Dosing is done once or twice daily. For children with ADHD, the usual dosage is 20 to 40 mg in the morning, supplemented with 20 mg in the early afternoon when needed.

Long-Duration. Three LD products are available. Their trade names are Concerta, Metadate CD, and Ritalin LA. With all three, dosing is done once daily in the morning; no afternoon dose is needed.

Concerta. Concerta is available in 18-, 27-, 36-, and 54-mg tablets. Each tablet has an outer coating of immediate-release methylphenidate and a special inner core that releases the remainder of each dose gradually. As a result, effects begin rapidly and last up to 14 hours. Because of their special architecture, Concerta tablets must be swallowed whole, not crushed or chewed. The tablet shell may not dissolve fully in the GI tract. Accordingly, patients should be warned they may see tablet "ghosts" in the stool.

Dosage depends on whether the patient is already taking methylphenidate (SD or ID). For children *not* already taking methylphenidate, the initial dosage is 18 mg once daily in the morning. Dosage can be increased to a maximum of 54 mg once daily. For children who *are* taking methylphenidate (SD or ID), the initial dosage of Concerta is as follows:

- For those taking 5 mg bid or tid of SD methylphenidate or 20 mg once daily of ID methylphenidate, start with 18 mg of Concerta.
- For those taking 10 mg bid or tid of SD or 40 mg once daily of ID, start with 36 mg of Concerta.
- For those taking 15 mg bid or tid of SD or 60 mg once daily of ID, start with 54 mg of Concerta.

Metadate CD. Metadate CD is available in 20-mg capsules that contain immediate-release and delayed-release beads. The beads release 30% of the dose rapidly, and the remaining 70% four hours later. As a result, plasma levels peak twice—at 1.5 and 4.5 hours. This is the same pattern produced by taking SD methylphenidate twice daily. For ADHD patients *not* already taking methylphenidate, the initial dosage is 20 mg once daily in the morning. This can be gradually increased to a maximum of 60 mg once daily. For patients who *are* already taking methylphenidate, start with 20 mg of Metadate once daily (for those taking 10 mg of SD methylphenidate bid), or with 40 mg of Metadate once daily (for those taking 20 mg of SD methylphenidate bid). If needed, Metadate CD capsules can be opened and sprinkled on a small amount of soft food (e.g., applesauce) just prior to ingestion.

Ritalin LA. Ritalin LA is available in 20-, 30-, and 40-mg extended-release capsules. This formulation is much like Metadate CD in that part of the dose is released immediately and the remainder is released 4 hours later. Dosing is done *once daily in the morning.* As with Metadate CD and Concerta, dosage depends on whether the patient is already taking methylphenidate (SD or ID). For children *not* already taking methylphenidate, the initial dosage is 20 mg. Dosage can be gradually increased to a maximum of 60 mg. For children who *are* taking methylphenidate (SD or ID), the initial dosage is as follows:

- For those taking 10 mg bid of SD methylphenidate or 20 mg qd of ID methylphenidate, start with 20 mg of Ritalin LA.
- For those taking 15 mg bid of SD, start with 30 mg of Ritalin LA.
- For those taking 20 mg bid of SD or 40 mg qd of ID, start with 40 mg of Ritalin LA.
- For those taking 30 mg bid of SD or 60 mg qd of ID, start with 60 mg of Ritalin LA.

Dexmethylphenidate

Dexmethylphenidate [Focalin], a new drug for ADHD, is simply the dextro isomer of methylphenidate. As noted, the dextro isomer accounts for most of the pharmacologic activity of methylphenidate, a 50:50 mixture of dextro and levo isomers. Accordingly, the pharmacology of dexmethylphenidate is nearly identical to that of methylphenidate. The only difference is that the dosage of dexmethylphenidate is one-half the dosage of methylphenidate. Dexmethylphenidate is available in 2.5-, 5-, and 10-mg tablets. For children currently being treated with methylphenidate, the initial dosage of dexmethylphenidate is one-half the methylphenidate dosage. For children who are not currently being treated, the initial dosage is 2.5 mg twice daily. The maximum dosage is 10 mg twice daily. Dexmethylphenidate is a Schedule II drug and must be dispensed accordingly.

METHYLXANTHINES

The methylxanthines are derivatives of xanthine—hence the family name. As shown in Figure 35–2, these compounds consist of a xanthine nucleus to which one or more methyl groups is attached. Caffeine, the most familiar member of the family, will serve as our prototype.

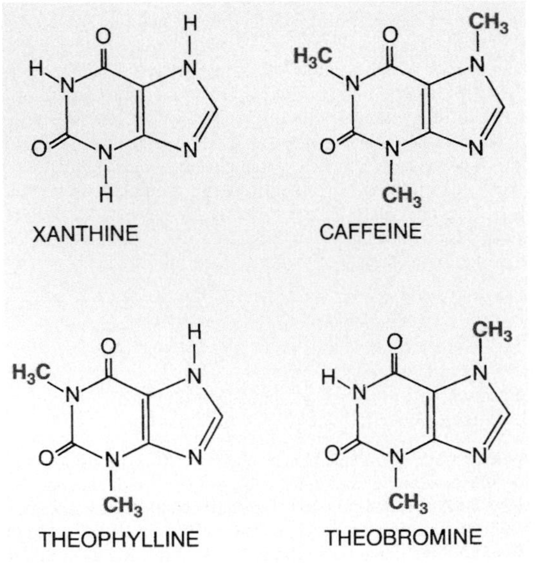

Figure 35–2 ■ **Structural formulas of the methylxanthines.**

Caffeine

Caffeine is consumed worldwide for its stimulant effects. In the United States, per capita consumption is about 200 mg/day—mostly in the form of coffee. Although clinical applications of caffeine are few, caffeine remains of interest because of its widespread ingestion for nonmedical purposes.

Dietary Sources

Caffeine can be found in chocolates, desserts, soft drinks, and beverages prepared from various natural products. Common dietary sources are coffee, tea, and cola drinks. The caffeine in cola drinks derives partly from the cola nut and partly from caffeine added by the manufacturer. Caffeine is also present in many noncola soft drinks. The caffeine content of some common foods and beverages is shown in Table 35–1.

TABLE 35–1 ■ Dietary Caffeine		
Product	**Amount**	**Caffeine (mg)**
Coffee		
Brewed	8 oz	135
Instant	8 oz	95
Expresso (Starbucks)	1 oz	89
Decaffeinated	8 oz	5
Tea		
Brewed (Lipton)	8 oz	35–40
Snapple ice tea	16 oz	48
Celestial Seasonings Herbal Tea, all varieties	8 oz	0
Lipton Natural Brew Iced Tea Mix, decaffeinated	8 oz	<5
Soda		
Jolt	12 oz	71
Josta	12 oz	58
Mountain Dew	12 oz	55
Diet Coke	12 oz	47
Coca-Cola	12 oz	45
Dr. Pepper	12 oz	41
Orange soda, Sunkist	12 oz	40
Pepsi-Cola	12 oz	37
7-UP	12 oz	0
Sprite	12 oz	0
Caffeinated Water		
Java Water	16.9 oz	125
Krank20	16.9 oz	100
Aqua Blast	16.9 oz	90
Water Joe	16.9 oz	60–70
Aqua Java	16.9 oz	50–60
Ice Cream and Yogurt		
Starbucks Coffee Ice Cream	1/2 cup	20–30
Häagen-Dazs Coffee Fudge Ice Cream	1/2 cup	15
Dannon Coffee Yogurt	4 oz	22
Miscellaneous		
Cocoa	8 oz	2–50
Chocolate milk	1.5 oz	3–11
Hershey's Bar (milk chocolate)	1.5 oz	10
Hershey's Special Dark Chocolate Bar	1.5 oz	31
Baker's chocolate	1.5 oz	38–53

Mechanism of Action

Several mechanisms of action have been proposed. These include (1) reversible blockade of adenosine receptors, (2) enhancement of calcium permeability in the sarcoplasmic reticulum, and (3) inhibition of cyclic nucleotide phosphodiesterase, resulting in accumulation of cyclic adenosine monophosphate (cyclic AMP). Blockade of adenosine receptors appears responsible for most of caffeine's effects.

Pharmacologic Effects

Central Nervous System. In low doses, caffeine decreases drowsiness and fatigue and increases the capacity for prolonged intellectual exertion. With increasing dosage, caffeine produces nervousness, insomnia, and tremors. When administered in very large amounts, the drug can cause convulsions. Despite popular belief, there is little evidence that caffeine can restore mental function during intoxication with alcohol.

Heart. High doses of caffeine stimulate the heart. When caffeine-containing beverages are consumed in excessive amounts, dysrhythmias may result.

Blood Vessels. Caffeine affects blood vessels in the periphery differently from those in the CNS. In the periphery, caffeine promotes *vasodilation,* whereas in the CNS, caffeine promotes *vasoconstriction.* Constriction of cerebral blood vessels is thought to underlie caffeine's ability to relieve headache.

Bronchi. Caffeine and other methylxanthines cause relaxation of bronchial smooth muscle, and thereby promote bronchodilation. Theophylline is an especially effective bronchodilator and, because of this action, can be used to treat asthma (see Chapter 71).

Kidney. Caffeine is a diuretic. The mechanism underlying increased urine formation is not fully understood.

Reproduction. Caffeine may pose a risk of birth defects and first-trimester abortion. When applied to cells in culture, caffeine can cause chromosomal damage and mutations. However, the concentrations required are much greater than can be achieved by drinking caffeine-containing beverages. Also, although there is clear proof that caffeine can cause birth defects in animals, studies have failed to document birth defects in humans. Nonetheless, there *is* good evidence that moderately heavy caffeine consumption (500 mg/day) increases the risk of first-trimester spontaneous abortion, especially among women who do *not* smoke. Accordingly, in order to reduce the risk of spontaneous abortion (and possibly a risk of birth defects), it would seem prudent to minimize caffeine consumption during pregnancy.

Pharmacokinetics

Caffeine is readily absorbed from the GI tract, and achieves peak plasma levels within 1 hour. Plasma half-life ranges from 3 to 7 hours. Elimination is by hepatic metabolism.

Therapeutic Uses

Neonatal Apnea. Premature infants may experience prolonged apnea (lasting 15 seconds or more) along with bradycardia. Hypoxemia and neurologic damage may result. Caffeine and other methylxanthines can reduce the number and duration of apnea episodes and can promote a more regular pattern of breathing.

Promoting Wakefulness. Caffeine is used commonly as an aid to staying awake. The drug is marketed in various over-the-counter preparations [Maximum Strength NoDoz, Vivarin, others] for this purpose. Of course, individuals desiring increased alertness needn't take a pill; they can get just as much caffeine by drinking coffee or some other caffeine-containing beverage.

Other Applications. Intravenous caffeine can help relieve headache induced by spinal puncture. The drug is used orally to enhance analgesia induced by opioids and non-narcotic agents (e.g., aspirin).

Acute Toxicity

Caffeine poisoning is characterized by intensification of the responses seen at low doses. Stimulation of the CNS results in excitement, restlessness, and insomnia; if the dosage is very high, convulsions may occur. Tachycardia and respiratory stimulation are likely. Sensory phenomena (ringing in the ears, flashing lights) are common. Death from caffeine overdose is rare. When fatalities have occurred, between 5 and 10 gm have been ingested.

Preparations, Dosage, and Administration

For Promoting Wakefulness. Caffeine is available in three formulations for promoting wakefulness: 200-mg tablets, 200-mg capsules, and 75-mg lozenges. The usual dosage for promoting alertness is 100 to 200 mg every 3 to 4 hours as needed.

For Neonatal Apnea. Caffeine citrate [Cafcit] is used for neonatal apnea. The drug is available in oral and IV solutions. Both have the same concentration: 20 mg/ml. Treatment consists of an IV loading dose (20 mg/kg) followed every 24 hours by an oral or IV maintenance dose (5 mg/kg). Note: The amount of caffeine *base* in a 20-mg dose of caffeine citrate is only 10 mg (i.e., one half of the total dose on a milligram basis).

Theophylline

Theophylline has pharmacologic actions much like those of caffeine. Like caffeine, theophylline is an effective CNS stimulant. However, in contrast to caffeine, theophylline is used to treat asthma; benefits derive from causing bronchodilation. Use in asthma is discussed in Chapter 71.

Theobromine

Theobromine is a methylxanthine that occurs naturally in the seeds of *Theobroma cacao,* from which cocoa and chocolate are made. The caffeine content of these seeds is relatively low. Although there are similarities between theobromine and caffeine, these compounds do differ. The most distinct difference is that caffeine is a CNS stimulant, whereas theobromine is not. Accordingly, any CNS excitation produced by ingestion of cocoa and chocolate derives from their caffeine content and not from theobromine.

MISCELLANEOUS CNS STIMULANTS

Pemoline

Actions, Uses, and Adverse Effects. Pemoline [Cylert] is a CNS stimulant with effects much like those of the amphetamines. However, the drug differs from the amphetamines in two major ways: (1) it causes less cardiac stimulation and vasoconstriction, and (2) it can cause liver failure. The drug's only approved indication is ADHD (see below). Pemoline has been used investigationally in narcolepsy but is not approved for this application. The abuse potential of pemoline is less than that of the amphetamines and methylphenidate. As a result, pemoline is a Schedule IV drug, compared with Schedule II for the amphetamines and methylphenidate. Adverse effects of pemoline are generally like those of other CNS stimulants.

Rarely, pemoline causes *acute liver failure.* Deaths have occurred. Patients should be taught about signs of liver failure (jaundice, dark urine, nausea, fatigue) and instructed to discontinue the drug if they develop. Liver function should be assessed prior to treatment and every 2 weeks thereafter. Unfortunately, since liver failure may develop suddenly, such routine testing may not be helpful.

Preparations, Dosage, and Administration. Pemoline [Cylert, PemADD] is dispensed in standard tablets (18.75, 37.5, and 75 mg) and chewable tablets (37.5 mg). The usual dosage for ADHD is 56.25 mg/day, administered as a single dose in the morning. Because of the risk of liver failure, physicians must obtain written informed consent prior to prescribing the drug.

Modafinil

Modafinil [Provigil] is a CNS stimulant indicated only for narcolepsy, a disorder characterized by excessive daytime sleepiness and sudden attacks of sleep. In patients with narcolepsy, modafinil increases wakefulness, but only to about 50% of the level seen in normal people. In contrast, methylphenidate and dextroamphetamine increase wakefulness to about 70% of normal. Modafinil is not an amphetamine, and its mechanism of action in narcolepsy is unknown. The drug has been used investigationally to augment the effects of antidepressants. In addition, modafinil is being used off-label to ward off sleepiness. Users have remained awake for 2 to 3 days with no apparent ill effects, including the cardiovascular and CNS stimulation associated with amphetamines.

Modafinil is rapidly absorbed from the GI tract. Plasma levels peak in 2 to 4 hours. Food decreases the rate of absorption but not the extent. Elimination is by hepatic metabolism followed by renal excretion. The half-life is about 15 hours.

Modafinil is generally well tolerated. The most common adverse effects are headache, nausea, nervousness, diarrhea, and rhinitis. Modafinil does not disrupt nighttime sleep. In clinical trials, only 5% of patients dropped out because of undesired effects. Subjective effects—euphoria; altered perception, thinking, and feeling—are like those of other CNS stimulants. Because of its subjective effects, modafinil is regulated as a Schedule IV substance. Physical dependence and withdrawal have not been reported.

Modafinil inhibits some forms of cytochrome P450 (CYP) and induces others. Induction of CYP3A4 may accelerate the metabolism of oral contraceptives, cyclosporine, and certain other drugs, thereby causing their levels to decline. Caution should be exercised.

Modafinil is available in 100- and 200-mg tablets. The usual dosage is 200 mg/day, given as a single dose in the morning. Dosage should be decreased by 50% in patients with severe hepatic dysfunction. Dosage reduction may also be needed in the elderly.

Strychnine

Strychnine was introduced in the 16th century as a rat poison. At one time the drug was also employed therapeutically. Although strychnine is no longer used as a medicine, it remains a source of accidental poisoning, and is of interest for that reason.

Strychnine is a powerful convulsant that stimulates the CNS at all levels. Stimulation results from blockade of receptors for glycine, an inhibitory neurotransmitter.

Strychnine Poisoning

Causes. A common cause of strychnine poisoning is accidental ingestion of strychnine-based rodenticides. Poisoning also occurs through the use of "street drugs" to which strychnine has been added. (Since strychnine does not enhance the effects of illicit drugs, the practice of mixing this agent with street drugs is not only dangerous, it also lacks any pharmacologic rationale.) The lethal dose is about 15 mg in children, and 50 to 100 mg in adults.

Symptoms. The first manifestation of poisoning is stiffness in the muscles of the face and neck. This is followed by a generalized increase in reflex excitability. During the early stages of poisoning, the victim is fully conscious. As poisoning progresses, convulsions occur. Strychnine-induced convulsions are characterized by tonic contraction of all voluntary muscles; contraction of the diaphragm, abdominal muscles, and thoracic muscles stops respiration. Convulsive episodes alternate with periods of depression until the victim dies or until the poisoning is successfully treated. Few patients survive beyond the fifth convulsive episode; some are killed by the first. Death is from respiratory arrest.

Treatment. Management is directed primarily at control of convulsions and support of respiration. Intravenous diazepam is the treatment of choice to suppress convulsions. If poisoning is severe, general anesthesia or neuromuscular blockade may be needed to eliminate convulsions. If anticonvulsant therapy fails to permit adequate breathing, mechanical support of respiration is indicated.

Doxapram

Doxapram [Dopram] stimulates the CNS at all levels. The drug is employed clinically to stimulate respiration. However, since the doses required are close to those that can produce generalized CNS stimulation and convulsions, doxapram must be used with great care. Furthermore, although doxapram is labeled for treatment of general CNS depressant poisoning, its use for this purpose should be discontinued: Experience has shown that respiratory depression from CNS depressant poisoning can be managed more safely and effectively with mechanical support of ventilation than with pharmacologic stimulation of respiration.

Cocaine

Cocaine is a powerful CNS stimulant with a high potential for abuse. The only clinical application of this drug—local anesthesia—is discussed in Chapter 25. The basic pharmacology of cocaine and cocaine abuse are discussed in Chapter 38.

ATTENTION-DEFICIT/ HYPERACTIVITY DISORDER

ADHD in Children

ADHD is the most common neuropsychiatric disorder of childhood. In the United States, over 2 million school-age children are affected—an average of one child with ADHD for every classroom. The incidence in boys is 2 to 3 times the incidence in girls. Symptoms begin between ages 3 and 7, and typically persist into the teens. The majority (60% to 70%) of children respond well to stimulant drugs. Methylphenidate [Ritalin, others] is the agent employed most.

Signs and Symptoms

ADHD is characterized by *inattention, hyperactivity,* and *impulsivity.* Affected children are fidgety, unable to concentrate on schoolwork, and unable to wait their turn; switch excessively from one activity to another; call out excessively in class; and never complete tasks. For a diagnosis to be made, symptoms must appear prior to age 7 and be present for at least 6 months. Since other disorders—especially anxiety and depression—may cause similar symptoms, diagnosis must be done carefully. Specific diagnostic criteria for ADHD, as described in the *Diagnostic and Statistical Manual of Mental Disorders, Fourth Edition,* are summarized in Table 35–2. Depending on the symptom profile, ADHD can be subclassified as predominately inattentive type, predominately hyperactive-impulsive type, or combined type. Former names for ADHD—*hyperkinetic syndrome and minimal brain dysfunction*—are misleading and have been abandoned.

Etiology

Although various theories have been proposed, the underlying pathophysiology of ADHD has not been established. Several theories implicate dysregulation in neuronal pathways that employ NE and DA as transmitters. These theories would be consistent with the beneficial effects of stimulant drugs (which promote release of these transmitters and, to some degree, block their reuptake) as well as atomoxetine (a new drug that blocks NE reuptake).

Management Overview

Multiple strategies may be employed to manage ADHD. In addition to drugs, the treatment program can include family therapy, parent training, and cognitive therapy for the child. Although many experts believe that a combination of cognitive therapy and stimulant drugs constitutes the most effective treatment, there is no proof that this is true. A large trial to test this assumption is in progress.

Drug Therapy I: CNS Stimulants

Stimulant drugs are the mainstay of therapy. Drugs with proven efficacy include *methylphenidate* [Ritalin, others], *dexmethylphenidate* [Focalin], *dextroamphetamine* [Dexedrine, others], an *amphetamine mixture* [Adderall], and *pemoline* [Cylert]. Of these, methylphenidate is by far the most commonly employed: Over 70% of children with ADHD receive this drug. Although pemoline is very effective, it can cause life-threatening liver failure, and hence is used only rarely. Although all of the stimulants are very similar, they are not identical. As a result, children who fail to respond to one agent may still respond to another.

Response to stimulants can be dramatic. These drugs can increase attention span and goal-oriented behavior while decreasing impulsiveness, distractibility, hyperactivity, and restlessness. Overall behavior becomes more tolerable to parents and teachers. Tests of cognitive function (memory, reading, arithmetic) often improve significantly.

Although reduction of impulsiveness and hyperactivity with a stimulant may seem paradoxical—it isn't. Stimulants don't suppress rowdy behavior directly. Rather, they improve attention and focus. Impulsiveness and hyperactivity decline because the child is now able to concentrate on the task at hand. It should be noted that stimulants do not create *positive* behavior; they only reduce *negative* behavior. Accordingly, these drugs cannot give a child good study skills and other appropriate behaviors. Rather, these must be learned once the disruptive behavior is no longer an impediment.

The dosing schedule employed is important, and determined by the time course of the formulation selected. As discussed above (and shown in Table 35–3), CNS stimulants are available in short-, intermediate-, and long-duration formulations. With the SD and ID formulations, the child usually takes two or three doses a day. In contrast, the LD formulations are taken just once a day. Not only is once-daily dosing more convenient, it saves the child from the embarrassment and stigma associated with taking medicine at school. Accordingly, LD formulations (e.g., Adderall-XR, Concerta) are generally preferred. Dosage is determined by monitoring for improvement in symptoms and appearance of side effects.

Principal adverse effects of the stimulants are *insomnia* and *growth suppression*. Insomnia results from CNS stimulation, and can be minimized by reducing the size of the afternoon dose and taking the afternoon dose no later than 4:00 PM. Growth suppression occurs secondary to appetite suppression. Growth suppression can be minimized by administering stimulants during or after meals, which reduces the impact of appetite suppression, and by taking "drug holidays" on weekends and in the summer, which creates the opportunity for growth to catch up. Once use of stimulants has ceased, a rebound increase in growth takes place; as a result, adult height is usually not affected. Other adverse effects include *headache* and *abdominal pain,* which have an incidence of 10%, and *lethargy* and *listlessness,* which can occur when dosage is excessive.

Stimulants should be interrupted periodically. The rationale for this practice is to (1) assess the need for continued treatment and (2) minimize suppression of growth. Many children can reduce or eliminate drug use on weekends and holidays. In no case should treatment continue for more than 1 school year without interruption. The summer school break is often a good opportunity for a prolonged drug holiday, with treatment resuming, if indicated, when school resumes.

Drug Therapy II: Atomoxetine

Description and Therapeutic Effects. Atomoxetine [Strattera] is a unique, new drug approved for ADHD in adults and children. It's the first *nonstimulant* approved for ADHD

and the only drug approved for ADHD in adults (along with children). Older nonstimulants, such as imipramine and bupropion, although *used* for ADHD, are not actually *approved* for ADHD. In contrast to the CNS stimulants, atomoxetine has no potential for abuse, and hence is not regulated as a controlled substance. As a result, prescriptions can be re-

---

TABLE 35–2 ■ DSM-IV-TR Diagnostic Criteria for ADHD

A. Either (1) or (2)

   (1) **Inattention.** Six (or more) of the following symptoms have persisted for at least 6 months:

   • Often fails to give close attention to details or makes careless mistakes in schoolwork, work, or other activities
   • Often has difficulty sustaining attention in tasks or play activities
   • Often does not seem to listen when spoken to directly
   • Often does not follow through on instructions and fails to finish schoolwork, chores, or duties in the workplace
   • Often has difficulty organizing tasks and activities
   • Often avoids, dislikes, or is reluctant to engage in tasks that require sustained mental effort (e.g., schoolwork, homework)
   • Often loses things necessary for tasks or activities (e.g., toys, school assignments, pencils, books, tools)
   • Is often easily distracted by extraneous stimuli
   • Is often forgetful in daily activities

   (2) **Hyperactivity-impulsivity.** Six (or more) of the following symptoms have persisted for at least 6 months:

   Hyperactivity
   • Often fidgets with hands or feet or squirms in seat
   • Often leaves seat in classroom or in other situations in which remaining seated is expected
   • Often runs about or climbs excessively in situations in which it is inappropriate (in adolescents or adults, may be limited to subjective feelings of restlessness)
   • Often has difficulty playing or engaging in leisure activities quietly
   • Is often "on the go" or often acts as if "driven by a motor"
   • Often talks excessively

   Impulsivity
   • Often blurts out answers before questions have been completed
   • Often has difficulty awaiting turn
   • Often interrupts or intrudes on others (e.g., butts into conversations or games)

B. Some hyperactive-impulsive or inattentive symptoms were present before age 7 years.

C. Symptoms are present in two or more settings (e.g., at school [or work] and at home).

D. There must be clear evidence of clinically significant impairment in social, academic, or occupational functioning.

E. The symptoms do not occur exclusively during the course of a pervasive developmental disorder, schizophrenia, or other psychotic disorder, and are not better accounted for by another mental disorder (e.g., mood disorder, anxiety disorder, dissociative disorder, or a personality disorder).

Modified from the Diagnostic and Statistical Manual of Mental Disorders, Fourth Edition, Text Revision. Washington, DC, American Psychiatric Press, 2000, with permission. Copyright © 2000 American Psychiatric Association.

TABLE 35–3 ▪■ Stimulant Drugs Used for Attention-Deficit/Hyperactivity Disorder

Drug	Trade Name	Duration (hr)	Dosing Schedule	Usual Dosage
Methylphenidate				
Short-duration	Ritalin Methylin	3–5	bid–tid	10 mg at 8 AM and noon, and 5 mg at 4 PM
Intermediate-duration	Ritalin SR Metadate ER Methylin ER	6–8	qd–bid	20 mg in AM plus an early afternoon dose if needed
Long-duration	Concerta	Up to 14	qd	36 mg in AM
	Metadate CD	6–8		40 mg in AM
	Ritalin LA	7–9	qd	60 mg in AM
Dexmethylphenidate				
Short-duration	Focalin	4–5	bid	5 mg at 8 AM and noon, and 2.5 mg at 4 PM
Dextroamphetamine				
Short-duration	Dexedrine Dextrostat	4–6	bid–tid	5 mg at 8 AM, noon, and 4 PM
Long-duration	Dexedrine Spansules	6–10	qd–bid	10 mg at 8 AM
Amphetamine Mixture				
Short-duration	Adderall	4–6	bid	5 mg in AM and 5 hours later
Long-duration	Adderall-XR	10–12	qd	20 mg in AM

filled over the phone, making atomoxetine more convenient than the stimulants. Like the long-acting stimulants, atomoxetine can be administered just once a day.

In clinical trials comparing atomoxetine with placebo in children or adults with ADHD, atomoxetine was clearly superior at reducing symptoms. Benefits were similar whether the drug was given once a day or in two divided doses. It should be noted that responses develop slowly: The initial response takes a few days to develop, and the maximal response takes 1 to 3 weeks. This contrasts with the CNS stimulants, whose effects are near-maximal with the first dose.

To date, there have been no well-controlled, blinded trials comparing atomoxetine directly with the CNS stimulants. Accordingly, we don't know if these treatments are equally effective, or if one is superior to the other.

Mechanism of Action. Atomoxetine is a *selective inhibitor of NE reuptake,* and hence causes NE to accumulate at synapses. Although the precise relationship between this neurochemical action and symptom relief is unknown, it would appear that *adaptive changes* that occur following uptake blockade underlie benefits. Why? Because uptake blockade occurs immediately, but full therapeutic effects are not seen for at least a week—suggesting that, after uptake blockade occurs, additional processes must take place before benefits can be seen.

Pharmacokinetics. Atomoxetine is rapidly and completely absorbed following oral administration. Plasma levels peak in 1 to 3 hours, depending on whether the drug was taken without or with food. Atomoxetine is metabolized in the liver, primarily by CYP2D6 (the 2D6 isozyme of cytochrome P450). For most patients, the half-life is 5 hours. However, for 5% to 10% of patients, the half-life is much longer: 24 hours. Why? Because they have an atypical form of CYP2D6, which metabolizes atomoxetine slowly. Dosage should be reduced in these people.

Adverse Effects. In Children. Like the CNS stimulants, atomoxetine is generally well tolerated. In clinical trials, the most common effects included GI reactions (dyspepsia, nausea, and vomiting), reduced appetite, dizziness, somnolence, mood swings, and trouble sleeping. Sexual dysfunction and urinary retention were seen in adults. Severe allergic reactions, including angioneurotic edema, occurred rarely. If allergy develops, patients should discontinue the drug and contact the physician immediately. Atomoxetine may cause a small increase in blood pressure and heart rate, and hence should be used with caution by patients with hypertension, tachycardia, and other cardiovascular disorders.

Perhaps the biggest concern is weight loss and growth retardation, which can occur secondary to suppression of appetite. Among children who used atomoxetine for 18 months or longer, mean height and weight percentiles declined. Because experience with the drug is limited, we don't know if expected adult height will be affected. Nor do we know if "drug holidays" would have an impact on growth.

Drug Interactions. Combining atomoxetine with an *MAO inhibitor* (e.g., isocarboxazid [Marplan], phenelzine [Nardil]) can cause hypertensive crisis (owing to accumulation of NE at synapses in the periphery). Accordingly, these drugs must not be used together or within 3 weeks of each other.

Inhibitors of CYP2D6 can increase levels of atomoxetine, and hence must be used with caution. Common examples include paroxetine [Paxil], fluoxetine [Prozac], and quinidine.

Role in ADHD Therapy. Because atomoxetine is a new drug, its role in ADHD has not been established. Yes, the drug appears both safe and effective, and it lacks the potential for abuse. However, well-controlled trials comparing it directly with the CNS stimulants have not been conducted. Furthermore, we have no information on the drug's long-term dangers, including effects on growth. Accordingly, because the

CNS stimulants have a long record of safety and efficacy, whereas atomoxetine does not, it would seem prudent to reserve the new drug for patients who are unresponsive to or intolerant of CNS stimulants—at least until much more is known. Certainly, in the absence of a compelling reason, patients doing well on the stimulants shouldn't switch.

Preparations, Dosage, and Administration. Atomoxetine [Strattera] is available in capsules (10, 18, 25, 40, and 60 mg) that should be swallowed whole, either with or without food. Dosage is based on body weight as follows:

- Children who weigh *less than 70 kg*—Start with 0.5 mg/kg/day and then, after at least 3 days, increase to the recommended target of 1.2 mg/kg/day. The maximum dosage is 1.4 mg/kg/day or 100 mg, whichever is smaller.
- Children who weigh *more than 70 kg* and *all adults*—Start with 40 mg/day and then, after at least 3 days, increase to the recommended target of 80 mg/day. Do not exceed 100 mg/day.

Two dosing schedules may be used: patients may either (1) take the total daily dose all at once in the morning or (2) divide the dosage up, taking half in the morning and half in the late afternoon or early evening. Note that, with either schedule, dosing during school hours is unnecessary.

Dosage should be reduced in patients who are slow metabolizers, either because of hepatic insufficiency or atypical CYP2D6.

Drug Therapy III: Antidepressants

Three antidepressants—desipramine, imipramine, and bupropion—can reduce behavioral symptoms in children with ADHD. However, these antidepressants are less effective than CNS stimulants and are not approved for ADHD. Accordingly, they are generally reserved for children who have not responded to trials with at least two different stimulants.

Tricyclic Antidepressants. Desipramine [Norpramin] and imipramine [Tofranil] can reduce symptoms in children with ADHD. These drugs decrease hyperactivity but have little effect on impulsivity and inattention. Responses develop slowly. Beneficial effects begin in 2 to 3 weeks and reach a maximum around 6 weeks. Tolerance frequently develops within a few months. In contrast to the stimulants, which can be discontinued on weekends, antidepressants must be taken continuously. Adverse effects include sedation and anticholinergic effects (e.g., dry mouth, blurred vision, urinary retention, constipation). More importantly, sudden death (from cardiotoxicity) has occurred in at least three children. Compared with stimulants, antidepressants have their benefits (no insomnia, abuse potential, or suppression of appetite and growth) as well as drawbacks (anticholinergic effects, delayed onset, tolerance, less efficacy, risk of sudden death). Since these antidepressants are less effective and more dangerous than the stimulants, they are considered second-choice drugs. Dosages for ADHD range from 2 to 5 mg/kg/day, administered in two or three divided doses. The basic pharmacology of the antidepressants is presented in Chapter 31.

Bupropion. Bupropion [Wellbutrin] can reduce behavioral symptoms of ADHD, but is less effective than stimulants. The drug lacks the adverse effects associated with tricyclic antidepressants (e.g., cardiotoxicity, anticholinergic effects), but does pose a risk of seizures. Like the tricyclic antidepressants, bupropion is considered a second-choice drug for ADHD. Dosage is 100 to 150 mg twice a day. The basic pharmacology of bupropion is presented in Chapter 31.

ADHD in Adults

Contrary to traditional assumptions, we now know that ADHD frequently persists into adulthood. Symptoms include poor concentration, stress intolerance, antisocial behavior, outbursts of anger, and inability to maintain a routine. Just how many children with ADHD are likely to exhibit symptoms as adults? The incidence is uncertain; estimates range widely—from just a few percent to as high as 70%. Much of this uncertainty stems from a lack of clearly defined diagnostic criteria.

As in childhood ADHD, stimulants are the principal drugs used in adults. Methylphenidate is prescribed most often. About 33% of adults fail to respond to stimulants or cannot tolerate their side effects. For these patients, a trial with desipramine or bupropion may be of help.

⠶ KEY POINTS

- The amphetamine family consists of dextroamphetamine, amphetamine (a racemic mixture of dextroamphetamine and levamphetamine), and methamphetamine.
- The amphetamines produce their effect primarily by causing release of NE and DA from neurons, and partly by blocking NE and DA reuptake.
- Through actions in the CNS, the amphetamines can increase wakefulness and alertness, reduce fatigue, elevate mood, stimulate respiration, and suppress appetite.
- By promoting release of norepinephrine from peripheral neurons, amphetamines can cause vasoconstriction and cardiac effects (increased heart rate, increased AV conduction, and increased force of contraction).
- The most common adverse effects of amphetamines are insomnia and weight loss. Amphetamines may also cause psychosis and adverse cardiovascular effects (dysrhythmias, angina, hypertension).
- The principal indications for amphetamines are ADHD and narcolepsy.
- The pharmacology of methylphenidate is nearly identical to that of the amphetamines.
- Methylphenidate is the drug most frequently prescribed for ADHD.
- Methylphenidate and other CNS stimulants reduce symptoms of ADHD by enhancing the child's ability to focus.
- Atomoxetine is the only nonstimulant approved for ADHD.
- Caffeine and other methylxanthines act primarily by blocking adenosine receptors.
- Responses to caffeine are dose dependent: low doses decrease drowsiness and fatigue; higher doses cause nervousness, insomnia, and tremors; and huge doses cause convulsions.
- Caffeine has two principal uses: treatment of apnea in premature infants and reversal of drowsiness.

Summary of Major Nursing Implications*

AMPHETAMINES, METHYLPHENIDATE, AND DEXMETHYLPHENIDATE

Preadministration Assessment

Therapeutic Goal

Reduction of symptoms in children and adults with ADHD. Reduction of sleep attacks in patients with narcolepsy.

Baseline Data

Children with ADHD. Document the degree of inattention, impulsivity, hyperactivity, and other symptoms of ADHD. Symptoms must be present for at least 6 months to allow a diagnosis of ADHD. Obtain baseline values of height and weight.

Narcolepsy. Document the degree of daytime sleepiness and the frequency and circumstances of sleep attacks.

Identifying High-Risk Patients

Amphetamines are *contraindicated* for patients with symptomatic cardiovascular disease, advanced arteriosclerosis, hypertension, hyperthyroidism, agitated states, and a history of drug abuse and in those who have taken monoamine oxidase inhibitors within the previous 2 weeks.

Implementation: Administration

Route

Oral.

Administration

Instruct the patient to swallow long-acting formulations intact, without crushing or chewing.

Children with ADHD should take the morning dose after breakfast and the last daily dose by 4:00 PM.

These drugs are classified under Schedule II of the Controlled Substances Act and must be dispensed accordingly.

Ongoing Evaluation and Interventions

Evaluating Therapeutic Effects

Children with ADHD. Monitor for reductions in symptoms (impulsiveness, hyperactivity, inattention) and for improvement in cognitive function. Periodic drug holidays are required to determine if therapy is still needed. Continuous treatment for longer than 1 school year should not be done.

Minimizing Adverse Effects

Excessive CNS Stimulation. These drugs can cause restlessness and insomnia. **Advise patients to use the smallest dose required and to avoid dosing late in the day. Advise patients to minimize or eliminate dietary caffeine (e.g., coffee, tea, caffeine-containing soft drinks).**

Weight Loss. Appetite suppression can cause weight loss. Administering the morning dose after breakfast and the last daily dose early in the afternoon will minimize interference with eating.

Cardiovascular Effects. Warn patients about cardiovascular responses (palpitations, hypertension, angina, dysrhythmias) and instruct them to notify the physician if these develop.

Psychosis. If amphetamine-induced psychosis develops, therapy should be discontinued. For most individuals, symptoms resolve within a week. For some patients, drug-induced psychosis may represent unmasking of latent schizophrenia; these patients require psychiatric care.

Withdrawal Reactions. Abrupt discontinuation can produce extreme fatigue and depression. Minimize by withdrawing amphetamines and methylphenidate gradually.

Minimizing Abuse

If the medical history reveals the patient is prone to drug abuse, monitor use of these drugs closely.

Avoid routine use of amphetamines for weight loss.

CAFFEINE

General Considerations

Caffeine is usually administered to promote wakefulness. **Warn patients against habitual caffeine use to compensate for chronic lack of sleep. Advise patients to consult the physician if fatigue is persistent or recurrent.**

Minimizing Adverse Effects

Cardiovascular Effects. Inform patients about cardiovascular responses to caffeine (palpitations, rapid pulse, dizziness) and instruct them to discontinue caffeine if these occur.

Excessive CNS Stimulation. Warn patients that overdose can cause convulsions. Advise them to ingest no more caffeine than needed.

Effects in Pregnancy. Caffeine can induce first-trimester abortion and, possibly, birth defects. **Advise pregnant women to minimize caffeine consumption.**

*Patient education is highlighted as blue text.

Drug Abuse I: Basic Considerations

DEFINITIONS
DIAGNOSTIC CRITERIA FOR SUBSTANCE ABUSE
AND SUBSTANCE DEPENDENCE
FACTORS THAT CONTRIBUTE TO DRUG ABUSE
NEUROBIOLOGY OF ADDICTION
PRINCIPLES OF ADDICTION TREATMENT
THE CONTROLLED SUBSTANCES ACT

Mind-altering drugs have intrigued human beings since the dawn of civilization. Throughout history, people have taken drugs to elevate mood, release inhibitions, distort perceptions, induce hallucinations, and modify thinking. Many of those who use mind-altering drugs restrict usage to socially approved patterns. However, many others self-administer drugs to excess. Excessive drug use is our focus in this chapter and the two that follow.

Drug abuse confronts clinicians in a variety of ways, making knowledge of abuse a necessity. Important areas in which expertise on drug abuse may be applied include (1) diagnosis and treatment of acute toxicity, (2) diagnosis and treatment of secondary medical complications of drug abuse, (3) facilitating drug withdrawal, and (4) educating and counseling drug abusers in hopes of maintaining long-term abstinence.

Our discussion of drug abuse occurs in two stages. In this chapter we discuss basic concepts that apply to drug abuse. In Chapters 37 and 38, we focus on the pharmacology of specific abused agents and on methods of treating individuals who abuse them.

DEFINITIONS

Drug Abuse

Drug abuse can be defined as *using a drug in a fashion inconsistent with medical or social norms.* Traditionally, the term also implies drug usage that is harmful to the individual or to society. As we shall see, although we can give abuse a general definition, deciding whether a particular instance of drug use constitutes "abuse" is often difficult.

Whether or not drug use is considered abuse depends, in part, on the purpose for which a drug is taken. Not everyone who takes large doses of psychoactive agents is an abuser. For example, we do not consider it abuse to take opioids in large doses on a long-term basis to relieve pain caused by cancer. However, we do consider it abusive for an otherwise healthy individual to take those same opioids in the same doses for the purpose of producing euphoria.

When we speak of drug abuse, we should be aware that abuse can have different degrees of severity. Some people, for example, use heroin only occasionally, whereas others use it habitually and compulsively. Although both patterns of drug use are socially condemned, and therefore constitute abuse, there is an obvious quantitative difference between taking heroin once or twice and taking it routinely and compulsively.

Note that, by the definition above, *drug abuse is culturally defined.* Because abuse is culturally defined, and because societies differ from one another and are changeable, there can be wide variations in what is labeled abuse. *What is defined as abuse can vary from one culture to another.* For example, in the United States, moderate consumption of alcohol is not usually considered abuse. In contrast, *any* ingestion of alcohol would be considered abuse in some Moslem societies. Furthermore, *what is defined as abuse can vary from one time to another within the same culture.* For example, when a few Americans first began to experiment with lysergic acid diethylamide (LSD) and other psychedelic drugs, these agents were legal and their use was not generally disapproved. However, when use of psychedelics became widespread, our societal posture changed and legislation was passed to make the manufacture, sale, and use of these drugs illegal.

Within the United States, there is divergence of opinion about what constitutes drug abuse. For example, some people would consider any use of marijuana to be drug abuse, whereas others would call smoking marijuana abusive only if it were done *habitually.* Similarly, although many Americans do not seem to consider cigarette smoking to be drug abuse (even though the practice is compulsive and clearly harmful to the individual and society), there are others who believe very firmly that cigarette smoking constitutes a blatant form of abuse.

As we can see, distinguishing between culturally acceptable drug use and drug use that is to be called abuse is more in the realm of social science than pharmacology. Accordingly, since this is a pharmacology text and not a sociology text, we will not attempt to define just what patterns of drug use do or do not constitute abuse. Instead, we will focus on the pharmacologic properties of abused drugs—leaving distinctions about what is and is not abuse to sociologists and legislators. Fortunately, we can identify the drugs that tend to be abused and discuss their pharmacology without having to resolve all arguments about what patterns of use should or should not be considered abusive.

As discussed later, the American Psychiatric Association has established diagnostic criteria for *substance abuse,* a specific substance use disorder. These objective criteria are largely independent of cultural bias, and should not be confused with the concept of drug abuse as just presented.

Addiction

The American Society of Addiction Medicine defines addiction as *a disease process characterized by the continued use of a specific psychoactive substance despite physical, psychologic, or social harm.* Please note that nowhere in this definition is addiction equated with physical dependence. As discussed below, although physical dependence can contribute to addictive behavior, it is neither necessary nor sufficient for addiction to occur. Addiction can be considered essentially equivalent to substance dependence as defined in the *Diagnostic and Statistical Manual of Mental Disorders, Fourth Edition* (DSM-IV) (see below).

Other Definitions

Tolerance results from regular drug use and can be defined as a state in which a particular dose elicits a smaller response than it did with initial use. As tolerance increases, higher and higher doses are needed to elicit desired effects.

Cross-tolerance is a state in which tolerance to one drug confers tolerance to another. Cross-tolerance generally develops among drugs within a particular class, and not between drugs in different classes. For example, tolerance to one opioid (e.g., heroin) confers cross-tolerance to other opioids (e.g., morphine), but not to central nervous system (CNS) depressants, psychostimulants, psychedelics, or nicotine.

Psychologic dependence can be defined as an intense subjective need for a particular psychoactive drug.

Physical dependence can be defined as a state in which an abstinence syndrome will occur if drug use is discontinued. Physical dependence is the result of neuroadaptive processes that take place in response to prolonged drug exposure.

Cross-dependence refers to the ability of one drug to support physical dependence on another drug. When cross-dependence exists between drug A and drug B, drug A will be able to prevent withdrawal in a patient physically dependent on drug B, and vice versa. As with cross-tolerance, cross-dependence generally exists among drugs in the same pharmacologic family, but not between drugs in different families.

A *withdrawal syndrome* is a constellation of signs and symptoms that occurs in physically dependent individuals when they discontinue drug use. Quite often, the symptoms seen during withdrawal are opposite to effects the drug produced before it was withdrawn. For example, discontinuation of a CNS depressant can cause CNS excitation.

DIAGNOSTIC CRITERIA FOR SUBSTANCE ABUSE AND SUBSTANCE DEPENDENCE

Diagnostic criteria for substance abuse and substance dependence are set forth in DSM-IV, published by the American Psychiatric Association. A summary appears in Table 36–1. As defined in DSM-IV, substance dependence, which can be equated with addiction, is a more severe disorder than substance abuse. Accordingly, individuals whose drug problem is not bad enough to meet the criteria for substance dependence might nonetheless meet the criteria for substance abuse.

As indicated in Table 36–1, tolerance and withdrawal are among the criteria for substance dependence. Please note, however, that tolerance and withdrawal, by themselves, are neither necessary nor sufficient for substance dependence (addiction) to exist. Put another way, the pattern of drug use that constitutes substance dependence can exist in persons who are not physically dependent on drugs and who have not developed tolerance. Since this distinction is extremely important, I will express it another way: *Being physically dependent on a drug is not the same as being addicted!* Many people are physically dependent but do not meet the criteria for substance dependence. These people are not considered addicts because they do not demonstrate the behavior pattern that constitutes substance dependence. Patients with terminal cancer, for example, are often physically dependent on opioids; however, since their lives are not disrupted by their medication (quite the contrary), their drug use does not meet the criteria for substance dependence (or substance abuse, for that matter). Similarly, some degree of physical dependence occurs in all patients who take phenobarbital to control epilepsy; despite their physical dependence, epileptics do not carry out stereotypic addictive behavior, and therefore cannot be considered substance dependent as defined in DSM-IV.

Having stressed that physical dependence and substance dependence (addiction) are different from each other, we must note that these two phenomena are not entirely unrelated. As discussed below, although physical dependence is not the same as addiction, physical dependence often contributes to addictive behavior.

FACTORS THAT CONTRIBUTE TO DRUG ABUSE

Drug abuse is the end result of a progressive involvement with drugs. Taking psychoactive drugs is usually initiated out of curiosity. From this initial involvement, the user can progress to occasional use. Occasional use can then evolve into compulsive use. Factors that play a role in the progression from experimental use to compulsive use are discussed below.

Reinforcing Properties of Drugs

Although there are several reasons for initiating drug use (e.g., curiosity, peer pressure), individuals would not continue drug use unless drugs produced desirable feelings or experiences. By making people feel "good," drugs reinforce the reasons for their use. Conversely, if drugs did not give people experiences that they found desirable, the reasons for initiating drug use would not be reinforced, and drug use would stop.

Reinforcement by drugs can occur in two ways. First, drugs can give the individual an experience that is pleasurable. Cocaine, for example, produces a state of euphoria. Second, drugs can reduce the intensity of unpleasant experience. For example, drugs can reduce anxiety and stress.

The reinforcing properties of drugs can be clearly demonstrated in experiments with animals. In the laboratory, animals will self-administer most of the drugs that are abused by humans (e.g., opioids, barbiturates, alcohol, cocaine, amphetamines, phencyclidine, nicotine, caffeine). When these drugs are made freely available, animals develop patterns of drug use that are similar to those of humans. Animals will self-administer these drugs (except for nicotine and caffeine) in preference to eating, drinking, and sex. When permitted, these animals often die from lack of food and fluid. These observations strongly suggest that pre-existing psychopathology is not necessary for drug abuse to take place. Rather, these studies suggest that drug abuse results, in large part, from the reinforcing properties of drugs themselves.

Physical Dependence

As defined above, physical dependence is a state in which an abstinence syndrome will occur if drug use is discontinued. The degree of physical dependence is determined largely by dosage size and duration of drug use. Physical dependence is greatest in people who take large doses for a long time. The more physically dependent a person is, the more intense the withdrawal syndrome. Substantial physical dependence develops to the opioids (e.g., morphine, heroin) and CNS depressants (e.g., barbiturates, alcohol). Physical dependence tends to be less prominent with other abused drugs (e.g., psychostimulants, psychedelics, marijuana).

Physical dependence can contribute to compulsive drug use. Once dependence has developed, the desire to avoid withdrawal becomes a motivator for continued drug administration. Furthermore, if the drug is administered after the onset of withdrawal, its ability to alleviate the discomfort of withdrawal can reinforce its desirability. It must be noted, however, that although physical dependence plays a role in the abuse of drugs, physical dependence should not be viewed as the primary cause of addictive behavior. Rather, physical dependence is just one of several factors that can contribute to the development and continuation of compulsive use.

Psychologic Dependence

Psychologic dependence is defined as *an intense subjective need for a drug*. Individuals who are psychologically dependent feel very strongly that their sense of well-being is dependent upon continued drug use; a sense of "craving" is felt when the drug is unavailable. There is no question that psychologic dependence can be a major factor in addictive behavior. For example, it is psychologic dependence—and not physical dependence—that plays the principal role in causing renewed use of opioids by addicts who had previously gone through withdrawal.

Social Factors

Social factors can play an important role in the development of drug abuse. The desire for social status and approval is a common reason for initiating drug use. Also, since initial drug experiences are frequently unpleasant, the desire for social approval can be one of the most compelling reasons for repeating drug use after the initial exposure. For example, most people do not especially enjoy their first cigarette; if it were not for peer pressure, many would quit before they had reached the point where they began to experience smoking as pleasurable. Similarly, initial use of heroin, with its associated nausea and vomiting, is often deemed unpleasant; peer pressure is a common reason for continuing heroin use long enough to develop tolerance to these undesirable effects.

Drug Availability

Drug availability is clearly a factor in the development and maintenance of abuse. Abuse can flourish only in environments where drugs can be readily obtained. In contrast, where procurement of drugs is difficult, abuse is minimal. The ready availability of drugs in hospitals and clinics is a major reason for the unusually high rate of addiction among pharmacists,

TABLE 36–1 ■ DSM-IV-TR Diagnostic Criteria for Substance Abuse and Substance Dependence

Substance Abuse

Substance abuse is a maladaptive pattern of substance use leading to clinically significant impairment or distress, as manifested by one (or more) of the following within a 12-month period:

- Recurrent substance use that results in a failure to fulfill major role obligations at work, school, or home
- Recurrent substance use in situations in which it is physically hazardous
- Recurrent substance-related legal problems
- Continued substance use despite persistent or recurrent social or interpersonal problems caused or exacerbated by the substance

Individuals who display tolerance, withdrawal, and other symptoms of substance dependence would be diagnosed under substance dependence, a more severe disorder, rather than under substance abuse.

Substance Dependence

Substance dependence is a maladaptive pattern of substance use, leading to clinically significant impairment or distress, as manifested by three (or more) of the following, occurring at any time in the same 12-month period:

- Tolerance to the substance
- Withdrawal, as manifested by either:
  –the characteristic withdrawal syndrome for the substance, *or*
  –the same (or closely related) substance is taken to relieve or avoid withdrawal symptoms
- The substance is often taken in larger amounts or over a longer time than intended
- Substance use continues despite a persistent desire or repeated efforts to cut down or control consumption
- A great deal of time is spent in activities necessary to obtain the substance, use the substance, or recover from its effects
- Important social, occupational, or recreational activities are given up or reduced because of substance use
- Substance use continues despite knowledge of a persistent or recurrent physical or psychologic problem that substance use probably caused or exacerbated (e.g., drinking despite knowing that alcohol made an ulcer worse)

Modified from the Diagnostic and Statistical Manual of Mental Disorders, Fourth Edition, Text Revision. Washington, DC, American Psychiatric Association, 2000, with permission. Copyright © 2000 American Psychiatric Association.

nurses, and physicians. It is the desire to reduce drug abuse through reducing drug availability that provides much of the rationale for law enforcement efforts directed at the manufacture and distribution of illicit drugs.

Vulnerability of the Individual

Some individuals are more prone to becoming drug abusers than others. By way of illustration, let's consider three individuals from the same social setting who have equal access to the same psychoactive drug. The first person experiments with the drug briefly and never uses it again. The second person progresses from experimentation to occasional use. The third goes on to take the drug compulsively. Since social factors, drug availability, and the properties of the drug itself are the same for all three people, these factors cannot explain the three different patterns of drug use that developed. We must conclude, therefore, that the three patterns developed because of differences in the users themselves: one individual was not prone to drug abuse, one had only moderate tendencies toward abuse, and the third was highly vulnerable to becoming an abuser.

Several psychologic factors have been associated with tendencies toward drug abuse. Drug abusers are frequently individuals who are impulsive, have a low tolerance for frustration, and are rebellious against social norms. Other psychologic factors that seem to predispose individuals to abusing drugs include depressive disorders, anxiety disorders, and antisocial personality. It is also clear that individuals who abuse one type of drug are likely to abuse other drugs.

There is speculation that some instances of drug abuse may actually be attempts at self-medication to relieve emotional discomfort. For example, some people may use alcohol and other depressants as a means of controlling severe anxiety. Although their drug use may appear excessive, it may be no more than is needed to prevent feelings that are deemed intolerable.

Genetics also contribute to drug abuse. Vulnerability to alcoholism, for example, may result from an inherited predisposition.

NEUROBIOLOGY OF ADDICTION

How does repeated use of an addictive drug eventually change a voluntary user into a compulsive user? By causing molecular changes in the brain. Each time the drug is taken, it causes changes that promote further drug use. With repeated drug exposure, these changes are reinforced, making drug use more and more difficult to control.

Where do these molecular changes occur? The most important site is the so-called *reward circuit*—a system that normally serves to reinforce behaviors essential for survival, such as eating and reproductive activities. Neurons of the reward circuit originate in the ventral tegmental area of the midbrain, and project to the nucleus accumbens. Their major transmitter is *dopamine.* Under normal circumstances, biologically critical behavior, such as sexual intercourse, activates the circuit. The resultant release of dopamine rewards and reinforces the behavior. Like natural positive stimuli, addictive drugs can also activate the system, causing synaptic levels of dopamine to rise. Whether the system is activated by use of drugs or by behavior essential for survival, the outcome is the same: a tendency to repeat the behavior that turned the system on. With repeated activation over time, the system eventually undergoes synaptic remodeling, thereby consolidating changes in brain function, and hence in addiction-related behavior. Remodeling persists after drug use has ceased.

PRINCIPLES OF ADDICTION TREATMENT

Drug addiction is a treatable disease. With therapy, between 40% and 60% of addicts can reduce drug use. In 1999, treatment underwent a significant advance when the National Institute on Drug Abuse published *Principles of Drug Addiction Treatment,* the first science-based guide on addiction therapy. The guide centers on 13 principles of effective treatment, which are summarized in Table 36–2.

Ideally, the goal of treatment is *complete cessation* of drug use. However, total abstinence is not the only outcome that can be considered successful. Treatment that changes drug use from compulsive to moderate will permit increased productivity, better health, and a decrease in socially unacceptable behavior. Clearly, this outcome is beneficial to both the individual and society—even though some degree of drug use continues. It must be noted, however, that in the treatment of some forms of abuse, nothing short of total abstinence can be considered a true success. Experience has shown that abusers of *cigarettes, alcohol,* and *opioids* are rarely capable of sustained moderation. Hence, for many of these individuals, abstinence must be complete if there is to be any hope of avoiding a return to compulsive use.

Recovery from addiction is a prolonged process that typically requires multiple treatment episodes. Why? Because addiction is a *chronic, relapsing* illness. As such, periods of treatment-induced abstinence will very likely be followed by relapse. This does not mean that treatment has failed. Rather, it simply means that at least one more treatment episode is needed. Eventually, many patients achieve stable, long-term abstinence, along with a more productive and rewarding life.

Because addiction is a complex illness that affects all aspects of life, the treatment program must be comprehensive and multifaceted. In addition to addressing drug use itself, the program should address any related medical, psychologic, social, vocational, and legal problems. Obviously, treatment must be tailored to the individual; no single approach works for all people. Multiple techniques are employed. Techniques with proven success include (1) therapy directed at resolving emotional problems that underlie drug use, (2) substitution of alternative rewards for the rewards of drug use, (3) threats and external pressure to discourage drug use, and (4) use of pharmacologic agents to modify the effects of abused drugs. The most effective treatment programs incorporate two or more of these methods.

THE CONTROLLED SUBSTANCES ACT

The *Comprehensive Drug Abuse Prevention and Control Act of 1970,* known informally as the *Controlled Substances Act,* is the principal federal legislation addressing drug abuse. One objective of the act is to reduce the chances that drugs originating from legitimate sources will become available to abusers. To accomplish this goal, the act sets forth regulations for the handling of controlled substances by manufacturers, distributors, pharmacists, nurses, and physicians. Enforcement of the act is the responsibility of the *Drug Enforcement Agency* (DEA), an arm of the U.S. Department of Justice.

Record Keeping

In order to keep track of controlled substances that originate from legitimate sources, a written record must be made of all transactions involving these agents. Every time a controlled substance is purchased or dispensed, the transfer must be recorded. Physicians, pharmacists, and hospitals must keep an inventory of all controlled substances in stock. This inventory must be reported to the DEA every 2 years. Although not specifically obliged to do so by the act, many hospitals require that floor stocks of controlled substances be counted at the beginning and end of each nursing shift.

TABLE 36–2 ■ Principles of Drug-Addiction Treatment

1. **No single treatment is appropriate for all individuals.** Matching treatment settings, interventions, and services to each patient's problems and needs is critical.

2. **Treatment needs to be readily available.** Treatment applicants can be lost if treatment is not immediately available or readily accessible.

3. **Effective treatment must attend to multiple needs of the individual, not just to his or her drug use.** In addition to addressing drug use, treatment must address the individual's medical, psychologic, social, vocational, and legal problems.

4. **Because needs of the individual can change, the treatment plan must be reassessed continually and modified as indicated.** At different times during treatment, a patient may develop a need for medical services, family therapy, vocational rehabilitation, and social and legal services.

5. **Remaining in treatment for an adequate time is critical for effectiveness.** The time depends on the individual's needs. For most patients, the threshold for significant improvement is reached at about 3 months. Additional treatment can produce further progress. Programs should include strategies to prevent patients from leaving prematurely.

6. **Individual and/or group counseling and other behavioral therapies are critical components of treatment.** In therapy, patients address motivation, build skills to resist drug use, replace drug-using activities with constructive and rewarding non–drug-related activities, and improve problem-solving abilities. Behavioral therapy also facilitates interpersonal relationships.

7. **Medication can be an important element of treatment, especially when combined with counseling and other behavioral therapies.** Methadone, LAAM, and naltrexone can help persons addicted to opiates. Nicotine replacement therapy (e.g., patches, gum) and/or bupropion can help patients addicted to nicotine.

8. **Addicted individuals who also have mental disorders should have both conditions treated in an integrated way.**

9. **Medical detoxification is only the first stage of addiction treatment and, by itself, does little to change long-term drug use.** Medical detoxification manages the acute physical symptoms of withdrawal—and can serve as a precursor to effective drug addiction treatment.

10. **Treatment needn't be voluntary to be effective.** Sanctions or enticements coming from the family, employer, or criminal justice system can significantly increase treatment entry, retention, and success.

11. **Individuals in treatment must undergo continuous monitoring for possible drug use.** Monitoring drug use (e.g., through urinalysis) can help the patient withstand urges to use drugs. Monitoring also can provide early evidence of drug use, thereby allowing appropriate adjustment of the treatment program.

12. **Treatment programs should provide assessment for HIV/AIDS, hepatitis B and C, tuberculosis, and other infectious diseases, along with counseling to help patients modify behaviors that place them or others at risk.**

13. **Recovery from drug addiction is typically a long-term process, and often requires multiple treatment episodes.** As with other chronic illnesses, relapses can occur during or after successful treatment episodes. Participation in self-help support programs during and following treatment can help maintain abstinence.

Adapted from National Institute on Drug Abuse. Principles of Drug Addiction Treatment: A Research-Based Guide (Publication No. 99-4180). Bethesda, MD, National Institutes of Health, 1999.
HIV/AIDS = human immunodeficiency virus/acquired immunodeficiency syndrome; LAAM = levomethadyl.

DEA Schedules

Each drug preparation regulated under the Controlled Substances Act has been assigned to one of five categories: Schedule I, II, III, IV, or V. Drugs in Schedule I have a high potential for abuse and no approved medical use in the United States. In contrast, drugs in Schedules II through V all have approved applications. Assignment of drugs to Schedules II through V is based on their abuse potential and their potential for causing physical or psychologic dependence. Drugs in Schedule II have the highest potential for abuse and dependence. Drugs in the remaining schedules have decreasing abuse and dependence liabilities. Table 36–3 lists the primary drugs that come under the five DEA Schedules.

Scheduling of drugs under the Controlled Substances Act undergoes periodic re-evaluation. With increased understanding of the abuse and dependence liabilities of a drug, the DEA may choose to reassign it to a different Schedule. For example, glutethimide (a general CNS depressant) was recently switched from Schedule III to Schedule II.

Prescriptions

The Controlled Substances Act places restrictions on prescribing drugs in Schedules II through V. (Drugs in Schedule I have no approved uses, and hence are not prescribed at all.) Only physicians registered with the DEA are authorized to prescribe controlled drugs. Regulations on prescribing controlled substances are summarized below.

TABLE 36–3 ▪■ Classification of Controlled Substances by the Drug Enforcement Agency

Schedule I Drugs	Schedule II Drugs	Schedule III Drugs	Schedule IV Drugs	Schedule V Drugs
Opioids	**Opioids**	**Opioids**	**Opioids**	**Opioids**
Acetylmethadol	Alfentanil	Buprenorphine	Butorphanol	Diphenoxylate plus
Heroin	Codeine	Hydrocodone syrup	Pentazocine	atropine
Normethadone	Fentanyl	Paregoric	Propoxyphene	
Many others	Hydromorphone	**Cannabinoids**	**Stimulants**	
Psychedelics	Levorphanol	Dronabinol (THC)	Diethylpropion	
Bufotenin	Meperidine	**Stimulants**	Fenfluramine	
Diethyltryptamine	Methadone	Benzphetamine	Mazindol	
Dimethyltryptamine	Morphine	Phendimetrazine	Pemoline	
Ibogaine	Opium tincture	**Barbiturates**	Phentermine	
d-Lysergic acid	Oxycodone	Aprobarbital	**Barbiturates**	
diethylamide (LSD)	Oxymorphone	Butabarbital	Mephobarbital	
Mescaline	Remifentanil	Metharbital	Methohexital	
3,4-Methylenedioxy-	Sufentanil	Talbutal	Phenobarbital	
methamphetamine	**Psychostimulants**	Thiamylal	**Benzodiazepines**	
(MDMA)	Amphetamine	Thiopental	Alprazolam	
Psilocin	Cocaine	**Miscellaneous**	Chlordiazepoxide	
Psilocybin	Dextroamphetamine	**Depressants**	Clonazepam	
Cannabis Derivatives	Methamphetamine	Gamma-hydroxybutyrate	Clorazepate	
Hashish	Methylphenidate	Methyprylon	Diazepam	
Marijuana	Phenmetrazine	**Anabolic Steroids**	Estazolam	
Others	**Barbiturates**	Fluoxymesterone	Flunitrazepam	
Methaqualone	Amobarbital	Methyltestosterone	Flurazepam	
Phencyclidine	Pentobarbital	Nandrolone	Halazepam	
	Secobarbital	Oxandrolone	Lorazepam	
	Miscellaneous	Stanozolol	Midazolam	
	Depressants	Testosterone	Oxazepam	
	Glutethimide		Prazepam	
			Quazepam	
			Temazepam	
			Triazolam	
			Miscellaneous	
			Depressants	
			Chloral hydrate	
			Dichloralphenazone	
			Ethchlorvynol	
			Ethinamate	
			Meprobamate	
			Paraldehyde	

Schedule II. All prescriptions for Schedule II drugs must be typed or filled out in ink or indelible pencil and signed by the prescribing physician. Oral prescriptions may be made, but only in emergencies, and a written prescription must follow within 72 hours. Prescriptions of Schedule II drugs cannot be refilled. Hence, a new prescription must be written if continued therapy is needed.

Schedules III and IV. Prescriptions for drugs in Schedules III and IV may be oral or written. If authorized by the physician, these prescriptions may be refilled up to 5 times. Refills must be made within 6 months of the original order. If additional medication is needed beyond the amount provided for in the original prescription, a new prescription must be written.

Schedule V. The same regulations for prescribing drugs in Schedules III and IV apply to drugs in Schedule V. In addition, Schedule V drugs may be dispensed without a prescription provided the following conditions are met: (1) the drug is dispensed by a pharmacist; (2) the amount dispensed is very limited; (3) the recipient is at least 18 years old and can prove

it; (4) the pharmacist writes and initials a record indicating the date, the name and amount of the drug, and the name and address of the recipient; and (5) state and local laws do not prohibit dispensing Schedule V drugs without a prescription.

Labeling

When drugs in Schedules II, III, and IV are dispensed, their containers must bear this label: *Caution—Federal law prohibits the transfer of this drug to any person other than the patient for whom it was prescribed.* The label must also indicate whether the drug belongs to Schedule II, III, or IV. The symbols C-II, C-III, and C-IV are used to indicate the Schedule.

State Laws

All states have their own laws regulating drugs of abuse. In many cases, the provisions of the state law are more stringent than those of the federal law. As a rule, whenever there is a difference between state and federal laws, the more restrictive of the two takes precedence.

⠠⠇ KEY POINTS

- Drug abuse can be defined as drug use that is inconsistent with medical or social norms.
- Drug abuse is a culturally defined term. Hence, what is considered abuse can vary from one culture to another and from one time to another within the same culture.
- Addiction can be defined as a disease process characterized by the continued use of a specific psychoactive substance despite physical, psychologic, or social harm.
- Addiction is largely equivalent to substance dependence as defined in DSM-IV.
- Tolerance is a state in which a particular drug dose elicits a smaller response than it formerly did.
- Cross-tolerance is a state in which tolerance to one drug confers tolerance to another drug.
- Psychologic dependence is defined as an intense subjective need for a particular psychoactive drug.
- Physical dependence is a state in which an abstinence syndrome will occur if drug use is discontinued. Physical dependence is *not* equivalent to addiction.
- Cross-dependence refers to the ability of one drug to support physical dependence on another drug.
- A withdrawal syndrome is a group of signs and symptoms that occur in physically dependent individuals when they discontinue drug use.
- As defined in DSM-IV, substance dependence is a more severe substance use disorder than substance abuse.

- Although tolerance and withdrawal are among the diagnostic criteria for substance dependence, they are neither necessary nor sufficient for a diagnosis.
- Although physical dependence is not the same as addiction (substance dependence), physical dependence can certainly contribute to addictive behavior.
- Drugs can reinforce their own use by providing pleasurable experiences, reducing the intensity of unpleasant experiences, and warding off a withdrawal syndrome.
- Addictive drugs activate the brain's reward circuit—and, over time, they cause molecular changes that make controlling their use more and more difficult.
- Some individuals, because of psychologic or genetic factors, are more prone to drug abuse than others.
- Because addiction is a chronic, relapsing illness, recovery is a prolonged process that typically requires multiple episodes of treatment.
- The ideal goal of treatment is complete abstinence. However, treatment that substantially reduces drug use can still be considered a success.
- Under the Controlled Substances Act, drugs in Schedule I have a high potential for abuse and no medically approved use in the United States. Drugs in Schedules II through V have progressively less abuse potential and are all medically approved.

CHAPTER
37

Drug Abuse II: Alcohol

BASIC PHARMACOLOGY OF ALCOHOL
ALCOHOL ABUSE
DRUGS EMPLOYED IN ALCOHOL
ABUSE TREATMENT
> Drugs Used to Facilitate Withdrawal
> Drugs Used to Maintain Abstinence
> Other Drugs Used in the Treatment
> of Alcohol Abuse

Alcohol (ethyl alcohol, ethanol) is the most commonly used and abused drug in the United States. Although alcohol does have some therapeutic applications, the drug is of primary interest because of its nonmedical use. When consumed in moderation, alcohol prolongs life; reduces the risk of dementia, heart failure, myocardial infarction, and ischemic stroke; and, many would argue, contributes to the joy of living. Conversely, when consumed in excess, alcohol does nothing but diminish life both in quality and quantity. These dose-related contrasts between the detrimental and beneficial effects of alcohol were aptly summed up by our 16th president, Abraham Lincoln, when he noted

> *"None seemed to think the injury arose from use of a bad thing, but from the abuse of a very good thing."*

In approaching our study of alcohol, we begin by discussing the basic pharmacology of this widely used drug. After that, we discuss alcohol abuse and the drugs employed for its treatment.

BASIC PHARMACOLOGY OF ALCOHOL

Central Nervous System Effects

Acute Effects. Alcohol is a central nervous system (CNS) depressant. Like the barbiturates, alcohol causes general (relatively nonselective) depression of CNS function. In addition to depressing CNS function, alcohol activates the brain's reward circuit—a system we first encountered in Chapter 36.

How does alcohol affect neuronal activity? For many years, we believed that alcohol simply dissolved into the neuronal membrane, thereby disrupting the ordered arrangement of membrane phospholipids. However, we now know that alcohol interacts with specific proteins (certain receptors, ion channels, and enzymes) that regulate neuronal excitability. Two target proteins are of particular importance, namely (1) receptors for gamma-aminobutyric acid (GABA) and (2) the 5-HT$_3$ subset of receptors for serotonin (5-hydroxytryptamine, 5-HT). The *depressant* effects of alcohol result from binding with recep-

tors for GABA, the principal inhibitory transmitter in the CNS. By binding with these receptors, alcohol enhances GABA-mediated inhibition, thereby causing widespread depression of CNS function. The *rewarding* effects of alcohol result from binding with 5-HT$_3$ receptors in the brain's reward circuit, which we discussed in Chapter 36. When these 5-HT$_3$ receptors are activated (by serotonin), they promote release of dopamine, the major transmitter of the reward system. When alcohol binds with these receptors, it enhances serotonin-mediated release of dopamine, and thereby intensifies the reward process.

The depressant effects of alcohol are dose dependent. When dosage is low, higher brain centers (cortical areas) are primarily affected. As dosage increases, more primitive brain areas (e.g., medulla) become depressed. With depression of cortical function, thought processes and learned behaviors are altered, inhibitions are released, and self-restraint is replaced by increased sociability and expansiveness. Cortical depression also impairs motor function. As CNS depression deepens, reflexes diminish greatly and consciousness becomes impaired. At very high doses, alcohol produces a state of general anesthesia. (Alcohol is not actually used for anesthesia because anesthetic doses are very close to lethal doses). Table 37–1 summarizes the effects of alcohol as a function of blood alcohol level and indicates the brain areas involved.

Chronic Effects. When consumed chronically and in excess, alcohol can produce severe neurologic and psychiatric disorders. Injury to the CNS is caused by the direct actions of alcohol and by the nutritional deficiencies frequently suffered by chronic heavy drinkers.

Two neuropsychiatric syndromes commonly seen in alcoholics are *Wernicke's encephalopathy* and *Korsakoff's psychosis*. Both disorders are caused by thiamin deficiency, which results from poor diet and alcohol-induced suppression of thiamin absorption. Wernicke's encephalopathy is characterized by confusion, nystagmus, and abnormal ocular movements. This syndrome is readily reversible with thiamin. Korsakoff's psychosis is characterized by polyneuropathy, inability to convert short-term memory into long-term memory, and confabulation (unconscious filling of gaps in memory with fabricated facts and experiences). Korsakoff's psychosis is not reversible.

Perhaps the most dramatic effect of long-term excessive alcohol consumption is enlargement of the cerebral ventricles, presumably in response to atrophy of the cerebrum itself. These gross anatomic changes are associated with impaired intellectual function and memory. With cessation of drinking, ventricular enlargement and cognitive deficits reverse (partially) in some individuals but not all.

Effect on Sleep. Although alcohol is commonly used as a sleep aid, it actually disrupts sleep. Drinking can alter sleep cycles, decrease total sleeping time, and reduce the quality of sleep. In addition, alcohol can intensify snoring and exacerbate obstructive sleep apnea. Having a drink with dinner won't affect sleep—but drinking late in the evening will.

Other Pharmacologic Effects

Cardiovascular System. When alcohol is consumed acutely and in moderate doses, cardiovascular effects are minor. The most prominent effect is *dilation of cutaneous blood vessels,* which increases blood flow to the skin. By increasing blood flow to the body surface, alcohol imparts a sensation of warmth—but at the same time promotes loss of heat. Hence, despite images of Saint Bernards with little barrels of whiskey about their necks, alcohol may do more harm than good for the individual stranded in the snow with hypothermia.

Although the cardiovascular effects of moderate alcohol consumption are unremarkable, chronic and excessive consumption is clearly harmful. Abuse of alcohol results in *direct damage to the myocardium,* thereby increasing the risk of heart failure. Some investigators believe that alcohol may be the major cause of cardiomyopathy in the Western world.

In addition to damaging the heart, alcohol produces a dose-dependent *elevation of blood pressure.* The cause is vasoconstriction in vascular beds of skeletal muscle brought on by increased activity of the sympathetic nervous system. Estimates suggest that heavy drinking may be responsible for 10% of all cases of hypertension.

Not all of the cardiovascular effects of alcohol are deleterious: There is clear evidence that people who drink *moderately* (2 drinks a day or less for men, 1 drink a day or less for women) experience less coronary artery disease (CAD), myocardial infarction (MI), and heart failure than do abstainers. It is important to note, however, that with heavy drinking (5 or more drinks/day) the risk of heart disease and stroke is increased. Available data suggest that alcohol protects against heart disease largely by raising levels of high-density lipoprotein (HDL) cholesterol. As discussed in Chapter 48, HDL cholesterol protects against CAD, whereas low-density lipoprotein (LDL) cholesterol promotes it. In addition to raising HDL cholesterol, alcohol may confer protection through three other mechanisms: decreasing platelet aggregation, increasing levels of tissue plasminogen activator (a clot-dissolving enzyme), and suppressing the inflammatory component of atherosclerosis. The degree of cardiovascular protection is nearly equal for beer, wine, and distilled spirits. That is, protection is determined primarily by the amount of alcohol consumed—not by the particular beverage the alcohol is in. Red wine may confer additional protection owing to its content of flavonoids and polyphenols—compounds that can (1) induce endothelium-dependent vasodilation, (2) suppress synthesis of endothelin-1 (a potent vasoconstrictor), and (3) protect LDL from oxidation (LDL must first be oxidized before it can promote atherosclerosis).

In addition to protecting against heart disease, moderate alcohol consumption protects against ischemic stroke. Presumably, the basis of protection is the same as for CAD: elevation of HDL cholesterol, possibly coupled with decreased platelet aggregation, increased fibrinolysis, and reduced intravascular inflammation.

Respiration. Like all other CNS depressants, alcohol depresses respiration. Respiratory depression from moderate drinking is negligible. However, when consumed in excess, alcohol can cause death by respiratory arrest. The respiratory

Blood Alcohol Level (%)	Pharmacologic Response	Brain Area Affected
–0.50		
	Peripheral collapse	Medulla
–0.45		
	Respiratory depression	
–0.40	Stupor, coma	Diencephalon
–0.35	Apathy, inertia	
–0.30	Altered equilibrium	Cerebellum
	Double vision	Occipital lobe
–0.25	Altered perception	
–0.20	↓ Motor skills	Parietal lobe
	Slurred speech	
–0.15	Tremors	
	Ataxia	
–0.10	↓ Attention	Frontal lobe
	Loquaciousness	
	Altered judgment	
–0.05	Increased confidence	
	Euphoria, ↓ inhibitions	

TABLE 37–1 ■ Central Nervous System Responses at Various Blood Alcohol Levels

depressant effects of alcohol are potentiated by other CNS depressants (e.g., benzodiazepines, opioids, barbiturates).

Liver. Alcohol-induced liver damage can progress from fatty liver to hepatitis to cirrhosis—depending on the amount consumed. Acute use of alcohol causes reversible accumulation of fat and protein in the liver. With more prolonged consumption, *hepatitis* develops in about 90% of heavy drinkers. In 8% to 20% of chronic alcoholics, hepatitis evolves into *cirrhosis*—a condition characterized by proliferation of fibrous tissue and destruction of liver parenchymal cells. Although various factors can cause cirrhosis, alcohol abuse is unquestionably the major cause of *fatal* cirrhosis.

Stomach. Immoderate use of alcohol can cause *erosive gastritis.* About one-third of alcoholics have this disorder. Alcohol causes gastritis by two mechanisms. First, it stimulates secretion of gastric acid. Second, when present in high concentrations, it can injure the gastric mucosa directly.

Kidney. Alcohol is a diuretic. The drug promotes urine formation by inhibiting the release of antidiuretic hormone (ADH) from the pituitary. Since ADH acts on the kidney to promote water reabsorption, thereby decreasing urine formation, a reduction in circulating ADH will increase urine formation.

Pancreas. Approximately 35% of cases of acute pancreatitis can be attributed to alcohol, making alcohol the second most common cause of this disorder. Flare-ups typically occur after a bout of heavy drinking. Only 5% of alcoholics develop pancreatitis, and then only after years of overindulgence.

Sexual Function. Alcohol has both psychologic and physiologic effects related to human sexual behavior. Although alcohol is not exactly an aphrodisiac, its ability to release people from their inhibitions has been known to motivate sexual activity. Ironically, the physiologic effects of alcohol may frustrate attempts at consummating the activity that the psychologic effects helped bring about: Objective measurements in males and females show that alcohol significantly decreases our physiologic capacity for sexual responsiveness. The opposing psychologic and physiologic effects of alcohol on sexual function were aptly described long ago by no less an authority than William Shakespeare. In *Macbeth* (Act II, Scene 1), Macduff inquires of a porter "What . . . does drink especially provoke?" To which the porter replies,

> *Lechery, sir, it provokes, and unprovokes; it provokes the desire, but it takes away the performance.*

In males, long-term use of alcohol may induce *feminization.* Symptoms include testicular atrophy, impotence, sterility, and breast enlargement.

Breast Cancer. Alcohol is associated with an increased risk of breast cancer. As alcohol consumption rises, so does the risk. Accordingly, women who drink on a regular basis can reduce their risk by drinking less. Although alcohol increases the risk of breast cancer, moderate drinking nonetheless *reduces* the overall risk of death.

Effects in Pregnancy and Lactation. Pregnancy. Consumption of alcohol during pregnancy can cause *fetal alcohol syndrome* (FAS). This syndrome develops in one in three children born to alcoholic mothers. FAS is characterized by mild to moderate mental retardation, slow growth rate, craniofacial malformations, and limb abnormalities. Also, resistance to infection is greatly reduced (apparently secondary to immune system derangement).

In addition to FAS, alcohol use during pregnancy can result in *stillbirth, spontaneous abortion, low birth weight,* and *mental retardation.* (Alcohol may be the greatest teratogenic cause of mental deficiency in the Western world.) Neonates whose mothers consumed large amounts of alcohol during pregnancy may be born with *physical dependence* on alcohol. These infants will need to undergo withdrawal therapy.

From the above, it is clear that pregnancy is a contraindication to use of alcohol. Mild FAS has been caused by as little as 30 ml of alcohol a day. Drinking 30 ml of alcohol twice weekly is associated with an increase in second-trimester spontaneous abortion. Although there may be some small amount of alcohol that can be consumed safely during pregnancy, we do not know what that amount is. Consequently, in the interests of fetal health, pregnant women should be advised to avoid alcohol entirely. Having said that, it is important to appreciate that a few drinks early in pregnancy are not likely to harm the fetus. Accordingly, if a woman consumes a small amount of alcohol before realizing she's pregnant, she should be reassured that the risk to her baby—if any—is extremely low.

Lactation. Unless alcohol consumption is heavy, alcohol in breast milk is not likely to reach levels that can affect the nursing infant. Yes, alcohol does enter breast milk, but significant amounts will not be present until maternal blood levels of alcohol reach 0.3%—a level associated with gross intoxication. Use of alcohol during lactation may inhibit the milk ejection reflex.

Impact on Longevity

The effects of alcohol on life span depend on the amount consumed. Heavy drinkers have a higher mortality rate than the population at large. Causes of increased mortality include cir-

TABLE 37–2 ■ People Who Should Avoid Alcohol*
• Women who are pregnant or trying to conceive.
• People who plan to drive or perform other activities that require unimpaired attention or muscular coordination.
• People taking antihistamines, sedatives, or other drugs that can intensify alcohol's effects.
• Recovering alcoholics.
• People under age 21.
Caution is indicated for people with a strong family history of alcoholism and for those with diabetes, peptic ulcer disease, and other medical conditions that can be exacerbated by alcohol.

*According to the National Institute on Alcohol Abuse and Alcoholism.

rhosis, respiratory disease, cancer, and fatal accidents. The risk of death associated with alcohol abuse increases markedly in individuals who consume six or more drinks a day.

Interestingly, people who consume *moderate* amounts of alcohol live longer than those who abstain. When compared with nondrinkers, moderate drinkers have a 30% lower mortality rate, a 50% lower incidence of MI, and a 59% lower incidence of heart failure. According to a study by the American Medical Association, if all Americans were to give up drinking, deaths from heart disease would increase by 81,000 a year. However, despite the apparent benefits of drinking—and the apparent health disadvantage of abstinence—no one is recommending that abstainers take up drinking. Furthermore, when the risks of alcohol outweigh any possible benefits—as in the examples listed in Table 37–2—then alcohol consumption should obviously be avoided.

Pharmacokinetics

Absorption. Alcohol is absorbed from the stomach and small intestine. About 20% of ingested alcohol is absorbed from the stomach. Gastric absorption is relatively slow and is delayed even further by the presence of food. Milk is especially effective at retarding absorption. Absorption from the small intestine is rapid and largely independent of the presence of food; about 80% of ingested alcohol is absorbed from this site. Because most alcohol is absorbed from the small intestine, gastric emptying time (the time required for the contents of the stomach to be released into the small intestine) is a major determinant of individual variation in alcohol absorption.

Distribution. Alcohol is distributed to all tissues and body fluids. The drug crosses the blood-brain barrier with ease, allowing alcohol in the brain to equilibrate rapidly with alcohol in the blood. Alcohol also crosses the placenta and can affect the developing fetus.

Metabolism. Alcohol is metabolized in both the liver and stomach. The liver is the primary site. The pathway for alcohol metabolism is shown in Figure 37–1. As depicted, the process begins with conversion of alcohol to acetaldehyde, a reaction catalyzed by *alcohol dehydrogenase.* This reaction is slow and puts a limit on the rate at which alcohol can be inactivated. Once formed, acetaldehyde undergoes *rapid* conversion to acetic acid. Through a series of reactions, acetic acid is then used to synthesize cholesterol, fatty acids, and other compounds.

The kinetics of alcohol metabolism differ from those of most other drugs. With most drugs, as plasma drug levels rise,

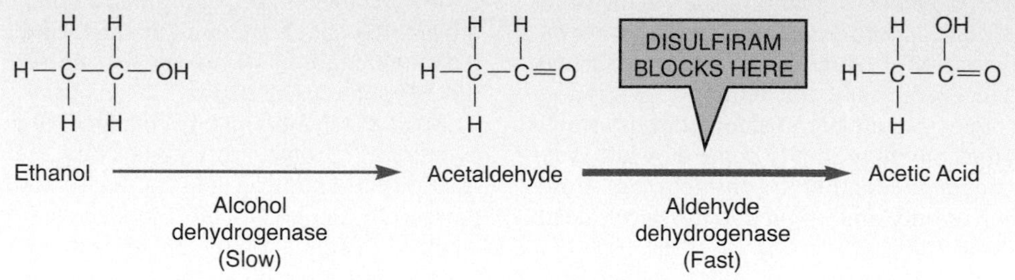

Figure 37-1 ■ Ethanol metabolism and the effect of disulfiram.
Conversion of ethanol into acetaldehyde takes place slowly (about 15 ml/hr). Consumption of more than 15 ml/hr will cause ethanol to accumulate. Effects of disulfiram result from accumulation of acetaldehyde secondary to inhibition of aldehyde dehydrogenase.

the amount of drug metabolized per unit time also increases. This is not true for alcohol: As the alcohol content of blood increases, there is almost no change in the speed of alcohol breakdown. That is, alcohol is metabolized at a relatively *constant rate*—regardless of how much alcohol is in the body. The average rate at which individuals can metabolize alcohol is about *15 ml (0.5 oz) per hour.*

Because alcohol is metabolized at a slow and constant rate, there is a limit to how much alcohol one can consume without having the drug accumulate. For practical purposes, that limit is about *one drink per hour.* Consumption of more than one drink per hour—be that drink beer, wine, straight whiskey, or a cocktail—will result in alcohol buildup.

The information in Table 37–3 helps explain why we can't metabolize more than one drink's worth of alcohol per hour. As the table indicates, beer, wine, and whiskey differ from one another with respect to alcohol concentration and usual serving size. However, despite these differences, it turns out that *the average can of beer, the average glass of wine, and the average shot of whiskey all contain the same amount of alcohol—namely, 18 ml (0.6 oz).* Since the liver can metabolize about 15 ml of alcohol per hour, and since the average alcoholic drink contains 18 ml of alcohol, one drink contains just about the amount of alcohol that the liver can comfortably process each hour. Consumption of more than one drink per hour will overwhelm the capacity of the liver for alcohol metabolism, and therefore will cause alcohol to accumulate.

When used on a regular basis, alcohol induces hepatic drug-metabolizing enzymes, thereby increasing the rate of its own metabolism and that of other drugs. As a result, individuals who consume alcohol routinely in high amounts can metabolize the drug faster than people who drink occasionally and moderately.

Males and females differ with respect to activity of alcohol dehydrogenase in the stomach. Specifically, women have much lower activity than men. As a result, gastric metabolism of alcohol in women is significantly less than in men. This difference partly explains why women achieve higher blood alcohol levels than men after consuming the same number of drinks.

Blood Levels of Alcohol. Since alcohol in the brain rapidly equilibrates with alcohol in the blood, blood levels of alcohol are predictive of CNS effects. The behavioral effects associated with specific blood levels are summarized in Table 37–1. The earliest effects (euphoria, reduced inhibitions, increased confidence) are seen when blood alcohol content is about 0.05%. As

TABLE 37–3 ■ Alcohol Content of Beer, Wine, and Whiskey

	Wine	Beer	Whiskey
Usual serving	1 glass	1 can or bottle	1 shot
Serving size	150 ml (5 oz)	360 ml (12 oz)	45 ml (1.5 oz)
Alcohol concentration	12%[a]	5%[c]	40%[e]
Alcohol per serving	18 ml[b] (0.6 oz)	18 ml[d] (0.6 oz)	18 ml[f] (0.6 oz)

[a]The alcohol content of wine varies from 8% to 20%; typical table wines contain 12%.
[b]The alcohol in a 5-ounce glass of wine varies from 12 to 30 ml, depending on the alcohol concentration in the wine. Wine with 12% alcohol has 18 ml of alcohol per 5-ounce glass.
[c]The alcohol content of beer varies: 5% alcohol is typical of American premium beers; cheaper American beers and light beers have less alcohol (2.4% to 5%); and imported beers may have more alcohol (6%). Beer sold in Europe may have 7% to 8% alcohol.
[d]The alcohol in a 12-ounce can of beer varies from 9 to 29 ml, depending on the alcohol concentration in the beer. Beer with 5% alcohol has 18 ml per 12-ounce can.
[e]Whiskeys and other distilled spirits (e.g., rum, vodka, gin) are usually 80 proof (40% alcohol) but may also be 100 proof (50% alcohol).
[f]The alcohol in a 1.5-ounce shot of whiskey can be either 18 or 22.5 ml, depending on the proof of the whiskey. Eighty-proof whiskey has 18 ml alcohol per 1.5-ounce serving.

blood alcohol rises, intoxication becomes more intense. When blood alcohol exceeds 0.4%, there is a substantial risk of respiratory depression, peripheral collapse, and death. In most states, a level of 0.1% defines intoxication.

Tolerance

Chronic consumption of alcohol produces tolerance. As a result, in order to alter consciousness, people who drink on a regular basis require larger amounts of alcohol than people who drink occasionally. Tolerance to alcohol confers cross-tolerance to general anesthetics, barbiturates, and other general CNS depressants. However, no cross-tolerance develops to opioids. Tolerance subsides within a few weeks following cessation of alcohol use.

Although tolerance develops to many of the effects of alcohol, *very little tolerance develops to respiratory depression.* Consequently, the lethal dose of alcohol for chronic, heavy drinkers is not much bigger than the lethal dose for non-drinkers. Alcoholics may tolerate blood alcohol levels as high as 0.4% (four times the amount normally defined by law as intoxicating) with no marked reduction in consciousness. However, if blood levels rise only slightly above this level, death may ensue.

Physical Dependence

Chronic use of alcohol produces physical dependence. If alcohol is withdrawn abruptly, an abstinence syndrome will result. The intensity of the abstinence syndrome is proportional to the degree of physical dependence. Individuals who are physically dependent on alcohol show cross-dependence with other general CNS depressants (e.g., barbiturates, chloral hydrate, benzodiazepines) but not with opioids. The alcohol withdrawal syndrome and its management are discussed in detail below.

Drug Interactions

CNS Depressants. The CNS effects of alcohol are additive with those of other CNS depressants (e.g., barbiturates, benzodiazepines, opioids). Consumption of alcohol with other CNS depressants intensifies the psychologic and physiologic manifestations of CNS depression. Combining alcohol with other CNS depressants greatly increases the risk of death from respiratory depression.

Nonsteroidal Anti-inflammatory Drugs. Like alcohol, aspirin, ibuprofen, and other nonsteroidal anti-inflammatory drugs (NSAIDs) can injure the GI mucosa. The combined effects of alcohol and NSAIDs can result in significant gastric bleeding.

Acetaminophen. The combination of acetaminophen [Tylenol, others] with alcohol poses a risk of potentially fatal liver injury. There is evidence that relatively modest alcohol consumption (2 to 4 drinks a day) can cause fatal liver damage when combined with acetaminophen taken in normal therapeutic doses. Accordingly, some authorities recommend that people who drink take no more than 2 gm of acetaminophen a day (i.e., half the normal dosage). The interaction between alcohol and acetaminophen is discussed further in Chapter 67.

Disulfiram. The combination of alcohol with disulfiram [Antabuse] can cause a variety of adverse effects, some of which are dangerous. These effects, and the use of disulfiram in the treatment of alcoholism, are discussed later.

Antihypertensive Drugs. Since alcohol raises blood pressure, it will tend to counteract the effects of antihypertensive medications. Elevation of blood pressure is most significant when the dosage of alcohol is high.

Acute Overdose

Acute overdose produces vomiting, coma, pronounced hypotension, and respiratory depression. The combination of vomiting and unconsciousness can result in aspiration, which in turn can result in pulmonary obstruction and pneumonia. Alcohol-induced hypotension results from a direct effect on peripheral blood vessels, and cannot be corrected with vasoconstrictors (e.g., epinephrine). Hypotension can lead to renal failure (secondary to compromised renal blood flow) and cardiovascular shock, a common cause of alcohol-related death. Although death can also result from respiratory depression, this is not the usual cause.

Since the symptoms of acute alcohol poisoning can mimic symptoms of other pathologies (e.g., diabetic coma, skull fracture), a definitive diagnosis may not be possible without measuring alcohol in the blood, urine, or expired air. The smell of "alcohol" on the breath is not a reliable means of diagnosis, since the breath odors we associate with alcohol are due to impurities in alcoholic beverages—and not to alcohol itself. Hence, these odors may or may not be present.

Alcohol poisoning is treated like poisoning with all other general CNS depressants. Details of management are discussed in Chapter 33. Alcohol can be removed from the body by gastric lavage and dialysis. Stimulants (e.g., caffeine, pentylenetetrazol) should not be given.

Summary of Precautions and Contraindications

Alcohol can injure the GI mucosa and should not be consumed by persons with *peptic ulcer disease.* Alcohol is harmful to the liver and should not be used by individuals with *liver disease.* Alcohol should be avoided during *pregnancy* because of the risk of fetal alcohol syndrome, mental retardation, reduced birth weight, stillbirth, and spontaneous abortion.

Alcohol must be used with caution by patients with *epilepsy.* During alcohol use, the CNS is depressed. When alcohol consumption ceases, the CNS undergoes rebound excitation; seizures can result.

Alcohol increases the risk of *breast cancer.* All women—and especially those at high risk—should minimize alcohol consumption.

Alcohol can cause serious adverse effects if combined with *CNS depressants, NSAIDs, acetaminophen, vasodilators,* and *disulfiram.* These combinations should be avoided.

Therapeutic Uses

Although our emphasis has been on the nonmedical use of alcohol, it should be remembered that alcohol does have therapeutic applications.

Topical. Alcohol applied to the skin can promote cooling in febrile patients. Topical alcohol is also a popular skin disinfectant. In addition, alcohol application can help prevent decubitus ulcers.

Oral. Because of its ability to promote gastric secretion, alcohol can serve as an aid to digestion in bedridden patients. Oral alcohol is frequently used as self-medication for insomnia—although it can actually disrupt sleep.

Intravenous. Solutions of alcohol (5% or 10%) in 5% dextrose are administered by slow IV infusion to provide calories and fluid replacement. Intravenous alcohol is also used to treat poisoning by methanol and ethylene glycol.

Local Injection. Injection of alcohol in the vicinity of nerves produces nerve block. This technique can relieve pain of trigeminal neuralgia, inoperable carcinoma, and other causes.

ALCOHOL ABUSE

Alcoholism is a chronic, relapsing disorder characterized by impaired control over drinking, preoccupation with alcohol consumption, use of alcohol despite awareness of adverse consequences, and distortions in thinking, especially as evidenced by denial of a drinking problem. The development and manifestations of alcoholism are influenced by genetic, psychosocial, and environmental factors.

The disease is progressive and often fatal. In the United States, about 8.1 million adults are alcoholics.

In the *Diagnostic and Statistical Manual of Mental Disorders, Fourth Edition* (DSM-IV), the pattern of alcohol use that constitutes alcoholism is termed *alcohol dependence* (if tolerance and withdrawal are present) or *alcohol abuse* (if tolerance and withdrawal are absent). Complete diagnostic criteria from DSM-IV for alcohol dependence and alcohol abuse are presented in Table 37–4.

Misuse of alcohol is responsible for 6 million nonfatal injuries each year—and 100,000 deaths. Causes of death range from liver disease to automobile wrecks. Fully 45% of all fatal highway crashes are alcohol related. Among teens, alcohol-related crashes are the leading cause of death. Alcohol also causes industrial accidents, and is responsible for 40% of industrial fatalities.

Alcohol abuse is a major public health problem, and its consequences are numerous. Alcoholism produces psychologic derangements, including anxiety, depression, and suicidal ideation. Malnutrition, secondary to inadequate diet and malabsorption, is common. Poor work performance and disruption of family life reflect the social deterioration suffered by alcoholics. Alcohol abuse during pregnancy can result in fetal alcohol syndrome, stillbirth, spontaneous abortion, low birth weight, and mental retardation. Lastly, chronic alcohol abuse is harmful to the body; consequences include liver disease, cardiomyopathy, and brain damage—not to mention injury and death from accidents.

Chronic alcohol consumption produces substantial tolerance. Tolerance is both pharmacokinetic (accelerated alcohol metabolism) and pharmacodynamic. Pharmacodynamic tolerance is evidenced by an increase in the blood alcohol level required to produce intoxication. Alcoholics may tolerate blood alcohol levels of 200 to 400 mg/dl—2 to 4 times the level that defines legal intoxication in most states—with no marked reduction in consciousness. It should be noted, however, that very little tolerance develops to respiratory depression. Hence, as the alcoholic consumes increasing amounts in an effort to produce desired psychologic effects, the risk of death from respiratory arrest gets increasingly high. Cross-tolerance exists with general anesthetics and other CNS depressants, but not with opioids.

Chronic use of alcohol produces physical dependence, and abrupt withdrawal produces an abstinence syndrome. When the degree of physical dependence is low, withdrawal symptoms are mild (disturbed sleep, weakness, nausea, anxiety, mild tremors) and last for less than a day. In contrast, the withdrawal syndrome experienced by individuals highly dependent upon alcohol is severe. Symptoms begin 12 to 72 hours after the last drink and continue for 5 to 7 days. Early manifestations include cramps, vomiting, hallucinations, and intense tremors; heart rate, blood pressure, and temperature may rise; and tonic-clonic seizures may develop. As the syndrome progresses, disorientation and loss of insight occur. A few alcoholics (less than 1%) experience *delirium tremens* (severe persecutory hallucinations). Hallucinations can be so vivid and lifelike that alcoholics often can't distinguish them from reality. In extreme cases, alcohol withdrawal can result in cardiovascular collapse and death. Drugs used to ease withdrawal are discussed below.

TABLE 37–4 ■ DSM-IV Diagnostic Criteria for Alcohol Dependence and Alcohol Abuse

Alcohol Dependence

Alcohol dependence is a maladaptive pattern of alcohol use, leading to clinically significant impairment or distress, as manifested by three (or more) of the following, occurring at any time in the same 12 month period:

- Tolerance to alcohol
- Withdrawal from alcohol
- Consumption of alcohol in larger amounts or over longer periods than intended
- Continued alcohol use despite a persistent desire or repeated efforts to cut down or control consumption
- A great deal of time is spent drinking alcohol or recovering from its effects
- Important social, occupational, or recreational activities are given up or reduced because of alcohol
- Alcohol use continues despite knowledge of a persistent or recurrent physical or psychologic problem that alcohol probably caused or exacerbated (e.g., drinking despite knowing that alcohol made an ulcer worse)

Alcohol Abuse

Alcohol abuse is a maladaptive pattern of alcohol use leading to clinically significant impairment or distress, as manifested by one (or more) of the following within a 12-month period:

- Recurrent alcohol use that results in a failure to fulfill major role obligations at work, school, or home
- Recurrent alcohol use in situations in which it is physically hazardous
- Recurrent alcohol-related legal problems
- Continued alcohol use despite persistent or recurrent social or interpersonal problems caused or exacerbated by alcohol

Individuals who display tolerance, withdrawal, and other symptoms of alcohol dependence would be diagnosed under alcohol dependence rather than alcohol abuse.

Adapted from the Diagnostic and Statistical Manual of Mental Disorders, Fourth Edition, Text Revision. Washington, DC, American Psychiatric Association, 2000, with permission. Copyright © 2000 American Psychiatric Association.

DRUGS EMPLOYED IN ALCOHOL ABUSE TREATMENT

About 1 million Americans seek treatment for alcoholism every year. Unfortunately, the success rate is discouraging: nearly 50% relapse during the first few months of treatment. The objective of therapy is to modify drinking patterns (i.e., to reduce or completely eliminate alcohol consumption). Drugs can help in two ways: they can facilitate withdrawal, and they can help maintain abstinence after withdrawal has been accomplished.

Drugs Used to Facilitate Withdrawal

Management of withdrawal depends on the degree of alcohol dependence. When dependence is mild, withdrawal can be accomplished on an outpatient basis without drugs. However, when dependence is great, withdrawal carries a risk of death. Accordingly, hospitalization and drug therapy are indicated. The goals of treatment are to minimize symptoms of withdrawal, prevent seizures and delirium tremens, and facilitate transition to a program for maintaining abstinence. In theory, any drug that has cross-dependence with alcohol (i.e., any of the general CNS depressants) should be effective. However, in actual practice, benzodiazepines are the drugs of choice. The benefits of benzodiazepines and other drugs used during withdrawal are summarized in Table 37–5.

Benzodiazepines

Of the drugs used to facilitate alcohol withdrawal, benzodiazepines are most effective. Furthermore, they are safe. In patients with severe alcohol dependence, benzodiazepines can stabilize vital signs, reduce symptom intensity, and decrease the risk of seizures and delirium tremens. Although all benzodiazepines are effective, agents with longer half-lives are generally preferred. Why? Because they provide the greatest protection against seizures and breakthrough symptoms. The benzodiazepines employed most often are chlordiazepoxide [Librium, others], diazepam [Valium], oxazepam [Serax], and lorazepam [Ativan]. Traditionally, benzodiazepines have been administered around-the-clock on a fixed schedule. However, PRN administration (in response to symptoms) is just as effective and permits speedier withdrawal.

Adjuncts to Benzodiazepines

Combining a benzodiazepine with another drug may improve withdrawal outcome. Agents that have been used with benzodiazepines include carbamazepine (an antiepileptic drug), clonidine (an alpha-adrenergic blocker), and atenolol and propranolol (beta-adrenergic blockers). Carbamazepine may reduce withdrawal symptoms and the risk of seizures, clonidine may reduce withdrawal symptoms, and the beta-blockers may improve vital signs and decrease craving. It should be stressed, however, that these drugs are not very effective as monotherapy. Hence, they should be viewed only as adjuncts to benzodiazepines—and not as substitutes.

Drugs Used to Maintain Abstinence

Once withdrawal has been accomplished, the goal is to prevent—or at least minimize—future drinking. The ideal goal is complete abstinence. However, if drinking must re-

TABLE 37–5 ■ Drugs Used to Facilitate Alcohol Withdrawal	
Drug	**Benefit During Withdrawal**
Benzodiazepines Chlordiazepoxide Diazepam Oxazepam Lorazepam	Decrease withdrawal symptoms; stabilize vital signs; prevent seizures and delirium tremens
Beta-Adrenergic Blockers Atenolol Propranolol	Improve vital signs; decrease craving
Alpha-Adrenergic Blocker Clonidine	Decreases withdrawal symptoms
Antiepileptic Drug Carbamazepine	Decreases withdrawal symptoms; prevents seizures

sume, keeping it to a minimum is still beneficial, since doing so will reduce alcohol-related morbidity.

In trials of drugs used to maintain abstinence, several parameters are used to measure efficacy. These include

- Proportion of patients who maintain complete abstinence
- Time to relapse
- Number of drinking days
- Number of drinks per drinking day

In the United States, two drugs—disulfiram and naltrexone—are approved for maintenance of abstinence. Disulfiram discourages drinking by causing an unpleasant reaction if alcohol is consumed. Naltrexone discourages drinking by blocking the pleasurable effects of alcohol and by decreasing craving. Naltrexone is more effective than disulfiram.

Disulfiram Aversion Therapy

Therapeutic Effects. Disulfiram [Antabuse] is taken by alcoholics to help them refrain from drinking. The drug discourages drinking by causing severe adverse effects if alcohol is ingested. Disulfiram has no applications outside the treatment of alcoholism.

Although disulfiram has been employed for over 50 years, its efficacy is only moderate. In clinical trials, the drug is no better than placebo at maintaining abstinence: The proportion of patients who relapse and the time to relapse are the same as with placebo. However, although disulfiram doesn't prevent drinking, it does decrease the frequency of drinking after relapse has occurred—presumably because of the unpleasant reaction that the patient is now familiar with. There is some indication that supervised administration of disulfiram may be more effective than when patients self-administer the drug.

Mechanism of Action. As indicated in Figure 37–1, disulfiram disrupts alcohol metabolism. Specifically, disulfiram causes *irreversible inhibition of aldehyde dehydrogenase,* the enzyme that converts acetaldehyde to acetic acid. As a result, if alcohol is ingested, *acetaldehyde* will accumulate to toxic levels, producing unpleasant and potentially harmful effects.

Pharmacologic Effects. The constellation of adverse effects caused by alcohol plus disulfiram is referred to as the *acetaldehyde syndrome.* The syndrome can be very dangerous—even fatal. In its "mild" form, the syndrome manifests as nausea, copious vomiting, flushing, palpitations, headache, sweating, thirst, chest pain, weakness, blurred vision, and hypotension; blood pressure may ultimately decline to shock levels. This reaction, which may last from 30 minutes to several hours, can be brought on by consuming as little as 7 ml of alcohol.

In its most severe manifestation, the acetaldehyde syndrome is life threatening. Potential reactions include marked respiratory depression, cardiovascular collapse, cardiac dysrhythmias, MI, acute congestive heart failure, convulsions, and death. Clearly, the acetaldehyde syndrome is not simply unpleasant; this syndrome can be extremely hazardous and must be avoided.

In the absence of alcohol, disulfiram rarely causes significant effects. Drowsiness and skin eruptions may occur during initial use, but they diminish with time.

Patient Selection. Because of the severity of the acetaldehyde syndrome, candidates must be carefully chosen. Alcoholics who lack the determination to stop drinking should not be given disulfiram. In other words, disulfiram must not be administered to alcoholics who are likely to attempt drinking while undergoing treatment.

Patient Education. Patient education is an extremely important component of disulfiram therapy. Patients must be thoroughly informed about the potential hazards of treatment. That is, they must be made aware that consumption of *any* alcohol while taking disulfiram may produce a severe, potentially fatal, reaction. Patients must be warned to avoid all forms of alcohol, including alcohol found in sauces and cough syrups, and alcohol applied to the skin in aftershave lotions, colognes, and liniments. Patients should be made aware that the effects of disulfiram will persist for about 2 weeks after the last dose is taken; hence, continued abstinence is necessary. Individuals using disulfiram should be encouraged to carry identification indicating their status.

Preparations, Dosage, and Administration. Disulfiram [Antabuse] is dispensed in tablets (250 and 500 mg) for oral use. At least 12 hours must elapse between the patient's last drink and initiation of treatment. The initial dosage is 500 mg once daily for 1 to 2 weeks. Maintenance dosages range from 125 to 500 mg/day, usually taken as a single dose in the morning. Therapy may last for months or even years.

Naltrexone

Naltrexone [ReVia] is a pure opioid antagonist that decreases craving for alcohol and blocks alcohol's reinforcing (pleasurable) effects. Alcoholics report that naltrexone decreases their "high." Although the mechanism underlying these effects is uncertain, one possibility is blockade of dopamine release secondary to blockade of opioid receptors. Naltrexone is generally well tolerated. Nausea is the most common adverse effect (10%), followed by headache (7%), anxiety (2%), and sedation (2%). Since naltrexone is an opioid antagonist, the drug will precipitate withdrawal if given to individuals with opioid dependence. Conversely, if a patient taking naltrexone needs emergency treatment with an opioid analgesic, high doses of the opioid will be required. The usual dosage of naltrexone is 50 mg once a day. Naltrexone is best used in combination with counseling.

Naltrexone was approved for alcoholism on the basis of randomized clinical trials that combined extensive counseling along with the drug. In these trials, naltrexone cut the relapse rate by 50%. Compared with patients taking placebo, those taking naltrexone reported less craving for alcohol, fewer days drinking, fewer drinks per occasion, and reduced severity of alcohol-related problems. In contrast to the original trials, a more recent trial, conducted by the U.S. Department of Veterans Affairs, failed to show any benefit of naltrexone in maintaining abstinence. Why did naltrexone work in the original trials but not in the more recent one? The most likely reason is that the subjects in the two trials were very different: The alcoholic veterans suffered from long-term alcoholism, had little or no social support, and received minimal counseling during the trial, whereas the subjects in the earlier studies were younger, had good support systems, and received extensive counseling along with naltrexone. Hence, the new study does not prove that naltrexone doesn't work. Rather, it only proves that naltrexone doesn't work for all drinkers, and doesn't work in the absence of adequate counseling. Until more is known, naltrexone should still be considered a useful agent for maintaining sobriety.

Acamprosate

Acamprosate, a drug used in Europe, decreases the frequency of drinking and helps maintain abstinence. In a 48-week clinical trial, abstinence was maintained in 43% of patients taking acamprosate compared with only 21% of those taking placebo. In a shorter trial (only 12 weeks), the abstinence rate was 60% with acamprosate versus 22% with placebo. Two mechanisms may underlie these benefits: reduced activity in excitatory (glutaminergic) pathways and enhanced activity in inhibitory (GABAergic) pathways. By altering transmission in these pathways, acamprosate may decrease craving and distress, and hence may decrease the desire for alcohol. The major side effects are headache (20%) and diarrhea (10%). The usual dosage is 2 to 3 gm/day in divided doses. Acamprosate is eliminated intact in the urine, and hence renal insufficiency may necessitate a dosage reduction. Acamprosate is undergoing clinical trials in the United States and may be available here soon.

Ondansetron

Ondansetron [Zofran], a selective 5-HT₃–receptor antagonist, is under investigation as an aid for maintaining sobriety. The drug was originally developed to suppress nausea and vomiting caused by anticancer drugs (see Chapter 75). Why give ondansetron to alcoholics? Because, by blocking 5-HT₃ receptors, the drug could, in theory, prevent alcohol from activating the brain's reward system, and hence could decrease the motivation for drinking. In a preliminary trial, ondansetron did help suppress alcohol ingestion—but only among certain alcoholics: The drug reduced drinking by people with *early-onset* alcoholism (alcoholism that began before age 25) but had no effect on people with *late-onset* alcoholism (alcoholism the began after age 25). Among those with early-onset alcoholism, ondansetron increased the proportion of days spent without drinking (by 40% compared with placebo) and decreased the number of drinks consumed on drinking days (by 39% compared with placebo). The most effective dosage was 4 mg/kg twice a day. These results are important in that they suggest that dysfunction of serotonergic transmission is different in early-onset alcoholism compared with late-onset alcoholism. This implies that, for treatment to be most effective, it should be tailored to the patient's clinical subtype: early-onset alcoholism or late-onset alcoholism.

Other Drugs Used in the Treatment of Alcohol Abuse

Malnutrition is a common problem in the chronic alcoholic. Poor nutrition results from two factors: (1) poor diet and (2) malabsorption of nutrients and vitamins. Malabsorption is caused by alcohol-induced damage to the GI mucosa. Poor diet occurs in part because alcoholics meet up to 50% of their caloric needs with alcohol, and therefore consume subnormal amounts of foods with high nutritional value. Because of their poor nutritional state, alcoholics are in need of fat, protein, and vitamins. The B vitamins (thiamin, folic acid, cyanocobalamin) are especially needed. To correct nutritional deficiencies, a program of dietary modification and vitamin supplements should be implemented.

Alcoholics frequently require fluid replacement therapy and antibiotics. Fluids are needed to replace fluids lost because of gastritis, or because of vomiting associated with withdrawal. Antibiotics may be needed to manage pneumonitis, a common complication of alcoholism.

⁖ KEY POINTS

- Alcohol is beneficial when consumed in moderation and detrimental when consumed in excess.
- As blood levels of alcohol rise, CNS depression progresses from cortical areas to more primitive brain areas (e.g., medulla).
- Long-term, excessive drinking actually reduces the size of the cerebrum.
- Alcohol produces a dose-dependent increase in blood pressure.
- Moderate drinking is defined as two drinks per day or less for men, and one drink per day or less for women.

- Moderate drinking significantly reduces the risk of CAD, MI, heart failure, and ischemic stroke—primarily by raising HDL cholesterol, and partly by suppressing platelet aggregation, enhancing fibrinolysis, and suppressing the inflammatory component of atherosclerosis.
- Excessive drinking causes direct damage to the myocardium.
- Like all other CNS depressants, alcohol depresses respiration.
- Chronic, heavy drinking can cause hepatitis and cirrhosis. People with liver disease should avoid alcohol.
- Heavy drinking can cause erosive gastritis.
- Alcohol is a diuretic.
- Alcohol increases the risk of breast cancer.
- Excessive drinkers die younger than the population at large.
- Because of the cardioprotective effects of alcohol, moderate drinkers live longer than those who abstain.
- Alcohol dehydrogenase is the rate-limiting enzyme in alcohol metabolism.
- Alcohol is metabolized at a constant rate, regardless of how high blood levels rise. In contrast, the rate of metabolism of most drugs increases as their blood levels rise.
- Most people can metabolize about one drink per hour—be it beer, wine, straight whiskey, or a cocktail. Consumption of more than one drink per hour causes alcohol to accumulate.

- Chronic consumption of alcohol produces tolerance to many of its effects—but not to respiratory depression.
- Tolerance to alcohol confers cross-tolerance to general anesthetics, barbiturates, and other general CNS depressants—but not to opioids.
- The CNS-depressant effects of alcohol are additive with those of other CNS depressants.
- The combined effects of alcohol and NSAIDs can cause significant gastric bleeding. People with peptic ulcer disease should avoid the drug.
- The combination of alcohol and acetaminophen can cause fatal hepatic failure.
- Alcohol use during pregnancy can result in fetal alcohol syndrome, stillbirth, spontaneous abortion, low birth weight, and mental retardation. Women who are pregnant or trying to conceive should not drink.
- Benzodiazepines (e.g., chlordiazepoxide, diazepam, lorazepam) are drugs of choice for facilitating withdrawal in alcohol-dependent individuals. Benzodiazepines suppress symptoms because of cross-dependence with alcohol.
- Disulfiram is given to help alcoholics refrain from drinking. The drug blocks aldehyde dehydrogenase; hence, if alcohol is consumed, acetaldehyde will accumulate, thereby causing a host of unpleasant and potentially dangerous symptoms.
- Naltrexone helps alcoholics refrain from drinking by decreasing their craving for alcohol and by blocking alcohol's reinforcing effects.

Summary of Major Nursing Implications*

DISULFIRAM

Preadministration Assessment

Therapeutic Goal

Facilitation of abstinence from alcohol.

Patient Selection

Candidates for therapy must be chosen carefully. Disulfiram must not be given to alcoholics who are likely to attempt drinking while taking this drug.

Identifying High-Risk Patients

Disulfiram is *contraindicated* for patients suspected of being incapable of abstinence from alcohol; for patients with myocardial disease, coronary occlusion, or psychosis; and for patients who have recently received alcohol, metronidazole, paraldehyde, or alcohol-containing medications (e.g., cough syrups, tonics).

Implementation: Administration

Route

Oral.

Administration

Instruct the patient not to administer the first dose until at least 12 hours after his or her last drink.

Dosing is done once daily and may continue for months or even years.

Inform patients that tablets may be crushed or mixed with liquid.

Implementation: Measures to Enhance Therapeutic Effects

Patient education is essential for safety. Inform patients about the potential hazards of treatment, and warn them to avoid all forms of alcohol, including alcohol in vinegar, sauces, and cough syrups, and alcohol applied to the skin in aftershave lotions, colognes, and liniments. Inform patients that the effects of disulfiram will persist for about 2 weeks after the last dose and that alcohol must not be consumed during this time. Encourage patients to carry identification to alert emergency health care personnel to their condition.

*Patient education information is highlighted as blue text.

Drug Abuse III: Major Drugs of Abuse (Other Than Alcohol)

OPIOIDS

GENERAL CNS DEPRESSANTS
  Barbiturates
  Benzodiazepines
  Alcohol and Miscellaneous CNS Depressants
PSYCHOSTIMULANTS
  Cocaine
  Amphetamines
MARIJUANA AND RELATED PREPARATIONS
PSYCHEDELICS
  d-Lysergic Acid Diethylamide (LSD)
  Mescaline, Psilocybin, Psilocin,
  and Dimethyltryptamine
3,4-METHYLENEDIOXYMETHAMPHETAMINE
(MDMA, ECSTASY)
PHENCYCLIDINE
INHALANTS
NICOTINE AND SMOKING
  Basic Pharmacology of Nicotine
  Pharmacologic Aids to Smoking Cessation
ANABOLIC STEROIDS

TABLE 38–1 ■ Pharmacologic Categorization of Abused Drugs	
Category	**Examples**
Opioids	Heroin
	Morphine
	Meperidine
	Hydromorphine
Psychostimulants	Cocaine
	Dextroamphetamine
	Methamphetamine
	Methylphenidate
Depressants	
Barbiturates	Amobarbital
	Secobarbital
	Pentobarbital
	Phenobarbital
Benzodiazepines	Diazepam
	Chlordiazepoxide
	Lorazepam
Miscellaneous	Alcohol
	Methaqualone
	Chloral hydrate
	Meprobamate
Psychedelics	LSD
	Mescaline
	Psilocybin
	Dimethyltryptamine
Anabolic Steroids	Nandrolone
	Oxandrolone
	Testosterone
Miscellaneous	Marijuana
	Phencyclidine
	Nicotine
	Nitrous oxide
	Amyl nitrite

In this chapter, we discuss all of the major drugs of abuse except alcohol, which is discussed in Chapter 37. As indicated in Table 38–1, abused drugs fall into six major pharmacologic categories: (1) opioids, (2) psychostimulants, (3) depressants, (4) psychedelics, (5) anabolic steroids, and (6) miscellaneous drugs of abuse. The basic pharmacology of many of these drugs has been presented in previous chapters, and hence their discussion here is brief. Agents that have not been addressed previously (e.g., marijuana, *d*-lysergic acid diethylamide [LSD], nicotine) are discussed in depth. Structural formulas of representative controlled substances are shown in Figure 38–1. Street names for some abused drugs are given in Table 38–2.

OPIOIDS

The opioids (e.g., heroin, morphine) are major drugs of abuse. This fact is underscored by the classification of most opioids as Schedule II substances. The basic pharmacology of the opioids is discussed in Chapter 27.

Patterns of Use

In the United States, about 3 million people have taken opioids. Of these, about 980,000 are long-term users. In the early 1990s, opioid use increased dramatically. However, use is currently in decline.

Opioid abuse is encountered in all segments of American society. Formerly, opioid use was limited almost exclusively to lower socioeconomic groups residing in cities. However, opioids are now used by people outside cities and by people of means.

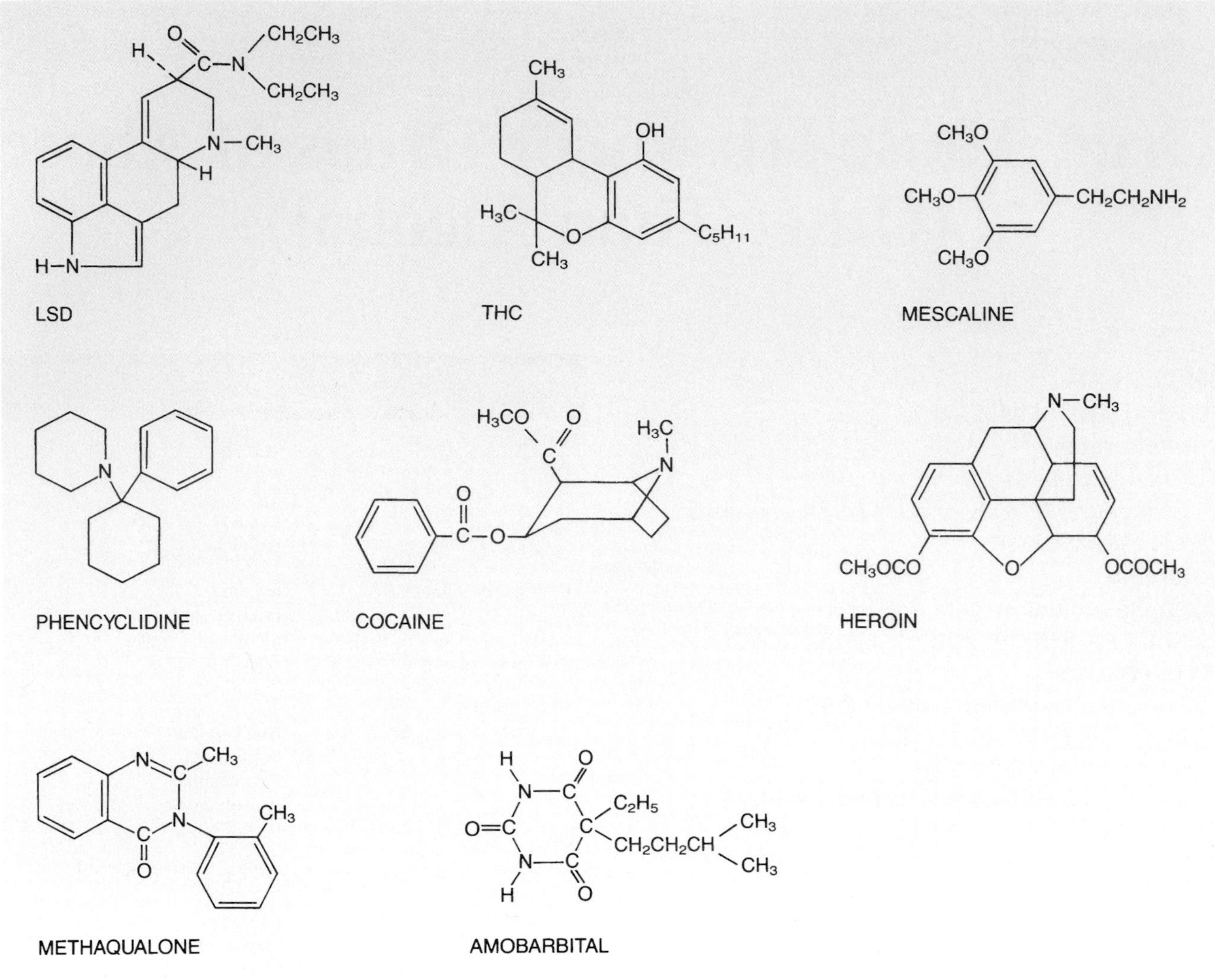

Figure 38–1 ■ **Structural formulas of representative drugs of abuse.**
(LSD = *d*-lysergic acid diethylamide; THC = tetrahydrocannabinol.)

For most abusers, initial exposure to opioids occurs either socially (i.e., illicitly) or in the context of pain management in a medical setting. The overwhelming majority of individuals who go on to abuse opioids begin their drug use illicitly. Only an exceedingly small percentage of those exposed to opioids therapeutically develop a pattern of compulsive drug use.

Opioid abuse by healthcare providers deserves special consideration. It is well established that physicians, nurses, and pharmacists, as a group, abuse opioids to a greater extent than all other groups with similar educational backgrounds. The vulnerability of healthcare professionals to opioid abuse is primarily the result of drug access.

Subjective and Behavioral Effects

Moments after IV injection, heroin produces a sensation in the lower abdomen similar to sexual orgasm. This initial reaction, known as a "rush" or "kick," persists for about 45 seconds. After this, the user experiences a prolonged sense of euphoria (well-being); there is a feeling that "all is well with the world." It is for these extended effects, rather than the initial rush, that most opioid abuse occurs.

Interestingly, when individuals first use opioids, nausea and vomiting are prominent, and an overall sense of *dysphoria* may be felt. In many cases, were it not for peer pressure, individuals would not continue opioid use long enough to allow these unpleasant reactions to be replaced by a more agreeable experience.

Preferred Drugs and Routes of Administration

Heroin. Among street users, *heroin* is the opioid of choice. This agent is easy to procure and is taken by about 90% of opioid abusers. The popularity of heroin is related to its high lipid solubility, which allows the drug to cross the blood-brain barrier with ease, thereby producing effects that are both immediate and intense. It is this combination of speed and intensity that sets heroin apart from other opioids, and makes it such a desirable drug of abuse.

Heroin can be administered in several ways. The most common method is IV injection, followed by smoking and nasal

TABLE 38–2 ■ Street Names for Abused Drugs

Drug	Street Names
Opioids	
Heroin	H, Harry, horse, junk, smack, skag
Hydromorphone	Juice
Methadone	Dolly
Psychedelics	
d-Lysergic acid diethylamide	LSD, LSD-25, acid, blotter, microdot
Dimethyltryptamine	DMT, businessman's trip
Mescaline	Peyote, cactus buttons
2,5-Dimethoxy-4-methylamphetamine	DOM, STP
Psilocybin	Magic mushrooms
Psilocin	Magic mushrooms
Psychostimulants	
Amphetamine	Bennies, hearts, whites, cartwheels
Dextroamphetamine	Dexies, oranges, footballs
Methamphetamine	Speed, bombita, crank, crystal meth, ice
Methylphenidate	Kiddie dope, R-ball, vitamin R
Biphetamine	Black beauties
Cocaine	Coke, crack, snow, blow, flake, nose candy, toot
General CNS Depressants	
Amobarbital	Blue devils
Flunitrazepam [Rohypnol]*	Forget-me pill, Roche, R2, roofies, rope, rophies
Gamma-hydroxybutyrate (GHB)*	Grievous bodily harm, Georgia home boy, liquid ecstasy
Pentobarbital	Yellow jackets
Secobarbital	Red devils
Methaqualone	Ludes, sopors
Miscellaneous Agents	
3,4-Methylenedioxymethamphetamine	MDMA, ecstasy, XTC, the love drug
Phencyclidine	PCP, angel dust, dummy dust, hog, horse tranquilizer, peace pill, rocket fuel, sheets
Marijuana	Pot, grass, reefer, weed, Panama red, Acapulco gold, many others
Combinations	
Heroin + cocaine	Speedball
Heroin + crack cocaine	Moon rock
Heroin + marijuana	Atom bomb

*Associated with sexual assault.

inhalation (known as sniffing or snorting). Intravenous injection produces effects with the greatest intensity and most rapid onset (7 to 8 seconds). When heroin is smoked or snorted, effects develop more slowing, reaching a peak in 10 to 15 minutes. Among users who seek addiction treatment, injection is the predominant method of administration. However, because sniffing and smoking are safer and easier than injection, these routes are becoming increasingly popular.

It should be noted that, when heroin is administered orally or subcutaneously, as opposed to intravenously, its effects cannot be distinguished from those of morphine and other opioids. This observation is not surprising given that, once in the brain, heroin is rapidly converted into morphine, its active form.

Meperidine. Nurses and physicians who abuse opioids often select *meperidine* [Demerol] as their drug of choice. This agent has distinct advantages for these users. First, unlike heroin, meperidine is highly effective when administered orally; hence, abuse need not be associated with telltale signs of repeated injections. Second, meperidine produces less pupillary constriction than other opioids, thereby minimizing awkward

questions about miosis. Lastly, meperidine has minimal effects on smooth muscle function; hence, constipation and urinary retention are less problematic than with other opioids.

Oxycodone. In some parts of the United States, people are abusing the *controlled-release* formulation of oxycodone [OxyContin], an opioid similar to morphine. The controlled-release tablets were designed to provide steady levels of oxycodone over an extended time, and are safe and effective when swallowed intact. However, abusers do not ingest the tablets whole. Rather, they crush the tablets, and then either snort the powder, or dissolve it in water and then inject it IV. As a result, the entire dose is absorbed *immediately,* producing blood levels that are dangerously high. At least 39 deaths have been reported. The risk of respiratory depression and death is greatest in people who have not developed tolerance to opioids.

Tolerance and Physical Dependence

Tolerance. With prolonged opioid use, tolerance develops to some pharmacologic effects, but not others. Effects to which tolerance does develop include euphoria, respiratory depression, and nausea. In contrast, little or no tolerance develops to constipation and miosis. Because tolerance to respiratory depression develops in parallel with tolerance to euphoria, respiratory depression does not increase as higher doses are taken to produce desired subjective effects. Persons tolerant to one opioid are cross-tolerant to other opioids. However, there is no cross-tolerance between opioids and general central nervous system (CNS) depressants (e.g., barbiturates, benzodiazepines, alcohol).

Physical Dependence. Long-term use produces substantial physical dependence. The abstinence syndrome resulting from opioid withdrawal is described in Chapter 27. It is important to note that, although the opioid withdrawal syndrome can be extremely unpleasant, it is rarely dangerous.

Following the acute abstinence syndrome, which takes about 10 days to run its course, opioid addicts may experience a milder but protracted phase of withdrawal. This second phase, which may persist for months, is characterized by insomnia, irritability, and fatigue. Gastrointestinal hyperactivity and premature ejaculation may also occur.

Treatment of Acute Toxicity

Treatment of acute opioid toxicity is discussed at length in Chapter 27 and summarized here. Overdose produces a classic triad of symptoms: *respiratory depression, coma,* and *pinpoint pupils. Naloxone* [Narcan], an opioid antagonist, is the treatment of choice. This agent rapidly reverses all signs of opioid poisoning. However, dosage must be titrated carefully, because, if too much is given, the addict will swing from a state of intoxication to one of withdrawal. Because of its short half-life, naloxone must be re-administered every few hours until opioid concentrations have dropped to nontoxic levels, which may take days. Failure to repeat naloxone dosing may result in the death of patients who had earlier been rendered symptom free.

Nalmefene [Revex], a long-acting opioid antagonist, is an alternative to naloxone. Because of its long half-life, nalmefene does not require repeated dosing—an obvious advantage. However, if the dose is excessive, nalmefene will put opioid-dependent patients into prolonged withdrawal—an obvious disadvantage.

Detoxification

Persons who are physically dependent on opioids experience unpleasant symptoms if drug use is abruptly discontinued. Techniques for minimizing discomfort are discussed below.

Methadone Substitution. Methadone, an oral opioid with a long duration of action, is the agent most commonly employed for easing withdrawal. The first step in methadone-aided withdrawal is to substitute methadone for the opioid upon which the addict is dependent. Because opioids display cross-dependence with one another, methadone will prevent an abstinence syndrome. Once the subject has been stabilized on methadone, withdrawal is accomplished by administering methadone in gradually smaller doses. The resultant abstinence syndrome is mild, with symptoms resembling those of moderate influenza. The entire process of methadone substitution and withdrawal takes about 10 days.

When substituting methadone for another opioid, suppression of the abstinence syndrome requires that methadone dosage be closely matched to the existing degree of physical dependence. Hence, to ensure that methadone dosing is adequate, the extent of physical dependence must be assessed. This can be accomplished by taking a history on the extent of drug use and by observing the patient for symptoms of withdrawal. Of the two approaches, observation is the more reliable. Estimates of drug use based on patient histories may be unreliable because (1) street users don't know the purity of the drugs they have taken, (2) claims of drug use may be inflated in hopes of receiving larger doses of methadone, and (3) addicts from the ranks of the healthcare professions may report minimal consumption to downplay the extent of abuse. Because information from addicts is not likely to permit accurate assessment of dependence, it is essential to observe the patient to make certain methadone dosage is sufficient to suppress withdrawal.

Use of methadone for *maintenance therapy* and *suppressive therapy* is discussed separately below.

Clonidine-Assisted Withdrawal. Clonidine is a centrally acting alpha$_2$-adrenergic agonist. When administered to an individual physically dependent on opioids, clonidine can suppress some symptoms of abstinence. Clonidine is most effective against symptoms related to autonomic hyperactivity (nausea, vomiting, diarrhea). Modest relief is provided from muscle aches, restlessness, anxiety, and insomnia. Opioid craving is not diminished. The basic pharmacology of clonidine is discussed in Chapter 19.

Rapid and Ultrarapid Withdrawal. In both procedures, the addict is given an opioid *antagonist* (naloxone or naltrexone) to precipitate immediate withdrawal, and thereby accelerate the withdrawal process. The ultrarapid procedure is carried out under general anesthesia or heavy sedation with IV midazolam [Versed]. In both procedures, clonidine may be added to ease symptoms. In theory, accelerated withdrawal reduces the risk of relapse. These procedures also permit a rapid switch to maintenance therapy with an opioid antagonist. Studies comparing rapid and ultrarapid withdrawal with more traditional withdrawal procedures are needed.

Drugs for Long-Term Management of Opioid Addiction

Two kinds of drugs are employed for long-term management: *opioid agonists* and *opioid antagonists.* Opioid agonists are employed as a substitute for the abused opioid. These drugs are given to patients who are not yet ready for detoxification. In contrast, opioid antagonists are used to discourage renewed opioid use after detoxication has been accomplished. Three opioid agonists—methadone, levomethadyl, and buprenorphine—are approved for treatment of addiction. Naltrexone is the only opioid antagonist suitable for addiction management.

Methadone. In addition to its role in facilitating opioid withdrawal, methadone can be used for *maintenance therapy* and *suppressive therapy.* These strategies are employed to modify drug-using behavior in addicts who are not ready to attempt withdrawal.

Methadone maintenance consists of transferring the addict from the abused opioid to oral methadone. By taking methadone, the addict avoids withdrawal and the need to procure illegal drugs. Maintenance dosing is done once a day. Maintenance is most effective when done in conjunction with nondrug measures directed at altering patterns of drug use.

Suppressive therapy is done to prevent the reinforcing effects of opioid-induced euphoria. Suppression is achieved by giving the addict progressively larger doses of methadone until a very high dose (120 mg/day) is reached. Building up to this dose creates a high degree of tolerance, and hence no subjective effects are experienced from the methadone itself. Since cross-tolerance exists among opioids, once the patient is tolerant to methadone, taking street drugs, even in high doses, cannot produce significant psychologic effects. As a result, individuals made tolerant with methadone will not experience the reinforcing effects of illicit opioids.

Use of methadone to treat opioid addicts is restricted to agencies approved by the Food and Drug Administration (FDA) and state authorities. These restrictions on the nonanalgesic use of methadone are needed to control methadone abuse, since the drug has about the same abuse liability as morphine and other strong opioids.

Levomethadyl. Levomethadyl [ORLAAM] is a long-acting analog of methadone approved only for managing addiction. The drug is not used to relieve pain. Like methadone, levomethadyl can be employed for maintenance therapy and suppressive therapy. The principal difference between the drugs is convenience: Because of its prolonged half-life, levomethadyl can be administered just 3 times a week, compared with once daily for methadone. Levomethadyl dosing is begun at 20 to 40 mg (or 1.2 to 1.3 times the existing dose of methadone for patients being switched from that drug). The maintenance dosage, which is achieved gradually, ranges between 70 and 100 mg 3 times a week. The most common adverse effects are excessive sweating, constipation, abdominal pain, decreased libido, and delayed or absent ejaculation. Some patients switching from methadone experience mood fluctuations and anxiety. Levomethadyl prolongs the QT interval, and can thereby cause life-threatening dysrhythmias. Accordingly, the drug should not be used by patients with congenital QT prolongation or by those taking other drugs that cause QT prolongation. Patients who develop signs of a dysrhythmia should seek immediate medical attention. Like methadone, levomethadyl is available only through programs for addiction treatment.

Buprenorphine. Buprenorphine, an agonist-antagonist opioid, was recently approved for use in addiction. As discussed in Chapter 27, the drug is a partial agonist at mu receptors and a full antagonist at kappa receptors. In clinical trials, buprenorphine—administered sublingually—has been used (1) for maintenance/suppressive therapy and (2) to facilitate detoxification. When used for maintenance, the drug alleviates craving, reduces use of illicit opioids, and increases retention in therapeutic programs. When used for detoxification, the drug decreases symptoms of withdrawal.

Buprenorphine has several properties that make it attractive for treating addiction. Because it is a partial agonist at mu receptors, it has a low potential for abuse—but can still suppress craving for heroin. If dosage is sufficiently high, the drug can completely block access of heroin to mu receptors, and can thereby prevent heroin-induced euphoria. With buprenorphine, there is a ceiling to respiratory depression, which makes the drug safer than methadone. Development of physical dependence is low, and hence withdrawal is relatively mild.

Buprenorphine is available in two sublingual formulations, marketed as *Subutex* (buprenorphine alone) and *Suboxone* (buprenorphine combined with naloxone). Subutex is used a few days to ease withdrawal. Suboxone is used long term for maintenance. Both products are classified under Schedule III of the Controlled Substances Act.

Opioid Antagonists. Once a patient has undergone opioid detoxification, an opioid antagonist can be used to discourage renewed opioid abuse. Benefits of the antagonist derive from blocking euphoria and all other opioid-induced effects. By preventing pleasurable effects, opioid antagonists eliminate the reinforcing properties of drug use. When the former addict learns that taking an opioid cannot produce the desired response, drug-using behavior will cease. Of the opioid antagonists available, *naltrexone* is best suited for this application. Why? Because naltrexone can be taken orally and because its long half-life permits alternate-day dosing. In contrast, naloxone has low oral efficacy and, because its half-life is very short, multiple daily doses would be needed. These properties make naloxone impractical.

Sequelae of Compulsive Opioid Use

Surprisingly, chronic opioid use has very few *direct* detrimental effects. Addicts in treatment programs have been maintained on high doses of methadone for a decade with no significant impairment of health. Furthermore, individuals on methadone maintenance can be successful socially and at work. It appears, then, that opioid use is not necessarily associated with poor health, lack of productivity, or inadequate social interaction.

Although opioids have few direct ill effects, there are many *indirect* hazards. These risks stem largely from the lifestyle of the opioid user and from impurities common to street drugs. Infections secondary to sharing nonsterile needles occur frequently. The infections that opioid abusers acquire include septicemia, subcutaneous ulcers, tuberculosis, hepatitis C, and HIV. Foreign-body emboli have resulted from impurities in opioid preparations. Opioid users suffer an unusually high death rate. Some deaths reflect the violent nature of the subculture in which opioid use often takes place. Many others result from accidental overdose.

GENERAL CNS DEPRESSANTS

The family of CNS depressants consists of barbiturates, benzodiazepines, alcohol, and other agents. With the exception of the benzodiazepines, all of these drugs are more alike than different. The benzodiazepines have properties that set them apart. The basic pharmacology of the benzodiazepines, barbiturates, and most other CNS depressants is presented in Chapter 33; the pharmacology of alcohol is presented in Chapter 37. Discussion here is limited to abuse of these drugs.

Barbiturates

The barbiturates, which embody all of the properties that typify general CNS depressants, can be considered the prototypes of the group. Depressant effects are dose dependent and range from mild sedation to sleep to coma to death. With prolonged use, barbiturates produce tolerance and physical dependence.

The abuse liability of the barbiturates stems from their ability to produce subjective effects similar to those of alcohol. The barbiturates with the highest potential for abuse have a short to intermediate duration of action. These agents—amobarbital, pentobarbital, and secobarbital—are classified under Schedule II of the Controlled Substances Act. Other barbiturates appear under Schedules III and IV (see Table 36–3). Despite legal restrictions, barbiturates are available cheaply and in abundance.

Tolerance. Regular use of barbiturates produces tolerance to some effects but not others. Tolerance to subjective effects is significant. As a result, progressively larger doses are needed to produce desired psychologic responses. Unfortunately, very little tolerance develops to *respiratory depression.* Consequently, as barbiturate use continues, the dose needed to produce subjective effects comes closer and closer to the dose that can cause fatal respiratory depression. (Note that this differs from the pattern seen with opioids, in which tolerance to subjective effects and respiratory depression develop in parallel.) Individuals tolerant to barbiturates show cross-tolerance with other CNS depressants (e.g., alcohol, benzodiazepines, general anesthetics). However, little or no cross-tolerance develops to opioids.

Physical Dependence and Withdrawal Techniques. Chronic barbiturate use can produce substantial physical dependence. Cross-dependence exists between barbiturates and other CNS depressants but not with opioids. When physical dependence is great, the associated abstinence syndrome can be severe—sometimes fatal (see Chapter 33). In contrast, the opioid abstinence syndrome, although unpleasant, is rarely life threatening.

One technique for easing barbiturate withdrawal employs phenobarbital, a barbiturate with a long half-life. Because of cross-dependence, substitution of phenobarbital for the abused barbiturate suppresses symptoms of abstinence. Once the patient has been stabilized, the dosage of phenobarbital is gradually tapered off, thereby minimizing symptoms of abstinence.

Acute Toxicity. Overdose with barbiturates produces a triad of symptoms: *respiratory depression, coma,* and *pinpoint pupils*—the same symptoms that accompany opioid poisoning. Treatment is directed at maintaining respiration and removing the drug from the body; endotracheal intubation and ventilatory assistance may be required. Details of management are presented in Chapter 33. Barbiturate overdose has no specific antidote; naloxone, which reverses poisoning by opioids, is *not* effective against poisoning by barbiturates.

Benzodiazepines

Benzodiazepines differ significantly from barbiturates. Benzodiazepines are much safer than the barbiturates and overdose with *oral* benzodiazepines *alone* is rarely lethal. However, the risk of death is greatly increased when oral benzodiazepines are combined with other CNS depressants (e.g., alcohol, barbiturates) or when benzodiazepines are administered IV. If severe overdose occurs, signs and symptoms can be reversed with *flumazenil,* a benzodiazepine antagonist. As a rule, tolerance and physical dependence are only moderate when benzodiazepines are taken for legitimate indications, but can be substantial when these drugs are abused. In patients who develop physical dependence, the abstinence syndrome can be minimized by withdrawing benzodiazepines very slowly—over a period of months. The abuse liability of the benzodiazepines is much lower than that of the barbiturates. As a result, all benzodiazepines but one are classified under Schedule IV. The exception—flunitrazepam [Rohypnol]—is classified under Schedule III (see Box 38–1). Benzodiazepines are discussed at length in Chapter 33.

Alcohol and Miscellaneous CNS Depressants

Alcohol is the topic of Chapter 37. Discussion there focuses on the basic pharmacology of alcohol, alcohol abuse, and drugs used in alcoholism treatment.

In addition to barbiturates, benzodiazepines, and alcohol, other CNS depressants (e.g., paraldehyde, meprobamate, chloral hydrate) are subject to abuse. As noted in Chapter 33, the pharmacologic properties of these drugs are similar to those of the barbiturates.

Methaqualone is unique among the CNS depressants and requires comment. At one time, methaqualone [Quaalude] was available legally for use as a sedative. However, because of its high abuse potential and the availability of superior alternatives (i.e., benzodiazepines), methaqualone was withdrawn from the market. This drug differs from other depressants in that overdose is not characterized by obvious signs of CNS depression; rather, poisoning can produce restlessness, hypertonia, and convulsions.

PSYCHOSTIMULANTS

Discussion here focuses on the CNS stimulants with the highest potential for abuse: amphetamines, cocaine, and related substances. Because of their considerable abuse liability, these drugs are classified as Schedule II agents. In addition to stimulating the CNS, the amphetamines and cocaine can stimulate the heart, blood vessels, and other structures under sympathetic control. Because of these peripheral actions, these agents are also referred to as *sympathomimetics.*

Stimulants that are not addressed in this chapter are the ones whose abuse potential is moderate, low, or nonexistent. Included in this group are Schedule III stimulants (e.g., benzphetamine), Schedule IV stimulants (e.g., diethylpropion), and stimulants that are not regulated at all (e.g., caffeine, ephedrine).

Cocaine

Cocaine is a stimulant extracted from the leaves of the coca plant. The drug has CNS effects similar to those of the amphetamines. In addition, cocaine can produce local anesthesia (see Chapter 25) as well as vasoconstriction and cardiac stimulation. Among abusers, a form of cocaine known as "crack" is used widely. Crack is extremely addictive and the risk of lethal overdose is high.

Estimates of cocaine use vary. According to the National Household Survey on Drug Abuse (NHSDA), the number of Americans using cocaine peaked at 5.7 million in 1985, and then declined to 1.5 million by 1997. In contrast, the Office of National Drug Control Policy estimates that 3.6 million Americans currently use cocaine—not the 1.5 million estimated by NHSDA.

Forms. Cocaine is available in two forms: *cocaine hydrochloride* and *cocaine base* (alkaloidal cocaine, freebase cocaine, "crack"). Cocaine base is heat stabile, whereas cocaine hydrochloride is not. Cocaine hydrochloride is available as a white powder that is frequently diluted ("cut") before sale. Cocaine base is sold in the form of crystals ("rocks") that consist of nearly pure cocaine. Cocaine base is widely known by the street name "crack," a term inspired by the sound the crystals make when heated.

Special Interest Topic

BOX 38–1 ■ DATE-RAPE DRUGS: ROHYPNOL AND GHB

Over the past decade, two drugs—Rohypnol and gamma-hydroxybutyrate (GHB)—have gained notoriety over their use to facilitate rape. Both agents are powerful sedative-hypnotics. Use of either drug to commit sexual assault is a federal crime, punishable under the Drug-Induced Rape Prevention and Punishment Act. Street names for Rohypnol include roofies, Roche, rope, rophies, R2, forget-me pill, and Mexican Valium. Street names for GHB include G, Georgia homeboy, grievous bodily harm, and liquid ecstasy.

Rohypnol

Rohypnol is the trade name for flunitrazepam, a potent benzodiazepine. Like diazepam [Valium] and other benzodiazepines, Rohypnol causes sedation, psychomotor slowing, muscle relaxation, and retrograde amnesia. When used to facilitate sexual assault, the drug is slipped into the victim's drink. The combination of alcohol and flunitrazepam produces a vulnerable state characterized by suggestibility, impaired judgment, loss of inhibition, extreme sleepiness, weakness, and inability to remember what happened after the drugs took effect; most victims eventually lose consciousness. Because an intoxicated person is considered legally incapable of consent, performing sex with such a person is considered an aggressive criminal act, and can be prosecuted as felony sexual assault. Unfortunately, because of Rohypnol-induced amnesia, the victim is often unsure that rape actually took place, and certainly can't attest to details. As a result, prosecution is difficult. Two precautions can reduce the risk of being secretly drugged: In public settings (parties, night clubs, etc.), never leave a drink unattended and never accept a drink from a person you don't know and trust.

Facilitation of rape is neither the only nor the principal reason for Rohypnol abuse. Most people take it just to get high. As a rule, the drug is combined with another abused substance, typically alcohol or heroin. Because Rohypnol is relatively cheap (about $5 a dose), it is especially popular among high school and college students. In the United States, abuse of Rohypnol is most common in the East and Southwest.

Rohypnol, manufactured by Hoffmann LaRoche, is available for medical use in several countries, but not the United States. In Europe, Rohypnol is the most widely prescribed drug for relieving insomnia. Effects begin within 30 minutes, peak in 2 hours, and persist for 8 hours. The principal difference between Rohypnol and other benzodiazepines is that Rohypnol is very potent—about 10 times more potent than diazepam. Hence, a small dose has a big effect. One source claims that taking 2 mg of Rohypnol is like drinking an entire six-pack of beer.

To make secretive use of Rohypnol more difficult, Hoffmann LaRoche has reformulated the pill. The new formulation dissolves more slowly than the old one and contains a dye that turns pale drinks bright blue and makes dark drinks murky. In addition, the pill contains insoluble particles that will float on top of all drinks. However, since flunitrazepam is also made in clandestine laboratories, not all formulations will produce these conspicuous effects.

Because of its abuse potential, the legal status of flunitrazepam has changed. Initially, the drug was classified under Schedule IV, like all other benzodiazepines. In 1995, the World Health Organization reclassified it under Schedule III. In the United States, importation of flunitrazepam has been banned, and the Drug Enforcement Agency is considering placing it in Schedule I.

In 1996, Congress passed the Drug-Induced Rape Prevention and Punishment Act. The law imposes a maximum prison term of 20 years for importing and distributing 1 gm or more of flunitrazepam. The act also stiffens the penalty for giving a controlled substance without consent and with the intent of committing rape or any other violent crime.

GHB

Gamma-hydroxybutyrate, or GHB, has two notable actions: it depresses CNS function and, by causing release of growth hormone, it promotes muscle growth. During the 1990s, GHB gained popularity as a drug of abuse, primarily among adolescents and young adults. The drug is taken in social settings (parties, raves, clubs, etc.) to produce relaxation, euphoria, and disinhibition. It is taken by athletes to increase strength. And it is administered clandestinely to facilitate sexual assault. When used for assault, GHB is much like Rohypnol: The perpetrator simply slips a few drops of the colorless, odorless, tasteless liquid into the intended victim's drink; within 20 minutes, the GHB produces incoordination, confusion, and deep sedation, along with amnesia about what has taken place.

The pharmacology of GHB is similar to that of other CNS depressants. This is no surprise given that GHB is a metabolite of gamma-aminobutyric acid, the major inhibitory transmitter in the brain. When taken in moderate doses, GHB produces sedation, relaxation, and mild euphoria. Overdose produces significant respiratory depression, which is made worse by concurrent use of alcohol. Seizures may occur, especially with combined use of methamphetamine. Overdose can also cause nausea, vomiting, bradycardia, hypothermia, agitation, delirium, unconsciousness, and coma. GHB has been linked to more than 60 deaths and thousands of emergency department admissions.

Repeated use of GHB appears to cause tolerance and physical dependence. Tolerance is indicated by the need for bigger and bigger doses to produce relaxation and euphoria. Physical dependence is indicated by signs of withdrawal—agitation, delirium, tachycardia, insomnia, anxiety, tremors, sweating—when regular use stops.

GHB has only one approved use: reduction of cateplexy in patients with narcolepsy (see Chapter 103). The drug is regulated as a Schedule III substance.

A precursor of GHB, known as *1,4-butanediol,* undergoes conversion to GHB in the body, and hence has effects identical to those of GHB itself. Butanediol is used as an industrial solvent, and is also available as a "dietary supplement." The supplements are claimed to enhance muscle growth, fight aging, increase sexual desire, promote relaxation, and elevate mood. Trade names for the supplements include Thunder Nectar, Inner G, and Zen.

Routes of Administration. Cocaine *hydrochloride* is usually administered *intranasally.* The drug is "snorted" and absorbed across the nasal mucosa into the bloodstream. In addition to intranasal administration, cocaine hydrochloride is often injected IV. Cocaine hydrochloride cannot be smoked because it is unstable at high temperature.

Cocaine *base* is administered by *smoking,* a process referred to as "freebasing." Smoking delivers large amounts of cocaine to the lungs, where absorption is very rapid. Subjective and physiologic effects are equivalent to those elicited by IV injection.

Subjective Effects and Addiction. At usual doses, cocaine produces euphoria similar to that produced by amphetamines. In a laboratory setting, individuals familiar with the effects of cocaine are unable to distinguish between cocaine and amphetamine. How does cocaine cause euphoria? The drug inhibits neuronal reuptake of dopamine, and thereby increases activation of dopamine receptors in the brain's reward circuit.

As with many other psychoactive drugs, the intensity of subjective responses depends on the rate at which plasma drug levels rise. Since cocaine levels rise relatively slowly with intranasal administration, this route produces responses of low intensity. In contrast, since IV administration and smoking cause nearly instantaneous elevations of plasma levels, these routes produce responses that are intense.

When crack cocaine is smoked, desirable subjective effects begin to fade within minutes and are often replaced by dysphoria. In an attempt to avoid dysphoria and regain euphoria, the user may administer repeated doses at short intervals. This usage pattern can rapidly lead to addiction.

Acute Toxicity: Symptoms and Treatment. Overdose is frequent and deaths have occurred. Mild overdose produces agitation, dizziness, tremor, and blurred vision. Severe overdose can produce hyperpyrexia, convulsions, ventricular dysrhythmias, and hemorrhagic stroke. Angina pectoris and myocardial infarction may develop secondary to coronary artery spasm. Psychologic manifestations of overdose include severe anxiety, paranoid ideation, and hallucinations (visual, auditory, or tactile). Because cocaine has a short half-life, symptoms subside in 1 to 2 hours.

Although there is no specific antidote to cocaine toxicity, most symptoms can be controlled with drugs. Intravenous *diazepam* or *lorazepam* can reduce anxiety and suppress seizures. *Diazepam* may also alleviate hypertension and dysrhythmias, since these result from increased central sympathetic activity. If hypertension is severe, it can be corrected with intravenous *nitroprusside* or *phentolamine.* Dysrhythmias associated with prolongation of the QT interval may respond to *hypertonic sodium bicarbonate.* Although beta blockers can suppress dysrhythmias, they can further compromise coronary perfusion (by preventing beta$_2$-mediated coronary vasodilation); hence, their use is controversial. Reduction of thrombus formation with aspirin can lower the risk of myocardial ischemia. Hyperthermia should be reduced with external cooling.

Chronic Toxicity. When administered intranasally on a long-term basis, cocaine can cause atrophy of the nasal mucosa and loss of sense of smell. In extreme cases, necrosis and perforation of the nasal septum have occurred. Nasal pathology results from local ischemia secondary to chronic vasoconstriction. Injury to the lungs can occur from smoking cocaine base.

Use During Pregnancy. Cocaine is highly lipid soluble and readily crosses the placenta, allowing it to accumulate in the fetal circulation. Until recently, it was assumed, but not proved, that cocaine exposure could cause significant harm to the fetus. However, a recent report in *JAMA* (March 28, 2001, pages 1613–1625), indicates that, if cocaine does harm the fetus, the injury is minimal—and, in all likelihood, considerably less than injury caused by tobacco or alcohol. Specifically, the report noted that there is no solid proof that *in utero* exposure to cocaine diminishes growth, affects developmental scores during the first 6 years, produces any lasting effect on motor development, or causes significant alterations in responses to behavioral stimuli. In short, available data fail to show that prenatal cocaine exposure has major adverse developmental effects.

Tolerance, Dependence, and Withdrawal. In animal models, regular administration of cocaine results in *increased* sensitivity to the drug, not tolerance. However, in humans, the opposite occurs. That is, when humans take cocaine on a regular basis, tolerance usually develops; hence, dosage must be increased to produce euphoria.

The degree of physical dependence produced by cocaine is in dispute. Some observers report little or no evidence of withdrawal following cocaine discontinuation. In contrast, others report symptoms similar to those associated with amphetamines: dysphoria, craving, fatigue, depression, and prolonged sleep.

Detoxification and Maintenance of Abstinence. Addiction to crack cocaine is very difficult to treat. The crack addict is typically unresponsive to persuasion and traditional psychotherapeutic techniques, although cognitive behavioral therapy may be beneficial. Benefits of acupuncture are minimal. If treatment on an outpatient basis is ineffective, admission to a treatment facility that prevents all access to cocaine may help.

Although various drugs have been given to help maintain abstinence following cocaine withdrawal, none is considered highly effective. Agents that have been tried include antidepressants (e.g., desipramine, bupropion, fluoxetine), dopamine agonists (bromocriptine, amantadine), opioid antagonists (e.g., naltrexone), and mood stabilizers (lithium, carbamazepine). Recent studies indicate that selegiline may help.

Amphetamines

The basic pharmacology of the amphetamines is discussed in Chapter 35. Discussion here is limited to amphetamine abuse.

Forms and Routes. The amphetamine family includes dextroamphetamine, methamphetamine, and amphetamine (a racemic mixture of dextroamphetamine and levamphetamine). When taken for purposes of abuse, amphetamines are usually administered orally or IV. In addition, a form of dextroamphetamine known as "ice" or "crystal meth" can be smoked.

Subjective and Behavioral Effects. Amphetamines produce arousal and elevation of mood. Euphoria is likely and talkativeness is prominent. A sense of increased physical strength and mental capacity occurs. Self-confidence rises. The amphetamine user feels little or no need for food and sleep. Orgasm is delayed, intensified, and more pleasurable.

Adverse CNS Effects. Amphetamines can produce a psychotic state characterized by hallucinations and paranoid ideation. This condition closely resembles paranoid schizophrenia. Although psychosis can be triggered by a single dose, it occurs more commonly in the context of long-term abuse. Amphetamine-induced psychosis usually resolves spontaneously following drug withdrawal. If needed, an antipsychotic agent (e.g., haloperidol) can be given to suppress symptoms.

Adverse Cardiovascular Effects. Because of their sympathomimetic actions, amphetamines can cause vasoconstriction and excessive stimulation of the heart. These actions can lead to hypertension, angina pectoris, and dysrhythmias. Overdose may also cause cerebral and systemic vasculitis and renal failure. Changes in cerebral blood vessels can lead to stroke. Vasoconstriction can be relieved with an alpha-adrenergic blocker (e.g., phentolamine). Cardiac stimulation can be reduced with a beta blocker (e.g., labetalol). Drug elimination can be accelerated by giving ammonium chloride to acidify the urine.

Tolerance, Dependence, and Withdrawal. Prolonged amphetamine use results in tolerance to mood elevation, appetite suppression, and cardiovascular effects. Although physical dependence is only moderate, psychologic dependence can be intense. Amphetamine withdrawal can produce dysphoria and a strong sense of craving. Other symptoms include fatigue, prolonged sleep, excessive eating, and depression. Depression can persist for months and is a common reason for resuming amphetamine use.

MARIJUANA AND RELATED PREPARATIONS

Cannabis sativa, the Source of Marijuana

Marijuana is prepared from *Cannabis sativa,* the Indian hemp plant—an unusual plant in that it has separate male and female forms. Psychoactive compounds are present in all parts of the male and female plants. However, the greatest concentration of psychoactive substances is found in the flowering tops of the females.

The two most common *Cannabis* derivatives are *marijuana* and *hashish.* Marijuana is a preparation consisting of leaves and flowers of male and female plants. Alternative names for marijuana include *grass, weed, pot,* and *dope.* The terms *joint* and *reefer* refer to marijuana cigarettes. Hashish is a dried preparation of the resinous exudate from female flowers. Hashish is considerably more potent than marijuana.

Marijuana use in the United States is on the rise again. Among youths ages 12 to 17, nearly 10% used marijuana in 1997—compared with less than 5% in 1992. However, current use is still below the 1979 value of 14.2%.

Psychoactive Component

The major psychoactive substance in *Cannabis sativa* is *delta-9-tetrahydrocannabinol* (THC), an oily chemical with high lipid solubility. The structure of THC appears in Figure 38–1.

The THC content of *Cannabis* preparations is variable. The highest concentrations are found in the flowers of the female plant. The lowest concentrations are in the seeds. Depending on growing conditions and the strain of the plant, THC in marijuana preparations may range from 1% to 11%.

Mechanism of Action

THC has several possible mechanisms. Perhaps the most important is activation of specific cannabinoid receptors found in various brain regions. The endogenous ligand for these receptors appears to be *anandamide,* a derivative of arachidonic acid unique to the brain. Other proposed mechanisms are (1) activation of phospholipase A_2 in the brain, resulting in increased production of prostaglandin E_2, and (2) augmentation of neuronal membrane fluidity through interaction with membrane lipids.

Recent evidence indicates that marijuana may act in part through the same reward system as opioids and cocaine. Both heroin and cocaine produce pleasurable sensations by promoting release of dopamine in the brain's reward circuit. In 1997, researchers demonstrated that, in rats, intravenous THC also causes dopamine release. Interestingly, release of dopamine by THC is blocked by naloxone, a drug that blocks the effects of opioids. This suggests that THC causes release of dopamine by first causing release of endogenous opioids.

Pharmacokinetics

Administration by Smoking. When marijuana or hashish is smoked, about 60% of the THC content is absorbed. Absorption from the lungs is rapid. Subjective effects begin in minutes and peak in 20 to 30 minutes. Effects from a single marijuana cigarette may persist 2 to 3 hours. Termination of effects results from metabolism of THC to inactive products.

Oral Administration. When marijuana or hashish is ingested, practically all of the THC undergoes absorption. However, the majority is inactivated on its first pass through the liver. Hence only 6% to 20% of absorbed drug actually reaches the general circulation. Because of this extensive first-pass metabolism, oral doses must be 3 to 10 times greater than smoked doses to produce equivalent effects. With oral administration, effects are delayed and prolonged; responses begin 30 to 50 minutes after administration and persist up to 12 hours.

Behavioral and Subjective Effects

Marijuana produces three principal subjective effects: *euphoria, sedation,* and *hallucinations.* This set of responses is unique to marijuana; no other psychoactive drug produces all three. Because of this singular pattern of effects, marijuana is in a class by itself.

Effects of Low to Moderate Doses. Responses to low doses of THC are variable and depend on several factors, including dosage size, route of administration, setting of drug use, and expectations and previous experience of the user. The following effects are common: euphoria and relaxation; gaiety and a heightened sense of the humorous; increased sensitivity to visual and auditory stimuli; enhanced sense of touch, taste, and smell; increased appetite and ability to appreciate the flavor of food; and distortion of time perception such that short spans seem much longer than they really are. In addition to these effects, which might be considered pleasurable (or at least innocuous), moderate doses can produce undesirable responses. These include impairment of short-term memory; decreased capacity to perform multistep tasks; impairment of driving skills (which can be substantially worsened by concurrent use of alcohol); temporal disintegration (inability to distinguish between past, present, and future); depersonalization (a sense of strangeness about the self); decreased ability to perceive the emotions of others; and reduced interpersonal interaction.

High-Dose Effects. In high doses, marijuana can have serious adverse psychologic effects. The user may experience hallucinations, delusions, and paranoia. Euphoria may be displaced by intense anxiety, and a dissociative state may occur in which the user feels "outside of himself or herself." In extremely high doses, marijuana can produce a state resembling toxic psychosis, which may persist for weeks. Because of the widespread use of marijuana, psychiatric emergencies caused by the drug are relatively common.

Not all users are equally vulnerable to the adverse psychologic effects of marijuana. Some individuals experience ill effects only at extremely high doses. In contrast, others routinely experience adverse effects at moderate doses. Schizophrenics are at unusually high risk for adverse reactions. In the stabilized schizophrenic, marijuana can precipitate an acute psychotic episode.

Effects of Chronic Use. Chronic, excessive use of marijuana is associated with a behavioral phenomenon known as an *amotivational syndrome,* characterized by apathy, dullness, poor grooming, reduced interest in achievement, and disinterest in the pursuit of conventional goals. The precise relationship between marijuana and development of the syndrome is not known, nor is it certain what other factors may contribute. Available data do not suggest that the amotivational syndrome is due to organic brain damage.

Physiologic Effects

Cardiovascular Effects. Marijuana produces a dose-related increase in heart rate. Increases of 20 to 50 beats/min are typical. However, rates up to 140 beats/min are not uncommon. Pretreatment with propranolol prevents marijuana-induced tachycardia but does not block the drug's subjective effects. Marijuana causes orthostatic hypotension and pronounced reddening of the conjunctivae. These responses apparently result from vasodilation.

Respiratory Effects. When used *acutely,* marijuana produces *bronchodilation.* However, when smoked chronically, the drug causes airway constriction. In addition, chronic use is closely associated with development of bronchitis, sinusitis, and asthma. Lung cancer is another possible outcome. Animal studies have shown that tar from marijuana smoke is a more potent carcinogen than tar from cigarettes.

Effects on Reproduction. Research in animals has shown multiple effects on reproduction. In males, marijuana decreases spermatogenesis and testosterone levels. In females, the drug reduces levels of follicle-stimulating hormone, luteinizing hormone, and prolactin. In some species, marijuana has caused birth defects. However, teratogenesis has not been proved in humans.

Tolerance and Dependence

When taken in extremely high doses, marijuana can produce tolerance and physical dependence. Neither effect, however, is remarkable. Some tolerance develops to the cardiovascular, perceptual, and motor effects of marijuana. Little or no tolerance develops to subjective effects.

To demonstrate physical dependence on marijuana, the drug must be given in very high doses—and even then the degree of dependence is only moderate. Symptoms brought on by abrupt discontinuation of high-dose marijuana include irritability, restlessness, nervousness, insomnia, reduced appetite, and weight loss. Tremor, hyperthermia, and chills may occur too. Symptoms subside in 4 to 5 days. With moderate marijuana use, no withdrawal symptoms occur.

Therapeutic Uses

Approved Uses. *Suppression of Emesis.* Intense nausea and vomiting are common side effects of cancer chemotherapy. In certain patients, these responses can be suppressed more effectively with cannabinoids than with traditional antiemetics (e.g., prochlorperazine, metoclopramide). At this time, only one cannabinoid—dronabinol (THC)—is available for antiemetic use. Dosage forms and dosages are presented in Chapter 75. Another cannabinoid—nabilone—has been withdrawn from the market.

Appetite Stimulation. Dronabinol (THC) is approved for stimulating appetite in patients with AIDS. By relieving anorexia, treatment may prevent or reverse loss of weight.

Potential Uses. Proponents of making marijuana available by prescription argue that smoked marijuana can reduce chronic pain, suppress nausea caused by chemotherapy, improve appetite in patients with AIDS, lower intraocular pressure in patients with glaucoma, and suppress spasticity associated with multiple sclerosis and spinal cord injury. However, the evidence in support of these claims is weak—largely because federal regulations effectively barred marijuana research.

In 1999, two developments opened the doors to marijuana research. First, an expert panel, convened by the National Academy of Sciences' Institute of Medicine, recommended that clinical trials on marijuana proceed. Because smoking marijuana poses a risk of lung cancer and other respiratory disorders, the panel also recommended development of a rapid-onset nonsmoked delivery system. In response to this report and to pressure from scientists and voters, the government created new guidelines that loosened restraints on marijuana research. Under the guidelines, researchers will be allowed to purchase marijuana directly from the government. (On behalf of the government, the University of Mississippi maintains a plot of marijuana on 1.8 closely guarded acres.) The only catch is that proposed research must first be reviewed and approved by the National Institutes of Health.

Comparison of Marijuana with Alcohol

In several important ways, responses to marijuana and alcohol are quite different. Whereas increased hostility and aggression are common sequelae of alcohol consumption, aggressive behavior is rare among marijuana users. Although loss of judgment and control can occur with either drug, these losses are greater with alcohol. For the marijuana user, increased appetite and food intake are typical. In contrast, heavy drinkers often suffer nutritional deficiencies. Lastly, whereas marijuana can cause toxic psychosis, dissociative phenomena, and paranoia, these severe adverse psychologic reactions rarely occur with alcohol.

PSYCHEDELICS

The psychedelics are a fascinating drug family for which LSD can be considered the prototype. Other family members include mescaline, dimethyltryptamine (DMT), and psilocin.

The psychedelics are so named because of their ability to produce what has been termed a *psychedelic state*. Individuals in this state show an increased awareness of sensory stimuli and are likely to perceive the world around them as beautiful and harmonious; the normally insignificant may assume exceptional meaning, the "self" may seem split into an "observer" and a "doer," and boundaries between "self" and "nonself" may fade, producing a sense of unity with the cosmos.

Psychedelic drugs are often referred to as *hallucinogens* or *psychotomimetics*. These names reflect an ability to produce hallucinations as well as mental states that resemble psychosis.

Although psychedelics can cause hallucinations and psychotic-like states, these are not their most characteristic effects. The characteristic that truly distinguishes the psychedelics from other agents is their *ability to bring on the same types of alterations in thought, perception, and feeling that otherwise occur only in dreams*. In essence, the psychedelics seem able to activate mechanisms for dreaming without causing unconsciousness.

d-Lysergic Acid Diethylamide (LSD)

History. The first person to experience LSD was a Swiss chemist named Albert Hofman. In 1943, 5 years after LSD was first synthesized, Hofman accidentally ingested a minute amount of the drug. The result was a dream-like state accompanied by perceptual distortions and vivid hallucinations. The high potency and unusual actions of LSD led to speculation the drug might provide a model for studying psychosis. Unfortunately, that speculation did not prove correct: Extensive research has revealed that the effects of LSD cannot be equated with idiopathic psychosis. With the realization that LSD did not produce a "model psychosis," medical interest in the drug declined. Not everyone, however, lost interest; during the 1960s, nonmedical experimentation with the drug flourished. This widespread use caused substantial societal concern, and, by 1970, LSD had been classified as a Schedule I substance. Despite regulatory efforts, street use of LSD continues.

Mechanism of Action. LSD acts at multiple sites in the brain and spinal cord. Effects are thought to result from activation of serotonin$_2$ receptors. This concept has been reinforced by the observation that *ritanserin*, a selective blocker of serotonin$_2$ receptors, can prevent the effects of LSD in animals.

Time Course. LSD is usually administered orally but can also be injected or smoked. With oral administration, initial effects can be felt in minutes. Over the next few hours, responses become progressively more intense. Effects subside in 8 to 12 hours.

Subjective and Behavioral Effects. Responses to LSD can be diverse, complex, and changeable. The drug can alter thinking, feeling, perception, sense of self, and sense of relationship with the environment and other people. LSD-induced experiences may be sublime or terrifying. Just what will be experienced during any particular "trip" cannot be predicted.

Perceptual alterations can be dramatic. Colors may appear iridescent or glowing, kaleidoscopic images may appear, and vivid hallucinations may occur. Sensory experiences may merge so that colors seem to be heard and sounds seem to be visible. Afterimages may occur, causing current perceptions to overlap with preceding perceptions. The LSD user may feel a sense of wonderment and awe at the beauty of commonplace things.

LSD can have a profound impact on affect. Emotions may range from elation, good humor, and euphoria to sadness, dysphoria, and fear. The intensity of emotion may be overwhelming.

Thoughts may turn inward. Attitudes may be re-evaluated, and old values assigned new priorities. A sense of new and important insight may be felt. However, despite the intensity of these experiences, enduring changes in beliefs, behavior, and personality are rare.

Physiologic Effects. LSD has few physiologic effects. Activation of the sympathetic nervous system can produce tachycardia, elevation of blood pressure, mydriasis, piloerection, and hyperthermia. Neuromuscular effects (tremor, incoordination, hyperreflexia, and muscular weakness) may also occur.

Tolerance and Dependence. Tolerance to LSD develops rapidly. Substantial tolerance can be seen after just three or four daily doses. Tolerance to subjective and behavioral effects develops to a greater extent than to cardiovascular effects. Cross-tolerance exists with LSD, mescaline, and psilocybin, but not with DMT. Since DMT is similar to LSD, the absence of cross-tolerance is surprising. There is no cross-tolerance with amphetamines or THC. Upon cessation of LSD use, tolerance fades rapidly. Abrupt withdrawal of LSD is not associated with an abstinence syndrome; hence, there is no evidence for physical dependence.

Toxicity. Toxic reactions are primarily psychologic. LSD has never been a direct cause of death, although fatalities have occurred from accidents and suicides.

Acute panic reactions are relatively common and may be associated with a fear of disintegration of the self. Such "bad trips" can usually be managed by a process of "talking down" (providing emotional support and reassurance in a nonthreatening environment). Panic episodes can also be managed with an antianxiety agent, such as *diazepam*. Neuroleptics (e.g., haloperidol, chlorpromazine) may actually intensify the experience; hence, their use is questionable.

A small percentage of former LSD users experience episodic visual disturbances, formerly referred to as "flashbacks." These disturbances may manifest as geometric pseudohallucinations, flashes of color, or positive afterimages. Visual disturbances may be precipitated by several factors, including marijuana use, fatigue, stress, and anxiety. Phenothiazines exacerbate these experiences rather than provide relief. These disturbances appear to be caused by permanent changes in the visual system.

In addition to panic reactions and visual disturbances, LSD can cause other adverse psychologic effects. Depressive episodes, dissociative reactions, and distortions of body image may occur. When an LSD experience has been intensely terrifying, the user may be left with persistent residual fear. The drug may also cause prolonged psychotic reactions. In contrast to acute effects, which differ substantially from symptoms of schizophrenia, prolonged psychotic reactions mimic schizophrenia faithfully.

Therapeutic Uses. LSD has no recognized therapeutic applications. The drug has been evaluated for possible use in treating alcoholism, opioid addiction, and psychiatric disorders. In addition, LSD has been studied as a possible means of promoting psychologic well-being in patients with terminal cancer. However, for all of these potential uses, LSD proved either ineffective or impractical.

Mescaline, Psilocybin, Psilocin, and Dimethyltryptamine

In addition to LSD, the family of psychedelic drugs includes mescaline, psilocin, psilocybin, dimethyltryptamine (DMT), and several related compounds (see Table 38–2). Some psychedelics are synthetic and some occur naturally. DMT and LSD represent the synthetic compounds. Mescaline, a constituent of the peyote cactus, and psilocin and psilocybin, constituents of "magic mushrooms," represent compounds found in nature.

The subjective and behavioral effects of the miscellaneous psychedelic drugs are similar to those of LSD. Like LSD, these drugs can elicit modes of thought, perception, and feeling that are normally restricted to dreams. In addition, they can cause hallucinations and induce mental states that resemble psychosis.

The miscellaneous psychedelics differ from LSD with respect to potency and time course. LSD is the most potent of the psychedelics, producing its full spectrum of effects at doses as low as 0.5 mg/kg. Psilocin and psilocybin are 100 times less potent than LSD, and mescaline is 4000 times less potent than LSD. Whereas the effects of LSD are prolonged (responses may last 12 or more hours), the effects of mescaline and DMT are shorter: responses to mescaline usually terminate within 8 to 12 hours, and responses to DMT terminate within 1 to 2 hours.

3,4-METHYLENEDIOXYMETHAMPHETAMINE (MDMA, ECSTASY)

MDMA, also known as "ecstasy," is a complex drug with stimulant and psychedelic properties. The drug is structurally related to methamphetamine (a stimulant) and mescaline (a hallucinogen). Low doses produce mild LSD-like psychedelic effects; higher doses produce amphetamine-like stimulant effects. Although MDMA can produce effects that are clearly pleasurable, it can also be dangerous; the biggest concerns are neurotoxicity, seizures, hyperthermia and its sequelae, and excessive cardiovascular stimulation. MDMA is classified as a Schedule I drug.

Time Course and Dosage. MDMA is usually administered orally, but may also be snorted, injected, or inserted as a rectal suppository. With oral administration, effects begin in 20 minutes, peak in 2 to 3 hours, and persist 4 to 5 hours. The usual dose is 100 mg or less.

Who Uses MDMA and Why? MDMA is used primarily by adolescents and young adults, who often take it at nightclubs and all-night dance parties, known as "raves." The drug is used by young people in cities, in the suburbs, and in the country. According to a survey conducted in 2000, 4.3% of 8th-graders, 7.3% of 10th-graders, and 11.0% of 12th-graders have used MDMA at least once in their lives.

Why do people take MDMA? Because it makes them feel really good. The drug can elevate mood, increase sensory awareness, and heighten sensitivity to music. It can also facilitate interpersonal relationships: Users report a sense of closeness with others, lowering of defenses, reduced anxiety, enhanced communication, and increased sociability.

Adverse Effects. Unfortunately, MDMA is not free of risks. The drug can injure serotonergic neurons, stimulate the heart, and raise body temperature to a dangerous level. In addition, it can cause neurologic effects (e.g., seizures, spasmodic jerking, jaw clenching, teeth grinding) and a host of adverse psychologic effects (e.g., confusion, anxiety, paranoia, panic attacks, visual hallucinations, and suicidal thoughts and behavior). In 2000, MDMA was associated with 4511 admissions to emergency departments, mainly because of seizures.

MDMA can damage serotonergic neurons, perhaps irreversibly. When administered to rats and primates in doses only 2 to 4 times greater than those that produce hallucinations in humans, MDMA causes *irreversible destruction of serotonergic neurons,* resulting in passivity and insomnia. At least three lines of evidence suggest that MDMA is also neurotoxic in humans. (1) MDMA causes dose-related impairment of memory, a brain function mediated in part by serotonin. Memory impairment persists long after MDMA was last taken. (2) The cerebrospinal fluid of long-term MDMA users contains abnormally low concentrations of serotonin metabolites, suggesting a loss of serotonergic neurons. (3) Using positron emission tomography to study former MDMA users, researchers demonstrated decreased binding of a ligand selective for the serotonin transporter, indicating damage to serotonergic neurons. In this study, reductions in ligand binding correlated with the extent of MDMA use, and not with the duration of abstinence.

MDMA can cause hyperthermia in association with dehydration, hyponatremia, and rhabdomyolysis (disintegration of muscle tissue). Treatment consists of rapid cooling, rehydration, and administering dantrolene [Dantrium], a drug that relaxes skeletal muscle, thereby reducing heat generation and the risk of rhabdomyolysis. The risk of hyperthermia and dehydration could be greatly reduced by providing ample fluids at raves and other events where MDMA is likely to be used.

Because of its amphetamine-like actions, MDMA can increase heart rate, blood pressure, and myocardial oxygen consumption. Remarkably, the increases in heart rate and blood pressure equal those produced by maximal doses of dobutamine, a powerful adrenergic agonist (see Chapter 17). Cardiovascular stimulation is a potential danger to users with heart disease.

PHENCYCLIDINE

Phencyclidine ("PCP," "angel dust," "peace pill") was originally developed as an anesthetic for animals. The drug was tried briefly as a general anesthetic for humans but was withdrawn because it produced severe emergence delirium. Although rejected for therapeutic use, phencyclidine has become widely used as a drug of abuse. Use has grown in large part because the drug can be synthesized easily by amateur chemists, making it cheap and abundant. The popularity of phencyclidine is disturbing in that the drug causes a high incidence of severe adverse effects—effects that make it one of the most dangerous abused substances.

Chemistry and Pharmacokinetics

Chemistry. Phencyclidine is a weak organic base with high lipid solubility. The drug is chemically related to ketamine, an unusual general anesthetic (see Chapter 26). The structural formula of phencyclidine appears in Figure 38–1.

Pharmacokinetics. Phencyclidine can be administered orally, intranasally, intravenously, and by smoking. For administration by smoking, the drug is usually sprinkled on plant matter (e.g., oregano, parsley, tobacco, marijuana). Because of its high lipid solubility, phencyclidine is readily absorbed from all sites.

Once absorbed, phencyclidine undergoes substantial gastroenteric recirculation. Because it is a base, phencyclidine in the blood can be drawn into the acidic environment of the stomach (by the pH partitioning effect); from the stomach, the drug re-enters the intestine, from which it is reabsorbed into the blood. This cycling from blood to GI tract and back prolongs the drug's sojourn in the body. Elimination occurs eventually through a combination of hepatic metabolism and renal excretion.

Mechanism of Action

The mechanism by which phencyclidine affects the CNS is not clear. The drug binds with high affinity to sites in the cerebral cortex and limbic system, and blocks certain glutamate receptors and binds certain receptors for opioids. However, the relationship between binding activity and psychologic effects has not been established.

Subjective and Behavioral Effects

Phencyclidine produces a unique set of effects. Hallucinations are prominent. In addition, the drug can produce CNS depression, CNS excitation, and analgesia. This complex response profile is not seen with any other drug of abuse. Because of its singular range of effects, phencyclidine is in a class by itself.

Effects of Low to Moderate Doses. At low doses, phencyclidine produces effects like those of alcohol. Low-dose intoxication is characterized by euphoria, release of inhibitions, and emotional lability. Nystagmus, slurred speech, and motor incoordination may occur too.

As dosage increases, the clinical picture becomes more variable and complex. Symptoms include excitation, disorientation, anxiety, disorganized thoughts, altered body image, and reduced perception of tactile and painful stimuli. Mood may be volatile and hostile. Bizarre behavior may develop. Heart rate and blood pressure are elevated.

High-Dose (Toxic) Effects. High doses can cause severe adverse physiologic and psychologic effects. Death may result from a variety of causes.

Psychologic effects include hallucinations, confusional states, combativeness, and psychosis. The psychosis closely resembles schizophrenia and may persist for weeks. Individuals with pre-existing psychoses are especially vulnerable to psychotogenic effects. Suicide has been attempted.

The physiologic effects of high-dose phencyclidine are varied. Extreme overdose can produce hypertension, coma, seizures, and muscular rigidity associated with severe hyperthermia and rhabdomyolysis.

Treatment of Toxicity. Treatment is primarily supportive. Psychotic reactions are best managed by isolation from external stimuli. "Talking down" is not effective, and the benefits of antipsychotic drugs, such as haloperidol, are limited. Physical restraint may be needed to prevent self-inflicted harm and protect others from assault. If respiration is depressed, mechanical support of ventilation may be needed. Severe hypertension can be managed with diazoxide, a vasodilator. Seizures can be controlled with IV diazepam. If fever is high, external cooling can lower temperature. By promoting muscle relaxation, dantrolene can reduce heat generation and rhabdomyolysis.

Elimination of phencyclidine can be accelerated by continuous gastric lavage and acidification of the urine with ammonium chloride. Continuous lavage is effective because gastroenteric recirculation keeps delivering drug to the stomach. Acidification of urine may promote phencyclidine excretion by reducing tubular reabsorption of this weak base.

INHALANTS

The inhalants are a diverse group of drugs that have only one characteristic in common: administration by inhalation. These drugs can be divided into three classes: anesthetics, volatile nitrites, and organic solvents.

Anesthetics

Provided that dosage is modest, anesthetics produce subjective effects similar to those of alcohol (euphoria, exhilaration, loss of inhibitions). The anesthetics that have been abused most are *nitrous oxide* ("laughing gas") and *ether.* One reason for the popularity of these drugs is ease of administration: Both agents can be used without exotic equipment. For nitrous oxide, ready availability also promotes use: Small cylinders of the drug, marketed for aerating whipping cream, can be purchased without restriction.

Volatile Nitrites

Four volatile nitrites—*amyl nitrite, butyl nitrite, isobutyl nitrite,* and *cyclohexyl nitrite*—are subject to abuse. These drugs are abused by homosexual males because of an ability to relax the anal sphincter, and by males in general because of a reputed ability to prolong and intensify sexual orgasm.

The most pronounced pharmacologic effect of volatile nitrites is *venodilation,* which causes pooling of blood in veins, which in turn causes a profound drop in systolic blood pressure. The result is dizziness, light-headedness, palpitations, and possibly pulsatile headache. Effects begin seconds after inhalation and fade rapidly. The primary toxicity is methemoglobinemia, which can be treated with methylene blue and supplemental oxygen.

Nitrites are available from medical and nonmedical sources. Amyl nitrite is a drug used for angina pectoris. Cyclohexyl nitrite is present in room odorizers. And butyl nitrite and isobutyl nitrite are present in products made solely for recreational use. Trade names for butyl nitrite and isobutyl nitrite include Climax, Rush, and Locker Room. On the street, preparations of amyl nitrite are known as "poppers" or "snappers." These terms reflect the fact that amyl nitrite is packaged in glass ampules that make a popping sound when snapped open to allow inhalation.

Organic Solvents

A wide assortment of solvents have been inhaled to induce intoxication. These compounds include *toluene, gasoline, lighter fluid, paint thinner, nail-polish remover, benzene, acetone, chloroform,* and *model-airplane glue.* These agents are used primarily by children and the very poor—people who, because of age or insufficient funds, lack access to more conventional drugs of abuse.

Administration. Solvents are administered by three processes, referred to as "bagging," "huffing," and "sniffing." Bagging is performed by pouring solvent in a plastic bag and inhaling the vapor. Huffing is performed by pouring the solvent on a rag and inhaling the vapor. Sniffing is performed by inhaling the solvent directly from its container.

Pharmacologic Effects. The acute effects of organic solvents are somewhat like those of alcohol (euphoria, impaired judgment, slurred speech, flushing, CNS depression). In addition, these compounds can cause visual hallucinations and disorientation with respect to time and place. High doses can cause sudden death. Possible causes include anoxia, respiratory depression, vagal stimulation (which slows heart rate), and dysrhythmias.

Prolonged use is associated with multiple toxicities. Gasoline can cause lead poisoning; chloroform is toxic to the heart, liver, and kidneys; and toluene can cause severe brain damage and bone marrow depression. Many solvents can damage the heart; fatal dysrhythmias have occurred secondary to drug-induced heart block.

Management. Management of acute toxicity is strictly supportive. The objective is to stabilize vital signs. We have no antidotes for volatile solvents.

NICOTINE AND SMOKING

Cigarette smoking remains the greatest single cause of preventable illness and premature death. In the United States, smoking kills more than 440,000 people each year—over 264,000 males and 178,000 females. On average, male smokers die 13.2 years prematurely, and females die 14.5 years prematurely. As shown in Table 38–3, most deaths result from lung cancer (128,813), heart disease (111,344), and chronic airway obstruction (64,735). Not only do cigarettes kill the people who smoke them, every year they also kill over 36,000 nonsmokers who inhaled secondhand smoke. The direct medical costs of smoking exceed $70 billion a year. Indirect costs, such as lost time from work and disability, add up to an additional $82 billion.

Although tobacco smoke contains many dangerous compounds, nicotine is of greatest concern. Other hazardous components in tobacco smoke include carbon monoxide, hydrogen cyanide, ammonia, nitrosamines, and tar. Tar is composed of various polycyclic hydrocarbons, some of which are proven carcinogens.

Basic Pharmacology of Nicotine
Mechanism of Action

The effects of nicotine result from actions at nicotinic receptors. Whether these receptors are activated or inhibited depends on nicotine dosage. *Low* doses *activate* nicotinic receptors; *high* doses *block* them. The amount of nicotine received from cigarettes is relatively low. Accordingly, cigarette smoking causes receptor *activation*.

Nicotine can activate nicotinic receptors at several locations. Most effects result from activating nicotinic receptors in autonomic ganglia and the adrenal medulla. In addition, nicotine can activate nicotinic receptors in the carotid body, aortic arch, and CNS. As discussed below, actions in the CNS mimic those of cocaine and other highly addictive substances. When present at the levels produced by smoking, nicotine has no significant effect on nicotinic receptors of the neuromuscular junction.

Pharmacokinetics

Absorption of nicotine depends on whether the delivery system is a cigarette, a cigar, or smokeless tobacco. Nicotine in cigarette smoke is absorbed primarily from the lungs. When cigarette smoke is inhaled, between 90% and 98% of nicotine in the lungs enters the blood. Unlike nicotine in cigarette smoke, nicotine in cigar smoke is absorbed primarily from the mouth, as is nicotine in smokeless tobacco.

Nicotine can cross membranes easily and is widely distributed throughout the body. The drug readily enters breast milk, reaching levels that can be toxic to the nursing infant. Nicotine also crosses the placental barrier and can cause fetal harm.

Nicotine is rapidly metabolized to inactive products. Nicotine and its metabolites are excreted by the kidney. The drug's half-life is 1 to 2 hours.

Pharmacologic Effects

The pharmacologic effects discussed in this section are associated with *low* doses of nicotine. These are the effects caused by smoking cigarettes. Responses to *high* doses are discussed under *Acute Poisoning.*

Cardiovascular Effects. The cardiovascular effects of nicotine result primarily from activating nicotinic receptors in *sympathetic ganglia* and the *adrenal medulla.* Activation of these receptors promotes release of norepinephrine from sympathetic nerves and release of epinephrine (and some norepinephrine) from the adrenals. Norepinephrine and epinephrine act on the cardiovascular system to constrict blood vessels, accelerate the heart, and increase the force of ventricular contraction. The net result is elevation of blood pressure and increased cardiac work. These effects underlie cardiovascular deaths.

GI Effects. Nicotine influences GI function primarily by activating nicotinic receptors in *parasympathetic* ganglia. The result is increased secretion of gastric acid and increased tone and motility of GI smooth muscle. In addition, nicotine can promote vomiting. Nicotine-induced vomiting results from a complex process that involves nicotinic receptors in the aortic arch, the carotid sinus, and CNS.

CNS Effects. Nicotine is a CNS stimulant. The drug stimulates respiration and produces an arousal pattern on the electroencephalogram. Moderate doses can cause tremors, and high doses can cause convulsions.

Nicotine has multiple psychologic effects. The drug increases alertness, facilitates memory, improves cognition, reduces aggression, and suppresses appetite. In addition, by promoting release of dopamine, nicotine activates the brain's "pleasure system" located in the mesolimbic area. The effects of nicotine on the pleasure system are identical to those of other highly addictive drugs, including cocaine, amphetamines, and opioids.

Effects During Pregnancy and Lactation. Exposure to nicotine can harm the developing fetus. Nicotine in breast milk can harm the nursing infant. Accordingly, therapeutic formulations of nicotine (e.g., nicotine chewing gum, nicotine transdermal patches, nicotine nasal spray) are contraindicated during pregnancy, and their use by nursing mothers is not recommended.

Tolerance and Dependence

Tolerance. Tolerance develops to some effects of nicotine but not to others. Tolerance does develop to nausea and dizziness, which are common in the unseasoned smoker. In contrast, *very little tolerance develops to the cardiovascular actions of nicotine: Veteran smokers continue to experience increased blood pressure and increased cardiac work whenever they smoke.*

Dependence. Chronic cigarette smoking results in dependence. By definition, this means that individuals who discontinue smoking will experience an abstinence syndrome. The tobacco withdrawal syndrome is characterized by craving, nervousness, restlessness, irritability, impatience, increased hostility, insomnia, impaired concentration, increased appetite, and weight gain. Symptoms begin about 24 hours after smoking has ceased, and can last for weeks to months. Women report more discomfort than men. Experience has shown that abrupt discontinuation may be preferable to gradual reduction. (All that gradual reduction seems to do is prolong suffering.)

Acute Poisoning

Nicotine is highly toxic. Doses as low as 40 mg can be fatal. The drug's toxicity is attested to by its use in insecticides. Common causes of nicotine poisoning include ingestion of tobacco by children and exposure to nicotine-containing insecticides.

Symptoms. The most prominent symptoms involve the cardiovascular, GI, and central nervous systems. Specific symptoms include nausea, salivation, vomiting, diarrhea, cold sweat, disturbed hearing and vision, confusion, and faintness; pulses may be rapid, weak, and irregular. Death results from respiratory paralysis, which is caused by direct effects of nicotine on the muscles of respiration, as well as by effects in the CNS.

Treatment. Management centers on reducing nicotine absorption and supporting respiration; there is no specific antidote to nicotine poisoning. To minimize absorption, patients should be given syrup of ipecac followed by activated charcoal. Ipecac induces vomiting, thereby removing any nicotine remaining in the stomach. Activated charcoal adsorbs nicotine, thereby preventing any nicotine that remains in the GI tract from being absorbed into the blood. If respiration is depressed, ventilatory assistance should be provided. Since nicotine undergoes rapid metabolic inactivation, recovery from the acute phase of poisoning can occur within hours.

Chronic Toxicity from Smoking

Adverse effects of chronic tobacco smoking range from vascular diseases (coronary artery disease, cerebrovascular disease, peripheral vascular disease) to chronic lung disease to cancers of the larynx, esophagus, oral cavity, lung, bladder, and pancreas. Smoking during pregnancy increases the risk of low birth weight, spontaneous abortion, perinatal mortality, and sudden infant death. Quantitatively, cardiovascular disease and lung disease are the greatest dangers.

Fortunately, many adverse effects of smoking are reversible. Within 5 to 10 years after smoking has ceased, the risks of smoking-related disease for the ex-smoker are only slightly higher than the risks for the person who has never smoked.

TABLE 38–3 ▪ ▪ Annual Smoking-Attributable Mortality in the United States, 1995–1999		
	Smoking-Related Deaths	
Disease Category	**Male**	**Female**
Neoplasms		
Lip, oral cavity, pharynx	3873	1264
Esophagus	6280	1613
Pancreas	3065	3415
Larynx	2525	602
Trachea, lung, bronchus	80,571	44,242
Cervix uteri	—	552
Urinary bladder	3699	1053
Kidney, other urinary	2799	236
TOTAL	**102,812**	**52,949**
Cardiovascular Diseases		
Hypertension	3320	2740
Ischemic heart disease		
Ages 35–64 yr	22,059	7069
Age ≥ 65 yr	29,312	23,536
Other heart diseases	18,822	10,546
Cerebrovascular disease		
Ages 35–64 yr	3898	3586
Age ≥65 yr	4697	5264
Atherosclerosis	1644	883
Aortic aneurysm	6489	3135
Other arterial disease	665	940
TOTAL	**90,906**	**57,699**
Respiratory Diseases		
Pneumonia, influenza	8802	6774
Bronchitis, emphysema	9944	7752
Chronic airways obstruction	34,919	29,816
TOTAL	**53,665**	**44,342**
Perinatal Conditions		
Short gestation/low birth weight	227	175
Respiratory distress syndrome	85	24
Other respiratory—newborn	84	33
Sudden infant death syndrome	202	175
TOTAL	**599**	**408**
Burn Deaths	589	377
Secondhand Smoke Deaths		
Lung cancer	1110	1890
Ischemic heart disease	14,407	20,646
Overall Total	**264,087**	**178,311**

Adapted from Centers for Disease Control and Prevention. Annual smoking-attributable mortality, years of potential life lost, and economic costs—United States, 1995–1999. MMWR Morb Mortal Wkly Rep 2002; 51:300–303.

Pharmacologic Aids to Smoking Cessation

Cigarettes are highly addictive, and hence giving them up is very hard. Nonetheless, abstinence *can* be achieved. Every year, about 45% of American smokers make one or more attempts to quit. Of those who try to quit without help, only 7% achieve long-term success. In contrast, when a combination of counseling and drugs is employed, the 1-year abstinence rate approaches 30%. However, even with the aid of counseling and drugs, the first attempt usually fails. In fact, most people try quitting 5 to 7 times before they ultimately succeed. As time without a cigarette increases, the chances of relapse get progressively smaller: Of those who quit for a year, only 15% smoke again; and of those who quit for 5 years, only 3% smoke again.

Long-term smokers should be assured that quitting still offers important health benefits. Regardless of how long one has smoked, quitting can (1) reduce the risk of developing a tobacco-related disease, (2) slow the progression of an established tobacco-related disease, and (3) increase life expectancy. These benefits apply not only to people who quit while they are young and healthy, but also to people who quit after the age of 65 and to those with established tobacco-related disease.

Seven drugs have been shown to aid smoking cessation (Table 38–4). Of these, five are specifically approved by the FDA for this use, and are considered first-line treatments. The other two—nortriptyline and clonidine—are considered second-line treatments. Of the five first-line drugs, four contain nicotine and one doesn't. The nicotine-based products—nicotine gum, nicotine patch, nicotine inhaler, and nicotine nasal spray—are employed as nicotine replacement therapy (NRT). The nicotine-free product—bupropion [Zyban]—is taken to decrease nicotine craving along with some symptoms of withdrawal. When used alone, all five first-line drugs are equally effective: they about double the rate of abstinence. Combining bupropion with a nicotine patch may provide some additional benefit. Similarly, combining a nicotine patch with nicotine nasal spray may be more effective than either product alone.

At this time, we cannot predict who will respond best to a particular product. Accordingly, selection among the first-line drugs should be based on patient preference, success with a particular product in the past, and side effects. The second-line drugs should be reserved for patients who cannot use the first-line drugs or who failed to quit while using them.

Effective strategies for smoking cessation can be found in *A Clinical Practice Guideline for Treating Tobacco Use and Dependence,* issued by the U.S. Public Health Service in 2000. As stated in the guideline, tobacco dependence is a chronic condition that warrants repeated intervention until long-term abstinence is achieved. This is the same philosophy that guides treatment of dependence on other highly addictive substances, including cocaine and heroin. The guideline strongly recommends that, in the absence of specific contraindications, every one who is trying to quit should use at least one first-line drug: bupropion or a nicotine-based product.

Nicotine Replacement Therapy

NRT allows smokers to substitute a pharmaceutical source of nicotine for the nicotine in cigarettes—and then gradually withdraw the replacement nicotine. This is analogous to using methadone to wean addicts from heroin.

Four formulations of nicotine are available: chewing gum, transdermal patches, a nasal spray, and an inhaler (see Table 38–4). With the gum, patches, and inhaler, blood levels of nicotine rise slowly and remain relatively steady. Because nicotine levels rise slowly, these delivery systems pro-

TABLE 38–4 ■ Pharmacologic Aids for Smoking Cessation

Product	Common Side Effects	Advantages	Disadvantages
Nicotine-Based Products			
Nicotine gum [Nicorette]	Mouth and throat irritation, aching jaw muscles, dyspepsia, hiccoughs	Nonprescription; user controls dose	Unpleasant taste; requires proper chewing technique; cannot eat or drink while chewing the gum; can damage dental work and is difficult for denture wearers to use
Nicotine patch [Habitrol, Nicotrol, Nicoderm CQ]	Transient itching, burning, and redness under the patch; insomnia	Nonprescription; provides a steady level of nicotine; easy to use; unobtrusive	User cannot adjust dose if craving occurs; nicotine released more slowly than in other products
Nicotine nasal spray [Nicotrol NS]	During 1st week: mouth and throat irritation, rhinitis, sneezing, coughing, teary eyes	User controls dose; fastest nicotine delivery and highest nicotine levels of all nicotine-based products	Prescription required; most irritating nicotine-based product; device visible when used
Nicotine inhaler [Nicotrol Inhaler]	Mouth and throat irritation, cough	User controls dose; mimics hand-to-mouth motion of smoking	Prescription required; slow onset and low nicotine levels; frequent puffing needed; device visible when used
Nicotine-Free Products			
Bupropion [Zyban]	Insomnia, dry mouth, agitation	Easy to use (pill); no nicotine; promotes weight loss, which may limit cessation-related weight gain; first-choice drug for smokers with depression	Prescription required; carries a small risk of seizures; unexplained deaths under investigation in Europe
Nortriptyline* [Aventyl, Pamelor]	Dry mouth, sedation, dizziness	Easy to use (pill); no nicotine	Prescription required; side effects are common; caution required in patients with heart disease
Clonidine* [Catapres]	Dry mouth, sedation, dizziness	Easy to use (pill); no nicotine	Prescription required; side effects limit use

*Not FDA-approved for use as a smoking cessation aid; considered a second-line treatment.

duce less pleasure than cigarettes, but nonetheless do relieve withdrawal symptoms. With the nasal spray, blood levels of nicotine rise rapidly, much as they do with smoking. Hence, the nasal spray provides some of the subjective pleasure that smoking does.

Long-term quitting rates are significantly greater with NRT than with placebo—although absolute success rates remain low. For example, the 1-year success with nicotine patches is about 25%, compared with 9% for placebo. Success rates are highest when replacement therapy is combined with counseling and behavioral therapy.

Nicotine Chewing Gum (Nicotine Polacrilex). Nicotine chewing gum [Nicorette] is composed of a gum base plus nicotine polacrilex, an ion exchange resin to which nicotine is bound. The gum must be chewed to release the nicotine. Following release, nicotine is absorbed across the oral mucosa into the systemic circulation. Like other forms of NRT, nicotine gum doubles the cessation success rate.

The most common adverse effects are mouth and throat soreness, jaw muscle ache, eructation (belching), and hiccups. Using optimal chewing technique minimizes these effects. Nicotine gum and all other nicotine-containing products should be avoided during pregnancy and lactation.

Patients should be advised to chew the gum slowly and intermittently for about 30 minutes. Rapid chewing can release too much nicotine at one time, resulting in effects similar to those of excessive smoking (e.g., nausea, throat irritation, hiccups). Since foods and beverages can reduce nicotine absorption, patients should not eat or drink while chewing or for 15 minutes before chewing.

Nicotine gum is available in two strengths: 2 mg/piece and 4 mg/piece. Dosing is individualized and based on the degree of nicotine dependence. For initial therapy, patients with low to moderate nicotine dependence should use the 2-mg strength; highly dependent patients (those who smoke more than 25 cigarettes a day) should use the 4-mg strength. The average adult dosage is 9 to 12 pieces of gum/day. The maximum daily dosage is 30 pieces of the 2-mg strength or 20 pieces of the 4-mg strength. Experience indicates that dosing on a fixed schedule (one piece every 2 to 3 hours) is more effective than PRN dosing for achieving abstinence.

After 3 months without cigarettes, patients should discontinue nicotine use. Withdrawal should be done gradually. Use of nicotine gum beyond 6 months is not recommended.

Nicotine Transdermal Systems (Patches). Nicotine transdermal systems are nicotine-containing adhesive patches that, after application to the skin, slowly release their nicotine content. The nicotine is absorbed into the skin and then into the blood, producing steady blood levels. Use of the patch about doubles the cessation success rate.

Three systems are available: Habitrol, Nicoderm CQ, and Nicotrol. All three can now be purchased without a prescription. As indicated in Table 38–4, the patches come in different sizes. The larger patches release greater amounts of nicotine.

Nicotine patches are applied once a day to clean, dry, nonhairy skin of the upper body or upper arm. The site should be changed daily and not reused for at least 1 week. With two products—Habitrol and Nicoderm CQ—the patch is left in place for 24 hours and then immediately replaced with a fresh one. With one product—Nicotrol—the patch is applied in the morning and removed 16 hours later at bedtime. This pattern is intended to simulate nicotine dosing produced by smoking.

Most patients begin treatment with a large patch and then progress to smaller patches over several weeks (Table 38–5). Certain patients (those with cardiovascular disease, those who weigh less than 100 pounds, or those who smoke less than one-half pack of cigarettes a day) should begin with a smaller patch.

Adverse effects are generally mild. Short-lived erythema, itching, and burning occur under the patch in 35% to 50% of users. In 14% to 17% of users, persistent erythema occurs, lasting up to 24 hours after patch removal. Patients who experience severe, persistent local reactions (e.g., severe erythema, itching, edema) should discontinue the patch and contact a physician. Nicotine patches and all other nicotine-containing products should be avoided during pregnancy and lactation.

Nicotine Inhaler. The nicotine inhaler [Nicotrol Inhaler] differs from other NRT products in that it looks much like a cigarette. Puffing on it delivers the nicotine. Because of this delivery method, using the inhaler can be a substitute for the hand-to-mouth behavior of smoking. In addition to nicotine, the inhaler contains menthol, whose purpose is to create a sensation in the back of the throat reminiscent of that caused by smoke. Like other forms of NRT, the inhaler doubles cessation success rates.

The nicotine inhaler consists of a mouthpiece and a sealed, tubular cartridge. Inside the cartridge is a porous plug containing 10 mg of nicotine. Insertion of the cartridge into the mouthpiece breaks the seal. Puffing on the mouthpiece draws air over the plug, and thereby draws nicotine vapor into the mouth. Most of the nicotine is absorbed through the *oral mucosa*—not in the lungs. As a result, blood levels rise slowly, and peak 10 to 15 minutes after puffing stops. Blood levels are less than half those achieved with cigarettes. Each cartridge can deliver 300 to 400 puffs. Benefits are greatest with frequent puffing over 20 minutes, after which the cartridge is discarded. Patients generally use 6 to 16 cartridges a day for 3 months, and then taper off over 2 to 3 months.

Adverse effects of the inhaler are mild. The most frequent are dyspepsia, coughing, throat irritation, oral burning, and

TABLE 38–5 ▪ Nicotine Transdermal Systems (Patches)					
	Surface	Hours/Day		Duration of Use	
Trade Name	Area (cm²)	in Place	Dose Absorbed	Per Patch Size	Total
Nicoderm CQ,	30	24	21 mg over 24 hr	First 4–6 wk	8–10 wk
Habitrol	20		14 mg over 24 hr	Next 2 wk	
	10		7 mg over 24 hr	Last 2 wk	
Nicotrol	30	16	15 mg over 16 hr	6 wk	6 wk

rhinitis. The inhaler should not be used by patients with asthma. Because the cartridges contain dangerous amounts of nicotine, they should be kept away from children and pets.

Nicotine Nasal Spray. Nicotine nasal spray [Nicotrol NS] differs from other NRT formulations in that blood levels of nicotine rise *rapidly* after each administration, thereby closely simulating smoking. Because nicotine levels rise rapidly, the spray provides some of the subjective pleasure associated with cigarettes. As with other forms of NRT, the spray doubles success rates.

The spray device delivers 0.5 mg of nicotine per activation. Two sprays (one in each nostril) constitute one dose and are equivalent to the amount of nicotine absorbed from one cigarette. Treatment should be started with 1 or 2 doses per hour—and never more than 5 doses per hour, or 40 doses a day. After 4 to 6 weeks, dosing should be gradually reduced and then stopped.

Quitting success with the spray has been good news and bad news. The good news, as reported in one study, is that 27% of users avoided smoking for 1 year—about twice the abstinence rate achieved with placebo. The bad news is that many patients continued to use the spray, being unwilling or unable to give it up. Nonetheless, since the spray delivers nicotine without the additional hazards in smoke, using the spray is clearly preferable to smoking.

Adverse effects are mild and temporary. At first, most users experience rhinitis, sneezing, coughing, watering eyes, and nasal and throat irritation. Fortunately, these effects abate in a few days. Nicotine nasal spray should be avoided by patients with sinus problems, allergies, or asthma.

Bupropion

Bupropion [Zyban], an atypical antidepressant, is the first and only non-nicotine drug approved as an aid to quit smoking. The drug is structurally similar to amphetamine and, like amphetamine, causes CNS stimulation and suppresses appetite. In people trying to quit cigarettes, bupropion reduces the urge to smoke and reduces some symptoms of nicotine withdrawal (e.g., irritability, anxiety). The drug is effective in the presence and absence of depression. Although the mechanism of action is uncertain, benefits may derive from blocking uptake of norepinephrine and dopamine. For use in depression, bupropion is sold under the trade name Wellbutrin.

Like other NRT products, bupropion doubles the cessation success rate. In one trial, patients were given bupropion (100, 150, or 300 mg/day) or placebo. At 7 weeks, abstinence rates were 19% with placebo, and 29%, 39%, and 44% with increasing dosages of bupropion. At 12 weeks, abstinence rates were lower: 12% with placebo and 20%, 23%, and 23% with increasing dosages of bupropion. There is some evidence that combining a nicotine patch with bupropion may be slightly more effective than bupropion alone.

Adverse effects are generally mild. The most common are dry mouth and insomnia. High doses (>450 mg/day) are associated with a 0.4% risk of seizures. However, at the doses employed for smoking cessation (300 mg/day), seizures have not been reported. Nonetheless, bupropion should be avoided in patients with seizure risk factors, such as head trauma, history of seizures, anorexia nervosa, cocaine use, and alcohol withdrawal. Because it suppresses appetite, bupropion can cause weight loss. However, since weight gain is common among ex-smokers, appetite reduction may be an added benefit rather than a drawback. Bupropion should not be combined with a monoamine oxidase inhibitor. Nor should it be given to patients taking Wellbutrin, which is just another name for bupropion itself.

The usual regimen is 150 mg in the morning for 3 days, followed by 150 mg twice a day for 7 to 12 weeks. To minimize interference with sleep, the second dose should be taken as early as possible—but at least 8 hours after the morning dose. Because onset of effects is delayed, dosing should begin 1 week before attempting to give up cigarettes.

The basic pharmacology of bupropion is discussed in Chapter 31.

Nortriptyline and Clonidine

Nortriptyline [Aventyl, Pamelor] and clonidine [Catapres] are second-line drugs for helping people quit smoking. Neither agent is approved by the FDA for this use. Nortriptyline is a tricyclic antidepressant (see Chapter 31). Clonidine is a centrally acting alpha$_2$ agonist used primarily to treat hypertension (see Chapter 19). Both drugs cause dry mouth, sedation, and dizziness—but the intensity is greater with clonidine. For nortriptyline, dosing is initiated at 25 mg/day starting 10 to 28 days before the quitting date, and then gradually increased to 75 to 100 mg/day. For clonidine, the dosage is 0.1 to 0.3 mg twice a day.

ANABOLIC STEROIDS

Many athletes take anabolic steroids (androgens) to enhance athletic performance. The principal benefit is increased muscle mass and strength. Because of the massive doses that are employed, the risk of adverse effects is substantial. With long-term steroid use, an addiction syndrome develops. Because of their abuse potential, most androgens are now classified as Schedule III drugs (see Table 38–2). The basic pharmacology of androgens and their abuse by athletes are discussed fully in Chapter 58.

⁙ KEY POINTS

- Because heroin is very lipid soluble, initial effects are more intense and occur faster than with other opioids. As a result, heroin is the opioid of choice among abusers.
- Among healthcare providers who abuse opioids, meperidine [Demerol] is a drug of choice. Why? Because meperidine is orally active, causes minimal pupillary constriction, and causes less constipation and urinary retention than other opioids.
- With opioids, tolerance to respiratory depression develops in parallel with tolerance to euphoria. As a result, respiratory depression does not increase as higher doses are taken to produce desired subjective effects.
- Persons tolerant to one opioid are cross-tolerant to all other opioids.
- Although the opioid withdrawal syndrome can be extremely unpleasant, it is rarely dangerous.
- Opioid overdose produces a classic triad of symptoms: respiratory depression, coma, and pinpoint pupils. Death can result.
- Naloxone, an opioid antagonist, is the treatment of choice for opioid overdose.

- Naloxone dosage must be titrated carefully, since too much naloxone will transport the patient from a state of intoxication to one of withdrawal. Also, since the half-life of naloxone is shorter than the half-lives of the opioids, naloxone must be administered repeatedly until the crisis is over.
- Because of cross-dependence, methadone can ease withdrawal symptoms in opioid-dependent individuals. To ease withdrawal, methadone is substituted for the abused opioid and then gradually tapered.
- In opioid abusers who are not ready for withdrawal, methadone can be used for maintenance therapy or suppressive therapy. In maintenance therapy, the methadone dosage is equivalent to the dosage of the abused opioid, thereby preventing withdrawal. In suppressive therapy, the abuser is rendered opioid tolerant with very high doses of methadone; as a result, use of street opioids can no longer produce subjective effects.
- With barbiturates, tolerance develops to subjective effects but not to respiratory depression. As a result, as increasingly large doses are taken to produce subjective effects, the risk of serious respiratory depression increases. (Note that this differs from the situation with opioids.)
- Individuals who are tolerant to barbiturates show cross-tolerance with other CNS depressants (e.g., alcohol, benzodiazepines, general anesthetics) but not with opioids.
- Individuals who are physically dependent on barbiturates show cross-dependence with other CNS depressants, but not with opioids.
- When physical dependence on barbiturates (and other CNS depressants) is great, the associated abstinence syndrome can be severe—sometimes fatal. (Note that this differs from the situation with opioids.)
- Overdose with barbiturates produces the same triad of symptoms seen with opioids: respiratory depression, coma, and pinpoint pupils. Death can result.
- In contrast to opioid overdose, barbiturate overdose has no antidote, and hence treatment is only supportive.
- In contrast to overdose with opioids or barbiturates, overdose with benzodiazepines alone is rarely fatal.
- If necessary, benzodiazepine overdose can be treated with flumazenil, a benzodiazepine antagonist.
- The psychologic effects of cocaine result from activation of dopamine receptors secondary to cocaine-induced blockade of dopamine reuptake.
- Severe overdose with cocaine can produce hyperpyrexia, convulsions, ventricular dysrhythmias, and hemorrhagic stroke; death has occurred. Psychologic effects of overdose include severe anxiety, paranoid ideation, and hallucinations.
- There is no specific antidote to cocaine overdose. Intravenous diazepam can suppress anxiety, seizures, hypertension, and dysrhythmias. Intravenous nitroprusside or phentolamine can treat severe hypertension.
- Regular use of cocaine produces tolerance. Whether significant physical dependence occurs is in dispute.

- Although various drugs have been given to help maintain abstinence following cocaine withdrawal, none is considered highly effective.
- In addition to CNS stimulation, amphetamines cause vasoconstriction and stimulate the heart. Cardiovascular stimulation may result in hypertension, angina, and dysrhythmias.
- Regular use of amphetamines can produce a state that closely resembles paranoid schizophrenia.
- Although physical dependence on amphetamines is only moderate, psychologic dependence can be intense. Withdrawal can produce dysphoria and a strong sense of craving.
- The major psychoactive substance in marijuana is delta-9-tetrahydrocannabinol (THC).
- THC acts through specific receptors in the brain.
- Marijuana has three principal subjective effects: euphoria, sedation, and hallucinations.
- Physiologic effects of marijuana, as well as tolerance and physical dependence, are minimal.
- Psychedelic drugs produce alterations in thought, perception, and feeling that otherwise occur only in dreams.
- Psychedelic drugs are also known as hallucinogens or psychotomimetics—names that reflect their ability to produce hallucinations and mental states that resemble psychosis.
- Lysergic acid diethylamide (LSD) can be considered the prototype of the psychedelic drugs.
- LSD produces its effects by activating serotonin$_2$ receptors in the brain.
- Although tolerance develops to LSD, physiologic effects and physical dependence are minimal.
- Acute panic reactions to LSD can be managed by "talking down" and by treatment with benzodiazepines. Neuroleptic drugs (e.g., haloperidol) may intensify the reaction.
- LSD users may experience episodic visual disturbances after discontinuing the drug. In many cases, the underlying cause is a permanent change in the visual system.
- Some LSD users experience prolonged psychotic reactions that closely resemble schizophrenia.
- Ecstasy (MDMA) produces psychedelic effects at low doses and amphetamine-like stimulation at higher doses.
- Ecstasy can cause irreversible destruction of serotonergic neurons.
- Phencyclidine produces alcohol-like effects at low doses and hallucinations and psychotic reactions at high doses.
- Extreme overdose with phencyclidine can produce hypertension, coma, seizures, and muscular rigidity associated with severe hyperthermia and rhabdomyolysis.
- There is no specific antidote to phencyclidine overdose. "Talking down" is not effective, and antipsychotic drugs are of limited help.
- Cigarette smoking kills over 440,000 Americans a year, making smoking the largest preventable cause of premature death.

- The principal cause of death among smokers is lung cancer, followed closely by heart disease.
- Nicotine in cigarette smoke is absorbed from the lung, whereas nicotine in cigar smoke and smokeless tobacco is absorbed from the mouth.
- By stimulating nicotinic receptors in sympathetic ganglia and the adrenal medulla, nicotine promotes vasoconstriction, acceleration of heart rate, and increased force of ventricular contraction, thereby elevating blood pressure and increasing cardiac work. These effects underlie cardiovascular deaths.
- Through actions in the CNS, nicotine increases alertness, facilitates memory, improves cognitive function, reduces aggression, and suppresses appetite. In addition, by promoting release of dopamine, nicotine activates the same pleasure circuit whose activation underlies addiction to cocaine, amphetamines, and opioids.
- Although tolerance develops to some effects of nicotine, very little tolerance develops to cardiovascular effects: Veteran smokers continue to experience an increase in blood pressure and cardiac work whenever they smoke.
- Nicotine causes physical dependence. Withdrawal is characterized by craving, nervousness, restlessness, irritability, impatience, increased hostility, insomnia, impaired concentration, increased appetite, and weight gain.
- Nicotine for replacement therapy is available in four delivery systems: chewing gum, transdermal patches, nasal spray, and inhaler.
- Bupropion [Zyban] is the only non-nicotine drug approved as an aid to smoking cessation.
- Use of NRT and/or bupropion doubles the chances of quitting smoking.
- With the aid of counseling and pharmacotherapy—NRT or bupropion—about 30% of smokers who attempt to quit can expect to achieve long-term abstinence.

Diuretics

Diuretics are drugs that increase the output of urine. These agents have two major applications: (1) treatment of hypertension and (2) mobilization of edematous fluid (associated with heart failure, cirrhosis, and kidney disease). In addition, because of their ability to maintain urine flow, diuretics are used to prevent renal failure.

REVIEW OF RENAL ANATOMY AND PHYSIOLOGY

Understanding the diuretic drugs requires a basic knowledge of the anatomy and physiology of the kidney. Accordingly, we will review these topics before discussing the diuretics themselves.

Anatomy

The basic functional unit of the kidney is the nephron. As indicated in Figure 39–1, the nephron has four functionally distinct regions: (1) the *glomerulus*, (2) the *proximal convoluted tubule*, (3) the *loop of Henle*, and (4) the *distal convoluted tubule*. All nephrons are oriented within the kidney such that the upper portion of Henle's loop is located within the renal cortex and the lower end of the loop descends toward the renal *medulla*. Without this orientation, the kidney could not produce concentrated urine.

In addition to the nephrons, the *collecting ducts* (the tubules into which the nephrons pour their contents) play a critical role in kidney function. As suggested by Figure 39–1, the final segment of the distal convoluted tubule plus the collecting duct into which it empties can be considered a single functional unit: the *distal nephron*.

Physiology
Overview of Kidney Functions

The kidney serves three basic functions: (1) cleansing of extracellular fluid (ECF) and maintenance of ECF volume and composition; (2) maintenance of acid-base balance; and (3) excretion of metabolic wastes and foreign substances (e.g., drugs, toxins). Of the three, maintenance of ECF volume and composition is the one most affected by diuretics.

The Three Basic Renal Processes

The effects of the kidney on ECF are the net result of three basic processes: (1) *filtration,* (2) *reabsorption,* and (3) *active secretion.* You should note that, in order to cleanse the entire ECF, huge volumes of plasma must be filtered. Furthermore, in order to maintain homeostasis, practically everything that has been filtered must be reabsorbed—leaving behind only a small volume of urine for excretion.

Filtration. Filtration occurs at the *glomerulus* and is the first step in urine formation. Virtually all small molecules (electrolytes, amino acids, glucose, drugs, metabolic wastes) that are present in plasma undergo filtration. In contrast, cells and large molecules (lipids, proteins) remain behind in the blood. The most prevalent constituents of the filtrate are sodium ions and chloride ions. Bicarbonate ions and potassium ions are also present, but in smaller amounts.

The filtration capacity of the kidney is huge. Each minute the kidney produces 125 ml of filtrate, which adds up to 180 L/day. Since the total volume of ECF is only 12.5 L, the kidney can process the equivalent of all the ECF in the body every 100 minutes. Hence, the ECF undergoes complete cleansing many times each day.

Be aware that filtration is a *nonselective process,* and therefore cannot regulate the composition of urine. Reabsorption and secretion—processes that display a significant degree of selectivity—are the primary determinants of what the urine ultimately contains. Of the two, reabsorption is by far the more important.

Reabsorption. Greater than 99% of the water, electrolytes, and nutrients that are filtered at the glomerulus undergo reabsorption. This conserves valuable constituents of the filtrate while allowing wastes to undergo excretion. Reabsorption of solutes (e.g., electrolytes, amino acids, glucose) takes

399

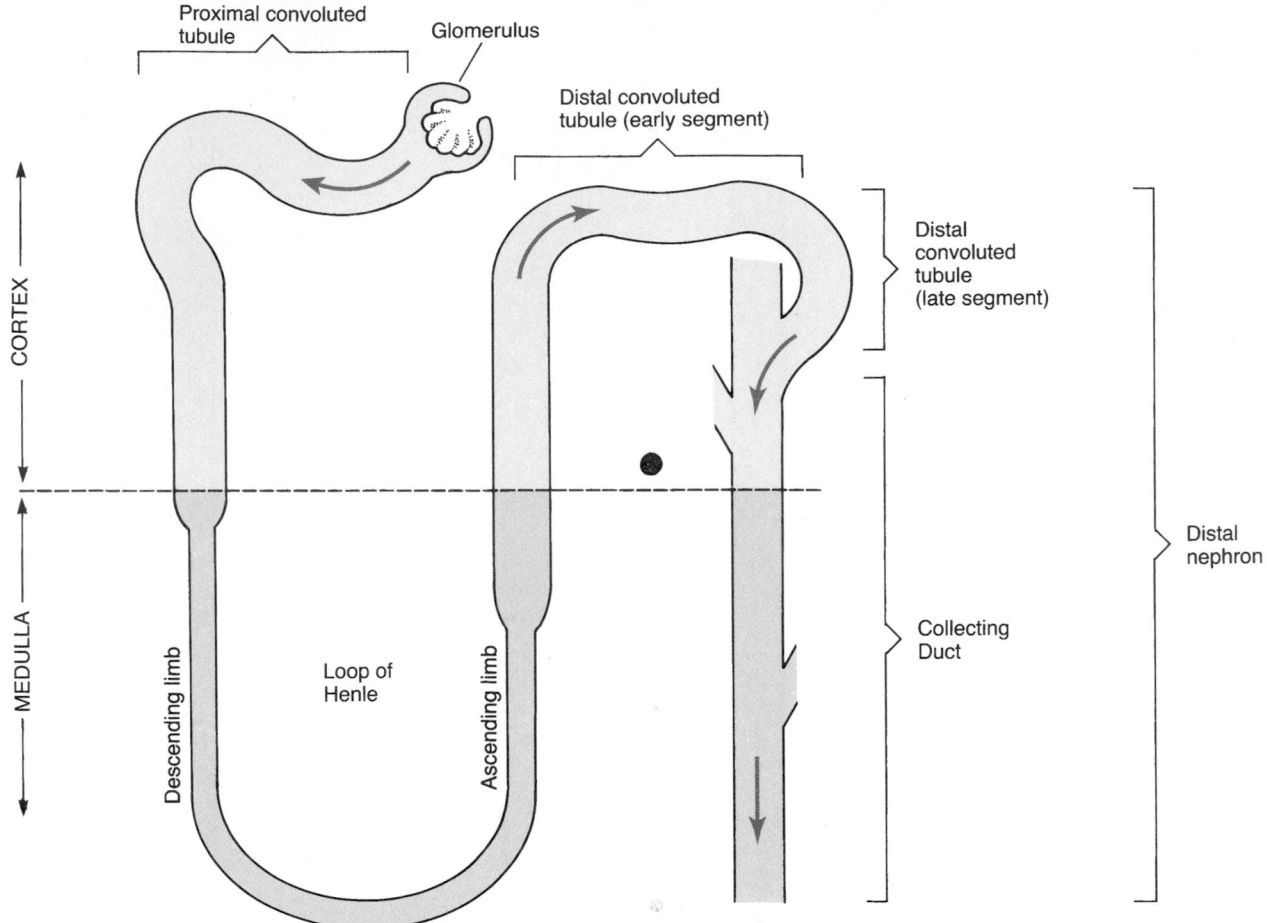

Figure 39–1 ■ **Schematic representation of a nephron and collecting duct.**

place by way of *active transport*. Water then follows passively along the osmotic gradient created by solute reuptake. Specific sites along the nephron at which reabsorption takes place are discussed below. It is primarily through interfering with reabsorption that diuretics produce their effects.

Active Tubular Secretion. The kidney has two kinds of "pumps" for active secretion. These pumps transport compounds from the plasma into the lumen of the nephron. One kind of pump is selective for *organic acids* and the other transports *organic bases*. Together, these pumps can promote the excretion of a wide assortment of molecules, including metabolic wastes, drugs, and toxins. The pumps for active secretion are located in the *proximal convoluted tubule*.

Processes of Reabsorption That Occur at Specific Sites Along the Nephron

Since most diuretics act by disrupting solute reabsorption, to understand the diuretics, we must first understand the major processes by which nephrons reabsorb filtered solutes. Since sodium and chloride ions are the predominant solutes in the filtrate, reabsorption of these ions is of greatest interest. As we discuss reabsorption, numeric values are given for the percentage of solute reabsorbed at specific sites along the nephron; bear in mind that these values are only approximate. Figure 39–2 provides a summary of the sites of sodium and chloride reabsorption, indicating the amount of reabsorption that occurs at each site.

Proximal Convoluted Tubule. The proximal convoluted tubule (PCT) has a high reabsorptive capacity. As indicated in Figure 39–2, *a large fraction (about 65%) of filtered sodium and chloride is reabsorbed at the PCT.* In addition, essentially all of the bicarbonate and potassium in the filtrate is reabsorbed here. As sodium, chloride, and other solutes are actively reabsorbed, water follows passively. Since solutes and water are reabsorbed to an equal extent, the tubular urine remains isotonic (300 mOsm/L). By the time the filtrate leaves the PCT, sodium and chloride are the only solutes that remain in significant amounts.

Loop of Henle. The *descending limb* of the loop of Henle is freely permeable to water. Hence, as tubular urine moves down the loop and passes through the hypertonic environment of the renal medulla, water is drawn from the loop into the interstitial space. This process decreases the volume of the tubular urine and causes the urine to become concentrated (tonicity increases to about 1200 mOsm/L).

Within the thick segment of the *ascending limb* of the loop of Henle, about *20% of filtered sodium and chloride is reabsorbed* (see Fig. 39–2). Since, unlike the descending limb, the ascending limb is not permeable to water, water must remain in the loop as reabsorption of sodium and chloride takes place. This process causes the tonicity of the tubular urine to return to that of the original filtrate (300 mOsm/L).

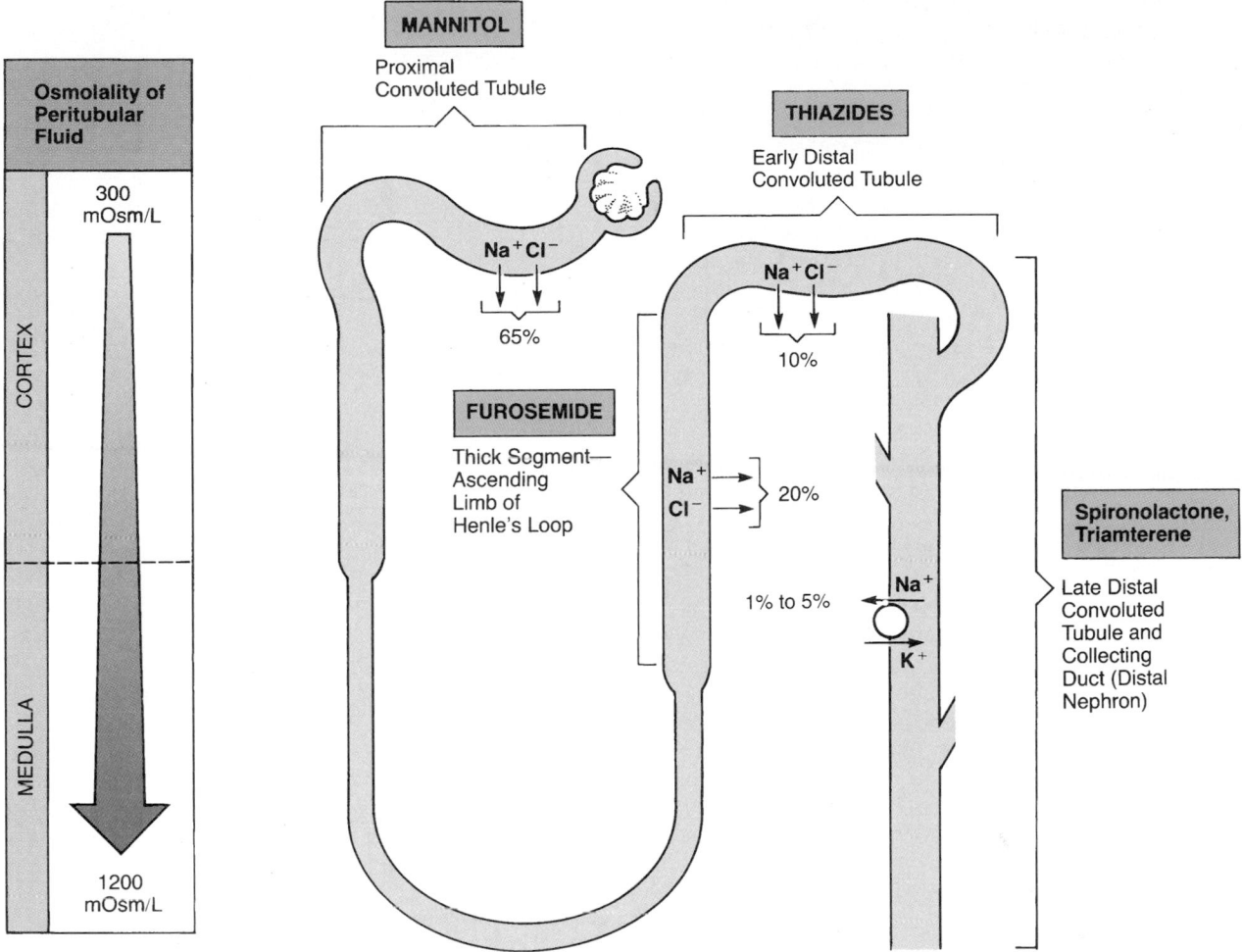

Figure 39–2 ■ **Schematic diagram of a nephron showing sites of sodium absorption and diuretic action.**
The percentages indicate how much of the filtered sodium and chloride is reabsorbed at each site.

Distal Convoluted Tubule (Early Segment). About 10% of filtered sodium and chloride is reabsorbed in the early segment of the distal convoluted tubule. Water follows passively.

Late Distal Convoluted Tubule and Collecting Duct (Distal Nephron). The distal nephron is the site of two important processes. The first involves exchange of sodium for potassium and is under the influence of aldosterone. The second determines the final concentration of the urine and is regulated by antidiuretic hormone (ADH).

Sodium-Potassium Exchange. Aldosterone, the principal mineralocorticoid of the adrenal cortex, stimulates reabsorption of sodium from the distal nephron. At the same time, aldosterone causes potassium to be secreted. Although not directly coupled, these two processes—sodium retention and potassium excretion—can be viewed as an exchange mechanism. This exchange is shown schematically in Figure 39–2. Aldosterone promotes sodium-potassium exchange by stimulating cells of the distal nephron to synthesize more of the pumps responsible for sodium and potassium transport.

Regulation of Urine Concentration by ADH. Although of great physiologic significance, ADH has little to do with the actions of diuretics. Hence, discussion of this physiologically important topic is presented in small type.

ADH acts on the collecting duct to regulate conservation of water. To understand the effects of ADH, we need to know four facts:

- In the absence of ADH, the collecting duct is impermeable to water.
- The collecting duct is oriented such that it begins in the cortex of the kidney and then passes down through the hypertonic renal medulla (see Fig. 39–2).
- Tubular urine entering the collecting duct is isotonic (300 mOsm/L).
- ADH acts on the collecting duct to increase its permeability to water.

By rendering the collecting duct permeable to water, ADH allows water to be drawn from the duct as it passes through the hypertonic renal medulla. Because of this water reabsorption, urine that entered the duct in a relatively dilute state becomes concentrated and reduced in volume.

In the absence of ADH, water cannot be reabsorbed in the collecting duct. As a result, large volumes of dilute urine are produced. The clinical syndrome resulting from ADH deficiency is known as *diabetes insipidus.*

INTRODUCTION TO DIURETICS

How Diuretics Work

Most diuretics share the same basic mechanism of action: blockade of sodium and chloride reabsorption. By blocking the reabsorption of these prominent solutes, diuretics create osmotic pressure within the nephron that prevents the passive reabsorption of water. Hence, diuretics cause water and solutes to be retained within the nephron, and thereby promote the excretion of both.

The increase in urine flow that a diuretic produces is directly related to the amount of sodium and chloride reabsorption that it blocks. Accordingly, drugs that block solute reabsorption to the greatest degree produce the most profound diuresis. Since the amount of solute in the nephron becomes progressively smaller as filtrate flows from the proximal tubule to the collecting duct, *drugs whose site of action is early in the nephron have the opportunity to block the greatest amount of solute reabsorption. Accordingly, these agents produce the greatest diuresis.* Conversely, since most of the filtered solute has already been reabsorbed by the time the filtrate reaches the distal parts of the nephron, diuretics that act at distal sites have very little reabsorption available to block. Consequently, distally acting agents produce relatively scant diuresis.

It is instructive to look at the quantitative relationship between blockade of solute reabsorption and production of diuresis. Recall that the kidney produces 180 L of filtrate a day, practically all of which is normally reabsorbed. With filtrate production at this volume, a diuretic will increase daily urine output by 1.8 L for each 1% of solute reabsorption that is blocked. A 3% blockade of solute reabsorption will produce 5.4 L of urine a day—a rate of fluid loss that would reduce body weight by 12 pounds in 24 hours. Clearly, with only a small blockade of reabsorption, diuretics can produce a profound effect on the fluid and electrolyte composition of the body.

Adverse Impact on Extracellular Fluid

In order to promote excretion of water, diuretics must compromise the normal operation of the kidney. By doing so, diuretics can cause *hypovolemia* (from excessive fluid loss), *acid-base imbalance,* and *disturbance of electrolyte levels.* These adverse effects can be minimized by using short-acting diuretics and by timing drug administration such that the kidney is allowed to operate in a drug-free manner between periods of diuresis. Both measures will give the kidney periodic opportunities to readjust the ECF so as to compensate for any undesired alterations produced under the influence of diuretics.

Classification of Diuretics

There are four major categories of diuretic drugs: (1) *high-ceiling (loop) diuretics* (e.g., furosemide); (2) *thiazide diuretics* (e.g., hydrochlorothiazide); (3) *osmotic diuretics* (e.g., mannitol); and (4) *potassium-sparing diuretics.* The last group, the potassium-sparing agents, can be subdivided into *aldosterone antagonists* (e.g., spironolactone) and *nonaldosterone antagonists* (e.g., triamterene).

In addition to the four major categories of diuretics, there is a fifth group: the *carbonic anhydrase inhibitors.* Although the carbonic anhydrase inhibitors are classified as diuretics, these drugs are employed primarily to lower intraocular pressure (IOP) and not to increase urine production. Consequently, the carbonic anhydrase inhibitors are discussed in Chapter 100 (Drugs for the Eye) rather than here.

HIGH-CEILING (LOOP) DIURETICS

The high-ceiling agents are the most effective diuretics available. These drugs produce more loss of fluid and electrolytes than any other diuretics. Because their site of action is in the loop of Henle, the high-ceiling agents are also known as *loop diuretics.*

Furosemide

Furosemide [Lasix] is the most frequently prescribed loop diuretic and will serve as our prototype for the family.

Mechanism of Action

Furosemide acts in the thick segment of the ascending limb of Henle's loop to block reabsorption of sodium and chloride (see Fig. 39–2). By blocking solute reabsorption, furosemide prevents passive reabsorption of water. Since a substantial amount (20%) of filtered NaCl is normally reabsorbed in the loop of Henle, interference with reabsorption can produce profound diuresis.

Pharmacokinetics

Furosemide can be administered orally, IV, and IM. With oral administration, diuresis begins in 60 minutes and persists for 8 hours. Oral therapy is used when rapid onset of effects is not required. Effects of intravenous furosemide begin within 5 minutes and last for 2 hours. Intravenous therapy is used in critical situations (e.g., pulmonary edema) that demand immediate mobilization of fluid. Furosemide undergoes hepatic metabolism followed by renal excretion.

Therapeutic Uses

Furosemide is a powerful drug that is generally reserved for situations that require rapid or massive mobilization of fluid. This drug should be avoided when less efficacious diuretics (thiazides) will suffice. Conditions that justify use of furosemide include (1) pulmonary edema associated with congestive heart failure (CHF); (2) edema of hepatic, cardiac, or renal origin that has been unresponsive to less efficacious diuretics; and (3) hypertension that cannot be controlled with other diuretics. Furosemide is especially useful in patients with severe renal impairment, since, unlike the thiazides (see below), this drug can promote diuresis even when renal blood flow and glomerular filtration rate are low. If treatment with furosemide alone is insufficient, a thiazide diuretic may be added to the regimen. There is no benefit to combining furosemide with another high-ceiling agent.

Adverse Effects

Hyponatremia, Hypochloremia, and Dehydration. Furosemide can produce excessive loss of sodium, chloride, and water. Severe dehydration can result. Signs of evolving dehydration include dry mouth, unusual thirst, and oliguria (scanty urine output). Impending dehydration can also be anticipated from excessive loss of weight. If dehydration occurs, furosemide should be withheld.

Dehydration can promote thrombosis and embolism. Symptoms include headache and pain in the chest, calves, or pelvis. The physician should be notified if these develop.

The risk of dehydration and its sequelae can be minimized by initiating therapy with low doses, adjusting the dosage carefully, monitoring weight loss every day, and administering furosemide on an intermittent schedule.

Hypotension. Furosemide can cause a substantial drop in blood pressure. At least two mechanisms are involved: (1) loss of volume and (2) relaxation of venous smooth muscle, which reduces venous return to the heart. Signs of hypotension include dizziness, lightheadedness, and fainting. If blood pressure falls precipitously, furosemide should be discontinued. Because of the risk of hypotension, blood pressure should be monitored routinely.

Outpatients should be taught to monitor their blood pressure and instructed to notify the physician if it drops substantially. Also, patients should be informed about symptoms of postural hypotension (dizziness, lightheadedness) and advised to sit or lie down if these occur. Patients should be taught that postural hypotension can be minimized by getting up slowly.

Hypokalemia. Potassium is lost through increased secretion in the distal nephron. If serum potassium falls below 3.5 mEq/L, fatal dysrhythmias may result. As discussed below under *Drug Interactions,* loss of potassium is of special concern for patients taking digoxin, a drug used for heart failure. Hypokalemia can be minimized by consuming potassium-rich foods (e.g., dried fruits, nuts, spinach, citrus fruits, potatoes, bananas), taking potassium supplements, or using a potassium-sparing diuretic.

Ototoxicity. Rarely, loop diuretics cause hearing impairment. With furosemide, deafness is transient. With ethacrynic acid (another loop diuretic), irreversible hearing loss has occurred. The ability to impair hearing is unique to the high-ceiling agents; diuretics in other classes are not ototoxic. Because of the risk of hearing loss, caution is needed when high-ceiling diuretics are used in combination with other ototoxic drugs (e.g., aminoglycoside antibiotics).

Hyperglycemia. Elevation of plasma glucose levels is a potential, albeit uncommon, complication of furosemide therapy. Hyperglycemia appears to result from inhibition of insulin release. Increased glycogenolysis and decreased glycogen synthesis may also contribute. When furosemide is taken by a diabetic patient, he or she should be especially diligent about monitoring blood glucose content.

Hyperuricemia. Elevation of plasma uric acid content is a frequent side effect of treatment. For most patients, furosemide-induced hyperuricemia is asymptomatic. However, for patients predisposed to gout, elevation of uric acid levels may precipitate a gouty attack. Patients should be informed about symptoms of gout (tenderness or swelling in joints) and instructed to notify the physician if these develop.

Use in Pregnancy. When administered to pregnant laboratory animals, high-ceiling diuretics have caused maternal death, abortion, fetal resorption, and other adverse effects. There are no definitive studies on loop diuretics during human pregnancy. However, given the toxicity displayed in animals, prudence dictates that pregnant women use these drugs only if absolutely required.

Impact on Lipids, Calcium, and Magnesium. Furosemide reduces high-density lipoprotein (HDL) cholesterol and raises low-density lipoprotein (LDL) cholesterol and triglycerides. Although these undesirable effects by themselves can increase the risk of coronary heart disease, they are more than balanced by the beneficial effects of the diuretic therapy on the heart. That is, despite adverse effects on lipids, high-ceiling diuretics reduce the risk of coronary mortality by 25%.

Furosemide increases urinary excretion of magnesium. Magnesium deficiency may result. Symptoms include muscle weakness, tremor, twitching, and dysrhythmias.

Furosemide increases urinary excretion of calcium. This action has been exploited to treat hypercalcemia.

Drug Interactions

Digoxin. Digoxin is used to treat heart failure (see Chapter 46) and cardiac dysrhythmias (see Chapter 47). In the presence of low potassium levels, the risk of serious digoxin-induced toxicity (ventricular dysrhythmias) is greatly increased. Since high-ceiling diuretics promote potassium loss, use of these drugs in combination with digoxin can increase the risk of dysrhythmias. This interaction is unfortunate in that most patients who take digoxin for heart failure must also take a diuretic as part of their therapy. To reduce the risk of toxicity, potassium levels should be monitored routinely, and, when indicated, potassium supplements or a potassium-sparing diuretic should be given.

Ototoxic Drugs. The risk of furosemide-induced hearing loss is increased by concurrent use of other ototoxic drugs—especially aminoglycoside antibiotics (e.g., gentamicin). Accordingly, combined use of these drugs should be avoided.

Potassium-Sparing Diuretics. The potassium-sparing diuretics (e.g., spironolactone, triamterene) can help counterbalance the potassium-wasting effects of furosemide, thereby reducing the risk of hypokalemia.

Lithium. Lithium is used to treat bipolar disorder (see Chapter 32). In the presence of low sodium levels, excretion of lithium is reduced. By lowering sodium levels, furosemide can cause lithium to accumulate to toxic levels. Accordingly, lithium levels should be monitored, and, if they climb too high, lithium dosage should be reduced.

Antihypertensive Agents. The hypotensive effects of furosemide add with those of other hypotensive drugs. To avoid excessive reduction of blood pressure, patients may need to reduce or eliminate use of other hypotensive medications.

Nonsteroidal Anti-inflammatory Drugs. The nonsteroidal anti-inflammatory drugs (NSAIDs; e.g., aspirin) can attenuate the diuretic effects of furosemide. The mechanism appears to be inhibition of prostaglandin synthesis in the kidney. (Part of the diuretic effect of furosemide results from increasing renal blood flow. Furosemide is thought to increase renal blood flow through a prostaglandin-mediated process. By inhibiting prostaglandin synthesis, NSAIDs prevent the increase in renal blood flow, and thereby partially blunt diuretic effects.)

Preparations, Dosage, and Administration

Oral. Furosemide [Lasix] is available in tablets (20, 40, and 80 mg) and in solution (8 and 10 mg/ml) for oral use. The initial dosage for adults is 20 to 80 mg/day as a single dose. The maximum daily dosage is 600 mg. Twice-daily dosing (8:00 AM and 2:00 PM) is common. Administration late in the day produces nocturia and should be avoided.

Parenteral. Furosemide is available as an injection (10 mg/ml) for IV and IM administration. The usual parenteral dose for adults is 20 to 40 mg, repeated in 1 or 2 hours if needed. Intravenous administration should be done slowly (over 1 to 2 minutes). For high-dose therapy, furosemide can be administered by continuous infusion at a rate of 4 mg/min or slower.

Other High-Ceiling Diuretics

In addition to furosemide, three other high-ceiling agents are available: *ethacrynic acid* [Edecrin], *bumetanide* [Bumex], and *torsemide* [Demadex]. All three are very similar to furosemide. They all promote diuresis by inhibiting sodium and chloride reabsorption in the thick ascending limb of the loop of Henle. All are approved for treating edema caused by heart failure, chronic renal disease, and cirrhosis, but only torsemide, like furosemide, is also approved for hypertension. All can cause ototoxicity, hypovolemia, hypotension, hypokalemia, hyperuricemia, hyperglycemia, and disruption of lipid metabolism (i.e., reduction of HDL cholesterol and elevation of LDL cholesterol and triglycerides). Lastly, they all share the same drug interactions: their effects can be blunted by NSAIDs, they can intensify ototoxicity caused by aminoglycosides, they can increase cardiotoxicity caused by digoxin, and they can cause lithium to accumulate to toxic levels. Routes, dosages, and time courses are summarized in Table 39–1.

TABLE 39–1 ⋮■ High-Ceiling (Loop) Diuretics: Routes, Time Course, and Dosage

Drug	Route	Onset (min)	Duration (hr)	Dosage (mg)	Doses/ Day
Furosemide	Oral	Within 60	6–8	20–80	1–2
[Lasix]	IV or IM	Within 5	2	20–40	
Ethacrynic acid	Oral	Within 30	6–8	50–100	1–2
[Edecrin]	IV	Within 5	2	50	1–2
Bumetanide	Oral	30–60	4–6	0.5–2	1
[Bumex]	IV	Within a few	0.5–1	0.5–1	1–3
Torsemide	Oral	Within 60	6–8	5–20	1
[Demadex]	IV	Within 10	6–8	5–20	1

THIAZIDES AND RELATED DIURETICS

The thiazide diuretics (also known as benzothiadiazides) have effects similar to those of the loop diuretics. Like the loop diuretics, thiazides increase renal excretion of sodium, chloride, potassium, and water. In addition, thiazides elevate plasma levels of uric acid and glucose. The principal difference between the thiazides and the high-ceiling diuretics is that the maximum diuresis produced by the thiazides is considerably lower than the maximum diuresis produced by the high-ceiling agents. In addition, whereas loop diuretics can be effective even when urine flow is scant, the thiazides cannot.

Hydrochlorothiazide

Hydrochlorothiazide [HydroDIURIL, others] is the most widely used thiazide diuretic and will serve as our prototype for the family. Because of its use in hypertension, a very common disorder, hydrochlorothiazide is one of our most widely used drugs.

Mechanism of Action

Hydrochlorothiazide promotes urine production by blocking the reabsorption of sodium and chloride in the *early segment of the distal convoluted tubule* (see Fig. 39–2). Retention of sodium and chloride in the nephron causes water to be retained as well, thereby producing an increased flow of urine. Since only 10% of filtered sodium and chloride is normally reabsorbed at the site where thiazides act, the maximum urine flow these drugs can produce is lower that the maximum flow that the high-ceiling diuretics produce.

The ability of thiazides to promote diuresis is dependent on adequate kidney function. These drugs are ineffective when glomerular filtration rate is low (less than 15 to 20 ml/min). Hence, in contrast to the high-ceiling agents, thiazides cannot be used to promote fluid loss in patients with severe renal impairment.

Pharmacokinetics

Diuresis begins about 2 hours after oral administration. Effects peak within 4 to 6 hours, and may persist up to 12 hours. Most of the drug is excreted unchanged in the urine.

Therapeutic Uses

Essential Hypertension. The primary indication for hydrochlorothiazide is hypertension, a condition for which thiazides are often drugs of first choice. For many hypertensive patients, blood pressure can be controlled with a thiazide alone, although many other patients require multiple-drug therapy. The role of thiazides in hypertension is discussed in Chapter 45.

Edema. Thiazides are preferred drugs for mobilizing *edema associated with mild to moderate heart failure.* These drugs are also given to mobilize *edema associated with hepatic or renal disease.*

Diabetes Insipidus. Diabetes insipidus is a rare condition characterized by excessive production of urine. In patients with this disorder, thiazides reduce urine production by 30% to 50%. The mechanism of this paradoxical effect is unclear.

Adverse Effects

The adverse effects of thiazide diuretics are similar to those of the high-ceiling agents. In fact, with the exception that thiazides lack ototoxic actions, the adverse effects of the thiazides and loop diuretics are nearly identical.

Hyponatremia, Hypochloremia, and Dehydration. Loss of sodium, chloride, and water can lead to *hyponatremia, hypochloremia,* and *dehydration.* It should be noted, however, that since the diuresis produced by thiazides is moderate, these drugs have a smaller impact on sodium, chloride, and water than do the loop diuretics. To evaluate fluid and electrolyte status, electrolyte levels should be determined periodically, and the patient should be weighed on a regular basis.

Hypokalemia. Like the high-ceiling diuretics, the thiazides can cause hypokalemia from excessive potassium excretion. As noted, potassium loss is of particular concern for patients taking digoxin. Potassium levels should be measured periodically, and, if serum potassium falls below 3.5 mEq/L, treatment with potassium supplements or a potassium-sparing diuretic should be instituted. Hypokalemia can be minimized by eating potassium-rich foods.

Use in Pregnancy and Lactation. The thiazides have direct and indirect effects on the developing fetus. By reducing blood volume, thiazides can decrease placental perfusion, and may thereby compromise fetal nutrition and growth. Furthermore, thiazides can cross the placental barrier to produce fetal harm directly; potential effects include electrolyte imbalance, hypoglycemia, jaundice, and hemolytic anemia. Because of the potential for fetal harm, *thiazides should not be used routinely during pregnancy.* Edema of pregnancy is not an indication for diuretic therapy—except when unusually severe. In contrast, edema from pathologic causes (e.g., heart failure, cirrhosis) does constitute a legitimate indication for thiazide use.

TABLE 39–2 ■ Thiazides and Related Diuretics: Dosages and Time Course of Effects

Generic Name	Trade Name	Onset (hr)	Duration (hr)	Optimal Oral Adult Dosage (mg/day)
Thiazides				
Chlorothiazide	Diuril, Diurigen	1–2	6–12	500–1000
Hydrochlorothiazide	Esidrix, Oretic, HydroDIURIL, others	2	6–12	12.5–25
Bendroflumethiazide	Naturetin	2	6–12	2.5–15
Benzthiazide	Exna	2	6–12	25–100
Hydroflumethiazide	Diucardin, Saluron	2	6–12	25–100
Methyclothiazide	Aquatensen, Enduron	2	24	2.5–5
Polythiazide	Renese	2	24–48	2–4
Trichlormethiazide	Metahydrin, Naqua Diurese	2	24	2–4
Related Drugs				
Chlorthalidone	Hygroton, Thalitone	2	24–72	50–100
Indapamide	Lozol	1–2	Up to 36	2.5–5
Metolazone	Zaroxolyn,* Mykrox*	1	12–24	2.5–20*
Quinethazone	Hydromox	2	18–24	50–100

*Zaroxolyn and Mykrox are not bioequivalent. Of the two, Mykrox is more rapidly and completely absorbed. As a result, dosages for Mykrox are 5 to 10 times lower than dosages for Zaroxolyn. The dosages presented are for Zaroxolyn.

Thiazides enter breast milk and can be hazardous to the nursing infant. Women who are taking thiazides should be cautioned against breast-feeding.

Hyperglycemia. Like the loop diuretics, the thiazides can elevate plasma levels of glucose. Significant hyperglycemia develops only in diabetic patients, who should therefore be especially diligent about monitoring blood glucose. To maintain normal glucose levels, the diabetic patient may require larger doses of insulin or an oral hypoglycemic drug.

Hyperuricemia. The thiazides, like the loop diuretics, can cause retention of uric acid, thereby elevating plasma uric acid levels. Although hyperuricemia is usually asymptomatic, it may precipitate gouty arthritis in patients with a history of the disorder. Plasma levels of uric acid should be measured periodically.

Impact on Lipids, Calcium, and Magnesium. Thiazides can increase levels of LDL cholesterol, total cholesterol, and triglycerides. In addition, thiazides reduce urinary excretion of calcium; because of this action, thiazides have been used to treat calcium-related kidney stones. Thiazides increase excretion of magnesium, sometimes causing magnesium deficiency; symptoms include muscle weakness, tremor, twitching, and dysrhythmias.

Drug Interactions

The important drug interactions of the thiazides are nearly identical to those of the loop diuretics. By promoting potassium loss, thiazides can increase the risk of toxicity from *digoxin.* By counterbalancing the potassium-wasting effects of the thiazides, the *potassium-sparing diuretics* can help prevent excessive potassium loss. By lowering blood pressure, thiazides can augment the effects of other *antihypertensive drugs.* By promoting sodium loss, thiazides can reduce renal excretion of *lithium,* thereby causing the drug to accumulate, possibly to toxic levels. *NSAIDs* may blunt the diuretic effects of thiazides. In contrast to the loop diuretics, the thiazides can be combined with *ototoxic agents* without an increased risk of hearing loss.

Preparations, Dosage, and Administration

Hydrochlorothiazide [HydroDIURIL, others] is dispensed in capsules (12.5 mg), tablets (25, 50, and 100 mg), and solution (10 mg/ml) for oral administration. Like most other thiazides, hydrochlorothiazide is administered only by mouth.

The usual adult dosage is 25 to 50 mg once or twice daily. To minimize nocturia, the drug should not be administered late in the day. To minimize electrolyte imbalance, the drug should be administered on an intermittent basis (e.g., every other day). In addition to being marketed alone, hydrochlorothiazide is available in fixed-dose combinations with potassium-sparing diuretics; trade names are Aldactazide, Dyazide, Maxzide, and Moduretic.

Other Thiazide-Type Diuretics

In addition to hydrochlorothiazide, 11 other thiazides (and related drugs) are approved for use in the United States (Table 39–2). All have pharmacologic properties similar to those of hydrochlorothiazide. With the exception of chlorothiazide, these drugs are administered only by mouth. Chlorothiazide can be administered intravenously as well as orally. Although the thiazides differ from one another in milligram potency (see Table 39–2), at therapeutically equivalent doses, all elicit the same degree of diuresis. Although most have the same onset time (1 to 2 hours), these drugs differ significantly with respect to duration of action. As with hydrochlorothiazide, disturbance of electrolyte balance can be minimized through alternate-day dosing. Nocturia can be minimized by avoiding dosing in the late afternoon.

Table 39–2 lists four drugs—chlorthalidone, indapamide, metolazone, and quinethazone—that are not true thiazides. However, these agents are very similar to thiazides both in structure and function, hence their inclusion in this group.

POTASSIUM-SPARING DIURETICS

The potassium-sparing diuretics can elicit two potentially useful responses. First, these drugs produce a modest increase in urine production. Second, they produce a substantial *decrease in potassium excretion.* Because their diuretic effects are limited, the potassium-sparing drugs are rarely employed alone to promote diuresis. However, because of their marked ability to decrease potassium excretion, these drugs are used with great regularity to counteract potassium loss caused by thiazide and loop diuretics.

There are two subcategories of potassium-sparing diuretics: aldosterone antagonists and nonaldosterone antagonists. Only one aldosterone antagonist—spironolactone—is approved for use in the United States. Two nonaldosterone antagonists—triamterene and amiloride—are currently employed.

Spironolactone
Mechanism of Action

Spironolactone [Aldactone] blocks the actions of aldosterone in the distal nephron. Since aldosterone acts to promote sodium uptake in exchange for potassium secretion (see Fig. 39–2), inhibition of aldosterone by spironolactone has the opposite effect: *retention of potassium and increased excretion of sodium.* The diuresis caused by spironolactone is scanty because most of the filtered sodium load has already been reabsorbed by the time the filtrate reaches the distal nephron. (Recall that the degree of diuresis a drug produces is directly proportional to the amount of sodium reuptake that it blocks.)

As indicated in Table 39–3, the effects of spironolactone are delayed, taking up to 48 hours to develop. To understand this delay, recall that aldosterone acts by stimulating cells of the distal nephron to synthesize the proteins required for sodium and potassium transport. By preventing aldosterone's action, spironolactone blocks the synthesis of new proteins, but does not stop existing transport proteins from doing their job. Hence, the effects of spironolactone are not visible until the existing proteins complete their normal life cycle—a process that takes one or two days to run its course.

Therapeutic Uses

Spironolactone is indicated primarily for patients with *hypertension* and *edema.* Although it can be employed alone, the drug is used most commonly in combination with a thiazide or loop diuretic. The purpose of spironolactone in these combinations is to counteract the potassium-wasting effects of the more powerful diuretics. Spironolactone also makes a small contribution to diuresis.

In 1999, researchers reported that spironolactone can benefit patients with severe *heart failure.* The drug greatly reduces mortality and hospital admissions. The use of spironolactone for heart failure is discussed further in Chapter 46.

In addition to its use in hypertension, edema, and heart failure, spironolactone can be given to block the effects of aldosterone in patients with *primary hyperaldosteronism.*

Adverse Effects

Hyperkalemia. The potassium-sparing effects of spironolactone can result in hyperkalemia, a condition that can produce fatal dysrhythmias. Although hyperkalemia is most likely when spironolactone is used alone, it can also develop when spironolactone is used in conjunction with potassium-wasting agents (thiazides and high-ceiling diuretics). If serum potassium rises above 5 mEq/L, or if signs of hyperkalemia develop (e.g., abnormal cardiac rhythm), spironolactone should be discontinued and potassium intake restricted. Injection of insulin can help lower potassium levels by promoting potassium uptake into cells.

Benign and Malignant Tumors. When given long-term to rats in doses 25 to 250 times those used in humans, spironolactone caused benign adenomas of the thyroid and testes, malignant mammary tumors, and proliferative changes in the liver. The risk of tumors in humans from use of normal doses is unknown.

Endocrine Effects. Spironolactone is a steroid derivative with a structure similar to that of steroid hormones (e.g., progesterone, estradiol, testosterone). As a result, spironolactone can cause a variety of endocrine effects, including *gynecomastia, menstrual irregularities, impotence, hirsutism,* and *deepening of the voice.*

Drug Interactions

Thiazide and Loop Diuretics. Spironolactone is frequently combined with thiazide and loop diuretics. The principal objective is to counteract the potassium-wasting effects of the more powerful diuretic.

Drugs That Raise Potassium Levels. Because of the risk of hyperkalemia, *spironolactone must never be combined with potassium supplements or with another potassium-sparing diuretic.* In addition, since *angiotensin-converting enzyme (ACE) inhibitors* can also elevate potassium levels (by suppressing aldosterone secretion), they should be combined with spironolactone only when clearly necessary.

Preparations, Dosage, and Administration

Spironolactone [Aldactone] is dispensed in tablets (25, 50, and 100 mg) for oral administration. The usual adult dosage is 25 to 100 mg/day. Spironolactone is also marketed in a fixed-dose combination with hydrochlorothiazide under the trade name Aldactazide.

Triamterene
Mechanism of Action

Like spironolactone, triamterene [Dyrenium] disrupts sodium-potassium exchange in the distal nephron. However, in contrast to spironolactone, which reduces ion transport indirectly through blockade of aldosterone, triamterene is a *direct inhibitor of the exchange mechanism itself.* The net effect of this inhibition is a decrease in sodium reuptake and a reduction in potassium secretion. Hence, sodium excretion is increased, while potassium is conserved. Because it inhibits ion transport directly, triamterene acts much more quickly than spironolactone. As indicated in Table 39–3, initial responses develop in hours, as compared with days for spironolactone. Like spironolactone, triamterene is unable to cause more than a scant diuresis.

TABLE 39–3 ■ Potassium-Sparing Diuretics: Names, Dosages and Time Course of Effects				
		Time Course		**Usual Adult**
Generic Name	**Trade Name**	**Onset (hr)**	**Duration (hr)**	**Dosage (mg/day)**
Spironolactone	Aldactone	24–48	48–72	25–200
Triamterene	Dyrenium	2–4	12–16	200–300
Amiloride	Midamor	2	24	5–20

Therapeutic Uses

Triamterene can be used alone or in combination with other diuretics to treat *hypertension* and *edema*. When used alone, triamterene produces mild diuresis. When combined with other diuretics (e.g., furosemide, hydrochlorothiazide), triamterene augments diuresis and helps counteract the potassium-wasting effects of the more powerful diuretic. It is the latter effect for which triamterene is principally employed.

Adverse Effects

Hyperkalemia. Excessive potassium accumulation is the most significant adverse effect. Hyperkalemia is most likely when triamterene is used alone, but can also occur when the drug is combined with thiazides or high-ceiling agents. Triamterene should never be used in conjunction with another potassium-sparing diuretic or with potassium supplements. In addition, caution is needed if the drug is combined with an ACE inhibitor.

Other Adverse Effects. Relatively common side effects include *nausea, vomiting, leg cramps,* and *dizziness.* Blood dyscrasias occur rarely.

Preparations, Dosage, and Administration

Triamterene [Dyrenium] is available in 50- and 100-mg capsules for oral use. The usual initial dosage is 100 mg twice a day. The maximum daily dosage is 300 mg. Triamterene is also marketed in fixed-dose combinations with hydrochlorothiazide under the trade names Dyazide and Maxzide.

Amiloride

Pharmacologic Properties. Amiloride [Midamor] has actions similar to those of triamterene. Both drugs inhibit potassium loss by direct blockade of sodium-potassium exchange in the distal nephron. Also, both drugs produce only modest diuresis. Although it can be employed alone as a diuretic, amiloride is used primarily to counteract potassium loss caused by more powerful diuretics (thiazides, high-ceiling agents). The major adverse effect of amiloride is hyperkalemia. Accordingly, concurrent use of other potassium-sparing diuretics or potassium supplements must be avoided. Caution is needed if the drug is combined with an ACE inhibitor.

Preparations, Dosage, and Administration. Amiloride [Midamor] is dispensed in 5-mg tablets for oral use. Dosing is begun at 5 mg/day and may be increased to a maximum of 20 mg. Amiloride is available in a fixed-dose combination with hydrochlorothiazide under the trade name Moduretic.

OSMOTIC DIURETICS

Four compounds—mannitol, urea, glycerin, and isosorbide—are classified as osmotic diuretics. However, of the four, only mannitol is used for its diuretic actions. The osmotic agents differ from other diuretics both in mechanism and indications.

Mannitol

Mannitol [Osmitrol] is a simple six-carbon sugar that possesses the four properties characteristic of an osmotic diuretic:

- It is freely filtered at the glomerulus.
- It undergoes minimal reabsorption.
- It is not metabolized to a significant degree.
- It is pharmacologically inert (i.e., it has no direct effects on the biochemistry or physiology of cells).

Mechanism of Diuretic Action

Mannitol promotes diuresis by creating an osmotic force within the lumen of the nephron. Unlike other solutes, mannitol undergoes minimal reabsorption after filtration. As a result, most of the drug remains within the nephron, creating an osmotic force that inhibits passive reabsorption of water. Hence, urine flow increases. The degree of diuresis produced is directly related to the concentration of mannitol in the filtrate; the more mannitol present, the greater the diuresis. Mannitol has no significant effect on the excretion of potassium and other electrolytes.

Pharmacokinetics

Mannitol does not diffuse across the GI epithelium and cannot be transported by the uptake systems that absorb dietary sugars. Accordingly, in order to reach the circulation, the drug must be given parenterally. Following IV injection, mannitol distributes freely to extracellular water. Diuresis begins in 30 to 60 minutes and persists 6 to 8 hours. Most of the drug is excreted intact in the urine.

Therapeutic Uses

Prophylaxis of Renal Failure. Under certain conditions (e.g., dehydration, severe hypotension, hypovolemic shock), blood flow to the kidney is decreased, causing a great reduction in filtrate volume. When the volume of filtrate is this low, the transport mechanisms of the nephron are able to reabsorb virtually all of the sodium and chloride present, causing complete reabsorption of water as well. As a result, urine production ceases, and kidney failure ensues. The risk of renal failure can be reduced with mannitol. Since filtered mannitol is not reabsorbed—even when filtrate volume is small—filtered mannitol will remain in the nephron, drawing water with it. Hence, mannitol can preserve urine flow and may thereby prevent renal failure. Thiazides and loop diuretics are not as effective for this application because, under conditions of low filtrate production, there is such an excess of reabsorptive capacity (relative to the amount of filtrate) that these drugs are unable to produce sufficient blockade of reabsorption to promote diuresis.

Reduction of Intracranial Pressure. Intracranial pressure (ICP) that has been elevated by cerebral edema can be reduced with mannitol. The drug lowers ICP because its presence in the cerebral vasculature creates an osmotic force that draws edematous fluid out of the brain. There is no risk of increasing cerebral edema because mannitol cannot exit the capillary beds of the brain.

Reduction of Intraocular Pressure. Mannitol and other osmotic agents can lower IOP. Mannitol reduces IOP by rendering the plasma hyperosmotic with respect to intraocular fluids, thereby creating an osmotic force that draws ocular fluid into the blood. Use of mannitol to lower IOP is reserved for patients who have not responded to more conventional treatment.

Adverse Effects

Edema. Mannitol can leave the vascular system at all capillary beds except those of the brain. When the drug exits capillaries, it draws water along, causing edema. Mannitol must be used with extreme caution in patients with heart disease, since it may precipitate CHF and fulminating pulmonary edema. If signs of pulmonary congestion or CHF develop, use of the drug must cease immediately. Mannitol must also be discontinued if patients with heart failure or pulmonary edema develop renal failure, since the resultant accumulation of mannitol would increase the risk of cardiac or pulmonary injury.

Other Adverse Effects. Common responses include *headache, nausea,* and *vomiting. Fluid and electrolyte imbalance* may also occur.

Preparations, Dosage, and Administration

Mannitol [Osmitrol] is administered by IV infusion. Solutions for IV use range in concentration from 5% to 25%. Dosing is complex and varies with the objectives of therapy (prevention of renal failure, lowering of ICP, lowering of IOP). The usual adult dosage for preventing renal failure is 50 to 100 gm over 24 hours. The infusion rate should be set to elicit a urine flow of at least 30 to 50 ml/hr. It should be noted that mannitol may crystallize out of solution if exposed to low temperature. Accordingly, preparations should be observed for crystals prior to use. Preparations that contain crystals should be warmed (to redissolve the mannitol) and then cooled to body temperature for administration. A filter needle is employed to withdraw mannitol from the vial; an in-line filter is used to prevent crystals from entering the circulation. If urine flow declines to a very low rate or ceases entirely, the infusion should be stopped.

Urea, Glycerin, and Isosorbide

In addition to mannitol, three other drugs—urea, glycerin, and isosorbide—are classified as osmotic diuretics. Like mannitol, these agents are freely filtered at the glomerulus and undergo limited reabsorption. These properties promote osmotic diuresis. It must be noted, however, that although urea, glycerin, and isosorbide can produce diuresis, none is actually used for this purpose. Rather, these agents are used only to reduce IOP and ICP. Urea [Ureaphil] is administered intravenously. Glycerin [Osmoglyn] and isosorbide [Ismotic] are administered orally.

⁂ KEY POINTS

- More than 99% of the water, electrolytes, and nutrients that are filtered at the glomerulus undergo reabsorption.
- Most diuretics block active reabsorption of sodium and chloride, which prevents passive reabsorption of water.
- The amount of diuresis that a drug produces is directly related to the amount of sodium and chloride reabsorption that it blocks.
- Drugs that act early in the nephron are in a position to block the greatest amount of solute reabsorption; hence, these agents produce the greatest diuresis.
- High-ceiling diuretics (loop diuretics) block sodium and chloride reabsorption in the loop of Henle.
- High-ceiling diuretics produce the greatest diuresis.
- In contrast to thiazide diuretics, high-ceiling diuretics are effective even when the glomerular filtration rate is low.
- High-ceiling diuretics can cause dehydration through excessive fluid loss.
- High-ceiling diuretics can cause hypotension by decreasing blood volume and relaxing venous smooth muscle.
- High-ceiling diuretics can cause hearing loss, which is usually reversible.
- Hypokalemia caused by high-ceiling diuretics is a special problem for patients taking digoxin.

- Thiazide diuretics block sodium and water reabsorption in the early distal convoluted tubule.
- Thiazide diuretics produce less diuresis than high-ceiling diuretics.
- Thiazide diuretics are ineffective when glomerular filtration rate is low.
- Like the high-ceiling diuretics, thiazide diuretics can cause dehydration and hypokalemia; however, thiazides do not cause hearing loss.
- Thiazide-induced hypokalemia is a special problem for patients taking digoxin.
- Potassium-sparing diuretics act by directly or indirectly blocking sodium-potassium "exchange" in the distal convoluted tubule.
- Potassium-sparing diuretics cause only modest diuresis.
- Potassium-sparing diuretics are used primarily to counteract potassium loss in patients taking high-ceiling diuretics or thiazides.
- The principal adverse effect of potassium-sparing diuretics is hyperkalemia.
- Because of the risk of hyperkalemia, potassium-sparing diuretics should not be combined with one another or with potassium supplements, and they should be used cautiously in patients taking ACE inhibitors.
- High-ceiling diuretics and thiazides are used to treat hypertension and edema associated with heart failure, cirrhosis, and kidney disease.

Summary of Major Nursing Implications*

HIGH-CEILING (LOOP) DIURETICS

Bumetanide
Ethacrynic Acid
Furosemide
Torsemide

Preadministration Assessment

Therapeutic Goal

High-ceiling diuretics are indicated for patients with (1) pulmonary edema associated with congestive heart failure; (2) edema of hepatic, cardiac, or renal origin that has been unresponsive to less effective diuretics; (3) hypertension that cannot be controlled with thiazide and potassium-sparing diuretics; and (4) all patients who need diuretic therapy but have low renal blood flow.

Baseline Data

For all patients, obtain baseline values for weight, blood pressure (sitting and supine), pulse, respiration, and electrolytes (sodium, potassium, chloride). For patients with edema, record sites and extent of edema. For patients with ascites, measure abdominal girth.

*Patient education information is highlighted as blue text.

Identifying High-Risk Patients

Use with *caution* in patients with cardiovascular disease, renal impairment, diabetes mellitus, or a history of gout, and in patients who are pregnant or taking digoxin, lithium, ototoxic drugs, NSAIDs, or antihypertensive drugs.

Implementation: Administration

Routes

Furosemide and Bumetanide. Oral, IV, IM.
Ethacrynic Acid and Torsemide. Oral, IV.

Administration

Oral. Dosing may be done once daily, twice daily, or on alternate days. **Instruct patients who are using once-a-day or alternate-day dosing to take their medication in the morning. Instruct patients using twice-a-day dosing to take their medication at 8:00 AM and 2:00 PM (to minimize nocturia).**

Advise patients to administer furosemide with food if GI upset occurs.

Parenteral. Administer IV injections slowly (over 1 to 2 minutes). For high-dose therapy, administer by continuous infusion. Discard discolored solutions.

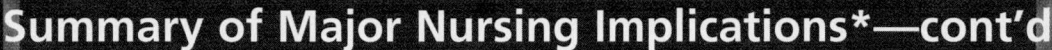

Summary of Major Nursing Implications*—cont'd

Promoting Compliance

Increased frequency of urination is inconvenient and can discourage compliance. **To promote compliance, forewarn patients that treatment will increase urine volume and frequency of voiding, and inform them that these effects will subside 6 to 8 hours after dosing. Inform patients that nighttime diuresis can be minimized by avoiding dosing late in the day.**

Ongoing Evaluation and Interventions

Evaluating Therapeutic Effects

Monitor blood pressure and pulse rate, weigh the patient daily, and evaluate for decreased edema.

Monitor intake and output. Notify the physician if oliguria (urine output less than 25 ml/hr) or anuria (no urine output) develops.

Instruct outpatients to weigh themselves daily, preferably in the morning before eating, and to maintain a weight record.

Minimizing Adverse Effects

Hyponatremia, Hypochloremia, and Dehydration. Loss of sodium, chloride, and water can cause hyponatremia, hypochloremia, and severe dehydration. Signs of dehydration include dry mouth, unusual thirst, and oliguria. Withhold the drug if these appear.

Dehydration can promote thromboembolism. Monitor the patient for symptoms (headache; pain in the chest, calves, or pelvis), and notify the physician if these develop.

The risk of dehydration and its sequelae can be minimized by (1) initiating therapy with low doses, (2) adjusting the dosage carefully, (3) monitoring weight loss daily, and (4) using an intermittent dosing schedule.

Hypotension. Monitor blood pressure. If it falls precipitously, withhold medication and notify the physician.

Teach patients to monitor their blood pressure and instruct them to notify the physician if it drops substantially.

Inform patients about signs of postural hypotension (dizziness, lightheadedness), and advise them to sit or lie down if these occur. Inform patients that postural hypotension can be minimized by getting up slowly.

Hypokalemia. If serum potassium falls below 3.5 mEq/L, fatal dysrhythmias may result. Hypokalemia can be minimized by consuming potassium-rich foods (e.g., nuts, dried fruits, spinach, citrus fruits, potatoes, bananas), taking potassium supplements, or using a potassium-sparing diuretic.

Ototoxicity. **Inform patients about possible hearing loss and instruct them to notify the physician if a hearing deficit develops.** Exercise caution when high-ceiling diuretics are used concurrently with other ototoxic drugs—especially aminoglycosides.

Hyperglycemia. High-ceiling diuretics may elevate blood glucose levels in diabetic patients. **Advise these patients to be especially diligent about monitoring blood glucose.**

Hyperuricemia. High-ceiling diuretics frequently cause *asymptomatic* hyperuricemia, although gout-prone patients may experience a gouty attack. **Inform patients about signs of gout (tenderness or swelling in joints), and instruct them to notify the physician if these occur.**

Minimizing Adverse Interactions

Digoxin. By lowering potassium levels, high-ceiling diuretics increase the risk of fatal dysrhythmias from digoxin. Serum potassium levels must be monitored and maintained above 3.5 mEq/L.

Lithium. High-ceiling diuretics can suppress lithium excretion, thereby causing the drug to accumulate, possibly to toxic levels. Plasma lithium content should be monitored routinely. If drug levels become elevated, lithium dosage should be reduced.

Ototoxic Drugs. The risk of hearing loss from high ceiling diuretics is increased in the presence of other ototoxic drugs—especially aminoglycosides. Exercise caution when such combinations are employed.

THIAZIDE DIURETICS

Thiazide diuretics have actions very similar to those of the high-ceiling diuretics. Hence, nursing implications for the thiazides are nearly identical to those of the high-ceiling agents.

Preadministration Assessment

Therapeutic Goal

Thiazide diuretics are used to treat hypertension and edema.

Baseline Data

For all patients, obtain baseline values for weight, blood pressure (sitting and supine), pulse, respiration, and electrolytes (sodium, chloride, potassium). For patients with edema, record sites and extent of edema.

Identifying High-Risk Patients

Use with *caution* in patients with cardiovascular disease, renal impairment, diabetes mellitus, or a history of gout and in patients taking digoxin, lithium, or antihypertensive drugs. *Generally avoid* in women who are pregnant or breast-feeding.

Implementation: Administration

Routes

Oral. *All* thiazide-type diuretics.
Intravenous. *Chlorothiazide.*

Administration

Dosing may be done once daily, twice daily, or on alternate days. **When once-a-day dosing is employed, instruct patients to take their medicine early in the day to minimize nocturia. When twice-a-day dosing is employed, instruct patients to take their medicine at 8:00 AM and 2:00 PM.**

*Patient education information is highlighted as blue text.

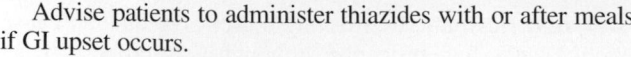

Summary of Major Nursing Implications*—cont'd

Advise patients to administer thiazides with or after meals if GI upset occurs.

Promoting Compliance

See nursing implications for *High-Ceiling (Loop) Diuretics.*

Ongoing Evaluation and Interventions

Evaluating Therapeutic Effects

See nursing implications for *High-Ceiling (Loop) Diuretics.*

Minimizing Adverse Effects

Like the high-ceiling diuretics, thiazides can cause *hyponatremia, hypochloremia, dehydration, hypokalemia, hypotension, hyperglycemia,* and *hyperuricemia.* For implications regarding these effects, see implications for *High-Ceiling (Loop) Diuretics.*

Thiazides can cause fetal harm and can enter breast milk. These drugs should be avoided during pregnancy unless absolutely required. **Caution women not to breast-feed.**

Minimizing Adverse Interactions

Like high-ceiling diuretics, thiazides can interact adversely with *digoxin* and *lithium.* For nursing implications regarding these interactions, see implications for *High-Ceiling (Loop) Diuretics.*

POTASSIUM-SPARING DIURETICS

Amiloride
Spironolactone
Triamterene

Preadministration Assessment

Therapeutic Goal

Potassium-sparing diuretics are given primarily to counterbalance the potassium-losing effects of thiazides and high-ceiling diuretics.

Baseline Data

Obtain baseline values for serum potassium.

*Patient education information is highlighted as blue text.

Identifying High-Risk Patients

Potassium-sparing diuretics are *contraindicated* for patients with hyperkalemia and for patients taking potassium supplements or another potassium-sparing diuretic. Use with *caution* in patients taking ACE inhibitors.

Implementation: Administration

Route

Oral.

Administration

Advise patients to take these drugs with or after meals if GI upset occurs.

Ongoing Evaluation and Interventions

Evaluating Therapeutic Effects

Monitor serum potassium levels on a regular basis. The objective is to maintain serum potassium levels between 3.5 and 5 mEq/L.

Minimizing Adverse Effects

Hyperkalemia. Hyperkalemia is the principal adverse effect. **Instruct patients to restrict intake of potassium-rich foods (e.g., nuts, dried fruits, spinach, citrus fruits, potatoes, bananas).** If serum potassium levels rise above 5 mEq/L, or if signs of hyperkalemia develop (e.g., abnormal cardiac rhythm), withhold medication and notify the physician. Insulin can be given to drive potassium levels down.

Endocrine Effects. Spironolactone may cause *menstrual irregularities* and *impotence.* **Inform patients about these effects, and instruct them to notify the physician if they occur.**

Minimizing Adverse Interactions

Drugs That Raise Potassium Levels. Because of the risk of hyperkalemia, don't combine a potassium-sparing diuretic with potassium supplements or with another potassium-sparing diuretic. Combine with ACE inhibitors only when clearly indicated.

Agents Affecting the Volume and Ion Content of Body Fluids

The drugs discussed in this chapter are used to correct disturbances in the volume and ionic composition of body fluids. Three groups of agents are considered: (1) drugs used to correct disorders of fluid volume and osmolality, (2) drugs used to correct disturbances of hydrogen ion concentration (acid-base status), and (3) drugs used to correct electrolyte imbalances.

DISORDERS OF FLUID VOLUME AND OSMOLALITY

Good health requires that both the volume and osmolality of extracellular and intracellular fluids remain within a normal range. If a substantial alteration in either the volume or osmolality of these fluids develops, significant harm can result.

Maintenance of fluid volume and osmolality is primarily the job of the kidneys, and, even under adverse conditions, renal mechanisms usually succeed in keeping the volume and composition of body fluids within acceptable limits. However, circumstances can arise in which the regulatory power of the kidneys is exceeded. When this occurs, disruption of fluid volume, osmolality, or both can result.

Abnormal states of hydration can be divided into two major categories: volume contraction and volume expansion. *Volume contraction* is defined as a *decrease* in total body water; conversely, *volume expansion* is defined as an *increase* in

total body water. States of volume contraction and volume expansion have three subclassifications based on alterations in extracellular osmolality. For volume contraction, the subcategories are *isotonic contraction, hypertonic contraction,* and *hypotonic contraction.* Volume expansion may also be subclassified as *isotonic, hypertonic,* or *hypotonic.* Descriptions and causes of these abnormal states are discussed below.

In the clinical setting, changes in osmolality are described in terms of the sodium content of plasma. Sodium is used as the reference for classification because this ion is the principal extracellular solute. (Recall that plasma sodium content ranges from 135 to 145 mEq/L.) In most cases, the total osmolality of plasma is equal to approximately twice the osmolality of sodium. That is, total plasma osmolality usually ranges from 280 to 300 mOsm/kg water.

Volume Contraction
Isotonic Contraction

Definition and Causes. Isotonic contraction is defined as volume contraction in which *sodium and water are lost in isotonic proportions.* Hence, although there is a decrease in the total volume of extracellular fluid, there is no change in osmolality. Causes of isotonic contraction include vomiting, diarrhea, kidney disease, and misuse of diuretics. Isotonic contraction is characteristic of cholera, an infection that produces vomiting and severe diarrhea.

Treatment. Lost volume should be replaced with fluids that are isotonic to plasma. This can be accomplished by infusing isotonic (0.9%) sodium chloride in sterile water, a solution in which both sodium and chloride are present at a concentration of 145 mEq/L. Volume should be replenished slowly to avoid pulmonary edema.

Hypertonic Contraction

Definition and Causes. Hypertonic contraction is defined as volume contraction in which *loss of water exceeds loss of sodium.* Hence, there is a reduction in extracellular fluid volume coupled with an increase in osmolality. Because of extracellular hypertonicity, water is drawn out of cells, thereby producing intracellular dehydration and partial compensation for lost extracellular volume.

Causes of hypertonic contraction include excessive sweating, osmotic diuresis, and feeding excessively concentrated foods to infants. Hypertonic contraction may also develop secondary to extensive burns or disorders of the central nervous system (CNS) that render the patient unable to experience or report thirst.

411

Treatment. Volume replacement in hypertonic contraction should be accomplished with hypotonic fluids (e.g., 0.11% sodium chloride) or with fluids that contain no solutes at all. Initial therapy may consist simply of drinking water. Alternatively, 5% dextrose can be infused intravenously; since dextrose is rapidly metabolized to carbon dioxide and water, dextrose solutions can be viewed as the osmotic equivalent of water alone. Volume replenishment should be done in stages. About 50% of the estimated loss should be replaced during the first few hours of treatment. The remainder should be replenished over 1 to 2 days.

Hypotonic Contraction

Definition and Causes. Hypotonic contraction is defined as volume contraction in which *loss of sodium exceeds loss of water.* Hence both the volume and osmolality of extracellular fluid are reduced. Since intracellular osmolality now exceeds extracellular osmolality, extracellular volume becomes diminished further by movement of water into cells.

The principal cause of hypotonic contraction is excessive loss of sodium through the kidneys. This may occur because of diuretic therapy, chronic renal insufficiency, or lack of aldosterone (the adrenocortical hormone that promotes renal retention of sodium).

Treatment. If hyponatremia is mild and if renal function is adequate, hypotonic contraction can be corrected by infusing *isotonic* sodium chloride solution for injection; plasma tonicity will be adjusted by the kidneys. However, if the sodium loss is severe, a *hypertonic* (e.g., 3%) solution of sodium chloride should be infused. Administration should continue until plasma sodium concentration has been raised to about 130 mEq/L. Patients should be monitored for signs of fluid overload (distention of neck veins, peripheral or pulmonary edema). When hypotonic contraction is due to aldosterone insufficiency, patients should receive hormone replacement therapy along with intravenous infusion of isotonic sodium chloride.

Volume Expansion

Volume expansion is defined as an *increase in the total volume of body fluid.* As with volume contraction, volume expansion may be *isotonic, hypertonic,* or *hypotonic.* Volume expansion may result from an overdose with therapeutic fluids (e.g., sodium chloride infusion) or may be associated with disease states (e.g., heart failure, nephrotic syndrome, cirrhosis of the liver with ascites). The principal drugs employed to correct volume expansion are *diuretics* and the *agents used for heart failure.* These drugs are discussed in Chapters 39 and 46, respectively.

ACID-BASE DISTURBANCES

Maintenance of acid-base balance is a complex process, the full discussion of which is beyond the scope of this text. Hence, consideration here is condensed.

Acid-base status is regulated by multiple systems. The most important are (1) the bicarbonate–carbonic acid buffer system, (2) the respiratory system, and (3) the kidneys. The respiratory system influences pH through control of CO_2 exhalation. Since CO_2 represents volatile carbonic acid, exhalation of CO_2 tends to elevate pH (reduce acidity), whereas CO_2 retention (secondary to respiratory slowing) tends to lower pH. The kidneys influence pH by regulating bicarbonate excretion. By retaining bicarbonate, the kidneys can raise pH. Conversely, by increasing the excretion of bicarbonate, the kidneys can compensate for alkalosis.

There are four principal types of acid-base imbalance: (1) respiratory alkalosis, (2) respiratory acidosis, (3) metabolic alkalosis, and (4) metabolic acidosis. The causes and treatments of these states are discussed below.

Respiratory Alkalosis

Causes. Respiratory alkalosis is produced by hyperventilation. Deep and rapid breathing increases loss of CO_2, which in turn lowers the pCO_2 of blood and thereby increases pH. Mild hyperventilation may result from a number of causes, including hypoxia, pulmonary disease, and drugs (especially aspirin and other salicylates). Severe hyperventilation can be caused by injury to the CNS and by hysteria.

Treatment. Management of respiratory alkalosis is dictated by the severity of pH elevation. When alkalosis is mild, no specific treatment is indicated. Severe respiratory alkalosis produced by hysteria can be controlled by having the patient rebreathe his or her CO_2-laden expired breath. This can be accomplished by holding a paper bag over the nose and mouth. A similar effect can be achieved by having the patient inhale a gas mixture containing 5% CO_2. A sedative (e.g., diazepam) can help suppress the hysteria.

Respiratory Acidosis

Causes. Respiratory acidosis results from retention of CO_2 secondary to hypoventilation. Reduced exhalation of CO_2 raises plasma pCO_2, which in turn causes plasma pH to fall. Primary causes of impaired ventilation are (1) depression of the medullary respiratory center, and (2) pathologic changes in the lungs (e.g., status asthmaticus, airway obstruction). With time, the kidneys compensate for respiratory acidosis by excreting less bicarbonate.

Treatment. Primary treatment of respiratory acidosis is directed at correcting respiratory impairment. The patient may also need oxygen and ventilatory assistance. Infusion of sodium bicarbonate solution may be indicated if acidosis is severe.

Metabolic Alkalosis

Causes. Metabolic alkalosis is characterized by increases in both the pH and bicarbonate content of plasma. Causes include excessive loss of gastric acid (through vomiting or suctioning) and administration of alkalinizing salts (e.g., sodium bicarbonate). The body compensates for metabolic alkalosis by (1) hypoventilation (causing retention of CO_2), (2) increased renal excretion of bicarbonate, and (3) accumulation of organic acids.

Treatment. In most cases, metabolic alkalosis can be corrected by infusing a solution of *sodium chloride plus potassium chloride.* This facilitates renal excretion of bicarbonate, and thereby promotes normalization of plasma pH. When alkalosis is severe, direct correction of pH is indicated. This can be accomplished by infusing dilute (0.1 N) *hydrochloric acid* through a central venous catheter or by administering an acid-forming salt, such as *ammonium chloride*. Ammonium chloride must not be given to patients with liver failure, since the drug is likely to cause hepatic encephalopathy in these patients.

Metabolic Acidosis

Causes. Principal causes of metabolic acidosis are chronic renal failure, loss of bicarbonate during severe diarrhea, and metabolic disorders that result in overproduction of lactic acid (lactic acidosis) or ketoacids (ketoacidosis). Metabolic acidosis may also result from poisoning by methanol and certain medications (e.g., aspirin and other salicylates).

Treatment. Treatment of metabolic acidosis consists of correcting the underlying cause, and, if the acidosis is severe, administering an alkalinizing salt (e.g., sodium bicarbonate, sodium carbonate).

When an alkalinizing salt is indicated, *sodium bicarbonate* is generally preferred. Administration may be oral or intravenous. If acidosis is mild, oral administration is preferred. Intravenous infusion is usually reserved for severe reductions of pH. When sodium bicarbonate is given IV to treat acute, severe acidosis, caution must be exercised to avoid excessive elevation of plasma pH, since rapid conversion from acidosis to alkalosis can be hazardous. Also, because of the sodium content of sodium bicarbonate, care should be taken to avoid hypernatremia.

POTASSIUM IMBALANCES

Potassium is the most abundant *intracellular* cation, having a concentration within cells of about 150 mEq/L. In contrast, *extracellular* concentrations are low (4 to 5 mEq/L). Potassium plays a major role in conducting nerve impulses and maintaining the electrical excitability of muscle. Potassium also helps regulate acid-base balance.

Regulation of Potassium Levels

Serum levels of potassium are regulated primarily by the kidneys. Under steady-state conditions, urinary output of potassium equals intake. Renal excretion of potassium is increased by aldosterone, an adrenal steroid that promotes conservation of sodium while increasing potassium loss. Potassium excretion is also increased by most diuretics. Potassium-sparing diuretics (e.g., spironolactone) are the exception.

Potassium levels are influenced by extracellular pH. In the presence of extracellular *alkalosis,* potassium uptake by cells is *enhanced,* causing a *reduction* in extracellular potassium levels. Conversely, extracellular *acidosis* promotes the exit of potassium from cells, thereby causing extracellular *hyperkalemia.*

Insulin has a profound effect on potassium: in high doses, insulin stimulates potassium uptake by cells. This ability has been exploited to treat hyperkalemia.

Hypokalemia
Causes and Consequences

Hypokalemia is defined as a deficiency of potassium in the blood. By definition, hypokalemia exists when serum potassium levels fall below 3.5 mEq/L. The most common cause of hypokalemia is treatment with thiazide or loop diuretics (see Chapter 39). Other causes include insufficient potassium intake; alkalosis and excessive insulin (both of which decrease extracellular potassium levels by driving potassium into cells); increased renal excretion of potassium (e.g., as caused by aldosterone); and potassium loss associated with vomiting, diarrhea, and abuse of laxatives. Hypokalemia may also occur because of excessive potassium loss in sweat. As a rule, potassium depletion is accompanied by loss of chloride. Insufficiency of both ions produces *hypokalemic alkalosis.*

Hypokalemia has adverse effects on skeletal muscle, smooth muscle, blood pressure, and the heart. Symptoms include weakness or paralysis of skeletal muscle, a risk of fatal dysrhythmias, and intestinal dilation and ileus. In patients taking digoxin (a cardiac drug), concurrent hypokalemia is the principal cause of digoxin toxicity. For all people, hypokalemia increases the risk of hypertension and stroke.

Prevention and Treatment

Potassium depletion can be treated with three potassium salts: potassium chloride, potassium phosphate, and potassium bicarbonate. These may also be used for prophylaxis against insufficiency. For either treatment or prophylaxis, the preferred salt is *potassium chloride*. Why? Because chloride deficiency frequently coexists with deficiency of potassium.

Potassium chloride may be administered orally or IV. Oral administration is preferred for prophylaxis and for treating mild deficiency. Intravenous therapy is reserved for severe deficiency and for patients who cannot take potassium orally.

Oral Potassium Chloride. Uses, Dosage, and Preparations. Oral potassium chloride may be used for both prevention and treatment of potassium deficiency. Dosages for prevention range from 16 to 24 mEq/day. Dosages for correcting deficiency range from 40 to 100 mEq/day.

Oral potassium chloride is available in solution and in several solid formulations: standard tablets, sustained-release tablets, effervescent tablets, and powders. *The sustained-release tablets (e.g., K-Dur, Micro-K, Slow-K) are preferred.* Why? Because they are more convenient and better tolerated than the other formulations, and hence offer the best chance of compliance.

Adverse Effects. Potassium chloride irritates the GI tract, frequently causing abdominal discomfort, nausea, vomiting, and diarrhea. With the exception of the sustained-release tablets, solid formulations can produce high local concentrations of potassium, resulting in severe intestinal injury (ulcerative lesions, bleeding, perforation); death has occurred. To minimize GI effects, oral potassium chloride should be taken with meals or a full glass of water. If symptoms of irritation occur, administration should be discontinued. Rarely, oral potassium chloride produces hyperkalemia. This dangerous development is much more likely with IV therapy.

Intravenous Potassium Chloride. Intravenous potassium chloride is indicated for prevention and treatment of hypokalemia. Intravenous solutions must be diluted (preferably to 40 mEq/L or less) and infused slowly (generally no faster than 10 mEq/hr in adults).

The principal complication is *hyperkalemia,* which can prove fatal. To reduce the risk of hyperkalemia, serum potassium levels should be measured prior to the infusion and periodically throughout the treatment interval. Also, renal function should be assessed before and during treatment to ensure adequate output of urine. If renal failure develops, the infusion should be stopped immediately. Changes in the electrocardiogram (EKG) can be an early indication that potassium toxicity is developing.

Contraindications to Potassium Use. Potassium should be avoided under conditions that predispose the patient to hyperkalemia (e.g., severe renal impairment, use of potassium-sparing diuretics, hypoaldosteronism). Potassium must also be avoided when hyperkalemia already exists.

Hyperkalemia
Causes and Consequences

Causes. Hyperkalemia (excessive elevation of serum potassium content) can result from a number of causes. These include severe tissue trauma, untreated Addison's disease, acute acidosis (which draws potassium out of cells), misuse of potassium-sparing diuretics, and overdose with IV potassium.

Consequences. The most serious consequence of hyperkalemia is disruption of the electrical activity of the heart. Because hyperkalemia alters the generation and conduction of cardiac impulses, alterations in the EKG and cardiac rhythm are usually the earliest signs that potassium levels are becoming dangerously high. With mild elevation of serum potassium (5 to 7 mEq/L), the T wave heightens and the PR interval becomes prolonged. When serum potassium reaches 8 to 9 mEq/L, cardiac arrest occurs, possibly preceded by ventricular tachycardia or fibrillation.

Effects of hyperkalemia are not limited to the heart. Noncardiac effects include confusion, anxiety, dyspnea, weakness or heaviness of the legs, and numbness or tingling of the hands, feet, and lips.

Treatment

Treatment is begun by withholding any foods that contain potassium and any medicines that promote potassium accumulation (e.g., potassium-sparing diuretics, potassium supplements). After this, management consists of measures that (1) counteract potassium-induced cardiotoxicity and (2) lower extracellular levels of potassium. Specific steps include (1) infusion of a *calcium salt* (e.g., calcium gluconate) to offset effects of hyperkalemia on the heart; (2) infusion of *glucose* and *insulin* to promote uptake of potassium by cells and thereby decrease extracellular potassium levels; and (3) if acidosis is present (which is likely), infusion of *sodium bicarbonate* to move pH toward alkalinity, and thereby increase cellular uptake of potassium. If these measures prove inadequate, steps can be taken to remove potassium. These include (1) oral or rectal administration of *sodium polystyrene sulfonate,* an exchange resin that absorbs potassium; and (2) peritoneal or extracorporeal dialysis.

MAGNESIUM IMBALANCES

Magnesium is required for the activity of many enzymes and for binding of messenger RNA to ribosomes. In addition, magnesium helps regulate neurochemical transmission and the excitability of muscle. The concentration of magne-

sium within cells is about 40 mEq/L, much higher than its concentration outside cells (about 2 mEq/L).

Hypomagnesemia
Causes and Consequences

Low levels of magnesium may result from a variety of causes, including diarrhea, hemodialysis, kidney disease, and prolonged intravenous feeding with magnesium-free solutions. Hypomagnesemia may also be seen in chronic alcoholics and people with diabetes or pancreatitis. Frequently, patients with magnesium deficiency also present with hypocalcemia and hypokalemia.

Prominent symptoms of hypomagnesemia involve cardiac and skeletal muscle. In the presence of low levels of magnesium, release of acetylcholine at the neuromuscular junction is enhanced. This can increase muscle excitability to the point of tetany. Hypomagnesemia also increases excitability of neurons in the CNS, causing disorientation, psychoses, and seizures.

In the kidneys, hypomagnesemia may lead to nephrocalcinosis (formation of minuscule calcium stones within nephrons). Renal injury occurs when the stones become large enough to block the flow of tubular urine.

Prevention and Treatment

Frank hypomagnesemia is treated with parenteral magnesium sulfate. For prophylaxis against magnesium deficiency, an oral preparation (magnesium gluconate, magnesium hydroxide) may be used.

Magnesium Gluconate and Magnesium Hydroxide. Tablets of magnesium gluconate or magnesium hydroxide may be taken as supplements to dietary magnesium to help prevent hypomagnesemia. Milk of magnesia (a liquid formulation of magnesium hydroxide) may also be used for prophylaxis. With any oral magnesium preparation, excessive doses may cause diarrhea. The adult and pediatric dosage for preventing deficiency is 5 mg/kg/day.

Magnesium Sulfate. Uses, Administration, and Dosage. Magnesium sulfate (IM or IV) is the preferred treatment for severe hypomagnesemia. The IM dosage is 0.5 to 1 gm 4 times a day. For IV therapy, a 10% solution can be used; the infusion rate is 1.5 ml/min or less.

Adverse Effects. Excessive levels of magnesium cause *neuromuscular blockade.* Paralysis of the respiratory muscles is of particular concern. By suppressing neuromuscular transmission, magnesium excess can intensify the effects of neuromuscular blocking agents (e.g., tubocurarine, succinylcholine). Hence, caution must be exercised in patients receiving these drugs. The neuromuscular blocking actions of magnesium can be counteracted with calcium. Accordingly, when parenteral magnesium is being employed, an injectable form of calcium (e.g., calcium gluconate) should be immediately available.

In the heart, excessive magnesium can suppress impulse conduction through the atrioventricular (AV) node. Accordingly, magnesium sulfate is contraindicated for patients with AV heart block.

To minimize the risk of toxicity, serum magnesium levels should be monitored. Respiratory paralysis occurs at 12 to 15 mEq/L. When magnesium levels exceed 25 mEq/L, cardiac arrest may take place.

Hypermagnesemia

Toxic elevation of magnesium levels is most common in patients with renal insufficiency, especially when magnesium-containing antacids or cathartics are being used. Symptoms of mild intoxication include muscle weakness (resulting from inhibition of acetylcholine release), hypotension, sedation, and EKG changes. As noted, respiratory paralysis is likely when plasma levels reach 12 to 15 mEq/L. At higher concentrations of magnesium, there is a risk of cardiac arrest. Muscle weakness and paralysis can be counteracted with an intravenous calcium preparation.

⠫ KEY POINTS

- Treat isotonic volume contraction with isotonic (0.9%) sodium chloride.
- Treat hypertonic volume contraction with hypotonic (e.g., 0.11%) sodium chloride.
- Treat hypotonic volume contraction with hypertonic (e.g., 3%) sodium chloride.
- Treat volume expansion with diuretics.
- Treat respiratory or metabolic acidosis with sodium bicarbonate.
- Treat respiratory alkalosis by having patients inhale 5% CO_2 or rebreathe their expired air.
- Treat metabolic alkalosis with an infusion of sodium chloride plus potassium chloride. For severe cases, infuse 0.1% hydrochloric acid or ammonium chloride.
- Treat moderate hypokalemia with potassium chloride in sustained-release tablets.
- Treat severe hypokalemia with IV potassium chloride.
- To treat hyperkalemia, begin by withdrawing potassium-containing foods and as well as drugs that promote potassium accumulation (e.g., potassium supplements, potassium-sparing diuretics). Subsequent measures include (1) infusing a calcium salt to offset the cardiac effects of potassium, (2) infusing glucose and insulin to promote potassium uptake by cells, and (3) infusing sodium bicarbonate if acidosis is present.
- Treat hypomagnesemia with IM or IV magnesium sulfate. For prophylaxis, give oral magnesium (e.g., magnesium gluconate).

Review of Hemodynamics

Hemodynamics is the study of the movement of blood throughout the circulatory system, as well as the regulatory mechanisms and driving forces involved. Concepts introduced here reappear throughout the chapters on cardiovascular drugs. Accordingly, I urge you to review these now. Because this is a pharmacology text, and not a physiology text, discussion is limited to hemodynamic factors that have particular relevance to the actions of drugs.

OVERVIEW OF THE CIRCULATORY SYSTEM

The circulatory system has two primary functions: (1) delivery of oxygen, nutrients, hormones, electrolytes, and other essentials to cells; and (2) removal of carbon dioxide, metabolic wastes, and other detritus from cells. In addition, the system helps fight infection.

The circulatory system has two divisions: the *pulmonary circulation* and the *systemic circulation*. The pulmonary circulation delivers blood to the lungs. The systemic circulation delivers blood to all other tissues. The systemic circulation is also known as the greater *circulation* or *peripheral circulation*.

Components of the Circulatory System

The circulatory system is composed of the *heart* and *blood vessels*. The heart is the pump that moves blood through the arterial tree. The blood vessels have several functions:

- *Arteries* transport blood under high pressure to tissues.
- *Arterioles* are control valves that regulate local blood flow.
- *Capillaries* are the sites for exchange of fluid, oxygen, carbon dioxide, nutrients, hormones, wastes, and so forth.
- *Venules* collect blood from the capillaries.
- *Veins* transport blood back to the heart. In addition, veins serve as a major reservoir for blood.

Arteries and veins differ from each other with respect to distensibility (elasticity). Arteries are very muscular, and hence do not readily stretch. As a result, large increases in arterial pressure (AP) cause only small increases in arterial diameter. Veins are much less muscular than arteries, and hence are 6 to 10 times more distensible. As a result, small increases in venous pressure cause large increases in venous diameter, which produces a large increase in venous volume.

Distribution of Blood

The adult circulatory system contains about 5 L of blood, which is distributed throughout the system. As indicated in Figure 41–1, 9% is in the pulmonary circulation, 7% is in the heart, and 84% is in the systemic circulation. Within the systemic circulation, however, distribution is uneven: most (64%) of the blood is in veins, venules, and venous sinuses; the remaining 20% is in arteries (13%) and arterioles or capillaries (7%). The large volume of blood in the venous system serves as a reservoir.

What Makes Blood Flow?

Blood moves within vessels because the force that drives flow is greater than the resistance to flow. As indicated in Figure 41–2, the force that drives blood flow is the pressure gradient between two points in a vessel. Obviously, blood will flow from the point where pressure is higher toward the point where pressure is lower. Resistance to flow is determined by the diameter and length of the vessel, and by blood viscosity. From a pharmacologic viewpoint, the most important determinant of resistance is vessel diameter: the larger the vessel, the smaller the resistance, and vice versa. Accordingly, when vessels dilate, resistance declines, causing blood flow to increase—and when vessels constrict, resistance rises, causing blood flow to decline. In order to maintain adequate flow when resistance rises, blood pressure must rise as well.

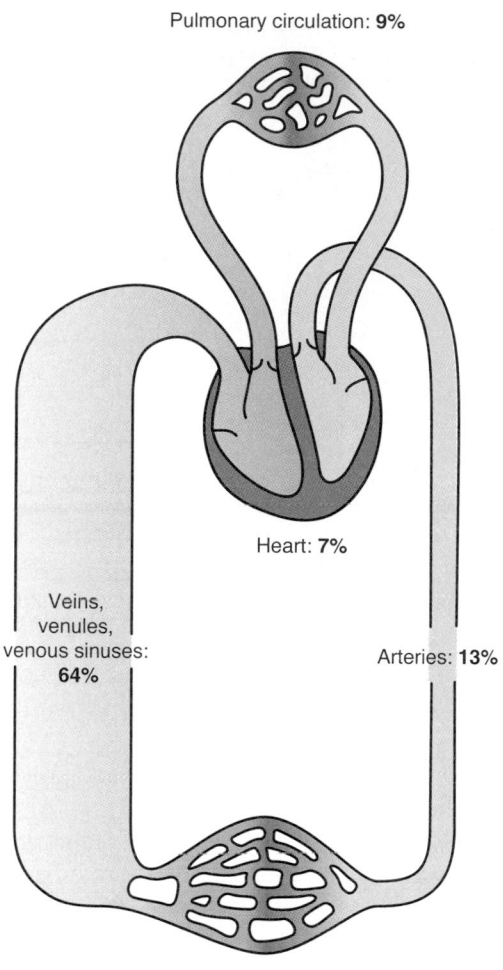

Figure 41–1 ▪ **Distribution of blood in the circulatory system.**
Note that a large percentage of the blood resides in the venous system.

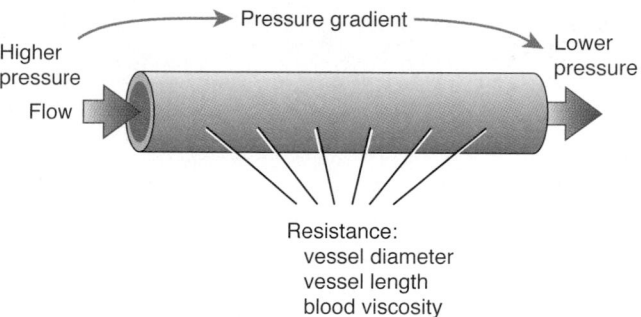

Figure 41–2 ▪ **Forces that promote and impede flow of blood.**
Blood flows from the point of higher pressure toward the point of lower pressure. Resistance to flow is determined by vessel diameter, vessel length, and blood viscosity.

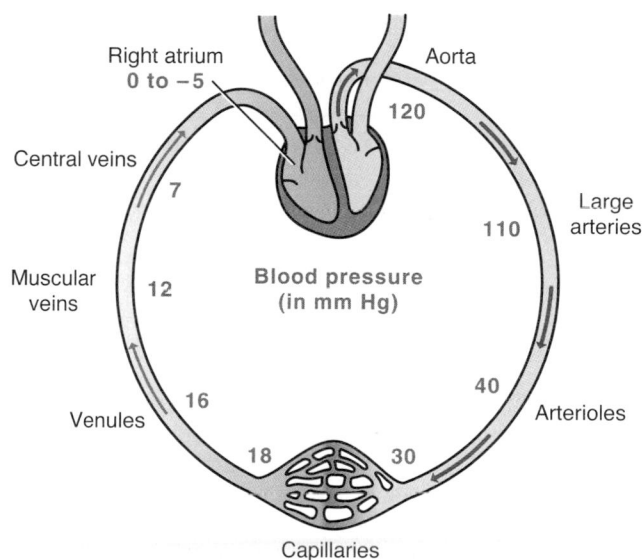

Figure 41–3 ▪ **Distribution of pressure within the systemic circulation.**
Note that pressure is highest when blood leaves the left ventricle, falls to only 18 mm Hg as blood exits capillaries, and reaches negative values within the right atrium.

How Does Blood Get Back to the Heart?

As indicated in Figure 41–3, pressure falls progressively as blood moves through the systemic circulation. Pressure is 120 mm Hg when blood enters the aorta, 30 mm Hg when blood enters capillaries, only 18 mm Hg when blood leaves capillaries, and then drops to negative values (0 to −5 mm Hg) in the right atrium. (Negative atrial pressure is generated by expansion of the chest during respiration.)

Given that pressure is only 18 mm Hg when blood leaves capillaries, we must ask, "How does blood get back to the heart? After all, a pressure of 18 mm Hg does not seem adequate to move blood from the feet all the way up to the thorax." The answer is that, in addition to the small pressure head in venules, three mechanisms help ensure venous return. First, negative pressure in the right atrium helps "suck" blood toward the heart. Second, constriction of smooth muscle in veins increases venous pressure, which helps drive blood toward the heart. Third, and most important, the combination of venous valves and skeletal muscle contraction constitutes an auxiliary "venous pump." As indicated in Figure 41–4A, the veins are equipped with a system of one-way valves. When skeletal muscles contract (Fig. 41–4B), venous blood is squeezed toward the heart—the only direction permitted by the valves.

REGULATION OF CARDIAC OUTPUT

In the average adult, cardiac output is about 5 L/min. Hence, every minute the heart pumps the equivalent of all the blood in the body. In this section, we consider the major factors that determine how much blood the heart pumps.

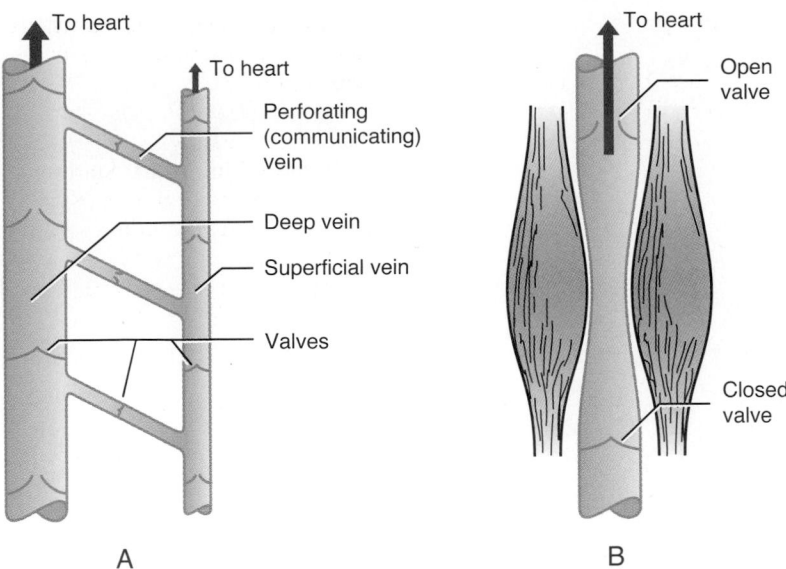

Figure 41–4 ■ **Venous valves and the auxiliary venous "pump."**
A, Veins and their one-way valves in the leg. Note that the arrangement of valves ensures that blood will move toward the heart. *B,* Contraction of skeletal muscle pumps venous blood toward the heart.

Determinants of Cardiac Output

The basic equation for cardiac output is

$$CO = HR \times SV$$

where CO is cardiac output, HR is heart rate, and SV is stroke volume. According to the equation, an increase in HR or SV will increase CO, whereas a decrease in HR or SV will decrease CO. For the average person, heart rate is about 70 beats/min and stroke volume is about 70 ml. Multiplying these, we get 4.9 L/min—the average value for CO.

Heart Rate. Heart rate is controlled primarily by the autonomic nervous system (ANS). Rate is increased by the sympathetic branch acting through beta$_1$-adrenergic receptors in the sinoatrial (SA) node. Rate is decreased by the parasympathetic branch acting through muscarinic receptors in the SA node. Parasympathetic impulses reach the heart via the vagus nerve.

Stroke Volume. Stroke volume is determined largely by three factors: (1) myocardial contractility, (2) cardiac afterload, and (3) cardiac preload. *Myocardial contractility* is defined as the force with which the ventricles contract. Contractility is determined primarily by the degree of cardiac dilation, which in turn is determined by the amount of venous return. The importance of venous return in regulating contractility and stroke volume is discussed separately below. In addition to regulation by venous return, contractility can be increased by the sympathetic nervous system, acting through beta$_1$-adrenergic receptors in the myocardium.

Preload. Preload is formally defined as the amount of tension (stretch) applied to a muscle prior to contraction. In the heart, stretch is determined by ventricular filling pressure, that is, the *force of venous return:* the greater filling pressure is, the greater the ventricles will stretch. Cardiac preload can be expressed as either *end-diastolic volume* or *end-diastolic pressure.* As discussed below, an increase in preload will in-crease stroke volume, whereas a decrease in preload will reduce stroke volume. Frequently, the terms *preload* and *force of venous return* are used interchangeably—although they are not truly equivalent.

Afterload. Afterload is formally defined as the load against which a muscle exerts its force (i.e., the load a muscle must overcome in order to contract). For the heart, afterload is the *arterial pressure* that the left ventricle must overcome to eject blood. Common sense tells us that, if afterload increases, stroke volume will decrease. Conversely, if afterload falls, stroke volume will rise. Cardiac afterload is determined primarily by the degree of peripheral resistance, which in turn is determined by constriction and dilation of arterioles: When arterioles constrict, peripheral resistance rises, causing AP (afterload) to rise as well; conversely, when arterioles dilate, peripheral resistance falls, causing AP to decline.

Control of Stroke Volume by Venous Return

Q: How much blood does the heart pump with each stroke?
A: Exactly the amount delivered to it by the veins!

Starling's Law of the Heart

Starling's law states that the force of ventricular contraction is proportional to muscle fiber length (up to a point). Accordingly, as fiber length (ventricular diameter) increases, there is a corresponding increase in contractile force (Fig. 41–5). Because of this built-in mechanism, when more blood enters the heart, more is pumped out. As a result, the healthy heart is able to precisely match its output with the volume of blood delivered by the veins: When venous return increases, cardiac output increases correspondingly; conversely, when venous return declines, cardiac output declines to precisely the same extent. Hence,

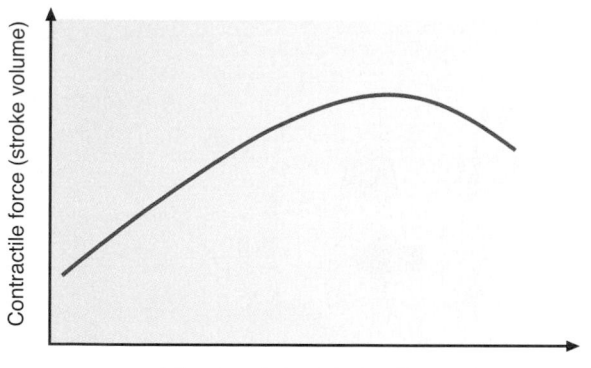

Figure 41–5 ▪ The Starling relationship between myocardial fiber length and contractile force.
Note that an increase in fiber length produces a corresponding increase in contractile force. Fiber length increases as the ventricles enlarge during filling. Increased contractile force is reflected by increased stroke volume.

under normal, nonstressed conditions, stroke volume is determined by factors that regulate venous return.

Why does contractile force change as a function of fiber length (ventricular diameter)? Recall that muscle contraction results from the interaction of two proteins: actin and myosin. As the heart stretches in response to increased ventricular filling, actin and myosin are brought into a more optimal alignment with each other, which allows them to interact with greater force.

Factors That Determine Venous Return

Having established that venous return is the primary determinant of stroke volume (and hence cardiac output), we need to understand the factors that determine venous return. With regard to pharmacology, the most important factor is *systemic filling pressure* (i.e., the force that returns blood to the heart). The normal value for filling pressure is 7 mm Hg. This value can be raised to 17 mm Hg by constriction of veins. Filling pressure can also be raised by an increase in blood volume. Conversely, filling pressure, and hence venous return, can be lowered by venodilation or by reducing blood volume. Blood volume and venous tone can both be altered with drugs.

In addition to systemic filling pressure, three other factors influence venous return: (1) the auxiliary muscle pumps discussed above, (2) resistance to flow between peripheral vessels and the right atrium, and (3) right atrial pressure, elevation of which will impede venous return. None of these factors can be directly influenced with drugs.

Starling's Law and Maintenance of Systemic-Pulmonary Balance

Because the myocardium operates in accord with Starling's law, the right and left ventricles always pump exactly the same amount of blood. When venous return increases, stroke volume of the right ventricle increases, thereby increasing delivery of blood to the pulmonary circulation, which in turn delivers more blood to the left ventricle; this increases filling of

the left ventricle, which causes *its* stroke volume to increase. Because an increase in venous return causes the output of *both* ventricles to increase, blood flow through the systemic and pulmonary circulations is always in balance, as long as the heart is healthy.

In the failing heart, Starling's law breaks down. That is, force of contraction no longer increases in proportion to increased ventricular filling. As a result, blood backs up behind the failing ventricle. The deadly consequences are illustrated in Figure 41–6. In this example, output of the left ventricle is 1% less than the output of the right ventricle, which causes blood to back up in the pulmonary circulation. In only 20 minutes, this small imbalance between left and right ventricular output shifts a liter of blood from the systemic circulation to the pulmonary circulation. In less than 40 minutes, death from pulmonary congestion would ensue. This example underscores the importance of systemic-pulmonary balance, and the critical role of Starling's mechanism in maintaining it.

REGULATION OF ARTERIAL PRESSURE

AP is the driving force that moves blood through the arterial side of the systemic circulation. The general formula for AP is

$$AP = PR \times CO$$

where AP is arterial pressure, PR is peripheral resistance, and CO is cardiac output. Accordingly, an increase in PR or CO will increase AP, whereas a decrease in PR or CO will decrease AP. Peripheral resistance is regulated primarily through constriction and dilation of arterioles. CO is regulated by the mechanisms discussed above. Regulation of AP through processes that alter PR and CO is discussed below.

Overview of Control Systems

Under normal circumstances, AP is regulated primarily by three systems: the ANS, the renin-angiotensin-aldosterone system (RAAS), and the kidneys. These systems differ greatly with regard to time frame of response. The ANS acts in two ways: (1) it responds rapidly (in seconds or minutes) to acute changes in blood pressure, and (2) it provides steady-state control. The RAAS responds more slowly, taking hours or days to influence AP. The kidneys are responsible for long-term control, and hence may take days or weeks to adjust AP.

Arterial pressure is also regulated by a fourth system: a family of natriuretic peptides. These peptides come into play primarily under conditions of volume overload.

Steady-State Control by the ANS

The ANS regulates AP by adjusting CO and peripheral resistance. Sympathetic tone to the heart increases heart rate and contractility, thereby increasing CO. In contrast, parasympathetic tone slows the heart, and thereby reduces CO. As discussed in Chapter 13, constriction of blood vessels is regulated exclusively by the sympathetic branch of the ANS; blood vessels have no parasympathetic innervation. Steady-

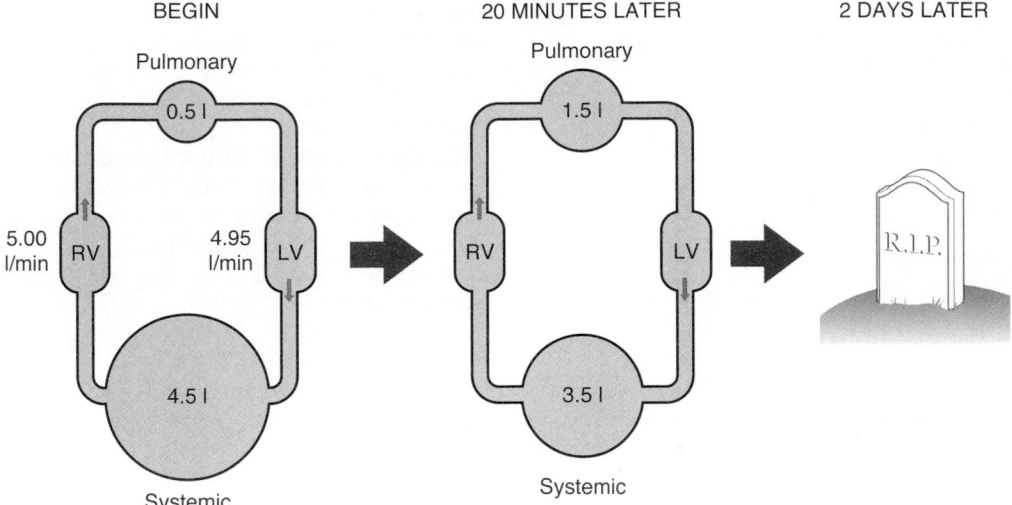

BEGIN   20 MINUTES LATER   2 DAYS LATER

Figure 41–6 ■ Systemic-pulmonary imbalance that develops when the output of the left and right ventricles is not identical.
In this example, the output of the left ventricle is 1% less than the output of the right ventricle. Hence, while the right ventricle pumps 5000 ml/min, the left pumps only 4950 ml/min—50 ml/min less than the right side. This causes blood to back up in the pulmonary circulation. After 20 minutes, 1000 ml of blood has shifted from the systemic circulation to the pulmonary circulation. Death would ensue in less than 40 minutes. The 2 days are an allowance for the undertaker and parson. Numbers in the pulmonary and systemic circulations indicate volume of blood in liters. (Adapted from Burton AC. Physiology and Biophysics of the Circulation. Chicago, Year Book Medical Publishers, 1968:144.)

state sympathetic tone provides a moderate level of vasoconstriction. The resultant resistance to blood flow maintains AP. Complete elimination of sympathetic tone would cause AP to fall by 50%.

Rapid Control by the ANS: The Baroreceptor Reflex

The baroreceptor reflex serves to maintain AP at a predetermined level. When AP changes, the reflex immediately attempts to restore AP to the preset value.

The reflex works as follows. Baroreceptors in the aortic arch and carotid sinus sense AP and relay this information to the vasoconstrictor center of the medulla. When AP changes, the vasoconstrictor center compensates by sending appropriate instructions to arterioles, veins, and the heart. For example, when AP drops, the vasoconstrictor center causes (1) constriction of nearly all arterioles, thereby increasing peripheral resistance; (2) constriction of veins, thereby increasing venous return; and (3) acceleration of heart rate (by increasing sympathetic impulses to the heart and decreasing parasympathetic impulses). The combined effect of these responses is to restore AP to the preset level. When AP rises too high, opposite responses occur: The reflex dilates arterioles and veins, and slows heart rate.

The baroreceptor reflex is poised for rapid action—but not for sustained action. When AP falls or rises, the reflex acts within seconds to restore the preset pressure. However, when AP *remains* elevated or lowered, the system resets to the new pressure within 1 to 2 days. After this, the system perceives the new (elevated or reduced) pressure as "normal," and hence ceases to respond.

Drugs that lower AP will trigger the baroreceptor reflex. For example, if we administer a drug that dilates arterioles, the resultant drop in peripheral resistance will reduce AP, causing the baroreceptor reflex to activate. The most noticeable response is *reflex tachycardia*. The baroreceptor reflex can temporarily negate efforts to lower AP with drugs.

The Renin-Angiotensin-Aldosterone System

The RAAS supports AP by causing (1) constriction of arterioles and veins, and (2) retention of water by the kidney. Vasoconstriction is mediated by a hormone named *angiotensin II;* water retention is mediated in part by *aldosterone*. Responses develop in hours (vasoconstriction) to days (water retention). The RAAS and its role in controlling blood pressure are discussed at length in Chapter 42.

Renal Retention of Water

When AP remains low for a long time, the kidney responds by retaining water, which in turn causes AP to rise. Pressure rises because fluid retention increases blood volume, which increases venous pressure, which increases venous return, which increases CO, which increases AP. Water retention is a mechanism for maintaining AP over long periods (weeks, months, years).

Why does a reduction in AP cause the kidney to retain water? First, low AP reduces renal blood flow (RBF), which in turn reduces glomerular filtration rate (GFR). Since less fluid is filtered, less urine is produced, and therefore more water is retained. Second, low AP activates the RAAS, causing levels of angiotensin II and aldosterone to rise. Angiotensin II causes constriction of renal blood vessels, and thereby further decreases RBF and GFR. Aldosterone promotes renal retention of sodium, which causes water to be retained along with it.

Postural Hypotension

Postural hypotension, also known as *orthostatic hypotension,* is a reduction in AP that can occur when we move from a supine or seated position to an upright position. The cause of hypotension is pooling of blood in veins, which decreases venous return, which in turn decreases CO. Between 300 and 800 ml of blood can pool in veins when we stand, causing CO to drop by as much as 2 L/min. Why does blood collect in veins? When we stand, gravity increases the pressure that blood exerts on veins. Since veins are not very muscular, they are unable to retain their shape when pressure increases, and hence they stretch. The resultant increase in venous volume allows blood to pool.

Two mechanisms help overcome postural hypotension. One is the system of auxiliary venous pumps, which promote venous return. In fact, in healthy individuals, these auxiliary pumps usually prevent postural hypotension from occurring in the first place. When postural hypotension does occur, the baroreceptor reflex can restore AP by (1) constricting veins and arterioles and (2) increasing heart rate.

What would happen if we gave a drug that promoted dilation of veins (or prevented them from constricting)? In patients taking drugs that interfere with venoconstriction, postural hypotension is more intense and more prolonged. Hypotension is more intense because venous pooling is greater. Hypotension is more prolonged because there is no venoconstriction to help reverse venous pooling. As with drugs that reduce AP by dilating arterioles, drugs that reduce AP by relaxing veins can trigger the baroreceptor reflex, and can thereby cause reflex tachycardia.

Natriuretic Peptides

Natriuretic peptides serve to protect the cardiovascular system under conditions of volume overload, a condition that increases preload, and thereby increases CO and AP. Volume overload is caused by excessive retention of sodium and water. Natriuretic peptides work primarily by (1) reducing blood volume and (2) promoting dilation of arterioles and veins. Both actions lower AP.

The family of natriuretic peptides has three principal members: *atrial natriuretic peptide* (ANP), *B-* or *brain natriuretic peptide* (BNP), and *C-natriuretic peptide* (CNP). ANP is produced by myocytes of the atria; BNP is produced by myocytes of the ventricles (and to a lesser extent by cells in the brain, where BNP was discovered); and CNP is produced by cells of the vascular endothelium. When blood volume is excessive, all three peptides are released. (Release of ANP and BNP is triggered by stretching of the atria and ventricles, which occurs because of increased preload.)

ANP and BNP have similar actions. Both peptides reduce blood volume and increase venous capacitance, and thereby reduce cardiac preload. Three processes are involved. First,

ANP and BNP shift fluid from the vasculature to the extravascular compartment; the underlying mechanism is increased vascular permeability. Second, they act on the kidney to cause diuresis (loss of water) and natriuresis (loss of sodium). Third, they promote dilation of arterioles and veins, in part by suppressing sympathetic outflow from the central nervous system. In addition to these actions, ANP and BNP help protect the heart during the early phase of heart failure. How? By suppressing both the RAAS and sympathetic outflow, and by inhibiting proliferation of myocytes. Although CNP shares some actions of ANP and BMP, its primary action is promotion of vasodilation.

■:■ KEY POINTS*

- Arterioles serve as control valves to regulate local blood flow.
- Veins are a reservoir for blood.
- Arteries are not very distensible. As a result, large increases in AP cause only small increases in arterial diameter.
- Veins are highly distensible. As a result, small increases in venous pressure cause large increases in venous diameter.
- The adult circulatory system contains 5 L of blood, 64% of which is in systemic veins.
- Vasodilation reduces resistance to blood flow, whereas vasoconstriction increases resistance to flow.
- In addition to the small pressure head in venules, three mechanisms help ensure venous return: (1) negative pressure in the right atrium sucks blood toward the heart; (2) constriction of veins increases venous pressure, and thereby drives blood toward the heart; and (3) contraction of skeletal muscles, in conjunction with one-way venous valves, pumps blood toward the heart.
- Heart rate is increased by sympathetic nerves and decreased by parasympathetic nerves.
- Stroke volume is determined by myocardial contractility, cardiac preload, and cardiac afterload.
- Preload is defined as the amount of tension (stretch) applied to a muscle prior to contraction. In the heart, preload is determined by the force of venous return.
- Afterload is defined as the load against which a muscle exerts its force. For the heart, afterload is the AP that the left ventricle must overcome to eject blood.
- Cardiac afterload is determined primarily by peripheral resistance, which in turn is determined by the degree of constriction in arterioles.
- Starling's law states that the force of ventricular contraction is proportional to myocardial fiber length. Because of this relationship, when more blood enters the heart, more is pumped out. As a result, the healthy heart is able to precisely match output with venous return.

---

*Key points are limited to concepts that might not have been stressed when you studied physiology (e.g., veins serve as a blood reservoir). Important but obvious concepts (e.g., the heart is a pump; arteries deliver blood to tissues under pressure) are not included in this summary.

- The most important determinant of venous return is systemic filling pressure, which can be raised by constricting veins and by increasing blood volume.
- Because cardiac muscle operates under Starling's law, the right and left ventricles always pump exactly the same amount of blood (assuming the heart is healthy). Hence, balance between the pulmonary and systemic circulations is maintained.
- AP is regulated by the ANS, the RAAS, the kidneys, and natriuretic peptides.
- The ANS regulates arterial pressure (1) through tonic control of heart rate and peripheral resistance and (2) through the baroreceptor reflex.
- The baroreceptor reflex is only useful for short-term control of AP. When pressure remains elevated or lowered, the system resets to the new pressure within 1 to 2 days, and hence ceases to respond.
- Drugs that lower AP trigger the baroreceptor reflex, and thereby cause reflex tachycardia. Hence, the baroreceptor reflex can temporarily negate efforts to lower AP with drugs.
- The RAAS supports AP by causing (1) constriction of arterioles and veins and (2) retention of water by the kidneys. Vasoconstriction is mediated by angiotensin II; water retention is mediated in part by aldosterone.
- The kidneys provide long-term control of blood pressure by regulating blood volume.
- Postural (orthostatic) hypotension is caused by decreased venous return secondary to pooling of blood in veins when we assume an erect posture.
- Drugs that dilate veins intensify and prolong postural hypotension. As with other drugs that reduce AP, venodilators can trigger the baroreceptor reflex, and can thereby cause reflex tachycardia.
- Natriuretic peptides defend the cardiovascular system from volume overload—primarily by reducing blood volume and promoting vasodilation.

Drugs Acting on the Renin-Angiotensin-Aldosterone System

In this chapter we consider three families of drugs: angiotensin-converting enzyme (ACE) inhibitors, angiotensin II receptor blockers (ARBs), and selective aldosterone receptor blockers. With all three groups, effects result from interfering with the renin-angiotensin-aldosterone system (RAAS). The ACE inhibitors, available for more than two decades, have established roles in the treatment of hypertension, heart failure, and diabetic nephropathy; in addition, these drugs are indicated for myocardial infarction and prevention of cardiovascular events in patients at risk. Indications for ARBs, which are relatively new drugs, are limited to hypertension, heart failure, and diabetic nephropathy. Eplerenone—the only selective aldosterone receptor antagonist available—is approved only for hypertension. We begin the chapter by reviewing the physiology of the RAAS, after which we discuss the drugs that affect it.

PHYSIOLOGY OF THE RENIN-ANGIOTENSIN-ALDOSTERONE SYSTEM

The RAAS plays an important role in regulating blood pressure, blood volume, and fluid and electrolyte balance. In addition, the system appears to mediate certain pathophysiologic changes associated with hypertension, heart failure, and myocardial infarction. The RAAS exerts its effects in large part through angiotensin II.

Types of Angiotensin

Before considering the physiology of the RAAS, we need to introduce the angiotensin family, which consists of angiotensin I, angiotensin II, and angiotensin III. All three compounds are small polypeptides. Angiotensin I is the precursor of angiotensin II (Fig. 42–1) and has very little biologic activity. In contrast, angiotensin II has very high biologic activity. Angiotensin III, which is formed by degradation of angiotensin II, has moderate biologic activity.

Actions of Angiotensin II

Angiotensin II mediates essentially all of the effects of the RAAS. The most prominent actions of angiotensin II are vasoconstriction and stimulation of aldosterone release. Both actions serve to raise blood pressure. In addition, angiotensin II can act on the heart and blood vessels to alter their morphology.

Vasoconstriction. Angiotensin II is a potent vasoconstrictor. The compound acts directly on vascular smooth muscle (VSM) to cause contraction. Vasoconstriction is prominent in arterioles and less so in veins. As a result of angiotensin-induced vasoconstriction, blood pressure rises. In addition to its direct action on blood vessels, angiotensin II can cause vasoconstriction indirectly by acting on (1) sympathetic neurons to promote norepinephrine release, (2) the adrenal medulla promote epinephrine release, and (3) the central nervous system to increase sympathetic outflow to blood vessels.

Release of Aldosterone. Angiotensin II acts on the adrenal cortex to promote synthesis and secretion of aldosterone. Aldosterone, in turn, acts on the kidney to cause retention of sodium and excretion of potassium and hydrogen. Because retention of sodium causes water to be retained as well, aldosterone increases plasma volume, and thereby increases blood pressure. The adrenal cortex is highly sensitive to angiotensin II; as a result, angiotensin II can stimulate aldosterone release even when angiotensin II levels are too low to induce vasoconstriction. Aldosterone secretion is enhanced when sodium levels are low and when potassium levels are high.

Alteration of Cardiac and Vascular Structure. Angiotensin II may cause pathologic structural changes in the heart and blood vessels. The compound is thought to cause both *hypertrophy* (increased mass of a structure) and *remodeling* (redistribution of mass within a structure). In hypertension, angiotensin II may be responsible for increasing the thickness of blood vessel walls; in atherosclerosis, it may be responsible for thickening the intimal surface of blood ves-

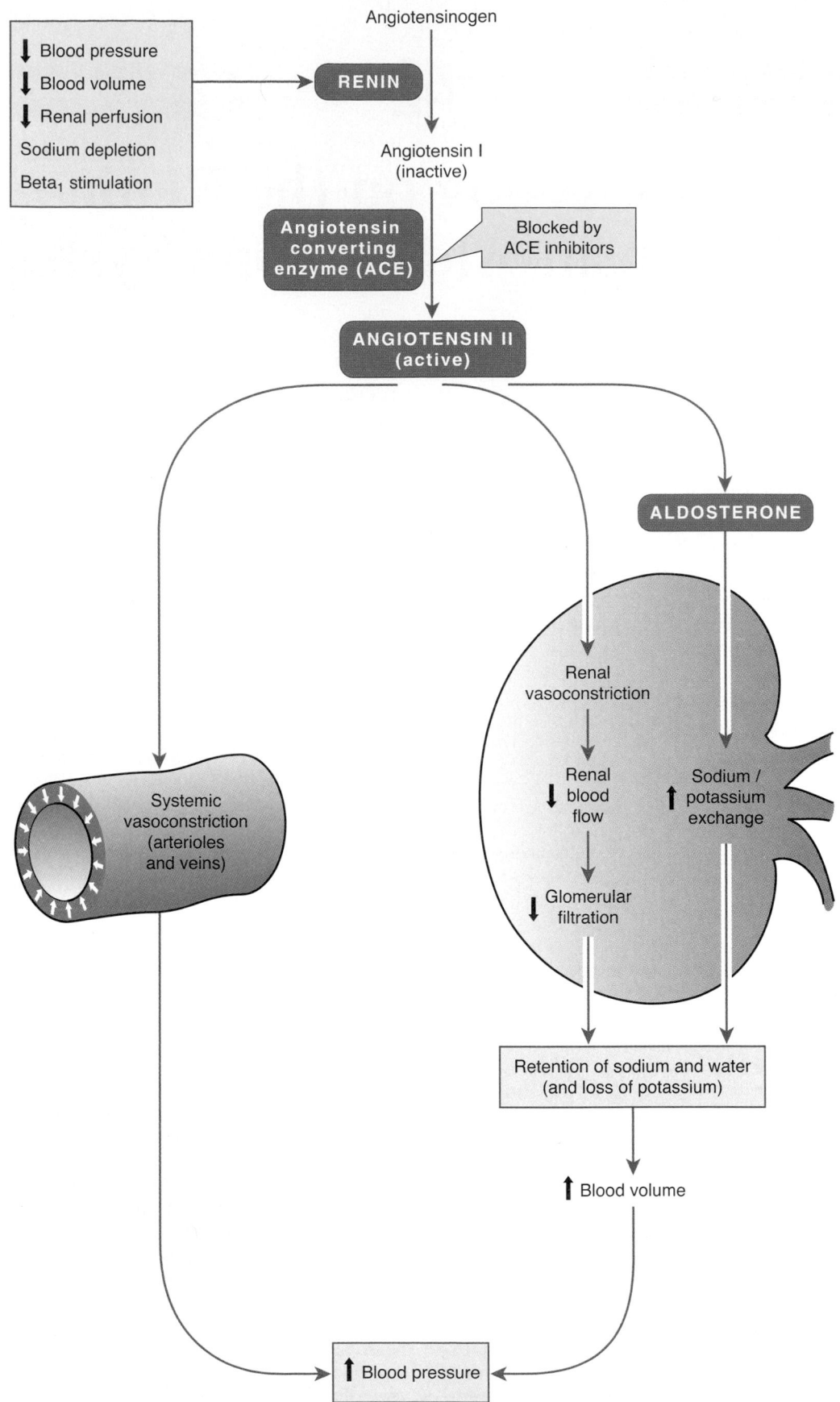

Figure 42–1 ■ **Regulation of blood pressure by the renin-angiotensin-aldosterone system.** In addition to the mechanisms depicted, angiotensin II can affect blood pressure by (1) promoting release of norepinephrine from sympathetic nerves, (2) promoting release of epinephrine from the adrenal medulla, and (3) acting in the central nervous system to increase sympathetic outflow to blood vessels. All three processes promote vasoconstriction, and hence can raise arterial pressure.

sels; and in heart failure and myocardial infarction, it may be responsible for causing cardiac hypertrophy and fibrosis. Known effects of angiotensin II that could underlie these pathologic changes include

- Increased migration, proliferation, and hypertrophy of VSM cells
- Increased production of extracellular matrix by VSM cells
- Hypertrophy of cardiac myocytes
- Increased production of extracellular matrix by cardiac fibroblasts

Formation of Angiotensin II by Renin and Angiotensin-Converting Enzyme

As indicated in Figure 42–1, angiotensin II is formed through two sequential reactions. The first is catalyzed by renin, the second by ACE.

Renin

Renin (pronounced "reenin") catalyzes the formation of *angiotensin I* from *angiotensinogen*. This reaction is the rate-limiting step in angiotensin II formation. Renin is produced by juxtaglomerular cells of the kidney and undergoes controlled release into the bloodstream, where it converts angiotensinogen into angiotensin I.

Regulation of Renin Release. Since renin catalyzes the rate-limiting step in angiotensin II formation, and since renin must be released into the blood in order to act, the factors that regulate renin release regulate the rate of angiotensin II formation.

As indicated in Figure 42–1, release of renin can be triggered by multiple factors. Release *increases* in response to a *decline* in blood pressure, blood volume, plasma sodium content, or renal perfusion pressure. Reduced renal perfusion pressure is an especially important stimulant of renin release and can occur in response to (1) stenosis of the renal arteries, (2) reduced systemic blood pressure, and (3) reduced plasma volume (brought on by dehydration, hemorrhage, or chronic sodium depletion). For the most part, these factors increase renin release through effects exerted locally in the kidney. However, some of these factors may also promote renin release through activation of the sympathetic nervous system. Sympathetic nerves increase secretion of renin by causing stimulation of beta$_1$-adrenergic receptors on juxtaglomerular cells.

Release of renin is *suppressed* by factors opposite to those that cause release. That is, renin secretion is inhibited by elevation of blood pressure, blood volume, and plasma sodium content. Hence, as blood pressure, blood volume, and plasma sodium content increase in response to renin release, further release of renin is suppressed. In this regard, we can view release of renin as being regulated by a classic negative feedback loop.

Angiotensin-Converting Enzyme (Kinase II)

ACE catalyzes the conversion of angiotensin I (inactive) into angiotensin II (highly active). ACE is located on the luminal surface of all blood vessels, the vasculature of the lungs being especially rich in the enzyme. Because ACE is abundant, conversion of angiotensin I into angiotensin II occurs almost instantaneously after angiotensin I has been

formed. ACE is a relatively nonspecific enzyme that can act on a variety of substrates in addition to angiotensin I.

Nomenclature regarding ACE can be confusing and requires comment. As just noted, ACE can act on several substrates. When the substrate is angiotensin I, we refer to the enzyme as ACE. However, when the enzyme is acting on other substrates, we refer to it by different names. Of relevance to us, when the substrate is a hormone known as *bradykinin,* we refer to the enzyme as *kinase II*. So, please remember, whether we call it ACE or kinase II, we're talking about the same enzyme.

Regulation of Blood Pressure by the Renin-Angiotensin-Aldosterone System

The RAAS is poised to help regulate blood pressure: factors that lower blood pressure turn the system on; factors that raise blood pressure turn it off. However, although the RAAS does indeed contribute to blood pressure control, its role in *normovolemic, sodium-replete* individuals is only modest. In contrast, the system can be a major factor in maintaining blood pressure in the presence of *hemorrhage, dehydration,* or *sodium depletion.*

As depicted in Figure 42–1, the RAAS, acting through angiotensin II, raises blood pressure through two basic processes: vasoconstriction and renal retention of water and sodium. Vasoconstriction raises blood pressure by increasing total peripheral resistance; retention of water and sodium raises blood pressure by increasing blood volume. Vasoconstriction occurs within minutes to hours of activating the system, and hence can raise blood pressure quickly. In contrast, days, weeks, or even months are required for the kidney to raise blood pressure by increasing blood volume.

As suggested by Figure 42–1, angiotensin II acts in two ways to promote renal retention of water. First, by constricting renal blood vessels, angiotensin II reduces renal blood flow, and thereby reduces glomerular filtration. Second, angiotensin II stimulates release of aldosterone from the adrenal cortex. Aldosterone then acts on the kidney to promote retention of sodium and water and excretion of potassium.

Tissue (Local) Angiotensin II Production

In addition to the traditional RAAS that we've been discussing, in which angiotensin II is produced in the blood and then carried to target tissues, angiotensin II can be produced in individual tissues. This permits discrete, local effects of angiotensin II independent of the main system. Interference with local production of angiotensin II may underlie some effects of the ACE inhibitors.

It is important to note that some angiotensin II is produced by pathways that do *not* involve ACE. As a result, drugs that inhibit ACE cannot completely block angiotensin II production.

ANGIOTENSIN-CONVERTING ENZYME INHIBITORS

The ACE inhibitors are important drugs for treating hypertension, heart failure, diabetic nephropathy, and myocardial infarction (MI). In addition, they are used to prevent adverse cardiovascular events in patients at risk. Their most prominent adverse effects are cough, first-dose hypotension, and hyperkalemia. For all of these agents, beneficial effects result largely from suppressing formation of angiotensin II. Because the similarities among ACE inhibitors are much more striking than their differences, we will discuss these drugs as a group, rather than selecting a prototype to represent them.

Mechanism of Action and Overview of Pharmacologic Effects

Beneficial effects derive from (1) reducing levels of angiotensin II (through inhibition of ACE) and (2) increasing levels of bradykinin (through inhibition of kinase II). By reducing levels of angiotensin II, ACE inhibitors can dilate blood vessels (primarily arterioles and to a lesser extent veins), reduce blood volume (through effects on the kidney), and, importantly, prevent or reverse angiotensin II–mediated pathologic changes in the heart and blood vessels. Elevation of bradykinin levels promotes vasodilation. (Bradykinin promotes vasodilation by stimulating production of prostaglandins and nitric oxide.)

Like beneficial effects, certain adverse effects result from inhibiting ACE/kinase II. Inhibition of ACE can cause hypotension, hyperkalemia, renal failure, and fetal injury. Inhibition of kinase II, with resultant accumulation of bradykinin, can cause cough and angioedema.

Pharmacokinetics

Regarding pharmacokinetics, the following generalizations apply:

- Nearly all ACE inhibitors are administered *orally*. The only exception is enalaprilat (the active form of enalapril), which is given IV.
- Except for captopril and moexipril, all oral ACE inhibitors can be administered with food.
- With the exception of captopril, all ACE inhibitors have prolonged half-lives, and hence can be administered just once or twice a day. Captopril is administered 2 or 3 times a day.
- With the exception of lisinopril, all ACE inhibitors are *prodrugs* that must undergo conversion to their active form in the small intestine and liver. Lisinopril is active as given.
- All ACE inhibitors are *excreted by the kidneys*. As a result, nearly all can accumulate to dangerous levels in patients with kidney disease, and hence *dosages must be reduced in these patients*. Only one agent—fosinopril—does not require a dosage reduction.

Therapeutic Uses

When the ACE inhibitors were introduced (over 20 years ago), their only indication was hypertension. Since then, we have learned that their benefits go far beyond reducing blood pressure: In addition to treating patients with hypertension, these drugs are now used for patients with heart failure, acute MI, left ventricular dysfunction, and diabetic and nondiabetic nephropathy; most recently, they have been used to prevent MI, stroke, and death in patients at high risk for cardiovascular events. It should be noted that no single ACE inhibitor is approved for all of these conditions (Table 42–1). However, given that all ACE inhibitors are very similar, it seems likely that all can produce similar therapeutic effects.

Hypertension. All ACE inhibitors are approved for treating hypertension. These drugs are especially effective against malignant hypertension and hypertension secondary to renal arterial stenosis. They are also useful against essential hypertension of mild to moderate intensity; in this disorder, maximal benefits may take several weeks to develop.

In patients with essential hypertension, the mechanism underlying blood pressure reduction is not fully understood. *Initial* responses are proportional to circulating angiotensin II levels and are clearly related to reduced formation of that compound. (By lowering angiotensin II levels, ACE inhibitors dilate blood vessels and reduce blood volume; both actions help lower blood pressure.) However, with *prolonged* therapy, blood pressure often undergoes additional decline. During this second phase, there is no correspondence between reductions in blood pressure and reductions in *circulating* angiotensin II. It may be that the delayed response is due to reductions in *local* angiotensin II levels—reductions that would not be revealed by measuring angiotensin II in the blood.

ACE inhibitors offer several advantages over most other antihypertensive drugs. In contrast to the sympatholytic agents, ACE inhibitors do not interfere with cardiovascular reflexes. Hence, exercise capacity is not impaired and orthostatic hypotension is minimal. In addition, these drugs can be used safely in patients with bronchial asthma, a condition that precludes the use of beta$_2$-adrenergic antagonists. ACE inhibitors do not promote hypokalemia, hyperuricemia, or hyperglycemia—side effects seen with thiazide diuretics. Furthermore, these drugs do not induce lethargy, weakness, or sexual dysfunction—responses that are common with other antihypertensive agents. Most importantly, *ACE inhibitors reduce the risk of cardiovascular mortality caused by hypertension*. The only other drugs proved to reduce hypertension-associated mortality are beta-adrenergic blockers and diuretics (see Chapter 45).

Heart Failure. ACE inhibitors produce multiple benefits in heart failure. By lowering arteriolar tone, these drugs improve regional blood flow, and, by reducing cardiac afterload, they increase cardiac output. By causing venous dilation, they reduce pulmonary congestion and peripheral edema. By dilating blood vessels in the kidney, they increase renal blood flow, and thereby promote excretion of sodium and water. This loss of fluid has two beneficial effects: (1) it helps reduce edema and (2) by lowering blood volume, it decreases venous return to the heart, thereby reducing right-heart size. Lastly, by reducing local production of angiotensin II in the heart, ACE inhibitors may suppress growth of myocytes, and may thereby prevent pathologic thickening of the ventricular wall. Although only six ACE inhibitors are approved for heart failure (see Table 42–1), both the American Heart Association and the American College of Cardiology have concluded that the ability to improve symptoms and prolong survival is a class effect. The use of ACE inhibitors in heart failure is discussed further in Chapter 46.

Myocardial Infarction. ACE inhibitors can reduce mortality following acute MI (heart attack). In addition, they decrease the chance of developing overt heart failure. Treatment should begin as soon as possible after infarction and should continue for at least 6 weeks. In patients who develop overt heart failure, treatment should continue long term. As for patients who do not develop heart failure, there are no data to indicate whether continued treatment would be beneficial or

TABLE 42–1 ▪▪ ACE Inhibitors: Indications and Dosages

Generic Name	Trade Name	Approved Indications*	Starting Dosage†	Usual Maintenance Dosage†
Benazepril	Lotensin	Hypertension	10 mg once/day	20–40 mg/day in 1 or 2 doses
Captopril	Capoten	Hypertension Heart failure LVD after MI Diabetic nephropathy	25 mg bid or tid 25 mg tid 12.5 mg tid 25 mg tid	25–50 mg bid or tid 50–100 mg tid 50 mg tid 25 mg tid
Enalapril	Vasotec	Hypertension Heart failure Asymptomatic LVD	5 mg once/day 2.5 mg bid 2.5 mg bid	10–40 mg/day in 1 or 2 doses 10–20 mg bid 10 mg bid
Enalaprilat	Vasotec I.V.	Hypertension	1.25 mg every 6 hours	
Fosinopril	Monopril	Hypertension Heart failure	10 mg once/day 10 mg once/day	20–40 mg/day in 1 or 2 doses 20–40 mg once/day
Lisinopril	Prinivil, Zestril	Hypertension Heart failure Acute MI	10 mg once/day 5 mg once/day 5 mg once/day	20–40 mg once/day 20–40 mg once/day 10 mg once/day
Moexipril	Univasc	Hypertension	7.5 mg once/day	7.5–30 mg/day in 1 or 2 doses
Perindopril	Aceon	Hypertension	4 mg once/day	4–8 mg/day in 1 or 2 doses
Quinapril	Accupril	Hypertension Heart failure	10–20 mg/day 5 mg bid	20–80 mg/day in 1 or 2 doses 20–40 mg bid
Ramipril	Altace	Hypertension Heart failure Prevention of MI, stroke, and death in people at high risk for CVD	2.5 mg once/day 2.5 mg bid 2.5 mg/day for 1 week	2.5–20 mg/day in 1 or 2 doses 5 mg bid 5 mg once/day for 3 weeks
Trandolapril	Mavik	Hypertension Heart failure after MI LVD after MI	1 mg once/day 1 mg once/day 1 mg once/day	2–4 mg once/day 4 mg once/day 4 mg once/day

*CVD = cardiovascular disease; LVD = left ventricular dysfunction; MI = myocardial infarction.
†For all ACE inhibitors except fosinopril, dosage must be reduced in patients with significant renal impairment.

not. At this time, only three ACE inhibitors—captopril, lisinopril, and trandolapril—are approved for patients with MI.

Diabetic and Nondiabetic Nephropathy. ACE inhibitors can benefit patients with diabetic nephropathy, the leading cause of end-stage renal disease in the United States. In patients with overt nephropathy, as indicated by proteinuria of more than 500 mg/day, these drugs can slow progression of renal disease. In patients with less advanced nephropathy (30 to 300 mg proteinuria/day), these drugs can delay onset of overt nephropathy. These benefits were first demonstrated in patients with type 1 diabetes (insulin-dependent diabetes mellitus) and were later demonstrated in patients with type 2 diabetes (non–insulin-dependent diabetes mellitus). More recently, ACE inhibitors have been shown to provide similar protection in patients with nephropathy unrelated to diabetes.

The principal protective mechanism appears to be reduction of glomerular filtration pressure. ACE inhibitors lower filtration pressure by reducing levels of angiotensin II, a compound that can raise filtration pressure by two mechanisms. First, angiotensin II raises systemic blood pressure, which raises pressure in the afferent arteriole of the glomerulus (Fig. 42–2). Second, it constricts the efferent arteriole, thereby generating backpressure in the glomerulus. The resultant increase in filtration pressure promotes injury. By reducing levels of angiotensin II, ACE inhibitors lower glomerular filtration pressure, and thereby slow development of renal injury.

At this time, the only ACE inhibitor actually approved for nephropathy is captopril. However, the American Diabetes Association considers benefits in diabetic nephropathy to be a class effect, and hence recommends choosing an ACE inhibitor based on its cost and likelihood of patient compliance.

Prevention of MI, Stroke, and Death in Patients at High Cardiovascular Risk. One ACE inhibitor—*ramipril* [Altace]—is approved for reducing the risk of MI, stroke, and death (from cardiovascular causes) in patients at high risk for a major cardiovascular event—high risk being defined by (1) a history of stroke, coronary artery disease, peripheral vascular disease, or diabetes, combined with (2) at least one other risk factor, such as hypertension, high LDL cholesterol, low HDL cholesterol, or cigarette smoking. Ramipril was approved for this use based on results of the Heart Outcomes Prevention Evaluation (HOPE) trial, a large study in which patients at high cardiovascular risk took either ramipril (10 mg/day) or placebo. Follow-up time was 5 years. The result? The combined endpoint of MI, stroke, or death from cardiovascular causes was significantly lower in the ramipril group (14% vs. 18%)—a 22% reduction in risk. Possible mechanisms underlying benefits include reduced vascular resistance and protection of the heart, blood vessels, and kidneys from the damage that angiotensin II and aldosterone can cause over time. Do other ACE inhibitors also reduce cardiovascular risk? Possibly. However, at this time there is insufficient evidence to say for sure.

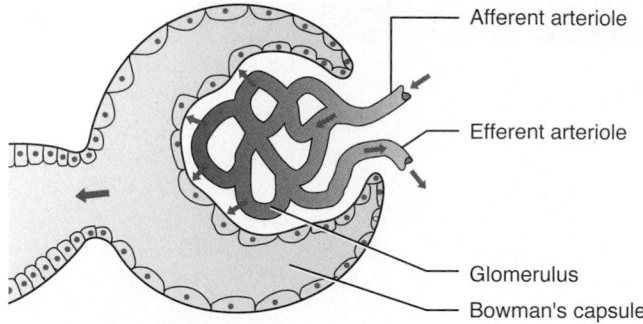

Afferent arteriole

Efferent arteriole

Glomerulus

Bowman's capsule

Figure 42–2 ▪ Elevation of glomerular filtration pressure by angiotensin II.
Angiotensin II increases filtration pressure by (1) increasing pressure in the afferent arteriole (secondary to increasing systemic arterial pressure), and by (2) constricting the efferent arteriole, thereby generating backpressure in the glomerulus.

Adverse Effects

ACE inhibitors are generally well tolerated. Some adverse effects (e.g., first-dose hypotension, hyperkalemia) are due to reduction in angiotensin II, whereas others (cough, angioedema) are due to elevation of bradykinin.

First-Dose Hypotension. A precipitous drop in blood pressure may occur following the first dose of an ACE inhibitor. This reaction is caused by widespread vasodilation secondary to abrupt lowering of angiotensin II levels. First-dose hypotension is most likely in patients with severe hypertension, in patients taking diuretics, and in patients who are sodium depleted or volume depleted. To minimize the first-dose effect, initial doses should be low. Also, diuretics should be temporarily discontinued, starting 2 to 3 days before initiating therapy with an ACE inhibitor. Blood pressure should be monitored for several hours following the first captopril dose. If hypotension develops, the patient should assume a supine position. If necessary, blood pressure can be raised with an infusion of normal saline.

Cough. Persistent, dry, irritating, nonproductive cough can develop with all ACE inhibitors. This reaction occurs in 5% of patients and is the most common reason for discontinuing therapy. Cough is more troublesome when the patient is supine, and occurs more in women than in men. Cough begins to subside 3 days after discontinuing ACE inhibitors and is gone within 10 days. Cough is caused by accumulation of bradykinin secondary to inhibition of kinase II (another name for ACE).

Hyperkalemia. Inhibition of aldosterone release (secondary to inhibition of angiotensin II production) can cause potassium retention by the kidney. As a rule, significant potassium accumulation is limited to patients taking potassium supplements or a potassium-sparing diuretic. For most other patients, hyperkalemia is rare. Patients should be instructed to avoid potassium supplements and potassium-containing salt substitutes unless they are prescribed by the physician.

Renal Failure. ACE inhibitors can cause severe renal insufficiency in patients with *bilateral renal artery stenosis or stenosis in the artery to a single remaining kidney*. In patients with renal artery stenosis, the kidneys release large amounts of renin. The resulting high levels of angiotensin II serve to maintain glomerular filtration by two mechanisms: elevation of blood pressure and constriction of efferent glomerular arterioles (see Fig. 42–2). When ACE is inhibited, causing angiotensin II levels to fall, the mechanisms that had been supporting glomerular filtration fail, causing urine production to drop precipitously. Not surprisingly, *ACE inhibitors are contraindicated for patients with bilateral renal artery stenosis (or stenosis in the artery to a single remaining kidney).*

Fetal Injury. Use of ACE inhibitors during the *second* and *third* trimesters of pregnancy can injure the developing fetus. Specific effects include hypotension, hyperkalemia, skull hypoplasia, anuria, renal failure (reversible and irreversible), and death. Women who become pregnant while using ACE inhibitors should discontinue treatment as soon as possible. Infants who have been exposed to ACE inhibitors during the second or third trimester should be closely monitored for hypotension, oliguria, and hyperkalemia. Exposure to ACE inhibitors during the first trimester is not associated with fetal injury; pregnant women who have taken ACE inhibitors during the first trimester should be told this.

Angioedema. Angioedema is a rare and potentially fatal reaction. Symptoms, which result from increased capillary permeability, include giant wheals and edema of the tongue, glottis, and pharynx. Severe reactions should be treated with subcutaneous epinephrine. If angioedema develops, ACE inhibitors should be discontinued and never used again. Angioedema is caused by accumulation of bradykinin (owing to inhibition of kinase II).

Dysgeusia and Rash. Dysgeusia (impaired or distorted sense of taste) and rash are relatively common with captopril, but can occur with other ACE inhibitors as well. For some patients, dysgeusia may result in anorexia and weight loss. If these complications arise, the ACE inhibitor should be withdrawn. Both reactions resolve following cessation of treatment. At one time, researchers believed rash and dysgeusia were related to the sulfhydryl group found in the structure of captopril and some other ACE inhibitors have. However, this appears to be untrue—because ACE inhibitors that lack a sulfhydryl group also cause these reactions.

Neutropenia. Neutropenia, with its associated risk of infection, is a rare but serious complication. Neutropenia is most likely in patients with renal impairment and in those with collagen vascular diseases (e.g., systemic lupus erythematosus, scleroderma). These patients should be followed closely. Fortunately, neutropenia is reversible when detected early. To promote early detection, a white blood cell count with differential should be obtained every 2 weeks during the first 3 months of therapy and periodically thereafter. If neutropenia develops, ACE inhibitors should be withdrawn immediately; neutrophil counts should normalize in approximately 2 weeks. In the absence of early detection, neutropenia may progress to fatal agranulocytosis. Patients should be informed about early signs of infection (e.g., fever, sore throat) and instructed to report them immediately. As with dysgeusia and rash, neutropenia is more common with captopril than with other ACE inhibitors.

Drug Interactions

Diuretics. Diuretics may intensify first-dose hypotension. To prevent this interaction, diuretics should be withdrawn 1 week prior to initiating ACE inhibitor treatment. Diuretic therapy can be resumed later if needed.

Antihypertensive Agents. The hypotensive effects of ACE inhibitors are often additive with those of other antihypertensive drugs (e.g., diuretics, sympatholytics, vasodilators, calcium channel blockers). When an ACE inhibitor is added to an antihypertensive regimen, dosages of other drugs may require reduction.

Drugs That Raise Potassium Levels. ACE inhibitors increase the risk of hyperkalemia caused by *potassium supplements* and *potassium-sparing diuretics*. The risk of hyperkalemia is increased because, by suppressing aldosterone secretion, ACE inhibitors can reduce excretion of potassium. To minimize the risk of hyperkalemia, potassium supplements and potassium-sparing diuretics should be employed only when clearly indicated.

Lithium. ACE inhibitors can make lithium accumulate to toxic levels. Lithium levels should be monitored frequently.

Preparations, Dosage, and Administration

Except for enalaprilat, all ACE inhibitors are administered PO. Of the oral products, all are available in single-drug formulations, and most are also available in fixed-dose combinations with hydrochlorothiazide, a thiazide diuretic. Except for captopril and moexipril, all oral formulations may be administered without regard to meals; captopril and moexipril should be administered 1 hour before meals. Dosages for all ACE inhibitors (except fosinopril) should be reduced in patients with renal impairment. Dosages for specific indications are summarized in Table 42–1. Formulations are described below.

- Benazepril is available alone (in 5-, 10-, 20-, and 40-mg tablets) as *Lotensin,* and combined with hydrochlorothiazide as *Lotensin HCT.*
- Captopril is available alone (in 12.5-, 25-, 50-, and 100-mg tablets) as *Capoten,* and combined with hydrochlorothiazide as *Capozide.*
- Enalapril is available alone (in 2.5-, 5-, 10-, and 20-mg tablets) as *Vasotec,* and combined with hydrochlorothiazide as *Vaseretic.*
- Enalaprilat [Vasotec I.V.], the active form of enalapril, is available in solution (1.25 mg/ml) for IV therapy of severe hypertension. Enalaprilat is the only ACE inhibitor that is not given PO.
- Fosinopril is available alone (in 10-, 20-, and 40-mg tablets) as *Monopril,* and combined with hydrochlorothiazide as *Monopril HCT.*
- Lisinopril is available alone (in 2.5-, 5-, 10-, 20-, and 40-mg tablets) as *Prinivil* and *Zestril,* and combined with hydrochlorothiazide as *Prinzide.*
- Moexipril is available alone (in 7.5- and 15-mg tablets) as *Univasc,* and combined with hydrochlorothiazide as *Uniretic.*
- Perindopril is available in tablets (2, 4, and 8 mg) as *Aceon.* The drug is not available in combination with hydrochlorothiazide.
- Quinapril is available alone (in 5-, 10-, 20-, and 40-mg tablets) as *Accupril,* and combined with hydrochlorothiazide as *Accuretic.*
- Ramipril is available in capsules (1.25, 2.5, 5, and 10 mg) as *Altace.* The drug is not available in combination with hydrochlorothiazide.
- Trandolapril is available in tablets (1, 2, and 4 mg) as *Mavik.* The drug is not available in combination with hydrochlorothiazide.

ANGIOTENSIN II RECEPTOR BLOCKERS

The angiotensin II receptor blockers (ARBs) are a relatively new family of drugs whose indications are continuing to evolve. Initially, ARBs were used only for patients with hypertension. Today, they are approved for patients with heart failure and diabetic nephropathy as well.

Like the ACE inhibitors, ARBs decrease the influence of angiotensin II. However, they do so by different mechanisms: Whereas ACE inhibitors block *production* of angiotensin II, ARBs block angiotensin II *actions*. Because both groups interfere with angiotensin II, they both have similar effects. The principal difference between them is that ARBs do not cause cough or hyperkalemia.

Seven ARBs are now available. All are very similar, and hence we will discuss them as a group, rather than choosing a prototype to represent them.

Mechanism of Action and Overview of Pharmacologic Effects

ARBs block access of angiotensin II to its receptors in blood vessels, the adrenals, and all other tissues. As a result, ARBs have effects much like those of the ACE inhibitors. By blocking angiotensin II receptors on blood vessels, ARBs cause dilation of arterioles and veins. By blocking angiotensin II receptors in the heart, ARBs can prevent angiotensin II from inducing pathologic changes in cardiac structure. By blocking angiotensin II receptors in the adrenals, ARBs decrease release of aldosterone, and can thereby increase renal excretion of sodium and water. Sodium and water excretion is further increased through dilation of renal blood vessels.

In contrast to the ACE inhibitors, ARBs do *not* increase levels of bradykinin (because ARBs do not inhibit kinase II). As a result, ARBs do not promote cough, the most common reason for discontinuing ACE inhibitors.

It should be noted that ARBs are even better at preventing the effects of angiotensin II than are the ACE inhibitors. Why? Recall that angiotensin II can be produced by pathways that do not involve ACE, and hence ACE inhibitors cannot completely block angiotensin II production and actions. In contrast, because ARBs block angiotensin II at its receptors, ARBs can completely eliminate the influence of this compound.

Therapeutic Uses

Hypertension. All ARBs are approved for hypertension. Reductions in blood pressure equal those seen with ACE inhibitors. Whether ARBs share the ability of ACE inhibitors to reduce mortality has not been established.

Heart Failure. At this time, only one ARB—*valsartan*—is approved for use in heart failure. In clinical trials, the drug reduced symptoms, decreased hospitalizations, improved functional capacity, and increased left-ventricular ejection fraction. More importantly, it prolonged survival. Because experience with valsartan is limited, the drug should be reserved for patients who cannot tolerate ACE inhibitors (because of cough). Although other ARBs are not yet approved for heart failure, most authorities believe they are effective.

Diabetic Nephropathy. Two ARBs—*irbesartan* and *losartan*—are approved for managing nephropathy in hypertensive patients with type 2 diabetes. In clinical trials, these drugs delayed development of overt nephropathy, and slowed progression of established renal disease. Benefits are due in part to reductions in blood pressure, and in part to mechanisms that have not been determined. To date, ARBs have not been compared directly with ACE inhibitors, so we can't say which is superior. Nonetheless, ARBs do represent an attractive alternative for who can't tolerate ACE inhibitors because of cough.

Adverse Effects

All of the ARBs are well tolerated. In contrast to ACE inhibitors, ARBs do not cause clinically significant hyperkalemia. Furthermore, because ARBs do not promote accumulation of bradykinin, they do not cause cough.

Angioedema. Like the ACE inhibitors, ARBs can cause angioedema—even though ARBs do not increase bradykinin levels. (Recall that elevation of bradykinin underlies angioedema caused by ACE inhibitors.) The mechanism underlying ARB-induced angioedema is unknown. If angioedema occurs,

ARBs should be withdrawn immediately and never used again. Severe reactions are treated with subcutaneous epinephrine.

Fetal Harm. Like the ACE inhibitors, ARBs can injure the developing fetus if taken during the second or third trimester of pregnancy. Accordingly, ARBs are contraindicated for use during that period.

Renal Failure. Like the ACE inhibitors, ARBs can cause renal failure in patients with bilateral renal artery stenosis or stenosis in the artery to a single remaining kidney. Accordingly, ARBs are contraindicated for patients with these conditions.

Drug Interactions

The hypotensive effects of ARBs are additive with those of other antihypertensive drugs. When an ARB is added to an antihypertensive regimen, dosages of the other drugs may require reduction.

Preparations, Dosage, and Administration

All ARBs are administered PO, and all may be taken with or without food. In addition, all are available in single-drug formulations, and, with one exception (olmesartan), all are also available in fixed-dose combinations with hydrochlorothiazide, a thiazide diuretic. Dosages for specific indications are summarized in Table 42–2. Formulations are described below.

- Candesartan is available alone (in 4-, 8-, 16-, and 32-mg tablets) as *Benicar*, and combined with hydrochlorothiazide as *Atacand HCT*.
- Eprosartan is available alone (in 400- and 600-mg tablets) as *Teveten*, and combined with hydrochlorothiazide as *Teveten HCT*.
- Irbesartan is available alone (in 75-, 150-, and 300-mg tablets) as *Avapro*, and combined with hydrochlorothiazide as *Avalide*.
- Losartan is available alone (in 25- and 50-mg tablets) as *Cozaar*, and combined with hydrochlorothiazide as *Hyzaar*.
- Olmesartan is available in tablets (5, 20, and 40 mg) as *Benicar*. The drug is not available combined with hydrochlorothiazide.
- Telmisartan is available alone (in 20-, 40-, and 80-mg tablets) as *Micardis*, and combined with hydrochlorothiazide as *Micardis HCT*.
- Valsartan is available alone (in 40-, 80-, 160-, and 320-mg tablets) as *Diovan*, and combined with hydrochlorothiazide as *Diovan HCT*.

SELECTIVE ALDOSTERONE RECEPTOR BLOCKER: EPLERENONE

Eplerenone [Inspra], approved in September 2002, is the first representative of a new class of drugs: selective aldosterone receptor blockers. A much older drug—spironolactone [Aldactone]—also blocks aldosterone receptors, but is less selective than eplerenone. Both agents have similar structures and actions. However, because eplerenone is more selective than aldosterone, it may cause fewer side effects. Spironolactone is discussed at length in Chapters 39 (Diuretics) and 46 (Drugs for Heart Failure).

Therapeutic Use

Eplerenone is approved only for *hypertension*. The drug may be used alone or in combination with other antihypertensive agents. In clinical trials, reductions in blood pressure were equivalent to those produced by spironolactone, and superior to those produced by losartan (an ARB). In patients already using an ACE inhibitor or an ARB, adding eplerenone to the regimen produced a further reduction in blood pressure. Although it is clear that eplerenone can reduce blood pressure, we have no information on what really matters: the drug's ability to reduce morbidity and mortality. Until more is known, eplerenone should be reserved for patients who have not responded to traditional antihypertensive drugs.

As discussed in Chapter 46, spironolactone can improve symptoms, reduce hospitalizations, and prolong life in patients with heart failure. At this time, we do not know if eplerenone shares these abilities. A trial examining the possibility is ongoing.

Mechanism of Action

Eplerenone produces selective blockade of aldosterone receptors, having little or no effect on receptors for other steroid hormones (e.g., glucocorticoids, progesterone, androgens). In the kidney, *activation* of aldosterone receptors promotes excretion of potassium and retention of sodium and water. Receptor *blockade* has the opposite effect: *retention of potassium and increased excretion of sodium and water.* Loss of sodium and water reduces blood pressure. The ability of eplerenone to block aldosterone receptors at nonrenal sites (e.g., heart, blood vessels) may also contribute to beneficial effects. Maximal reductions in blood pressure take about 4 weeks to develop.

Pharmacokinetics

Eplerenone is administered orally. Absorption is not affected by food. Plasma levels peak about 1.5 hours after ingestion. Absolute bioavailability is unknown. Eplerenone

TABLE 42–2 ■ Angiotensin II Receptor Blockers: Indications and Dosages				
Generic Name	**Trade Name**	**Approved Indications**	**Initial Dosage**	**Dosage Range**
Candesartan	Atacand	Hypertension	16 mg once/day	8–32 mg/day in 1 or 2 doses
Eprosartan	Teveten	Hypertension	600 mg once/day	400–800 mg/day in 1 or 2 doses
Irbesartan	Avapro	Hypertension Diabetic nephropathy*	150 mg once/day 300 mg once/day	150–300 once/day 300 mg once/day
Losartan	Cozaar	Hypertension Diabetic nephropathy*	25–50 mg once/day 50 mg once/day	25–100 mg/day in 1 or 2 doses 50–100 mg once/day
Olmesartan	Benicar	Hypertension	20 mg once/day	20–40 mg once/day
Telmisartan	Micardis	Hypertension	40 mg once/day	20–80 mg once/day
Valsartan	Diovan	Hypertension Heart failure	80–160 mg once/day 40 mg twice/day	80–320 mg once/day 80–160 mg twice/day

*In patients with type 2 diabetes.

undergoes metabolism by CYP3A4 (the 3A4 isozyme of cytochrome P450), followed by excretion in the urine (67%) and feces (32%). The elimination half-life is 4 to 6 hours.

Adverse Effects

Eplerenone is well tolerated. The incidence of adverse effects is nearly identical to that seen with placebo. A few adverse effects—diarrhea, abdominal pain, cough, fatigue, gynecomastia, flu-like syndrome—occurred slightly (1% to 2%) more often with eplerenone than with placebo.

Hyperkalemia. The greatest risk with eplerenone is hyperkalemia, which can occur secondary to potassium retention. Because of this risk, combined use with potassium supplements or potassium-sparing diuretics (e.g., spironolactone, triamterene) is contraindicated. Combined use with ACE inhibitors or ARBs is permissible, but should be done with caution. Eplerenone is contraindicated for patients with high serum potassium (>5.5 mEq/L), and for patients with either impaired renal function or type 2 diabetes with microalbuminuria, both of which can promote hyperkalemia. Monitoring of potassium levels is recommended for patients at risk (e.g., those taking ACE inhibitors or ARBs).

Drug Interactions

Inhibitors of CYP3A4 can increase levels of eplerenone, thereby posing a risk of toxicity. Weak inhibitors (e.g., erythromycin, saquinavir, verapamil, fluconazole) can double eplerenone levels. Strong inhibitors (e.g., ketoconazole, itraconazole) can increase levels fivefold. If eplerenone is combined with a weak inhibitor, eplerenone dosage should be reduced. *Eplerenone should not be combined with strong inhibitors.*

Drugs that raise potassium levels can increase the risk of hyperkalemia. Eplerenone should not be combined with potassium supplements or potassium-sparing diuretics. Combining the drug with ACE inhibitors or ARBs should be done with caution.

Drugs similar to eplerenone (e.g., ACE inhibitors and diuretics) are known to increase levels of *lithium.* Although the combination of eplerenone and lithium has not been studied, caution is nonetheless advised. Lithium levels should be measured frequently.

Preparations, Dosage, and Administration

Eplerenone [Inspra] is available in 25-, 50-, and 100-mg tablets. The usual starting dosage is 50 mg PO once a day, taken with or without food. After 4 weeks, dosage can be increased to 50 mg twice daily (if the hypotensive response has been inadequate). Raising the dosage above 100 mg/day is not recommended. Why? Because doing so is unlikely to increase the therapeutic response—but *will* increase the risk of hyperkalemia. In patients taking weak inhibitors of CYP3A4, the initial dosage should be reduced by 50% (to 25 mg once a day).

⠏ KEY POINTS

- The RAAS helps regulate blood pressure, blood volume, and fluid and electrolyte balance.
- The RAAS acts through production of angiotensin II and aldosterone.
- Angiotensin II has much greater biologic activity than angiotensin I or angiotensin III.
- Angiotensin II is formed by the actions of two enzymes: renin and ACE.
- Angiotensin II causes vasoconstriction (primarily in arterioles) and release of aldosterone. In addition, angiotensin II can promote pathologic changes in the heart and blood vessels.
- The RAAS raises blood pressure by causing vasoconstriction and increasing blood volume (secondary to renal retention of sodium and water).
- In addition to the traditional RAAS, in which angiotensin II is produced in the blood and then carried to target tissues, angiotensin II can be produced locally by individual tissues.
- Beneficial effects of ACE inhibitors result largely from inhibition of ACE and partly from inhibition of kinase II (the name for ACE when the substrate is bradykinin).
- By inhibiting ACE, ACE inhibitors decrease production of angiotensin II. The result is vasodilation, decreased blood volume, and prevention or reversal of angiotensin II–mediated pathologic changes in the heart and blood vessels.
- ACE inhibitors are used to treat patients with hypertension, heart failure, myocardial infarction (MI), and nephropathy, both diabetic and nondiabetic. In addition, they are used to prevent MI, stroke, and death (from cardiovascular causes) in patients at high risk for a cardiovascular event.
- ACE inhibitors can produce serious first-dose hypotension by causing a sharp drop in circulating angiotensin II.
- Cough, secondary to accumulation of bradykinin, is the most common reason for discontinuing ACE inhibitors.
- By suppressing aldosterone release, ACE inhibitors can cause hyperkalemia. Exercise caution in patients taking potassium supplements or potassium-sparing diuretics.
- ACE inhibitors are dangerous to the fetus during the second and third trimesters, but not during the first trimester.
- ACE inhibitors can cause a precipitous drop in blood pressure in patients with bilateral renal artery stenosis (or stenosis in the artery to a single remaining kidney).
- Angiotensin II receptor blockers (ARBs) block the actions of angiotensin II in blood vessels, the adrenals, and all other tissues.
- ARBs are similar to ACE inhibitors in that they cause vasodilation, suppress aldosterone release, promote excretion of sodium and water, reduce blood pressure, and cause birth defects and angioedema.
- ARBs differ from ACE inhibitors in that they do not cause hyperkalemia or cough.

Summary of Major Nursing Implications*

ANGIOTENSIN-CONVERTING ENZYME INHIBITORS

Benazepril
Captopril
Enalapril
Enalaprilat
Fosinopril
Lisinopril
Moexipril
Perindopril
Quinapril
Ramipril
Trandolapril

Unless indicated otherwise, the implications summarized below pertain to all of the ACE inhibitors.

Preadministration Assessment

Therapeutic Goal

Reduction of blood pressure in patients with hypertension (*all ACE inhibitors*).

Hemodynamic improvement in patients with heart failure (*captopril, enalapril, fosinopril, lisinopril, moexipril, quinapril*).

Slowed progression of diabetic nephropathy (*captopril*).
Reduction of mortality following acute MI (*lisinopril*).
Treatment of heart failure after MI (*ramipril, trandolapril*).
Reduction of risk of MI, stroke, or death from cardiovascular causes in patients at high risk (*ramipril*).

Baseline Data

Determine blood pressure and obtain a white blood cell count and differential.

Identifying High-Risk Patients

ACE inhibitors are *contraindicated* during the second and third trimesters of pregnancy and for patients with (1) bilateral renal artery stenosis (or stenosis in the artery to a single remaining kidney) or (2) a history of hypersensitivity reactions (especially angioedema) to ACE inhibitors.

Exercise *caution* in patients with salt or volume depletion, renal impairment, or collagen disease, and in those taking potassium supplements, potassium-sparing diuretics, or lithium.

Implementation: Administration

Routes

Oral. All ACE inhibitors (except enalaprilat).
Intravenous. Enalaprilat.

Dosage and Administration

Begin therapy with low doses and then gradually increase the dosage.

Instruct patients to administer captopril and moexipril at least 1 hour before meals. All other oral ACE inhibitors can be administered with food.

Ongoing Evaluation and Interventions

Monitoring Summary

Monitor blood pressure closely for 2 hours after the first dose and periodically thereafter. Obtain a white blood cell count and differential every 2 weeks for the first 3 months of therapy and periodically thereafter.

Evaluating Therapeutic Effects

Hypertension. Monitor for reduced blood pressure. The usual target pressure is systolic/diastolic of 140/90 mm Hg.
Heart Failure. Monitor for lessening of signs and symptoms (e.g., dyspnea, cyanosis, jugular vein distention, edema).
Diabetic Nephropathy. Monitor for proteinuria.

Minimizing Adverse Effects

First-Dose Hypotension. Severe hypotension can occur with the first dose. Minimize hypotension by (1) withdrawing diuretics 1 week before initiating ACE inhibitors and (2) using low initial doses. Monitor blood pressure for 2 hours following the first dose. Instruct patients to lie down if hypotension develops. If necessary, infuse normal saline to restore pressure.

Cough. Warn patients about the possibility of persistent, dry, irritating, nonproductive cough. Instruct them to consult the physician if cough is bothersome. It may be necessary to discontinue the ACE inhibitor.

Hyperkalemia. ACE inhibitors may increase potassium levels. Instruct patients to avoid potassium supplements and potassium-containing salt substitutes unless they are prescribed by the physician. Potassium-sparing diuretics must also be avoided.

Fetal Injury. Warn women of child-bearing age that ACE inhibitors taken during the *second* and *third* trimesters of pregnancy can cause fetal injury (hypotension, hyperkalemia, skull hypoplasia, anuria, reversible and irreversible renal failure, death). If the patient becomes pregnant, withdraw ACE inhibitors as soon as possible. Closely monitor infants who have been exposed to ACE inhibitors during the second or third trimester for hypotension, oliguria, and hyperkalemia. Reassure women who took ACE inhibitors during the *first* trimester that this does not represent a risk to the fetus.

Angioedema. This rare and potentially fatal reaction is characterized by giant wheals and edema of the tongue, glottis, and pharynx. If angioedema occurs, discontinue the ACE inhibitor and never use it again. Treat severe reactions with subcutaneous epinephrine.

Renal Failure. Renal failure is a risk for patients with bilateral renal artery stenosis or stenosis in the artery to a single remaining kidney. ACE inhibitors are contraindicated for these people.

Rash and Dysgeusia (Mainly with Captopril). Minimize these reactions by avoiding high doses. Instruct patients to notify the physician if rash or dysgeusia persists. If dysgeusia results in anorexia and weight loss, withdraw the drug. Rash and dysgeusia resolve with cessation of treatment.

*Patient education information is highlighted as blue text.

Neutropenia (Mainly with Captopril). Neutropenia poses a high risk of infection. **Inform patients about early signs of infection (fever, sore throat, mouth sores) and instruct them to notify the physician if these occur.** Obtain white blood cell counts and differential every 2 weeks during the first 3 months of therapy and periodically thereafter. If neutropenia develops, withdraw the drug immediately; neutrophil counts should normalize in approximately 2 weeks. Neutropenia is most likely in patients with renal impairment and collagen vascular diseases (e.g., systemic lupus erythematosus, scleroderma); monitor these patients closely.

Minimizing Adverse Interactions

Diuretics. Diuretics may intensify first-dose hypotension. Withdraw diuretics 1 week prior to beginning an ACE inhibitor. Diuretics may be resumed later if needed.

Antihypertensive Agents. The antihypertensive effects of ACE inhibitors are additive with those of other antihypertensive drugs (e.g., diuretics, sympatholytics, vasodilators, calcium channel blockers). When an ACE inhibitor is added to an antihypertensive regimen, dosages of the other drugs may require reduction.

Drugs That Elevate Potassium Levels. ACE inhibitors increase the risk of hyperkalemia associated with *potassium supplements* and *potassium-sparing diuretics.* Risk can be minimized by avoiding potassium supplements and potassium-sparing diuretics except when they are clearly indicated.

Lithium. ACE inhibitors can increase serum levels of lithium, causing toxicity. Monitor lithium levels frequently.

ANGIOTENSIN II RECEPTOR BLOCKERS

Candesartan
Eprosartan
Irbesartan
Losartan
Olmesartan
Telmisartan
Valsartan

Unless indicated otherwise, the implications summarized below pertain to all of the ARBs.

Preadministration Assessment

Therapeutic Goal

Reduction of blood pressure in patients with hypertension (*all ARBs*).

Treatment of heart failure (*valsartan*).

Slowed progression of diabetic nephropathy (*irbesartan, losartan*).

Baseline Data

Determine blood pressure.

*Patient education information is highlighted as blue text.

Identifying High-Risk Patients

ARBs are *contraindicated* during the second and third trimesters of pregnancy and for patients with either (1) bilateral renal artery stenosis (or stenosis in the artery to a single remaining kidney) or (2) a history of hypersensitivity reactions (especially angioedema) to ARBs.

Implementation: Administration

Route

Oral.

Dosage and Administration

Inform patients that ARBs may be taken with or without food.

Ongoing Evaluation and Interventions

Evaluating Therapeutic Effects

Hypertension. Monitor for reduced blood pressure. The usual target pressure is systolic/diastolic of 140/90 mm Hg.

Heart Failure. Monitor for lessening of signs and symptoms (e.g., dyspnea, cyanosis, jugular vein distention, edema).

Diabetic Nephropathy. Monitor for proteinuria.

Minimizing Adverse Effects

Angioedema. This rare and potentially fatal reaction is characterized by giant wheals and edema of the tongue, glottis, and pharynx. If angioedema occurs, discontinue the ARB and never use it again. Treat severe reactions with subcutaneous epinephrine.

Fetal Injury. **Warn women of child-bearing age that ARBs taken during the *second* and *third* trimesters of pregnancy can cause fetal injury.** If the patient becomes pregnant, withdraw ARBs as soon as possible. Closely monitor infants who have been exposed to ARBs during the second or third trimester for hypotension, oliguria, and hyperkalemia. **Reassure women who took ARBs during the *first* trimester that this does not represent a risk to the fetus.**

Renal Failure. Renal failure is a risk for patients with bilateral renal artery stenosis or stenosis in the artery to a single remaining kidney. ARBs inhibitors are contraindicated for these people.

Minimizing Adverse Interactions

Antihypertensive Agents. The antihypertensive effects of ARBs are additive with those of other antihypertensive drugs (e.g., diuretics, sympatholytics, vasodilators, calcium channel blockers). When an ARB is added to an antihypertensive regimen, dosages of the other drugs may require reduction.

CHAPTER
43

Calcium Channel Blockers

Calcium channel blockers (CCBs) are drugs that prevent calcium ions from entering cells. These drugs have their greatest effects on the heart and blood vessels. CCBs are used widely to treat hypertension, angina pectoris, and cardiac dysrhythmias. Since 1995, there has been controversy about the safety of CCBs, especially in patients with hypertension and diabetes. Alternative names for CCBs are *calcium antagonists* and *slow channel blockers*.

CALCIUM CHANNELS: PHYSIOLOGIC FUNCTIONS AND CONSEQUENCES OF BLOCKADE

Calcium channels are gated pores in the cytoplasmic membrane that regulate entry of calcium ions into cells. Calcium entry plays a critical role in the function of vascular smooth muscle (VSM) and the heart.

Vascular Smooth Muscle

In VSM, calcium channels regulate contraction. When an action potential travels down the surface of a smooth muscle cell, calcium channels open and calcium ions flow inward, thereby initiating the contractile process. If calcium channels are blocked, contraction will be prevented and vasodilation will result.

At therapeutic doses, CCBs act selectively on *peripheral arterioles* and *arteries and arterioles of the heart.* CCBs have no significant effect on veins.

Heart

In the heart, calcium channels help regulate function of the myocardium, the sinoatrial (SA) node, and the atrio-ventricular (AV) node. Calcium channels at all three sites are coupled to beta$_1$-adrenergic receptors.

Myocardium. In cardiac muscle, calcium entry has a positive inotropic effect. That is, calcium increases force of contraction. If calcium channels in atrial and ventricular muscle are blocked, contractile force will diminish.

SA Node. Pacemaker activity of the SA node is regulated by calcium influx. When calcium channels are open, spontaneous discharge of the SA node increases. Conversely, when calcium channels close, pacemaker activity declines. Hence, the effect of calcium channel blockade is to reduce heart rate.

AV Node. Impulses that originate in the SA node must pass through the AV node on their way to the ventricles. Because of this arrangement, regulation of AV conduction plays a critical role in coordinating contraction of the ventricles with contraction of the atria.

The excitability of AV nodal cells is regulated by calcium entry. When calcium channels are open, calcium entry increases and cells of the AV node discharge more readily. Conversely, when calcium channels are closed, discharge of AV nodal cells is suppressed. Hence, the effect of calcium channel blockade is to decrease velocity of conduction through the AV node.

Coupling of Cardiac Calcium Channels to Beta$_1$-Adrenergic Receptors. In the heart, calcium channels are coupled to beta$_1$-adrenergic receptors (see Fig. 43–1). As a result, when cardiac beta$_1$ receptors are activated, calcium influx is enhanced. Conversely, when beta$_1$ receptors are blocked, calcium influx is suppressed. Because of this relationship between calcium channels and beta$_1$ receptors, CCBs and beta blockers have identical effects on the heart. That is, they both reduce force of contraction, slow heart rate, and suppress conduction through the AV node.

CALCIUM CHANNEL BLOCKERS: CLASSIFICATION AND SITES OF ACTION

Classification

The CCBs used in the United States belong to three chemical families (Table 43–1). The largest family is the *dihydropyridines,* for which *nifedipine* is the prototype. This family name is encountered frequently and hence is worth remembering. The other two families consist of orphans: *verapamil* is the only *phenylalkylamine,* and *diltiazem* is the only *benzothiazepine.* The drug names are important; the family names are not.

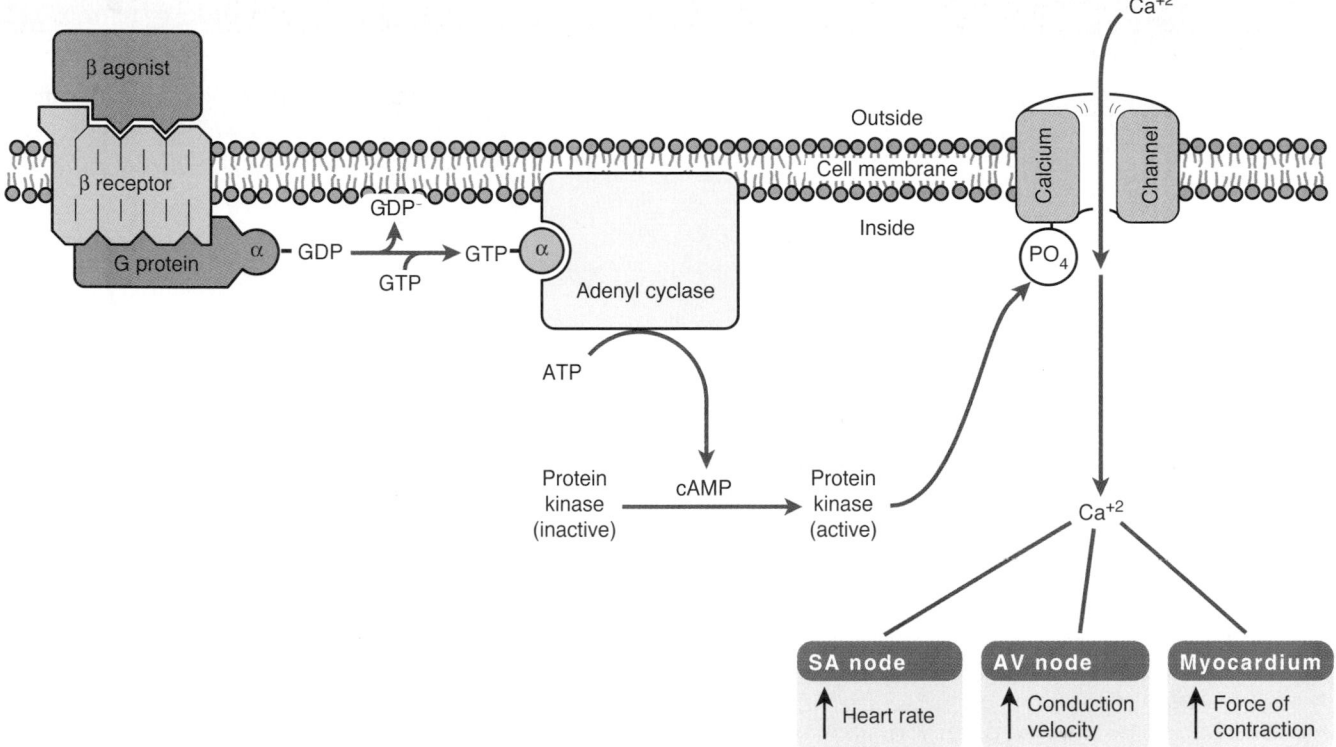

Figure 43–1 ■ **Coupling of cardiac calcium channels with beta$_1$-adrenergic receptors.**
In the heart, beta$_1$ receptors are coupled to calcium channels. As a result, when cardiac beta$_1$ receptors are activated, calcium influx is enhanced. The process works as follows. Binding of an agonist (e.g., norepinephrine) causes a conformational change in the beta receptor, which in turn causes a change in G protein, converting it from an inactive state (in which GDP is bound to the alpha subunit) to an active state (in which GTP is bound to the alpha subunit). (G protein is so named because it binds guanine nucleotides: GDP and GTP.) Following activation, the alpha subunit dissociates from the rest of G protein and activates adenylyl cyclase, an enzyme that converts ATP to cyclic AMP (cAMP). Cyclic AMP then activates protein kinase, an enzyme that phosphorylates proteins—in this case, the calcium channel. Phosphorylation changes the channel such that calcium entry is enhanced when the channel opens. (Opening of the channel is triggered by a change in membrane voltage [i.e., by passage of an action potential].)

The effect of calcium entry on cardiac function is determined by the type of cell involved. If the cell is in the SA node, heart rate increases; if the cell is in the AV node, impulse conduction through the node accelerates; and if the cell is part of the myocardium, force of contraction is increased.

Since binding of a single agonist molecule to a single beta receptor stimulates the synthesis of many cAMP molecules, with the subsequent activation of many protein kinase molecules, causing the phosphorylation of many calcium channels, this system can greatly amplify the signal initiated by the agonist.

Sites of Action

At therapeutic doses, the dihydropyridines act primarily on arterioles; in contrast, verapamil and diltiazem act on arterioles *and* the heart (see Table 43–1). However, although dihydropyridines don't affect the heart at therapeutic doses, *toxic* doses can produce dangerous cardiac suppression (just like verapamil and diltiazem can). The differences in selectivity among CCBs are based on structural differences among the drugs themselves and structural differences among calcium channels.

VERAPAMIL AND DILTIAZEM: AGENTS THAT ACT ON VASCULAR SMOOTH MUSCLE AND THE HEART

Verapamil

Verapamil [Calan, Covera-HS, Isoptin, Verelan] blocks calcium channels in blood vessels and in the heart. Major indications are angina pectoris, essential hypertension, and cardiac dysrhythmias. Verapamil was the first CCB available and will serve as our prototype for the group.

TABLE 43–1 ■ Calcium Channel Blockers: Classification, Sites of Action, and Indications

Classification*	Sites of Action	Indications			
		Hypertension	Angina	Dysrhythmias	Others
Dihydropyridines					
Nifedipine [Adalat, Nifedical, Procardia]	Arterioles	✔	✔		†,‡
Amlodipine [Norvasc]	Arterioles	✔	✔		
Felodipine [Plendil]	Arterioles	✔			
Isradipine [DynaCirc]	Arterioles	✔			
Nicardipine [Cardene]	Arterioles	✔	✔		
Nimodipine [Nimotop]	Arterioles				†,§
Nisoldipine [Sular]	Arterioles	✔			
Phenylakylamines					
Verapamil [Calan, Covera-HS, Isoptin, Verelan]	Arterioles/heart	✔	✔	✔	†
Benzothiazepines					
Diltiazem [Cardizem, Cartia XT, Dilacor, Diltia XT, Tiazac]	Arterioles/heart	✔	✔	✔	

*A fourth class—diarylaminopropylamine ethers—has one member: *bepridil* [Vascor]. Bepridil can cause serious dysrhythmias, and hence is reserved for patients who have not responded to safer CCBs.
†Migraine headache (investigational use).
‡Suppression of preterm labor (investigational use).
§Prophylaxis of neurologic injury after rupture of an intracranial aneurysm.

Hemodynamic Effects

The overall hemodynamic response to verapamil is the net result of (1) direct effects on the heart and blood vessels and (2) reflex responses.

Direct Effects. By blocking calcium channels in the heart and blood vessels, verapamil has five direct effects:

- Blockade at peripheral arterioles causes dilation, and thereby reduces arterial pressure.
- Blockade at arteries and arterioles of the heart increases coronary perfusion.
- Blockade at the SA node reduces heart rate.
- Blockade at the AV node decreases AV nodal conduction.
- Blockade in the myocardium decreases force of contraction.

Of the direct effects on the heart, reduced AV conduction is the most important.

Indirect (Reflex) Effects. Verapamil-induced lowering of blood pressure activates the baroreceptor reflex, causing increased firing of sympathetic nerves to the heart. Norepinephrine released from these nerves acts to increase heart rate, AV conduction, and force of contraction. However, since these same three parameters are suppressed by the direct actions of verapamil, the direct and indirect effects tend to negate each other.

Net Effect. Since the direct effects of verapamil on the heart are counterbalanced by indirect effects, the drug has little or no net effect on cardiac performance: For most patients, heart rate, AV conduction, and contractility are not noticeably altered. Consequently, the overall cardiovascular effect of verapamil is simply vasodilation accompanied by reduced arterial pressure and increased coronary perfusion.

Pharmacokinetics

Verapamil may be administered orally and intravenously. The drug is well absorbed following oral administration, but undergoes extensive metabolism on its first pass through the liver. Consequently, only about 20% of an oral dose reaches the systemic circulation. Effects begin in 30 minutes and peak within 5 hours. Elimination is primarily by hepatic metabolism. Because the drug is eliminated by the liver, doses must be reduced substantially in patients with liver dysfunction.

Therapeutic Uses

Angina Pectoris. Verapamil is used widely to treat angina pectoris. The drug is approved for vasospastic angina and effort-induced angina. Benefits in both derive from vasodilation. The role of verapamil in antianginal therapy is discussed further in Chapter 49.

Essential Hypertension. Verapamil is a first-line agent for chronic hypertension. The drug lowers blood pressure by promoting dilation of arterioles. The role of verapamil and other CCBs in hypertension is discussed in Chapter 45.

Cardiac Dysrhythmias. Verapamil is used to slow ventricular rate in patients with atrial flutter, atrial fibrillation, and paroxysmal supraventricular tachycardia. Benefits derive from suppressing impulse conduction through the AV node, which prevents the atria from driving the ventricles at an excessive rate. Antidysrhythmic applications are discussed in Chapter 47.

Migraine. Verapamil can reduce symptoms of migraine headache. This application is discussed in Chapter 29.

Adverse Effects

Common Effects. Verapamil is generally well tolerated. *Constipation* occurs frequently and is the most common cause of complaints. This problem, which can be especially severe in the elderly, can be minimized by increasing dietary fluids and fiber. Constipation results from blockade of calcium channels in smooth muscle of the intestine. Other common effects—*dizziness, facial flushing, headache,* and *edema of the ankles and feet*—occur secondary to vasodilation. *Gingival hyperplasia* (overgrowth of gum tissue) may also develop.

Cardiac Effects. Blockade of calcium channels in the heart can compromise cardiac function. In the SA node, calcium channel blockade can cause bradycardia; in the AV node, blockade can cause partial or complete AV block; and in the myocardium, blockade can decrease contractility. When the heart is healthy, these effects are minimal. However, in patients with certain cardiac diseases, verapamil can seriously exacerbate dysfunction. Accordingly, the drug must be used with special caution in patients with cardiac failure, and must not be used at all in patients with sick sinus syndrome or second-degree or third-degree AV block.

Drug Interactions

Digoxin. Like verapamil, digoxin suppresses impulse conduction through the AV node. Accordingly, when these drugs are used concurrently, the risk of AV block is increased. Patients receiving the combination should be monitored closely.

Verapamil increases plasma levels of digoxin by about 60%, thereby increasing the risk of digoxin toxicity. If signs of toxicity appear, digoxin dosage should be reduced.

Beta-Adrenergic Blocking Agents. Beta blockers and verapamil have the same effects on the heart: decreases in heart rate, AV conduction, and contractility. Hence, when a beta blocker and verapamil are used concurrently, there is a risk of excessive cardiosuppression. To minimize this risk, administration of beta blockers and IV verapamil should be separated by several hours.

Toxicity

Clinical Manifestations. Overdose can produce severe hypotension and cardiotoxicity (bradycardia, AV block, ventricular tachydysrhythmias).

Treatment. General Measures. Verapamil can be removed from the GI tract with an emetic or with gastric lavage followed by a cathartic. Intravenous calcium gluconate can counteract both vasodilation and negative inotropic effects, but will not reverse AV block.

Hypotension. Hypotension can be treated with IV norepinephrine, which promotes vasoconstriction (by activating alpha$_1$ receptors on blood vessels) and increases cardiac output (by activating beta$_1$ receptors in the heart). Placing the patient in Trendelenburg's position (inclined with the head down) and administering IV fluids may also help.

Bradycardia and AV Block. Bradycardia and AV block can be treated with isoproterenol (a beta-adrenergic agonist) and with atropine (an anticholinergic drug that can block parasympathetic influences on the heart). If pharmacologic measures are inadequate, electronic pacing may be required.

Ventricular Tachydysrhythmias. The preferred treatment is direct current (DC) cardioversion. Antidysrhythmic drugs (procainamide, lidocaine) may also be tried.

Preparations, Dosage, and Administration

Oral. Verapamil is available in regular tablets (40, 80, and 120 mg) as Calan; in sustained-release tablets (120, 180, and 240 mg) as Calan SR, Covera-HS, and Isoptin SR; and in sustained-release capsules (120, 180, 240, and 360 mg) as Verelan. In addition, verapamil is available as Verelan PM (100-, 200-, and 300-mg capsules), a timed-release formulation that, when administered at bedtime, produces maximum verapamil levels in the morning. The sustained-, timed-, and extended-release formulations are approved only for hypertension. Instruct patients to swallow these formulations intact, without crushing or chewing.

The usual initial dosage for *angina pectoris* is 80 to 120 mg 3 times a day. The usual initial dosage for *essential hypertension* is 80 mg 3 times a day (using standard tablets), 240 mg of a sustained-release formulation (administered once a day in the morning with food), or 200 mg of Verelan PM (administered once a day at bedtime). Dosages should be reduced for elderly patients and for patients with advanced renal or liver disease. Dosages for dysrhythmias are presented in Chapter 47.

Intravenous. Intravenous verapamil is used for dysrhythmias. Since IV verapamil can cause severe adverse cardiovascular effects, blood pressure and the electrocardiogram (EKG) should be monitored and equipment for resuscitation should be immediately available. Intravenous dosages for dysrhythmias are presented in Chapter 47.

Diltiazem

Actions and Uses. Like verapamil, diltiazem [Cardizem, Cartia XT, Dilacor, Diltia XT, Tiazac] blocks calcium channels in the heart and blood vessels. As a result, the actions and applications of the two drugs are very similar. Diltiazem has the same effects on cardiovascular function as verapamil. Both drugs lower blood pressure through arteriolar dilation and, because their direct suppressant actions are balanced by reflex cardiac stimulation, both have little net effect on the heart. Like verapamil, diltiazem is used for angina pectoris, essential hypertension, and cardiac dysrhythmias (atrial flutter, atrial fibrillation, paroxysmal supraventricular tachycardia).

Pharmacokinetics. Oral diltiazem is well absorbed and then extensively metabolized on its first pass through the liver. As a result, bioavailability is only about 50%. Effects begin rapidly (within a few minutes) and peak within half an hour. The drug undergoes nearly complete metabolism prior to elimination in the urine and feces.

Adverse Effects. The adverse effects of diltiazem are like those of verapamil, except that diltiazem causes less constipation. The most common effects are dizziness, flushing, headache, and edema of the ankles and feet. Like verapamil, diltiazem can exacerbate cardiac dysfunction in patients with bradycardia, sick sinus syndrome, heart failure, or second-degree or third-degree AV block.

Drug Interactions. Like verapamil, diltiazem can exacerbate digoxin-induced suppression of AV conduction, and can intensify the cardiosuppressant effects of beta blockers. Patients receiving diltiazem concurrently with digoxin or a beta blocker should be monitored closely for cardiac status.

Preparations, Dosage, and Administration. Oral diltiazem is available in standard tablets (30, 60, 90, and 120 mg) as Cardizem and in sustained-release capsules (60, 90, 120, 180, 240, 300, 360, and 420 mg) as Cardizem SR, Cardizem CD, Cartia XT, Dilacor XR, Diltia XT, and Tiazac. The drug is also available in solution (5 mg/ml) for IV administration under the trade name Cardizem. The usual initial dosage for hypertension is 180 mg once a day with Cardizem CD or 60 to 120 mg twice a day with Cardizem SR or Dilacor XR. Angina pectoris can be treated with standard tablets (30 mg 4 times a day initially and 60 mg 4 times a day for maintenance).

DIHYDROPYRIDINES: AGENTS THAT ACT MAINLY ON VASCULAR SMOOTH MUSCLE

All of the drugs discussed in this section belong to the *dihydropyridine* family. At therapeutic doses, these drugs produce significant blockade of calcium channels in blood

Special Interest Topic

BOX 43-1 ■ ARE CALCIUM CHANNEL BLOCKERS SAFE?

There is controversy over the safety of CCBs. The controversy began when researchers concluded that nifedipine increases the risk of mortality in patients with myocardial infarction and unstable angina. Subsequent studies concluded that CCBs increase the risk of mortality in patients with hypertension. There is conflicting evidence on the dangers of CCBs in patients with left ventricular dysfunction—and data from several large studies indicate that CCBs are no danger at all. Hence, the issue of CCB safety is unresolved.

In 1995, a study reported that *rapid-acting* nifedipine is associated with increased mortality in patients with myocardial infarction and unstable angina. However, a cause-and-effect relationship has not been established. Furthermore, there is no evidence that *sustained-release* nifedipine represents any risk. In response to this study, the National Heart, Lung, and Blood Institute recommended that rapid-acting nifedipine, especially in higher doses, be used with great caution, if at all.

CCBs may (or may not) represent a risk for hypertensive patients with type 2 diabetes. In the Appropriate Blood Pressure Control in Diabetes (ABCD) trial, patients received either nisoldipine (a CCB) or enalapril (an ACE inhibitor). Patients taking nisoldipine experienced more cardiovascular events than did patients taking enalapril. Among 470 patients in the trial, the combined incidence of fatal and nonfatal myocardial infarction was 5% with nisoldipine versus only 1% with enalapril. However, since the trial was not placebo controlled, it is impossible to tell whether the CCB *increased* the incidence of cardiovascular events, or the ACE inhibitor *protected* against cardiovascular events. That is, it is possible that nisoldipine had a neutral impact on cardiovascular events, whereas the ACE inhibitor actually reduced them. If the CCB did indeed increase cardiovascular risk, this would be the first evidence that a *long-acting* CCB can do so. In a study published after the ABCD trial, researchers concluded that nitrendipine, another long-acting CCB, was *not* harmful to hypertensive diabetics.

Are CCBs dangerous for other patients with hypertension? Two large, randomized, controlled trials, suggest the answer is "No." One study—the Nordic Diltiazem (NORDIL) study—which enrolled 10,916 patients, compared diltiazem with di-uretics, beta-blockers, or both. The other study—the International Nifedipine GITS study—which enrolled 6575 patients, compared sustained-release nifedipine with diuretic-based regimens. In both studies, CCBs failed to increase cardiovascular risk. However, although these studies were large, they were not large enough to detect small increases in risk.

The Systolic Hypertension in Europe (Syst-Eur) trial adds more proof that CCBs are probably safe. In this study, elderly patients with isolated systolic hypertension were treated with nitrendipine (a CCB). Compared with patients taking placebo, the experimental subjects experienced significantly fewer cardiovascular events, including fatal myocardial infarction. Hence, in this study, CCBs seem to have *reduced* the risk of cardiovascular complications.

Are CCBs a hazard for patients with left ventricular dysfunction? Analysis of data from two studies—the Studies of Left Ventricular Dysfunction (SOLVD) trial and the Survival and Ventricular Enlargement (SAVE) trial—has yielded opposing answers. Data from the SOLVD study suggest that CCBs increase the risk of myocardial infarction in patients with left ventricular dysfunction. However, data from the SAVE study indicate no increase in risk.

The ongoing Antihypertensive and Lipid Lowering Treatment to Prevent Heart Attack Trial (ALLHAT) will help resolve the question of CCB safety. This huge trial, which has 40,000 subjects, was designed to compare four antihypertensive drugs: amlodipine (a CCB), lisinopril (an ACE inhibitor), doxazosin (a vasodilator), and chlorthalidone (a diuretic). One objective is to determine if these drugs increase the risk of adverse cardiovascular outcomes. Although final results are not yet available, an interim analysis indicated that one of the drugs—doxazosin—did indeed increase cardiovascular risk, and hence that arm of the study was stopped. Since the amlodipine arm was not stopped, we can conclude that, at least up to this point in the study, amlodipine did *not* increase cardiovascular risk. When the final results are available, we should have a much more solid understanding of CCB safety—or lack thereof. Until then, it seems reasonable to continue using these drugs for appropriate indications.

---

vessels and minimal blockade of calcium channels in the heart. The dihydropyridines are similar to verapamil in some respects but quite different in others. Beginning in 1995, controversy developed about the safety of these drugs (see Box 43–1).

Nifedipine

Nifedipine [Adalat, Nifedical, Procardia] was the first dihydropyridine available and will serve as our prototype for the family. Like verapamil, nifedipine blocks calcium channels in VSM and thereby promotes vasodilation. However, in contrast to verapamil, nifedipine produces very little blockade of calcium channels in the heart. As a result, nifedipine cannot be used to treat dysrhythmias, does not cause adverse cardiac suppression, and is less likely than verapamil to exacerbate pre-existing cardiac disorders. Nifedipine also differs from verapamil in that nifedipine is more likely to cause reflex tachycardia. Contrasts between nifedipine and verapamil are summarized in Table 43–2.

Hemodynamic Effects

Direct Effects. The direct effects of nifedipine on the cardiovascular system are limited to blockade of calcium channels in VSM. Blockade of calcium channels in peripheral arterioles causes vasodilation, and thereby lowers arterial pressure. Blockade of calcium channels in arteries and arterioles of the heart increases coronary perfusion. Since nifedipine does not block cardiac calcium channels at usual

TABLE 43–2 ▦ Comparisons and Contrasts Between Nifedipine and Verapamil

Property	Drug	
	Nifedipine	Verapamil
Direct Effects on the Heart and Arterioles		
Arteriolar dilation	Yes	Yes
Effects on the heart	No	Yes
Reduced automaticity	No	Yes
Reduced AV conduction	No	Yes
Reduced contractile force		
Major Indications		
Hypertension	Yes	Yes
Angina pectoris (classic and variant)	Yes	Yes
Dysrhythmias	No	Yes
Adverse Effects		
Exacerbation of		
AV block	No	Yes
Sick sinus syndrome	No	Yes
Heart failure	No	Yes
Effects secondary to vasodilation		
Edema (ankles and feet)	Yes	Yes
Flushing	Yes	Yes
Headaches	Yes	Yes
Dizziness	Yes	Yes
Reflex tachycardia	Yes	No
Constipation	No	Yes
Drug Interactions		
Intensifies digoxin-induced AV block	No	Yes
Intensifies cardiosuppressant effects of beta blockers	No	Yes
Often combined with a beta blocker to suppress reflex tachycardia	Yes	No

therapeutic doses, the drug does not significantly reduce automaticity, AV conduction, or contractile force.

Indirect (Reflex) Effects. By lowering blood pressure, nifedipine activates the baroreceptor reflex, thereby causing sympathetic stimulation of the heart. Since nifedipine has minimal direct cardiosuppressant actions, cardiac stimulation is unopposed; hence, heart rate and contractile force increase.

It is important to note that reflex effects occur primarily with the *fast-acting* formulation of nifedipine—not with the sustained-release formulation. Why? Because the baroreceptor reflex is turned on only by a *rapid* fall in blood pressure; a gradual decline will not activate the reflex. With the fast-acting formulation, blood levels of nifedipine rise quickly; hence blood pressure drops quickly and the reflex is activated. Conversely, with the sustained-release formulation, blood levels of nifedipine rise slowly; hence blood pressure falls slowly and the reflex is blunted.

Net Effect. The overall hemodynamic response to nifedipine is simply the sum of its direct effect (vasodilation) and indirect effect (reflex cardiac stimulation). Hence, nifedipine (1) lowers blood pressure, (2) increases heart rate, and (3) increases contractile force. Please note, however, that the reflex increases in heart rate and contractile force are transient and occur primarily with the rapid-acting formulation.

Pharmacokinetics

Nifedipine is well absorbed following oral administration, but undergoes extensive first-pass metabolism. As a result, only about 50% of an oral dose reaches the systemic circulation. With the fast-acting formulation, effects begin rapidly and peak in 30 minutes; with the sustained-release formulation, effects begin in 20 minutes and peak in 6 hours. Nifedipine is fully metabolized prior to excretion in the urine.

Therapeutic Uses

Angina Pectoris. Nifedipine is indicated for vasospastic angina and for angina of effort. The drug is usually combined with a beta blocker to prevent reflex stimulation of the heart, which could intensify anginal pain. The role of nifedipine in angina is discussed further in Chapter 49.

Hypertension. Nifedipine is used widely to treat *essential hypertension.* In addition, it can be used for *hypertensive emergencies,* although other drugs are safer. For essential hypertension, only the sustained-release formulation is approved. The rapid-acting formulation is used for hypertensive emergencies. The use of CCBs in hypertensive states is discussed further in Chapter 45.

Investigational Uses. Nifedipine has been used on an investigational basis to relieve *migraine headache* (see Chapter 29) and to *suppress preterm labor* (see Chapter 62).

Adverse Effects

Some adverse effects of nifedipine are like those of verapamil; others are quite different. Like verapamil, nifedipine can cause *flushing, dizziness, headache, peripheral edema,* and *gingival hyperplasia.* In contrast to verapamil, nifedipine does not cause much constipation. Also, since nifedipine causes minimal blockade of calcium channels in the heart, the drug is not likely to exacerbate AV block, heart failure, bradycardia, or sick sinus syndrome. Accordingly, nifedipine is preferred to verapamil for patients with these disorders.

A response that occurs with nifedipine that does not occur with verapamil is *reflex tachycardia.* This response is problematic in that it increases cardiac oxygen demand and can thereby increase pain in patients with angina. To prevent reflex tachycardia, nifedipine can be combined with a beta blocker (e.g., propranolol).

Rapid-acting nifedipine has been associated with increased mortality in patients with myocardial infarction and unstable angina. Other rapid-acting CCBs have been associated with an increased risk of myocardial infarction in patients with hypertension. However, in both cases, a cause-and-effect relationship has not been established. Nonetheless, the National Heart, Lung, and Blood Institute has recommended that rapid-acting nifedipine, especially in higher doses, be used with great caution, if at all. It is important to note that these adverse effects have not been associated with *sustained-release* nifedipine or with any other long-acting CCB.

Drug Interactions

Beta-Adrenergic Blockers. Beta blockers are combined with nifedipine to prevent reflex tachycardia. It is important to note that, whereas beta blockers can *decrease* the adverse cardiac effects of *nifedipine,* they can *intensify* the adverse cardiac effects of *verapamil* and *diltiazem.*

Toxicity

When taken in excessive dosage, nifedipine loses selectivity. Hence, toxic doses affect the heart in addition to blood vessels. Consequently, the manifestations and treatment of nifedipine overdose are the same as described above for verapamil.

Preparations, Dosage, and Administration

Nifedipine is available in capsules (10 and 20 mg) as Adalat and Procardia and in sustained-release tablets (30, 60, and 90 mg) as Adalat CC, Nifedical XL, and Procardia XL. Instruct patients to swallow sustained-release tablets whole, without crushing or chewing.

For treatment of *angina pectoris,* the usual initial dosage is 10 mg 3 times a day. The usual maintenance dosage is 10 to 20 mg 3 times a day. The maximum recommended dosage is 180 mg/day.

For *essential hypertension,* only the sustained-release tablets are approved. The usual initial dosage is 30 mg once a day.

Other Dihydropyridines

In addition to nifedipine, six other dihydropyridines are available. All are similar to nifedipine. Like nifedipine, these drugs produce greater blockade of calcium channels in VSM than in the heart.

Nicardipine. At therapeutic doses, nicardipine [Cardene, Cardene SR, Cardene I.V.] produces selective blockade of calcium channels in blood vessels and has minimal direct effects on the heart. The drug has two indications: essential hypertension and effort-induced angina pectoris. The most common adverse effects are flushing, headache, asthenia (weakness), dizziness, palpitations, and edema of the ankles and feet. Gingival hyperplasia (overgrowth of gum tissue) has been reported. Like nifedipine, nicardipine can be combined with a beta-adrenergic blocker to promote therapeutic effects and sup-

press reflex tachycardia. Nicardipine is available in standard capsules (20 and 30 mg), sustained-release capsules (30, 45, and 60 mg), and an IV formulation (2.5 mg/ml). The usual initial dosage for *angina pectoris* is 20 mg 3 times a day using the standard capsules. The usual initial dosage for *essential hypertension* is 20 mg 3 times a day (using standard capsules) or 30 mg twice a day (using sustained-release capsules).

Amlodipine. At therapeutic doses, amlodipine [Norvasc] produces "selective" blockade of calcium channels in blood vessels, having minimal direct effects on the heart. Approved indications are essential hypertension and angina pectoris (effort induced and vasospastic). Amlodipine is administered orally and absorbed slowly; peak levels develop in 6 to 12 hours. The drug has a long half-life (30 to 50 hours) and therefore is effective with once-a-day dosing. Principal adverse effects are peripheral and facial edema. Flushing, dizziness, and headache may also occur. In contrast to other dihydropyridines, amlodipine causes little reflex tachycardia. Amlodipine is available in 2.5-, 5-, and 10-mg tablets. The usual initial dosage for hypertension or angina pectoris is 5 mg once a day. A fixed-dose combination with benazepril (an angiotensin-converting enzyme [ACE] inhibitor) is available under the trade name *Lotrel.*

Isradipine. Like nifedipine, isradipine [DynaCirc, DynaCirc CR] produces relatively selective blockade of calcium channels in blood vessels. In the United States, the drug is approved only for hypertension. Isradipine is rapidly absorbed following oral administration, but undergoes extensive metabolism on its first pass through the liver. Parent drug and metabolites are excreted in the urine. The most common side effects are facial flushing (11%), headache (14%), dizziness (7%), and ankle edema (7%). In contrast to nifedipine, isradipine causes minimal reflex tachycardia. The drug is available in capsules (2.5 and 5 mg) and controlled-release tablets (5 and 10 mg). The usual antihypertensive dosage is 2.5 to 5 mg twice a day.

Felodipine. Felodipine [Plendil] produces "selective" blockade of calcium channels in blood vessels. In the United States, the drug is approved only for essential hypertension. Felodipine is well absorbed following oral administration but undergoes extensive first-pass metabolism. As a result, bioavailability is low—only 20%. Plasma levels peak in 2.5 to 5 hours and then decay with a half-life of 24 hours. Because of its prolonged half-life, felodipine is effective with once-a-day dosing. Characteristic adverse effects are reflex tachycardia, peripheral edema, headache, facial flushing, and dizziness. Gingival hyperplasia has been reported. Felodipine is available in extended-release tablets (2.5, 5, and 10 mg). The usual dosage for hypertension is 5 to 10 mg once a day. A fixed-dose combination with enalapril (an ACE inhibitor) is available under the trade name *Lexxel.*

Nimodipine. Nimodipine [Nimotop] produces selective blockade of calcium channels in *cerebral blood vessels.* The only approved application is prophylaxis of neurologic injury following rupture of an intracranial aneurysm. Benefits derive from preventing the cerebral arterial spasm that follows subarachnoid hemorrhage (SAH) and can result in ischemic neurologic injury. Dosing (60 mg every 4 hours) should begin within 96 hours of SAH and continue for 21 days. As discussed in Chapter 29, nimodipine may also be useful against migraine. The drug is available in 30-mg liquid-filled capsules.

Nisoldipine. Like nifedipine, nisoldipine [Sular] produces selective blockade of calcium channels in blood vessels; the drug has minimal direct effects on the heart. The only approved indication is hypertension. Nisoldipine is well absorbed following oral administration, but the first-pass effect limits bioavailability to 5%. Plasma levels peak 6 hours after administration. The most common side effects are dizziness, headache, and peripheral edema. Reflex tachycardia may also occur. Nisoldipine is dispensed in extended-release tablets (10, 20, 30, and 40 mg). The dosage for hypertension is 20 to 60 mg once a day.

⠿ KEY POINTS

- Calcium channels are gated pores in the cytoplasmic membrane that regulate entry of calcium into cells.
- In blood vessels, calcium entry causes vasoconstriction; calcium channel blockade causes vasodilation.
- In the heart, calcium entry increases heart rate, AV conduction, and myocardial contractility; calcium channel blockade has the opposite effect.
- In the heart, calcium channels are coupled to beta$_1$ receptors, activation of which enhances calcium entry.

As a result, calcium channel blockade and beta block-ade have identical effects on cardiac function.

■ At therapeutic doses, nifedipine and the other dihy-dropyridines act primarily on VSM; in contrast, verap-amil and diltiazem act on VSM *and* the heart.

■ All CCBs promote vasodilation, and hence are useful in hypertension and angina pectoris.

■ Because they suppress AV conduction, verapamil and diltiazem are useful against cardiac dysrhythmias (in addition to hypertension and angina pectoris).

■ Because of their cardiosuppressant effects, verapamil and diltiazem can cause bradycardia, partial or com-plete AV block, and exacerbation of heart failure.

■ Beta blockers intensify cardiosuppression caused by verapamil and diltiazem.

■ Nifedipine and other dihydropyridines can cause re-flex tachycardia. Tachycardia is most intense with rapid-acting formulations, and much less intense with sustained-release formulations.

■ Beta blockers can be used to suppress reflex tachycar-dia caused by nifedipine and other dihydropyridines.

■ Because they cause vasodilation, all CCBs can cause dizziness, headache, and peripheral edema.

■ In toxic doses, nifedipine and other dihydropyridines can cause cardiosuppression, just like verapamil and diltiazem.

■ Rapid-acting nifedipine has been associated with in-creased mortality in patients with myocardial infarc-tion and unstable angina, although a cause-and-effect relationship has not been established. The National Heart, Lung, and Blood Institute has recommended that rapid-acting nifedipine, especially in higher doses, be used with great caution, if at all.

Summary of Major Nursing Implications*

VERAPAMIL AND DILTIAZEM

Preadministration Assessment

Therapeutic Goal

Verapamil and diltiazem are indicated for *hypertension, angina pectoris,* and *cardiac dysrhythmias.*

Baseline Data

For *all patients,* determine blood pressure and pulse rate, and obtain laboratory evaluations of liver and kidney function. For patients with *angina pectoris,* obtain base-line data on the frequency and severity of anginal attacks. For baseline data relevant to *hypertension,* refer to Chapter 45.

Identifying High-Risk Patients

Verapamil and diltiazem are *contraindicated* for patients with severe hypotension, sick sinus syndrome (in the ab-sence of electronic pacing), and second-degree or third-degree AV block. Use with *caution* in patients with heart failure or liver dysfunction and in patients taking digoxin or beta blockers.

Implementation: Administration

Routes

Oral, IV.

Administration

Oral. Verapamil and *diltiazem* may be used for angina pectoris and essential hypertension. *Verapamil* may be used with digoxin to control ventricular rate in patients with atrial fibrillation and atrial flutter.

Sustained-release formulations are reserved for essential hypertension. **Instruct patients to swallow sustained-release formulations whole, without crushing or chewing.**

Prior to administration, measure blood pressure and pulse rate. If hypotension or bradycardia is detected, withhold medication and notify the physician.

Intravenous. Intravenous therapy is used for cardiac dys-rhythmias. Perform injections slowly (over 2 to 3 minutes). Monitor the EKG for AV block, sudden reduction in heart rate, and prolongation of the PR or QT interval. Have facilities for cardioversion and cardiac pacing immediately available.

Ongoing Evaluation and Interventions

Evaluating Therapeutic Effects

Angina Pectoris. Keep an ongoing record of anginal at-tacks, noting the time and intensity of each attack and the likely precipitating event. **Teach outpatients to chart the time, intensity, and circumstances of their attacks.**

Essential Hypertension. Monitor blood pressure peri-odically. The goal is to reduce systolic/diastolic pressure to 140/90 mm Hg. **Teach patients to self-monitor their blood pressure and to maintain a blood pressure record.**

Minimizing Adverse Effects

Cardiosuppression. Verapamil and diltiazem can cause bradycardia, AV block, and heart failure. **Inform patients about manifestations of cardiac effects (e.g., slow heart beat, shortness of breath, weight gain) and instruct them to notify the physician if these occur.** If cardiac impairment is severe, drug use should stop.

Peripheral Edema. **Inform patients about signs of edema (swelling in ankles or feet) and instruct them to no-tify the physician if these occur.** If necessary, edema can be reduced with a diuretic.

Constipation. Constipation occurs primarily with *verap-amil.* **Advise patients that constipation can be minimized by increasing dietary fluid and fiber.**

*Patient education is highlighted as blue text.

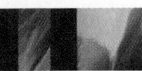

Summary of Major Nursing Implications*—cont'd

Minimizing Adverse Interactions

Digoxin. The combination of digoxin with verapamil or diltiazem increases the risk of partial or complete AV block. Monitor for indications of impaired AV conduction.

Verapamil (and possibly diltiazem) can increase plasma levels of digoxin. Digoxin dosage should be reduced.

Beta Blockers. Concurrent use of a beta blocker with verapamil or diltiazem can cause bradycardia, AV block, or heart failure. Monitor closely for cardiac suppression. Administer *intravenous verapamil* and beta blockers several hours apart from each other.

Managing Acute Toxicity

Remove unabsorbed drug with an emetic or with gastric lavage followed by a cathartic. Give intravenous calcium to help counteract excessive vasodilation and reduced myocardial contractility.

To raise blood pressure, give IV norepinephrine. Intravenous fluids and placing the patient in Trendelenburg's position can also help.

Bradycardia and AV block can be reversed with isoproterenol and atropine. If these are inadequate, electronic pacing may be required.

Ventricular tachydysrhythmias can be treated with DC cardioversion. Antidysrhythmic drugs (lidocaine or procainamide) may also be used.

DIHYDROPYRIDINES

Amlodipine
Felodipine
Isradipine
Nicardipine
Nifedipine
Nimodipine
Nisoldipine

Preadministration Assessment

Therapeutic Goal

Amlodipine, nifedipine, and *nicardipine* are approved for essential hypertension and angina pectoris.

*Patient education is highlighted as blue text.

Isradipine, felodipine, and *nisoldipine* are approved for hypertension only.

Nimodipine is used only for subarachnoid hemorrhage.

Baseline Data

See Nursing Implications for verapamil and diltiazem.

Identifying High-Risk Patients

Use dihydropyridines with *caution* in patients with hypotension, sick sinus syndrome (in the absence of electronic pacing), angina pectoris (because of reflex tachycardia), heart failure, and second-degree or third-degree AV block.

Implementation: Administration

Route

Oral. All dihydropyridines.
Intravenous. *Nicardipine.*

Administration

Instruct patients to swallow sustained-release formulations whole, without crushing or chewing.

Ongoing Evaluation and Interventions

Evaluating Therapeutic Effects

See Nursing Implications for verapamil and diltiazem.

Minimizing Adverse Effects

Reflex Tachycardia. Reflex tachycardia can be suppressed with a beta blocker.

Peripheral Edema. **Inform patients about signs of edema (swelling in ankles or feet) and instruct them to notify the physician if these occur.** If necessary, edema can be reduced with a diuretic.

Managing Acute Toxicity

See Nursing Implications for verapamil and diltiazem.

Vasodilators

BASIC CONCEPTS IN VASODILATOR PHARMACOLOGY
    Selectivity of Vasodilatory Effects
    Overview of Therapeutic Uses
    Adverse Effects Related to Vasodilation
PHARMACOLOGY OF INDIVIDUAL VASODILATORS
    Hydralazine
    Minoxidil
    Diazoxide
    Sodium Nitroprusside
    Angiotensin-Converting Enzyme Inhibitors
    Angiotensin II Receptor Blockers
    Organic Nitrates
    Calcium Channel Blockers
    Sympatholytics

TABLE 44–1 ▐▪ Types of Vasodilators	
Category	**Examples**
Angiotensin-Converting Enzyme Inhibitors	Captopril
	Enalapril
	Lisinopril
Angiotensin II Receptor Blockers	Losartan
	Valsartan
Organic Nitrates	Nitroglycerin
	Isosorbide dinitrate
Calcium Channel Blockers	Verapamil
	Nifedipine
	Diltiazem
Sympatholytics	
Alpha-adrenergic blockers	Phentolamine
	Phenoxybenzamine
	Prazosin
	Terazosin
Ganglionic blockers	Mecamylamine
	Trimethaphan
Adrenergic neuron blockers	Reserpine
	Guanethidine
	Guanadrel
Centrally acting agents	Clonidine
	Guanabenz
	Methyldopa
Other Important Vasodilators	Hydralazine
	Minoxidil
	Nitroprusside
	Diazoxide

Vasodilation can be produced with a variety of drugs. The major classes of vasodilators, along with representative agents, are listed in Table 44–1. Some of these drugs act primarily on arterioles, some act primarily on veins, and some dilate both types of vessel. The vasodilators are widely used, with indications ranging from hypertension to angina pectoris to heart failure. Many of the vasodilators have been discussed in previous chapters. Four agents—hydralazine, minoxidil, diazoxide, and nitroprusside—are introduced here.

In approaching the vasodilators, we begin by considering concepts that apply to the vasodilators as a group. After that we discuss the pharmacology of individual agents.

BASIC CONCEPTS IN VASODILATOR PHARMACOLOGY

Selectivity of Vasodilatory Effects

It is important to appreciate that vasodilators differ from one another with respect to the types of blood vessels they affect. Some agents (e.g., hydralazine) produce selective dilation of arterioles. Others (e.g., nitroglycerin) produce selective dilation of veins. Still others (e.g., prazosin) dilate arterioles *and* veins. The selectivity of some important vasodilators is summarized in Table 44–2.

The selectivity of a vasodilator determines its hemodynamic effects. For example, drugs that dilate *resistance vessels* (arterioles) cause a decrease in cardiac *afterload* (the force against which the heart must work to pump blood). By decreasing afterload, arteriolar dilators reduce cardiac work while causing cardiac output and tissue perfusion to increase. In contrast, drugs that dilate *capacitance vessels* (veins) reduce the force with which blood is returned to the heart, which reduces ventricular filling. This reduction in filling decreases cardiac *preload* (the degree of stretch of the ventricular muscle prior to contraction), which in turn decreases the force of ventricular contraction. Hence, by decreasing preload, venous dilators cause a decrease in cardiac work, along with a decrease in cardiac output and tissue perfusion.

Because hemodynamic responses to dilation of arterioles and veins differ, the selectivity of a vasodilator is a major determinant of its effects, both therapeutic and undesired. Undesired effects related to selective dilation of arterioles and veins are discussed below. Therapeutic implications of selective dilation are discussed in Chapters 45, 46, 49, and 51—the chapters in which the primary uses of the vasodilators are presented.

TABLE 44–2 ▪ Vasodilator Selectivity		
	Site of Vasodilation	
Vasodilator	**Arterioles**	**Veins**
Hydralazine	+	
Minoxidil	+	
Diltiazem	+	
Nifedipine	+	
Verapamil	+	
Prazosin	+	+
Terazosin	+	+
Phentolamine	+	+
Nitroprusside	+	+
Captopril	+	+
Enalapril	+	+
Lisinopril	+	+
Losartan	+	+
Nitroglycerin		+
Isosorbide dinitrate		+

Overview of Therapeutic Uses

The vasodilators, as a group, have a broad spectrum of applications. Principal indications are *essential hypertension, hypertensive crisis, angina pectoris, heart failure,* and *myocardial infarction.* Additional indications include *pheochromocytoma, peripheral vascular disease,* and *production of controlled hypotension during surgery.* The specific applications of any particular agent are determined by its pharmacologic profile. Important facets of that profile are route of administration, site of vasodilation (arterioles, veins, or both), and intensity and duration of effects.

Adverse Effects Related to Vasodilation
Postural Hypotension

Postural (orthostatic) hypotension is defined as a fall in blood pressure brought on by moving from a supine or seated position to an upright position. The underlying cause of orthostatic hypotension is relaxation of smooth muscle in *veins*. Because of venous relaxation, gravity causes blood to "pool" in veins, thereby decreasing venous return to the heart. This reduction in venous return causes a decrease in cardiac output and a corresponding drop in blood pressure. Hypotension from venous dilation is minimal in recumbent subjects because, when we are lying down, the impact of gravity on venous return is small.

Patients receiving vasodilators should be informed about symptoms of hypotension (lightheadedness, dizziness) and advised to sit or lie down if these occur. Why? Because failure to do so may result in fainting. In addition, patients should be informed that they can minimize hypotension by avoiding abrupt transitions from a supine or seated position to an upright position.

Reflex Tachycardia

Reflex tachycardia can be produced by dilation of *arterioles* or *veins*. The mechanism of reflex tachycardia is as follows: (1a) *arteriolar* dilation causes a direct decrease in arterial pressure or (1b) *venous* dilation reduces cardiac output, which

in turn reduces arterial pressure; (2) baroreceptors in the aortic arch and carotid sinus sense the drop in pressure and relay this information to the vasomotor center of the medulla; and (3) in an attempt to bring blood pressure back up, the medulla sends impulses along sympathetic nerves instructing the heart to beat faster.

Reflex tachycardia is undesirable for two reasons. First, tachycardia can put an unacceptable burden on the heart. Second, if the vasodilator was given to reduce blood pressure, tachycardia would raise pressure and thereby counteract beneficial effects.

To help prevent vasodilator-induced reflex tachycardia, patients can be pretreated with a beta blocker (e.g., propranolol), which will block sympathetic stimulation of the heart.

Expansion of Blood Volume

Prolonged use of *arteriolar* or *venous* dilators can cause an increase in blood volume (secondary to prolonged reduction of blood pressure). This increase in blood volume represents an attempt by the body to restore blood pressure to pretreatment levels.

Blood volume is increased by two mechanisms. First, reduced blood pressure triggers secretion of aldosterone by the adrenal glands. Aldosterone then acts on the kidney to promote retention of sodium and water, thereby increasing blood volume. The second mechanism also involves the kidney: By reducing arterial pressure, vasodilators decrease renal blood flow and glomerular filtration rate; because filtrate volume is decreased, the kidney is able to reabsorb an increased fraction of filtered sodium and water, which causes blood volume to expand.

Increased plasma volume can negate the beneficial effects of vasodilator therapy. For example, if plasma volume increases during the treatment of hypertension, blood pressure will rise and the benefits of therapy will be canceled. To prevent the kidney from neutralizing the beneficial effects of vasodilation, patients often receive concurrent therapy with a diuretic, which prevents fluid retention and volume expansion.

PHARMACOLOGY OF INDIVIDUAL VASODILATORS

In this section we focus on four drugs: hydralazine, minoxidil, diazoxide, and sodium nitroprusside. All of the other vasodilators are discussed at length in other chapters, and hence their discussion here is brief.

Hydralazine
Cardiovascular Effects

Hydralazine [Apresoline] causes selective dilation of arterioles. The drug has little or no effect on veins. Arteriolar dilation results from a direct action on vascular smooth muscle (VSM); the precise mechanism is unknown. In response to arteriolar dilation, peripheral resistance and arterial blood pressure fall. In addition, heart rate and myocardial contractility increase, largely by reflex mechanisms. Since hydralazine acts selectively on arterioles, postural hypotension is minimal.

Pharmacokinetics

Absorption and Time Course of Action. Hydralazine is readily absorbed following oral administration. Effects are apparent within 45 minutes and persist for 6 hours or more. With parenteral administration, effects begin rapidly (within 10 minutes) and last for 2 to 4 hours.

Metabolism. Hydralazine is inactivated by a metabolic process known as *acetylation*. The ability to acetylate hydralazine and other drugs is genetically determined. Some people are rapid acetylators, and some are slow acetylators. The distinction between rapid and slow acetylators can be clinically significant. Why? Because individuals who acetylate hydralazine slowly are likely to have higher blood levels of the drug. These high levels can result in excessive vasodilation and other undesired effects. To avoid hydralazine accumulation, dosage should be reduced in slow acetylators.

Therapeutic Uses

Essential Hypertension. Oral hydralazine can be used to lower blood pressure in patients with essential hypertension. The regimen almost always includes a beta blocker, and may also include a diuretic. Although commonly employed in the past, hydralazine has been largely replaced by newer antihypertensive agents (see Chapter 45).

Hypertensive Crisis. Parenteral hydralazine is used to lower blood pressure rapidly in severe hypertensive episodes. The drug should be administered in small, incremental doses. If dosage is excessive, severe hypotension may replace the hypertension. Treatment of hypertensive emergencies is discussed in Chapter 45.

Heart Failure. As discussed in Chapter 46, hydralazine can be used short term to reduce afterload in patients with heart failure. With prolonged therapy, tolerance to hydralazine develops.

Adverse Effects

Reflex Tachycardia. By lowering arterial blood pressure, hydralazine can trigger reflex stimulation of the heart, thereby causing cardiac work and myocardial oxygen demand to increase. Because hydralazine-induced reflex tachycardia is frequently severe, the drug is usually combined with a beta blocker.

Increased Blood Volume. Hydralazine-induced hypotension can cause sodium and water retention and a corresponding increase in blood volume. Volume expansion can be prevented with a diuretic.

Systemic Lupus Erythematosus–like Syndrome. Hydralazine can cause an acute rheumatoid syndrome that closely resembles systemic lupus erythematosus (SLE). The syndrome is characterized by muscle pain, joint pain, fever, nephritis, pericarditis, and the presence of antinuclear antibodies. The syndrome occurs most frequently in slow acetylators and is rare when dosage is kept below 200 mg/day. If an SLE-like reaction occurs, hydralazine should be discontinued. Symptoms are usually reversible but may take 6 or more months to resolve. In some cases, rheumatoid symptoms persist for years.

Other Adverse Effects. Common responses include *headache, dizziness, weakness,* and *fatigue.* These reactions are related to hydralazine-induced hypotension.

Drug Interactions

Hydralazine is combined with a *beta blocker* to protect against reflex tachycardia, and with *diuretics* to prevent sodium and water retention and expansion of blood volume. Drugs that lower blood pressure will intensify hypotensive responses to hydralazine. Accordingly, if hydralazine is used with other *antihypertensive agents,* care is needed to avoid excessive hypotension.

Preparations, Dosage, and Administration

Preparations. Hydralazine [Apresoline] is dispensed in tablets (10, 25, 50, and 100 mg) for oral use and in solution (20 mg/ml in 1-ml ampules) for parenteral administration. Hydralazine is also available in fixed-dose combinations with hydrochlorothiazide (a diuretic) under the trade name *Apresazide.*

Oral Therapy. Dosage should be low initially (10 mg 4 times a day) and then gradually increased. Rapid increases may produce excessive hypotension. Usual maintenance dosages for adults range from 25 to 100 mg 2 times a day. Daily doses greater than 200 mg are associated with an increased incidence of adverse effects and should be avoided.

Parenteral Therapy. Parenteral administration (IV and IM) is reserved for hypertensive crises. The usual dose is 20 to 40 mg, repeated as needed. Blood pressure should be monitored frequently to minimize excessive hypotension. In most cases, patients can be switched from hydralazine injections to oral therapy within 48 hours.

Minoxidil

Minoxidil [Loniten] produces more intense vasodilation than hydralazine but also causes more severe adverse reactions. Because it is both very effective and very dangerous, minoxidil is reserved for patients with severe hypertension that has been refractory to safer drugs.

Cardiovascular Effects

Like hydralazine, minoxidil produces selective dilation of *arterioles.* Little or no venous dilation occurs. Arteriolar dilation decreases peripheral resistance and arterial blood pressure. In response, reflex mechanisms increase in heart rate and myocardial contractility. These responses can increase cardiac oxygen demand, and can thereby exacerbate angina pectoris.

Vasodilation results from a direct action on VSM. In order to relax VSM, minoxidil must first be metabolized to minoxidil sulfate. This metabolite then causes potassium channels in VSM to open. The resultant efflux of potassium hyperpolarizes VSM cells, thereby reducing their ability to contract.

Pharmacokinetics

Minoxidil is rapidly and completely absorbed following oral administration. Vasodilation is maximal within 2 to 3 hours and then gradually declines. Residual effects may persist for 2 days or more. Minoxidil is extensively metabolized. Metabolites and parent drug are eliminated in the urine.

Therapeutic Uses

The only cardiovascular indication for minoxidil is *severe hypertension.* Because of its serious adverse effects, minoxidil is reserved for patients who have failed to respond to safer drugs. To minimize adverse cardiovascular responses (reflex tachycardia, expansion of blood volume, pericardial effusion), minoxidil should be used with a beta blocker plus intensive diuretic therapy.

Topical minoxidil [Rogaine, Minoxidil for Men] is used to promote hair growth in balding men (see Chapter 101).

Adverse Effects

Reflex Tachycardia. Blood pressure reduction triggers reflex tachycardia. Tachycardia is a serious side effect and can be minimized by concurrent use of a beta blocker.

Sodium and Water Retention. Fluid retention is both common and serious. Volume expansion may be so severe as to cause cardiac decompensation. Management of fluid retention requires a high-ceiling diuretic (e.g., furosemide) used alone or in combination with a thiazide diuretic. If diuretics are inadequate, dialysis must be employed, or minoxidil must be withdrawn.

Hypertrichosis. About 80% of patients taking minoxidil for 4 weeks or more develop hypertrichosis (excessive growth of hair). Hair growth begins on the face and later develops on the arms, legs, and back. Hypertrichosis appears to result from proliferation of epithelial cells at the base of the hair follicle; vasodilation may also be involved. Overgrowth of hair is a cosmetic problem and can be controlled by shaving or using a depilatory. However, many patients (primarily women) find hypertrichosis both unmanageable and intolerable and refuse to continue treatment.

Pericardial Effusion. Rarely, minoxidil-induced fluid retention results in pericardial effusion (fluid accumulation beneath the pericardium). In most cases, pericardial effusion is asymptomatic. However, in some cases, fluid accumulation becomes so great as to cause cardiac tamponade (compression of the heart with a resultant decrease in cardiac performance). If tamponade occurs, it must be treated by pericardiocentesis or surgical drainage.

Other Adverse Effects. Minoxidil may cause *nausea, headache, fatigue, breast tenderness, glucose intolerance, thrombocytopenia,* and *skin reactions* (rashes, Stevens-Johnson syndrome). In addition, the drug has caused *hemorrhagic cardiac lesions* in experimental animals.

Preparations, Dosage, and Administration

Minoxidil [Loniten] is dispensed in 2.5- and 10-mg tablets for oral administration. The initial dosage is 5 mg once a day; the maximum dosage is 100 mg/day. The usual adult dosage is 10 to 40 mg/day administered in single or divided doses. When a rapid response is needed, a loading dose of 5 to 20 mg is given followed by doses of 2.5 to 10 mg every 4 hours.

As noted, a topical formulation [Rogaine, Minoxidil for Men] is available for treating baldness (see Chapter 101).

Diazoxide

Diazoxide [Hyperstat IV] is a close relative of the thiazide diuretics but lacks diuretic effects. The drug is indicated for hypertensive emergencies.

Cardiovascular Effects

Like hydralazine and minoxidil, diazoxide produces selective dilation of *arterioles;* the drug does not dilate veins. Intravenous diazoxide causes a rapid drop in diastolic and systolic pressure. Reduced arterial pressure triggers reflex tachycardia along with an increase in myocardial contractility; these effects combine to increase cardiac output. Arteriolar dilation also promotes substantial salt and water retention.

Vasodilation results from a direct effect on VSM. Diazoxide activates potassium channels in VSM, which results in hyperpolarization and a reduced ability to contract.

Pharmacokinetics

Diazoxide is administered intravenously, either as a bolus injection or by infusion. Bolus injection is generally preferred. Effects begin within minutes and may persist for hours. Most of the drug is eliminated unchanged in the urine.

Therapeutic Uses

Parenteral diazoxide is reserved for acute treatment of hypertensive emergencies (e.g., malignant hypertension, hypertensive encephalopathy). Oral antihypertensive agents should be instituted as soon as possible. In most cases, diazoxide can be discontinued within 4 to 5 days.

Adverse Effects

Reflex Tachycardia. Reflex tachycardia occurs in response to lowering of blood pressure. If necessary, tachycardia can be blunted with a beta blocker.

Salt and Water Retention. Diazoxide causes substantial retention of salt and water. The primary cause is reduced glomerular filtration. If fluid retention is severe, edema and even congestive heart failure can result. Edema and expansion of blood volume can be prevented with a diuretic; a high-ceiling agent (e.g., furosemide) is preferred.

Hyperglycemia. Like the thiazide diuretics, diazoxide can suppress release of insulin, and can thereby cause blood glucose to rise. For most patients, the degree of hyperglycemia is insignificant. However, for patients with diabetes, hyperglycemia may be substantial. If hyperglycemia develops, insulin dosage should be increased.

Hyperuricemia. Like the thiazide diuretics, diazoxide can decrease renal excretion of uric acid, thereby raising uric acid levels in blood. For most patients, hyperuricemia is asymptomatic. However, in gout-prone individuals, uric acid retention may precipitate a gouty attack.

Other Adverse Effects. Diazoxide may cause *GI effects* (nausea, vomiting, anorexia), *headache, flushing, hypotension,* and *temporary interruption of labor.* Rapid injection of large doses may produce *severe hypotension, anginal symptoms,* and *myocardial infarction.*

Drug Interactions

Diuretics. High-ceiling diuretics are used to counteract diazoxide-induced retention of salt and water. Since *thiazide diuretics* might potentiate the hyperglycemic and hyperuricemic effects of diazoxide, these diuretics should be avoided.

Antihypertensive Drugs. With the exception of high-ceiling diuretics, antihypertensive drugs should not be routinely combined with diazoxide. The concurrent use of diazoxide with other hypotensive agents may cause excessive lowering of blood pressure.

Preparations, Dosage, and Administration

Diazoxide [Hyperstat IV] is dispensed in solution (15 mg/ml) for IV administration. In the past, it was common practice to administer diazoxide as a single, large (300-mg) IV bolus. This is no longer recommended. Experts now consider it safer and more effective to use a series of "minibolus" injections, rather than one large injection. Accordingly, treatment should begin with a dose of 1 to 3 mg/kg injected by rapid (30 seconds or less) IV push. Dosing is then repeated every 5 to 15 minutes until the desired drop in blood pressure has been achieved. Once hypertension has been controlled, injections can be made every 4 to 24 hours. Blood pressure should be monitored closely until an acceptable and stable level has been produced; hourly monitoring should be performed thereafter. The patient should remain recumbent for at least 30 minutes after diazoxide injection. After 4 or 5 days of treatment, the patient can usually be switched to oral antihypertensive therapy.

Sodium Nitroprusside

Sodium nitroprusside [Nitropress] is a potent and efficacious vasodilator. It is also the fastest acting antihypertensive agent available. Because of these qualities, nitroprusside is a drug of choice for hypertensive emergencies.

Cardiovascular Effects

In contrast to hydralazine, minoxidil, and diazoxide, nitroprusside causes *venous* dilation in addition to *arteriolar* dilation. Curiously, although nitroprusside is an effective arteriolar dilator, reflex tachycardia is minimal. Administration is by IV infusion. Onset of effects is immediate. By adjusting the infusion rate, blood pressure can be depressed to almost any level desired. When the infusion is stopped, blood pressure returns to pretreatment levels in minutes. Nitroprusside can trigger retention of sodium and water; furosemide can help offset this effect.

Mechanism of Action

Once in the body, nitroprusside breaks down to release *nitric oxide* (Fig. 44–1), which then activates *guanylate cyclase,* an enzyme present in VSM. Guanylate cyclase catalyzes the production of *cyclic GMP,* which, through a series of reactions, causes vasodilation. This mechanism is similar to that of nitroglycerin.

Metabolism

As shown in Figure 44–1, nitroprusside contains five *cyanide groups,* which are split free in the first step of nitroprusside metabolism. *Nitric oxide,* the active component of the drug, is released next. Both reactions take place in smooth muscle. Once freed, the cyanide groups are converted to *thiocyanate* in the liver; *thiosulfate* is a required co-factor for the reaction. Thiocyanate is eliminated by the kidneys over several days.

Therapeutic Uses

Hypertensive Emergencies. Nitroprusside is used to lower blood pressure rapidly in hypertensive emergencies. Oral antihypertensive medication should be initiated simultaneously. During nitroprusside treatment, furosemide may be needed to prevent excessive retention of fluid.

Other Uses. Nitroprusside is approved for production of controlled hypotension during surgery (to reduce bleeding in the surgical field). In addition, the drug has been employed investigationally to treat severe, refractory congestive heart failure and myocardial infarction.

Adverse Effects

Excessive Hypotension. If administered too rapidly, nitroprusside can cause a precipitous fall in blood pressure, resulting in headache, palpitations, nausea, vomiting, and sweating. Blood pressure should be monitored continuously.

Cyanide Poisoning. Rarely, lethal amounts of cyanide have accumulated. Cyanide buildup is most likely in patients with liver disease and in those with low stores of thiosulfate, the co-factor for cyanide detoxification. The chances of cyanide poisoning can be minimized by avoiding rapid infusion (faster than 5 μg/kg/min) for a prolonged time and by coadministration of thiosulfate. If cyanide toxicity occurs, nitroprusside should be discontinued.

Thiocyanate Toxicity. When nitroprusside is given for several days, thiocyanate (a metabolite of nitroprusside) may accumulate. Although much less hazardous than cyanide, thiocyanate can also cause adverse effects. These effects, which involve the central nervous system (CNS), include disorientation, psychotic behavior, and delirium. To minimize toxicity, patients receiving nitroprusside for more than 3 days should be monitored for plasma levels of thiocyanate. These levels should not be allowed to exceed 0.1 mg/ml.

Preparations, Dosage, and Administration

Sodium nitroprusside [Nitropress] is dispensed in powdered form (50 mg) to be dissolved and then diluted for IV infusion. Fresh solutions may have a faint brown coloration; solutions that are deeply colored (blue, green, dark red) should be discarded. Solutions of nitroprusside can be degraded by light, and hence should be protected with an opaque material.

Blood pressure can be adjusted to practically any level by increasing or decreasing the rate of infusion. The initial infusion rate is 0.3 μg/kg/min. The maximal rate is 10 μg/kg/min. If infusion at the maximal rate for 10 minutes

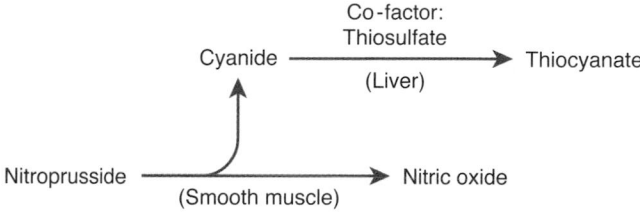

Figure 44–1 ■ **Structure and metabolism of sodium nitroprusside.**
Note the five cyanide groups in nitroprusside and their liberation during metabolism. Note also the release of nitric oxide, the active component of nitroprusside.

fails to produce an adequate drop in blood pressure, administration should be discontinued. During the infusion, blood pressure should be monitored continuously, with either an arterial line or an electronic monitoring device. No other drugs should be mixed with the infusion solution.

Angiotensin-Converting Enzyme Inhibitors

Inhibitors of angiotensin-converting enzyme (ACE) promote vasodilation by preventing the conversion of angiotensin I (a weak vasoconstrictor) into angiotensin II (a powerful vasoconstrictor). The primary indications for ACE inhibitors are essential hypertension and heart failure. In addition, these drugs can help preserve renal function in people with diabetes. The basic pharmacology of the ACE inhibitors is presented in Chapter 42. Their use in hypertension and heart failure is discussed in Chapters 45 and 46, respectively.

Angiotensin II Receptor Blockers

Angiotensin II receptor blockers (ARBs) are relatively new drugs with effects similar to those of the ACE inhibitors. However, instead of preventing formation of angiotensin II, these drugs block receptors for angiotensin II. Like the ACE inhibitors, ARBs dilate arterioles and veins. Currently, these drugs have three indications: hypertension, heart failure, and diabetic nephropathy. The basic pharmacology of the ARBs is discussed in Chapter 42.

Organic Nitrates

The organic nitrates (e.g., nitroglycerin, isosorbide dinitrate) produce selective dilation of veins; dilation of arterioles is minimal. The primary indication for these drugs is angina pectoris. In addition, nitroglycerin is given to treat heart failure and myocardial infarction, and to provide controlled hypotension during surgery. The pharmacology of the organic nitrates is discussed in Chapter 49.

Calcium Channel Blockers

The calcium channel blockers (e.g., verapamil, nifedipine) produce vasodilation by preventing calcium entry into VSM. At therapeutic doses, these drugs produce selective dilation of arterioles; very little venous dilation occurs. The vasodilating ability of these drugs is exploited in the treatment of hypertension and angina pectoris. The calcium channel blockers are the subject of Chapter 43.

Sympatholytics

Sympatholytics are drugs that promote vasodilation by preventing the sympathetic nervous system from causing vasoconstriction. Some of these drugs act by direct blockade of adrenergic receptors on blood vessels. Others act on sympathetic ganglia, adrenergic neurons, or the CNS.

Alpha-Adrenergic Blocking Agents. The alpha blockers (e.g., phentolamine, prazosin) promote vasodilation by preventing activation of alpha-adrenergic receptors on veins and arterioles. In their capacity as vasodilators, these drugs have multiple therapeutic applications, including hypertension, peripheral vascular disease, and pheochromocytoma. The alpha blockers are discussed in Chapter 18.

Ganglionic Blocking Agents. Ganglionic blocking agents interrupt impulse transmission through all ganglia of the autonomic nervous system. By doing so, they prevent sympathetic stimulation of arterioles and veins, and thereby cause vasodilation. Ganglionic blockers can be used for hypertensive emergencies and severe cases of essential hypertension. In addition, they can be given to produce hypotension during surgery. Prominent side effects—dry mouth, blurred vision, urinary retention, and paresis of the bowel—result from parasympathetic blockade. At this time, only two ganglionic blockers are available: trimethaphan and mecamylamine. Their pharmacology is discussed in Chapter 16.

Adrenergic Neuron Blocking Agents. Adrenergic neuron blockers (e.g., reserpine, guanethidine) act within terminals of adrenergic neurons to reduce norepinephrine release. By decreasing the release of norepinephrine from sympathetic nerves that control vasomotor tone, these drugs promote vasodilation. Their principal indication is hypertension. The adrenergic neuron blockers are discussed in Chapter 19.

Centrally Acting Agents. The centrally acting sympatholytics (e.g., clonidine, methyldopa) act within the CNS to inhibit impulse outflow along sympathetic nerves. These agents are used primarily for hypertension. Their pharmacology is discussed in Chapter 19.

⁙ KEY POINTS

- Some vasodilators are selective for arterioles, some are selective for veins, and some dilate both types of vessel.
- Drugs that dilate arterioles reduce cardiac afterload, and can thereby reduce cardiac work while increasing cardiac output and tissue perfusion.
- Drugs that dilate veins reduce cardiac preload, and can thereby reduce cardiac work, cardiac output, and tissue perfusion.
- Principal indications for vasodilators are essential hypertension, hypertensive crisis, angina pectoris, heart failure, and myocardial infarction.
- Drugs that dilate veins can cause orthostatic hypotension.
- Drugs that dilate arterioles or veins can cause reflex tachycardia, which increases cardiac work and elevates blood pressure. Reflex tachycardia can be blunted with a beta blocker.
- Drugs that dilate arterioles or veins can cause fluid retention. This response can be blunted with a diuretic.
- Hydralazine causes selective dilation of arterioles.
- Hydralazine can cause a syndrome that resembles SLE.
- Minoxidil causes selective and profound dilation of arterioles.
- Minoxidil can cause hypertrichosis.
- Sodium nitroprusside dilates arterioles and veins.
- Prolonged infusion of nitroprusside can result in toxic accumulation of cyanide and thiocyanate.

Drugs for Hypertension

Hypertension (elevated blood pressure [BP]) is a common, chronic disorder that affects 50 million Americans, and over 1 billion people worldwide. Left untreated, hypertension can lead to heart disease, kidney disease, and stroke. Conversely, a treatment program of lifestyle modifications and drug therapy can reduce both BP and the risk of long-term complications. However, it is important to appreciate that we cannot cure hypertension, we can only reduce symptoms. As a result, treatment must continue lifelong, making noncompliance a significant problem. Despite advances in management, hypertension remains underdiagnosed and undertreated: Among Americans with the disease, 70% have been diagnosed, 59% undergo treatment, and only 34% take sufficient medicine to bring their blood pressure under control.

Thirteen drug classes are used for treatment. All have been introduced in previous chapters. Hence, in this chapter, rather than struggling with a huge array of new drugs, we simply discuss the antihypertensive applications of drugs you already know about.

On May 14, 2003, the National Heart, Lung, and Blood Institute issued revised clinical guidelines on hypertension.

The new document—*The Seventh Report of the Joint National Committee on Prevention, Detection, Evaluation, and Treatment of High Blood Pressure,* known simply as *JNC 7*—was prepared by a special committee of the National High Blood Pressure Education Program. Recommendations in JNC 7 update and simplify those of JNC 6, published in 1997. Important changes include a new blood-pressure classification scheme, increased emphasis on controlling systolic blood pressure, and the recommendation to use thiazide diuretics as initial therapy for most patients. Throughout this chapter, clinical practice recommendations reflect those in JNC 7.

CLASSIFICATION OF BLOOD PRESSURE

JNC 7 defines four blood pressure categories: normal, prehypertension, stage 1 hypertension, and stage 2 hypertension (Table 45-1). This scheme differs from that of JNC 6 in three ways:

- The cutoff values for normal blood pressure have been reduced.
- A new category—prehypertension—has been added.
- Two classes of hypertension—stages 2 and 3 from JNC 6—have been combined into one—stage 2 in JNC 7—because management of both is much the same.

Normal. In JNC 7, normal blood pressure is defined as systolic BP <120 mm Hg and diastolic BP <80 mm Hg, compared with <130/<85 in JNC 6. Why were the cutoff values reduced? Because the values from JNC 6 are not as safe as previously believed.

Prehypertension. The classification of prehypertension indicates increased risk of cardiovascular disease—even though outright hypertension has not yet developed. Data from the Framingham Heart Study show that, relative to people with normal blood pressure, those with pressure in the prehypertension range have a 2- to 3-fold increased risk of cardiovascular events. To reduce risk, these people should adopt certain health-promoting lifestyle changes (see below). Prehypertension affects about 22% of American adults, which equals 45 million people.

Hypertension. Hypertension is defined as systolic BP >140 mm Hg or diastolic BP >90 mm Hg. If systolic BP is above 140 mm Hg and diastolic BP is below 90 mm Hg, a diagnosis of *isolated systolic hypertension* (ISH) applies. When systolic BP and diastolic BP fall in different categories, classification is based on the higher category. For example, a reading of 160/92 mm Hg indicates stage 2 hypertension, and a reading of 170/82 indicates stage 2 ISH.

449

TABLE 45–1 ▪■ Classification of Blood Pressure for Adults Age 18 and Older			
Classification*	Systolic (mm Hg)		Diastolic (mm Hg)
Normal	<120	*and*	<80
Prehypertension	120–139	*or*	80–89
Stage 1 Hypertension	140–159	*or*	90–99
Stage 2 Hypertension	≥160	*or*	≥100

*Not taking any antihypertensive drugs and not acutely ill. When systolic and diastolic blood pressures fall into different categories, the higher category should be selected to classify blood pressure status. For example, 160/92 mm Hg should be classified as stage 2 hypertension. Isolated systolic hypertension is defined as systolic BP of 140 mm Hg or higher and diastolic BP below 90 mm Hg and staged appropriately (e.g., 170/82 is defined as stage 2 isolated systolic hypertension).
Data from The Seventh Report of the Joint National Committee on Detection, Evaluation, and Treatment of High Blood Pressure. JAMA 2003;289:2560–2572.

TABLE 45–2 ▪■ Types of Hypertension and Their Frequency	
Type of Hypertension	Frequency (%)
Primary (Essential) Hypertension	92
Secondary Hypertension	
Chronic renal disease	4
Renovascular disease	2
Oral contraceptive–induced	1
Coarctation of the aorta	0.3
Primary aldosteronism	0.2
Cushing's syndrome	0.1
Pheochromocytoma	0.1
Sleep apnea	?
Thyroid or parathyroid disease	?

Diagnosis of hypertension should be based on several blood pressure readings, not just one. If an initial screen shows that blood pressure is elevated (but does not represent an immediate danger), measurement should be repeated on two subsequent visits. At each visit, two measurements should be made, at least 5 minutes apart. The patient should be seated in a chair—not on an examination table—with his or her feet on the floor. High readings should be confirmed in the contralateral arm. If the mean of all readings shows that systolic BP is indeed greater than 140 mm Hg or that diastolic BP is greater than 90 mm Hg, a diagnosis of hypertension can be made.

TYPES OF HYPERTENSION

There are two broad categories of hypertension: *primary hypertension* and *secondary hypertension*. As indicated in Table 45–2, primary hypertension is by far the most common form of hypertensive disease. Less than 10% of people with hypertension have a secondary form.

Primary (Essential) Hypertension

Primary hypertension is defined as hypertension that has no identifiable cause. A diagnosis of primary hypertension is made by ruling out probable specific causes of blood pressure elevation. Primary hypertension is a chronic, progressive disorder. In the absence of treatment, patients will experience a continuous, gradual rise in blood pressure over the remainder of their lives.

In the United States, primary hypertension affects about 25% of adults. However, not all groups are at equal risk: older people are at higher risk than younger people; African Americans and Mexican Americans are at higher risk than white Americans; postmenopausal women are at higher risk than premenopausal women; and obese people are at higher risk than lean people.

Although the cause of primary hypertension is unknown, the condition can be successfully treated. It should be un-

derstood, however, that treatment is not curative: drugs can lower blood pressure, but they do not eliminate the underlying pathology. Consequently, treatment must continue lifelong.

Primary hypertension is also referred to as *essential hypertension*. This alternative name preceded the term *primary hypertension* and reflects our ignorance about the cause of the problem. Historically, it had been noted that, as people grew older, their blood pressure rose. Why older people had elevated blood pressure was (and remains) unknown. One hypothesis noted that, as people aged, their vascular systems offered greater resistance to blood flow. In order to move blood against this increased resistance, a compensatory increase in blood pressure was required. Therefore, the hypertension that occurred with age was seen as being "essential" for providing adequate perfusion of tissues—hence, the term *essential hypertension*. Over time, the term *essential hypertension* came to be applied to all cases of hypertension for which an underlying cause could not be found.

Secondary Hypertension

Secondary hypertension is defined as an elevation of blood pressure brought on by an identifiable primary cause. The most common causes are listed in Table 45–2.

Because secondary hypertension results from an identifiable cause, it may be possible to treat that cause directly, rather than relying on drugs for symptomatic relief. As a result, some individuals can actually be cured. For example, if hypertension occurs secondary to pheochromocytoma (a catecholamine-secreting tumor), surgical removal of the tumor may produce permanent cure. When cure is not possible, secondary hypertension can be managed with the same drugs used for primary hypertension.

CONSEQUENCES OF HYPERTENSION

Chronic hypertension is associated with increased morbidity and mortality. Left untreated, prolonged elevation of blood pressure can lead to heart disease (myocardial infarction [MI], heart failure, angina pectoris), kidney disease, and stroke. The

Special Interest Topic

BOX 45–1 ▦■ ISOLATED SYSTOLIC HYPERTENSION: THE REAL KILLER OF AGING AMERICANS

Over the past decade, several large randomized clinical trials involving older hypertensive patients have produced unequivocal evidence that, compared with elevated *diastolic* BP, elevated *systolic* BP is the stronger predictor of cardiovascular disease, kidney disease, stroke, and death. Additional studies have shown that, when elevated systolic BP is reduced, there is a corresponding reduction in the incidence of kidney failure, heart failure, MI, stroke, and death. Accordingly, in 2000, the Coordinating Committee of the National High Blood Pressure Education Program issued a clinical advisory recommending that systolic BP—rather than diastolic BP—be used as the major clinical end point for the detection, evaluation, and treatment of hypertension, especially in middle-aged and older Americans. The importance of elevated systolic pressure is reflected in the recommendations of JNC 7, released in 2003.

Some readers may be asking, "What's new here? I mean, hasn't elevated systolic BP always been a concern?" Well, no, it hasn't. In fact, until recently, isolated systolic hypertension (ISH)—defined as systolic BP above 140 mm Hg and diastolic BP below 90 mm Hg—was considered a relatively benign condition that did not merit treatment. After all, most experts agreed that, in people with hypertension, elevated diastolic BP—not elevated systolic BP—was the principal cause of morbidity and mortality. Of course, this view has been proven dead wrong.

ISH is primarily a disease of the elderly. As we grow older, systolic BP gradually rises. The underlying cause is increased stiffness (reduced compliance) in large arteries—owing to progressive replacement of elastin with collagen in the arterial wall. Among older Americans, ISH is the most common form of hypertension: According to the National Health and Nutrition Examination Survey (NHANES), of all hypertensive individuals over the age of 60, fully 65% have ISH. Because of their ISH, older people are at increased risk, as demonstrated in the Multiple Risk Factor Intervention Trial (MRFIT), which

evaluated over 316,000 men and found a nearly linear relationship between increased systolic BP and increased risk of adverse cardiovascular events.

Does lowering elevated systolic BP reduce cardiovascular risk? You bet! The benefits of treating ISH have been documented in several large, randomized controlled trials. Important among these are the Systolic Hypertension in the Elderly Program (SHEP) and the Systolic Hypertension in Europe (Syst-Eur) trial. An analysis of the results of these trials indicated that lowering systolic BP decreased overall mortality by 13%, cardiovascular mortality by 18%, cardiovascular complications by 26%, coronary events by 23%, and stroke by 30%.

Unfortunately, among people with ISH, control of blood pressure is generally poor. For most hypertensive people, the target BP is 140/90 mm Hg. However, among elderly African Americans, only 25% achieve this goal. And among white Americans, the success rate is even worse: Only 18% achieve the goal. This low success rate is both sad and troubling, in that it means many people will experience unnecessary morbidity and mortality.

The low rate of blood pressure control in the elderly, coupled with our heightened appreciation of the dangers of ISH, led the Coordinating Committee to issue its advisory. As noted, the Committee recommended that systolic BP, rather than diastolic BP, be the major consideration in the detection, evaluation, and treatment of hypertension—especially in older Americans. The Committee recommended using either a low-dose thiazide diuretic (with or without a beta blocker) or a long-acting dihydropyridine CCB for initial treatment. These recommendations were based in part on the successful use of these drugs in the SHEP and Syst-Eur trials. Although ACE inhibitors were not recommended by the Committee, recent evidence indicates that these drugs too can reduce the risk of stroke, MI, heart failure, and death in older hypertensive people.

---

degree of injury is directly related to the degree of pressure elevation: the higher the pressure, the greater the risk. Among people 40 to 70 years old, the risk of cardiovascular disease is doubled for each 20 mm Hg increase in systolic BP or each 10 mm Hg increase in diastolic BP—beginning at 115/75 mm Hg and continuing through 185/155 mm Hg. For people over the age of 50, elevated *systolic* BP poses a greater risk than elevated diastolic BP (see Box 45-1). For patients of all ages, hypertension-related deaths result largely from cerebral hemorrhage, renal failure, heart failure, and MI.

Unfortunately, despite its potential for serious harm, hypertension usually remains asymptomatic until long after injury has begun to develop. As a result, the disease can exist for years before overt pathology is evident. Because injury develops slowly and progressively, and because hypertension rarely causes discomfort, many people who have the disease don't know it. Furthermore, many who do know it forgo treatment, largely because hypertension doesn't make them feel bad—that is, until it's too late.

MANAGEMENT OF CHRONIC HYPERTENSION I: BASIC CONSIDERATIONS

Benefits of Lowering Blood Pressure

Multiple clinical trials have demonstrated unequivocally that, when the blood pressure of hypertensive individuals is lowered, morbidity is decreased and life is prolonged. Treatment reduces the incidence of stroke by 35% to 40%, MI by 20% to 25%, and heart failure by more than 50%. Although reductions in morbidity are not as dramatic, they are nonetheless significant: Among patients with stage 1 hypertension plus additional cardiovascular risk factors, one death would be prevented for every 11 patients who reduced systolic pressure by 12 mm Hg for a period of 10 years—and among those with hypertension plus cardiovascular disease or target-organ damage, 1 death would be prevented for every 9 patients who achieved a sustained 12 mm Hg reduction in pressure.

Patient Evaluation

Evaluation of patients with hypertension has 2 major objectives. Specifically, we must assess for (1) identifiable causes of hypertension, and (2) factors that increase cardiovascular risk. To aid evaluation, certain diagnostic tests are required.

Hypertension with a Treatable Cause. As discussed above, some forms of hypertension result from treatable causes, such as Cushing's syndrome, pheochromocytoma, and oral contraceptive use (Table 45-2). Patients should be evaluated for these causes and managed appropriately. In many cases, direct treatment of the underlying cause can control blood pressure, thereby eliminating the need for further antihypertensive therapy.

Factors That Increase Cardiovascular Risk. Two types of factors—existing target-organ damage and major cardiovascular risk factors—increase the risk of cardiovascular events in patients with hypertension. When these factors are present, aggressive therapy is indicated. Accordingly, in order to select appropriate interventions, we must identify patients with the following types of *target-organ damage*

- Heart diseases
  - Left ventricular hypertrophy
  - Angina pectoris
  - Prior MI
  - Prior coronary revascularization
  - Heart failure
- Stroke or transient ischemic attack
- Chronic kidney disease
- Peripheral arterial disease
- Retinopathy

as well as patients with the following *major cardiovascular risk factors* (other than hypertension)

- Cigarette smoking
- Obesity
- Inadequate exercise
- Dyslipidemia
- Diabetes
- Microalbuminuria
- Advancing age (>55 years for men, >65 years for women)
- Family history of premature cardiovascular disease

Diagnostic Tests. The following tests should be done in all patients: electrocardiogram; complete urinalysis; hemoglobin and hematocrit; and blood levels of sodium, potassium, calcium, creatinine, glucose, uric acid, triglycerides, and cholesterol (total, LDL, and HDL cholesterol).

Treatment Goals

The ultimate goal in treating hypertension is to reduce cardiovascular and renal morbidity and mortality. Hopefully, this can be accomplished without decreasing quality of life with the drugs employed. For most patients with stage 1 or stage 2 hypertension, the goal is to maintain systolic BP below 140 mm Hg and diastolic BP *below* 90 mm Hg. For patients with diabetes or chronic kidney disease, the target blood pressure is lower: <130/<80 mm Hg. For patients over the age of 50, reducing *systolic* pressure is the primary goal; however, although treatment is focused on systolic pressure, interventions that achieve the systolic goal will likely achieve the diastolic goal too.

Therapeutic Interventions

We can reduce blood pressure in two ways: We can implement healthy lifestyle changes and we can treat with antihypertensive drugs. As shown in Table 45-3, for people with *prehypertension,* lifestyle changes are all that is needed. In contrast, for those with *hypertension*—either stage 1 or stage 2—a *combination* of lifestyle changes and drugs is indicated. Lifestyle changes and drug therapy are discussed in detail below.

TABLE 45–3 ■ Overview of Blood Pressure Management in Adults 18 Years and Older				
		Bood Pressure Goal	
Blood Pressure Classification	**Therapeutic Interventions**	**Patient *Without* Diabetes or Chronic Kidney Disease**	**Patients *With* Diabetes or Chronic Kidney Disease**
Normal	Encourage lifestyle changes	Prevent increase	Prevent increase
Prehypertension	Initiate lifestyle changes	Prevent increase/ promote decrease	Prevent increase/ promote decrease
Stage 1 Hypertension	Initiate or continue lifestyle changes and begin antihypertensive drug therapy	<140/<90 mm Hg	<130/<80 mm Hg
Stage 2 Hypertension	Initiate or continue lifestyle changes and begin or intensify antihypertensive drug therapy	<140/<90 mm Hg	<130/<80 mm Hg

SBP = systolic blood pressure, DBP = diastolic blood pressure.
Recommendations from The Seventh Report of the Joint National Committee on Detection, Evaluation, and Treatment of High Blood Pressure. JAMA 2003;289:2560–2572.

MANAGEMENT OF CHRONIC HYPERTENSION II: LIFESTYLE MODIFICATIONS

Lifestyle changes offer multiple cardiovascular benefits—and they do so with little cost and minimal risk. When implemented before hypertension develops, they may actually prevent hypertension. When implemented after hypertension has developed, they can lower blood pressure, thereby decreasing or eliminating the need for drugs. Lastly, lifestyle modifications can decrease other cardiovascular risk factors. Accordingly, all patients should be strongly encouraged to adopt a healthy lifestyle. Key components are discussed below.

Weight Loss. There is a direct relationship between obesity and elevation of blood pressure. Studies indicate that weight loss can reduce blood pressure in 60% to 80% of overweight hypertensive individuals. In addition, weight loss can enhance responses to antihypertensive drugs. Consequently, a program of calorie restriction and exercise is recommended for all patients who are overweight. The goal is to achieve a body mass index in the normal range (18.5–24.9).*

Sodium Restriction. Reduction of sodium chloride (salt) intake can lower blood pressure in people with hypertension. In addition, salt restriction can enhance the hypotensive effects of drugs. However, recent data indicate that the benefits of sodium restriction are short lasting: Over time, blood pressure returns to its original level, despite continued salt restriction. Nonetheless, it is recommended that all people with hypertension consume no more than 6 gm of sodium chloride (2.4 gm of sodium) a day. To facilitate salt restriction, patients should be given information on the salt content of foods.

Experts disagree about the relationship between salt intake and blood pressure in *normotensive* patients. In particular, they disagree as to whether a high-salt diet *causes* hypertension. Hence, for people with normal blood pressure, a low-salt diet may be considered healthy or unnecessary, depending on which expert you consult.

The DASH Eating Plan. Two studies have shown that we can reduce blood pressure by adopting a healthy diet, known as the Dietary Approaches to Stop Hypertension (DASH) eating plan. This diet is rich in fruits, vegetables, and lowfat dairy products, and low in total fat, saturated fats, and cholesterol. In addition, the plan encourages intake of whole grain products, fish, poultry, and nuts, and recommends minimal intake of red meat and sweets. Details are available online at *www.nhlbi.nih.gov/health/public/heart/hbp/dash.*

Alcohol Restriction. Excessive alcohol consumption can raise blood pressure and create resistance to antihypertensive drugs. Accordingly, patients should limit alcohol intake: Most men should consume no more than 1 ounce/day; women and lighter men should consume no more than 0.5 ounce/day. (One ounce of ethanol is equivalent to about two mixed drinks, two glasses of wine, or two cans of beer.)

Aerobic Exercise. Regular aerobic exercise (e.g., jogging, walking, swimming, bicycling) can reduce blood pressure by about 10 mm Hg. In addition, exercise facilitates weight loss, reduces the risk of cardiovascular disease, and reduces all-cause mortality. In normotensive people, exercise decreases the risk of developing hypertension. Accordingly, all people with a sedentary lifestyle should be encouraged to develop an exercise program. An activity as simple as brisk walking 30 to 45 minutes most days of the week is beneficial.

Smoking Cessation. Smoking is a major risk factor for cardiovascular disease. Each time a cigarette is smoked, blood pressure rises. In patients with hypertension, smoking may reduce the effects of antihypertensive drugs. Clearly, all patients who smoke should be strongly encouraged to quit. (Pharmacologic aids to smoking cessation are discussed in Chapter 38.) As a rule, use of nicotine-replacement products (e.g., nicotine gum, nicotine patch) does not elevate blood pressure. The cardiovascular benefits of quitting become evident within a year.

Maintenance of Potassium and Calcium Intake. Potassium has a beneficial effect on blood pressure. In patients with hypertension, potassium can lower blood pressure. In normotensive people, high potassium intake helps protect against hypertension, whereas low intake elevates blood pressure. For optimal cardiovascular effects, all people should take in 50 to 90 mmol of potassium a day. Preferred sources are fresh fruits and vegetables. If hypokalemia develops secondary to diuretic therapy, dietary intake may be insufficient to correct the problem. In this case, the patient may need to use a potassium supplement, a potassium-sparing diuretic, or a potassium-containing salt substitute.

Although adequate calcium is needed for overall good health, the impact of calcium on blood pressure is only modest. In epidemiologic studies, high calcium intake is associated with a reduced incidence of hypertension. Among patients with hypertension, a few may be helped by increasing calcium intake. To maintain good health, calcium intake should be 1000 mg/day for adults under the age of 50, and 1200 mg/day for those 51 and older.

MANAGEMENT OF CHRONIC HYPERTENSION III: PHARMACOLOGIC THERAPY

Drug therapy, together with lifestyle modifications, can control blood pressure in all patients with chronic hypertension. The decision to use drugs should be the result of collaboration between clinician and patient. A wide range of antihypertensive drugs is available, permitting versatility in the regimen. Consequently, for the majority of patients, it should be possible to establish a program that is effective and yet devoid of objectionable side effects.

Review of Blood Pressure Control

Before discussing the antihypertensive drugs, we need to review the major mechanisms by which blood pressure is controlled. This information will help us understand the mechanisms by which drugs lower blood pressure.

---

*The definition and calculation of body mass index are presented in Chapter 78 (Drugs for Obesity).

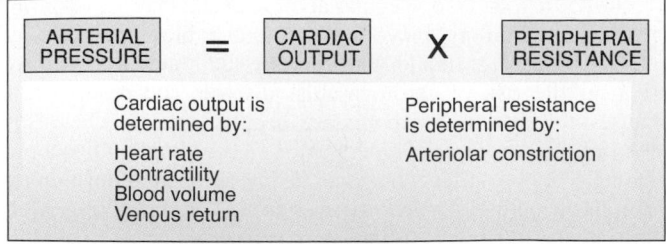

Figure 45–1 ■ **Primary determinants of arterial blood pressure.**

Principal Determinants of Blood Pressure

The principal determinants of blood pressure are summarized in Figure 45–1. As indicated, arterial pressure is the product of cardiac output and peripheral resistance. An increase in either will increase blood pressure.

As shown in the figure, cardiac output is influenced by four factors: (1) heart rate, (2) myocardial contractility (force of contraction), (3) blood volume, and (4) venous return of blood to the heart. An increase in any of these factors will increase cardiac output, thereby causing blood pressure to rise. Conversely, by reducing these factors, we can make blood pressure fall. Drugs that affect these factors are (1) beta blockers, verapamil, and diltiazem and other drugs that decrease heart rate and contractile force; (2) diuretics and other drugs that decrease blood volume; and (3) venodilators, which reduce venous return.

Peripheral vascular resistance is regulated by arteriolar constriction. Accordingly, we can reduce blood pressure with drugs that promote arteriolar dilation.

Systems That Help Regulate Blood Pressure

Having established that blood pressure is determined by heart rate, myocardial contractility, blood volume, venous return, and arteriolar constriction, we will now examine how these factors are regulated. Three regulatory systems are of particular significance: (1) the sympathetic nervous system, (2) the renin-angiotensin-aldosterone system (RAAS), and (3) the kidney.

Sympathetic Baroreceptor Reflex. The sympathetic nervous system employs a reflex circuit—the baroreceptor reflex—to keep blood pressure at a preset level. This circuit operates as follows: (1) Baroreceptors in the aortic arch and carotid sinus sense blood pressure and relay this information to the brainstem. (2) When blood pressure is perceived as too low, the brainstem sends impulses along sympathetic nerves to stimulate the heart and blood vessels. (3) Blood pressure is then elevated by (a) activation of beta$_1$ receptors in the heart, resulting in increased cardiac output; and (b) activation of vascular alpha$_1$ receptors, resulting in vasoconstriction. (4) When blood pressure has been restored to an acceptable level, sympathetic stimulation of the heart and vascular smooth muscle subsides.

The baroreceptor reflex frequently opposes our attempts to reduce blood pressure with drugs. Opposition occurs because the "set point" of the baroreceptors is high in people with hypertension. That is, the baroreceptors are set to perceive excessively high blood pressure as "normal" (i.e., appropriate). As a result, the system operates to maintain blood pressure at pathologic levels. Consequently, when we at-

tempt to lower blood pressure using drugs, the reduced (healthier) pressure is interpreted by the baroreceptors as below what it should be, and, in response, signals are sent along sympathetic nerves to "correct" the reduction. These signals produce reflex tachycardia and vasoconstriction—responses that can counteract the hypotensive effects of drugs. Clearly, if treatment is to succeed, the regimen must compensate for the resistance offered by the baroreceptor reflex. Inclusion of a *beta blocker,* which will block reflex tachycardia, can be an effective method of compensation. Fortunately, when blood pressure has been suppressed with drugs for an extended time, the baroreceptors become reset at a lower level. Consequently, as therapy proceeds, sympathetic reflexes offer progressively less resistance to the hypotensive effects of medication.

Renin-Angiotensin-Aldosterone System. The RAAS can elevate blood pressure, thereby negating the hypotensive effects of our drugs. The RAAS is discussed at length in Chapter 42 and reviewed briefly here.

How does the RAAS elevate blood pressure? The process begins with the release of renin from juxtaglomerular cells of the kidney. These cells release renin in response to reduced renal blood flow, reduced blood volume, reduced blood pressure, and activation of beta$_1$-adrenergic receptors on the cell surface. Following its release, renin promotes the conversion of angiotensinogen into angiotensin I, a weak vasoconstrictor. After this, *angiotensin-converting enzyme* (ACE) acts on angiotensin I to form *angiotensin II,* a compound that constricts systemic and renal blood vessels. Constriction of systemic blood vessels elevates blood pressure by increasing peripheral resistance. Constriction of renal blood vessels elevates blood pressure by reducing glomerular filtration, which causes retention of salt and water, which in turn increases blood volume and blood pressure. In addition to causing vasoconstriction, angiotensin II causes release of *aldosterone* from the adrenal cortex. Aldosterone acts on the kidneys to further increase retention of sodium and water.

Since drug-induced reductions in blood pressure can activate the RAAS, this system can counteract the effect we are trying to achieve. We have four ways to cope with this problem. First, we can suppress renin release with *beta blockers.* Second, we can prevent the conversion of angiotensin I into angiotensin II with an *ACE inhibitor.* Third, we can block receptors for angiotensin II with an *angiotensin II receptor blocker.* And fourth, we can block receptors for aldosterone with an *aldosterone receptor blocker.*

Renal Regulation of Blood Pressure. As discussed in Chapter 41, the kidney plays a central role in long-term regulation of blood pressure. When blood pressure falls, glomerular filtration rate (GFR) falls as well, thereby promoting retention of sodium, chloride, and water. The resultant increase in blood volume increases venous return to the heart, causing an increase in cardiac output, which in turn increases arterial pressure. We can neutralize renal effects on blood pressure with *diuretics.*

Antihypertensive Mechanisms: Sites of Drug Action and Effects Produced

As discussed, drugs can lower blood pressure by reducing heart rate, myocardial contractility, blood volume, venous return, and the tone of arteriolar smooth muscle. In this section

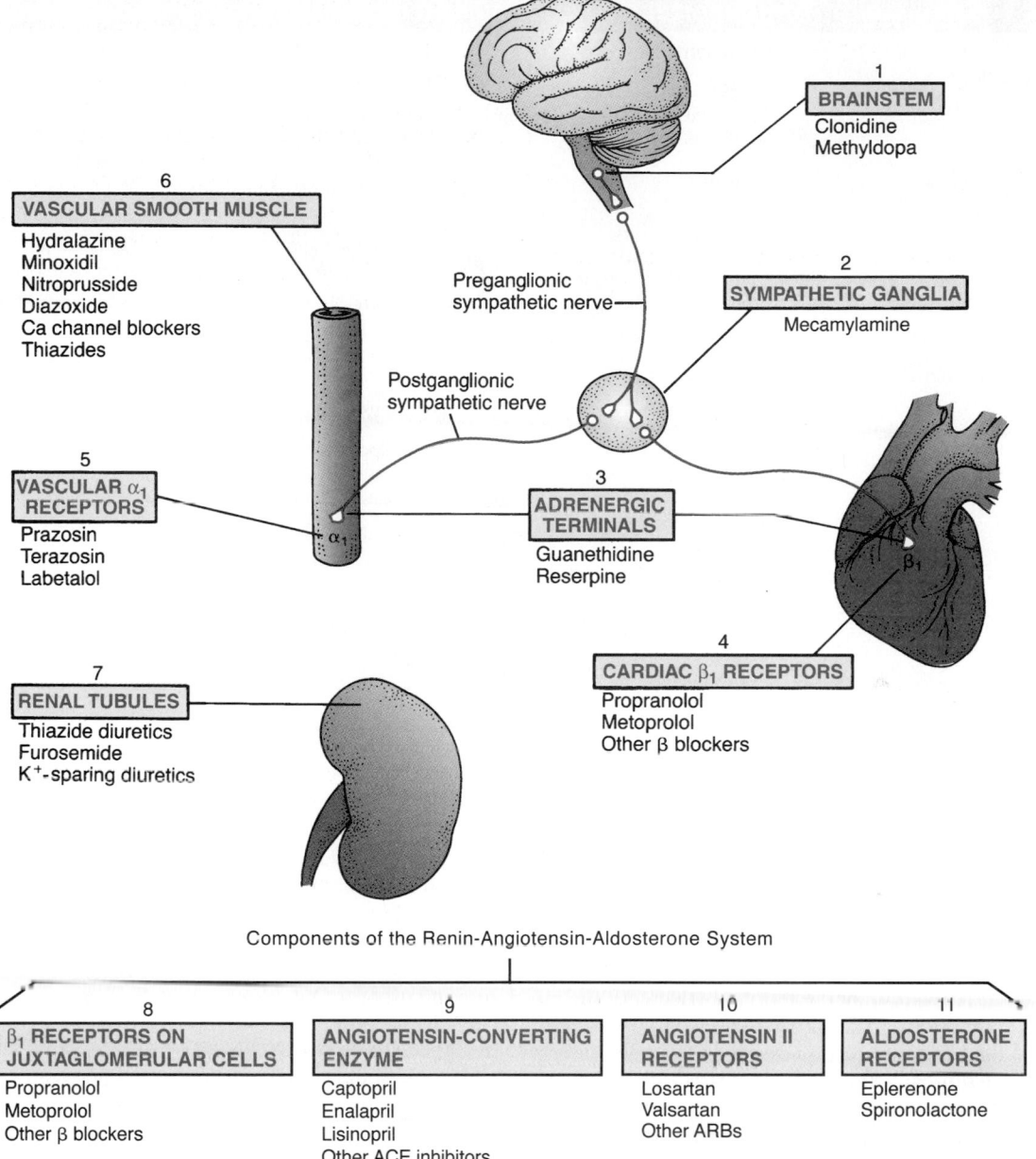

Figure 45–2 ■ Sites of action of antihypertensive drugs.
Note that some antihypertensive agents act at more than one site: beta blockers act at sites 4 and 8, and thiazides act at sites 6 and 7. The hemodynamic consequences of drug actions at the sites depicted are summarized in Table 45–4.
(ACE = angiotensin-converting enzyme, ARB = angiotensin II receptor blocker.)

we survey the principal mechanisms by which drugs produce these effects.

The major mechanisms for lowering blood pressure are summarized in Figure 45–2 and Table 45–4. The figure depicts the 11 principal sites at which antihypertensive drugs act. The table summarizes the effects elicited by drug actions at these sites. The sites of drug action and resultant effects are described briefly in the following section. Sites numbered 1 through 11 below correspond with sites 1 through 11 in the figure and table.

1—Brainstem. Antihypertensive drugs acting in the brainstem suppress sympathetic outflow to the heart and blood vessels, resulting in decreased heart rate, decreased myocardial contractility, and vasodilation. Vasodilation contributes the most to reductions in blood pressure. Dilation of arterioles reduces blood pressure by decreasing vascular resistance. Dilation of veins decreases blood pressure by decreasing venous return to the heart.

2—Sympathetic Ganglia. Ganglionic blockade reduces sympathetic stimulation of the heart and blood vessels. Anti-

TABLE 45–4 ■ Summary of Antihypertensive Effects Elicited by Drug Actions at Specific Sites

Site of Drug Action*	Representative Drug	Drug Effects
1. Brainstem	Clonidine	Suppression of sympathetic outflow decreases sympathetic stimulation of the heart and blood vessels.
2. Sympathetic ganglia	Trimethaphan	Ganglionic blockade reduces sympathetic stimulation of the heart and blood vessels.
3. Adrenergic nerve terminals	Guanethidine	Reduced norepinephrine release decreases sympathetic stimulation of the heart and blood vessels.
4. Cardiac beta$_1$ receptors	Propranolol	Beta$_1$ blockade decreases heart rate and myocardial contractility.
5. Vascular alpha$_1$ receptors	Prazosin	Alpha$_1$ blockade causes vasodilation.
6. Vascular smooth muscle	Hydralazine	Relaxation of vascular smooth muscle causes vasodilation.
7. Renal tubules	Chlorothiazide	Promotion of diuresis results in decreased blood volume.
8. Beta$_1$ receptors on juxtaglomerular cells	Propranolol	Beta$_1$ blockade suppresses renin release, resulting in (1) vasodilation secondary to reduced production of angiotensin II, and (2) prevention of aldosterone-mediated volume expansion.
9. Angiotensin-converting enzyme (ACE)	Captopril	Inhibition of ACE decreases formation of angiotensin II and thereby prevents (1) vasoconstriction, and (2) aldosterone-mediated volume expansion.
10. Angiotensin II receptors	Losartan	Blockade of angiotensin II receptors prevents angiotensin-mediated vasoconstriction and aldosterone-mediated volume expansion.
11. Aldosterone receptors	Eplerenone	Blockade of aldosterone receptors in the kidney promotes excretion of sodium and water, and thereby reduces blood volume.

*Sites 1 through 11 in this table correspond to sites 1 through 11 in Figure 45–2.

hypertensive effects result primarily from dilation of arterioles and veins. Ganglionic blocking agents produce such a profound reduction in blood pressure that they are used rarely, and then only for hypertensive emergencies.

3—Terminals of Adrenergic Nerves. Antihypertensive agents that act at adrenergic nerve terminals decrease the release of norepinephrine, resulting in decreased sympathetic stimulation of the heart and blood vessels.

4—Beta$_1$-Adrenergic Receptors on the Heart. Blockade of cardiac beta$_1$ receptors prevents sympathetic stimulation of the heart. As a result, heart rate and myocardial contractility decline.

5—Alpha$_1$-Adrenergic Receptors on Blood Vessels. Blockade of vascular alpha$_1$ receptors promotes dilation of arterioles and veins. Arteriolar dilation reduces peripheral resistance. Venous dilation reduces venous return to the heart.

6—Vascular Smooth Muscle. Several antihypertensive drugs (see Fig. 45–2) act directly on vascular smooth muscle to cause relaxation. Two of these agents—sodium nitroprusside and diazoxide—are used only for hypertensive emergencies. The rest are used for chronic hypertension.

7—Renal Tubules. Diuretics act on renal tubules to promote salt and water excretion. As a result, blood volume declines, causing blood pressure to fall.

8—Beta$_1$ Receptors on Juxtaglomerular Cells. Blockade of beta$_1$ receptors on juxtaglomerular cells suppresses release of renin. The resultant decrease in angiotensin II levels has three effects: peripheral vasodilation, renal vasodilation, and suppression of aldosterone-mediated volume expansion.

9—Angiotensin-Converting Enzyme. Inhibitors of ACE suppress formation of angiotensin II. The result is peripheral vasodilation, renal vasodilation, and suppression of aldosterone-mediated volume expansion.

10—Angiotensin II Receptors. Blockade of angiotensin II receptors prevents the actions of angiotensin II. Hence blockade results in peripheral vasodilation, renal vasodilation, and suppression of aldosterone-mediated volume expansion.

11—Aldosterone Receptors. Blockade of aldosterone receptors in the kidney promotes excretion of sodium and water, and thereby reduces blood volume.

Classes of Antihypertensive Drugs

In this section we consider the principal drugs employed to treat *chronic hypertension*. Drugs for *hypertensive emergencies* and *hypertensive disorders of pregnancy* are considered separately.

Individual antihypertensive drugs and their classes are summarized in Table 45–5. Combination products are summarized in Table 45–6. All of these drugs have been discussed in previous chapters. Accordingly, discussion here is limited to their use in hypertension. Of primary interest are mechanisms of antihypertensive action and major adverse effects.

Diuretics

Diuretics are a mainstay of antihypertensive therapy. These drugs reduce blood pressure when used alone, and they can enhance the effects of other hypotensive drugs. The basic pharmacology of the diuretics is discussed in Chapter 39.

Thiazide Diuretics. The thiazide diuretics (e.g., hydrochlorothiazide) are among the most commonly used antihy-

TABLE 45–5 ▪▪ Drugs for Chronic Hypertension

Diuretics	Sympatholytics	Others
Thiazides and Related Diuretics	**Beta Blockers**	**ACE Inhibitors**
Bendroflumethiazide	Acebutolol (has ISA)	Benazepril
Benzthiazide	Atenolol	Captopril
Chlorothiazide	Betaxolol	Enalapril
Chlorthalidone	Bisoprolol	Fosinopril
Cyclothiazide	Carteolol (has ISA)	Lisinopril
Hydrochlorothiazide	Metoprolol	Moexipril
Hydroflumethiazide	Nadolol	Quinapril
Indapamide	Penbutolol (has ISA)	Ramipril
Methyclothiazide	Pindolol (has ISA)	Trandolapril
Metolazone	Propranolol	
Polythiazide	Timolol	**Aldosterone Receptor Blockers**
Quinethazone		Eplerenone
Trichlormethiazide	**Alpha₁ Blockers**	Spironolactone
Loop Diuretics	Doxazosin	**Angiotensin II Receptor Blockers**
Furosemide	Prazosin	Candesartan
Ethacrynic acid	Terazosin	Eprosartan
Bumetanide		Irbesartan
Torsemide	**Alpha/Beta Blockers**	Losartan
	Carvedilol	Olmesartan
Potassium-Sparing Diuretics	Labetalol	Telmisartan
Spironolactone		Valsartan
Triamterene	**Centrally Acting Alpha₂ Agonists**	
Amiloride	Clonidine	**Calcium Channel Blockers**
	Methyldopa	Amlodipine
	Guanabenz	Diltiazem (non-DHP)
	Guanfacine	Felodipine
		Isradipine
	Adrenergic Neuron Blockers	Nifedipine
	Guanethidine	Nicardipine
	Guanadrel	Nimodipine
	Reserpine	Nisoldipine
		Verapamil (non-DHP)
		Direct-Acting Vasodilators
		Hydralazine
		Minoxidil

DHP = dihydropyridine, ISA = intrinsic sympathomimetic activity.

pertensive drugs. Thiazides reduce blood pressure by two mechanisms: reduction of blood volume and reduction of arterial resistance. Reduced blood volume is responsible for initial antihypertensive effects. Reduced vascular resistance develops over time and is responsible for long-term antihypertensive effects. The mechanism by which thiazides reduce vascular resistance has not been determined.

The principal adverse effect of thiazides is *hypokalemia*. This can be minimized by consuming potassium-rich foods (e.g., bananas, citrus fruits) and using potassium supplements or a potassium-sparing diuretic. Other side effects include *dehydration, hyperglycemia,* and *hyperuricemia.*

As discussed in Box 45–2, thiazides are superior to calcium channel blockers and ACE inhibitors, and hence are preferred to these more expensive drugs.

High-Ceiling (Loop) Diuretics. High-ceiling diuretics (e.g., furosemide) produce much greater diuresis than the thiazides. For most individuals with chronic hypertension, the amount of fluid loss that loop diuretics can produce is greater than needed or desirable. Consequently, loop diuretics are not used routinely. Rather, they are reserved for (1) patients

who need greater diuresis than can be achieved with thiazides and (2) patients with a low GFR (because thiazides won't work when GFR is low). Like the thiazides, the loop diuretics lower blood pressure by reducing blood volume and promoting vasodilation.

Most adverse effects are like those of the thiazides: *hypokalemia, dehydration, hyperglycemia,* and *hyperuricemia.* In addition, high-ceiling agents can cause *hearing loss.*

Potassium-Sparing Diuretics. The degree of diuresis induced by the potassium-sparing agents (e.g., spironolactone) is small. Consequently, these drugs have only modest hypotensive effects. However, because of their ability to conserve potassium, these drugs can play an important role in an antihypertensive regimen. That role is to balance potassium loss caused by thiazides or loop diuretics. The most significant adverse effect of the potassium-sparing agents is *hyperkalemia.* Because of the risk of hyperkalemia, potassium-sparing diuretics must not be used in combination with one another or with potassium supplements. Also, they should not be used routinely with ACE inhibitors or angiotensin II receptor blockers, both of which promote hyperkalemia.

TABLE 45–6 ■ Combination Products for Chronic Hypertension

Generic Name	Trade Name
Combinations with a Thiazide Diuretic	
Thiazide Plus a Beta Blocker	
Hydrochlorothiazide + propranolol	Inderide
Hydrochlorothiazide + metoprolol	Lopressor HCT
Hydrochlorothiazide + timolol	Timolide
Hydrochlorothiazide + bisoprolol	Ziac
Bendroflumethiazide + nadolol	Corzide
Chlorthalidone + atenolol	Tenoretic
Thiazide Plus an ACE Inhibitor	
Hydrochlorothiazide + captopril	Capozide
Hydrochlorothiazide + benazepril	Lotensin HCT
Hydrochlorothiazide + enalapril	Vaserectic
Hydrochlorothiazide + fosinopril	Monopril HCT
Hydrochlorothiazide + lisinopril	Prinzide, Zestoretic
Hydrochlorothiazide + moexipril	Uniretic
Hydrochlorothiazide + quinipril	Accuretic
Thiazide Plus an Angiotensin II Receptor Blocker	
Hydrochlorothiazide + losartan	Hyzaar
Hydrochlorothiazide + valsartan	Diovan HCT
Hydrochlorothiazide + candesartan	Atacand HCT
Hydrochlorothiazide + eprosartan	Teveten HCT
Hydrochlorothiazide + irbesartan	Avalide
Hydrochlorothiazide + telmisartan	Micardis HCT
Thiazide Plus a Centrally Acting Alpha$_2$ Agonist	
Chlorothiazide + methyldopa	Aldoclor
Chlorthalidone + clonidine	Combipres
Hydrochlorothiazide + methyldopa	Aldoril
Thiazide Plus an Adrenergic Neuron Blocker	
Chlorthalidone + reserpine	Demi-Regroton
Hydrochlorothiazide + guanethidine	Esimil
Hydrochlorothiazide + reserpine	Hydropres
Thiazide Plus a Direct Acting Vasodilator	
Hydrochlorothiazide + hydralazine	Apresazide
Thiazide Plus an Alpha Blocker	
Polythiazide + prazosin	Minizide
Thiazide Plus a Potassium-Sparing Diuretic	
Hydrochlorothiazide + spironolactone	Aldactazide
Hydrochlorothiazide + triamterene	Dyazide, Maxzide
Hydrochlorothiazide + amiloride	Moduretic
Calcium Channel Blocker/ACE Inhibitor Combinations	
Amlodipine + benazepril	Lotrel
Diltiazem + enalapril	Teczem
Verapamil + trandolapril	Tarka
Felodipine + enalapril	Lexxel

Sympatholytics (Adrenergic Antagonists)

Sympatholytic drugs suppress the influence of the sympathetic nervous system on the heart, blood vessels, and other structures. These drugs are used widely in the treatment of hypertension.

As indicated in Table 45–5, there are five subcategories of sympatholytic drugs: (1) beta blockers, (2) alpha$_1$ blockers, (3) alpha/beta blockers, (4) centrally acting alpha$_2$ agonists, and (5) adrenergic neuron blockers.

Beta-Adrenergic Blockers. The beta blockers (e.g., propranolol, metoprolol) are among the most widely used antihypertensive drugs. However, despite their efficacy and frequent use, the exact mechanism by which they reduce blood pressure is somewhat uncertain. Beta blockers are less effective in African American patients than in white patients.

The beta blockers have at least four useful actions in hypertension. First, blockade of cardiac beta$_1$ receptors decreases heart rate and contractility, thereby decreasing cardiac output. Second, beta blockers can suppress reflex tachycardia caused by vasodilators in the regimen. Third, blockade of beta₁ receptors on juxtaglomerular cells of the kidney reduces release of renin, thereby reducing angiotensin II–mediated vasoconstriction and aldosterone-mediated volume expansion. Fourth, long-term use of beta blockers reduces peripheral vascular resistance—by a mechanism that is unknown. This action could readily account for most of their antihypertensive effects.

Four beta blockers have *intrinsic sympathomimetic activity* (see Table 45–5). That is, they can produce mild stimulation of beta receptors while blocking receptor stimulation by strong agonists (e.g., norepinephrine). As a result, heart rate at rest is slowed less than with other beta blockers. Accordingly, if a patient develops symptomatic bradycardia with another beta blocker, switching to one of these may help.

Beta blockers can produce a variety of adverse effects. Blockade of cardiac beta₁ receptors can produce *bradycardia, decreased atrioventricular (AV) conduction,* and *reduced contractility.* Consequently, beta blockers should not be used by patients with sick sinus syndrome or second- or third-degree AV block—and must be used with care in patients with heart failure. Blockade of beta₂ receptors in the lung can promote *bronchoconstriction.* Accordingly, beta blockers should be avoided by patients with asthma. If an asthmatic individual absolutely must use a beta blocker, a beta₁-selective agent (e.g., metoprolol) should be employed. Beta blockers can mask signs of hypoglycemia, and therefore must be used with caution in patients with diabetes. Through actions exerted in the central nervous system, beta blockers can cause *depression, insomnia, bizarre dreams,* and *sexual dysfunction.*

The basic pharmacology of the beta blockers is discussed in Chapter 18.

Alpha₁ Blockers. The alpha₁ blockers (e.g., doxazosin, terazosin) prevent stimulation of alpha₁ receptors on arterioles and veins, thereby preventing sympathetically mediated vasoconstriction. The resultant vasodilation reduces both peripheral resistance and venous return to the heart.

The most disturbing side effect of alpha blockers is *orthostatic hypotension.* Hypotension can be especially severe with the initial dose. Significant hypotension continues with subsequent doses but is less profound.

The American College of Cardiology recommends that alpha blockers *not* be used as first line therapy for hypertension. Why? Because in a huge clinical trial, known as ALLHAT, in which doxazosin was compared with chlorthalidone (a thiazide diuretic), patients taking doxazosin experienced 25% more cardiovascular events and were twice as likely to be hospitalized for heart failure. It is not clear whether doxazosin *increased* cardiovascular risk or whether chlorthalidone *decreased* risk. Either way, the diuretic is clearly preferred to the alpha blocker.

The basic pharmacology of the alpha blockers is discussed in Chapter 18.

Alpha/Beta Blockers: Carvedilol and Labetalol. Carvedilol and labetalol are unusual in that they can block alpha₁ receptors as well as beta receptors. Blood pressure reduction results from a combination of actions: (1) alpha₁ blockade promotes dilation of arterioles and veins, (2) blockade of cardiac beta₁ receptors reduces heart rate and contractility, and (3) blockade of beta₁ receptors on juxtaglomerular cells suppresses release of renin. Presumably, these drugs also share the ability of other beta blockers to reduce peripheral vascular resistance. Like other nonselective beta blockers, labetalol and carvedilol can exacerbate bradycardia, AV heart block, and asthma. Blockade of venous alpha₁ receptors can produce postural hypotension.

Centrally Acting Alpha₂ Agonists. As discussed in Chapter 19, these drugs (e.g., clonidine, methyldopa) act within the brainstem to suppress sympathetic outflow to the heart and blood vessels. The result is vasodilation and reduced cardiac output, both of which help lower blood pressure. All central alpha₂ agonists can cause *dry mouth* and *sedation.* In addition, clonidine can cause severe *rebound hypertension* if treatment is abruptly discontinued. Additional adverse effects of methyldopa are *hemolytic anemia* (accompanied by a positive direct Coombs' test) and *liver disorders.*

Adrenergic Neuron Blockers. This group consists of three drugs: guanethidine, guanadrel, and reserpine. All three decrease blood pressure through actions in the terminals of postganglionic sympathetic neurons. Guanethidine and guanadrel inhibit release of norepinephrine, whereas reserpine causes norepinephrine depletion. Both actions result in decreased sympathetic stimulation of the heart and blood vessels.

The major adverse effect of *guanethidine* and *guanadrel* is *severe orthostatic hypotension* resulting from decreased sympathetic tone to veins. Because of the risk of postural hypotension, these drugs are last-choice agents for chronic hypertension.

The major adverse effect of *reserpine* is *depression.* Accordingly, reserpine is absolutely contraindicated for patients with a history of depressive illness.

The basic pharmacology of reserpine and guanethidine is discussed in Chapter 19.

Direct-Acting Vasodilators: Hydralazine and Minoxidil

Hydralazine and minoxidil reduce blood pressure by promoting dilation of *arterioles.* Neither drug causes significant dilation of veins. Because venous dilation is minimal, these agents produce very little orthostatic hypotension. With both drugs, lowering of blood pressure may be followed by reflex tachycardia, renin release, and fluid retention. Reflex tachycardia and release of renin can be prevented with a beta blocker. Fluid retention can be prevented with a diuretic.

The most disturbing adverse effect of *hydralazine* is a syndrome resembling *systemic lupus erythematosus* (SLE). Fortunately, this reaction is rare at recommended doses. If an SLE-like reaction occurs, hydralazine should be withdrawn. Hydralazine is considered a third-choice drug for chronic hypertension.

Minoxidil is substantially more toxic than hydralazine. By causing fluid retention, minoxidil can promote *pericardial effusion* (accumulation of fluid beneath the myocardium) that in some cases progresses to *cardiac tamponade* (compression of the heart). A less serious effect is *hypertrichosis* (excessive hair growth). Because of its capacity for significant harm, minoxidil is not used routinely in chronic hypertension. Instead, the drug is reserved for patients with severe hypertension who have not responded to less dangerous drugs.

The basic pharmacology of hydralazine and minoxidil is discussed in Chapter 44.

Calcium Channel Blockers

The calcium channel blockers (CCBs) fall into two groups: dihydropyridines (e.g., nifedipine) and nondihydropyridines (verapamil and diltiazem). Drugs in both groups promote dilation of arterioles. In addition, verapamil and diltiazem have direct suppressant effects on the heart.

Like other vasodilators, CCBs can cause *reflex tachycardia*. This reaction is greatest with the dihydropyridines and minimal with verapamil and diltiazem. Reflex tachycardia is low with verapamil and diltiazem because of cardiosuppression. Since nifedipine does not block cardiac calcium channels, reflex tachycardia with this drug can be substantial.

Because of their ability to compromise cardiac performance, verapamil and diltiazem must be used cautiously in patients with bradycardia, heart failure, or AV heart block. These precautions do not apply to nifedipine.

The *rapid-acting* formulation of nifedipine has been associated with increased mortality in patients with MI and unstable angina. As a result, the National Heart, Lung, and Blood Institute has recommended that rapid-acting nifedipine be used with great caution, if at all.

The basic pharmacology of the CCBs is discussed in Chapter 43.

ACE Inhibitors

The ACE inhibitors (e.g., captopril, enalapril) lower blood pressure by preventing formation of angiotensin II, and thereby prevent angiotensin II–mediated vasoconstriction and aldosterone-mediated volume expansion. In hypertensive diabetic patients with renal damage, these actions slow progression of kidney injury. Like the beta blockers, ACE inhibitors are less effective in African Americans than in white patients. Principal adverse effects are *persistent cough, first-dose hypotension, angioedema,* and *hyperkalemia* (secondary to suppression of aldosterone release). Because of the risk of hyperkalemia, combined use with potassium supplements or potassium-sparing diuretics is generally avoided. ACE inhibitors can cause *fetal harm* during the second and third trimesters of pregnancy, and hence must not be given to pregnant women. ACE inhibitors and angiotensin receptor blockers are the only antihypertensives specifically contraindicated during pregnancy. The basic pharmacology of the ACE inhibitors is discussed in Chapter 42.

Angiotensin II Receptor Blockers

Angiotensin II receptor blockers (ARBs) are relatively new drugs for use in hypertension. These agents lower blood pressure in much the same way as do the ACE inhibitors. Like the ACE inhibitors, ARBs prevent angiotensin II–mediated vasoconstriction and release of aldosterone. The only difference is that ARBs do so by blocking the *actions* of angiotensin II, whereas ACE inhibitors block the *formation* of angiotensin II. Like the ACE inhibitors, ARBs can cause *fetal harm* and must not be used during pregnancy. In contrast to ACE inhibitors, ARBs do not induce cough or significant hyperkalemia but they do cause angioedema. Because ARBs are relatively new, their niche in antihypertensive therapy has not been established. The basic pharmacology of these drugs is discussed in Chapter 42.

Aldosterone Receptor Blockers

Aldosterone receptor blockers lower blood pressure by promoting renal excretion of sodium and water. Only two agents are available: eplerenone and spirolactone. (In case you're confused about spironolactone, yes, it's the same drug we discussed above under *potassium-sparing diuretics*. We're also discussing it here because it produces diuresis through aldosterone receptor blockade.) Both spironolactone and eplerenone promote renal retention of potassium, and hence pose a risk of *hyperkalemia*. Accordingly, they should not be given to patients with existing hyperkalemia, and should not be combined with potassium-sparing diuretics or potassium supplements. Combined use with ACE inhibitors and ARBs is permissible, but must be done with caution. Spironolactone is discussed in Chapters 39 (Diuretics) and 46 (Drugs for Heart Failure); eplerenone is discussed in Chapter 42 (Drugs Acting on the Renin-Angiotensin-Aldosterone System).

Fundamentals of Hypertension Drug Therapy
Treatment Algorithm

The basic approach to treating hypertension is outlined in Figure 45–3. As shown, lifestyle changes should be instituted first. If these fail to lower blood pressure enough, drug therapy should be initiated—and the lifestyle changes should continue. Treatment often begins with a single drug. If needed, another drug may be *added* (if the initial drug was well tolerated but inadequate) or *substituted* (if the initial drug was poorly tolerated). However, before another drug is considered, possible reasons for failure of the initial drug should be assessed. Among these are insufficient dosage, poor compliance, excessive salt intake, and the presence of secondary hypertension. If treatment with two drugs is unsuccessful, a third and even fourth may be added.

Initial Drug Selection

Initial drug selection is determined by the presence or absence of a *compelling indication*, defined as a comorbid condition for which a specific class of antihypertensive drugs has been shown to improve outcomes. Initial drugs for patients with and without compelling indications are discussed below.

Patients WITHOUT Compelling Indications. For initial therapy in the absence of a compelling indication, a *thiazide diuretic* is recommended for most patients. This preference is based on long-term controlled trials showing conclusively that thiazides can reduce morbidity and mortality in hypertensive patients, and are well tolerated and inexpensive too (see Box 45-2). *Beta blockers*, also proved to reduce morbidity and mortality, are a good alternative. Other options for initial therapy—*ACE inhibitors, ARBs, CCBs,* and *alpha/beta blockers*—equal diuretics and beta blockers in their ability to lower blood pressure. However, they may not be as effective at reducing morbidity and mortality. Accordingly, these drugs should be reserved for special indications and for patients who have not responded to thiazide diuretics and beta blockers. Another group of drugs—*centrally acting sympatholytics, adrenergic neuron blockers,* and *direct-acting vasodilators*—are associated with a high incidence of undesirable effects, and hence are not well suited for initial monotherapy. One last

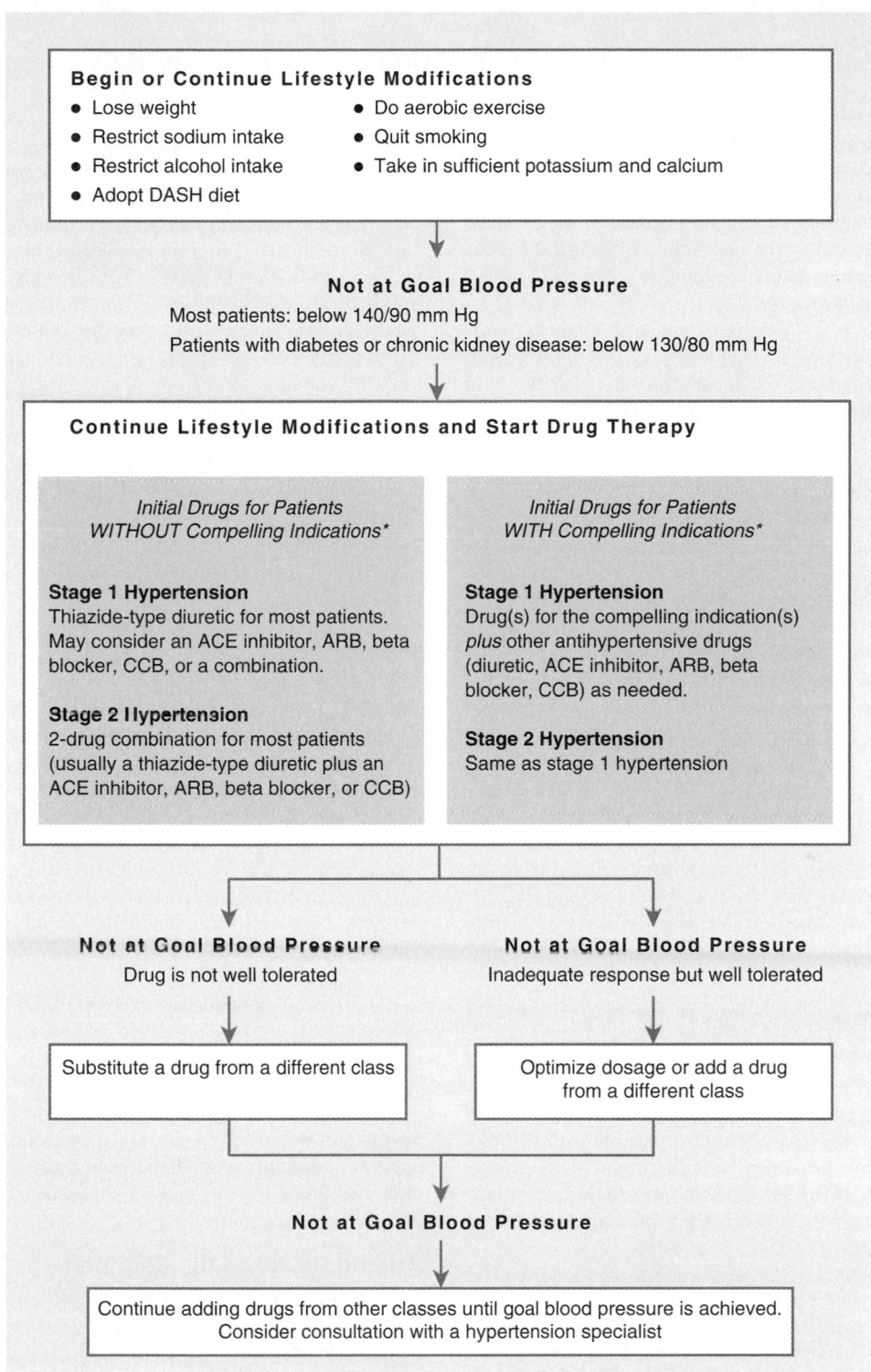

Begin or Continue Lifestyle Modifications
- Lose weight
- Restrict sodium intake
- Restrict alcohol intake
- Adopt DASH diet
- Do aerobic exercise
- Quit smoking
- Take in sufficient potassium and calcium

Not at Goal Blood Pressure

Most patients: below 140/90 mm Hg

Patients with diabetes or chronic kidney disease: below 130/80 mm Hg

Continue Lifestyle Modifications and Start Drug Therapy

Initial Drugs for Patients WITHOUT Compelling Indications*

Stage 1 Hypertension
Thiazide-type diuretic for most patients. May consider an ACE inhibitor, ARB, beta blocker, CCB, or a combination.

Stage 2 Hypertension
2-drug combination for most patients (usually a thiazide-type diuretic plus an ACE inhibitor, ARB, beta blocker, or CCB)

Initial Drugs for Patients WITH Compelling Indications*

Stage 1 Hypertension
Drug(s) for the compelling indication(s) *plus* other antihypertensive drugs (diuretic, ACE inhibitor, ARB, beta blocker, CCB) as needed.

Stage 2 Hypertension
Same as stage 1 hypertension

Not at Goal Blood Pressure
Drug is not well tolerated

Not at Goal Blood Pressure
Inadequate response but well tolerated

Substitute a drug from a different class

Optimize dosage or add a drug from a different class

Not at Goal Blood Pressure

Continue adding drugs from other classes until goal blood pressure is achieved. Consider consultation with a hypertension specialist

Figure 45–3 ■ **Algorithm for treating hypertension.** (ACE = angiotensin-converting enzyme, ARB = angiotensin II receptor blocker, CCB = calcium channel blocker).

*A "compelling indication" is a comorbid condition (e.g., heart failure, diabetes) for which a specific class of antihypertensive drugs has been shown to improve outcomes. See text for details.

Modified from The Seventh Report of the Joint National Committee on Detection, Evaluation, and Treatment of High Blood Pressure, JAMA 2003;289:2560-2572.

Special Interest Topic

BOX 45–2 ■ AND THE BEST DRUG IS . . . THE CHEAP ONE!

Results from the Antihypertensive and Lipid-Lowering Treatment to Prevent Heart Attack Trial (ALLHAT),[1] published December 18, 2002, show unequivocally that the least expensive drugs for hypertension, the thiazide diuretics, are also the most effective—a welcome revelation in these cost-conscious times. ALLHAT is arguably the most important clinical trial to date on hypertension therapy, and hence these results should have a profound impact on clinical practice.

ALLHAT is a large, double-blind, trial that compared the impact of four antihypertensive drugs—chlorthalidone (a thiazide diuretic), amlodipine (a CCB), lisinopril (an ACE inhibitor), and doxazosin (an alpha blocker)—on the incidence of adverse cardiovascular (CV) events. The study enrolled 33,357 patients, including more women (47%), blacks (32%), and Hispanics (19%) than most earlier trials. All participants had stage 1 or stage 2 hypertension plus at least one additional risk factor for coronary heart disease (CHD). The mean follow-up time was 4.9 years.

The results? With one drug—doxazosin—the incidence of adverse CV events was substantially higher than with the others, and hence this arm of the study was terminated early. Effects of the remaining three drugs—chlorthalidone, amlodipine, and lisinopril—were similar in some respects but significantly different in others. With all three, rates of (1) fatal CHD or nonfatal heart attacks and (2) all-cause mortality were identical. However, in other ways, chlorthalidone was clearly superior. Specifically, chlorthalidone was slightly better at reducing systolic blood pressure. More importantly, chlorthalidone was associated fewer adverse CV events: Compared with patients taking chlorthalidone, those taking amlodipine experienced a higher 6-year rate of heart failure (10.2% vs 7.7%), and those taking lisinopril experienced higher 6-year rates of stroke (6.3% vs 5.6%), heart failure (8.7% vs 7.7%), and combined CV disease (33.3% vs 30.9%).

You might ask "Can the results seen with chlorthalidone, lisinopril, and amlodipine be extended to other members of the drug families they represent?" The answer is a qualified "Yes." All thiazide diuretics are very similar, and hence the results seen with chlorthalidone are likely to be seen with all other thiazides. Similarly, all ACE inhibitors are much the same, and hence the results seen with lisinopril are probably representative. The story with amlodipine is different. Amlodipine belongs to a subclass of CCBs known as dihydropyridines (DHPs), which differ significantly from CCBs in other subclasses. Accordingly, extrapolation of the results seen with amlodipine should probably be limited to CCBs in the DHP subclass.

How do thiazides compare with beta blockers? Unfortunately, beta blockers were not included in ALLHAT. However, data from other large studies indicate that beta blockers are certainly no more effective than thiazides, and may well be less effective.

The message from ALLHAT is both clear and compelling: Thiazide diuretics should be the initial drugs of choice for most patients with hypertension. These drugs are at least as effective as the alternatives, and they cost *much* less. Hydrochlorothiazide, for example, costs about 10 cents a day, compared with about $1 a day for amlodipine, a drug that Americans now spend about $1.6 billion on annually. Clearly, if most patients were to switch from amlodipine (and other expensive drugs) to the thiazides, the savings for our healthcare system would be huge—and would quickly offset the $120 million that tax payers invested on ALLHAT. Wouldn't it be great if more clinical studies led to the same good news: The best drug for what ails you is also the cheapest.

[1]The ALLHAT Officers and Coordinators for the ALLHAT Collaborative Research Group. Major outcomes in high-risk hypertensive patients randomized to angiotensin-converting enzyme inhibitor or calcium channel blocker vs diuretic: the Antihypertensive and Lipid-Lowering Treatment to Prevent Heart Attack Trial (ALLHAT). JAMA 2002;288:2981–2997.

group—*alpha₁ blockers*—is no longer recommended as first-line therapy. As noted above, when an the alpha blocker doxazosin was compared with the diuretic chlorthalidone, doxazosin was associated with a much higher incidence of adverse cardiovascular events.

How many drugs should be used for initial therapy? The answer depends on the hypertension stage. For patients with stage 1 hypertension, treatment with just 1 drug—usually a thiazide diuretic—is recommended. For patients with stage 2 hypertension, initial therapy should consist of two drugs—typically a thiazide combined with either a beta blocker, ACE inhibitor, ARB, or CCB.

Patients WITH Compelling Indications. For patients with hypertension plus certain comorbid conditions (e.g., heart failure, diabetes) there is strong evidence that specific antihypertensive drugs can reduce morbidity and mortality. Drugs shown to improve outcomes for 6 comorbid conditions are indicated in Table 45-7. Clearly, these drugs should be used for initial therapy. If needed, other antihypertensive agents can be added to the regimen. Management of hypertension in patients with diabetes and renal disease—two specific comorbid conditions—is discussed further under *Individualizing Therapy*.

Adding Drugs to the Regimen

Rationale for Drug Selection. When using two or more drugs to treat hypertension, each drug should come from a different class. That is, each drug should have a different mechanism of action. In accord with this guideline, it would be appropriate to combine a beta blocker, a diuretic, and a vasodilator, since each lowers blood pressure by a different mechanism. In contrast, it would be inappropriate to combine two thiazide diuretics or two beta blockers or two vasodilators.

Benefits of Multidrug Therapy. Treatment with multiple drugs offers significant benefits. First, by employing drugs that have different mechanisms, we can increase the chance of success: Attacking blood pressure control at several sites is

TABLE 45–7 ▪■ Classes of Antihypertensive Drugs Recommended for Initial Therapy of Hypertension in Patients with Certain High-Risk Comorbid Conditions

High-Risk Comorbid Conditions That Constitute Compelling Indications for the Drugs Checked	Drug Classes Recommended for Initial Therapy of Hypertension					
	Diuretic	Beta Blocker	ACE Inhibitor	ARB	CCB	Aldosterone Antagonist
Heart Failure	✓	✓	✓	✓		✓
Post-myocardial infarction		✓	✓			✓
High coronary disease risk	✓	✓	✓		✓	
Diabetes	✓	✓	✓	✓	✓	
Chronic kidney disease			✓	✓		
Recurrent stroke prevention	✓		✓			

ACE = angiotensin-converting enzyme; ARB = angiotensin II receptor blocker; CCB = calcium channel blocker.
Adapted from The Seventh Report of the Joint National Committee on Detection, Evaluation, and Treatment of High Blood Pressure. JAMA 2003;289:2560–2572.

more likely to be effective than attacking at one site. Second, when drugs are used in combination, each can be administered in a lower dosage than would be possible if it were used alone; as a result, both the frequency and the intensity of side effects are reduced. Third, when proper combinations are selected, one agent can offset the adverse effects of another. For example, if a vasodilator is used alone, reflex tachycardia is likely. However, if a vasodilator is combined with a beta blocker, reflex tachycardia will be minimal.

Dosing

For each drug in the regimen, *dosage should be low initially and then gradually increased.* There are several reasons for this approach. First, for most people with chronic hypertension, the disease poses no immediate threat. Hence there is no need to lower blood pressure rapidly using large doses. Second, when blood pressure is reduced slowly, baroreceptors gradually reset to the new, lower pressure. As a result, sympathetic reflexes offer less resistance to the hypotensive effects of therapy. Third, since there is no need to drop blood pressure rapidly, and since higher doses carry a higher risk of adverse effects, use of high initial doses would needlessly increase the risk of unpleasant responses.

Step-Down Therapy

After blood pressure has been controlled for at least 1 year, an attempt should be made to reduce dosages and the number of drugs in the regimen. Of course, lifestyle modifications should continue. When reductions are made slowly and progressively, many patients are able to maintain blood pressure control with less medication—and some can be maintained with no medication at all. If drugs are discontinued, regular follow-up is essential, since blood pressure usually returns to hypertensive levels—although it may take years to do so.

Individualizing Therapy
Patients with Comorbid Conditions

Comorbid conditions complicate treatment of hypertension. Two conditions that are especially problematic—renal disease and diabetes—are discussed below. Preferred drugs for patients with these and other comorbid conditions are summarized in Table 45–7. Drugs to avoid in patients with specific comorbid conditions are summarized in Table 45–8.

Renal Disease. Nephrosclerosis (hardening of the kidney) secondary to hypertension is among the most common causes of progressive renal disease. Pathophysiologic changes include degeneration of renal tubules and fibrotic thickening of the glomeruli, both of which contribute to renal insufficiency. Nephrosclerosis sets the stage for a downward spiral: Renal insufficiency causes water retention, which in turn causes blood pressure to rise higher, which in turn promotes even more renal injury, and so on. Accordingly, early detection and treatment are essential. To retard progression of renal damage, the most important action is to lower blood pressure. The target pressure is less than 130/80 mm Hg. Achieving this goal often requires 3 or more drugs. Although all classes of antihypertensive agents are effective in nephrosclerosis, ACE inhibitors and ARBs work best. Hence, in the absence of contraindications, all patients should get one of these drugs. As a rule, a diuretic is used too. In patients with advanced renal insufficiency, thiazide diuretics are ineffective, hence a loop diuretic should be employed. Potassium-sparing diuretics should be avoided.

Diabetes. In patients with diabetes, the target blood pressure is 130/80 mm Hg or less. Preferred antihypertensive drugs are ACE inhibitors, ARBs, CCBs, and diuretics (in low doses). In patients with diabetic nephropathy, ACE inhibitors and ARBs can slow progression of renal damage and reduce albuminuria. In diabetic patients, as in nondiabetics, beta blockers and diuretics can decrease morbidity and mortality. Keep in mind, however, that beta blockers can suppress glycogenolysis and mask early signs of hypoglycemia, and therefore must be used with caution. Thiazides and high-ceiling diuretics promote hyperglycemia, and hence should be used with care.

A recent study compared a long-acting dihydropyridine CCB (nisoldipine) with an ACE inhibitor (enalapril) for treating hypertension in people with diabetes. The result? Patients taking the CCB had a higher incidence of MI than the patients taking the ACE inhibitor. Because the study was not placebo controlled, it was impossible to distinguish between two possible interpretations: (1) the CCB increased the risk of MI or (2) the ACE inhibitor protected against MI. Either way, it seems clear that ACE inhibitors are better than CCBs for patients with hypertension and diabetes.

Patients in Special Populations

African Americans. Hypertension is a major health problem for African American adults. Hypertension develops earlier in blacks than in whites, has a much higher incidence, and is likely to be more severe. As a result, African Americans face a greater risk of heart disease, end-stage renal disease, and stroke. Compared with the general population, African Americans experience a 50% higher rate of death from heart disease, an 80% higher rate of death from stroke, and a 320% higher rate of hypertension-related end-stage renal disease.

With timely treatment, the disparity between blacks and nonblacks can be greatly reduced, if not eliminated. We know that blacks and whites respond equally to treatment (although not always to the same drugs). The problem is that, among blacks, hypertension often goes untreated until after significant organ damage has developed. If hypertension were diagnosed and treated earlier, the prognosis would be greatly improved. Accordingly, it is important that African Americans undergo routine monitoring of blood pressure. If hypertension is diagnosed, treatment should begin at once. Because African Americans have a high incidence of salt sensitivity, obesity, and cigarette use, lifestyle modifications are an important component of treatment.

African Americans respond better to some antihypertensive drugs than to others. Controlled trials have shown that *diuretics* can decrease morbidity and mortality in blacks. Accordingly, diuretics are drugs of first choice. *CCBs* and *alpha/beta blockers* are also effective. In contrast, monotherapy with *beta blockers* or *ACE inhibitors* is less effective in blacks than in whites. Nonetheless, beta blockers and ACE inhibitors should be used if they are strongly indicated for a comorbid condition. For example, ACE inhibitors should be used in black patients who have type 1 diabetes with proteinuria. Also, ACE inhibitors should be used in patients with hypertensive nephrosclerosis, a condition for which ACE inhibitors are superior to CCBs.

Children and Adolescents. The incidence of secondary hypertension in children is much higher than in adults. Accordingly, efforts to diagnose and treat an underlying cause should be especially diligent. For children with primary hypertension, treatment is the same as for adults—although doses are lower and should be adjusted with care. Because ACE inhibitors and ARBs can cause fetal harm, they should be avoided in girls who are sexually active or pregnant.

The Elderly. The incidence of hypertension in people over age 60 is about 65%, and the prevalence of isolated systolic hypertension is greater than in younger adults. In clinical trials, antihypertensive treatment has reduced the incidence of stroke by 36% and MI by 27%. Although all antihypertensive drugs are effective in older adults, only *beta blockers* and *diuretics* have been shown in controlled trials to reduce morbidity and mortality. Hence, these drugs are generally preferred. In patients with isolated systolic hypertension, diuretics are preferred. Since cardiovascular reflexes are blunted in the elderly, treatment carries a significant risk of orthostatic hypotension. Accordingly, initial doses should be low—about one-half those used for younger adults. Drugs that are especially likely to cause orthostatic hypotension (e.g., guanethidine, alpha$_1$ blockers, alpha/beta blockers) should be used with caution, as should clonidine and methyldopa (central alpha$_2$ agonists), both of which can cause cognitive dysfunction.

Minimizing Adverse Effects

Antihypertensive drugs can produce many unwanted effects, including hypotension, sedation, and sexual dysfunction. (Although not stressed previously, practically all antihypertensive drugs can interfere with sexual feelings or performance.)

The fundamental strategy for decreasing side effects is to tailor the regimen to the sensitivities of the patient. Simply put, if one drug causes effects that are objectionable, a more acceptable drug should be substituted. The best way to identify unacceptable responses is to encourage the patient to report them.

Adverse effects caused by exacerbation of comorbid diseases are both predictable and avoidable. We know, for example, that beta blockers can intensify asthma and AV block, and hence should not be taken by people with these disorders. Other conditions that can be aggravated by antihypertensive drugs are listed in Table 45–8. To help avoid drug-disease mismatches, the medical history should identify all comorbid conditions. With this information, the prescriber can choose drugs that are least likely to make the comorbid condition worse.

High initial doses and rapid dosage escalation can increase the incidence and severity of adverse effects. Accordingly, doses should be low initially and then gradually increased. Remember, there is usually no need to reduce blood pressure rapidly. Hence, it makes no sense to give large initial doses that can produce a rapid fall in blood pressure but that also produce intense undesired responses.

Promoting Compliance

The major cause of treatment failure in patients with chronic hypertension is lack of adherence to the therapeutic regimen. In this section we consider the causes of noncompliance and discuss some solutions.

Why Compliance Can Be Difficult to Achieve

Much of the difficulty in promoting compliance stems from the nature of hypertension itself. Hypertension is a chronic, slowly progressing disease that, through much of its course, is devoid of overt symptoms. Because symptoms are absent, it can be difficult to convince patients that they are ill and need treatment. In addition, since there are no symptoms to relieve, drugs cannot produce an obvious therapeutic response. In the absence of such a response, it can be difficult for patients to believe that their medication is doing anything useful.

Because hypertension progresses very slowly, the disease tends to encourage procrastination. For most people, the adverse effects of hypertension will not become manifest for many years. Realizing this, patients may reason (incorrectly) that they can postpone therapy without significantly increasing their risk.

The negative aspects of treatment also contribute to noncompliance. Antihypertensive regimens can be complex and expensive. In addition, treatment must continue lifelong. Lastly, antihypertensive drugs can cause a number of adverse effects, ranging from sedation to hypotension to disruption of sexual function. It is difficult to convince people who are feeling good to take drugs that may make them feel worse. Some people may decide that exposing themselves to the negative effects of therapy today is paying too high a price to avoid the adverse consequences of hypertension at some indefinite time in the future.

TABLE 45–8 ▪ Comorbid Conditions That Require Cautious Use or Complete Avoidance of Certain Antihypertensive Drugs

Comorbid Condition	Drugs to Be Avoided or Used with Caution	Reason for Concern
Cardiovascular Disorders		
Heart failure	Verapamil Diltiazem	These drugs act on the heart to decrease myocardial contractility and can thereby further reduce cardiac output.
AV heart block	Beta blockers Labetalol Verapamil Diltiazem	These drugs act on the heart to suppress AV conduction and can thereby intensify AV block.
Coronary artery disease	Guanethidine Hydralazine	Reflex tachycardia induced by these drugs can precipitate an anginal attack.
Post–myocardial infarction	Guanethidine Hydralazine	Reflex tachycadia induced by these drugs can increase cardiac work and oxygen demand.
Other Disorders		
Dyslipidemia	Beta blockers Diuretics	These drugs may exacerbate dyslipidemia.
Renal insufficiency	K^+-sparing diuretics K^+ supplements	Use of these agents can lead to dangerous accumulations of potassium.
Asthma	Beta blockers Labetalol	$Beta_2$ blockade promotes bronchoconstriction.
Depression	Reserpine Beta blockers	These drugs can cause depression.
Diabetes mellitus	Thiazides Furosemide Beta blockers	Thiazides and furosemide promote hyperglycemia, beta blockers suppress glycogenolysis and can mask signs of hypoglycemia.
Gout	Thiazides Furosemide	These diuretics promote hyperuricemia.
Hyperkalemia	K^+-sparing diuretics ACE inhibitors Aldosterone receptor blockers	These drugs cause potassium accumulation.
Hypokalemia	Thiazides Furosemide	These drugs cause potassium loss.
Collagen diseases	Hydralazine	Hydralazine can precipitate a lupus erythematosus–like syndrome.
Liver disease	Methyldopa	Methyldopa is hepatotoxic.
Pre-eclampsia	ACE inhibitors ARBs	These drugs can injure the fetus.

ACE = angiotensin-converting enzyme, ARBs = angiotensin II receptor blockers, AV = atrioventricular.

Ways to Promote Compliance

Educate the Patient. Compliance requires motivation; patient education can help provide it. Patients should be taught about the consequences of hypertension and the benefits of treatment. Because hypertension does not cause discomfort, it may not be clear to patients that their condition is indeed serious. Patients must be made to understand that, left untreated, hypertension can cause heart disease, kidney disease, and stroke. In addition, patients should appreciate that, with proper therapy, the risks of these long-term complications can be minimized, resulting in a longer and healthier life. Lastly, patients must understand that drugs do not cure hypertension—they only control symptoms. Hence, for treatment to be effective, medication must be taken lifelong.

Teach Self-Monitoring. Patients should be taught the goal of treatment (usually maintenance of blood pressure below 140/90 mm Hg), and they should be taught to monitor and record their blood pressure daily. This increases patient involvement and provides positive feedback that can help promote compliance.

Minimize Side Effects. Common sense dictates that, if we expect patients to comply with long-term treatment, we must keep undesired effects to a minimum. As discussed above, adverse effects can be minimized by (1) encouraging patients to report side effects, (2) discontinuing objectionable drugs and substituting more acceptable ones, (3) avoiding drugs that can exacerbate comorbid conditions, and (4) using doses that are low initially and then gradually increased.

Establish a Collaborative Relationship. The patient who feels like a collaborative partner in the treatment program is more likely to comply than is the patient who feels that treatment is being imposed. Collaboration allows the patient to help set treatment goals, create the treatment program, and evaluate progress. In addition, a collaborative relationship facilitates communication about side effects. This is especially important with respect to drug-induced sexual dysfunction, which patients may be reluctant to discuss.

Simplify the Regimen. Antihypertensive regimens may consist of several drugs taken multiple times a day. Such complex regimens deter compliance. Therefore, in order to promote compliance, steps should be taken to make the dosing schedule as simple as possible. Once an effective regimen has been established, an attempt should be made to switch to once-a-day or twice-a-day dosing. If an appropriate combination product is available (e.g., a fixed-dose combination of a thiazide diuretic plus a beta blocker), the combination product may be substituted for its components.

Other Measures. Compliance can be promoted by giving positive reinforcement when therapeutic goals are achieved. Involvement of family members in the program can be helpful. Also, compliance can be promoted by scheduling office visits at convenient times and by following up when appointments are missed. For many patients, antihypertensive therapy represents a significant economic burden; devising a regimen that is effective and yet keeps costs low will certainly encourage compliance.

DRUGS FOR HYPERTENSIVE EMERGENCIES

A hypertensive emergency exists when diastolic blood pressure exceeds 120 mm Hg. The severity of the emergency is determined by the likelihood of organ damage. When excessive blood pressure is associated with papilledema (edema of the retina), intracranial hemorrhage, MI, or acute congestive heart failure, a severe emergency exists—and blood pressure must be lowered rapidly (within 1 hour). If severe hypertension is present but does not yet pose an immediate threat of organ damage, it is preferable to reduce blood pressure more slowly (over 24 to 48 hours). Why? Because rapid reductions in blood pressure can cause cerebral ischemia, MI, and renal failure. Hence, pressure should be reduced gradually whenever possible.

The major drugs used for hypertensive emergencies are discussed below. All reduce blood pressure by causing vasodilation, and all are administered IV.

Sodium Nitroprusside. When acute, severe hypertension demands a rapid but controlled reduction in blood pressure, IV nitroprusside [Nitropress] is usually the drug of first choice. Nitroprusside is a direct-acting vasodilator that relaxes smooth muscle of arterioles and veins. Effects begin in seconds and then fade rapidly when administration ceases. Nitroprusside is administered by continuous IV infusion using a pump to control the rate. The usual rate is 0.5 to 8 μg/kg/min. To avoid overshoot, continuous monitoring of blood pressure is required. Because nitroprusside has an extremely short duration of action, overshoot can be corrected quickly by reducing the rate of the infusion. Prolonged infusion (longer than 72 hours) can produce toxic accumulation of

thiocyanate and should be avoided. The basic pharmacology of nitroprusside is discussed in Chapter 44.

Fenoldopam. Fenoldopam [Corlopam] is an IV drug indicated for short-term management of hypertensive emergencies. Benefits equal those of nitroprusside. Fenoldopam lowers blood pressure by activating dopamine$_1$ receptors on arterioles, and thereby promotes vasodilation. In animal models, the drug dilates renal, coronary, mesenteric, and peripheral vessels.

Fenoldopam differs from other antihypertensives in that it helps maintain (or even improve) renal function. Two mechanisms are involved. First, the drug dilates renal blood vessels, and thereby increases renal blood flow (despite reducing arterial pressure). Second, fenoldopam promotes sodium and water excretion through direct effects on renal tubules.

Fenoldopam has a rapid onset and short duration. Effects begin in less than 5 minutes. The drug undergoes rapid hepatic metabolism followed by renal excretion. The plasma half-life is only 5 minutes.

Fenoldopam is generally well tolerated. The most common side effects are hypotension, headache, flushing, dizziness, and reflex tachycardia—all of which occur secondary to vasodilation. Tachycardia may cause ischemia in patients with angina. Combined used with a beta blocker can minimize tachycardia, but may also result in excessive lowering of blood pressure. Fenoldopam can elevate intraocular pressure, and hence should be used with caution in patients with glaucoma.

Fenoldopam is administered by continuous IV infusion. To minimize tachycardia, the initial dosage should be low. The typical infusion rate is 0.1 to 0.3 μg/kg/min. With continuous 24-hour infusion, no tolerance develops to antihypertensive effects, and there is no rebound increase in blood pressure when the infusion is stopped. With a 48-hour infusion, some tolerance may develop. Oral antihypertensive therapy can be added as soon as blood pressure has stabilized.

Labetalol. Labetalol [Trandate, Normodyne] blocks alpha- and beta-adrenergic receptors. Blood pressure is reduced by arteriolar dilation secondary to alpha blockade. Beta blockade prevents reflex tachycardia in response to reduced arterial pressure, and hence the drug is probably safe for patients with angina or MI. Beta blockade can aggravate bronchial asthma, heart failure, AV block, cardiogenic shock, and bradycardia. Accordingly, labetalol should not be given to patients with these disorders. Administration is by slow IV injection.

Diazoxide. Diazoxide [Hyperstat IV] causes selective dilation of arterioles. Effects begin within minutes and may persist for hours. The drug can be administered by IV bolus or slow IV infusion (over 15 to 30 minutes). Diazoxide can cause reflex tachycardia and hence should be avoided in patients with angina. Reflex tachycardia can be reduced with a beta blocker. Fluid retention may occur and can be controlled with a diuretic. Hyperglycemia may be a complication for patients with diabetes. The basic pharmacology of diazoxide is discussed in Chapter 44.

Trimethaphan. Trimethaphan [Arfonad] is a ganglionic blocking agent that dilates arterioles and veins. Effects begin and end within minutes. Like nitroprusside, trimethaphan must be administered by continuous IV infusion, using a pump to control the flow rate. Constant monitoring is required. Prominent side effects—dry mouth, blurred vision, urinary retention, paresis of the bowel—result from parasympathetic blockade. The basic pharmacology of trimethaphan is discussed in Chapter 16.

DRUGS FOR HYPERTENSIVE DISORDERS OF PREGNANCY

Hypertension is the most common complication of pregnancy, with an incidence of about 10%. When hypertension develops, it is essential to distinguish between chronic hypertension and preeclampsia. Why? Because chronic hypertension is relatively benign, whereas preeclampsia can lead to life-threatening complications for the mother and fetus.

Chronic Hypertension

Chronic hypertension, which occurs in 5% of pregnancies, is defined as hypertension that was present before pregnancy or that developed prior to the 20th week of gestation. Persistent hypertension carries a risk to both the mother and fetus. Potential adverse outcomes include placental abruption, maternal cardiac decompensation, premature birth, growth retardation, central nervous system hemorrhage, and renal failure. The goal of treatment is to minimize the risk of hypertension to the mother and fetus while avoiding drug-induced harm to the fetus. With the exception of the ACE inhibitors and ARBs, antihypertensive drugs that were being taken before pregnancy can be continued. *ACE inhibitors and ARBs are contraindicated because of their potential for harm* (fetal growth retardation, congenital malformations, neonatal renal failure, neonatal death). When drug therapy is initiated *during* pregnancy, *methyldopa* is the traditional agent of choice. The drug has limited effects on uteroplacental and fetal hemodynamics, and does not affect the fetus or neonate. *Labetalol,* a combination alpha- and beta-blocker, is a good alternative. Regardless of the drug selected, treatment should not be too aggressive. Why? Because an excessive drop in blood pressure could compromise uteroplacental blood flow.

How high can blood pressure rise before drug therapy is indicated? According to guidelines issued in 2001 by the American College of Obstetricians and Gynecologists (ACOG), "severe" hypertension requires treatment, whereas "mild" hypertension generally does not. (The ACOG defines severe hypertension as systolic BP >180 mm Hg or diastolic BP >110 mm Hg, and mild hypertension as systolic BP 140 to 179 mm Hg or diastolic BP 90 to 109 mm Hg.) There is good evidence that treating severe hypertension reduces risk. In contrast, there is little evidence that treating mild hypertension offers significant benefit.

Women who have chronic hypertension during pregnancy are at increased risk of developing preeclampsia (see below). Unfortunately, reducing blood pressure does *not* lower this risk.

Preeclampsia and Eclampsia

Preeclampsia is characterized by elevated blood pressure (greater than 140/90 mm Hg) and proteinuria (300 mg or more in 24 hours) that develop after the 20th week of gestation. The disorder occurs in 5% to 8% of pregnancies. Rarely, women with preeclampsia develop seizures. If seizures do develop, the condition is then termed *eclampsia.* Risk factors for preeclampsia include obesity, black race, chronic hypertension, diabetes, collagen vascular disorders, and previous preeclampsia.

Management of preeclampsia is based on the severity of the disease, the status of mother and fetus, and the length of gestation. The objective is to preserve the health of the mother and deliver an infant that will not require intensive and prolonged neonatal care. Success requires close maternal and fetal monitoring. Although drugs can help reduce blood pressure, delivery is the only cure.

Management of *mild* preeclampsia is controversial and depends on the duration of gestation. If preeclampsia develops near term, and if fetal maturity is certain, induction of labor is advised. However, if mild preeclampsia develops earlier in gestation, experts disagree about what to do. Suggested measures include bed rest, prolonged hospitalization, treatment with antihypertensive drugs, and prophylaxis with an anticonvulsant. Studies to evaluate these strategies have generally failed to demonstrate benefits from any of them, including treatment with antihypertensive drugs.

The definitive intervention for *severe* preeclampsia is delivery. However, making the choice to induce labor presents a dilemma. Since preeclampsia can deteriorate rapidly, with grave consequences for mother and fetus, immediate delivery is recommended. However, if the fetus is not sufficiently mature, immediate delivery could threaten its life. Hence the dilemma: Do we deliver the fetus immediately, which would eliminate risk for the mother but present a serious risk for the fetus—or do we postpone delivery, which would reduce risk for the fetus but greatly increase risk for the mother? If the patient elects to postpone delivery, then blood pressure can be lowered with drugs. Because severe preeclampsia can be life threatening, treatment must be done in a tertiary care center to permit close monitoring of mother and fetus. The major objective is to prevent cerebral complications (e.g., hemorrhage, encephalopathy). The drug of choice for lowering blood pressure is *hydralazine* (5 mg by IV bolus); dosing may be repeated 3 times at 20-minute intervals.

Because preeclampsia can (rarely) evolve into eclampsia, an anticonvulsant may be given for prophylaxis. *Magnesium sulfate* is the drug of choice. In a recent study, prophylaxis with magnesium sulfate reduced the risk of eclampsia by 58% and the risk of death by 45%. Dosing consists of a 10-gm IM loading dose followed by 5 gm IM every 4 hours for maintenance.

If eclampsia develops, magnesium sulfate is the preferred drug for seizure control. Dosing consists of a 4-gm IV loading dose followed by 5 gm IM every 4 hours for maintenance. To ensure therapeutic effects and prevent toxicity, blood levels of magnesium should be monitored. The target range is 4 to 7 mEq/L (the normal range for magnesium is 1.5 to 2 mEq/L).

Recent evidence indicates that vitamins C and E may prevent development of preeclampsia. In high-risk women, these vitamins appear to reduce the risk of preeclampsia by 76%. Effective daily dosages are 1000 mg for vitamin C and 400 IU for vitamin E. Treatment is begun between 18 and 22 weeks of gestation. How do these vitamins work? Both are antioxidants, and hence can scavenge free radicals that are believed to trigger preeclampsia.

⸪ KEY POINTS

- Hypertension is defined as systolic BP greater than 140 mm Hg or diastolic BP greater than 90 mm Hg.
- Primary hypertension (essential hypertension), which is defined as hypertension that has no identifiable cause, is the most common form of hypertension.
- Untreated hypertension can lead to heart disease, kidney disease, and stroke.
- In patients older than 50, elevated systolic BP represents a greater cardiovascular risk than elevated diastolic BP.
- The goal of antihypertensive therapy is to decrease morbidity and mortality without decreasing quality of life. For most patients, this goal is achieved by maintaining blood pressure below 140/90 mm Hg, or below 130/80 mm Hg for those with diabetes or chronic kidney disease.

- To reduce blood pressure, two kinds of treatment may be used: drug therapy and lifestyle modification (weight reduction, smoking cessation, reduction of salt and alcohol intake, following the DASH diet, and increasing aerobic exercise).
- The baroreceptor reflex, the kidneys, and the RAAS can oppose our attempts to lower blood pressure with drugs. We can counteract the baroreceptor reflex with a beta blocker, the kidneys with a diuretic, and the RAAS with an ACE inhibitor, ARB, or aldosterone receptor blocker.
- Thiazide diuretics (e.g., hydrochlorothiazide) and loop diuretics (e.g., furosemide) reduce blood pressure in two ways: they reduce blood volume (by promoting diuresis) and they reduce arterial resistance (by an unknown mechanism).
- Loop diuretics should be reserved for (1) patients who need greater diuresis than can be achieved with thiazides and (2) patients with a low GFR (because thiazides won't work when GFR is low).
- Beta blockers (e.g., propranolol) appear to lower blood pressure primarily by reducing peripheral vascular resistance; the mechanism is unknown. They may also lower blood pressure by decreasing myocardial contractility and suppressing reflex tachycardia (through $beta_1$ blockade in the heart), and by decreasing renin release (through $beta_1$ blockade in the kidney).
- Calcium channel blockers (e.g., diltiazem, nifedipine) reduce blood pressure by promoting dilation of arterioles.
- ACE inhibitors and ARBs lower blood pressure by preventing angiotensin II–mediated vasoconstriction and aldosterone-mediated volume expansion. ACE inhibitors work by blocking formation of angiotensin II, whereas ARBs block the actions of angiotensin II.
- Aldosterone receptor blockers lower blood pressure by preventing aldosterone-mediated retention of sodium and water in the kidney.
- Patients with stage 1 hypertension can often be treated with 1 drug, whereas those with stage 2 hypertension usually require 2 or more drugs.
- Thiazide diuretics are preferred drugs for initial therapy of uncomplicated hypertension.
- When a combination of drugs is used for hypertension, each drug should have a different mechanism of action.
- Dosages of antihypertensive drugs should be low initially and then gradually increased. This approach minimizes adverse effects and permits baroreceptors to reset to a lower pressure.
- Lack of patient compliance is the major cause of treatment failure in antihypertensive therapy.
- Compliance is difficult to achieve because (1) hypertension has no symptoms (so drug benefits aren't obvious); (2) hypertension progresses slowly (so patients think they can postpone treatment); and (3) treatment is complex and expensive, continues lifelong, and can cause adverse effects.
- A hypertensive emergency exists when diastolic blood pressure exceeds 120 mm Hg.
- Nitroprusside (IV) is a drug of choice for hypertensive emergencies.
- Hypertension is the most common complication of pregnancy.
- Methyldopa is a drug of choice for treating chronic hypertension of pregnancy.

Summary of Major Nursing Implications*

ANTIHYPERTENSIVE DRUGS

Preadministration Assessment

Therapeutic Goal

The goal of antihypertensive therapy is to prevent the long-term sequelae of hypertension (heart disease, kidney disease, stroke) while minimizing drug effects that can reduce quality of life. For most patients, blood pressure should be reduced to less than 140/90 mm Hg or less than 130/80 mm Hg for those with diabetes or chronic kidney disease.

Baseline Data

The following tests should be done in all patients: blood pressure; electrocardiogram; complete urinalysis; hemoglobin and hematocrit; and blood levels of sodium, potassium, calcium, creatinine, glucose, uric acid, triglycerides, and cholesterol (total, LDL, and HDL cholesterol).

Identifying High-Risk Patients

When taking the patient's drug history, attempt to identify drugs that can raise blood pressure or that can interfere with the effects of antihypertensive drugs. Some drugs of concern are listed below under *Minimizing Adverse Interactions.*

The patient history should identify comorbid conditions that either contraindicate use of specific agents (e.g., asthma and AV block contraindicate use of beta blockers) or require that drugs be used with special caution (e.g., thiazide diuretics must be used with caution in patients with gout or diabetes). For risk factors that pertain to specific antihypertensive drugs, refer to the chapters in which those drugs are discussed.

Implementation: Administration

Routes

All drugs for chronic hypertension are administered orally. None are injected.

Dosage

To minimize adverse effects, dosages should be low initially and then gradually increased. It is counterproductive to employ high initial dosages that produce a rapid fall in pressure while also producing intense undesired responses that can discourage compliance. After 12 months of successful treat-

*Patient education information is highlighted as blue text.

Summary of Major Nursing Implications*—cont'd

ment, an attempt should be made to reduce dosages to their lowest effective level.

Implementation: Measures to Enhance Therapeutic Effects

Lifestyle Modifications

In hypertensive patients, lifestyle changes can reduce blood pressure and increase responsiveness to antihypertensive drugs. These changes should be tried for 6 to 12 months before implementing drug therapy and should continue even if drug therapy is required.

Weight Reduction. **Help overweight patients develop an exercise program and a restricted-calorie diet. The goal is a body mass index in the normal range (18.5–24.9).**

Sodium Restriction. **Encourage patients to consume no more than 6 gm of salt (2.4 gm of sodium) daily and provide them with information on the salt content of foods.**

DASH Diet. **Encourage patients to adopt a diet rich in fruits, vegetables, and lowfat dairy products, and low in total fat, unsaturated fat, and cholesterol.**

Alcohol Restriction. **Encourage patients to limit alcohol consumption to 1 ounce/day (for most men) and 0.5 ounce/ day (for women and small men). One ounce of ethanol is equivalent to about two mixed drinks, two glasses of wine, or two cans of beer.**

Exercise. **Encourage patients with a sedentary lifestyle to perform 30 to 45 minutes of aerobic exercise (e.g., walking, jogging, swimming, bicycling) most days of the week.**

Smoking Cessation. **Strongly encourage patients to quit smoking. Teach patients about aids for smoking cessation (e.g., nicotine patch, bupropion).**

Promoting Compliance

Noncompliance is the major cause of treatment failure. Compliance can be difficult to achieve for several reasons: hypertension is devoid of overt symptoms; drugs do not make people feel better—and may make them feel worse; regimens can be complex and expensive; complications of hypertension take years to develop, thereby providing a misguided rationale for postponing treatment; and treatment usually lasts lifelong.

Provide Patient Education. **Educate patients about the long-term consequences of hypertension and the ability of lifestyle changes and drug therapy to decrease morbidity and prolong life. Inform patients that drugs do not cure hypertension, and therefore must usually be taken lifelong.**

Encourage Self-Monitoring. **Make certain that patients know the treatment goal (usually reduction of blood pressure to <140/90 mm Hg) and teach them to monitor and chart their own pressure. This will increase their involvement and help them see the benefits of treatment.**

Minimize Side Effects. Adverse drug effects are an obvious deterrent to compliance. Measures to reduce undesired effects are discussed below, under *Minimizing Adverse Effects*.

Establish a Collaborative Relationship. **Encourage patients to be active partners in setting treatment goals, creating a treatment program, and evaluating progress.**

Simplify the Regimen. An antihypertensive regimen can consist of several drugs taken multiple times a day. Once an effective regimen has been established, attempt to switch to once-a-day or twice-a-day dosing. If an appropriate combination product is available (e.g., a fixed-dose combination of a thiazide diuretic plus a beta blocker), substitute the combination product for its components.

Other Measures. Additional measures to promote compliance include providing positive reinforcement when treatment goals are achieved, involving family members in the treatment program, scheduling office visits at convenient times, following up on patients who miss an appointment, and devising a program that is effective but keeps costs low.

Ongoing Evaluation and Interventions

Evaluating Treatment

Monitor blood pressure periodically. The usual goal is to reduce it to less than 140/90 mm Hg. **Teach patients to self-monitor their blood pressure and to maintain a blood pressure record.**

Minimizing Adverse Effects

General Considerations. The fundamental strategy for decreasing adverse effects is to tailor the regimen to the sensitivities of the patient. If a drug causes objectionable effects, a more acceptable drug should be substituted.

Inform patients about the potential side effects of treatment and encourage them to report objectionable responses.

Avoid drugs that can exacerbate comorbid conditions. For example, don't give beta blockers to patients who have bradycardia, AV block, or asthma. A list of pathologies and drugs to avoid is given in Table 45–8.

Initiate therapy with low doses and increase them gradually.

Adverse Effects of Specific Drugs. For measures to minimize adverse effects of specific antihypertensive drugs (e.g., beta blockers, diuretics, ACE inhibitors), refer to the chapters in which those drugs are discussed.

Minimizing Adverse Interactions

When taking the patient history, identify drugs that can raise blood pressure or interfere with the effects of antihypertensive drugs. Drugs of concern include oral contraceptives, nasal decongestants and other cold remedies, nonsteroidal anti-inflammatory drugs, glucocorticoids, appetite suppressants, tricyclic antidepressants, monoamine oxidase inhibitors, cyclosporine, erythropoietin, and alcohol (in large quantities).

Antihypertensive regimens frequently contain two or more drugs, thereby posing a potential risk of adverse interactions (e.g., ACE inhibitors can increase the risk of hyperkalemia caused by potassium-sparing diuretics). For interactions that pertain to specific antihypertensive drugs, refer to the chapters in which those drugs are discussed.

*Patient education information is highlighted as blue text.

Drugs for Heart Failure

Heart failure (HF) is a serious, progressive disorder characterized by ventricular dysfunction, reduced cardiac output, insufficient tissue perfusion, and signs of fluid retention (e.g., peripheral edema, shortness of breath). Of the estimated 4.8 million Americans who have HF, 24% are likely to die within 1 year, and 65% within 5 years. Among adults over 65, HF is the leading reason for hospitalization, resulting in 680,000 admissions a year. In 1998, HF contributed to 260,000 American deaths. With improved evaluation and care, many hospitalizations could be prevented, quality of life could be improved, and life expectancy could be extended.

Until recently, HF was commonly referred to as *congestive heart failure.* This term was used because HF frequently causes fluid accumulation (congestion) in the lungs and peripheral tissues. However, because many patients do not have signs of pulmonary or systemic congestion, the term *heart failure* is preferred.

The principal drugs employed for treatment are *angiotensin-converting enzyme (ACE) inhibitors, diuretics, beta blockers,* and *digoxin.* A new drug for HF—*spironolactone*—may also be used. Except for digoxin and spironolactone, all of these drugs are discussed at length in other chapters; hence, their consideration here is brief. Discussion of digoxin and spironolactone is more extensive.

In order to understand HF and the drugs used for treatment, you need a basic understanding of hemodynamics. In particular, you need to understand the contribution of venous pressure, afterload, and the Starling mechanism in determining cardiac output. You also need to understand the roles of the baroreceptor reflex, renin-angiotensin-aldosterone system (RAAS), and kidneys in regulating arterial pressure. If your understanding of these concepts is a little hazy, you can refresh your memory by reading Chapter 41 (Review of Hemodynamics).

PATHOPHYSIOLOGY OF HEART FAILURE

Heart failure is a syndrome in which the heart is unable to pump sufficient blood to meet the metabolic needs of tissues. The syndrome is characterized by signs of *inadequate tissue perfusion* (fatigue, shortness of breath, exercise intolerance) and/or signs of *volume overload* (venous distention, peripheral and pulmonary edema). The major underlying causes of HF are chronic hypertension and myocardial infarction. Other causes include valvular disease, coronary artery disease, congenital heart disease, dysrhythmias, and aging of the myocardium. In its earliest stage, HF is asymptomatic. As failure progresses, fatigue and shortness of breath develop. With further decline in cardiac performance, blood backs up behind the failing ventricles, causing venous distention, peripheral edema, and pulmonary edema. Heart failure is a chronic disorder that requires continuous treatment with drugs.

Cardiac Remodeling

In the initial phase of failure, the heart undergoes remodeling, a process in which the ventricles dilate (grow larger), hypertrophy (increase in wall thickness), and become more spherical (less cylindrical). These alterations in cardiac geometry increase wall stress and reduce left ventricular (LV) ejection fraction. Remodeling occurs in response to cardiac injury, brought on by infarction and other causes. The remodeling process is driven primarily by neurohormonal systems, including the sympathetic nervous system and RAAS. In addition to promoting remodeling, neurohormonal factors promote cardiac fibrosis and myocyte death. The net result of these pathologic changes—remodeling, fibrosis, and cell death—is progressive decline in cardiac output. As a rule, cardiac remodeling precedes development of symptoms, and continues after symptoms appear. As a result, cardiac performance continues to decline.

Physiologic Adaptations to Reduced Cardiac Output

In response to reductions in the pumping ability of the heart, the body undergoes several adaptive changes. Some of these help improve tissue perfusion, whereas others compound existing problems.

Cardiac Dilation. Dilation of the heart is characteristic of HF. Cardiac dilation results from a combination of increased venous pressure (see below) and reduced contractile force. Reduced contractility lowers the amount of blood ejected during systole, causing end-systolic volume to rise. The increase in venous pressure increases diastolic filling, which causes the heart to expand even further.

Because of the Starling mechanism, the increase in heart size that occurs during HF helps improve cardiac output. That is, as the heart fails and its volume expands, contractility increases, causing a corresponding increase in stroke volume. However, it must be noted that the maximal contractile force that can be developed by the failing heart is considerably lower than the maximal force of the healthy heart. This limitation is reflected in the curve for the failing heart shown in Figure 46–1.

If cardiac dilation is insufficient to maintain cardiac output, other factors come into play. As discussed below, these are not always beneficial.

Increased Sympathetic Tone. Heart failure causes arterial pressure to fall. In response, the baroreceptor reflex increases sympathetic output to the heart, veins, and arterioles. At the same time, parasympathetic effects on the heart are reduced. The consequences of increased sympathetic tone are summarized below.

- *Increased heart rate.* Acceleration of heart rate increases cardiac output, thereby helping improve tissue perfusion. However, if heart rate increases too much, there will be insufficient time for complete ventricular filling, and hence cardiac output will fall.
- *Increased contractility.* Increased myocardial contractility has the obvious benefit of increasing cardiac output. The only detriment is an increase in cardiac oxygen demand.
- *Increased venous tone.* Elevation of venous tone increases venous pressure, and thereby increases ventricular filling. Because of the Starling mechanism, increased filling increases stroke volume. Unfortunately, if venous pressure is excessive, blood will back up behind the failing ventricles, thereby aggravating pulmonary and peripheral edema. Furthermore, excessive filling pressure can dilate the heart so much that stroke volume will begin to decline (see Fig. 46–1).
- *Increased arteriolar tone.* Elevation of arteriolar tone increases arterial pressure, thereby increasing perfusion of vital organs. Unfortunately, increased arterial pressure also means that the heart must pump against greater resistance. Since cardiac reserve is minimal in HF, the heart may be unable to meet this challenge, and cardiac output may fall.

Water Retention and Increased Blood Volume. *Mechanisms.* Water retention results from two mechanisms. First, reduced cardiac output causes a reduction in renal blood flow, which in turn decreases glomerular filtration rate (GFR). As a result, urine production is decreased and water is retained. Retention of water increases blood volume.

Second, HF activates the RAAS. Activation occurs in response to reduced blood pressure and reduced renal blood flow. Once activated, the RAAS promotes water retention by increasing circulating levels of *aldosterone* and *angiotensin II.* Aldosterone acts directly on the kidneys to promote retention of sodium and water.* Angiotensin II causes constriction of renal blood vessels, which decreases renal blood flow, and thereby further decreases urine production. In addition to promoting water retention, angiotensin II causes constriction of systemic arterioles and veins, and thereby increases venous and arterial pressure.

---

*In addition to promoting sodium and water retention, aldosterone acts directly on the heart and blood vessels to cause injury. These additional harmful effects are discussed under the heading *Spironolactone: An Aldosterone Receptor Blocker.*

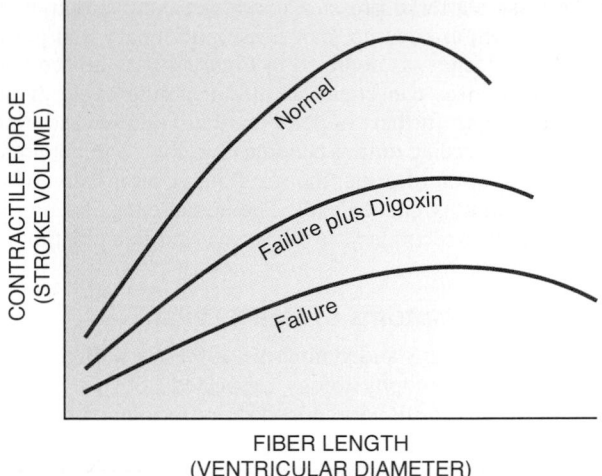

Figure 46–1 ■ Relationship of ventricular diameter to contractile force.
In the normal heart and the failing heart, increased fiber length produces increased contractile force. However, for any given fiber length, contractile force in the failing heart is much less than in the healthy heart. By increasing cardiac contractility, digoxin shifts the relationship between fiber length and stroke volume in the failing heart toward that in the normal heart.

Consequences. As with other adaptive responses to HF, increased blood volume can be both beneficial and harmful. Increased blood volume increases venous pressure, and thereby increases venous return. As a result, ventricular filling and stroke volume are increased. The resultant increase in cardiac output can improve tissue perfusion. However, as noted, if venous pressure is too high, edema of the lungs and periphery may result. More importantly, *if the increase in cardiac output is insufficient to maintain adequate kidney function, renal retention of water will progress unabated. The resultant accumulation of fluid will cause severe cardiac, pulmonary, and peripheral edema—and, ultimately, death.*

Natriuretic Peptides. In response to stretching of the atria and dilation of the ventricles, the heart releases two natriuretic peptides: atrial natriuretic peptides (ANP) and B-natriuretic peptide (BNP). As discussed in Chapter 41, these hormones promote dilation of arterioles and veins, as well as loss of sodium and water through the kidneys. Hence, they tend to counterbalance vasoconstriction caused by the sympathetic nervous system and angiotensin II, as well as retention of sodium and water caused by the RAAS. However, as HF progresses, the effects of ANP and BNP eventually become overwhelmed by the effects of the sympathetic nervous system and RAAS.

The Vicious Cycle of "Compensatory" Physiologic Responses

As discussed above, reduced cardiac output leads to compensatory responses: (1) cardiac dilation, (2) activation of the sympathetic nervous system, (3) activation of the RAAS, and (4) retention of water and expansion of blood volume. Although these responses represent the body's attempt to compensate for reduced cardiac output, they can actually make matters worse: excessive heart rate can reduce ventricular filling; excessive arterial pressure can lower cardiac output; and excessive venous pressure can cause pulmonary and peripheral edema. Hence, as depicted in Figure 46–2, the "compensatory" responses can create a self-sustaining cycle of maladaptation that further impairs cardiac output and tissue perfusion. If cardiac output becomes too low to maintain sufficient production of urine, the resultant accumulation of water will eventually cause death. The actual cause is complete cardiac failure secondary to excessive cardiac dilation and cardiac edema.

Signs and Symptoms of Heart Failure

The prominent signs and symptoms of HF are a direct consequence of the pathophysiology described above. Decreased tissue perfusion results in reduced exercise tolerance, fatigue, and shortness of breath; shortness of breath may also stem from pulmonary edema. Increased sympathetic tone produces tachycardia. Increased ventricular filling, reduced systolic ejection, and myocardial hypertrophy result in cardiomegaly (increased heart size). The combination of increased venous tone plus increased blood volume helps cause pulmonary edema, peripheral edema, hepatomegaly (increased liver size), and distention of the jugular veins. Weight gain results from fluid retention.

Classification of Heart Failure Severity

There are two major schemes for classifying HF severity. One scheme, established by the New York Heart Association (NYHA), classifies HF based on the functional limitations it causes. A much newer scheme, proposed jointly by the American College of Cardiology (ACC) and the American Heart Association (AHA), is based on the fact that HF is a progressive disease that moves through stages of increasing severity.

The NYHA scheme, which has four classes, can be summarized as follows:

- Class I—No limitation of ordinary physical activity
- Class II—Slight limitation of physical activity: normal activity produces fatigue, dyspnea, palpitations, or angina
- Class III—Marked limitation of physical activity: even mild activity produces symptoms
- Class IV—Symptoms occur at rest

The ACC/AHA scheme, which also has four stages, can be summarized as follows:

- Stage A—At high risk for HF but without structural heart disease or symptoms of HF
- Stage B—Structural heart disease but without symptoms of HF
- Stage C—Structural heart disease with prior or current symptoms of HF
- Stage D—Advanced structural heart disease with marked symptoms of HF at rest, and requiring specialized interventions (e.g., heart transplant, mechanical assist device).

This new staging scheme was unveiled in 2001 in an updated clinical guideline titled *ACC/AHA Guidelines for the Evaluation and Management of Chronic Heart Failure in the Adult,* which is available free online at *www.acc.org/clinical/guidelines/failure/hf_index.htm* and *www.americanheart.org/presenter.jhtml?identifier=11841.*

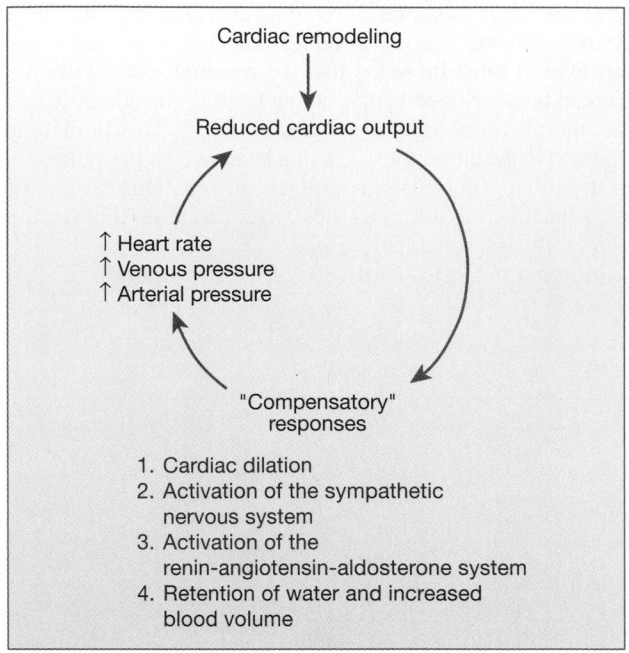

Figure 46–2 ■ **The vicious cycle of maladaptive compensatory responses to a failing heart.**

Please note that the ACC/AHA scheme is intended to complement the NYHA scheme, not replace it. The relationship between the two is shown graphically in Figure 46–3.

OVERVIEW OF DRUGS USED TO TREAT HEART FAILURE

Heart failure is treated with four major classes of drugs: (1) vasodilators, (2) diuretics, (3) beta blockers, and (4) inotropic agents. In addition, spironolactone, an aldosterone antagonist, can offer significant benefits.

ACE Inhibitors and Other Vasodilators

Vasodilators—especially ACE inhibitors—are important drugs for treatment of HF. In addition to improving symptoms, some vasodilators can prolong life.

Vasodilators differ with respect to route of administration (oral versus IV) and site of action (arterioles, veins, or both). Route of administration determines whether a drug is used long term (oral agents) or just acutely (IV agents). Site of action determines specific hemodynamic benefits.

Drugs that dilate *veins* increase venous capacitance, and thereby decrease venous pressure. As a result, venodilators reduce venous return and cardiac filling, which in turn decreases excessive ventricular stretching and cardiac oxygen demand. In addition to their beneficial effects on the heart, venodilators decrease pulmonary congestion and peripheral edema.

Drugs that dilate *arterioles* have three beneficial effects: (1) arteriolar dilation reduces cardiac afterload, and thereby allows stroke volume and cardiac output to increase; (2) by

ACC/AHA Stage   NYHA Functional Classification

A At high risk for HF but without structural heart disease or symptoms of HF	
B Structural heart disease but without symptoms of HF	I Asymptomatic
C Structural heart disease with prior or current symptoms of HF	II Symptomatic with moderate exertion
	III Symptomatic with minimal exertion
D Advanced structural heart disease with marked symptoms of HF at rest despite maximal medical therapy. Specialized interventions (e.g., heart transplant, mechanical assist device) required	IV Symptomatic at rest

Figure 46–3 ■ American College of Cardiology/American Heart Association (ACC/AHA) Stage and New York Heart Association (NYHA) Classification of Heart Failure.

increasing cardiac output and dilating arterioles in the kidney, these drugs increase renal perfusion, and thereby promote loss of fluid; and (3) in skeletal muscle, arteriolar dilation increases local perfusion.

ACE Inhibitors

ACE inhibitors (e.g., captopril, enalapril) are a cornerstone of HF treatment. These drugs can improve functional status and prolong life. In one trial, the 2-year mortality rate for patients taking enalapril was 47% lower than the mortality rate for patients taking placebo. Other large, controlled trials have shown similar benefits. Accordingly, in the absence of specific contraindications, all patients with HF should receive one of these drugs. Although ACE inhibitors can be used alone, they are usually combined with a beta blocker, a diuretic, and digoxin.

How do ACE inhibitors help? These drugs block production of angiotensin II, and thereby *dilate arterioles and veins and decrease release of aldosterone.* Arteriolar dilation improves regional blood flow and, by reducing afterload, increases stroke volume and cardiac output. Venous dilation reduces venous pressure, and thereby reduces pulmonary congestion, peripheral edema, and cardiac dilation. By dilating renal blood vessels, ACE inhibitors improve renal blood flow, and thereby enhance excretion of sodium and water. Suppression of aldosterone release further enhances excretion of sodium, while causing retention of potassium. From the foregoing, we can see that giving an ACE inhibitor is much like giving three different drugs: an arteriolar dilator, a venodilator, and a diuretic.

In addition to blocking angiotensin II production, ACE inhibitors suppress degradation of kinins, and thereby enhance the effects of these compounds. Long-term benefits of ACE inhibitors, including reduced mortality, are probably due more to preservation of kinins, rather than to reduced production of angiotensin II production. This statement is based in part on the observation that long-term therapy reduces mortality, even though angiotensin II levels are not suppressed during prolonged treatment.

The principal adverse effects of the ACE inhibitors are *hypotension* (secondary to arteriolar dilation), *hyperkalemia* (secondary to decreased aldosterone release), *intractable cough,* and *angioedema.* Because of their ability to elevate potassium levels, ACE inhibitors should be used with caution in patients taking potassium supplements or a potassium-sparing diuretic (e.g., spironolactone). ACE inhibitors can cause *fetal injury* if taken during the second or third trimester, and hence are contraindicated for use during pregnancy. In addition, they can cause *renal failure in patients with bilateral renal artery stenosis.*

Adequate dosing is critical: Higher doses are associated with increased survival. Early results of the Assessment of Treatment with Lisinopril and Survival (ATLAS) trial indicate that the doses needed to increase survival are higher than the doses needed to produce hemodynamic changes. Unfortunately, in everyday practice, dosages are often too low: Physicians frequently prescribe doses that are large enough to produce hemodynamic benefits, but are still too low to prolong life. Target doses associated with increased survival are summarized in Table 46–1. These doses should be used unless side effects make them intolerable.

The basic pharmacology of the ACE inhibitors is discussed in Chapter 42.

Angiotensin II Receptor Blockers

Hemodynamic effects of the angiotensin II receptor blockers (ARBs) are nearly identical to those of the ACE inhibitors. Clinical trials have shown that ARBs improve LV ejection fraction, reduce HF symptoms, increase exercise tolerance, decrease hospitalization, enhance quality of life, and, most importantly, reduce mortality. However, ARBs should *not* be combined with ACE inhibitors. Why? Because doing so appears to *increase* mortality. At this time, only one ARB—valsartan [Diovan]—is approved for treating HF. Nonetheless, other ARBs are probably effective too. Until more is known, ARBs should not be used as first-line therapy. Rather, they should be reserved for patients who cannot tolerate ACE inhibitors (because of intractable cough). The pharmacology of the ARBs is discussed in Chapter 42.

TABLE 46-1 ■ ACE Inhibitor Dosages for Heart Failure

ACE Inhibitor	Initial Dose (mg)	Target Dose (mg)	Maximum Dose (mg)
Captopril [Capoten]	6.25 tid	50 tid	50 tid
Enalapril [Vasotec]	2.5 bid	10 bid	20 bid
Lisinopril [Zestril, Prinvil]	2.5–5 qd	10–20 qd	40 qd
Quinapril [Accupril]	10 bid	20 bid	40 bid
Fosinopril [Monopril]	5–10 qd	20 qd	40 qd
Ramipril [Altace]	1.25–2.5 qd	5 qd	10 qd

Isosorbide Dinitrate Plus Hydralazine

For treatment of HF, isosorbide dinitrate (ISDN) and hydralazine are usually combined. The combination represents an alternative to using an ACE inhibitor or an ARB. However, ACE inhibitors and ARBs are generally preferred.

Isosorbide dinitrate [Isordil, Sorbitrate] belongs to the same drug family as nitroglycerin. Like nitroglycerin, ISDN causes selective dilation of *veins*. In patients with severe, refractory HF, the drug can reduce congestive symptoms and improve exercise capacity. In addition to its hemodynamic actions, ISDN may inhibit abnormal myocyte growth, and hence may retard cardiac remodeling. Principal adverse effects are *orthostatic hypotension* and *reflex tachycardia*. The basic pharmacology of ISDN and other organic nitrates is discussed in Chapter 49.

Hydralazine [Apresoline] causes selective dilation of *arterioles*. By doing so, the drug can improve cardiac output and renal blood flow. For treatment of HF, hydralazine is always used in combination with ISDN, since hydralazine by itself is not very effective. Principal adverse effects are *hypotension, tachycardia*, and a syndrome that resembles *systemic lupus erythematosus*. The basic pharmacology of hydralazine is discussed in Chapter 44.

Intravenous Agents for Acute Care

Nitroglycerin. Intravenous nitroglycerin is a powerful *venodilator* that produces a dramatic reduction in venous pressure. Effects have been described as being equivalent to "pharmacologic phlebotomy." In HF, nitroglycerin is used to relieve acute severe pulmonary edema. Principal adverse effects are *hypotension* and resultant *reflex tachycardia*. The basic pharmacology of nitroglycerin is discussed in Chapter 49.

Sodium Nitroprusside. Sodium nitroprusside [Nitropress] acts rapidly to dilate *arterioles* and *veins*. Arteriolar dilation reduces afterload and thereby increases cardiac output. Venodilation reduces venous pressure and thereby decreases pulmonary and peripheral congestion. The drug is indicated for short-term therapy of severe refractory HF. The principal adverse effect is *profound hypotension*. Blood pressure must be monitored continuously. The basic pharmacology of nitroprusside is discussed in Chapter 44.

Nesiritide. Nesiritide [Natrecor] is a synthetic form of human B-type natriuretic peptide (BNP) indicated for short-term, IV therapy of acutely decompensated HF, characterized by increased pulmonary capillary wedge pressure (PCWP) and dyspnea at rest. Nesiritide is produced by recombinant DNA technology and has the same amino acid sequence as naturally occurring BNP. Hemodynamic benefits of the drug equal those of nitroglycerin. However, nesiritide costs much more than nitroglycerin, and hypotension, which can be caused by both drugs, lasts much longer.

Mechanism of Action. Nesiritide affects hemodynamics by three mechanisms: suppression of the RAAS, suppression of sympathetic outflow from the central nervous system (CNS), and direct dilation of arterioles and veins. In patients with HF, benefits derive primarily from direct vasodilation. To promote vasodilation, nesiritide binds to receptors on vascular smooth muscle (VSM), and thereby stimulates production of cyclic GMP (cGMP), a second messenger that causes VSM to relax. This mechanism is similar to that of nitroglycerin, which also stimulates cGMP production. However, whereas nitroglycerin acts primarily on veins, nesiritide dilates arterioles as well. By dilating arterioles and veins, nesiritide reduces both preload and afterload. The net result is a decrease in PCWP and increased cardiac output. Also, by dilating afferent renal arterioles, nesiritide increases GFR, and thereby increases excretion of sodium and water. The result is a reduction in blood volume, which further reduces cardiac preload.

Clinical Effects. Nesiritide has been studied in several clinical trials, including the Vasodilation in the Management of Acute Congestive Heart Failure (VMAC) trial, which compared nesiritide with IV nitroglycerin and placebo. The result? Three hours after the start of treatment, nesiritide produced a significant reduction in PCWP and a significant improvement in dyspnea. The effect was equivalent to that of IV nitroglycerin and superior to that of placebo.

Pharmacokinetics. With continuous infusion, nesiritide achieves steady levels that are 3 to 6 times greater than the level of endogenous BNP present at baseline. Nesiritide is eliminated by three mechanisms: (1) proteolytic cleavage by endopeptidases present on the luminal surface of blood vessels; (2) binding to clearance receptors on the surface of cells, followed by cellular uptake and proteolytic cleavage; and (3) renal filtration. The drug's half-life is 18 minutes.

Adverse Effects. The principal adverse effect is symptomatic *hypotension*. In the VMAC trial, hypotension developed in 4% of patients, about the same rate seen with nitroglycerin. However, because nesiritide has a longer half-life than nitroglycerin, the duration of hypotension was also longer (2.2 hours vs. 0.7 hours with nitroglycerin). The risk of hypotension is increased by high doses of nesiritide and by concurrent use of ACE inhibitors and other vasodilators. In addition to causing hypotension, nesiritide can cause tachycardia (3%), bradycardia (1%), headache (8%), back pain (4%), dizziness (3%), and nausea (4%).

Preparations, Dosage, and Administration. Nesiritide [Natrecor] is available in 1.5-mg, single-use vials. The powder must be dissolved and then diluted to a final concentration of 6 μg/ml. Dosing consists of an initial IV bolus (2 μg/kg) followed by continuous infusion (0.01 μg/kg/min), typically lasting 48 hours or less. If symptomatic hypotension develops, the infusion should be slowed or stopped.

Diuretics

Diuretics are first-line drugs for all patients with signs of volume overload (or with a history of volume overload). By reducing blood volume, these drugs can decrease venous pressure, arterial pressure (afterload), pulmonary edema, peripheral edema, and cardiac dilation. It is important to note, however, that excessive diuresis is hazardous and must be avoided: If blood volume drops too low, cardiac output and blood pressure may fall precipitously, thereby further compromising tissue perfusion. Nonetheless, for most patients, diuretics offer a high benefit-to-risk ratio. The basic pharmacology of the diuretics is discussed in Chapter 39.

Thiazide Diuretics. The thiazide diuretics (e.g., hydrochlorothiazide) produce moderate diuresis. These oral agents are used for long-term therapy of HF when edema is not too great. Since thiazides are ineffective when GFR is low, these drugs cannot be used if cardiac output is greatly reduced. The principal adverse effect of the thiazides is *hypokalemia*, which increases the risk of *digoxin-induced dysrhythmias* (see below).

High-Ceiling (Loop) Diuretics. The loop diuretics (e.g., furosemide) produce profound diuresis. In contrast to the thiazides, these drugs can promote fluid loss even when GFR is low. Hence, loop diuretics are preferred to thiazides when cardiac output is greatly reduced. Administration may be oral or

IV. Because they can mobilize large volumes of water, and because they work when GFR is low, loop diuretics are drugs of choice for patients with severe HF. Like the thiazides, these drugs can cause *hypokalemia,* thereby increasing the risk of *digoxin toxicity.* In addition, loop diuretics can cause severe *hypotension* secondary to excessive volume reduction.

Potassium-Sparing Diuretics. In contrast to the thiazides and loop diuretics, the potassium-sparing diuretics (e.g., spironolactone, triamterene) promote only scant diuresis. In patients with HF, these drugs are employed to counteract potassium loss caused by thiazide and loop diuretics, thereby lowering the risk of digoxin-induced dysrhythmias. Not surprisingly, the principal adverse effect of the potassium-sparing drugs is *hyperkalemia.* Because *ACE inhibitors* also carry a risk of hyperkalemia, caution is needed if they are combined with a potassium-sparing diuretic. Accordingly, when therapy with an ACE inhibitor is initiated, the potassium-sparing diuretic should be discontinued. It can be resumed later if needed.

One potassium-sparing diuretic—spironolactone—prolongs survival in patients with HF primarily by blocking receptors for aldosterone, not by causing diuresis. This drug is discussed separately under the heading *Spironolactone: An Aldosterone Receptor Blocker.*

Beta Blockers

The role of beta blockers in HF continues to evolve. Until recently, HF was considered an absolute contraindication to use of beta blockers. After all, blockade of cardiac beta$_1$-adrenergic receptors *reduces* contractility—an effect that is clearly detrimental, given that contractility is already compromised in the failing heart. However, it is now clear that, with careful control of dosage, beta blockers can improve patient status. Controlled trials have shown that three beta blockers—*carvedilol, metoprolol,* and *bisoprolol*—when added to conventional therapy, can improve LV ejection fraction, increase exercise tolerance, slow progression of HF, reduce the need for hospitalization, and, most importantly, prolong survival. Accordingly, beta blockers are now recommended for most patients. These drugs can even be used in patients with severe disease (NYHA class IV), provided they are euvolemic and hemodynamically stable. Although the mechanism underlying benefits is uncertain, likely possibilities include protecting the heart from excessive sympathetic stimulation and protecting against dysrhythmias. Because excessive beta blockade can reduce contractility, doses must be very low initially and then gradually increased. Full benefits may not be seen for 1 to 3 months. Among patients with heart failure, the principal adverse effects are (1) fluid retention and worsening of HF, (2) fatigue, (3) hypotension, and (4) bradycardia or heart block. Currently, carvedilol [Coreg] and metoprolol [Lopressor, Toprol XL] are the only beta blockers approved by the Food and Drug Administration for use in HF. The basic pharmacology of the beta blockers is discussed in Chapter 18.

Inotropic Agents

Inotropic agents are drugs that increase the force of myocardial contraction. These drugs are given to improve performance of the failing heart. Three types of inotropic drugs are available: *cardiac glycosides, sympathomimetics,* and *phosphodiesterase (PDE) inhibitors.* The sympathomimetics and PDE inhibitors currently available must be administered by IV infusion. Accordingly, their use is generally restricted to acute care of hospitalized patients. At this time, the cardiac glycosides are the only inotropic agents that can be used orally. Hence, they are the only inotropics suited for long-term therapy.

Cardiac Glycosides

The cardiac glycosides (e.g., digoxin) are the oldest and most frequently prescribed inotropic drugs. These agents are used widely for long-term therapy of HF. Unfortunately, although these drugs reduce symptoms, they do not prolong life. The pharmacology of the cardiac glycosides is discussed at length later.

Sympathomimetic Drugs: Dopamine and Dobutamine

The basic pharmacology of dopamine and dobutamine is presented in Chapter 17. Discussion here is limited to their use in HF.

Dopamine. Dopamine [Intropin] is a catecholamine that can activate (1) beta$_1$-adrenergic receptors in the heart, (2) dopamine receptors in the kidney, and (3) at high doses, alpha$_1$-adrenergic receptors in blood vessels. Activation of beta$_1$ receptors increases myocardial contractility, thereby improving cardiac performance. Beta$_1$ activation also increases heart rate, creating a risk of tachycardia. Activation of dopamine receptors dilates renal blood vessels, thereby increasing renal blood flow and urine output. Activation of alpha$_1$ receptors increases vascular resistance (afterload), and can thereby reduce cardiac output. Dopamine is administered by continuous infusion. Constant monitoring of blood pressure, the electrocardiogram (EKG), and urine output is required. Dopamine is employed as a short-term rescue measure for patients with severe, acute cardiac failure.

Dobutamine. Dobutamine [Dobutrex] is a synthetic catecholamine that causes selective activation of beta$_1$-adrenergic receptors. By doing so, the drug can increase myocardial contractility, thereby improving cardiac performance. Like dopamine, dobutamine can cause tachycardia. In contrast to dopamine, dobutamine does not activate alpha$_1$ receptors, and therefore does not increase vascular resistance. As a result, the drug is generally preferred to dopamine for short-term treatment of acute HF. Administration is by continuous infusion.

Phosphodiesterase Inhibitors

Inamrinone. Inamrinone [Inocor], formerly known as *amrinone,* has been called an *inodilator,* because it increases myocardial contractility and promotes vasodilation. Increased contractility results from intracellular accumulation of cyclic AMP (cAMP) secondary to inhibition of PDE-3, the enzyme that normally degrades cAMP. The mechanism underlying vasodilation is unclear. Comparative studies indicate that improvements in cardiac function elicited by amrinone are superior to those elicited by dopamine or dobutamine. Like dopamine and dobutamine, inamrinone is administered by IV infusion, and hence is not suited for outpatient use. Inamrinone is indicated only for short-term (2- to 3-day) treatment of HF in patients who have not responded to vasodilators, diuretics, and digoxin. The drug should be protected from light and should not be mixed with glucose-containing solutions. Constant monitoring is required. The initial dose is 0.75 mg/kg (intravenously) administered over 2 to 3 minutes. The maintenance infusion is 5 to 10 µg/kg/min.

Milrinone. Like inamrinone, milrinone [Primacor] is an inodilator. Increased contractility results from accumulation of cAMP secondary to inhibition of PDE-3. Milrinone is administered by IV infusion and is indicated only for short-term therapy of severe HF. Dosing is complex.

Spironolactone: An Aldosterone Receptor Blocker

Results of the Randomized Aldactone Evaluation Study (RALES) indicate that spironolactone [Aldactone] can reduce symptoms, decrease hospitalizations, and prolong life in patients with moderate to severe HF (NYHA class III or IV). The RALES trial involved 1663 patients at 195 centers in 15 countries on five continents. Half of the patients received standard therapy (ACE inhibitors, diuretics, and, sometimes, digoxin) plus spironolactone (25 mg/day); the other half received standard therapy plus placebo. After 2 years, the mortality rate in the spironolactone group was 30% lower than the mortality rate in the placebo group. Because of these dramatic results, some authorities believe that spironolactone should be added to the regimens of all patients (in the absence of specific contraindications).

Spironolactone helps patients with HF by blocking receptors for aldosterone. Although we usually think of spironolactone as a potassium-sparing diuretic (see Chapter 39), benefits in HF do not result primarily from diuresis and potassium retention. Rather, they result from blockade of receptors for aldosterone, primarily in the heart and blood vessels. To understand the effects of spironolactone, we need to understand the role of aldosterone in HF. Until recently, understanding of aldosterone's role was limited to effects on the kidney—namely, retention of sodium (and water) in exchange for excretion of potassium. As discussed above, aldosterone-mediated water retention contributes to volume overload. However, we now know that aldosterone has additional—and more harmful—effects. Among these are

- Promotion of myocardial remodeling (which impairs pumping)
- Promotion of myocardial fibrosis (which increases the risk of dysrhythmias)
- Activation of the sympathetic nervous system and suppression of norepinephrine uptake in the heart (both of which can promote dysrhythmias and ischemia)
- Promotion of vascular fibrosis (which decreases arterial compliance)
- Promotion of baroreceptor dysfunction

During HF, activation of the RAAS causes levels of aldosterone to rise. In some patients, levels reach 20 times normal. As aldosterone levels grow higher, harmful effects increase, and prognosis becomes progressively worse.

Drugs can reduce the impact of aldosterone in two ways: they can decrease formation of aldosterone or they can block the actions of aldosterone. ACE inhibitors decrease aldosterone formation; spironolactone blocks aldosterone's actions. Although ACE inhibitors reduce aldosterone production, they do not block it entirely. Hence, when ACE inhibitors are used alone, some detrimental effects persist. However, when spironolactone is added to the regimen, these residual effects are nearly eliminated. As a result, symptoms of HF are improved and life is prolonged.

Spironolactone has two adverse effects of concern: *gynecomastia* and *hyperkalemia*. Gynecomastia (breast enlargement), which develops in men, is both cosmetically troublesome and painful. Spironolactone causes gynecomastia by blocking receptors for testosterone. In the RALES trial, 10% of males experienced painful breast enlargement. Hyperkalemia was less common, occurring in only 2% of patients. Spironolactone promotes hyperkalemia by decreasing renal excretion of potassium. To minimize the risk of hyperkalemia, potassium levels should be monitored. In addition, caution is needed in patients taking potassium supplements, ACE inhibitors, or ARBs, and in patients with renal insufficiency, since all of these factors can cause potassium levels to rise.

CARDIAC (DIGITALIS) GLYCOSIDES

The cardiac glycosides are naturally occurring compounds that have profound effects on the mechanical and electrical properties of the heart. By improving mechanical function of the heart, these drugs can reduce symptoms of HF. By altering electrical properties of the heart, these drugs can suppress dysrhythmias—or cause them. Because they are prepared by extraction from *Digitalis purpurea* (purple foxglove) and *Digitalis lanata* (Grecian foxglove), the cardiac glycosides are also known as *digitalis glycosides*.

The cardiac glycosides are among the most widely used prescription drugs, and they are also among the most dangerous. Their frequent use stems from an ability to improve cardiac performance in patients with HF. The high incidence of toxicity results from their propensity to cause dysrhythmias—at doses that are close to therapeutic. There is no question that the cardiac glycosides are a mixed blessing, having the potential for life-enhancing benefits as well as life-threatening harm. Accordingly, it is essential that we use these drugs with respect, caution, and skill.

In the United States, digoxin is the only cardiac glycoside available. Another cardiac glycoside—digitoxin—was recently withdrawn from the U.S. market.

Digoxin

Digoxin [Lanoxin, Lanoxicaps, Digitek] is indicated for HF and dysrhythmias. Treatment of HF is discussed here; treatment of dysrhythmias is discussed in Chapter 47. When used for HF, digoxin can reduce symptoms, increase exercise tolerance, and decrease hospitalizations. However, the drug does not prolong life. Furthermore, when used by *women*, it may actually *shorten* life (see Box 46–1).

Chemistry

Digoxin consists of three components: a steroid nucleus, a lactone ring, and three molecules of digitoxose (a sugar). It is because of the sugars that digoxin is known as a glycoside. The region of the molecule composed of the steroid nucleus plus the lactone ring (i.e., the region without the sugar molecules) is responsible for the pharmacologic effects of digoxin. The sugars only increase solubility.

Mechanical Effects on the Heart

Digoxin exerts a *positive inotropic action* on the heart. That is, the drug *increases the force of ventricular contraction,* and thereby increases cardiac output.

Special Interest Topic

BOX 46–1 ■ ATTENTION LADIES: DIGOXIN MAY BE HAZARDOUS TO YOUR HEALTH

A new analysis of older data indicates that, for *women* with heart failure, digoxin may do more harm than good. In 1997, the Digitalis Investigation Group[1] (DIG) reported the results of a large, randomized, placebo-controlled trial designed to assess the impact of digoxin on morbidity and mortality in patients with heart failure. The study enrolled 6801 patients (men and women) with heart failure and followed them for an average of 37 months. They all took an ACE inhibitor and a diuretic; half also received digoxin and the other half received a placebo. The result? Digoxin improved symptoms and decreased hospitalizations, but did not reduce mortality. The overall death rate was 35%, regardless of whether patients took digoxin or placebo. However, the data were not analyzed for possible gender-related effects. Accordingly, in 2002, Rathore et al.[2] performed a retrospective analysis of the DIG data to determine whether digoxin had different effects in men and women. What did their analysis reveal? Among men, digoxin had no significant impact on mortality, mirroring the overall mortality seen in 1997. However, among *women*, digoxin produced a small, but significant *increase* in mortality: After 37 months, the death rate was 28.9% for women taking placebo compared with 33.1% for those taking digoxin—an increase of 4.2%.

Why did digoxin increase the mortality rate in women, but not in men? The answer is unknown. Theoretical possibilities include sex-based differences in autonomic function, muscle metabolism, signal transduction, or myocardial cell growth and function. However, there may be a more simple answer: In the women who died, digoxin plasma levels may have been excessive. It is well established that digoxin can be lethal at high levels. In the DIG trial, digoxin levels were measured only in randomly selected patients, and hence Rathore et al. lacked the data needed to determine whether deaths were related to high drug levels. If high digoxin levels were indeed responsible for the observed mortality increase, then the take-home message is obvious: We must keep digoxin doses low.

The Rathore et al. study suggests that, for female patients, the benefits of digoxin therapy (primarily a small [4%] decrease in the risk of hospitalization) may not justify the risk (possible drug-induced death). Until more is known, prudence dictates using digoxin in women with increased caution. As a rule, the drug should be reserved for patients who have not responded adequately to first-line medicines: ACE inhibitors, diuretics, and beta blockers. Furthermore, digoxin levels should be kept as low as possible (0.5 to 1 ng/ml is a reasonable initial target). Finally, although the new analysis underscores the potential dangers of digoxin, we mustn't forget that the drug *can* benefit many patients—especially those with heart failure combined with atrial fibrillation. Accordingly, we shouldn't withhold digoxin indiscriminately. Nor should we discontinue it without careful consideration, since doing so might lead to hemodynamic decompensation.

[1]The Digitalis Investigation Group. The effect of digoxin on mortality and morbidity in patients with heart failure. N Engl J Med 1997;336:525–533.
[2]Rathore SS, Wang Y, Krumholz H. Sex-based differences in the effect of digoxin for the treatment of heart failure. N Engl J Med 2002;347:1403–1411.

Mechanism of Inotropic Action. Digoxin increases myocardial contractility by inhibiting an enzyme known as *sodium potassium ATPase* (Na^+,K^+-ATPase). By way of an indirect process (see below), inhibition of Na^+,K^+-ATPase promotes calcium accumulation inside myocytes. The calcium then augments contractile force by facilitating the interaction of myocardial contractile proteins: actin and myosin.

To understand how inhibition of Na^+,K^+-ATPase causes intracellular calcium to rise, we must first understand the normal role of Na^+,K^+-ATPase in myocytes. That role is illustrated in Figure 46–4. As indicated, when an action potential passes along the myocyte membrane (sarcolemma), Na^+ ions and Ca^{++} ions enter the cell, and K^+ ions exit. Once the action potential has passed, these ion fluxes must be reversed so that the original ionic balance of the cell can be restored. Na^+,K^+-ATPase is critical to this process. As shown in Figure 46–4, Na^+,K^+-ATPase acts as a "pump" to draw extracellular K^+ ions into the cell, while simultaneously extruding intracellular Na^+. The energy required for pumping Na^+ and K^+ is provided by the breakdown of ATP—hence the name Na^+,K^+-ATPase. To complete the normalization of cellular ionic composition, Ca^{++} ions must leave the cell. Extrusion of Ca^{++} is accomplished through an exchange process in which extracellular Na^+ ions are taken into the cell while Ca^{++} ions exit. This exchange of Na^+ for Ca^{++} is a passive (energy-independent) process.

We can now answer the question, how does digoxin's ability to inhibit Na^+,K^+-ATPase produce an increase in intracellular Ca^{++} levels? By inhibiting Na^+,K^+-ATPase, digoxin prevents the myocyte from restoring its proper ionic composition following the passage of an action potential. Inhibition of Na^+,K^+-ATPase blocks uptake of K^+ and extrusion of Na^+. Hence, with each successive action potential, intracellular K^+ levels decline and intracellular

Na^+ levels rise. It is this rise in Na^+ that leads to the rise in intracellular Ca^{++}. In the presence of excess intracellular Na^+, further Na^+ entry is suppressed. Since Na^+ entry is suppressed, the passive exchange of Ca^{++} for Na^+ cannot take place; hence, Ca^{++} accumulates within the cell.

Relationship of Potassium to Inotropic Action. Potassium ions compete with digoxin for binding to Na^+,K^+-ATPase. This competition is of great clinical significance. Because potassium competes with digoxin, when potassium levels are low, binding of digoxin to Na^+,K^+-ATPase increases. This increase can produce excessive inhibition of Na^+,K^+-ATPase with resultant toxicity. Conversely, when levels of potassium are high, inhibition of Na^+,K^+-ATPase by digoxin is reduced, causing a reduction in the therapeutic response. Because an increase in potassium can impair therapeutic responses, whereas a decrease in potassium can cause toxicity, it is imperative that potassium levels be kept within the normal physiologic range: 3.5 to 5 mEq/L.

Beneficial Effects in Heart Failure

Increased Cardiac Output. The primary effect of digoxin is to increase myocardial contractility, which in turn increases cardiac output. As shown in Figure 46–1, by increasing contractility, digoxin shifts the relationship of fiber length to stroke volume in the failing heart toward that in the healthy heart. Consequently, at any given heart

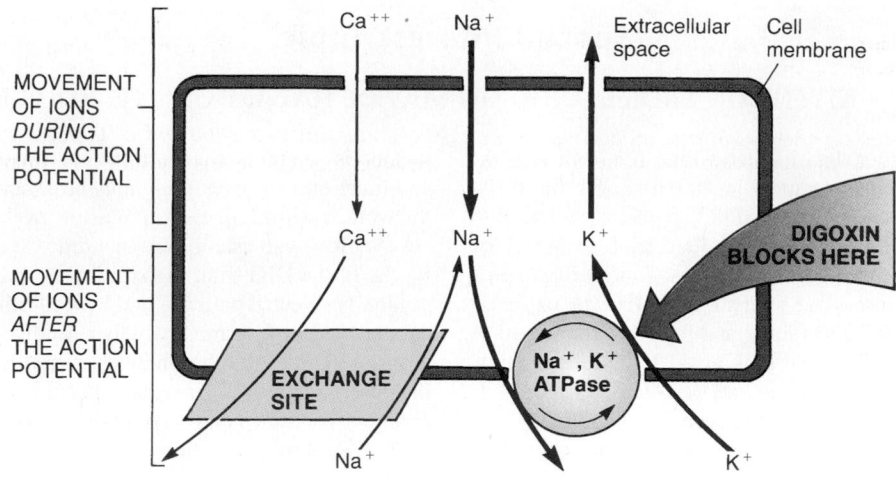

Figure 46–4 ■ Ion fluxes across the cardiac cell membrane.
During the action potential, Na^+ and Ca^{++} enter the cardiac cell and K^+ exits. Following the action potential, Na^+,K^+-ATPase pumps Na^+ out of the cell and takes up K^+. Ca^{++} leaves the cell in exchange for the uptake of Na^+. By inhibiting Na^+,K^+-ATPase, digoxin prevents the extrusion of Na^+, causing Na^+ to accumulate inside the cell. The resulting buildup of intracellular Na^+ suppresses the Na^+-Ca^{++} exchange process, thereby causing intracellular levels of Ca^{++} to rise.

size, the stroke volume of the failing heart increases, causing cardiac output to rise.

Consequences of Increased Cardiac Output. As a result of increased cardiac output, three major secondary responses occur: (1) sympathetic tone declines, (2) urine production increases, and (3) renin release declines. These responses can lead to reversal of virtually all signs and symptoms of HF. However, they do nothing to correct the underlying problem of cardiac remodeling.

Decreased Sympathetic Tone. By increasing contractile force and cardiac output, digoxin increases arterial pressure. In response, sympathetic nerve traffic to the heart and blood vessels is reduced via the baroreceptor reflex. (Recall that a compensatory *increase* in sympathetic tone had taken place because of HF.)

The decrease in sympathetic tone has several beneficial effects. First, heart rate is reduced, thereby allowing more complete ventricular filling. Second, afterload is reduced (because of reduced arteriolar constriction), thereby allowing more complete ventricular emptying. Third, venous pressure is reduced (because of reduced venous constriction), thereby reducing cardiac distention, pulmonary congestion, and peripheral edema.

Increased Urine Production. The increase in cardiac output increases renal blood flow, and thereby increases production of urine. The resultant loss of water reduces blood volume, which in turn reduces cardiac distention, pulmonary congestion, and peripheral edema.

Decreased Renin Release. In response to increased arterial pressure, renin release declines, causing levels of aldosterone and angiotensin II to decline as well. The decrease in angiotensin II decreases vasoconstriction, thereby further reducing afterload and venous pressure. The decrease in aldosterone reduces retention of sodium and water, which reduces blood volume, which in turn further reduces venous pressure.

Summary of Effects in Heart Failure. In summary, we can see that, through direct and indirect mechanisms, digoxin has the potential to reverse all of the overt manifestations of HF: cardiac output improves, heart rate decreases, heart size declines, constriction of arterioles and veins decreases, water retention reverses, blood volume declines, peripheral and pulmonary edema decrease, and weight is lost (because of water loss). In addition, exercise tolerance improves and fatigue is reduced. There is, however, one important caveat to keep in mind: Although digoxin can produce substantial improvement in symptoms, the drug does not alter the natural course of HF, and does not prolong life.

Electrical Effects on the Heart

The effects of digoxin on the electrical activity of the heart are of therapeutic and toxicologic importance. It is because of its electrical effects that digoxin is useful for treating dysrhythmias (see Chapter 47). Ironically, these same electrical effects are responsible for *causing* dysrhythmias—the most serious toxicity of digoxin.

The electrical effects of digoxin can be bewildering in their complexity. Through a combination of actions, digoxin can alter the electrical activity in noncontractile tissue (sinoatrial [SA] node, atrioventricular [AV] node, Purkinje fibers) as well as in ventricular muscle. In these various regions, digoxin can alter automaticity, refractoriness, and impulse conduction. Whether these parameters are increased or decreased depends on cardiac status, digoxin dosage, and the particular region involved.

Although the electrical effects of digoxin are many and varied, only a few are clinically significant. These are discussed below.

Mechanisms for Altering Electrical Activity of the Heart. Digoxin alters the electrical properties of the heart by *inhibiting Na^+,K^+-ATPase* and by *enhancing vagal influences on the heart.* By inhibiting Na^+,K^+-ATPase, digoxin alters the distribution of ions (Na^+, K^+, Ca^{++})

across the cardiac cell membrane. This change in ion distribution can alter the electrical responsiveness of the cells involved. Since hypokalemia intensifies inhibition of Na$^+$,K$^+$-ATPase, hypokalemia intensifies alterations in cardiac electrical properties.

Digoxin acts in two ways to enhance vagal effects on the heart. First, the drug acts in the CNS to increase the firing rate of vagal fibers that innervate the heart. Second, digoxin increases the responsiveness of the SA node to acetylcholine (the neurotransmitter released by the vagus). The net result of these vagotonic effects is (1) decreased automaticity of the SA node, and (2) decreased conduction through the AV node.

Effects on Specific Regions of the Heart. In the SA node, digoxin decreases automaticity (by the vagotonic mechanisms just mentioned). In the AV node, digoxin decreases conduction velocity and prolongs the effective refractory period; these effects, which can promote varying degrees of AV block, result primarily from the drug's vagotonic actions. In Purkinje fibers, digoxin-induced inhibition of Na$^+$,K$^+$-ATPase results in increased automaticity; this increase can generate ectopic foci that, in turn, can cause ventricular dysrhythmias. In the ventricular myocardium, digoxin acts to shorten the effective refractory period and to (possibly) increase automaticity.

Cardiotoxicity: Generation of Dysrhythmias

Dysrhythmias are the most serious adverse effect of digoxin. The drug causes dysrhythmias by altering the electrical properties of the heart. Fortunately, when used in the dosages recommended today, dysrhythmias are uncommon.

Because serious dysrhythmias are a potential consequence of therapy, all patients should be evaluated frequently for changes in heart rate and rhythm. If significant changes occur, digoxin should be withheld and the physician consulted. Outpatients should be taught to monitor their pulses and instructed to report any significant changes in rate or regularity.

Types of Digoxin-Induced Dysrhythmias. Digoxin can mimic practically all types of dysrhythmias. Atrioventricular block with escape beats is among the most common. Ventricular flutter and ventricular fibrillation are the most dangerous.

Mechanism of Ventricular Dysrhythmia Generation. Digoxin-induced ventricular dysrhythmias result from a combination of four factors:

- Decreased automaticity of the SA node
- Decreased impulse conduction through the AV node
- Spontaneous discharge of Purkinje fibers (caused in part by increased automaticity)
- Shortening of the effective refractory period in ventricular muscle.

Increased Purkinje fiber discharge and shortening of the ventricular effective refractory period predispose the ventricles to developing ectopic beats. Potential ectopic beats become manifest because the effects of digoxin on the SA and AV nodes decrease the ability of the normal pacemaker to drive the ventricles, thereby allowing ventricular ectopic beats to take over.

Predisposing Factors. Hypokalemia. The most common cause of dysrhythmias in patients receiving digoxin is hypokalemia secondary to the use of diuretics. Less common causes include vomiting and diarrhea. Hypokalemia promotes dysrhythmias by increasing digoxin-induced inhibition of Na$^+$,K$^+$-ATPase, which in turn leads to increased automaticity of Purkinje fibers. Because low potassium can precipitate dysrhythmias, *it is imperative that serum potassium levels be kept within a normal range.* If diuretic therapy causes potassium levels to fall, a potassium-sparing diuretic (e.g., spironolactone) can be prescribed to correct the problem. Potassium supplements may also be used. Patients should be taught to

recognize symptoms of hypokalemia (e.g., muscle weakness) and instructed to notify the physician if these develop.

Elevated Digoxin Levels. Digoxin has a narrow therapeutic range: Drug levels only slightly higher than therapeutic greatly increase the risk of toxicity. Possible causes of excessive digoxin levels include (1) intentional or accidental overdose, (2) increased digoxin absorption, and (3) decreased digoxin elimination.

If digoxin levels are kept within the therapeutic range (0.5 to 1.1 ng/ml), the chances of a dysrhythmia will be reduced. However, it is important to note that careful control over drug levels does not eliminate the risk entirely. As discussed above, there is only a loose relationship between digoxin levels and clinical effects. As a result, some patients may experience dysrhythmias even when drug levels are well within what is normally considered the therapeutic range.

Heart Disease. The ability of digoxin to cause dysrhythmias is greatly increased by the presence of heart disease. Doses of digoxin that have no adverse effects on healthy volunteers can precipitate serious dysrhythmias in patients with HF. The probability and severity of a dysrhythmia are directly related to the severity of the underlying disease. Since heart disease is the reason for taking digoxin, it should be no surprise that people taking the drug are at risk of dysrhythmias.

Diagnosis of Cardiotoxicity. Diagnosis of digoxin-induced dysrhythmias is not easy. Much of the difficulty stems from the fact that the failing heart is prone to developing dysrhythmias spontaneously. Hence, when a dysrhythmia occurs, we cannot simply assume that digoxin is the cause: The possibility that the dysrhythmia is the direct result of heart disease must be considered. Compounding diagnostic difficulties is the poor correlation between plasma digoxin levels and dysrhythmia onset. Because of this loose correspondence, the presence of an apparently excessive digoxin level does not necessarily indicate that digoxin is responsible for the problem. Laboratory data required for diagnosis include digoxin level, serum electrolytes, and an EKG. Ultimately, diagnosis is based on experience and clinical judgment. Resolution of the dysrhythmia following digoxin withdrawal confirms the diagnosis.

Management of Digoxin-Induced Dysrhythmias. With proper treatment, digoxin-induced dysrhythmias can almost always be controlled. Basic management measures are as follows:

- *Withdraw digoxin and potassium-wasting diuretics.* For many patients, no additional treatment is needed. To help ensure that medication is stopped, a written order to withhold digoxin should be made.
- *Monitor serum potassium.* If the potassium level is low or nearly normal, potassium (IV or PO) should be administered. Potassium displaces digoxin from Na$^+$,K$^+$-ATPase and thereby helps reverse toxicity. However, if potassium levels are high or if AV block is present, no more potassium should be given. Under these conditions, more potassium may cause complete AV block.
- Some patients may require an antidysrhythmic drug. *Phenytoin* and *lidocaine* are most effective. Quinidine, another antidysrhythmic drug, can cause plasma levels of digoxin to rise, and hence should not be used.
- Patients who develop bradycardia or AV block can be treated with atropine. (Atropine blocks the vagal influ-

ences that underlie bradycardia and AV block.) Alternatively, electronic pacing may be employed.

■ When overdose is especially severe, digoxin levels can be lowered using *Fab antibody fragments* [Digibind]. Following IV administration, these fragments bind digoxin, and thereby prevent it from acting. Treatment is expensive: A full neutralizing dose costs $2000 to $3000. *Cholestyramine* and *activated charcoal,* agents that also bind digoxin, can be administered orally to suppress absorption of digoxin from the GI tract.

Noncardiac Adverse Effects

The principal noncardiac toxicities of digoxin concern the GI system and the CNS. Since adverse effects on these systems frequently precede development of dysrhythmias, symptoms involving the GI tract and CNS can provide advance warning of more serious toxicity. Accordingly, patients should be taught to recognize these effects and instructed to notify the physician if they occur.

Anorexia, nausea, and *vomiting* are the most common GI effects of digoxin. These responses result primarily from stimulation of the chemoreceptor trigger zone of the medulla. Digoxin rarely causes diarrhea.

Fatigue is the most frequent CNS effect. *Visual disturbances* (e.g., blurred vision, yellow tinge to vision, appearance of halos around dark objects) are also relatively common.

TABLE 46–2 ■ Drug Interactions with Digoxin

Drug	Effect
Pharmacodynamic Interactions	
Thiazide diuretics Loop diuretics	Promote potassium loss and thereby increase the risk of digoxin-induced dysrhythmias
Beta blockers Verapamil Diltiazem	Decrease contractility and heart rate
Sympathomimetics	Increase contractility and heart rate
Pharmacokinetic Interactions	
Cholestyramine Kaolin-pectin Neomycin Sulfasalazine	Decrease digoxin levels by decreasing digoxin absorption or bioavailability
Aminoglycosides Antacids Colestipol Erythromycin Omeprazole Tetracycline	Increase digoxin levels by increasing digoxin absorption or bioavailability
Alprazolam Amiodarone Captopril Diltiazem Nifedipine Nitrendipine Propafenone Quinidine Verapamil	Increase digoxin levels by decreasing excretion of digoxin, altering distribution of digoxin, or both

Reducing the Risk of Toxicity

Patient education can help reduce the incidence of toxicity. Patients should be warned about digoxin-induced dysrhythmias and instructed to take their medication exactly as prescribed. In addition, they should be informed about symptoms of developing toxicity (altered heart rate or rhythm, visual or GI disturbances) and instructed to notify the physician if these develop. If a potassium supplement or potassium-sparing diuretic is part of the regimen, it should be taken exactly as prescribed.

Drug Interactions

Digoxin is subject to a large number of significant drug interactions. Some are pharmacodynamic and some are pharmacokinetic. Several important interactions are discussed below. A summary of interactions is presented in Table 46–2.

Diuretics. *Thiazide diuretics* and *loop diuretics* promote loss of potassium, and thereby increase the risk of digoxin-induced dysrhythmias. Accordingly, when digoxin and these diuretics are used concurrently, serum potassium levels must be monitored and maintained within a normal range (3.5 to 5 mEq/L). If hypokalemia develops, potassium levels can be restored with potassium supplements, a potassium-sparing diuretic, or both.

ACE Inhibitors. These drugs can increase potassium levels, and can thereby decrease therapeutic responses to digoxin. Exercise caution if an ACE inhibitor is combined with potassium supplements or a potassium-sparing diuretic.

Sympathomimetics. Sympathomimetic drugs (e.g., dopamine, dobutamine) act on the heart to increase the rate and force of contraction. The increase in contractile force can add to the positive inotropic effects of digoxin. These complementary actions can be beneficial. In contrast, the ability of sympathomimetics to increase heart rate may be detrimental in that the risk of a tachydysrhythmia is increased.

Quinidine. Quinidine is an antidysrhythmic drug that can cause plasma levels of digoxin to rise. Quinidine increases digoxin levels by (1) displacing digoxin from tissue binding sites and (2) reducing the renal excretion of digoxin. By elevating levels of free digoxin, quinidine can promote digoxin toxicity. Accordingly, concurrent use of quinidine and digoxin should be avoided.

Verapamil. Verapamil, a calcium channel blocker, can significantly increase plasma levels of digoxin. If the combination is employed, digoxin dosage must be reduced. In addition, verapamil can suppress myocardial contractility, and can thereby counteract the benefits of digoxin.

Pharmacokinetics

Absorption. Absorption of oral digoxin can be variable. The extent of absorption is lowest and most variable with digoxin *tablets,* ranging between 60% and 80%. Absorption from digoxin capsules [Lanoxicaps] is more complete and less variable, ranging between 90% and 100%. However, although digoxin capsules permit excellent absorption, they do have one drawback: they are much more expensive than the tablets. Hence, it may be preferable to reserve the capsules for patients in whom stable drug levels cannot be achieved with tablets.

Several factors can decrease digoxin bioavailability. For example, meals high in bran can decrease absorption significantly. Bioavailability can also be decreased by cholestyramine, kaolin-pectin, and certain other drugs (see Table 46–3). Taking digoxin with meals slows the rate of absorption, but does not decrease the extent of absorption.

In the past, there was considerable variability in the absorption of digoxin from tablets prepared by different manufacturers. This variability resulted from differences in the rate and extent of tablet dissolution. Because of this variable bioavailability, it had been recommended that patients not switch between different digoxin brands. Today, bioavailability of digoxin in tablets produced by different companies is fairly uniform, making brands of digoxin more interchangeable than in the past. However, given the narrow therapeutic range of the digoxin, some authorities still recommend that patients not switch between brands of digoxin tablets—even when prescriptions are written generically—except with the approval and supervision of the physician.

Distribution. Digoxin is distributed widely and crosses the placenta. High levels are achieved in cardiac and skeletal muscle, owing largely to binding to Na$^+$,K$^+$-ATPase. About 23% of digoxin in plasma is bound to proteins, mainly albumin.

Elimination. Digoxin is eliminated primarily by *renal excretion.* Hepatic metabolism is minimal. Because digoxin is eliminated by the kidneys, alterations in renal function can have a significant impact on digoxin blood levels: If kidney function declines, digoxin may accumulate to levels that are toxic. Accordingly, dosage must be reduced in patients with renal impairment. Because digoxin is not metabolized to a significant extent, changes in liver function do not affect plasma digoxin levels.

Half-Life and Time to Plateau. The half life of digoxin is about 1.5 days. Hence, in the absence of a loading dose, about 6 days (four half-lives) are required for plateau levels to be achieved. When use of the drug is discontinued, another 6 days are required for digoxin stores to be eliminated.

Single-Dose Time Course. Effects of a single oral dose begin 30 minutes to 2 hours after administration and peak within 4 to 6 hours. Effects of intravenous digoxin begin rapidly (within 5 to 30 minutes) and peak in 1 to 4 hours.

A Note on Plasma Digoxin Levels. Most hospitals are equipped to measure plasma levels of digoxin. The therapeutic range is 0.5 to 1.1 ng/ml. Levels above 2.0 ng/ml are toxic. Knowledge of plasma levels can be useful for

- Establishing dosage
- Monitoring compliance
- Diagnosing toxicity
- Determining the cause of therapeutic failure

Once a stable blood level has been achieved, routine measurement of digoxin levels is unnecessary; rather, an annual determination is usually sufficient. Additional measurements may be useful when

- Digoxin dosage is changed
- Symptoms of HF intensify
- Kidney function deteriorates
- Signs of toxicity appear
- Drugs that can affect digoxin levels are added to or deleted from the regimen

Although knowledge of digoxin plasma levels can aid the clinician, it must be understood that the extent of this aid is limited. The correlation between plasma levels of digoxin and clinical effects—both therapeutic and adverse—is not very tight: Drug levels that are safe and effective for patient A may be subtherapeutic for patient B and toxic for patient C. Because of interpatient variability, knowledge of digoxin levels does not permit precise predictions of therapeutic effects or toxicity. Hence, information regarding drug levels must not be relied upon too heavily. Rather, this information should be seen as but one factor among several to be considered when evaluating clinical responses.

Preparations, Dosage, and Administration

Preparations. Digoxin is available in four formulations:

- Tablets—0.125 and 0.25 mg [Lanoxin, Digitek]
- Pediatric elixir—0.05 mg/ml [Lanoxin]
- Solution for injection—0.1 and 0.25 mg/ml [Lanoxin]
- Capsules with digoxin in solution—0.05, 0.1, and 0.2 mg [Lanoxicaps]

Administration. Digoxin can be administered *orally* and *intravenously.* *Intramuscular* administration causes severe pain and tissue damage and should be avoided. Prior to administration, the rate and regularity of the heart beat should be determined. If heart rate is less than 60 beats/min or if a change in rhythm is detected, digoxin should be withheld and the physician notified. When digoxin is given intravenously, cardiac status should be monitored continuously for 1 to 2 hours.

Dosage in Heart Failure. Most patients can be treated with initial and maintenance dosages in the range of 0.125 to 0.25 mg/day. Low doses (0.125 mg daily or every other day) are needed for patients who are older than 70 or especially lean, or who have renal dysfunction. Doses above 0.25 mg/day are rarely used or needed. The target plasma drug level is 0.5 to 1.1 ng/ml.

Digitalization. The term *digitalization* refers to the use of a loading dose to achieve high plasma levels of digoxin quickly. (As noted, 6 days are needed for drug levels to reach plateau if no loading dose is employed.) Although digitalization was common in the past, the practice is now considered both unnecessary and inappropriate.

Digitoxin

Digitoxin, a drug no longer available in the United States, is similar to digoxin in most respects. These drugs have the same mechanism of action (inhibition of Na$^+$,K$^+$-ATPase), the same clinical applications (treatment of HF and dysrhythmias), and the same major toxicities (dysrhythmias). The principal differences between them are pharmacokinetic: Absorption of digitoxin is complete, whereas absorption of digoxin is both incomplete and variable; digitoxin is eliminated by the liver, whereas digoxin is eliminated by the kidneys; and digitoxin has a longer half-life (7 days vs. 1.6 days). Because digitoxin has a prolonged half-life, management of toxicity is much harder than with digoxin. For more information on digitoxin, refer to the fourth edition of this book.

MANAGEMENT OF HEART FAILURE

Our discussion of HF management reflects recommendations in the 2001 revision of the *ACC/AHA Guidelines for the Evaluation and Management of Chronic Heart Failure in the Adult.* As noted earlier, these guidelines approach HF as a progressive disease that advances through four stages of increasing severity. Management for each stage is discussed below.

Stage A

By definition, patients in ACC/AHA Stage A have no symptoms of HF and no structural or functional cardiac abnormalities—but they do have behaviors or conditions strongly associated with developing HF. Important among these factors are hypertension, coronary artery disease, diabetes, family history of cardiomyopathy, and a personal history of alcohol abuse, rheumatic fever, or treatment with a cardiotoxic drug (e.g., doxorubicin, trastuzumab).

Management is directed at reducing risk. Hypertension, hyperlipidemia, and diabetes should be controlled, as should ventricular rate in patients with supraventricular tachycardias. An ACE inhibitor is recommended for patients with diabetes, atherosclerosis, or hypertension. Patients should cease behaviors that increase HF risk, especially smoking and alcohol abuse. (Excessive, chronic consumption of alcohol is a leading cause of cardiomyopathy. In patients with HF, acute alcohol consumption can suppress contractility.) There is no evidence that development of symptomatic HF can be avoided by reducing salt intake, using dietary supplements, or getting regular exercise.

Stage B

Like patients in Stage A, those in Stage B have no signs or symptoms of HF—but they do have structural heart disease that is strongly associated with development of HF. Among these structural changes are LV hypertrophy or fibrosis, LV dilation or hypocontractility, valvular heart disease, and previous myocardial infarction.

The goal of management is to prevent development of symptomatic HF. The approach is to implement measures that can prevent further cardiac injury and thereby retard the progression of remodeling and LV dysfunction. Specific measures include all those discussed above for Stage A. In addition, treatment with an ACE inhibitor plus a beta blocker is recommended for all patients with a reduced ejection fraction, history of myocardial infarction, or both. As in Stage A, there is no evidence that reducing salt intake, using dietary supplements, or getting regular exercise can help prevent progression to symptomatic HF.

Stage C

Patients in Stage C have symptoms of HF and also have structural heart disease. As discussed earlier, symptoms include dyspnea, fatigue, peripheral edema, and distention of the jugular vein. Treatment has four major goals: (1) relief of pulmonary and peripheral congestive symptoms, (2) improvement of functional capacity and quality of life, (3) slowing of cardiac remodeling and progression of LV dysfunction, and (4) prolongation of life. Treatment measures include those recommended for Stages A and B, along with those discussed below.

Drug Therapy

Drug therapy of HF has changed dramatically in the past decade. Formerly, cardiac glycosides (usually digoxin) were the mainstay of treatment. Today, their role is secondary. First-line therapy now consists of three drugs: a diuretic, an ACE inhibitor, and a beta blocker. Digoxin is used primarily when symptoms cannot be managed with these preferred agents.

Diuretics. All patients with evidence of fluid retention (or a history of fluid retention) should receive a diuretic. These drugs are the only reliable means of correcting fluid overload. Furthermore, they produce symptomatic improvement faster than any other drugs. If renal function is good, a thiazide diuretic will work. However, if renal function is significantly

impaired, as it is in most patients, a loop diuretic will be needed. Efficacy of diuresis is best assessed by daily measurement of body weight. Once fluid overload has been corrected, diuretic therapy should continue to prevent recurrence. Diuretics should not be used alone. Rather, for most patients, they should be combined with an ACE inhibitor and a beta blocker (and usually digoxin). Since aspirin and other nonsteroidal anti-inflammatory drugs (NSAIDs) can decrease the effects of diuretics, these drugs should be avoided.

ACE Inhibitors. In the absence of specific contraindications (e.g., pregnancy), all patients with Stage C HF should receive an ACE inhibitor. If fluid retention is evident, a diuretic should be used as well. Symptomatic improvement may take weeks or even months to develop. However, even in the absence of symptomatic improvement, ACE inhibitors may prolong life. Dosages should be sufficient to reduce mortality (see Table 46–1).

For patients who cannot tolerate ACE inhibitors (owing to intractable cough or angioedema), an ARB may be used instead. However, it is important to note that, at this time, ARBs are considered neither equivalent nor superior to ACE inhibitors.

Beta Blockers. In the absence of specific contraindications, all patients with Stage C HF should receive a beta blocker—usually in combination with an ACE inhibitor and diuretic. As with ACE inhibitors, symptomatic improvement may not be evident for months; nonetheless, life may be prolonged even in the absence of clinical improvement.

Digoxin. Digoxin may be used in combination with ACE inhibitors, diuretics, and beta blockers to improve clinical status. However, although digoxin can reduce symptoms, it does not prolong life. Dosing is based on clinical response. The drug may be started early to help improve symptoms, or it may be reserved for patients who have not responded adequately to a diuretic, ACE inhibitor, and beta blocker.

Spironolactone. Spironolactone is a new treatment for HF and its role has not been established. The ACC/AHA guidelines recommend reserving the drug for patients who have symptoms at rest despite treatment with an ACE inhibitor, diuretic, beta blocker, and digoxin. Spironolactone should not be used if kidney function is impaired or serum potassium is abnormal.

Drugs to Avoid

Patients in Stage C should avoid three classes of drugs: antidysrhythmics, calcium channel blockers, and NSAIDs (e.g., aspirin). Reasons for not using these drugs are as follows:

- *Antidysrhythmic agents*—These drugs have cardiosuppressant and prodysrhythmic actions that can make HF worse. Only one agent—amiodarone [Cordarone]—has been proven to not reduce survival.
- *Calcium channel blockers*—These drugs can make HF worse and may increase the risk of adverse cardiovascular events. Only one agent—amlodipine [Norvasc]—has been shown not to reduce survival.
- *NSAIDs*—These drugs promote sodium retention and peripheral vasoconstriction, actions that can make HF worse. In addition, they can reduce the efficacy and intensify the toxicity of diuretics and ACE inhibitors. Hence, even though aspirin has beneficial effects on coagulation, it should still not be used.

Exercise Training

In the past, bed rest was recommended owing to concern that physical activity might accelerate progression of LV dysfunction. However, we now know that inactivity is actually detrimental: it reduces conditioning, worsens exercise intolerance, and contributes to HF symptoms. Conversely, studies have shown that exercise training can improve clinical status, increase exercise capacity, and improve quality of life. Accordingly, exercise training should be considered for all stable patients.

Evaluating Treatment

Evaluation is based on symptoms and physical findings. Reductions in dyspnea on exertion, paroxysmal nocturnal dyspnea, and orthopnea (difficulty breathing, except in the upright position) indicate success. The physical examination should assess for reductions in jugular distention, edema, and rales. Success is also indicated by increased capacity for physical activity. Accordingly, patients should be interviewed to determine improvements in the maximal activity they can perform without symptoms, the type of activity that regularly produces symptoms, and the maximal activity that they can tolerate. (Activity is defined as walking, stair climbing, activities of daily living, or any other activity that is appropriate for the patient.) Successful treatment should also improve health-related quality of life in general. Hence the interview should look for improvements in sleep, sexual function, outlook on life, cognitive function (alertness, memory, concentration), and ability to participate in usual social, recreational, and work activities.

Routine measurement of ejection fraction or maximal exercise capacity is not recommended. Although the degree of reduction in ejection fraction measured at the beginning of therapy is predictive of outcome, improvement in the ejection fraction does not necessarily indicate that the prognosis has changed.

Stage D

Patients in Stage D have advanced structural heart disease and marked symptoms of HF at rest—despite treatment with maximal doses of medications used in Stage C. Repeated and prolonged hospitalization is common. For eligible candidates, the best long-term solution is a heart transplant.

Management focuses largely on control of fluid retention, which underlies most signs and symptoms. Intake and output should be monitored closely, and the patient should be weighed daily. Fluid retention can usually be treated with a loop diuretic, perhaps combined with a thiazide diuretic. If volume overload becomes severe, the patient should be hospitalized and given an IV diuretic. If needed, IV dopamine or dobutamine can be added to increase renal blood flow, thereby enhancing diuresis. Patients should not be discharged until a stable and effective oral diuretic regimen has been established.

What other measures should be considered? Beta blockers and ACE inhibitors may be tried, but doses should be low and responses monitored with care. Why? Because, in Stage D, beta blockers pose a significant risk of making HF worse, and ACE inhibitors may induce profound hypotension or renal failure.

∴ KEY POINTS

- Heart failure is characterized by ventricular dysfunction, reduced cardiac output, signs of inadequate tissue perfusion (fatigue, shortness of breath, exercise intolerance), and signs of fluid overload (venous distention, peripheral edema, pulmonary edema).
- The initial phase of HF consists of cardiac remodeling—a process in which the ventricles dilate (grow larger), hypertrophy (increase in wall thickness), and become more spherical—coupled with cardiac fibrosis and myocyte death. As a result of these changes, cardiac output is reduced.
- Reduced cardiac output leads to compensatory responses: (1) activation of the sympathetic nervous system, (2) activation of the renin-angiotensin-aldosterone system, and (3) retention of water and expansion of blood volume. As a result of volume expansion, cardiac dilation increases.
- If the compensatory responses are insufficient to maintain adequate production of urine, water will continue to accumulate, eventually causing death (from complete cardiac failure secondary to excessive cardiac dilation and cardiac edema).
- Drugs that dilate veins decrease venous pressure, and thereby decrease excessive ventricular stretching and cardiac oxygen demand. The decrease in venous pressure also reduces pulmonary and peripheral edema.
- Drugs that dilate arterioles reduce afterload, and thereby allow stroke volume and cardiac output to increase. By increasing cardiac output and dilating arterioles in the kidney, arteriolar dilators increase renal perfusion, and thereby promote loss of fluid.
- ACE inhibitors block formation of angiotensin II and reduce release of aldosterone. As a result, they cause dilation of veins and arterioles, promote renal excretion of water, and help blunt the damaging effects of aldosterone.
- In patients with HF, ACE inhibitors improve functional status and reduce mortality. In the absence of specific contraindications, all patients should get one.
- ACE inhibitors can cause hypotension, hyperkalemia, cough, and angioedema.
- The combination of isosorbide dinitrate (which dilates veins) and hydralazine (which dilates arterioles) can be used in place of an ACE inhibitor for patients who cannot tolerate them.
- Diuretics are first-line drugs for all patients with fluid overload. By reducing blood volume, these drugs can decrease venous pressure, arterial pressure, pulmonary edema, peripheral edema, and cardiac dilation.
- Thiazide diuretics are ineffective when GFR is low, and hence cannot be used if cardiac output is greatly reduced.
- Loop diuretics are effective even when GFR is low, and hence are preferred to thiazides for most patients.
- Thiazide diuretics and loop diuretics can cause hypokalemia, and can thereby increase the risk of digoxin-induced dysrhythmias.

- Potassium-sparing diuretics are used to counteract potassium loss caused by thiazide diuretics and loop diuretics.
- Potassium-sparing diuretics can cause hyperkalemia. By doing so, they can increase the risk of hyperkalemia in patients taking ACE inhibitors.
- Although beta blockers can harm patients with HF, when used properly, they can decrease mortality. To minimize risk, doses must be very low initially and then gradually increased.
- In patients with HF, spironolactone reduces symptoms and prolongs life. Benefits derive from blocking aldosterone receptors in the heart and blood vessels.
- Inotropic agents (e.g., cardiac glycosides, sympathomimetics) increase the force of myocardial contraction, and thereby increase cardiac output.
- Of the available inotropic agents, digoxin is the only one that is both effective and safe when used orally, and hence the only one suitable for long-term use.
- Digoxin increases contractility by inhibiting myocardial Na^+,K^+-ATPase, thereby (indirectly) increasing intracellular calcium content, which in turn facilitates the interaction of actin and myosin.
- Potassium competes with digoxin for binding to Na^+,K^+-ATPase. Hence, if potassium levels are low, excessive inhibition of Na^+,K^+-ATPase can occur, resulting in toxicity. Conversely, if potassium levels are high, insufficient inhibition can occur, resulting in loss of therapeutic effects. Accordingly, it is imperative to keep potassium levels in the normal physiologic range: 3.5 to 5 mEq/L.
- By increasing cardiac output, digoxin can reverse all of the overt manifestations of HF: cardiac output improves, heart rate decreases, heart size declines, constriction of arterioles and veins decreases, water retention reverses, blood volume declines, peripheral and pulmonary edema decrease, weight is lost (because of water loss), and exercise tolerance improves.

- Unfortunately, although digoxin can improve symptoms, it does not alter the natural course of HF, and does not prolong life.
- Digoxin causes dysrhythmias by altering the electrical properties of the heart (secondary to inhibition of Na^+,K^+-ATPase).
- The most common reason for digoxin-related dysrhythmias is diuretic-induced hypokalemia.
- If a severe digoxin overdose is responsible for dysrhythmias, digoxin levels can be lowered using Fab antibody fragments [Digibind].
- In addition to dysrhythmias, digoxin can cause GI effects (anorexia, nausea, vomiting) and CNS effects (fatigue, visual disturbances). Gastrointestinal and CNS effects often precede dysrhythmias, and therefore can provide advance warning of serious toxicity.
- Digoxin has a narrow therapeutic range.
- Digoxin is eliminated by renal excretion.
- Although routine monitoring of digoxin levels is generally unnecessary, monitoring can be helpful when dosage is changed, symptoms of HF intensify, kidney function declines, signs of toxicity appear, or drugs that affect digoxin levels are added to or deleted from the regimen.
- Maintenance doses of digoxin are based primarily on observation of the patient: Doses should be large enough to minimize symptoms of HF but not so large as to cause adverse effects.
- Maintenance doses of digoxin must be reduced if renal function declines.
- Therapy of Stage C HF has four major goals: (1) relief of pulmonary and peripheral congestion, (2) improvement of functional status and quality of life, (3) retarding progression of cardiac remodeling and LV dysfunction, and (4) prolongation of life.
- Most patients with Stage C HF are treated with four drugs: a diuretic, an ACE inhibitor, a beta blocker, and digoxin.

Summary of Major Nursing Implications*

DIGOXIN

Preadministration Assessment

Therapeutic Goal

Digoxin is used to treat HF and cardiac dysrhythmias. Be sure to confirm which disorder the drug has been prescribed for.

Baseline Data

Assess for signs and symptoms of HF, including fatigue, weakness, cough, breathing difficulty (orthopnea, dyspnea on exertion, paroxysmal nocturnal dyspnea), jugular distention, and edema.

Determine baseline values for maximal activity without symptoms, activity that regularly causes symptoms, and maximal tolerated activity.

Laboratory tests should include an EKG, serum electrolytes, measurement of ejection fraction, and evaluation of kidney function.

Identifying High-Risk Patients

Digoxin is *contraindicated* for patients experiencing ventricular fibrillation, ventricular tachycardia, or digoxin toxicity. Exercise *caution* in the presence of conditions that can predispose the patient to serious adverse responses to digoxin, such as hypokalemia, partial AV block, advanced HF, or renal impairment.

Implementation: Administration

Routes

Oral, slow IV injection.

*Patient education information is highlighted as blue text.

Summary of Major Nursing Implications*—cont'd

Administration

Oral. Determine heart rate and rhythm prior to administration. If heart rate is less than 60 beats/min or if a change in rhythm is detected, withhold digoxin and notify the physician.

Warn patients not to "double up" on doses in attempts to compensate for missed doses.

Intravenous. Monitor cardiac status closely for 1 to 2 hours following IV injection.

Promoting Compliance

Since digoxin has a narrow therapeutic range, rigid adherence to the prescribed dosage is essential. **Inform patients that failure to take digoxin exactly as prescribed may lead to toxicity or therapeutic failure.** If poor compliance is suspected, serum drug levels may help in assessing the extent of noncompliance.

Implementation: Measures to Enhance Therapeutic Effects

Advise patients to limit salt intake to 2 gm/day, and to avoid excessive fluids. Advise patients who drink alcohol to consume no more than one drink each day. Advise obese patients to adopt a reduced-calorie diet. Help patients establish an appropriate program of regular, mild exercise (e.g., walking, cycling). Precipitating factors for HF (e.g., hypertension, valvular heart disease) should be corrected.

Ongoing Evaluation and Interventions

Evaluating Therapeutic Effects

Evaluation is based on symptoms and physical findings. Assess for reductions in orthopnea, dyspnea on exertion, paroxysmal nocturnal dyspnea, neck vein distention, edema, and rales, and for increased capacity for physical activity. In addition, assess for improvements in sleep, sexual function, outlook on life, cognitive function, and ability to participate in social, recreational, and work activities.

Measurement of plasma drug levels can help determine the cause of therapeutic failure. The therapeutic range for digoxin is 0.5 to 1.1 ng/ml.

Minimizing Adverse Effects

Cardiotoxicity. Dysrhythmias are the most serious adverse effect of digoxin.

Monitor hospitalized patients for alterations in heart rate or rhythm, and withhold digoxin if significant changes develop.

Inform outpatients about the danger of dysrhythmias. Teach them to monitor their pulses for rate and rhythm, and instruct them to notify the physician if significant changes

occur. Provide the patient with an EKG rhythm strip; this can be used by physicians unfamiliar with the patient (e.g., when the patient is traveling) to verify suspected changes in rhythm.

Hypokalemia, usually diuretic induced, is the most frequent underlying cause of dysrhythmias. Monitor serum potassium concentrations. If hypokalemia develops, potassium levels can be raised with potassium supplements, a potassium-sparing diuretic, or both. **Teach patients to recognize early signs of hypokalemia (e.g., muscle weakness), and instruct them to notify the physician if these develop.** Severe vomiting and diarrhea can increase potassium loss; exercise caution if these events occur.

To treat digoxin-induced dysrhythmias: (1) withdraw digoxin and diuretics (make sure that a written order for digoxin withdrawal is made); (2) administer potassium (unless potassium levels are above normal or AV block is present); (3) administer an antidysrhythmic drug (phenytoin or lidocaine, but not quinidine) if indicated; (4) manage bradycardia with atropine or electrical pacing; and (5) treat with Fab fragments if toxicity is life threatening.

Noncardiac Effects. Nausea, vomiting, diarrhea, fatigue, and visual disturbances (blurred or yellow vision) frequently foreshadow more serious toxicity (dysrhythmias) and should be reported immediately. **Inform patients about these early indications of toxicity, and instruct them to notify the physician if they develop.**

Minimizing Adverse Interactions

Diuretics. Thiazide diuretics and loop diuretics increase the risk of dysrhythmias by promoting potassium loss. Monitor potassium levels. If hypokalemia develops, it should be corrected with potassium supplements, a potassium-sparing diuretic, or both.

ACE Inhibitors. These drugs can elevate potassium levels, and can thereby decrease therapeutic responses to digoxin. Exercise caution if an ACE inhibitor is combined with potassium supplements or a potassium-sparing diuretic.

Sympathomimetic Agents. Sympathomimetic drugs (e.g., dopamine, dobutamine) stimulate the heart, thereby increasing the risk of tachydysrhythmias and ectopic pacemaker activity. When sympathomimetics are combined with digoxin, monitor closely for dysrhythmias.

Quinidine. Quinidine can elevate plasma levels of digoxin. If quinidine is employed concurrently with digoxin, digoxin dosage must be reduced. Do not use quinidine to treat digoxin-induced dysrhythmias.

*Patient education information is highlighted as blue text.

Antidysrhythmic Drugs

There are two basic types of dysrhythmias: *tachydysrhythmias* (dysrhythmias in which heart rate is increased) and *bradydysrhythmias* (dysrhythmias in which heart rate is slowed). In this chapter, we only consider the tachydysrhythmias. This is by far the largest group of dysrhythmias and the group that responds best to drugs. We do not discuss the bradydysrhythmias because they are few in number and are commonly treated with electronic pacing. When drugs are indicated, atropine (see Chapter 14) and isoproterenol (see Chapter 17) are usually the agents of choice.

It is important to appreciate that virtually all of the drugs used to treat dysrhythmias can also *cause* dysrhythmias. These drugs can create new dysrhythmias and worsen existing ones. Because of these prodysrhythmic actions, antidysrhythmic drugs should be employed only when the benefits of treatment clearly outweigh the risks.

For two reasons, use of antidysrhythmic drugs is declining. First, research has shown that some of these agents actually *increase* the risk of death. Second, nonpharmacologic therapies—especially implantable defibrillators and radiofrequency ablation—have begun to replace drugs as the preferred treatment for many types of dysrhythmias.

A note on terminology: Dysrhythmias are also known as *arrhythmias*. Since the term *arrhythmia* denotes an *absence* of cardiac rhythm, whereas *dysrhythmia* denotes an *abnormal* rhythm, dysrhythmia would seem the more appropriate term.

ELECTRICAL PROPERTIES OF THE HEART

Dysrhythmias result from alteration of the electrical impulses that regulate cardiac rhythm—and antidysrhythmic drugs control rhythm by correcting or compensating for these alterations. Accordingly, in order to understand both the generation and treatment of dysrhythmias, we must first understand the electrical properties of the heart. Accordingly, we begin the chapter by reviewing (1) pathways and timing of impulse conduction, (2) cardiac action potentials, and (3) basic elements of the electrocardiogram (EKG).

Impulse Conduction: Pathways and Timing

For the heart to pump effectively, contraction of the atria and ventricles must be coordinated. Coordination is achieved through precise timing and routing of impulse conduction. In the healthy heart, impulses originate in the sinoatrial (SA) node, spread rapidly through the atria, pass slowly through the atrioventricular (AV) node, and then spread rapidly through the ventricles via the His-Purkinje system (Fig. 47–1).

A dysrhythmia is defined as *an abnormality in the rhythm of the heartbeat.* In their mildest forms, dysrhythmias have only modest effects on cardiac output. However, in their most severe forms, dysrhythmias can so disable the heart that no blood is pumped at all. Because of their ability to compromise cardiac function, dysrhythmias are associated with a high degree of morbidity and mortality.

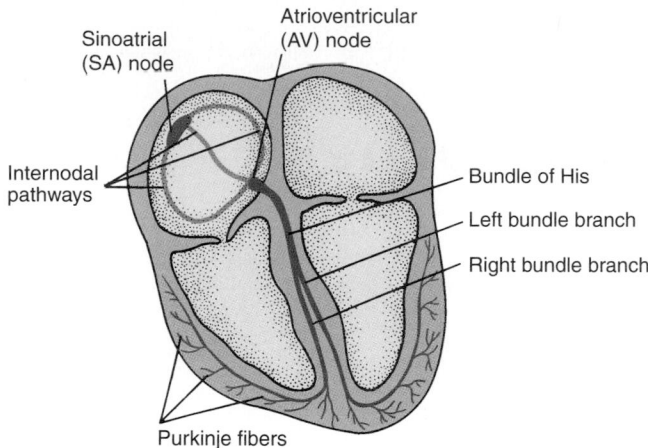

Sinoatrial (SA) node

Atrioventricular (AV) node

Internodal pathways

Bundle of His

Left bundle branch

Right bundle branch

Purkinje fibers

Figure 47–1 ■ Cardiac conduction pathways.

SA Node. Under normal circumstances, the SA node serves as the pacemaker for the heart. Pacemaker activity results from spontaneous phase 4 depolarization (see below). Because cells of the sinus node usually discharge faster than other cells that display automaticity, the SA node normally dominates all other potential pacemakers.

After the SA node discharges, impulses spread rapidly through the atria along the *internodal pathways.* This rapid conduction allows the atria to contract in unison.

AV Node. Impulses originating in the atria must travel through the AV node to reach the ventricles. In the healthy heart, impulses arriving at the AV node are delayed before going on to excite the ventricles. This delay provides time for blood to fill the ventricles prior to ventricular contraction.

His-Purkinje System. The fibers of the His-Purkinje system consist of specialized conducting tissue. The function of these fibers is to conduct electrical excitation very rapidly to all parts of the ventricles. Stimulation of the His-Purkinje system is caused by impulses leaving the AV node. These impulses are conducted rapidly down the bundle of His, enter the right and left bundle branches, and then distribute to the many fine branches of the Purkinje fibers (see Fig. 47–1). Because impulses travel quickly through this system, all regions of the ventricles are stimulated almost simultaneously, producing synchronized ventricular contraction with resultant forceful ejection of blood.

Cardiac Action Potentials

Cardiac cells can initiate and conduct action potentials, consisting of self-propagating waves of depolarization followed by repolarization. As in neurons, cardiac action potentials are generated by the movement of ions into and out of cells. These ion fluxes take place by way of specific channels in the cell membrane. In the resting cardiac cell, negatively charged ions cover the inner surface of the cell membrane while positively charged ions cover the external surface. Because of this separation of charge, the cell membrane is said to be *polarized.* Under proper conditions, channels in the cell membrane open, allowing positively charged ions to rush in. This influx eliminates the charge difference across the cell membrane; hence, the cell is said to depolarize. Following depolarization,

positively charged ions are extruded from the cell, causing the cell to return to its original polarized state.

In the heart, two kinds of action potentials occur: *fast potentials* and *slow potentials.* These potentials differ with respect to the mechanisms by which they are generated, the kinds of cells in which they occur, and the drugs to which they respond.

Profiles of fast and slow potentials are depicted in Figure 47–2. Please note that action potentials in this figure represent the electrical activity of *single cardiac cells.* Such single-cell recordings, which are made using experimental preparations, should not be confused with the EKG, which is made using surface electrodes, and reflects the electrical activity of the entire heart.

Fast Potentials

Fast potentials occur in fibers of the *His-Purkinje system* and in *atrial and ventricular muscle.* These responses serve to conduct electrical impulses rapidly throughout the heart.

As indicated in panel *A* of Figure 47–2, fast potentials have five distinct phases, labeled 0, 1, 2, 3, and 4. As we discuss each phase, we will focus on its ionic basis and its relationship to the actions of antidysrhythmic drugs.

Phase 0. In phase 0, the cell undergoes *rapid depolarization* in response to *influx of sodium ions.* Phase 0 is important in that the speed of phase 0 depolarization determines the velocity of impulse conduction. Drugs that decrease the rate of phase 0 depolarization (by blocking sodium channels) slow impulse conduction though the His-Purkinje system and myocardium.

Phase 1. During phase 1, rapid (but partial) repolarization takes place. Phase 1 has no relevance to antidysrhythmic drugs.

Phase 2. Phase 2 consists of a prolonged plateau in which the membrane potential remains relatively stable. During this phase, *calcium* enters the cell and promotes contraction of atrial and ventricular muscle. Drugs that reduce calcium entry during phase 2 do *not* influence *cardiac rhythm.* However, since calcium influx is required for contraction, these drugs *can* reduce myocardial contractility.

Phase 3. In phase 3, rapid repolarization takes place. This repolarization is caused by *extrusion of potassium* from the cell. Phase 3 is relevant in that delay of repolarization prolongs the action potential duration, and thereby prolongs the effective refractory period (ERP). (The ERP is the time during which a cell is unable to respond to excitation and initiate a new action potential. Hence, extending the ERP prolongs the minimum interval between two propagating responses.) Phase 3 repolarization can be delayed by drugs that block potassium channels.

Phase 4. During phase 4, two types of electrical activity are possible: (1) the membrane potential may remain *stable* (solid line in Fig. 47–2A), or (2) the membrane may undergo *spontaneous depolarization* (dotted line). In cells undergoing spontaneous depolarization, the membrane potential gradually rises until a threshold potential is reached. At this point, rapid phase 0 depolarization takes place, setting off a new action potential. Hence, it is phase 4 depolarization that gives cardiac cells *automaticity* (the ability to initiate an action potential through self-excitation). The capacity for self-excitation makes potential pacemakers of all cells that have it.

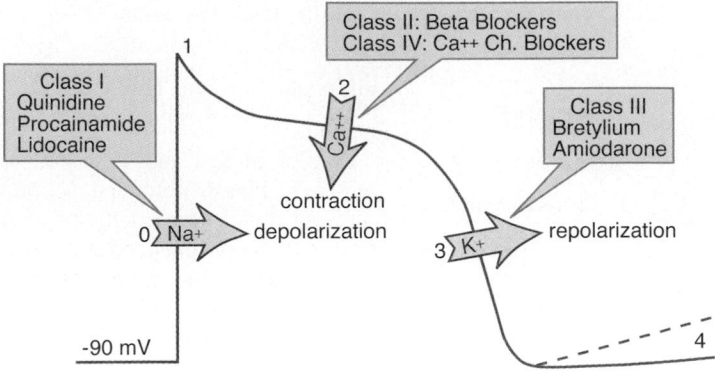

A **Myocardium and His-Purkinje System**

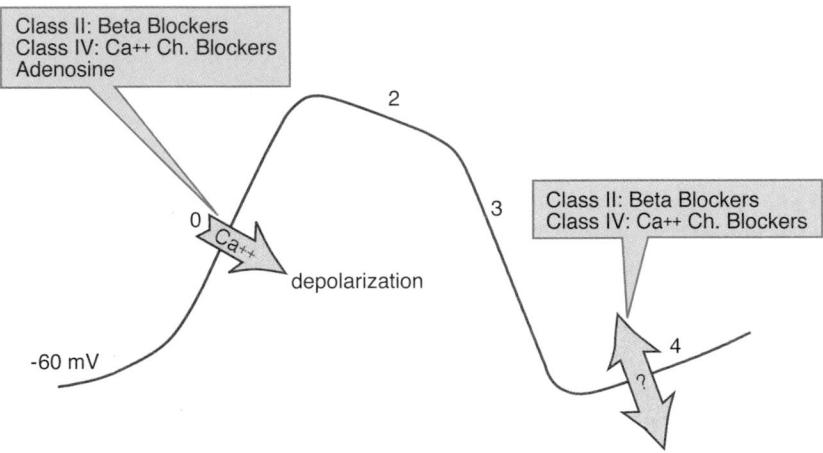

B **SA Node and AV Node**

Figure 47–2 ■ **Ion fluxes during cardiac action potentials and effects of antidysrhythmic drugs.**
A, Fast potential of the His-Purkinje system and atrial and ventricular myocardium. Blockade of sodium influx by class I drugs slows conduction in the His-Purkinje system. Blockade of calcium influx by beta blockers and calcium channel blockers decreases contractility. Blockade of potassium efflux by class III drugs delays repolarization and thereby prolongs the effective refractory period. *B,* Slow potential of the sinoatrial (SA) node and atrioventricular (AV) node. Blockade of calcium influx by beta blockers, calcium channel blockers, and adenosine slows AV conduction. Beta blockers and calcium channel blockers decrease SA nodal automaticity (phase 4 depolarization); the ionic basis of this effect is not understood.

Under normal conditions, His-Purkinje cells undergo very slow spontaneous depolarization, and myocardial cells do not undergo any. However, under pathologic conditions, significant phase 4 depolarization may occur in all of these cells, and especially in Purkinje fibers. When this happens, a dysrhythmia can result.

Slow Potentials

Slow potentials occur in cells of the *SA node* and *AV node.* The profile of a slow potential is depicted in Figure 47–2B. Like fast potentials, slow potentials are generated by ion fluxes. However, the specific ions involved are not the same for every phase.

From a physiologic and pharmacologic perspective, slow potentials have three features of special significance: (1) phase 0 depolarization is slow and mediated by calcium influx, (2) these potentials conduct slowly, and (3) spontaneous phase 4 depolarization in the SA node normally determines heart rate.

Phase 0. Phase 0 (depolarization phase) of slow potentials differs significantly from phase 0 of fast potentials. As we can see from Figure 47–2, whereas phase 0 of fast potentials is caused by an *inward rush of sodium,* phase 0 of slow potentials is caused by *slow influx of calcium.* Because calcium influx is slow, the rate of depolarization is slow; and because depolarization is slow, these potentials conduct slowly. This explains why impulse conduction through the AV node is de-

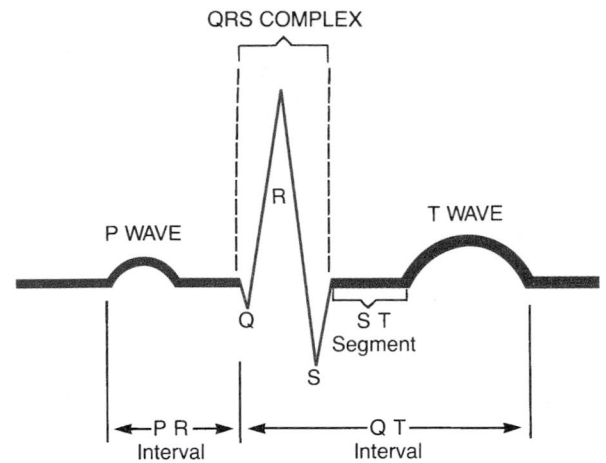

Figure 47–3 ■ The electrocardiogram.

layed. Phase 0 of the slow potential is of therapeutic significance in that drugs that suppress calcium influx during phase 0 can slow (or stop) AV conduction.

Phases 1, 2, and 3. Slow potentials lack a phase 1 (see Fig. 47–2*B*). Phases 2 and 3 of the slow potential are not significant with respect to the actions of antidysrhythmic drugs.

Phase 4. Cells of the SA node and AV node undergo spontaneous phase 4 depolarization. The ionic basis of this phenomenon is complex and incompletely understood.

Under normal conditions, the rate of phase 4 depolarization in cells of the SA node is faster than in all other cells of the heart. As a result, the SA node discharges first and determines heart rate. Hence, the SA node is referred to as the cardiac *pacemaker.*

As indicated in Figure 47–2*B,* two classes of drugs (beta blockers and calcium channel blockers) can suppress phase 4 depolarization. By doing so, these agents can decrease automaticity in the SA node.

The Electrocardiogram

The EKG provides a graphic representation of cardiac electrical activity. The EKG can be used to identify dysrhythmias and monitor responses to therapy. (*Note:* In referring to the electrocardiogram, two abbreviations may be used: EKG and ECG. Many people prefer EKG over ECG. Why? Because ECG sounds much like EEG [electroencephalogram] when spoken aloud.)

The major components of an EKG are illustrated in Figure 47–3. As we can see, three features are especially prominent: the P wave, the QRS complex, and the T wave. The P wave is caused by *depolarization in the atria.* Hence, the P wave corresponds to atrial contraction. The QRS complex is caused by *depolarization of the ventricles.* Hence, the QRS complex corresponds to ventricular contraction. If conduction through the ventricles is slowed, the QRS complex will widen. The T wave is caused by *repolarization of the ventricles.* Hence, this wave is not associated with overt physical activity of the heart.

In addition to the features just described, the EKG has three other components of interest: the PR interval, the QT interval, and the ST segment. The PR interval is defined as

the time between the onset of the P wave and the onset of the QRS complex. Lengthening of this interval indicates a delay in conduction through the AV node. Several drugs increase the PR interval. The QT interval is defined as the time between the onset of the QRS complex and the completion of the T wave. This interval is prolonged by drugs that delay ventricular repolarization. The ST segment is the portion of the EKG that lies between the end of the QRS complex and the beginning of the T wave. Digoxin depresses the ST segment.

GENERATION OF DYSRHYTHMIAS

Dysrhythmias arise from two fundamental causes: *disturbances of impulse formation* (automaticity) and *disturbances of impulse conduction.* One or both of these disturbances underlie all dysrhythmias. Factors that may alter automaticity or conduction include hypoxia, electrolyte imbalance, cardiac surgery, reduced coronary blood flow, myocardial infarction, and antidysrhythmic drugs.

Disturbances of Automaticity

Disturbances of automaticity can occur in any area of the heart. Cells normally capable of automaticity (cells of the SA node, AV node, and His-Purkinje system) can produce dysrhythmias if their normal rate of discharge changes. In addition, dysrhythmias may be produced if tissues that do not normally express automaticity (atrial and ventricular muscle) develop spontaneous phase 4 depolarization.

Altered automaticity in the SA node can produce tachycardia or bradycardia. Excessive discharge of sympathetic neurons that innervate the SA node can augment automaticity to such a degree that sinus tachycardia results. Excessive vagal (parasympathetic) discharge can suppress automaticity to such a degree that sinus bradycardia results.

Increased automaticity of Purkinje fibers is a common cause of dysrhythmias. The increase can be brought on by injury and by excessive stimulation of Purkinje fibers by the sympathetic nervous system. If Purkinje fibers begin to discharge faster than the SA node, they will escape control by the SA node; potentially serious dysrhythmias may result.

Under special conditions, automaticity may develop in cells of atrial and ventricular muscle. Dysrhythmias will result if these cells begin to fire faster than the SA node.

Disturbances of Conduction

Atrioventricular Block. Impaired conduction through the AV node produces varying degrees of AV block. If impulse conduction is delayed (but not prevented entirely), the block is termed *first degree.* If some impulses pass through the node but others do not, the block is termed *second degree.* If all traffic through the AV node stops, the block is termed *third degree.*

Reentry (Recirculating Activation). Reentry, also referred to as recirculating activation, is a generalized mechanism by which dysrhythmias can be produced. Reentry causes dysrhythmias by establishing a localized, self-sustaining circuit capable of repetitive cardiac stimulation. Reentry results from a unique form of conduction disturbance. The mechanism of reentrant activation and the effects of drugs on this process are described below.

The mechanism for establishing a reentrant circuit is depicted in Figure 47–4, panels *A* and *B*. In the figure, the inverted Y-shaped structure represents a branched Purkinje fiber terminating on a strip of ventricular muscle, which appears as a horizontal bar. Normal impulse conduction is shown in Figure 47–4*A*. As indicated by the arrows, impulses travel down both branches of the Purkinje fiber to cause excitation of the muscle at two locations. Impulses created within the muscle travel in both directions (to the right and to the left) away from their sites of origin. Those impulses that are moving toward each other meet midway between the two branches of the Purkinje fiber. Since the muscle in the wake of both impulses is in a refractory state, neither impulse can proceed further, and hence both impulses stop.

Figure 47–4*B* depicts a reentrant circuit. The shaded area in branch 1 of the Purkinje fiber represents a region of one-way conduction block. This region prevents conduction of impulses downward (toward the muscle) but does not prevent impulses from traveling upward. (Impulses can travel back up the block because impulses in muscle are very strong, and hence are able to pass

the block, whereas impulses in the Purkinje fiber are weaker, and hence are unable to pass.) A region of one-way block is essential for reentrant activation.

How does one-way block lead to reentrant activation? As an impulse travels down the Purkinje fiber, it is stopped in branch 1 but continues unimpeded in branch 2. Upon reaching the tip of branch 2, the impulse stimulates the muscle. As described above, the impulse in the muscle travels to the right and to the left away from its site of origin. However, in this new situation, as the impulse travels toward the impaired branch of the Purkinje fiber, it meets no impulse coming from the other direction; hence, the impulse continues on, resulting in the stimulation of the terminal end of branch 1. This stimulation causes an impulse to travel backward up the Purkinje fiber. Since blockade of conduction is unidirectional, the impulse passes through the region of block and then back down into branch 2, causing reentrant activation of this branch. Under proper conditions, the impulse will continue to cycle indefinitely, resulting in repetitive ectopic beats.

There are two mechanisms by which drugs can abolish a reentrant dysrhythmia. First, drugs can improve conduction in the sick branch of the Purkinje fiber, and can thereby eliminate the one-way block (Fig. 47–4*C*). Alternatively, drugs can suppress conduction in the sick branch, thereby converting unidirectional block into two-way block (Fig. 47–4*D*).

A Normal Conduction

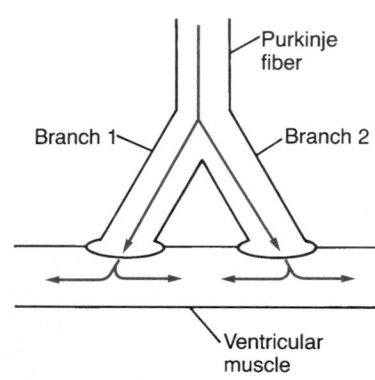

B Reentrant Activation

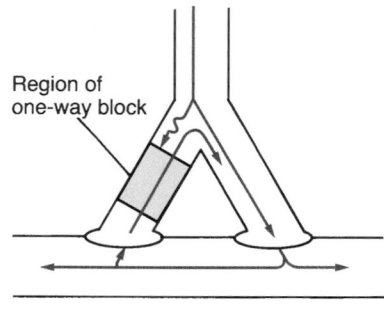

C Drug Effect I

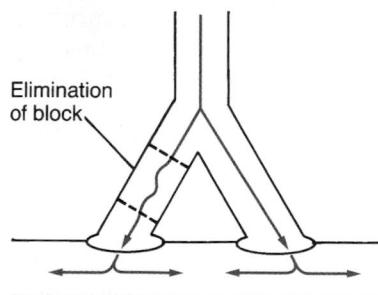

D Drug Effect II

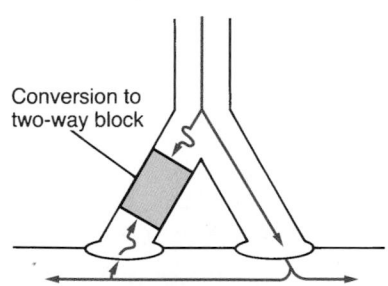

Figure 47–4 ■ Reentrant activation: mechanism and drug effects.
A, In normal conduction, impulses from the branched Purkinje fiber stimulate the strip of ventricular muscle in two places. Within the muscle, waves of excitation spread from both points of excitation, meet between the Purkinje fibers, and cease further travel. *B,* In the presence of one-way block, the strip of muscle is excited at only one location. Impulses spreading from this area meet no impulses coming from the left and, therefore, can travel far enough to stimulate branch 1 of the Purkinje fiber. This stimulation passes back up the fiber, past the region of one-way block, and then stimulates branch 2, causing reentrant activation. *C,* Elimination of reentry by a drug that improves conduction in the sick branch of the Purkinje fiber. *D,* Elimination of reentry by a drug that further suppresses conduction in the sick branch, thereby converting one-way block into two-way block.

CLASSIFICATION OF ANTIDYSRHYTHMIC DRUGS

According to the Vaughan Williams classification scheme, the antidysrhythmic drugs fall into five groups (Table 47–1). As the table shows, there are four major classes of antidysrhythmic drugs (classes I, II, III, and IV) and a fifth group that includes adenosine, digoxin, and magnesium. Membership in classes I through IV is determined by effects on ion movements during slow and fast potentials (see Fig. 47–2).

Class I: Sodium Channel Blockers

Class I drugs block cardiac sodium channels (see Fig. 47–2). By doing so, these drugs slow impulse conduction in the atria, ventricles, and His-Purkinje system. Class I constitutes the largest group of antidysrhythmic drugs.

Class II: Beta Blockers

Class II consists of beta-adrenergic blocking agents. As suggested by Figure 47–2, these drugs reduce calcium entry (during fast and slow potentials) and they depress phase

---

TABLE 47–1 ■ Vaughan Williams Classification of Antidysrhythmic Drugs

Class I: Sodium Channel Blockers

Class IA
  Quinidine
  Procainamide [Pronestyl, others]
  Disopyramide [Norpace]

Class IB
  Lidocaine [Xylocaine]
  Phenytoin [Dilantin]
  Mexiletine [Mexitil]
  Tocainide [Tonocard]

Class IC
  Flecainide [Tambocor]
  Propafenone [Rythmol]

Other Class I
  Moricizine [Ethmozine]

Class II: Beta Blockers
  Propranolol [Inderal]
  Acebutolol [Sectral]
  Esmolol [Brevibloc]

Class III: Potassium Channel Blockers (Drugs That Delay Repolarization)
  Amiodarone [Cordarone, Pacerone]
  Dofetilide [Tikosyn]
  Bretylium
  Sotalol [Betapace]

Class IV: Calcium Channel Blockers
  Diltiazem [Cardizem, others]
  Verapamil [Isoptin, Calan, Verelan]

Other Antidysrhythmic Drugs
  Adenosine [Adenocard]
  Digoxin [Lanoxin, Lanoxicaps]
  Ibutilide [Corvert]

---

4 depolarization (in slow potentials only). Beta blockers have three prominent effects on the heart:

- In the SA node they reduce automaticity.
- In the AV node they slow conduction velocity.
- In the atria and ventricles they reduce contractility.

Cardiac effects of the beta blockers are nearly identical to those of the calcium channel blockers.

Class III: Potassium Channel Blockers (Drugs That Delay Repolarization)

Class III drugs block potassium channels (Fig. 47–2A), and thereby delay repolarization of fast potentials. By delaying repolarization, these drugs prolong both the action potential duration and the effective refractory period.

Class IV: Calcium Channel Blockers

Only two calcium channel blockers—verapamil and diltiazem—are employed as antidysrhythmics. As indicated in Figure 47–2, calcium channel blockade has the same impact on cardiac action potentials as beta blockade. Accordingly, verapamil, diltiazem, and beta blockers have nearly identical effects on cardiac function—namely, reduction of automaticity in the SA node, delay of conduction through the AV node, and reduction of myocardial contractility. Antidysrhythmic effects derive from suppressing AV nodal conduction.

Other Antidysrhythmic Drugs

Adenosine, digoxin, and ibutilide do not fit into the four major classes of antidysrhythmic drugs. Adenosine and digoxin decrease conduction through the AV node and reduce automaticity in the SA node. Ibutilide prolongs the action potential duration, but, unlike class III drugs, does not block potassium channels.

PRODYSRHYTHMIC EFFECTS OF ANTIDYSRHYTHMIC DRUGS

Virtually all of the drugs used to treat dysrhythmias have prodysrhythmic (proarrhythmic) effects. That is, *all of these drugs can worsen existing dysrhythmias and generate new ones.* This ability was documented dramatically in the Cardiac Arrhythmia Suppression Trial (CAST), in which use of class IC drugs (encainide and flecainide) to prevent dysrhythmias after myocardial infarction actually *doubled the rate of mortality.* Because of their prodysrhythmic actions, antidysrhythmic drugs should be used only when dysrhythmias are symptomatically significant, and only when the potential benefits clearly outweigh the risks. Applying this guideline, it would be inappropriate to give antidysrhythmic drugs to a patient with nonsustained ventricular tachycardia, since this dysrhythmia does not significantly reduce cardiac output. Conversely, when a patient is facing death from ventricular fibrillation, any therapy that might work must be tried; in this case, the risk of prodysrhythmic effects is clearly outweighed by the potential benefits of stopping the fibrillation. Regardless of the particular circumstances of drug use, all patients must be followed closely.

Of the mechanisms by which drugs can cause dysrhythmias, one deserves special mention: prolongation of the QT interval. As discussed in Chapter 7, drugs that prolong the QT interval increase the risk of *torsades de pointes,* a dysrhythmia that can progress to fatal ventricular fibrillation. All class IV and class IA antidysrhythmic drugs cause QT prolongation, and hence must be used with special caution.

OVERVIEW OF COMMON DYSRHYTHMIAS AND THEIR TREATMENT

The common dysrhythmias can be divided into two major groups: *supraventricular dysrhythmias* and *ventricular dysrhythmias.* In general, ventricular dysrhythmias are more dangerous than supraventricular dysrhythmias. With either type, intervention is required only if the dysrhythmia interferes with effective ventricular pumping. Treatment usually proceeds in two phases: (1) *termination* of the dysrhythmia (with electrical countershock, drugs, or both), followed by (2) *long-term suppression* with drugs. Dysrhythmias can also be treated with an implantable cardioverter/defibrillator or by destroying small areas of cardiac tissue using radiofrequency catheter ablation (see below).

Therapy of the common dysrhythmias is summarized in Table 47–2. As indicated, drugs are not always the preferred treatment. In fact, drugs constitute the first line of treatment for only two of the common dysrhythmias: ventricular premature beats (VPBs) and digoxin-induced ventricular dysrhythmias. For several dysrhythmias, direct current (DC) cardioversion (electrical countershock) is the preferred therapy. In one case (supraventricular tachycardia [SVT]), maneuvers that increase vagal tone are the treatment of choice.

It is important to appreciate that drug therapy of dysrhythmias is highly empiric (i.e., based largely on the response of the patient and not on scientific principles). In practice, this means that, even after a dysrhythmia has been identified, we cannot predict with certainty just which drugs will be effective. Frequently, trials with several drugs are required before control of rhythm is achieved. In the discussion below, only first-choice drugs are considered.

Supraventricular Dysrhythmias

Supraventricular dysrhythmias are dysrhythmias that arise in areas of the heart above the ventricles (atria, SA node, AV node). Supraventricular dysrhythmias per se are not especially harmful. Why? Because dysrhythmic activity within the atria does not significantly reduce cardiac output (except in patients with valvular disorders and heart failure). Supraventricular tachydysrhythmias *can* be dangerous, however, in that atrial impulses are likely to traverse the AV node, resulting in

TABLE 47–2 ■ Treatment of Common Dysrhythmias

| Type of Dysrhythmia | Acute Treatment | | Long-Term Suppression |
	Preferred	Alternatives	
Supraventricular			

Supraventricular tachycardia	Vagotonic maneuvers	*To terminate:*
		  Beta blocker (II)
		  Verapamil (IV)
		  Diltiazem (IV)
		  Adenosine
		  Digoxin
			Quinidine (IA)*
			Procainamide (IA)
			Other drugs

Atrial flutter and atrial fibrillation	DC cardioversion	*To slow ventricular response:*
		  Beta blocker (II)
		  Verapamil (IV)
		  Diltiazem (IV)
		  Digoxin
			Quinidine (IA)*
			Procainamide (IA)
			Other drugs

Ventricular			
Sustained ventricular tachycardia	DC cardioversion	Lidocaine (IB) Procainamide (IA) Amiodarone (III) Bretylium (III)	Quinidine (IA) Procainamide (IA) Sotalol (III) Other drugs
Ventricular fibrillation	Defibrillation	Lidocaine (IB)† Procainamide (IA)† Amiodarone (III) Bretylium (III)†	Amiodarone (III)
Ventricular premature beats	Asymptomatic patients need no treatment	Beta blocker (II)‡	
Digoxin-induced ventricular dysrhythmias	Digoxin-immune Fab (digoxin antibody fragments)	Lidocaine (IB) Phenytoin (IB)	

*Quinidine may *increase* mortality in these patients.
†Defibrillation is the treatment of choice. Drugs are given to prevent recurrence.
‡Beta blockers are used only if the dysrhythmia is symptomatic.

excitation of the ventricles. If the atria drive the ventricles at an excessive rate, diastolic filling will be incomplete and cardiac output will decline. Hence, when treating supraventricular tachydysrhythmias, the objective is frequently one of *blocking impulse conduction through the AV node* and not elimination of the dysrhythmia itself. Of course, if treatment did abolish the dysrhythmia, this outcome would be welcome. As indicated in Table 47–2, acute treatment of supraventricular dysrhythmias is accomplished with vagotonic maneuvers, DC cardioversion, and certain drugs: class II agents, class IV agents, adenosine, and digoxin.

Sustained SVT. SVT is usually caused by an AV nodal reentrant circuit. Heart rate is increased to 150 to 250 beats/min. SVT is best treated by maneuvers that increase vagal tone, such as carotid sinus massage or the Valsalva maneuver. If vagal maneuvers are ineffective, intravenous adenosine or verapamil should be given. If these drugs fail, others may be tried (see Table 47–2). Once the dysrhythmia has been controlled, long-term prophylaxis with quinidine may prevent its recurrence.

Atrial Flutter. Atrial flutter is caused by an ectopic atrial focus discharging at a rate of 250 to 350 times a minute. Ventricular rate is considerably slower, however, because the AV node is unable to transmit impulses at such a high rate. Typically, one atrial impulse out of three manages to reach the ventricles. The treatment of choice is DC cardioversion, which almost always converts atrial flutter to normal sinus rhythm. If cardioversion is ineffective, drugs may be employed; the objective is to decrease the number of atrial impulses that pass to the ventricles. The drug of choice for atrial flutter is digoxin. Verapamil, diltiazem, or a beta blocker may also be effective. Long-term therapy with quinidine has been used to prevent the dysrhythmia from recurring. However, recent analysis of older data indicates that quinidine can actually increase mortality in these patients. It is not known whether other drugs used for prophylaxis pose a similar danger.

Atrial Fibrillation. Atrial fibrillation is caused by multiple atrial ectopic foci firing randomly; each focus stimulates a small area of atrial muscle. This chaotic excitation produces a highly irregular atrial rhythm. Depending upon the extent of impulse transmission through the AV node, ventricular rate may be rapid or nearly normal.

Treatment is the same as for atrial flutter. DC cardioversion is the preferred therapy. If DC cardioversion is ineffective, ventricular rate can be controlled with a beta blocker, calcium channel blocker, or digoxin. Long-term quinidine therapy may prevent the dysrhythmia from recurring, but may also increase the risk of mortality.

Atrial fibrillation carries a high risk of intracardiac thrombus formation. This occurs because some blood can become trapped in the atria, rather than flowing straight through to the ventricles. When normal sinus rhythm is restored, intracardiac thrombi may become dislodged, creating a risk of embolism. To reduce this risk, patients are usually given warfarin (an anticoagulant drug) for 3 to 4 weeks prior to treating the dysrhythmia, and for another 4 weeks after normal rhythm has been restored.

Ventricular Dysrhythmias

In contrast to atrial dysrhythmias, which are generally benign, ventricular dysrhythmias can cause significant disruption of cardiac pumping. Accordingly, the usual objective is to abolish the dysrhythmia. Cardioversion is often the treatment of choice. When antidysrhythmic drugs are indicated, agents in class I or class III are usually employed.

Sustained Ventricular Tachycardia. Ventricular tachycardia arises from a single, rapidly firing ventricular ectopic focus, typically located at the border of an old infarction. The focus drives the ventricles at a rate of 150 to 250 beats/min. Since the ventricles cannot pump effectively at these rates, immediate treatment is required. Cardioversion is the treatment of choice. If cardioversion fails to normalize rhythm, lidocaine should be administered. If lidocaine is also ineffective, bretylium, procainamide, or amiodarone should be tried. For long-term management, drugs (e.g., sotalol) or an implantable cardioverter/defibrillator (ICD) may be employed.

Ventricular Fibrillation. Ventricular fibrillation is a life-threatening emergency that requires immediate treatment. This dysrhythmia results from the asynchronous discharge of multiple ventricular ectopic foci. Because many different foci are firing, and because each focus initiates contraction in its immediate vicinity, localized twitching takes place all over the ventricles, making coordinated ventricular contraction impossible. As a result, the pumping action of the heart stops. In the absence of blood flow, the patient becomes unconscious and cyanotic. If heartbeat is not restored rapidly, death soon follows. Electrical countershock (defibrillation) is applied to eliminate fibrillation and restore cardiac function. If necessary, lidocaine can be used to enhance the effects of defibrillation. Procainamide and bretylium may also be helpful. Amiodarone can be used for long-term suppression. As an alternative, an ICD may be employed.

Ventricular Premature Beats. VPBs are beats that occur before they should in the cardiac cycle. These beats are caused by ectopic ventricular foci. VPBs may arise from a single ectopic focus or from several foci. In the absence of additional signs of heart disease, VPBs are benign and not usually treated. However, in the presence of acute myocardial infarction, VPBs may predispose the patient to ventricular fibrillation. In this case, therapy is required. A beta blocker is the agent of choice. Because VPBs are associated with a premature QRS complex on the EKG, this dysrhythmia is also known as *premature ventricular complexes*.

Digoxin-Induced Ventricular Dysrhythmias. Digoxin toxicity can mimic practically all types of dysrhythmias. Varying degrees of AV block are among the most common. Ventricular flutter and ventricular fibrillation are the most dangerous. Digoxin causes dysrhythmias by increasing automaticity in the atria, ventricles, and His-Purkinje system, and by decreasing conduction through the AV node.

With proper treatment, digoxin-induced dysrhythmias can almost always be controlled. Treatment is discussed at length in Chapter 46. If antidysrhythmic drugs are required, lidocaine and phenytoin are the agents of choice. In patients with digoxin toxicity, DC cardioversion may bring on ventricular fibrillation. Accordingly, this procedure should be used only when absolutely required.

Torsades de Pointes. Torsades de pointes is an atypical, rapid, undulating, ventricular tachydysrhythmia that can evolve into potentially fatal ventricular fibrillation. The main factor associated with development of torsades de pointes is prolongation of the QT interval, which can be caused by a variety of drugs (see Table 7–2 in Chapter 7), including class IA and class III antidysrhythmic agents. The preferred treatment is intravenous magnesium.

CLASS I: SODIUM CHANNEL BLOCKERS

Class I antidysrhythmic drugs block cardiac sodium channels. By doing so, these drugs decrease conduction velocity in the atria, ventricles, and His-Purkinje system.

There are three subgroups of class I agents. Drugs in all three groups block sodium channels. In addition, class IA agents delay repolarization, whereas class IB agents accelerate repolarization. Class IC agents have pronounced prodysrhythmic actions.

The class I drugs are similar in action and structure to the local anesthetics. In fact, one of these drugs—lidocaine—has both local anesthetic and antidysrhythmic applications. Because of their relationship to the local anesthetics, class I agents are sometimes referred to as *local anesthetic antidysrhythmic agents.*

Some important properties of the class I drugs (and other antidysrhythmics) are summarized in Table 47–3.

Class IA Agents
Quinidine

Quinidine is the oldest and most thoroughly studied of the class IA drugs. Accordingly, quinidine will serve as our prototype for the group. Quinidine is the most frequently

---

TABLE 47–3 ▪■ Properties of Antidysrhythmic Drugs

Drug	Usual Route	Effects on the EKG	Major Antidysrhythmic Applications
Class IA			
Quinidine	PO	Widens QRS, prolongs QT	Broad spectrum: used for long-term suppression of ventricular and supraventricular dysrhythmias
Procainamide	PO	Widens QRS, prolongs QT	Broad spectrum: similar to quinidine, but toxicity makes it less desirable for long-term use
Disopyramide	PO	Widens QRS, prolongs QT	Ventricular dysrhythmias
Class IB			
Lidocaine	IV	No significant change	Ventricular dysrhythmias
Mexiletine	PO	No significant change	Ventricular dysrhythmias
Tocainide	PO	No significant change	Life-threatening ventricular dysrhythmias
Phenytoin	PO	No significant change	Digoxin-induced ventricular dysrhythmias
Class IC			
Flecainide	PO	Widens QRS, prolongs PR	Life-threatening ventricular dysrhythmias
Propafenone	PO	Widens QRS, prolongs PR	Life-threatening ventricular dysrhythmias
Other Class I			
Moricizine	PO	Widens QRS, prolongs PR	Life-threatening ventricular dysrhythmias
Class II			
Propranolol	PO	Prolongs PR, bradycardia	Dysrhythmias caused by excessive sympathetic activity; control of ventricular rate in patients with supraventricular tachydysrhythmias
Acebutolol	PO	Prolongs PR, bradycardia	Premature ventricular beats
Esmolol	IV	Prolongs PR, bradycardia	Control of ventricular rate in patients with supraventricular tachydysrhythmias
Class III			
Amiodarone	PO	Prolongs QT and PR, widens QRS	Life-threatening ventricular dysrhythmias
Bretylium	IV	Prolongs QT	Life-threatening ventricular dysrhythmias
Sotalol	IV	Prolongs QT and PR, bradycardia	Life-threatening ventricular dysrhythmias
Dofetilide	PO	Prolongs QT	Highly symptomatic atrial dysrhythmias
Class IV			
Verapamil	PO	Prolongs PR, bradycardia	Control of ventricular rate in patients with supraventricular tachydysrhythmias
Diltiazem	IV	Prolongs PR, bradycardia	Same as verapamil
Others			
Adenosine	IV	Prolongs PR	Termination of paroxysmal supraventricular tachycardia
Digoxin	PO	Prolongs PR, depresses ST	Control of ventricular rate in patients with supraventricular tachydysrhythmias
Ibutilide	IV	Prolongs QT	Atrial flutter, atrial fibrillation

used oral antidysrhythmic agent. Like other antidysrhythmic drugs, quinidine has prodysrhythmic actions.

Chemistry and Source. Quinidine is similar to quinine in structure and actions. The natural source of both drugs is the bark of the South American cinchona tree. Accordingly, these agents are referred to as *cinchona alkaloids.* Like quinine, quinidine has antimalarial and antipyretic properties.

Effects on the Heart. By blocking sodium channels, quinidine *slows impulse conduction* in the atria, ventricles, and His-Purkinje system. In addition, the drug *delays repolarization* at these sites, apparently by blocking potassium channels. Both actions contribute to suppression of dysrhythmias.

Quinidine is strongly *anticholinergic* (atropine-like) and blocks vagal input to the heart. The resultant *increase* in SA nodal automaticity and AV conduction can drive the ventricles at an excessive rate. To prevent excessive ventricular stimulation, patients are usually pretreated with digoxin, verapamil, or a beta blocker, all of which suppress AV conduction.

Effects on the EKG. Quinidine has two pronounced effects on the EKG. The drug *widens the QRS complex* (by slowing depolarization of the ventricles) and *prolongs the QT interval* (by delaying ventricular repolarization).

Therapeutic Uses. Quinidine is a broad-spectrum agent active against *supraventricular* and *ventricular dysrhythmias.* The drug's principal indication is long-term suppression of dysrhythmias, including SVT, atrial flutter, atrial fibrillation, and sustained ventricular tachycardia. To prevent quinidine from increasing ventricular rate, patients are usually pretreated with an AV nodal blocking agent (digoxin, verapamil, beta blocker). An analysis of older studies indicates that quinidine may actually *increase* mortality in patients with *atrial flutter* and *atrial fibrillation.*

Pharmacokinetics. Quinidine is rapidly absorbed following oral administration. Peak responses to *quinidine sulfate* develop in 30 to 90 minutes; responses to *quinidine gluconate* develop more slowly, peaking after 3 to 4 hours. Elimination is by hepatic metabolism. Accordingly, patients with liver dysfunction may require a reduction in dosage. Therapeutic plasma levels are 2 to 5 μg/ml.

Adverse Effects. *Diarrhea.* Diarrhea and other GI symptoms develop in about 33% of patients. These reactions can be immediate and intense, frequently forcing discontinuation of treatment. Gastric upset can be reduced by administering quinidine with food.

Cinchonism. Cinchonism is characterized by tinnitus (ringing in the ears), headache, nausea, vertigo, and disturbed vision. These symptoms can develop with just one quinidine dose.

Cardiotoxicity. At high concentrations, quinidine can cause severe cardiotoxicity (sinus arrest, AV block, ventricular tachydysrhythmias, asystole). These reactions occur secondary to increased automaticity of Purkinje fibers and reduced conduction throughout all regions of the heart.

As cardiotoxicity develops, the EKG changes. Important danger signals are *widening of the QRS complex* (by 50% or more) and *excessive prolongation of the QT interval.* The physician should be notified immediately if these changes occur.

Arterial Embolism. Embolism is a potential complication of treating *atrial fibrillation.* During atrial fibrillation, thrombi may form in the atria. When sinus rhythm is restored, these thrombi may be dislodged and cause embolism. To reduce the risk of embolism, warfarin (an anticoagulant) is given for 3 to 4 weeks prior to quinidine, and is maintained

for an additional 4 weeks. Signs of embolism (e.g., sudden chest pain, dyspnea) should be reported immediately.

Other Adverse Effects. Quinidine can cause alpha-adrenergic blockade, resulting in vasodilation and subsequent *hypotension.* This reaction is much more serious with IV therapy than with oral therapy. Rarely, quinidine has caused *hypersensitivity reactions,* including fever, anaphylactic reactions, and thrombocytopenia.

Drug Interactions. *Digoxin.* Quinidine can double digoxin levels. The increase is caused by displacing digoxin from plasma albumin and by decreasing digoxin elimination. When these drugs are used concurrently, digoxin dosage must be reduced. Also, patients should be monitored closely for digoxin toxicity (dysrhythmias). Because of its interaction with digoxin, quinidine is a last-choice drug for treating digoxin-induced dysrhythmias.

Other Interactions. Because of its anticholinergic actions, quinidine can intensify the effects of other atropine-like drugs; one possible result is excessive tachycardia. Phenobarbital, phenytoin, and other drugs that induce hepatic drug metabolism can shorten the half-life of quinidine by as much as 50%. Quinidine can intensify the effects of warfarin by a mechanism that is not known.

Preparations, Dosage, and Administration. *Preparations.* Quinidine is available as three salts: *quinidine sulfate, quinidine gluconate,* and *quinidine polygalacturonate.* Because these salts have different molecular weights, equal doses of these preparations (on a milligram basis) do not provide equal amounts of quinidine. A 200-mg dose of quinidine sulfate is equivalent to 275 mg of either quinidine gluconate or quinidine polygalacturonate. Quinidine sulfate [Quinora, Quinidex Extentabs] is available in standard tablets (200 and 300 mg) and sustained-release tablets (300 mg). Quinidine gluconate [Quinalan, Quinaglute Dura-Tabs] is available in sustained-release tablets (324 mg) and as an injection (80 mg/ml). Quinidine polygalacturonate [Cardioquin] is available in 275-mg tablets.

Dosage. The usual dosage of quinidine sulfate is 200 to 400 mg every 4 to 6 hours. The usual dosage of quinidine gluconate is 324 to 648 mg every 8 to 12 hours. Dosage is adjusted to produce plasma quinidine levels between 2 and 5 μg/ml.

Administration. Quinidine is almost always administered by mouth. If time permits, a small test dose (200 mg orally or intramuscularly) should be given prior to the full therapeutic dose to assess for hypersensitivity. Intramuscular administration is painful and produces erratic absorption. Intravenous injection carries a high risk of adverse cardiovascular reactions, and hence continuous cardiovascular monitoring is required.

Procainamide

Procainamide [Pronestyl, Procanbid] is similar to quinidine in actions and applications. Like quinidine, procainamide is active against a broad spectrum of dysrhythmias. Unfortunately, serious side effects frequently limit its use.

Effects on the Heart and EKG. Like quinidine, procainamide blocks cardiac sodium channels, thereby decreasing conduction velocity in the atria, ventricles, and His-Purkinje system. Also, the drug delays repolarization. In contrast to quinidine, procainamide is only weakly anticholinergic. Hence, procainamide is not likely to increase ventricular rate. Effects on the EKG are the same as with quinidine: widening of the QRS complex and prolongation of the QT interval.

Therapeutic Uses. Procainamide is effective against a broad spectrum of atrial and ventricular dysrhythmias. Like quinidine, the drug can be used for long-term suppression. However, since prolonged therapy is often associated with serious adverse effects (see below), procainamide is less desirable than quinidine for long-term use. In contrast to quinidine, procainamide can be used to terminate ventricular tachycardia and ventricular fibrillation.

Pharmacokinetics. Routes are oral, IV, and IM. Peak plasma levels develop 1 hour after oral administration. Procainamide has a short half-life and requires more frequent dosing than quinidine.

Elimination is by hepatic metabolism and renal excretion. The major metabolite—*N*-acetylprocainamide (NAPA)—has antidysrhythmic properties of its own. NAPA is excreted by the kidneys and can accumulate to toxic levels in patients with renal impairment.

Adverse Effects. *Systemic Lupus Erythematosus–like Syndrome.* Prolonged treatment with procainamide is associated with severe immunologic reactions. Within a year, about 70% of patients develop antinuclear antibodies (ANAs)—antibodies directed against the patient's own nucleic acids. If procainamide is continued, between 20% and 30% of patients with ANAs go on to develop symptoms resembling those of systemic lupus erythematosus (SLE). These symptoms include pain and inflammation of the joints, pericarditis, fever, and hepatomegaly. When procainamide is withdrawn, symptoms usually subside. If the patient has a life-threatening dysrhythmia for which no alternative drug is available, procainamide can be continued and the symptoms of SLE can be controlled with a nonsteroidal anti-inflammatory agent (e.g., aspirin) or a glucocorticoid. All patients taking procainamide chronically should be tested for ANAs. If the ANA titer rises, discontinuation of treatment should be considered.

Blood Dyscrasias. About 0.5% of patients develop blood dyscrasias, including neutropenia, thrombocytopenia, and agranulocytosis. Fatalities have occurred. These reactions usually develop during the first 12 weeks of treatment. Complete blood counts should be obtained weekly during this time and periodically thereafter. Also, complete blood counts should be obtained promptly at the first sign of infection, bruising, or bleeding. If blood counts indicate bone marrow suppression, procainamide should be withdrawn. Hematologic status usually returns to baseline within 1 month.

Cardiotoxicity. Procainamide has cardiotoxic actions like those of quinidine. Danger signs are QRS widening (>50%) and excessive prolongation of the QT interval. If these develop, the drug should be withheld and the physician informed.

Other Adverse Effects. Like quinidine, procainamide can cause *GI symptoms* and *hypotension*. However, these are much less prominent than with quinidine. Procainamide is a derivative of procaine (a local anesthetic), and patients with a history of procaine allergy are at high risk of having an *allergic response* to procainamide. As with quinidine, *arterial embolism* may occur during treatment of atrial fibrillation.

Preparations, Dosage, and Administration. *Oral.* Procainamide [Pronestyl, Procanbid] is available in tablets and capsules (250, 375, and 500 mg) and sustained-release tablets (250, 500, 750, and 1000 mg). The usual maintenance dosage is 50 mg/kg/day in divided doses. Standard tablets and capsules are administered every 3 to 4 hours and sustained-release tablets every 6 hours. Dosage is adjusted to maintain plasma drug levels between 4 and 10 µg/ml.

Parenteral. Procainamide solution (100 and 500 mg/ml) is available for IM and IV administration. Intramuscular injection is made deep into the gluteal muscle; dosage is 0.5 to 1.0 gm repeated every 4 to 8 hours.

Intravenous infusion may be performed at an initial rate of 20 mg/min (maximal loading dose is 500 to 600 mg). After the loading period, an infusion rate of 2 to 6 mg/min should be employed. Once the dysrhythmia has been controlled, the patient should be switched to oral procainamide. Three hours should elapse between terminating the infusion and the first oral dose.

Disopyramide

Disopyramide [Norpace] is a class I drug with actions like those of quinidine. However, because of prominent side effects, indications for disopyramide are limited.

Effects on the Heart and EKG. Cardiac effects are similar to those of quinidine. By blocking sodium channels, disopyramide decreases conduction velocity in the atria, ventricles, and His-Purkinje system. In addition, the drug delays repolarization. Anticholinergic actions are greater than those of quinidine. In contrast to quinidine, disopyramide causes a pronounced reduction in contractility. Like quinidine, disopyramide causes widening of the QRS complex and prolongation of the QT interval.

Adverse Effects. *Anticholinergic responses* are most common. These include dry mouth, blurred vision, constipation, and urinary hesitancy or retention. Urinary retention frequently requires discontinuation of treatment.

Because of its negative inotropic effects, disopyramide can cause *severe hypotension* (secondary to reduced cardiac output) and can *exacerbate congestive heart failure* (CHF). The drug should not be administered to patients with CHF or to patients taking beta blockers. Whenever disopyramide is used, pressor drugs should be immediately available.

Therapeutic Uses. Disopyramide is indicated only for ventricular dysrhythmias (VPBs, ventricular tachycardia, ventricular fibrillation). The drug is reserved for patients who cannot tolerate safer medications (e.g., quinidine, procainamide).

Preparations, Dosage, and Administration. Disopyramide [Norpace] is available in standard and extended-release capsules (100 and 150 mg). An initial loading dose (200 to 300 mg) is followed by maintenance doses (100 to 200 mg) every 6 hours.

Class IB Agents

As a group, class IB agents differ from quinidine and the other class IA agents in two respects: (1) whereas class IA agents *delay* repolarization, class IB agents *accelerate* repolarization; and (2) class IB agents have little or no effect on the EKG.

Lidocaine

Lidocaine [Xylocaine], an intravenous agent, is used only for ventricular dysrhythmias. In addition to its antidysrhythmic applications, lidocaine is employed as a local anesthetic (see Chapter 25).

Effects on the Heart and EKG. Lidocaine has three significant effects on the heart: (1) like other class I drugs, lidocaine blocks cardiac sodium channels and thereby *slows conduction* in the atria, ventricles, and His-Purkinje system; (2) the drug *reduces automaticity* in the ventricles and His-Purkinje system by a mechanism that is not understood; and (3) lidocaine *accelerates repolarization* (shortens action potential duration and the ERP). In contrast to quinidine and procainamide, lidocaine is devoid of anticholinergic properties. Also, lidocaine has no significant impact on the EKG: A small reduction in the QT interval may occur, but there is no widening of the QRS complex.

Pharmacokinetics. Lidocaine undergoes rapid metabolism by the liver. If the drug were administered orally, most of each dose would be inactivated on its first pass through the liver. For this reason, administration is by IV infusion.

Because lidocaine is rapidly degraded, plasma drug levels can be easily controlled: If levels climb too high, the infusion can be slowed and the liver will quickly remove excess drug from the circulation. The therapeutic range for lidocaine is 1.5 to 5 µg/ml.

Antidysrhythmic Use. Antidysrhythmic use of lidocaine is limited to short-term therapy of *ventricular dysrhythmias*. Because its levels can be easily controlled, lidocaine is the drug of choice for several ventricular dysrhythmias, including those associated with myocardial infarction, cardiac surgery, and digoxin toxicity. Lidocaine is not active against supraventricular dysrhythmias.

Adverse Effects. Lidocaine is generally well tolerated. However, adverse central nervous system (CNS) effects can occur. High therapeutic doses can cause *drowsiness, confusion,* and *paresthesias*. Toxic doses may produce *convulsions* and *respiratory arrest*. Consequently, whenever lidocaine is used, equipment for resuscitation must be available. Convulsions can be managed with diazepam or phenytoin.

Preparations, Dosage, and Administration. Administration is parenteral only. The usual route is IV. Intramuscular injection can be used in emergencies. Blood pressure and the EKG should be monitored for signs of toxicity.

Intravenous. Lidocaine [Xylocaine] preparations intended for IV administration are clearly labeled as such. They contain no preservatives or catecholamines. (Lidocaine used for local anesthesia frequently contains epinephrine.) *Preparations that contain epinephrine or another catecholamine must never be administered intravenously, since doing so can cause severe hypertension and life-threatening dysrhythmias.*

Intravenous therapy is initiated with a loading dose followed by continuous infusion for maintenance. The usual loading dose is 50 to 100 mg (1 mg/kg) administered at a rate of 25 to 50 mg/min. An infusion rate of 1 to 4 mg/min is used for maintenance; the rate is adjusted on the basis of cardiac response. Intravenous lidocaine should be discontinued as soon as possible, usually within 24 hours. Lidocaine for IV administration is dispensed in concentrated and dilute formulations. The concentrated formulations must be diluted with 5% dextrose in water.

To avoid toxicity, dosage should be reduced in patients with impaired hepatic function or impaired hepatic blood flow (e.g., elderly patients; patients with cirrhosis, shock, or CHF).

Intramuscular. Lidocaine is dispensed in an automatic injection device [LidoPen Auto-Injector] for IM administration. A dose of 300 mg is injected into the deltoid muscle. This dose can be repeated in 60 to 90 minutes if necessary. The patient should be switched to IV lidocaine as soon as possible.

Phenytoin

Phenytoin [Dilantin] is an antiseizure drug that is also used to treat digoxin-induced dysrhythmias. The basic pharmacology of phenytoin is presented in Chapter 23 (Drugs for Epilepsy). Discussion here is limited to antidysrhythmic applications.

Effects on the Heart and EKG. Like lidocaine, phenytoin reduces automaticity (especially in the ventricles), and has little or no effect on the EKG. In contrast to lidocaine (and practically all other antidysrhythmic agents), phenytoin increases AV nodal conduction.

Pharmacokinetics. Phenytoin has two unfortunate kinetics properties. First, metabolism of the drug is subject to wide interpatient variation. Second, doses only slightly greater than therapeutic are likely to cause toxicity. Because of these characteristics, maintenance of therapeutic plasma levels (5 to 20 μg/ml) is difficult.

Adverse Effects and Interactions. The most common adverse reactions are sedation, ataxia, and nystagmus. With too-rapid IV administration, phenytoin can cause hypotension, dysrhythmias, and cardiac arrest. Gingival hyperplasia is a frequent complication of long-term treatment. Phenytoin is subject to multiple undesirable drug interactions (see Chapter 23).

Antidysrhythmic Applications. Phenytoin is a second-choice drug after lidocaine for treating digoxin-induced dysrhythmias. The ability of phenytoin to increase AV nodal conduction can help counteract the reduction in AV conduction caused by digoxin intoxication. Phenytoin should not be used to treat atrial fibrillation or atrial flutter. Why? Because enhanced AV conduction could increase the number of atrial impulses reaching the ventricles, thereby driving the ventricles at an excessive rate.

Dosage and Administration. Phenytoin [Dilantin] is administered orally and intravenously. For oral therapy, a loading dose (14 mg/kg) is followed by daily maintenance doses (200 to 400 mg).

Intravenous administration is reserved for severe, acute dysrhythmias. Blood pressure and the EKG must be monitored continuously. Phenytoin is not soluble in water and must be diluted in the medium supplied by the manufacturer. This medium is highly alkaline (pH 12) and will cause phlebitis if given by continuous infusion. Consequently, administration is by intermittent injections. Intravenous injections must be performed slowly (50 mg/min or less), since rapid injection can cause cardiovascular collapse. Treatment is begun with a series of loading doses (50 to 100 mg every 5 minutes until the dysrhythmia has been controlled or until toxicity appears). Maintenance dosages range from 200 to 400 mg/day.

Mexiletine

Mexiletine [Mexitil] is an oral congener of lidocaine used to treat symptomatic ventricular dysrhythmias. Principal indications are VPBs and sustained ventricular tachycardia. Like lidocaine, mexiletine does not alter the EKG. The drug is eliminated by hepatic metabolism; hence, effects may be prolonged in patients with liver disease or reduced hepatic blood flow. The most common adverse effects are GI (nausea, vomiting, diarrhea, constipation) and neurologic (tremor, dizziness, sleep disturbances, psychosis, convulsions). About 40% of patients find these intolerable. Like other class I agents, mexiletine has prodysrhythmic properties. The initial dosage is 100 to 200 mg every 8 hours. The maintenance dosage is 100 to 300 mg every 6 to 12 hours. All doses should be taken with food.

Mexiletine is also used to alleviate persistent pain of diabetic neuropathy. Benefits derive from lidocaine-like anesthetic actions. Because mexiletine can *cause* arrhythmias, it should not be used by diabetic patients with heart disease.

Tocainide

Like mexiletine, tocainide [Tonocard] is an oral analog of lidocaine used to treat ventricular dysrhythmias. Effects on the EKG are minimal. Elimination is by hepatic metabolism and renal excretion. As with mexiletine, the most common side effects are GI (especially nausea) and neurologic (especially tremor). In addition, tocainide can cause serious blood dyscrasias, including a 2% incidence of agranulocytosis; hence, blood counts should be monitored. The drug can also cause pulmonary fibrosis and pneumonitis. Because of its serious adverse effects, tocainide should be reserved for patients with severe ventricular dysrhythmias that have not responded to safer drugs. The initial dosage is 200 to 400 mg every 8 hours. The maintenance dosage is 200 to 600 mg every 8 hours.

Class IC Agents

Class IC antidysrhythmics block cardiac sodium channels and thereby reduce conduction velocity in the atria, ventricles, and His-Purkinje system. In addition, these drugs delay ventricular repolarization, causing a small increase in the effective refractory period. All class IC agents can exacerbate existing dysrhythmias and create new ones. Currently, only two class IC agents are available: flecainide and propafenone. A third agent—encainide [Enkaid]—was voluntarily withdrawn from the market.

Flecainide

Flecainide [Tambocor] is employed for oral therapy of severe ventricular dysrhythmias. Like other class IC agents, the drug decreases cardiac conduction and increases the effective refractory period. Prominent effects on the EKG are prolongation of the PR interval and widening of the QRS complex. Excessive QRS widening indicates a need for dosage reduction. Flecainide has prodysrhythmic effects. As a result, the drug can intensify existing dysrhythmias and provoke new ones. In patients with asymptomatic ventricular tachycardia associated with acute myocardial infarction, flecainide has caused a twofold increase in mortality. Flecainide decreases myocardial contractility and can thereby exacerbate or precipitate heart failure. Accordingly, the drug should not be combined with other agents that can decrease contractile force (e.g., beta blockers, verapamil, diltiazem). Elimination is by hepatic metabolism and renal excretion. Dosage is low initially (100 mg every 12 hours) and then gradually increased to a maximum of 400 mg/day. Because of its potential for serious side effects, flecainide should be reserved for severe ventricular dysrhythmias that have not responded to safer drugs. Patients should be monitored closely.

Propafenone

Propafenone [Rythmol] is similar to flecainide in actions and uses. By blocking cardiac sodium channels, the drug decreases conduction velocity in the atria, ventricles, and His-Purkinje system. In addition, it causes a small increase in the ventricular ERP. Prominent effects on the EKG are QRS widening and PR prolongation. Like flecainide, propafenone has prodysrhythmic actions that can exacerbate existing dysrhythmias and create new ones. It is not known if propafenone, like flecainide, increases mortality in patients with asymptomatic ventricular dysrhythmias after myocardial infarction. Propafenone has beta adrenergic blocking properties and can thereby decrease myocardial contractility and promote bronchospasm. Accordingly, the drug should be used with caution in patients with heart failure, AV block, or asthma. Noncardiac adverse effects are generally mild and include dizziness, altered taste, blurred vision, and GI symptoms (abdominal discomfort, anorexia, nausea, vomiting). Because of its prodysrhythmic actions, propafenone should be reserved for patients with life-threatening ventricular dysrhythmias that have not responded to safer drugs. Propafenone is dispensed in tablets (150, 225, and 300 mg) for oral use. The dosage is 150 mg every 8 hours initially, and can be gradually increased to 300 mg every 8 hours.

Other Class I: Moricizine

Moricizine [Ethmozine] is a class I antidysrhythmic drug approved for oral therapy of life-threatening ventricular dysrhythmias. This agent shares properties with other class I drugs but doesn't quite fit any of the existing subclasses (IA, IB, and IC). Like other class I agents, moricizine blocks cardiac sodium channels and thereby decreases conduction velocity in the atria, ventricles, and His-Purkinje system. Prominent effects on the EKG are QRS widening and PR prolongation. The most common adverse effects are dizziness, nausea, and headache. Like other antidysrhythmic drugs, moricizine is prodysrhythmic. In addition, moricizine can cause bradycardia, AV block, and heart failure. Interactions with digoxin, diuretics, beta blockers, calcium channel blockers, angiotensin-converting enzyme inhibitors, and warfarin have not been reported. Because of its potential for adverse cardiac effects, moricizine should be reserved for life-threatening ventricular dysrhythmias that have not responded to safer drugs. Moricizine is available in 200-, 250-, and 300-mg tablets. The dosage is 200 mg every 8 hours initially, and may be gradually increased to a maximum of 300 mg every 8 hours.

CLASS II: BETA BLOCKERS

Class II consists of beta-adrenergic blocking agents. At this time only four beta blockers—propranolol, acebutolol, esmolol, and sotalol—are approved for treating dysrhythmias. One of these drugs—sotalol—also blocks potassium channels, and hence is discussed under class III. The basic pharmacology of the beta blockers is presented in Chapter 18. Discussion here is limited to use for dysrhythmias.

Propranolol

Propranolol [Inderal] is considered a nonselective beta-adrenergic antagonist, in that it blocks both beta$_1$- and beta$_2$-adrenergic receptors. As discussed in Chapter 18, beta$_1$ blockade affects the heart and beta$_2$ blockade affects the bronchi.

Effects on the Heart and EKG. Blockade of cardiac beta$_1$ receptors attenuates sympathetic stimulation of the heart. The result is (1) decreased automaticity of the SA node, (2) decreased velocity of conduction through the AV node, and (3) decreased myocardial contractility. The reduction in AV conduction velocity translates to a prolonged PR interval on the EKG.

It is worth noting that cardiac beta$_1$ receptors are functionally coupled to calcium channels, and that beta$_1$ blockade causes these channels to close. Hence, the effects of beta blockers on heart rate, AV conduction, and contractility all result from decreased calcium influx. Because beta blockers and calcium channel blockers both decrease calcium entry, the cardiac effects of these drugs are very similar.

Therapeutic Use. Propranolol is especially useful for treating dysrhythmias caused by excessive sympathetic stimulation of the heart. Among these are sinus tachycardia, severe recurrent ventricular tachycardia, exercise-induced tachydysrhythmias, and paroxysmal atrial tachycardia provoked by emotion or exercise. In patients with supraventricular tachydysrhythmias, propranolol has two beneficial effects: (1) suppression of excessive discharge of the SA node, and (2) slowing of ventricular rate by decreasing transmission of atrial impulses through the AV node.

Adverse Effects. Beta blockers are generally well tolerated. Principal adverse effects concern the heart and bronchi. By blocking cardiac beta$_1$ receptors, propranolol can cause *heart failure, AV block,* and *sinus arrest.* Hypotension can occur secondary to reduced cardiac output. In patients with asthma, blockade of beta$_2$ receptors in the lung can cause *bronchospasm.* Because of its cardiac and pulmonary effects, propranolol is contraindicated for patients with asthma, sinus bradycardia, high-degree heart block, and heart failure.

Dosage and Administration. Propranolol can be administered orally and, in life-threatening emergencies, by IV injection. Dosages with either route show wide individual variation. Oral dosages range from 10 to 80 mg every 6 to 8 hours. The usual IV dose is 1 to 3 mg injected at a rate of 1 mg/min.

Acebutolol

Acebutolol [Sectral] is a cardioselective beta blocker approved for oral therapy of VPBs. Adverse effects are like those of propranolol: bradycardia, heart failure, AV block, and—despite cardioselectivity—bronchospasm. Accordingly, acebutolol is contraindicated for patients with heart failure, severe bradycardia, AV block, and asthma. Acebutolol can also cause adverse immunologic reactions; titers of antinuclear antibodies may rise, resulting in myalgia, arthralgia, and arthritis. For suppression of VPBs, the initial dosage is 200 mg twice daily. Usual maintenance dosages range from 600 to 1200 mg/day.

Esmolol

Esmolol [Brevibloc] is a cardioselective beta blocker with a very short half-life (9 minutes). Administration is by IV infusion. The drug is employed for immediate control of ventricular rate in patients with atrial flutter and atrial fibrillation. Use is short term only (e.g., in patients with dysrhythmias associated with surgery). The most common adverse reaction is hypotension. However, like other beta blockers, esmolol can also cause bradycardia, heart block, heart failure, and bronchospasm (at higher doses). In addition, pain can occur at the infusion site. Esmolol is available in two concentrations: 10 mg/ml and 250 mg/ml. *The concentrated formulation must be diluted prior to use.* Treatment is begun with a loading dose of 500 μg/kg infused over 1 minute. The usual maintenance infusion rate is 100 μg/kg/min.

CLASS III: POTASSIUM CHANNEL BLOCKERS (DRUGS THAT DELAY REPOLARIZATION)

Four class III antidysrhythmics are available: bretylium, amiodarone, dofetilide, and sotalol (which is also a beta blocker). All four drugs delay repolarization of fast potentials. Hence, all four prolong the action potential duration and ERP. By doing so, they prolong the QT interval. In addition, each drug can affect the heart in other ways. Hence, these agents are not interchangeable.

Bretylium

Bretylium is used only for short-term therapy of severe ventricular dysrhythmias. The drug's principal adverse effect is profound hypotension.

Effects on the Heart and EKG. Therapeutic effects result from blockade of potassium channels in Purkinje fibers and ventricular muscle (see Fig. 47–2A). By doing so, bretylium delays repolarization and thereby prolongs both the action potential duration and ERP. Because ventricular repolarization is delayed, the QT interval is prolonged.

When first administered, bretylium is taken up by sympathetic neurons, where it causes a transient increase in catecholamine release, followed by blockade of further release. In the heart, the initial increase in release can briefly exacerbate dysrhythmias. In blood vessels, the extended blockade of release produces hypotension.

Adverse Effects. Profound and persistent hypotension is the most troubling side effect. This reaction is common, occurring in up to 66% of patients. Blood pressure may fall in patients who are supine as well as in those who are standing. Hypotension results from blockade of norepinephrine release in sympathetic neurons that promote contraction of vascular smooth muscle. Continuous monitoring of blood pressure is required. If hypotension develops, blood pressure may be raised with dopamine or norepinephrine.

Therapeutic Use. Bretylium is indicated for short-term therapy of ventricular fibrillation and recurrent ventricular tachycardia in patients who have been refractory to more conventional therapy (cardioversion, lidocaine). For these patients, bretylium may be life saving.

Preparations, Dosage, and Administration. Bretylium is dispensed in solution (2, 4, and 50 mg/ml). The drug must be diluted for certain applications. In all cases, the EKG and blood pressure should be monitored continuously.

Intravenous. For nonemergency treatment, bretylium is administered by slow IV infusion. Rapid injection is reserved for emergencies. To manage ventricular fibrillation, the following protocol may be employed: (1) rapid IV injection of a 5-mg/kg dose, (2) rapid IV injection of additional doses (10 mg/kg) until the dysrhythmia has been controlled, and (3) slow IV infusion of maintenance doses (5 to 10 mg/kg) every 6 hours. (Maintenance doses are infused slowly because rapid administration results in nausea and vomiting. Initial doses are injected rapidly, despite the risk of nausea and vomiting, because of the need for rapid control of rhythm.)

Intramuscular. Bretylium is used undiluted for IM injection. The initial dose is 5 to 10 mg/kg. Dosing may be repeated every 6 to 8 hours. The injection site should be rotated.

Amiodarone

Amiodarone [Cordarone, Pacerone] is a class III antidysrhythmic drug that has complex effects on the heart. The drug is highly effective against both atrial and ventricular dysrhythmias. Unfortunately, serious toxicities (e.g., lung damage, visual impairment) are common, and may persist for months after treatment has stopped. Because of toxicity, amiodarone is *approved* only for life-threatening ventricular dysrhythmias that have been refractory to safer agents. Nonetheless, because of its efficacy, amiodarone is being used with increasing frequency against a variety of atrial and ventricular dysrhythmias.

Amiodarone is available for oral and IV use. Indications, electrophysiologic effects, time course of action, and adverse effects are different for each route. Accordingly, oral and IV therapy are considered separately.

Oral Therapy

Therapeutic Use. Although amiodarone is very effective, concerns about toxicity limit its indications. In the United States, oral amiodarone is approved only for long-term therapy of two life-threatening ventricular dysrhythmias: *recurrent ventricular fibrillation* and *recurrent hemodynamically unstable ventricular tachycardia*. Treatment should be reserved for patients who have not responded to safer drugs.

In addition to its approved uses, oral amiodarone has been used with success to convert *atrial fibrillation* to normal sinus rhythm, and to maintain normal sinus rhythm following conversion.

Effects on the Heart and EKG. Amiodarone has complex effects on the heart. Like bretylium, amiodarone delays repolarization, and thereby prolongs the action potential duration and ERP. The underlying cause of these effects may be blockade of potassium channels. Additional cardiac effects include reduced automaticity in the SA node, reduced contractility, and reduced conduction velocity in the AV node, ventricles, and His-Purkinje system. These occur secondary to blockade of sodium channels, calcium channels, and beta receptors. Prominent effects on the EKG are QRS widening and prolongation of the PR and QT intervals. Amiodarone also acts on coronary and peripheral blood vessels to promote dilation.

Pharmacokinetics. Amiodarone is highly lipid soluble and accumulates in many tissues, especially the liver and lungs. Elimination is by hepatic metabolism and excretion in the bile. Amiodarone has an extremely long half-life, ranging from 25 to 110 days. Because of its slow elimination, amiodarone continues to act long after administration has ceased.

Adverse Effects. Amiodarone produces many serious adverse effects. Since the drug's half-life is protracted, toxicity can continue for weeks or months after drug withdrawal.

Pulmonary toxicity (pneumonitis, alveolitis, pulmonary fibrosis) is the most serious adverse effect. Symptoms (dyspnea, cough, chest pain) resemble those of heart failure and pneumonia. Pulmonary toxicity develops in 2% to 17% of patients and carries a 10% risk of mortality. Patients at highest risk are those receiving long-term, high-dose therapy. A baseline chest x-ray and pulmonary function test are required. Pulmonary function should be monitored throughout treatment.

Amiodarone may cause a paradoxical *increase in dysrhythmic activity*. In addition, by suppressing the SA and AV nodes, the drug can cause *sinus bradycardia* and *AV block*. By reducing contractility, amiodarone can precipitate *heart failure*.

Virtually all patients develop *corneal microdeposits*, which may cause photophobia or blurred vision. *Optic neuropathy,* sometimes progressing to *blindness,* may also occur. Between 2% and 5% of patients experience *blue-gray discoloration of the skin. Gastrointestinal reactions* (anorexia, nausea, vomiting) are common. Possible *CNS reactions* include ataxia, dizziness, tremor, mood alteration, and hallucinations. *Hepatitis* and *thyroid dysfunction* (hypothyroidism, hyperthyroidism) have occurred; hence, all patients should undergo periodic liver and thyroid tests.

Drug Interactions. Amiodarone can increase plasma levels of several drugs, including quinidine, procainamide, phenytoin, digoxin, diltiazem, and warfarin. Dosages of these agents often require reduction.

Dosage. Amiodarone for oral use is available in 200- and 400-mg tablets. Treatment should be initiated in a hospital. The following schedule is used for loading: 800 to 1600 mg daily for 1 to 3 weeks followed by 600 to 800 mg daily for 4 weeks. The daily maintenance dosage is 100 to 400 mg.

Intravenous Therapy

Therapeutic Use. Intravenous amiodarone is approved only for initial treatment and prophylaxis of *recurrent ventricular fibrillation* and *hemodynamically unstable ventricular tachycardia* in patients refractory to safer drugs. For these indications, amiodarone may be more effective than IV bretylium.

In addition to its approved uses, IV amiodarone has been used with success against other dysrhythmias, including *atrial fibrillation, AV nodal reentrant tachycardia,* and *shock-resistant ventricular fibrillation.*

Effects on the Heart and EKG. In contrast to oral amiodarone, which affects multiple aspects of cardiac function, IV amiodarone affects primarily the AV node. Specifically, the drug slows AV conduction and prolongs AV refractoriness. Both effects probably result from antiadrenergic actions. The mechanism underlying antidysrhythmic effects is unknown.

Adverse Effects. The most common adverse effects are hypotension and bradydysrhythmias. Hypotension develops in 15% to 20% of patients, and may require discontinuation of treatment. Bradycardia or AV block occurs in 5% of patients; discontinuation of treatment or insertion of a pacemaker may be needed. Infused concentrations above 3 mg/ml (in 5% dextrose in water) produce a high incidence of phlebitis, and hence should be administered through a central venous catheter. Torsades de pointes in association with QT prolongation occurs rarely.

Dosage. Dosing is complex. During the first 24 hours, a total dose of 1050 mg is infused. After that, a maintenance infusion (0.5 mg/min) is given around the clock. The usual duration of treatment is 2 to 4 days. However, maintenance infusions may be continued for up to 3 weeks before switching to oral amiodarone.

Sotalol

Actions and Uses. Sotalol [Betapace] is a beta blocker that also delays repolarization. Hence, the drug has combined class II and class III properties. Prodysrhythmic properties are pronounced. Sotalol was initially approved only for ventricular dysrhythmias, such as sustained ventricular tachycardia, that are considered life threatening. In 1999, it was also approved for prophylaxis and treatment of atrial flutter and fibrillation, but only if symptoms are severe. The drug is not approved for hypertension or angina pectoris (the primary indications for other beta blockers).

Pharmacokinetics. Sotalol is administered orally and undergoes nearly complete absorption. The drug is excreted unchanged in the urine. Its half-life is 12 hours.

Adverse Effects. The major adverse effect is torsades de pointes, a serious dysrhythmia that develops in about 5% of patients. The risk of this dysrhythmia is increased by hypokalemia and by other drugs that prolong the QT interval.

At therapeutic doses, sotalol produces substantial beta blockade. Hence, it can cause bradycardia, AV block, heart failure, and bronchospasm. Accordingly, the usual contraindications to beta blockers apply.

Preparations, Dosage, and Administration. Sotalol is dispensed in tablets (80, 120, 160, and 240 mg) for oral use. Treatment should start in a hospital. The initial dosage is 80 mg twice daily. The usual maintenance dosage is 160 to 320 mg/day in two or three divided doses. The dosing interval should be increased in patients with renal impairment.

Dofetilide

Therapeutic Use. Dofetilide [Tikosyn] is an oral class III antidysrhythmic indicated for restoring and maintaining normal sinus rhythm in patients with atrial flutter or atrial fibrillation. The drug causes dose-related QT prolongation and thereby poses a serious risk of torsades de pointes. Accordingly, it should be reserved for patients with highly symptomatic atrial dysrhythmias. Initiation of treatment requires continuous EKG monitoring in a hospital. Dosage must be carefully titrated on the basis of renal function tests. Dofetilide is available only through authorized hospitals and prescribers.

Effects on the Heart and the EKG. Like other class III agents, dofetilide blocks cardiac potassium channels, and thereby delays repolarization, and hence prolongs the QT interval on the EKG. Dofetilide does not affect the PR interval or widen the QRS complex, and has no effect on cardiac beta receptors or sodium channels.

Pharmacokinetics. Dofetilide is well absorbed (90%) both in the presence and absence of food. Very little of the drug is metabolized. About 80% of each dose is excreted in the urine, primarily unchanged. Renal excretion results largely from active tubular secretion, mediated by *cationic pumps* (i.e., pumps specific for molecules that are cations). In patients with normal renal function, the drug's half-life is about 10 hours. However, in patients with renal impairment, the half-life is increased. In patients with moderate impairment, dosage must be reduced; in patients with severe impairment, dofetilide must not be used.

Adverse Effects. By increasing the QT interval, dofetilide predisposes patients to *torsades de pointes,* which can progress to fatal ventricular fibrillation. The risk is directly related to dofetilide blood levels, and is increased by hypokalemia and by other drugs that cause QT prolongation. To assess risk, an EKG should be obtained at baseline, and EKG monitoring should be continuous during the initial phase of treatment. Dofetilide is contraindicated for patients with a baseline QT interval greater than 440 milliseconds (or greater than 500 milliseconds in patients with ventricular conduction abnormalities). Other side effects include headache (11%), chest pain (10%), and dizziness (8%).

Drug Interactions. Drugs that are excreted by renal cation pumps can interfere with the excretion of dofetilide, thereby causing its levels to rise. Accordingly, concurrent use of these drugs (e.g., cimetidine, trimethoprim, ketoconazole, prochlorperazine, megestrol) is contraindicated.

Drugs that prolong the QT interval may increase the risk of dysrhythmias, and hence should be avoided. Among these are class I and class III antidysrhythmics, phenothiazines, tricyclic antidepressants, and some macrolide antibiotics.

Combining verapamil with dofetilide increases the risk of torsades de pointes, and hence should be avoided.

Preparations, Dosage, and Administration. Dofetilide [Tikosyn] is available in capsules (125, 250, and 500 mg) for oral administration. Because of the risk of dysrhythmias, treatment must be initiated in a hospital with *continuous EKG monitoring for at least 3 days.* Because the risk of dysrhythmias is directly related to plasma drug levels, which in turn are directly related to cre-

atinine clearance (a measure of renal function), *creatinine clearance must be monitored.* Dosage declines with decreasing creatinine clearance as follows: For patients with normal renal function (creatinine clearance greater than 60 ml/min), give 500 mg twice a day; for creatinine clearance 40 to 60 ml/min, give 250 mg twice a day; for creatinine clearance 20 to 39.9 ml/min, give 125 mg twice a day; and for creatinine clearance below 20 ml/min, withhold dofetilide. If the QT interval becomes excessively prolonged (greater than 500 milliseconds, or greater than 550 milliseconds in patients with ventricular conduction abnormalities) dosage should be reduced.

CLASS IV: CALCIUM CHANNEL BLOCKERS

Only two calcium channel blockers—verapamil [Calan, Isoptin, Verelan] and diltiazem [Cardizem, others]—are able to block calcium channels in the heart. Hence, these are the only calcium channel blockers used to treat dysrhythmias. The basic pharmacology of these drugs is discussed in Chapter 43. Consideration here is limited to their use against dysrhythmias.

Effects on the Heart and EKG. Blockade of cardiac calcium channels has three effects:

- Slowing of SA nodal automaticity
- Delay of AV nodal conduction
- Reduction of myocardial contractility

Note that these are identical to the effects of beta blockers (which makes sense in that beta blockers promote calcium channel closure in the heart). The principal effect on the EKG is prolongation of the PR interval, reflecting delayed AV conduction.

Therapeutic Uses. Verapamil and diltiazem have two antidysrhythmic uses. First, they can slow ventricular rate in patients with atrial fibrillation or atrial flutter. Second, they can terminate SVT caused by an AV nodal reentrant circuit. In both cases, benefits derive from suppressing AV nodal conduction. With IV administration, effects can be seen in 2 to 3 minutes. Verapamil and diltiazem are not active against ventricular dysrhythmias.

Adverse Effects. Although generally safe, these drugs *can* cause undesired effects. Blockade of cardiac calcium channels can cause *bradycardia, AV block,* and *heart failure.* Blockade of calcium channels in vascular smooth muscle can cause vasodilation, resulting in *hypotension* and *peripheral edema.* Blockade of calcium channels in intestinal smooth muscle can produce *constipation.*

Drug Interactions. Both verapamil and diltiazem can elevate levels of *digoxin,* thereby increasing the risk of digoxin toxicity. Also, since digoxin shares with verapamil and diltiazem the ability to decrease AV conduction, combining digoxin with either drug increases the risk of AV block.

Because verapamil, diltiazem, and *beta blockers* have nearly identical suppressant effects on the heart, combining verapamil or diltiazem with a beta blocker increases the risk of bradycardia, AV block, and heart failure.

Preparations, Dosage, and Administration. *Verapamil.* Administration may be IV or oral. Intravenous therapy is preferred for initial treatment. Oral therapy is used for maintenance.

Verapamil for *intravenous* use is dispensed in solution (5 mg/2 ml). The initial dose is 5 to 10 mg injected slowly (over 2 to 3 minutes). If the dysrhythmia persists, an additional 10 mg may be administered in 30 minutes. An IV infusion (0.375 mg/min) can be used for maintenance. Intravenous verapamil can cause serious cardiovascular effects. Accordingly, blood pressure and the EKG should be monitored, and equipment for resuscitation should be immediately available.

Verapamil for *oral* use is available in standard and sustained-release tablets. The maintenance dosage is 40 to 120 mg 3 or 4 times a day.

Diltiazem. For treatment of dysrhythmias, diltiazem is administered IV. Therapy is initiated with an IV bolus (0.25 mg/kg). If the response is inadequate, a second bolus (0.35 mg/kg) may be administered in 15 minutes. If appropriate, initial therapy may be followed with a continuous IV infusion (up to 24 hours' duration) at a rate of 5 to 15 mg/hr.

OTHER ANTIDYSRHYTHMIC DRUGS

Adenosine

Adenosine [Adenocard], a naturally occurring nucleotide, is the current drug of choice for terminating paroxysmal SVT. The drug has an extremely short half-life, and hence must be administered IV. Adverse effects are minimal because the drug is rapidly cleared from the blood.

Effects on the Heart and EKG. Adenosine decreases automaticity in the SA node and greatly slows conduction through the AV node. The most prominent EKG change is prolongation of the PR interval, brought on by delayed AV conduction. Adenosine works in part by inhibiting cyclic AMP–induced calcium influx, thereby suppressing calcium-dependent action potentials in the SA and AV nodes.

Therapeutic Use. Adenosine is approved only for termination of paroxysmal SVT, including Wolff-Parkinson-White syndrome. The drug is not active against atrial fibrillation, atrial flutter, or ventricular dysrhythmias.

Pharmacokinetics. Adenosine has an extremely short plasma half life (less than 10 seconds) owing primarily to rapid uptake by cells, and partly to deactivation by circulating adenosine deaminase. Because of its rapid clearance from the blood, adenosine must be administered by IV bolus, as close to the heart as possible.

Adverse Effects. Adverse effects are short lived, lasting for less than 1 minute. The most common are sinus bradycardia, dyspnea (from bronchoconstriction), hypotension and facial flushing (from vasodilation), and chest discomfort (perhaps from stimulation of pain receptors in the heart).

Drug Interactions. *Methylxanthines* (aminophylline, theophylline, caffeine) block receptors for adenosine. Hence, asthma patients taking aminophylline or theophylline need larger doses of adenosine, and even then adenosine may not work.

Dipyridamole, an antiplatelet drug, blocks cellular uptake of adenosine, and can thereby intensify its effects.

Preparations, Dosage, and Administration. Adenosine [Adenocard] is dispensed in solution (3 mg/ml) for bolus IV administration. The injection should be made as close to the heart as possible, and should be followed by a saline flush. The initial dose is 6 mg. If there is no response in 1 or 2 minutes, 12 mg may be tried and repeated once. If a response is going to occur, it should happen as soon as the drug reaches the AV node.

Digoxin

Although its primary indication is heart failure, digoxin [Lanoxin] is also used to treat supraventricular dysrhythmias. The basic pharmacology of digoxin is discussed in Chapter 46. Consideration here is limited to treatment of dysrhythmias.

Effects on the Heart. Digoxin suppresses dysrhythmias by decreasing conduction through the AV node and by decreasing automaticity in the SA node. The drug decreases AV conduction by (1) a direct depressant effect on the AV node and (2) acting in the CNS to increase vagal (parasympathetic) impulses to the AV node. Digoxin decreases automaticity of the SA node by increasing vagal traffic to the node and by decreasing sympathetic traffic. It should be noted that, although digoxin decreases auto-

maticity in the SA node, it can *increase* automaticity in *Purkinje* fibers. The latter effect contributes to dysrhythmias *caused* by digoxin.

Effects on the EKG. By slowing AV conduction, digoxin prolongs the PR interval. The QT interval may be shortened, reflecting accelerated repolarization of the ventricles. Depression of the ST segment is common. The T wave may be depressed or even inverted. There is little or no change in the QRS complex.

Adverse Effects and Interactions. The major adverse effect is *cardiotoxicity* (dysrhythmias). The risk of dysrhythmias is increased by hypokalemia, which can result from concurrent therapy with diuretics (thiazides and high-ceiling agents). Accordingly, it is essential that potassium levels be kept within the normal range (3.5 to 5 mEq/L). The most common adverse effects are GI disturbances (anorexia, nausea, vomiting, abdominal discomfort). CNS responses (fatigue, visual disturbances) are also relatively common.

Antidysrhythmic Uses. Digoxin is used only for supraventricular dysrhythmias. The drug is inactive against ventricular dysrhythmias.

Atrial Fibrillation and Atrial Flutter. Digoxin is used to slow ventricular rate in patients with atrial fibrillation and atrial flutter. Ventricular rate is decreased by reducing the number of atrial impulses that pass through the AV node. It should be noted that, although atrial fibrillation and flutter respond to digoxin and other drugs, cardioversion is the treatment of choice.

Supraventricular Tachycardia. Digoxin may be employed acutely and chronically to treat SVT. Acute therapy is used to abolish the dysrhythmia. Chronic therapy is used to prevent its return. Digoxin suppresses SVT by increasing cardiac vagal tone and by decreasing sympathetic tone.

Dosage and Administration. Oral therapy is generally preferred. The initial dosage is 1 to 1.5 mg administered in three or four doses over 24 hours. The maintenance dosage is 0.125 to 0.5 mg/day.

Ibutilide

Ibutilide [Corvert] is an IV agent used to terminate atrial flutter and atrial fibrillation of recent onset (i.e., that has been present no longer than 90 days). Conversion to sinus rhythm occurs during the infusion or within 90 minutes of its termination. Ibutilide is more effective against atrial flutter (48% to 70% success) than atrial fibrillation (22% to 43% success). Like class III agents, ibutilide prolongs the action potential duration; however, the mechanism does not involve blockade of potassium channels. Because it prolongs action potential duration, ibutilide prolongs the QT interval. Up to 8% of patients develop torsades de pointes, frequently in association with QT prolongation. Oral doses are teratogenic and embryocidal in rats. For patients who weigh over 60 kg, the dosage is 1 mg infused over 10 minutes. If the dysrhythmia does not convert within 10 minutes of terminating the infusion, a second 1-mg infusion may be made.

PRINCIPLES OF ANTIDYSRHYTHMIC DRUG THERAPY

Balancing Risks and Benefits

Therapy with antidysrhythmic drugs is based on a simple but important concept: Treat only if there is a clear benefit—and then only if the benefit outweighs the risks. As a rule, this means that intervention is needed only when the dysrhythmia interferes with ventricular pumping.

Treatment offers two potential benefits: reduction of symptoms and reduction of mortality. Symptoms that can be reduced include palpitations, angina, dyspnea, and faintness. For most antidysrhythmic drugs, there is little or no evidence of reduced mortality; in fact, mortality may actually increase.

Antidysrhythmic therapy carries considerable risk. Because of their *prodysrhythmic actions,* antidysrhythmic drugs can exacerbate existing dysrhythmias and generate new ones. Examples abound: toxic doses of digoxin can generate a wide variety of dysrhythmias; drugs that prolong the QT interval can cause torsades de pointes; many drugs can cause ventricular ectopic beats; several drugs (quinidine, encainide, flecainide, propafenone) can cause atrial flutter; and two drugs—encainide and flecainide—can produce incessant ventricular tachycardia. Because of their prodysrhythmic actions, antidysrhythmic drugs can *increase mortality*. Other adverse effects include heart failure and third-degree AV block (caused by calcium channel blockers and beta blockers), as well as many noncardiac effects, including severe diarrhea (quinidine), a lupus-like syndrome (procainamide), and pulmonary toxicity (amiodarone).

Properties of the Dysrhythmia to Be Considered

Sustained Versus Nonsustained Dysrhythmias. As a rule, nonsustained dysrhythmias require intervention only when they are symptomatic; in the absence of symptoms, treatment is usually unnecessary. In contrast, sustained dysrhythmias can be dangerous; hence, the benefits of treatment generally outweigh the risks.

Asymptomatic Versus Symptomatic Dysrhythmias. No study has demonstrated a benefit to treating dysrhythmias that are asymptomatic or minimally symptomatic. In contrast, therapy may be beneficial for dysrhythmias that produce symptoms (palpitations, angina, dyspnea, faintness).

Supraventricular Versus Ventricular Dysrhythmias. Supraventricular dysrhythmias are generally benign. The primary harm comes from driving the ventricles too rapidly to allow adequate filling. The goal of treatment is to either (1) terminate the dysrhythmia or (2) prevent excessive atrial beats from reaching the ventricles (using a beta blocker, calcium channel blocker, or digoxin). In contrast to supraventricular dysrhythmias, ventricular dysrhythmias frequently interfere with pumping. Accordingly, the goal of treatment is to terminate the dysrhythmia and prevent its recurrence.

Phases of Treatment

Treatment has two phases: acute and long term. The goal of acute treatment is to terminate the dysrhythmia. For many dysrhythmias, termination is accomplished with DC cardioversion (electrical countershock) or vagotonic maneuvers (e.g., carotid sinus massage), rather than drugs. The goal of long-term therapy is to prevent dysrhythmias from recurring. Quite often, the risks of long-term prophylactic therapy outweigh the benefits.

Long-Term Treatment: Drug Selection and Evaluation

Selecting a drug for long-term therapy is largely empiric. There are many drugs that might be employed, and we usually can't predict which one is going to work. Hence, finding an effective drug is done by trial and error.

Drug selection can be aided with electrophysiologic testing. In these tests, a dysrhythmia is generated artificially by programmed electrical stimulation of the heart. If a candidate drug is able to suppress the electrophysiologically induced dysrhythmia, it may also work against the real thing.

Holter monitoring can be used to evaluate treatment. A Holter monitor is a portable EKG device that is worn by the patient around the clock. If Holter monitoring indicates that dysrhythmias are still occurring with the present drug, a different drug should be tried.

Minimizing Risks

Several measures can help minimize risk. These include

- Starting with low doses and increasing them gradually
- Using a Holter monitor during initial therapy to detect danger signs—especially QT prolongation, which can precede torsades de pointes

- Monitoring plasma drug levels. Unfortunately, although drug levels can be good predictors of noncardiac toxicity (e.g., quinidine-induced nausea), they are less helpful for predicting adverse cardiac effects.

NONDRUG TREATMENT OF DYSRHYTHMIAS

Implantable Cardioverter/Defibrillators

ICDs are surgically implanted devices that monitor and analyze cardiac rhythm, and, by delivering electrical shocks to the heart, terminate any dysrhythmias that develop. Termination is accomplished with either (1) a series of pacing stimuli, which are usually imperceptible; or (2) a defibrillating shock, which can be painful. It is important to note that ICDs do not prevent dysrhythmias; rather, they neutralize the ones that occur. ICDs are indicated for patients with recurrent ventricular fibrillation or sustained ventricular tachycardia. For these patients, ICDs significantly reduce the risk of sudden death. The major complication associated with ICDs is mortality during surgical implantation. The mortality rate had been as high as 8%, but is declining due to use of newer techniques. ICDs cost about $20,000 to $25,000. The cost for implantation, including hospitalization, adds another $30,000 to $50,000.

Radiofrequency Catheter Ablation

Radiofrequency (RF) catheter ablation is a technique in which cardiac tissue responsible for causing a dysrhythmia is identified and destroyed; the result is often permanent cure. In preparation for RF ablation, the patient undergoes electrophysiologic cardiac testing to identify the small region of the heart that is generating the dysrhythmia. Next, an RF catheter is placed at the site. Activation of the catheter generates RF energy, which heats (and thereby destroys) all tissue within 5 to 8 mm of the catheter tip. Destruction of the offending tissue eliminates the dysrhythmia. Success rates depend on the dysrhythmia being treated. In patients with atrial tachycardia, AV nodal reentrant tachycardia, or dysrhythmias associated with Wolff-Parkinson-White syndrome, the rate of permanent cure is between 90% and 100%. In patients with atrial flutter, initial responses are generally good, but recurrence is common. Complications develop in less than 5% of procedures. The most common complications are AV block and myocardial perforation. Complications that require intervention or that result in long-term injury occur in only 1% of patients. When RF catheter ablation is done on an outpatient basis, the cost is about $10,000.

⁙ KEY POINTS

- Dysrhythmias result from alteration of the electrical impulses that regulate cardiac rhythm. Antidysrhythmic drugs control rhythm by correcting or compensating for these alterations.
- In the healthy heart, the SA node is the pacemaker.
- Impulses originating in the SA node must travel through the AV node to reach the ventricles. Impulses arriving at the AV node are delayed before going on to excite the ventricles.

- The His-Purkinje system conducts impulses rapidly throughout the ventricles, thereby causing all parts of the ventricles to contract in near-synchrony.
- The heart employs two kinds of action potentials: fast potentials and slow potentials.
- Fast potentials occur in the His-Purkinje system, atrial muscle, and ventricular muscle.
- Slow potentials occur in the SA node and AV node.
- Phase 0 of fast potentials (depolarization) is generated by rapid influx of sodium. Because depolarization is fast, these potentials conduct rapidly.
- During phase 2 of fast potentials, calcium enters myocardial cells, thereby promoting contraction.
- Phase 3 of fast potentials (repolarization) is generated by rapid extrusion of potassium.
- Phase 0 of slow potentials (depolarization) is caused by slow influx of calcium. Because depolarization is slow, these potentials conduct slowly.
- Spontaneous phase 4 depolarization (of fast or slow potentials) confers automaticity upon cells. Spontaneous phase 4 depolarization of cells in the SA node normally determines heart rate.
- The P wave of an EKG is caused by depolarization of the atria.
- The QRS complex is caused by depolarization of the ventricles. Widening of the QRS complex indicates slowed conduction through the ventricles.
- The T wave is caused by repolarization of the ventricles.
- The PR interval represents the time between onset of the P wave and onset of the QRS complex. PR prolongation indicates delayed AV conduction.
- The QT interval represents the time between onset of the QRS complex and completion of the T wave. QT prolongation indicates delayed ventricular repolarization.
- Dysrhythmias arise from disturbances of impulse formation (automaticity) or impulse conduction.
- Reentrant dysrhythmias result from a localized, self-sustaining circuit capable of repetitive cardiac stimulation.
- Dysrhythmias can be divided into two major groups: supraventricular dysrhythmias and ventricular dysrhythmias. In general, ventricular dysrhythmias disrupt cardiac pumping more than do supraventricular dysrhythmias.
- Treatment of supraventricular tachydysrhythmias is often directed at blocking impulse conduction through the AV node, rather than at eliminating the dysrhythmia.
- Treatment of ventricular dysrhythmias is usually directed at eliminating the dysrhythmia.
- All antidysrhythmic drugs are also prodysrhythmic (proarrhythmic). That is, they all can worsen existing dysrhythmias and generate new ones.
- Class I antidysrhythmic drugs block cardiac sodium channels, and thereby slow impulse conduction through the atria, ventricles, and His-Purkinje system.
- Slowing ventricular conduction widens the QRS complex.
- Quinidine (a class IA drug) blocks sodium channels and delays ventricular repolarization. Delaying ventricular repolarization prolongs the QT interval.
- Quinidine causes diarrhea and other GI symptoms in 33% of patients. These effects frequently force drug withdrawal.
- Quinidine can cause dysrhythmias. Widening of the QRS complex (by 50% or more) and excessive prolongation of the QT interval are warning signs.
- Quinidine elevates digoxin levels. If the drugs are used together, digoxin dosage must be reduced.
- Class IB agents differ from class IA agents in two ways: they accelerate repolarization and have little or no effect on the EKG.
- Lidocaine (a class IB agent) is used only for ventricular dysrhythmias. The drug is not active against supraventricular dysrhythmias.
- Lidocaine undergoes rapid inactivation by the liver. As a result, the drug must be administered by continuous IV infusion.
- Propranolol and other class II drugs block cardiac beta$_1$ receptors.
- By blocking cardiac beta$_1$ receptors, propranolol attenuates sympathetic stimulation of the heart, and thereby decreases SA nodal automaticity, AV conduction velocity, and myocardial contractility.
- By decreasing AV conduction velocity, propranolol prolongs the PR interval.
- The effects of propranolol on the heart result (ultimately) from suppressing calcium entry. Hence, the effects of propranolol and the effects of calcium channel blockade are nearly identical.
- Propranolol is especially useful for treating dysrhythmias caused by excessive sympathetic stimulation of the heart.
- In patients with supraventricular tachydysrhythmias, propranolol helps by (1) slowing discharge of the SA node and (2) decreasing conduction through the AV node, which prevents the atria from driving the ventricles at an excessive rate.
- Class III antidysrhythmics block potassium channels, and thereby delay repolarization of fast potentials. As a result, they prolong the action potential duration and the effective refractory period. By delaying ventricular repolarization, they prolong the QT interval.
- Bretylium (a class III agent) is used only for short-term therapy of severe ventricular dysrhythmias that have been refractory to safer treatments.
- Bretylium blocks release of norepinephrine from sympathetic nerves, and thereby causes profound and persistent hypotension in up to 66% of patients.
- Amiodarone (a class III agent) is highly effective against atrial and ventricular dysrhythmias, but can cause multiple serious adverse effects, including damage to the lungs, eyes, liver, and thyroid.
- Verapamil and diltiazem (class IV antidysrhythmics) block cardiac calcium channels, and thereby reduce automaticity of the SA node, slow conduction through the AV node, and decrease myocardial con-

tractility. These effects are identical to those of the beta blockers.
■ By suppressing AV conduction, verapamil and diltiazem prolong the PR interval.
■ Verapamil and diltiazem are used to slow ventricular rate in patients with atrial fibrillation or atrial flutter and to terminate SVT caused by an AV nodal reentrant

circuit. In both cases, benefits derive from suppressing AV nodal conduction.
■ Adenosine is the drug of choice for terminating paroxysmal SVT.
■ Adenosine has a very short half-life (less than 10 seconds), and hence must be given by IV bolus.

Summary of Major Nursing Implications*

Summaries are limited to the major antidysrhythmic drugs. Summaries for beta blockers (propranolol, acebutolol, and esmolol), phenytoin, calcium channel blockers (verapamil and diltiazem), and digoxin appear in Chapters 18, 23, 43, and 46, respectively.

QUINIDINE

Preadministration Assessment

Therapeutic Goal

The usual goal is long-term suppression of atrial and ventricular dysrhythmias.

Baseline Data

Obtain a baseline EKG and laboratory evaluation of liver function. Determine blood pressure.

Identifying High-Risk Patients

Quinidine is *contraindicated* for patients with a history of hypersensitivity to quinidine or other cinchona alkaloids and for patients with complete heart block, digoxin intoxication, or conduction disturbances associated with marked QRS widening and QT prolongation. Exercise *caution* in patients with partial AV block, heart failure, hypotensive states, and hepatic dysfunction.

Implementation: Administration

Routes

Usual Route. Oral.
Rare Routes. IM and IV.

Administration

Before giving full therapeutic doses, assess for hypersensitivity by giving a small test dose (200 mg PO or IM).

Advise patients to take quinidine with meals. Warn patients not to crush or chew sustained-release formulations.

Dosing must account for the particular quinidine salt being used: 200 mg of quinidine sulfate is equivalent to 275 mg of quinidine gluconate or quinidine polygalacturonate.

Ongoing Evaluation and Interventions

Evaluating Therapeutic Effects

Monitor for beneficial changes in the EKG. Plasma drug levels should be kept between 2 and 5 μg/ml.

Minimizing Adverse Effects

Diarrhea. Diarrhea and other GI disturbances occur in one third of patients and frequently force drug withdrawal. to reduce these effects, administer quinidine with meals.

Cinchonism. Inform patients about symptoms of cinchonism (tinnitus, headache, nausea, vertigo, disturbed vision), and instruct them to notify the physician if these develop.

Cardiotoxicity. Monitor the EKG for signs of cardiotoxicity, especially widening of the QRS complex (by 50% or more) and excessive prolongation of the QT interval. Monitor pulses for significant changes in rate or regularity. If signs of cardiotoxicity develop, withhold quinidine and notify the physician.

Arterial Embolism. Embolism may occur during therapy of atrial fibrillation. The risk can be reduced with warfarin (an anticoagulant). Observe for signs of thromboembolism (e.g., sudden chest pain, dyspnea) and report these immediately.

Minimizing Adverse Interactions

Digoxin. Quinidine can double digoxin levels. When these drugs are combined, digoxin dosage should be reduced. Monitor patients for digoxin toxicity (dysrhythmias).

PROCAINAMIDE

Preadministration Assessment

Therapeutic Goal

Procainamide is indicated for acute and long-term management of ventricular and supraventricular dysrhythmias. Because of toxicity associated with long-term use, quinidine is preferred to procainamide for chronic suppression.

Baseline Data

Obtain a baseline EKG, complete blood count, and laboratory evaluations of liver and kidney function. Determine blood pressure.

Identifying High-Risk Patients

Procainamide is *contraindicated* for patients with systemic lupus erythematosus, complete AV block, and second- or third-degree AV block in the absence of an electronic pacemaker. Exercise *caution* in patients with hepatic or renal dysfunction or a history of procaine allergy.

*Patient education information is highlighted as blue text.

Summary of Major Nursing Implications*—cont'd

Implementation: Administration

Routes

Oral, IM, IV.

Administration

Instruct patients to administer procainamide at evenly spaced intervals around the clock. Warn patients not to crush or chew sustained-release preparations.

When switching from IV procainamide to oral procainamide, allow 3 hours to elapse between stopping the infusion and giving the first oral dose.

Give IM injections deep into the gluteal muscle.

Ongoing Evaluation and Interventions

Evaluating Therapeutic Effects

Monitor the EKG for beneficial changes. Plasma drug levels should be kept between 3 and 10 µg/ml.

Minimizing Adverse Effects

SLE-like Syndrome. Prolonged therapy can produce a syndrome resembling SLE. **Inform patients about manifestations of SLE (joint pain and inflammation; hepatomegaly; unexplained fever; soreness of the mouth, throat, or gums), and instruct them to notify the physician if these develop.** If SLE is diagnosed, procainamide should be discontinued. If discontinuation is impossible, signs and symptoms can be controlled with a nonsteroidal anti-inflammatory drug (e.g., aspirin) or a glucocorticoid. The ANA titer should be measured periodically and, if it rises, procainamide withdrawal should be considered.

Blood Dyscrasias. Procainamide can cause agranulocytosis, thrombocytopenia, and neutropenia. Deaths have occurred. Obtain complete blood counts weekly during the first 3 months of treatment and periodically thereafter. **Instruct patients to inform the physician at the first sign of infection (fever, chills, sore throat), bruising, or bleeding.** If subsequent blood counts indicate hematologic disturbance, discontinue procainamide immediately.

Cardiotoxicity. Procainamide can cause dysrhythmias. Monitor pulses for changes in rate or regularity. Monitor the EKG for excessive QRS widening (greater than 50%) and for PR prolongation. If these occur, withhold procainamide and notify the physician.

Arterial Embolism. Embolism may occur during therapy of atrial fibrillation. The risk can be reduced with warfarin. Observe for signs of thromboembolism (e.g., sudden chest pain, dyspnea) and report these immediately.

LIDOCAINE

Preadministration Assessment

Therapeutic Goal

Acute management of ventricular dysrhythmias.

Baseline Data

Obtain a baseline EKG and determine blood pressure.

Identifying High-Risk Patients

Lidocaine is *contraindicated* for patients with Stokes-Adams syndrome, Wolff-Parkinson-White syndrome, and severe degrees of SA, AV, or intraventricular block in the absence of electronic pacing. Exercise *caution* in patients with hepatic dysfunction or impaired hepatic blood flow.

Implementation: Administration

Routes

Usual. IV.
Emergencies. IM.

Administration

Intravenous. Make certain the lidocaine preparation is labeled for IV use (i.e., is devoid of preservatives and catecholamines). Dilute concentrated preparations with 5% dextrose in water.

The initial dose is 50 to 100 mg (1 mg/kg) infused at a rate of 25 to 50 mg/min. For maintenance, monitor the EKG and adjust the infusion rate on the basis of cardiac response. The usual rate is 1 to 4 mg/min.

Intramuscular. Reserve for emergencies. The usual dose is 300 mg injected into the deltoid muscle. Switch to IV lidocaine as soon as possible.

Ongoing Evaluation and Interventions

Evaluating Therapeutic Effects

Continuous EKG monitoring is required. Plasma drug levels should be kept between 1.5 and 5 µg/ml.

Minimizing Adverse Effects

Excessive doses can cause convulsions and respiratory arrest. Equipment for resuscitation should be available. Convulsions can be managed with diazepam or phenytoin.

*Patient education information is highlighted as blue text.

Prophylaxis of Coronary Heart Disease: Drugs That Lower LDL Cholesterol Levels

Our main topic in this chapter is cholesterol and its impact on coronary artery atherosclerosis (thickening of the coronary arteries), also known as coronary heart disease (CHD). Moderate CHD manifests as anginal pain. Severe CHD sets the stage for myocardial infarction (MI; heart attack). In the United States, CHD is the leading killer of both men and women, causing over 515,000 deaths in 2000. According to the American Heart Association, at least 12,900,000 Americans alive today have a history of coronary events (angina, MI, or both). More than half of these people are women.

Atherosclerosis begins with development of a fatty streak in the arterial wall. This is followed by deposition of fibrous plaque. As atherosclerotic plaque grows, it impedes coronary blood flow, causing anginal pain. Worse yet, coronary atherosclerosis encourages formation of thrombi, which can block flow entirely, thereby causing MI.

The risk of developing CHD is directly related to increased levels of blood cholesterol, in the form of low-density lipoproteins (LDLs). By reducing levels of LDL cholesterol, we can slow progression of atherosclerosis, reduce the risk of serious CHD, and prolong life. The preferred method for lowering LDL cholesterol is modification of diet. Drugs are employed only when diet modification is insufficient.

We approach our topic—cholesterol and its impact on CHD—in three stages. First, we discuss cholesterol itself, plasma lipoproteins (structures that transport cholesterol in blood), and the process of atherogenesis. Second, we discuss guidelines for cholesterol screening and management of high cholesterol. Third, we discuss the pharmacology of the cholesterol-lowering drugs.

CHOLESTEROL

Cholesterol has multiple physiologic roles. Of greatest importance, cholesterol is a component of all cell membranes, as well as the membranes of intracellular organelles. In addition to these structural roles, cholesterol is required for synthesis of certain hormones (estrogen, progesterone, testosterone, adrenal corticosteroids) and for synthesis of bile salts, which are needed for digestion and absorption of fats. Also, cholesterol is deposited in stratum corneum of the skin, where it reduces evaporation of water and blocks transdermal absorption of water-soluble compounds.

Some of our cholesterol comes from dietary sources (exogenous cholesterol) and some is manufactured by cells (endogenous cholesterol), primarily in the liver. More cholesterol comes from endogenous production than from the diet. A critical step in hepatic synthesis of cholesterol is catalyzed by an enzyme named hydroxymethylglutaryl coenzyme A (HMG-CoA) reductase. Drugs that inhibit this enzyme constitute our most widely used class of cholesterol-lowering agents. During the night, endogenous synthesis of cholesterol increases. Hence, HMG-CoA reductase inhibitors are most effective when given in the evening.

An increase in dietary cholesterol produces only a small increase in cholesterol in the blood, primarily because increased ingestion of cholesterol inhibits endogenous cholesterol synthesis. Interestingly, an increase in dietary saturated fats produces a substantial (15% to 25%) increase in circulating cholesterol. Why? Because saturated fats are a substrate for cholesterol production by the liver. Accordingly, when we want to reduce cholesterol levels, it is more important to reduce intake of saturated fats than to reduce intake of cholesterol itself, although cholesterol intake should definitely be lowered.

PLASMA LIPOPROTEINS

Structure and Function of Lipoproteins

Function. Lipoproteins serve as carriers for transporting lipids—cholesterol and triglycerides—in blood. Like all other nutrients and metabolites, lipids use the bloodstream to move throughout the body. However, since cholesterol and triglycerides are not water soluble, these substances cannot dissolve directly in plasma. Lipoproteins represent a means of solubilizing these lipids, thereby permitting transport.

Basic Structure. The basic structure of lipoproteins is depicted in Figure 48–1. As indicated, lipoproteins are tiny, spherical structures that consist of a *hydrophobic core,* composed of cholesterol and triglycerides, surrounded by a *hydrophilic shell,* composed primarily of phospholipids arranged in a monolayer. Because the hydrophilic (water-soluble) shell completely covers the lipid core, the entire structure is soluble in plasma.

Apolipoproteins. All lipoproteins have one or more *apolipoprotein* molecules embedded in their shell (see Fig. 48–1). Apolipoproteins, which constitute the protein component of lipoproteins, have three functions:

- They serve as recognition sites for cell-surface receptors, and thereby allow cells to bind with and ingest lipoproteins.
- They activate enzymes that metabolize lipoproteins.
- They increase the structural stability of lipoproteins.

The apolipoproteins of greatest clinical interest are labeled A-I, A-II, and B-100. All lipoproteins that deliver cholesterol and triglycerides to nonhepatic tissues contain *apolipoprotein B-100.* Conversely, all lipoproteins that transport lipids from nonhepatic tissues back to the liver (i.e., that remove lipids from tissues) contain *apolipoprotein A-I.*

Classes of Lipoproteins

There are six major classes of plasma lipoproteins. Distinctions among classes are based on size, density, apolipoprotein content, transport function, and primary core lipids (choles-

terol or triglycerides). From a pharmacologic perspective, the features of greatest interest are *lipid content, apolipoprotein content,* and *transport function.*

The topic of lipoprotein density deserves comment for two reasons. First, naming of lipoproteins is based on their density. Second, differences in density provide the basis for the physical isolation and subsequent measurement of plasma lipoproteins. The various classes of lipoproteins differ in density as a result of dissimilarities in their percent composition of lipid and protein. Because protein is more dense than lipid, lipoproteins that have a high percentage of protein (and a low percentage of lipid) have a relatively high density. Conversely, lipoproteins with a lower percentage of protein have a lower density.

Of the six major classes of lipoproteins, three are of particular relevance to coronary atherosclerosis. These classes are named (1) very-low-density lipoproteins (VLDLs), (2) low-density lipoproteins (LDLs), and (3) high-density lipoproteins (HDLs). Properties of these classes are summarized in Table 48–1.

Very-Low-Density Lipoproteins

VLDLs contain *triglycerides* (and some cholesterol) as their core lipids, and account for nearly all of the triglycerides in blood. The physiologic role of VLDLs is *delivery of triglycerides* from the liver to adipose tissue and muscle. Each VLDL particle contains one molecule of *apolipoprotein*

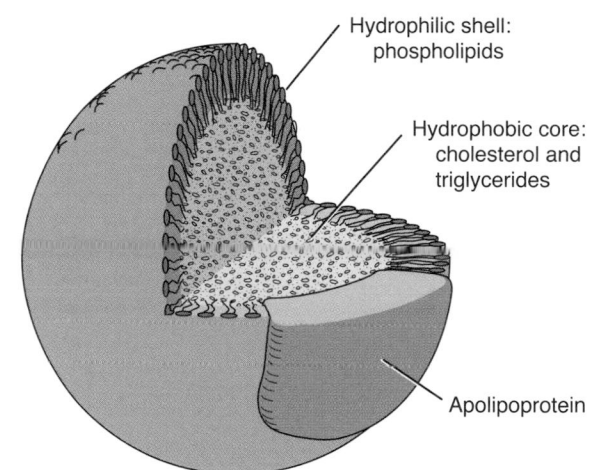

Hydrophilic shell: phospholipids

Hydrophobic core: cholesterol and triglycerides

Apolipoprotein

Figure 48–1 ■ Basic structure of plasma lipoproteins.

TABLE 48–1 ■ Properties of the Plasma Lipoproteins That Affect Atherosclerosis				
Lipoprotein Class*	**Major Core Lipids**	**Apolipoproteins**	**Transport Function**	**Influence on Atherosclerosis**
VLDL	Triglycerides	B-100, E, others	Delivery of triglycerides to nonhepatic tissues	*Probably contribute* to atherosclerosis
LDL	Cholesterol	B-100	Delivery of cholesterol to nonhepatic tissues	*Definitely contribute* to atherosclerosis
HDL	Cholesterol	A-I, A-II, A-IV	Transport of cholesterol from nonhepatic tissues back to the liver	*Protect* against atherosclerosis

*VLDL = very-low-density lipoproteins, LDL = low-density lipoproteins, HDL = high-density lipoproteins.

B-100, which allows VLDLs to bind with cell-surface receptors and thereby transfer their lipid content to cells.

The role of VLDLs in atherosclerosis is unclear. Although several studies suggest a link between elevated levels of VLDLs and development of atherosclerosis, this link has not been firmly established. However, we do know that elevation of triglyceride levels (>500 mg/dl) increases the risk of *pancreatitis.*

Low-Density Lipoproteins

LDLs contain *cholesterol* as their primary core lipid, and account for the majority (60% to 70%) of all cholesterol in blood. The physiologic role of LDLs is *delivery of cholesterol to nonhepatic tissues.* Each LDL particle contains one molecule of *apolipoprotein B-100,* which is needed for binding of LDL particles to LDL receptors on cells. LDLs can be looked on as by-products of VLDL metabolism, in that the lipids and apolipoproteins that compose LDLs are remnants of VLDL degradation.

Cells that require cholesterol meet their needs through endocytosis (engulfment) of LDLs, a process that begins with binding of LDL particles to LDL receptors on the cell surface. When cellular demand for cholesterol increases, cells synthesize more LDL receptors, and thereby increase their capacity for LDL uptake. Cells that are unable to make more LDL receptors are unable to increase cholesterol absorption. An important mechanism by which drugs reduce LDL levels is to increase the number of LDL receptors on cells.

Of all lipoproteins, LDLs make the greatest contribution to coronary atherosclerosis. The probability of developing CHD is directly related to the level of LDLs in blood. Conversely, by reducing LDL levels, we decrease the risk of CHD. Accordingly, when cholesterol-lowering drugs are used, the primary goal is to reduce LDL levels. Multiple studies have shown that, by reducing LDL levels, we can arrest or reverse atherosclerosis, and can thereby reduce mortality from CHD. For individuals with elevated levels of LDLs, a 25% reduction may reduce the risk of serious coronary events by 50%.

High-Density Lipoproteins

Like LDLs, HDLs contain *cholesterol* as their primary core lipid, and account for 20% to 30% of all cholesterol in blood. In contrast to LDLs, whose function is delivery of cholesterol to peripheral tissues, HDLs carry cholesterol from peripheral tissues back to the liver. That is, *HDLs promote cholesterol removal.*

The influence of HDLs on CHD is dramatically different from that of LDLs. Whereas elevation of LDLs *increases* the risk of CHD, elevation of HDLs *reduces* the risk of CHD. That is, high HDL levels actively protect against CHD.

Not all HDL particles are the same. Some contain only apolipoprotein A-I, whereas others contain apolipoproteins A-I *and* A-II. Available data suggest that cardioprotection is conferred by the HDLs that contain only *apolipoprotein A-I.*

LDL Cholesterol Versus HDL Cholesterol

From the foregoing, it is clear that not all cholesterol in plasma has the same impact on CHD. As discussed, a rise in cholesterol associated with LDLs increases the risk of CHD.

In contrast, a rise in cholesterol associated with HDLs lowers the risk of CHD. Consequently, when speaking of plasma cholesterol levels, we need to distinguish between cholesterol that is associated with HDLs and cholesterol that is associated with LDLs. To make this distinction, we use the terms *HDL cholesterol* and *LDL cholesterol.* Because it promotes atherosclerosis, LDL cholesterol has been dubbed "bad cholesterol." Conversely, because it protects against atherosclerosis, HDL cholesterol is known as "good cholesterol."

ROLE OF LDL CHOLESTEROL IN ATHEROSCLEROSIS

LDLs initiate and fuel development of atherosclerosis. The process begins with transport of LDLs from the arterial lumen into endothelial cells and from there into the space that underlies the arterial epithelium. Once in the subendothelial space, components of LDLs undergo *oxidation.* This step is critical in that oxidized LDLs

- Attract monocytes from the circulation into the subendothelial space, after which the monocytes undergo conversion to macrophages
- Inhibit macrophage mobility, thereby keeping macrophages at the site of atherogenesis
- Undergo uptake by macrophages (macrophages do not take up LDLs that have not been oxidized)
- Are cytotoxic, and hence can damage the vascular endothelium directly

As macrophages engulf more and more cholesterol, they become large and vacuolated. When macrophages assume this form, they are referred to as *foam cells.* Accumulation of foam cells beneath the arterial epithelium produces a fatty streak, which makes the surface of the arterial wall lumpy. Continued accumulation of foam cells can eventually cause rupture of the endothelium, thereby exposing the underlying tissue to the blood. This results in platelet adhesion and formation of microthrombi. As the process continues, smooth muscle cells migrate to the site, synthesis of collagen increases, and there can be repeated rupturing and healing of the endothelium. The end result is a mature atherosclerotic lesion, characterized by a large lipid core and a tough fibrous cap. In less mature lesions, the fibrous cap is not strong, and hence the lesions are unstable. As a result, arterial pressure and shear forces from moving blood can cause the cap to rupture; accumulation of platelets at the site of rupture can rapidly cause thrombosis, and can thereby cause infarction. Infarction is less likely at sites of mature atherosclerotic lesions.

It is important to appreciate that atherogenesis involves more than just deposition of lipids. In fact, atherogenesis is now considered primarily a chronic *inflammatory process.* When LDLs penetrate the arterial wall, they cause mild injury. The injury, in turn, triggers an inflammatory response, causing infiltration of macrophages, T lymphocytes, and other mediators of inflammation (e.g., C-reactive protein). In the late stage of the disease process, inflammation can weaken atherosclerotic plaque, leading to rupture and subsequent thrombosis. The role of inflammation in atherothrombosis is discussed further in Box 48–1.

DETECTION, EVALUATION, AND TREATMENT OF HIGH CHOLESTEROL: RECOMMENDATIONS FROM ATP III

It is well established that high cholesterol levels cause substantial morbidity and mortality, and that aggressive treatment can save lives. Accordingly, periodic cholesterol screening and risk assessment is recommended. If the assessment indicates CHD risk, lifestyle changes—especially diet and exercise—should be implemented. If CHD risk is especially high, LDL-lowering drugs should be added to the regimen.

Since 1988, the National Cholesterol Education Program (NCEP) has been issuing guidelines on cholesterol detection and management. The most recent update was published in 2001. A summary of the new guidelines—*Executive Summary of the Third Report of the National Cholesterol Education Program Expert Panel on Detection, Evaluation, and Treatment of High Blood Cholesterol in Adults* (also known as Adult Treatment Panel III or simply ATP III)—was published in *JAMA* (Vol. 285, No. 19, 2486-2497, 2001) and is available online at *www.nhlbi.nih.gov/guidelines/cholesterol/atp_iii.htm*. A quick-reference document—*ATP III Guidelines At-A-Glance Quick Desk Reference*—is available online at *www.nhlbi.nih.gov/guidelines/cholesterol/dskref.htm*. Previous NCEP guidelines were issued in 1988 (ATP I) and 1993 (ATP II). The discussion below reflects recommendations in ATP III.

Like earlier NCEP guidelines, ATP III focuses on the role of high cholesterol in CHD and stresses the importance of treatment. However, owing to revised risk assessment criteria, ATP III recommends drug therapy for many more Americans: about 36 million, compared with only 13 million under ATP II. In addition, ATP III addresses two new concerns: *elevated triglycerides* and *metabolic syndrome* (formerly known as syndrome X or insulin resistance syndrome).

Cholesterol Screening

Management of high LDL cholesterol begins with screening, which should be done every 5 years for all adults over the age of 20. Under ATP II, only LDL and total cholesterol were usually measured. In contrast, ATP III recommends a more thorough screen, consisting of total cholesterol, LDL cholesterol, HDL cholesterol, and triglycerides (TGs). Blood for these tests should be drawn after fasting. Classification of total cholesterol and LDL cholesterol (Table 48–2) is nearly identical to the classification in ATP II. The only change is that optimal LDL cholesterol is now defined as <100 mg/dl, compared with <130 mg/dl under ATP II. In addition, the cutoff for *low* HDL cholesterol is now <40 mg/dl, up from <35 mg/dl under ATP II. (Recall that low HDL cholesterol is detrimental, whereas high HDL cholesterol is protective.)

CHD Risk Assessment

Under ATP III, CHD risk assessment differs from prior guidelines in that assessment is now directed at determining the patient's *absolute risk of developing clinical coronary disease over the next 10 years.* The LDL goal and the mode of intervention are determined by the individual's degree of risk.

Factors in Risk Assessment

In order to assess the CHD risk for an individual, we need three kinds of information. Specifically we need to (1) identify CHD risk factors, (2) calculate 10-year CHD risk, and (3) identify CHD risk equivalents.

Identifying CHD Risk Factors. Major risk factors that modify LDL treatment goals are summarized in Table 48–3. The table lists five positive risk factors (advancing age, family history of premature CHD, hypertension, cigarette smoking, and low HDL cholesterol) and one negative risk factor (high HDL cholesterol). (LDL itself is not listed because the reason for counting these risk factors is to modify treatment of high LDL.) For the purpose of CHD risk assessment, each

TABLE 48–2 ▪ ATP III Classification of LDL, Total, and HDL Cholesterol

Cholesterol Type	Level (mg/dL)	Classification
LDL cholesterol	<100	Optimal
	100–129	Near optimal/above optimal
	130–159	Borderline high
	160–189	High
	≥190	Very high
Total cholesterol	<200	Desirable
	200–239	Borderline high
	≥240	High
HDL cholesterol	<40	Low
	≥60	High

From the Executive Summary of the Third Report of the National Cholesterol Education Program (NCEP) Expert Panel on Detection, Evaluation, and Treatment of High Blood Cholesterol in Adults (Adult Treatment Panel III). JAMA 2001;285:2486–2497.

TABLE 48–3 ▪ Major Risk Factors (Other Than High LDL Cholesterol) That Modify LDL Treatment Goals

Positive Risk Factors*

- Age:
  Men ≥45 yr
  Women ≥55 yr
- Family history of premature CHD in a first-degree relative:
  Male first-degree relative <55 yr old *or*
  Female first-degree relative <65 yr old
- Hypertension: blood pressure ≥140/90 *or* taking antihypertensive medication
- Current cigarette smoking (smoked at least 1 in the last month)
- Low HDL cholesterol (<40 mg/dl)

Negative Risk Factor

- High HDL cholesterol (≥60 mg/dL)†

*In ATP II, diabetes was listed a risk factor. However, in ATP III, diabetes is considered a CHD risk *equivalent,* not simply a risk *factor.*
†High HDL cholesterol (≥60 mg/dL) is protective, and hence counts as a "negative" risk factor; its presence removes one risk factor from the total count.
From the Executive Summary of the Third Report of the National Cholesterol Education Program (NCEP) Expert Panel on Detection, Evaluation, and Treatment of High Blood Cholesterol in Adults (Adult Treatment Panel III). JAMA 2001;285:2486–2497.

positive factor counts as 1 point; if the patient has high HDL cholesterol (a negative risk factor), 1 point is subtracted. For example, if the subject were a 62-year old female hypertensive smoker with an HDL level of 62 mg/dl, her point total score would be 2 (3 points for the three positive risk factors minus 1 point for the one negative risk factor).

It should be noted that, in ATP III, diabetes carries more weight in risk assessment than in ATP II. Why? Because we now know that diabetes is a very strong predictor of developing clinical CHD. Accordingly, diabetes is no longer listed as a risk *factor* (as it was in ATP II). Instead, for the purpose of risk assessment, diabetes is now considered a CHD risk *equivalent*. That is, having diabetes is now considered equivalent to having CHD as a predictor of a major coronary event.

Box 48–1 discusses three additional factors that could aid with CHD risk prediction: inflammation, homocysteine, and infection. A marker for inflammation—C-reactive protein—appears to be a good predictor of coronary events. The predictive value of homocysteine levels and infection has not been established.

Calculating 10-Year CHD Risk. ATP III defines three 10-year risk categories: >20%, 10% to 20%, and <10%. Some people are automatically in the highest (>20%) risk group—specifically, those with existing CHD (or other forms of atherosclerotic disease) and those with diabetes. For all other people, 10-year risk must be calculated. The instrument employed is the Framingham Risk Prediction Score, which takes five factors into account: age, total cholesterol, HDL cholesterol, smoking status, and systolic blood pressure. Framingham scores can determined using either (1) the tables for men and women shown in Figure 48–2 or (2) a web-based risk calculator, such as the one at *hin.nhlbi.nih.gov/ atpiii/calculator.asp.*

Identifying CHD Risk Equivalents. A CHD risk equivalent is a condition that poses the same risk of a major coronary event as does established CHD (i.e., >20% risk of a major event within 10 years). There are three basic CHD risk equivalents:

- Diabetes
- Atherosclerotic disease other than CHD (peripheral arterial disease, abdominal aortic aneurysm, and symptomatic carotid artery disease)
- The presence of multiple risk factors that confer a Framingham Risk Score of >20%

Identifying an Individual's CHD Risk Category

Under ATP III, there are four categories of CHD risk, labeled I, II, III, and IV (Table 48–4). People in category I are at highest risk: Their risk of a major coronary event within 10 years is over 20%. In comparison, the 10-year risk for people in category IV is low—less than 10%.

Category assignment is based on (1) the presence or absence of CHD (or a CHD risk equivalent, such as diabetes), (2) the number of risk factors the individual has (other than high LDL cholesterol), and (3) the individual's 10-year Framingham Risk Prediction Score. Although this assessment sounds complicated, it's not. Let's consider the case of Ralph Jones. Ralph is 62 years old, hypertensive, and smokes—but, remarkably, his HDL cholesterol is high (>60 mg/dl). Mr. Jones has no family history of premature CHD, does not have CHD himself, and does not have diabetes. His 10-year Framingham Risk Prediction Score is 11%. What CHD risk category does he belong in? Well, his age, blood pressure, and use of cigarettes represent three major risk factors, but his high (healthy) HDL cholesterol allows subtraction of one risk factor, leaving a net of two ma-

TABLE 48–4 ■ LDL Cholesterol Goals and Therapeutic Interventions for People in Specific CHD Risk Categories			
CHD Risk Category	**LDL Goal**	**LDL Level at Which to Initiate TLCs***	**LDL Level at Which to Consider Drug Therapy**
I *Highest Risk:* Has CHD or a CHD risk equivalent† (10-year risk is >20%)	<100 mg/dL	≥100 mg/dL	≥130 mg/dL (between 100 and 129 mg/dL, LDL-lowering drugs are optional)‡
II *Next Highest Risk:* Has 2 or more risk factors, but not CHD, and 10-year risk is 10%-20%	<130 mg/dL	≥130 mg/dL	≥130 mg/dL
III *Moderate Risk:* Has 2 or more risk factors, but not CHD, and 10-year risk is <10%	<130 mg/dL	≥130 mg/dL	≥160 mg/dL
IV *Low to Moderate Risk:* Has 0 to 1 risk factor, but not CHD (10-year risk is probably <10%)§	<160 mg/dL	≥160 mg/dL	≥190 mg/dL (between 160 and 189 mg/dL, LDL-lowering drugs are optional)

*TLCs = therapeutic lifestyle changes.
†CHD risk equivalents include diabetes, forms of atherosclerosis other than CHD (e.g., peripheral arterial disease, symptomatic coronary artery disease), and any combination of risk factors that creates a 10-year Framingham Risk Score of greater than 20%.
‡For patients in this LDL cholesterol range, some authorities recommend LDL-lowering drugs, others recommend drugs that primarily modify levels of triglycerides and HDL cholesterol (e.g., nicotinic acid or a fibrate), and still others might defer drug therapy.
§Almost all people with 0 to 1 risk factor and no CHD have a 10-year risk below 10%, and hence formal evaluation of 10-year risk is not needed.
Modified from the Executive Summary of the Third Report of the National Cholesterol Education Program (NCEP) Expert Panel on Detection, Evaluation, and Treatment of High Blood Cholesterol in Adults (Adult Treatment Panel III). JAMA 2001;285:2486–2497.

Estimate of 10-year risk for MEN

Age	Points
20-34	−9
35-39	−4
40-44	0
45-49	3
50-54	6
55-59	8
60-64	10
65-69	11
70-74	12
75-79	13

Total Cholesterol	Points Age 20-39	Age 40-49	Age 50-59	Age 60-69	Age 70-79
<160	0	0	0	0	0
160-199	4	3	2	1	0
200-239	7	5	3	1	0
240-279	9	6	4	2	1
≥280	11	8	5	3	1

	Points Age 20-39	Age 40-49	Age 50-59	Age 60-69	Age 70-79
Nonsmoker	0	0	0	0	0
Smoker	8	5	3	1	1

HDL (mg/dL)	Points
≥60	−1
50-59	0
40-49	1
<40	2

Systolic BP (mmHg)	If Untreated	If Treated
<120	0	0
120-129	0	1
130-139	1	2
140-159	1	2
≥160	2	3

Point Total	10-Year Risk %
<0	<1
0	1
1	1
2	1
3	1
4	1
5	2
6	2
7	3
8	4
9	5
10	6
11	8
12	10
13	12
14	16
15	20
16	25
≥17	≥30

10-Year risk _____ %

Estimate of 10-year risk for WOMEN

Age	Points
20-34	−7
35-39	−3
40-44	0
45-49	3
50-54	6
55-59	8
60-64	10
65-69	12
70-74	14
75-79	16

Total Cholesterol	Points Age 20-39	Age 40-49	Age 50-59	Age 60-69	Age 70-79
<160	0	0	0	0	0
160-199	4	3	2	1	1
200-239	8	6	4	2	1
240-279	11	8	5	3	2
≥280	13	10	7	4	2

	Points Age 20-39	Age 40-49	Age 50-59	Age 60-69	Age 70-79
Nonsmoker	0	0	0	0	0
Smoker	9	7	4	2	1

HDL (mg/dL)	Points
≥60	−1
50-59	0
40-49	1
<40	2

Systolic BP (mmHg)	If Untreated	If Treated
<120	0	0
120-129	1	3
130-139	2	4
140-159	3	5
≥160	4	6

Point Total	10-Year Risk %
<9	<1
9	1
10	1
11	1
12	1
13	2
14	2
15	3
16	4
17	5
18	6
19	8
20	11
21	14
22	17
23	22
24	27
≥25	≥30

10-Year risk _____ %

Figure 48–2 ■ Tables for calculating Framingham Risk Prediction Scores.
To determine an individual's 10-year risk of developing clinical coronary disease, simply circle the appropriate points for each of the five risk factors considered (age, total cholesterol, smoking status, HDL cholesterol, and systolic blood pressure) and then add the points up. The point total indicates the 10-year risk. For example, a total of 13 points indicates a 10-year risk of 12%.

Special Interest Topic

BOX 48–1 ■ THE *UN*USUAL SUSPECTS: INFLAMMATION, INFECTION, AND HOMOCYSTEINE

Although we know about some risk factors for CHD—advancing age, obesity, hypertension, diabetes, smoking, high LDL cholesterol, and sedentary lifestyle—it is clear that other risk factors must exist. Why? Because many young, lean, active, normotensive, nondiabetic, nonsmokers with low cholesterol still manage to die from MI. Obviously, additional risk factors must be involved. The leading candidates are inflammation, infection, and homocysteine.

Inflammation and C-Reactive Protein

There is good evidence that inflammation plays a central role in atherosclerosis. Although inflammation normally protects tissues, it can also do harm. For example, inflammation in the lungs leads to bronchospasm in asthma, and inflammation of joints underlies tissue injury in arthritis. In arteries, inflammation appears to set the stage for atherogenesis. In addition, inflammation may weaken the surface of atherosclerotic plaques, thereby increasing the risk of plaque rupture. Factors that might evoke an inflammatory response include smoking, diabetes, high levels of homocysteine (see below), and infection (see below).

The strongest evidence implicating inflammation in CHD comes from measuring plasma levels of C-reactive protein (CRP), a marker for vascular inflammation. This protein is produced in large amounts by the liver in response to inflammation, infection, and other pathologic events. CRP has multiple actions that can contribute to atherothrombosis: It promotes inflammation, increases lipid accumulation in atherosclerotic plaques, activates complement, stimulates coagulation, and disrupts the normal function of vascular endothelial cells.

In clinical studies, elevation of CRP has been associated with increased cardiovascular risk. For example, in the *Physician's Health Study,* high levels of CRP predicted danger 6 to 8 years *in advance:* Among people with no prior cardiovascular events, high levels of CRP were associated with a threefold increased risk of heart attacks and a twofold increased risk of stroke. In the *Women's Health Study,* similar results were obtained: Over an 8-year period, women with the highest levels of CRP experienced 4.5 times as many heart attacks or strokes as did women with the lowest levels. Furthermore, not only did elevated CRP predict cardiovascular risk, it did so for women whose LDL cholesterol was *normal*—not just those whose LDL cholesterol was high. This is important. Why? Because it means that elevated CRP is an *independent* risk factor for cardiovascular events; it's not simply a surrogate for LDL cholesterol. Hence, measuring CRP *and* LDL cholesterol might identify different risk groups.

Cardiovascular protection conferred by aspirin and statins may result in part from anti-inflammatory actions. It is well known that aspirin suppresses platelet aggregation, and thereby helps protect against MI. However, recent evidence indicates that aspirin is most beneficial in patients with high levels of CRP, suggesting that aspirin's anti-inflammatory actions may also contribute to cardiovascular benefits. Likewise, it is well known that statins reduce LDL cholesterol levels, and thereby protect against CHD. However, in patients with *normal* cholesterol levels and high levels of CRP, pravastatin still offers protection. Specifically, the drug can lower CRP levels by 17% and

reduce the risk of recurrent MI—again suggesting that anti-inflammatory actions may partly explain clinical benefits.

Given that elevated CRP may predict cardiovascular events, should we screen people to see if their CRP is high? Yes, we should, according to a 2003 statement issued by an expert panel convened jointly by the American Heart Association (AHA) and Centers for Disease Control and Prevention (CDC). However, the AHA/CDC panel does not recommend screening for everyone. Rather, screening should be limited to patients deemed at *intermediate* cardiovascular risk (i.e., having a 10% to 20% risk of developing CHD in the next 10 years) as indicated by their age, LDL cholesterol level, and other traditional risk criteria. The panel does not recommend screening for patients considered at high or low risk. Why? Because the test results are unlikely to reveal information that would alter treatment decisions: With people at high risk, we already have sufficient information to guide treatment; with people at low risk, CRP tests are unlikely to reveal a previously unknown risk that would indicate a need for treatment.

How should CRP be tested? The AHA/CDC panel recommends testing for a specific form of CRP, known as *high-sensitivity CRP* (hs-CRP). Because levels of hs-CRP can vary over time, two tests should be done, about 2 weeks apart. The degree of cardiovascular risk associated with specific hs-CRP levels is as follows:

- Less than 1.0 mg/L = low risk
- 1.0 to 3.0 mg/L = average risk
- More than 3.0 mg/L = high risk

People in the high-risk group have a twofold greater risk of an adverse cardiovascular event compared with people in the low-risk group.

If the hs-CRP level indicates high risk, what should be done? Recall that hs-CRP testing is recommended only for patients already classified as having intermediate risk, as determined by traditional risk criteria. For these people, a high level of hs-CRP would signal a need for more intensive intervention.

It is important to note that hs-CRP should not be tested in the presence of trauma, infection, or systemic inflammatory disorders. Why? Because these conditions can raise hs-CRP levels substantially. Hence, if hs-CRP levels tested as high, we couldn't tell if these conditions or vascular inflammation were the cause.

Does lowering CRP reduce cardiovascular risk? No one knows. Randomized controlled trials (RCTs) designed to answer this question are in progress, but have not been completed.

Infection

Chlamydia pneumoniae, an obligate intracellular bacterium and a common cause of pneumonia, may help initiate and promote atherosclerosis. Several lines of evidence implicate the bug:

- Patients with CHD often have high titers of antibodies against *C. pneumoniae.*
- *C. pneumoniae* is present in 59% of atheromatous arteries and only 3.1% of healthy arteries.

- *In vitro* studies indicate that *C. pneumoniae* can alter the function of atheroma-associated cells in a way that could promote atherogenesis.
- Rabbits inoculated with *C. pneumoniae* and fed a high-cholesterol diet developed evidence of atherosclerosis within 3 months—but not if they were given azithromycin [Zithromax], an antibiotic that suppresses growth of *C. pneumoniae*.
- Patients with a prior MI and a high antibody titer to *C. pneumoniae* are 4 times more likely to experience recurrent MI, compared with patients who have low antibody titers to *C. pneumoniae*.

These data indicate that *C. pneumoniae* is frequently present in atherosclerotic plaque and is there early, suggesting a possible causative role.

How might *C. pneumoniae* contribute to CHD? The most likely mechanism is promotion of inflammation. One theory suggests that macrophages in the lungs or elsewhere ingest the bacterium, and then migrate to a site where plaque is developing. Once inside the plaque, the bacteria multiply, causing chronic infection. An immune response to the infection then causes inflammation of the arterial wall, which could promote further atherogenesis and destabilize established plaque.

Can antibiotics directed at *C. pneumoniae* protect against coronary events? Research into this question has produced inconsistent results. In preliminary trials, giving antibiotics to patients with coronary artery disease reduced the incidence of recurrent coronary events. Unfortunately, more rigorous studies failed to confirm these results. Does this failure mean that *C. pneumoniae* is *not* involved? No. The inability of antibiotics to confer protection may simply mean that the drugs employed were unable to eradicate *C. pneumoniae*. Or the results may mean that, by the time atherosclerosis is well established, it may be too late for patients to benefit from killing the bug. Ongoing studies should help resolve the issue.

Homocysteine

Homocysteine, a sulfur-containing amino acid, has long been suspected as a contributor to CHD. However, despite years of research, definitive proof of its involvement is still lacking.

Homocysteine is formed from methionine, an essential amino acid found in proteins. Clearance of homocysteine is facilitated by three vitamins: folic acid, vitamin B_6 (pyridoxine), and vitamin B_{12} (cyanocobalamin). If intake of these vitamins is inadequate, blood levels of homocysteine will rise. (Normal blood levels range between 5 and 15 mmol/L).

The homocysteine story began in 1969, when Dr. Kilmer S. McCully, a Harvard pathologist, reported autopsy evidence of extensive arterial thrombosis in two children with homocystinuria, an inborn error of metabolism that results in high blood levels of homocysteine. On the basis of this evidence, Dr. McCully suggested that excessive homocysteine may equal excessive cholesterol as a risk factor for CHD.

There is now a large body of evidence relating homocysteine to heart disease. More than 75 *observational* studies (as opposed to *randomized controlled trials*) have shown an association between high levels of homocysteine and increased risk of cardiovascular disease. For example, a 1998 study involving 21,520 men found that, in men with the highest levels of homocysteine, the risk of ischemic heart disease was 3.7 times greater than in men with the lowest levels of homocysteine. The authors estimated that raising homocysteine levels by 5 mmol/L increased the risk of death from CHD by 33%.

Results of the *Nurse's Health Study,* published in 1998, add support to the homocysteine theory. In this 14-year observational study, a diet high in folic acid and vitamin B_6 was associated with a significant reduction in the risk of heart disease. Participants who consumed 400 mg of folic acid and 3 mg of vitamin B_6 daily reduced their risk of MI by about 50%, compared with those who consumed the lowest amounts of these vitamins. Presumably, ingesting these vitamins reduced levels of homocysteine, and thereby reduced the risk of CHD. However, another interpretation is possible: Folic acid and vitamin B_6 are directly protective, and benefits had nothing to do with homocysteine. Nonetheless, because of the apparent protection conferred by these vitamins, the authors recommended consuming at least 400 mg of folic acid daily (the current recommended dietary allowance [RDA]) and 3 mg of vitamin B_6 daily (twice the current RDA).

Although nearly all observational studies have shown an association between high homocysteine levels and increased risk of CHD, results of RCTs have been mixed. (As discussed in Chapter 3, RCTs are much more reliable than observational studies.) One small RCT, the *Swiss Heart Study,* provides strong support for the homocysteine theory. In this trial, 533 patients who had undergone coronary angioplasty were given either placebo or homocysteine-lowering therapy (folic acid, vitamin B_6, and vitamin B_{12}). The result? Rates of coronary restenosis in the treatment group were much lower than in the placebo group. Furthermore, the degree of vessel occlusion was lowest in the patients with the lowest homocysteine levels. Another RCT, the *Women's Health Study,* also supports the homocysteine theory—but only slightly. This 3-year, prospective study enrolled 28,263 healthy postmenopausal women. High levels of homocysteine at the beginning of the study were associated with an increased risk of cardiovascular events. However, the increase was only modest—considerably lower than the risk posed by conventional CHD risk factors (e.g., hypertension, diabetes, high cholesterol).

How might homocysteine promote CHD? There is evidence for several possible mechanisms, including activation of the coagulation system, increased adhesiveness of platelets, increased growth of vascular smooth muscle, direct toxicity to the vascular endothelium, and impaired responses to nitric oxide (an endogenous vascular relaxing agent).

In summary, we know that:

- High levels of homocysteine are associated with an increased risk of CHD.
- People who take homocysteine-lowering vitamins (folic acid, vitamin B_6, and vitamin B_{12}) have a reduced risk of CHD.
- Some RCTs indicate that high levels of homocysteine predict an increased risk of CHD.

- One small RCT has shown that homocysteine-lowering therapy reduces the risk of coronary restenosis.
- There are plausible mechanisms by which homocysteine could promote CHD.

These data are intriguing, but do not prove a causal relationship between homocysteine and CHD. To prove this relationship, we need large RCTs that confirm and extend the results of the Swiss Heart Study. That is, we need more evidence indicating that interventions that reduce high levels of homocysteine also reduce the risk of CHD. Until these data are available, the question will remain open. In the meantime, it would seem prudent for individuals with high homocysteine levels (above 10 to 12 mmol/L) to ensure adequate intake of folic acid, vitamin B_6, and vitamin B_{12}.

A final note: Since January 1, 1998, manufacturers of enriched grain products (e.g., enriched bread, pasta, flour, breakfast cereal, grits, rice) have been required to fortify these foods with folic acid. As a result, the incidence of folic acid deficiency in the United States has declined sharply, and the percentage of people with high levels of homocysteine has dropped as well (from 19% down to 10%). Hence, even if homocysteine really is a risk factor for CHD, increased folate in the American diet may render the issue moot.

jor risk factors. The presence of two major risk factors plus the 11% Framingham score place Mr. Jones in CHD risk category II (the next to highest risk group). Pretty easy, huh?

Category IV deserves comment. People assigned to this group have one CHD risk factor or less, and do not have CHD. As a rule, their 10-year CHD risk is not calculated. Why? Because there's no need: With so few risk factors, their 10-year risk is almost always below 10%.

Treatment of High LDL Cholesterol

Treatment of high LDL cholesterol is based on the individual's CHD risk category: The greater the 10-year risk, the more aggressive treatment should be. As CHD risk increases, the target LDL goal gets lower, as does the LDL level at which treatment should commence. For example, among individuals in risk category I, the LDL goal is quite low (<100 mg/dl), compared with the higher goal (<160 mg/dl) for people in category IV. Similarly, for individuals in category I, drugs are recommended if the LDL level is 130 mg/dl or above, compared with a much higher value (190 mg/dl or above) for those in category IV. Table 48–4 summarizes the LDL goal and the LDL levels at which to initiate treatment for all four CHD risk categories.

To reduce LDL levels, ATP III recommends two forms of intervention: (1) therapeutic lifestyle changes (TLCs) and (2) drug therapy. For some people, cholesterol can be reduced adequately with TLCs alone. Others require TLCs *plus* cholesterol-lowering drugs. Please note: Drugs should be used only as an *adjunct* to TLCs—not as a *substitute*.

Therapeutic Lifestyle Changes

Therapeutic lifestyle changes are nondrug measures used to lower LDL cholesterol. TLCs focus on three main issues: diet, weight control, and exercise.

The TLC Diet. The TLC diet has two objectives: (1) reducing LDL cholesterol and (2) establishing and maintaining a healthy weight. As in ATP II, the central feature of the diet is reduced intake of cholesterol and saturated fats. However, recommended limits have been lowered: Individuals should now limit cholesterol intake to 200 mg/day or less (down from 300 mg/day or less) and saturated fat intake to 7% or less of total calories (down from 10% or less of total calories). Intake of *trans* fats—found primarily in crackers, commercial

TABLE 48–5 ■ Nutrient Composition of the TLC Diet Described in ATP III	
Nutrient	**Recommended Intake**
Cholesterol	<200 mg/day
Saturated fat*	<7% of total calories
Polyunsaturated fat	Up to 10% of total calories
Monounsaturated fat	Up to 20% of total calories
Total fat	25%–35% of total calories
Carbohydrates†	50%–60% of total calories
Protein	About 15% of total calories
Fiber	20–30 gm/day
Total calories‡	Balance energy intake and expenditure to maintain a desirable body weight or prevent weight gain

TLC = therapeutic lifestyle changes.
Trans fatty acids should be kept to a minimum.
†Carbohydrates should be derived mainly from foods rich in complex carbohydrates, such as fruits, vegetables, and grains (especially whole grains).
‡Daily energy expenditure should include at least moderate physical activity (contributing about 200 kcal/day).
From the Executive Summary of the Third Report of the National Cholesterol Education Program (NCEP) Expert Panel on Detection, Evaluation, and Treatment of High Blood Cholesterol in Adults (Adult Treatment Panel III). JAMA 2001;285:2486–2497.

baked goods, and french fries—should be minimized. ATP III recommendations for cholesterol, fats, and other nutrients are summarized in Table 48–5. A list of specific foods to choose or avoid appears in Table 48–6.

If the basic TLC diet fails to lower LDL cholesterol adequately, ATP III recommends two additional measures: increased intake of soluble fiber (10 to 25 gm/day) and increased intake of plant stanols and sterols (2 gm/day). Oatmeal is a good source of soluble fiber. Plant stanols and sterols are available in the form of cholesterol-lowering margarines (see below under *Plant Stanol and Sterol Esters*).

Weight Control. Being overweight or obese is a major risk factor for CHD. Conversely, weight loss can reduce both LDL cholesterol and CHD risk. Weight loss is especially important

TABLE 48–6 ■ Recommended Dietary Modifications to Lower Serum Cholesterol

Food Type	Recommendation	
	Choose	**Decrease**
Fish, chicken, turkey, and lean meats	Fish; poultry without skin; lean cuts of beef, lamb, pork, or veal; shellfish	Fatty cuts of beef, lamb, or pork; spareribs; organ meats; regular cold cuts; sausage; hot dogs
Skim and low-fat milk, cheese, yogurt, and dairy products	Skim and 1% fat milk (liquid, powdered, evaporated), buttermilk	4% fat milk (regular, evaporated, condensed), 2% fat milk, cream, half and half, imitation milk products, most nondairy creamers, whipped toppings
	Nonfat (%) or low-fat yogurt	Whole-milk yogurt
	Low-fat cottage cheese (1% or 2% fat)	Whole-milk cottage cheese (4%)
	Low-fat cheeses, farmer or pot cheeses (all of these cheeses should have no more than 2–6 gm of fat per ounce)	All natural cheeses (e.g., blue, Roquefort, Camembert, cheddar, Swiss)
		Cream cheese (including low-fat and "light" types), sour cream (including low-fat and "light" types)
	Sherbert, sorbet	Ice cream
Eggs	Egg whites (2 whites = 1 whole egg in recipes), cholesterol-free egg substitutes	Egg yolks†
Fruits and vegetables	Fresh, frozen, canned, and dried fruits and vegetables	Vegetables prepared in butter, cream, and other sauces
Breads and cereals	Homemade baked goods using unsaturated oils sparingly, angel food cake, low-fat crackers, low-fat cookies	Commercial baked goods: pies, cakes, muffins, doughnuts, croissants, biscuits, high-fat crackers, high-fat cookies
	Rice, pasta	Egg noodles
	Whole-grain breads and cereals (oatmeal, whole wheat, rye, bran, multigrain, etc.)	Breads in which eggs are a major ingredient
Fats and oils	Unsaturated vegetable oils: corn, olive, rapeseed (canola oil), safflower, sesame, soybean, sunflower	Butter, coconut oil, palm oil, palm kernel oil, lard, bacon fat
	Margarine (regular or diet),* shortening made from one of the unsaturated oils listed above	
	Mayonnaise, salad dressings made with one of the unsaturated oils listed above, low-fat dressings	Dressings made with egg yolk
	Seeds and nuts	Coconut
	Baking cocoa	Chocolate

Author's note: Since the publication of this table in 1988, new evidence indicates that *stick* margarine (but probably not newer low-fat spreads), which contains 17% *trans* fat, raises LDL cholesterol and lowers HDL cholesterol, and hence should not be recommended.

†*Author's note:* Consuming up to 1 egg/day is not associated with an increased risk of fatal or nonfatal MI or ischemic or hemorrhagic stroke, except possibly in people with diabetes.

From the National Cholesterol Education Program Adult Treatment Panel report. Arch Intern Med 1988;148:36.

for people with metabolic syndrome (see below). In ATP III, achieving a healthy weight is encouraged for all people.

Exercise. A sedentary lifestyle carries an increased risk of CHD. Conversely, regular exercise lowers CHD risk. Running and swimming, for example, can decrease LDL cholesterol and elevate HDL cholesterol, thereby reducing risk. In addition, exercise can reduce blood pressure, decrease insulin resistance, and improve overall cardiovascular performance. Accordingly, ATP III encourages regular physical activity (defined as 30 minutes of activity on most days, if not all days).

Smoking Cessation. Cigarette smoking raises LDL cholesterol and lowers HDL cholesterol, thereby increasing the risk of CHD. All people should be forcefully encouraged to quit.

Drug Therapy

Drugs are not the first-line therapy for lowering LDL cholesterol. Rather, drugs should be employed only if TLCs fail to reduce LDL cholesterol to an acceptable level—and then only if the combination of elevated LDL cholesterol and the patient's CHD risk category justify drug use (see Table 48–4). When drugs are employed, it is essential that dietary modification continues. Why? Because the beneficial effects of diet and drugs are additive; drugs alone may be unable to achieve the LDL goal.

Table 48–7 summarizes properties of the drug families used to lower LDL cholesterol. The most effective agents are the *HMG-CoA reductase inhibitors* (e.g., lovastatin), also known as *statins*. Principal alternatives are *bile-acid seques-*

trants (e.g., cholestyramine) and *nicotinic acid* (niacin). (Although fibrates are listed in Table 48–7, these drugs are used primarily to reduce levels of TGs—not LDLs.) Treatment is initiated with a single drug, almost always a statin. If the statin is ineffective, a bile-acid sequestrant or nicotinic acid can be added to the regimen. Because LDL cholesterol levels will return to pretreatment values if drugs are withdrawn, *treatment must continue lifelong.* Patients should be made aware of this requirement. It is important to note that the primary benefit of drug therapy is *primary prevention:* Drugs are much better at preventing or retarding CHD than at promoting regression of established coronary atherosclerosis.

In addition to lowering LDL cholesterol, drugs may be used to raise HDL cholesterol. The most effective agents are nicotinic acid and the fibrates. However, as indicated in Table 48–7, virtually all of the drugs that we use to lower LDL cholesterol have the added benefit of increasing HDL cholesterol, at least to some degree.

Secondary Treatment Targets
Metabolic Syndrome

Metabolic syndrome, thought to arise from insulin resistance, is now recognized as a risk factor for CHD. According to ATP III, the syndrome is diagnosed when three or more of the following are present:

- Abdominal obesity (waist circumference >40 inches for men; >35 inches for women)
- High blood pressure (≥130/≥85 mm Hg)
- Hyperglycemia (fasting blood glucose ≥110 mg/dl)
- High TG levels (≥150 mg/dl)
- Low HDL cholesterol (<40 mg/dl for men; <50 mg/dl for women)

Primary therapy consists of weight reduction and increased physical activity, which, together, can reduce all signs of metabolic syndrome. In addition, specific treatment should be directed at lowering blood pressure and TG levels. Patients should take aspirin to reduce the risk of thrombosis.

High Triglycerides

High TG levels (>200 mg/dl) are an independent risk factor for CHD. In clinical practice, high TGs are seen most often in patients with metabolic syndrome. However, high levels may also be associated with obesity, sedentary lifestyle, cigarette smoking, excessive alcohol intake, type 2 diabetes, genetic disorders, and high carbohydrate intake (more than 60% of total calories). In patients with high TG levels, the principal aim of treatment is to achieve the original LDL goal. Drugs known to lower triglycerides—nicotinic acid and fibrates—may also be used.

DRUGS AND OTHER PRODUCTS USED TO ALTER PLASMA LIPIDS

Drugs that lower LDL cholesterol levels include HMG-CoA reductase inhibitors, bile-acid sequestrants, and nicotinic acid. All are effective to varying degrees. The HMG-CoA reductase inhibitors cause the fewest adverse effects and are tolerated best.

TABLE 48–7 ■ Drugs Used to Alter Plasma Levels of LDL, HDL, and Triglycerides

Drug Class	Effect on LDL, HDL, and TGs	Adverse Effects	Contraindications	Clinical Trial Results
HMG-CoA reductase inhibitors (statins)	LDL ↓ 18%–55% HDL ↑ 5%–15% TG ↓ 7%–30%	• Myopathy • Hepatotoxicity	*Absolute:* • Active or chronic liver disease • Pregnancy *Relative:* • Concurrent use of certain drugs*	Reduced major coronary events, stroke, CHD deaths, need for coronary procedures, and total mortality
Bile-acid sequestrants	LDL ↓ 15%–30% HDL ↑ 3%–5% TG ↓/no change	• GI distress • Constipation • Reduced drug absorption	*Absolute:* • Dysbetalipoproteinemia • TG >400 mg/dL *Relative:* • TG >200 mg/dL	Reduced major coronary events and CHD deaths
Nicotinic acid	LDL ↓ 5%–25% HDL ↑ 15%–35% TG ↓ 20%–50%	• Flushing • Hyperglycemia • Hyperuricemia • Upper GI distress • Hepatotoxicity	*Absolute:* • Chronic liver disease • Severe gout *Relative:* • Diabetes • Hyperuricemia • Peptic ulcer disease	Reduced major coronary events and, possibly, reduced mortality
Fibrates	LDL ↓ 5%–20%, but may increase if TGs are high HDL ↑ 10%–20% TG ↓ 20%–50%	• Dyspepsia • Gallstones • Myopathy	*Absolute:* • Severe renal disease • Severe liver disease	Reduced major coronary events

*Use caution in patients taking nicotinic acid, fibrates, and agents that inhibit cytochrome P450 isozyme 3A4, including cyclosporine, macrolide antibiotics (e.g., erythromycin), azole antifungal drugs (e.g., ketoconazole), and HIV protease inhibitors (e.g., ritonavir).
Modified from the Executive Summary of the Third Report of the National Cholesterol Education Program (NCEP) Expert Panel on Detection, Evaluation, and Treatment of High Blood Cholesterol in Adults (Adult Treatment Panel III). JAMA 2001;285:2486–2497.

HMG-CoA Reductase Inhibitors (Statins)

HMG-CoA reductase inhibitors, also known as statins, are the most effective drugs for lowering LDL cholesterol levels, and they cause few adverse effects. As a result, statins are the most widely used cholesterol-lowering agents. At this time, five statins are available: atorvastatin, fluvastatin, lovastatin, pravastatin, and simvastatin. In 2001, two of them—atorvastatin [Lipitor] and simvastatin [Zocor]—were ranked first and third among the top 10 best-selling drugs in the United States.

Beneficial Actions

The statins have multiple actions that can benefit patients with atherosclerosis. The most obvious is reduction of LDL cholesterol. However, other actions are also involved.

Reduction of LDL Cholesterol. Statins have a profound effect on LDL cholesterol. Low doses decrease LDL cholesterol by about 25%, and large doses decrease levels by as much as 55% (Table 48–8). Reductions are significant within 2 weeks and maximal within 4 to 6 weeks. Because cholesterol synthesis normally increases during the night, statins are most effective when given in the evening. If statins are withdrawn, serum cholesterol will return to pretreatment levels. Hence, treatment must continue lifelong.

Elevation of HDL Cholesterol. Statins can increase levels of HDL cholesterol. Recall that low levels of HDL cholesterol (<40 mg/dl) are an independent risk factor for CHD. Hence, by raising HDL cholesterol, statins can help reduce the risk of cardiovascular events. The objective is to raise levels to 50 mg/dl or more.

Nonlipid Beneficial Cardiovascular Actions. There is increasing evidence that statins do more than just alter lipid levels. Specifically, they can promote plaque stability (by decreasing plaque cholesterol content), reduce inflammation at the plaque site, slow progression of coronary artery calcification, improve abnormal endothelial function, enhance the ability of blood vessels to dilate, reduce the risk of atrial fibrillation, and reduce the risk of thrombosis (by inhibiting

platelet deposition and aggregation, and by suppressing production of thrombin, a key enzyme in clot formation). All of these actions help reduce the risk of cardiovascular events.

Increased Bone Formation. There is evidence that statins can promote bone formation, and may thereby reduce the risk of osteoporosis and related fractures. In animal studies, statins have increased bone formation, apparently by enhancing the activity of osteoblasts (the cells that lay down new bone). Several case-control studies in humans have shown an association between statin use and reduced risk of osteoporotic fractures. However, other case-control studies have failed to demonstrate a protective effect. The reason for this discrepancy could lie with the inherent weaknesses of case-control studies. Hence, the issue is likely to remain unresolved until data from randomized controlled trials are available. In the meantime, osteoporosis should be managed with bisphosphonates and other drugs of proven efficacy (see Chapter 70, Drugs That Affect Calcium Levels and Bone Mineralization).

Mechanism of Cholesterol-Lowering Action

The mechanism by which statins decrease LDL cholesterol levels is complex, and depends ultimately on *increasing the number of LDL receptors on hepatocytes* (liver cells). The process begins with inhibition of hepatic HMG-CoA reductase, the rate-limiting enzyme in cholesterol biosynthesis. In response to decreased cholesterol production, hepatocytes synthesize more HMG-CoA reductase. As a result, cholesterol synthesis is largely restored to pretreatment levels. However, for reasons that are not fully understood, inhibition of cholesterol synthesis causes hepatocytes to synthesize more LDL receptors. As a result, hepatocytes are able to remove more LDLs from the blood. In patients who are genetically unable to synthesize LDL receptors, statins fail to reduce LDL levels, indicating that (1) inhibition of cholesterol synthesis, by itself, is not sufficient to explain cholesterol-lowering effects; and (2) in order for statins to be effective, production of LDL receptors must increase.

In addition to inhibiting HMG-CoA reductase, statins decrease production of apolipoprotein B-100. As a result, hepatocytes decrease production of VLDLs. This lowers VLDL levels along with LDL levels. Statins also raise HDL levels by 5% to 16%.

	% Change in Serum Lipids*				Effect of CYP3A4 Inhibitors on Statin Levels‡
Drug	LDL	HDL	TGs	LFT Monitoring†	
Atorvastatin [Lipitor]	↓29–55	↑2–8	↓19–52	At 12 wk and then every 6 mo	Moderate increase
Fluvastatin [Lescol]	↓21–34	↑3–9	↓3–11	At 12 wk and then every 6 mo	No effect
Lovastatin [Mevacor]	↓24–40	↑7–10	↓6–10	At 6 and 12 wk and then every 6 mo	Dramatic increase
Pravastatin [Pravachol]	↓18–37	↑5–15	↓11–24	At 12 wk and then every 6 mo	No effect
Simvastatin [Zocor]	↓23–46	↑6–12	↓10–36	At 6 and 12 mo (and also at 3 mo if 80 mg/day is used)	Dramatic increase

TABLE 48–8 ■ HMG-CoA Reductase Inhibitors: Selected Aspects of Clinical Pharmacology

*LDL = low-density lipoprotein cholesterol, HDL = high-density lipoprotein cholesterol, TGs = triglycerides.
†LFT = liver function test. LFTs should be performed at baseline and at the indicated times after the first dose and after any change in dosage.
‡CYP3A4 is an enzyme in the cytochrome P450 family. Inhibitors of CYP3A4 include itraconazole, ketoconazole, erythromycin, clarithromycin, HIV protease inhibitors, cyclosporine, nefazodone, and grapefruit juice.

Clinical Trials

Statins slow progression of CHD and decrease the risk of stroke, hospitalization, cardiac events, peripheral vascular disease, and death. Benefits are seen in men and in women, and in apparently healthy people as well as those with a history of cardiac events. Hence, the statins are useful for both primary and secondary prevention. Furthermore, these drugs can even help people with *normal* LDL levels, in addition to those whose LDL is high.

Secondary Prevention Studies. In patients with evidence of existing CHD (angina pectoris or previous MI), statins reduce the risk of death from cardiac causes. This was first demonstrated conclusively in the landmark *Scandinavian Simvastatin Survival Study* (4S). After 4.9 to 6.3 years of follow-up, the death rate was 12% among patients taking placebo and 8% among those taking simvastatin—a 30% decrease in overall mortality. Benefits were due to a decrease in cardiac-related mortality; deaths from noncardiac causes were the same in both groups.

The *Cholesterol and Recurrent Events* (CARE) trial demonstrated the ability of statins to reduce the risk of stroke in addition to coronary events. In this study, 4159 people with a history of MI were given pravastatin (40 mg daily) or placebo. After 5 years, the incidence of MI (fatal or nonfatal) was 13.2% in those taking placebo and 10.2% in those taking the drug. Pravastatin also produced a 26% decrease in the risk of stroke.

Primary Prevention Studies. Two studies have demonstrated the ability of statins to reduce mortality in people with no previous history of coronary events. In the first trial—the *West of Scotland Coronary Prevention Study* (WOSCOPS)—6595 men with high cholesterol were given either pravastatin (40 mg/day) or placebo. During an average follow-up of 4.9 years, 4.1% of those taking placebo died, compared with only 3.2% of those taking the drug. The second trial—the *Air Force/Texas Coronary Atherosclerosis Prevention Study* (AFCAPS/TexCAPS)—enrolled 6605 low-risk patients: men and women with average cholesterol levels (221 mg/dl) and no history of cardiovascular events. The subjects were randomly assigned to receive lovastatin (20 to 40 mg/day) or placebo. After an average follow-up of 5.5 years, the incidence of first major coronary events was 5.5% for those taking placebo and 3.5% for those taking the drug—representing a 36% decrease in risk.

Prevention in Patients with Normal Cholesterol Levels. The landmark *Heart Protection Study,* published in 2002, was the first major trial to demonstrate that statins can reduce the risk of major coronary events in people who have normal levels of cholesterol. This double-blind, placebo-controlled trial enrolled 20,536 high-risk British patients: men and women with diabetes, prior MI, stroke, or angioplasty. Some had high levels of LDL and total cholesterol; others had normal levels. Subjects were randomly assigned to receive either simvastatin (40 mg/day) or placebo. After 5 years, the incidence of death was 12.9% in the treatment group, compared with 14.7% in the placebo group. Death from CHD was reduced by 18%. In addition, simvastatin reduced the risk of nonfatal MI by 38%, stroke by 25%, and the need for coronary revascularization (e.g., angioplasty) by 30%. Most strikingly, benefits were seen in patients whose LDL cholesterol was *normal* or *low,* as well as in those whose levels were high. These data suggest a radical shift in practice. Specifically, they suggest *we should treat people at high CHD risk—not simply those with high cholesterol levels.* Obviously, doing so would greatly expand the number of patients receiving statin therapy.

Indications

Indications for the statins keep expanding. When these drugs first became available, they were approved only for hypercholesterolemia. As our understanding of their benefits has grown, so has the list of indications. Today, statins have eight approved applications. The most recent additions are primary prevention of coronary events and elevation of HDL cholesterol. Indications for individual statins are summarized in Table 48–9.

Pharmacokinetics

Statins are administered orally. The amount absorbed ranges between 30% and 90%, depending on the drug. Regardless of how much is absorbed, most of an absorbed dose is extracted from the blood on its first pass through the liver, the

TABLE 48–9 ▪ HMG-CoA Reductase Inhibitors: FDA-Approved Indications

Indication	Atorvastatin	Fluvastatin	Lovastatin	Pravastatin	Simvastatin
Primary hypercholesterolemia	✔	✔	✔	✔	✔
Homozygous familial hyperlipidemia	✔				✔
Mixed dyslipidemia (Fredrickson types IIa and IIb)	✔	✔		✔	✔
Primary dysbetalipoproteinemia (Fredrickson type III)	✔			✔	✔
Hypertriglyceridemia (Fredrickson type IV)	✔			✔	✔
Primary prevention of coronary events			✔	✔	
Secondary prevention of cardiovascular events		✔	✔	✔	✔
Increasing HDL cholesterol in primary hypercholesterolemia	✔			✔	✔

principal site at which statins act. Only a small fraction of each dose reaches the general circulation. Statins undergo rapid hepatic metabolism followed by excretion in primarily the bile. Only three agents—*lovastatin, pravastatin,* and *simvastatin*—undergo clinically significant (10% to 20%) excretion in the urine.

Three statins—*atorvastatin, lovastatin,* and *simvastatin*—are metabolized by the 3A4 isozyme of cytochrome P450 (CYP3A4). As a result, levels of these drugs can be lowered by agents that induce synthesis of CYP3A4. More importantly, their levels can be increased—sometimes dramatically—by agents that inhibit CYP3A4 (see below).

Adverse Effects

Statins are generally well tolerated. Side effects are uncommon. Some patients develop headache, rash, or GI disturbances (dyspepsia, cramps, flatulence, constipation, abdominal pain). However, these effects are usually mild and transient. Serious adverse effects—hepatotoxicity and myopathy—are rare.

Hepatotoxicity. Liver injury, as evidenced by elevations in serum transaminase levels, develops in 0.5% to 2% of patients treated 1 year or longer. However, jaundice and other clinical signs are rare. Progression to outright liver failure is extremely rare—if it occurs at all. Because of the risk of liver injury, liver function tests (LFTs) should be done before treatment and every 6 to 12 months thereafter. (Timing of LFTs for patients taking specific statins is summarized in Table 48–8.) If serum transaminase levels rise to 3 times normal and remain there, statins should be discontinued. Transaminase levels decline to pretreatment levels following drug withdrawal. Because of the risk for liver injury, statins are contraindicated for patients with active liver disease. Exercise caution in patients who consume alcohol in excess.

Myopathy. Statins can injure muscle tissue. Mild injury, manifesting as muscle ache or weakness, occurs in 1% to 5% of patients. Rarely, muscle injury progress to *myositis,* defined as muscle inflammation associated with moderate elevation of creatine kinase (CK), an enzyme released from injured muscle. Myositis, in turn, may progress to potentially fatal *rhabdomyolysis,* defined as muscle disintegration or dissolution, associated with marked elevation of CK (greater than 10 times the upper limit of normal [ULN]) and possibly with renal failure. Fortunately, fatal rhabdomyolysis is extremely rare: the incidence is less than 0.15 cases per 1 million prescriptions. Patients should be informed about the risk of myopathy and instructed to notify the physician if unexplained muscle pain or tenderness occurs. How statins cause myopathy is unknown.

Several factors increase the risk of myopathy. Among these are advanced age, small body frame, frailty, multisystem disease (e.g., chronic renal insufficiency, especially associated with diabetes), use of statins in high doses, concurrent use of fibrates (which can cause myopathy by themselves), and concurrent use of drugs that can raise statin levels (see below). In addition, hypothyroidism increases risk. Accordingly, if muscle pain develops, thyroid function should be assessed.

Measurement of CK levels can facilitate diagnosis. The level should be determined at baseline, and again if symptoms of myopathy appear. If the CK level is more than 10 times the ULN, the statin should be discontinued. If the level is less than 10 times the ULN, the statin can be continued, provided myopathy symptoms and the CK level are followed weekly. Routine monitoring of CK in asymptomatic patients is unnecessary.

The risk of rhabdomyolysis is equal for the five statins available today. A sixth agent—cerivastatin [Baycol]—was withdrawn in 2001 because the risk of death was 16 to 80 times higher than with other statins.

Peripheral Neuropathy. Very rarely, peripheral neuropathy develops in statin users. Symptoms include weakness, difficulty walking, and tingling and pain in the hands and feet. The underlying mechanism could be disruption of neuronal integrity secondary to inhibition of cholesterol synthesis. Statin-related neuropathy is often reversible, but may take 3 to 12 months to resolve. At this time, solid proof that statins cause neuropathy is lacking—although the available data are strongly suggestive. Hence, if symptoms of neuropathy develop, the statin should be suspected.

Drug Interactions

Fibrates. Like the statins, gemfibrozil and fenofibrate can cause myopathy. Accordingly, if these drugs are combined with a statin, the risk of myopathy is greater than with either agent alone. Clearly, the combination should be used with caution.

Agents That Inhibit CYP3A4. Agents that inhibit CYP3A4 can raise levels of lovastatin and simvastatin substantially, and can raise levels of atorvastatin moderately. Important inhibitors of CYP3A4 include cyclosporine, macrolide antibiotics (e.g., erythromycin), azole antifungal drugs (e.g., ketoconazole), and HIV protease inhibitors (e.g., ritonavir). If these drugs are combined with a statin, caution is advised. Some authorities recommend an automatic reduction in statin dosage. In addition to drugs, grapefruit juice can inhibit CYP3A4. However, to produce significant inhibition, the patient would have to drink about 1 quart a day.

Use in Pregnancy

Statins are classified in Food and Drug Administration Pregnancy Risk Category X: the risks to the fetus outweigh any potential benefits of treatment. When administered to pregnant rats in doses 500 times greater than the maximal recommended dosage for humans, lovastatin produced fetal skeletal malformations. Teratogenic effects in humans have not been reported. However, because statins inhibit synthesis of cholesterol, and since cholesterol is required for synthesis of cell membranes as well as several hormones, concern regarding human fetal injury remains. Moreover, there is no compelling reason to continue lipid-lowering drugs during pregnancy. Women of child-bearing age should be informed about the potential for fetal harm and warned against becoming pregnant. If pregnancy occurs, statins should be withdrawn.

Preparations, Dosage, and Administration

Five statins are available: atorvastatin, fluvastatin, lovastatin, pravastatin, and simvastatin. Information on their preparations, dosage, and administration is summarized in Table 48–10. Note that lovastatin should be administered with the evening meal, whereas the other four may be administered without regard to meals. Note also that with three

TABLE 48–10 ■ HMG-CoA Reductase Inhibitors: Preparations, Dosage, and Administration

Drug	Dosage	Administration with Regard to Meals	Dosage Change for Renal Impairment	Preparations*
Atorvastatin [Lipitor]	*Initial:* 10 mg at bedtime *Maximum:* 80 mg at bedtime	Take without regard to meals	No change needed	10-, 20-, 40-, 80-mg tablets
Fluvastatin [Lescol, Lescol XL]	*Initial:* 20 mg at bedtime *Maximum:* 40 mg twice a day (Lescol); 80 mg at bedtime (Lescol XL)	Take without regard to meals	No change needed	*Lescol:* 20-, 40-mg capsules *Lescol XL:* 80-mg ER tablets
Lovastatin [Altocor, Mevacor]	*Initial:* 20 mg with the evening meal *Maximum:* 40 mg twice daily or 80 mg at bedtime	Take with evening meal to increase absorption	Reduce dosage for severe renal impairment	*Mevacor:* 10-, 20-, 40-mg tablets *Altocor:* 10-, 20-, 40-, 60-mg ER tablets
Pravastatin [Pravachol]	*Initial:* 20 mg at bedtime *Maximum:* 40 mg at bedtime	Take without regard to meals	Reduce dosage for moderate to severe renal impairment	10-, 20-, 40-, 80-mg tablets
Simvastatin [Zocor]	*Initial:* 20 mg at bedtime *Maximum:* 40 mg twice daily or 80 mg at bedtime	Take without regard to meals	Reduce dosage for severe renal impairment	5-, 10-, 20-, 40-, 80-mg tablets

*ER = extended-release.

statins—lovastatin, pravastatin, and simvastatin—dosage should be reduced in patients with renal impairment.

Nicotinic Acid (Niacin)

Nicotinic acid [Niaspan, Niacor, Slo-Niacin, others] reduces LDL and TG levels. In addition, it increases HDL levels better than any other drug. In patients with high LDL levels, nicotinic acid reduces the risk of major coronary events and may also reduce total mortality. Unfortunately, although nicotinic acid is effective, it causes a variety of side effects. For example, nearly all patients experience flushing. Because of its side effect profile, nicotinic acid has limited clinical utility.

Mechanism of Action. The primary effect of nicotinic acid is to decrease production of VLDLs. Since LDLs are by-products of VLDL degradation, the fall in VLDL levels causes LDL levels to fall as well. There appear to be several mechanisms by which nicotinic acid decreases VLDL production. Notable among these is inhibition of lipolysis in adipose tissue.

Effect on Plasma Lipoproteins. Nicotinic acid reduces LDL cholesterol by 5% to 25% and TGs by 20% to 50%. In addition, it raises HDL cholesterol by 15% to 35%. Triglyceride levels begin to fall within the first 4 days of therapy. LDL levels decline more slowly, taking 3 to 5 weeks for maximum reductions. Combining nicotinic acid with lovastatin can reduce LDL cholesterol by 45% and can raise HDL cholesterol by 41%. Triple therapy (nicotinic acid plus a statin plus a bile-acid sequestrant) can decrease LDL cholesterol by 70% or more.

Therapeutic Use. Nicotinic acid is a drug of choice for lowering TG levels in patients at risk of pancreatitis. Additional uses include mixed elevation of LDLs and TGs, and elevation of TGs in combination with low levels of HDLs. One formulation—Niaspan—is approved for elevating HDL cholesterol.

Nicotinic acid (niacin) also has a role as a vitamin. The doses employed to correct niacin deficiency are much smaller than those employed to reduce lipoprotein levels. The role of nicotinic acid as a vitamin is discussed in Chapter 76.

Adverse Effects. The most frequent adverse reactions involve the skin (flushing, itching) and GI tract (gastric upset, nausea, vomiting, diarrhea). *Intense flushing* of the face, neck, and ears occurs in practically all patients receiving nicotinic acid in pharmacologic doses. This reaction diminishes in several weeks, and can be attenuated by taking 325 mg of aspirin 30 minutes before each dose. (Aspirin reduces flushing by preventing synthesis of prostaglandins, which mediate the flushing response.)

Nicotinic acid is *hepatotoxic.* Severe liver damage has occurred. Liver injury is most likely with older *sustained-release* formulations, especially in high doses (above 2 gm/day). Liver injury is less likely with Niaspan, a new extended-release formulation. Because of the risk of hepatotoxicity, liver function should be assessed before treatment and periodically thereafter.

Nicotinic acid can *raise blood levels of homocysteine,* and may thereby *increase* CHD risk (see Box 48–1). Homocysteine levels can increase by 17% with a dose of 1 gm/day, and by 55% with a dose of 3 gm/day. Treatment with folic acid can help lower homocysteine levels.

Additional adverse effects are *hyperglycemia* and *gouty arthritis.*

Preparations, Dosage, and Administration. Nicotinic acid (niacin) is marketed generically and under multiple trade names. The drug is available in tablets (standard, timed-release, controlled-release, sustained-release), capsules (timed-release, controlled-release, sustained-release), and an elixir. The usual maintenance dosage is 1 to 2 gm 3 times a day, administered with or after meals. With Niaspan, the recommended dosage is 1 to 2 gm once daily in the evening. (*Note:* When nicotinic acid is taken as a vitamin, the dosage is only about 25 mg/day—much lower than the dosages employed to lower plasma lipoproteins.)

Niacin-Lovastatin Combination

Actions and Uses. Niacin (extended-release) and lovastatin (immediate release) are now available in a fixed-dose combination under the trade name *Advicor.* Lovastatin serves primarily to lower LDL cholesterol; niacin raises HDL cholesterol and lowers TGs. In one clinical trial, using the combination for 12 months lowered LDL cholesterol by 45%, raised HDL cholesterol by 41%, and lowered TGs by 42%. The product has two indications: primary hypercholesterolemia and mixed dyslipidemia. However, it should not be used for initial therapy of either condition. Rather, it should be reserved for patients who have not responded adequately to lovastatin or niacin alone.

Adverse Effects. The principal concerns are *flushing* (from the niacin) and *hepatotoxicity* (from both drugs). Flushing can be reduced by taking aspirin or ibuprofen 30 minutes before dosing. To monitor liver injury, LFTs should be obtained at baseline, every 6 to 12 weeks for the first 6 months of treatment, and every 6 months thereafter.

Lovastatin poses a very small risk of *myopathy.* Advise patients to report any muscle pain or weakness. Adding a fibrate to the regimen increases the risk of muscle injury.

Preparations, Dosage, and Administration. Advicor is available in three niacin/lovastatin strengths: 500/20 mg, 750/20 mg, and 1000/20 mg. The recommended initial dosage is 500/20 mg once a day at bedtime. At 4-week intervals, the niacin dosage can be increased by 500 mg/day. The maximum dosage is 2000/40 mg. All doses should be taken with a low-fat snack, which can enhance absorption and reduce GI distress.

Bile-Acid Sequestrants

Bile-acid sequestrants reduce LDL cholesterol levels. In the past, these drugs were a mainstay of lipid-lowering therapy. Today, they are used primarily as adjuncts to the statins. Three agents are available: cholestyramine, colestipol, and colesevelam. Colesevelam is newer than the other two and better tolerated.

Older Agents: Cholestyramine and Colestipol

Cholestyramine [Questran, Prevalite, LoCHOLEST] and colestipol [Colestid] have been available for years. These drugs are alike in practically all respects, and hence we will discuss them together. Both are unusually safe, although they frequently cause constipation, abdominal discomfort, and bloating.

Effect on Plasma Lipoproteins. The principal response to bile-acid sequestrants is a reduction in LDL cholesterol. LDL levels begin to fall during the first week of therapy, and become maximal (about a 20% drop) within 1 month. When these drugs are discontinued, LDL cholesterol returns to pretreatment levels in 3 to 4 weeks.

Bile-acid sequestrants may increase VLDL levels in some patients. In most cases, the elevation is transient and mild. However, if VLDL levels are elevated prior to treatment, the increment induced by bile-acid sequestrants may be sustained and substantial. Accordingly, bile-acid sequestrants are not drugs of choice for lowering LDL cholesterol in patients with high VLDL levels.

Pharmacokinetics. Bile-acid sequestrants are biologically inert. They are insoluble in water, cannot be absorbed from the GI tract, and are impervious to digestive enzymes. Following oral administration, they simply pass through the intestine and become excreted in the feces.

Mechanism of Action. The bile-acid sequestrants lower LDL cholesterol through a mechanism that ultimately depends on increasing LDL receptors on hepatocytes. Following ingestion, these drugs form an insoluble complex with bile acids present in the intestine; this complex prevents the reabsorption of bile acids, and thereby accelerates their excretion. Because bile acids are normally reabsorbed, the increase in excretion creates a demand for increased synthesis, which takes place in the liver. Since bile acids are made from cholesterol, liver cells must have an increased cholesterol supply in order to increase bile acid production. The required cholesterol is provided by LDL. To avail themselves of more LDL cholesterol, liver cells increase their number of LDL receptors, thereby increasing their capacity for LDL uptake. The resultant increase in LDL uptake from plasma decreases circulating LDL levels. Individuals who are genetically incapable of increasing LDL receptor synthesis are unable to benefit from these drugs.

Therapeutic Use. Bile-acid sequestrants are used to reduce LDL cholesterol. In current practice, these drugs are usually combined with a statin. When taken alone (in conjunction with a low-cholesterol diet), the sequestrants can reduce LDL cholesterol by 15% to 30%. In contrast, combined therapy with a statin can reduce LDL cholesterol by up to 50%. Similar results can be obtained by combining a sequestrant with nicotinic acid.

Adverse Effects. The bile-acid sequestrants are not absorbed from the GI tract, and hence are devoid of systemic effects. Accordingly, they are safer than all other lipid-lowering drugs.

Adverse effects are limited to the GI tract. *Constipation* is the principal complaint. This can be minimized by increasing dietary fiber and fluids. If necessary, a mild laxative may be used. Other GI effects include *bloating, indigestion,* and *nausea.* Rarely, these drugs decrease fat absorption, and may thereby *decrease uptake of fat-soluble vitamins* (vitamins A, D, E, and K). Vitamin supplements may be required.

Drug Interactions. The bile-acid sequestrants can form complexes with other drugs. Medications that undergo binding cannot be absorbed, and hence are not available for systemic effects. Drugs known to form complexes with the sequestrants include thiazide diuretics, digoxin, warfarin, and some antibiotics. To reduce formation of sequestrant-drug complexes, oral medications should be administered either 1 hour before the sequestrant or 4 hours after.

Preparations, Dosage, and Administration. Cholestyramine. Cholestyramine [Questran, Questran Light, Prevalite, LoCHOLEST, LoCHOLEST Light] is dispensed in powdered form. Patients should be instructed to mix the powder with fluid, because swallowing it dry can cause esophageal irritation and impaction. Appropriate liquids for mixing include water, fruit juices, and soups. Pulpy fruits with a high fluid content (e.g., applesauce, crushed pineapple) may also be used. The dosage range is 4 to 16 gm/day.

Colestipol. Colestipol hydrochloride [Colestid] is dispensed in granular form (5 gm) and 1-gm tablets. The dosage for the *granules* is 5 to 30 gm/day administered in one or more doses. Patients should be instructed to mix the granules with fluids or pulpy fruits before ingestion. The dosage for the *tablets* is 2 to 16 gm/day administered in one or more doses. Tablets should be swallowed whole and taken with fluid.

New Agent: Colesevelam

Colesevelam [Welchol] is an oral, nonabsorbable bile-acid sequestrant similar to cholestyramine and colestipol. However, there are three important differences: (1) colesevelam is better tolerated than the older drugs (it causes less constipation, flatulence, bloating, and cramping); (2) it does not reduce the absorption of fat-soluble vitamins (A, D, E, and K); and (3) it does not significantly reduce the absorption of statins, digoxin, warfarin, and most other drugs studied. Because of these differences, colesevelam is likely to become the bile-acid sequestrant of choice.

Colesevelam is indicated as adjunctive therapy to diet and exercise for reducing LDL cholesterol in patients with primary hypercholesterolemia. The drug may be used alone or in combination with a statin. Colesevelam can lower LDL cholesterol by 19%, but treatment is expensive: a 1-month supply costs over $100. The drug is available in 625-mg tablets for oral use. The initial dosage is 3 tablets (1.9 gm) twice daily or 6 tablets (3.8 gm) once daily. All doses are taken with food and water. Please note that the dosage of colesevelam is much smaller than the dosage of cholestyramine (8 to 24 gm/day) or colestipol (5 to 30 gm/day), which probably explains why colesevelam is better tolerated.

Fibric Acid Derivatives (Fibrates)

The fibric acid derivatives, also known as fibrates, are the most effective drugs available for lowering triglyceride levels. In addition, they can raise HDL cholesterol. These drugs have little or no effect on LDL cholesterol. Fibrates can increase the risk of bleeding in patients taking warfarin (an anticoagulant) and the risk of rhabdomyolysis in patients taking statins. In the United States, two fibrates are available: gemfibrozil [Lopid] and fenofibrate [Tricor]. A third agent—clofibrate [Atromid-S]—is no longer available in the United States.

Gemfibrozil

Gemfibrozil [Lopid] decreases triglyceride (VLDL) levels and raises HDL cholesterol levels. The drug does not reduce LDL cholesterol. Its principal indication is hypertriglyceridemia.

Effects on Plasma Lipoproteins. Gemfibrozil decreases plasma triglyceride content by lowering VLDL levels. Maximum reductions in VLDLs range from 40% to 55%, and are achieved within 3 to 4 weeks of treatment. Gemfibrozil can raise HDL cholesterol by 6% to 10%. In patients with normal TG levels, the drug can produce a small reduction in LDL levels. However, if TG levels are high, gemfibrozil may actually increase LDL levels.

Mechanism of Action. Recent studies suggest that gemfibrozil and other fibrates produce their effects by interacting with specific receptors—known as peroxisome proliferator-activated receptors (PPARs)—present in the liver and brown adipose tissue. Activation of PPARs leads to (1) increased synthesis of lipoprotein lipase (LPL) and (2) reduced production of apolipoprotein C-III (an inhibitor of LPL). Both actions accelerate the clearance of VLDLs, and thereby reduce levels of TGs. How do fibrates elevate HDL levels? By activating PPARs, fibrates increase production of apolipoproteins A-I and A-II, which in turn facilitates HDL formation.

Therapeutic Use. Gemfibrozil is used primarily to *reduce high levels of plasma triglycerides* (VLDLs). Treatment is limited to patients who have not responded adequately to weight loss and diet modification. Although gemfibrozil can also reduce LDL cholesterol, other drugs (statins, cholestyramine, colestipol) are more effective.

Gemfibrozil can be used to *raise HDL cholesterol,* although it is not approved for this application. When tested in patients with normal LDL cholesterol and low HDL cholesterol, gemfibrozil reduced the risk of major cardiovascular events (e.g., stroke, fatal and nonfatal MI) by 20%. Because LDL cholesterol was normal, it appears that benefits were due primarily to elevation of HDL cholesterol, along with reduction of plasma triglycerides.

Adverse Effects. Gemfibrozil is generally well tolerated. The most common reactions are rashes and GI disturbances (nausea, abdominal pain, diarrhea).

Gallstones. Gemfibrozil increases biliary cholesterol saturation, thereby increasing the risk of gallstones. Patients should be informed about manifestations of gallbladder disease (e.g., upper abdominal discomfort, intolerance of fried foods, bloating) and instructed to notify the physician if these develop. Patients with pre-existing gallbladder disease should not take the drug.

Myopathy. Like the statins, gemfibrozil (and other fibrates) can cause myopathy. Warn patients to report any signs of muscle injury, such as tenderness, weakness, or unusual muscle pain.

Liver Injury. Gemfibrozil is hepatotoxic. The drug can disrupt liver function and may also pose a risk of liver cancer. Periodic tests of liver function are required.

Drug Interactions. *Gemfibrozil displaces warfarin from plasma albumin,* thereby increasing anticoagulant effects. Prothrombin time should be measured frequently to assess coagulation status. Warfarin dosage may need to be reduced.

Gemfibrozil increases the risk of *statin-induced myopathy.* Accordingly, the combination of a statin with gemfibrozil should be used with great caution, if at all.

Preparations, Dosage, and Administration. Gemfibrozil [Lopid] is available in 600-mg tablets. The adult dosage is 600 mg twice a day. Dosing is done 30 minutes before the morning and evening meals.

Fenofibrate

Actions and Uses. Fenofibrate [Tricor, Lofibra] is indicated for hypertriglyceridemia in patients who have not responded to dietary measures. The drug lowers triglycerides by decreasing levels of VLDLs. Fenofibrate was approved for American use in 1998, but has been available in other countries for years.

Pharmacokinetics. Fenofibrate is well absorbed from the GI tract, especially in the presence of food. Once absorbed, the drug is rapidly converted to fenofibric acid, its active form. In the blood, the drug is 98% protein bound. Elimination is the result of hepatic metabolism followed by renal excretion. The plasma half-life is about 20 hours.

Adverse Effects and Interactions. The most common adverse effects are rash and GI disturbances. Like gemfibrozil, fenofibrate can cause gallstones and liver injury. In animal models, doses 1 to 6 times the maximum human dose caused cancers of the pancreas and liver. Like gemfibrozil, fenofibrate can increase the risk of bleeding with warfarin and the risk of myopathy with statins.

Preparations, Dosage, and Administration. Fenofibrate is available in standard tablets (54 and 160 mg) sold as Tricor, and in micronized capsules (67, 134, and 200 mg) sold as Lofibra. The usual dosage is 160 mg once a day using Tricor, or 200 mg once a day using Lofibra. All doses should be taken with food.

Ezetimibe

Ezetimibe [Zetia] is a new and unique drug for reducing plasma cholesterol. Benefits derive from blocking cholesterol absorption.

Mechanism of Action and Impact on Plasma Lipids.
Ezetimibe acts on cells of the brush border of the small intestine to inhibit cholesterol absorption. The drug blocks absorption of dietary cholesterol as well as cholesterol secreted in the bile. Treatment reduces plasma levels of total cholesterol, LDL cholesterol, triglycerides, and apolipoprotein B. In addition, ezetimibe can produce a small *increase* in HDL cholesterol.

Therapeutic Use. Ezetimibe is indicated as an adjunct to diet modification for reducing total cholesterol, LDL cholesterol, and apolipoprotein B in patients with primary hypercholesteremia. The drug is approved for monotherapy and for combined use with a statin. In clinical trials, ezetimibe alone reduced LDL cholesterol by about 19%, and increased HDL cholesterol by about 4%. When ezetimibe was combined with a statin, the reduction in LDL cholesterol was about 25% greater than with the statin alone. Because ezetimibe is new, we do yet not know if it reduces cardiovascular morbidity or mortality.

Pharmacokinetics. Ezetimibe is administered orally, and the amount absorbed is not affected by food. In the small intestine and liver, ezetimibe undergoes extensive conversion to ezetimibe glucuronide, an active metabolite. Both compounds—parent drug and metabolite—are eliminated primarily in the bile. The elimination half-life is about 22 hours.

Adverse Effects. Ezetimibe is well tolerated. When the drug is used alone or combined with a statin, the incidence of side effects is nearly identical to that seen with placebo. In contrast to the bile-acid sequestrants, ezetimibe does not cause constipation and other adverse GI effects.

Drug Interactions. Statins. In patients taking a statin, adding ezetimibe slightly increases the risk of liver damage (as indicated by elevated transaminase levels). If the drugs are combined, transaminase levels should be carefully monitored.

Fibrates. Both ezetimibe and fibrates (gemfibrozil and fenofibrate) can increase the cholesterol content of bile, and can thereby increase the risk of gallstones. Therefore, combined use is not recommended.

Bile-Acid Sequestrants. Cholestyramine (and probably colestipol) can significantly decrease the absorption of ezetimibe. To minimize effects on absorption, ezetimibe should be administered at least 2 hours before a sequestrant or 4 hours after.

Cyclosporine. Cyclosporine may greatly increase levels of ezetimibe. If the drugs are combined, careful monitoring is needed.

Caution. In patients with hepatic impairment, availability of ezetimibe is significantly increased. At this time, we do not know if increased availability is harmful. Until more is known, patients with moderate or severe hepatic insufficiency should not be given the drug.

Preparations, Dosage, and Administration. Ezetimibe [Zetia] is available in 10-mg tablets for oral use. The recommended dosage is 10 mg once a day, taken with or without food. If ezetimibe is combined with a statin, both drugs can be taken at the same time. If ezetimibe is combined with a bile-acid sequestrant, ezetimibe should be taken 2 hours before the sequestrant or 4 hours after.

Plant Stanol and Sterol Esters

Stanol esters and sterol esters derived from plant material can reduce intestinal absorption of cholesterol, and can thereby reduce levels of LDL cholesterol. Chemically, these compounds are structural analogs of cholesterol. Where can you get plant stanols and sterols? Two good sources are margarines sold under the names *Benecol* and *Take Control*. As indicated in Table 48–11, Benecol contains plant stanols derived from pine pulp and Take Control contains plant sterols derived from soybeans. In clinical trials, use of these products (2 to 3 tablespoons/day instead of regular margarine) reduced LDL levels by about 10%. Neither product affects HDL levels. ATP III recommends adding plant stanols or sterols to the diet if the basic TLC diet fails to reduce LDL cholesterol to the target level.

Estrogen

In postmenopausal women, estrogen replacement (0.625 mg/day) reduces LDL cholesterol by 15% to 25% and increases HDL cholesterol by 10% to 15%. However, despite these beneficial effects on plasma lipids, estrogen replacement does not reduce cardiovascular morbidity or mortality. In fact, recent data indicate that, when estrogen is combined with a progestin for replacement therapy, the risk of MI and other cardiovascular events actually goes up. Accordingly, estrogen replacement is no longer recommended for cardiovascular protection in postmenopausal women. The risk and benefits of estrogen replacement are discussed at length in Chapter 59 (Estrogens and Progestins).

Cholestin

Cholestin is the trade name for a dietary supplement that can lower cholesterol levels. The product is made from rice fermented with red yeast. Its principal active ingredient—*lovastatin*—is identical to the active ingredient in Mevacor, a brand-name cholesterol-lowering drug. In addition to lovastatin, Cholestin contains at least seven other HMG-CoA reductase inhibitors (statins).

Several clinical trials have demonstrated that Cholestin can lower cholesterol levels, although none has studied its effects on cardiovascular events. In a trial conducted at the Tufts University School of Medicine, Cholestin reduced total cholesterol by 11.4% and LDL cholesterol by 21%, and increased HDL cholesterol by 14.6%. Similarly, in a study conducted at the University of California at Los Angeles Medical School, Cholestin reduced total cholesterol by 16% and LDL cholesterol by 22%. Whether Cholestin also reduces the incidence of CHD is unknown.

Information on Cholestin is lacking in four important areas: clinical benefits, adverse effects, drug interactions, and precise mechanism of action. As noted, there are no data on the ability of Cholestin to reduce the risk of MI, stroke, or any other cardiovascular event. In contrast, the clinical benefits of prescription statins are fully documented. There is little or no information on the adverse effects or drug interactions of Cholestin. In contrast, the safety (and hazards) of prescription statins, as well as their drug interactions, have been studied extensively.

The mechanism by which Cholestin lowers cholesterol levels is only partly understood. The recommended daily dose of Cholestin contains only 5 mg of lovastatin and other HMG-CoA reductase inhibitors, compared with 10 mg for the lowest recommended dose of Mevacor. Hence, it seems unlikely that the statins in Cholestin can fully account for the supplement's ability to reduce cholesterol levels. This implies that Cholestin must have one or more active ingredients that have not yet been identified. What they are and how they may work is a complete mystery.

Until more is known about Cholestin, it would seem prudent to stick with statins—medications of proven safety and efficacy. Furthermore, for people with health insurance, using statins is cheaper: Most insurers will cover the cost of statins, but will not pay for Cholestin.

TABLE 48–11 ■ Cholesterol-Lowering Margarines

	Benecol		Take Control	
	Regular	**Light**	**Regular**	**Light**
Serving size	1 tsp (14 gm)		1 tbsp (14 gm)	
Servings/day	3		2	
Active ingredient				
Type	Plant stanol esters		Plant sterol esters	
Source	Pine pulp		Soybean extract	
Amount/serving	1.5 gm		1.7 gm	
Amount/day	4.5 gm		3.4 gm	
Calories				
Per serving	80	45	80	45
Per day	240	135	160	90
Fat content				
Total fat (gm)				
Per serving	9	5	8	5
Per day	27	15	16	10
Saturated fat (gm)				
Per serving	1	0.5	1	0.5
Per day	3	1.5	2	1
Polyunsaturated fat (gm)				
Per serving	3	2	2	2
Per day	9	6	4	4
Monounsaturated fat (gm)				
Per serving	4	2.5	4.5	2
Per day	12	7.5	9	4
Trans fatty acids (gm)				
Per serving	<0.5	<0.5	0	0
Per day	<1.5	<1.5	0	0
Cholesterol (mg)				
Per serving	0	0	<5	<5
Per day	0	0	<10	<10
Usable in cooking	Yes	?	No	No
Can be frozen	Yes	Yes	No	No

⸪ KEY POINTS

- Lipoproteins are structures that transport lipids (cholesterol and triglycerides [TGs]) in blood.
- Lipoproteins consist of a hydrophobic core, a hydrophilic shell, plus at least one apolipoprotein, which serves as a recognition site for receptors on cells.
- Lipoproteins that contain apolipoprotein B-100 transport cholesterol and/or TGs from the liver to peripheral tissues.
- Lipoproteins that contain apolipoproteins A-I or A-II transport cholesterol from peripheral tissues back to the liver.
- VLDLs transport TGs to peripheral tissues.
- The contribution of VLDLs to CHD is unclear.
- LDLs transport cholesterol to peripheral tissues.
- Elevation of LDL cholesterol greatly increases the risk of CHD.

- By reducing LDL cholesterol levels, we can arrest or reverse atherosclerosis, and can thereby reduce morbidity and mortality from CHD.
- HDLs transport cholesterol back to the liver.
- HDLs protect against CHD.
- Atherogenesis is a chronic inflammatory process that begins with accumulation of LDLs beneath the arterial endothelium, followed by oxidation of LDLs.
- Under ATP III, all adults over the age of 20 should be screened every 5 years for total cholesterol, LDL cholesterol, HDL cholesterol, and TGs.
- Under ATP III, treatment of high LDL cholesterol is based on the individual's 10-year risk of having a major coronary event.
- Individuals with established CHD or a CHD risk equivalent (e.g., diabetes) are in the highest (>20%) 10-year risk group.

- The higher the 10-year risk, the lower the LDL goal and the LDL levels at which therapeutic lifestyle changes (TLCs) and drug therapy should be implemented.
- Diet modification (along with exercise) is the primary method for reducing LDL cholesterol. Drugs are employed only if diet modification and exercise fail to reduce LDL cholesterol to the target level.
- Therapy with cholesterol-lowering drugs must continue lifelong. If these drugs are withdrawn, cholesterol levels will return to pretreatment values.
- Statins (HMG-CoA reductase inhibitors) are the most effective drugs for lowering LDL cholesterol, and they cause few adverse effects.
- Statins can slow progression of CHD, decrease the number of adverse cardiac events, and reduce mortality.
- Statins reduce LDL cholesterol levels by increasing the number of LDL receptors on hepatocytes, thereby enabling hepatocytes to remove more LDLs from the blood. The process by which LDL receptor number is increased begins with inhibition of HMG-CoA reductase, the rate-limiting enzyme in cholesterol synthesis.
- Three statins—atorvastatin, lovastatin, and simvastatin—are metabolized by CYP3A4, and hence their levels can be increased by CYP3A4 inhibitors (e.g., cycloserine, erythromycin, ketoconazole, ritonavir).
- Rarely, statins cause liver damage. Tests of liver function should be done at baseline and every 6 to 12 months thereafter.
- Rarely, statins cause myopathy. Patients who experience unusual muscle pain or soreness should inform the physician. A marker for muscle injury—creatine kinase (CK)—should be measured at baseline and again if signs of myopathy develop.
- Statins should not be used during pregnancy.
- Bile-acid sequestrants (e.g., cholestyramine) reduce LDL cholesterol levels by increasing the number of LDL receptors on hepatocytes. The mechanism is complex and begins with preventing reabsorption of bile acids in the intestine.
- Bile-acid sequestrants are not absorbed from the GI tract, and hence do not cause systemic adverse effects. However, they do cause constipation and other GI effects. (GI effects with one agent—colesevelam—are minimal).
- Bile-acid sequestrants form complexes with other drugs, and thereby prevent their absorption. Accordingly, oral medications should be administered 1 hour before the sequestrant or 4 hours after. (Interactions of colesevelam with other drugs are minimal.)
- Ezetimibe lowers LDL cholesterol by reducing cholesterol absorption in the small intestine.
- Gemfibrozil and other fibrates are the most effective drugs for lowering TG levels.
- Nicotinic acid reduces LDL and TG levels and raises HDL levels. Unfortunately, the drug also causes adverse effects in nearly all patients. As a result, its clinical utility is limited.
- Nicotinic acid causes intense flushing of the face, neck, and ears in most patients. Flushing can be reduced by taking aspirin or ibuprofen 30 minutes before dosing with nicotinic acid.
- Nicotinic acid can cause liver injury. The risk is greatest with older sustained-release formulations.

Summary of Major Nursing Implications*

IMPLICATIONS THAT APPLY TO ALL DRUGS THAT LOWER LDL CHOLESTEROL

Preadministration Assessment

Baseline Data

Obtain laboratory values for total cholesterol, LDL cholesterol, HDL cholesterol, and TGs (VLDLs).

Identifying CHD Risk Factors

The patient history and physical examination should identify CHD risk factors. These include smoking, obesity, advancing age (men >45 years, women >55 years), family history of premature CHD, a personal history of cerebrovascular or peripheral vascular disease, reduced levels of HDL cholesterol (<40 mg/dl), and hypertension.

In the past, diabetes was considered a CHD risk factor. However, because the association between diabetes and CHD is so strong, diabetes is now considered a CHD risk *equivalent* (i.e., it poses the same 10-year risk of a major coronary event as does CHD itself).

Measures to Enhance Therapeutic Effects

Diet Modification

Diet modification should precede and accompany drug therapy for elevated LDL cholesterol. **Inform patients about the importance of diet in controlling cholesterol levels and arrange for dietary counseling. Advise patients to limit consumption of cholesterol (to <200 mg/day) and saturated fat (to <7% of caloric intake) and to follow the other dietary recommendations listed in Table 48–5. If these measures fail to reduce LD cholesterol to the target level, advise patients to add soluble fiber and plant stanols or sterols to the regimen.**

Exercise

Regular exercise can reduce LDL cholesterol and elevate HDL cholesterol, thereby reducing the risk of CHD. **Help the patient establish an appropriate exercise program.**

*Patient education information is highlighted as blue text.

Summary of Major Nursing Implications*—cont'd

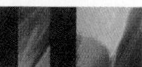

Reduction of CHD Risk Factors

Correctable CHD risk factors should be addressed. **Encourage cigarette smokers to quit. Encourage obese patients to lose weight.** Disease states that promote CHD—diabetes mellitus and hypertension—must be treated.

Promoting Compliance

Drug therapy for elevated LDL cholesterol must continue lifelong; if drugs are withdrawn, cholesterol levels will return to pretreatment values. **Inform patients about the need for continuous therapy, and encourage them to adhere to the prescribed regimen.**

HMG-COA REDUCTASE INHIBITORS (STATINS)

Atorvastatin
Fluvastatin
Lovastatin
Pravastatin
Simvastatin

In addition to the implications discussed below, *see above* for implications that apply to all drugs that lower LDL cholesterol.

Preadministration Assessment

Therapeutic Goal

Statins, in combination with diet modification and exercise, are used primarily to lower levels of LDL cholesterol. Additional indications are shown in Table 48–9.

Baseline Data

Obtain a baseline lipid profile, consisting of total cholesterol, LDL cholesterol, HDL cholesterol, and TGs (VLDLs). Also, obtain baseline LFTs and a CK level.

Identifying High-Risk Patients

Statins are *contraindicated* for patients with active or chronic liver disease and for women who are pregnant. Exercise *caution* in patients who consume alcohol to excess and in those taking fibrates (gemfibrozil or fenofibrate), or agents that inhibit CYP3A4 (e.g., cyclosporine, erythromycin, ketoconazole, ritonavir).

Implementation: Administration

Route

Oral.

Administration

Instruct patients to take lovastatin with the evening meal; all other statins can be administered without regard to meals. Advise patients that dosing in the evening is preferred for all statins.

*Patient education information is highlighted as blue text.

Ongoing Evaluation and Interventions

Evaluating Therapeutic Effects

Cholesterol levels should be monitored monthly early in treatment and at longer intervals thereafter.

Minimizing Adverse Effects

Statins are very well tolerated. Side effects are uncommon, and serious adverse effects—hepatotoxicity and myopathy—are rare.

Hepatotoxicity. Statins can injure the liver, but jaundice and other clinical signs are rare. Liver function should be assessed before treatment and every 6 to 12 months thereafter (see Table 48–8). If serum transaminase becomes persistently excessive (more than 3 times normal), statins should be discontinued. Statins should be avoided in patients with active or chronic liver disease.

Myopathy. Statins can cause muscle injury. If statins are not withdrawn, injury may progress to severe myositis or potentially fatal rhabdomyolysis. **Inform patients about the risk of myopathy, and instruct them to notify the physician if unexplained muscle pain or tenderness develops.** If muscle pain does develop, the CK level should be measured, and, if it is more than 10 times the ULN, the statin should be withdrawn.

Minimizing Adverse Interactions

The risk of myopathy is increased by gemfibrozil and fenofibrate, which promote myopathy themselves, and by inhibitors of CYP3A4—cyclosporine, macrolide antibiotics (e.g., erythromycin), azole antifungal drugs (e.g., ketoconazole), and HIV protease inhibitors (e.g., ritonavir)—which can cause statin levels to rise. The combination of a statin with any of these drugs should be used with caution.

Use in Pregnancy

Statins are contraindicated during pregnancy. **Inform women of child-bearing age about the potential for fetal harm and warn them against becoming pregnant.** If pregnancy occurs, statins should be withdrawn.

NICOTINIC ACID (NIACIN)

In addition to the implications discussed below, *see above* for implications that apply to all drugs that lower LDL cholesterol.

Preadministration Assessment

Therapeutic Goal

Nicotinic acid, in conjunction with diet modification and exercise, is used to reduce levels of LDL cholesterol, VLDLs, and TGs. It is also used to raise HDL cholesterol.

Baseline Data

Obtain laboratory values for total cholesterol, LDL cholesterol, HDL cholesterol, and TGs (VLDLs). Obtain a baseline test of liver function.

Summary of Major Nursing Implications*—cont'd

Identifying High-Risk Patients

Nicotinic acid is *contraindicated* for patients with active liver disease or severe gout. Exercise *caution* in patients with diabetes mellitus, hyperuricemia, mild gout, and peptic ulcer disease.

Implementation: Administration

Route

Oral.

Administration

Instruct patients to take nicotinic acid with meals to reduce GI upset.

Measures to Enhance Therapeutic Effects

Dietary Therapy

Diet modification should precede and accompany drug therapy for elevated TGs and VLDLs. **Inform patients about the importance of diet in controlling lipid levels and arrange for dietary counseling.** In addition to following the guidelines presented above for all drugs that reduce LDL cholesterol, patients with hypertriglyceridemia should restrict consumption of alcohol and other sources of triglycerides.

Ongoing Evaluation and Interventions

Evaluating Therapeutic Effects

Blood lipid levels should be monitored monthly early in treatment and at longer intervals thereafter.

Minimizing Adverse Effects

Flushing. Nicotinic acid causes flushing of the face, neck, and ears in most patients. **Advise patients that flushing can be reduced by taking 325 mg of aspirin 30 minutes before each dose.**

Hepatotoxicity. Nicotinic acid (primarily the older sustained-release formulation) may injure the liver, causing jaundice or other symptoms. Liver function should be assessed before treatment and periodically thereafter. Hepatotoxicity is less likely with Niaspan, a new extended-release formulation.

Elevation of Homocysteine. Nicotinic acid raises homocysteine levels, and may thereby increase the risk of CHD. Homocysteine levels can be lowered with folic acid.

Hyperglycemia. Nicotinic acid may cause hyperglycemia and reduced glucose tolerance. Blood glucose should be monitored frequently. Exercise caution in patients with diabetes.

Hyperuricemia. Nicotinic acid can elevate blood levels of uric acid. Exercise caution in patients with gout.

BILE-ACID SEQUESTRANTS

Cholestyramine
Colestipol
Colesevelam

*Patient education information is highlighted as blue text.

In addition to the implications discussed below, *see above* for implications that apply to all drugs that lower LDL cholesterol.

Preadministration Assessment

Therapeutic Goal

Bile-acid sequestrants, in conjunction with diet modification and exercise, are used to reduce elevated levels of LDL cholesterol.

Baseline Data

Obtain laboratory values for total cholesterol, LDL cholesterol, HDL cholesterol, and TGs (VLDLs).

Implementation: Administration

Route

Oral.

Administration

Instruct patients to mix cholestyramine powder and colestipol granules with water, fruit juice, soup, or pulpy fruit (e.g., applesauce, pineapple) to reduce the risk of esophageal irritation and impaction. Inform patients that the sequestrants are not water soluble, and hence mixtures will be cloudy suspensions, not clear solutions.

Ongoing Evaluation and Interventions

Evaluating Therapeutic Effects

Cholesterol levels should be monitored monthly early in treatment and at longer intervals thereafter.

Minimizing Adverse Effects

Constipation. **Inform patients that constipation can be minimized by increasing dietary fiber and fluids. A mild laxative may be used if needed. Instruct patients to notify the physician if constipation becomes bothersome.**

Vitamin Deficiency. Cholestyramine and colestipol can impair absorption of fat-soluble vitamins (A, D, E, and K). Vitamin supplements may be required. Colesevelam does not reduce vitamin absorption.

Minimizing Adverse Interactions

Cholestyramine and colestipol can bind with other drugs and prevent their absorption. **Advise patients to administer other medications 1 hour before these sequestrants or 4 hours after.** Interaction of colesevelam with other drugs is minimal.

GEMFIBROZIL

Preadministration Assessment

Therapeutic Goal

Gemfibrozil, in conjunction with diet modification, is used to reduce elevated levels of TGs (VLDLs). The drug is not very effective at lowering LDL cholesterol. It may also be used to raise low levels of HDL cholesterol.

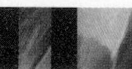

Summary of Major Nursing Implications*—cont'd

Baseline Data

Obtain laboratory values for total cholesterol, LDL cholesterol, HDL cholesterol, and TGs (VLDLs).

Identifying High-Risk Patients

Gemfibrozil is *contraindicated* for patients with liver disease, severe renal dysfunction, and gallbladder disease. Use with *caution* in patients taking statins or warfarin.

Implementation: Administration

Route

Oral.

Administration

Instruct patients to administer gemfibrozil 30 minutes before the morning and evening meals.

Ongoing Evaluation and Interventions

Evaluating Therapeutic Effects

Obtain periodic tests of blood lipids.

*Patient education information is highlighted as blue text.

Minimizing Adverse Effects

Gallstones. Gemfibrozil increases gallstone development. Inform patients about symptoms of gallbladder disease (e.g., upper abdominal discomfort, intolerance of fried foods, bloating), and instruct them to notify the physician if these develop.

Myopathy. Gemfibrozil can cause muscle damage. Warn patients to report any signs of muscle injury, such as tenderness, weakness, or unusual muscle pain.

Liver Disease. Gemfibrozil may disrupt liver function. Cancer of the liver may also be a risk. Obtain periodic tests of liver function.

Minimizing Adverse Interactions

Warfarin. Gemfibrozil enhances the effects of warfarin, thereby increasing the risk of bleeding. Obtain frequent measurements of prothrombin time and observe the patient for signs of bleeding. Reduction of warfarin dosage may be required.

Statins. Gemfibrozil and statins both cause muscle injury. Use the combination with caution.

Drugs for Angina Pectoris

Angina pectoris is defined as sudden pain beneath the sternum, often radiating to the left shoulder and arm. Anginal pain is precipitated when the oxygen supply to the heart is insufficient to meet oxygen demand. Most often, angina occurs secondary to atherosclerosis of the coronary arteries. Hence, angina should be seen as a symptom of a disease and not as a disease in its own right. In the United States, over 7 million people have chronic stable angina; about 350,000 new cases develop annually.

Drug therapy of angina has two goals: (1) prevention of myocardial infarction (MI) and death and (2) prevention of myocardial ischemia and anginal pain. Two types of drugs are used to decrease the risk of MI and death: cholesterol-lowering drugs and antiplatelet drugs. These agents are discussed in Chapters 48 and 50, respectively.

In this chapter, our focus is on antianginal drugs (i.e., drugs that prevent myocardial ischemia and anginal pain). There are three families of antianginal agents: *organic nitrates* (e.g., nitroglycerin), *beta blockers* (e.g., propranolol), and *calcium channel blockers* (e.g., verapamil). Most of the chapter focuses on the organic nitrates. Beta blockers and calcium channel blockers are discussed at length in previous chapters; hence, consideration here is limited to their use in angina.

DETERMINANTS OF CARDIAC OXYGEN DEMAND AND OXYGEN SUPPLY

Before discussing angina pectoris, we need to review the major factors that determine cardiac oxygen demand and oxygen supply.

Oxygen Demand. The principal determinants of cardiac oxygen demand are heart rate, myocardial contractility, and, most importantly, intramyocardial wall tension. Wall tension is determined by two factors: cardiac preload and cardiac afterload. (Preload and afterload are defined in Chapter 41.) In summary, cardiac oxygen demand is determined by four major factors: (1) heart rate, (2) contractility, (3) preload, and (4) afterload. Drugs that reduce these factors reduce oxygen demand.

Oxygen Supply. Cardiac oxygen supply is determined by myocardial blood flow. Under resting conditions, the heart extracts nearly all of the oxygen delivered to it by the coronary vessels. Hence, the only way to accommodate an increase in oxygen demand is to increase blood flow. When oxygen demand increases, coronary arterioles dilate; the resultant decrease in vascular resistance allows blood flow to increase. During exertion, coronary blood flow increases to 4 to 5 times the flow rate at rest. It is important to note that myocardial perfusion takes place only during diastole (i.e., when the heart relaxes). Perfusion does not take place during systole. Why? Because the vessels that supply the myocardium are squeezed shut when the heart contracts.

ANGINA PECTORIS: PATHOPHYSIOLOGY AND TREATMENT STRATEGY

Angina pectoris has three forms: (1) *chronic stable angina* (exertional angina), (2) *variant angina* (Prinzmetal's or vasospastic angina), and (3) *unstable angina.* Our focus is on stable angina and variant angina. Consideration of unstable angina is brief.

Chronic Stable Angina (Exertional Angina)

Pathophysiology. Stable angina is triggered most often by an increase in physical activity. Emotional excitement, large meals, and cold exposure may also precipitate an attack. Because stable angina usually occurs in response to strain, this condition is also known as *exertional angina* or *angina of effort.*

The underlying cause of exertional angina is coronary artery disease (CAD), a condition characterized by deposition of fatty plaque on the arterial wall. If an artery is only partially occluded by plaque, blood flow will be reduced and angina pectoris will result. However, if complete vessel blockage occurs, blood flow will stop and MI (heart attack) will result.

The impact of CAD on the balance between myocardial oxygen demand and oxygen supply is illustrated in Figure 49–1. As depicted, in both the healthy heart and the heart with CAD, oxygen supply and oxygen demand are in balance during rest. (In the presence of CAD, resting oxygen demand is met through dilation of arterioles distal to the partial occlusion. This dilation reduces resistance to blood flow and thereby compensates for the increase in resistance created by plaque.)

The picture is very different during exertion. In the healthy heart, as cardiac oxygen demand rises, coronary arterioles dilate, causing blood flow to increase. The increase keeps oxygen supply in balance with oxygen demand. By contrast, in people with CAD, arterioles in the affected region are already fully dilated during rest. Hence, when exertion occurs, there is no way to increase blood flow to compensate for the increase

in oxygen demand. The resultant imbalance between oxygen supply and oxygen demand is the cause of anginal pain.

Treatment Strategy. The goal of antianginal therapy is to reduce the intensity and frequency of anginal attacks. Because anginal pain results from an imbalance between oxygen supply and oxygen demand, logic dictates two possible remedies: (1) increase cardiac oxygen supply or (2) decrease oxygen demand. Since the underlying cause of stable angina is occlusion of the coronary arteries, there is little we can do to increase cardiac oxygen supply. Hence, the first remedy is not a real option. Consequently, the principal way we can relieve the pain of stable angina is to *decrease cardiac oxygen demand*. As discussed above, we can reduce oxygen demand with drugs that decrease heart rate, contractility, afterload, and preload.

Overview of Therapeutic Agents. Stable angina can be treated with three types of drugs: *organic nitrates, beta blockers,* and *calcium channel blockers.* All three relieve the pain of stable angina primarily by decreasing cardiac oxygen demand (Table 49–1). It should be noted that drugs only pro-

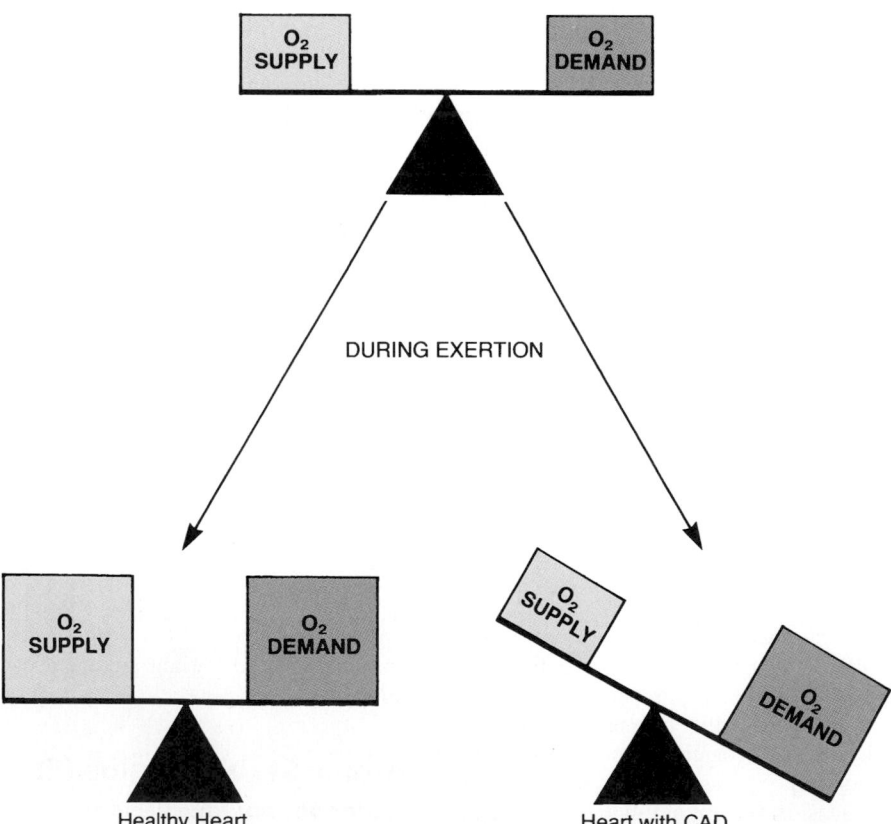

Figure 49–1 ■ **Effect of exertion on the balance between oxygen supply and oxygen demand in the healthy heart and the heart with CAD.**
In the healthy heart, O₂ supply and O₂ demand are always in balance; during exertion, coronary arteries dilate, producing an increase in blood flow to meet the increase in O₂ demand. In the heart with CAD, O₂ supply and demand are in balance only during rest. During exertion, dilation of coronary arteries cannot compensate for the increase in O₂ demand, and an imbalance results.

vide symptomatic relief; they do not affect the underlying pathology (CAD). To reduce the risk of MI, all patients should receive an antiplatelet drug (e.g., aspirin) unless it is contraindicated. Other measures to reduce the risk of infarction are discussed later under *Drugs Used to Prevent Myocardial Infarction and Death.*

Nondrug Therapy. Patients should attempt to avoid factors that can precipitate angina. These include overexertion, heavy meals, emotional stress, and exposure to cold.

Risk factors for stable angina should be corrected. Important among these are smoking, obesity, hypertension, hyperlipidemia, and a sedentary lifestyle. Patients should be strongly encouraged to quit smoking. Overweight patients should be given a restricted-calorie diet; the diet should be low in saturated fats, and total fat content should not exceed 30% of caloric intake. The target weight is 110% of ideal or less. Patients with a sedentary lifestyle should be encouraged to establish a regular program of aerobic exercise (e.g., walking, jogging, swimming, bicycling). Hypertension and hyperlipidemia are major risk factors and should be treated. These disorders are discussed in Chapters 45 and 48, respectively.

Variant Angina (Prinzmetal's Angina, Vasospastic Angina)

Pathophysiology. Variant angina is caused by *coronary artery spasm,* which restricts blood flow to the myocardium. Hence, as in stable angina, pain is secondary to insufficient oxygenation of the heart. In contrast to stable angina, whose symptoms occur primarily at times of exertion, variant angina can produce pain at any time, even during rest and sleep. Frequently, variant angina occurs in conjunction with stable angina. Alternative names for variant angina are *vasospastic angina* and *Prinzmetal's angina.*

Treatment Strategy. The goal of therapy is to reduce the incidence and severity of attacks. In contrast to stable angina, which is treated primarily by reducing oxygen demand, variant angina is treated by *increasing cardiac oxygen supply.* This makes sense in that the pain is caused by a reduction in oxygen supply, rather than by an increase in demand. Oxygen supply is increased with vasodilators, which prevent or relieve coronary artery spasm.

Overview of Therapeutic Agents. Vasospastic angina is treated with two groups of drugs: *calcium channel blockers* and *organic nitrates.* Both act by relaxing coronary artery spasm. Beta blockers, which are effective in stable angina, are not effective in variant angina. As with stable angina, therapy is symptomatic only; drugs do not alter the underlying pathology.

Unstable Angina

Pathophysiology. Unstable angina is a medical emergency. Symptoms result from severe CAD complicated by vasospasm, platelet aggregation, and transient coronary thrombi or emboli. The patient may present with either (1) symptoms of angina at rest, (2) new-onset exertional angina, or (3) intensification of existing angina. Unstable angina poses a much greater risk of death than stable angina, but a smaller risk of death than MI. The risk of dying is greatest initially and then declines to baseline in about 2 months (unless death occurs first).

Treatment. In March of 2002, the American College of Cardiology (ACC) and the American Heart Association (AHA) issued updated guidelines for the diagnosis and management of unstable angina. The document—*ACC/AHA 2002 Guideline Update for the Management of Patients with Unstable Angina and Non–ST-Segment Elevation Myocardial Infarction*—is available free online at *www.acc.org* and *www.americanheart.org.* According to the guideline, the treatment strategy is to *maintain oxygen supply* and *decrease oxygen demand.* The goal is to reduce pain and prevent progression to MI or death. All patients should be hospitalized. Acute management consists of anti-ischemic therapy combined with antiplatelet and anticoagulation therapy.

Anti-ischemic therapy consists of

■ Nitroglycerin—give the first dose sublingually (tablet or spray) and follow with IV therapy
■ A beta blocker—give the first dose IV if chest pain is ongoing. If beta blockers are contraindicated, substitute a nondihydropyridine calcium channel blocker (verapamil or diltiazem).
■ Supplemental oxygen—for patients with cyanosis or respiratory distress
■ IV morphine sulfate—if pain is not relieved immediately by nitroglycerin, or if pulmonary congestion or severe agitation is present
■ An angiotensin-converting enzyme inhibitor—but only for patients with persistent hypertension, and only if they have left ventricular dysfunction or congestive heart failure

Antiplatelet therapy, which should be started promptly, consists of

■ Aspirin—continue indefinitely
■ Clopidogrel [Plavix]—continue for at least 1 month

	Mechanism of Pain Relief	
Drug Class	**Stable Angina**	**Variant Angina**
Nitrates	*Decrease oxygen demand* by dilating veins, which decreases preload	*Increase oxygen supply* by relaxing coronary vasospasm
Beta Blockers	*Decrease oxygen demand* by decreasing heart rate and contractility	Not used
Calcium Channel Blockers	*Decrease oxygen demand* by dilating arterioles, which decreases afterload (all calcium blockers), and by decreasing heart rate and contractility (verapamil and diltiazem)	*Increase oxygen supply* by relaxing coronary vasospasm

TABLE 49–1 ■ Mechanisms of Antianginal Action

■ Abciximab [ReoPro], a glycoprotein IIb/IIIa inhibitor—but only if angioplasty is planned
■ Eptifibatide [Integrilin] or tirofiban [Aggrastat] (both are glycoprotein IIb/IIIa inhibitors)—but only in high-risk patients with continuing ischemia, and only if angioplasty is *not* planned

Anticoagulant therapy consists of subcutaneous low-molecular-weight heparin (e.g., dalteparin [Fragmin]) or intravenous unfractionated heparin.

ORGANIC NITRATES

The organic nitrates are the oldest and most frequently used antianginal drugs. These agents relieve angina by causing vasodilation. Nitroglycerin, the most familiar organic nitrate, will serve as our prototype for the family. A complete list of organic nitrates appears in Table 49–2.

Nitroglycerin

Nitroglycerin has been used to treat angina since 1879. The drug is effective, fast acting, and inexpensive. Despite availability of newer antianginal agents, nitroglycerin remains the drug of choice for relieving acute anginal attacks.

Vasodilator Actions

Nitroglycerin acts directly on vascular smooth muscle (VSM) to promote vasodilation. At usual therapeutic doses, the drug acts primarily on *veins;* dilation of arterioles is only modest.

The biochemical events that lead to vasodilation are outlined in Figure 49–2. The process begins with uptake of nitrate by VSM, followed by conversion of nitrate to its active form: *nitric oxide.* As indicated, this conversion requires the presence of *sulfhydryl groups.* Nitric oxide then activates guanylate cyclase, an enzyme that catalyzes the formation of cyclic GMP. Through a series of reactions that are poorly understood, elevation of cyclic GMP leads to dephosphorylation of myosin light chain in VSM. (Recall that, in all muscles, phosphorylated myosin interacts with actin to produce contraction.) As a result of dephosphorylation, myosin is unable to interact with actin, and hence VSM relaxes, causing vasodilation. For our purposes, the most important aspect of this sequence is the conversion of nitrate to its active form—nitric oxide—in the presence of a sulfhydryl source.

Mechanism of Antianginal Effects

Stable Angina. Nitroglycerin decreases the pain of exertional angina primarily by *decreasing cardiac oxygen demand.* Oxygen demand is decreased as follows: By dilating veins, nitroglycerin decreases venous return to the heart, and thereby decreases ventricular filling; the resultant decrease in wall tension (preload) decreases oxygen demand.

TABLE 49–2 ■ Trade Names for Organic Nitrates	
Generic Name	**Trade Name(s)**
Nitroglycerin	
Sublingual tablets	Nitrostat, NitroQuick
Translingual spray	Nitrolingual
Transmucosal tablets	Nitrogard
Oral tablets, SR	Nitrong
Oral capsules, SR	Nitroglyn, Nitro-Time
Transdermal patches	Deponit, Minitran, Nitrodisc Nitro-Dur, Nitrek, Transderm-Nitro
Topical ointment	Nitro-Bid, Nitrol
Intravenous	Nitro-Bid IV, Tridil
Isosorbide Mononitrate	
Oral tablets, IR	ISMO, Monoket
Oral tablets, ER	Isotrate ER, Imdur
Isosorbide Dinitrate	
Sublingual tablets	Isordil, Sorbitrate
Chewable tablets	Sorbitrate
Oral tablets, IR	Isordil Titradose, Sorbitrate
Oral tablets, SR	Isordil Tembids
Oral capsules, SR	Dilatrate-SR, Isordil Tembids
Amyl Nitrite	
Inhalant	Generic only

ER = extended release, IR = immediate release, SR = sustained release.

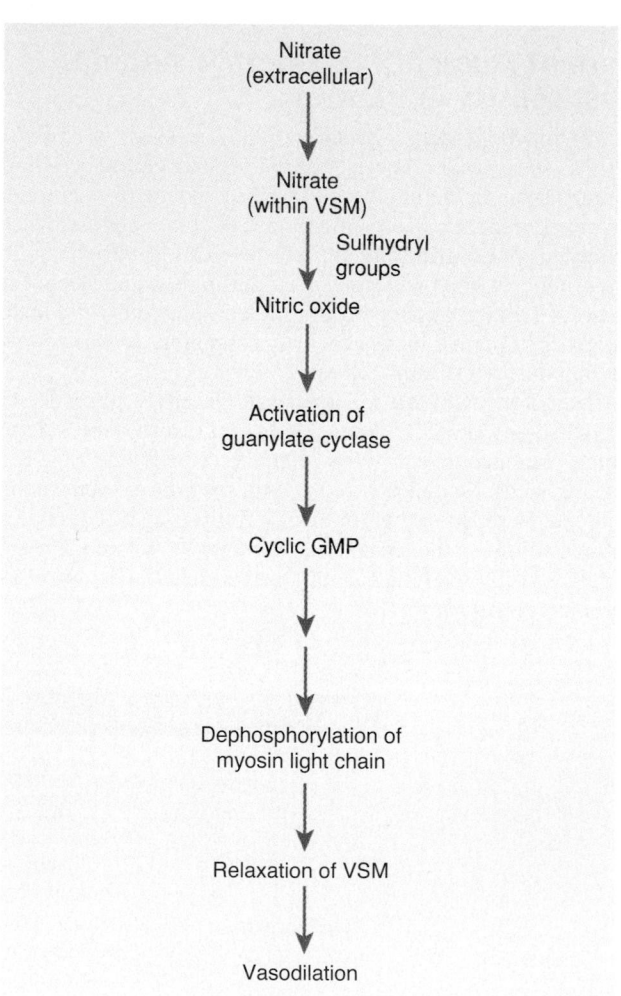

Figure 49–2 ■ Biochemistry of nitrate-induced vasodilation. Note that sulfhydryl groups are needed to catalyze the conversion of nitrate to its active form, nitric oxide. If sulfhydryl groups are depleted from VSM, tolerance to nitrates will occur.

In patients with stable angina, nitroglycerin does not appear to increase blood flow to ischemic areas of the heart. This statement is based on two observations. First, nitroglycerin does not dilate atherosclerotic coronary arteries. Second, when nitroglycerin is injected directly into coronary arteries during an anginal attack, it does not relieve pain. Both observations suggest that pain relief results from effects of nitroglycerin on peripheral blood vessels—and not from effects on coronary blood flow.

Variant Angina. In patients with variant angina, nitroglycerin acts by relaxing or preventing spasm in coronary arteries. Hence, the drug *increases oxygen supply*. It does not reduce oxygen demand.

Pharmacokinetics

Absorption. Nitroglycerin is *highly lipid soluble* and crosses membranes with ease. Because of this property, nitroglycerin can be administered by uncommon routes (sublingual, buccal, transdermal) as well as by more conventional routes (oral, intravenous).

Metabolism. Nitroglycerin undergoes *rapid inactivation* by hepatic enzymes (organic nitrate reductases). As a result, the drug has a plasma half-life of only 5 to 7 minutes. When nitroglycerin is administered orally, most of each dose is destroyed on its first pass through the liver.

Adverse Effects

Nitroglycerin is generally well tolerated. Principal adverse effects—headache, hypotension, and tachycardia—occur secondary to vasodilation.

Headache. Initial therapy can produce severe headache. This response diminishes over the first few weeks of treatment. In the meantime, headache can be reduced with aspirin, acetaminophen, or some other mild analgesic.

Orthostatic Hypotension. Relaxation of VSM causes blood to pool in veins when the patient assumes an erect posture. Pooling decreases venous return to the heart, which reduces cardiac output, causing blood pressure to fall. Symptoms of orthostatic hypotension include lightheadedness and dizziness. Patients should be instructed to sit or lie down if these occur. Lying with the feet elevated promotes venous return, and can thereby help restore blood pressure.

Reflex Tachycardia. Nitroglycerin lowers blood pressure—primarily by decreasing venous return, and partly by dilating arterioles. By lowering blood pressure, the drug can activate the baroreceptor reflex, thereby causing sympathetic stimulation of the heart. The resultant increase in both heart rate and contractile force increases cardiac oxygen demand, which negates the benefits of therapy. Pretreatment with a beta blocker or verapamil (a calcium channel blocker that directly suppresses the heart) can prevent sympathetic cardiac stimulation.

Drug Interactions

Hypotensive Drugs. Nitroglycerin can intensify the effects of other hypotensive agents. Consequently, care should be exercised when nitroglycerin is used concurrently with beta blockers, calcium channel blockers, diuretics, and all other drugs that can lower blood pressure. Also, patients should be advised to avoid alcohol.

Beta Blockers, Verapamil, and Diltiazem. These drugs can suppress nitroglycerin-induced tachycardia. Beta blockers do so by preventing sympathetic activation of beta$_1$-adrenergic receptors on the heart. Verapamil and diltiazem prevent tachycardia through direct suppression of pacemaker activity in the sinoatrial node.

Sildenafil. Sildenafil [Viagra], a drug for erectile dysfunction, can greatly intensify nitroglycerin-induced vasodilation. Life-threatening hypotension can result. (In volunteers, combining sildenafil with nitroglycerin has caused systolic pressure to drop by 25 mm Hg or more.) To minimize risk, patients should be warned not to take sildenafil within 24 hours of taking any nitroglycerin preparation.

What's the mechanism of the interaction? Sildenafil inhibits phosphodiesterase 5, the enzyme that inactivates cyclic GMP. Hence, when we combine nitroglycerin (which stimulates cyclic GMP production) with sildenafil (which inhibits cyclic GMP degradation), levels of cyclic GMP can rise dangerously high, thereby causing excessive vasodilation and a precipitous drop in blood pressure.

Tolerance

Tolerance to nitroglycerin-induced vasodilation can develop rapidly (over the course of a single day). One possible mechanism is depletion of sulfhydryl groups in VSM; in the absence of sulfhydryl groups, nitroglycerin cannot be converted to nitric oxide, its active form. Another possible mechanism, suggested by recent data, is reversible oxidative injury to mitochondrial aldehyde dehydrogenase, an enzyme needed to convert nitroglycerin into nitric oxide. Patients who develop tolerance to nitroglycerin display cross-tolerance to all other nitrates and vice versa. Development of tolerance is most likely with high-dose therapy and uninterrupted therapy. To prevent tolerance, nitroglycerin and other nitrates should be used in the lowest effective dosages; long-acting formulations (e.g., patches, sustained-release preparations) should be used on an intermittent schedule that allows at least 8 drug-free hours every day, usually during the night. If pain occurs during the nitrate free interval, it can be managed with sparing use of a short-acting nitrate (e.g., sublingual nitroglycerin) or by adding a beta blocker or calcium channel blocker to the regimen. Tolerance can be reversed by withholding nitrates for a short time.

Preparations and Routes of Administration

Nitroglycerin is available in an assortment of formulations for administration by a variety of routes. This proliferation of dosage forms reflects efforts to delay hepatic metabolism, and thereby prolong therapeutic effects.

All nitroglycerin preparations produce qualitatively similar responses; differences relate only to onset and duration of action (Table 49–3). With some preparations, effects begin rapidly (in 1 to 5 minutes) and then fade in less than 1 hour. With others, effects begin slowly but last several hours. Only three preparations have both a rapid onset *and* long duration.

Applications of specific preparations are based on their time course. Preparations with a *rapid onset* are employed to *terminate an ongoing anginal attack*. When used for this purpose, rapid-acting preparations are administered as soon as pain begins. Rapid-acting preparations can also be used for *acute prophylaxis of angina*. For this purpose, these preparations are taken just prior to anticipated exertion. *Long-acting preparations* are used to provide *sustained protection* against

TABLE 49–3 ■ Organic Nitrates: Time Course of Action

Drug and Dosage Form	Onset*	Duration†
Nitroglycerin		
Sublingual tablets	Rapid (1–3 min)	Brief (30–60 min)
Translingual spray	Rapid (2–3 min)	Brief (30–60 min)
Transmucosal tablets	Rapid (1–2 min)	Long (3–5 hr)
Oral tablets, SR	Slow (20–45 min)	Long (3–8 hr)
Oral capsules, SR	Slow (20–45 min)	Long (3–8 hr)
Transdermal patches	Slow (30–60 min)	Long (24 hr)‡
Topical ointment	Slow (30–60 min)	Long (2–12 hr)
Isosorbide Mononitrate		
Oral tablets, IR	Slow (30–60 min)	Long (6–10 hr)
Oral tablets, SR	Slow (30–60 min)	Long (7–12 hr)
Isosorbide Dinitrate		
Sublingual tablets	Rapid (2–5 min)	Long (1–3 hr)
Chewable tablets	Rapid (2–5 min)	Long (1–3 hr)
Oral tablets, IR	Slow (20–40 min)	Long (4–6 hr)
Oral tablets, SR	Slow (30 min)	Long (6–8 hr)
Oral capsules, SR	Slow (30 min)	Long (6–8 hr)

IR = immediate release, SR = sustained release.

*Nitrates with a *rapid* onset have two uses: (1) termination of an ongoing anginal attack and (2) short-term prophylaxis prior to anticipated exertion. Of the rapid-acting nitrates, nitroglycerin (sublingual or spray) is preferred to the others for terminating an ongoing attack.

†*Long-acting* nitrates are used for sustained prophylaxis (prevention) of anginal attacks. All cause tolerance if used without interruption.

‡Although patches can release nitroglycerin for up to 24 hours, they should be removed after 12 to 14 hours to avoid tolerance.

anginal attacks. To provide protection, these preparations are administered on a fixed schedule (but one that permits at least 8 drug-free hours each day).

Dosages for nitroglycerin preparations are summarized in Table 49–4. Trade names are shown in Table 49–2.

Sublingual Tablets. When administered sublingually (beneath the tongue), nitroglycerin is absorbed directly through the oral mucosa and into the bloodstream. Hence, unlike orally administered drugs, which must pass through the liver on their way to the systemic circulation, sublingual nitroglycerin bypasses the liver, and thereby temporarily avoids metabolism. Because the liver is bypassed, sublingual doses can be low (between 0.3 and 0.6 mg). These doses are about 10 times lower than those required when nitroglycerin is taken orally.

Effects of sublingual nitroglycerin begin rapidly—in 1 to 3 minutes—and persist up to 1 hour. Because sublingual administration works fast, this route is ideal for (1) termination of an ongoing anginal attack and (2) short-term prophylaxis when exertion is anticipated.

To terminate an acute anginal attack, sublingual nitroglycerin should be administered as soon as pain begins. Administration should not be delayed until the pain has become severe. If 1 tablet is insufficient, 1 or 2 additional tablets should be taken at 5-minute intervals. If pain persists, the patient should contact a physician or report to an emergency department, since anginal pain that is unresponsive to nitroglycerin may indicate MI.

Sublingual administration is unfamiliar to most patients. Accordingly, education is needed. The patient should be instructed to place the tablet under the tongue and leave it there while it dissolves. Nitroglycerin tablets formulated for sublingual use are ineffective if swallowed.

Nitroglycerin tablets are chemically unstable and can lose effectiveness over time. Shelf life can be prolonged by storing tablets in a tightly closed, dark container. Under these conditions, tablets should remain effective for at least 6 months after the container is first opened. As a rule, nitroglycerin tablets should be discarded after this time. Patients should be instructed to write the date of opening on the container and to discard unused tablets 6 months later.

Sustained-Release Oral Tablets and Capsules. Sustained-release oral formulations are intended for long-term prophylaxis only; these formulations cannot act rapidly enough to terminate an ongoing anginal attack. Sustained-release tablets and capsules contain a large dose of nitroglycerin that is slowly absorbed across the GI wall. In theory, doses are large enough so that amounts of nitroglycerin sufficient to produce a therapeutic response will survive passage through the liver. Because they produce sustained blood levels of nitroglycerin, these formulations can cause tolerance. To reduce the risk of tolerance, these products should be taken only once or twice daily. Patients should be instructed to swallow sustained-release formulations intact.

Transdermal Delivery Systems. Nitroglycerin patches look like Band-Aids and contain a reservoir from which nitroglycerin is slowly released. Following release, the drug is absorbed through the skin and then into the blood. The rate of release is constant for any particular transdermal patch and, depending upon the patch used, can range from 0.1 to 0.8 mg/hr. Effects begin within 30 to 60 minutes and persist as long as the patch remains in place (up to 14 hours). Patches

TABLE 49–4 ■ Organic Nitrate Dosages

Drug and Formulation	Usual Dosage
Nitroglycerin	
Sublingual tablets	0.3–0.6 mg as needed
Translingual spray	0.4 mg as needed
Transmucosal tablets	1–3 mg 3 times daily
Oral tablets and capsules, SR	2.5–6.5 mg 3 or 4 times daily; to avoid tolerance, administer only once or twice daily; do not crush or chew
Transdermal patches	1 patch a day; to avoid tolerance, remove after 12–14 hr, allowing 10–12 patch-free hr each day. Patches come in sizes that release 0.1–0.8 mg/hr.
Topical ointment	1–2 inches (7.5–40 mg) every 4–8 hr
Intravenous	5 μg/min initially, then increased gradually as needed (max 200 μg/min); tolerance develops with prolonged continuous infusion
Isosorbide Mononitrate	
Oral tablets, IR	20 mg twice daily; to avoid tolerance, take the first dose upon awakening and the second dose 7 hr later
Oral tablets, SR	60–240 mg once a day; do not crush or chew
Isosorbide Dinitrate	
Sublingual tablets	2.5–15 mg every 4–6 hr; do not crush or chew
Chewable tablets	5 mg every 2–3 hr
Oral tablets, IR	5–80 mg every 6 hr; to avoid tolerance, take only 2 or 3 times daily, with the last dose no later than 7 PM
Oral tablets and capsules, SR	40 mg every 6–12 hr; to avoid tolerance, take only once or twice daily (at 8 AM and 2 PM)
Amyl Nitrite	
Inhalant	0.18 or 0.3 ml

IR = immediate release, SR = sustained release.

are applied once daily to a hairless area of skin. The site should be rotated to avoid local irritation.

Tolerance develops if patches are used continuously (24 hours a day every day). Accordingly, a daily "patch-free" interval of 10 to 12 hours is recommended. This can be accomplished by applying a new patch each morning, leaving it in place for 12 to 14 hours, and then removing it in the evening.

Because of their long duration, patches are well suited for sustained prophylaxis. Since patches have a delayed onset, they cannot be used to abort an ongoing attack.

Translingual Spray. Nitroglycerin can be delivered to the oral mucosa using a metered-dose spray device. Each activation delivers a 0.4-mg dose. Indications for nitroglycerin spray are the same as for sublingual tablets: suppression of an acute anginal attack and prophylaxis of angina when exertion is anticipated. As with sublingual tablets, no more than three doses should be administered within a 15-minute interval. *Patients should be instructed not to inhale the spray.*

Transmucosal (Buccal) Tablets. Administration of transmucosal nitroglycerin tablets consists of placing the tablet between the upper lip and the gum, or in the buccal area between the cheek and the gum. The tablet adheres to the oral mucosa and slowly dissolves over 3 to 5 hours. As the tablet dissolves, nitroglycerin is absorbed directly through the oral mucosa and then into the blood, thereby bypassing the liver. Like sublingual nitroglycerin, transmucosal nitroglycerin has a rapid onset. Hence, transmucosal administration can be used to terminate an ongoing anginal attack and to provide short-term pro-

phylaxis prior to exertion. In addition, since the effects of transmucosal nitroglycerin are prolonged, this formulation can be used for sustained prophylaxis. Patients should be instructed not to chew or swallow these tablets.

Topical Ointment. Topical nitroglycerin ointment is used for sustained protection against anginal attacks. The ointment is applied to the skin of the chest, back, abdomen, or anterior thigh. (Since nitroglycerin acts primarily by dilating peripheral veins, there is no mechanistic advantage to applying topical nitroglycerin directly over the heart.) Following topical application, nitroglycerin is absorbed through the skin and then into the blood. Effects begin within 20 to 60 minutes and may persist up to 12 hours.

Nitroglycerin ointment (2%) is dispensed from a tube, and the length of the ribbon squeezed from the tube determines dosage. (One inch contains about 15 mg of nitroglycerin.) The usual adult dosage is 1 to 2 inches applied every 4 to 8 hours. The ointment should be spread over a 6-inch by 6-inch area and then covered with a plastic wrap. Sites of application should be rotated to minimize skin irritation. As with other long-acting formulations, uninterrupted use can cause tolerance.

Intravenous Infusion. Intravenous nitroglycerin is employed only rarely to treat angina pectoris. When used for angina, IV nitroglycerin is limited to patients who have failed to respond to other medications. Additional uses of IV nitroglycerin include treatment of heart failure associated with acute MI, treatment of perioperative hypertension, and production of controlled hypotension for surgery.

Intravenous nitroglycerin has a very short duration of action, and hence continuous infusion is required. The rate is 5 μg/min initially and then increased gradually until an adequate response has been achieved. Heart rate and blood pressure must be monitored continuously.

Stock solutions of nitroglycerin must be diluted for IV therapy. Since ampules of nitroglycerin prepared by different manufacturers can differ in both volume and nitroglycerin concentration, the label must be read carefully when dilutions are made.

Administration should be performed using a glass IV bottle and the administration set provided by the manufacturer. Nitroglycerin absorbs into standard polyvinyl chloride tubing, and hence this tubing should be avoided.

Discontinuing Nitroglycerin

Long-acting preparations (transdermal patches, topical ointment, sustained-release oral tablets or capsules) should be discontinued slowly. If they are withdrawn abruptly, vasospasm may result.

Summary of Therapeutic Uses

Acute Therapy of Angina. For acute treatment of angina pectoris, nitroglycerin is administered in sublingual tablets, transmucosal tablets, and a translingual spray. All three formulations can be used to abort an ongoing anginal attack and to provide prophylaxis in anticipation of exertion.

Sustained Therapy of Angina. For sustained prophylaxis against angina, nitroglycerin is administered in the following formulations: transdermal patches, topical ointment, transmucosal tablets, and sustained-release oral tablets or capsules.

Intravenous Therapy. Intravenous nitroglycerin is indicated for perioperative control of blood pressure, production of controlled hypotension during surgery, and treatment of heart failure associated with acute MI. In addition, IV nitroglycerin is used to treat unstable angina and chronic angina when symptoms cannot be controlled with preferred medications.

Other Organic Nitrates

Isosorbide Mononitrate and Isosorbide Dinitrate. Both drugs have pharmacologic actions identical to those of nitroglycerin. Both drugs are used for angina, both are taken orally, and both produce headache, hypotension, and reflex tachycardia. Differences between them relate only to route of administration and time course of action. Time course determines whether a particular drug or dosage form will be used for acute therapy, sustained prophylaxis, or both. As with nitroglycerin, tolerance can develop to long-acting preparations. To avoid tolerance, long-acting preparations should be used on an intermittent schedule that allows at least 8 drug-free hours a day. Trade names, time courses, and dosages are summarized in Tables 49–2, 49–3, and 49–4, respectively.

Erythrityl Tetranitrate and Pentaerythritol Tetranitrate. These drugs have pharmacologic actions identical to those of nitroglycerin. Both have been withdrawn from the market in the United States. Information on dosage and time course can be found in prior editions of this text.

Amyl Nitrite

Amyl nitrite is an ultrashort-acting agent used to treat acute episodes of angina pectoris. The drug has the same mechanism as nitroglycerin. Amyl nitrite is a volatile liquid dispensed in glass ampules. For administration, an ampule is crushed, allowing the volatile compound to be inhaled. Effects begin within 30 seconds and terminate in 3 to 5 minutes. Amyl nitrite is highly flammable and hence should not be used near flame. The drug is reputed to intensify sexual orgasm and has been abused for that purpose (see Chapter 38).

BETA BLOCKERS

Beta blockers (e.g., propranolol, metoprolol) are important drugs for *stable angina,* but are *not* effective against vasospastic angina. When administered on a fixed schedule, beta blockers can provide sustained protection against effort-induced anginal pain. Exercise tolerance is increased and the frequency and intensity of anginal attacks are lowered. All of the beta blockers appear equally effective. In addition to reducing anginal pain, beta blockers decrease the risk of death, especially in patients with a prior MI.

Beta blockers reduce anginal pain primarily by *decreasing cardiac oxygen demand.* This is accomplished mainly through blockade of $beta_1$ receptors in the heart, which decreases heart rate and contractility. Beta blockers reduce oxygen demand further by causing a modest reduction in arterial pressure (afterload). In addition to decreasing oxygen demand, beta blockers help increase oxygen supply. How? By slowing heart rate, these drugs increase time in diastole, and thereby increase the time during which blood flows through myocardial vessels. (Recall that blood does not flow in these vessels during systole.) In patients taking vasodilators (e.g., nitroglycerin), beta blockers provide the additional benefit of blunting reflex tachycardia.

For treatment of stable angina, dosage should be low initially and then gradually increased. The dosing goal is to reduce resting heart rate to 50 to 60 beats/min, and limit exertional heart rate to about 100 beats/min. Beta blockers should not be withdrawn abruptly, since doing so can increase the incidence and intensity of anginal attacks, and may even precipitate MI.

Beta blockers can produce a variety of adverse effects. Blockade of cardiac $beta_1$ receptors can produce *bradycardia, decreased atrioventricular (AV) conduction,* and *reduction of contractility.* Consequently, beta blockers should not be used by patients with sick sinus syndrome, heart failure, or second- or third-degree AV block. Blockade of $beta_2$ receptors in the lung can promote bronchoconstriction. Accordingly, beta blockers should be avoided by patients with asthma. If an asthmatic individual absolutely must use a beta blocker, a $beta_1$-selective agent (e.g., metoprolol) should be selected. Beta blockers can mask signs of hypoglycemia, and therefore must be used with caution in patients with diabetes. Through effects on the central nervous system, these drugs can cause *insomnia, depression, bizarre dreams,* and *sexual dysfunction.*

The basic pharmacology of the beta blockers is discussed in Chapter 18.

CALCIUM CHANNEL BLOCKERS

The calcium channel blockers used most frequently are *verapamil, diltiazem,* and *nifedipine* (a dihydropyridine-type calcium channel blocker). Accordingly, our discussion focuses on these three drugs. *All three* can block calcium channels in VSM, primarily in arterioles. The result is arteriolar dilation and reduction of peripheral resistance (afterload). In addition, all three can relax coronary vasospasm. *Verapamil* and *diltiazem* also block calcium channels in the heart, and can thereby decrease heart rate, AV conduction, and contractility.

Calcium channel blockers are used to treat both stable angina and variant angina. In *variant angina,* these drugs promote relaxation of coronary artery spasm, thereby *increasing cardiac oxygen supply.* In *stable angina,* these drugs promote relaxation of peripheral arterioles; the resultant decrease in afterload *reduces cardiac oxygen demand.* Verapamil and diltiazem can produce modest additional reductions in oxygen demand by suppressing heart rate and contractility.

The major adverse effects of the calcium channel blockers are cardiovascular. Dilation of peripheral arterioles lowers blood pressure, and can thereby induce *reflex tachycardia.* This reaction is greatest with nifedipine and minimal with verapamil and diltiazem. Because of their suppressant effects on the heart, verapamil and diltiazem must be used cautiously in patients taking beta blockers and in patients with bradycardia, heart failure, or AV block. These precautions do not apply to nifedipine or other dihydropyridines.

The basic pharmacology of the calcium-channel blockers is discussed in Chapter 43.

REVASCULARIZATION THERAPY: CABG AND PTCA

If drug therapy of angina fails to control symptoms, surgical revascularization should be considered. The two principal forms of revascularization are coronary artery bypass grafting (CABG) and percutaneous transluminal coronary angioplasty (PTCA).

Coronary Artery Bypass Graft Surgery

CABG surgery is used to increase blood flow to ischemic areas of the heart. In this procedure, one end of a segment of healthy blood vessel (internal mammary artery or saphenous vein) is grafted onto the aorta, and the other end is connected to the diseased coronary artery at a point distal to the region of atherosclerotic plaque. Hence, the graft constitutes a shunt whereby blood flow can circumvent the occluded section of a diseased coronary vessel. Following surgery, most patients remain in the hospital for a week, and then recuperate for another 6 weeks at home. Once considered exotic, CABG surgery is now commonplace; more than 300,000 Americans undergo the procedure each year.

Vessel blockage can recur over time, thereby requiring repeat surgery. When an artery is used for the graft, the incidence of reblockage is only 4% after 10 years. In contrast, when a vein is used, the incidence of reblockage is nearly 50% after 10 years.

A relatively new procedure, called *minimally invasive direct coronary artery bypass* (MIDCAB) surgery, is an alternative to CABG surgery for some patients. MIDCAB surgery is much less invasive than CABG surgery, and therefore faster and cheaper. Furthermore, MIDCAB surgery is performed on the beating heart; hence, heart-lung bypass machinery is not needed. At this time, MIDCAB surgery is used only to bypass blockage in the left ascending coronary artery.

Percutaneous Transluminal Coronary Angioplasty

PTCA is an alternative to CABG surgery for patients with stable angina. In the most common form of PTCA, known as balloon angioplasty, a miniature catheter containing a deflated balloon is inserted into the femoral artery, threaded up into the aorta, and then manipulated into the occluded coronary artery. The balloon is then inflated, thereby flattening the obstruction and allowing blood to flow. In the vast majority of these procedures, the cardiologist implants a stent (a tiny tube made of stainless steel mesh) to help prevent restenosis. (Restenosis is caused by hyperplasia of neointimal cells and constrictive remodeling of the injured artery.) Unfortunately, even with stenting, restenosis remains a troublesome problem. Recent studies indicate that restenosis can be significantly reduced by localized intracoronary irradiation. PTCA is performed on over 500,000 North Americans each year.

Comparison of CABG Surgery with PTCA

CABG surgery and PTCA are equally safe and almost equally effective. The 5-year survival rate after either procedure is about 90%. However, in other respects, the procedures differ substantially. Compared with PTCA, CABG surgery is more traumatic and more expensive, requires a longer hospital stay, and recovery is slower. On the other hand, CABG surgery is more effective: coronary blood flow is better, relief of angina is superior, exercise tolerance is higher, and patients require less antianginal medication. Moreover, the incidence of reblockage after CABG surgery is far less. For example, in one study, the rate of reblockage 5 years after PTCA was 54%, compared with only 8% 5 years after CABG surgery. At this time, CABG surgery is considered the treatment of choice for patients with multivessel disease. For patients with single-vessel disease, either procedure is generally appropriate; the choice between them is based on patient preference.

SUMMARY OF TREATMENT MEASURES

Guidelines for Management of Chronic Stable Angina

In 1999, three organizations—the American Heart Association, the American College of Cardiology, and the American College of Physicians–American Society of Internal Medicine—joined forces to produce the first national guidelines on the management of chronic stable angina. In the fall of 2002, the guidelines were updated. The update, titled *ACC/AHA 2000 Guideline Update for the Management of Patients with Chronic Stable Angina,* is available free online at *www.acc.org* and *www.americanheart.org.* The discussion below reflects recommendations in these guidelines.

Treatment of stable angina has two objectives: (1) prevention of MI and death, and (2) reduction of cardiac ischemia and associated anginal pain. Although both goals are desirable, prevention of MI and death is clearly more important. Hence, if two treatments are equally effective at decreasing anginal pain, but one also decreases the risk of death, then the one that decreases the risk of death is preferred.

Drugs Used to Prevent Myocardial Infarction and Death

We now have medical treatments that can decrease the risk of MI and death in patients with chronic stable angina. Therapy directed at prevention of MI and death is a new paradigm in the management of stable angina, and all practitioners should become familiar with it.

Antiplatelet Drugs. These agents decrease platelet aggregation and thereby decrease the risk of thrombus formation in coronary arteries. The most effective agents are *aspirin* and *clopidogrel.* In patients with stable angina, low-dose aspirin produces a 33% decrease in the risk of adverse cardiovascular events. Benefits of clopidogrel seem equal to those of aspirin, although they are not as well documented. The guidelines recommend that all patients with stable angina take 75 to 325 mg of aspirin daily, unless there is a specific reason not to. Aspirin, clopidogrel, and other antiplatelet drugs are discussed in Chapter 50.

Cholesterol-Lowering Drugs. Elevated cholesterol is a major risk factor for coronary atherosclerosis. Drugs that lower cholesterol can slow the progression of CAD, stabilize atherosclerotic plaques, and even cause plaque regression. Therapies that reduce cholesterol are associated with decreased mortality from coronary heart disease. For example, in patients with established CAD, treatment with simvastatin decreased the risk of mortality by 35%. Because of the well-established benefits of cholesterol-lowering therapy, the guidelines recommend that all patients with stable angina receive a cholesterol-lowering drug. The pharmacology of the cholesterol-lowering drugs is discussed in Chapter 48.

Angiotensin-Converting Enzyme (ACE) Inhibitors. There is strong evidence that, in patients with CAD, ACE inhibitors greatly reduce the incidence of adverse outcomes. In the Heart Outcomes Prevention Evaluation (HOPE) trial, for example, ramipril reduced the incidence of stroke, MI, and cardiovascular death. Among one subset of patients—those with diabetes—benefits were particularly striking. Ramipril decreased the risk of stroke by 33%, MI by 22%, and cardiovascular death by 37%; in addition, the drug reduced the risk of nephropathy, retinopathy, and other microvascular complications of diabetes. Because of these well-documented benefits, the guidelines now recommend ACE inhibitors for most patients with established CAD, and especially for those with diabetes. The pharmacology of the ACE inhibitors is discussed in Chapter 42.

Antianginal Agents: Drugs Used to Reduce Anginal Pain

The goal of antianginal therapy is to achieve complete (or nearly complete) elimination of anginal pain—along with a return to normal activities. This should be accomplished with a minimum of adverse drug effects.

The basic strategy of antianginal therapy is to provide baseline protection using one or more long-acting drugs (beta blocker, calcium channel blocker, long-acting nitrate) supplemented with sublingual nitroglycerin when breakthrough pain occurs. A flow plan for drug selection is shown in Figure 49–3. As indicated, treatment is approached sequentially. Progression from one step to the next is based on patient response. Some patients can be treated with a single long-acting drug, some require two or three, and some require revascularization.

Initial treatment consists of sublingual nitroglycerin plus a long-acting antianginal drug. As indicated in Figure 49–3, beta blockers are the preferred agents for baseline therapy. Why? Because they can decrease mortality, especially in patients with a prior MI. In addition to providing prophylaxis, beta blockers suppress nitrate-induced reflex tachycardia.

If a beta blocker is inadequate, or if there are contraindications to beta blockade, a long-acting calcium channel blocker should be added or substituted. Since calcium channel blockers do not promote bronchoconstriction, they are preferred to beta blockers for patients with asthma. Dihydropyridine-type calcium channel blockers (e.g., nifedipine) lack cardiosuppressant actions, and hence are safer than beta blockers for patients with bradycardia, AV block, or heart failure. When a calcium channel blocker is to be *combined* with a beta

blocker, a dihydropyridine is preferred to verapamil or diltiazem. Why? Because verapamil and diltiazem will intensify the cardiosuppressant actions of the beta blocker, whereas a dihydropyridine will not.

If a calcium channel blocker is inadequate, or if there are contraindications to calcium channel blockade, a long-acting

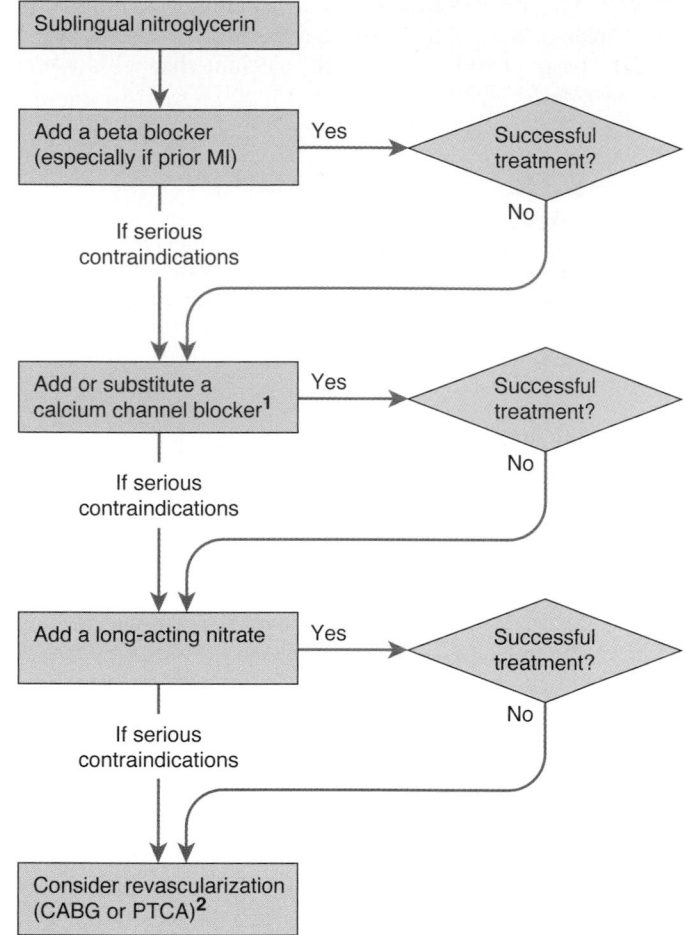

Figure 49–3 ■ **Flow plan for antianginal drug selection in patients with chronic stable angina.**
[1]Avoid short-acting dihydropyridines.
[2]At any point in this process, based on coronary anatomy, severity of angina symptoms, and patient preference, it is reasonable to consider evaluation for coronary revascularization (PTCA or CABG). Unless a patient is documented to have left main, three-vessel, or two-vessel CAD with significant stenosis of the proximal left anterior descending coronary artery, there is no demonstrated survival advantage associated with CABG or PTCA in low-risk patients with chronic stable angina. Accordingly, medical therapy should be attempted in most patients before considering PTCA or CABG. (Adapted from Gibbons RJ, Chatterjee K, Daley J, et al. ACC/AHA 2002 guideline update for the management of patients with chronic stable angina: A report of the American College of Cardiology/ American Heart Association Task Force on Practice Guidelines [Committee to Update the 1999 Guidelines for the Management of Patients with Chronic Stable Angina]. 2002. Available at *www.acc.org/clinical/guidelines/stable/stable.pdf*)

nitrate (e.g., transdermal nitroglycerin) should be added or substituted. However, because tolerance can develop quickly, these preparations are less well suited than beta blockers or calcium channel blockers for continuous protection.

Note that, as we proceed along the drug-selection flow plan, drugs are *added* to the regimen, resulting in treatment with two or more agents. Combination therapy increases our chances of success because oxygen demand is decreased by multiple mechanisms: beta blockers reduce heart rate and contractility; calcium channel blockers reduce afterload (by dilating arterioles); and nitrates reduce preload (by dilating veins).

If combined treatment with a beta blocker, calcium channel blocker, and long-acting nitrate fails to provide relief, CABG surgery or PTCA may be indicated. Note that these invasive procedures should be considered only after more conservative treatment has been tried.

How should we treat angina in patients who have a coexisting condition? The antianginal drugs employed—nitrates, beta blockers, and calcium channel blockers—are the same ones used in patients who have angina alone. However, when selecting among these drugs, we must consider the coexisting disorder as well as the angina. For example, as noted above, in patients with asthma, calcium channel blockers are preferred to beta blockers (because beta blockers promote bronchoconstriction, whereas calcium channel blockers do not). Table 49–5 lists over 20 coexisting conditions, and indicates which antianginal agents to use as well as which ones to avoid.

TABLE 49–5 ■ Choosing Between Beta Blockers and Calcium Channel Blockers for Treating Angina in Patients Who Have a Coexisting Condition

Coexisting Condition	Recommended Treatment (Alternative Treatment)	Drugs to Avoid
Medical Conditions		
Systemic hypertension	Beta blockers (long-acting, slow-release CCBs)	
Migraine or vascular headache	Beta blockers (verapamil or diltiazem)	
Asthma or COPD with bronchospasm	Verapamil or diltiazem	Beta blockers
Hyperthyroidism	Beta blockers	
Raynaud's syndrome	Long-acting, slow-release CCBs	Beta blockers
Type 1 diabetes	Beta blockers, particularly if prior MI, or long-acting, slow-release CCBs	
Type 2 diabetes	Beta blockers or long-acting, slow-release CCBs	
Depression	Long-acting, slow-release CCBs	Beta blockers
Mild peripheral vascular disease	Beta blockers or long-acting, slow-release CCBs	
Severe peripheral vascular disease with ischemia at rest	Long-acting, slow-release CCBs	Beta blockers
Cardiac Dysrhythmias and Conduction Abnormalities		
Sinus bradycardia	Long-acting, slow-release CCBs that do not decrease heart rate	Beta blockers, diltiazem, verapamil
Sinus tachycardia (not due to heart failure)	Beta blockers	
Supraventricular tachycardia	Verapamil, diltiazem, or beta blockers	
AV block	Long-acting, slow-release CCBs that do not slow AV conduction	Beta blockers, diltiazem, verapamil
Rapid atrial fibrillation (with digoxin)	Verapamil, diltiazem, or beta blockers	
Ventricular dysrhythmias	Beta blockers	
Left Ventricular Dysfunction		
Congestive heart failure		
Mild (LVEF ≥40%)	Beta blockers	
Moderate to severe (LVEF <40%)	Amlodipine or felodipine (nitrates)	Diltiazem, verapamil
Left-sided valvular heart disease		
Mild aortic stenosis	Beta blockers	
Aortic insufficiency	Long-acting, slow-release dihydropyridine CCBs	
Mitral regurgitation	Long-acting, slow-release dihydropyridine CCBs	
Mitral stenosis	Beta blockers	
Hypertropic cardiomyopathy	Beta blockers, verapamil, diltiazem	Dihydropyridine CCBs, nitrates

AV = atrioventricular, CCB = calcium channel blocker, COPD = chronic obstructive pulmonary disease, LVEF = left ventricular ejection fraction, MI = myocardial infarction.
Adapted from Gibbons RJ, Chatterjee K, Daley J, et al. ACC/AHA 2002 guideline update for the management of patients with chronic stable angina: A report of the American College of Cardiology/American Heart Association Task Force on Practice Guidelines (Committee to Update the 1999 Guidelines for the Management of Patients With Chronic Stable Angina). 2002. Available at *www.acc.org/clinical/guidelines/stable/stable.pdf*

Reduction of Risk Factors

The treatment program should reduce anginal risk factors: smokers should quit; obese patients should lose weight; sedentary patients should get aerobic exercise; and patients with diabetes, hypertension, or high cholesterol should receive appropriate therapy.

Smoking. Smoking increases the risk of cardiovascular mortality by 50%. Fortunately, smoking cessation greatly decreases cardiovascular risk. Accordingly, all patients who smoke should be strongly encouraged to quit. Drugs employed as an aid to smoking cessation are discussed in Chapter 38.

High Cholesterol. As noted, high cholesterol levels increase the risk of adverse cardiovascular events, and therapies that reduce cholesterol reduce that risk. Accordingly, all patients with high cholesterol levels should receive cholesterol-lowering therapy.

Hypertension. High blood pressure increases the risk of cardiovascular mortality, and lowering blood pressure reduces the risk. Accordingly, all patients with hypertension should receive treatment. Blood pressure should be reduced to 140/90 mm Hg or less. In patients with additional risk factors (e.g., diabetes, heart failure, retinopathy), the target blood pressure is 130/80 mm Hg or less. Management of hypertension is discussed at length in Chapter 45.

Diabetes. Both type 1 (insulin-dependent) and type 2 (non–insulin-dependent) diabetes increase the risk of cardiovascular mortality. Type 1 increases the risk 3- to 10-fold; type 2 increases the risk 2- to 4-fold. Although there is good evidence that tight glycemic control decreases the risk of microvascular complications of diabetes, there is little evidence to show that tight glycemic control decreases the risk of cardiovascular complications. Nonetheless, it is prudent to strive for optimal glycemic control.

Obesity. Obesity is associated with an increased risk of coronary disease and mortality; weight reduction is likely to reduce that risk. Accordingly, a program of diet and exercise is recommended for all patients whose body weight exceeds 120% of ideal. Weight reduction is especially important for patients with diabetes, hypertension, and hypertriglyceridemia. Obesity and its management are discussed at length in Chapter 78.

Physical Inactivity. Increased physical activity has multiple benefits. In patients with chronic stable angina, exercise increases exercise tolerance and the sense of well-being, and decreases anginal symptoms, cholesterol levels, and objective measures of ischemia. Accordingly, the guidelines recommend that patients perform 30 to 60 minutes of a moderate-intensity activity 3 to 4 times a week. Such activities include walking, jogging, cycling, and other aerobic exercises. Exercise by moderate- to high-risk patients should be medically supervised.

Management of Variant Angina

Treatment of vasospastic angina can proceed in three steps. For initial therapy, either a calcium channel blocker or a long-acting nitrate is selected. If either drug alone is inadequate, then combined therapy with a calcium channel blocker *plus* a nitrate should be tried. If the combination fails to control symptoms, CABG surgery may be indicated. Beta blockers are not effective in vasospastic angina.

⠿ KEY POINTS

- Anginal pain occurs when cardiac oxygen supply is insufficient to meet oxygen demand.
- Cardiac oxygen demand is determined by heart rate, contractility, preload, and afterload. Drugs that reduce these factors will help relieve anginal pain.
- Cardiac oxygen supply is determined by myocardial blood flow. Drugs that increase oxygen supply will reduce anginal pain.
- Angina pectoris has three forms: chronic stable angina, variant (vasospastic) angina, and unstable angina.
- The underlying cause of stable angina is coronary artery atherosclerosis.
- The underlying cause of variant angina is coronary artery spasm.
- Drugs relieve pain of stable angina by decreasing cardiac oxygen demand. They do not increase oxygen supply.
- Drugs relieve pain of variant angina by increasing cardiac oxygen supply. They do not decrease oxygen demand.
- Nitroglycerin and other organic nitrates are vasodilators.
- To cause vasodilation, nitroglycerin must first be converted to nitric oxide, its active form. This reaction requires a sulfhydryl source.
- Nitroglycerin relieves pain of stable angina by dilating veins, which decreases venous return, which decreases preload, which decreases oxygen demand.
- Nitroglycerin relieves pain of variant angina by relaxing coronary vasospasm, which increases oxygen supply.
- Nitroglycerin is highly lipid soluble, and therefore readily absorbed through the oral mucosa and skin.
- Nitroglycerin undergoes very rapid inactivation in the liver. Hence, when the drug is administered orally, most of each dose is destroyed before reaching the systemic circulation.
- When nitroglycerin is administered sublingually, it is absorbed directly into the systemic circulation, and therefore temporarily bypasses the liver. Hence, to produce equivalent effects, sublingual doses can be much smaller than oral doses.
- Nitroglycerin causes three characteristic side effects: headache, orthostatic hypotension, and reflex tachycardia. All three occur secondary to vasodilation.
- Reflex tachycardia from nitroglycerin can be prevented with a beta blocker, verapamil, or diltiazem.
- Continuous use of nitroglycerin can produce tolerance within 24 hours. The mechanism may be depletion of sulfhydryl groups.
- To prevent tolerance, nitroglycerin should be used in the lowest effective dosage, and long-acting formulations should be used on an intermittent schedule that allows at least 8 drug-free hours every day, usually during the night.
- Nitroglycerin preparations that have a rapid onset (e.g., sublingual nitroglycerin) are used to abort an ongoing anginal attack and to provide acute prophylaxis when exertion is expected. Administration is PRN.

- Nitroglycerin preparations that have a long duration (e.g., patches, sustained-release oral tablets) are used for extended protection against anginal attacks. Administration is on a fixed schedule (but one that allows at least 8 drug-free hours each day).
- Beta blockers prevent pain of stable angina primarily by decreasing heart rate and contractility, which reduces cardiac oxygen demand.
- Beta blockers are administered on a fixed schedule, not PRN.
- Beta blockers are not used for variant angina.
- Calcium channel blockers relieve pain of stable angina by reducing cardiac oxygen demand. Two mechanisms are involved. First, all calcium channel blockers relax peripheral arterioles, and thereby decrease afterload. Second, verapamil and diltiazem reduce heart rate and contractility (in addition to decreasing afterload).
- Calcium channel blockers relieve pain of variant angina by increasing cardiac oxygen supply. The mechanism is relaxation of coronary artery spasm.

- When a calcium channel blocker is combined with a beta blocker, a dihydropyridine (e.g., nifedipine) is preferred to verapamil or diltiazem. Why? Because verapamil and diltiazem will intensify cardiosuppression caused by the beta blocker, whereas a dihydropyridine will not.
- In patients with chronic stable angina, treatment has two objectives: (1) prevention of MI and death and (2) prevention of anginal pain.
- The risk of MI and death can be decreased with two types of drugs: (1) antiplatelet agents (e.g., aspirin) and (2) cholesterol-lowering drugs.
- Anginal pain is prevented with one or more long-acting antianginal drugs (beta blocker, calcium channel blocker, long-acting nitrate) supplemented with sublingual nitroglycerin when breakthrough pain occurs.
- As a rule, revascularization with CABG surgery or PTCA is indicated only after treatment with two or three antianginal drugs has failed.

Summary of Major Nursing Implications*

NITROGLYCERIN

Preadministration Assessment

Therapeutic Goal

Reduction of the frequency and intensity of anginal attacks.

Baseline Data

Obtain baseline data on the frequency and intensity of anginal attacks, the location of anginal pain, and the factors that precipitate attacks.

The patient interview and physical examination should identify risk factors for angina pectoris, including treatable contributing pathophysiologic conditions (e.g., hypertension, hyperlipidemia).

Identifying High-Risk Patients

Use with *caution* in hypotensive patients and patients taking drugs that can lower blood pressure, including alcohol and antihypertensive medications. Do not combine with sildenafil [Viagra].

Implementation: Administration

Routes and Administration

Sublingual Tablets. Use: prophylaxis or termination of an acute anginal attack.

Instruct patients to place the tablet under the tongue and leave it there until fully dissolved; the tablet should not be swallowed.

Inform patients that if 1 tablet fails to relieve pain, 1 or 2 additional tablets should be taken at 5-minute intervals. Instruct patients to seek medical help immediately if pain is not relieved within 15 minutes.

Instruct patients to store tablets in a dark, tightly closed bottle that contains no other medications. Instruct patients to write the date of opening on the bottle and to discard unused medication after 6 months.

Sustained-Release Oral Tablets and Capsules. Use: sustained protection against anginal attacks.

To avoid tolerance, administer only once or twice daily.

Instruct patients to swallow these preparations intact, without chewing or crushing.

Transdermal Delivery Systems. Use: sustained protection against anginal attacks.

Instruct patients to apply transdermal patches to a hairless area of skin, using a new patch and a different site each day.

Instruct patients to remove the patch after 12 to 14 hours, allowing 10 to 12 "patch-free" hours each day. This will prevent tolerance.

Intravenous. Uses: (1) angina pectoris refractory to more conventional therapy, (2) perioperative control of blood pressure, (3) production of controlled hypotension during surgery, and (4) heart failure associated with acute MI.

Technique of administration: Perform IV administration using a glass IV bottle and the administration set provided by the manufacturer; avoid standard IV tubing. Dilute stock solutions before use.

Administer by continuous infusion. The rate is slow initially (5 μg/min) and then gradually increased until an adequate response is achieved.

Monitor cardiovascular status constantly.

Translingual Spray. Use: prophylaxis or termination of an acute anginal attack.

*Patient education information is highlighted as blue text.

Summary of Major Nursing Implications*—cont'd

Technique of administration: Instruct patients to direct the spray against the oral mucosa. Warn patients not to inhale the spray.

Transmucosal (Buccal) Tablets. *Uses:* (1) prophylaxis or termination of an acute anginal attack and (2) sustained prophylaxis.

Technique of administration: Instruct patients to place the transmucosal tablet between the upper lip and the gum or in the buccal area between the cheek and the gum. Inform patients that the tablet will adhere to the oral mucosa and slowly dissolve over 3 to 5 hours. To achieve sustained prophylaxis, a tablet should be administered every 3 to 8 hours.

Topical Ointment. *Use:* sustained protection against anginal attacks.

Before applying a new dose, remove ointment remaining from the previous dose.

Technique of administration: (1) squeeze a ribbon of ointment of prescribed length onto the applicator paper provided; (2) using the applicator paper, spread the ointment over a 6-inch by 6-inch area (application may be made to the chest, back, abdomen, upper arm, or anterior thigh); and (3) cover the ointment with plastic wrap. Avoid touching the ointment.

Rotate the application site to minimize local irritation.

Terminating Therapy

Warn patients against abrupt withdrawal of long-acting preparations (transdermal systems, topical ointment, sustained-release tablets and capsules).

Implementation: Measures to Enhance Therapeutic Effects

Reducing Risk Factors

Precipitating Factors. Advise patients to avoid activities that are likely to elicit an anginal attack (e.g., overexertion, heavy meals, emotional stress, cold exposure).

Weight Reduction. Help overweight patients develop a restricted-calorie diet. The diet should be low in saturated fats, and total fat should not exceed 30% of caloric intake. Target weight is 110% of ideal or less.

Exercise. Encourage patients who have a sedentary lifestyle to establish a regular program of aerobic exercise (e.g., walking, jogging, swimming, bicycling).

Smoking Cessation. Strongly encourage patients to quit smoking.

*Patient education information is highlighted as blue text.

Contributing Disease States. Ensure that patients with contributing pathology (especially hypertension or hypercholesterolemia) are receiving appropriate treatment.

Ongoing Evaluation and Interventions
Evaluating Therapeutic Effects

Have the patient keep a record of the frequency and intensity of anginal attacks, the location of anginal pain, and the factors that precipitate attacks.

Minimizing Adverse Effects

Headache. Inform patients that headache will diminish with continued drug use. Advise patients that headache can be relieved with aspirin, acetaminophen, or some other mild analgesic.

Orthostatic Hypotension. Inform patients about symptoms of hypotension (e.g., dizziness, lightheadedness), and advise them to sit or lie down if these occur. Inform patients that hypotension can be minimized by moving slowly when changing from a sitting or supine position to an upright posture.

Reflex Tachycardia. This reaction can be suppressed by concurrent treatment with a beta blocker, verapamil, or diltiazem.

Minimizing Adverse Interactions

Hypotensive Agents. Nitroglycerin can interact with other hypotensive drugs to produce excessive lowering of blood pressure. Advise patients to avoid alcohol. Exercise caution when nitroglycerin is used in combination with beta blockers, calcium channel blockers, diuretics, and all other drugs that can lower blood pressure. One hypotensive agent—sildenafil [Viagra]—should not be taken within 24 hours of nitroglycerin.

ISOSORBIDE MONONITRATE AND ISOSORBIDE DINITRATE

Both drugs have pharmacologic actions identical to those of nitroglycerin. Differences relate only to dosage forms, routes of administration, and time course of action. Hence, the implications presented for nitroglycerin apply to these drugs as well.

Anticoagulant, Antiplatelet, and Thrombolytic Drugs

The drugs discussed in this chapter are used to prevent formation of thrombi (intravascular blood clots) and to dissolve thrombi that have already formed. These drugs act in several ways: some suppress coagulation, some inhibit platelet aggregation, and some promote clot dissolution. All of these drugs interfere with normal hemostasis. As a result, all carry a significant risk of hemorrhage.

PHYSIOLOGY AND PATHOPHYSIOLOGY OF COAGULATION

Hemostasis

Hemostasis is the physiologic process by which bleeding is stopped. Hemostasis occurs in two stages: (1) formation of a platelet plug, followed by (2) reinforcement of the platelet plug with fibrin. Both processes are set in motion by blood vessel injury.

Stage One: Formation of a Platelet Plug. Platelet aggregation is initiated when platelets come in contact with collagen on the exposed surface of a damaged blood vessel. In response to contact with collagen, platelets adhere to the site of vessel injury. Adhesion initiates platelet *activation,* which in turn leads to massive platelet *aggregation.*

Platelet aggregation is a complex process that ends with formation of *fibrinogen bridges* between *glycoprotein IIb/IIIa (GP IIb/IIIa) receptors* on adjacent platelets (Fig. 50–1). In order for these bridges to form, GP IIb/IIIa receptors must first undergo activation—that is, they must undergo a configurational change that allows them to bind with fibrinogen. As indicated in Figure 50–1A, activation of GP IIb/IIIa can be stimulated by multiple factors, including thromboxane A$_2$ (TXA$_2$), thrombin, collagen, platelet activating factor, and ADP. Under the influence of these factors, GP IIb/IIIa changes its shape, binds with fibrinogen, and thereby causes aggregation (Fig. 50–1B). The aggregated platelets constitute a plug that stops bleeding. This plug is unstable, however, and must be reinforced with fibrin if protection is to last.

Stage Two: Coagulation. Coagulation is defined as production of fibrin, a protein that reinforces the platelet plug. Fibrin is produced by way of two convergent pathways (Fig. 50–2). Both consist of a series of cascading reactions. These pathways are referred to as the *intrinsic system* and the *extrinsic system.* The intrinsic system is so named because all necessary clotting factors are present within the vascular system. The extrinsic system is so named because tissue thromboplastin, a factor from outside the vascular system, is required for the extrinsic system to work. As Figure 50–2 indicates, the two systems converge at factor Xa, after which they employ the same final series of reactions. Both systems are required for optimal production of fibrin.

Characteristic of both the intrinsic and extrinsic systems is the fact that each reaction in these sequences serves to enhance the reaction that follows (see Fig. 50–2). Looking at the intrinsic system, we can see that the reaction cascade

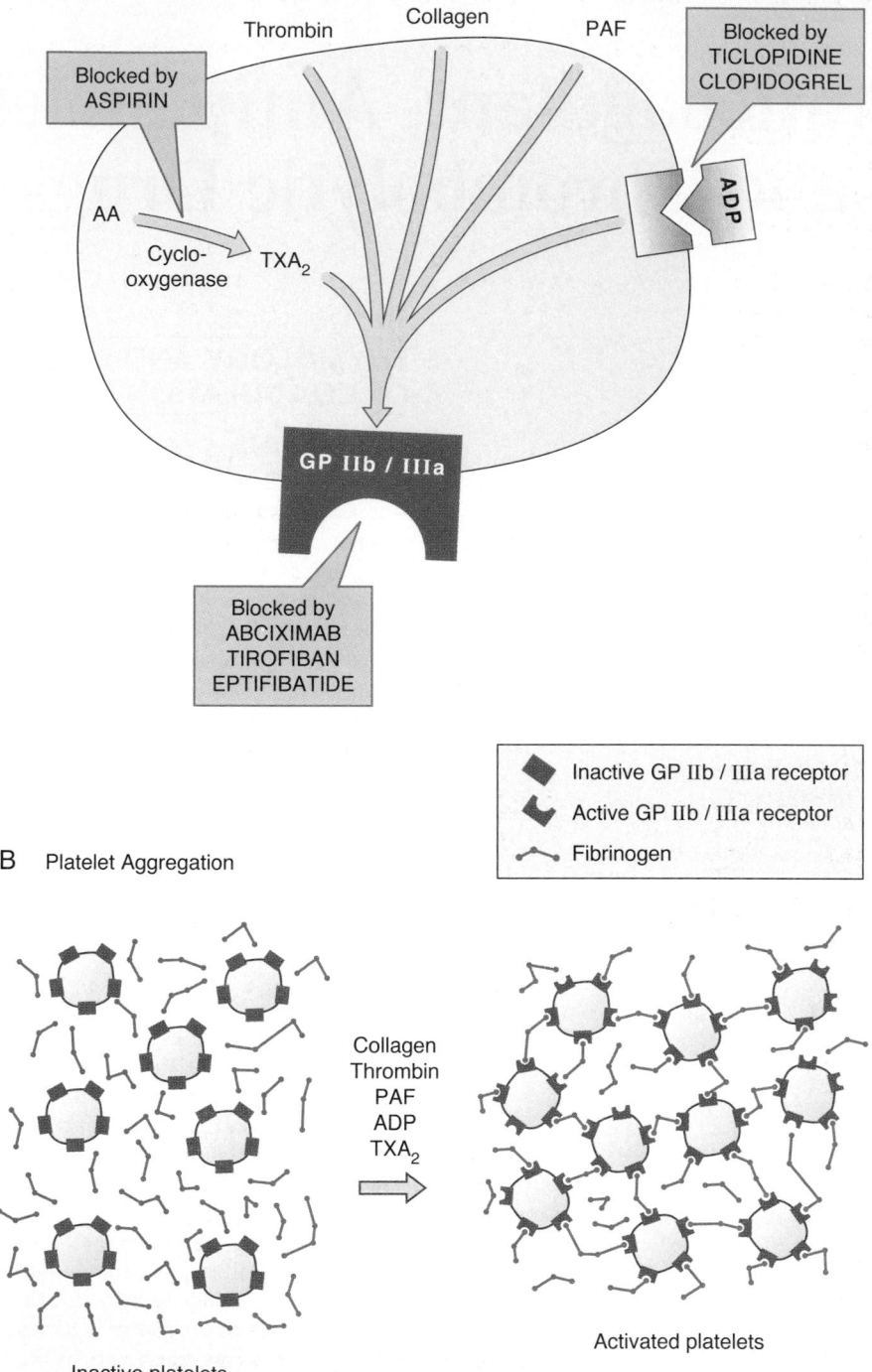

Figure 50–1 ■ **Mechanism of platelet aggregation and actions of antiplatelet drugs.**
A, Multiple factors—TXA$_2$, thrombin, collagen, PAF, ADP—promote activation of the GP IIb/IIIa receptor. Each platelet has 50,000 to 80,000 GP IIb/IIIa receptors, although only one is shown. *B,* Activation of the GP IIb/IIIa receptor permits binding of fibrinogen, which then causes aggregation by forming cross-links between platelets.

(AA = arachidonic acid, ADP = adenosine diphosphate, GP IIb/IIIa = glycoprotein IIb/IIIa receptor, PAF = platelet activation factor, TXA$_2$ = thromboxane A2.)

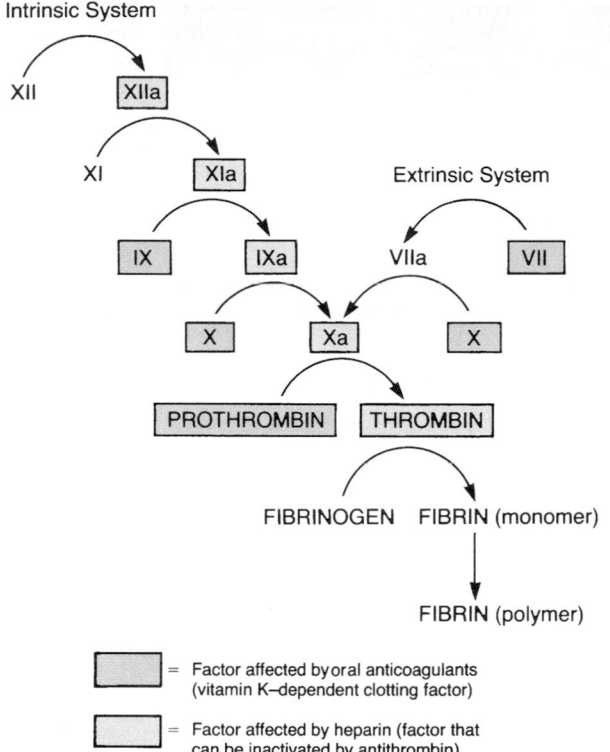

Figure 50–2 ▪ Outline of the coagulation cascade showing factors affected by anticoagulant drugs.
Common names for factors shown: VII = proconvertin, IX = Christmas factor, X = Stuart factor, XI = plasma thromboplastin antecedent, and XII = Hageman factor.

begins with the conversion of clotting factor XII into its active form, XIIa. The active form of factor XII then stimulates the conversion of factor XI into its active form (XIa), and so on. Hence, once the sequence is initiated, it becomes self-sustaining and self-reinforcing.

Important to our understanding of anticoagulant drugs is the fact that *four coagulation factors—factors VII, IX, X, and prothrombin—require vitamin K for their synthesis.* These factors appear in green boxes in Figure 50–2. The significance of the vitamin K–dependent factors will become apparent when we discuss warfarin, an oral anticoagulant.

Keeping Hemostasis Under Control. To protect against widespread coagulation, the body must inactivate any clotting factors that stray from the site of vessel injury. This inactivation is accomplished with *antithrombin* (formerly known as *antithrombin III*), a protein that forms a complex with clotting factors, and thereby inhibits their activity. The clotting factors that can be neutralized by antithrombin appear in amber-colored boxes in Figure 50–2. As we shall see, antithrombin is intimately involved in the action of *heparin*, an injectable anticoagulant drug.

Physiologic Removal of Clots. As healing of an injured vessel proceeds, removal of the clot is eventually necessary. The body accomplishes this with *plasmin*, an enzyme that digests the fibrin meshwork of the clot. Plasmin is produced through the activation of its precursor, *plasminogen.* The *thrombolytic drugs*—streptokinase, uro-

kinase, alteplase, and anistreplase—act by promoting conversion of plasminogen into plasmin.

Thrombosis

A thrombus is a blood clot formed within a blood vessel or within the heart. Thrombosis (thrombus formation) reflects pathologic functioning of hemostatic mechanisms.

Arterial Thrombosis. Formation of an arterial thrombus begins with adhesion of platelets to the arterial wall. (Adhesion is stimulated by damage to the wall or rupture of an atherosclerotic plaque.) Following adhesion, platelets release ADP and TXA_2, and thereby attract additional platelets to the evolving thrombus. With continued platelet aggregation, occlusion of the artery takes place. As blood flow comes to a stop, the coagulation cascade is initiated, causing the original plug to undergo reinforcement with fibrin. The consequence of an arterial thrombus is localized tissue injury owing to lack of perfusion.

Venous Thrombosis. Venous thrombi develop at sites where blood flow is slow. Stagnation of blood initiates the coagulation cascade, resulting in the production of fibrin, which enmeshes red blood cells and platelets to form the thrombus. The typical venous thrombus has a long tail that can break off to produce an *embolus.* Such emboli travel within the vascular system and become lodged at faraway sites, frequently the pulmonary arteries. Hence, unlike an arterial thrombus, whose harmful effects are localized, injury from a venous thrombus occurs secondary to embolization at a site distant from the original thrombus.

OVERVIEW OF DRUGS USED TO TREAT THROMBOEMBOLIC DISORDERS

The drugs considered in this chapter fall into three major categories: (1) anticoagulants, (2) antiplatelet drugs, and (3) thrombolytic drugs. *Anticoagulants* (e.g., heparin, warfarin) are drugs that disrupt the coagulation cascade, and thereby suppress production of fibrin. *Antiplatelet drugs* (e.g., aspirin, tirofiban) inhibit platelet aggregation. *Thrombolytic drugs* (e.g., alteplase, streptokinase) promote lysis of fibrin, and thereby cause dissolution of thrombi. Characteristic features of these classes are summarized in Table 50–1.

Although the anticoagulants and the antiplatelet drugs both suppress thrombosis, they do so by different mechanisms. As a result, these drugs differ in their effects and applications. The *antiplatelet drugs* are most effective at preventing *arterial* thrombosis. Conversely, *anticoagulants* (heparin and warfarin) are most effective against *venous* thrombosis.

PARENTERAL ANTICOAGULANTS I: HEPARIN AND RELATED DRUGS

All of the anticoagulants discussed in this section share the same mechanism of action. Specifically, they greatly enhance the activity of antithrombin, a protein that inactivates two major clotting factors: thrombin and factor Xa. In the absence of thrombin and factor Xa, production of fibrin is reduced, and hence clotting is suppressed.

TABLE 50–1 ■ Overview of Drugs Used to Treat Thromboembolic Disorders			
Drug Class	**Prototype**	**Drug Action**	**Therapeutic Effect**
Anticoagulants: parenteral	Heparin	↓ Fibrin formation (by promoting inactivation of clotting factors)	Prevention of venous thrombosis
Anticoagulants: oral	Warfarin	↓ Fibrin formation (by decreasing synthesis of clotting factors)	Prevention of venous thrombosis
Antiplatelet drugs	Aspirin	↓ Platelet aggregation	Prevention of arterial thrombosis
Thrombolytic drugs	Streptokinase	Promotion of fibrin digestion	Removal of newly formed thrombi

Heparin (Unfractionated)

Heparin is a rapid-acting anticoagulant administered only by injection. Heparin differs from the oral anticoagulants in several respects, including mechanism of action, time course of effects, indications, and management of overdose.

Source

Heparin is present in a variety of mammalian tissues. The heparin employed clinically is prepared from two sources: lungs of cattle and intestines of pigs. The anticoagulant activity of heparin from either source is equivalent. Although heparin occurs naturally, its physiologic role is unknown.

Chemistry

Heparin is not a single molecule, but rather a mixture of long polysaccharide chains, with molecular weights that range from 3000 to 30,000. The active region is a unique pentasaccharide (five-sugar) sequence found randomly along the chain. An important feature of heparin's structure is the presence of many negatively charged groups. Because of these negative charges, heparin is highly polar, and hence cannot readily cross membranes.

Mechanism of Anticoagulant Action

Heparin suppresses coagulation by helping antithrombin inactivate clotting factors, primarily thrombin and factor Xa. As shown in Figure 50–3, binding of heparin to antithrombin produces a conformational change in antithrombin that greatly enhances its ability to inactivate both thrombin and factor Xa. However, the process of inactivating these two clotting factors is not identical. In order to inactivate thrombin, heparin must simultaneously bind with both thrombin and antithrombin, thereby forming a ternary complex (Fig. 50–3). In contrast, in order to inactivate factor Xa, heparin binds only with antithrombin, and not with factor Xa.

By promoting the inactivation of thrombin and factor Xa, heparin ultimately suppresses formation of fibrin. Since fibrin forms the framework of thrombi in *veins,* heparin is especially useful for prophylaxis of *venous thrombosis.* Because heparin, in combination with antithrombin, acts directly to inhibit clotting factor activity, the anticoagulant effects of heparin develop *quickly* (within minutes of IV administration). This contrasts with the oral anticoagulants, whose full effects take *days* to develop.

Pharmacokinetics

Absorption and Distribution. Because of its polarity and large size, heparin is unable to cross membranes, including those of the GI tract. Consequently, heparin cannot be absorbed if given orally, and therefore must be given by injection (IV or SC). Since it cannot cross membranes, heparin does not traverse the placenta and does not enter breast milk.

Protein and Tissue Binding. Heparin chains bind nonspecifically to plasma proteins, mononuclear cells, and endothelial cells. As a result, plasma levels of free heparin can be highly variable following IV or SC administration. Because of this variability, intensive monitoring is required (see below).

Metabolism and Excretion. Heparin undergoes hepatic metabolism followed by renal excretion. Under normal conditions, the half-life of heparin is short (about 1.5 hours). However, in patients with hepatic or renal disease, the half-life is increased.

Time Course of Effects. Therapy is initiated with a bolus IV injection and effects begin immediately. Duration of action is brief (hours) and varies with dosage. Effects are prolonged in patients with hepatic or renal impairment.

Therapeutic Uses

Heparin is a preferred anticoagulant for use during *pregnancy* and in situations that require rapid onset of anticoagulant effects, including *pulmonary embolism, evolving stroke,* and *massive deep vein thrombosis* (DVT). In addition, heparin is used for patients undergoing *open heart surgery* and *renal dialysis;* during these procedures, heparin serves to prevent coagulation in devices of extracorporeal circulation (heart-lung machines, dialyzers). Low-dose therapy is used to *prevent postoperative venous thrombosis.* Heparin may also be useful for treating *disseminated intravascular coagulation,* a complex disorder in which fibrin clots form throughout the vascular system and in which bleeding tendencies may be present; bleeding can occur because massive fibrin production consumes available supplies of clotting factors. Heparin is also used as an adjunct to thrombolytic therapy of *acute myocardial infarction* (MI).

Adverse Effects

Hemorrhage. Bleeding develops in about 10% of patients and is the principal complication of treatment. Hemorrhage can occur at any site and may be fatal. Patients should be

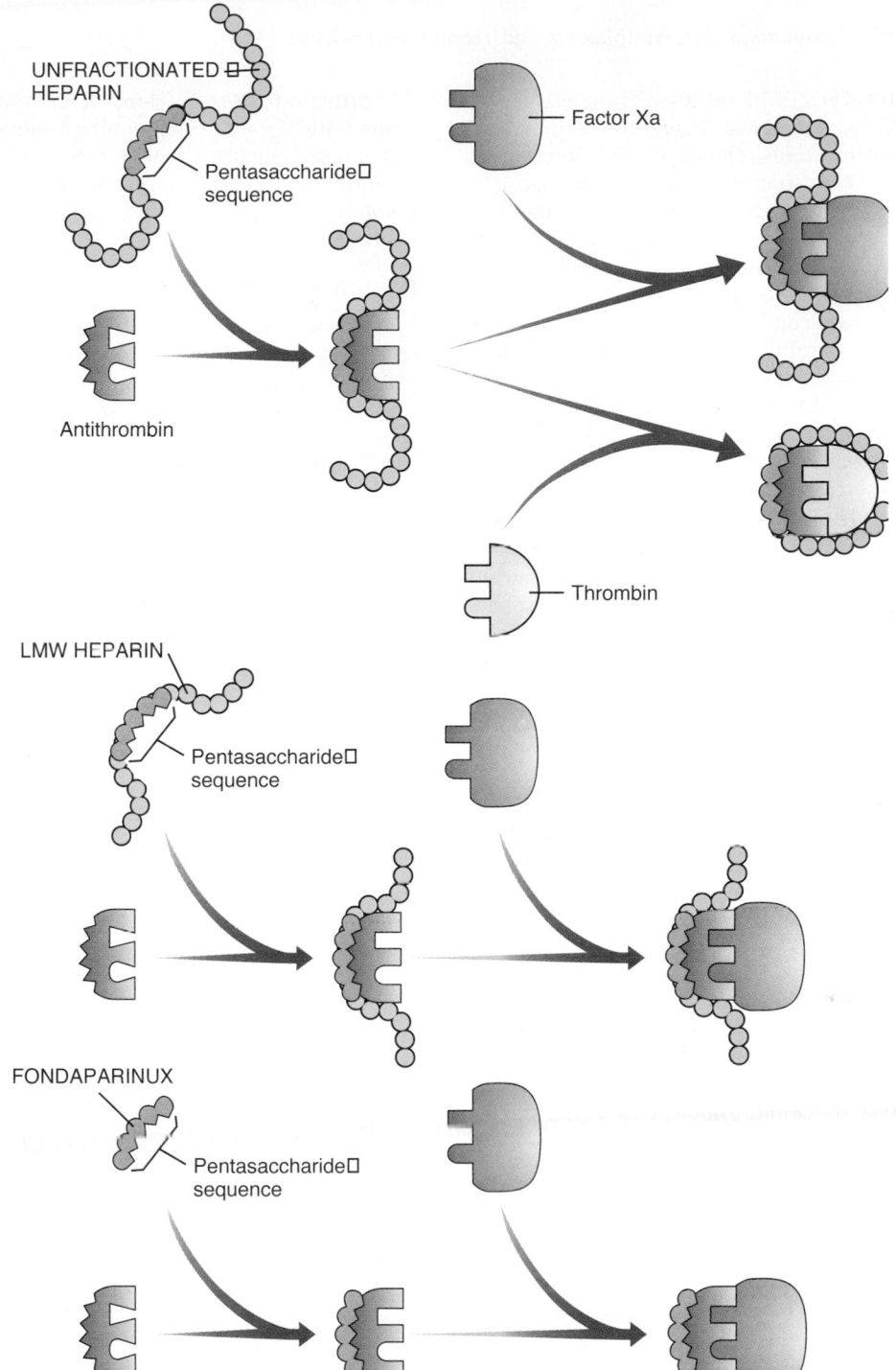

Figure 50–3 ■ Mechanism of action of heparin, LMW heparins, and fondaparinux.
All three drugs share a pentasaccharide sequence that allows them to bind with—and thereby activate—antithrombin, a protein that inactivates two major clotting factors: thrombin and factor Xa. All three drugs enable antithrombin to inactivate factor Xa, but only heparin also facilitates inactivation of thrombin.

Upper Panel: Unfractionated heparin binds with antithrombin, thereby causing a conformational change in antithrombin that greatly increases its ability to interact with factor Xa and thrombin. As shown, when the heparin-antithrombin complex binds with thrombin, heparin changes its conformation such that both heparin and antithrombin come in contact with thrombin. Formation of this ternary complex is necessary for thrombin inactivation. Inactivation of factor Xa is different: it only requires contact between activated antithrombin and factor Xa; contact between heparin and factor Xa is unnecessary.

Middle Panel: Low-molecular-weight (LMW) heparins have the same pentasaccharide sequence as unfractionated heparin, and hence can bind with and thereby activate antithrombin. However, in contrast to unfractionated heparin, which promotes inactivation of both thrombin and factor Xa, most molecules of LMW heparin can only inactivate factor Xa; they are unable to inactivate thrombin. Why? Because most molecules of LMW heparin are too small to form a ternary complex with thrombin and antithrombin.

Lower Panel: Fondaparinux is a synthetic pentasaccharide identical in structure to the antithrombin binding sequence found in unfractionated heparin and LMW heparins. Being even smaller than LMW heparins, fondaparinux is too small to form a ternary complex with thrombin, and hence can only inactivate factor Xa.

monitored closely for signs of blood loss. These include reduced blood pressure, increased heart rate, bruises, petechiae, hematomas, red or black stools, cloudy or discolored urine, pelvic pain (suggesting ovarian hemorrhage), headache or faintness (suggesting cerebral hemorrhage), and lumbar pain (suggesting adrenal hemorrhage). If bleeding develops, heparin should be withdrawn. Severe overdose can be treated with *protamine sulfate* (see below).

The risk of hemorrhage can be decreased in several ways. First, dosage should be carefully controlled so that the activated partial thromboplastin time (see below) does not exceed 2 times the control value. In addition, candidates for heparin therapy should be screened for risk factors (see *Warnings and Contraindications*). Finally, antiplatelet drugs (e.g., aspirin) should be avoided.

Heparin-Induced Thrombocytopenia. Heparin-induced thrombocytopenia (HIT) is a potentially fatal immune-mediated disorder characterized by reduced platelet counts (thrombocytopenia) and a seemingly paradoxical *increase* in thrombotic events. The underlying cause is development of antibodies against heparin-platelet protein complexes. These antibodies activate platelets and damage the vascular endothelium, thereby promoting both thrombosis and a rapid loss of circulating platelets. Thrombus formation poses a risk of DVT, pulmonary embolism, cerebral thrombosis, and MI. Ischemic injury secondary to thrombosis in the limbs may require amputation of an arm or leg. Coronary thrombosis can be fatal. The primary treatment for HIT is discontinuation of heparin and, if anticoagulation is still needed, substitution of a nonheparin anticoagulant, typically lepirudin or argatroban. The incidence of HIT is between 1% and 3% among patients who receive heparin for more than 4 days.

HIT should be suspected whenever platelet counts fall significantly or when thrombosis develops despite adequate anticoagulation. Accordingly, to reduce the risk of HIT, patients should be monitored for signs of thrombosis and for reductions in platelets. Platelet counts should be determined frequently (2 to 3 times a week) during the first 3 weeks of heparin use, and monthly thereafter. If severe thrombocytopenia develops (platelet count <100,000/mm³), heparin should be discontinued.

Hypersensitivity Reactions. Because commercial heparin is extracted from animal tissues, these preparations may be contaminated with antigens that can promote allergy. Possible allergic responses include chills, fever, and urticaria. Anaphylactic reactions are rare. To minimize the risk of severe reactions, patients should receive a small test dose of heparin prior to the full therapeutic dose.

Other Adverse Effects. Subcutaneous administration may produce *local irritation* and *hematoma*. *Vasospastic reactions* that persist for several hours may develop after 1 or more weeks of treatment. Long-term, high-dose therapy may cause *osteoporosis*.

Warnings and Contraindications

Warnings. Heparin must be used with extreme caution in all patients for whom there is a high likelihood of bleeding. Among these are individuals with *hemophilia, increased capillary permeability, dissecting aneurysm, peptic ulcer disease, severe hypertension,* or *threatened abortion.* Heparin must also be used cautiously in patients with *severe disease of the liver or kidneys.*

Contraindications. Heparin is contraindicated for patients with *thrombocytopenia* and *uncontrollable bleeding.* In addition, heparin should be avoided both *during and immediately after surgery of the eye, brain, or spinal cord. Lumbar puncture* and *regional anesthesia* are additional contraindications.

Drug Interactions

In heparin-treated patients, platelet aggregation is the major remaining defense against hemorrhage. Drugs that depress platelet function (e.g., aspirin) will weaken this defense and must be employed with caution.

Protamine Sulfate for Heparin Overdose

Protamine sulfate is an antidote to severe heparin overdose. Protamine is a small protein that has multiple positively charged groups. These charged groups bond ionically with the negatively charged groups on heparin, thereby forming a heparin-protamine complex that is devoid of anticoagulant activity. Neutralization of heparin occurs immediately and lasts for 2 hours, after which additional protamine may be needed. Protamine is administered by slow IV injection (no faster than 20 mg/min or 50 mg in 10 min). Dosage is based on the fact that 1 mg of protamine will inactivate 100 units of heparin. Hence, for each 100 units of heparin in the body, 1 mg of protamine should be injected.

Laboratory Monitoring

The objective of anticoagulant therapy is to reduce blood coagulability to a level that is low enough to prevent thrombosis, but not so low as to promote spontaneous bleeding. Because heparin levels can be highly variable, achieving this goal is difficult, and requires careful control of dosage based on frequent tests of coagulation. The laboratory test employed most commonly is the *activated partial thromboplastin time* (aPTT). The normal value for aPTT is 40 seconds. At therapeutic levels, heparin *increases* the aPTT by a factor of 1.5 to 2, making the aPTT 60 to 80 seconds. Since heparin has a rapid onset and brief duration, if an aPTT value should fall outside the therapeutic range, coagulability can be quickly corrected through an adjustment in dosage: if the aPTT is too long (>80 seconds), the dosage should be lowered; conversely, if the aPTT is too short (<60 seconds), the dosage should be increased. Measurements of aPTT should be made frequently (every 4 to 6 hours) during the initial phase of therapy. Once an effective dosage has been established, one aPTT measurement a day will suffice.

Unitage and Preparations

Unitage. Heparin is prescribed in units, not in milligrams. The heparin unit is an index of anticoagulant activity, and is defined as the amount of heparin that will prevent 1.0 ml of sheep plasma from coagulating for 1 hour. Heparin is prescribed in units because heparin preparations tend to differ from one another in anticoagulant activity when compared on a milligram basis.

Preparations. Heparin sodium is dispensed in single-dose vials; multiple-dose vials; and unit-dose, preloaded syringes that have their own needles. Concentrations range from 1000 to 40,000 units/ml. Heparin sodium for use in heparin locks [Hep-Lock] is dispensed in dilute solutions (10 and 100 units/ml) that are too weak to produce systemic anticoagulant effects.

Dosage and Administration

General Considerations. Heparin is administered by injection only. Two routes are employed: *intravenous* (either intermittent or continuous) and *subcutaneous.* Intramuscular injection causes hematoma and must not be used. Heparin is not administered orally because heparin is too large and too polar to permit intestinal absorption.

Dosage varies with the application. Postoperative prophylaxis of thrombosis, for example, requires relatively small doses. In other situations, such as open heart surgery, much larger doses are required. The dosages given below are for "general anticoagulant therapy." As a rule, the aPTT should be employed as a guideline for dosage titration; increases in aPTT of 1.5- to 2-fold are therapeutic. Since heparin is dispensed in widely varying concentrations, the label must be read carefully to ensure that dosing is correct.

Intermittent IV Therapy. Intermittent IV heparin is administered via an indwelling rubber-capped needle (heparin lock). Therapy is initiated with a dose of 10,000 units. Subsequent doses of 5000 to 10,000 units are given every 4 to 6 hours. The aPTT should be taken 1 hour before each injection until dosage is stabilized. To avoid venous injury, the site of the heparin lock should be moved every 2 or 3 days. When heparin is administered intermittently, plasma levels of the drug will fluctuate, possibly causing alternating periods of excessive and insufficient anticoagulation.

Continuous IV Infusion. Intravenous infusion provides steady levels of heparin, and therefore is preferred to intermittent injections. Dosing is begun with a bolus of 5000 to 10,000 units; this loading dose is followed by infusion at a rate of 1000 units/hr. During the initial phase of treatment, the aPTT should be measured once every 4 hours and the infusion rate adjusted accordingly. To decrease the risk of overdose, when heparin solutions are prepared, the amount made up should be sufficient for no more than a 6-hour infusion. Heparin should be infused using an electric pump, and the rate should be checked every 30 to 60 minutes.

Deep SC Injection. Subcutaneous injections are made deep into the fatty layer of the abdomen (but not within 2 inches of the umbilicus). The heparin solution should be withdrawn using a 20- to 22-gauge needle. This needle is then discarded and replaced with a small needle (1/2 to 5/8 inch, 25- or 26-gauge) to make the injection. Following administration, firm but gentle pressure should be applied to the injection site for 1 to 2 minutes. The initial SC dose is 10,000 to 20,000 units (preceded immediately by an IV loading dose of 5000 units). The initial SC dose is followed by either (1) 8000 to 10,000 units every 8 hours or (2) 15,000 to 20,000 units every

12 hours. Dosage is adjusted on the basis of aPTTs taken 4 to 6 hours after each injection. The injection site should be rotated.

Low-Dose Therapy. Heparin in low doses is given for prophylaxis against postoperative thromboembolism. The initial dose (5000 units SC) is given 2 hours prior to surgery. Additional doses of 5000 units are given every 8 to 12 hours for 7 days (or until the patient is ambulatory). Low-dose heparin is also employed as adjunctive therapy for patients with MI. During low-dose therapy, monitoring of aPTT is not usually required.

Low-Molecular-Weight Heparins
Group Properties

Low-molecular-weight (LMW) heparins are simply heparin preparations composed of molecules that are shorter than those found in unfractionated heparin. LMW heparins are as effective as unfractionated heparin, and offer several advantages. Most importantly, LMW heparins can be given on a fixed-dose schedule and don't require aPTT monitoring. As a result, LMW heparins can be used at home, whereas unfractionated heparin must be given in a hospital. In addition, LMW heparins are much less likely to cause thrombocytopenia. Because of their advantages, LMW heparins are now considered first-line therapy for prevention and treatment of DVT. In the United States, three LMW heparins are available: enoxaparin [Lovenox], dalteparin [Fragmin], and tinzaparin [Innohep]. A fourth agent—ardeparin [Normiflo]—was withdrawn. Differences between LMW heparins and unfractionated heparin are summarized in Table 50–2.

Production. LMW heparins are made by depolymerizing unfractionated heparin (i.e., breaking unfractionated heparin into smaller pieces). Molecular weights in LMW preparations range between 1000 and 9000, with a mean of 4000 to 5000. In comparison, molecular weights in unfractionated heparin range between 3000 and 30,000, with a mean of 12,000 to 15,000.

Mechanism of Action. Anticoagulant activity of LMW heparin is mediated by the same active pentasaccharide sequence that mediates anticoagulant action of standard heparin. However, because LMW heparin molecules are short, they do not have quite the same effect as standard heparin.

TABLE 50–2 ■ Comparison of Unfractionated Heparin with Low-molecular-weight Heparin

Property	Type of Heparin	
	Unfractionated	**Low Molecular Weight**
Molecular weight range	3000–30,000	1000–9000
Mean molecular weight	12,000–15,000	4000–5000
Mechanism of action	Inactivation of factor Xa and thrombin	Preferential inactivation of factor Xa
Routes	IV, SC	SC only
Nonspecific binding	Widespread	Minimal
Laboratory monitoring	aPTT monitoring is essential	No aPTT monitoring required
Dosage	Dosage must be adjusted on basis of aPTT	Dosage is fixed
Setting for use	Hospital	Hospital or home
Cost	$3/day for heparin itself, but hospitalization and aPTT monitoring greatly increase the real cost	$14/day for LMW heparin, but home use and absence of aPTT monitoring greatly reduce the real cost

Specifically, whereas standard heparin is equally good at inactivating factor Xa *and* thrombin, *LMW heparins preferentially inactivate factor Xa,* being much less able to inactivate thrombin. Why the difference? In order to inactivate thrombin, a heparin chain must not only contain the pentasaccharide sequence that activates antithrombin, it must also be long enough to provide a binding site for thrombin. This binding site is necessary because inactivation of thrombin requires simultaneous binding of thrombin with heparin and antithrombin (see Fig. 50–3). In contrast to standard heparin chains, most LMW heparin chains are too short to allow thrombin binding, and hence are unable to inactivate thrombin.

Therapeutic Use. *Approved* uses of LMW heparins are limited. All three agents used in the United States are approved for *prevention of DVT* following hip replacement or knee replacement surgery. However, these drugs have also been used extensively to prevent DVT after general surgery and in patients with multiple trauma and acute spinal injury. In addition, LMW heparins have been used safely and effectively to *treat established DVT,* although only dalteparin and enoxaparin are approved for this use. LMW heparins are also given to treat patients with ischemic stroke, pulmonary embolism, and non–Q-wave MI. When used for prophylaxis or treatment of DVT, LMW heparins are at least as effective as unfractionated heparin, and possibly more effective.

Pharmacokinetics. Compared with unfractionated heparin, LMW heparins have higher bioavailability and longer half-lives. Bioavailability is higher because LMW heparins do not undergo nonspecific binding to proteins and tissues, and hence are more available for anticoagulant effects. Half-lives are prolonged (up to 6 times longer than that of unfractionated heparin) because LMW heparins undergo less binding to macrophages, and hence undergo slower clearance by the liver. Because of increased bioavailability, plasma levels of LMW heparin are highly predictable. As a result, these drugs can be given on a fixed schedule with no need for routine monitoring of coagulation. Because of their long half-lives, LMW heparins can be given just once or twice a day.

Administration, Dosing, and Monitoring. LMW heparins are administered SC. Dosage is based on body weight. Because plasma levels of LMW heparin are predictable for any given dose, these preparations can be administered on a fixed schedule without the need for laboratory monitoring. This contrasts with unfractionated heparin, which requires adjusting the dosage on the basis of aPTT measurements. Because LMW heparins have an extended half-life, dosing can be done once or twice daily. For prophylaxis of DVT, dosing is begun in the perioperative period and continued 5 to 10 days.

Adverse Effects and Interactions. *Bleeding* is the major adverse effect of LMW heparins. However, the incidence of bleeding complications is less than with unfractionated heparin. Despite the potential for bleeding, LMW heparins are considered safe for outpatient use. Like unfractionated heparin, LMW heparins can cause immune-mediated *thrombocytopenia.* However, the incidence is about 10 times lower. As with unfractionated heparin, overdose with LMW heparins can be treated with protamine sulfate.

Like unfractionated heparin, LMW heparins can cause *severe neurologic injury,* including permanent paralysis, when given to patients undergoing spinal puncture or spinal or epidural anesthesia. Neurologic injury results from pressure on the spinal cord generated by an epidural or spinal bleed. The risk of serious harm is increased by concurrent use of antiplatelet drugs (e.g., aspirin, ticlopidine) or warfarin. Patients should be monitored closely for signs of neurologic impairment.

Cost. LMW heparins cost more than unfractionated heparin (e.g., about $63/day for dalteparin vs. $8/day for unfractionated heparin). However, since LMW heparins can be used at home and don't require monitoring of aPTT, the overall cost of treatment is far less than with unfractionated heparin.

Individual Preparations

In the United States, three LMW heparins are available: enoxaparin, dalteparin, and tinzaparin. Other LMW heparins are available outside this country. Each preparation is unique. Hence clinical experience with one may not apply fully to the others.

Enoxaparin. Enoxaparin [Lovenox] was the first LMW heparin available in the United States. The drug is prepared by depolymerization of unfractionated porcine heparin. Molecular weights range between 2000 and 8000.

Enoxaparin is approved for prevention of DVT following hip and knee replacement surgery or abdominal surgery in patients considered at high risk of thromboembolic complications (e.g., obese patients, those over 40, and those with malignancy or a history of DVT or pulmonary embolism). The drug is also approved for prevention of ischemic complications in patients with unstable angina or non–Q-wave MI. Administration is by deep SC injection. The following dosages are employed:

- *Prevention of DVT after hip or knee replacement surgery*—30 mg every 12 hours starting 12 to 24 hours after surgery and continuing for 7 to 10 days
- *Prevention of DVT after abdominal surgery*—40 mg once daily, beginning 2 hours before surgery and continuing for 7 to 10 days
- *Treatment of established DVT*—1 mg/kg every 12 hours for 7 days
- *Patients with unstable angina or non–Q-wave MI*—1 mg/kg every 12 hours (in conjunction with oral aspirin, 100 to 325 mg once daily) for 2 to 8 days.

In the event of overdose, hemorrhage can be controlled with protamine sulfate. The dosage is 1 mg of protamine sulfate for each milligram of enoxaparin administered.

Dalteparin. Dalteparin [Fragmin] was the second LMW heparin to be marketed in the United States. The drug is prepared by depolymerization of porcine heparin. Molecular weights range between 2000 and 9000, the mean being 5000. Approved indications are much like those of enoxaparin: prevention of DVT following hip replacement surgery or abdominal surgery in patients considered at high risk of thromboembolic complications, and prevention of ischemic complications in patients with unstable angina or non–Q-wave MI. Administration is by deep SC injection. Dosages are as follows:

- *Prevention of DVT after hip replacement surgery*—2500 anti–factor Xa IU 1 or 2 hours before surgery, 2500 IU that evening (at least 6 hours after the first dose), and then 5000 IU once daily for 5 to 10 days
- *Prevention of DVT after abdominal surgery*—2500 IU once daily for 5 to 10 days, starting 1 to 2 hours before surgery
- *Patients with unstable angina or non–Q-wave MI*—120 IU/kg (but not more than 10,000 IU total) every 12 hours for 5 to 8 days. Concurrent therapy with aspirin (75 to 165 mg/day) is required.

Overdose is treated with 1 mg of protamine sulfate for every 100 anti–factor Xa IU of dalteparin administered.

Tinzaparin. Tinzaparin [Innohep] is the newest LMW heparin approved for use in the United States. The drug is indicated for acute symptomatic DVT (with or without pulmonary embolism) and should be used in conjunction with warfarin. Tinzaparin has a mean molecular weight of 6500 and a half-life of 3 to 4 hours. Excretion is via the urine. In clinical trials, bleeding developed in 0.8% of patients and thrombocytopenia in 1%. Eight men experienced priapism (persistent erection). Tinzaparin is supplied in 2-ml vials containing 20,000 anti–factor Xa IU/ml. Administration is by SC injection in the abdominal region. The recommended dosage is 175 anti-Xa IU/kg once daily for 6 or more days. Warfarin should be initiated when appropriate, usually 1 to 3 days after starting tinzaparin. When warfarin has taken effect, as indicated by an international normalized ratio (INR; see below) of 2 or more for 2 consecutive days, tinzaparin can be discontinued. Overdose is treated with 1 mg of protamine sulfate for every 100 anti–factor Xa IU of dalteparin administered.

Fondaparinux

Actions. Fondaparinux [Arixtra] is a synthetic anticoagulant that enhances the activity of antithrombin, and thereby causes *selective inhibition of activated factor X* (factor Xa). As a result, production of thrombin is inhibited, and hence coagulation is suppressed. Although fondaparinux inhibits thrombin production indirectly (by inactivating factor Xa), it is unable to inhibit thrombin directly.

Fondaparinux is closely related in structure and function to heparin and the LMW heparins. Structurally, fondaparinux is a pentasaccharide identical to the antithrombin-binding region of the heparins. Hence, like the heparins, fondaparinux is able to induce a conformational change in antithrombin, thereby increasing antithrombin's activity—but only against factor Xa, not against thrombin. Why is fondaparinux selective for factor Xa? Because the drug is quite small—even smaller than the LMW heparins. As a result, it is too small to form a complex with both antithrombin and thrombin, and hence cannot reduce thrombin activity (see Fig. 50–3).

Fondaparinux has no effect on prothrombin time, aPTT, bleeding time, or platelet aggregation.

Therapeutic Use. Fondaparinux is approved only for prevention of DVT following hip fracture surgery, hip replacement surgery, or knee replacement surgery. The drug is somewhat more effective than enoxaparin (an LMW heparin) at preventing DVT, but may also cause slightly more bleeding. Fondaparinux is administered just once a day, and routine laboratory monitoring is unnecessary. Anticoagulation may persist for 2 to 4 days after the last dose.

Pharmacokinetics. Fondaparinux is administered SC and bioavailability is 100%. Plasma levels peak 2 hours after injection. The drug is eliminated by the kidneys with a half-life of 17 to 21 hours. The half-life is increased in patients with renal dysfunction.

Adverse Effects. As with other anticoagulants, *bleeding* is the biggest concern. The risk is increased by advancing age and renal impairment. Fondaparinux should be used with caution in patients with moderate renal impairment (creatinine clearance 30 to 50 ml/min) and avoided in patients with severe renal impairment (creatinine clearance <30 ml/min). The drug should also be avoided in patients weighing less than 50 kg. Why? Because low body weight increases bleeding risk. Aspirin and other drugs that interfere with hemostasis should be used with caution. In contrast to overdose with heparin or LMW heparins, overdose with fondaparinux cannot be treated with protamine sulfate.

Fondaparinux does not promote immune-mediated HIT, although it still can lower platelet counts. During clinical trials, *thrombocytopenia* developed in 3% of patients. Platelet counts should be monitored and, if they fall below 100,000/mm³, fondaparinux should be discontinued.

In patients undergoing anesthesia using an epidural or spinal catheter, fondaparinux (as well as other anticoagulants) can cause *spinal or epidural hematoma,* which can result in permanent paralysis. However, in clinical trials, when fondaparinux was administered no sooner than 2 hours after catheter removal, no hematomas were reported.

Preparations, Dosage, and Administration. Fondaparinux [Arixtra] is available in 2.5-mg, single-dose, prefilled syringes. The recommended dosage is 2.5 mg SC once a day, starting 6 to 8 hours after surgery. The usual duration is 5 to 9 days.

Danaparoid

Danaparoid [Orgaran] is very similar to the LMW heparins, although it doesn't have heparin in its structure. Rather, it contains *haparin,* a molecule that acts like heparin. Because it lacks heparin, danaparoid is referred to as an *LMW heparinoid,* rather than an LMW heparin. Danaparoid is prepared by extraction from porcine intestinal mucosa and has an average molecular weight of 5500. Like the LMW heparins, danaparoid facilitates inactivation of factor Xa by antithrombin. The drug has little impact on thrombin activity and does not suppress platelet aggregation. Danaparoid has good bioavailability and a prolonged half-life. Hence, as with the LMW heparins, dosing is relatively infrequent (twice daily) and routine laboratory monitoring is unnecessary. At this time, danaparoid is approved only for prevention of DVT following hip replacement surgery. The dosage is 750 anti-Xa units SC twice daily, starting 1 to 4 hours before surgery and continuing 7 to 10 days. The most important adverse effect is bleeding. Side effects include pain (8.2%), fever (7.3%), nausea (4.1%), constipation (3.5%), rash (2.1%), and infection (2.1%). HIT has not been observed. As with other heparins, caution is required in patients taking warfarin or antiplatelet drugs. There is no known antidote to overdose; protamine sulfate, which can reverse the effects of heparin and the LMW heparins, cannot reverse the effects of danaparoid.

PARENTERAL ANTICOAGULANTS II: DIRECT THROMBIN INHIBITORS

The anticoagulants discussed in this section—bivalirudin, lepirudin, and argatroban—work by direct inhibition of thrombin. Hence, they differ from the heparin-like anticoagulants, which inhibit thrombin indirectly (by enhancing the activity of antithrombin). All three are administered by continuous IV infusion, and are not suited for outpatient use.

Bivalirudin

Therapeutic Use. Bivalirudin [Angiomax], formerly known as *hirulog,* is an IV anticoagulant given in combination with aspirin to prevent clot formation in patients with unstable angina who are undergoing coronary angioplasty. At this time, the standard therapy for these patients is aspirin combined with a platelet GP IIb/IIIa inhibitor combined with low-dose, unfractionated heparin. Bivalirudin, an alternative to heparin in this regimen, has been studied only in combination with aspirin; it has not been studied in combination with GP IIb/IIIa inhibitors. In one clinical trial—the Hirulog Angioplasty Study—bivalirudin plus aspirin was compared with heparin plus aspirin. Bivalirudin was at least as effective as heparin at preventing ischemic complications (MI, abrupt vessel closure, death), and caused fewer bleeding complications. In a subgroup of patients—those with postinfarction angina—bivalirudin was significantly *more* effective than heparin.

Mechanism of Action. Bivalirudin is a *direct,* reversible inhibitor of thrombin—in contrast to heparin, which acts *indirectly* by facilitating the actions of antithrombin. Bivalirudin binds with and inhibits thrombin that is free in the blood as well as thrombin that is bound to clots. In contrast, heparin inhibits only free thrombin—being inactive against thrombin bound to clots. By inhibiting thrombin, bivalirudin prevents (1) the conversion of fibrinogen into fibrin and (2) the activation of factor XIIIa, thereby preventing the conversion of soluble fibrin into insoluble fibrin. Bivalirudin is a synthetic, 20-amino acid peptide chemically related to *hirudin,* an anticoagulant isolated from the saliva of leeches.

Adverse Effects. The most common side effects are back pain (42%), nausea (15%), hypotension (12%), and headache (12%). Other relatively common effects (incidence greater than 5%) include vomiting, abdominal pain, pelvic pain, anxiety, nervousness, insomnia, bradycardia, and fever.

Bleeding is the adverse effect of greatest concern. However, compared with heparin, bivalirudin causes fewer incidents of major bleeding (3.7% vs. 9.3%) and fewer patients require transfusions (2% vs. 5.7%). Coadministration of bivalirudin with heparin, warfarin, or thrombolytic drugs increases the risk of bleeding.

Pharmacokinetics. Bivalirudin is administered IV and anticoagulation begins immediately. Drug levels are maintained by continuous infusion. Bivalirudin is eliminated primarily by renal excretion, and partly by proteolytic cleavage. The half-life is short (25 minutes) in patients with normal renal function, but may be longer in those with renal impairment. Coagulation returns to baseline about 1 hour after stopping the infusion. Anticoagulation can be monitored by measuring activated clotting time.

Comparison with Heparin. Bivalirudin is just as effective as heparin and has several advantages: it works independently of antithrombin, inhibits clot-bound thrombin as well as free thrombin, and causes less bleeding and fewer ischemic events. However, the drug also has two disadvantages. First, there is little information on using bivalirudin with GP IIb/IIIa inhibitors, the antiplatelet drugs employed most commonly during angioplasty. In the absence of such data, cardiologists will be reluctant to switch from heparin. Second, bivalirudin is more expensive than heparin: one single-use vial, good for a full course of treatment, costs about $420, compared with $10 for an equivalent course of heparin. However, the manufacturer estimates that reductions in bleeding and ischemic complications would save, on average, $500 to $1000 per patient, which would more than offset the greater cost of bivalirudin. The bottom line? Bivalirudin works as well as heparin, is safer, and may be equally cost-effective, but more clinical experience is needed before the drug is likely to replace heparin as the preferred anticoagulant in patients undergoing angioplasty.

Preparations, Dosage, and Administration. Bivalirudin [Angiomax] is dispensed as lyophilized powder (250 mg) for reconstitution in sterile water. Dosing consists of an initial IV bolus (1 mg/kg) followed by a 4-hour infusion (2.5 mg/kg/hr). If necessary, the drug may be infused for up to 20 additional hours at a rate of 0.2 mg/kg/hr. Treatment should begin just prior to angioplasty. Dosage should be reduced in patients with severe renal impairment. All patients should take aspirin (300 to 325 mg).

Lepirudin

Like bivalirudin, lepirudin [Refludan] is an intravenous anticoagulant that works by direct inhibition of thrombin. The drug is indicated for prophylaxis and treatment of thrombosis in patients with heparin-induced thrombocytopenia (HIT). As discussed above, when HIT develops, the primary treatment is to withdraw heparin and substitute a nonheparin anticoagulant—usually lepirudin or argatroban. In clinical trials, lepirudin produced effective anticoagulation in about 80% of patients, and thereby significantly reduced the risk of death and new thrombotic complications. Like other anticoagulants, lepirudin poses a risk of bleeding. The risk is increased by liver dysfunction, renal insufficiency, recent stroke or surgery, and recent therapy with thrombolytic drugs. Dosing consists of an initial IV bolus (0.4 mg/kg infused over 15 to 20 seconds) followed by a continuous infusion (0.15 mg/kg/hr) for 2 to 10 days. Dosage should be titrated to achieve an aPTT ratio (i.e., the ratio between the patient's aPTT and a reference aPTT) of 1.5 to 2.5. Treatment is expensive: One week of therapy costs about $4700.

Argatroban

Like bivalirudin and lepirudin, argatroban [Acova] is an intravenous anticoagulant that works by direct inhibition of thrombin. Like lepirudin, the drug is indicated for prophylaxis and treatment of thrombosis in patients with HIT. In clinical trials, argatroban reduced development of new thrombosis and permitted restoration of platelet counts. Like other anticoagulants, argatroban poses a risk of hemorrhage. About 12% of patients experience hematuria. Allergic reactions (dyspnea, cough, rash), which develop in 10% of patients, occur almost exclusively in those receiving either thrombolytic drugs (e.g., streptokinase) or contrast media for coronary angioplasty. Argatroban has a short half-life—about 45 minutes—owing to rapid metabolism by the liver. Treatment is monitored by measuring aPTT. When infusion of argatroban is discontinued, aPTT returns to baseline in 2 to 4 hours.

Argatroban is supplied in 2.5-ml single-dose vials (100 mg/ml) intended for dilution followed by continuous IV infusion. In patients with normal liver function, the initial infusion rate is 2 µg/kg/min. In patients with liver dysfunction, the initial rate is only 0.5 µg/kg/min. Dosage is adjusted to maintain the aPTT at 1.5 to 3 times the baseline value. As with lepirudin, treatment is expensive: The cost for the first day alone is over $550.

ORAL ANTICOAGULANTS

Oral anticoagulants are similar to heparin in some respects and quite different in others. Like heparin, oral anticoagulants are used to prevent thrombosis. In contrast to heparin, oral agents have a delayed onset of action, which makes them inappropriate for emergency use. However, because they don't require injection, these drugs are well suited for long-term prophylaxis. As with heparin, oral anticoagulants carry a significant risk of hemorrhage. This risk is amplified by the many drug interactions to which the oral agents are subject. In the United States, only two oral anticoagulants are available: warfarin and anisindione. Of these, warfarin is by far the most frequently prescribed.

Warfarin

Warfarin [Coumadin] is the oldest member of the oral anticoagulant family and will serve as our prototype for the group.

History

The history of warfarin underscores the potential hazards of oral anticoagulants. The warfarin story began with the observation that ingestion of spoiled clover silage could induce bleeding in cattle; the causative agent was identified as bishydroxycoumarin (dicumarol). Research into derivatives of dicumarol resulted in the synthesis of warfarin. When warfarin was first developed, clinical use was ruled out because

of concerns about hemorrhage. Instead of becoming a medicine, warfarin was used to kill rats. The drug proved especially effective in this application and remains one of our most widely used rodenticides. Clinical interest in warfarin was renewed following the report of a failed suicide attempt using huge doses of a warfarin-based rat poison. The clinical trials triggered by that event soon demonstrated that warfarin could be employed safely in humans.

Mechanism of Action

Warfarin suppresses coagulation by acting as an *antagonist of vitamin K.* Four clotting factors (factors VII, IX, X, and prothrombin) require vitamin K for their synthesis. By antagonizing vitamin K, warfarin blocks the biosynthesis of these vitamin K–dependent factors.

Pharmacokinetics

Absorption, Distribution, and Elimination. Warfarin is readily absorbed following oral administration. Once in the blood, about 99% of warfarin becomes bound to albumin. This binding provides the basis of several drug interactions. Warfarin molecules that remain free (unbound) can readily cross membranes, including those of the placenta and milk-producing glands. Warfarin undergoes hepatic metabolism followed by excretion in the urine and feces.

Time Course of Effects. Although warfarin acts quickly to inhibit clotting factor *synthesis,* noticeable *anticoagulant effects* are delayed. Why? Because warfarin has no effect on clotting factors already in circulation. Hence, until these clotting factors decay, coagulation remains unaffected. Since decay of clotting factors occurs with a half-life of 6 hours to 2.5 days (depending on the clotting factor under consideration), initial responses may not be evident until 8 to 12 hours after the first dose. Peak effects take several days to develop.

After warfarin is discontinued, coagulation remains inhibited for 2 to 5 days. This residual effect is due to the long half-life of warfarin (1.5 to 2 days). Because warfarin leaves the body slowly, synthesis of new clotting factors remains suppressed, despite stopping drug administration.

Therapeutic Uses

Warfarin is employed most frequently for long-term prophylaxis of thrombosis. Specific indications are (1) prevention of venous thrombosis and associated pulmonary embolism, (2) prevention of thromboembolism in patients with prosthetic heart valves, and (3) prevention of thrombosis during atrial fibrillation. For all of these indications, warfarin is the oral anticoagulant of choice. The drug has also been used to reduce the risk of recurrent transient ischemic attacks (TIAs) and recurrent MI. Because onset of effects is delayed, warfarin is not useful in emergencies. When rapid action is needed, anticoagulant therapy can be initiated with heparin.

Monitoring Treatment

The anticoagulant effects of warfarin are evaluated by monitoring *prothrombin time* (PT)—a coagulation test that is especially sensitive to alterations in vitamin K–dependent factors. The average pretreatment value for PT is 12 seconds. Treatment with warfarin prolongs PT.

Traditionally, PT test results have been reported as a *PT ratio,* which is simply the ratio of the patient's PT to a control PT. However, there is a serious problem with this form of reporting: test results can vary widely among laboratories. The underlying cause of variability is thromboplastin, a critical reagent employed in the PT test. To ensure that test results from different laboratories are comparable, results are now reported in terms of an *international normalized ratio* (INR). The INR is determined by multiplying the observed PT ratio by a correction factor specific to the particular thromboplastin preparation employed for the test.

The objective of treatment is to raise the INR to an appropriate value. Recommended INR ranges are summarized in Table 50–3. As indicated, an INR of 2 to 3 is appropriate for most patients—although for some the target INR is 3 to 4.5. If the INR is below the recommended range, warfarin dosage should be increased. Conversely, if the INR is above the recommended range, dosage should be reduced. Unfortunately, since warfarin has a delayed onset and prolonged duration of action, the INR cannot be altered quickly: Once the dosage has been changed, it may take a week or more to reach the desired INR.

PT must be determined frequently during warfarin therapy. PT should be measured daily during the first 5 days of treatment, twice a week for the next 1 to 2 weeks, once a week for the next 1 to 2 months, and every 2 to 4 weeks thereafter. In addition, PT should be determined whenever a drug that interacts with warfarin is added to or deleted from the regimen.

Concurrent therapy with heparin can influence PT values. To minimize this influence, blood for PT determinations should be drawn no sooner than 5 hours after an IV injection of heparin, and no sooner than 24 hours after an SC injection.

PT can now be monitored at home. Currently, two monitoring devices are available: *CoaguChek* and the *ProTime Microcoagulation System.* These small, hand-held machines are easy to use and provide reliable results. Both devices determine PT and INR values. In addition, the ProTime meter can be programmed by the physician with upper and lower INR values appropriate for the individual patient. When this is done, the meter will display either *In Range, INR High,* or *INR Low,* depending on the degree of anticoagulation. Home monitoring is more convenient than laboratory monitoring and gives patients a sense of empowerment. In addition, it improves anticoagulation control. We don't know yet if home monitoring reduces the incidence of bleeding (from excessive anticoagulation) or thrombosis (from insufficient anticoagulation). The CoaguChek meter costs about $1300 and the ProTime meter costs about $2000. Each test costs about $10.

Adverse Effects

Hemorrhage. Bleeding is the major complication of warfarin therapy. Hemorrhage can occur at any site. Patients should be monitored closely for signs of bleeding. (For specific signs, refer to the discussion of heparin-induced hemorrhage above.) If bleeding develops, warfarin should be discontinued. Severe overdose can be treated with *vitamin K* (see below). Patients should be encouraged to carry identification (e.g., Medic Alert bracelet) to inform emergency personnel of warfarin use.

Several measures can reduce the risk of bleeding. Candidates for treatment must be carefully screened for risk factors (see *Warnings and Contraindications*). Prothrombin time must be measured frequently. A variety of drugs can potentiate warfarin's effects (see below), and hence must be used with extreme care. Patients should be given detailed verbal and written instructions regarding signs of bleeding, dosage

	TABLE 50–3 ▪ Monitoring Oral Anticoagulant Therapy: Recommended Ranges of Prothrombin Time-Derived Values	
	Recommended Ranges	
Condition Being Treated	**Observed PT Ratio***	**INR†**
Acute myocardial infarction‡	1.3–1.5	2.0–3.0
Atrial fibrillation‡	1.3–1.5	2.0–3.0
Valvular heart disease‡	1.3–1.5	2.0–3.0
Pulmonary embolism	1.3–1.5	2.0–3.0
Venous thrombosis§	1.3–1.5	2.0–3.0
Tissue heart valves‡	1.3–1.5	2.0–3.0
Mechanical heart valves	1.5–2.0	3.0–4.5
Systemic embolism		
Prevention	1.3–1.5	2.0–3.0
Recurrent	1.5–2.0	3.0–4.5

*Observed PT ratio = ratio of patient's PT to a control PT value. In this particular case, the reagent used to determine the control PT value is one of the preparations of rabbit brain thromboplastin employed in the United States. Had a different preparation of thromboplastin been used, the observed PT ratio could be very different.
†INR = international normalized ratio. This value is calculated from the observed PT ratio. The INR is equivalent to the PT ratio that would have been obtained if the patient's PT has been compared to a PT value obtained using the International Reference Preparation, a standardized human brain thromboplastin prepared by the World Health Organization. In contrast to PT ratios, INR values are comparable from one laboratory to the next throughout the United States and the rest of the world.
‡For prevention of systemic embolism.
§Prophylaxis in high-risk surgery; treatment.

size and timing, and scheduling of PT tests. When a patient is incapable of accurate self-medication, a responsible individual must supervise therapy. Patients should be advised to record administration of each dose, rather than relying on memory. A soft toothbrush can reduce gingival bleeding. An electric razor can reduce cuts from shaving.

Warfarin intensifies bleeding during surgery and dental procedures. Accordingly, surgeons and dentists must be informed of warfarin use. Patients anticipating elective procedures should discontinue warfarin several days prior to the appointment. If an emergency procedure must be performed, injection of vitamin K will help suppress bleeding.

Fetal Hemorrhage and Teratogenesis from Use During Pregnancy. Warfarin can cross the placenta and affect the developing fetus. Fetal hemorrhage and death have occurred. In addition, warfarin can cause gross malformation, central nervous system (CNS) defects, and optic atrophy. Accordingly, *warfarin is classified in Food and Drug Administration Pregnancy Risk Category X: The risks to the developing fetus outweigh any possible benefits of treatment.* Women of child-bearing age should be informed about the potential for teratogenesis and advised to postpone pregnancy. If pregnancy occurs, the possibility of termination should be discussed. If an anticoagulant is needed during pregnancy, heparin, which does not cross the placenta, should be employed.

Use During Lactation. Warfarin enters breast milk. Women should be advised against breast-feeding.

Other Adverse Effects. Adverse effects other than hemorrhage are uncommon. Possible undesired responses include skin necrosis, alopecia, urticaria, dermatitis, fever, GI disturbances, and red-orange discoloration of urine, which must not be confused with hematuria. Recent evidence indicates that long-term warfarin use (more than 12 months) may weaken bones, and thereby increase the risk of fractures.

Drug Interactions

General Considerations. Warfarin is subject to a large number of clinically significant adverse interactions—perhaps more than any other drug. As a result of these interactions, anticoagulant effects may be reduced to the point of permitting thrombosis, or they may be increased to the point of causing hemorrhage. Patients must be informed about the potential for hazardous interactions and instructed to avoid all drugs not specifically approved by the physician. This prohibition includes prescription drugs and over-the-counter agents.

Interactions between warfarin and other drugs are summarized in Table 50–4. As indicated, the interactants fall into three major categories: (1) *drugs that increase anticoagulant effects,* (2) *drugs that promote bleeding,* and (3) *drugs that decrease anticoagulant effects.* The major mechanisms by which anticoagulant effects can be *increased* are (1) displacement of warfarin from plasma albumin and (2) inhibition of the hepatic enzymes that degrade warfarin. The major mechanisms for *decreasing* anticoagulant effects are (1) acceleration of warfarin degradation through induction of hepatic drug-metabolizing enzymes, (2) increased synthesis of clotting factors, and (3) inhibition of warfarin absorption. Mechanisms by which drugs can *promote bleeding,* and thereby complicate anticoagulant therapy, include (1) inhibition of platelet aggregation, (2) inhibition of the coagulation cascade, and (3) generation of GI ulcers.

The existence of an interaction between warfarin and another drug does not absolutely preclude using the combination. Such an interaction does mean, however, that the combination must be used with due caution. The potential for harm is greatest when an interacting drug is being added to or deleted from the regimen. At these times, prothrombin time must be monitored, and the dosage of warfarin adjusted to compensate for the impact of removing or adding an interacting drug.

TABLE 50–4 ■ Interactions Between Warfarin and Other Drugs

Drug Category	Mechanism of Interaction	Representative Interacting Drugs
Drugs that *increase* the effects of warfarin	Displacement of warfarin from albumin	Aspirin and other salicylates Chloral hydrate Sulfonamides
	Inhibition of warfarin degradation	Acetaminophen Amiodarone Azole antifungal agents Cimetidine Disulfiram Sulfonamides
	Decreased synthesis of clotting factors	Certain parenteral cephalosporins, including cefoperazone and cefamandole
Drugs that *promote bleeding*	Inhibition of platelet aggregation	Abciximab Aspirin and other salicylates Cilostazol Clopidogrel Dipyridamole Eptifibatide Ticlopidine Tirofiban
	Inhibition of clotting factors	Antimetabolites Heparin
	Promotion of ulcer formation	Aspirin Indomethacin Glucocorticoids Phenylbutazone
Drugs that *decrease* the effects of warfarin	Induction of drug-metabolizing enzymes	Carbamazepine Phenobarbital Phenytoin Rifampin
	Promotion of clotting factor synthesis	Oral contraceptives Vitamin K_1
	Reduction of warfarin absorption	Cholestyramine Colestipol

Specific Interacting Drugs. Of the many drugs listed in Table 50–4, a few are especially likely to produce interactions of clinical significance. Three are discussed below.

Heparin. The interaction of heparin with warfarin is obvious: Being an anticoagulant itself, heparin directly increases the bleeding tendencies brought on by warfarin. Combined therapy with heparin plus warfarin must be performed with care.

Aspirin. Aspirin inhibits platelet aggregation. By blocking aggregation, aspirin can suppress formation of the platelet plug that initiates hemostasis. To make matters worse, aspirin can act directly on the GI tract to cause ulcers, thereby initiating bleeding. Hence, when the antifibrin effects of warfarin are coupled with the antiplatelet and ulcerogenic effects of aspirin, the potential for hemorrhagic disaster is substantial. Accordingly, patients should be warned specifically against using any product that contains aspirin, unless the physician has prescribed aspirin therapy. Drugs similar to aspirin (e.g., indomethacin, ibuprofen) should be avoided as well.

Acetaminophen. Until recently, acetaminophen was considered safe for patients on warfarin. In fact, acetaminophen was routinely recommended as an aspirin substitute for patients who need a mild analgesic. Now, however, it appears that acetaminophen can increase the risk of bleeding: Compared with nonusers of acetaminophen, those who take just 4 regular-strength tablets a day for a week are 10 times more likely to have a dangerously high INR. Unlike aspirin, which promotes bleeding by inhibiting platelet aggregation, acetaminophen is believed to act by inhibiting warfarin degradation, thereby raising warfarin levels. At this time, the interaction between acetaminophen and warfarin has not been proved. Nonetheless, when the drugs are combined, the INR should be monitored closely.

Other Notable Interactions. Several drugs, including *phenobarbital, carbamazepine,* and *rifampin,* are powerful inducers of hepatic drug-metabolizing enzymes. As a result, these drugs can accelerate warfarin degradation, thereby decreasing anticoagulant effects. Accordingly, if one of these drugs is added to the regimen, warfarin dosage must be increased. Of equal importance, when an inducer is withdrawn, causing rates of drug metabolism to decline, a compensatory decrease in warfarin dosage must be made.

Intravaginal miconazole can intensify the anticoagulant effects of warfarin. (Miconazole is the antifungal agent found in Monistat brand vaginal suppositories and cream, used for vaginal candidiasis [yeast infection].) One woman using the combination reported bruising, bleeding gums, and a nosebleed. We have long known that *systemic* miconazole (as well as other azole antifungal agents) can inhibit the metabolism of warfarin, and can thereby cause warfarin levels to rise. Apparently, intravaginal miconazole can be absorbed in amounts sufficient to do the same thing. Because of this interaction, women taking warfarin should not use intravaginal miconazole. If the drugs must be used concurrently, anticoagulation should be monitored closely and warfarin dosage reduced as indicated.

Like the azole antifungal agents, *cimetidine* (a drug for ulcers) and *disulfiram* (a drug for alcoholism) can inhibit warfarin metabolism, and can thereby increase anticoagulant effects.

Vitamin K increases clotting factor synthesis, and can thereby decrease anticoagulant effects.

Sulfonamide antibacterial drugs can displace warfarin from albumin, and thereby increase anticoagulant effects.

Warnings and Contraindications

Like heparin, warfarin is contraindicated for patients with *severe thrombocytopenia* or *uncontrollable bleeding* and for patients undergoing *lumbar puncture, regional anesthesia,* or *surgery of the eye, brain, or spinal cord.* Also like heparin, warfarin must be used with extreme caution in patients at high risk of bleeding, including those with *hemophilia, increased capillary permeability, dissecting aneurysm, GI ulcers,* and *severe hypertension,* and in *women anticipating abortion.* In addition, warfarin is contraindicated in the presence of *vitamin K deficiency, liver disease,* and *alcoholism*—conditions that can disrupt hepatic synthesis of clotting factors. Warfarin is also contraindicated during *pregnancy* and *lactation.*

Vitamin K₁ for Warfarin Overdose

The effects of warfarin overdose can be overcome with vitamin K_1 (phytonadione). Vitamin K_1 antagonizes warfarin's actions and can thereby reverse warfarin-induced inhibition of clotting factor synthesis. (Vitamin K_3—menadione—has no effect on warfarin.)

Vitamin K may be given orally or IV; SC administration should be avoided. Intravenous vitamin K can cause severe anaphylactoid reactions, characterized by flushing, hypotension, and cardiovascular collapse. To reduce this risk, vitamin K should be diluted and infused slowly.

As a rule, small doses—2.5 mg PO or 0.5 to 1 mg IV—are preferred. Why? Because large doses (e.g., 10 mg) can cause prolonged resistance to warfarin, thereby hampering restoration of anticoagulation once bleeding is under control.

If vitamin K fails to control bleeding, levels of clotting factors can be raised quickly by infusing fresh whole blood, fresh-frozen plasma, or plasma concentrates of vitamin K–dependent clotting factors.

Contrasts Between Warfarin and Heparin

Although heparin and warfarin are both anticoagulants, they differ in important ways. Whereas administration of warfarin is oral, heparin must be given by injection. Although both drugs decrease fibrin formation, they do so by different mechanisms: heparin inactivates thrombin and factor Xa, whereas warfarin inhibits synthesis of clotting factors. Heparin and warfarin differ markedly with respect to time course of action: effects of heparin begin and fade rapidly, whereas effects of warfarin begin slowly but then persist for several days. Different tests are used to monitor therapy: changes in aPTT are used to monitor heparin treatment; changes in PT are used to monitor warfarin. Finally, these drugs differ with respect to management of overdose: protamine is given to counteract heparin; vitamin K_1 is given to counteract warfarin. These differences are summarized in Table 50–5.

TABLE 50–5 ■ Summary of Contrasts Between Heparin and Warfarin

	Heparin	Warfarin
Mechanism of action	Promotes action of antithrombin	Inhibits synthesis of vitamin K–dependent clotting factors
Route	IV or SC	PO
Onset	Rapid (minutes)	Slow (hours)
Duration	Brief (hours)	Prolonged (days)
Monitoring	aPTT*	PT†
Antidote for overdose	Protamine	Vitamin K_1

*Activated partial thromboplastin time.
†Prothrombin time. Test results are reported in terms of a PT ratio or in terms of an INR (international normalized ratio).

Preparations, Dosage, and Administration

Warfarin sodium [Coumadin] is dispensed in tablets (1, 2, 2.5, 3, 4, 5, 6, 7.5, and 10 mg) for oral use. The initial dosage is 10 mg/day. Maintenance dosages range from 2 to 10 mg/day and are determined by the target INR value: For most patients, dosage should be adjusted to produce an INR between 2 and 3.

Anisindione

Anisindione [Miradon] has actions and uses like those of warfarin. However, since the incidence of severe side effects with this drug is much greater than with warfarin, use of anisindione is rare. The drug is dispensed in 50-mg tablets for oral administration. The initial dose is 300 mg. Maintenance dosages range from 25 to 250 mg/day.

ANTIPLATELET DRUGS

Antiplatelet drugs are agents that suppress platelet aggregation. Since a platelet core constitutes the bulk of an *arterial thrombus*, the principal indication for the antiplatelet drugs is prevention of thrombosis in *arteries*. In contrast, the principal indication for heparin and warfarin is prevention of thrombosis in veins.

There are three major groups of antiplatelet drugs: aspirin (a "group" with one member), ADP receptor antagonists, and GP IIb/IIIa receptor antagonists. As indicated in Figure 50–1, aspirin and the ADP antagonists affect only one pathway in platelet activation, and hence their antiplatelet effects are limited. In contrast, the GP IIb/IIIa antagonists block the final common step in platelet activation, and therefore have powerful antiplatelet effects. Properties of the major classes of antiplatelet drugs are summarized in Table 50–6.

Aspirin

The basic pharmacology of aspirin is discussed in Chapter 67. Consideration here is limited to aspirin's role in preventing arterial thrombosis.

Mechanism of Antiplatelet Action. Aspirin suppresses platelet aggregation by causing *irreversible inhibition of cyclooxygenase,* an enzyme required by platelets to synthesize thromboxane A_2 (TXA_2). As noted earlier, TXA_2 is one of the factors that can promote platelet activation. In addition to activating platelets, TXA_2 acts on vascular smooth muscle to promote vasoconstriction. Both actions promote hemostasis.

By inhibiting cyclooxygenase, aspirin suppresses both TXA_2-mediated vasoconstriction and platelet aggregation, thereby reducing the risk of arterial thrombosis. Since inhibition of cyclooxygenase by aspirin is irreversible, and since platelets lack the machinery to synthesize new cyclooxygenase, the effects of a single dose of aspirin persist for the life of the platelet (7 to 10 days).

In addition to inhibiting the synthesis of TXA_2, aspirin can inhibit synthesis of *prostacyclin* by the blood vessel wall. Since prostacyclin has effects that are exactly opposite to those of TXA_2—namely, suppression of platelet aggregation and promotion of vasodilation—suppression of prostacyclin synthesis can partially offset the beneficial effects of aspirin therapy. Fortunately, aspirin is able to inhibit synthesis of TXA_2 at doses that are lower than those needed to inhibit synthesis of prostacyclin. Accordingly, if we keep the dosage of aspirin *low* (325 mg/day or less), we can minimize inhibition of prostacyclin production, while maintaining inhibition of TXA_2 production.

Indications for Antiplatelet Therapy. Antiplatelet therapy with aspirin has three applications of proven efficacy: (1) primary prevention of MI (i.e., prevention of a first MI), (2) secondary prevention of MI (i.e., prevention of reinfarction in patients who have already had an MI), and (3) prevention of stroke in patients with a history of TIAs. In all three situations, prophylactic therapy with aspirin can reduce morbidity, and possibly mortality.

Primary Prevention of MI. In January of 2002, the United States Preventive Services Task Force (USPSTF) issued updated guidelines on the use of aspirin for primary prevention of MI. The USPSTF noted that the benefit/risk ratio is most favorable for people at high risk of MI, defined as a 3% (or higher) risk of a cardiovascular event within the next 5 years. For these people, daily aspirin lowers the risk of MI by 28%. Unfortunately, although aspirin lowers the risk of MI, it does *not* reduce the risk of death. Cardiovascular risk is based on five factors—age, gender, cholesterol levels, blood pressure, and smoking status—and can be calculated using an online risk-assessment tool, such as those at *www.med-decisions.com* and *www.intmed.mcw.edu/clincalc/heartrisk.html.* Although the optimal aspirin dosage for primary prevention is unknown, low doses (e.g., 81 mg/day) appear as effective as higher ones.

Adverse Effects. Even in low doses, aspirin increases the risk of GI bleeding and hemorrhagic stroke. Among middle-aged people taking aspirin for 5 years, the estimated rate of

TABLE 50–6 ■ Properties of the Major Classes of Antiplatelet Drugs			
	Aspirin	**ADP Receptor Blockers**	**Glycoprotein IIb/IIIa Receptor Blockers**
Representative drug	Aspirin	Clopidogrel [Plavix]	Tirofiban [Aggrastat]
Mechanism of antiplatelet action	Irreversibly inhibits cyclooxygenase, and thereby blocks synthesis of TXA_2	Irreversibly blocks receptors for ADP	Reversibly blocks receptors for GP IIb/IIIa
Route	PO	PO	IV infusion
Duration of effects	Effects persist 7–10 days after the last dose	Effects persist 7–10 days after the last dose	Effects stop within 4 hr of stopping the infusion
Cost	$3/month	$87/month	$1000/course

major GI bleeding episodes is 2 to 4 per 1000 patients, and the rate of hemorrhagic stroke is 0 to 2 episodes per 1000 patients. Use of enteric-coated or buffered aspirin may *not* reduce the risk of GI bleeding. Benefits of treatment must be weighed against bleeding risks.

Dosing. Dosage for preventing cardiovascular events should be low. Maximal inhibition of platelet cyclooxygenase, and hence maximal effects on platelet function, can be produced in a few days by taking 81 mg/day. Dosages above 81 mg/day offer no increase in benefits, but do increase the risk of GI bleeding and stroke. Accordingly, for *chronic therapy,* a dosage of 81 mg/day is probably adequate. A higher dosage (e.g., 325 mg/day) is indicated for *initial* treatment of an acute event, such as MI, in order to establish full antiplatelet effects rapidly—after which 81 mg/day can be taken for maintenance.

Adenosine Diphosphate Receptor Antagonists

Two ADP receptor antagonists are now available: ticlopidine and clopidogrel. Both drugs cause irreversible blockade of ADP receptors on the platelet surface, and thereby prevent ADP-stimulated aggregation (see Fig. 50–1). Ticlopidine is approved for prevention of ischemic stroke. Clopidogrel is approved for prevention of stroke and MI. Both drugs are taken orally and both can cause potentially fatal hematologic effects, although the risk is much higher with ticlopidine.

Ticlopidine

Actions. Ticlopidine [Ticlid] is an oral antiplatelet drug with effects similar to those of aspirin. However, unlike aspirin, which acts by inhibiting synthesis of TXA_2, ticlopidine inhibits ADP-mediated aggregation. As with aspirin, antiplatelet effects are irreversible, and hence persist for the life of the platelet.

Uses. Ticlopidine has only one approved indication: prevention of thrombotic stroke. The drug is at least as beneficial as aspirin, but is much more expensive. More importantly, ticlopidine can cause life-threatening adverse effects (see below). Accordingly, the drug should be reserved for patients who have not responded to aspirin or cannot use aspirin because of intolerance.

Since 1995, ticlopidine, in combination with aspirin, has been the primary therapy for preventing thrombus formation in coronary artery stents. About 500,000 stent recipients take the drug each year, although it is not formally approved for this use.

Pharmacokinetics. Ticlopidine is well absorbed following oral administration. Antiplatelet effects begin within 48 hours and become maximal in about a week. The drug undergoes extensive hepatic metabolism followed by renal excretion. Ticlopidine has a long half-life (4 to 5 days). Effects persist for 7 to 10 days after drug withdrawal (i.e., until new platelets have been synthesized).

Adverse Effects. Hematologic Effects. Ticlopidine can cause life-threatening hematologic reactions, including *neutropenia/agranulocytosis* and *thrombotic thrombocytopenic purpura* (TTP).

Neutropenia develops in 2.4% of patients, and is sometimes severe. Rarely, agranulocytosis develops. Both effects reverse within 1 to 3 weeks after drug withdrawal.

TTP occurs in 0.02% of patients with coronary stents who are taking ticlopidine. The mortality rate is 20% to 30%. TTP is characterized by thrombocytopenia, fever, anemia, renal dysfunction, and neurologic disturbances. The risk is highest during the first few weeks of treatment. After 12 weeks, the risk is very low. Patients should be instructed to report potential signs of TTP (e.g., unusual bleeding, bruising, rash).

To reduce the risk of harm from hematologic reactions, complete blood counts and a white cell differential should be obtained every 2 weeks during the first 12 weeks of treatment, and at any sign of infection. Ticlopidine should be withdrawn if neutropenia, agranulocytosis, or TTP develops.

Other Adverse Effects. The most common side effects are *GI disturbances* (diarrhea, abdominal pain, flatulence, nausea, dyspepsia) and *dermatologic reactions* (rash, purpura, pruritus).

Preparations and Dosage. Ticlopidine [Ticlid] is dispensed in 250-mg tablets for oral administration. The recommended dosage is 250 mg twice a day, taken with food.

Clopidogrel

Clopidogrel [Plavix] is a chemical relative of ticlopidine, but causes far fewer adverse hematologic effects. The drug is indicated for secondary prevention of MI, ischemic stroke, and other vascular events.

Antiplatelet Actions. Like ticlopidine, clopidogrel causes irreversible blockade of ADP receptors on platelets, and thereby prevents ADP-stimulated aggregation. The drug undergoes extensive metabolism on its first pass through the liver. Antiplatelet effects begin 2 hours after the first dose, and plateau after 3 to 7 days of use. At the recommended dosage, platelet aggregation is inhibited by 40% to 60%. Platelet function and bleeding time return to baseline about 7 to 10 days after drug withdrawal.

Pharmacokinetics. Clopidogrel is rapidly absorbed from the GI tract, both in the presence and absence of food. Bioavailability is about 50%. Clopidogrel is inactive as administered and must be converted to its active form in the body. The primary metabolite found in blood is a carboxylic acid derivative. However, neither the parent drug nor this derivative affects platelet aggregation. The metabolite responsible for inhibiting aggregation has not been identified. The carboxylic acid derivative is eliminated in the feces and urine. Its half-life is 8 hours.

Therapeutic Use. Clopidogrel is used to reduce the risk of thrombotic events—MI, ischemic stroke, vascular death—in patients with atherosclerosis documented by recent MI, recent stroke, or established peripheral arterial disease. In the Clopidogrel Versus Aspirin in Patients at Risk of Ischemic Events (CAPRIE) trial, which enrolled 19,185 high-risk patients, clopidogrel (75 mg once daily) was slightly better than aspirin (325 mg once daily) at reducing the combined risk of MI, ischemic stroke, or vascular death. The trial indicated that, for every 1000 patients treated for 1 year, clopidogrel would prevent 24 vascular events, compared with 19 for aspirin. However, even though clopidogrel is slightly more effective than aspirin, it is much more expensive: A 1-month supply costs about $87, compared with $3 for aspirin. Accordingly, it would seem best to reserve clopidogrel for patients who cannot tolerate aspirin or haven't responded to it adequately.

Adverse Effects and Interactions. Clopidogrel is generally well tolerated. Adverse effects are about the same as with aspirin. The most common effects are abdominal pain (6%), dyspepsia (5%), diarrhea (5%), and rash (4%). Compared with aspirin, clopidogrel causes less intracranial hemorrhage (ICH) (0.4% vs. 0.5%) and less GI bleeding (2.0% vs. 2.7%). In contrast to ticlopidine, clopidogrel does not cause neutropenia or granulocytopenia. However, it *can* cause TTP, usually during the first 2 weeks of treatment. To date, 11 cases have been reported, including one that was fatal. Fortunately, the risk of TTP is low—even lower than with ticlopidine. Clopidogrel should be used with caution in patients taking other drugs that promote bleeding (e.g., heparin, warfarin, aspirin and other nonsteroidal anti-inflammatory drugs).

Preparations, Dosage, and Administration. Clopidogrel [Plavix] is available in 75-mg tablets. The dosage is 75 mg once a day, taken with or without food. Dosage needn't be changed for elderly patients or those with renal dysfunction.

Glycoprotein IIb/IIIa Receptor Antagonists
Group Properties

The GP IIb/IIIa receptor antagonists, sometimes called "super aspirins," are the most effective antiplatelet drugs on the market. Three agents are currently available: abciximab, tirofiban, and eptifibatide. All three are administered IV, usually in combination with aspirin and low-dose heparin. Treatment is expensive, costing $1000 or more for a brief course. Dosages are summarized in Table 50–7.

Actions. The GP IIb/IIIa antagonists cause *reversible* blockade of platelet GP IIb/IIIa receptors, and thereby inhibit the final step in aggregation (see Fig. 50–1). As a result, they can prevent aggregation stimulated by any and all factors, including collagen, TXA_2, ADP, thrombin, and platelet activating factor.

TABLE 50-7 ■ Dosages for Glycoprotein IIb/IIIa Receptor Antagonists

Application	GPIIb/IIIa Inhibitor		
	Tirofiban [Aggrastat]	Eptifibatide [Integrelin]	Abciximab [ReoPro]
Acute coronary syndromes (ACSs)	0.4 μg/kg/min for 30 min, then 0.1 μg/kg/min for 48–108 hr	180-μg/kg bolus, then 2 μg/kg/min for up to 72 hr	0.25-mg/kg bolus, then 10 μg/kg/min for 18–24 hr
Percutaneous coronary intervention* (PCI) following treatment for ACSs	Continue 0.1 μg/kg/min for the procedure and 12–24 hr after	Consider decreasing the infusion rate to 0.5 μg/kg/min for the procedure and 20–24 hr after	Continue 10 μg/kg/min for the procedure and 1 hr after
PCI without prior treatment for ACSs	Not FDA approved for this application	135-μg/kg bolus prior to procedure, then 0.5 μg/kg/min for 20–24 hr	0.25-mg/kg bolus 10–60 min before the procedure, then 0.125 μg/kg/min (max 10 μg/min) for 12 hr

*Balloon or laser angioplasty, or atherectomy.

Therapeutic Use. The GP IIb/IIIa antagonists are used short-term to prevent ischemic events in patients with acute coronary syndromes (ACSs) and those undergoing percutaneous coronary intervention (PCI).

Acute Coronary Syndromes. ACSs have two major manifestations: unstable angina and non–Q-wave MI. In both cases, symptoms result from thrombosis triggered by disruption of atherosclerotic plaque. When added to traditional drugs for ACSs (heparin and aspirin), GP IIb/IIIa antagonists reduce the risk of ischemic complications.

Percutaneous Coronary Intervention. GP IIb/IIIa antagonists reduce the risk of rapid reocclusion following coronary artery revascularization with PCI (balloon or laser angioplasty, or atherectomy using an intra-arterial rotating blade). Reocclusion is common because PCI damages the arterial wall, and thereby encourages platelet aggregation.

Properties of Individual GP IIb/IIIa Antagonists

Abciximab. Description and Use. Abciximab [ReoPro] is a purified Fab fragment of a monoclonal antibody. The drug binds to platelets in the vicinity of GP IIb/IIIa receptors, and thereby prevents the receptor from binding fibrinogen. Abciximab, in conjunction with aspirin and heparin, is approved for IV therapy of ACSs and for patients undergoing PCI. In addition, clinical studies indicate it can accelerate revascularization in patients undergoing thrombolytic therapy for acute MI. Antiplatelet effects persist for 24 to 48 hours after stopping the infusion. The cost of a single course of treatment is about $1200. Dosages for ACSs and PCI are summarized in Table 50–7.

Adverse Effects and Interactions. Abciximab doubles the risk of major bleeding, especially at the PCI access site in the femoral artery. The drug may also cause GI, urogenital, and retroperitoneal bleeds. However, it does not increase the risk of fatal hemorrhage or hemorrhagic stroke. In the event of severe bleeding, infusion of abciximab and heparin should be discontinued. Other drugs that impede hemostasis will increase the risk of bleeding.

Eptifibatide. Eptifibatide [Integrilin] is a small peptide that causes reversible and highly selective inhibition of GP IIb/IIIa receptors. The drug is approved for use in ACSs and patients undergoing PCI. Antiplatelet effects reverse by 4 hours after stopping the infusion. The most important adverse effect is bleeding, which occurs most often at the site of PCI catheter insertion, and in the GI and urinary tracts. As with other GP IIb/IIIa inhibitors, the risk of bleeding is increased by concurrent use of other drugs that impede hemostasis. Dosages are summarized in Table 50–7.

Tirofiban. Tirofiban [Aggrastat] causes selective and reversible inhibition of GP IIb/IIIa receptors. The drug—neither an antibody nor a peptide—was modeled after a platelet inhibitor isolated from the venom of the saw-scaled viper, a snake indigenous to Africa. Like other GP IIb/IIIa inhibitors, tirofiban is used to reduce ischemic events associated with ACSs and PCI. Platelet function returns to baseline within 4 hours of stopping the infusion. Bleeding is the primary adverse effect. The risk of bleeding can be increased by other drugs that suppress hemostasis. Dosages for ACSs and PCI are summarized in Table 50–7.

Other Antiplatelet Drugs
Dipyridamole

Dipyridamole [Persantine] suppresses platelet aggregation, perhaps by increasing plasma levels of adenosine. The drug is approved only for prevention of thromboembolism following heart valve replacement surgery. For this application, dipyridamole is always combined with warfarin. The recommended dosage is 75 to 100 mg 4 times a day. A new combination product containing dipyridamole and aspirin is indicated for recurrent stroke (see below).

Dipyridamole plus Aspirin

Actions and Use. Dipyridamole combined with aspirin is now available in a fixed-dose formulation under the trade name *Aggrenox*. The product is used to prevent recurrent ischemic stroke in patients who have had a previous stroke or TIA. Both drugs—aspirin and dipyridamole—suppress platelet aggregation. However, since they do so by different mechanisms, the combination is more effective than either drug alone.

Clinical Trial. The benefit of combining aspirin and dipyridamole was demonstrated in the second *European Stroke Prevention Trial* (ESPS-2), a randomized controlled trial involving over 6000 patients who had suffered a prior ischemic stroke or TIA. Some patients took aspirin alone (25 mg twice daily), some took dipyridamole alone (200 mg twice daily), some took both drugs, and some took placebo. The result? After 24 months, the incidence of fatal or nonfatal ischemic stroke was reduced by 16% with dipyridamole alone, 18% with aspirin alone, and 37% with the combination. Unfortunately, ESPS-2 was tainted by scientific scandal (one investigator, who later resigned, was charged with creating and falsifying data). Although all fraudulent data were discarded prior to publication, some authorities remain skeptical of the results.

Adverse Effects. The most common adverse effects of the combination are headache, dizziness, and GI disturbances (nausea, vomiting, diarrhea, abdominal pain, dyspepsia). Of course, bleeding is a concern: The drug can cause hemorrhage (3.2% vs. 1.5% with placebo), nose bleed (2.4% vs. 1.5%), and purpura (1.4% vs. 0.4%). The aspirin in Aggrenox poses a risk of GI bleeding from peptic ulcer disease.

Preparations, Dosage, and Administration. Aggrenox capsules contain 25 mg of aspirin and 200 mg of extended-release dipyridamole. The recommended dosage is 2 capsules a day—one in the morning and one at night. The cost of treatment is about $90 a month, compared with $3 a month for aspirin alone. It is important to note that the daily dose of aspirin (50 mg) is lower than the dose recommended for prevention of MI (at least 80 mg/day). Accordingly, supplemental aspirin may be necessary for some patients.

TABLE 50–8 ■ Properties of Thrombolytic Drugs

Property	Drug					
	Streptokinase	**Alteplase (tPA)**	**Tenecteplase**	**Reteplase**	**Anistreplase**	**Urokinase**
Trade name	Streptase	Activase	TNKase	Retavase	Eminase	Abbokinase
Description	A compound that forms an active complex with plasminogen	A compound identical to human tPA	Modified form of tPA with a prolonged half-life	A compound that contains the active sequence of amino acids present in tPA	An equimolar complex of acetylated streptokinase and human plasminogen	An enzyme that converts plasminogen to plasmin
Source	Streptococcal culture	Recombinant DNA technology	Recombinant DNA technology	Recombinant DNA technology	Streptococcal culture and human plasma	Cultured human fetal kidney cells
Mechanism	All six drugs act directly or indirectly to convert plasminogen to plasmin, an enzyme that degrades the fibrin matrix of thrombi					
Adverse effects						
Bleeding	Yes	Yes	Yes	Yes	Yes	Yes
Allergic reactions	Yes	No	No	No	Yes	No
Half-life (min)	40–80	5	20–24	13–16	40–60	15–20
Dosage and administration for acute MI	*Intravenous:* 1.5 million IU infused over 30–60 min *Intracoronary:* 20,000 IU bolus, then 2000 IU/min for 60 min	*Intravenous:* 15-mg bolus, then 50 mg infused over 30 min, then 35 mg infused over 60 min	*Intravenous:* Bolus based on body weight (see text)	*Intravenous:* 10-IU bolus 2 times, separated by 30 min	*Intravenous:* 30 IU injected over 2–5 min	*Intracoronary:* 6000 IU/min for 2 hr or less
Cost	$540	$2750	$3750	$2750	$2000	$3800

Cilostazol

Actions and Therapeutic Use. Cilostazol [Pletal], a platelet inhibitor and vasodilator, is indicated for intermittent claudication. (Intermittent claudication is a syndrome characterized by pain, cramping, and weakness of the calf muscles brought on by walking and relieved by resting a few minutes. The underlying cause is atherosclerosis in the legs.) Cilostazol suppresses platelet aggregation by inhibiting type 3 phosphodiesterase (PDE-3) in platelets, and promotes vasodilation by inhibiting PDE-3 in blood vessels (primarily in the legs). Inhibition of platelet aggregation is greater than with aspirin, ticlopidine, or dipyridamole. Full effects take up to 12 weeks to develop, but reverse quickly (within 48 hours) following drug withdrawal.

Adverse Effects. Cilostazol causes a variety of untoward effects. The most common is headache (34%). Other side effects include diarrhea (19%), abnormal stools (15%), palpitations (10%), dizziness (10%), and peripheral edema (7%).

Other drugs that inhibit PDE-3 have increased mortality in patients with heart failure. Whether cilostazol represents a risk is unknown. Nonetheless, heart failure is a contraindication to cilostazol use.

Drug and Food Interactions. Cilostazol is metabolized by the 3A4 isozyme of cytochrome P450 (CYP3A4), and hence cilostazol levels can be increased by CYP3A4 inhibitors (e.g., ketoconazole, itraconazole, erythromycin, fluoxetine, fluvoxamine, nefazodone, sertraline, and grapefruit juice). Metabolism of cilostazol can also be inhibited by omeprazole.

Preparations, Dosage, and Administration. Cilostazol [Pletal] is available in 50- and 100-mg tablets. The usual dosage is 100 mg twice daily, taken 30 minutes before or 2 hours after breakfast and the evening meal. Dosage should be reduced to 50 mg twice daily in patients taking omeprazole and drugs or foods that inhibit CYP3A4.

THROMBOLYTIC DRUGS

As their name implies, thrombolytic drugs are given to remove thrombi that have already formed. This contrasts with the anticoagulants, which are given to prevent thrombus for-

mation. Six thrombolytic drugs are available: streptokinase, alteplase, reteplase, urokinase, anistreplase, and tenecteplase. All carry a risk of serious bleeding, and hence should be administered only by clinicians skilled in their use. Thrombolytic agents are employed acutely and only for severe thrombotic disease. Because of their mechanism of action, these agents are also known as *fibrinolytics* (and informally as *clot busters*). Properties of individual agents are summarized in Table 50–8.

Streptokinase

Streptokinase [Streptase] was the first thrombolytic drug available and will serve as our prototype for the group.

Mechanism of Action

Streptokinase acts by an indirect mechanism. The drug first binds to *plasminogen* to form an active complex. The streptokinase-plasminogen complex then catalyzes the conversion of other plasminogen molecules into plasmin, an enzyme that digests the fibrin meshwork of clots. In addition to digesting fibrin in clots, plasmin degrades fibrinogen and other clotting factors; these actions do not contribute to lysis of thrombi, but they do increase the risk of hemorrhage.

Therapeutic Uses

Streptokinase has three major indications: (1) acute coronary thrombosis (acute MI), (2) DVT, and (3) massive pulmonary emboli. In all three situations, timely intervention is essential. For example, in patients with acute MI, results are best when thrombolytic therapy is started within 4 to 6 hours of symptom onset, and preferably sooner. Thrombolytic therapy of acute MI is discussed further in Chapter 51.

Pharmacokinetics

Streptokinase may be administered by IV infusion or by infusion directly into an occluded coronary artery. Because of rapid inactivation, the drug's half-life is only 40 to 80 minutes.

Adverse Effects

Bleeding. Bleeding is the major complication of treatment. Intracranial hemorrhage (ICH), which occurs in 1% of patients, is by far the most serious concern. Bleeding occurs for two reasons: (1) plasmin can destroy pre-existing clots, and can thereby promote recurrence of bleeding at sites of recently healed injury; and (2) by degrading clotting factors, plasmin can disrupt the coagulation cascade, and can thereby interfere with new clot formation in response to vascular injury. Likely sites of bleeding include recent wounds, sites of needle puncture, and sites at which invasive procedures have been performed. Anticoagulants (heparin, warfarin) and antiplatelet drugs (e.g., aspirin) further increase the risk of hemorrhage. Accordingly, high-dose therapy with these drugs must be avoided until thrombolytic effects of streptokinase have abated.

Management of bleeding depends on severity. Oozing at sites of cutaneous puncture can be controlled with a pressure dressing. If severe bleeding occurs, streptokinase should be discontinued. Patients who require blood replacement can be given whole blood or blood products (packed red blood cells, fresh-frozen plasma). As a rule, blood replacement restores hemostasis. However, if this approach fails, excessive fibrinolysis can be reversed with IV *aminocaproic acid* [Amicar], a compound that prevents activation of plasminogen and directly inhibits plasmin.

The risk of bleeding can be lowered by

- Minimizing physical manipulation of the patient
- Avoiding SC and IM injections
- Minimizing invasive procedures
- Minimizing concurrent use of anticoagulants (heparin, warfarin)
- Minimizing concurrent use of antiplatelet drugs (e.g., aspirin)

Because of the risk of hemorrhage, streptokinase and other thrombolytic drugs must be avoided by patients at high risk for bleeding complications, and must be used with great caution in patients at lower risk of bleeding. A list of absolute and relative contraindications to thrombolytic therapy is presented in Table 50–9.

Antibody Production. Streptokinase is a foreign protein extracted from cultures of streptococci. As a result, antibodies may form. Two consequences are possible: *allergic reactions* and *neutralization of streptokinase.* The most common allergic reactions are urticaria, itching, flushing, and headache. These can be treated with antihistamines. Severe anaphylaxis is rare. Because neutralizing antibodies may develop within a few days of streptokinase administration, repeat courses of streptokinase may be ineffective. Hence, if a repeat course is needed, a different thrombolytic agent (e.g., alteplase) should be used.

Hypotension. Streptokinase may cause significant hypotension soon after administration. The incidence is between 1% and 10%. Hypotension is not related to bleeding or allergic reactions. Blood pressure should be monitored. If hypotension develops, it may be necessary to slow the streptokinase infusion.

Fever. Temperature elevation of 1.5°F or more occurs in one-third of patients. Only 3.5% of patients develop temperatures above 104°F. Acetaminophen—not aspirin—should be used to lower temperature.

Preparations, Dosage, and Administration

Streptokinase [Streptase] is dispensed as a powder and must be reconstituted for use. Solutions are prepared with either 0.9% saline or 5% dextrose. Dosage is prescribed in international units (IU).

For treatment of *pulmonary embolism, DVT,* and *arterial thrombosis or embolism,* streptokinase is administered by IV infusion. Therapy is usually initiated with an IV loading dose of 250,000 IU infused over 30 minutes. After the loading dose, the infusion is continued for 1 to 3 days at a rate of 100,000 IU/hr.

For treatment of an *evolving MI,* streptokinase may be infused through a catheter placed in the occluded coronary artery. This technique offers two benefits: (1) high levels of streptokinase are achieved at the site where the drug is needed, and (2) high levels are avoided at other sites, thereby minimizing generalized bleeding. Timing of therapy is critical: Streptokinase is most effective when therapy is begun within 6 hours of symptom onset, and preferably sooner.

TABLE 50–9 ■ Contraindications and Cautions Regarding Thrombolytic Use for Myocardial Infarction

Absolute Contraindications

- Previous hemorrhagic stroke at any time; other strokes or cerebrovascular events within 1 year
- Known intracranial neoplasm
- Active internal bleeding (other than menses)
- Suspected aortic dissection

Relative Contraindications/Cautions

- Severe uncontrolled hypertension on presentation (blood pressure >180/110 mm Hg)
- History of chronic hypertension
- History of prior cerebrovascular accident of known intracerebral pathology not covered in contraindications
- Current use of anticoagulants in therapeutic doses (INR ≥2–3); known bleeding diathesis
- Recent trauma (within 2–4 wk), including head trauma
- Recent internal bleeding (within 2–4 wk)
- Noncompressible vascular punctures
- For streptokinase/anistreplase: prior exposure (especially within 5 days to 2 yr) or prior allergic reaction
- Pregnancy
- Active peptic ulcer

Adapted from Ryan TJ, Antman EM, Brooks NH, et al. 1999 update: ACC/AHA guidelines for the management of patients with acute myocardial infarction. A report of the American College of Cardiology/American Heart Association Task Force on Practice Guidelines (Committee on Management of Acute Myocardial Infarction). J Am Coll Cardiol 1999;34:890–911.

Alteplase (tPA)

Alteplase [Activase], also known as tissue plasminogen activator (tPA), is produced commercially by recombinant DNA technology. The commercial preparation is identical to naturally occurring human tPA, an enzyme that promotes conversion of plasminogen to plasmin, an enzyme that digests the fibrin matrix of clots. Low therapeutic doses produce selective activation of plasminogen that is bound to fibrin in thrombi. As a result, activation of plasminogen in the general circulation is minimized. However, despite selective activation of fibrin-bound plasminogen, bleeding tendencies with alteplase are equivalent to those seen with the other thrombolytic drugs. Furthermore, the risk of intracranial bleeding is higher with alteplase than with streptokinase. Since alteplase is devoid of foreign proteins, it does not cause allergic reactions. In contrast to streptokinase, alteplase does not induce hypotension. Alteplase has a short half-life (about 5 minutes) owing to rapid hepatic inactivation.

Like streptokinase, alteplase is indicated for acute MI and pulmonary embolism. In addition, alteplase is now approved for treating ischemic stroke. As discussed below, the GUSTO-I trial has shown that alteplase is slightly better than streptokinase for treating acute MI. Unfortunately, alteplase is also much more expensive: A single course of alteplase costs about $2750, compared with $540 for streptokinase.

Alteplase is now given by an "accelerated" or "front-loaded" schedule. In this schedule, the infusion time is only 90 minutes, compared with the 3-hour infusion employed previously. For patients who weigh over 67 kg, the total dose for treating acute MI is 100 mg. Administration is divided into three phases: a 15-mg IV bolus, followed by 50 mg infused over 30 minutes, followed in turn by 35 mg infused over 60 minutes. Total doses in excess of 100 mg are associated with an increased risk of intracranial bleeding and should be avoided.

Tenecteplase

Tenecteplase [TNKase], a variant of human tissue plasminogen activator (tPA, alteplase), has been approved for treating patients undergoing acute MI. Except for the substitution of three amino acids, the drug is structurally identical to tPA. However, because of this small structural change, the pharmacokinetics of tenecteplase are much different from those of tPA. Specifically, tenecteplase is 80 times more resistant than tPA to circulating inhibitors and has a much longer half-life (20 to 24 minutes vs. 5 minutes for tPA). Like tPA, tenecteplase acts by converting plasminogen into plasmin, an enzyme that digests fibrin clots. *Tenecteplase is just as safe and effective as tPA, but much is easier to use: Whereas tPA must be infused over 90 minutes, tenecteplase is given by bolus injection.* As a result, thrombolysis develops faster, and emergency room personnel are spared the work of monitoring a prolonged infusion. Because tenecteplase is so easy to administer, it has the potential to allow dosing before the patient reaches a hospital.

Tenecteplase was compared with tPA in the second Assessment of the Safety and Efficacy of a New Thrombolytic (ASSENT-2) study, which enrolled 16,949 patients. Tenecteplase was given as a 5-second IV bolus; tPA was infused over 90 minutes. The median time between symptom onset and starting treatment was 2.7 hours for tenecteplase and 2.8 hours for tPA. Thirty days after treatment, responses

were equivalent with respect to mortality (6.2% with each drug), intracranial hemorrhage (0.93% with tenecteplase vs. 0.94% with tPA), and total stroke (1.78% vs. 1.66% with tPA). Of significance, the incidence of major hemorrhage (other than intracranial) was *lower* with tenecteplase (4.7% vs. 5.9%).

Dosage of tenecteplase is based on body weight (BW) as follows:

- BW <60 kg: dose 30 mg
- BW 60 to 69.9 kg: dose 35 mg
- BW 70 to 79.9 kg: dose 40 mg
- BW 80 to 89.9 kg: dose 45 mg
- BW >90 kg: dose 50 mg

Note that no one is given more than 50 mg. Interestingly, the current price of tenecteplase ($2750/dose) is identical to that of tPA [Activase] and reteplase [Retavase].

Other Thrombolytic Drugs

Urokinase, anistreplase, and reteplase are similar to streptokinase with regard to mechanism of action, indications, and ability to promote bleeding. Principal differences among these drugs relate to half-life, source, antigenicity, cost, and specific indications.

Urokinase

Urokinase [Abbokinase] is an enzyme that occurs naturally in human urine. Commercial urokinase is prepared by extraction from cultures of human fetal kidney cells. Like streptokinase, urokinase promotes the conversion of plasminogen into plasmin, its active form. As with other thrombolytics, bleeding is the principal adverse effect. Since urokinase is human derived, it is not antigenic, and hence allergic reactions do not occur. Urokinase has a short half-life (15 to 20 minutes) owing to rapid inactivation by the liver. The drug is approved for acute MI, DVT, and clearance of IV catheters. For treatment of acute MI, urokinase is infused for 2 hours or less at a rate of 6000 IU/hr. Because of its high cost (see Table 50–8), urokinase is used much less frequently than streptokinase.

Anistreplase (APSAC)

Anistreplase [Eminase] is an acylated complex of streptokinase plus human plasminogen. The streptokinase portion is obtained from streptococcal culture; the human plasminogen portion is obtained by extraction from human plasma. Because it is acylated, the plasminogen in anistreplase is inactive. Once in the body, the drug undergoes gradual deacylation followed by conversion to plasmin, which then acts to digest fibrin in clots. In addition to degrading fibrin in clots, anistreplase can degrade circulating fibrinogen. Both actions (digestion of fibrin and degradation of fibrinogen) promote bleeding. The risk of bleeding complications with anistreplase is the same as with the other thrombolytic drugs. Since anistreplase contains streptokinase (a foreign protein), the drug can cause allergic reactions. Like streptokinase, anistreplase may cause hypotension. Anistreplase differs from the other thrombolytics in that it can be administered by slow IV injection instead of infusion. This makes anistreplase more convenient. The recommended dosage for acute MI is 30 units injected over 2 to 5 minutes. Like urokinase and alteplase, anistreplase is expensive, costing over $2000 for one course of treatment. An alternative name for anistreplase is *anisoylated plasminogen-streptokinase activator complex,* or *APSAC.*

Reteplase

Reteplase [Retavase] is a derivative of tPA produced by recombinant DNA technology. In contrast to tPA itself, which contains 527 amino acids, reteplase is composed of only 355 amino acids. Like tPA, reteplase converts plasminogen to plasmin, which in turn digests the fibrin matrix of the thrombus. Reteplase has a short half-life (13 to 16 minutes) because of rapid clearance by the liver and kidneys. As with other thrombolytic drugs, bleeding is the major adverse effect. The risk of bleeding is increased by concurrent use of heparin and aspirin. Allergic reactions have not been reported.

Reteplase was compared with front-loaded alteplase in the RAPID II (Reteplase Versus Alteplase Patency Investigation During Myocardial Infarction Study). The results indicate that reteplase produces higher rates of early reperfusion than alteplase without increasing the risk of hemorrhagic stroke or other complications.

Reteplase is approved only for acute MI. Treatment consists of two 10-unit doses separated by 30 minutes. Each dose is given by IV bolus injected over a 2-minute interval. Reteplase should not be administered through a line that contains heparin. If a heparin-containing line must be used, it should be flushed prior to giving reteplase.

Streptokinase Versus Alteplase: The GUSTO-I Trial

The GUSTO-I (Global Utilization of Streptokinase and tPA for Occluded Coronary Arteries) trial is the largest study ever conducted on the treatment of acute MI. Over 41,000 patients from 15 countries participated. The results indicate that *mortality* from MI in patients receiving alteplase (tPA) is somewhat lower than in patients receiving streptokinase (SK)—although the risk of *hemorrhagic stroke* with tPA is higher. However, as discussed below, the apparent superiority of tPA as seen in GUSTO may not be relevant to everyday clinical practice.

In GUSTO-I, each participant received one of the following treatments (30-day mortality rates are in parentheses):

- tPA + IV heparin (6.3%)
- SK + IV heparin (7.4%)
- SK + SC heparin (7.2%)
- SK + tPA + IV heparin (7.0%)

As the mortality figures indicate, 7.4 of each 100 patients who received streptokinase (plus IV heparin) died within 30 days. In contrast, only 6.3 of each 100 patients who received tPA (plus IV heparin) died within 30 days. Hence, by using tPA instead of streptokinase, we might expect to save one additional life for each 100 patients.

What the above figures don't indicate is the timing of tPA administration with respect to onset of MI symptoms. In GUSTO-I, nearly 90% of patients received treatment within 2 to 4 hours of symptom onset. Among patients who received tPA within 2 hours of symptom onset, the death rate was only 5.4%; among those treated 2 to 4 hours after symptom onset, the rate increased to 6.6%; and among those treated 4 to 6 hours after symptom onset, the rate jumped to 9.4%. Not only do these figures underscore the importance of early treatment of MI, they bring into question the relevance of GUSTO-I to ordinary clinical practice. Why? Because, in usual practice, very few patients are treated as early as those in GUSTO. Furthermore, among patients who are treated *after* 4 hours, GUSTO-I showed no significant difference in mortality between treatment with tPA and treatment with streptokinase. Hence, although tPA may be superior to streptokinase when these drugs are employed under *ideal* conditions, tPA may not be superior in everyday practice. When this observation is coupled with two others—the much higher cost of tPA and the greater incidence of hemorrhagic stroke with tPA—the desirability of tPA over streptokinase is less obvious. Regardless of whether tPA is significantly better than streptokinase, there is no question that treatment with either drug is much better than no treatment at all. Put another way, selecting some thrombolytic drug is much more important than which one is selected.

KEY POINTS

- Hemostasis occurs in two stages: formation of a platelet plug, followed by coagulation (i.e., production of fibrin, a protein that reinforces the platelet plug).
- Platelet aggregation depends upon activation of GP IIb/IIIa receptors, which bind fibrinogen to form cross-links between platelets.
- Fibrin is produced by two pathways, known as the intrinsic and extrinsic systems. These pathways converge with production of factor Xa, which catalyzes formation of thrombin, which in turn catalyzes formation of fibrin.
- Four factors in the coagulation pathways require vitamin K for synthesis.
- Plasmin, the active form of plasminogen, serves to dissolve the fibrin meshwork of clots.
- A thrombus is a blood clot formed within a blood vessel or within the heart.
- Arterial thrombi begin with formation of a platelet plug, which is then reinforced with fibrin.
- Venous thrombi begin with formation of fibrin, which then enmeshes red blood cells and platelets.
- Arterial thrombi are best prevented with antiplatelet drugs (e.g., aspirin), whereas venous thrombi are best prevented with anticoagulants (warfarin, heparin).
- Heparin is a large polymer (molecular weight range = 3000 to 30,000) that carries many negative charges.
- Heparin suppresses coagulation by helping antithrombin inactivate thrombin and factor Xa.
- Heparin is administered IV or SC. Because of its large size and negative charges, heparin is unable to cross membranes, and hence cannot be administered PO.
- Anticoagulant effects of heparin develop within minutes of IV administration.
- The major adverse effect of heparin is bleeding.
- Severe heparin-induced bleeding can be treated with protamine sulfate, a drug that binds heparin and thereby stops it from working.
- Heparin-induced thrombocytopenia is a potentially fatal condition caused by development of antibodies against heparin-platelet protein complexes.
- Heparin is contraindicated for patients with thrombocytopenia or uncontrollable bleeding, and must be used with extreme caution in all patients for whom there is a high likelihood of bleeding.
- Heparin therapy is monitored by measuring aPTT (activated partial thromboplastin time). The target aPTT is 60 to 80 seconds (i.e., 1.5 to 2 times the normal value of 40 seconds).
- Low-molecular-weight (LMW) heparins are produced by breaking molecules of unfractionated heparin into smaller pieces.
- In contrast to unfractionated heparin, which inactivates factor Xa and thrombin equally, LMW heparins preferentially inactivate factor Xa.
- In contrast to unfractionated heparin, LMW heparins do not bind nonspecifically to plasma proteins and tissues. As a result, their bioavailability is high, making their plasma levels predictable.

- Because plasma levels of LMW heparins are predictable, these drugs can be administered on a fixed schedule with no need for routine laboratory monitoring. As a result, LMW heparins can be used at home.
- Warfarin is the prototype of the oral anticoagulants.
- Warfarin antagonizes vitamin K, and thereby blocks the biosynthesis of vitamin K–dependent clotting factors.
- Anticoagulant responses to warfarin develop slowly and persist for several days after warfarin is discontinued.
- Warfarin therapy is monitored by measuring pro-thrombin time (PT). Results are expressed as an international normalized ratio (INR). An INR of 2 to 3 is the target for most patients.
- Bleeding is the major complication of warfarin therapy.
- Moderate warfarin overdose is treated with vitamin K.
- Warfarin must not be used during pregnancy. The drug can cause fetal malformation, CNS defects, and optic atrophy.
- Warfarin is subject to a large number of clinically significant drug interactions. Drugs can increase anticoagulant effects by displacing warfarin from plasma albumin and by inhibiting hepatic enzymes that degrade warfarin. Drugs can decrease anticoagulant effects by inducing hepatic drug-metabolizing enzymes, increasing synthesis of clotting factors, and inhibiting warfarin absorption. Drugs that promote bleeding, such as heparin and aspirin, will obviously increase the risk of bleeding in patients taking warfarin. Instruct patients to avoid all drugs—prescription and nonprescription—that have not been specifically approved by the physician.

- Aspirin and other antiplatelet drugs suppress thrombus formation in arteries.
- Aspirin inhibits platelet aggregation by causing irreversible inhibition of cyclooxygenase. Since platelets are unable to synthesize new cyclooxygenase, inhibition persists for the life of the platelet (7 to 10 days).
- In its role as an antiplatelet drug, aspirin is given for primary prophylaxis of MI, prevention of MI recurrence, and prevention of stroke in patients with a history of TIAs.
- When used to suppress platelet aggregation, aspirin is administered in low doses—typically 80 to 325 mg/day.
- The GP IIb/IIIa receptor blockers (e.g., abciximab) inhibit the final common step in platelet aggregation, and hence are the most effective antiplatelet drugs available.
- Thrombolytic drugs (e.g., streptokinase, alteplase [tPA]) are used to dissolve existing thrombi (rather than prevent thrombi from forming).
- Thrombolytic drugs work by converting plasminogen to plasmin, an enzyme that degrades the fibrin matrix of thrombi.
- Thrombolytic therapy is most effective when started early (i.e., within 4 to 6 hours of symptom onset, and preferably sooner).
- Thrombolytic drugs carry a significant risk of bleeding. Intracranial hemorrhage is the greatest concern.
- For patients with acute MI, tPA is slightly more effective than streptokinase, but costs much more and causes more intracranial bleeding.

Summary of Major Nursing Implications*

HEPARIN

Preadministration Assessment

Therapeutic Goal

The objective of treatment is to prevent thrombosis without inducing spontaneous bleeding.

Heparin is the preferred anticoagulant for use during pregnancy and in situations that require rapid onset of effects, including pulmonary embolism, evolving stroke, and massive DVT. Other indications include open heart surgery, renal dialysis, and disseminated intravascular coagulation. Low doses are used to prevent postoperative venous thrombosis and to enhance thrombolytic therapy of MI.

Baseline Data

Obtain baseline values for blood pressure, heart rate, complete blood cell counts, platelet counts, hematocrit, and aPTT.

Identifying High-Risk Patients

Heparin is *contraindicated* for patients with severe thrombocytopenia or uncontrollable bleeding and for patients undergoing lumbar puncture, regional anesthesia, or surgery of the eye, brain, or spinal cord.

Use with *extreme caution* in patients at high risk of bleeding, including those with hemophilia, increased capillary permeability, dissecting aneurysm, GI ulcers, or severe hypertension. Caution is also needed in patients with severe hepatic or renal dysfunction.

Implementation: Administration

Routes

Intravenous (continuous infusion or intermittent) and subcutaneous. Avoid IM injections!

Administration

General Considerations. Dosage is prescribed in units, not milligrams. Heparin preparations vary widely in concentration; read the label carefully to ensure correct dosing.

Intermittent IV Administration. Administer through a heparin lock every 4 to 6 hours. aPTT should be determined before each dose during the early phase of treatment, and daily thereafter. Rotate the injection site every 2 to 3 days.

*Patient education information is highlighted as blue text.

Summary of Major Nursing Implications*—cont'd

Continuous IV Infusion. Administer with a constant infusion pump or some other approved volume control unit. Policy may require that dosage be double-checked by a second person. Check the infusion rate every 30 to 60 minutes. During the early phase of treatment, aPTT should be determined every 4 hours. Check the site of needle insertion periodically for extravasation.

Deep SC Injection. Perform SC injections into the fatty layer of the abdomen (but not within 2 inches of the umbilicus). Withdraw heparin solution using a 20- to 22-gauge needle, and then discard that needle and replace it with a small needle (1/2 to 5/8 inch, 25- or 26-gauge) to make the injection. Apply firm but gentle pressure to the injection site for 1 to 2 minutes following administration. Rotate and record injection sites.

Ongoing Evaluation and Interventions

Evaluating Treatment

Periodic determinations of aPTT are used to evaluate treatment. Heparin should increase the aPTT by 1.5- to 2-fold above baseline.

Minimizing Adverse Effects

Hemorrhage. Heparin overdose may cause hemorrhage. Monitor closely for signs of bleeding. These include lowering of blood pressure, elevation of heart rate, discoloration of urine or stool, bruises, petechiae, hematomas, persistent headache or faintness (suggestive of cerebral hemorrhage), pelvic pain (suggestive of ovarian hemorrhage), and lumbar pain (suggestive of adrenal hemorrhage). Laboratory data suggesting hemorrhage include reductions in the hematocrit and blood cell counts. If bleeding occurs, heparin should be discontinued. Severe overdose can be treated with *protamine sulfate* administered by slow IV injection. The risk of bleeding can be reduced by ensuring that the aPTT does not exceed 2 times the baseline value.

Heparin-Induced Thrombocytopenia. HIT, characterized by reduced platelet counts and increased thrombotic events, poses a risk of DVT, pulmonary embolism, cerebral thrombosis, MI, and ischemic injury to the arms and legs. To reduce risk, monitor platelet counts 2 to 3 times a week during the first 3 weeks of heparin use, and monthly thereafter. If severe thrombocytopenia develops (platelet count <100,000/mm^3), discontinue heparin and, if anticoagulation is still needed, substitute lipirudin or argatroban.

Hypersensitivity Reactions. Allergy may develop to antigens in heparin preparations. To minimize the risk of severe reactions, administer a small test dose prior to the full therapeutic dose.

Minimizing Adverse Interactions

Antiplatelet Drugs. Concurrent use of antiplatelet drugs (e.g., aspirin, ticlopidine) increases the risk of bleeding. Use these agents with caution.

WARFARIN

Preadministration Assessment

Therapeutic Goal

The goal of therapy is to prevent thrombosis without inducing spontaneous bleeding. Specific indications include prevention of venous thrombosis and associated pulmonary embolism, prevention of thromboembolism in patients with prosthetic heart valves, and prevention of thrombosis during atrial fibrillation.

Baseline Data

Obtain a thorough medical history. Be sure to identify use of any medications that might interact adversely with warfarin. Obtain baseline values of vital signs and PT.

Identifying High-Risk Patients

Warfarin is *contraindicated* in the presence of vitamin K deficiency, liver disease, alcoholism, thrombocytopenia, uncontrollable bleeding, pregnancy, and lactation, and for patients undergoing lumbar puncture, regional anesthesia, or surgery of the eye, brain, or spinal cord.

Use with *extreme caution* in patients at high risk of bleeding, including those with hemophilia, increased capillary permeability, dissecting aneurysm, GI ulcers, and severe hypertension.

Implementation: Administration

Route

Oral.

Administration

For most patients, dosage is adjusted to maintain an INR value of 2 to 3. Maintain a flow chart for hospitalized patients indicating INR values and dosage size and timing.

Implementation: Measures to Enhance Therapeutic Effects

Promoting Compliance

Safe and effective therapy requires rigid adherence to the dosing schedule. Achieving adherence requires active and informed participation by the patient. Provide the patient with detailed written and verbal instructions regarding the purpose of treatment, dosage size and timing, and the importance of strict adherence to the dosing schedule. Also, provide the patient with a chart on which to keep an ongoing record of warfarin use. If the patient is incompetent (e.g., mentally ill, alcoholic, senile), ensure that a responsible individual supervises treatment.

Nondrug Measures

Advise the patient to (1) avoid prolonged immobility, (2) elevate the legs when sitting, (3) avoid garments that can restrict blood flow in the legs, (4) participate in exercise activities, and (5) wear support hose. These measures will reduce venous stasis, and will thereby reduce the risk of thrombosis.

*Patient education information is highlighted as blue text.

Summary of Major Nursing Implications*—cont'd

Ongoing Evaluation and Interventions

Evaluating Therapeutic Effects

Monitoring Prothrombin Time. Evaluate therapy by monitoring PT. Test results are reported as an INR. For most patients, the target INR is 2 to 3. If the INR is below this range, dosage should be increased. Conversely, if the INR is above this range, dosage should be reduced.

PT should be measured frequently: daily during the first 5 days, twice a week for the next 1 to 2 weeks, once a week for the next 1 to 2 months, and every 2 to 4 weeks thereafter. In addition, PT should be determined whenever a drug that interacts with warfarin is added to or deleted from the regimen.

If heparin is being employed concurrently, blood for PT determinations should be drawn no sooner than 5 hours after IV administration of heparin, and no sooner than 24 hours after SC administration.

If appropriate, teach patients how to monitor their PT and INR at home.

Minimizing Adverse Effects

Hemorrhage. Hemorrhage is the major complication of warfarin therapy. **Warn patients about the danger of hemorrhage, and inform them about signs of bleeding. These include lowering of blood pressure, elevation of heart rate, discoloration of urine or stools, bruises, petechiae, hematomas, persistent headache or faintness (suggestive of cerebral hemorrhage), pelvic pain (suggestive of ovarian hemorrhage), and lumbar pain (suggestive of adrenal hemorrhage).** Laboratory data suggesting hemorrhage include reductions in the hematocrit and blood cell counts.

Instruct the patient to withhold warfarin and notify the physician if signs of bleeding are noted. Advise the patient to wear some form of identification (e.g., Medic Alert bracelet) indicating warfarin use.

To reduce the incidence of bleeding, advise the patient to avoid excessive consumption of alcohol. Suggest use of a soft toothbrush to prevent bleeding from the gums. Advise patients to shave with an electric razor.

Warfarin intensifies bleeding during surgical or dental procedures. **Instruct the patient to make certain the surgeon or dentist is aware that warfarin is being used.** Warfarin should be discontinued several days prior to elective procedures. If emergency surgery must be performed, vitamin K_1 can help reduce bleeding.

Warfarin-induced bleeding can be controlled with vitamin K_1. For most patients, oral vitamin K will suffice. For patients with severe bleeding or a very high INR, vitamin K is given by injection (usually IV). The physician may advise the patient to keep a supply of vitamin K on hand for use in emergencies, but only after consultation with a physician.

Use in Pregnancy and Lactation. Warfarin can cross the placenta, causing fetal hemorrhage and malformation. **Inform women of child-bearing age about potential risks to the fetus, and warn them against becoming pregnant.** If pregnancy develops, termination should be considered.

Warfarin enters breast milk and may harm the nursing infant. **Warn women against breast-feeding.**

Minimizing Adverse Interactions

Inform patients that warfarin is subject to a large number of potentially dangerous drug interactions. Instruct them to avoid all drugs—prescription and nonprescription—that have not been specifically approved by the physician. Prior to treatment, take a complete medication history to identify any drugs that might interact adversely with warfarin.

THROMBOLYTIC DRUGS

Alteplase (tPA)
Anistreplase
Reteplase
Streptokinase
Tenecteplase
Urokinase

Preadministration Assessment

Therapeutic Goal

Thrombolytic drugs are used to treat acute MI, massive pulmonary emboli, ischemic stroke, and DVT.

Baseline Data

Obtain baseline values for blood pressure, heart rate, platelet counts, hematocrit, aPTT, PT, and fibrinogen level.

Identifying High-Risk Patients

Thrombolytic drugs are *contraindicated* for patients with active bleeding, aortic dissection, acute pericarditis, cerebral neoplasm, cerebral vascular disease, or a history of intracranial bleeding. Use with *great caution* in patients with relative contraindications, including pregnancy, severe hypertension, ischemic stroke within the prior 6 months, and major surgery within the prior 2 to 4 weeks. See Table 50–9 for a complete list of absolute and relative contraindications.

Implementation: Administration

Routes

Intracoronary, intravenous (see Table 50–8).

Administration

Depending on the drug employed and the specific application, administration may be by IV infusion, slow IV injection, IV bolus, intracoronary infusion, or intracoronary bolus. (See Table 50–8 for administration during acute MI.)

Do not administer heparin and streptokinase through the same IV line.

Ongoing Evaluation and Interventions

Minimizing Adverse Effects

Hemorrhage. Thrombolytics may cause bleeding; ICH is the greatest concern. To reduce the risk of major bleeding, minimize manipulation of the patient, avoid SC and IM in-

*Patient education information is highlighted as blue text.

Summary of Major Nursing Implications*—cont'd

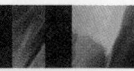

jections, minimize invasive procedures, and minimize concurrent use of anticoagulants (heparin, warfarin) and antiplatelet drugs (e.g., aspirin). Manage oozing at cutaneous puncture sites with a pressure dressing.

For severe bleeding, discontinue streptokinase and give whole blood or blood products (packed red blood cells, fresh-frozen plasma). If bleeding continues, give IV aminocaproic acid.

*Patient education information is highlighted as blue text.

Minimizing Adverse Interactions

Anticoagulants and Antiplatelet Drugs. Anticoagulants (heparin, warfarin) and antiplatelet drugs (e.g., aspirin) increase the risk of bleeding from antithrombotics. Avoid high-dose therapy with these drugs until thrombolytic effects have subsided.

Management of Myocardial Infarction

Myocardial infarction (MI) is defined as necrosis of the myocardium resulting from acute occlusion of a coronary artery. Risk factors include advanced age, a family history of MI, sedentary lifestyle, obesity, high serum cholesterol, hypertension, smoking, and diabetes. In the United States, MI strikes about 1.5 million people each year and is the most common cause of death. Between 20% and 30% of MI victims die before reaching the hospital, another 9.9% die in the hospital, and 7.1% die within a year of being discharged. The objectives of this chapter are to describe the pathophysiology of MI and to discuss interventions that can help reduce morbidity and mortality.

PATHOPHYSIOLOGY OF MYOCARDIAL INFARCTION

MI occurs when blood flow to a region of the myocardium (heart muscle) is stopped because of platelet plugging and thrombus formation in a coronary artery—almost always at a site of a fissured or ruptured atherosclerotic plaque. Myocardial injury is ultimately the result of an imbalance between oxygen demand and oxygen supply.

In response to local ischemia (insufficient oxygen), a dramatic redistribution of ions takes place. Hydrogen ions accumulate in the myocardium and calcium ions become sequestered in mitochondria. The resultant acidosis and functional calcium deficiency alter the distensibility of cardiac muscle. Sodium ions accumulate in myocardial cells and promote edema. Potassium ions are lost from myocardial cells, thereby setting the stage for dysrhythmias.

Local metabolic changes begin rapidly following coronary artery occlusion. Within seconds, metabolism shifts from aerobic to anaerobic. High energy stores of ATP and creatine phosphate become depleted. As a result, contraction ceases in the affected region.

If blood flow is not restored, cell death occurs within 2 to 6 hours. Clear indices of cell death—myocyte disruption, coagulative necrosis, elevation of serum enzymes—are present by 24 hours. By 4 days, monocyte infiltration and removal of dead myocytes weaken the infarcted area, making it vulnerable to expansion and rupture. Healing begins in 10 to 12 days with deposition of collagen, and is usually complete with dense scar formation in 4 to 6 weeks.

The degree of residual cardiac dysfunction depends on how much of the myocardium was damaged. With infarction of 10% of left ventricular (LV) mass, the ejection fraction is reduced. With 25% LV infarction, cardiac dilation and congestive heart failure (CHF) occur. With 40% LV infarction, cardiogenic shock and death are likely.

DIAGNOSIS OF MYOCARDIAL INFARCTION

Myocardial infarction is diagnosed by the presence of chest pain, characteristic electrocardiographic (EKG) changes, and elevated serum levels of myocardial cellular components (creatine kinase, troponin). Other symptoms include sweating, weakness, and a sense of impending doom. About 20% of people with MI experience no symptoms.

Chest Pain. Patients undergoing acute MI typically experience severe substernal pressure that they characterize as unbearable crushing or constricting pain. The pain often radiates down the arms and up to the jaw. Acute MI can be differentiated from angina pectoris in that pain caused by MI lasts longer (20 to 30 minutes) and is not relieved by nitroglycerin. Some patients confuse the pain of MI with indigestion.

EKG Changes. Myocardial infarction often produces characteristic changes in the EKG (Fig. 51–1). These changes occur because conduction of electrical impulses through the heart becomes altered in the region of myocardial injury. Elevation of the ST segment occurs almost immediately in response to acute ischemia. Following a period of ST elevation, a prominent Q wave (>0.04-second duration) develops in the majority of patients. (Q waves are small or absent in the normal EKG.) Over time, the ST segment returns to baseline, after which a symmetric inverted T wave appears. This T wave inversion may resolve within weeks to months. Q waves may resolve over a period of years.

Biochemical Markers for MI. Components of damaged myocardial cells are released into the blood following an acute MI. Hence elevations in these cellular components can be diagnostic. The component measured most commonly is the *MB isozyme of creatine kinase* (CK-MB). Since CK-MB is found primarily in cardiac muscle rather than skeletal muscle, an increase in serum CK-MB is highly suggestive of cardiac injury. Following MI, serum levels of CK-MB begin to rise in 4 to 8 hours, peak in 24 hours, and return to baseline in 36 to 72 hours. In some patients, the increase in CK-MB may be too small to allow a definitive diagnosis, even though significant myocardial injury has occurred.

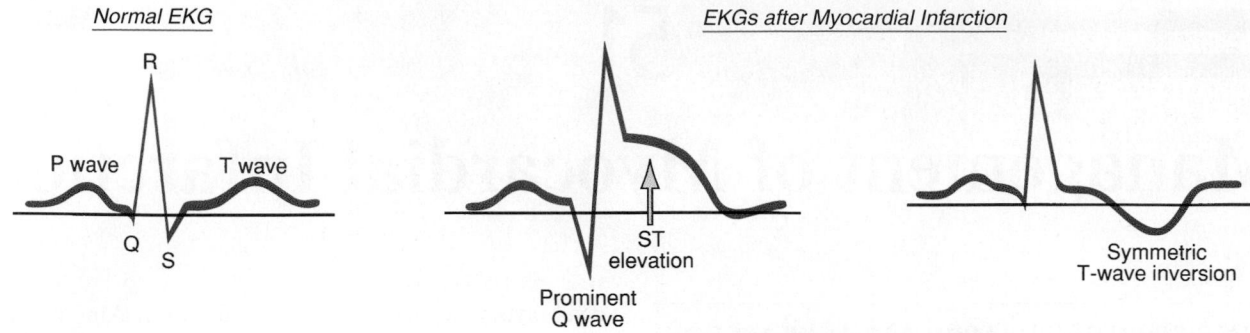

Normal EKG

R

P wave   T wave

Q S

EKGs after Myocardial Infarction

ST elevation

Prominent Q wave

Symmetric T-wave inversion

Figure 51–1 ■ EKG changes associated with myocardial infarction.

Like CK-MB, *troponin I* and *troponin T* are released by injured myocardial cells. Studies show a strong correlation between the degree of troponin elevation and the risk of MI complications. Compared with measurements of CK-MB, measurements of troponin I and troponin T are more sensitive and produce fewer false-positive or false-negative results.

MANAGEMENT OF MYOCARDIAL INFARCTION

The acute phase of management refers to the interval between the onset of symptoms and discharge from the hospital (usually in 6 to 10 days). The goal is to bring cardiac oxygen supply back in balance with oxygen demand. This can be accomplished by reperfusion therapy, which restores blood flow to the myocardium, and by reducing myocardial oxygen demand. The first few hours of treatment are the most critical. The major threats to life during acute MI are ventricular dysrhythmias, cardiogenic shock, and CHF.

In 1999, the American College of Cardiology (ACC), in conjunction with the American Heart Association (AHA), issued revised guidelines for the management of acute MI. The guidelines—ACC/AHA Guidelines for the Management of Patients with Acute Myocardial Infarction: A Report of the American College of Cardiology/American Heart Association Task Force on Practice Guidelines—are available online at *www.acc.org* and *www.americanheart.org*. The discussion below reflects guideline recommendations.

Reperfusion Therapy

The goal of reperfusion therapy is to restore blood flow through the blocked coronary artery. Reperfusion therapy is the most effective way to preserve myocardial function and limit infarct size. Reperfusion can be accomplished with thrombolytic drugs or with angioplasty. Both techniques are equally effective. With either approach, maximum benefits are achieved when treatment is instituted rapidly, ideally within 1 to 2 hours of symptom onset. The advantages of thrombolytic therapy versus those of primary angioplasty are summarized in Table 51–1.

Thrombolytic Therapy

Thrombolytic drugs dissolve clots. They accomplish this by converting plasminogen into plasmin, a proteolytic enzyme that digests the fibrin meshwork that holds clots together. Five

TABLE 51–1 ■ Comparison of Thrombolytic Therapy with Primary PTCA

Advantages of Thrombolytic Therapy
- More universal access
- Shorter time to treatment
- Greater clinical trial evidence of (1) reduction of infarct size and (2) improvement of LV function
- Results less dependent on physician experience
- Lower system cost

Advantages of Primary PTCA
- Higher inital reperfusion rates
- Less residual stenosis
- Lower recurrence rates of ischemia/infarction
- Does not promote intracranial bleeding
- Defines coronary anatomy and LV function
- Can be used when thrombolytic therapy is contraindicated

LV = left ventricular, PTCA = percutaneous transluminal coronary angioplasty.

thrombolytic drugs are used: *alteplase* (tissue plasminogen activator, or tPA), *reteplase, streptokinase, anistreplase,* and *tenecteplase.* The basic pharmacology of these drugs is presented in Chapter 50. Discussion here is limited to their use in MI.

Thrombolytic therapy is considered standard treatment for early MI. When thrombolytics are given soon enough, the occluded artery can be opened in 80% of patients. Clinical trials have shown that timely therapy improves ventricular function, limits infarct size, and reduces mortality. Restoration of blood flow reduces or eliminates chest pain, and often reduces ST elevation too. Treatment should be initiated within 4 to 6 hours of the symptom onset—and preferably much sooner (within 1 to 2 hours). Current guidelines restrict thrombolytic therapy to patients younger than 75 and to those whose ischemic pain has been present no more than 12 hours. Patients in whom thrombolytic therapy is contraindicated are listed in Table 51–2. Under *typical* conditions, all of the available thrombolytics are equally beneficial. However, under *ideal* conditions (i.e., treatment within 4 to 6 hours of pain onset), alteplase is most effective, especially in patients under the age of 75 (see discussion of the GUSTO-I trial in Chapter 50). Unfortunately, alteplase is also very expensive. With two drugs—streptokinase and anistreplase—neutralizing antibodies may develop within 5 days of initial use. Because these antibodies prevent anistre-

TABLE 51–2 ▪ Contraindications and Cautions Regarding Thrombolytic Therapy for Myocardial Infarction

Absolute Contraindications

- Previous hemorrhagic stroke at any time; other strokes or cerebrovascular events within 1 year
- Known intracranial neoplasm
- Active internal bleeding (other than menses)
- Suspected aortic dissection

Relative Contraindications/Cautions

- Severe uncontrolled hypertension on presentation (blood pressure >180/110 mm Hg)
- History of chronic hypertension
- History of prior cerebrovascular accident of known intracerebral pathology not covered in contraindications
- Current use of anticoagulants in therapeutic doses (INR ≥2–3); known bleeding diathesis
- Recent trauma (within 2–4 wk), including head trauma
- Recent internal bleeding (within 2–4 wk)
- Noncompressible vascular punctures
- For streptokinase/anistreplase: prior exposure (especially within 5 days to 2 yr) or prior allergic reaction
- Pregnancy
- Active peptic ulcer

INR = international normalized ratio.
Adapted from Ryan TJ, Antman EM, Brooks NH, et al. 1999 update: ACC/AHA guidelines for the management of patients with acute myocardial infarction. A report of the American College of Cardiology/American Heart Association Task Force on Practice Guidelines (Committee on Management of Acute Myocardial Infarction). J Am Coll Cardiol 1999;34:890–911.

plase and streptokinase from acting, a different agent must be used if thrombolytic therapy must be repeated.

The major complication of thrombolytic therapy is bleeding, which occurs in 1% to 5% of patients. Intracranial hemorrhage (ICH) is the greatest concern. ICH has an incidence of 0.5% to 1%, and is most likely in the elderly. Nonetheless, the benefits of thrombolysis generally outweigh the risks. ICH occurs slightly more often with alteplase than with streptokinase.

Primary Coronary Angioplasty

The term *primary angioplasty* refers to the use of angioplasty, rather than thrombolytic therapy, to recanalize an occluded coronary artery. In the most common type of angioplasty, a catheter containing a deflated balloon is worked into the affected coronary artery, and then the balloon is inflated. This opens the vessel, allowing blood to flow. Placement of a stent (a small mesh tube) in the artery helps prevent reocclusion. The success rate with primary angioplasty is somewhat higher than with thrombolytic therapy. Moreover, studies indicate that the benefits of angioplasty last longer. After 30 days, the rate of death, reinfarction, or disabling stroke following angioplasty is 9.6%, versus 13.6% following tPA. After 5 years, the rate of all-cause mortality following angioplasty is 13%, versus 24% with streptokinase—the difference being due entirely to lower cardiovascular mortality in angioplasty-treated patients.

Adjunctive Drug Therapy

Morphine

Intravenous morphine controls the pain of MI and improves hemodynamics. By promoting venodilation, the drug reduces cardiac preload. By promoting modest arterial dilation, morphine may cause some reduction in afterload. The combined reductions in preload and afterload lower cardiac oxygen demand, thereby helping preserve the ischemic myocardium.

Antiplatelet Drugs

Aspirin. Low-dose aspirin suppresses platelet aggregation. In the Second International Study of Infarct Survival (ISIS-2), aspirin produced a substantial reduction in mortality. Moreover, benefits were synergistic with thrombolytic drugs: mortality was 13.2% with thrombolytics alone, and dropped to 8% with the addition of aspirin. Because of these benefits, virtually all patients with evolving MI should get aspirin. Therapy should begin immediately after onset of symptoms, and should continue indefinitely. The first tablet (325 mg) should be crushed or chewed—not swallowed whole—to accelerate absorption. Prolonged therapy with aspirin (81 mg/day) reduces the risk of reinfarction, stroke, and death.

Glycoprotein (GP) IIb/IIIa Inhibitors. As discussed in Chapter 50, the GP IIb/IIIa inhibitors (e.g., tirofiban [Aggrastat], abciximab [ReoPro]), are powerful, intravenous antiplatelet drugs that inhibit the final step in platelet aggregation. These drugs can be used as adjuncts to both thrombolytic therapy and primary angioplasty. In patients undergoing thrombolytic therapy, the GP IIb/IIIa inhibitors accelerate vessel opening, permit a significant reduction in thrombolytic dosage, and reduce rates of reocclusion and reinfarction. In patients undergoing primary angioplasty, they reduce early complications of the procedure, but do *not* reduce rates of reocclusion.

Anticoagulants

Heparin. Heparin is a parenteral anticoagulant that was used widely to treat MI before thrombolytics became available. The drug was shown to decrease mortality, reinfarction, stroke, pulmonary embolism, and deep vein thrombosis. However, among patients who receive thrombolytic therapy, indications for heparin are limited. Heparin offers no additional benefits to patients treated with *streptokinase* or *anistreplase;* hence, the drug is not recommended following these thrombolytics. In contrast, heparin does reduce the risk of coronary artery reocclusion following therapy with *alteplase* or *reteplase,* both of which have short half-lives. Accordingly, follow-up therapy with IV heparin is recommended. Heparin is also recommended after primary angioplasty because the procedure causes vascular trauma that can encourage thrombus formation. For all patients, the main complication of heparin therapy is bleeding. The basic pharmacology of heparin is discussed in Chapter 50.

Warfarin. Warfarin [Coumadin] is an oral anticoagulant with benefits much like those of aspirin. That is, like aspirin, warfarin can reduce the risk of reinfarction, thromboembolism, and early death. However, since aspirin is cheaper, safer (causes less bleeding), and doesn't require monitoring of prothrombin time, aspirin is preferred. Among patients with acute MI, the principal indications for warfarin are (1) a large anterior infarction and (2) a left ventricular thrombus. In both cases, warfarin can decrease the risk of thrombotic embolization. Treatment should begin immediately and continue for 3 to 6 months.

Nitroglycerin

Nitroglycerin reduces preload, and thereby reduces oxygen demand. The drug may also increase collateral blood flow in the ischemic region of the heart. When given IV during acute MI, nitroglycerin limits infarct size and improves LV function. However, combining nitroglycerin with thrombolytics does not offer any mortality advantage over thrombolytic therapy alone. Nonetheless, since nitroglycerin is easily administered, offers hemodynamic benefits, and helps relieve ischemic chest pain, it continues to be used.

Beta-Adrenergic Blocking Agents

When given to patients undergoing acute MI, beta blockers (e.g., atenolol, metoprolol) reduce cardiac pain, infarct size, and short-term mortality. Recurrent ischemia and reinfarction are also decreased. Reduction in myocardial wall tension may decrease the risk of myocardial rupture. Continued use of an oral beta blocker increases long-term survival. Unfortunately, although nearly all patients can benefit from beta blockers, many patients don't receive them.

Benefits result from several mechanisms. As an MI evolves, traffic along sympathetic nerves to the heart increases greatly, as does the number of beta receptors in the heart. As a result, heart rate and force of contraction rise substantially, thereby increasing cardiac oxygen demand. By preventing beta receptor activation, beta blockers reduce heart rate and contractility, and thereby reduce oxygen demand. They reduce oxygen demand further by lowering blood pressure. By prolonging diastolic filling time, beta blockers increase coronary blood flow and myocardial oxygen supply. Additional benefits derive from antidysrhythmic actions.

Beta blockers should be used routinely in the absence of specific contraindications (e.g., bradycardia, significant LV dysfunction). For patients who reach the hospital within 24 hours of symptom onset, administration should be IV. Otherwise, oral therapy is recommended. Treatment should continue for at least 2 to 3 years, and perhaps longer. Beta blockers are especially good for patients with reflex tachycardia, systolic hypertension, atrial fibrillation, and atrioventricular conduction abnormalities. Contraindications include overt severe heart failure, pronounced bradycardia, persistent hypotension, advanced heart block, and cardiogenic shock. The basic pharmacology of the beta blockers is presented in Chapter 18.

Angiotensin-Converting Enzyme Inhibitors

In patients with acute MI, angiotensin-converting enzyme (ACE) inhibitors (e.g., captopril, enalapril, lisinopril) decrease mortality, severe heart failure, and recurrent MI. As discussed in Chapter 46, ACE inhibitors are now standard therapy for patients with heart failure. Benefits derive from reducing preload and afterload, and from promoting water loss. In MI patients who develop LV dysfunction, ACE inhibitors slow progression of heart failure and decrease mortality. Mortality is also reduced in patients who do not have LV dysfunction. Because of their benefits, ACE inhibitors should be given to all MI patients in the absence of specific contraindications. Treatment should start within 24 hours of symptom onset and should continue 4 to 6 weeks; in patients with signs of LV dysfunction, treatment should continue for at least

3 years, and perhaps indefinitely. The possibility that long-term therapy may also benefit patients who do not have LV dysfunction is being evaluated in large-scale trials. The major adverse effects of ACE inhibitors are hypotension and cough. Contraindications to ACE inhibitors are hypotension, bilateral renal artery stenosis, renal failure, and a history of ACE inhibitor–induced cough or angioedema. The basic pharmacology of the ACE inhibitors is presented in Chapter 42.

Lidocaine

Lidocaine, a class I antidysrhythmic agent (see Chapter 47), is a drug of choice for treating ischemic ventricular dysrhythmias. Among patients with acute MI, 4% to 8% experience potentially fatal ventricular fibrillation within the first 24 to 48 hours of symptom onset. In the past, lidocaine was given prophylactically to prevent dysrhythmias from occurring. However, *prophylactic* treatment is no longer recommended. Why? Because even though lidocaine does indeed reduce the incidence of serious ventricular dysrhythmias, prophylactic use actually *increases* mortality, probably because of the drug's prodysrhythmic actions (see Chapter 47). Accordingly, lidocaine is now reserved for *treating* serious ventricular dysrhythmias once they occur. Specific indications include ventricular fibrillation, ventricular tachycardia (sustained or nonsustained), and ventricular premature beats (more than 6 per minute). Small clinical studies suggest that prophylaxis with *amiodarone,* an antidysrhythmic drug with complex actions, can prevent dysrhythmias without increasing mortality. Larger trials are needed to confirm this possibility.

Magnesium

Magnesium has several potential cardioprotective effects. The drug decreases platelet aggregation, increases coronary blood flow, reduces cardiac afterload, and lowers the risk of serious ventricular dysrhythmias. In several small trials, magnesium infusion decreased mortality from MI. However, in ISIS-4, a trial involving over 58,000 patients, adding magnesium to thrombolytic therapy failed to reduce mortality—and actually *increased* the incidence of bradycardia, CHF, and death from cardiogenic shock. Accordingly, magnesium is not recommended for routine use. In patients who are not candidates for reperfusion therapy, magnesium may offer some benefit.

Calcium Channel Blockers

Because of their antianginal, vasodilatory, and antihypertensive actions, calcium channel blockers were presumed beneficial for patients with acute MI, and hence have been used widely. However, in large-scale controlled trials, these drugs have failed to decrease mortality either during or after an acute MI. Accordingly, calcium channel blockers are not recommended for treatment.

COMPLICATIONS OF MYOCARDIAL INFARCTION

Myocardial infarction predisposes the heart and vascular system to serious complications. Among the most severe are ventricular dysrhythmias, cardiogenic shock, and CHF.

Ventricular Dysrhythmias. These develop frequently and are the major cause of death following MI. Sudden death from dysrhythmias occurs in 15% of patients during the first hour. Ultimately, ventricular dysrhythmias cause 60% of infarction-related deaths. Acute management of ventricular fibrillation consists of defibrillation followed by IV lidocaine for 24 to 48 hours. Programmed ventricular stimulation with guided antidysrhythmic therapy may be lifesaving for some patients.

Attempts to prevent dysrhythmias by giving antidysrhythmic drugs *prophylactically* have failed to reduce mortality. Worse yet, attempted prophylaxis of ventricular dysrhythmias with two drugs—encainide and flecainide—actually increased mortality. Similarly, when quinidine was employed to prevent supraventricular dysrhythmias, it too increased mortality. Therefore, since prophylaxis with antidysrhythmic drugs does not reduce mortality—and may in fact increase mortality—antidysrhythmic drugs should be withheld until a dysrhythmia actually occurs.

Cardiogenic Shock. Shock results from greatly reduced tissue perfusion secondary to impaired cardiac function. Shock develops in 7% to 15% of patients during the first few days after MI and has a mortality rate of up to 90%. Patients at highest risk are those with large infarcts, a previous infarct, a low ejection fraction (less than 35%), diabetes, and advanced age. Drug therapy includes inotropic agents (e.g., dopamine, dobutamine) to increase cardiac output and vasodilators (nitroglycerin, nitroprusside) to improve tissue perfusion and reduce cardiac work and oxygen demand. Unfortunately, although these drugs can improve hemodynamic status, they do not seem to reduce mortality. Restoration of cardiac perfusion with angioplasty or coronary artery bypass grafting may be of value.

Congestive Heart Failure. CHF secondary to acute MI can be treated with a combination of drugs. A diuretic (e.g., furosemide) is given to decrease preload and pulmonary congestion. Inotropic agents (e.g., digoxin) increase cardiac output by enhancing contractility. Vasodilators (e.g., nitroglycerin, nitroprusside) improve hemodynamic status by reducing preload, afterload, or both. ACE inhibitors, which reduce both preload and afterload, can be especially helpful. Beta blockers may also improve outcome. Drug therapy of heart failure is discussed at length in Chapter 46.

Cardiac Rupture. Weakening of the myocardium predisposes the heart wall to rupture. Following rupture, shock and circulatory collapse develop rapidly. Death is often immediate. Fortunately, cardiac rupture is relatively rare (less than 2% incidence). Patients at highest risk are those with a large anterior infarction. Cardiac rupture is most likely within the first days after MI. Early treatment with vasodilators and beta blockers may reduce the risk of wall rupture.

Arterial Embolism and Deep Venous Thrombosis. Arterial embolism occurs when a thrombus in the heart breaks free and becomes lodged in a systemic artery. The incidence of embolism is 2% to 6%. Deep venous thrombosis of the legs develops in 17% to 38% of patients, usually within a few days of the MI. The incidence of embolism and thrombosis can be reduced with heparin. Treatment should begin soon (within 12 to 18 hours) after the onset of MI symptoms and should continue for 10 days.

Pericarditis. About 10% of patients with acute MI develop pericarditis, usually within 2 to 4 days. Inflammation develops in response to transmural necrosis. Symptoms can be reduced with anti-inflammatory doses of aspirin.

SECONDARY PREVENTION

As a rule, patients who survive the acute phase of MI can be discharged from the hospital after 6 to 10 days. However, they are still at risk of reinfarction (5% to 15% incidence within the first year) and other complications (e.g., dysrhythmias, heart failure). Outcome can be improved with risk-factor reduction, exercise, and long-term therapy with drugs. The discussion below reflects recommendations in the *AHA/ACC Guidelines for Preventing Heart Attack and Death in Patients with Atherosclerotic Cardiovascular Disease: 2001 Update,* available online at *www.acc.org.*

Reduction of risk factors for MI can increase long-term survival. Patients who smoke must be encouraged to quit. Patients with high serum cholesterol should be given an appropriate dietary plan and, if necessary, treated with a cholesterol-lowering drug (usually one of the statins). Patients with high triglyceride levels should be given niacin or a "fibrate" (e.g., gemfibrozil). Overweight patients should reduce; the goal is a body mass index of 18.5 to 29.4 kg/m^2 (see Chapter 78). Hypertension and diabetes increase the risk of mortality and must be controlled.

Exercise training can be valuable for two reasons: (1) it reduces complications associated with prolonged bed rest and (2) it accelerates return to an optimal level of functioning. The goal is 30 minutes of exercise at least 3 to 4 days a week, and preferably 7. Although exercise is safe for most patients, there is concern about cardiac risk and impairment of infarct healing in patients whose infarct is large.

All post-MI patients should take three drugs: (1) a beta blocker, (2) an ACE inhibitor, and (3) either an antiplatelet drug (e.g., aspirin, clopidogrel) or warfarin (an anticoagulant). Use of all three should continue indefinitely.

Hormone replacement therapy (HRT) for postmenopausal women is not effective as secondary prevention, and hence should not be initiated post-MI. However, women who had been taking HRT prior to having an MI may continue to use it.

⋰ KEY POINTS

- MI is defined as necrosis of the myocardium secondary to acute occlusion of a coronary artery. The usual cause is platelet plugging and thrombus formation at the site of a ruptured atherosclerotic plaque.
- Myocardial infarction is diagnosed by the presence of chest pain, characteristic EKG changes, and elevated serum levels of myocardial cellular components: CK MB, troponin I, or troponin T.
- Reperfusion therapy, which restores blood flow through blocked coronary arteries, is the most beneficial treatment for MI.
- Reperfusion can be accomplished with thrombolytic drugs or primary angioplasty. Both techniques are highly and equally effective.
- Thrombolytic drugs dissolve clots by converting plasminogen into plasmin, an enzyme that digests the fibrin meshwork that holds clots together.
- Under typical conditions, all thrombolytic drugs are equally effective. However, when treatment is initiated within 4 to 6 hours of pain onset, alteplase is most effective (but also very expensive).
- The major complication of thrombolytic therapy is bleeding. Intracranial hemorrhage is the greatest concern.
- Aspirin suppresses platelet aggregation, and thereby decreases mortality, reinfarction, and stroke. All patients should receive a 325-mg dose upon hospital admission, and should take 81 mg/day indefinitely after discharge.
- Aspirin and warfarin offer similar benefits, but aspirin is cheaper, safer, and easier to use. Accordingly, aspirin is preferred.

- Glycoprotein IIb/IIIa inhibitors (e.g., tirofiban, abciximab) are powerful IV antiplatelet drugs that can enhance the benefits of thrombolytic therapy and primary angioplasty.
- Heparin offers no additional benefits to patients treated with streptokinase or anistreplase, but does reduce the risk of coronary reocclusion following primary angioplasty or treatment with alteplase or reteplase.
- In patients undergoing acute MI, beta blockers reduce cardiac pain, infarct size, short-term mortality, recurrent ischemia, and reinfarction. Continued use increases long-term survival. All patients should receive a beta blocker in the absence of specific contraindications.
- In patients with acute MI, ACE inhibitors decrease mortality, severe heart failure, and recurrent MI. All patients should receive an ACE inhibitor in the absence of specific contraindications.
- Lidocaine is a drug of choice for treating severe ischemic ventricular dysrhythmias (e.g., ventricular fibrillation). However, neither lidocaine nor any other drug is currently recommended for *prophylaxis* of ischemic dysrhythmias.
- To lower the risk of a second MI, all patients should decrease cardiovascular risk factors (e.g., smoking, hypercholesterolemia, hypertension, obesity, diabetes), exercise for 30 minutes at least 3 or 4 days a week, and undergo long-term therapy with three drugs: a beta blocker, an ACE inhibitor, and either an antiplatelet drug (e.g., aspirin) or warfarin.

Drugs for Deficiency Anemias

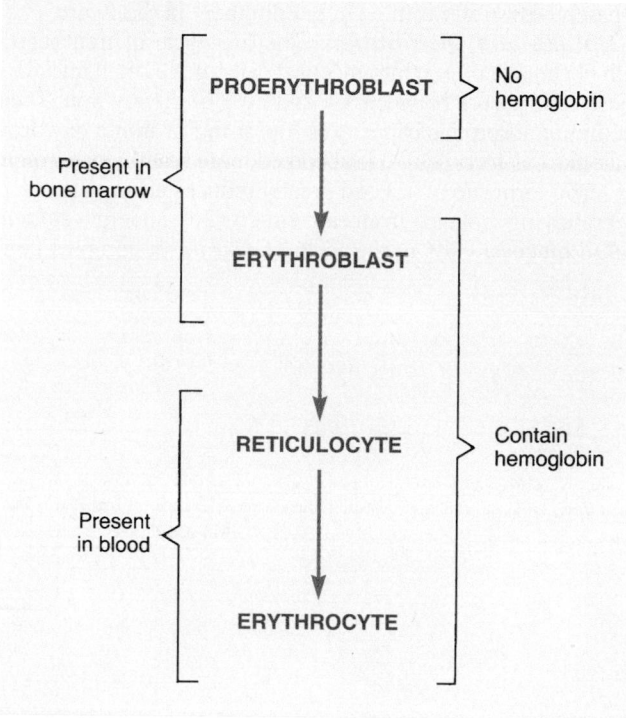

Figure 52–1 ■ Stages of red blood cell development.

Anemia is defined as a decrease in erythrocyte (red blood cell [RBC]) number, size, or hemoglobin content. Causes include blood loss, hemolysis, bone marrow dysfunction, and deficiencies of substances essential for RBC formation and maturation. Most deficiency anemias result from deficiency of iron, vitamin B$_{12}$, or folic acid. Accordingly, the chapter focuses on these three areas. To facilitate discussion, we begin by reviewing RBC development.

RED BLOOD CELL DEVELOPMENT

RBCs begin developing in the bone marrow and mature in the blood. As developing RBCs grow and divide, they evolve through four stages (Fig. 52–1). In their earliest stage, RBCs lack hemoglobin and are known as *proerythroblasts*. In the next stage, they gain hemoglobin and are called *erythroblasts*. Both the erythroblasts and the proerythroblasts reside in the bone marrow. After the erythroblast stage, RBCs evolve into *reticulocytes* (immature erythrocytes) and enter the systemic circulation. Following the reticulocyte stage, circulating RBCs reach full maturity and are referred to as *erythrocytes*.

Development of RBCs requires the cooperative interaction of several factors: the bone marrow must be healthy; erythropoietin (a stimulant of RBC maturation) must be present; iron must be available for hemoglobin synthesis; and other factors, including vitamin B$_{12}$ and folic acid, must be available to support synthesis of DNA. If any of these is absent or amiss, anemia will result.

IRON DEFICIENCY

Iron deficiency is the most common form of nutritional deficiency, and the most common cause of nutrition-related anemia. Worldwide, people with iron deficiency number in the hundreds of millions. In the United States, between 5% and 10% of the population is iron deficient.

Biochemistry and Physiology of Iron

In order to understand the consequences of iron deficiency as well as the rationale behind iron therapy, we must first understand the biochemistry and physiology of iron. This information is reviewed below.

Metabolic Functions

Iron is essential to the function of hemoglobin, myoglobin (the oxygen-storing molecule of muscle), and a variety of iron-containing enzymes. Most (70% to 80%) of the body's iron is present in hemoglobin. A much smaller amount (10%) is present in myoglobin and iron-containing enzymes.

Fate in the Body

The major pathways for iron movement and utilization are shown in Figure 52–2. In the discussion below, the numbers in parentheses refer to the circled numbers in the figure.

Uptake and Distribution. The life cycle of iron begins with (1) uptake of iron into mucosal cells of the small intestine. These cells absorb between 5% and 20% of dietary iron. Their maximum absorptive capacity is 3 to 4 mg of iron a day. Iron in the ferrous form (Fe^{++}) is absorbed more readily than iron in the ferric form (Fe^{+++}). Food greatly reduces absorption.

Following uptake, iron can either (2a) undergo storage within mucosal cells in the form of *ferritin* (a complex con-

sisting of iron plus a protein used for iron storage) or (2b) undergo binding to *transferrin* (the iron transport protein) for distribution throughout the body.

Utilization and Storage. Iron that is bound to transferrin can undergo one of three fates. The majority of transferrin-bound iron is (3a) taken up by cells of the bone marrow for incorporation into hemoglobin. Small amounts are (3b) taken up by the liver and other tissues for storage as ferritin. Lastly (3c), some of the iron in plasma is taken up by muscle (for production of myoglobin) and some is taken up by all tissues (for production of iron-containing enzymes).

Recycling. As Figure 52–2 depicts, iron associated with hemoglobin undergoes continuous recycling. After hemoglobin is made in bone marrow, iron re-enters the circulation (4) as a component of hemoglobin in erythrocytes. (The iron in circulating erythrocytes accounts for about 70% of total body iron.) After 120 days of useful life, RBCs are catabolized (5). Iron released by this process re-enters the plasma bound to transferrin (6)—and then the cycle begins anew.

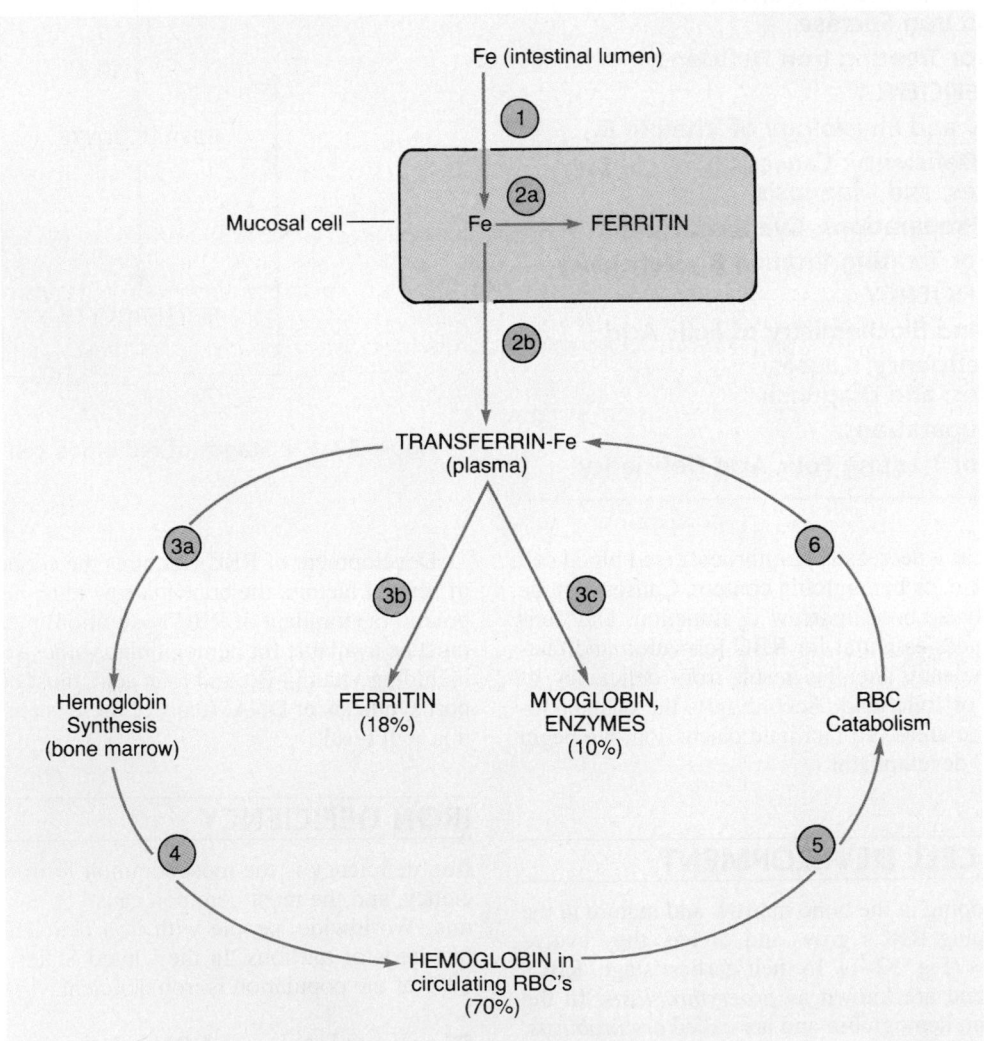

Figure 52–2 ■ Fate of iron in the body.
Pathways labeled with circled numbers are explained in the text. Values in parentheses indicate percentage of total body stores. Elimination of iron is not shown since most iron is rigidly conserved. (Fe = iron, RBC = red blood cell.)

Elimination. Excretion of iron is minimal. Under normal circumstances, only 1 mg of iron is excreted each day. At this rate, if none of the lost iron was replaced, body stores would decline by only 10% a year.

Iron leaves the body by several routes. Most excretion occurs via the bowel: Iron in ferritin is lost as mucosal cells slough off; iron also enters the bowel in the bile. Small amounts are excreted in the urine and sweat.

It should be noted that, although very little iron leaves the body as a result of excretion (i.e., normal physiologic loss), substantial amounts can leave because of blood loss. Hence, menorrhagia (excessive menstrual flow), hemorrhage, and blood donations can all cause iron deficiency.

Regulation of Body Iron Content. The amount of iron in the body is regulated through control of intestinal absorption. As noted, most of the iron that enters the body stays in the body. Hence, if all dietary iron were readily absorbed, body iron content would rapidly accumulate to toxic levels. However, *excessive buildup is prevented through control of iron uptake: As body stores rise, uptake of iron declines; conversely, as body stores become depleted, uptake increases.* For example, when body stores of iron are high, only 2% to 3% of dietary iron is absorbed. In contrast, when body stores are depleted, iron absorption may climb to 20%.

Daily Requirements

Requirements for iron are determined largely by the rate of erythrocyte production. When RBC production is low, iron needs are small. Conversely, when RBC production is high, iron needs are high too. Accordingly, infants and children—individuals whose rapid growth rate requires massive RBC synthesis—have iron requirements that are high (relative to body weight). In contrast, the daily iron needs of adults are relatively low. Adult males need only 10 mg of dietary iron each day. Adult females need somewhat more—to replace iron lost through menstruation.

During pregnancy, requirements for iron increase dramatically. This increase results from (1) expansion of maternal blood volume and (2) production of red blood cells by the fetus. In most cases, the iron needs of pregnant women are too great to be met by diet alone. Consequently, iron supplements (about 30 mg/day) are recommended during pregnancy and for 2 to 3 months after parturition.

Table 52–1 summarizes the recommended dietary allowances (RDAs) of iron as a function of age. For each age, the table presents two iron values. The first is the actual physiologic need for iron; the second is the RDA. Note that RDA values are about 10 times greater than the values for physiologic need. This disparity reflects the fact that, on average, only 10% of dietary iron is absorbed. Hence, if physiologic requirements are to be met, the diet must contain 10 times more iron than the body actually needs.

Dietary Sources

Iron is available in foods of plant and animal origin. Foods especially rich in iron include liver, egg yolk, brewer's yeast, and wheat germ. Other foods with a high iron content include muscle meats, fish, fowl, cereal grains, beans, and green leafy vegetables. Foods that do not provide much iron include milk and most nongreen vegetables. Since iron can be extracted from cooking utensils, using iron pots and pans can augment dietary iron. Except for individuals who have very high iron requirements (infants, pregnant women, those undergoing chronic blood loss), the average diet is sufficient to meet iron needs.

Iron Deficiency: Causes, Consequences, and Diagnosis

Causes

Iron deficiency results when there is an imbalance between iron uptake and iron demand. As a rule, this imbalance results from increased demand and not from reduced uptake. The most common causes of increased iron demand (and resulting iron deficiency) are (1) blood volume expansion during pregnancy coupled with red blood cell synthesis by the growing fetus, (2) blood volume expansion during infancy and early childhood, and (3) chronic blood loss, which is usually of GI or uterine origin. Rarely, iron deficiency results from reduced iron uptake; potential causes include gastrectomy and sprue.

Consequences

Iron deficiency has multiple effects, the most conspicuous being *iron deficiency anemia*. In the absence of iron for hemoglobin synthesis, red blood cells become *microcytic* (small) and *hypochromic* (pale). The reduced oxygen-carrying capac-

TABLE 52–1 ■ Recommended Dietary Allowances (RDAs) for Iron			
	Age (years)	Physiologic Requirement for Iron (mg/day)	RDA* for Iron (mg/day)
Infants	0–0.5	0.6	6
	0.5–1	1.0	10
Children	1–10	1.0	10
Males	11–18	1.2	12
	18+	1.0	10
Females	11–50	1.5	15
	50+	1.0	10
Pregnant and 2–3 mo postpartum	—	5	30†

*Since only a small fraction of dietary iron is absorbed, the RDA is higher than the actual physiologic need.
†Iron requirements during pregnancy cannot be met through dietary sources alone; supplements are recommended.

ity of blood results in listlessness, fatigue, and pallor of the skin and mucous membranes. If tissue oxygenation is severely compromised, tachycardia, dyspnea, and angina may result. In addition to causing anemia, iron deficiency impairs myoglobin production and reduces synthesis of iron-containing enzymes. In young children, iron deficiency can cause developmental problems, and in school-age children, iron deficiency may impair cognition.

Diagnosis

The hallmarks of iron deficiency anemia are (1) the presence of microcytic, hypochromic erythrocytes, and (2) the absence of hemosiderin (aggregated ferritin) in bone marrow. Additional laboratory data that can help confirm a diagnosis of iron deficiency anemia include reduced RBC count, reduced reticulocyte hemoglobin content, reduced hemoglobin and hematocrit values, reduced serum iron content, and increased serum iron-binding capacity (IBC).*

When a diagnosis of iron deficiency anemia is made, it is imperative that the underlying cause be determined. This is especially true when the suspected cause is blood loss of GI origin. Why? Because GI blood loss may be indicative of peptic ulcer disease or GI cancer, conditions that demand immediate treatment.

Oral Iron Preparations I: Iron Salts

Three oral iron salts are available: ferrous sulfate, ferrous gluconate, and ferrous fumarate. All three are equally effective. And with all three, GI disturbances are the major adverse effect.

Ferrous Sulfate

Ferrous sulfate is the least expensive oral iron preparation and the standard against which the others are measured. Accordingly, ferrous sulfate will be our prototype for the group.

Indications. Ferrous sulfate is the drug of choice for treating iron deficiency anemia. This compound is also employed for prophylaxis of iron deficiency in people whose need for iron cannot be met by diet alone (e.g., pregnant women, individuals experiencing chronic blood loss).

Adverse Effects. GI Disturbances. The most significant adverse effects of oral iron involve the GI tract. These effects, which are dose dependent, include nausea, pyrosis (heartburn), bloating, constipation, and diarrhea. Gastrointestinal reactions are most intense during initial therapy, and become less disturbing with continued drug use. Because of their effects on the GI tract, oral iron preparations can aggravate peptic ulcers, regional enteritis, and ulcerative colitis. Accordingly, patients with these disorders should not take iron orally. In addition to its other GI effects, oral iron may impart a dark green or black coloration to stools. This effect is harmless and should not be interpreted as a sign of bleeding.

Staining of Teeth. Liquid iron preparations can stain the teeth. This can be prevented by (1) diluting liquid preparations with juice or water, (2) administering the iron through a straw or with a dropper, and (3) rinsing the mouth after administration.

***

*Serum IBC measures iron binding by transferrin. An increase in IBC indicates an increase in the amount of transferrin that is *not* carrying any iron, and hence signals reduced iron availability.

Toxicity. Iron in large amounts is toxic. Poisoning is almost always the result of accidental or intentional overdose; poisoning from proper therapeutic use of iron is rare. Death from iron ingestion is rare in adults. By contrast, in young children, iron-containing products are the leading cause of poisoning fatalities. For children, the lethal dose of elemental iron is 2 to 10 gm. To reduce the risk of pediatric poisoning, iron should be stored in childproof containers and kept out of reach.

Symptoms. The effects of iron poisoning are complex. Early reactions include nausea, vomiting, diarrhea, and shock. These are followed by acidosis, gastric necrosis, hepatic failure, pulmonary edema, and vasomotor collapse.

Diagnosis and Treatment. With rapid diagnosis and treatment, mortality from iron poisoning is low (about 1%). Serum iron should be measured and the intestine x-rayed to determine if unabsorbed tablets are present. Induction of vomiting will remove iron from the stomach. Acidosis and shock should be treated as required.

If the plasma level of iron is high (above 500 mg/dl), it should be lowered with *deferoxamine.* Deferoxamine absorbs iron and thereby prevents toxic effects. The pharmacology of deferoxamine is discussed in Chapter 105 (Management of Poisoning).

Drug Interactions. Interaction of iron with other drugs can alter the absorption of iron, the other agent, or both. *Antacids* reduce the absorption of iron. Coadministration of iron with *tetracyclines* decreases absorption of both agents. *Ascorbic acid* (vitamin C) promotes iron absorption but also increases its adverse effects. Accordingly, attempts to enhance iron uptake by combining iron with ascorbic acid offer no advantage over a simple increase in iron dosage.

Formulations. Ferrous sulfate is available in several formulations. Some of these (timed- or sustained-release capsules and tablets) are intended to reduce gastric disturbances. Unfortunately, although side effects may be lowered, these formulations have disadvantages: iron may be released at variable rates, causing variable and unpredictable absorption. In addition, these preparations are expensive. Ordinary tablets do not have these drawbacks.

Dosage and Administration. General Considerations. Dosing with oral iron can be complicated in that oral iron salts differ from one another with regard to percentage of elemental iron (Table 52–2). Ferrous *sulfate,* for example, contains 20% iron by weight. In contrast, ferrous *gluconate* contains only 11.6% iron. Consequently, in order to provide equivalent amounts of elemental iron, we must use different doses of these iron preparations. For example, if we want to provide 100 mg of elemental iron, we need to administer a 500-mg dose of ferrous *sulfate.* To provide this same amount of elemental iron using ferrous *fumarate,* the dose would be only 300 mg. In the discussion below, dosage values refer to milligrams of *elemental iron,* and not to milligrams of any particular iron preparation needed to provide that amount of elemental iron.

Food affects therapy with oral iron in two ways. First, food helps protect against iron-induced GI distress. Second, food decreases absorption of iron by 50% to 70%. Hence, we have a dilemma: *Absorption is best* when iron is taken *between* meals, but *side effects are lowest* when iron is taken *with meals.* As a rule, iron should be administered between meals, thereby maximizing absorption; if necessary, the dosage can be lowered to render GI effects more acceptable.

For two reasons, it may be desirable to take iron *with* food during *initial* therapy. First, since the GI effects of iron

TABLE 52–2 ░■ Oral Iron Preparations		
Iron Preparation	% Iron (by weight)	Dose Providing 100 mg Iron
Iron Salts		
Ferrous sulfate	20	500 mg
Ferrous sulfate (dried)	~30	330 mg
Ferrous fumarate	33	300 mg
Ferrous gluconate	11.6	860 mg
Elemental Iron		
Carbonyl iron	100	100 mg

are most intense when treatment commences, the salving effects of food can be especially beneficial at this time. Second, by reducing GI discomfort during the early phase of therapy, administering iron with food can help promote compliance.

Use in Iron Deficiency Anemia. Dosing with oral iron represents a compromise between a desire to replenish lost iron rapidly and a desire to keep adverse GI effects to a minimum. For most adults, this compromise can best be achieved by giving 65 mg 3 times a day, yielding a total daily dose of about 200 mg. Since there is a ceiling to intestinal absorption of iron, doses above this amount provide only a modest increase in therapeutic effect. On the other hand, at dosages greater than 200 mg/day, GI disturbances become disproportionately high. Hence, elevation of the daily dosage above 200 mg would augment adverse effects without offering a significant increase in benefits. When treating iron deficiency in infants and children, a typical dosage is 5 mg/kg/day administered in three or four divided doses.

Timing of administration is important: Doses should be spaced evenly throughout the day. This schedule provides the bone marrow with a continuous iron supply, thereby maximizing RBC production.

Duration of therapy is determined by the therapeutic objective. If correction of anemia is the sole objective, a few months of therapy is sufficient. However, if the objective also includes replenishing ferritin, treatment must continue 4 to 6 months longer. It should be noted, however, that drugs are usually unnecessary for ferritin replenishment; in most cases, diet alone can do the job. Accordingly, once anemia has been corrected, pharmaceutical iron can usually be discontinued.

Prophylactic Use. Pregnant women are the principal candidates for prophylactic therapy. A total daily dose of 30 mg taken between meals is recommended. Other candidates include infants, children, and women experiencing menorrhagia.

Ferrous Gluconate and Ferrous Fumarate

In addition to ferrous sulfate, two other oral iron salts are available: ferrous gluconate and ferrous fumarate. Except for differences in percentage of iron content (see Table 52–2), all of these preparations are equivalent. Hence, when dosage is adjusted to provide equal amounts of elemental iron, ferrous gluconate and ferrous fumarate produce pharmacologic effects identical to those of ferrous sulfate: All three agents produce equivalent therapeutic responses, and all three cause the same degree of GI distress. Patients who fail to respond to one will not respond to the others. Patients who cannot tolerate the GI effects of one agent will find the others intolerable too.

Oral Iron Preparations II: Carbonyl Iron

Carbonyl iron is pure, elemental iron in the form of microparticles. Because of these microparticles, the iron has good bioavailability. Therapeutic efficacy of carbonyl iron equals that of the iron salts. Carbonyl iron is reputed to be less toxic than the iron salts, and hence should pose less risk to children in the event of poisoning. Two formulations are available: (1) 50-mg tablets, marketed as *Feosol;* and (2) a suspension (15 mg/1.25 ml), marketed as *Icar.* Because these products contain 100% iron, rather than an iron salt, there should be no confusion about dosage: 100 mg of either product provides 100 mg of elemental iron. The usual dosage is 50 mg 3 times a day.

Parenteral Iron I: Iron Dextran

Iron dextran [INFeD, DexFerrum] is the most frequently used parenteral iron preparation. This drug is a complex consisting of ferric hydroxide and dextrans (polymers of glucose). The rate of response to parenteral iron is equal to that of oral iron. Iron dextran is dangerous—fatal anaphylactic reactions have occurred—and hence should be used only when circumstances demand.

Indications

Iron dextran is reserved for patients with a clear diagnosis of iron deficiency and for whom oral iron is either ineffective or intolerable. Primary candidates for parenteral iron are patients who, because of intestinal disease, are unable to absorb iron taken orally. Iron dextran is also indicated when blood loss is so great (500 to 1000 ml/week) that oral iron cannot be absorbed fast enough to meet hematopoietic needs. Parenteral iron may also be employed when there is concern that oral iron might exacerbate pre-existing disease of the stomach or bowel. Lastly, parenteral iron can be given to the rare patient for whom the GI effects of oral iron are intolerable.

Adverse Effects

Anaphylactic Reactions. Potentially fatal anaphylaxis is the most serious adverse effect. These reactions are triggered by the dextran in the product, not by the iron. Although anaphylactic reactions are rare, their possible occurrence demands that iron dextran be used only when clearly required. Whenever iron dextran is administered, injectable epinephrine and facilities for resuscitation should be at hand. Furthermore, each full dose should be preceded by a small test dose.

Other Adverse Effects. Hypotension is common in patients receiving parenteral iron. In addition, iron dextran can cause headache, fever, urticaria, and arthralgia. More serious reactions—circulatory failure and cardiac arrest—may also occur. When administered IM, iron dextran can cause persistent pain and prolonged, localized discoloration. Very rarely, tumors have developed at sites of IM injection. Intravenous administration may result in lymphadenopathy and phlebitis.

Preparations, Dosage, and Administration

Preparations. Iron dextran [INFeD, DexFerrum] is dispensed in 2-ml, single-dose vials that contain 50 mg/ml of elemental iron.

Dosage. Dosage determination is complex. Dosage depends on the degree of anemia, the weight of the patient, and the presence of persistent bleeding. For patients with iron deficiency anemia who are not losing blood, the equation in Figure 52–3 provides a guideline for estimating total iron dosage.

Administration. Iron dextran may be administered IM or IV. Intravenous administration is preferred. This route is just as effective as IM administration but causes fewer anaphylactic reactions and other adverse effects.

Intravenous. To minimize anaphylactic reactions, intravenous iron dextran should be administered by the following protocol: (1) administer a tiny test dose (25 mg over 5 minutes) and observe the patient for at least 15 minutes; (2) if the test dose appears safe, slowly administer a larger dose (500 mg

$$\text{mg iron} = 0.66 \times \text{kg body weight} \times \left(100 - \frac{\text{hemoglobin value in g/dl}}{14.8}\right)$$

Figure 52–3 ■ **Formula for estimating total dosage of parenteral iron dextran.**

over a 10- to 15-minute interval); and (3) if the 500-mg dose is uneventful, additional doses may be given as needed.

Intramuscular. Intramuscular iron dextran has significant drawbacks and should be avoided. Disadvantages include persistent pain and discoloration at the injection site, possible development of tumors, and a greater risk of anaphylaxis. When IM administration must be performed, iron dextran should be injected deep into each buttock using the Z-track technique. (Z-track injection keeps the iron dextran deep in the muscle, thereby minimizing leakage and surface discoloration.) As with IV iron dextran, a small test dose should precede the full therapeutic dose.

Parenteral Iron II: Sodium–Ferric Gluconate Complex and Iron Sucrose

Iron sucrose and sodium–ferric gluconate complex (SFGC) represent alternatives to iron dextran for parenteral iron therapy. With both drugs, the risk of anaphylaxis is very low, and hence a test dose is not required before each use. As a result, both drugs are more convenient than iron dextran. At this time, iron sucrose and SFGC have only one indication: treatment of iron deficiency in patients undergoing chronic hemodialysis.

Sodium–Ferric Gluconate Complex

SFGC, sold under the trade name *Ferrlecit,* is a parenteral iron product indicated for iron deficiency anemia in patients undergoing chronic hemodialysis. The drug is always used in conjunction with erythropoietin, a compound that stimulates RBC production (see Chapter 53). SFGC can cause transient flushing and hypotension, associated with lightheadedness, malaise, fatigue, weakness, and severe pain in the chest, back, flanks, or groin. This reaction can be minimized by infusing the drug slowly. In contrast to iron dextran, SFGC poses little risk of anaphylaxis. Accordingly, *repeated* test doses are unnecessary—although a test dose *is* required the first time the drug is used. SFGC is dispensed in 5-ml ampules that contain 62.5 mg of elemental iron. Dilution is no longer required before the infusion. For most patients, a single dose consists of 125 mg infused slowly (over 10 minutes or more). The typical patient requires a cumulative dose of 1 gm (eight 125-mg infusions on separate days). A small test dose (25 mg infused over 60 minutes) should precede the first full dose. In addition, every time the drug is administered, facilities for cardiopulmonary resuscitation should be immediately available.

Iron Sucrose

Iron sucrose [Venofer] is a parenteral form of iron indicated for iron deficiency anemia in patients undergoing chronic hemodialysis. All patients must also receive erythropoietin. Although iron sucrose is new to the United States, it has been used in Europe for over 40 years.

The most common adverse effects are hypotension (36%) and cramps (23%). Life-threatening hypersensitivity reactions are very rare: None were observed during clinical trials, and only 27 cases (out of 450,000 patients) were reported during postmarketing surveillance. Nonetheless, facilities for cardiopulmonary resuscitation should be available during administration. However, in contrast to iron dextran, test doses are unnecessary.

Iron sucrose is available in 5-ml single-dose vials that contain 100 mg of elemental iron. For treating iron deficiency anemia in dialysis patients, the usual regimen is 5 ml (100 mg elemental iron) administered IV during dialysis on each of 10 consecutive dialysis sessions (total cumulative dose of 1000 mg). Iron sucrose should be administered directly into the dialysis line, and should not be mixed with other drugs or with peripheral nutrition solutions. Administration may be done by (1) slow injection (1 ml/min) or (2) infusion (dilute iron sucrose in up to 100 ml of 0.9% saline and infuse over 15 minutes or longer).

Guidelines for Treating Iron Deficiency

Assessment. Prior to starting therapy, the cause of iron deficiency must be determined. Without this information, appropriate treatment is not possible. Potential causes of deficiency include pregnancy, bleeding, inadequate diet, and, rarely, reduced intestinal absorption.

The objective is to increase the production of hemoglobin and erythrocytes. When therapy is successful, reticulocytes will increase within 4 to 7 days; within 1 week, increases in hemoglobin and the hematocrit will be apparent; and within 1 month, hemoglobin levels will rise by at least 2 gm/dl. If these responses fail to occur, the patient should be evaluated for (1) compliance, (2) continued bleeding, (3) inflammatory disease (which can interfere with hemoglobin production), and (4) malabsorption of oral iron.

Routes of Administration. Iron preparations are available for oral, IV, and IM administration. Oral iron is preferred. Why? Because oral administration is safer than parenteral administration and just as effective. Parenteral iron should be used only when oral iron is ineffective or intolerable. Of the two parenteral routes, IV is safer and preferred.

Duration of Therapy. Therapy with oral iron should be continued until hemoglobin levels become normal (about 15 gm/dl). This phase of treatment may require 1 to 2 months. After this time, continued treatment can help replenish stores of ferritin. However, for most patients, diet alone is sufficient to replenish these stores.

Therapeutic Combinations. As a rule, combinations of antianemic agents should be avoided. Combining oral iron with parenteral iron can lead to iron toxicity. Accordingly, use of oral iron should cease prior to giving iron injections. Combinations of iron with vitamin B_{12} or folic acid should be avoided; as discussed in the following sections, these combinations can confuse interpretation of hematologic responses.

VITAMIN B_{12} DEFICIENCY

The term *vitamin B_{12}* refers not to a single compound but rather to a group of compounds that have similar structures. These compounds are large molecules that contain an atom of cobalt. Because of the cobalt atom, members of the vitamin B_{12} family are known as *cobalamins.*

The most prominent consequences of vitamin B_{12} deficiency are *anemia* and *injury to the nervous system.* Anemia reverses rapidly following vitamin B_{12} administration. Neurologic damage takes longer to repair and, in some cases, may never fully recover. Additional effects of B_{12} deficiency include GI disturbances and impaired production of white blood cells and platelets.

Biochemistry and Physiology of Vitamin B_{12}

In order to understand the consequences of vitamin B_{12} deficiency and the rationale behind therapy, we must first understand the normal biochemistry and physiology of B_{12}. This information is reviewed below.

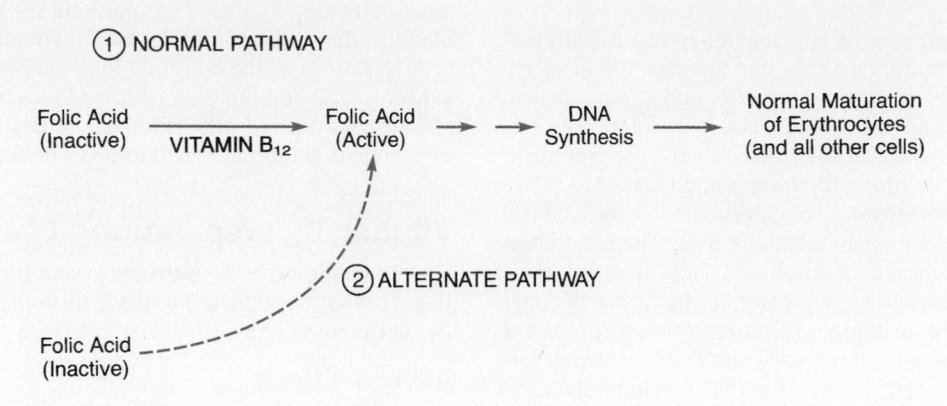

Figure 52–4 ■ Relationship of folic acid and vitamin B$_{12}$ to DNA synthesis and cell maturation.
Folic acid requires activation to be of use. Normally, activation occurs via a vitamin B$_{12}$–dependent pathway. However, when folic acid is present in large amounts, activation can occur via an alternate pathway, thereby bypassing the need for B$_{12}$.

Metabolic Function

Vitamin B$_{12}$ is essential for synthesis of DNA, and hence is required for the growth and division of virtually all of our cells. The mechanism by which the vitamin influences DNA synthesis is depicted in Figure 52–4. As indicated, vitamin B$_{12}$ helps catalyze the conversion of folic acid to its active form. Active folic acid then participates in several reactions essential for DNA synthesis. Hence, *it is by permitting utilization of folic acid that vitamin B$_{12}$ influences cell growth and division*—and it is the absence of usable folic acid that underlies the blood cell abnormalities seen during B$_{12}$ deficiency.

Fate in the Body

Absorption. Efficient absorption of B$_{12}$ requires *intrinsic factor*, a compound secreted by parietal cells of the stomach. Following ingestion, vitamin B$_{12}$ forms a complex with intrinsic factor. Upon reaching the ileum, the B$_{12}$–intrinsic factor complex interacts with specific receptors on the intestinal wall, causing the complex to be absorbed. In the absence of intrinsic factor, absorption of vitamin B$_{12}$ is greatly reduced. However, about 1% of the amount present can still be absorbed by passive diffusion; no intrinsic factor is required.

Distribution and Storage. Following absorption, the vitamin B$_{12}$–intrinsic factor complex dissociates. Free B$_{12}$ then binds to *transcobalamin II* for transport to tissues. Most vitamin B$_{12}$ goes to the liver and is stored. Total body stores of B$_{12}$ are minute, ranging from 2 to 3 mg by most estimates.

Elimination. Excretion of vitamin B$_{12}$ takes place very slowly; daily losses are about 0.1% of total body stores. Because B$_{12}$ is excreted so slowly, years are required for B$_{12}$ deficiency to develop—even when virtually no replenishment of lost B$_{12}$ has been taking place.

Daily Requirements

Because very little vitamin B$_{12}$ is excreted, and because body stores are small to begin with, daily requirements for this vitamin are minuscule. The average adult needs about 2.4 mg of B$_{12}$ per day. Children need even less.

Dietary Sources

The ability to biosynthesize vitamin B$_{12}$ is limited to microorganisms; higher plants and animals are unable to make this compound. The microorganisms that make B$_{12}$ reside in the soil, sewage, and the intestines of humans and other animals. Unfortunately, vitamin B$_{12}$ produced in the human GI tract is unavailable for absorption. Consequently, humans must obtain the majority of their B$_{12}$ by consuming animal products. Liver and dairy products are especially good sources. Between 10% and 30% of adults over age 50 are unable to absorb vitamin B$_{12}$ found naturally in foods. Accordingly, these people should meet their requirements by consuming B$_{12}$-fortified foods or a B$_{12}$-containing vitamin supplement.

Vitamin B$_{12}$ Deficiency: Causes, Consequences, and Diagnosis

Causes

In the majority of cases, vitamin B$_{12}$ deficiency is the result of impaired absorption. Insufficient B$_{12}$ in the diet is rarely a cause of deficiency. Potential causes of poor absorption include (1) regional enteritis, (2) celiac disease (a malabsorption syndrome involving abnormalities in the intestinal villi), and (3) development of antibodies directed against the vitamin B$_{12}$–intrinsic factor complex. In addition, because stomach acid is required to release vitamin B$_{12}$ from foods, it cannot be absorbed if acid secretion is significantly reduced, as often happens in the elderly.

Most frequently, impaired absorption of vitamin B$_{12}$ occurs secondary to a lack of intrinsic factor. The principal causes of intrinsic factor deficiency are atrophy of gastric parietal cells and surgery of the stomach (total gastric resection).

When vitamin B$_{12}$ deficiency is caused by an absence of intrinsic factor, the resulting syndrome is called *pernicious anemia*—a term suggesting a highly destructive or fatal condition. Pernicious anemia is an old term that refers back to the days when, for most patients, vitamin B$_{12}$ deficiency had no effective therapy. Hence, the condition was uniformly fatal. Today, vitamin B$_{12}$ deficiency secondary to lack of intrinsic factor can be managed successfully. Hence, the label *pernicious* no longer bears its original ominous connotation.

Consequences

Many of the consequences of B_{12} deficiency result from disruption of DNA synthesis. Tissues that are affected most are those that have a high proportion of cells undergoing growth and division. Accordingly, B_{12} deficiency has profound effects on the bone marrow (the site where blood cells are produced) and the epithelial cells lining the mouth and GI tract.

Megaloblastic Anemia. The most conspicuous consequence of B_{12} deficiency is an anemia in which large numbers of *megaloblasts* (oversized erythroblasts) appear in the bone marrow, and in which *macrocytes* (oversized erythrocytes) appear in the blood. These strange cells are produced because of impaired DNA synthesis: lacking sufficient DNA, growing cells are unable to divide; hence, as erythroblasts mature and their division is prevented, oversized cells result. Most megaloblasts die within the bone marrow; only a few evolve into the macrocytes that can be seen in the blood. Because of these unusual cells, the anemia associated with vitamin B_{12} deficiency is often referred to as either *megaloblastic* or *macrocytic* anemia.

Severe anemia is the principal cause of mortality from B_{12} deficiency. Anemia produces peripheral and cerebral hypoxia. Heart failure and dysrhythmias are the most frequent cause of death.

It is important to note that the hematologic effects of vitamin B_{12} deficiency can be reversed with large doses of *folic acid*. As indicated in Figure 52–4, when folic acid is present in large amounts, some of it can be activated by an alternate pathway that is independent of vitamin B_{12}. This pathway bypasses the metabolic block caused by B_{12} deficiency, thereby permitting DNA synthesis to proceed.

Neurologic Damage. Deficiency of vitamin B_{12} causes demyelination of neurons, primarily in the spinal cord and brain. A variety of signs and symptoms can result. Early manifestations include paresthesias (tingling, numbness) of the hands and feet and a reduction in deep tendon reflexes. Late-developing responses include loss of memory, mood changes, hallucinations, and psychosis. If vitamin B_{12} deficiency is prolonged, neurologic damage can become permanent.

The precise mechanism by which B_{12} deficiency results in neuronal damage is unknown. We do know, however, that *neuronal damage is not related to effects on folic acid or DNA*. That is, the mechanism that underlies neuronal damage is different from the mechanism that underlies disruption of hematopoiesis. Consequently, although administering large doses of folic acid can correct the hematologic consequences of B_{12} deficiency, folic acid will not affect the neurologic picture.

Other Effects. As noted, vitamin B_{12} deficiency can adversely affect virtually all tissues in which a high proportion of cells are undergoing growth and division. Hence, in addition to disrupting the production of erythrocytes, lack of B_{12} also prevents the bone marrow from making leukocytes (white blood cells) and thrombocytes (platelets). Loss of these blood elements can lead to infection and spontaneous bleeding. Disruption of DNA synthesis can also suppress division of the cells that form the epithelial lining of the mouth, stomach, and intestine, thereby causing oral ulceration and a variety of GI disturbances.

Diagnosis

When megaloblastic anemia occurs, it may be due to vitamin B_{12} deficiency or other causes, especially a lack of folic acid. Hence, if therapy is to be appropriate, a definitive diagnosis must be made. Two tests are particularly helpful. The first is obvious: measurement of plasma B_{12} content. The second procedure, known as the Schilling test, measures vitamin B_{12} absorption. The combination of megaloblastic anemia plus low plasma vitamin B_{12} plus evidence of B_{12} malabsorption permits a clear diagnosis of vitamin B_{12} deficiency.

Vitamin B_{12} Preparations: Cyanocobalamin

Cyanocobalamin is a purified, crystalline form of vitamin B_{12}. This compound is the drug of choice for all forms of B_{12} deficiency.

Adverse Effects

Cyanocobalamin is generally devoid of serious adverse effects. One potential response, *hypokalemia,* may occur as a natural consequence of increased erythrocyte production. Erythrocytes incorporate significant amounts of potassium. Hence, as large numbers of new erythrocytes are produced, levels of free potassium may fall.

Dosage and Administration

Cyanocobalamin can be given orally, intranasally, and by IM or SC injection. Most pharmacology texts, including prior editions of this one, will tell you that oral therapy is appropriate only for people who absorb B_{12} well; all others (i.e., those with impaired absorption) should use intranasal or parenteral therapy. However, this statement is not correct. Although it *is* true that various conditions—including lack of intrinsic factor, low gastric acidity, and regional enteritis—severely impair B_{12} absorption, these conditions do not prevent absorption entirely. Hence, even people with impaired absorption can still be treated orally; the only catch is that doses must be very high. Is there any advantage to oral therapy compared with parenteral therapy? Yes. First, oral therapy is more comfortable (injections sometimes hurt). Second, oral therapy is much more convenient (regular trips to the physician for injections are avoided).

Oral. Oral cyanocobalamin is appropriate for most people with mild to moderate B_{12} deficiency, regardless of the cause. (The principal exception is patients with severe neurologic involvement.) If the B_{12} deficiency is due to malabsorption, dosages must be high—ranging between 1000 and 10,000 μg a day. To ensure that absorption has been adequate, B_{12} levels should be measured periodically.

In addition to treating patients with B_{12} deficiency, oral cyanocobalamin can be used as a dietary supplement. The usual dosage is 6 μg/day.

Parenteral. Parenteral cyanocobalamin can be administered by *IM or deep SC injection. Cyanocobalamin must NOT be given intravenously.* Intramuscular and SC injections are generally well tolerated, although they occasionally cause pain and other local reactions.

Parenteral administration is indicated for patients with impaired B_{12} absorption—although most of these people can be treated with oral cyanocobalamin instead. If the cause of malabsorption is irreversible (e.g., parietal cell atrophy, total gastrectomy), therapy must continue lifelong. A typical dosing schedule for megaloblastic anemia is 30 μg/day for 5 to 10 days followed by 100 to 200 μg monthly until remission is complete. After anemia has been corrected, doses of 100 μg are administered monthly for life.

Intranasal. Cyanocobalamin for nasal administration is available in a metered-dose device under the trade name *Nascobal.* One actuation of the device delivers 500 μg of cyanocobalamin gel. Nasal administration represents a convenient alternative to IM or SC injection for people who cannot take cyanocobalamin orally. Efficacy of intranasal cyanocobalamin has not been determined for patients with nasal congestion, allergic rhinitis, or upper respiratory infections. Accordingly, until more is known, patients with these disorders should not use this formulation. Hot foods or liquids can increase nasal secretions, which might flush cyanocobalamin gel from the nose. Accordingly, administration should be done no sooner than 1 hour after eating hot foods, and hot foods should be eaten no sooner than 1 hour after administering the drug. For patients with B_{12} malabsorption, the recommended initial dose is 500 μg once a week.

Guidelines for Treating Vitamin B_{12} Deficiency

Route of B_{12} Administration. As discussed above, oral therapy can be used for most patients, including those with conditions that impair B_{12} absorption. The major exception is patients with severe neurologic deficits caused by B_{12} deficiency. For these people, parenteral cyanocobalamin is indicated.

Treatment of Moderate B_{12} Deficiency. The primary manifestations of moderate B_{12} deficiency are megaloblasts in the bone marrow and macrocytes in peripheral blood. Moderate deficiency does not cause leukopenia, thrombocytopenia, or neurologic complications. Moderate deficiency can be managed with vitamin B_{12} alone; no other measures are required.

Treatment of Severe B_{12} Deficiency. Severe deficiency produces multiple effects, all of which must be attended to. Unlike mild B_{12} deficiency, in which erythrocytes are the only blood cells affected, severe deficiency disrupts production of all blood cells. Loss of erythrocytes leads to hypoxia, cerebrovascular insufficiency, and heart failure. Loss of leukocytes encourages infection. And loss of thrombocytes promotes bleeding. In addition to causing serious hematologic deficits, severe B_{12} deficiency has adverse effects on the nervous system and GI tract.

Treatment of severe deficiency involves the following: (1) IM injection of vitamin B_{12} and folic acid (the folic acid accelerates recovery of hematologic deficits); (2) administration of 2 to 3 units of packed red blood cells (to correct anemia quickly); (3) transfusion of platelets (to suppress bleeding); and (4) therapy with antibiotics if infection has developed.

Following treatment with vitamin B_{12} plus folic acid, recovery from anemia occurs quickly. Within 1 to 2 days, megaloblasts disappear from the bone marrow; within 3 to 5 days, reticulocyte counts become elevated; by day 10, the hematocrit begins to rise; and within 14 to 21 days, the hematocrit becomes normal.

Recovery from neurologic damage is slow and depends on how long the damage had been present. When deficits have been present for only 2 to 3 months, recovery is relatively fast. When deficits have been present for many months or for years, recovery is slow: Months may pass before any improvement is apparent, and complete recovery may never occur.

Long-Term Treatment. For patients who lack intrinsic factor or who suffer from some other permanent cause of vitamin B_{12} malabsorption, lifelong treatment is required. Traditional therapy consists of monthly IM or SC injections. However, weekly intranasal doses or *large* daily oral doses can be just as effective. During prolonged therapy, treatment should be periodically assessed: plasma levels of vitamin B_{12} should be measured every 3 to 6 months, blood samples should be examined for the return of macrocytes, and blood counts should be performed.

Potential Hazard of Folic Acid. Treatment with folic acid can exacerbate the neurologic consequences of B_{12} deficiency. Recall that folic acid, by itself, can reverse the *hematologic* effects of B_{12} deficiency—but will not alleviate *neurologic* deficits. Hence, by correcting the most obvious manifestation of B_{12} deficiency (anemia), folic acid can obscure the fact that a deficiency of B_{12} still exists. As a result, *use of folic acid can lead to undertreatment with B_{12} itself,* and can thereby permit neurologic damage to progress. Clearly, folic acid is not a substitute for vitamin B_{12}, and vitamin B_{12} deficiency should never be treated with folic acid alone. Whenever folic acid is employed during treatment of vitamin B_{12} deficiency, extra care must be taken to ensure that B_{12} dosage is adequate.

FOLIC ACID DEFICIENCY

In one respect, folic acid deficiency is identical to a vitamin B_{12} deficiency: in both states, *megaloblastic anemia* is the most conspicuous pathology. However, in other important ways, folic acid deficiency and vitamin B_{12} deficiency are dissimilar (Table 52–3 provides a summary). Consequently, when a patient presents with megaloblastic anemia, it is essential to determine whether the cause is deficiency of folic acid, vitamin B_{12}, or both.

Physiology and Biochemistry of Folic Acid
Metabolic Function

As noted when we discussed vitamin B_{12}, folic acid (also known as *folate*) is an essential factor for DNA synthesis. Without folic acid, DNA replication and cell division become disrupted.

In order to be usable, dietary folic acid must first be converted to an active form. Under normal conditions, activation occurs via a pathway employing vitamin B_{12} (see Fig. 52–4). However, when large amounts of folate are ingested, some can be activated via an alternate pathway—one that does not employ vitamin B_{12}. Hence, even in the absence of vitamin B_{12}, if sufficient amounts of folic acid are consumed, active folate will be available for DNA synthesis.

Fate in the Body

Folic acid is absorbed in the early segment of the small intestine. Following absorption, folic acid is transported to the liver and other tissues, where it is either used or stored.

Folic acid in the liver undergoes extensive enterohepatic recirculation. That is, folate from the liver is excreted into the intestine, after which it is reabsorbed and then returned to the liver through the hepatic-portal circulation. This enterohe-

TABLE 52–3 ⁍■ Vitamin B₁₂ Deficiency Versus Folic Acid Deficiency

	Vitamin B$_{12}$ Deficiency	Folic Acid Deficiency
Usual Cause	Vitamin B$_{12}$ malabsorption from lack of intrinsic factor	Low dietary folic acid
Primary Hematologic Effect	Megaloblastic anemia	Megaloblastic anemia
Neurologic Effect	Damage to brain and spinal cord	None*
Diagnosis	Low plasma vitamin B$_{12}$; low B$_{12}$ absorption (Schilling test)	Low plasma folic acid
Treatment (Usual Route)	Cyanocobalamin (IM)	Folic acid (PO)
Usual Duration of Therapy	Lifelong	Short term

*Folic acid deficiency in pregnancy can cause neural tube defects in the fetus.

patic recirculation helps salvage up to 200 μg of folate per day. Accordingly, this process is an important means of maintaining folic acid stores.

In contrast to vitamin B$_{12}$, folic acid is not conserved rigidly: every day, significant amounts are excreted. As a result, if intake of folic acid were to cease, signs of deficiency would develop rapidly (within weeks if body stores were already low).

Daily Requirements

The RDA of folic acid is now 400 μg for adult males and females. RDAs during pregnancy and lactation are 600 μg and 500 μg, respectively. Individuals with malabsorption syndromes (e.g., tropical sprue) may require as much as 2000 μg (2 mg) per day; at these high doses, folate will be taken up in sufficient quantity despite impaired absorption.

Dietary Sources

Folic acid is present in all foods. Good sources include liver, peas, lentils, oranges, whole-wheat products, asparagus, beets, broccoli, and spinach. Also, many grain products (e.g., cereals, bread, pasta, rice, flour) are now fortified with folic acid.

Folic Acid Deficiency: Causes, Consequences, and Diagnosis

Causes

Folic acid deficiency has two principal causes: (1) poor diet (especially as seen in alcoholics), and (2) malabsorption secondary to intestinal disease. Rarely, certain drugs may cause folate deficiency.

Alcoholism. Alcoholism, either acute or chronic, may be the most common cause of folate deficiency. Deficiency results for two reasons: (1) insufficient folic acid in the diet and (2) derangement of enterohepatic recirculation secondary to alcohol-induced injury to the liver. Fortunately, with improved diet and reduced alcohol consumption, alcohol-related folate deficiency can often be reversed.

Sprue. Sprue is an intestinal malabsorption syndrome that decreases folic acid uptake. Since sprue does not block folate absorption entirely, deficiency can be corrected by giving large doses of folic acid orally.

Consequences

All People. With the important exception that folic acid deficiency does not injure the nervous system, the effects of folate deficiency are identical to those of vitamin B$_{12}$ deficiency. Hence, as with B$_{12}$ deficiency, the most prominent consequence of folate deficiency is *megaloblastic anemia.* In addition, like B$_{12}$ deficiency, lack of folic acid may result in

leukopenia, thrombocytopenia, and injury to the oral and GI mucosa. Since we already noted that many of the consequences of vitamin B$_{12}$ deficiency result from depriving cells of active folic acid, the similarities between folate deficiency and vitamin B$_{12}$ deficiency should be no surprise.

The Developing Fetus. Folic acid deficiency *very early* in pregnancy can cause neural tube defects (e.g., spina bifida, anencephaly). Accordingly, it is imperative that all women of reproductive age ensure adequate folate levels *before* pregnancy occurs. Because folate present naturally in foods has relatively low bioavailability, women capable of becoming pregnant should consume 400 μg/day of *synthetic* folate (either from fortified foods, supplements, or both). If pregnancy occurs, folate intake should increase to 600 μg/day.

Other Consequences. As discussed in Chapter 76 (Vitamins) folic acid deficiency may increase the risk of colorectal cancer and atherosclerosis.

Diagnosis

When patients present with megaloblastic anemia, it is essential to distinguish between folic acid deficiency and vitamin B$_{12}$ deficiency as the cause. We can make this distinction by comparing plasma levels of folate and vitamin B$_{12}$. If folic acid levels are low and vitamin B$_{12}$ levels are normal, a diagnosis of folic acid deficiency is suggested. Conversely, if folate levels are normal and B$_{12}$ is low, B$_{12}$ deficiency would be the likely diagnosis. A decision against folic acid deficiency would be strengthened if neurologic deficits were observed.

Folic Acid Preparations
Nomenclature

Nomenclature regarding folic acid preparations can be confusing and hence deserves comment. Two forms of folic acid are available. One form is inactive as administered (but undergoes activation once it has been absorbed). The second form is active to start with. Both forms have several generic names: the *inactive form* is referred to as *folacin, folate, pteroylglutamic acid,* and *folic acid;* the *active form* is referred to as *leucovorin calcium, folinic acid,* and *citrovorum factor.* The inactive form is by far the most commonly used preparation.

Folic Acid (Pteroylglutamic Acid)

Chemistry. Folic acid is inactive as administered and cannot support DNA synthesis. Activation takes place rapidly following absorption.

Indications. Folic acid has three uses: (1) treatment of megaloblastic anemia resulting from folic acid deficiency; (2) prophylaxis of folate deficiency, especially during pregnancy and lactation; and (3) initial treatment of severe megaloblastic anemia resulting from vitamin B_{12} deficiency.

Adverse Effects. Oral folic acid is nontoxic. Massive dosages (e.g., as much as 15 mg/day) have been taken with no ill effects.

Warning. If taken in sufficiently large doses, folic acid can correct the hematologic consequences of vitamin B_{12} deficiency, thereby masking the fact that a deficiency in vitamin B_{12} still exists. Since folic acid will not prevent the neurologic consequences of B_{12} deficiency (despite correcting the hematologic picture), this masking effect may allow the development of irreversible damage to the nervous system. To reduce the chances of this problem, folate should not be used indiscriminately: Unless specifically indicated, consumption of folic acid should not exceed 1000 μg/day. Furthermore, whenever folic acid is given to patients known to have a deficiency in vitamin B_{12}, special care must be taken to ensure that the vitamin B_{12} dosage is adequate.

Formulations and Routes of Administration. Folic acid is available in tablets (0.4, 0.8, and 1.0 mg) for oral use and in a 0.5-mg/ml solution [Folvite] for IM, IV, or SC injection. As a rule, injections are reserved for patients with severely impaired GI absorption.

Dosage. For treatment of folate-deficient megaloblastic anemia in adults, the usual oral dosage is 1000 to 2000 μg/day. Once symptoms have resolved, a maintenance dosage of 400 μg/day is given. For prophylaxis during pregnancy and lactation, doses up to 1000 μg/day may be used.

Leucovorin Calcium (Folinic Acid)

Leucovorin calcium is an active form of folic acid used primarily as an adjunct to cancer chemotherapy (see Chapter 98). Leucovorin is not used routinely to correct folic acid deficiency. Why? Because folic acid is just as effective and less expensive.

Guidelines for Treating Folic Acid Deficiency

Choice of Treatment Modality. The modality for treating folic acid deficiency should be matched with the cause. If folic acid deficiency is due to poor diet, the deficiency should be corrected by dietary measures—not with drugs (except for women who may become pregnant). Ingestion of one fresh vegetable or one glass of fruit juice a day will often suffice. In contrast, when folate deficiency is the result of malabsorption, diet alone cannot correct the deficiency, and hence a pharmaceutical preparation of folate will be needed.

Route of Administration. Oral administration is preferred for most patients. Unlike vitamin B_{12}, folic acid is rarely administered by injection. Even in the presence of intestinal disease, oral folic acid can be effective, providing the dosage is big enough.

Prophylactic Use of Folic Acid. Folic acid should be taken prophylactically only when clearly appropriate. The principal indications are pregnancy and lactation. Since folic acid may mask vitamin B_{12} deficiency, indiscriminate use of folate should be avoided.

Treatment of Severe Deficiency. Folic acid deficiency can produce severe megaloblastic anemia. To ensure a rapid response, therapy should be initiated with an IM injection of folic acid and vitamin B_{12}. (Because of the metabolic interrelationship between folic acid and vitamin B_{12}, combining these agents accelerates recovery.) After the initial injection, treatment should be continued with folic acid alone. Folic acid should be given orally in a dosage of 1000 to 2000 μg/day for 1 to 2 weeks. After this, maintenance doses of 400 μg/day may be required.

Therapy is evaluated by monitoring the hematologic picture. When treatment has been effective, megaloblasts will disappear from the bone marrow within 48 hours; the reticulocyte count will increase measurably within 2 to 3 days; and the hematocrit will begin to rise in the second week.

▪▪ KEY POINTS

- The principal cause of iron deficiency is increased iron demand secondary to (1) maternal and fetal blood volume expansion during pregnancy, (2) blood volume expansion during infancy and early childhood, or (3) chronic blood loss, usually of GI or uterine origin.
- The major consequence of iron deficiency is microcytic, hypochromic anemia.
- Ferrous sulfate, given PO, is the drug of choice for iron deficiency.
- Iron-deficient patients who cannot tolerate or absorb oral ferrous salts are treated with parenteral iron—usually iron dextran administered IV.
- The major adverse effects of ferrous sulfate are GI disturbances. These are best managed by reducing the dosage (rather than by administering the drug with food, which would greatly reduce its absorption).
- Parenteral iron dextran carries a significant risk of fatal anaphylactic reactions. The risk is much lower with other parenteral iron products (e.g., iron sucrose).
- The principal cause of vitamin B_{12} deficiency is impaired absorption secondary to lack of intrinsic factor.
- The principal consequences of B_{12} deficiency are megaloblastic (macrocytic) anemia and neurologic injury.
- Vitamin B_{12} deficiency caused by malabsorption is treated lifelong with cyanocobalamin. Traditional treatment consists of IM injections administered monthly. However, intranasal doses administered weekly or large oral doses administered daily are also effective.
- For initial therapy of *severe* vitamin B_{12} deficiency, parenteral folic acid is given along with cyanocobalamin.
- When folic acid is combined with vitamin B_{12} to treat B_{12} deficiency, it is essential that the dosage of B_{12} be adequate. Why? Because folic acid can mask continued B_{12} deficiency (by improving the hematologic picture), while allowing the neurologic consequences of B_{12} deficiency to progress.
- The principal causes of folic acid deficiency are poor diet (usually in alcoholics) and malabsorption secondary to intestinal disease.
- The principal consequences of folic acid deficiency are megaloblastic anemia and neural tube defects (in the developing fetus).
- To prevent neural tube defects, all women who may become pregnant should ingest 400 μg of folate daily, in the form of folate supplements or folate-fortified foods.

Summary of Major Nursing Implications*

IRON PREPARATIONS

Carbonyl iron
Ferrous fumarate
Ferrous gluconate
Ferrous sulfate
Iron dextran
Iron sucrose
Sodium–ferric gluconate complex (SFGC)
Except where indicated, the implications summarized below apply to all of the iron preparations.

Preadministration Assessment

Therapeutic Goal

Prevention or treatment of iron deficiency anemias.

Baseline Data

Prior to treatment, assess the degree of anemia. Fatigue, listlessness, and pallor indicate mild anemia; dyspnea, tachycardia, and angina suggest severe anemia. Laboratory findings indicative of anemia are subnormal hemoglobin levels, subnormal hematocrit, subnormal hemosiderin in bone marrow, and the presence of microcytic, hypochromic erythrocytes.

The cause of iron deficiency (e.g., pregnancy, occult bleeding, menorrhagia, inadequate diet, malabsorption) must be determined.

Identifying High-Risk Patients

All iron preparations are *contraindicated* for patients with anemias other than iron deficiency anemia.

Parenteral preparations are *contraindicated* for patients who have had a severe allergic reaction to them in the past.

Use *oral* preparations with *caution* in patients with peptic ulcer disease, regional enteritis, and ulcerative colitis.

Implementation: Administration

Routes

Oral. Ferrous sulfate, ferrous fumarate, ferrous gluconate, carbonyl iron.

Parenteral. Iron dextran, SFGC, iron sucrose.

Oral Administration

Food reduces GI distress from oral iron but also greatly reduces absorption. **Instruct patients to administer oral iron between meals to maximize uptake.** If GI distress is intolerable, the dosage may be reduced. If absolutely necessary, oral iron may be administered with meals.

Liquid preparations can stain the teeth. **Instruct patients to dilute liquid preparations with juice or water, administer them through a straw, and rinse the mouth after.**

Warn patients not to crush or chew sustained-release preparations.

Warn patients against ingesting iron salts together with antacids or tetracyclines.

Inform patients that oral iron preparations are not identical and warn them against changing from one to another.

Parenteral Administration: Iron Dextran

Iron dextran may be given intravenously or intramuscularly. Intravenous administration is safer and preferred.

Intravenous. To minimize anaphylactic reactions, follow this protocol: (1) Inject 1 or 2 drops as a test dose and observe the patient for at least 15 minutes. (2) If the test dose appears safe, infuse 500 mg over 10 to 15 minutes. (3) If the 500-mg dose proves uneventful, give additional doses as needed.

Intramuscular. Intramuscular injection can cause significant adverse reactions (anaphylaxis, persistent pain, localized discoloration, promotion of tumors) and is generally avoided. Make injections deep into each buttock using the Z-track technique. Give a small test dose before giving the full therapeutic dose.

Parenteral Administration: SFGC

To minimize adverse reactions, precede the first full dose with a test dose (25 mg infused IV over 60 minutes). Administer therapeutic doses by slow IV infusion (no faster than 12.5 mg/min).

Parenteral Administration: Iron Sucrose

Administer iron sucrose directly into the dialysis line. Do not mix with other drugs or with parenteral nutrition solutions. Administer by either (1) slow injection (1 ml/min) or (2) infusion (dilute iron sucrose in up to 100 ml of 0.9% saline and infuse over 15 minutes or longer).

Implementation: Measures to Enhance Therapeutic Effects

If diet is poor in iron, advise the patient to increase consumption of iron-rich foods (e.g., liver, egg yolks, brewer's yeast, wheat germ, muscle meats, fish, fowl).

Ongoing Evaluation and Interventions

Evaluating Therapeutic Responses

Evaluate treatment by monitoring hematologic status. Reticulocyte number should increase within 4 to 7 days, hemoglobin content and the hematocrit should begin to rise within 1 week, and hemoglobin levels should rise by at least 2 gm/dl within 1 month. If these responses do not occur, evaluate the patient for compliance, persistent bleeding, inflammatory disease, and malabsorption.

Minimizing Adverse Effects

GI Disturbances. **Forewarn patients about possible GI reactions (nausea, vomiting, constipation, diarrhea) and inform them these will diminish over time.** If GI distress is severe, the dosage may be reduced, or, if absolutely necessary, iron may be administered with food.

Forewarn patients that iron will impart a harmless dark green or black color to stools.

*Patient education information is highlighted as blue text.

Summary of Major Nursing Implications*—cont'd

Anaphylactic Reactions. Parenteral iron dextran (and, rarely, SFGC and iron sucrose) can cause potentially fatal anaphylaxis. Before giving parenteral iron, ensure that injectable epinephrine and facilities for resuscitation are immediately available. After administration, observe the patient for 60 minutes. Give test doses as described above. Precede all doses of iron dextran and the first dose of SFGC with a test dose; test doses are unnecessary with iron sucrose.

Managing Acute Toxicity. Iron poisoning can be fatal to young children. **Instruct parents to store iron out of reach and in childproof containers.** If poisoning occurs, rapid treatment is imperative. Induce vomiting to remove iron from the stomach. Administer deferoxamine if plasma levels of iron exceed 500 mg/ml. Manage acidosis and shock as required.

CYANOCOBALAMIN (VITAMIN B$_{12}$)

Preadministration Assessment

Therapeutic Goal

Correction of megaloblastic anemia and other sequelae of vitamin B$_{12}$ deficiency.

Baseline Data

Assess the extent of vitamin B$_{12}$ deficiency. Record signs and symptoms of anemia (e.g., pallor, dyspnea, palpitations, fatigue). Determine the extent of neurologic damage. Assess GI involvement.

Baseline laboratory data include plasma vitamin B$_{12}$ levels, erythrocyte and reticulocyte counts, and hemoglobin and hematocrit values. Bone marrow may be examined for megaloblasts. A Schilling test may be ordered to assess vitamin B$_{12}$ absorption.

Identifying High-Risk Patients

Use with *caution* in patients receiving folic acid.

Implementation: Administration

Routes and Administration

Administration may be IM, SC, oral, or intranasal. For most patients, lifelong treatment is required. Traditional therapy consists of IM or SC injections administered monthly. However, intranasal doses administered weekly or large oral doses administered daily can be equally effective.

Implementation: Measures to Enhance Therapeutic Effects

Promoting Compliance

Patients with permanent impairment of B$_{12}$ absorption require lifelong B$_{12}$ therapy. To promote compliance, **educate patients about the nature of their condition and impress upon them the need for monthly injections or weekly intranasal therapy.** Schedule appointments for injections at convenient times.

*Patient education information is highlighted as blue text.

Improving Diet

When B$_{12}$ deficiency is not due to impaired absorption, a change in diet may accelerate recovery. **Advise the patient to increase consumption of B$_{12}$-rich foods (e.g., muscle meats, dairy products).**

Ongoing Evaluation and Interventions

Evaluating Therapeutic Effects

Assess for improvements in hematologic and neurologic status. Over a period of 2 to 3 weeks, megaloblasts should disappear, reticulocyte counts should rise, and the hematocrit should normalize. Neurologic damage may take months to improve; in some cases, full recovery may never occur.

For patients receiving long-term therapy, vitamin B$_{12}$ levels should be measured every 3 to 6 months, and blood counts should be performed.

Minimizing Adverse Effects

Hypokalemia may develop during the first days of therapy. Monitor serum potassium levels and observe the patient for signs of potassium insufficiency (e.g., muscle weakness, dysrhythmias).

Minimizing Adverse Interactions

Folic acid can mask hematologic symptoms of vitamin B$_{12}$ deficiency, resulting in undertreatment and progression of neurologic injury caused by B$_{12}$ insufficiency. When folic acid and cyanocobalamin are used concurrently, special care must be taken to ensure that the cyanocobalamin dosage is adequate.

FOLIC ACID (FOLACIN, FOLATE, PTEROYLGLUTAMIC ACID)

Preadministration Assessment

Therapeutic Goal

Folic acid is used for (1) treatment of megaloblastic anemia resulting from folic acid deficiency, (2) initial treatment of severe megaloblastic anemia resulting from vitamin B$_{12}$ deficiency, and (3) prevention of folic acid deficiency (especially during pregnancy).

Baseline Data

Assess the extent of folate deficiency. Record signs and symptoms of anemia (e.g., pallor, dyspnea, palpitations, fatigue). Determine the extent of GI damage.

Baseline laboratory data include serum folate levels, erythrocyte and reticulocyte counts, and hemoglobin and hematocrit values. In addition, bone marrow may be evaluated for megaloblasts. To rule out vitamin B$_{12}$ deficiency, vitamin B$_{12}$ determinations and a Schilling test may be ordered.

Summary of Major Nursing Implications*—cont'd

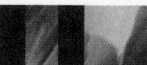

Identifying High-Risk Patients

Folic acid is *contraindicated* for patients with pernicious anemia (except during the acute phase of treatment). Inappropriate use of folic acid by these patients can mask signs of vitamin B_{12} deficiency, thereby allowing further neurologic deterioration.

Implementation: Administration

Routes

Oral, SC, IV, and IM. Oral administration is most common and preferred. Injections are employed only when intestinal absorption is severely impaired.

*Patient education information is highlighted as blue text.

Implementation: Measures to Enhance Therapeutic Effects

Improving Diet

If the diet is deficient in folic acid, advise the patient to increase consumption of folate-rich foods (e.g., green vegetables, liver). If alcoholism underlies dietary deficiency, counseling should be offered.

Ongoing Evaluation and Interventions

Evaluating Therapeutic Effects

Monitor hematologic status. Within 2 weeks, megaloblasts should disappear, reticulocyte counts should increase, and the hematocrit should begin to rise.

Hematopoietic and Thrombopoietic Growth Factors

HEMATOPOIETIC GROWTH FACTORS
  Epoetin Alfa (Erythropoietin)
  Darbepoetin Alfa (Erythropoietin, Long Acting)
  Filgrastim (Granulocyte
  Colony-Stimulating Factor)
  Pegfilgrastim (Granulocyte
  Colony-Stimulating Factor, Long Acting)
  Sargramostim (Granulocyte-Macrophage
  Colony-Stimulating Factor)
THROMBOPOIETIC GROWTH FACTORS
  Oprelvekin (Interleukin-11)

Our topic for this chapter is drugs that act on the bone marrow to stimulate formation of blood cells and platelets. The drugs that stimulate formation of blood cells (erythrocytes and leukocytes) are known as *hematopoietic growth factors,* whereas the drugs that stimulate formation of platelets (thrombocytes) are known as *thrombopoietic growth factors.*

HEMATOPOIETIC GROWTH FACTORS

Hematopoiesis is the process by which new blood cells are produced. This process is regulated in part by hematopoietic growth factors—naturally occurring hormones that (1) stimulate the proliferation and differentiation of hematopoietic stem cells, and (2) enhance function in the mature forms of those cells (neutrophils, monocytes, macrophages, and erythrocytes). In a laboratory setting, hematopoietic growth factors can cause stem cells to form colonies of mature blood cells. Because of this action, hematopoietic growth factors are also known as *colony-stimulating factors.* Therapeutic applications of hematopoietic growth factors include (1) acceleration of neutrophil repopulation after cancer chemotherapy, (2) acceleration of bone marrow recovery after autologous bone marrow transplant (BMT), and (3) stimulation of erythrocyte production in patients with chronic renal failure (CRF).

The names used for the hematopoietic growth factors are a potential source of confusion. Why? Because each product has a biologic name, a generic name, and one or more proprietary (trade) names. The biologic, generic, and proprietary names for the five available products are listed in Table 53–1.

Epoetin Alfa (Erythropoietin)

Epoetin alfa [Epogen, Procrit] is a hematopoietic growth factor produced by recombinant DNA technology. Chemically, the compound is a glycoprotein containing 165 amino acids. The protein portion of epoetin alfa is identical to that of human erythropoietin, a naturally occurring hormone. Epoetin alfa is used to maintain erythrocyte counts in (1) patients with CRF, (2) HIV-infected patients taking zidovudine, and (3) patients with nonmyeloid malignancies who have anemia secondary to chemotherapy. In addition, the drug can be used to elevate erythrocyte counts in anemic patients prior to elective surgery.

Physiology

Erythropoietin is a glycoprotein hormone that stimulates production of red blood cells (erythrocytes). The hormone is produced by peritubular cells in the proximal tubules of the kidney. In response to anemia or hypoxia, circulating levels of erythropoietin rise dramatically, triggering an increase in erythrocyte synthesis. However, since production of erythrocytes requires iron, folic acid, and vitamin B_{12}, the response to erythropoietin is minimal if any of these factors is deficient.

Therapeutic Uses

Anemia of Chronic Renal Failure. Epoetin alfa can reverse anemia associated with CRF. The drug is effective in patients on dialysis and in those who do not yet require dialysis. Effective treatment virtually eliminates the need for transfusions. Initial effects can be seen within 1 to 2 weeks. The hematocrit reaches target levels (30% to 36%) in 2 to 3 months. Patients experience an improved quality of life and increased energy levels. Unfortunately, treatment does not prevent progressive renal deterioration.

For therapy to be effective, iron stores must be adequate. Transferrin saturation should be at least 20%, and ferritin concentration should be at least 100 ng/ml. If pretreatment assessment indicates these values are low, they must be restored with iron supplements.

HIV-Infected Patients Taking Zidovudine. Epoetin alfa is approved for treating anemia caused by therapy with zidovudine (AZT) in patients with AIDS. For these patients, treatment can maintain or elevate erythrocyte counts and reduce the need for transfusions. However, if endogenous levels of erythropoietin are at or above 500 mU/ml, raising them further with epoetin is unlikely to help.

Chemotherapy-Induced Anemia. Epoetin alfa is used to treat chemotherapy-induced anemia in patients with *nonmyeloid malignancies,* thereby reducing or eliminating the

TABLE 53–1 ■ Nomenclature for Hematopoietic and Thrombopoietic Growth Factors

Biologic Name	Pharmacologic Names	
	Generic Name	Trade Name
Hematopoietic Growth Factors		
Granulocyte colony-stimulating factor (G-CSF)	Filgrastim	Neupogen
	Pegfilgrastim	Neulasta
Granulocyte-macrophage colony-stimulating factor (GM-CSF)	Sargramostim	Leukine
Erythropoietin	Darbepoetin alfa	Aranesp
	Epoetin alfa	Epogen, Procrit
Thrombopoietic Growth Factor		
Interleukin-11	Oprelvekin	Neumega

need for periodic transfusions. Since transfusions require hospitalization, whereas epoetin can be self-administered at home, epoetin therapy can spare patients considerable inconvenience. Because epoetin works slowly (the hematocrit may take 2 to 4 weeks to recover), transfusions are still indicated when rapid replenishment of red blood cells is required. Please note that epoetin is not approved for patients with *leukemias* and *other myeloid malignancies*. Why? Because the drug may stimulate proliferation of these cancers.

Anemia in Patients Facing Surgery. Epoetin may be given to increase erythrocyte levels in anemic patients scheduled for elective surgery. The drug should be used only when significant blood loss is anticipated—but should not be used prior to cardiac or vascular surgery. For surgical patients, epoetin offers two benefits: (1) it decreases the need for transfusions, and (2) by increasing erythrocyte synthesis, it allows patients to predeposit more blood in anticipation of transfusion needs.

Pharmacokinetics

Epoetin alfa is administered parenterally (IV or SC). The drug cannot be given orally because, being a glycoprotein, it would be degraded in the GI tract. The plasma half-life is highly variable and unchanged by dialysis.

Adverse Effects and Interactions

Epoetin alfa is generally well tolerated. Although the drug is a protein, no serious allergic reactions have been reported. The most significant adverse effect is hypertension. There are no significant drug interactions.

Hypertension. In patients with CRF, epoetin is frequently associated with an increase in blood pressure. The extent of hypertension is directly related to the rate of rise in the hematocrit. To minimize the risk of hypertension, blood pressure should be monitored and, if necessary, controlled with antihypertensive drugs. If hypertension cannot be controlled, epoetin dosage should be reduced. In patients with pre-existing hypertension (a common complication of CRF), it is imperative that blood pressure be under control prior to epoetin use. About 30% of dialysis patients receiving epoetin require an adjustment in their antihypertensive therapy once the hematocrit has been normalized.

Autoimmune Red-Cell Aplasia. Very, very rarely, treatment with epoetin leads to red-cell aplasia, a condition characterized by severe anemia and a complete absence of erythrocyte precursor cells in bone marrow. The cause is production of neutralizing antibodies directed against epoetin itself as well as any erythropoietin the body is still able to produce. In the absence of epoetin and erythropoietin, production of red blood cells ceases. Because patients can no longer make erythrocytes, transfusions are required for survival.

Monitoring

The hematocrit should be determined prior to treatment and twice weekly thereafter until the target level has been reached and a maintenance dose established. Complete blood counts with a differential should be done routinely. Blood chemistry—blood urea nitrogen (BUN), uric acid, creatinine, phosphorus, and potassium—should be monitored. Iron should be measured periodically and maintained at an adequate level.

Preparations, Dosage, and Administration

Epoetin alfa [Epogen, Procrit] is dispensed in 1-ml vials (2000, 3000, 4000, 10,000, and 20,000 units) for SC and IV injection. Vials should not be shaken because epoetin is a protein that can be denatured by agitation. Don't mix epoetin with other drugs. Store at 2°C to 8°C; don't freeze.

Patients with Chronic Renal Failure. Route. Administration may be IV or SC. Until recently, IV administration was preferred, in part because SC administration was reputedly painful, and in part because bioavailability following SC injection is reduced—although the half-life is prolonged. In 1998, a study comparing IV therapy with SC therapy indicated that both produce equivalent effects. Furthermore, with SC administration, 30% less epoetin is required—and reported discomfort at the injection site is minimal. Because epoetin is expensive, and because SC therapy is equivalent to IV therapy and cheaper, it seems likely that SC therapy will become the new standard.

Dosage. The initial dosage is 50 to 100 U/kg 3 times a week. Administration is by IV bolus for dialysis patients and by IV bolus or SC injection for nondialysis patients. The dosage should be reduced when the therapeutic endpoint is reached (hematocrit of 30% to 33%) or if the rate of rise in the hematocrit exceeds 4 units in 2 weeks. Once the target hematocrit has been achieved, an individualized maintenance dosage should be established: For dialysis patients, the median maintenance dosage is 75 U/kg 3 times a week; for nondialysis patients, the median maintenance dosage is 75 to 100 U/kg once a week. If the hematocrit rises above 36%, epoetin should be temporarily withheld.

HIV-Infected Patients Taking Zidovudine. Prior to treatment, measure the endogenous erythropoietin level. If this level is already at or above 500 mU/ml, epoetin alfa is unlikely to be helpful.

Therapy is begun at 100 U/kg (IV or SC injection) 3 times a week. If the response is insufficient, the dosage may be increased by increments of 50 to 100 U/kg until a maximum of 300 U/kg 3 times a week has been reached. When the hematocrit has been restored to the desired level, an individualized maintenance dosage should be established.

Patients Receiving Cancer Chemotherapy. The initial dosage is 150 U/kg SC 3 times a week. If the response is inadequate by 8 weeks, the dosage may be increased to 300 U/kg 3 times a week.

Anemic Patients Scheduled for Surgery. The recommended dosage is 300 U/kg/day SC for 15 days starting 10 days before surgery.

Darbepoetin Alfa (Erythropoietin, Long Acting)

Darbepoetin alfa [Aranesp], also known as novel erythrocyte stimulation protein or NESP, is a long-acting analog of epoetin [Epogen, Procrit]. Both drugs act on erythroid progenitor cells to stimulate production of erythrocytes. Darbepoetin differs structurally from epoetin in that it has two additional carbohydrate chains. Because of these chains, darbepoetin is cleared more slowly than epoetin, and hence has a longer half-life (49 hours vs. 18 to 24 hours). As a result, darbepoetin can be administered less frequently, and thus is more convenient. At this time, darbepoetin has only one approved indication: maintenance of erythrocyte counts in patients with CRF. As discussed above, epoetin has additional indications.

Darbepoetin is generally well tolerated. As with epoetin, the most common problem is hypertension. The risk can be minimized by ensuring that the rate of rise in hemoglobin does not exceed 1 gm/dl every 2 weeks. If hypertension develops, it should be controlled with antihypertensive drugs. Patients already taking antihypertensive drugs may need to increase their dosage.

Preparations, Dosage, Administration, and Monitoring

Preparations and Storage. Darbepoetin alfa [Aranesp] is available 1-ml, single-dose vials (25, 40, 60, 100, and 200 μg) for SC and IV injection. Don't dilute darbepoetin or mix it with other drugs. Because darbepoetin is a protein that can be denatured by agitation, don't shake the vials. Discard preparations that are discolored or contain particles. Store at 2°C to 8°C; don't freeze.

Dosage and Administration. For management of anemia associated with CRF, the initial dosage is 0.45 μg/kg, given IV or SC once a week. The target hemoglobin level is 12 gm/dl. Because responses develop gradually, dosage should be adjusted no more than once every 4 weeks. Quite often, the maintenance dosage is less than the initial dosage.

When switching from epoetin to darbepoetin, the new dosage and dosing frequency are based on the existing epoetin usage. For example, patients receiving 5000 to 11,000 units of epoetin each week should be given 25 μg of darbepoetin each week. If the epoetin dosing frequency was 2 to 3 times a week, darbepoetin should be given once a week; if epoetin was given once a week, darbepoetin should be given once every 2 weeks.

Monitoring. When initiating darbepoetin or changing dosage, the hemoglobin level should be measured weekly until it stabilizes. Thereafter, hemoglobin should be measured at least once a month.

Filgrastim (Granulocyte Colony-Stimulating Factor)

Filgrastim [Neupogen] is a hematopoietic growth factor produced by recombinant DNA technology. The drug is essentially identical in structure and actions to human granulocyte colony-stimulating factor (G-CSF), a naturally occurring hormone. Filgrastim has two principal uses: elevation of neutrophil counts in cancer patients and treatment of severe chronic neutropenia.

Physiology

G-CSF acts on cells in bone marrow to increase production of neutrophils (granulocytes). In addition, it enhances phagocytic and cytotoxic actions of mature neutrophils. The hormone is produced by monocytes, fibroblasts, and endothelial cells in response to inflammation and allergic challenge. This suggests that the hormone's natural role is to help fight infection and cancer.

Therapeutic Uses

Cancer. Patients Undergoing Myelosuppressive Chemotherapy. Filgrastim is given to reduce the risk of infection in patients undergoing cancer chemotherapy. Many anticancer drugs act on the bone marrow to suppress production of neutrophils, thereby greatly increasing the risk of infection. By stimulating production of neutrophils, filgrastim can decrease the risk of infection. Clinical trials have shown that treatment (1) reduces the incidence of severe neutropenia, (2) produces a dose-dependent increase in circulating neutrophils, (3) reduces the incidence of infection, (4) reduces the need for hospitalization, and (5) reduces the need for intravenous antibiotics. Unfortunately, this useful drug is very expensive: The cost to the pharmacist for a single course of treatment is $1800 to $2800. Because filgrastim stimulates proliferation of bone marrow cells, it should be used with great caution in patients with cancers that originated in the marrow.

Patients Undergoing Bone Marrow Transplant. Filgrastim is given to shorten the duration of neutropenia in patients who have undergone high-dose chemotherapy followed by a BMT. As noted, the drug is not used when the cancer is of myeloid origin.

Harvesting of Peripheral Blood Progenitor Cells. Peripheral blood progenitor cells (PBPCs) are harvested prior to bone marrow ablation with high-dose chemotherapy. Following chemotherapy, the PBPCs are infused back into the patient to accelerate repopulation of the bone marrow. Treatment with filgrastim prior to harvesting increases the number of circulating PBPCs, and therefore facilitates collection.

Severe Chronic Neutropenia. Filgrastim provides effective treatment for *congenital neutropenia* (Kostmann's syndrome), a condition characterized by pronounced neutropenia and frequent, severe infections. Therapy helps resolve existing infections and decreases the incidence of subsequent infections. Because treatment is chronic, the cost is extremely high. In addition to congenital neutropenia, filgrastim is used in patients with *idiopathic neutropenia* and *cyclic neutropenia*.

Investigational Uses. Filgrastim can reverse *zidovudine-induced neutropenia* in HIV-infected patients. However, the drug does not reduce the incidence of opportunistic infections. In patients with *acute myelogenous leukemia*, filgrastim has been given to stimulate division of cancer cells, thereby making them more sensitive to chemotherapeutic agents. Filgrastim has also been employed in patients with *aplastic anemia* and *myelodysplasia*.

Pharmacokinetics

Administration is parenteral (IV or SC). Filgrastim cannot be used orally because, being a protein, it would be destroyed in the GI tract. The drug is eliminated by renal excretion. Its serum half-life is about 3.5 hours.

Adverse Effects and Interactions

When used short-term, filgrastim is generally devoid of serious adverse effects. There are no drug interactions of note.

Bone Pain. Filgrastim causes bone pain in about 25% of patients. Pain is dose related and usually mild to moderate. In most cases, relief can be achieved with a nonopioid analgesic (e.g., acetaminophen). If not, an opioid may be tried.

Leukocytosis. When administered in doses greater than 5 mg/kg/day, filgrastim has caused white cell counts to rise above 100,000/mm³ in 2% of patients. Although no adverse effects were associated with this degree of leukocytosis, avoidance of leukocytosis would nonetheless be prudent. Excessive white cell counts can be avoided by obtaining complete blood counts twice weekly during treatment and by reducing filgrastim dosage if leukocytosis develops.

Other Adverse Effects. Treatment frequently causes elevation of plasma uric acid, lactate dehydrogenase (LDH), and alkaline phosphatase. Increases are usually moderate and reverse spontaneously. Long-term therapy has caused splenomegaly.

Preparations, Dosage, and Administration

Preparations and Storage. Filgrastim [Neupogen] is dispensed in solution (300 mg/ml) in 1- and 1.6-ml single-dose vials. The drug is stored at 2°C to 8°C—not frozen.

Dosage and Administration. *General Considerations.* Prior to administration, filgrastim can be kept at room temperature for up to 6 hours. It should not be agitated. Only one dose per vial should be used, and the vial should not be re-entered.

Cancer Chemotherapy. The usual dosage is 5 mg/kg once daily, administered IV or SC. Therapy should start no sooner than 24 hours after termination of chemotherapy, and should continue up to 2 weeks after the expected chemotherapy-induced nadir, or until the absolute neutrophil count has reached 10,000/mm³. Administer by SC bolus, short IV infusion, or continuous IV or SC infusion. A complete blood count and platelet count should be obtained prior to treatment and twice weekly during treatment.

Bone Marrow Transplant. The initial dosage is 10 mg/kg/day, administered by slow IV or SC infusion. During the period of neutrophil recovery, dosage is titrated against the neutrophil count.

Severe Chronic Neutropenia. Dosage is 6 mg/kg SC administered twice a day every day.

Pegfilgrastim (Granulocyte Colony-Stimulating Factor, Long Acting)

Pegfilgrastim [Neulasta] is a long-acting derivative of filgrastim [Neupogen]. Both drugs stimulate myeloid cells to increase production of neutrophils. Pegfilgrastim is made by conjugating filgrastim with polyethylene glycol (PEG), in a process known as pegylation. Pegylation increases the size of filgrastim, and thereby delays its excretion by the kidneys. As a result, the drug's half-life is greatly increased—from 3.5 hours (for native filgrastim) up to about 17 hours. Because pegfilgrastim has a longer half-life than filgrastim, the drug is easier to use: A course of treatment consists of just one dose, rather than one dose every day for 2 weeks. At this time, pegfilgrastim has only one approved application: prevention of febrile neutropenia in patients undergoing chemotherapy of nonmyeloid malignancies. As discussed above, filgrastim has additional uses.

Adverse effects are much like those of filgrastim. Bone pain is the most common, occurring in 26% of patients. About 6% require an opioid analgesic for relief. Other side effects include reversible elevations of LDH, alkaline phosphatase, and uric acid.

Preparations, Dosage, and Administration. Pegfilgrastim [Neulasta] is available in 6-mg, prefilled, single-dose syringes. For all patients, treatment consists of one 6-mg SC dose, injected 24 hours after each round of chemotherapy. Because stimulated myeloid cells are highly vulnerable to anticancer drugs, and because pegfilgrastim has a prolonged duration of action, at least 14 days must elapse between injecting pegfilgrastim and the next round of chemotherapy. Accordingly, if the scheduled interval between rounds of chemotherapy is less than 15 days (24 hours plus 14 days), pegfil-

grastim cannot be used. Instead, filgrastim, with its shorter duration of action, should be chosen. Pegfilgrastim has not been evaluated in infants, children, or adolescents who weigh less than 45 kg. Accordingly, the drug should not be used in these patients. Pegfilgrastim is expensive, costing nearly $3000 per dose. A comparable course of filgrastim costs about the same.

Sargramostim (Granulocyte-Macrophage Colony-Stimulating Factor)

Sargramostim [Leukine], like filgrastim, epoetin, and darbepoetin, is a hematopoietic growth factor produced by recombinant DNA technology. The drug is nearly identical in structure and actions to human granulocyte-macrophage colony-stimulating factor (GM-CSF), a naturally occurring hormone. Sargramostim is given to accelerate bone marrow recovery following a BMT.

Physiology

GM-CSF acts on cells in bone marrow to increase production of neutrophils, monocytes, macrophages, and eosinophils. In addition, the hormone acts on the mature forms of these cells to enhance their function. For example, GM-CSF acts on neutrophils and macrophages to increase their chemotactic, antifungal, and antiparasitic actions. Also, the hormone acts on monocytes and polymorphonuclear leukocytes to enhance their actions against cancer cells. GM-CSF is synthesized by T lymphocytes, monocytes, fibroblasts, and endothelial cells. Like G-CSF, GM-CSF is produced in response to inflammation and allergic challenge, suggesting that its natural role is to help fight infection and cancer.

Therapeutic Uses

Adjunct to Autologous Bone Marrow Transplantation. Sargramostim can accelerate myeloid recovery in cancer patients who have undergone an autologous BMT following high-dose chemotherapy (with or without concurrent irradiation). The drug is approved for promoting myeloid recovery following BMT in patients with acute lymphoblastic leukemia, non-Hodgkin's lymphoma, and Hodgkin's disease. In these patients, sargramostim can (1) accelerate neutrophil engraftment, (2) reduce the duration of antibiotic use, (3) reduce the duration of infectious episodes, and (4) reduce the duration of hospitalization. Therapy is expensive: The cost to the pharmacist for a 21-day course of sargramostim is more than $4000.

Treatment of Failed Bone Marrow Transplants. Sargramostim is approved for patients in whom an autologous or allogenic BMT has failed to take. For these patients, the drug can produce a significant increase in survival time.

Investigational Uses. In *HIV-infected patients,* sargramostim can reverse neutropenia caused by zidovudine (a drug that inhibits HIV replication) and by ganciclovir (a drug for cytomegalovirus retinitis).

In patients with *aplastic anemia* (a syndrome characterized by pancytopenia and high mortality from infection and bleeding), sargramostim can increase neutrophil counts and reduce the incidence and severity of infections.

Sargramostim is beneficial for patients with *myelodysplastic syndrome* (MDS), a chronic disorder characterized by greatly reduced hematopoiesis. Patients with MDS are neutropenic, thrombocytopenic, and anemic, putting them at high risk for serious infections and bleeding. The syndrome has a mortality rate of 66%—and those who survive often develop leukemia. Treatment with sargramostim can increase counts of neutrophils, eosinophils, and monocytes. However, the premalignant clone still exists and may eventually cause leukemia.

Pharmacokinetics

Sargramostim is administered by IV infusion. Since the drug is a protein and hence would be degraded in the digestive tract, it cannot be administered by mouth. Other aspects of its kinetics are unremarkable.

Adverse Effects and Interactions

Sargramostim is generally well tolerated. A variety of acute reactions have been observed, including *diarrhea, weakness, rash, malaise,* and *bone pain* that can be managed with non-opioid analgesics (e.g., acetaminophen). *Pleural and pericardial effusions* have occurred, but only when sargramostim dosage was massive (16 times the recommended dosage). There are no drug interactions of note.

Leukocytosis and Thrombocytosis. Stimulation of the bone marrow can cause excessive production of white blood cells and platelets. Complete blood counts should be done twice weekly during therapy. If the white cell count rises above $50,000/mm^3$, if the absolute neutrophil count rises above $20,000/mm^3$, or if the platelet count rises above $500,000/mm^3$, sargramostim should be interrupted or the dosage reduced.

Preparations, Dosage, and Administration

Preparations. Sargramostim [Leukine] is dispensed in solution (500 µg/ml) and as a powder (250 and 500 µg) to be reconstituted for IV infusion. To reconstitute the powder, add 1 ml of sterile water and swirl gently; don't shake.

Dilution. To prepare the final solution for infusion, dilute the concentrated solution in either (1) 0.9% sodium chloride (if the final concentration of sargramostim is to be 10 mg/ml or more) or (2) 0.9% sodium chloride plus 0.1% albumin (if the final concentration is to be less than 10 mg/ml). Since the solution contains no antibacterial preservatives, it should be used as soon as possible—and no later than 6 hours after preparation.

Storage. All sargramostim preparations, concentrated or dilute, should be stored at 2°C to 8°C (never frozen).

Dosage and Administration. To accelerate myeloid recovery after an autologous BMT, the recommended dosage is 250 µg/m² (as a 2-hour IV infusion) administered once daily for 21 days beginning 2 to 4 hours after the bone marrow infusion.

For patients in whom an autologous or allogenic BMT has failed or in whom engraftment has been delayed, the recommended dosage is 250 µg/m² (as a 2-hour IV infusion) administered once daily for 14 days. After a 7-day hiatus, the 14-day series of infusions can be repeated if needed. After another 7-day hiatus, the 14-day series can be repeated once more if needed. If the graft still has not taken, further treatment is unlikely to help.

THROMBOPOIETIC GROWTH FACTORS

Thrombopoietic growth factors are compounds that stimulate production of thrombocytes (platelets). At this time, oprelvekin is the only thrombopoietic growth factor available.

Oprelvekin (Interleukin-11)

Oprelvekin [Neumega] is a thrombopoietic growth factor produced by recombinant DNA technology. The drug is a protein nearly identical in structure and actions to human *interleukin-11,* a cytokine produced in bone marrow. Oprelvekin is given to stimulate platelet production in patients undergoing myelosuppressive chemotherapy for nonmyeloid cancers.

Actions

Oprelvekin acts on platelet progenitor cells to increase platelet production. Specifically, it stimulates proliferation of hematopoietic stem cells and megacaryocyte progenitor cells, and thereby increases synthesis of megacaryocytes, the cells that synthesize platelets. In addition to promoting megacaryocyte *synthesis,* oprelvekin induces megacaryocyte *maturation.* The net result is increased platelet production. In patients treated with oprelvekin daily for 14 days, platelet counts begin to increase 5 to 9 days after the first injection, peak about 7 days after the last injection, and return to baseline 14 days after that.

Therapeutic Use

Oprelvekin is administered to patients undergoing myelosuppressive chemotherapy to minimize thrombocytopenia (platelet deficiency) and to decrease the need for platelet transfusions. Because it stimulates the bone marrow, oprelvekin should *not* be given to patients with cancers of myeloid origin.

In clinical trials, oprelvekin was effective for some patients but not for others. To assess its benefits, oprelvekin was given to patients who had required platelet transfusions following earlier rounds of chemotherapy. Some were on moderately myelosuppressive regimens and some were on highly suppressive regimens. Among the patients on moderately suppressive regimens, 30% were spared the need for platelet transfusions by combining oprelvekin with chemotherapy. Among the patients on highly suppressive regimens, only 13% were spared the need for platelet transfusions. Hence, although oprelvekin can increase platelet counts and decrease the need for platelet transfusions, not all patients benefit equally. As these data indicate, the more myelosuppressive the regimen, the less effective oprelvekin is likely to be.

Pharmacokinetics

Oprelvekin is administered by SC injection. (Because the drug is a protein, it cannot be administered by mouth.) Serum levels peak about 3 hours after administration. Elimination is by a combination of hepatic and renal tubular metabolism, followed by excretion of the metabolites in urine. Children eliminate the drug faster than adults.

Adverse Effects

Fluid Retention. Oprelvekin causes retention of sodium and water by the kidney. The result is *peripheral edema* and a 10% to 15% *expansion of plasma volume.* Expansion of plasma volume decreases both the hematocrit and hemoglobin concentration, thereby causing anemia. As a result, about 48% of patients experience dyspnea (shortness of breath on exertion). Because of fluid retention, oprelvekin should be used with caution in patients with a history of heart failure or pleural effusion. Fluid balance should be monitored throughout treatment. Following oprelvekin withdrawal, fluid balance normalizes within days.

Cardiac Dysrhythmias. Tachycardia, atrial fibrillation, and *atrial flutter* are common. The incidence of tachycardia is higher in children (46%) than in adults. Conversely, atrial flutter and fibrillation are most likely in older adults. The cause of cardiac effects is unclear, although expansion of plasma volume is suspected. Oprelvekin does not affect the heart directly.

Effects on the Eye. *Conjunctival injection* is common. The incidence is 50% in children and 19% in adults. Other ophthalmic effects are transient visual blurring and papilledema (edema of the optic disk).

Sudden Death. Two patients have died. Both had severe hypokalemia, and both had been treated with a diuretic and high doses of ifosfamide (an anticancer drug). Although oprelvekin is suspected, its precise role in these deaths is unknown.

Preparations, Dosage, and Administration

Preparation. Oprelvekin [Neumega] is dispensed as a powder in 5-mg single-dose vials. To reconstitute the powder, add 1 ml of Sterile Water for Injection (supplied with the drug) and gently swirl; don't shake. Neither the powder nor the diluent contains preservatives, hence the solution must be used within 3 hours to avoid infection. Oprelvekin and its diluent should be kept refrigerated at 2°C to 8°C.

Dosage and Administration. Oprelvekin is administered by SC injection into the abdomen, thigh, hip, or upper arm. The recommended adult dosage is 50 mg/kg once daily; the pediatric dosage is 75 to 100 mg/kg once daily. Dosing should begin 4 to 6 hours after chemotherapy and should continue until the platelet count rises above 50,000/mm³—but should not exceed 21 days. Treatment should cease 2 days before the next round of chemotherapy.

⠇⠇ KEY POINTS

- Epoetin alfa is given to increase red blood cell counts. Specific indications include anemia associated with (1) chronic renal failure, (2) zidovudine therapy in AIDS patients, and (3) cancer chemotherapy.
- By increasing the hematocrit, epoetin alfa can cause or exacerbate hypertension.
- Filgrastim is given to elevate neutrophil counts, and thereby reduce the risk of infection. Specific indications are chronic severe neutropenia and neutropenia associated with cancer chemotherapy or a BMT.
- The principal adverse effects of filgrastim are bone pain and leukocytosis.
- Sargramostim is used to accelerate recovery from a BMT and to treat patients in whom a BMT has failed.
- The principal adverse effect of sargramostim is leukocytosis.
- Oprelvekin is given to stimulate platelet production in patients undergoing myelosuppressive chemotherapy for nonmyeloid cancers. The goal is to minimize thrombocytopenia and platelet transfusions.
- The principal adverse effects of oprelvekin are fluid retention (which causes edema and anemia) and cardiac dysrhythmias (tachycardia, atrial fibrillation, and atrial flutter).
- Since epoetin alfa, filgrastim, sargramostim, and oprelvekin stimulate proliferation of bone marrow cells, these drugs should be used with great caution, if at all, in patients with cancers of bone marrow origin.

Summary of Major Nursing Implications*

EPOETIN ALFA (ERYTHROPOIETIN)

Preadministration Assessment

Therapeutic Goal

Restoration and maintenance of erythrocyte counts in (1) patients with chronic renal failure, (2) HIV-infected patients receiving zidovudine, (3) patients receiving cancer chemotherapy, and (4) anemic patients facing elective surgery.

Baseline Data

All Patients. Obtain blood pressure; blood chemistry (BUN, uric acid, creatinine, phosphorus, potassium); complete blood counts with differential and platelet count; hematocrit; degree of transferrin saturation (should be at least 20%); and ferritin concentration (should be at least 100 ng/ml).

HIV-Infected Patients. Obtain an erythropoietin level. If the level is above 500 mU/ml, epoetin is unlikely to help.

Identifying High-Risk Patients

Epoetin alfa is *contraindicated* for patients with uncontrolled hypertension or hypersensitivity to mammalian cell-derived products or albumin. Use with *caution* in patients with cancers of myeloid origin.

Implementation: Administration

Routes

SC, IV.

Handling and Storage

Epoetin alfa is dispensed in single-use and multiuse vials; don't re-enter the single-use vials. Don't agitate. Don't mix with other drugs. Store at 2°C to 8°C; don't freeze.

Administration

Chronic Renal Failure. Administer by IV bolus or SC injection.

Zidovudine-Induced Anemia. Administer by IV or SC injection.

Chemotherapy-Induced Anemia. Administer by SC injection.

Surgery Patients. Administer by SC injection.

Ongoing Evaluation and Interventions

Monitoring Summary

Determine the hematocrit twice weekly until the target level has been reached and a maintenance dosage established. Obtain complete blood counts with a differential and platelet counts routinely. Monitor blood chemistry, including BUN, uric acid, creatinine, phosphorus, and potassium. Monitor iron stores and maintain at an adequate level. Monitor blood pressure.

Minimizing Adverse Effects

Hypertension. Monitor blood pressure and, if necessary, control with antihypertensive drugs. If hypertension cannot be controlled, reduce epoetin dosage. In patients with

---

*Patient education information is highlighted as blue text.

Summary of Major Nursing Implications*—cont'd

pre-existing hypertension (a common complication of CRF), make certain that blood pressure is controlled prior to epoetin use.

FILGRASTIM (GRANULOCYTE COLONY-STIMULATING FACTOR)

Preadministration Assessment

Therapeutic Goal

Filgrastim is given to promote neutrophil recovery in cancer patients following myelosuppressive chemotherapy or a BMT. The drug is also used to treat severe chronic neutropenia.

Baseline Data

Obtain complete blood counts and platelet counts.

Identifying High-Risk Patients

Filgrastim is *contraindicated* for patients with hypersensitivity to *Escherichia coli*–derived proteins. Use with *caution* in patients with cancers of bone marrow origin.

Implementation: Administration

Routes

SC, IV.

Handling and Storage

Filgrastim is dispensed in single-use vials. Don't re-enter the vial; discard the unused portion. Don't agitate. Store at 2°C to 8°C; don't freeze. Prior to administration, filgrastim may be kept at room temperature for up to 6 hours.

Administration

Cancer Chemotherapy. Administer by SC bolus, short IV infusion, or continuous IV or SC infusion.

Bone Marrow Transplant. Administer by slow IV or SC infusion.

Chronic Severe Neutropenia. Inject SC twice daily every day.

Ongoing Evaluation and Interventions

Evaluating Therapeutic Effects

Obtain complete blood counts twice weekly. Discontinue treatment when the absolute neutrophil count reaches 10,000/mm³.

Minimizing Adverse Effects

Bone Pain. Evaluate for bone pain and treat with a nonopioid analgesic (e.g., acetaminophen). Consider a more powerful (opioid) analgesic if the nonopioid is insufficient.

Leukocytosis. Massive doses can cause leukocytosis (white blood cell counts above 100,000/mm³). If leukocytosis develops, reduce filgrastim dosage.

SARGRAMOSTIM (GRANULOCYTE-MACROPHAGE COLONY-STIMULATING FACTOR)

Preadministration Assessment

Therapeutic Goal

Acceleration of myeloid recovery in cancer patients who have undergone an autologous BMT following high-dose chemotherapy (with or without concurrent irradiation).

Treatment of patients for whom an autologous or allogenic BMT has failed to take.

Baseline Data

Obtain complete blood counts with differential and platelet count.

Identifying High-Risk Patients

Sargramostim is *contraindicated* in the presence of hypersensitivity to yeast-derived products and excessive leukemic myeloid blasts in bone marrow or peripheral blood. Exercise *caution* in patients with cardiac disease, hypoxia, peripheral edema, pleural or pericardial effusion, or cancers of bone marrow origin.

Implementation: Administration

Route

IV (by infusion).

Handling and Storage

Sargramostim is dispensed in single-use vials; don't re-enter the vial, and discard the unused portion. Don't agitate. Don't mix with other drugs. Administer as soon as possible—and no later than 6 hours after reconstitution. Store sargramostim (liquid concentrate, powder, reconstituted powder, final IV solution) at 2°C to 8°C until used.

Administration

Administer by 2-hour IV infusion.

Ongoing Evaluation and Interventions

Minimizing Adverse Effects

Leukocytosis and Thrombocytosis. Obtain complete blood counts with a differential and platelet counts twice weekly. If the white blood cell count rises above 50,000/mm³, if the absolute neutrophil count rises above 20,000/mm³, or if the platelet count rises above 500,000/mm³, temporarily interrupt sargramostim or reduce its dosage.

OPRELVEKIN (INTERLEUKIN-11)

Preadministration Assessment

Therapeutic Goal

Oprelvekin is given to minimize thrombocytopenia and the need for platelet transfusions in patients undergoing myelosuppressive therapy for nonmyeloid cancers.

*Patient education information is highlighted as blue text.

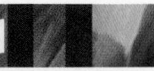

Summary of Major Nursing Implications*—cont'd

Baseline Data

Determine baseline blood cell counts and platelet count, hematocrit, and fluid and electrolyte status.

Identifying High-Risk Patients

Use with *caution* in patients with cancers of myeloid origin; patients taking diuretics or ifosfamide; and patients with a history of atrial dysrhythmias, heart failure, pleural effusion, or papilledema.

Implementation: Administration

Route

SC.

Handling and Storage

Oprelvekin is dispensed in single-use vials; don't re-enter the vial. Don't agitate. Don't mix with other drugs. Store at 2°C to 8°C; don't freeze.

*Patient education information is highlighted as blue text.

Administration

Administer once daily beginning 4 to 6 hours after chemotherapy. Continue for 21 days or until platelet counts exceed 50,000/mm³—whichever comes first.

Ongoing Evaluation and Interventions

Monitoring Summary

Monitor platelet counts from the time of the expected nadir until the count exceeds 50,000/mm³. Monitor blood cell counts, fluid status, and electrolyte status.

Minimizing Adverse Effects

Fluid Retention. Fluid retention can result in edema, expanded plasma volume, anemia, and dyspnea. **Warn patients with a history of congestive heart failure or pleural effusion to contact the physician if dyspnea worsens.**

Cardiac Dysrhythmias. Oprelvekin can cause tachycardia, atrial flutter, and atrial fibrillation. Use caution in patients with a history of these disorders.

Drugs for Diabetes Mellitus

DIABETES MELLITUS: OVERVIEW OF THE DISEASE AND ITS TREATMENT

The term *diabetes mellitus* is derived from the Greek word for *fountain* and the Latin word for *honey*. Hence, the name *diabetes mellitus* describes one of the prominent symptoms of untreated diabetes: production of large volumes of glucose-rich urine. In this chapter we use the terms *diabetes mellitus* and *diabetes* interchangeably.

Diabetes is primarily a disorder of carbohydrate metabolism. Symptoms result from a deficiency of insulin or from resistance to insulin's actions. The principal sign of diabetes is sustained hyperglycemia, which rapidly causes polyuria, polydipsia, ketonuria, and weight loss. Over time, hyperglycemia can lead to hypertension, heart disease, renal failure, blindness, neuropathy, amputations, impotence, and stroke.

Diabetes is a major public health concern. In the United States, diabetes is the most common endocrine disorder, and the fifth leading cause of death by disease. About 17 million Americans have diabetes, but only 11 million are diagnosed. In 2002, diabetes cost the U.S. economy an estimated $132 billion ($92 billion in direct medical expenditures and $40 billion in lost productivity). These costs represent a 35% increase over estimated costs for 1997.

Types of Diabetes Mellitus

There are two principal forms of diabetes: type 1 diabetes and type 2 diabetes. Several other types, including gestational diabetes, have been described. The distinguishing characteristics of type 1 and type 2 diabetes are summarized in Table 54–1 and discussed immediately below. Gestational diabetes is discussed below under *Diabetes and Pregnancy*.

Type 1 Diabetes

Type 1 diabetes accounts for 5% to 10% of all cases of diabetes. Approximately 850,000 Americans have this disorder. Until recently, type 1 diabetes was called *insulin-dependent diabetes mellitus (IDDM)* or *juvenile-onset diabetes mellitus*. As a rule, type 1 diabetes develops during childhood or adolescence. Onset of symptoms is relatively abrupt.

The primary defect in type 1 diabetes is destruction of pancreatic beta cells—the cells responsible for insulin synthesis. Insulin levels are reduced early in the disease and fall to zero later. Beta cell destruction is the result of an autoimmune process (i.e., development of antibodies against the patient's own beta cells). Although the trigger for this immune response is unknown, infection with Coxsackie virus is a leading candidate.

Type 2 Diabetes

Type 2 diabetes is the most prevalent form of diabetes. Approximately 16 million Americans have this disease. Until recently, type 2 diabetes was called *non–insulin-dependent diabetes mellitus (NIDDM)* or *adult-onset diabetes mellitus*. The disease usually begins in middle age and progresses gradually. Obesity is almost always present. In contrast to type 1 diabetes, type 2 diabetes carries little risk of ketoacidosis. However, type 2 diabetes does carry the same long-term risks as type 1 diabetes (see below).

Symptoms result from a combination of *insulin resistance* and *impaired insulin secretion*. In contrast to patients with type 1 diabetes, patients with type 2 diabetes are capable of insulin synthesis. In fact, insulin levels tend to be normal or slightly elevated. However, although insulin is still produced, its secretion is no longer tightly coupled to plasma glucose content: release of insulin is delayed and peak output is subnormal. More importantly, the target tissues of insulin (liver,

TABLE 54–1 ■ Characteristics of the Major Forms of Diabetes Mellitus

| Characteristics | Types of Diabetes Mellitus | |
	Type 1	Type 2
Alternative names	Insulin-dependent diabetes mellitus, juvenile-onset diabetes mellitus, ketosis-prone diabetes mellitus	Non–insulin-dependent diabetes mellitus, adult-onset diabetes mellitus
Age of onset	Usually childhood or adolescence	Usually over 40
Speed of onset	Abrupt	Gradual
Family history	Usually negative	Frequently positive
Prevalence	5% to 10% of diabetics have type 1 diabetes	90% to 95% of diabetics have type 2 diabetes
Etiology	Autoimmune process	Unknown—but there is a strong familial association, suggesting heredity as the underlying cause
Primary defect	Loss of pancreatic beta cells	Insulin resistance and inappropriate insulin secretion
Insulin levels	Reduced early in the disease and completely absent later	Levels may be low (indicating deficiency), normal, or high (indicating resistance)
Treatment	Insulin replacement is mandatory, along with strict dietary control; oral hypoglycemic drugs are *not* effective	Exercise and a reduced-calorie diet may be sufficient; if not, an oral hypoglycemic agent and/or insulin is required
Blood glucose	Levels fluctuate widely in response to infection, exercise, and changes in caloric intake and insulin dose	Levels are more stable than in type 1 diabetes
Symptoms	Polyuria, polydipsia, polyphagia, weight loss	May be asymptomatic
Body composition	Usually thin and undernourished	Frequently obese
Ketosis	Common, especially if insulin dosage is insufficient	Uncommon

muscle, adipose tissue) exhibit insulin resistance. Resistance appears to result from three causes: reduced binding of insulin to its receptors, reduced receptor number, and reduced receptor responsiveness. Over time, hyperglycemia leads to destruction of pancreatic beta cells, and hence insulin production and secretion eventually decline.

Although the underlying cause of type 2 diabetes is unknown, there is a strong familial association, suggesting that heredity may be a major factor. This possibility was reinforced by a study that implicated the gene for *insulin receptor substrate-2* (IRS-2), a compound that helps mediate intracellular responses to insulin. Mice that lack a functional IRS-2 gene develop symptoms identical to those of type 2 diabetes (e.g., insulin resistance in muscle and liver, fasting hypoglycemia, and gradual beta-cell failure).

Short-Term Complications of Diabetes

Acute complications are seen primarily in patients with type 1 diabetes. Principal concerns are *hyperglycemia* and *hypoglycemia*. Hyperglycemia results when insulin dosage is insufficient. Conversely, hypoglycemia results when insulin dosage is excessive. *Ketoacidosis,* a potentially fatal acute complication, develops when hyperglycemia is allowed to persist. All three complications are discussed below.

Long-Term Complications of Diabetes

The long-term sequelae of type 1 and type 2 diabetes take years to develop. More than 90% of diabetic deaths result from long-term complications, not from hypoglycemia or ketoacidosis. Most complications occur secondary to disruption of blood flow, owing to either macrovascular or microvascular damage. Ironically, insulin therapy can be viewed as having made long-term complications possible: Prior to the discovery of insulin, diabetic people died long before chronic complications could arise.

Two landmark studies—the *Diabetes Control and Complications Trial* (DCCT) and the *United Kingdom Prospective Diabetes Study* (UKPDS)—demonstrated that, with rigorous control of blood glucose, development of long-term complications can be greatly reduced. Subjects in the DCCT had type 1 diabetes; subjects in the UKPDS had type 2 diabetes. The DCCT demonstrated that, compared with patients whose glucose was only moderately controlled, patients whose glucose was tightly controlled experienced 76% less retinopathy, 60% less neuropathy, and 35% to 56% less nephropathy. The UKPDS demonstrated similar, albeit less dramatic, benefits for patients with type 2 diabetes.

Macrovascular Disease. Cardiovascular complications are the leading cause of death among diabetic patients. Diabetes carries an increased risk of *hypertension, heart disease,* and *stroke.* Much of this pathology is due to atherosclerosis, which develops earlier in diabetics than in nondiabetics and progresses at an accelerated rate. Macrovascular complications result from a combination of hyperglycemia and altered lipid metabolism.

Microvascular Disease. Microangiopathy is common. The basement membrane of capillaries thickens, causing blood flow in the microvasculature to decline. Destruction of small blood vessels leads to kidney damage and blindness. Microvascular complications are directly related to the degree and duration of hyperglycemia.

Retinopathy. Diabetes is the major cause of blindness among American adults. Every year, 12,000 to 24,000 diabetics lose their sight. Visual losses result most commonly from damage to retinal capillaries. Microaneurysms may occur, followed by scarring and proliferation of new vessels; the overgrowth of new retinal capillaries reduces visual acuity. Capillary damage may also impair vision by causing local ischemia, which can kill retinal cells. Retinopathy is accelerated by hyperglycemia, hypertension, and smoking. Accordingly, these risk factors should be controlled or eliminated.

Nephropathy. Diabetic nephropathy is characterized by proteinuria, reduced glomerular filtration, and increased arterial blood pressure. Diabetic nephropathy is the most common cause of end-stage renal disease, a condition that requires dialysis or a kidney transplant for survival. Between 10% and 21% of people with diabetes have kidney disease. The risk of nephropathy among patients with type 1 diabetes is 12 times higher than among patients with type 2 diabetes. Nephropathy is the primary cause of morbidity and mortality in patients with type 1 diabetes. If the injured kidney is replaced with a transplant, the new kidney is likely to fail within a few years unless tight control of diabetes is established.

Onset of diabetic nephropathy can be delayed and the extent of injury can be reduced. The DCCT revealed that tight glucose control decreases the risk of nephropathy by 35% to 56%. As discussed in Chapter 42, treatment with an *angiotensin-converting enzyme inhibitor* or an *angiotensin receptor blocker* can delay the onset of overt nephropathy and retard progression of nephropathy that is already present.

Neuropathy. Nerve degeneration often begins early in the course of diabetes, but symptoms are usually absent for years. Sensory and motor nerves may be affected. Symptoms of diabetic neuropathy include tingling sensations in the fingers and toes, pain, suppression of reflexes, and loss of sensation (especially vibratory sensation). Nerve damage is directly related to sustained hyperglycemia. In the DCCT, tight glycemic control reduced the incidence of neuropathy by 60%.

Amputations. Diabetes is responsible for more than 50% of lower limb amputations in the United States. Each year, 54,000 diabetic patients lose a foot or leg because of their disease. Amputations result in part because of severe nerve damage.

Impotence. The combination of blood vessel injury and neuropathy can cause impotence. About 13% of men with type 1 diabetes and 8% of men with type 2 diabetes suffer diabetes-related impotence.

Gastroparesis. Diabetic gastroparesis affects 20% to 30% of patients with long-standing diabetes. Manifestations include nausea, vomiting, delayed gastric emptying, and abdominal distention secondary to atony of the GI tract. Injury to the autonomic nerves that control GI motility may be the underlying cause. Symptoms can be reduced with metoclopramide [Reglan], a drug that promotes gastric emptying (see Chapter 75).

Diabetes and Pregnancy

Before the discovery of insulin, virtually all babies born to diabetic mothers died during infancy. Although insulin therapy has greatly improved outcomes, successful management of the diabetic pregnancy remains a challenge. Three factors contribute to the problem. First, the placenta produces hormones that can antagonize insulin's actions. Second, production of cortisol, a hormone that promotes hyperglycemia, increases threefold during pregnancy. Both of these factors increase the need for insulin. Third, since glucose can pass freely from the maternal circulation to the fetal circulation, hyperglycemia in the mother will stimulate secretion of fetal insulin; the resultant hyperinsulinemia can have multiple adverse effects on the developing fetus.

Successful management of the diabetic pregnancy demands that proper glucose levels be maintained in both the fetus and mother; failure to do so may be teratogenic or otherwise detrimental to the fetus. Achieving glucose control requires diligence on the part of the mother and her physician. Blood glucose levels must be monitored 6 to 7 times a day. Insulin dosage and food intake must be adjusted accordingly.

Because fetal death frequently occurs near term, it is desirable that delivery take place as soon as development of the fetus will permit. Hence, when tests indicate sufficient fetal maturation, it is common practice to deliver the infant early—either by cesarean section or by induction of labor with drugs.

Gestational diabetes is defined as diabetes that appears during pregnancy and then subsides rapidly after delivery. Gestational diabetes is managed in much the same manner as any other diabetic pregnancy: blood glucose should be monitored and then controlled with insulin and diet. In most cases, the diabetic state disappears almost immediately after delivery, permitting discontinuation of insulin. However, if the diabetic condition persists beyond parturition, it is no longer considered gestational and should be rediagnosed and treated accordingly.

Diagnosis of Diabetes

Excessive plasma glucose is diagnostic of diabetes. Three tests may be employed: a fasting plasma glucose (FPG) test, a casual plasma glucose test, and an oral glucose tolerance test (OGTT). Values diagnostic of diabetes are summarized in Table 54–2. To make a diagnosis, the patient must be tested on two separate days, and both tests must be positive. Any combination of two tests (e.g., two FPG tests, one FPG test and one OGTT) may be used.

FPG Test. To determine fasting plasma glucose levels, blood is drawn at least 8 hours after the last meal. In normoglycemic individuals, FPG levels are less than 110 mg/dl. If FPG glucose levels are 126 mg/dl or higher, diabetes is indicated. Of the tests employed to diagnose diabetes, the FPG test is preferred.

Casual Plasma Glucose Test. For this test, blood can be drawn at any time, without regard to meals. Fasting is not required. A plasma glucose level that is 200 mg/ml or higher

TABLE 54-2 ■ Criteria for the Diagnosis of Diabetes Mellitus
Fasting plasma glucose ≥126 mg/dl*
or
Casual plasma glucose ≥200 mg/dl *plus* symptoms of diabetes†
or
Oral glucose tolerance test (OGTT): 2-hr plasma glucose ≥200 mg/dl‡

*Fasting is defined as no caloric intake for at least 8 hours.
†*Casual* is defined as any time of day without regard to meals. Classic symptoms of diabetes include polyuria, polydipsia, and unexplained weight loss.
‡In this OGTT, plasma glucose content is measured 2 hours after ingesting the equivalent of 75 gm of anhydrous glucose dissolved in water. The OGTT is not recommended for routine clinical use.
Adapted from Expert Committee on the Diagnosis and Classification of Diabetes Mellitus. Report of the Expert Committee on the Diagnosis and Classification of Diabetes Mellitus. Diabetes Care 2003;26(Suppl 1): S5–S24.

suggests diabetes. However, to make a diagnosis, the patient must also display classic signs and symptoms of diabetes (polyuria, polydipsia, ketonuria, rapid weight loss).

Oral Glucose Tolerance Test. This test is used when diabetes is suspected but could not be definitively diagnosed by measuring fasting or casual plasma glucose. The OGTT is performed by giving an oral glucose load (equivalent to 75 gm of anhydrous glucose) and measuring plasma glucose levels 2 hours later. In normoglycemic individuals, 2-hour glucose levels will be below 140 mg/dl. Diabetes is suggested if 2-hour plasma glucose levels are 200 mg/dl or higher. The OGTT should not be used for routine screening.

Overview of Treatment
Type 1 Diabetes

The goal of therapy is to maintain glucose levels within an acceptable range. This will prevent acute complications and reduce or prevent long-term complications. Glycemic control is accomplished with an integrated program of *diet, self-monitoring of blood glucose (SMBG), exercise, and insulin replacement.*

Proper diet, balanced by insulin replacement, is the cornerstone of treatment. Because patients with type 1 diabetes are usually thin, the dietary goal is to maintain weight—not lose it. Dietary recommendations from the American Diabetes Association (ADA), released in January 2003, are as follows:

- Carbohydrates and monounsaturated fats, together, should provide 60% to 70% of daily energy intake.
- Protein should provide 15% to 20% of energy intake.
- Polyunsaturated fat should provide about 10% of energy intake.
- Saturated fats should provide less than 10% of energy intake.
- Cholesterol intake should be limited to 300 mg/day.

Total caloric intake should be spread evenly throughout the day, with meals spaced 4 to 5 hours apart.

For people who like sweets, the new ADA recommendations have good news: You can eat foods that contain sucrose (table sugar)—provided you reduce intake of other car-

bohydrates. This recommendation is based on the observation that, when taken in isocaloric amounts, ordinary sugar and all other carbohydrates raise blood sugar to the same extent. Hence, what really matters is the total amount of carbohydrate ingested—not the type of carbohydrate or its source.

Unless specifically contraindicated, regular exercise should be part of the management program. Exercise increases cellular responsiveness to insulin, and may also increase glucose tolerance. Because strenuous exercise can produce hypoglycemia, close oversight is needed to establish a safe balance between exercise, glucose intake, and insulin dosage. Exercise should be avoided if glycemic control is unstable.

Survival requires daily administration of insulin. Before insulin replacement became available, people with type 1 diabetes invariably died within a few years after disease onset. The cause of death was ketoacidosis. It is essential to coordinate insulin dosage with caloric intake. If caloric intake is too great or too small with respect to insulin dosage, hyperglycemia or hypoglycemia will result.

It should be noted that *oral hypoglycemic agents,* which can help patients with type 2 diabetes, are *not* effective for patients with type 1 diabetes.

Type 2 Diabetes

Basic Strategy. As with type 1 diabetes, the goal of therapy is to maintain blood glucose levels within an acceptable range. However, for patients with type 2 diabetes, the core of treatment is *diet and exercise;* insulin or oral hypoglycemics are employed only as adjuncts. Because patients are often obese, the usual dietary goal is to promote weight loss, and thereby establish leaner body composition. Clinical experience has shown that dietary measures, by themselves, often normalize insulin release and decrease insulin resistance. Frequently, these beneficial responses precede loss of weight. Exercise provides the additional benefit of promoting glucose uptake by muscle, even when insulin is low or absent.

If diet and exercise fail to produce adequate glycemic control, pharmacotherapy is indicated. An *oral hypoglycemic agent* and/or *insulin* is employed. It must be stressed, however, that drugs should be used only as a supplement to caloric restriction and exercise; drugs are not a substitute for nondrug measures.

In addition to lowering glucose levels, the management program should address other factors that can increase morbidity and mortality. Accordingly, all patients with type 2 diabetes should be screened and treated for hypertension, nephropathy, retinopathy, and neuropathy. In addition, dyslipidemias (high LDL cholesterol, low HDL cholesterol, and high triglycerides) should be corrected.

Drug Selection. Drug selection in type 2 diabetes is complex, due in large part to the recent introduction of new drugs. Furthermore, because the disease is progressive, therapy needs to be more aggressive as time passes. For example, after 3 years of treatment, 50% of patients who responded to monotherapy initially require a second drug; and after 9 years, 75% require a second drug.

To achieve glycemic control, a stepwise approach can be used. Lack of glycemic control (or a decline in control) indicates a need to move up a step.

- *Step 1.* Implement lifestyle changes: caloric restriction, exercise, and weight loss.
- *Step 2.* Initiate therapy with just *one* oral hypoglycemic drug. Drug selection is based on the patient's body composition and degree of hyperglycemia. For lean patients, use a sulfonylurea. Why? Lean patients are

usually insulin deficient; the sulfonylurea will promote insulin release. For obese patients, use metformin. Why? Obese patients are usually insulin resistant; metformin will reduce insulin resistance.

■ *Step 3.* Treat with *two* oral hypoglycemic drugs. As a rule, hypoglycemic effects are additive. Of course, the drugs employed should have different mechanisms. Accordingly, using a sulfonylurea plus metformin would make sense, whereas using two sulfonylureas would be irrational. The three most popular combinations are (1) metformin plus a sulfonylurea, (2) metformin plus a thiazolidinedione, and (3) a sulfonylurea plus a thiazolidinedione.

■ *Step 4a.* Treat with *three* oral hypoglycemic drugs (e.g., metformin plus a sulfonylurea plus a thiazolidinedione). There is no proof than any particular combination is superior to others at lowering glucose levels or preventing complications.

■ *Step 4b.* Treat with an oral hypoglycemic *plus* insulin. For lean patients, use a sulfonylurea plus insulin. For obese patients, use metformin plus insulin.

■ *Step 5.* Treat with insulin alone. Increase the dose as needed.

Monitoring Treatment

The goal of monitoring is to determine whether glucose levels are being maintained in a safe range. Self-measurement of blood glucose levels has become the standard method for routine monitoring. Measurement of urinary glucose is reserved for patients who cannot or will not monitor their blood glucose. Glycated hemoglobin is measured to assess long-term success. Target levels for these tests are summarized in Table 54–3.

Self-Monitoring of Blood Glucose

SMBG is now the standard way to monitor diabetes therapy. As a rule, the test is performed by placing a drop of blood on a chemically treated strip, which is then read by a small machine. The test is rapid and can be performed in almost any setting. Information on blood glucose content provides a basis for "fine tuning" insulin dosage. For patients with type 1 diabetes, SMBG should be done 3 or more times a day. Target values for blood glucose are 80 to 120 mg/dl before meals and 100 to 140 mg/dl at bedtime.

SMBG does have certain drawbacks. These tests are more expensive than urine tests and are more difficult to perform. Also, the machines employed require periodic calibration and patients require education on how to apply test results. Because of these disadvantages, SMBG may not be practical for patients with limited economic resources or for patients who are unable or unwilling to learn how to use the device and apply the results.

SMBG is far superior to measuring glucose in urine: With SMBG, hyperglycemia can be detected long before blood glucose levels are high enough to cause spilling of glucose into urine. Furthermore, SMBG can detect *hypoglycemia,* something that urinary measurements simply can't do.

Urine Glucose Monitoring

In the past, this procedure was the mainstay for assessing glycemic control. Urine testing is inexpensive and easy. Unfortunately, urine testing has limited utility. There is a poor correlation between urine glucose concentration and blood glucose levels. Furthermore, a negative urine glucose test tells us only that blood glucose is below 180 mg/dl, the usual threshold for spilling glucose from blood to urine. What a negative test does not tell us is how much below the threshold the glucose level is. Hence, a patient with a negative urine glucose test could be hypoglycemic, normoglycemic, or even slightly hyperglycemic; without some other means of evaluation, we cannot distinguish among these possibilities. Accordingly, although urine testing is superior to no testing at all, it is clearly inferior to SMBG.

Glycated Hemoglobin (Hemoglobin HbA$_{1c}$)

Measurement of glycated hemoglobin provides an index of average glucose levels over the prior *2 to 3 months.* Glucose interacts spontaneously with hemoglobin in red blood cells to form glycated derivatives. The most prevalent is named *hemoglobin A$_{1c}$* (HbA$_{1c}$). With *prolonged hyperglycemia,* levels of HbA$_{1c}$ gradually increase. Since red blood cells have a long life span (120 days), levels of HbA$_{1c}$ reflect *average* glucose levels over an extended time. Hence, by measuring HbA$_{1c}$ every few months, we can get a picture of *long-term* glycemic control. These measurements are a useful adjunct to daily blood glucose monitoring, but are definitely not a substitute. For patients with diabetes, the target value for HbA$_{1c}$ is less than 7%. Hemoglobin A$_{1c}$ should be measured at least twice a year (for patients who are meeting treatment goals and have stable glycemic control) or 4 times a year (for patients who are not meeting glycemic goals or whose therapy has changed).

Fructosamine

Measurement of fructosamine provides an index of average glucose levels over the prior *1 to 3 weeks.* Fructosamine is formed when glucose combines with albumin and other proteins in plasma. Fructosamine has a much shorter life span than HbA$_{1c}$, and hence fructosamine levels reflect glycemic control over a relatively short time (1 to 3 weeks instead of 2 to 3 months). Results of fructosamine tests are expressed in micromoles per liter (μmol/L). For patients with diabetes, a result of 310 μmol/L or less indicates good glycemic control. Fructosamine determinations are not a substitute for daily SMBG or for semiannual or quarterly measurements of HbA$_{1c}$.

INSULIN

Physiology

Structure. The structure of insulin is depicted in Figure 54–1. As indicated, insulin consists of two amino acid chains: the "A" (acidic) chain and the "B" (basic) chain. The A and B chains are linked to each other by two disulfide bridges.

TABLE 54–3 ■ Targets for Glycemic Control in Diabetes		
Monitoring Parameter	Target Value for Diabetics*	Normal Value for Nondiabetics
Premeal plasma glucose	90–130 mg/dl	<110 mg/dl
Peak postmeal plasma glucose	<180 mg/dl	<140 mg/dl
Hemoglobin A$_{1c}$	<7%	<6%

*Values from American Diabetes Association. Standards of medical care for patients with diabetes mellitus. Diabetes Care 2003;26(Suppl 1): S33–S50.

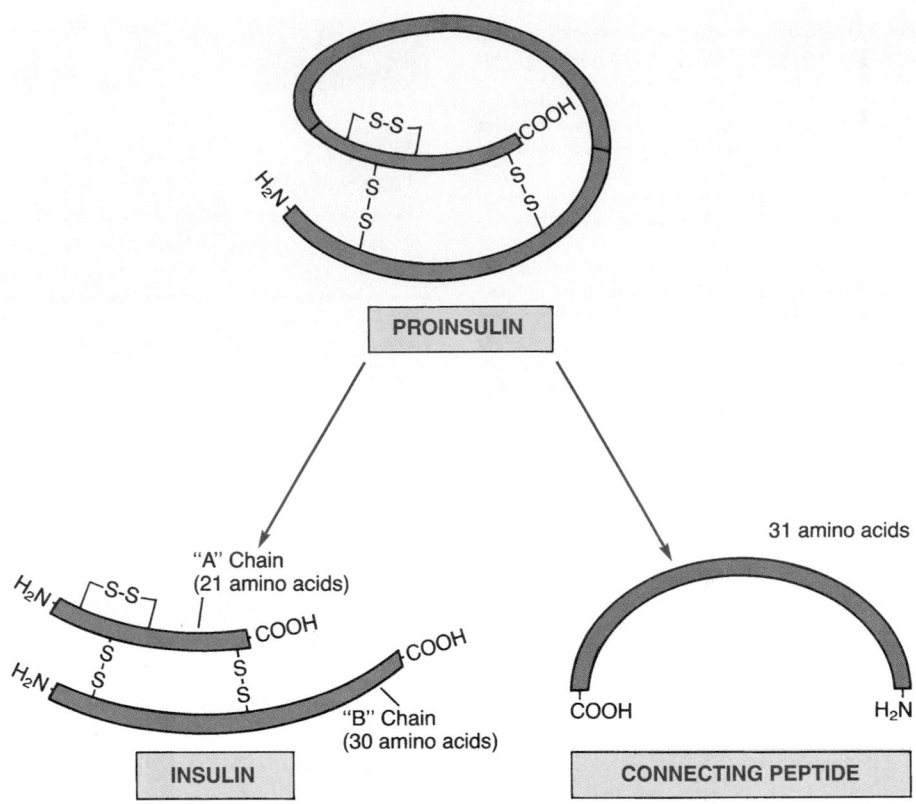

Figure 54–1 ■ Conversion of proinsulin to insulin.

Biosynthesis. Insulin is synthesized in the pancreas by beta cells within the islets of Langerhans. The immediate precursor of insulin is called proinsulin (see Fig. 54–1).

Proinsulin consists of insulin itself plus a peptide loop that runs from the A chain to the B chain. This loop is referred to as *connecting peptide* or *C-peptide*. In the final step of insulin synthesis, C-peptide is enzymatically clipped from the proinsulin molecule.

Measurement of plasma C-peptide levels offers a way to assess residual capacity for insulin synthesis. Since commercial insulin preparations are devoid of C-peptide, and since endogenous C-peptide is only present as a by-product of insulin biosynthesis, the presence of C-peptide in the blood indicates the pancreas is still producing some insulin of its own.

Secretion. The principal stimulus for insulin release is glucose. Under normal conditions, there is tight coupling between elevation of blood glucose content and increased secretion of insulin. Insulin release may also be triggered by amino acids, fatty acids, and ketone bodies.

The sympathetic nervous system provides additional control of insulin release. Activation of beta$_2$-adrenergic receptors in the pancreas *promotes* secretion of insulin. Conversely, activation of alpha-adrenergic receptors on the pancreas *inhibits* insulin release.

Metabolic Actions. The metabolic actions of insulin are primarily *anabolic* (i.e., conservative or constructive). Insulin promotes conservation of energy and buildup of energy stores. The hormone also promotes cell growth and division.

Insulin acts in two ways to promote anabolic effects. First, insulin stimulates cellular transport (uptake) of glu-cose, amino acids, nucleotides, and potassium. Second, insulin promotes synthesis of complex organic molecules. Under the influence of insulin and other factors, glucose is converted into glycogen, amino acids are assembled into proteins, and fatty acids are incorporated into triglycerides. The principal metabolic actions of insulin are summarized in Table 54–4.

Metabolic Consequences of Insulin Deficiency

Insulin deficiency puts the body into a *catabolic* mode (i.e., a metabolic state that favors the breakdown of complex molecules into their simple constituents). Hence, in the absence of insulin, glycogen is converted into glucose, proteins are degraded into amino acids, and fats are converted to glycerol (glycerin) and free fatty acids. These catabolic effects contribute to the signs and symptoms of diabetes. Note that the catabolic effects resulting from insulin deficiency are opposite to the anabolic effects seen when insulin levels are normal.

Insulin deficiency promotes *hyperglycemia* by three mechanisms: (1) increased glycogenolysis, (2) increased gluconeogenesis, and (3) reduced glucose utilization. *Glycogenolysis,* by definition, generates free glucose by breaking down glycogen. The raw materials that allow increased *gluconeogenesis* are the amino acids and fatty acids produced by degradation of proteins and fats. *Reduced glucose utilization* occurs because insulin deficiency decreases cellular uptake of glucose, and decreases conversion of glucose to glycogen.

TABLE 54–4 ▓■ Metabolic Actions of Insulin		
Substances Affected	Insulin Action	Site of Action
Carbohydrates	↑ Glucose uptake	Muscle, adipose tissue
	↑ Glucose oxidation	Muscle
	↑ Glucose storage	Muscle, liver
	↑ Glycogen synthesis	
	↓ Glycogenolysis	
	↓ Gluconeogenesis*	Liver
Amino acids and proteins	↑ Amino acid uptake	Muscle
	↓ Amino acid release	Muscle
	↑ Protein synthesis	Muscle
Lipids	↑ Triglyceride synthesis	Adipose tissue
	↓ Release of FFA† and glycerol	Adipose tissue
	↓ Oxidation of FFA to ketoacids‡	Liver

*Because of decreased delivery of substrate (fatty acids and amino acids) to the liver.
†Free fatty acids.
‡Because of decreased delivery of FFA to the liver.

Diabetic ketoacidosis occurs secondary to disruption of glucose and fat metabolism. This potentially fatal syndrome is discussed separately later.

Therapeutic Uses

The principal indication for insulin is *diabetes mellitus*. Insulin is required by all patients with type 1 diabetes and by some with type 2 diabetes. Intravenous insulin is used to treat *diabetic ketoacidosis*. Because of its ability to promote cellular uptake of potassium and thereby lower plasma potassium levels, insulin infusion is employed to treat *hyperkalemia*. The use of insulin in diabetes is discussed further below.

Preparations

Insulin is available in several forms. These differ with respect to time course of action, route of administration, and source.

Types of Insulin

There are seven types of insulin: "natural" insulin and six modified insulins. Two of the modified insulins—lispro insulin and insulin aspart—act more rapidly than natural insulin but have a shorter duration of action. The other modified insulins act more slowly than natural insulin but have a longer duration. Three processes have been used to prolong insulin effects: (1) complexing natural insulin with a protein, (2) altering the physical state of natural insulin by mixing it with zinc, and (3) altering the insulin molecule itself such that it has reduced solubility. When classified according to time course, insulin preparations fall into three major groups: short acting, intermediate acting, and long acting (Table 54–5). The short-acting insulins can be subdivided into two groups: rapid acting (lispro insulin and aspart insulin) and slower acting (regular insulin).

Regular (Natural) Insulin. Regular insulin is unmodified crystalline insulin. As shown in Table 54–5, regular insulin has a relatively rapid onset and short duration. Regular insulin is dispensed as a *clear solution* and is the only form of insulin that can be administered *intravenously*. The usual route, however, is subcutaneous. Following SC injection, molecules of regular insulin form small aggregates (dimers and hexamers). As a result, absorption is slightly delayed.

In the past, preparations of regular insulin were unstable at room temperature, and therefore required constant refrigeration. The stability of formulations available today is greatly improved. As a result, the insulin bottle in current use (usually a 2- to 4-week supply) does not have to be kept cold, although exposure to sunlight and extreme heat must be avoided.

Lispro Insulin. Lispro insulin [Humalog] is a rapid-acting analog of regular insulin. Effects begin within 15 to 30 minutes of SC injection and persist for 3 to 6 hours. Lispro insulin acts faster than regular insulin but has a shorter duration of action. Because of its rapid onset, lispro insulin can be administered immediately before eating—and even after eating. In contrast, regular insulin is generally administered 30 to 60 minutes before meals. Because of its short duration, lispro insulin should be used in combination with an intermediate- or long-acting insulin to provide basal glycemic control between meals and during the night. Unlike most other insulins, which are available over the counter, lispro insulin is available only by prescription.

The structure of lispro insulin is nearly identical to that of natural insulin. The only difference is that the position of two amino acids has been switched. In lispro insulin, lysine occupies position 28 in the B chain and proline occupies position 29—the reverse of their natural order. Because of this change, molecules of lispro insulin aggregate less than do molecules of regular insulin, which explains why lispro insulin acts more rapidly. Lispro insulin is produced by recombinant DNA technology.

Insulin Aspart. Insulin aspart [NovoLog] is an analog of human insulin with a rapid onset (10 to 20 minutes) and short duration (3 to 5 hours). The drug is structurally identical to human insulin except that one amino acid—proline in position 28 of the B chain—has been changed to aspartic acid. Production is by recombinant DNA technology. Insulin aspart is very similar to insulin lispro.

Insulin aspart (100 U/ml) is available in 10-ml vials and 3-ml *PenFill* cartridges. Administration is SC. Because of its rapid onset, the drug should be injected immediately before meals (eating should begin within 5 to 10 minutes of administration) or immediately after. Like insulin lispro, insulin aspart should be used in combination with an intermediate-acting or long-acting insulin to provide basal glycemic control between meals and during the night. Insulin aspart can be mixed with NPH insulin (provided mixing is done just before administration). There are no data on mixing the drug with lente or ultralente insulin. Like lispro insulin, insulin aspart is available only by prescription.

Neutral Protamine Hagedorn (NPH) Insulin. NPH insulin is prepared by conjugating regular insulin with protamine (a large protein). The presence of protamine decreases the solubility of NPH insulin and thereby retards absorption. As a result, onset of action is delayed and duration of action is extended. NPH insulin is classified as intermediate acting. Because protamine is a foreign protein, allergic reactions are possible.

TABLE 54–5 ▪ Types of Insulin: Source and Time Course of Action

Generic Name	Trade Name	Source*	Onset (min)	Peak (hr)	Duration (hr)
Short Duration: Rapid Acting					
Lispro insulin	Humalog	Human analog	15–30	0.5–2.5	3–6.5
Aspart insulin	NovoLog	Human analog	10–20	1–3	3–5
Short Duration: Slower Acting					
Regular insulin	Humulin R	Human	30–60	1–5	6–10
	Novolin R	Human	30–60	1–5	6–10
	Velosulin BR†	Human	30–60	1–3	8
	Iletin II Regular	Pork	30–60	1–5	4–12
Intermediate Duration					
Lente insulin	Humulin L	Human	60–180	6–14	16–24
	Novolin L	Human	60–180	6–14	16–24
	Iletin II Lente	Pork	60–180	6–14	24+
NPH insulin	Humulin N	Human	60–120	6–14	16–24+
	Novolin N	Human	60–120	6–14	16–24+
	Iletin II NPH	Pork	60–120	6–14	16–24+
Long Duration					
Ultralente insulin	Humulin U	Human	240–360	8–20	24–28
Glargine insulin	Lantus	Human analog	70	None‡	24

*Insulins listed as *human* or *human analog* are produced by recombinant DNA technology.
†Phosphate buffered; preferred for use in insulin pumps.
‡Levels are steady with no discernible peak.

Lente Insulin and Ultralente Insulin. The lente series of insulins consists of *semilente insulin, lente insulin,* and *ultralente insulin.* These are produced by complexing regular insulin with zinc, which changes the physical state of insulin, thereby reducing solubility. Semilente insulin is the most rapid-acting member of the series. Insulin in this preparation is amorphous (noncrystalline) and present as particles of small size. Semilente insulin is no longer available by itself. In *ultralente insulin,* insulin is present as large crystals that dissolve slowly, and thereby give ultralente insulin a long duration of action. *Lente insulin* is a stable mixture composed of 70% ultralente insulin and 30% semilente insulin. This preparation has an intermediate duration of action. Because no proteins are added, the lente insulins are less allergenic than NPH insulin.

Insulin Glargine. Insulin glargine [Lantus] is a modified human insulin with a prolonged duration of action (at least 24 hours). The drug is indicated for once-daily SC administration to treat adults and children with type 1 diabetes and adults with type 2 diabetes. According to package labeling, the daily injection should be made at bedtime. However, administration at other times of day (e.g., in the morning or after dinner) produces equivalent glycemic control.

Insulin glargine, which is produced by recombinant DNA technology, differs from natural human insulin by three amino acids. Specifically, the amino acid at position 21 has been replaced with glycine, and two arginines have been added to the C terminus of the B chain. Because of these modifications, insulin glargine has low solubility at physiologic pH. Hence, when injected SC, it forms microprecipitates that slowly dissolve, and thereby release insulin glargine in small amounts over an extended time. In contrast to other long-acting insulins (e.g., NPH insulin, ultralente insulin), whose blood levels rise to a distinct peak and then fall to a trough, insulin glargine achieves blood levels that are relatively steady over 24 hours. As a result, there is less risk of hypoglycemia (from excessive levels) or hyperglycemia (from insufficient levels).

Insulin glargine is supplied as a *clear solution* in 5- and 10-ml vials containing 100 U/ml, and in 3-ml cartridges for use in an *OptiPen One Insulin Delivery Device.* As with other long-acting insulins, administration is *subcutaneous.* Despite being a clear solution, *insulin glargine cannot be mixed with other insulins.* In addition, it *must not be injected IV,* because doing so could produce severe hypoglycemia owing to excessive insulin levels in blood. When educating patients, be sure to stress that insulin glargine should not be mixed with other insulins, should not be given IV, and *should* be given SC. This education is important. Why? Because patients have learned to associate clear solutions (of regular insulin) with both mixability and IV administration, and they have learned to associate cloudy suspensions with prolonged action. Accordingly, the idea that a clear solution can provide prolonged effects, but cannot be mixed with other insulins or injected IV is new, and hence needs reinforcement.

Sources of Insulin

Insulins are prepared by recombinant DNA technology and by extraction from pork and beef pancreas. Table 54–5 indicates the source of insulins available in the United States.

Recombinant DNA Technology. Human Insulin. In this process, the genetic code for human proinsulin is inserted into *Escherichia coli* or yeast, which then produce large amounts of proinsulin. The proinsulin is converted to insulin by enzymatic cleavage of C-peptide from proinsulin. The insulin made by this process is identical to insulin produced by the human pancreas.

Human Insulin Analogs. Three analogs of human insulin are available: lispro insulin, aspart insulin, and glargine insulin. The analogs are made by processes much like that used to produce human insulin.

Pork Pancreas. Some commercial insulin is prepared by extraction from pork pancreas. Pork insulin is structurally identical to human insulin with the exception of one amino acid. Because of this small structural difference, the immune system may consider the molecule as foreign, and hence may form antibodies against it.

Beef Pancreas. Insulin extracted from beef pancreas contains three amino acids that differ from those of human insulin. As a result, the body may produce antibodies directed against the molecule.

Insulin derived from beef pancreas is no longer produced in the United States. Hence, when existing stocks are gone, patients using beef insulin will have to switch to insulin from another source. Patients who are unwilling to switch will be allowed to import beef insulin, but the paperwork required is daunting. Information on importation is available on the Internet at *www.fda.gov/cder/drug/beefinsulin/faq-full.htm.*

Concentration

In the United States, insulin is available in two concentrations: 100 U/ml (U-100) and 500 U/ml (U-500). Preparations containing 40 U/ml are available in other countries but are no longer used here. U-100 insulins are employed for routine replacement therapy. U-500 insulin, which is available from the manufacturer by special request, is reserved for emergencies and for patients with severe insulin resistance, defined as needing more than 200 U/day.

Administration and Storage
Usual Routes of Administration

Insulin is given by injection. Because of its peptide structure, insulin would be inactivated by the digestive system if it were given by mouth. All insulins may be injected subcutaneously. Only *regular insulin* may also be administered *intravenously* and *intramuscularly.*

In emergencies, *regular* insulin (and only regular insulin) may be administered IV. Because regular insulin forms a true *solution,* it is safe for IV use. In contrast, all other insulin preparations (except insulin lispro and insulin glargine) consist of particles in suspension; introduction of these particles into the bloodstream could produce serious adverse effects. When administered by IV infusion, insulin can adsorb to the infusion set, thereby reducing the dose received. Because the extent of adsorption is not predictable, monitoring the glycemic response is essential. If emergency treatment by the IV route is impossible, regular insulin may be administered IM instead.

Preparing for Injection

With the exception of regular, lispro, and glargine insulin, all insulin preparations consist of particles in suspension. Hence, to ensure correct dosing, these particles must be evenly dispersed prior to loading the syringe. Dispersion is accomplished by rolling the insulin vial between the palms of the hands. Mixing must be gentle, because vigorous agitation will

TABLE 54-6 ■ Compatibility of Short-Acting Insulins with Intermediate-Acting and Long-Acting Insulins

Short-Acting Insulins	Longer Acting Insulins†			
	NPH	Lente	Ultralente	Glargine
Regular*	Yes	Yes	Yes	No
Lispro	Yes	Yes	Yes	No
Aspart	Yes	?	?	No

*Phosphate-buffered regular insulin should not be mixed with any other insulin types.
†Yes = can be mixed, No = should not be mixed, ? = no data on mixing available.

cause frothing and render accurate dosing impossible. If granules or clumps remain after gentle agitation, the vial should be discarded.

Unlike insulin suspensions, which are cloudy, three products—regular, lispro, and glargine insulin—are dispensed as clear, colorless solutions. Because they are in solution, these preparations can be administered without prior agitation. If one of these preparations becomes cloudy or discolored, or if a precipitate develops, it should be discarded.

Before loading the syringe, the bottle cap should be swabbed with alcohol. Air bubbles should be eliminated from the syringe and needle after loading. The skin should be cleaned with alcohol prior to injection.

Sites of Injection

The most common sites of SC injection are the upper arms, thighs, and abdomen. Because rates of absorption vary among sites, it is recommended that injections be made using only one general locale (e.g., thigh or abdomen). Regardless of whether one general locale or several are used, specific sites of injection within the locale should be rotated. This practice reduces the incidence of lipohypertrophy (see below). About 1 inch should be allowed between sites of injection. Ideally, each site should be used only once a month.

Mixing Insulins

When the treatment plan calls for the use of two different insulin preparations (e.g., regular insulin plus NPH insulin), it is usually desirable to mix the preparations rather than inject them separately, so as to eliminate the need for an additional shot. However, although mixing offers convenience, it can alter the time course of the response. Therefore, to ensure a consistent response, insulins should be mixed according to established guidelines (see below). Also, only insulins that are compatible with each other should be combined. Compatibility of short-acting insulins with intermediate- and long-acting insulins is summarized in Table 54-6. Commercially available premixed combinations are described in Table 54-7.

Regular Insulin. Regular insulin is compatible with NPH, lente, and ultralente insulins, but not with glargine insulin. When preparing a mixture of regular insulin with another insulin preparation, the regular insulin should be drawn into the syringe first. This sequence will avoid contaminating the stock vial of regular insulin with insulin of another type.

TABLE 54–7 ■ Premixed Insulin Combinations

Description	Trade Name	Time Course		
		Onset (min)	Peak (hr)	Duration (hr)
70% NPH insulin/	Humulin 70/30	30–60	1.5–16	Up to 24
30% regular insulin	Novolin 70/30	30–60	2–12	Up to 24
50% NPH insulin/	Humulin 50/50	30–60	2–5.5	Up to 24
50% regular insulin				
70% insulin aspart protamine/	NovoLog Mix 70/30	Rapid*	1–4	Up to 24
30% insulin aspart				
75% insulin lispro protamine/	Humalog Mix 75/25	Rapid*	1–6.5	Up to 24
25% insulin lispro				

*Faster than Humulin 70/30, Humulin 50/50, or Novolin 70/30.

Lispro Insulin. Lispro insulin can be mixed with NPH, lente, and ultralente insulins, but not with glargine insulin. When mixtures are prepared, lispro insulin should be drawn into the syringe first to avoid contaminating the lispro bottle with the longer acting insulin. As a rule, mixtures with lispro insulin should be administered within 15 minutes. Mixtures with NPH insulin are stable for 28 days.

Aspart Insulin. Data on mixing aspart insulin are limited. We do know that aspart insulin *can* be mixed with NPH insulin and should *not* be mixed with glargine insulin. Compatibility with lente and ultralente insulins has not been determined.

NPH Insulin. This preparation is compatible with regular, lispro, and aspart insulins. Mixtures of NPH and regular insulin may be prepared by the patient or may be purchased premixed (70% NPH/30% regular or 50% NPH/50% regular). Mixtures of regular and NPH insulin are stable and do not alter the kinetics of either component. It is best to inject mixtures with insulin lispro within 15 minutes.

Lente Insulins. Lente, semilente, and ultralente insulin may be mixed with one another, with regular insulin, or with lispro insulin. When the lente insulins are mixed with one another, no change in time course occurs. In contrast, when lente insulins are mixed with regular insulin, zinc present in the lente-type insulin can complex with the regular insulin, thereby delaying and prolonging its actions. Since this reaction begins soon after mixing, these mixtures should be injected immediately to avoid altering the regular insulin.

Insulin Glargine. Insulin glargine should not be mixed with any other types of insulin.

Storage

Insulin in *unopened vials* should be stored *under refrigeration* until needed. Vials should not be frozen. When stored unopened under refrigeration, insulin can be used up to the expiration date on the vial.

The vial in current use can be kept at room temperature for up to 1 month without significant loss of activity. Direct sunlight and extreme heat must be avoided. Partially filled vials should be discarded after several weeks if left unused. Injecting insulin stored at room temperature causes less pain than injecting cold insulin.

Mixtures of insulin prepared in *vials* are stable for 1 month at room temperature and for 3 months under refrigeration.

Mixtures of insulin in *prefilled syringes* (plastic or glass) should be stored in a refrigerator, where they will be stable for at least 1 week and perhaps 2. The syringe should be stored vertically with the needle pointing up to avoid clogging the needle. Prior to administration, the syringe should be agitated gently to resuspend the insulin.

Alternative Methods of Insulin Delivery

Insulin is usually administered subcutaneously using a syringe and needle. The devices discussed below represent alternatives to the traditional method of insulin administration.

Jet Injectors. These devices shoot insulin directly through the skin into subcutaneous tissue. No needle is used. Hence, for patients who dislike needles, a jet injector may be attractive. However, these devices do have a downside. They're expensive ($500 to $900) and can be difficult to use. Moreover, because insulin is delivered under high pressure, these devices can cause stinging, burning, and pain. In addition, bruising can occur in people with reduced subcutaneous fat (children, the elderly, thin people).

Pen Injectors. These devices are similar to a syringe and needle but more convenient. Pen injectors look like a fountain pen but have a disposable needle (where the writing tip would be) and a disposable insulin-filled cartridge inside. Administration is accomplished by sticking the needle under the skin and injecting the insulin manually. Dosage can be adjusted in 2-unit increments.

Portable Insulin Pumps. These computerized devices deliver a basal infusion of insulin (regular, lispro, or aspart) plus bolus doses before each meal. The basal infusion is usually about 1 U/hr and can be programmed to match the patient's metabolism. Mealtime boluses are calculated to match caloric intake. The pumps are about the size of a call-pager, weigh only 4 ounces, and are worn on the belt or in a pocket. An infusion set delivers insulin from the pump to a subcutaneous needle, usually located on the abdomen. The infusion set should be replaced every 1 to 3 days, at which time the needle should be moved to a new site (at least 1 inch away from the old one). Because the pump delivers short-acting insulin, insulin levels will drop quickly if the pump is removed. Accordingly, the pump should remain in place most of the day. However, it can be removed for an hour or two on special occasions. External insulin pumps cost between $3000 and $5000. Infusion sets, insulin, and glucose monitoring materials add another $300/month to the bill. Aside from expense, the main drawback of the pumps is underdelivery of insulin owing to formation of insulin microdeposits.

Implantable Insulin Pumps. These devices are surgically implanted in the abdomen and deliver insulin either intraperitoneally or intravenously. Like external pumps, internal pumps deliver a basal insulin infusion plus bolus doses with meals. Insulin delivery is adjusted by external telemetry. Compared with multiple daily injections, implantable pumps produce superior glycemic control, cause less hypoglycemia and weight gain, and improve quality of life. As with external pumps, delivery of insulin can be impeded by formation of insulin microprecipitates. Implantable pumps are experimental and not yet available for general use.

Intranasal Insulin. Intranasal administration of insulin is experimental. When insulin is administered by this route, effects have a rapid onset and brief duration. Hence, intranasal administration is suitable for delivery of mealtime insulin supplements, but cannot meet basal insulin needs. Therefore, long-acting SC insulin is still required. Additional problems are discomfort and expense. In order for absorption to occur, insulin must be administered with surfactants, which irritate the nasal mucosa. Intranasal insulin is expensive because only 10% of each dose is absorbed, which means the dose must be 10 times greater than an SC dose to produce equivalent effects.

Insulin Therapy of Diabetes

Insulin is given to all patients who have type 1 diabetes and to many who have type 2 diabetes. In addition, insulin is employed to manage gestational diabetes. In treating these disorders, the objective is to maintain levels of blood glucose within an acceptable range (see Table 54–3). When therapy is successful, both hyperglycemia and hypoglycemia are avoided, and the long-term complications of diabetes are minimized.

TABLE 54–8 ▪▪ Insulin Therapy of Diabetes Mellitus: Conventional Versus Intensive Conventional Therapy

Regimen	Insulin Type and Dosing Schedule			
	Breakfast	Lunch	Supper	Bedtime
Conventional therapy*	Regular + lente	None	Regular + lente	None
Intensive conventional therapy†	Regular	Regular	Regular	Ultralente

*Dosage is *fixed* (2/3 daily total in AM, 1/3 daily total in PM). As a result, flexibility of timing and composition of meals is not possible.

†Dosage of regular insulin is *adjusted for each meal;* hence, timing and composition of meals can be varied.

Tight Glucose Control: Benefits and Drawbacks

The process of maintaining glucose levels within a normal range is referred to as tight glucose control. Maintaining tight glucose control is difficult, but greatly reduces morbidity and mortality as compared with conventional therapy.

Benefits of Tight Control. The benefits of tight glucose control were demonstrated conclusively in two landmark studies: (1) the Diabetes Control and Complications Trial, a 9-year study published in 1993, and (2) the United Kingdom Prospective Diabetes Study, a 20-year study published in 1998. The DCCT evaluated tight control in patients with type 1 diabetes; the UKPDS evaluated tight control in patients with type 2 diabetes.

In the DCCT, patients received either *conventional insulin therapy* (i.e., one or two injections/day) or *intensive insulin therapy* (four injections/day). The patients who received intensive therapy experienced a 50% decrease in clinically significant kidney disease, a 35% to 56% decrease in neuropathy, and a 76% decrease in serious ophthalmic complications. Moreover, onset of ophthalmic problems was delayed and progression of existing problems was slowed. All of these benefits were correlated with improved glycemic control. Hence, with rigorous control of blood glucose, the high degree of morbidity traditionally associated with type 1 diabetes can be markedly reduced.

In the UKPDS, the principal benefit of tight glucose control was a reduction in microvascular complications. In one branch of the study, nonobese patients were given either intensive therapy or conventional therapy. Intensive therapy consisted of drugs (insulin or a sulfonylurea) in doses sufficient to keep FPG below 108 mg/dl. Conventional therapy consisted primarily of dietary counseling; drugs were used only if FPG exceeded 270 mg/dl. Mean values for HbA$_{1c}$ were 7% in the intensive group and 7.9% in the conventional group. Compared with patients in the conventional group, patients in the intensive group had a 12% reduction in total diabetes-related endpoints (cardiovascular, retinal, and renal damage). However, a reduction in microvascular complications (especially retinal damage) accounted for most of the benefit. In a parallel branch of the study, obese patients were given either conventional therapy or intensive therapy with metformin. Outcomes were similar to those seen with nonobese patients. Overall, the UKPDS study has shown that intensive treatment of type 2 diabetes is more beneficial than conventional treatment—although the benefits do not seem to be as great as in type 1 diabetes.

Drawbacks of Tight Control. Unfortunately, intensive therapy does have drawbacks. The greatest concern is *hypo-glycemia.* Because glucose levels are kept relatively low, the possibility of hypoglycemia secondary to a modest overdose with insulin or an oral hypoglycemic agent is significantly increased. In the DCCT, compared with patients using conventional therapy, those using intensive insulin experienced 3 times as many hypoglycemic events requiring the assistance of another person, and 3 times as many episodes of hypoglycemia-induced coma or seizures. In addition, patients on intensive insulin therapy gained more weight (about 10 pounds, on average). Other disadvantages are greater inconvenience, increased complexity, and a need for greater patient motivation. Finally, for patients treated with insulin, the expense is much higher: Whereas traditional therapy costs about $1700/year, intensive therapy costs about $4000/year (for multiple daily injections) or $5800 (for continuous infusion with a pump).

Dosage

To achieve tight glucose control, insulin dosage must be closely matched with insulin needs. If caloric intake is increased, insulin dosage must be increased as well. When a meal is missed or is low in calories, the dosage of insulin must be decreased. Dosage must undergo additional adjustments to meet specialized needs. For example, insulin needs are *increased* by infection, stress, obesity, the adolescent growth spurt, and pregnancy (after the first trimester). Conversely, insulin needs are *decreased* by exercise and pregnancy (during the first trimester). To ensure that insulin dosage is coordinated with insulin requirements, the patient and the healthcare team must work together to establish an integrated program of nutrition, exercise, blood glucose monitoring, and insulin replacement therapy.

Total daily dosages may range from 0.1 U/kg body weight to more than 2.5 U/kg. For patients with type 1 diabetes, initial dosages typically range from 0.5 to 0.6 U/kg/day. For patients with type 2 diabetes, initial dosages typically range from 0.2 to 0.6 U/kg/day.

Dosing Schedules

The schedule of insulin administration helps determine the extent to which tight glucose control is achieved. Three dosing schedules are compared below. These modes are referred to as (1) conventional therapy, (2) intensive conventional therapy, and (3) continuous subcutaneous insulin infusion.

Conventional Therapy. Several dosing schedules fall under the heading of conventional therapy. A representative schedule is summarized in Table 54–8. In this schedule, a combination of regular insulin (a short-acting, fast-onset preparation) plus lente insulin (an intermediate-acting preparation) is administered 15 to 30 minutes before breakfast and again before the evening meal. No insulin is administered with the noon meal. Typically, two-thirds of the total daily dose is given in the morning and the remainder is given late in the day. Dosage remains rigidly fixed from one day to the next.

Conventional therapy does not provide tight glucose control. The weak point of this schedule is that there is no provision for adjusting insulin dosage in response to ongoing changes in insulin needs. Hence, if a meal is abnormally large, insulin levels will be insufficient, causing hyperglycemia. Conversely, if a meal is delayed, reduced in size, or missed entirely, hypoglycemia will follow.

Intensive Conventional Therapy (ICT). This form of therapy is designed to provide tight glucose control. A representative regimen is presented in Table 54–8. In this regimen, the patient injects ultralente insulin (a long-acting preparation) in the evening and also injects regular insulin (a short-acting, fast onset preparation) 15 to 30 minutes before each meal.* The *ultralente* preparation provides a *basal* level of insulin throughout the night and the following day. The mealtime doses of *regular* insulin accommodate the acute needs that occur at times of caloric loading. Note that insulin is injected *four times each day,* rather than just twice as in conventional therapy.

The most significant feature of ICT is *adaptability.* Unlike conventional therapy, in which doses never change, the *prandial doses in ICT are adjusted to match the caloric content of each meal:* if no meal is eaten, no insulin is administered; if a meal is delayed, so is the dose of regular insulin; if a meal is larger than usual, the insulin dose is increased proportionately. Because insulin dosage is determined by the timing and size of each meal, ICT offers patients a degree of glycemic control and dietary flexibility that is not possible with conventional therapy.

SMBG is an essential component of ICT. Blood glucose should be measured 3 to 5 times a day. SMBG is discussed above under *Monitoring Treatment.*

Continuous Subcutaneous Insulin Infusion. Continuous subcutaneous insulin infusion (CSII) is accomplished using a portable infusion pump connected to an indwelling subcutaneous catheter. Three types of insulin may be used: regular, lispro, and aspart insulin. To provide a basal level of insulin, the pump is set to infuse insulin continuously at a slow but steady rate. To accommodate insulin needs created by eating, the pump is triggered manually to provide a bolus dose matched in size to the caloric content of each meal. Hence, like ICT, CSII can adapt to altered insulin needs. As with ICT, SMBG is essential. CSII is equivalent to ICT for achieving tight glucose control. Portable infusion pumps are discussed above under *Alternative Methods of Insulin Delivery.*

Achieving Tight Glucose Control

As we have seen, the primary requirement for achieving tight glucose control is a method of insulin delivery that permits adjustments in dosage to accommodate ongoing variations in insulin needs. ICT and CSII meet this crite-

rion. In addition to an adaptable method of insulin delivery, achieving tight glucose control requires the following:

- Careful attention to all elements of the treatment program (diet, exercise, insulin replacement therapy)
- A defined glycemia target (see Table 54–3)
- Self-monitoring of blood glucose 3 to 5 times daily
- A high degree of patient motivation
- Extensive patient education

Tight glucose control cannot be achieved without the informed participation of the patient. Accordingly, patients must receive thorough instruction on the following:

- The nature of diabetes
- The importance of tight glucose control
- The major components of the treatment routine (insulin replacement, SMBG, diet, exercise)
- Procedures for purchasing insulin, syringes, and needles
- The importance of avoiding arbitrary changes between human and pork insulins
- The importance of avoiding arbitrary changes between insulins from different manufacturers
- Methods of insulin storage
- Procedures for mixing insulins
- Calculation of dosage adjustments
- Techniques of insulin administration
- Methods for monitoring blood glucose

In the final analysis, responsibility for managing diabetes rests with the patient. The healthcare team can design a treatment program and provide education and guidance. However, tight glucose control can be achieved only if the patient is actively involved in his or her own therapy.

Complications of Insulin Treatment
Hypoglycemia

Hypoglycemia (blood glucose <50 mg/dl) occurs when insulin levels exceed insulin needs. A major cause of insulin excess is overdose. Imbalance between insulin levels and insulin needs can also result from reduced intake of food, vomiting and diarrhea (which reduce absorption of nutrients), excessive consumption of alcohol (which promotes hypoglycemia), unaccustomed exercise (which promotes glucose uptake and utilization), and parturition (which reduces insulin requirements).

Diabetic patients and their families should be familiar with the signs and symptoms of hypoglycemia. Some symptoms result from activation of the sympathetic nervous system, whereas others arise from the central nervous system (CNS). When glucose levels fall *rapidly,* activation of the sympathetic nervous system occurs, resulting in tachycardia, palpitations, sweating, and nervousness. However, if glucose declines *gradually,* symptoms may be limited to those of CNS origin. Mild CNS symptoms include headache, confusion, drowsiness, and fatigue. If hypoglycemia is severe, convulsions, coma, and death may follow.

Rapid treatment of hypoglycemia is mandatory; if hypoglycemia is allowed to persist, irreversible brain damage or even death may result. In conscious patients, glucose levels can be restored with a fast-acting oral sugar (e.g., glucose tablets, orange juice, sugar cubes, honey, corn syrup, nondiet soda). How-

---

*Lispro insulin or aspart insulin can be used instead of regular insulin. The advantage of lispro and aspart insulin is that they can be administered just a few minutes before eating—or immediately after.

ever, if the swallowing reflex or the gag reflex is suppressed, nothing should be administered by mouth. In cases of severe hypoglycemia, IV glucose is the preferred therapy. Parenteral *glucagon* is an alternative method of treatment. (The pharmacology of glucagon is discussed at the end of the chapter.)

In anticipation of hypoglycemic episodes, diabetic patients should always have an oral carbohydrate available (e.g., Life Savers, candy, glucose tablets, sugar cubes). Many physicians recommend that patients keep glucagon on hand as well. Patients should carry some sort of identification (e.g., Medic Alert bracelet) to inform emergency personnel of their condition.

In some patients, hypoglycemia occurs without producing the symptoms noted above. As a result, the patient remains unaware of hypoglycemia until blood sugar has become dangerously low. Hypoglycemia unawareness is a particular problem among patients practicing tight glucose control. The risk of dangerous hypoglycemia can be minimized by frequently monitoring blood glucose.

Severe hypoglycemia and diabetic ketoacidosis (see below) can both produce coma. Of the two causes, hypoglycemia is the more common. Since treatment of these two conditions is very different (hypoglycemia involves withholding insulin, whereas ketoacidosis requires giving insulin), it is essential that coma from these causes be differentiated. The most definitive diagnosis is made by measuring plasma or urinary glucose levels: in hypoglycemic coma, glucose levels are very low; in ketoacidosis, glucose levels are very high.

Other Complications

Lipodystrophies. Altered deposition of subcutaneous fat (lipodystrophy) can occur at sites of insulin injection. Two types of change may be seen: (1) *lipoatrophy* (loss of subcutaneous fat), and (2) *lipohypertrophy* (accumulation of subcutaneous fat).

Lipoatrophy produces a depression in the skin at the site of insulin injection. The cause of atrophy appears to be immunologic. Accordingly, fat atrophy is most likely with use of insulin preparations that have a high concentration of antigenic contaminants. Because the insulin preparations in use today are much purer than those used in the past, lipoatrophy is now rare. When lipoatrophy occurs, subcutaneous fat can often be restored by injecting a highly purified insulin preparation (e.g., human insulin) directly into the site of fat loss. Some improvement can be seen in 4 weeks, but full recovery can take 3 to 6 months.

Lipohypertrophy occurs at sites of frequent insulin injection. Fat accumulates because insulin stimulates fat synthesis. When use of the site is discontinued, excess fat is eventually lost. Lipohypertrophy can be minimized through systematic rotation of injection sites.

Allergic Reactions. Insulin injection can produce local and systemic allergic responses. Fortunately, allergic reactions are rare.

With local reactions, the injection site becomes red and hardened. These reactions are usually delayed, taking several hours to develop. Local reactions occur in response to a contaminant in the insulin preparation—not to the insulin itself. Because insulins in use today are highly purified, local reactions are uncommon.

Systemic reactions take place rapidly, and are characterized by the widespread appearance of red and intensely itchy welts. Breathing difficulty may develop. Systemic reactions occur in response to insulin itself, not to a contaminant. Beef insulin, which differs from human insulin by three amino acids, is the most frequent cause of systemic allergy. Generalized reactions are least likely with pork and human insulins. If severe allergy develops in a patient who nonetheless must continue insulin use, a desensitization procedure can be performed. This process entails giving small initial doses of purified pork or human insulin, followed by a series of progressively larger doses.

Drug Interactions

Hypoglycemic Agents. Drugs that lower blood glucose levels can intensify hypoglycemia induced by insulin. Among these drugs are *sulfonylureas, meglitinides, beta-adrenergic*

blocking agents, and *alcohol* (used acutely). When these drugs are combined with insulin, special care must be taken to ensure that blood glucose does not fall too low.

Hyperglycemic Agents. Drugs that raise blood glucose (e.g., *thiazide diuretics, glucocorticoids, sympathomimetics*) can counteract the therapeutic effects of insulin. When these agents are combined with insulin, insulin dosage may need to be increased.

Beta-Adrenergic Blocking Agents. Beta blockers can delay awareness of insulin-induced hypoglycemia by masking signs that are associated with stimulation of the sympathetic nervous system (e.g., tachycardia, palpitations). Furthermore, since beta blockade impairs glycogenolysis, and since glycogenolysis is one means by which the body can counteract a fall in blood glucose, beta blockers can make insulin-induced hypoglycemia even worse.

ORAL HYPOGLYCEMICS FOR TYPE 2 DIABETES

There are five families of oral hypoglycemic drugs: sulfonylureas, meglitinides, biguanides, thiazolidinediones, and alpha-glucosidase inhibitors. Oral hypoglycemics are indicated only for type 2 diabetes; they are not used for type 1 diabetes. These drugs should be employed only after a program of diet modification and exercise has failed to produce glycemic control. Actions and adverse effects of the oral hypoglycemics are summarized in Table 54–9.

Sulfonylureas

The sulfonylureas were the first oral hypoglycemics available. They work by promoting insulin release. Sulfonylureas are derivatives of the sulfonamide antibiotics, but lack antimicrobial activity. All of the sulfonylureas may be used alone or in combination with other hypoglycemic drugs. Dosages are summarized in Table 54–10.

The sulfonylureas fall into two groups: *first-generation agents* and *second-generation agents*. Both generations reduce glucose levels to the same extent. The principal difference between the generations is that the second-generation agents are more potent. That is, second-generation agents produce their effects at much lower doses than do the first-generation agents. However, although the differences in potency are large, these differences are of minimal clinical significance. More important than differences in potency are differences in duration of action (see Table 54–10), since agents with longer durations can be given once daily.

Tolbutamide

Tolbutamide [Orinase], a first-generation agent, will serve as our prototype for the sulfonylurea family. As with the other oral hypoglycemics, use of tolbutamide is restricted to patients with type 2 diabetes.

Mechanism of Action. Tolbutamide acts primarily by stimulating the release of insulin from pancreatic islets. If the pancreas is incapable of insulin synthesis, tolbutamide will be ineffective—which is why tolbutamide is ineffective in patients with type 1 diabetes. With prolonged use, tolbutamide may increase cellular sensitivity to insulin.

TABLE 54–9 ■ Oral Hypoglycemics for Type 2 Diabetes

Class and Specific Agents	Actions	Major Adverse Effects
Sulfonylureas Tolbutamide [Orinase] Glipizide [Glucotrol] Glyburide [Micronase] (See Table 54–10 for other sulfonylureas)	Promote insulin secretion by the pancreas; may also increase tissue response to insulin	Hypoglycemia
Meglitinides Repanglinide [Prandin] Nateglinide [Starlix]	Promote insulin secretion by the pancreas	Hypoglycemia
Biguanide Metformin [Glucophage]	Decreases glucose production by liver and increases glucose uptake by muscle	GI symptoms: decreased appetite, nausea, diarrhea Lactic acidosis (rarely)
Thiazolidinediones Rosiglitazone [Avandia] Pioglitazone [Actos]	Decrease insulin resistance, and thereby increase glucose uptake by muscle and decrease glucose production by the liver	Hypoglycemia, but only in the presence of excessive insulin
Alpha-Glucosidase Inhibitors Acarbose [Precose] Miglitol [Glyset]	Inhibit carbohydrate digestion and absorption, thereby decreasing the postprandial rise in blood glucose	GI symptoms: flatulence, cramps, abdominal distention, borborygmus

How does tolbutamide promote insulin release? It binds with and thereby blocks ATP-sensitive potassium channels in the cell membrane. As a result, the membrane depolarizes, thereby permitting influx of calcium, which in turn causes insulin release. The extent of release is glucose dependent, and diminishes at low glucose levels.

Pharmacokinetics. Tolbutamide is readily absorbed following oral administration. Plasma levels peak within 3 to 5 hours. The drug undergoes extensive hepatic metabolism followed by urinary excretion. Because of its mode of elimination, tolbutamide must be used with caution in patients with hepatic or renal impairment. Tolbutamide has a relatively short half-life (about 6 hours), and hence must be administered 2 to 3 times a day.

Therapeutic Use. Sulfonylureas are indicated only for type 2 diabetes. These drugs are of no help to patients with type 1 diabetes. Sulfonylureas should be employed only if blood glucose cannot be lowered by a program of caloric restriction and exercise. When these agents are to be used, they should be employed as an *adjunct* to nondrug therapy—not as a substitute. Tolbutamide and other sulfonylureas may be used alone or together with other hypoglycemic drugs.

Adverse Effects. Hypoglycemia. Tolbutamide and all other sulfonylureas can cause excessive lowering of blood glucose. Although hypoglycemia is usually mild, fatalities have occurred. Hypoglycemia is sometimes persistent, requiring infusion of dextrose for several days. Hypoglycemic reactions are most likely in patients with kidney or liver dysfunction, because accumulation of tolbutamide may occur. If signs of hypoglycemia develop (fatigue, excessive hunger, profuse sweating, palpitations), the physician should be notified.

Use in Pregnancy and Lactation. *Sulfonylureas should be avoided during pregnancy.* Although adequate studies in humans are lacking, sulfonylureas are teratogenic in animals. Furthermore, since sulfonylurea therapy during pregnancy often fails to provide good glycemic control, and since even mild hyperglycemia may be hazardous to the fetus, insulin is generally preferred for managing the diabetic pregnancy.

It is especially important to avoid tolbutamide near term. Newborns exposed to sulfonylureas at the time of delivery have experienced severe hypoglycemia lasting as long as 4 to 10 days. Hence, if a sulfonylurea has been taken during pregnancy, it should be discontinued at least 48 hours prior to the anticipated time of delivery.

Tolbutamide should not be taken by women who are nursing. The drug is excreted into breast milk, posing a risk of hypoglycemia to the infant. If a woman wishes to breast-feed, she should substitute insulin for the sulfonylurea.

Cardiovascular Toxicity. There has been controversy regarding the possibility of adverse cardiovascular reactions to oral hypoglycemics. In 1970, the University Group Diabetes Program (UGDP) published results indicating that sulfonylureas carried an increased risk of mortality from cardiovascular causes. In the UGDP study, cardiovascular mortality was 2.5 times greater among subjects treated with a combination of diet plus tolbutamide than among control subjects who received diet therapy alone. The UGDP study has been criticized on several grounds, including design, patient selection, dosing, and compliance. Subsequent clinical trials, including the UKPDS, have failed to confirm the conclusions of the UGDP report. The American Diabetes Association, which initially endorsed the UGDP study, has since withdrawn its support.

Drug Interactions. Alcohol. When alcohol is combined with tolbutamide, a disulfiram-like reaction may occur. This syndrome includes flushing, palpitations, and nausea. Disulfiram reactions are discussed fully in Chapter 37. Also, alcohol can potentiate the hypoglycemic effects of tolbutamide. Accordingly, patients using the drug must be warned against alcohol consumption.

Drugs That Can Intensify Hypoglycemia. A variety of drugs, acting by diverse mechanisms, can intensify hypoglycemic responses to sulfonylureas. Included are *nonsteroidal anti-inflammatory drugs, sulfonamide antibiotics, ethanol* (used acutely), *ranitidine,* and *cimetidine.* Caution must be exercised when a sulfonylurea is used in combination with these drugs.

TABLE 54–10 ▪■ Sulfonylureas: Time Course and Dosage

Generic Name [Trade Name]	Duration (hr)	Dosage*
First-Generation Agents		
Tolbutamide [Orinase]	6–12	Initial: 1–2 gm/day in 1–3 doses Maximum: 2–3 gm/day in 1–3 doses
Acetohexamide [Dymelor]	12–24	Initial: 0.25–1.5 gm/day in 1 or 2 doses Maximum: 1.5 gm/day in 1 or 2 doses
Tolazamide [Tolinase]	12–24	Initial: 100–250 mg/day with breakfast Maximum: 0.75–1 gm in 2 divided doses
Chlorpropamide [Diabinese]	24–72	Initial: 250 mg/day with breakfast Maximum: 750 mg once a day
Second-Generation Agents		
Glipizide		
Standard [Glucotrol]	12–24	Initial: 5 mg/day with breakfast Maximum: 40 mg/day in 2 divided doses
Sustained release [Glucotrol XL]	24	Initial 5 mg/day with breakfast Maximum: 20 mg/day with breakfast
Glyburide		
Nonmicronized [DiaBeta, Micronase]	12–24	Initial: 2.5–5 mg day with breakfast Maximum: 20 mg/day in 1 or 2 doses
Micronized [Glynase PresTab]	24	Initial: 1.5–3 mg/day with breakfast Maximum: 12 mg/day in 1 or 2 doses
Glimepiride [Amaryl]	24	Initial: 1–2 mg/day with breakfast Maximum: 8 mg/day with breakfast

*The dosages listed are for nonelderly patients. Elderly patients should use a smaller dose.

Beta-Adrenergic Blocking Agents. Beta blockers can interfere with tolbutamide's action by suppressing insulin release. (Recall that activation of beta receptors is one way to promote insulin release.) Because beta blockers can also mask sympathetic responses (e.g., tachycardia, tremors) to declining blood glucose, use of beta blockers can delay awareness of tolbutamide-induced hypoglycemia.

Other Sulfonylureas

In addition to tolbutamide, six other sulfonylureas are available (see Table 54–10). All have similar actions and side effects, and they all share the same application: treatment of type 2 diabetes. All sulfonylureas can cause hypoglycemia.

The sulfonylureas differ significantly from one another with respect to duration of action. For example, effects of tolbutamide, the shortest acting sulfonylurea, last only 6 to 12 hours. In contrast, effects of chlorpropamide, the longest acting oral hypoglycemic, last as long as 3 days. Time courses and dosages are summarized in Table 54–10.

One sulfonylurea—glyburide—is available in fixed-dose combination with metformin (see below).

Meglitinides

Meglitinides are relatively new hypoglycemic agents that have the same mechanism as the sulfonylureas: stimulation of pancreatic insulin release. At this time, only two meglitinides are available: repaglinide and nateglinide.

Repaglinide

Actions and Uses. Like the sulfonylureas, repaglinide [Prandin] blocks ATP-sensitive potassium channels on pancreatic beta cells, and thereby facilitates calcium influx, which leads to increased insulin release. In clinical trials, repaglinide was about as effective as glyburide and glipizide (sulfonylureas). Over time, repaglinide can lower HbA_{1c} levels by about 1.7%. The drug is approved only for type 2 diabetes. Because repaglinide has the same mechanism of action as the sulfonylureas, patients who do not respond to sulfonylureas will not respond to this agent either.

Pharmacokinetics. Repaglinide undergoes rapid absorption followed by rapid elimination. Blood levels peak within 1 hour of oral administration and return to baseline about 4 hours later. Elimination results from hepatic metabolism followed by biliary excretion. The drug's half-life is only 1 hour. Blood levels of insulin rise and fall in parallel with levels of repaglinide.

Adverse Effects. Repaglinide is generally well tolerated. The only significant adverse effect is *hypoglycemia.* In patients with liver dysfunction, metabolism of repaglinide may be slowed, and hence the risk of hypoglycemia may be increased. Because of possible hypoglycemia, it is imperative that patients eat no later than 30 minutes after drug administration.

Preparations, Dosage, and Administration. Repaglinide [Prandin] is available in 0.5-, 1-, and 2-mg tablets for oral use. Administration must always be associated with a meal. For patients who have not used another oral hypoglycemic, the initial dosage is 0.5 mg taken 0 to 30 minutes before each meal. Patients who *have* used another oral hypoglycemic may take 1 or 2 mg before each meal. The maximum daily dosage is 16 mg (4 mg with each meal for up to four meals).

Nateglinide

Basic Pharmacology. The pharmacology of nateglinide [Starlix] is nearly identical to that of repaglinide. Both drugs have the same indication (treatment of type 2 diabetes), mechanism action (promotion of insulin release), and major adverse effect (hypoglycemia). The drugs differ primarily with respect to time course. Specifically, nateglinide has a slightly faster onset (30 minutes vs. 1 hour) and a significantly shorter duration (2 hours vs.

4 hours). Because of its more rapid onset, nateglinide may be better suited than repaglinide for controlling the postprandial rise in glucose. However, because of its shorter duration, nateglinide is less effective than repaglinide (or metformin or a sulfonylurea) for controlling fasting glucose. Because the meglitinides and sulfonylureas have the same mechanism of action, nateglinide, like repaglinide, will not work in patients who have not responded to a sulfonylurea (e.g., tolbutamide). Nateglinide undergoes extensive metabolism by cytochrome P450 enzymes, followed by rapid and complete excretion, primarily in the urine.

Preparations, Dosage, and Administration. Nateglinide [Starlix] is available in 60- and 120-mg tablets. The initial dosage is 120 mg 3 times a day taken 0 to 30 minutes before a meal. For patients with HbA$_{1c}$ concentrations close to the target value, the initial dosage is lower: 60 mg three times a day taken 0 to 30 minutes before a meal. Please note that dosing must always be associated with a meal. Otherwise, nateglinide-induced insulin release could cause hypoglycemia. Nateglinide costs a little more than repaglinide ($85.50 for a 30-day supply vs. $68.40) and *much* more than sulfonylureas (e.g., generic glipizide costs only $9.60 for a 30-day supply).

Biguanides: Metformin

Metformin [Glucophage, Glucophage XR] was approved for treatment of type 2 diabetes in the United States in 1994. The drug has been available in Canada and Europe since 1959. Phenformin, a chemical relative of metformin, was withdrawn from the U.S. market in 1977 because of a high incidence of lactic acidosis. Both metformin and phenformin are classified chemically as biguanides. Metformin frequently causes GI disturbances; lactic acidosis is rare.

Mechanism of Action. Metformin lowers blood glucose primarily by decreasing production of glucose in the liver. The underlying mechanism appears to be suppression of gluconeogenesis. In addition to reducing glucose production, the drug enhances glucose uptake and utilization by muscle. In contrast to sulfonylureas, metformin does not promote insulin release from the pancreas and does not cause hypoglycemia.

Pharmacokinetics. Metformin is administered by mouth and absorbed slowly from the small intestine. Of particular interest, the drug is excreted unchanged by the kidneys. Hence, in the event of renal insufficiency, metformin can accumulate to toxic levels.

Therapeutic Uses. Glycemic Control. Metformin is used to lower blood sugar in type 2 diabetics who have not responded adequately to a program of diet modification and exercise. The drug may be used alone or in combination with a sulfonylurea. When used alone, metformin lowers basal and postprandial blood glucose levels. When metformin is combined with a sulfonylurea, the combination lowers blood sugar more effectively than either drug alone—which is to be expected in that metformin and sulfonylureas act by different mechanisms. Because benefits of metformin do not depend on insulin release, the drug is able to reduce blood sugar in patients who can no longer produce insulin. This contrasts with the sulfonylureas, which require pancreatic insulin to work.

Prevention of Type 2 Diabetes. Recent data from the Diabetes Prevention Program (DPP), a large study sponsored by the National Institutes of Health, indicate that metformin can delay development of type 2 diabetes in high-risk individuals. The DPP enrolled 3234 people ages 25 to 85. All participants had impaired glucose tolerance (as determined by an oral glucose tolerance test) and all were severely overweight. Participants were randomly assigned to one of three protocols:

(1) intensive lifestyle changes with the aim of reducing body weight by 7% through moderate exercise (e.g., vigorous walking 30 minutes a day 5 days a week) combined with a low-fat diet, (2) treatment with metformin (850 mg twice daily), or (3) treatment with placebo. The results? Metformin reduced the risk of developing type 2 diabetes by 31%. However, benefits were limited primarily to younger patients and to those who were most overweight; the drug was relatively ineffective in older patients and those less overweight. It must be stressed, however, that metformin is not a substitute for diet and exercise. In fact, the DPP showed that lifestyle changes are even more effective than metformin: the combination of moderate exercise plus weight loss (5% to 7% of initial weight) reduced the average risk of type 2 diabetes by 58%. Benefits were greatest (71%) for people over 60.

Side Effects. The most common side effects are decreased appetite, nausea, and diarrhea. These generally subside over time. However, in 3% to 5% of patients, GI effects lead to discontinuation of treatment. Metformin decreases absorption of vitamin B$_{12}$ and folic acid, which can result in deficiency. In contrast to sulfonylureas, metformin does not cause weight gain. In fact, patients *lose* an average of 7 to 8 pounds—probably because metformin causes nausea and decreases appetite.

Toxicity: Lactic Acidosis. Metformin and other biguanides inhibit mitochondrial oxidation of lactic acid, and can thereby cause lactic acidosis. This condition is a medical emergency and has a mortality rate of about 50%. Fortunately, lactic acidosis is rare (about 3 cases/100,000 patient years) when metformin is used at recommended doses in patients with good renal function. However, in patients with renal insufficiency, metformin can rapidly accumulate to toxic levels. Accordingly, the drug must never be used by these people. In addition, metformin must be avoided in patients who are prone to increased lactic acid production. Among these are patients with liver disease, severe infection, or a history of lactic acidosis; patients who consume alcohol to excess; and patients with heart failure, shock, and other conditions that can result in hypoxemia. All patients should be informed about early signs of lactic acidosis—hyperventilation, myalgia, malaise, and unusual somnolence—and instructed to report these to the physician. Metformin should be withdrawn until lactic acidosis has been ruled out. If lactic acidosis is present, hemodialysis can correct the acidosis and remove accumulated metformin.

Drug Interactions. As noted, alcohol increases the risk of lactic acidosis. Accordingly, alcohol must be avoided.

Preparations, Dosage, and Administration. Metformin is available alone in standard tablets (500 and 850 mg) as *Glucophage,* and in extended-release tablets (500 mg) as *Glucophage XR.* In addition, the drug is available combined with glyburide (as *Glucovance*), with glipizide (as *Metaglip*), and with rosiglitazone (as *Avandamet*). These combination products are discussed below.

With standard metformin tablets, the recommended initial dosage is 500 mg twice daily, taken with the morning and evening meals. The usual maintenance dosage is 850 mg twice daily. The maximum dosage is 850 mg 3 times a day.

With extended-release metformin tablets, dosing is done once daily with the *evening* meal. Why the evening meal? Because this timing may enhance absorption owing to slower GI transit time at night. For previously untreated patients, the initial dosage is 500 mg. For patients already taking metformin, the total daily dosage remains the same; it's simply taken all at once. The maximum daily dosage is 4 tablets (2000 mg).

Thiazolidinediones ("Glitazones")

The thiazolidinediones, also known as "glitazones," reduce glucose levels by decreasing insulin resistance. These agents are not related chemically or functionally to sulfonylureas, biguanides, or alpha-glucosidase inhibitors. Their only use is type 2 diabetes. At this time, two glitazones are available: rosiglitazone [Avandia] and pioglitazone [Actos]. A third agent—troglitazone [Rezulin]—can cause severe liver injury and has been withdrawn. All three glitazones can expand blood volume and cause edema, thereby posing a risk for patients with heart failure.

Rosiglitazone

Actions and Use. Rosiglitazone [Avandia] acts primarily by decreasing insulin resistance. That is, the drug increases the ability of target cells to respond to insulin. Accordingly, insulin must be present for rosiglitazone to work. Benefits take several weeks to develop. In animal models of diabetes, glitazones increase uptake of glucose by muscle and decrease glucose production by the liver. In clinical trials, rosiglitazone (4 mg/day) decreased fasting plasma glucose by 76 mg/dl and reduced HbA_{1c} by about 1%. Rosiglitazone is approved for use as monotherapy, and for use in combination with metformin, a sulfonylurea, or insulin.

Pharmacokinetics. Rosiglitazone is well absorbed, both in the presence and absence of food. Plasma levels peak 1 hour after ingestion. The drug undergoes hepatic metabolism followed by excretion in the urine and feces. Its half-life is 3 to 4 hours.

Adverse Effects and Interactions. Rosiglitazone is generally well tolerated. The most prominent side effect is *fluid retention,* with resultant edema and weight gain (2 to 3 kg). For most patients, fluid retention is not a significant concern. However, in patients with heart failure, fluid retention can make symptoms worse. Accordingly, rosiglitazone should be used with caution in patients with *mild* heart failure, and should not be used at all in those with *severe* failure. Patients using the drug should be informed about signs of heart failure (dyspnea, edema, weight gain, fatigue), and instructed to consult the physician if these develop. Insulin increases the risk of heart failure (by promoting fluid retention). Accordingly, using rosiglitazone and insulin together should be done with caution.

Rosiglitazone has mixed *effects on plasma lipid levels:* it (1) raises levels of low-density lipoprotein (LDL) cholesterol, which is bad, (2) raises levels of high-density lipoprotein (HDL) cholesterol, which is good, and (3) lowers levels of triglycerides, which is also good.

Monitoring. Although there is no proof that rosiglitazone is hepatotoxic, liver function should nonetheless be monitored. Why? Because rosiglitazone is in the same family as troglitazone, a drug whose hepatotoxicity is well documented. Accordingly, serum alanine aminotransferase (ALT) should be determined before treatment, every 2 months for the first year of treatment, and periodically thereafter. If baseline ALT is more than 2.5 times the upper limit of normal, rosiglitazone should not be used. If, during treatment, ALT rises to more than 3 times the upper limit of normal, rosiglitazone should be withdrawn. Patients should be informed about symptoms of liver injury (nausea, vomiting, abdominal pain, fatigue, anorexia, dark urine, jaundice) and instructed to notify the physician if these develop.

Preparations, Dosage, and Administration. Rosiglitazone is available alone as *Avandia,* and in combination with metformin as *Avandamet* (see below). As Avandia, metformin is formulated in 2-, 4-, and 8-mg tablets. The recommended starting dosage is either 4 mg once a day or 2 mg twice a day, administered with or without food. If the response is inadequate after 12 weeks, the dosage may doubled—to 8 mg once a day or 4 mg twice a day.

Pioglitazone

Pioglitazone [Actos] is the newest member of the "glitazone" family. Like rosiglitazone—and unlike troglitazone—pioglitazone appears devoid of hepatotoxicity. In addition, pioglitazone has a more favorable effect on plasma lipids than does rosiglitazone.

Actions and Uses. Like rosiglitazone, pioglitazone increases insulin sensitivity, and thereby promotes glycemic control in patients with type 2 diabetes. In clinical trials, monotherapy with pioglitazone decreased fasting blood glucose 30 to 56 mg/dl, and lowered HbA_{1c} by about 0.9%. Combining pioglitazone with insulin, metformin, or a sulfonylurea further improved glycemic control. Pioglitazone is approved for monotherapy or combined therapy with insulin, metformin, or a sulfonylurea.

Adverse Effects. Adverse effects are generally mild. The most common reactions are upper respiratory tract infection (13%), headache (9%), sinusitis (6%), and myalgia (5%). There is no proof that pioglitazone is hepatotoxic. In addition, the drug does not elevate plasma levels of triglycerides or LDL cholesterol, but it does raise levels of HDL cholesterol, which is beneficial. Like rosiglitazone, pioglitazone promotes water retention, and can thereby cause weight gain (0.5 to 2.8 kg) and edema. Hence, as with rosiglitazone, the drug should be used with caution in patients with mild heart failure, and should be avoided by those with severe failure. In addition, since insulin increases the risk of fluid retention, combining the two drugs should be done with caution. The incidence of hypoglycemia is low with pioglitazone alone, but rises to between 8% and 15% when the drug is combined with insulin.

Monitoring. As with rosiglitazone, liver function should be monitored, even though there is no proof that either drug is hepatotoxic. The same monitoring program employed for rosiglitazone (see above) is recommended for pioglitazone. Patients should be informed about symptoms of liver injury (nausea, vomiting, abdominal pain, fatigue, anorexia, dark urine, jaundice) and instructed to notify the physician if these develop.

Preparations, Dosage, and Administration. Pioglitazone [Actos] is available in 15-, 30-, and 45-mg tablets. The initial dosage for monotherapy is 15 or 30 mg once a day, taken with or without food. Dosage may be increased to 45 mg once a day if needed.

Alpha-Glucosidase Inhibitors

The alpha-glucosidase inhibitors—acarbose and miglitol—act in the intestine to delay absorption of carbohydrates. The drugs are indicated for type 2 diabetes.

Acarbose

Mechanism of Action. Acarbose [Precose] delays absorption of dietary carbohydrates, and thereby reduces the rise in blood glucose that occurs after meals. In order to be absorbed, oligosaccharides and complex carbohydrates must be broken down to monosaccharides by alpha-glucosidase, an enzyme located on the brush border of intestinal cells. Acarbose inhibits this enzyme. As a result, the drug slows digestion of carbohydrates, and hence reduces the postprandial rise in blood glucose.

Therapeutic Use. Acarbose is indicated for patients with type 2 diabetes whose hyperglycemia is not controlled by diet modification and exercise. The drug may be used alone or in combination with insulin, metformin, or a sulfonylurea. In clinical trials, 24 weeks of therapy with acarbose alone reduced mean peak postprandial glucose levels by 56 mg/dl, compared with 71 mg/dl for tolbutamide alone and 85 mg/dl for acarbose plus tolbutamide. In addition to lowering glucose levels after meals, acarbose lowers glycated hemoglobin levels, indicating an overall improvement in glycemic control.

Adverse Effects and Interactions. Acarbose frequently causes *flatulence, cramps, abdominal distention, borborygmus* (rumbling bowel sounds), and *diarrhea.* These responses result from bacterial fermentation of unabsorbed carbohydrates in the colon. In addition to its GI effects, acarbose can decrease absorption of iron, thereby posing a risk of anemia.

Hypoglycemia does not occur with acarbose alone, but may develop when acarbose is combined with *insulin* or a *sulfonylurea.* When hypoglycemia develops, sucrose cannot be used for oral therapy. Why? Because acarbose will impede its hydrolysis and thereby delay absorption. Accordingly, in patients taking acarbose, oral therapy of hypoglycemia must be accomplished with glucose.

Long-term, high-dose therapy may cause *liver dysfunction.* Asymptomatic elevation of plasma transaminases occurs in about 15% of patients. However, overt jaundice is rare. Liver function tests should be monitored every 3 months for the first year, and periodically thereafter. Liver dysfunction reverses when acarbose is discontinued.

The combination of metformin and acarbose should probably be avoided. Both drugs cause significant GI side effects, hence the combination could be very unpleasant. Furthermore, acarbose decreases metformin absorption.

Preparations, Dosage, and Administration. Acarbose [Precose] is available in 50- and 100-mg tablets. The drug is taken before meals. The initial dosage is 25 mg 3 times a day, prior to each meal. Depending on tolerability and postprandial blood glucose levels, the dosage may be increased at 4- to 8-week intervals. The maximum dosage is 50 mg 3 times a day (for patients under 60 kg) and 100 mg 3 times a day (for patients over 60 kg).

Miglitol

Miglitol [Glyset] is the second alpha-glucosidase inhibitor approved for use in the United States. Like acarbose, miglitol delays conversion of oligosaccharides and complex carbohydrates to glucose and other monosaccharides, and thereby reduces the postprandial rise in blood glucose. In clinical trials, the drug was especially effective among Hispanics and African Americans. Hypoglycemia does not occur with miglitol monotherapy, but may occur if the drug is combined with insulin or a sulfonylurea. Like acarbose, miglitol causes flatulence, abdominal discomfort, and other GI effects. In contrast to acarbose, miglitol has not been associated with liver dysfunction. As with acarbose therapy, oral sucrose cannot be used to treat hypoglycemia. Rather, oral glucose must be given. Miglitol is available in 25-, 50-, and 100-mg tablets. The initial dosage is 25 mg 3 times daily before meals. The maintenance dosage is 50 or 100 mg 3 times a day.

Combination Products

Many patients with type 2 diabetes take two different oral hypoglycemic drugs, often metformin combined with either a sulfonylurea or a glitazone. To simplify dosing, patients can now use one of the combination products that have recently become available.

Glyburide/Metformin

Glyburide (a sulfonamide) and metformin (a biguanide) are available in a combination sold as *Glucovance.* Glyburide acts primarily by increasing insulin secretion; metformin acts primarily by decreasing hepatic glucose production, and partly by increasing glucose uptake and utilization by muscle. Glucovance is indicated for initial therapy for patients with type 2 diabetes and for previously treated patients when glucose control has been inadequate with metformin or a sulfonylurea alone. The only advantage of the combination (over taking separate doses of metformin and a sulfonylurea) is convenience. Although Glucovance is approved for initial therapy, it would seem prudent to try either component alone initially, reserving the combination for patients who don't respond adequately. After all, why expose patients to the adverse effects of *two* drugs if treatment with just one would suffice?

Adverse effects of Glucovance are simply the sum of the adverse effects of glyburide and metformin. Glyburide poses a risk of *hypoglycemia.* Metformin can cause *GI disturbances* (nausea, diarrhea) and *appetite reduction.* Of greater concern, metformin poses a risk of *lactic acidosis.* Because of this risk, the combination is contraindicated for patients with renal insufficiency, metabolic acidosis, and heart failure that requires treatment.

Glucovance tablets are available in three glyburide/metformin strengths: 1.25/250 mg, 2.5/500 mg, and 5/500 mg. For previously untreated patients, the initial dosage is 1.25/250 mg once or twice daily. For previously treated patients, the recommended dosage is either 2.5/500 mg or 5/500 mg twice daily. The maximum dosage is 20/2000 mg/day. All doses are taken with meals.

Glipizide/Metformin

Glipizide (a sulfonylurea) and metformin are available in a combination sold as *Metaglip.* The product is nearly identical to glyburide/metformin [Glucovance], having the same indications, actions, and adverse effects.

Metaglip tablets are available in three glipizide/metformin strengths: 2.5/250 mg, 2.5/500 mg, and 5/500 mg. For previously untreated patients, the initial dosage is 2.5/250 mg once a day. For previously treated patients, the recommended dosage is either 2.5/500 mg or 5/500 mg twice daily. The maximum dosage is 20/2000 mg/day, administered in divided doses. All doses are taken with meals.

Rosiglitazone/Metformin

Rosiglitazone (a thiazolidinedione) and metformin are available in combination as *Avandamet.* Rosiglitazone acts by decreasing insulin resistance; metformin acts primarily by decreasing hepatic glucose production, and partly by increasing glucose uptake and utilization by muscle. Avandamet is indicated for treating type 2 diabetes in previously treated patients who (1) have not responded adequately to rosiglitazone or metformin alone or (2) *have* responded adequately to rosiglitazone *plus* metformin, but want to simplify dosing. The combination is not approved for initial therapy of type 2 diabetes.

Adverse effects of Avandamet are simply the sum of the adverse effects of rosiglitazone and metformin. With rosiglitazone, the principal concern is *fluid retention,* which can exacerbate heart failure. Accordingly, Avandamet should be used with caution in patients with *mild* heart failure, and should be avoided in those with *severe* failure. Insulin increases the risk of heart failure, and hence Avandamet and insulin should not be combined. With metformin, the principal concern is *lactic acidosis.* Accordingly, Avandamet should be avoided by patients prone to developing acidosis, including those with renal insufficiency, metabolic acidosis, and heart failure. In addition to lactic acidosis, metformin can cause *GI disturbances* (nausea, diarrhea) and *appetite reduction.*

Avandamet tablets are available in three rosiglitazone/metformin strengths: 1/500 mg, 2/500 mg/ and 4/500 mg. The maximum dosage is 8/2000 mg/day. Recommendations for initial dosages are as follows:

- *Patients already taking metformin alone:* Start with 4 mg rosiglitazone/day plus the dose of metformin already being used. Specifically, for patients taking 1000 mg metformin/day, give one 2/500-mg tablet twice daily, and for patients taking 2000 mg metformin/day, give two 1/500-mg tablets twice daily.
- *Patients already taking rosiglitazone alone:* Start with 1000 mg metformin/day plus the dose of rosiglitazone already being used. Specifically, for patients taking 4 mg rosiglitazone/day, give one 2/500-mg tablet twice daily, and for patients taking 8 mg rosiglitazone/day, give one 4/500-mg tablet twice daily.
- *Patients switching from rosiglitazone and metformin taken separately:* Start with the same dosage of each already in use.

DIABETIC KETOACIDOSIS

Ketoacidosis is the most severe manifestation of insulin deficiency. This syndrome is characterized by hyperglycemia, production of ketoacids, hemoconcentration, acidosis, and coma. Before insulin became available, practically all patients with type 1 diabetes died from ketoacidosis.

Pathogenesis

Diabetic ketoacidosis is brought on by derangements of glucose and fat metabolism. Altered glucose metabolism causes hyperglycemia, water loss, and hemoconcentration. Altered fat metabolism causes production of ketoacids. Figure 54–2 outlines the sequence of metabolic events by which ketoacidosis develops. Note that, in its final stages, the syndrome consists of hemoconcentration and shock in addition to ketoacidosis itself. The alterations in fat and glucose metabolism that lead to ketoacidosis are described in detail below.

Altered Fat Metabolism. Alterations in fat metabolism lead to production of ketoacids. As indicated in Figure 54–2, insulin deficiency promotes lipolysis (breakdown of fats) in adipose tissue. The products of lipolysis are glycerol and free fatty acids (FFA). Both of these metabolites are transported to the liver. In the liver, oxidation of FFA results in the production of two ketoacids (beta-hydroxybutyric acid and acetoacetic acid), also known as ketone bodies. Accumulation of ketoacids puts the body in a state of ketosis. Ketosis can be detected by an odor of decaying apples that ketones impart to the urine. As buildup of ketoacids increases, frank acidosis develops. At this point, the patient's condition changes from ketosis to ketoacidosis. (Ketoacidosis can be distinguished from ketosis by the presence of hyperventilation.) Acidosis contributes to the development of shock.

Altered Glucose Metabolism. Deranged glucose metabolism leads to hyperglycemia, water loss, and hemoconcentration. As shown in Figure 54–2, insulin deficiency has two direct effects on the metabolism of glucose: (1) an increase in glucose production and (2) a decrease in glucose utilization. (The glycerol released by lipolysis is a substrate for glucose synthesis, and therefore helps increase glucose production.) Because more glucose is being made, and less is being used, plasma levels of glucose rise, causing hyperglycemia. Glycosuria develops when plasma glucose content becomes so high that the amount of glucose filtered by the glomeruli exceeds the capacity of the renal tubules for glucose reuptake. As the concentration of glucose in the urine increases, osmotic diuresis develops, resulting in the loss of large volumes of water. Dehydration is worsened owing to vomiting brought on by ketosis. Vomiting is a direct source of fluid loss and, more importantly, is an impediment to rehydration with oral fluids. (It should be noted that, along with loss of water, sodium and potassium are also lost. These positive ions are excreted in conjunction with ketone bodies, compounds that carry a negative charge.) As dehydration becomes more severe, hemoconcentration develops. Hemoconcentration causes cerebral dehydration, which, together with acidosis, leads to shock.

Treatment

Diabetic ketoacidosis is a life-threatening emergency. Treatment is directed at the following: restoration of insulin levels, correction of acidosis, replacement of lost water and sodium, and normalization of potassium and glucose levels. Details of therapy are presented below.

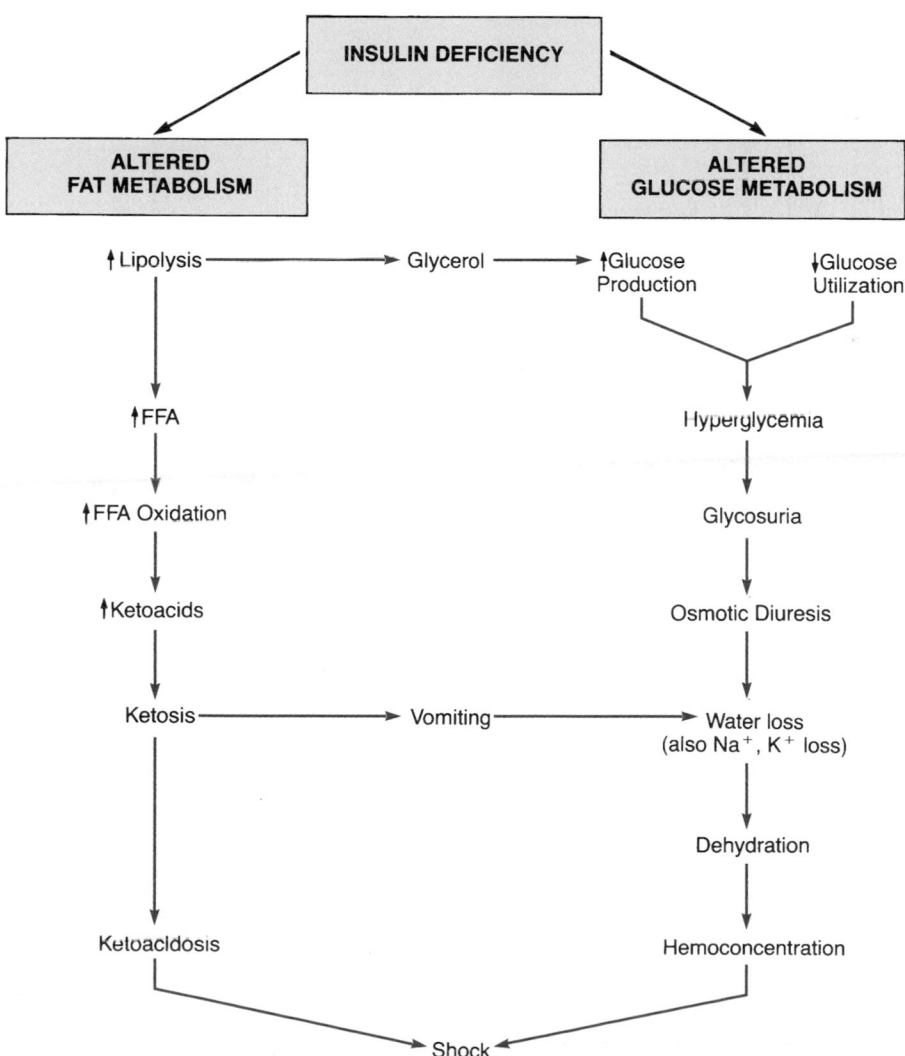

Figure 54–2 ■ Pathogenesis of diabetic ketoacidosis.
The syndrome of ketoacidosis is caused by derangements of fat and glucose metabolism that occur in response to lack of insulin. (FFA = free fatty acids.)

Insulin Replacement. Insulin levels are restored with an initial IV bolus of regular insulin (0.1 U/kg body weight) followed by continuous infusion at 0.1 U/kg/hr. When plasma glucose has fallen to 250 mg/dl, the infusion rate should be reduced to 0.05 U/kg/hr, and a dextrose solution (5% in half-normal saline) should be infused at a rate of 150 to 200 ml/hr. Thereafter, the insulin dosage should be adjusted as needed to maintain plasma glucose levels at 200 mg/dl until acidosis has resolved.

Intravenous infusion of insulin is preferred to SC injection. When insulin is administered SC, insulin levels cannot be lowered quickly in response to excessive dosing; hence, avoiding hypoglycemia may be difficult. In contrast, since insulin levels will drop quickly when an infusion is terminated, infusion permits better regulation of blood glucose content.

Bicarbonate for Acidosis. Treating acidosis with bicarbonate is controversial. Studies have failed to demonstrate any benefit of giving bicarbonate to patients with severe acidosis (blood pH 6.9 to 7.1). Nonetheless, some authorities recommend empiric therapy with bicarbonate if blood pH is below 6.9. The dose is 44.6 mEq of sodium bicarbonate (dissolved in 500 ml of 0.45% saline) infused over 1 hour. Because bicarbonate promotes hypokalemia, potassium should be infused along with the bicarbonate, unless hyperkalemia (serum potassium >5.5 mEq/L) is present.

Water and Sodium Replacement. Dehydration and sodium loss are both corrected with IV saline. Depending on the specific needs of the patient, either 0.9% or 0.45% saline is employed. Adults usually require between 8 and 10 L of fluid during the first 12 hours of treatment. In elderly patients and patients with heart disease, central venous pressure should be monitored.

Potassium Replacement. Loss of potassium is a serious problem and must be corrected. As a rule, potassium is replenished by IV administration. Because hypokalemia predisposes the patient to dysrhythmias, electrocardiographic monitoring is essential.

Treatment of potassium loss is tricky. Why? Because plasma potassium levels may be normal even though intracellular potassium is very low. When insulin is administered, causing cellular uptake of potassium to increase, severe hypokalemia can develop as plasma potassium rushes into potassium-depleted cells. Because of this relationship between insulin administration and plasma potassium levels, the following guidelines apply: (1) if plasma potassium is normal, no potassium should be administered until plasma levels decline in response to insulin; (2) if plasma potassium is low, potassium should be given immediately (and then re-administered if potassium levels fall following insulin administration).

Normalization of Glucose Levels. Treatment of ketoacidosis with insulin may convert hyperglycemia into hypoglycemia. Because cellular uptake of glucose is impaired by insulin deficiency, ketoacidosis is likely to be associated with a reduction in intracellular glucose—despite elevations in plasma glucose content. Under these conditions, insulin administration will cause plasma glucose to rush into the glucose-depleted cells, thereby causing plasma levels of glucose to drop precipitously. If insulin therapy induces hypoglycemia, plasma glucose can be restored by administering glucagon or glucose itself.

GLUCAGON FOR INSULIN OVERDOSE

Glucagon is a polypeptide hormone produced by alpha cells of the pancreatic islets. The hormone increases plasma levels of glucose and relaxes smooth muscle of the GI tract. The drug can be used to elevate blood glucose levels following insulin overdose.

Glucagon has effects on carbohydrate metabolism that are exactly opposite to those of insulin. Specifically, glucagon promotes the breakdown of glycogen, reduces glycogen synthesis, and stimulates biosynthesis of glucose. Hence, whereas insulin acts to lower plasma glucose content, glucagon causes glucose levels to rise. In addition, glucagon acts on GI smooth muscle to promote relaxation.

Glucagon is used to treat hypoglycemia resulting from insulin overdose. However, in patients with severe hypoglycemia, IV glucose is preferred; glucagon should be used only if IV glucose cannot be given. In unconscious patients, glucagon usually produces arousal within 20 minutes. Once consciousness has been restored, oral carbohydrates should be given; these will help prevent recurrence of hypoglycemia and will help replenish hepatic glycogen stores.

Glucagon cannot correct hypoglycemia resulting from starvation. Why? Because glucagon acts in large part by promoting glycogen breakdown, and people who are starved don't have any glycogen left to break down.

Glucagon is administered parenterally (IM, SC, and IV). The drug is dispensed in powder form and must be reconstituted to a concentration of 1 mg/ml (or less) using the diluent supplied by the manufacturer. A dose of 0.5 to 1 mg is usually effective.

⬗ KEY POINTS

- Diabetes mellitus (diabetes) is characterized by sustained hyperglycemia.
- Diabetes has two major forms: type 1 diabetes (formerly insulin-dependent diabetes mellitus) and type 2 diabetes (formerly non–insulin-dependent diabetes mellitus).
- Symptoms of type 1 diabetes result from a complete absence of insulin. The underlying cause is autoimmune destruction of pancreatic beta cells.
- Symptoms of type 2 diabetes result primarily from cellular resistance to insulin's actions, and not from insulin deficiency.
- Type 1 and type 2 diabetes share the same long-term complications: hypertension, heart disease, stroke, blindness, renal failure, neuropathy, lower limb amputations, impotence, and gastroparesis.
- Diabetes is diagnosed if (1) fasting plasma glucose is 126 mg/dl or higher, (2) casual blood glucose is 200 mg/dl or higher, or (3) blood glucose exceeds 200 mg/dl 2 hours after an oral glucose challenge.
- Type 1 diabetes is treated with insulin replacement. Oral hypoglycemics are not used.
- Type 2 diabetes is treated with oral hypoglycemics and/or insulin—but only in conjunction with a program of diet modification and exercise, and only if glycemic control cannot be maintained by diet and exercise alone.
- Self-monitoring of blood glucose (SMBG) is the standard method for day-to-day monitoring of diabetes therapy. The premeal target is 90 to 130 mg/dl, and the peak postmeal target is 180 mg/dl or lower.
- Glycated hemoglobin (HbA$_{1c}$) can be measured every few months to assess long-term glycemic control. The target value is 7% or lower.
- Insulin is anabolic. That is, the hormone promotes conservation of energy and buildup of energy stores.
- Insulin has two basic effects: it (1) stimulates uptake of glucose, amino acids, nucleotides, and potassium; and (2) promotes synthesis of complex organic molecules (glycogen, proteins, triglycerides).
- Insulin deficiency puts the body into a catabolic mode. As a result, glycogen is converted to glucose, proteins are degraded to amino acids, and fats are converted to glycerol (glycerin) and free fatty acids.
- Insulin deficiency promotes hyperglycemia by increasing glycogenolysis and gluconeogenesis and decreasing glucose utilization.
- Seven forms of insulin are used in the United States: regular insulin, lispro insulin, aspart insulin, NPH insulin, lente insulin, ultralente insulin, and glargine insulin.
- Lispro insulin and aspart insulin have a very rapid onset and short duration.
- Regular insulin has a rapid onset and short duration.
- NPH insulin and lente insulin have intermediate durations.
- Ultralente insulin and glargine insulin have prolonged durations.

- All insulins can be injected SC. Regular insulin can be administered IV and IM in addition to SC.
- Insulin suspensions (NPH insulin, lente insulin, ultralente insulin) should be gently agitated before use. Insulin solutions (regular insulin, lispro insulin, glargine insulin) do not need agitation.
- Insulin is used to treat all patients with type 1 diabetes and some patients with type 2 diabetes.
- When insulin therapy produces tight glucose control, it can markedly reduce the long-term complications of diabetes, as demonstrated in the Diabetes Complications and Control Trial (DCCT) and the United Kingdom Prospective Diabetes Study (UKPDS).
- To achieve tight glucose control, patients with type 1 diabetes must practice intensive insulin therapy, consisting of either (1) an evening injection of ultralente insulin or glargine insulin supplemented with mealtime injections of regular, lispro, or aspart insulin; or (2) continuous SC infusion of regular, lispro, or aspart insulin supplemented with mealtime bolus doses. With both approaches, the mealtime dose is adjusted to match caloric intake. Tight glucose control cannot be achieved with conventional insulin therapy (i.e., one or two injections a day).
- SMBG is an essential component of intensive therapy. Blood glucose should be measured 3 to 5 times a day.
- Compared with conventional therapy, intensive insulin therapy carries a greater risk of hypoglycemia. Other drawbacks are greater cost, inconvenience, complexity, and weight gain.
- The principal adverse effect of insulin is hypoglycemia (blood glucose <50 mg/dl), which occurs whenever insulin levels exceed insulin needs. Symptoms include tachycardia, palpitations, sweating, headache, confusion, drowsiness, and fatigue. If hypoglycemia is severe, convulsions, coma, and death may follow.

- Beta blockers can delay awareness of hypoglycemia by masking signs that are caused by activation of the sympathetic nervous system (e.g., tachycardia, palpitations).
- Insulin-induced hypoglycemia can be treated with a fast-acting oral sugar (e.g., glucose tablets, orange juice, sugar cubes), IV glucose, or parenteral glucagon.
- Oral hypoglycemic drugs—sulfonylureas, meglitinides, metformin, thiazolidinediones, and alpha-glucosidase inhibitors—are indicated only for type 2 diabetes. They are not used for type 1 diabetes.
- Sulfonylureas stimulate release of insulin from the pancreas. They may also increase cellular sensitivity to insulin.
- The major adverse effect of sulfonylureas is hypoglycemia.
- Metformin (a biguanide) decreases glucose production by the liver and increases glucose uptake by muscle.
- The major adverse effects of metformin are GI disturbances: decreased appetite, nausea, and diarrhea.
- Rarely, metformin causes lactic acidosis, which can be fatal. The risk of lactic acidosis is greatly increased by renal impairment, which decreases metformin excretion and thereby causes drug levels to rise rapidly.
- Acarbose (an alpha-glucosidase inhibitor) inhibits digestion and absorption of carbohydrates, and thereby reduces the postprandial rise in blood glucose. To be effective, the drug must be taken with every meal.
- The major adverse effects of acarbose are GI disturbances: flatulence, cramps, and abdominal distention.
- Rosiglitazone (a thiazolidinedione) increases insulin sensitivity in patients with type 2 diabetes, and thereby increases glucose uptake by muscle and decreases glucose production by the liver.
- Rosiglitazone promotes water retention, and can thereby cause weight gain and edema. Water retention can cause heart failure, and can exacerbate symptoms in those who already have the disease.

Summary of Major Nursing Implications*

INSULIN

Preadministration Assessment

Therapeutic Goal

Insulin is required by all patients with type 1 diabetes and by some with type 2 diabetes. The goal of insulin therapy is to maintain plasma glucose levels within an acceptable range (see Table 54–3).

Baseline Data

Assess for clinical manifestations of diabetes (e.g., polyuria, polydipsia, polyphagia, weight loss) and for indications of hyperglycemia. Baseline laboratory tests may include casual plasma glucose, FPG, an OGTT, HbA$_{1c}$, urinary glucose and ketones, and serum electrolytes.

Identifying High-Risk Patients

Special care is needed in patients taking drugs that can raise or lower blood glucose levels, including sympathomimetics, beta blockers, glucocorticoids, sulfonylureas, metformin, repaglinide, and thiazolidinediones (e.g., troglitazone).

Patients with a history of severe allergic reactions to insulin derived from pork pancreas should be treated with a human insulin or a human insulin analog.

Implementation: Administration

Routes

All insulins may be administered SC. None are given PO. Regular insulin may be administered IM and IV in addition to SC.

*Patient education information is highlighted as blue text.

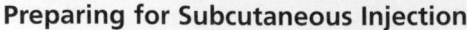

Summary of Major Nursing Implications*—cont'd

Preparing for Subcutaneous Injection

Teach the patient to prepare for SC injections as follows:

- Before loading the syringe, disperse insulin suspensions (i.e., all forms of insulin except lispro, regular, and glargine insulin) by rolling the vial gently between the palms. Vigorous agitation causes frothing and must be avoided. If granules or clumps remain after mixing, discard the vial.
- Regular, lispro, and glargine insulin are clear solutions, and hence can be administered without mixing. If a preparation becomes cloudy or discolored, or if a precipitate develops, discard the vial.
- Before loading the syringe, swab the bottle cap with alcohol.
- Eliminate air bubbles from the syringe and needle after loading.
- Cleanse the skin with alcohol prior to injection.

Sites of Injection

- Provide the patient with the following instruction regarding sites of SC injection:
- Usual sites of injection are the upper arms, thighs, and abdomen. To minimize variability in responses, make all injections in just one of these areas.
- Rotate the injection site within the general area employed (i.e., abdomen, thigh, or upper arm).
- Allow about 1 inch between sites. If possible, use each site just once a month.

Insulin Storage

Teach the patient the following about insulin storage:

- Store unopened vials of insulin in the refrigerator, but do not freeze. When stored under these conditions, insulin can be used up to the expiration date on the vial.
- The vial in current use can be stored at room temperature for up to 1 month, but must be kept out of direct sunlight and extreme heat. Discard partially filled vials after several weeks if left unused.
- Mixtures of insulin prepared in vials may be stored for 1 month at room temperature, and for 3 months under refrigeration.
- Mixtures of insulin in prefilled syringes (plastic or glass) should be stored in a refrigerator, where they will be stable for at least 1 week, and perhaps 2. Store the syringe vertically (needle pointing up) to avoid clogging the needle. Gently agitate the syringe prior to administration to resuspend the insulin.

Dosage Adjustment

The dosing goal is to maintain blood glucose levels within an acceptable range. Dosage must be adjusted to balance changes in caloric intake and other factors that can decrease insulin needs (strenuous exercise, pregnancy during the first trimester) or increase insulin needs (illness, trauma, stress, adolescent growth spurt, pregnancy after the first trimester).

Regular insulin can adsorb in varying amounts onto IV infusion sets. Dosage adjustments made to compensate for losses are based on the therapeutic response.

Patient and Family Education

Patient and family education is an absolute requirement for safe and successful glycemic control. Provide patients and their families with thorough instruction on

- The nature of diabetes
- The importance of tight glucose control
- The major components of the treatment routine (insulin, SMBG, diet, exercise)
- Procedures for purchasing insulin, syringes, and needles
- Methods of insulin storage
- Procedures for mixing insulins
- Calculation of dosage adjustments
- Techniques of insulin injection
- Rotation of injection sites
- Measurement of blood glucose content
- Signs and management of hypoglycemia
- Signs and management of hyperglycemia
- Special problems of diabetic pregnancy
- The procedure for obtaining Medic Alert registration
- The importance of not making arbitrary switches between insulins made by different manufacturers and between human and pork insulins

Ongoing Evaluation and Interventions
Evaluating Therapeutic Effects

Whenever practical, SMBG should be employed to evaluate treatment. Teach patients how to use the blood glucose measuring device, and encourage them to monitor blood glucose daily. Urinary glucose may be monitored as an alternative, but these measurements are much less useful than SMBG. The physician may request tests of hemoglobin A_{1c} to assess long-term glycemic control.

Minimizing Adverse Effects

Hypoglycemia. Hypoglycemia occurs whenever insulin levels exceed insulin needs. Inform the patient about potential causes of hypoglycemia (e.g., insulin overdose, reduced food intake, vomiting, diarrhea, excessive consumption of alcohol, unaccustomed exercise, termination of pregnancy), and teach the patient and family members to recognize the early signs and symptoms of hypoglycemia (tachycardia, palpitations, sweating, nervousness, headache, confusion, drowsiness, fatigue).

Rapid treatment is mandatory. If the patient is conscious, oral carbohydrates are indicated (e.g., glucose tablets, orange juice, sugar cubes, honey, corn syrup, nondiet soda). However, if the swallowing or gag reflex is suppressed, nothing should be administered PO. For unconscious patients, IV glucose is the treatment of choice. Parenteral glucagon is an alternative.

Hypoglycemic coma must be differentiated from coma of diabetic ketoacidosis (DKA). The differential diagnosis is

---

*Patient education information is highlighted as blue text.

Summary of Major Nursing Implications*—cont'd

made by measuring plasma or urinary glucose content: Hypoglycemic coma is associated with very low levels of glucose, whereas high levels signify DKA.

Lipohypertrophy. Accumulation of subcutaneous fat can occur at sites of frequent insulin injection. **Inform the patient that lipohypertrophy can be minimized by systematic rotation of the injection site.**

Systemic Allergic Reactions. Systemic reactions (widespread urticaria, impairment of breathing) are rare. Systemic allergy is most common with beef insulin (no longer sold in the United States) and less likely with pork or human insulin. If systemic allergy develops, it can be reduced through desensitization (i.e., administration of small initial doses of purified pork or human insulin followed by a series of progressively larger doses).

Minimizing Adverse Interactions

Hypoglycemic Agents. Several drugs, including *sulfonylureas, meglitinides, alcohol* (used acutely), and *beta blockers,* can intensify hypoglycemia induced by insulin. When any of these drugs is combined with insulin, special care must be taken to ensure that blood glucose content does not fall too low.

Hyperglycemic Agents. Several drugs, including thiazide diuretics, glucocorticoids, and sympathomimetics, can elevate blood glucose, and can thereby counteract the beneficial effects of insulin. When these agents are combined with insulin, increased insulin dosage may be required.

Beta Blockers. Beta blockade can mask sympathetic responses (e.g., tachycardia, palpitations, tremors) to declining blood glucose, and can thereby delay awareness of insulin-induced hypoglycemia. Also, because beta blockade impairs glycogenolysis, beta blockers can make insulin-induced hypoglycemia even worse.

SULFONYLUREAS

Acetohexamide
Chlorpropamide
Glimepiride
Glipizide
Glyburide
Tolazamide
Tolbutamide

*Patient education information is highlighted as blue text.

Preadministration Assessment
Therapeutic Goal

Sulfonylureas are used as an adjunct to caloric restriction and exercise to maintain glycemic control in patients with type 2 diabetes. These drugs do not work in patients with type 1 diabetes.

Identifying High-Risk Patients

Sulfonylureas are *contraindicated* during pregnancy and breast-feeding. Use with *caution* in patients with kidney or liver dysfunction. Sulfonylureas should not be used in conjunction with alcohol.

Implementation: Administration
Route

Oral.

Administration

Advise patients to administer with food if GI upset occurs.

Note that dosages for the second-generation agents are much lower than dosages for first-generation agents (see Table 54–10).

Sulfonylureas are intended only as supplemental therapy of type 2 diabetes. Encourage patients to maintain their established program of exercise and caloric restriction.

Ongoing Evaluation and Interventions
Minimizing Adverse Effects

Hypoglycemia. **Inform patients about signs of hypoglycemia (palpitations, tachycardia, sweating, fatigue, excessive hunger), and instruct them to notify the physician if these occur.** Treat severe hypoglycemia with IV glucose.

Use in Pregnancy and Lactation

Pregnancy. Discontinue sulfonylureas during pregnancy. If a hypoglycemic agent is needed, insulin is the drug of choice.

Lactation. Sulfonylureas are excreted into breast milk, posing a risk of hypoglycemia to the nursing infant. Women who choose to breast-feed should substitute insulin for the sulfonylurea.

CHAPTER 55

Drugs for Thyroid Disorders

THYROID PHYSIOLOGY
THYROID PATHOPHYSIOLOGY
- Hypothyroidism
- Hyperthyroidism

THYROID FUNCTION TESTS
THYROID HORMONE PREPARATIONS FOR HYPOTHYROIDISM
- Levothyroxine (T_4)
- Liothyronine (T_3)
- Other Thyroid Preparations

DRUGS FOR HYPERTHYROIDISM
- Propylthiouracil
- Methimazole
- Radioactive Iodine (^{131}I)
- Nonradioactive Iodine
- Propranolol

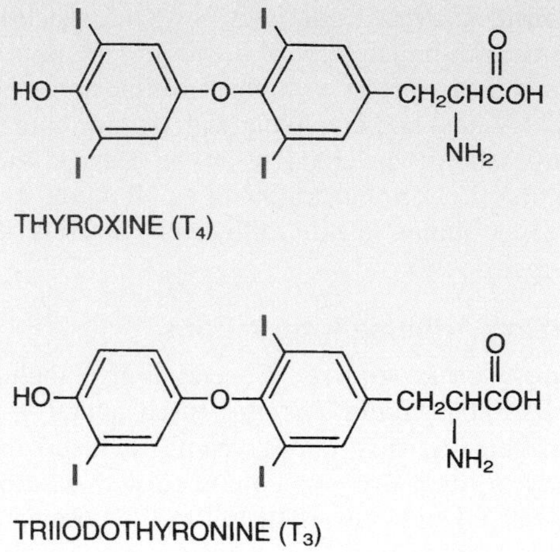

Figure 55–1 ■ **Structural formulas of the thyroid hormones.**

Thyroid hormones have profound effects on metabolism, cardiac function, growth, and development. These hormones stimulate the metabolic rate of most cells, and increase the force and rate of cardiac contraction. During infancy and childhood, thyroid hormones promote maturation; severe deficiency can produce dwarfism and permanent mental impairment. Fortunately, most abnormalities of thyroid function can be effectively treated.

We begin our study of thyroid drugs by reviewing thyroid physiology. Next we review the pathophysiology of hypothyroid and hyperthyroid states. Having established this background, we then discuss the agents used for thyroid disorders.

THYROID PHYSIOLOGY

Chemistry and Nomenclature

The thyroid gland produces two active hormones: triiodothyronine (T_3) and thyroxine (T_4, tetraiodothyronine). As shown in Figure 55–1, the structures of these hormones are nearly identical. The only difference is that T_4 contains four atoms of iodine, whereas T_3 contains three. The biologic effects of T_3 and T_4 are qualitatively similar. However, when compared on a molar basis, T_3 is more potent than T_4.

The preparations of T_3 and T_4 employed clinically, although synthetic, are identical in structure to the naturally occurring hormones. The generic name of synthetic T_3 is *liothyronine,* and the generic name of synthetic T_4 is *levothyroxine.* A fixed-ratio mixture of T_3 plus T_4, known as *liotrix,* is also available.

Thyroid Hormone Actions

Thyroid hormones have three principal actions: (1) stimulation of energy use, (2) stimulation of the heart, and (3) promotion of growth and development. Stimulation of energy use elevates the basal metabolic rate, resulting in increased oxygen consumption and increased heat production. Stimulation of the heart increases both the rate and force of contraction, resulting in increased cardiac output and increased oxygen demand. Thyroid effects on growth and development are profound: thyroid hormones are essential for normal development of the brain and other components of the nervous system, and they have a significant impact on maturation of skeletal muscle.

Synthesis and Fate of Thyroid Hormones

Synthesis. Synthesis of thyroid hormones takes place in four basic steps (Fig. 55–2). The circled numbers in the figure correspond with the steps below.

- *Step 1.* Formation of thyroid hormone begins with the active transport of *iodide* into the thyroid. Under normal conditions, this uptake process produces concentrations of iodide within the thyroid that are 20 to 50 times greater than the concentration of iodide in plasma. When plasma iodide levels are extremely low, intrathyroid iodide content may reach levels that are more than 100 times greater than those in plasma.
- *Step 2.* Following uptake, iodide undergoes oxidation to *iodine,* the active form of iodide. Oxidation of iodide is catalyzed by an enzyme called *peroxidase.*

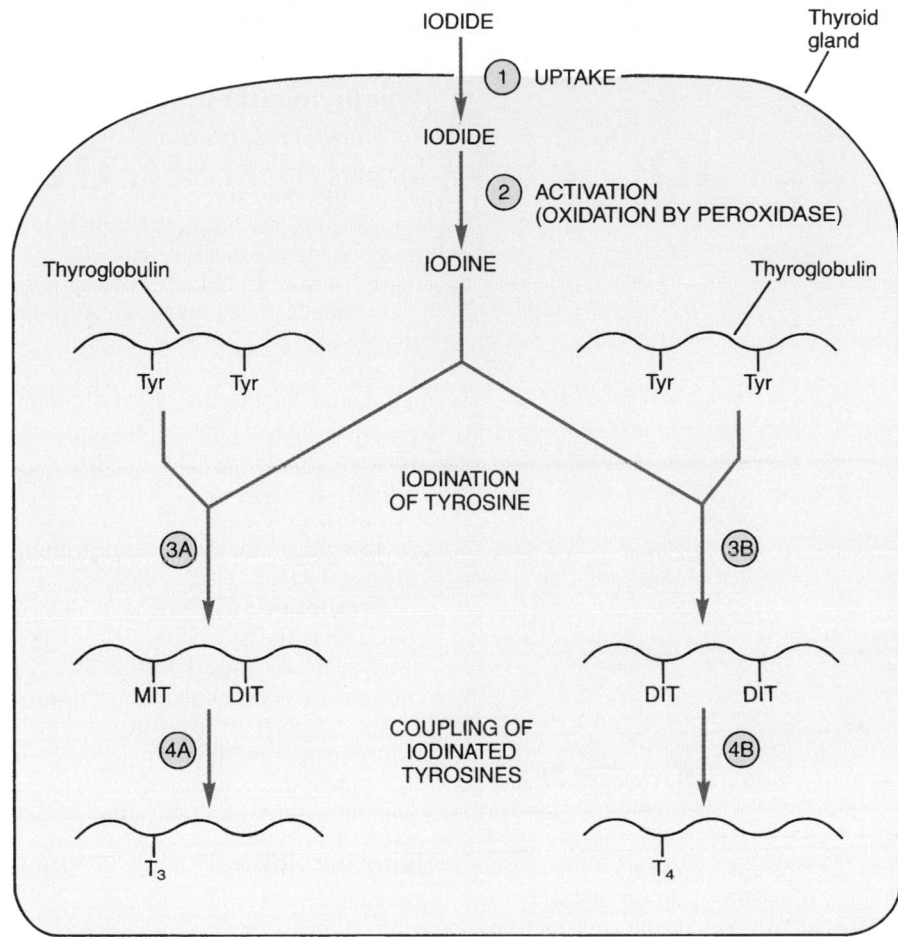

Figure 55–2 ■ Steps in thyroid hormone synthesis.
The reactions at each step (circled numbers) are explained in the text. (DIT = diiodotyrosine, MIT = monoiodotyrosine, T_3 = triiodothyronine, T_4 = thyroxine, Tyr = tyrosine.)

■ *Step 3.* In this step, activated iodine becomes incorporated into tyrosine residues that are bound to *thyroglobulin,* a large glycoprotein molecule. As indicated in Figure 55–2, one tyrosine molecule may receive either one or two iodine atoms, resulting in the production of monoiodotyrosine (MIT) and diiodotyrosine (DIT), respectively.

■ *Step 4.* In the final step of thyroid hormone synthesis, iodinated tyrosine molecules are coupled. Coupling of one DIT with one MIT forms T_3 (step 4A); coupling of one DIT with another DIT forms T_4 (step 4B).

Fate. Thyroid hormones are released from the thyroid gland by a proteolytic process. The amount of T_4 released is substantially greater than the amount of T_3. However, much of the T_4 that is released undergoes conversion to T_3 by enzymes in peripheral tissues. In fact, conversion of T_4 to T_3 accounts for the majority (about 80%) of the T_3 found in plasma.

More than 99.5% of the T_3 and T_4 in plasma is bound to plasma proteins. Consequently, only a tiny fraction of circulating thyroid hormone is free to produce biologic effects.

Thyroid hormones are eliminated primarily by hepatic metabolism. Because T_3 and T_4 are extensively bound to plasma proteins, metabolism takes place slowly. As a result, the half-lives of these hormones are prolonged. Triiodothyronine has a half-life of 1.5 days and T_4 has a half-life of 1 week.

Regulation of Thyroid Function by the Hypothalamus and Anterior Pituitary

The functional relationship between the hypothalamus, anterior pituitary, and thyroid is depicted in Figure 55–3. As indicated, thyrotropin-releasing hormone (TRH), secreted by the hypothalamus, acts on the pituitary to cause secretion of thyrotropin (thyroid-stimulating hormone; [TSH]). TSH then acts on the thyroid to stimulate all aspects of thyroid function: thyroid size is enlarged, iodine uptake is augmented, and synthesis and release of thyroid hormones are increased. In response to rising plasma levels of T_3 and T_4, further release of TSH is suppressed. The stimulatory effect of TSH on the thyroid, followed by the inhibitory effect of thyroid hormones on the pituitary, constitutes a negative feedback loop.

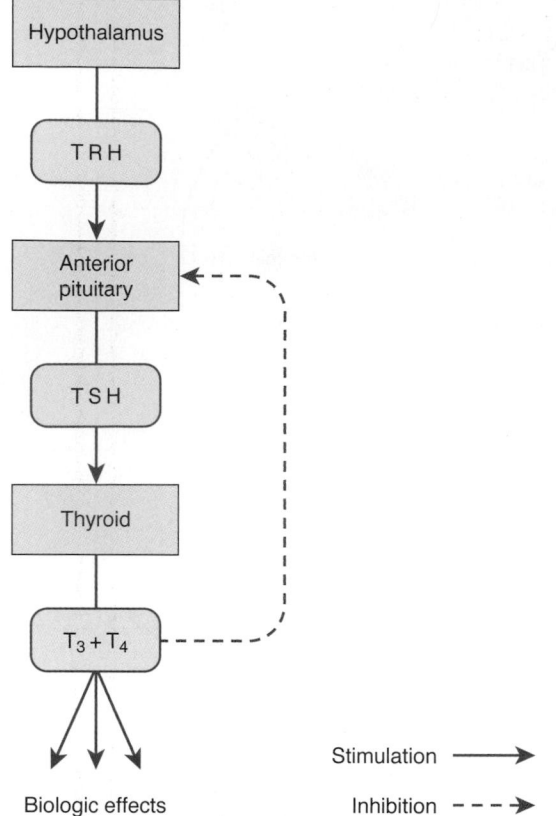

Figure 55–3 ■ **Regulation of thyroid function.**
TRH from the hypothalamus stimulates release of TSH from the pituitary. TSH stimulates all aspects of thyroid function, including release of T_3 and T_4. T_3 and T_4 act on the pituitary to suppress further TSH release. (T_3 = triiodothyronine, T_4 = thyroxine, TRH = thyrotropin-releasing hormone, TSH = thyrotropin [thyroid-stimulating hormone].)

Influence of Iodine Levels on Thyroid Function

Low Iodine. When iodine availability is diminished, production of thyroid hormones decreases. The ensuing drop in thyroid hormone levels promotes release of TSH. In response to increased levels of TSH, thyroid size increases (causing goiter), and the ability of the thyroid to concentrate iodine increases as well. If the iodine deficiency is not too severe, the increased capacity for iodine uptake will permit production of thyroid hormones in amounts sufficient to return plasma levels of T_3 and T_4 to normal.

High Iodine. The effect of extremely high iodine levels on thyroid function is opposite to that of low iodine: uptake of iodide is suppressed, and synthesis and release of thyroid hormones decline. The mechanisms underlying these effects are not fully understood.

THYROID PATHOPHYSIOLOGY

Hypothyroidism

Hypothyroidism can occur at any age. In the adult, mild deficiency of thyroid hormone is referred to simply as *hypothyroidism.* Severe deficiency in adults is called *myx-*

edema. When hypothyroidism occurs in infancy, the resulting condition is called *cretinism.*

Hypothyroidism in Adults

Clinical Presentation. Hypothyroidism in adults produces a characteristic set of signs and symptoms. The face is pale, puffy, and expressionless. The skin is cold and dry. The hair is brittle, and hair loss occurs. Heart rate and temperature are lowered. The patient may complain of lethargy, fatigue, and intolerance to cold. Mentality may be impaired. Thyroid enlargement (goiter) may occur if reduced levels of T_3 and T_4 promote excessive release of TSH.

Causes. Hypothyroidism in the adult is usually due to malfunction of the thyroid itself. In iodine-sufficient countries, the principal cause of thyroid malfunction is *chronic autoimmune thyroiditis* (Hashimoto's disease). Other causes are insufficient iodine in the diet, surgical removal of the thyroid, and destruction of the thyroid by radioactive iodine. Adult hypothyroidism may also result from insufficient secretion of TSH and TRH.

Therapeutic Strategy. Hypothyroidism in adults requires replacement therapy with thyroid hormones. In almost all cases, treatment must continue lifelong. Today, the standard replacement regimen consists of *levothyroxine* (T_4) alone. However, as discussed in Box 55–1, combined therapy with levothyroxine plus liothyronine (T_3) may be superior. When replacement doses are adequate, they eliminate all signs and symptoms of thyroid deficiency.

Hypothyroidism During Pregnancy

Maternal hypothyroidism can result in permanent neuropsychologic deficits in the child. We have long known that *congenital* hypothyroidism can cause mental retardation and other developmental problems (see below under *Hypothyroidism in Infants*). However, it was not until 1999 that researchers demonstrated that *maternal* hypothyroidism—in the absence of fetal hypothyroidism—can decrease IQ and other aspects of neuropsychologic function. The impact of maternal hypothyroidism is limited largely to the first trimester, a time during which the fetus is unable to produce thyroid hormones of its own. By the second trimester, the fetal thyroid gland is fully functional, and hence the fetus can supply its own hormones from then on. Therefore, to help ensure healthy fetal development, maternal hypothyroidism must be diagnosed and treated very early. Unfortunately, symptoms of hypothyroidism are often nonspecific (irritability, tiredness, poor concentration, etc.)—or there may be no symptoms at all. Accordingly, some authorities now recommend routine screening for hypothyroidism as soon as pregnancy is confirmed. If hypothyroidism is diagnosed, replacement therapy should begin immediately. In addition, because thyroid hormone requirements typically increase over the course of pregnancy, thyroid hormone levels should be monitored and dosage increased as needed.

Hypothyroidism in Infants

Clinical Presentation. Thyroid deficiency in infants (cretinism) causes mental retardation and derangement of growth. In the absence of thyroid hormones, the child develops a large and protruding tongue, potbelly, and dwarfish stature. Development of the nervous system, bones, teeth, and muscles is impaired.

Special Interest Topic

BOX 55-1 ■■ T₃ OR NOT T₃? . . . THAT IS THE QUESTION

Since the mid-1970s, the standard treatment for hypothyroidism has been replacement therapy with levothyroxine (T_4) alone. However, although this approach is satisfactory for most patients, a significant minority complain that they just don't feel right: They're depressed, fatigued, and can't concentrate. Recent evidence suggests that, for these patients, combined therapy with levothyroxine *plus* liothyronine (T_3) may produce a more desirable result.

Why do we treat hypothyroidism with just one hormone (T_4), when the thyroid itself produces two (T_3 and T_4)? The rationale is simple: When patients take T_4, enzymes in target tissues convert some of it to T_3. As a result, treatment with T_4 alone produces normal blood levels of both hormones. Therefore, giving T_3 appears unnecessary. However, studies with thyroidectomized rats suggest that the picture is more complex. Specifically, these studies indicate that conversion of exogenous T_4 to T_3 does not take place to the same extent in all tissues. For example, less T_3 is formed in the liver and kidneys than in other tissues. Hence, although replacement therapy with T_4 may produce normal *blood* levels of T_3, levels of T_3 in some *tissues* may be inadequate. This raises the possibility that low levels of T_3 in the *brain* may underlie the neuropsychologic deficits experienced by some hypothyroid patients when they are treated with T_4 alone. This, in turn, raises the possibility that treatment with a combination of T_3 and T_4 might work better.

In 1999, researchers reported in the *New England Journal of Medicine* that partial substitution of T_3 for T_4 can improve mood and neuropsychologic function in hypothyroid patients.[1] In this double-blind, crossover study, 33 patients were evaluated at the end of two 5-week periods. During one period, they took their normal dose of T_4 alone. During the other period, the dose of T_4 was reduced by 50 mg, and 12.5 mg of T_3 was added. After each 5-week period, patients underwent a battery of biochemical and psychologic tests. The results? The biochemical tests indicated that, with either regimen, indices of thyroid function were within the normal range. However, the psychologic tests indicated that most patients fared better when a low dose of T_3 was substituted for some of their T_4: scores for depression, fatigue, and anger declined, and overall scores for mood improved. Of the 33 patients, 20 preferred the combination of T_3 plus T_4, 11 had no preference, and 2 preferred T_4 alone (because adding T_3 made them feel nervous). The authors concluded that treating hypothyroidism with a combination of T_3 plus T_4 may produce a better quality of life than treatment with T_4 alone.

Should combined treatment with T_3 and T_4 become the new standard of care? For now, at least, the answer is "No"—for two reasons. First, most patients treated with T_4 alone have no complaints, and hence there is no compelling reason to alter their therapy. Second, currently available formulations of thyroid hormones are not suited for combination therapy. To mimic daily production of thyroid hormones, the ideal regimen would contain about 10 mg of T_3 and 100 mg of T_4. Furthermore, to avoid adverse cardiac effects, the T_3 should be in a *slow-release* formulation. None of the thyroid products available today, if used alone or in combination, can deliver the appropriate doses of T_3 and T_4 over an appropriate time span. However, when an acceptable formulation *does* become available, patients who are unsatisfied with T_4 alone may do well to consider a switch to combination therapy.

[1]Bunevicius R, Kazanavicius G, Zalinkevicius R, Prange AJ Jr. Effects of thyroxine as compared with thyroxine plus triiodothyronine in patients with hypothyroidism. N Engl J Med 1999;340:424–429.

Causes. Cretinism usually results from a failure in thyroid development. Other causes include autoimmune disease, severe iodine deficiency, TSH deficiency, and exposure to radioactive iodine *in utero*.

Therapeutic Strategy. Hypothyroidism in newborns requires replacement therapy with thyroid hormones. If treatment is initiated within a few days of birth, physical and mental development will be normal. However, if therapy is delayed for several months, some permanent retardation will be evident, although the physical effects of thyroid deficiency will reverse. Replacement therapy must continue for life.

Hyperthyroidism

There are two major forms of hyperthyroidism: *Graves' disease* and *toxic nodular goiter* (also known as *Plummer's disease*). Of the two, Graves' disease is more common. Signs and symptoms of both disorders are similar. The principal difference is that Graves' disease may cause exophthalmos, whereas toxic nodular goiter does not. If levels of thyroid hormone rise extremely high, patients with either form of hyperthyroidism may experience *thyrotoxic crisis*.

Graves' Disease

Graves' disease is the most common cause of excessive thyroid hormone secretion. This disorder occurs most frequently in women 20 to 40 years of age. The incidence in females is 6 times greater than in males.

Clinical Presentation. Most clinical manifestations of Graves' disease result from elevated levels of thyroid hormone. Heartbeat is rapid and strong, and dysrhythmias and angina may develop. The central nervous system is stimulated, resulting in rapid thought flow and rapid speech, nervousness, and insomnia. Skeletal muscles may weaken and atrophy. Metabolic rate is raised, resulting in increased heat production, increased body temperature, intolerance to heat, and skin that is warm and moist. Appetite is increased; however, despite increased food consumption, weight loss occurs if caloric intake fails to match the increase in metabolic rate. Collectively, the above signs and symptoms are referred to as *thyrotoxicosis*.

In addition to thyrotoxicosis, patients with Graves' disease often present with *exophthalmos* (protrusion of the eyeballs). The cause is obscure. However, we do know the condition is not caused by increased levels of thyroid hormones.

Cause. Thyroid stimulation in Graves' disease is caused by thyroid-stimulating immunoglobulins (TSIs). These immunoglobulins are antibodies produced by an autoimmune process. TSIs increase thyroid activity by stimulating receptors for TSH on the thyroid gland. That is, TSIs mimic the effects of TSH on thyroid function. TSIs are not responsible for exophthalmos.

Treatment. Treatment for Graves' disease is directed at decreasing the production of thyroid hormones. Three modalities are employed: (1) surgical removal of thyroid tissue, (2) destruction of thyroid tissue with radioactive iodine, and (3) suppression of thyroid hormone synthesis with antithyroid drugs (e.g., propylthiouracil, methimazole). In the United States, radiation is the preferred treatment for adults, whereas antithyroid drugs are preferred for younger patients.

Propranolol and nonradioactive iodine may be used as adjunctive therapy. Propranolol suppresses tachycardia by blocking beta-adrenergic receptors on the heart. Nonradioactive iodine inhibits synthesis and release of thyroid hormones.

Since exophthalmos is not the result of hyperthyroidism per se, this condition is not improved by lowering thyroid hormone production. If exophthalmos is severe, it can be treated with high doses of oral glucocorticoids.

Toxic Nodular Goiter (Plummer's Disease)

Toxic nodular goiter is the result of thyroid adenoma. Clinical manifestations are much like those of Graves' disease, except exophthalmos is absent. Toxic nodular goiter is a persistent condition that rarely undergoes spontaneous remission. Treatment modalities are the same as for Graves' disease. However, if antithyroid drugs are used, symptoms return rapidly when the drugs are withdrawn. Accordingly, surgery and radiation, which provide long-term control, are often preferred.

Thyrotoxic Crisis (Thyroid Storm)

Thyrotoxic crisis occurs when levels of thyroid hormone become extremely high. The syndrome is characterized by hyperthermia, severe tachycardia, and profound weakness. Unconsciousness, coma, and heart failure may ensue. Thyrotoxic crisis can be caused by excessive production of endogenous thyroid hormones or by overdose with thyroid hormones during replacement therapy.

Thyrotoxic crisis can be life threatening and requires immediate treatment. High doses of potassium iodide or strong iodine solution are given to suppress thyroid hormone release. Propylthiouracil is given to suppress thyroid hormone synthesis and conversion of T_4 to T_3 in the periphery. Propranolol is given to reduce heart rate. Additional measures include sedation, cooling, and giving glucocorticoids and IV fluids.

THYROID FUNCTION TESTS

Several laboratory tests can be used to evaluate thyroid function. Three are described below. Normal values are summarized in Table 55–1.

Serum T_4 Test. The serum T_4 test measures total (bound plus free) *thyroxine*. Because serum T_4 levels reflect overall thyroid activity, this test is useful for initial screening of thyroid function: levels of T_4 will be low in hypothyroid patients and high in hyperthyroid patients. The test can also be used to monitor thyroid hormone replacement therapy: All thyroid preparations, except liothyronine, should cause T_4 levels to rise.

Serum T_3 Test. The T_3 test measures total (bound plus free) *triiodothyronine*. This test is useful for diagnosing hyperthyroidism, because in this disorder levels of T_3 often rise sooner and to a greater extent than levels of T_4. T_3 determinations can also be employed to monitor thyroid hormone replacement therapy; all thyroid preparations should increase levels of T_3.

Serum TSH. Measurement of serum TSH is the most sensitive method for diagnosing hypothyroidism. Why? Because very small reductions in serum T_3 and T_4 cause a dramatic rise in serum TSH. Hence, even when the degree of hypothyroidism is minimal, it will be reflected by an abnormally high TSH level. When replacement therapy is instituted, TSH levels should return to normal.

Serum TSH determinations can also be used to distinguish primary hypothyroidism from secondary hypothyroidism. In primary (thyroidal) hypothyroidism, TSH levels are high, whereas in secondary hypothyroidism (hypothyroidism resulting from anterior pituitary dysfunction), TSH levels are low.

THYROID HORMONE PREPARATIONS FOR HYPOTHYROIDISM

Thyroid hormones are available as pure, synthetic compounds and as extracts of animal thyroid glands. All preparations have qualitatively similar effects. The synthetic preparations are more stable and better standardized than the animal gland extracts. As a result, the synthetics are preferred to the natural products. Properties of thyroid hormone preparations are summarized in Table 55–2.

TABLE 55–1 ■ Normal Values for Thyroid Function Tests

Test	Traditional Units	SI Units
Serum thyrotropin (TSH)	0.4–4.8 μU/ml	0.4–4.8 mU/L
Serum total thyroxine (T_4)	4.5–12.0 μg/dl	58–154 nmol/L
Serum free thyroxine (FT_4)	0.9–2.1 ng/dl	12–27 pmol/ml
Thyroxine-binding globulin (TBG)	15–34 μg/ml	15–34 mg/L
Serum total triiodothyronine (T_3)	70–190 ng/dl	1.1–2.9 nmol/L

Levothyroxine (T₄)

Levothyroxine [Levothroid, Levoxyl, Synthroid, Unithroid, others] is a synthetic preparation of thyroxine (T₄), a naturally occurring thyroid hormone. The structure of levothyroxine is identical to that of the natural hormone. Levothyroxine is the drug of choice for most patients who require thyroid hormone replacement. Consequently, levothyroxine will serve as our prototype for the thyroid hormone preparations.

Pharmacokinetics

Conversion to T₃. Much of an administered dose of levothyroxine is converted to T₃ in the body. As a result, levothyroxine can produce nearly normal levels of both T₃ and T₄. Hence, for most patients, there is no need to give T₃ along with levothyroxine.

Half-Life and Plasma Levels. Because levothyroxine is highly protein bound (about 99.97%), the hormone has a prolonged half-life (about 7 days). From a clinical perspective, this long half-life has advantages as well as disadvantages. On the negative side, about 1 month (four half-lives) is required for plasma levels of levothyroxine to reach plateau. As a result, onset of full effects is delayed. On the positive side, a long half-life causes hormone levels to remain steady between doses. This property permits once-a-day dosing, which makes levothyroxine well suited for lifelong therapy.

Therapeutic Uses

Levothyroxine is indicated for all forms of hypothyroidism, regardless of cause. The drug is used for cretinism, myxedema coma, ordinary hypothyroidism in adults and children, and simple goiter. Levothyroxine is also used to treat hypothyroidism resulting from insufficient TSH (secondary to pituitary malfunction) and from insufficient TRH (secondary to hypothalamic malfunction). In addition, levothyroxine is used to maintain proper levels of thyroid hormones following thyroid surgery, irradiation, and treatment with antithyroid drugs.

Levothyroxine and other thyroid hormones should not be taken to treat obesity. These hormones will accelerate metabolism and promote weight reduction only if the dosage is high enough to establish a pathologic (hyperthyroid) state.

Adverse Effects

When administered in appropriate dosage, levothyroxine rarely causes adverse effects. If the dosage is excessive, *thyrotoxicosis* may result. Signs and symptoms include tachycardia, angina, tremor, nervousness, insomnia, hyperthermia,

heat intolerance, and sweating. The patient should be informed about these signs and instructed to notify the physician if they develop. If the dosage is especially large, thyrotoxic crisis may occur.

Drug Interactions

Drugs That Reduce Levothyroxine Absorption. Absorption of levothyroxine can be reduced by the following drugs:

- Cholestyramine [Questran]
- Colestipol [Colestid]
- Calcium supplements (e.g., Tums, Os-Cal)
- Sucralfate [Carafate]
- Aluminum-containing antacids (e.g., Maalox, Mylanta)
- Iron supplements (e.g., ferrous sulfate)

To ensure adequate absorption of levothyroxine, patients should separate administration of levothyroxine and these drugs by 3 to 4 hours.

Drugs That Accelerate Levothyroxine Metabolism. Several drugs can accelerate the metabolism of levothyroxine. Among these are phenytoin [Dilantin], carbamazepine [Tegretol, Carbatrol], rifampin [Rifadin, Rimactane], sertraline [Zoloft], and phenobarbital. Accordingly, in order to maintain adequate levothyroxine levels, patients taking these drugs may need to increase their levothyroxine dosage.

Warfarin. Levothyroxine accelerates the degradation of vitamin K–dependent clotting factors. As a result, effects of warfarin, an anticoagulant, are enhanced. If thyroid hormone replacement therapy is instituted in a patient who has been taking warfarin, the dosage of warfarin should be reduced.

Catecholamines. Thyroid hormones increase cardiac responsiveness to catecholamines (epinephrine, dopamine, dobutamine), thereby increasing the risk of catecholamine-induced dysrhythmias. Caution must be exercised when administering catecholamines to patients receiving levothyroxine and other thyroid preparations.

Other Interactions. Levothyroxine can increase requirements for *insulin* and *digitalis*. Hence, when converting patients from a hypothyroid to a euthyroid state, dosages of insulin and digitalis may need to be increased.

Bioequivalence of Levothyroxine Preparations

For many years, the manufacturer of *Synthroid,* an expensive brand of levothyroxine, claimed that its product was more effective than levothyroxine made by its competitors. However,

TABLE 55–2 ■ Thyroid Hormone Preparations

Generic Name	Trade Names	Dosage Forms	Equivalent Dosage	Description
Levothyroxine	Levothroid, Synthroid, Eltroxin, Levoxyl, Levo-T, Unithroid	Tablets, injection	50–60 µg	Synthetic preparation of T₄ identical to the naturally occurring hormone
Liothyronine	Cytomel, Triostat	Tablets, injection	15–37 µg	Synthetic preparation of T₃ identical to the naturally occurring hormone
Liotrix	Thyrolar	Tablets	60 µg	Synthetic T₄ plus synthetic T₃ in a 4:1 fixed ratio
Thyroid	S-P-T, Thyrar, Thyroid USP, Thyroid Strong	Tablets, capsules	60 mg	Desiccated animal thyroid glands

a study published in 1997 (after being suppressed by the manufacturer of Synthroid) revealed that the most popular brands of levothyroxine—*Levothroid, Levoxyl,* and *Synthroid*—are all bioequivalent, and that switching among these drugs does not cause clinical problems. Although the study did not include other brands of levothyroxine, it is very likely that they, too, are equivalent to Synthroid. Switching from Synthroid to Levothroid or Levoxyl will save money: These alternatives cost about half as much as Synthroid.

Dosage and Administration I: General Considerations

Routes of Administration. Levothyroxine is almost always administered by mouth. Oral doses should be taken on an empty stomach to enhance absorption. Dosing is usually done in the morning before breakfast.

Intravenous administration is used for myxedema coma and for patients who cannot take levothyroxine orally. Intravenous doses are about one-half the size of oral doses.

Evaluation. The goal of thyroid hormone replacement therapy is to provide a dosage that will compensate precisely for the existing thyroid deficit. This dosage is determined using a combination of clinical judgment and laboratory tests. When therapy is successful in adults, clinical evaluation should reveal a reversal of the signs and symptoms of thyroid deficiency—and an absence of signs of thyroid excess. Successful therapy of infants is reflected in normalization of intellectual function and normalization of growth and development. Monthly determinations of height provide a good index of success.

Laboratory determinations of serum TSH are an important means of evaluation. Successful therapy will cause elevated TSH levels to fall. These levels will begin their decline within hours of the onset of therapy and will continue to drop as plasma levels of thyroid hormone build up. If an adequate dosage is established, TSH levels will remain suppressed for the duration of treatment. A TSH target of 1 to 3 mU/L is appropriate for most patients.

For some patients, serum T_4 must be used to evaluate levothyroxine therapy. In young children, TSH secretion may remain high even though levels of thyroid hormone have been restored. In such patients, TSH determinations are not helpful. For these patients, serum T_4 levels can be employed to evaluate dosage; when the dosage is appropriate, T_4 levels will be in the normal to high-normal range.

Duration of Therapy. For most hypothyroid patients, replacement therapy must be continued for life. Treatment provides symptomatic relief but does not produce cure. The patient must be made fully aware of the chronic nature of the condition. In addition, the patient should be forewarned that, although therapy will cause symptoms to improve, these improvements do not constitute a reason to interrupt or discontinue drug use.

Dosage and Administration II: Specific Applications

Hypothyroidism in Adults. The dosage should be low initially and then increased gradually until full replacement doses have been achieved. A typical dosing schedule consists of 50 μg daily (PO) for 2 weeks followed by 100 μg daily for 2 additional weeks. Thereafter, daily doses of 100 to 150 μg are taken for life. When calculated on a body weight basis, the average adult dose is about 1.7 μg/kg/day.

Myxedema Coma. Myxedema coma is a rare but serious condition that requires rapid treatment. Levothyroxine is administered IV in a dose of 200 to 500 μg. If required, an additional dose of 100 to 300 μg can be given 1 day later. Glucocorticoids (e.g., hydrocortisone) are also required.

Cretinism. In cretinism, thyroid hormone dosage decreases with age. For infants less than 6 months old, the dosage is 10 μg/kg/day; for children ages 6 to 8 months, 8 μg/kg/day; for children ages 1 to 5 years, 6 μg/kg/day; and for children ages 5 to 10 years, 4 μg/kg/day.

Simple Goiter. In simple goiter, the thyroid is enlarged and levels of thyroid hormones are reduced. Thyroid enlargement is caused by TSH that has been released in response to low levels of thyroid hormone. When treating simple goiter, the goal is to provide full replacement doses of thyroid hormone so as to suppress further TSH release. This can usually be achieved with 100 to 200 μg of levothyroxine per day.

Liothyronine (T₃)

Liothyronine [Cytomel, Triostat] is a synthetic preparation of triiodothyronine (T_3), a naturally occurring thyroid hormone. The structure of liothyronine is identical to that of thyroid-derived T_3. The effects of liothyronine are qualitatively similar to those of levothyroxine.

Contrasts with Levothyroxine. Liothyronine differs from levothyroxine in three important ways: (1) liothyronine has a shorter half-life and shorter duration of action, (2) liothyronine has a more rapid onset, and (3) liothyronine is more expensive. Because of its high price and relatively brief duration of action, liothyronine is less desirable than levothyroxine for long-term use. However, because its effects develop quickly, liothyronine may be superior to levothyroxine in situations that require speedy results, especially myxedema coma.

Evaluation. As with levothyroxine, the dosage of liothyronine is adjusted on the basis of clinical evaluation and laboratory data. Two laboratory tests are useful: serum T_3 and serum TSH. Since liothyronine is not converted into T_4, plasma levels of T_4 remain low. Hence, T_4 levels cannot be used to assess treatment.

Dosage and Administration. Liothyronine is usually administered by mouth, although IV administration may also be used. Dosage is about one half the dosage of levothyroxine.

Other Thyroid Preparations
Liotrix

Liotrix [Thyrolar] is a mixture of synthetic T_4 plus synthetic T_3 in a 4:1 fixed ratio. (This ratio is similar to the ratio of these hormones in plasma.) The rationale for using liotrix is that the mixture can produce plasma levels of T_4 and T_3 similar to those that occur naturally. However, since levothyroxine alone produces the same ratio of T_4 to T_3, liotrix offers no advantage over levothyroxine for most indications.

Thyroid

Thyroid consists of desiccated animal thyroid glands. Standardization of this preparation is based on content of iodine, levothyroxine, and liothyronine; the ratio of levothyroxine to liothyronine is not less than 5:1. Thyroid is dispensed in tablets ranging from 16 to 300 mg. Capsules are also available. For practical purposes, thyroid is obsolete: use is limited to those patients who have been taking the preparation for years. Thyroid is rarely prescribed for patients starting therapy today.

DRUGS FOR HYPERTHYROIDISM
Propylthiouracil

Propylthiouracil (PTU) inhibits thyroid hormone synthesis. The drug is a member of the thionamide category of antithyroid drugs and will serve as prototype for the group. Only one other thionamide—methimazole—is available in the United States.

Mechanism of Action

Therapeutic responses to PTU result primarily from blockade of thyroid hormone synthesis. Blockade occurs in two ways: (1) PTU prevents the oxidation of iodide, thereby inhibiting incorporation of iodine into tyrosine; and (2) PTU prevents iodinated tyrosines from coupling. Both effects result from inhibiting peroxidase, the enzyme that catalyzes both reactions.

In addition to blocking thyroid hormone synthesis, PTU acts in the periphery to suppress conversion of T_4 to T_3, the more active form of thyroid hormone.

Please note that, although PTU prevents thyroid hormone synthesis, it does not destroy existing stores of thyroid hormone. Hence, once therapy has begun, it may take 3 to 12 weeks to produce a euthyroid state.

Pharmacokinetics

Propylthiouracil is rapidly absorbed following oral administration. Therapeutic actions begin within 30 minutes. The plasma half-life of PTU is short (about 75 minutes). As a result, PTU must be administered several times a day. The drug can cross the placenta and can enter breast milk.

Therapeutic Uses

Propylthiouracil has four applications in hyperthyroidism. First, PTU can be used alone as the sole form of therapy for Graves' disease. Second, PTU can be employed as an adjunct to radiation therapy; PTU is administered to control hyperthyroidism until the effects of radiation become manifest. Third, PTU can be given to suppress thyroid hormone synthesis in preparation for thyroid gland surgery (subtotal thyroidectomy). Fourth, PTU is given to patients experiencing thyrotoxic crisis; benefits derive from suppressing thyroid hormone synthesis and from preventing conversion of T_4 to T_3.

Adverse Effects

Adverse responses to PTU are relatively rare. However, severe adverse effects can occur.

Agranulocytosis. Agranulocytosis is the most serious toxicity. This reaction is rare (about 3 cases per 10,000 patients) and usually develops during the first 2 months of therapy. Sore throat and fever may be the earliest indications; patients should be instructed to report these immediately. Because agranulocytosis often develops rapidly, periodic blood counts cannot guarantee early detection. If agranulocytosis occurs, PTU should be discontinued. Agranulocytosis will then reverse. Treatment with granulocyte colony-stimulating factor [Neupogen] may accelerate recovery.

Hypothyroidism. When given in high doses, PTU can convert the patient from a hyperthyroid state to a hypothyroid state. If this occurs, dosage should be reduced. Temporary administration of thyroid hormone may be required.

Pregnancy and Lactation. Propylthiouracil crosses the placenta and has caused neonatal hypothyroidism and goiter. Accordingly, the drug must be used judiciously during pregnancy. To minimize effects on the fetus, the dosage should be kept as low as possible. As an alternative, some physicians recommend treatment with full doses of PTU combined with thyroid hormone replacement therapy. However, this practice is controversial. Propylthiouracil enters breast milk and is contraindicated for nursing mothers.

Other Adverse Effects. The most common undesired effect of PTU is rash. The drug may also cause nausea, arthralgia, headache, dizziness, and paresthesias.

Preparations, Dosage, and Administration

Propylthiouracil is available in 50-mg tablets for oral administration. Because of its short half-life, PTU must be given in multiple daily doses.

Treatment of Graves' Disease. High doses (100 to 300 mg 3 times a day) are used initially. Lower doses (e.g., 50 mg 3 times a day) are used for maintenance. As a rule, treatment continues for 1 to 2 years. When PTU is discontinued, some 30% to 40% of patients remain euthyroid, indicating remission. Others become hyperthyroid in 1 to 4 weeks, indicating relapse. If relapse occurs, another round of PTU can be tried. Alternatively, the patient can opt for radiation therapy or surgery.

Methimazole

Methimazole [Tapazole] is very similar to PTU. Both drugs belong to the same chemical class (thionamides), both have the same mechanism of action (inhibition of peroxidase with subsequent inhibition of thyroid hormone synthesis), and both can produce the same serious toxicity (agranulocytosis). However, the drugs do have three important differences. First, methimazole has a longer half-life than PTU (4 to 6 hours vs. 75 minutes). As a result, most patients need only one dose a day, compared with 3 doses a day for PTU. Second, in contrast to PTU, methimazole does not block conversion of T_4 to T_3 in the periphery, and hence onset of effects may be slower. Third, methimazole crosses the placenta more readily than PTU. Accordingly, if a thionamide must be used in pregnancy, PTU is preferred. Like PTU, methimazole is contraindicated for nursing mothers. Methimazole is dispensed in 5- and 10-mg tablets. As with PTU, doses are high initially (30 to 40 mg once a day) and then decreased for maintenance (5 to 15 mg once a day).

Radioactive Iodine (^{131}I)
Physical Properties

Iodine-131 [Iodotope], a radioactive isotope of stable iodine, emits a combination of beta particles and gamma rays. Radioactive decay of ^{131}I takes place with a half-life of 8 days. Hence, after 56 days (seven half-lives), less than 1% of the radioactivity in a dose of ^{131}I remains.

Use in Graves' Disease

Iodine-131 can be used to destroy thyroid tissue in patients with hyperthyroidism. The objective is to produce clinical remission without causing complete destruction of the gland. Unfortunately, delayed hypothyroidism, due to excessive thyroid damage, is a frequent complication.

Effect on the Thyroid. Like stable iodine, ^{131}I is concentrated in the thyroid gland. Destruction of thyroid tissue is produced primarily by emission of beta particles. (The gamma rays from ^{131}I are relatively harmless.) Because beta particles have a very limited ability to penetrate any type of physical barrier, these particles do not travel outside the thyroid. Hence, damage to surrounding tissue is minimal.

Reduction of thyroid function is gradual. Initial effects become apparent in days or weeks. Full effects develop in 2 to 3 months.

Not all patients respond satisfactorily to a single ^{131}I treatment. About 66% of patients with Graves' disease are cured with a single exposure to ^{131}I. Others require two or more treatments.

Advantages and Disadvantages of ^{131}I Therapy. The advantages of ^{131}I treatment are considerable: (1) low cost; (2) patients are spared the risks, discomfort, and expense of thyroid surgery; (3) death from ^{131}I treatment has never occurred, nor is it ever likely to; and (4) no tissue other than the thyroid is injured (patients should be reassured of this).

Treatment with ^{131}I is not without drawbacks. First, the effect of treatment is delayed, taking several months to become maximal. Second, and more important, treatment is associated with a significant incidence of delayed hypothyroidism. Hypothyroidism results from excessive dosage and occurs in 10% of patients within the first year following ^{131}I exposure. An additional 2% to 3% develop hypothyroidism each year thereafter.

Who Should Be Treated and Who Should Not. Patients over the age of 30 may be candidates for ^{131}I therapy. Iodine-131 also is indicated for patients who have not responded adequately to antithyroid drugs or to subtotal thyroidectomy.

Children are considered inappropriate candidates. The likelihood of delayed hypothyroidism is higher than in adults. Also, there is concern that administration of ^{131}I to young patients may carry a slight risk of cancer. It should be noted, however, that there is no evidence that the use of ^{131}I in Graves' disease has ever caused cancer of the thyroid or any other tissue.

Iodine-131 is *contraindicated in pregnancy and lactation.* Exposure of the fetus to ^{131}I after the first trimester may damage the immature thyroid, and exposure to radiation at any point in fetal life carries a risk of generalized developmental harm. Because ^{131}I enters breast milk, women receiving this agent should not breast-feed.

Dosage. Dosage of ^{131}I is determined by thyroid size and by the rate of thyroidal iodine uptake. For Graves' disease, the dosage usually ranges between 4 and 10 millicuries (mCi).

Use in Thyroid Cancer

Iodine-131 can be used to destroy malignant thyroid cells. However, since most forms of thyroid cancer do not accumulate iodine, only a small percentage of patients are candidates for ^{131}I therapy.

The doses of ^{131}I used to treat cancer are large, ranging from 50 to 150 mCi. These doses are much higher than those used in Graves' disease. Because high amounts of radioactivity are involved, body wastes must be disposed of properly. In addition, adverse effects from large doses of ^{131}I can be severe: radiation sickness may occur; leukemia may be produced; and bone marrow function may be depressed, resulting in leukopenia, thrombocytopenia, and anemia.

Diagnostic Use

Iodine-131 is employed to diagnose a variety of thyroid disorders, including hyperthyroidism, hypothyroidism, and goiter. Following ^{131}I administration, the thyroid is scanned for uptake of radioactivity; the amount and location of ^{131}I uptake reveals the extent of thyroid activity. Doses used for diagnosis are minuscule (less than 1 μCi for children and less than 10 μCi for adults). These tracer doses pose virtually no threat to health.

Preparations

Iodine-131 is dispensed in capsules and solution for oral administration. Both preparations are odorless and tasteless. Capsules contain between 0.8 and 100 mCi of ^{131}I. Vials of oral solution contain between 3.5 and 150 mCi of ^{131}I. Capsules and oral solutions are available generically (as sodium iodide ^{131}I) and under the trade name Iodotope.

Nonradioactive Iodine

Three preparations of nonradioactive iodine are available. All three have the same mechanism of action and similar pharmacologic effects, although their specific applications may differ.

Strong Iodine Solution (Lugol's Solution)

Description. Lugol's solution is a mixture containing 5% elemental iodine and 10% potassium iodide. The iodine undergoes reduction to iodide within the GI tract prior to absorption.

Mechanism of Action. When present in high concentrations, iodide has a paradoxical suppressant effect on the thyroid. Suppression is brought about in three ways. First, high concentrations of iodide decrease iodine uptake by the thyroid. Second, high concentrations of iodide inhibit thyroid hormone synthesis by suppressing both the iodination of tyrosine and the coupling of iodinated tyrosine residues. Third, high concentrations of iodide inhibit release of thyroid hormone into the bloodstream. All three actions combine to decrease circulating levels of T_3 and T_4.

Unfortunately, the effects of iodide on thyroid function cannot be sustained indefinitely. With long-term iodide administration, suppressant effects become weaker. Accordingly, iodide is rarely used alone to produce thyroid suppression.

Therapeutic Use. Strong iodine solution can be given to hyperthyroid individuals to suppress thyroid function in preparation for thyroidectomy. Initial effects develop within 24 hours. Peak effects develop in 10 to 15 days. In most cases, plasma levels of thyroid hormone are reduced with PTU before initiating strong iodine solution. Then iodine solution (along with more PTU) is administered for the last 10 days prior to surgery. In addition to its use prior to thyroidectomy, strong iodine solution is employed in thyrotoxic crisis and as an antiseptic (see Chapter 92).

Adverse Effects. Chronic ingestion of iodine can produce *iodism.* Signs and symptoms include a brassy taste, a burning sensation in the mouth and throat, soreness of the teeth and gums, frontal headache, coryza (nasal inflammation and sneezing), salivation, and various skin eruptions. All of these fade rapidly upon discontinuation of iodine use.

Overdose. Iodine is corrosive, and overdose will injure the GI tract. Symptoms include abdominal pain, vomiting, and diarrhea. Swelling of the glottis may cause asphyxiation. Treatment consists of gastric lavage (to remove iodine from the stomach) and administration of sodium thiosulfate (to reduce iodine to iodide).

Dosage and Administration. When used to prepare hyperthyroid patients for thyroidectomy, strong iodine solution is administered in a dosage of 2 to 6 drops 3 times daily for 10 days immediately preceding surgery. Iodine solution should be mixed with juice or some other beverage to mask its unpleasant taste. The dosage for thyrotoxic crisis is 5 to 8 drops every 6 hours.

Sodium Iodide (IV)

Intravenous sodium iodide can be used for acute management of *thyrotoxic crisis.* Benefits derive from the ability of high concentrations of iodide to rapidly suppress thyroid hormone release. In the treatment of thyrotoxic crisis, sodium iodide is used in combination with propylthiouracil and propranolol. Sodium iodide for IV use is dispensed as a 10% solution in 10-ml ampules. The dosage is 0.5 to 1 gm every 12 hours.

Although IV sodium iodide rarely causes adverse effects, *severe hypersensitivity reactions* have occurred. These may develop immediately or may be delayed by several hours. The most characteristic feature is angioedema. Skin eruptions, serum sickness, and edema of the larynx may also develop. Death has occurred. There is no specific antidote to these hypersensitivity reactions. Hence, treatment is purely supportive.

Potassium Iodide

Use in Radiation Emergencies. Potassium iodide [Thyro-Block, Iostat, ThyroSafe] taken orally can be used to protect the thyroid gland in a radiation emergency. If a nuclear accident should release radioactive iodine into the environment, uptake by the thyroid would damage the gland. By administering large doses of nonradioactive iodide, uptake of radioactive material can be blocked. The dosage of potassium iodide is 130 mg/day for all people over the age of 1 year; children less than 1 year old should receive 65 mg daily. Duration of use is likely to last from 3 to 10 days.

Use in Thyroid Disease. A concentrated solution of potassium iodide, containing 1 gm of potassium iodide per milliliter, can be used to treat Graves' disease and thyrotoxic crisis.

In Graves' disease, potassium iodide has the same effect as Lugol's solution: suppression of iodine uptake by the thyroid, inhibition of thyroid hormone synthesis, and inhibition of thyroid hormone release. All three actions reduce circulating levels of T_3 and T_4. The dosage is 1 to 3 drops of concentrated potassium iodide solution PO 3 times a day.

In patients experiencing thyrotoxic crisis, potassium iodide is given to suppress thyroid hormone release. The dosage is 5 to 8 drops PO every 6 hours.

Propranolol

Propranolol [Inderal] can suppress tachycardia and other symptoms of *Graves' disease.* Benefits derive from beta-adrenergic blockade, not from reducing levels of T_3 or T_4. One advantage of propranolol is that its benefits occur rapidly, unlike those of PTU, methimazole, or ^{131}I. The dosage for hyperthyroidism is highly individualized, ranging from 40 to 240 mg/day in divided doses.

Propranolol is also beneficial in *thyrotoxic crisis.* In the absence of contraindications (e.g., asthma, heart failure), all patients should receive propranolol immediately. Administration may be oral or IV. The dosage is 80 to 120 mg PO every 6 hours or 2 to 4 mg IV every 4 hours.

The basic pharmacology of propranolol is discussed in Chapter 18.

.·. KEY POINTS

- The thyroid gland produces two active hormones: triiodothyronine (T_3), which is highly active, and thyroxine (T_4, tetraiodothyronine), which is less active.
- Thyroid hormones have three principal actions: stimulation of energy use, stimulation of the heart, and promotion of growth and development.
- Hormonal regulation of thyroid function occurs as follows: TRH from the hypothalamus causes the pituitary to release TSH, which causes the thyroid to make and release T_3 and T_4, which then act on the pituitary to suppress further release of TSH.
- The four steps in thyroid hormone synthesis are (1) uptake of iodide by the thyroid, (2) conversion of iodide to iodine, (3) linking of iodine to tyrosine, and (4) coupling of two iodinated tyrosines to form T_3 or T_4.
- Much of the T_4 released by the thyroid is converted to T_3 in the periphery.
- Low plasma levels of iodine stimulate synthesis of T_3 and T_4, whereas high levels suppress synthesis of T_3 and T_4.
- In iodine-sufficient areas, the major cause of hypothyroidism is chronic autoimmune thyroiditis (Hashimoto's disease).
- A goiter is an enlargement of the thyroid.
- Testing serum for elevated levels of TSH is the most sensitive way to diagnose hypothyroidism.
- Most patients with hypothyroidism require lifelong replacement therapy with thyroid hormones.
- Maternal hypothyroidism during the first trimester of pregnancy can result in permanent neuropsychologic deficits in the child.
- Levothyroxine (synthetic T_4) is the drug of choice for most patients who require thyroid hormone replacement.
- Cholestyramine [Questran], colestipol [Colestid], sucralfate [Carafate], aluminum-containing antacids, ferrous sulfate, and calcium supplements can significantly reduce levothyroxine absorption. Three to four hours should separate administration of levothyroxine and these drugs.
- Levothyroxine can intensify the anticoagulant effects of warfarin.
- The most common form of hyperthyroidism is Graves' disease.
- Thyrotoxic crisis (thyroid storm) occurs if levels of thyroid hormone rise exceptionally high.
- Graves' disease can be treated by surgical removal of thyroid tissue, destruction of thyroid tissue with radioactive iodine (^{131}I), or treatment with antithyroid drugs (propylthiouracil).
- Propylthiouracil, an antithyroid drug, benefits patients with hyperthyroidism by suppressing thyroid hormone synthesis and by inhibiting conversion of T_4 to T_3 in the periphery.
- Full benefits of propylthiouracil may take 3 to 12 weeks to develop.
- The most serious adverse effect of propylthiouracil is agranulocytosis.
- Propylthiouracil is contraindicated for nursing mothers and must be used with caution during pregnancy.
- Full effects of ^{131}I require 2 to 3 months to develop.
- Iodine-131 is contraindicated during pregnancy and lactation.
- Strong iodine solution (Lugol's solution) can be used to suppress thyroid hormone synthesis.

Summary of Major Nursing Implications*

LEVOTHYROXINE

Preadministration Assessment

Therapeutic Goal

Resolution of signs and symptoms of hypothyroidism and restoration of normal laboratory values for serum TSH and thyroid hormones.

Baseline Data

Obtain plasma levels of TSH and T_4.

Implementation: Administration

Routes

Oral, IV.

Administration

Oral. Instruct the patient to take levothyroxine on an empty stomach, preferably in the morning before breakfast.

Make certain the patient understands that replacement therapy must continue for life. Caution the patient against discontinuing treatment without consulting the physician.

Intravenous. Intravenous administration is reserved for treating myxedema coma and for patients who cannot take levothyroxine orally.

Ongoing Evaluation and Interventions

Evaluating Therapeutic Effects

Adults. Clinical evaluation should reveal reversal of signs of thyroid deficiency and an absence of signs of thyroid excess (e.g., tachycardia). Laboratory tests should indicate normal plasma levels of TSH and T_4.

Infants. Clinical evaluation should reveal normalization of intellectual function, growth, and development. Monthly measurements of height provide a good index of thyroid sufficiency. Laboratory tests should show normal plasma levels

*Patient education information is highlighted as blue text.

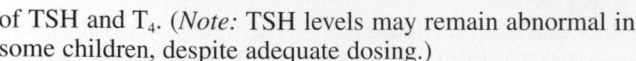

Summary of Major Nursing Implications*—cont'd

of TSH and T_4. (*Note:* TSH levels may remain abnormal in some children, despite adequate dosing.)

Minimizing Adverse Effects

Thyrotoxicosis. Overdose may cause thyrotoxicosis. Inform patients about symptoms of thyrotoxicosis (tachycardia, angina, tremor, nervousness, insomnia, hyperthermia, heat intolerance, sweating) and instruct them to notify the physician if these develop.

Minimizing Adverse Interactions

Drugs That Reduce Levothyroxine Absorption. Absorption of levothyroxine can be reduced by cholestyramine, colestipol, sucralfate, aluminum-containing antacids, ferrous sulfate, and calcium supplements. Allow several hours to separate administration of levothyroxine and these drugs.

Drugs That Accelerate Levothyroxine Metabolism. Several drugs, including carbamazepine, rifampin, phenytoin, phenobarbital, and sertraline, can accelerate metabolism of levothyroxine, and can thereby reduce its effects. An increase in levothyroxine dosage may be needed.

Warfarin. Levothyroxine can intensify the effects of warfarin. Warfarin dosage should be reduced.

Catecholamines. Thyroid hormones sensitize the heart to catecholamines (epinephrine, dopamine, dobutamine) and may thereby promote dysrhythmias. Exercise caution when catecholamines and levothyroxine are used together.

LIOTHYRONINE (T_3)

With the exceptions noted below, the nursing implications for liothyronine are the same as those for levothyroxine.

Evaluating Therapeutic Effects

Success is indicated by resolution of the signs and symptoms of hypothyroidism and by normalization of plasma T_3 and TSH levels. T_4 levels cannot be used to evaluate therapy.

PROPYLTHIOURACIL

Preadministration Assessment

Therapeutic Goals

Propylthiouracil has four indications: (1) reduction of thyroid hormone production in Graves' disease, (2) control of hyperthyroidism until the effects of radiation on the thyroid become manifest, (3) suppression of thyroid hormone production prior to subtotal thyroidectomy, and (4) treatment of thyrotoxic crisis.

Baseline Data

Obtain plasma levels of T_3 and T_4.

Identifying High-Risk Patients

Propylthiouracil is *contraindicated* for nursing mothers. Use with *caution* during pregnancy.

Implementation: Administration

Route

Oral.

Administration

Instruct the patient to take PTU at regular intervals around the clock (usually every 8 hours).

Ongoing Evaluation and Interventions

Summary of Monitoring

Evaluate treatment by monitoring for weight gain, decreased heart rate, and other indications that levels of thyroid hormone have declined. Laboratory tests should indicate a decrease in plasma T_3 and T_4.

Minimizing Adverse Effects

Agranulocytosis. Inform patients about early signs of agranulocytosis (fever, sore throat) and instruct them to notify the physician if these develop. If follow-up blood tests reveal leukopenia, PTU should be withdrawn. Giving granulocyte colony-stimulating factor may accelerate recovery.

Hypothyroidism. Propylthiouracil may cause excessive reductions in thyroid hormone synthesis. If signs of hypothyroidism develop or if plasma levels of T_3 and T_4 become subnormal, PTU dosage should be reduced. Supplemental thyroid hormone may be needed.

Use in Pregnancy and Lactation. Propylthiouracil can cause fetal hypothyroidism and goiter. Therefore, use with caution during pregnancy. Propylthiouracil is contraindicated for nursing mothers.

RADIOACTIVE IODINE (^{131}I)

Use in Graves' Disease

Therapeutic Goal. Suppression of thyroid hormone production.

Identifying High-Risk Patients. Iodine-131 is *contraindicated* during pregnancy and lactation.

Dosage and Administration. Iodine-131 is administered in capsules or an oral liquid. The dosing objective is to reduce thyroid hormone production without causing complete thyroid destruction. The dosage for Graves' disease is 4 to 10 mCi.

Promoting Therapeutic Effects. Responses take 2 to 3 months to develop fully. Propylthiouracil or methimazole may be required during this interval.

Minimizing Adverse Effects. Excessive thyroid destruction can cause hypothyroidism. Patients who develop thyroid insufficiency need thyroid hormone supplements.

Use in Thyroid Cancer

High doses (50 to 150 mCi) are required. These doses can cause radiation sickness, leukemia, and bone marrow depression. Monitor for these effects. Body wastes will be contaminated with radioactivity and must be disposed of appropriately.

*Patient education information is highlighted as blue text.

Summary of Major Nursing Implications*—cont'd

Diagnostic Use

Iodine-131 is used to diagnose hyperthyroidism, hypothyroidism, and goiter. Diagnostic doses are so small (less than 10 μCi) as to be virtually harmless.

STRONG IODINE SOLUTION (LUGOL'S SOLUTION)

Preadministration Assessment

Therapeutic Goal

Suppression of thyroid hormone production in preparation for subtotal thyroidectomy. Also used to suppress thyroid hormone release in patients experiencing thyroid storm.

Baseline Data

Obtain tests of thyroid function.

Implementation: Administration

Route

Oral.

*Patient education information is highlighted as blue text.

Administration

Advise the patient to dilute strong iodine solution with fruit juice or some other beverage to increase palatability.

Ongoing Evaluation and Interventions

Minimizing Adverse Effects

Mild Toxicity. Inform patients about symptoms of iodism (brassy taste, burning sensations in the mouth, soreness of gums and teeth) and instruct them to discontinue treatment and notify the physician if these occur. Symptoms fade upon drug withdrawal.

Severe Toxicity. Iodine solution can cause corrosive injury to the GI tract. Instruct patients to discontinue the drug and notify the physician immediately if severe abdominal distress develops. Treatment includes gastric lavage and administration of sodium thiosulfate.

Drugs Related to Hypothalamic and Pituitary Function

The hypothalamus and pituitary are intimately related both anatomically and functionally. Working together, these structures help regulate practically all bodily processes. To achieve their widespread effects, the hypothalamus and pituitary employ at least 15 hormones and regulatory factors (Fig. 56–1). The endocrinology of these two structures is exceedingly complex. Fortunately, from the perspective of therapeutics, the picture is much less imposing. Why? Because the clinical applications of the hypothalamic and pituitary hormones are limited. In this chapter, we emphasize three agents: growth hormone (GH), antidiuretic hormone (ADH), and prolactin. Additional hypothalamic and pituitary hormones of therapeutic interest are considered briefly here and discussed at greater length in other chapters.

OVERVIEW OF HYPOTHALAMIC AND PITUITARY ENDOCRINOLOGY

Anatomic Considerations

The pituitary sits in a depression in the skull located just below the third ventricle of the brain; the hypothalamus is located immediately above (see Fig. 56–1). The pituitary has two divisions: the *anterior pituitary* (or *adenohypophysis*) and the *posterior pituitary* (or *neurohypophysis*). Both divisions are under hypothalamic control. As indicated in Figure 56–1, the hypothalamus communicates with the *anterior* pituitary by way of release-regulating factors delivered through a system of portal blood vessels. In contrast, communication with the *posterior* pituitary is neuronal.

Hormones of the Anterior Pituitary

The anterior pituitary produces six major hormones. Production and release of these hormones is controlled largely by the hypothalamus. Functions of the anterior pituitary hormones are summarized briefly as follows:

- *Growth hormone* (GH) stimulates growth in practically all tissues and organs.
- *Corticotropin* (adrenocorticotropic hormone; ACTH) acts on the adrenal cortex to promote synthesis and release of adrenocortical hormones.
- *Thyrotropin* (thyroid-stimulating hormone; TSH) acts on the thyroid gland to promote synthesis and release of thyroid hormones.
- *Follicle-stimulating hormone* (FSH) acts on the ovaries to promote follicular growth and development. In the testes, FSH promotes spermatogenesis.
- *Luteinizing hormone* (LH) acts in women to promote ovulation and development of the corpus luteum. In men, LH, which is also known as *interstitial cell–stimulating hormone (ICSH),* acts on the testes to promote androgen production.
- *Prolactin* stimulates milk production after parturition.

Hormones of the Posterior Pituitary

The posterior pituitary has only two hormones: *oxytocin* and *antidiuretic hormone* (ADH). The principal function of oxytocin is to facilitate uterine contractions at term. ADH promotes renal conservation of water.

Although oxytocin and ADH are considered hormones of the posterior pituitary, these agents are actually synthesized in the hypothalamus. The cells that make oxytocin and ADH are called neurosecretory cells. As indicated in Figure 56–1, these cells originate in the hypothalamus and project their axons to the posterior pituitary. Oxytocin and ADH are produced within the bodies of these cells and then transported down the axons to the axon terminals for storage. When appropriate stimuli impinge upon the bodies of the neurosecretory cells, impulses are sent down the axon, causing hormone release.

Hypothalamic Release-Regulating Factors

The hypothalamus has the primary responsibility for regulating the release of hormones from the *anterior* pituitary. To accomplish this, the hypothalamus employs eight different release-regulating factors (see Fig. 56–1). Most of these factors *stimulate* the release of anterior pituitary hormones. However, two of these factors regulate release by an in-

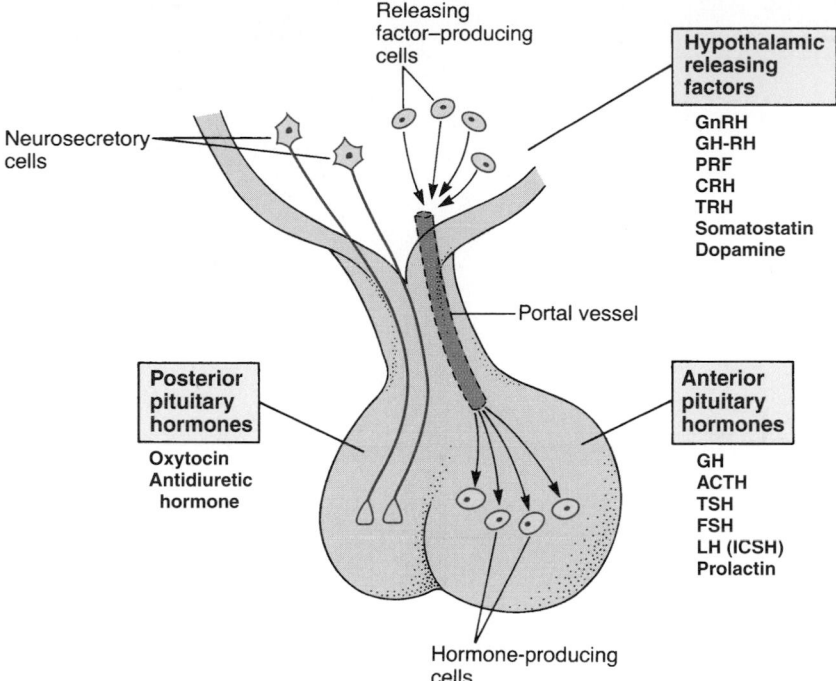

Figure 56–1 ■ Hormones and releasing factors of the hypothalamus and pituitary.

Hypothalamic releasing factors: GnRH = gonadotropin-releasing hormone, GH-RH = growth hormone–releasing hormone, PRF = prolactin-releasing factor, CRH = corticotropin-releasing hormone, TRH = thyrotropin-releasing hormone.

Anterior pituitary hormones: GH = growth hormone, ACTH = adrenocorticotropic hormone, TSH = thyroid-stimulating hormone, FSH = follicle-stimulating hormone, LH (ICSH) = luteinizing hormone (interstitial cell–stimulating hormone).

hibitory influence. As indicated in Figure 56–1, the hypothalamic release-regulating factors are delivered to the anterior pituitary via portal blood vessels. Although the hypothalamic releasing factors are of extreme *physiologic* importance, only three of these factors—growth hormone–releasing hormone, thyrotropin-releasing hormone, and gonadotropin-releasing hormone—have clinical applications. These are the only hypothalamic release-regulating factors that we will discuss.

Feedback Regulation of the Hypothalamus and Anterior Pituitary

With few exceptions, the release of hypothalamic and anterior pituitary hormones is regulated by a *negative feedback loop*. Such a loop is illustrated in Figure 56–2. In this example, the loop begins with the secretion of releasing-factor X from the hypothalamus. Factor X then acts on the anterior pituitary to stimulate release of hormone A. Hormone A then acts on its target gland to promote release of hormone B. Hormone B has two actions: (1) it produces its designated biologic effects and (2) it acts on the hypothalamus and pituitary to inhibit further release of factor X and hormone A. This feedback inhibition of the hypothalamus and pituitary suppresses further release of hormone B itself, thereby keeping levels of hormone B within an appropriate range.

GROWTH HORMONE

Growth hormone (GH) is a large polypeptide hormone (191 amino acids) produced by the anterior pituitary. As its name suggests, GH helps regulate growth. Childhood deficiency of GH results in *dwarfism*. Excessive GH results in *giantism* (when too much GH is present prior to puberty) and *acromegaly* (when too much GH is present during adulthood).

Physiology
Regulation of Release

The factors regulating GH release are summarized in Figure 56–3. As indicated, the hypothalamus first releases growth hormone–releasing hormone (GH-RH), which stimulates release of GH from the pituitary. Growth hormone then acts on the liver and other tissues to cause release of insulin-like growth factor-1 (IGF-1). IGF-1 has two actions: (1) it mediates increases in growth and (2) it acts on the hypothalamus and pituitary to suppress release of GH-RH and GH, thereby completing a negative feedback loop.

One additional hormone—somatostatin (SST)—helps regulate GH release. As shown in Figure 56–3, SST is produced in the hypothalamus and acts on the pituitary to inhibit GH release.

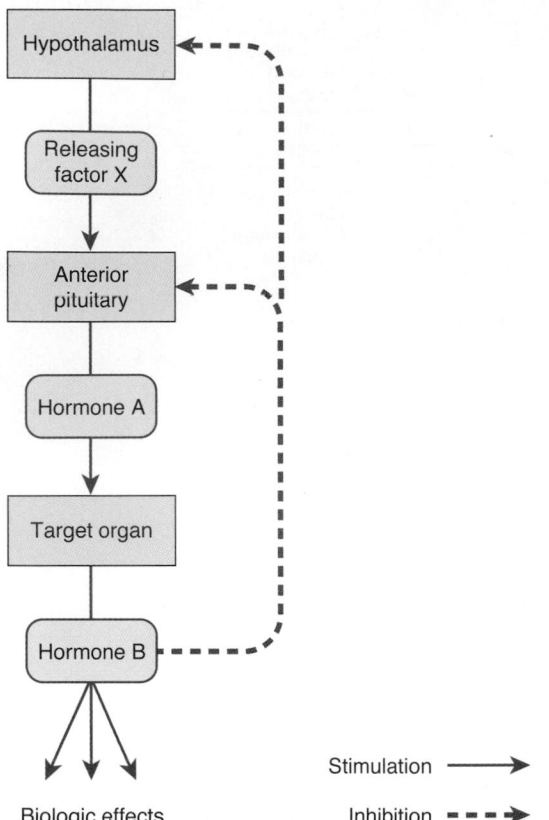

Figure 56–2 ■ **Negative feedback regulation of the hypothalamus and anterior pituitary.**
The feedback loop works as follows: Factor X stimulates the pituitary to release hormone A, which stimulates its target organ, causing release of hormone B. Hormone B then acts on the hypothalamus and pituitary to suppress further release of factor X and hormone A, thereby suppressing further release of hormone B itself.

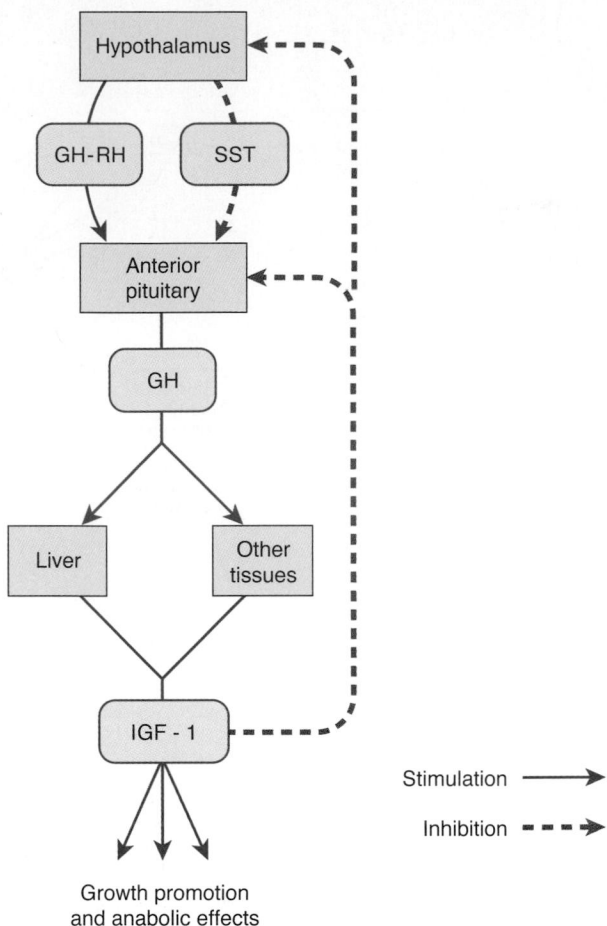

Figure 56–3 ■ **Regulation of growth hormone release.**
(GH-RH = growth hormone–releasing hormone, SST = somatostatin, GH = growth hormone, IGF-1 = insulin-like growth factor-1.)

Biologic Effects

Promotion of Growth. GH, acting through IGF-1, stimulates the growth of practically all organs and tissues. If administered to a GH-deficient subject prior to epiphyseal closure, GH will increase bone length, producing a corresponding increase in height. The size and number of muscle cells is increased, resulting in enlargement of muscle mass, and the internal organs are stimulated to grow in proportion to overall body growth. The only structures that do not respond noticeably to GH are the brain and eyes.

Promotion of Protein Synthesis. For growth to occur, cells must increase production of protein. GH facilitates this process by increasing amino acid uptake and utilization. Since amino acids have substantial nitrogen content, increased protein synthesis results in net nitrogen retention, which is reflected in reduced urinary nitrogen excretion. Increased amino acid utilization also causes blood urea nitrogen to fall.

Effect on Carbohydrate Metabolism. Administration of GH reduces glucose utilization. Hence, plasma levels of glucose tend to rise. When GH is administered to nondiabetics, elevation of blood glucose stimulates release of insulin, thereby maintaining glucose levels within a normal range. In

contrast, when GH is administered to diabetic patients, insulin cannot be released. As a result, the hyperglycemic action of GH goes unopposed, allowing plasma glucose levels to climb dramatically.

Pathophysiology
Growth Hormone Deficiency

Growth hormone is essential for normal growth of children, and GH deficiency results in *dwarfism*. In children who are GH deficient, growth is retarded to an equal extent in all parts of the body. Hence, the dwarf, although small, has normal proportions. Dwarfism is not associated with mental impairment. In contrast to normal individuals, whose growth ceases at puberty, dwarves continue to grow throughout life. The only treatment for GH deficiency is replacement therapy with human GH itself (see below under *Therapeutic Uses*).

Growth Hormone Excess

Consequences. When GH excess occurs in children, the resulting syndrome is called *giantism* (or *gigantism*), and when the excess occurs in adults, the syndrome is called *acromegaly*. The pathophysiology of both syndromes is similar. The principal difference is that GH excess causes children to grow

TABLE 56–1 ■ Growth Hormone Preparations: Approved Indications and Dosages

Drug (TRADE NAME)	Approved Indications	Dosage
Somatrem		
PROTROPIN	Pediatric GH deficiency	0.3 mg/kg/wk SC or IM divided into 3–7 once-a-day doses
Somatropin		
GENOTROPIN	Pediatric GH deficiency	0.16–0.24 mg/kg/wk SC divided into 6 or 7 once-a-day doses
	Adult GH deficiency	0.04 mg/kg/wk
HUMATROPE	Pediatric GH deficiency	0.18 mg/kg wk SC or IM divided into either (a) 6 once-a-day doses or (b) once-a-day doses on 3 alternate days
	Somatropin deficiency syndrome	0.006 mg/kg/day SC initially, increased to 0.0125 mg/kg/day (max)
	Turner's syndrome	0.375 mg/kg/wk (max) SC divided into either (a) 7 once-a-day doses or (b) once-a-day doses given on 3 alternate days
NUTROPIN	Pediatric GH deficiency	0.3 mg/kg/wk SC
	Chronic renal insufficiency	0.35 mg/kg/wk SC
	Turner's syndrome	0.375 mg/kg/wk SC divided into 3–7 once-a-day doses
	Adult GH deficiency	0.006 mg/kg/day SC initially, increased to 0.025 mg/kg/day (max) in patients <35 yr, or to 0.0125 mg/kg/day (max) in patients >35 yr
NUTROPIN DEPOT	Pediatric GH deficiency	15 mg/kg/mo *or* 0.75 mg/kg twice a month
SEROSTIM	Cachexia or wasting in AIDS	4–6 mg SC daily HS (dose depends on patient's weight)
SAIZEN	Pediatric GH deficiency	0.06 mg/kg SC or IM 3 days/wk
NORDITROPIN	Pediatric GH deficiency	0.024–0.034 mg/kg SC 6–7 days/wk

very tall—as much as 7 to 9 feet—owing to stimulation of long bones prior to epiphyseal closure. In adults, effects on bone growth result in coarse facial features, splayed teeth, and large hands and feet. However, because the epiphyses have already closed, height is not increased. Other manifestations, seen in adults *and* children, include cardiomegaly, hypertension, arthralgias, hyperglycemia, and headache. Levels of IGF-1 are elevated in all patients. In almost all cases, the cause of GH excess is a pituitary adenoma.

Treatment. Treatment of giantism requires surgical removal of the pituitary. In contrast, acromegaly may be treated with three modalities: surgery, radiation, or drugs. Surgical excision of the pituitary adenoma is the preferred initial treatment for most patients. Radiation therapy may be used as primary treatment or as an adjunct to surgery. When used as primary treatment, radiation takes 10 to 20 years to produce a full response.

Octreotide [Sandostatin, Sandostatin LAR Depot], a synthetic analog of somatostatin, is our most effective agent for suppressing GH release. The drug works by mimicking the suppressant actions of somatostatin on the pituitary (see Fig. 56–3). Octreotide can be used as primary therapy for acromegaly or as an adjunct to surgery or radiation. The usual dosage is 100 μg SC 3 times a day (for Sandostatin) and 10 to 30 mg IM once a month (for Sandostatin LAR Depot). Unfortunately, although octreotide is effective, it is also very expensive. Gastrointestinal side effects (nausea, cramps, diarrhea, flatulence) are common initially, but subside in 1 to 2 weeks. Within a year, cholesterol gallstones develop in about 25% of patients, although they usually are not symptomatic.

Clinical Pharmacology
Therapeutic Uses

Pediatric Growth Hormone Deficiency. Who Should Be Treated? GH replacement therapy is approved only for children whose growth has been retarded because of *proven GH deficiency.* Treatment should begin early in life and must stop prior to epiphyseal closure. To ensure timely termination of treatment, epiphyseal status should be assessed annually.

Expected Response. Treatment is prolonged and responses are usually satisfactory. When treatment is started early, adult height may be increased by as much as 6 inches. To monitor treatment, height and weight should be measured

monthly. Therapy should continue until a satisfactory adult height has been achieved, until epiphyseal closure occurs, or until a response can no longer be elicited. Efficacy of therapy declines as the patient grows older and is usually lost entirely by age 20 to 24 years. If treatment fails to promote growth, GH should be discontinued and the diagnosis of GH deficiency re-evaluated.

What About Children Who Have Normal GH Levels but Are Nonetheless Very Short? As a rule, short children with normal GH levels are considered inappropriate for GH therapy: In the absence of GH deficiency, the American Academy of Pediatrics recommends GH therapy only if short stature limits a child's ability to participate in normal activities of daily living. Furthermore, it should be noted that GH therapy is not very effective in children with normal GH levels: The average increase in expected height is only 2 inches.

Other Uses. GH has four approved uses in addition to GH deficiency. These are *somatropin deficiency syndrome in adults, pediatric growth failure associated with chronic renal insufficiency, cachexia or wasting in patients with AIDS,* and *Turner's syndrome.* Individual GH preparations that are approved for these indications are indicated in Table 56–1.

Adverse Effects and Interactions

Hyperglycemia. GH is diabetogenic. When used in patients with pre-existing diabetes, significant hyperglycemia may result. Glucose levels should be monitored and insulin dosage should be adjusted accordingly.

Hypothyroidism. GH causes hypothyroidism in about 5% of patients. Thyroid function should be assessed periodically. If thyroid hormone levels are insufficient, replacement therapy should be instituted.

Antibodies to GH. Two forms of GH are used clinically: somatropin and somatrem. Although antibodies may develop to either form, they are much more common with somatrem. Fortunately, these antibodies rarely decrease the effectiveness of treatment.

Interaction with Glucocorticoids. Glucocorticoids can oppose the growth-stimulating effects of GH. Patients receiving GH should not be given glucocorticoids in doses that exceed the equivalent of 10 to 15 mg/m^2 of hydrocortisone.

Preparations and Dosage

Somatrem. Somatrem [Protropin] is a form of GH produced by recombinant DNA technology. With the exception of one amino acid, the structure of somatrem is identical to that of GH produced by the human pituitary. The biologic activity of somatrem is indistinguishable from that of naturally occurring GH. The only approved use for somatrem is pediatric GH deficiency. The dosage is 0.3 mg/kg/wk (SC or IM) divided into 3 to 7 once-a-day doses.

Somatropin. Like somatrem, somatropin [Humatrope, Nutropin, others] is produced by recombinant DNA technology. The structure and actions of somatropin are identical to those of GH produced by the human pituitary. At this time, six preparations of somatropin are available. As indicated in Table 56–1, they differ with respect to approved indications and dosages.

Administration

GH is dispensed as a lyophilized powder for reconstitution with 1 to 5 ml of diluent. *Mix gently; do not shake.* Do not inject the drug if the preparation is cloudy or contains particulate matter.

Administration is parenteral—IM or SC. Subcutaneous administration is preferred because it is less painful than IM while being just as safe and effective. Subcutaneous administration can be done using either (1) a traditional syringe and needle, or (2) for some products, a needle-free device.

PROLACTIN

Prolactin is a polypeptide hormone produced by the anterior pituitary. The principal function of prolactin is stimulation of milk production after parturition. Prolactin deficiency is generally without symptoms, except for disturbance of lactation. In contrast, overproduction of prolactin causes multiple adverse effects.

Regulation of Release

Regulation of prolactin release is predominantly *inhibitory*. Under the influence of dopamine released from the hypothalamus, release of prolactin by the pituitary is suppressed. When release of dopamine declines, release of prolactin is allowed to increase. Another hypothalamic factor, known as prolactin-releasing factor (PRF), promotes prolactin release. However, the stimulatory influence of PRF is usually dominated by dopamine-mediated inhibition. The most powerful stimulus to prolactin release is suckling, an action that presumably suppresses release of dopamine from the hypothalamus.

Prolactin Hypersecretion

Excessive secretion of prolactin produces adverse effects in males and females. Women may experience amenorrhea, galactorrhea (excessive milk flow), and infertility. In men, li-

bido and potency are reduced; galactorrhea occurs on occasion. Puberty may be delayed in boys and girls. Causes of prolactin hypersecretion include pituitary adenoma, injury to the hypothalamus, and certain drugs (e.g., antipsychotic drugs, estrogens).

Bromocriptine for Suppression of Prolactin Release

Excessive secretion of prolactin can be reduced with bromocriptine, a dopamine agonist. By binding to dopamine receptors in the pituitary, bromocriptine exerts the same inhibitory influence on prolactin release as does dopamine released from the hypothalamus. The usual dosage is 2.5 mg administered 2 to 3 times daily. Adverse effects are common early in therapy and include nausea, vomiting, dizziness, and hypotension. Other uses of bromocriptine include management of infertility (see Chapter 61) and treatment of Parkinson's disease (see Chapter 21). In the past, bromocriptine was used to inhibit prolactin release in postpartum women, but this practice is rare today.

THYROTROPIN

Thyrotropin (thyroid-stimulating hormone; TSH) is a hormone produced by the anterior pituitary. The physiologic role of thyrotropin is stimulation of thyroid gland function. In promoting thyroid function, thyrotropin promotes (1) thyroidal uptake of iodine, (2) synthesis and release of thyroid hormones, and (3) thyroid growth. Clinical application of thyrotropin is limited to diagnostic evaluation of patients with thyroid cancer.

CORTICOTROPIN

Corticotropin (adrenocorticotropic hormone; ACTH) is a polypeptide hormone produced by the anterior pituitary. This hormone acts on the adrenal cortex to stimulate production and release of adrenocortical hormones (e.g., cortisol, aldosterone). The principal use of corticotropin is diagnosis of adrenocortical dysfunction. A synthetic analog of corticotropin, called cosyntropin, is available. Corticotropin and cosyntropin, along with the hormones of the adrenal cortex, are discussed in Chapter 57.

GONADOTROPINS

The anterior pituitary produces two gonadotropic hormones: *follicle-stimulating hormone* (FSH) and *luteinizing hormone* (LH). (Note: LH is also known as *interstitial cell–stimulating hormone* or ICSH.) LH and FSH are produced by the pituitaries of males and females and serve to regulate gonadal function in both sexes. In women, FSH acts on the ovaries to promote follicular growth and development. In men, FSH supports sperm production. The role of LH in women is to promote ovulation and formation of the corpus luteum. In men, LH stimulates testosterone synthesis by Leydig cells of the testicular interstitium. Plasma levels of LH and FSH are relatively stable in males. In females, levels of both hormones vary with the phase of the menstrual cycle. The physiology of LH and FSH in females is discussed further in Chapter 59.

LH and FSH are employed clinically to treat infertility in men and women. In women, fertility is increased by promoting follicular development and ovulation. In men, fertility is increased through enhanced spermatogenesis.

Four preparations of gonadotropins are used clinically: menotropins, urofollitropin, follitropin alfa, and follitropin beta. Menotropins [Pergonal, Repronex] is a 50:50 mixture of LH and FSH. Urofollitropin [Fertinex, Metrodin] is primarily FSH. Follitropin alfa [Gonal-F] and follitropin beta [Follistim] are human FSH preparations produced by recombinant DNA technology. The use of gonadotropins to treat infertility is discussed in Chapter 61.

ANTIDIURETIC HORMONE

ADH is a nine-peptide hormone that acts on the kidney to cause reabsorption (conservation) of water. Deficiency of ADH produces *hypothalamic diabetes insipidus,* a condition in which large volumes of dilute urine are produced.

Physiology

Actions. ADH promotes renal conservation of water. How? By acting on the collecting ducts of the kidney to increase their permeability to water, which results in increased water reabsorption. Because water is withdrawn from the tubular urine (back into the extracellular space), urine that entered the collecting ducts in a relatively dilute state becomes highly concentrated by the time it leaves.

In addition to its renal actions, ADH can stimulate contraction of vascular smooth muscle and smooth muscle of the GI tract. Because of its ability to cause vasoconstriction, ADH is also known as *vasopressin.* It should be noted that the plasma levels of ADH required to cause smooth muscle contraction are higher than those that occur physiologically.

Production, Storage, and Release. ADH is produced within neurosecretory cells of the hypothalamus, transported down their axons, and then stored in their terminals until released. Release is regulated by the hypothalamus—the brain center responsible for maintaining body fluids at their proper osmolality. When the hypothalamus senses that osmolality has risen too high, it instructs the posterior pituitary to release ADH. The resultant increase in water reabsorption dilutes body fluids, causing osmolality to decline. Release of ADH can also be stimulated by hypotension and by reduced plasma volume.

Pathophysiology: Hypothalamic Diabetes Insipidus

Causes, Signs, and Symptoms. Hypothalamic diabetes insipidus is a syndrome caused by partial or complete deficiency of ADH. The syndrome is characterized by polydipsia (excessive thirst) and excretion of large volumes of dilute urine. Deficiency of ADH may be inherited or it may result from head trauma, neurosurgery, cancer, and other causes. (In contrast to hypothalamic diabetes insipidus, *nephrogenic diabetes insipidus* results from a failure of the kidney to produce concentrated urine despite adequate levels of ADH.)

Treatment. The best treatment for hypothalamic diabetes insipidus is replacement therapy with ADH. (Although two other drugs—chlorpropamide and clofibrate—are effective, they are not recommended owing to side effects.) Of the ADH preparations available, *desmopressin* is the agent of choice. Desmopressin is preferred because of its prolonged action, ease of administration, and lack of significant side effects, especially vasoconstriction. The response to treatment is rapid, and urine volume quickly drops to normal. Desmopressin is administered by nasal spray, usually twice daily. Because desmopressin is expensive, and because excessive dosing can result in water intoxication (see below), the smallest effective dosage should be employed.

Antidiuretic Hormone Preparations

Two preparations with ADH activity are available: *vasopressin* and *desmopressin.* Vasopressin is identical in structure to naturally occurring ADH; desmopressin is a structural analog of natural ADH. The preparations differ from each other with respect to route of administration, duration of action, and therapeutic applications (Table 56–2). They also differ in their ability to cause vasoconstriction (see *Cardiovascular Effects*).

Therapeutic Uses

Diabetes Insipidus. Desmopressin and vasopressin may be employed to treat diabetes insipidus. However, because of its prolonged effects, convenient routes (oral and intranasal), and freedom from significant side effects, *desmopressin* is the drug of choice.

Other Uses. Vasopressin is indicated for postoperative abdominal distention and preparation for abdominal radiography.

Desmopressin is indicated for nocturnal enuresis (bedwetting), hemophilia A, and von Willebrand's disease. The drug decreases enuresis by reducing urine production, and helps patients with hemophilia A and von Willebrand's disease by increasing production of clotting factor VIII.

TABLE 56–2 ■ ADH Preparations

Generic Name (TRADE NAME)	Routes	Duration of Antidiuretic Action (hr)	Therapeutic Uses	Usual Dosage
Desmopressin DDAVP, STIMATE	Intranasal, SC, IV, PO	8–20	Diabetes insipidus	*Adults:* 0.1 ml (10 µg) intranasally 2 times/day or 0.25–0.5 ml SC or IV twice daily *Children:* 0.05–0.3 ml intranasally daily either as a single dose or in 2 doses
			Hemophilia	0.3 µg/kg IV over 15–30 min
			Nocturnal enuresis	10–40 µg intranasally HS
Vasopressin PITRESSIN SYNTHETIC	IM, SC*	2–8	Diabetes insipidus	5–10 units IM or SC 3–4 times/day
			Postoperative abdominal distention	5 units IM initially; then 10 units IM every 3–4 hr
			Abdominal radiography (to dispel gas shadows)	10 units 2 hr before and again 30 min before the procedure

*Sometimes administered intranasally or IV.

Adverse Effects

Water Intoxication. Excessive water retention can cause water intoxication. Early signs include drowsiness, listlessness, and headache. Severe intoxication progresses to convulsions and terminal coma. Patients experiencing early symptoms of intoxication should notify the physician. Treatment includes restriction of fluid intake and diuretic therapy.

A major cause of intoxication is failure to reduce water intake once ADH therapy has begun. Since treatment prevents continued fluid loss, failure to decrease fluid intake will result in water buildup. Hence, at the onset of treatment, patients should be instructed to reduce their accustomed fluid intake.

Cardiovascular Effects. Because of its powerful vasoconstrictor actions, *vasopressin* can cause severe adverse cardiovascular effects. (Desmopressin is a weak pressor agent, and hence does not adversely affect hemodynamics.) By constricting arteries of the heart, vasopressin can cause angina pectoris and even myocardial infarction—especially in patients with coronary insufficiency. In addition, vasopressin may cause gangrene by decreasing blood flow in the periphery. Because it can reduce cardiac perfusion, vasopressin must be used with extreme caution in patients with coronary artery disease. This warning does not apply to desmopressin.

OXYTOCIN

Oxytocin is produced by neurosecretory cells of the hypothalamus and is then transported down the axons of these cells for storage in the posterior pituitary. Oxytocin has two physiologic roles: (1) promotion of uterine contraction during labor and (2) stimulation of milk ejection during breast-feeding. The principal therapeutic application of the drug is induction of labor near term. The physiology, pharmacology, and applications of oxytocin are discussed in Chapter 62.

DRUGS RELATED TO HYPOTHALAMIC FUNCTION

Of the seven regulatory factors found in the hypothalamus, only four—growth hormone–releasing hormone (GH-RH), gonadotropin-releasing hormone (GnRH), thyrotropin-releasing hormone (TRH), and somatostatin—have clinical applications. GH-RH is used to diagnose the cause of growth hormone deficiency. GnRH and its synthetic analogs are used to treat prostatic cancer and endometriosis, and to induce ovulation. TRH is used to diagnose thyroid disorders. As discussed above, somatostatin is used to treat acromegaly.

Sermorelin (Growth Hormone–Releasing Factor)

Sermorelin [Geref] is a synthetic *growth hormone–releasing factor* that acts just like natural GH-RH. That is, sermorelin acts on the pituitary to stimulate release of GH, which in turn causes release of insulin-like growth factor-1. The structure of sermorelin is identical to the final 29-amino-acid sequence of GH-RH. Sermorelin has only one clinical application: diagnosis of the ability of the pituitary to secrete GH.

Gonadotropin-Releasing Hormone

Gonadotropin-releasing hormone is produced by the hypothalamus and promotes release of gonadotropins (LH and FSH) from the pituitary. Four preparations of GnRH are available: *leuprolide, goserelin, nafarelin,* and *gonadorelin*. Leuprolide and goserelin are discussed in Chapter 99 (Anticancer Drugs II). Nafarelin is discussed in Chapter 61 (Drugs for Infertility). Gonadorelin is used to evaluate anterior pituitary function.

Thyrotropin-Releasing Hormone

Thyrotropin-releasing hormone is produced by the hypothalamus and acts on the pituitary to stimulate release of thyrotropin (thyroid-stimulating hormone; TSH). A synthetic preparation of TRH, called *protirelin,* is used clinically. Protirelin is thought to be identical to TRH made by the hypothalamus. Protirelin is employed in the diagnosis of thyroid, pituitary, and hypothalamic disorders. Testing is performed by injecting protirelin IV and then sampling the blood for increases in TSH content. Interpretation of test findings can be difficult and is beyond the scope of this text. Protirelin is marketed under the trade names *Thypinone, Relefact TRH,* and *Thyrel TRH.* For a general discussion of thyroid physiology and pharmacology, refer to Chapter 55.

⋅ KEY POINTS

- Release of hormones from the anterior pituitary is stimulated by releasing factors from the hypothalamus and inhibited by negative feedback loops.
- The growth-promoting actions of growth hormone (GH) are mediated by insulin-like growth factor-1 (IGF-1).
- GH deficiency causes dwarfism.
- GH replacement is approved only for children who are GH deficient; GH is not approved for children who are short simply because of their genetic heritage.
- Exogenous glucocorticoids can inhibit responses to GH.
- GH can elevate glucose levels in children with diabetes.
- Prolactin stimulates milk production after delivery.
- Excessive production of prolactin can be suppressed with bromocriptine, a drug that mimics the inhibitory action of hypothalamic dopamine on the pituitary.
- Antidiuretic hormone (ADH) acts on the kidney to cause reabsorption (conservation) of water.
- ADH deficiency results in hypothalamic diabetes insipidus.
- Hypothalamic diabetes insipidus can be treated by replacement therapy with desmopressin, a synthetic form of ADH.
- When initiating ADH replacement therapy, warn the patient to decrease water intake, because failure to do so can cause water intoxication.
- Vasopressin, a drug identical to natural ADH, can cause profound vasoconstriction.

Summary of Major Nursing Implications*

GROWTH HORMONE: SOMATREM AND SOMATROPIN

The nursing implications summarized here apply only to the use of GH for *pediatric growth hormone deficiency.*

Preadministration Assessment

Therapeutic Goal

Normalization of growth and development in children with proven GH deficiency.

Baseline Data

Assess developmental status (height, weight, etc.). Obtain thyroid function tests.

Identifying High-Risk Patients

GH is *contraindicated* during and after epiphyseal closure. Use with *caution* in patients with diabetes mellitus and hypothyroidism.

Implementation: Administration

Routes

SC (preferred) or IM.

Administration

Reconstitute the lyophilized powder with 1 to 5 ml of diluent. *Mix gently; do not shake.* Do not inject if the preparation is cloudy or contains particulate matter.

Ongoing Evaluation and Interventions

Evaluating Treatment

Monitor height and weight monthly. Continue therapy until a satisfactory adult height has been achieved, until epiphyseal closure occurs, or until a response can no longer be elicited (usually by age 20 to 24).

If no stimulation of growth occurs, discontinue treatment and re-evaluate the diagnosis of GH deficiency.

Minimizing Adverse Effects and Interactions

Hyperglycemia. GH can elevate plasma glucose levels in diabetics. Increase insulin dosage as needed.

Hypothyroidism. GH may suppress thyroid function. Assess thyroid function before treatment and periodically thereafter. If levels of thyroid hormone fall, institute replacement therapy.

Interaction with Glucocorticoids. Glucocorticoids can oppose the growth-stimulating effects of GH. Dosage of glucocorticoids should not exceed the equivalent of 10 to 15 mg/m² of hydrocortisone.

*Patient education information is highlighted as blue text.

ANTIDIURETIC HORMONE

Desmopressin
Vasopressin

The nursing implications summarized here apply only to the use of ADH preparations for *hypothalamic diabetes insipidus.*

Preadministration Assessment

Therapeutic Goal

Normalization of urinary water excretion in patients with hypothalamic diabetes insipidus.

Baseline Data

Determine fluid and electrolyte status.

Identifying High-Risk Patients

Use *vasopressin* with *caution* in patients with coronary artery disease and other vascular diseases.

Implementation: Administration

Routes

Desmopressin. Intranasal, PO, SC, IV.
Vasopressin. IM, SC.

Administration

Teach the patient the technique for intranasal administration. To promote compliance, make certain the patient understands that treatment is lifelong.

Ongoing Evaluation and Interventions

Evaluating Therapeutic Effects

Teach the patient to monitor and record daily intake and output of fluid. If ADH dosage is correct, urine volume should rapidly drop to normal.

Minimizing Adverse Effects

Water Intoxication. Excessive retention of water can produce water intoxication—most often at the beginning of therapy. Instruct patients to decrease their accustomed fluid intake at the start of treatment. Inform patients about early signs of water intoxication (drowsiness, listlessness, and headache) and instruct them to notify the physician if these occur. Treatment includes fluid restriction and diuretic therapy.

Cardiovascular Effects. Vasopressin, but not desmopressin, is a powerful vasoconstrictor. Excessive vasoconstriction can produce angina pectoris, myocardial infarction, and gangrene (from extravasation of IV vasopressin). Use vasopressin with caution, especially in patients with coronary insufficiency.

Drugs for Disorders of the Adrenal Cortex

The hormones of the adrenal cortex affect multiple physiologic processes, including maintenance of glucose availability, regulation of water and electrolyte balance, development of sexual characteristics, and life-preserving responses to stress. As you might guess, when production of adrenal hormones goes awry, the consequences can be profound. The two most familiar forms of adrenocortical dysfunction are *Cushing's syndrome,* caused by adrenal hormone excess, and *Addison's disease,* caused by adrenal hormone deficiency.

In approaching the drugs used for disorders of the adrenal cortex, we begin by reviewing adrenocortical endocrinology. After that, we discuss the disease states associated with adrenal hormone excess and adrenal hormone insufficiency. Having established this background, we discuss the agents used for diagnosis and treatment of adrenocortical disorders.

PHYSIOLOGY OF THE ADRENOCORTICAL HORMONES

The adrenal cortex produces three classes of steroid hormones: *glucocorticoids, mineralocorticoids,* and *androgens.* Glucocorticoids influence carbohydrate metabolism and other processes; mineralocorticoids modulate salt and water balance; and adrenal androgens contribute to expression of sexual characteristics. When referring to either the glucocorticoids or the mineralocorticoids, three terms may be used: *corticosteroids, adrenocorticoids,* or simply *corticoids.* These terms are not used in reference to adrenal androgens.

Glucocorticoids

Glucocorticoids are so named because they increase the availability of glucose. Of the several glucocorticoids produced by the adrenal cortex, *cortisol* is the most important. The structural formula of cortisol is shown in Figure 57–1.

When considering the glucocorticoids, it is important to distinguish between *physiologic effects* and *pharmacologic effects. Physiologic effects* occur at *low* levels of glucocorticoids (i.e., the levels produced by release of glucocorticoids from healthy adrenals or by administration of exogenous glucocorticoids in low doses). *Pharmacologic effects* occur at *high* levels of glucocorticoids. These are the levels achieved when exogenous glucocorticoids are administered in the large doses required to treat disorders unrelated to adrenocortical function (e.g., allergic reactions, asthma, inflammation). In this chapter, discussion is limited to the *physiologic* role of glucocorticoids. The use of glucocorticoids for nonendocrine purposes (which is the major application of these agents) is discussed in Chapter 68.

Physiologic Effects

Carbohydrate Metabolism. Supplying the brain with glucose is essential for survival. Glucocorticoids help meet this need. Glucocorticoids promote glucose availability in three ways: (1) stimulation of gluconeogenesis, (2) reduction of peripheral glucose utilization, and (3) promotion of glucose storage (in the form of glycogen). All three actions increase glucose availability during fasting, and thereby help ensure the brain will not be deprived of its primary source of energy.

The effects of glucocorticoids on carbohydrate metabolism are opposite to those of insulin. That is, whereas insulin lowers

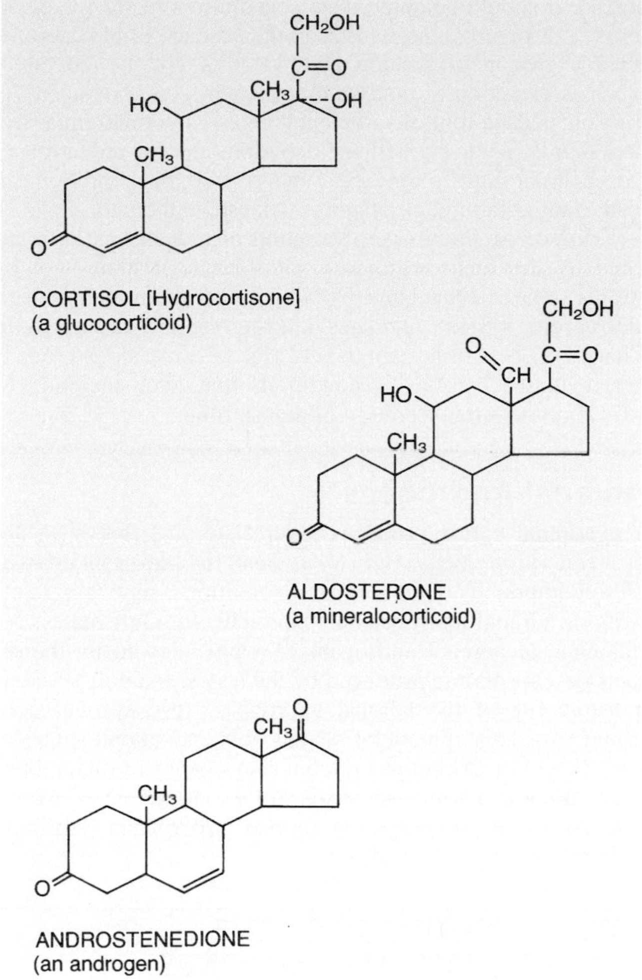

Figure 57–1 ■ **Structural formulas of representative adrenocortical hormones.**

plasma levels of glucose, glucocorticoids raise them. When present chronically in high concentrations, glucocorticoids produce symptoms much like those of diabetes.

Protein Metabolism. Glucocorticoids promote protein catabolism (breakdown). This action, which is opposite to that of insulin, provides amino acids for glucose synthesis. If present at high levels for a prolonged time, glucocorticoids will cause thinning of the skin, muscle wasting, and negative nitrogen balance.

Fat Metabolism. Glucocorticoids promote lipolysis (fat breakdown). When present at high levels for an extended time, as occurs in Cushing's syndrome, glucocorticoids cause fat redistribution, giving the patient a potbelly, "moon face," and "buffalo hump" on the back.

Cardiovascular System. Glucocorticoids are required to maintain the functional integrity of the vascular system. When levels of glucocorticoids are depressed, capillary permeability is increased, the ability of vessels to constrict is reduced, and blood pressure falls.

Glucocorticoids have multiple effects on blood cells. These hormones increase red blood cell counts and levels of hemo-

globin. Of the white blood cells, only the polymorphonuclear leukocytes increase; in contrast, lymphocytes, eosinophils, basophils, and monocytes decrease.

Skeletal Muscle. Glucocorticoids support function of striated muscle, primarily by maintaining circulatory competence. In the absence of sufficient levels of glucocorticoids, muscle perfusion decreases, causing work capacity to decrease as well.

Central Nervous System. Glucocorticoids affect mood, central nervous system (CNS) excitability, and the electroencephalogram. Glucocorticoid insufficiency is associated with depression, lethargy, and irritability. Rarely, outright psychosis occurs. In contrast, when present in excess, glucocorticoids can produce generalized excitation and euphoria.

Stress. In response to stress (e.g., anxiety, exercise, trauma, infection, surgery), the adrenal cortex secretes increased amounts of glucocorticoids, and the adrenal medulla secretes increased amounts of epinephrine. Working together, glucocorticoids and epinephrine serve to maintain blood pressure and blood glucose content. If glucocorticoid levels are inadequate, hypotension and hypoglycemia can occur. If the stress is extreme (e.g., trauma, surgery, severe infection), glucocorticoid deficiency can result in circulatory collapse and death. Accordingly, it is imperative that patients with adrenal insufficiency receive glucocorticoid supplements when severe stress occurs.

Respiratory System in Neonates. During labor and delivery, the adrenals of the full-term fetus release a burst of glucocorticoids. Within hours, these steroids act on the lungs to accelerate maturation. In the premature infant, the adrenals only produce small amounts of glucocorticoids. As a result, preterm infants experience a high incidence of respiratory distress syndrome.

Regulation of Synthesis and Secretion

Adrenal storage of glucocorticoids is minimal; hence glucocorticoids must be synthesized as they are needed. Accordingly, the amount of glucocorticoid released from the adrenals per unit time closely approximates the amount being made.

Synthesis and release of glucocorticoids are regulated by a negative feedback loop (Fig. 57–2). The loop begins with the release of corticotropin-releasing factor (CRF) from the hypothalamus. CRF acts on the anterior pituitary to promote release of adrenocorticotropic hormone (ACTH), which stimulates the zona fasciculata of the adrenal cortex, causing synthesis and release of cortisol and other glucocorticoids. Following release, cortisol acts in two ways: (1) it promotes its designated biologic effects and (2) it acts on the hypothalamus and pituitary to suppress further release of CRF and ACTH. Hence, as cortisol levels rise, they act to suppress further stimulation of glucocorticoid production, thereby keeping plasma levels of glucocorticoids within an appropriate range.

The hypothalamic-pituitary-adrenal system is activated by signals from the CNS. These signals turn the system on by causing the hypothalamus to release CRF. As indicated in Figure 57–2, two modes of activation are involved. One mode provides a basal level of stimulation. Basal stimulation follows a circadian rhythm, peaking in the early morning and reaching a nadir late in the evening. The second mode of activation is

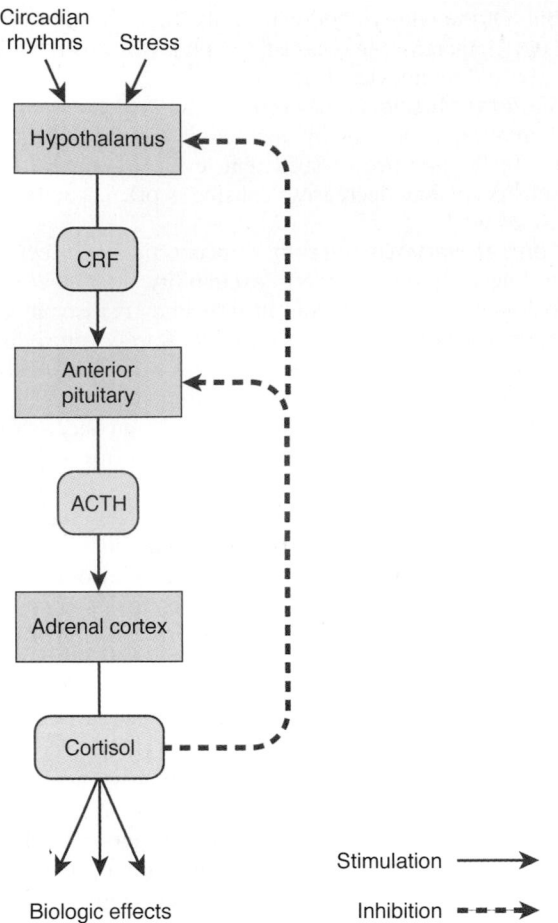

Figure 57–2 ■ **Negative feedback regulation of glucocorticoid synthesis and secretion.**
(CRF = corticotropin-releasing factor, ACTH = adrenocorticotropic hormone.)

stress. Stressful events that can activate the loop include injury, infection, and surgery. The signals generated by stress produce intense stimulation of the hypothalamus. The resultant release of CRF and ACTH can cause plasma levels of cortisol to increase by a factor of 10. Because stress is such a powerful stimulus, it overrides feedback inhibition by cortisol.

How much cortisol do the adrenals produce? Basal production ranges between 5 and 10 mg/m²/day (which is equivalent to 20 to 30 mg/day of hydrocortisone or 5 to 7 mg/day of prednisone). When severe stress occurs, production increases 5- to 10-fold—to a maximum of 100 mg/m²/day.

Mineralocorticoids

The mineralocorticoids influence renal processing of sodium, potassium, and hydrogen. Of the mineralocorticoids made by the adrenal cortex, *aldosterone* is the most important.

Physiologic Effects. Aldosterone promotes sodium and potassium hemostasis, and helps maintain intravascular volume. Specifically, the hormone acts on the collecting ducts of the nephron to promote sodium reabsorption in exchange for secretion of potassium and hydrogen. The total amount of hydrogen and potassium lost equals the amount of sodium reab-

sorbed. It should be noted that, as sodium is reabsorbed, water is reabsorbed along with it. In the absence of aldosterone, renal excretion of sodium and water is greatly increased, whereas excretion of potassium and hydrogen is reduced. As a result, aldosterone insufficiency causes hyponatremia, hyperkalemia, acidosis, cellular dehydration, and reduction of extracellular fluid volume. Left uncorrected, the condition can lead to renal failure, circulatory collapse, and death.

Control of Secretion. Secretion of aldosterone is regulated by the renin-angiotensin-aldosterone system—not by ACTH. The mechanisms by which the renin-angiotensin-aldosterone system regulates aldosterone are discussed in Chapter 42. It is important to note that, because aldosterone is not regulated by ACTH, conditions that alter secretion of ACTH do not alter secretion of aldosterone.

Adrenal Androgens

The adrenal cortex produces several steroids that have androgenic properties. *Androstenedione* is representative of these compounds. Under normal conditions, physiologic effects of adrenal androgens are minimal. In adult males, the influence of adrenal androgens is overshadowed by the effects of testosterone produced by the testes. In adult females, a metabolite of the adrenal androgens (testosterone) contributes to development of sexual hair and maintenance of normal libido. Although adrenal androgens normally have very little effect, when secretion of these hormones is excessive, as occurs in congenital adrenal hyperplasia, virilizing actions can be pronounced.

PATHOPHYSIOLOGY OF THE ADRENOCORTICAL HORMONES

Adrenal Hormone Excess
Cushing's Syndrome

Causes. Signs and symptoms of Cushing's syndrome result from excess levels of circulating glucocorticoids. Principal causes are (1) hypersecretion of ACTH by pituitary adenomas (Cushing's disease), (2) hypersecretion of glucocorticoids by adrenal adenomas and carcinomas, and (3) administration of exogenous glucocorticoids in the large doses used to treat arthritis and other nonendocrine disorders (see Chapter 68).

Clinical Presentation. Cushing's syndrome is characterized by obesity, hyperglycemia, glycosuria, hypertension, fluid and electrolyte disturbances, osteoporosis, muscle weakness, myopathy, hirsutism, menstrual irregularities, and decreased resistance to infection. The skin is weakened, resulting in striae (stretch marks) and increased susceptibility to injury. Fat undergoes redistribution to the abdomen, face, and upper back, giving the patient a characteristic potbelly, "moon face," and "buffalo hump." Psychiatric changes are common.

Treatment. Treatment of Cushing's syndrome is directed at the cause. The treatment of choice for adrenal adenoma and carcinoma is surgical removal of the diseased adrenal gland. If bilateral adrenalectomy is performed, replacement therapy with glucocorticoids and mineralocorticoids will be needed. For patients with inoperable adrenal carcinoma, treatment with *mitotane* is indicated. Mitotane is an anticancer drug that produces selective destruction of adrenocortical cells. The pharmacology of mitotane is discussed in Chapter 98.

When Cushing's syndrome is caused by pituitary adenoma, surgery is the preferred form of treatment. Partial removal of the pituitary often lowers ACTH secretion to safe levels, while leaving other pituitary functions intact. If partial adenectomy is unsuccessful, the remainder of the pituitary may be removed. As an alternative, pituitary irradiation may be employed.

The role of drugs in treating Cushing's syndrome is limited. Most commonly, drugs are employed as adjuncts to radiation and surgery; they are rarely the primary therapeutic modality. Drugs can relieve symptoms by inhibiting corticosteroid synthesis. Two drugs that act by this mechanism—*aminoglutethimide* and *ketoconazole*—are discussed below.

Primary Hyperaldosteronism

Clinical Presentation and Causes. Hyperaldosteronism (excessive secretion of aldosterone) causes hypokalemia, metabolic alkalosis, and hypertension. Muscle weakness and changes in the electrocardiogram develop secondary to hypokalemia. Hyperaldosteronism is frequently caused by an aldosterone-producing adrenal adenoma. The condition may also result from bilateral adrenal hyperplasia.

Treatment. Management of hyperaldosteronism depends on the cause. When an adrenal adenoma is responsible, surgical resection of the adrenal is usually curative. When bilateral adrenal hyperplasia is the cause, an aldosterone antagonist is the preferred treatment. The antagonist employed most frequently is *spironolactone,* a drug we normally think of as a potassium-sparing diuretic. Under the influence of spironolactone, potassium levels may normalize in 2 weeks. To achieve full control of hypertension, an additional diuretic may be required. The basic pharmacology of spironolactone is discussed in Chapter 39 (Diuretics). Pharmacologic alternatives to spironolactone are *amiloride* (another potassium-sparing diuretic) or an *angiotensin-converting enzyme inhibitor* (e.g., captopril).

Adrenal Hormone Insufficiency
General Therapeutic Considerations

Adrenal hormone insufficiency can result from multiple causes, including destruction of the adrenals, inborn deficiencies of the enzymes required for corticosteroid synthesis, and reduced secretion of ACTH and CRF. Regardless of the cause, adrenal insufficiency requires lifelong replacement therapy with appropriate corticosteroids. All patients require a *glucocorticoid.* Some may require a *mineralocorticoid* as well. Of the glucocorticoids available, *cortisone* and *hydrocortisone* are drugs of first choice. When a mineralocorticoid is indicated, *fludrocortisone* is the drug of choice.

Replacement therapy should mimic normal patterns of corticosteroid secretion. For glucocorticoids, this can be accomplished by dividing the daily dosage, giving two-thirds in the morning and one-third in the evening. Mineralocorticoids can be administered once a day. Doses of glucocorticoids and mineralocorticoids should approximate the amounts normally secreted by the adrenals. It is important to note that, when glucocorticoids are employed for replacement therapy, doses are much smaller than the doses employed to treat nonendocrine disorders.

At times of stress, patients must increase their glucocorticoid dosage. I cannot overemphasize the importance of doing so: *failure to increase the dosage can be fatal.* Recall that healthy adrenals increase their output of glucocorticoids in response to stress. For patients with adrenal insufficiency, the extra glucocorticoids that would normally be supplied by the adrenals must instead be supplied through supplemental dosing. Dosing guidelines related to specific medical conditions and surgical procedures are summarized in Table 57–1.

To ensure availability of glucocorticoids in emergencies, the patient should carry an adequate supply at all times. This supply should include an injectable preparation plus an oral preparation. Furthermore, the patient should wear some form of identification (e.g., Medic Alert bracelet) to inform emergency healthcare personnel about his or her glucocorticoid needs.

Addison's Disease (Primary Adrenocortical Insufficiency)

Clinical Presentation and Causes. Addison's disease is characterized by weakness, emaciation, hypoglycemia, and increased pigmentation of the skin and mucous membranes. Hyperkalemia, hyponatremia, and hypotension are present as well. These symptoms result from a deficiency of glucocorticoids and mineralocorticoids that occurs secondary to adrenal atrophy. Potential causes of adrenal atrophy include carcinoma, infection, and autoimmune disease.

Treatment. Replacement therapy with adrenocorticoids is required. *Hydrocortisone* and *cortisone* are drugs of choice. Both agents exert a combination of mineralocorticoid and glucocorticoid activity. Hence, therapy with either agent alone may suffice. If additional mineralocorticoid activity is needed, *fludrocortisone,* the only mineralocorticoid available, can be added to the regimen.

Secondary and Tertiary Adrenocortical Insufficiency

Secondary adrenocortical insufficiency results from decreased secretion of ACTH, while tertiary insufficiency results from decreased secretion of CRF. In both cases, adrenal secretion of glucocorticoids is diminished, whereas secretion of mineralocorticoids is usually not affected. Glucocorticoid insufficiency produces a characteristic set of symptoms: hypoglycemia, malaise, loss of appetite, and reduced capacity to respond to stress. For secondary and tertiary insufficiency, treatment consists of replacement therapy with a glucocorticoid (e.g., hydrocortisone, cortisone). Rarely, a mineralocorticoid is needed too.

Acute Adrenal Insufficiency (Adrenal Crisis)

Clinical Presentation. Acute adrenal insufficiency is characterized by hypotension, dehydration, weakness, lethargy, and GI symptoms (e.g., vomiting, diarrhea). Left untreated, the syndrome progresses to shock and then death.

Causes. Adrenal crisis may be brought on by adrenal failure, pituitary failure, or failure to provide patients receiving replacement therapy with adequate doses of corticosteroids. Adrenal crisis may also be triggered by abrupt withdrawal from chronic, high-dose glucocorticoid therapy.

Treatment. Patients require rapid replacement of fluid, salt, and glucocorticoids. They also need glucose for energy. These needs are met by injecting 100 mg of hydrocortisone

Table 57–1 ■ Guidelines for Giving Supplemental Doses of Glucocorticoids at Times of Stress Related to Medical Conditions and Surgical Procedures

Medical Condition or Surgical Procedure	Supplemental Glucocorticoid Dosage
Minor Inguinal hernia repair Colonoscopy Mild febrile illness Mild to moderate nausea/vomiting Gastroenteritis	25 mg of hydrocortisone (or 5 mg of methylprednisolone) IV on day of procedure
Moderate Open cholecystectomy Hemicolectomy Significant febrile illness Pneumonia Severe gastroenteritis	50–75 mg of hydrocortisone (or 10–15 mg of methylprednisolone) IV on day of procedure Taper quickly over 1–2 days to usual replacement dose
Severe Major cardiothoracic surgery Whipple procedure Liver resection Pancreatitis	100–150 mg of hydrocortisone (or 20–30 mg of methylprednisolone) IV on day of procedure Rapid taper to usual replacement dose over next 1–2 days
Critically Ill Sepsis-induced hypotension or shock	50–100 mg of hydrocortisone IV every 6–8 hr (or 0.18 mg/kg/hr as continuous infusion) *plus* 50 mg of fludrocortisone until shock resolves, which may take several days to a week or more Then, gradually taper to usual replacement dose, following vital signs and serum sodium

Adapted from Coursin DB, Wood KE. Corticosteroid supplementation for adrenal insufficiency. JAMA 2002;287:236–240.

(as an IV bolus) followed by IV infusion of normal saline with dextrose. Additional hydrocortisone is given by infusion at a rate of 100 mg every 8 hours.

Congenital Adrenal Hyperplasia

Clinical Presentation and Causes. Congenital adrenal hyperplasia results from an inborn deficiency of enzymes needed for glucocorticoid synthesis. The capacity to make glucocorticoids is reduced, but not eliminated. In an attempt to enhance glucocorticoid synthesis, the pituitary releases ACTH in amounts that are much greater than normal. The resultant high levels of ACTH produce powerful stimulation of the adrenals, causing growth of the adrenals (hyperplasia) and increased synthesis of glucocorticoids and androgens. (Synthesis of mineralocorticoids is minimally affected.) Frequently, stimulation of glucocorticoid synthesis may be sufficient to bring levels of cortisol up to normal. Unfortunately, the amounts of ACTH required to normalize glucocorticoid production are so large that synthesis of adrenal androgens becomes excessive. In girls, increased androgen levels cause masculinization of the external genitalia; the ovaries, uterus, and fallopian tubes are not affected. Increased androgen levels in boys may cause precocious penile enlargement. In children of both sexes, linear growth is accelerated. However, because androgens cause premature closure of the epiphyses, adult height is usually diminished.

Treatment. The therapeutic objective is to ensure adequate levels of glucocorticoids while preventing excessive production of adrenal androgens. This goal is achieved through lifelong administration of glucocorticoids. *Hydrocortisone* and *cortisone* are drugs of choice. By supplying glucocorticoids exogenously, we can suppress secretion of ACTH; because ACTH release is diminished, the adrenals are no longer stimulated to produce excessive quantities of androgens. As a rule, suppression of ACTH secretion can be achieved with daily doses of hydrocortisone equivalent to twice the amount secreted each day by normal adrenals. To assess the efficacy of therapy, children should be monitored every 3 months for growth rate and signs of virilization.

AGENTS FOR REPLACEMENT THERAPY IN ADRENOCORTICAL INSUFFICIENCY

Patients with adrenocortical insufficiency require replacement therapy with corticosteroids. A glucocorticoid is always required, and some patients require a mineralocorticoid as well.

The principal glucocorticoids employed are *hydrocortisone* and *cortisone*. *Fludrocortisone* is the only mineralocorticoid available.

It should be noted that classification of a drug as a "glucocorticoid" or "mineralocorticoid" may be an oversimplification. That is, a drug that we classify as a glucocorticoid may also exhibit salt-retaining (mineralocorticoid) activity. Conversely, a drug that we classify as a mineralocorticoid may also display typical glucocorticoid activity.

Hydrocortisone

Hydrocortisone is a synthetic steroid whose structure is identical to that of cortisol, the principal glucocorticoid produced by the adrenal cortex (see Fig. 57–1). Hydrocortisone is a drug of choice for adrenocortical insufficiency and will serve as our prototype of the glucocorticoids employed clinically. It should be noted that, despite its classification as a glucocorticoid, hydrocortisone also has mineralocorticoid properties.

Therapeutic Uses

Replacement Therapy. Hydrocortisone is a preferred drug for all forms of adrenocortical insufficiency. Oral hydrocortisone is ideal for chronic replacement therapy. Parenteral administration is used for acute adrenal insufficiency and to supplement oral doses at times of stress. Because of its mineralocorticoid actions, hydrocortisone can sometimes suffice as sole therapy for adrenal insufficiency, even when salt loss is a symptom.

Nonendocrine Applications. Hydrocortisone and other glucocorticoids are used to treat a broad spectrum of nonendocrine disorders, ranging from allergic reactions to inflammation to cancer. The doses required in these disorders are considerably higher than those employed for replacement therapy. The use of glucocorticoids for nonendocrine diseases is discussed in Chapter 68.

Adverse Effects

When given in the low doses required for replacement therapy, hydrocortisone and other glucocorticoids are devoid of adverse effects. In contrast, when taken chronically in the large doses employed to treat nonendocrine disorders, glucocorticoids are highly toxic. The adverse effects of chronic, high-dose therapy include adrenal suppression and production of Cushing's syndrome. These and other adverse effects are discussed in Chapter 68.

Preparations, Dosage, and Administration

Preparations. For replacement therapy, four hydrocortisone preparations are used: *hydrocortisone base, hydrocortisone cypionate, hydrocortisone sodium phosphate,* and *hydrocortisone sodium succinate.* The base and the cypionate salt can be administered orally. Because they are insoluble, these preparations must not be administered IV. The sodium phosphate and sodium succinate salts are water soluble and can be used IV and IM.

Dosage and Administration. The oral route is employed for chronic treatment. Intravenous and IM administration are reserved for emergencies. For oral therapy of chronic adrenal insufficiency, the total daily dose ranges from 20 to 30 mg/m². This dose should be divided, giving two-thirds in the morning and one-third in the afternoon. For emergency treatment, IV doses of 50 to 100 mg are employed (see Table 57–1). When IV injections can't be used, IM doses of 100 to 250 mg may be given instead. Doses for nonendocrine disorders are given in Chapter 68.

Cortisone

Cortisone is a prodrug that undergoes conversion to its active form—hydrocortisone (cortisol)—within the body. Like hydrocortisone itself, cortisone has both glucocorticoid and mineralocorticoid activity, and is a drug of choice for chronic adrenal insufficiency. In contrast to hydrocortisone, which can be administered PO, IV, or IM, cortisone can only be given PO or IM. Cortisone is insoluble in water and must never be administered IV. Absorption of IM cortisone is unpredictable; hence, cortisone injections are not recommended for acute adrenal insufficiency. For management of chronic adrenal insufficiency, the usual oral dosage is 12 to 15 mg/m²/day.

Fludrocortisone

Fludrocortisone [Florinef] is a potent mineralocorticoid that also possesses significant glucocorticoid activity. Fludrocortisone is the only mineralocorticoid available and is the drug of choice for chronic mineralocorticoid replacement.

Therapeutic Uses. Fludrocortisone is a preferred drug for treating Addison's disease, primary hypoaldosteronism, and congenital adrenal hyperplasia (when salt wasting is a feature of the syndrome). In most cases, fludrocortisone must be used in combination with a glucocorticoid (e.g., hydrocortisone, cortisone).

Adverse Effects. Adverse effects are a direct consequence of mineralocorticoid actions. When dosage is too high, salt and water are retained in excess, while excessive amounts of potassium are lost. These effects on salt and water can result in expansion of blood volume, hypertension, edema, cardiac enlargement, and hypokalemia. Patients should be monitored for weight gain and elevation of blood pressure. If these changes occur, fludrocortisone should be temporarily withdrawn. Fluid and electrolyte imbalance should resolve spontaneously within days.

Preparations, Dosage, and Administration. Fludrocortisone acetate [Florinef Acetate] is available in 0.1-mg tablets for oral administration. The usual daily dose is 0.1 mg. If excessive salt retention occurs, the daily dose should be decreased to 0.05 mg.

AGENTS FOR DIAGNOSTIC TESTING OF ADRENOCORTICAL FUNCTION
Corticotropin and Cosyntropin

Corticotropin and cosyntropin mimic the effects of human ACTH. That is, both compounds act on the adrenal cortex to stimulate synthesis and secretion of cortisol and other adrenal corticosteroids. Corticotropin is prepared from animal pituitary glands and is nearly identical in structure to human ACTH. Cosyntropin is a synthetic polypeptide whose structure corresponds to the first 24 amino acids of ACTH. Because corticotropin, cosyntropin, and ACTH all produce equivalent stimulation of the adrenal cortex, we will use the term *ACTH* in reference to all three compounds.

Clinical Applications

ACTH is used primarily for diagnostic tests. For reasons discussed below, ACTH has only limited utility as a medication.

Diagnosis of Adrenal Insufficiency. Suspected adrenal insufficiency can be assessed by administering ACTH and then measuring plasma cortisol content. In patients with primary adrenocortical insufficiency, ACTH is unable to promote cortisol synthesis. Hence, plasma levels of the hormone will not rise. If ACTH succeeds in elevating cortisol levels, primary adrenal insufficiency can be ruled out.

Therapeutic Uses. Because of its ability to stimulate glucocorticoid production, ACTH can, in theory, be used to treat a variety of conditions responsive to glucocorticoids. In practice, however, ACTH is rarely used for therapeutics. Why? Because (1) responses to ACTH are highly variable; (2) ACTH cannot be given orally, whereas glucocorticoids can; (3) ACTH can produce undesired side effects by stimulating production of adrenal androgens, and possibly aldosterone too; (4) since the therapeutic effects of ACTH derive from enhanced glucocorticoid production, ACTH is only useful in patients with functioning adrenal glands; and (5) there is no evidence that treatment with ACTH offers any benefit over treatment with glucocorticoids themselves. Consequently, in most cases where ACTH might be employed, it is preferable to treat with a glucocorticoid directly.

Preparations

There are two preparations of corticotropin and one of cosyntropin. *Corticotropin injection* [Acthar, ACTH] is dispensed in 25- and 40-unit vials; routes are IM, SC, and IV. *Repository corticotropin injection* [H.P. Acthar Gel, ACTH-80] is dispensed in 40- and 80-unit vials; routes are IM and SC. Cosyntropin [Cortrosyn] is dispensed in 0.25-mg vials; routes are IM and IV.

Dexamethasone

Dexamethasone is a synthetic steroid that has pronounced glucocorticoid properties and very little mineralocorticoid activity. The drug is used primarily to treat nonendocrine disorders. Dexamethasone is also employed in the diagnostic tests described below.

Overnight Dexamethasone Suppression Test

The overnight dexamethasone suppression test is used to diagnose Cushing's syndrome. This test is performed by administering 1 mg of dexamethasone at 11:00 PM followed by measurement of plasma cortisol levels at 8:00 the following morning. In normal individuals, dexamethasone acts on the pituitary to suppress release of ACTH, thereby suppressing synthesis and release of cortisol. If the patient has Cushing's syndrome, little or no suppression of cortisol production will occur.

Prolonged Dexamethasone Suppression Test

Once Cushing's syndrome has been diagnosed, the prolonged dexamethasone suppression test can be used to distinguish between excessive ACTH release as the cause versus dysfunction of the adrenal cortex as the cause. This test is performed as follows: (1) baseline measurement of urinary 17-hydroxycorticosteroids is made (these compounds provide an index of adrenal corticosteroid production); (2) dexamethasone is administered in 2-mg doses every 6 hours for 48 hours; and (3) 24-hour urine is collected for determination of 17-hydroxycorticosteroids. If primary adrenal dysfunction is responsible for the symptoms of Cushing's syndrome, no suppression of 17-hydroxycorticosteroid production will occur. In contrast, if excessive ACTH release underlies Cushing's syndrome, prolonged administration of dexamethasone should produce some suppression of ACTH secretion, and therefore should cause a small but measurable reduction in urinary 17-hydroxycorticosteroids.

It should be noted that the dexamethasone suppression test is not the best method for determining the underlying cause of Cushing's syndrome. The preferred procedure is to measure plasma ACTH and cortisol content directly. If plasma cortisol levels are high and ACTH levels are normal, adrenal dysfunction is responsible for the observed signs. If levels of both ACTH and cortisol are high, excessive ACTH secretion is the likely underlying problem.

INHIBITORS OF CORTICOSTEROID SYNTHESIS

Several drugs have been employed to inhibit excessive corticosteroid synthesis in patients with Cushing's disease. Two of these—ketoconazole and aminoglutethimide—are discussed below. Although these agents can help relieve hypercortisolism, they are not a preferred form of therapy. Instead, they are used primarily as adjuncts to radiation therapy during the period required for irradiation of the pituitary to produce its effects (usually several months).

Ketoconazole

Ketoconazole [Nizoral] is an antifungal drug that also inhibits glucocorticoid synthesis. In fact, ketoconazole is the most effective inhibitor of glucocorticoid synthesis available. In patients with Cushing's syndrome, the drug may be used as an adjunct to surgery or radiation, but not as primary treatment. The dosage for suppression of steroid synthesis is 600 to 800 mg/day—much higher than doses employed for antifungal therapy. At these doses, ketoconazole can cause significant liver dysfunction. The basic pharmacology of ketoconazole is discussed in Chapter 88 (Antifungal Agents).

Aminoglutethimide

Actions. Aminoglutethimide [Cytadren] blocks the conversion of cholesterol to pregnenolone, the first step in the synthesis of all adrenal steroids. As a result, production of glucocorticoids, mineralocorticoids, and androgens declines.

Therapeutic Use. Aminoglutethimide has been employed as temporary therapy to decrease excessive corticosteroid production in patients awaiting more definitive therapy (e.g., surgery). Duration of treatment is seldom greater than 3 months. In patients with adrenal adenoma, adrenal carcinoma, and ectopic ACTH-secreting tumors, morning plasma levels of cortisol are reduced by about 50%. Aminoglutethimide does not affect the underlying disease process; hence, if therapy is stopped, excessive production of adrenal corticoids will resume.

Adverse Effects. Untoward effects are common. The most frequent are drowsiness, nausea, anorexia, and morbilliform rash. Additional effects include headache, dizziness, hematologic abnormalities, hypothyroidism, muscle pain, and fever. Masculinization may occur in females. Precocious sexual development may occur in males.

Preparations, Dosage, and Administration. Aminoglutethimide [Cytadren] is available in 250-mg tablets for oral use. The initial dosage is 250 mg every 6 hours. If steroid synthesis remains excessive, dosage may be gradually increased, but should not exceed 2 gm/day.

⁘ KEY POINTS

- The adrenal cortex produces three classes of steroid hormones: glucocorticoids, mineralocorticoids, and androgens.
- Glucocorticoids influence the metabolism of carbohydrates, proteins, and fats. In addition, they affect skeletal muscle, the cardiovascular system, and the CNS. At times of stress, glucocorticoids are essential for survival.
- Synthesis and release of glucocorticoids is regulated by a negative feedback loop involving CRF from the hypothalamus, ACTH from the pituitary, and cortisol from the adrenal cortex.

- Aldosterone, the major mineralocorticoid, acts on the kidney to promote retention of sodium and water and excretion of potassium and hydrogen.
- Glucocorticoid excess causes Cushing's syndrome.
- The principal treatment for Cushing's syndrome is surgical removal of the adrenals (if adrenal cancer is the cause) or part of the pituitary (if pituitary cancer is the cause).
- Ketoconazole can be used to suppress synthesis of adrenal steroids in patients with Cushing's syndrome. However, this drug is employed only as an adjunct to surgery or radiation.
- Adrenal insufficiency causes Addison's disease.
- Adrenal insufficiency is treated by replacement therapy with glucocorticoids—usually cortisone or hydrocortisone. Fludrocortisone, a pure mineralocorticoid,

may be added if the mineralocorticoid actions of cortisone or hydrocortisone are inadequate.
- In patients with adrenal insufficiency, it is absolutely essential to increase glucocorticoid doses at times of stress (e.g., surgery, trauma). Failure to do so may be fatal.
- When used in the low (physiologic) doses needed for replacement therapy, glucocorticoids have no adverse effects. In contrast, when used chronically in the high (pharmacologic) doses needed to treat nonendocrine diseases (e.g., arthritis), glucocorticoids can cause severe adverse effects (see Chapter 68).
- Corticotropin and cosyntropin are drugs that act like ACTH (i.e., they stimulate the synthesis and release of corticosteroids).
- Corticotropin and cosyntropin are used only for diagnosis of adrenal insufficiency—not for treatment.

Summary of Major Nursing Implications*

GLUCOCORTICOIDS: HYDROCORTISONE AND CORTISONE

The nursing implications summarized here apply only to the use of glucocorticoids for *replacement therapy*. Nursing implications that apply to use of glucocorticoids for *nonendocrine disorders* are summarized in Chapter 68.

Use in Addison's Disease

Administration. Instruct the patient to take two-thirds of the daily dose in the morning and one-third in the afternoon. Make certain the patient understands that replacement therapy must continue lifelong.

Emergency Preparedness. Warn the patient that the dosage must be increased at times of stress (e.g., infection, surgery, trauma). Advise the patient to carry an emergency supply of glucocorticoids at all times. This supply should include an injectable glucocorticoid plus an oral preparation. Advise the patient to wear identification (e.g., Medic Alert bracelet) to inform emergency medical personnel of his or her glucocorticoid requirements.

Use in Congenital Adrenal Hyperplasia

To assess therapy, monitor the child at 3-month intervals for signs of excess androgen production (e.g., excessive growth rate, virilization in girls, precocious penile enlargement in boys). Suppression of these effects indicates success.

*Patient education information is highlighted as blue text.

Minimizing Adverse Effects

Excessive doses can produce symptoms of Cushing's syndrome. Observe the patient for signs of Cushing's syndrome and notify the physician if these develop.

FLUDROCORTISONE (A MINERALOCORTICOID)

Route

Oral.

Minimizing Adverse Effects

Excessive doses cause retention of sodium and water and excessive excretion of potassium, resulting in expansion of blood volume, hypertension, cardiac enlargement, edema, and hypokalemia. **Inform patients about signs of salt and water retention (e.g., unusual weight gain, swelling of the feet or lower legs), and instruct them to notify the physician if these occur.** Treatment consists of temporary withdrawal of fludrocortisone; fluid and electrolyte balance should normalize within days.

Androgens

The androgen hormones are produced by the testes, ovaries, and adrenal cortex. The major endogenous androgen is testosterone. Androgens are noted most for their ability to promote expression of male sex characteristics. However, androgens also influence sexuality in females. In addition, androgens have significant physiologic and pharmacologic effects unrelated to sex. The primary clinical application of the androgens is management of androgen deficiency in males. Principal adverse effects are virilization and hepatotoxicity.

TESTOSTERONE

Testosterone is the prototype of the androgen hormones. This compound is the principal endogenous androgen in both males and females. In addition to its physiologic role, testosterone is representative of the androgens employed clinically. The structural formula of testosterone is shown in Figure 58–1.

Biosynthesis and Secretion

Males. Testosterone is made by Leydig cells of the testes. Daily production in men ranges from 2.5 to 10 mg. Synthesis of testosterone is promoted by two hormones of the anterior pituitary: follicle-stimulating hormone (FSH) and luteinizing hormone (LH), also known as interstitial cell–stimulating hormone. Production of testosterone is under negative feedback control: Rising plasma levels of testosterone act on the pituitary to suppress further release of FSH and LH, thereby reducing the stimulus for further testosterone formation.

Some of the testosterone present in plasma is produced by the adrenals. However, androgenic activity of adrenal origin is much less than that of testicular origin. Hence, in males, adrenal androgens have minimal functional significance.

Females. In women, preandrogens (precursors of testosterone) are secreted by the adrenal cortex and the ovaries. Conversion into testosterone takes place in peripheral tissues. Synthesis of preandrogens by the adrenals is regulated by adrenocorticotropic hormone (ACTH), whereas ovarian production of preandrogens is under the control of LH. Total daily secretion of testosterone is about 0.3 mg—that is, 10 to 40 times less than the amount produced in men. In the event of ovarian or adrenocortical pathology (e.g., adenoma, carcinoma, hyperplasia), secretion of androgens can be greatly increased, and may be sufficient to produce virilization.

Mechanism of Action

Effects of testosterone on its target tissues are mediated by specific receptors located in the cell cytoplasm. Following binding of testosterone to its receptor, the hormone-receptor complex migrates to the cell nucleus, and then acts on DNA to promote synthesis of specific messenger RNA molecules. These, in turn, serve as templates for production of specific proteins. It is through these proteins that the effects of testosterone become manifest. It should be noted that in some tissues—prostate, seminal vesicles, and hair follicles—androgen receptors do not interact with testosterone itself; rather, they interact with dihydrotestosterone, a metabolite of testosterone.

Physiologic and Pharmacologic Effects
Effects on Sex Characteristics in Males

Pubertal Transformation. Increased production of testosterone brings on the transformations that signal puberty in males. Under the influence of testosterone, the testes enlarge, followed by growth of the penis and scrotum. Pubic and axillary hair appear, and hair on the trunk, arms, and legs assumes adult male patterns. Testosterone stimulates growth of bone and skeletal muscle, causing height and weight to increase rapidly. Testosterone also accelerates epiphyseal closure, causing bone growth to cease within a few years. The larynx enlarges, thereby deepening the voice. Sebaceous glands increase in number, causing the skin to become oily; acne results if the glands become clogged and infected. The final pubertal change is beard development. Several years are required for all of these transformations to take place.

Spermatogenesis. Androgens are necessary for production of sperm by the seminiferous tubules, and for maturation of sperm as they pass through the epididymis and vas deferens. Androgen deficiency causes sterility.

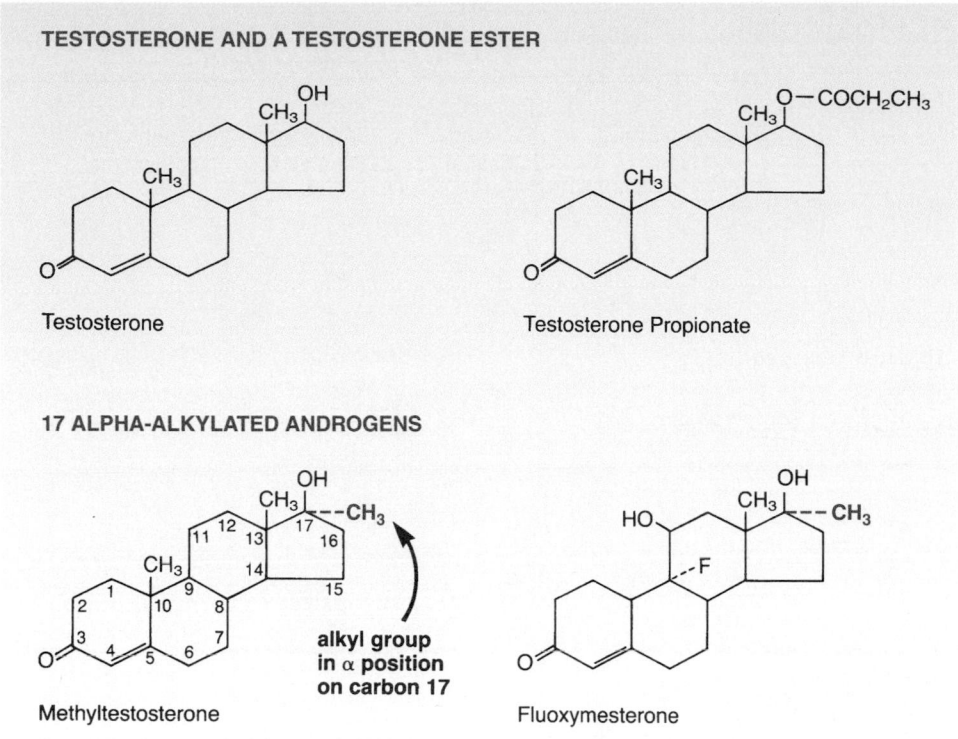

Figure 58–1 ■ **Structural formulas of representative androgens.**

Effects on Sex Characteristics in Females

Under physiologic conditions, endogenous androgens have only moderate effects in females. Principal effects are promotion of clitoral growth and, perhaps, maintenance of normal libido. However, when production of androgens becomes excessive (e.g., in girls with congenital adrenal hyperplasia), virilization can take place. Virilization can also occur in response to therapeutic use of androgens (see below).

Anabolic Effects

Testosterone promotes growth of skeletal muscle. This anabolic effect results from binding of androgens to the same type of receptor that mediates androgen actions in other tissues. Effects in young males and in females of any age can be dramatic. In contrast, effects in healthy adult males are modest—because the testes of adult males already produce enough testosterone to cause near-maximal stimulation of the musculature. Hence, in adult males, the increment in muscle mass that can be achieved with exogenous androgens is relatively small.

Erythropoietic Effects

Testosterone promotes synthesis of erythropoietin, a hormone that acts on bone marrow to increase production of erythrocytes. This action of testosterone, together with the high levels of testosterone present in males, explains why men have a greater hematocrit than women. When women are given testosterone, the hematocrit rises and hemoglobin levels increase by an average of 4.3 gm/dl. In contrast, since men have high testosterone levels to begin with, the in-

crease in plasma hemoglobin content that can be elicited with exogenous androgens is smaller—only 1 gm/dl.

CLINICAL PHARMACOLOGY OF THE ANDROGENS

In addition to testosterone, several other androgens are employed clinically. All of these agents can bind to androgen receptors, and therefore all can elicit similar responses. Major differences among individual androgens pertain to route of administration, pharmacokinetics, adverse effects, and specific applications.

Classification

The androgens fall into three basic categories: (1) testosterone and testosterone esters, (2) 17-alpha-alkylated compounds (noted for their hepatotoxicity), and (3) miscellaneous androgens. The androgens that belong to each class are listed in Table 58–1.

When speaking of testosterone-like compounds, it is traditional to distinguish between "androgens" and "anabolic steroids." However, we will not make this distinction. Why? Because it is now clear that the receptor type that mediates the androgenic actions of the androgens is the same receptor type that mediates the anabolic actions of these hormones. Consequently, it has not been possible to separate anabolic activity from androgenic activity: Virtually all anabolic hormones are also androgenic. Accordingly, rather than creating two categories—androgens versus anabolic steroids—and as-

TABLE 58–1 ■ Uses of Individual Androgens					
	Approved Indications				
Angrogen	**Hypogonadism (Male)**	**Delayed Puberty (Male)**	**Breast Cancer (Female)**	**Hereditary Angioedema**	**Catabolic States**
Testosterone and Testosterone Esters					
Testosterone	✔	✔	✔		
Testosterone cypionate	✔	✔	✔		
Testosterone enanthate	✔	✔	✔		
17-Alpha-Alkylated Androgens					
Fluoxymesterone	✔	✔	✔		
Methyltestosterone	✔	✔	✔		
Oxandrolone					✔
Stanozolol				✔	
Other Androgens					
Danazol				✔	
Testolactone			✔		

signing some agents to one category and some to the other, we will simply refer to all of the testosterone-like drugs as androgens.

Therapeutic Uses

Individual androgens differ from one another in their applications. No single androgen is employed for all of the uses discussed below. Specific applications of individual androgens are summarized in Table 58–1.

Male Hypogonadism. Hypogonadism in males is the principal indication for androgens. In this condition, the testes fail to produce adequate amounts of testosterone, and hence replacement therapy is required. Male hypogonadism may be hereditary or it may result from other causes, including pituitary failure, hypothalamic failure, and primary dysfunction of the testes.

When complete hypogonadism occurs in boys, puberty will not take place (unless exogenous androgens are supplied). To induce puberty, a long-acting parenteral preparation (usually *testosterone enanthate* or *testosterone cypionate*) is chosen; injections are given IM every 2 to 4 weeks for 3 to 4 years. Under the influence of these androgens, the normal sequence of pubertal changes occurs: growth is accelerated, the penis enlarges, the voice deepens, and other secondary sex characteristics become expressed. As in normal males, these changes take place over several years.

Androgen replacement therapy is also beneficial when testicular failure occurs in adult males. Treatment restores libido, increases ejaculate volume, and supports expression of secondary sex characteristics. However, treatment will not restore fertility. The principal drugs employed for testosterone replacement are testosterone itself and two testosterone esters: testosterone enanthate and testosterone cypionate. Preparations and dosages for replacement therapy are summarized in Table 58–2 and discussed below under *Androgen Preparations for Male Hypogonadism.*

Delayed Puberty. In some boys, puberty fails to occur at the usual age (i.e., prior to 15). Most often, this failure reflects a familial pattern of delayed puberty and is not indicative of pathology. Puberty can be expected to occur spontaneously, but at an age somewhat older than is normal. Hence, although androgen therapy can be employed, treatment is not an absolute necessity. However, although therapy is not required, the psychologic pressures of delayed sexual maturation are sometimes greater than a boy (or his parents) can tolerate. In these cases, a limited course of androgen therapy is indicated. If delayed puberty is the result of true hypogonadism, long-term replacement therapy should be instituted.

Breast Cancer. Testosterone and other androgens have been used to provide palliation in women with advanced and metastatic breast carcinoma. The mechanism of palliation is unknown. For treatment of breast cancer, high doses of androgens are required. As a result, some virilization is inevitable; the patient should be forewarned of this likelihood. In contrast to their beneficial effects in women, androgens *exacerbate* breast cancer in males, and hence are contraindicated.

Replacement Therapy in Menopausal Women. Testosterone replacement therapy can alleviate some menopausal symptoms, especially fatigue, reduced libido, and reduced genital sensitivity. Testosterone replacement therapy is discussed in Box 58–1.

Wasting in Patients with AIDS. Testosterone levels often decline in patients with AIDS, putting them at risk of wasting and loss of muscle mass. Testosterone replacement therapy decreases this risk.

Hereditary Angioedema. Hereditary angioedema is a disorder in which an inhibitor of the complement system is deficient. Lack of the inhibitor allows uncontrolled activation of the complement cascade, resulting in increased vascular permeability and angioedema (localized swelling of the subcutaneous tissue of the face, hands, feet, and genitalia). Androgens provide prophylaxis against this response by elevating plasma levels of the deficient inhibitor. For treatment of hereditary angioedema, *stanozolol* and *danazol* are the androgens of choice.

TABLE 58–2 ■ Products for Androgen Replacement Therapy in Hypogonadal Males

Formulation	Drug	Trade Name	Dosage	Comments
Oral	Fluoxymesterone Methyltestosterone	Halotestin Oreton Methyl	5–20 mg/day 10–50 mg/day	These 17-alpha-alkylated androgens are hepatotoxic and androgenic effects are erratic.
Intramuscular	Testosterone cypionate Testosterone enanthate	Depo-Testosterone Delatestryl	50–400 mg q 2–4 wk 50–400 mg q 2–4 wk	Safe, but require an office visit every 2 to 4 weeks. Blood levels fluctuate widely (high after dosing and low before the next dose) and thereby cause variations in libido, energy, and mood.
Transdermal Patch	Testosterone	Testoderm	One 10- or 15-mg patch/day (delivers 4 or 6 mg/24 hr)	Applied to the scrotum, which must be shaved weekly. Hard to apply and tends to fall off.
		Testoderm TTS	One 328-mg patch/day (delivers 5 mg/24 hr)	Applied to the arm, back, or upper buttocks, but *not* the scrotum. Stays in place, but causes local irritation.
		Androderm	One 12- or 24-mg patch/day (delivers 2.5 or 5 mg/24 hr)	Applied to the arm, back, abdomen, or thigh, but *not* the scrotum. Stays in place, but causes local irritation.
Transdermal Gel	Testosterone	AndroGel	5–10 gm of 1% gel/day (delivers 50–100 mg/day)	Applied to upper arm, shoulder, or abdomen, but *not* the scrotum. Easier to use and better tolerated than testosterone patches. Can transfer to others via intimate contact.
Implantable Pellets	Testosterone	Testopel	150–450 mg (2–6 pellets) SC q 3–4 mo	Implanted SC. Long lasting. Produce steady blood levels.

Anemias. Androgens may be used in men and women to treat anemias that have been refractory to other therapy. Anemias that may respond include aplastic anemia, anemia associated with renal failure, Fanconi's anemia, and anemia caused by cancer chemotherapy. Androgens help relieve anemia by promoting synthesis of erythropoietin, the renal hormone that stimulates production of red blood cells. In addition to increasing erythrocyte count, androgens may stimulate production of white blood cells and platelets.

Adverse Effects

Virilization. This is the most common complication of androgen therapy. When taken in high doses by women, androgens can cause acne, deepening of the voice, proliferation of facial and body hair, male-pattern baldness, increased libido, clitoral enlargement, and menstrual irregularities. Clitoral growth, hair loss, and lowering of the voice may be irreversible. Masculinization can also occur in children. Boys may experience growth of pubic hair, penile enlargement, increased frequency of erections, and even priapism (persistent erection). In girls, growth of pubic hair and clitoral enlargement may occur. To prevent irreversible masculinization, androgens must be discontinued when virilizing effects first appear. In the treatment of breast carcinoma, some virilization should be tolerated.

Premature Epiphyseal Closure. When given to children, androgens can accelerate epiphyseal closure, thereby decreasing adult height. To evaluate androgen effects on the epiphyses, x-ray examination of the hand and wrist should be performed every 6 months.

Hepatotoxicity. Androgens can cause *cholestatic hepatitis* and other disorders of the liver. Clinical *jaundice* may occur, but this is rare. Patients receiving androgens should undergo periodic tests of liver function. If jaundice develops, it will reverse following discontinuation of androgen use. Androgens may also be carcinogenic: *Hepatocellular carcinoma* has developed in some patients following prolonged use of these drugs.

It must be emphasized that not all androgens are hepatotoxic: Liver damage is associated primarily with *the 17-alpha-alkylated androgens.* As indicated in Figure 58–1 (see methyltestosterone), these androgens all share a structural feature in common: an alkyl group substituted on carbon 17 of the steroid nucleus. Because of their capacity to cause liver damage, *the 17-alpha-alkylated compounds should not be used long term.* In contrast to the 17-alpha-alkylated androgens, the testosterone esters (testosterone propionate, testosterone cypionate, testosterone enanthate) have never been associated with liver disease.

Effects on Cholesterol Levels. Androgens can lower plasma levels of high-density lipoprotein (HDL) cholesterol ("good cholesterol") and elevate plasma levels of low-density lipoprotein (LDL) cholesterol ("bad cholesterol"). These actions may increase the risk of atherosclerosis.

Use in Pregnancy. Because of their ability to induce masculinization of the female fetus, androgens are contraindicated during pregnancy. Potential fetal changes include vaginal malformation, clitoral enlargement, and formation of a structure resembling the male scrotum. Virilization is most likely when androgens are taken during the first trimester. Women who become pregnant while using androgens should be informed about the possible impact on the fetus. Androgens are classified in Food and Drug Administration Pregnancy Risk Category X: The ability to cause fetal harm outweighs any possible therapeutic benefit.

Edema. Edema can result from androgen-induced retention of salt and water. This complication is of concern for patients with heart failure and for those with a predisposition to developing edema from other causes. Treatment consists of discontinuing the androgen; a diuretic may also be needed.

BOX 58-1 ■ TESTOSTERONE REPLACEMENT THERAPY IN WOMEN?

Testosterone replacement is a relatively new and promising method to relieve some menopausal symptoms. As noted in the discussion of androgen physiology, women produce about 0.3 mg of testosterone daily. However, in the perimenopausal period, testosterone production falls. As a result, women may experience fatigue, loss of bone and muscle mass, and a decline in libido, genital sensitivity, and sense of well-being. Testosterone replacement therapy can improve some of these symptoms. Most notably, testosterone can reduce fatigue, increase sexual motivation, heighten genital sensitivity, and improve the sense of well-being. In addition, testosterone may reduce hot flushes as well as the breast pain that occurs in women taking estrogen supplements.

Because experience with testosterone replacement therapy is limited, we have no firm guidelines regarding dosage, dosing schedule, or route of administration. What we do know is that doses should be low, since the goal is to mimic premenopausal testosterone production—and not to supply testosterone in pharmacologic doses. Unfortunately, most commercial testosterone preparations are formulated for men, and hence contain doses that are much too high for women. As a result, formulations for women have to be custom compounded by the pharmacist.

Both topical and oral administration have been tried. For *oral* therapy, *methyltestosterone* and *testosterone* have been used. The recommended dosage for methyltestosterone is 0.25 to 0.75 mg/day. Formulations for *topical* therapy include *testosterone propionate (1% to 2%) in petrolatum* and *2% micronized testosterone gel.* The testosterone propionate formulation is applied to the genital mucosa. The micronized testosterone formulation is applied to the skin of the arm, thigh, or abdomen. For both formulations, the initial dosage is one-quarter teaspoon or less daily. Over time, the frequency of topical administration (genital or dermal) can be reduced to 3 or 4 times per week. Alternatively, topical therapy can be replaced with oral therapy.

Adverse effects are uncommon when testosterone dosages are kept appropriately low. However, if topical or oral dosing is excessive, typical androgenic side effects can result. Among these are acne, deepening of the voice, hirsutism, clitoral enlargement, and reduction of HDL cholesterol.

At this time, our understanding of testosterone replacement therapy is limited. We do not know the optimal dosage, dosing schedule, or route of administration, nor do we know what the full benefits or long-term risks of treatment may be. Hopefully, future research will resolve these uncertainties.

Gynecomastia. Breast enlargement may occur in males receiving androgen replacement therapy. This effect results from conversion of certain androgens into estrogen.

Abuse Potential. As discussed below, androgens are frequently misused (abused) to enhance athletic performance. Because of their abuse potential, most androgens are now regulated under the Controlled Substances Act. Of the androgens listed in Table 58–1, all but danazol are classified as Schedule III drugs; danazol remains unregulated.

Androgen Preparations for Male Hypogonadism

In recent years, treatment options for androgen replacement therapy have expanded. In the past, IM therapy with a long-acting testosterone ester was the major form of treatment. Today, we have three attractive alternatives: transdermal testosterone patches, a transdermal testosterone gel, and implantable testosterone pellets. Table 58–2 presents a summary of these and other androgen preparations used for replacement therapy in hypogonadal males.

Oral Androgens. Only two androgens are approved for oral therapy of male hypogonadism. Both drugs—*fluoxymesterone* [Halotestin] and *methyltestosterone* [Oreton Methyl]—are *17-alpha-alkylated androgens,* and hence pose a risk of hepatotoxicity. Accordingly, they should not be used long-term, and hence are not first-line agents.

Depot Preparations: Intramuscular Testosterone Esters. Two testosterone esters are available: *testosterone cypionate* [Depo-Testosterone] and *testosterone enanthate* [Delatestryl]. Both drugs are formulated in oil, and both are long

acting. Following IM injection, these drugs are slowly absorbed and then hydrolyzed to release free testosterone. For replacement therapy in hypogonadal males, the usual dosage for both is 50 to 400 mg IM every 2 to 4 weeks. Unfortunately, these preparations produce testosterone blood levels that fluctuate widely. Specifically, testosterone levels are higher than normal shortly after dosing, and decline to lower than normal prior to the next dose. As a result, patients may experience significant variations in libido, energy, and mood.

Testosterone Transdermal Patches. Testosterone is available in three transdermal patches: Testoderm, Testoderm TTS, and Androderm. All three products are indicated for replacement therapy in males with hypogonadism. The patches are replaced once every 24 hours.

Testoderm is applied once daily to the *scrotum.* (Because scrotal skin is very thin, absorption from this site is more efficient than from other sites.) To help the patch adhere, the scrotum must be shaved at least once a week. However, despite shaving, the patch may fall off during exercise. Also, in men with primary hypogonadism, the scrotum may be too small to accept the patch. The principal adverse effect is scrotal rash. Testoderm patches are available in two strengths: 10 mg (which delivers 4 mg of testosterone in 24 hours) and 15 mg (which delivers 6 mg of testosterone in 24 hours). For male hypogonadism, the usual dosage is one patch (10 or 15 mg) daily.

Testoderm TTS differs from Testoderm in that Testoderm TTS is designed for application to the arm, back, or upper buttocks—but *not* the scrotum. To ensure that testosterone blood levels are sufficient, Testoderm TTS patches contain much more testosterone than do Testoderm patches (328 mg

TABLE 58–3 ▪ Impact of Testosterone on Muscle Mass and Strength in Normal Men		
Regimen	Increase in Muscle Mass (pounds)	Increase in Bench-Press (pounds)
Testosterone* alone	7	20
Exercise alone	4	20
Testosterone* + exercise	13	48

*Testosterone dosage = 600 mg testosterone enanthate, IM, daily for 10 weeks.
Data from Bhasin S, Storer TW, Berman N. The effects of supraphysiologic doses of testosterone on muscle size and strength in normal men. N Engl J Med 1996;335:1.

vs. only 10 or 15 mg). Like Testoderm, Testoderm TTS can cause local irritation, but is better tolerated than Testoderm. Because Testoderm TTS patches are not applied to the scrotum, they adhere better than Testoderm.

Androderm patches are applied to the upper arm, thigh, back, or abdomen—but *not* the scrotum. Two sizes are available: 12 mg (which delivers 2.5 mg of testosterone in 24 hours) and 24 mg (which delivers 5 mg in 24 hours). The usual dosage is 12 or 24 mg once daily. The principal adverse effect—rash at the site of application—is more intense than with Testoderm or Testoderm TTS.

Testosterone Transdermal Gel. Testosterone is now available in a 1% gel [AndroGel] for once-daily topical therapy of male hypogonadism. After the gel is applied, testosterone is absorbed rapidly into the skin, and then slowly into the blood over the next 24 hours. Compared with transdermal patches, the gel has three advantages: (1) it causes less local irritation, (2) it can't fall off (as the patches often do), and (3) it produces more consistent blood levels of testosterone.

The principal disadvantage of the gel is that testosterone can be transferred to another person by skin-to-skin contact. This is possible because only 10% of an applied dose is absorbed; the other 90% remains on the skin after the gel dries. In one study, blood levels of testosterone were doubled in female partners of gel users following 15 minutes of intimate contact that had taken place 2 to 12 hours after gel application. Testosterone transfer is a concern because the drug can cause virilization of female partners and fetal harm.

AndroGel is dispensed in 2.5- and 5-gm unit-dose foil packets. The 2.5-gm packet contains 25 mg of testosterone (of which 2.5 mg becomes absorbed), and the 5.0-mg packet contains 50 mg of testosterone (of which 5.0 mg becomes absorbed). The gel is applied once daily (preferably in the morning) to clean, dry skin of the shoulders, upper arms, or abdomen—but *not* to the genitalia. Instruct patients to squeeze the entire contents of the packet into the palms, and then immediately apply the gel to the skin and rub it in. To prevent the transfer of testosterone to others, patients should wash their hands and, once the gel has dried, keep the treated area covered with clothing. Because testosterone can be washed off, patients should wait 5 to 6 hours before showering or swimming. To ensure safe and effective dosing, blood levels of testosterone should be measured 14 days after initiating therapy and periodically thereafter.

Testosterone Implantable Pellets. Testosterone pellets [Testopel] are long-acting formulations indicated for male hypogonadism and delayed puberty. The pellets are implanted subdermally in the abdominal wall lateral to the umbilicus. Each pellet contains 75 mg of testosterone. The usual dosage is 150 to 450 mg (2 to 6 pellets) every 3 to 4 months. About one-third of the dose is absorbed in the first month, one-quarter in the second month, and one-sixth in the third month. For patients switching from IM testosterone propionate or testosterone enanthate, the recommended dosage is 2 pellets for each 25 mg of IM testosterone used weekly. For example, a patient receiving 75 mg of IM testosterone enanthate each week would be switched to 6 implanted pellets every 3 to 4 months.

ANDROGEN (ANABOLIC STEROID) ABUSE BY ATHLETES

Many athletes take androgens (anabolic steroids) to enhance athletic performance. The potential benefits of this practice, although substantial, are accompanied by substantial risks. The drugs taken most commonly by athletes are nandrolone [Durabolin], stanozolol [Winstrol], and methenolone (not available in the United States). All of these drugs are regulated under the Controlled Substances Act, making their use by athletes illegal.

Who takes steroids? Steroid use is especially prevalent among football players, weight lifters, discus throwers, shot-putters, and body builders. The drugs are also used by sprinters and by athletes in endurance sports (e.g., cycling, Nordic skiing). Steroids are used by athletes of all ages (professionals as well as athletes in college, high school, and junior high). Use is not limited to males: Some females also take them, despite masculinizing effects.

What can anabolic steroids do for the athlete? The answer depends partly on the age and gender of the athlete, and partly on whether an athlete or a scientist is answering the question. Scientists and athletes have agreed for years that steroids can increase muscle mass in *young males* and in *females of all ages*. However, it was not until 1996 that scientists finally demonstrated what athletes have claimed for years: Exogenous androgens can significantly increase muscle mass and strength in *sexually mature males*. In order to demonstrate these effects, scientists gave normal men *large* daily injections of testosterone enanthate for 10 weeks. Some subjects did regular strength training while receiving the drug, and some did not. As indicated in Table 58–3, testosterone treatment produced a 7-pound increase in muscle mass in the subjects who did not exercise, and a 13-pound increase in the subjects who exercised along with taking the drug. In contrast, exercise in the absence of exogenous testosterone produced only a 4-pound increase in muscle mass. Similar in-

Special Interest Topic

BOX 58–2 ■ ANDRO STRIKES OUT

Androstenedione ("Andro"), available as a dietary supplement, is taken by athletes with the expectation of enhancing performance. However, when evaluated in a recent experiment, Andro had virtually no beneficial effects. Worse yet, it produced side effects that could be harmful.

Thanks to Mark McGwire, first baseman for the St. Louis Cardinals, Andro received national attention in the summer of 1998. That was the season in which McGwire and Sammy Sosa (of the Chicago Cubs) were competing to break baseball's single-season home run record, set at 61 by Roger Maris 37 years earlier. Both players surpassed Maris' record, and McGwire went on to set the new record at 70 homers (which Sosa surpassed the next season). Along the way, McGwire revealed that he took Andro to help maintain his health—and thereby set off a national debate about the drug. Although androstenedione use is allowed by major league baseball, the drug is banned by the International Olympic Committee, National Football League, and National Collegiate Athletic Association.

When McGwire and Sosa were battling for a place in baseball history, our knowledge of Andro was very limited. We knew that androstenedione is produced naturally by the adrenal glands and gonads, and that it undergoes conversion to testosterone in peripheral tissues. In males, the amount of testosterone derived from endogenous androstenedione is insignificant compared with testosterone produced by the testes. In females, testosterone derived from endogenous androstenedione may have two functions: promotion of clitoral growth and maintenance of normal libido. In the summer of 1998, we had no information about *exogenous* Andro in *males*—although we did know, from a 1962 study,[1] that exogenous Andro could raise serum testosterone in *females* by four- to sevenfold.

A study published in 1999 greatly increased our knowledge of Andro.[2] The objective of the study was to determine the effects of oral Andro on three parameters: sex hormone levels, cholesterol levels, and adaptation of muscle to resistance training. Twenty young men, ages 19 to 29, participated in the 8-week study. Resistance training (e.g., biceps curls, bench-press, leg-press) was directed at all major muscle groups. The dosing schedule was 300 mg of oral Andro per day on days 1 to 14, 21 to 35, and 43 to 56. The results were surprising:

- Andro failed to increase blood levels of testosterone.
- Andro failed to enhance muscle responses to exercise (i.e., subjects taking Andro or placebo had identical increases in muscle size and strength after 8 weeks of training).

- Andro substantially increased blood levels of two estrogens: estradiol (up 40%) and estrone (up 44%).
- Andro produced a small (12%) decrease in HDL cholesterol (good cholesterol).

A study published the following year presented similar findings regarding the effects of Andro on levels of sex hormones.[3] In this study, 42 healthy men, ages 20 to 40, were given either placebo or oral Andro (100 or 300 mg daily for 7 days). Blood levels of testosterone and estradiol were measured at baseline and at the end of the treatment period. The result? After 7 days, testosterone levels in men given the low dose of Andro were no higher than in men given placebo. The 300-mg dose, however, did raise testosterone levels, but the increase was only modest (34%). Both doses increased levels of estradiol (up 42% with the low Andro dose and 128% with the high dose). Looking at the results of both studies, it is clear that Andro can increase levels of estradiol, and, if the dosage is sufficiently large, may produce a small increase in levels of testosterone.

In Chapter 1, we noted that effectiveness is the most important property of an ideal drug: If a drug is not effective, there is no justification for using it. From the two studies cited, it appears that Andro is not very effective: It didn't enhance skeletal muscle adaptation to resistance training, it didn't raise testosterone levels when taken in low dosage, and, when taken in high dosage, it produced a small increase in testosterone levels in one study and no increase in the other. That is, the drug largely failed to provide the benefits for which it was taken. On this basis alone, use of Andro would seem ill advised.

Not only did Andro fail to do anything beneficial, it produced effects that are potentially harmful. By raising estrogen levels in males, Andro can produce gynecomastia (breast enlargement). Although gynecomastia was not observed in these studies, it could have developed if the studies had lasted longer. Of greater concern, Andro decreased levels of HDL cholesterol—the form of cholesterol that helps protect against atherosclerosis. Hence, with prolonged use, Andro can increase the risk of coronary artery disease. Lastly, elevation of estrogen and androstenedione levels is associated with an increased risk of pancreatic cancer.

Since Andro offers little or no apparent benefit but does present risks, why is it available? Because Andro is marketed as a *dietary supplement*—not as a drug. Accordingly, Andro is not required to meet the efficacy and safety standards the Food and Drug Administration sets for medications. As long as manufacturers do not make unsubstantiated claims that Andro can be used to prevent, diagnose, or treat disease, they may continue to sell it as a supplement. Although this doesn't make pharmacologic sense, it is, nonetheless, entirely legal.

[1]Mahesh SM, Greenblatt RB. The in vivo conversion of dehydroepiandrosterone and androstenedione to testosterone in the human. Acta Endocrinol 1962;41:400–496.

[2]King DS, Sharp RL, Vukovich MD, et al. Effect of oral androstenedione on serum testosterone and adaptations to resistance training in young men: A randomized controlled trial. JAMA 1999;281:2020–2028.

[3]Leder BZ, Longcope C, Catlin DH, et al. Oral androstenedione administration and serum testosterone concentrations in young men. JAMA 2000;283:779–782.

creases were shown in the subjects' ability to bench-press weights (Table 58–3). Why has it taken so long for scientists to agree with the athletes? The principal reason is that, in studies performed prior to 1996, the doses of androgens employed were too small to elicit a clear response. When sufficiently large doses were finally given, the results were unequivocal. (In the 1996 study, the testosterone dosage was equivalent to 6 to 8 times the amount produced by the testes.)

The potential for adverse effects of androgens is significant. Salt and water retention can lead to hypertension. When administered in the high doses used by athletes, androgens suppress release of LH and FSH, resulting in testicular shrinkage, sterility, and gynecomastia (breast development). Acne is common. Reduction of HDL cholesterol and elevation of LDL cholesterol may accelerate development of atherosclerosis (although no effect was seen on lipids in the study just noted). Because most of the androgens that athletes take are 17-alpha-alkylated compounds, hepatotoxicity (cholestatic hepatitis, jaundice, hepatocellular carcinoma) is an ever-present risk. In females, androgens can cause menstrual irregularities and virilization (growth of facial hair, deepening of the voice, decreased breast size, uterine atrophy, clitoral enlargement, and male-pattern baldness); hair loss, growth of facial hair, and voice change may be irreversible. In boys and girls, androgens promote premature epiphyseal closure, thereby reducing attainable adult height. In boys, androgens can induce premature puberty.

What about psychologic effects? Interestingly, although androgens are reputed to cause depression, manic episodes, and aggressiveness ('roid rage), none of these effects was observed in the 1996 study. The authors suggested that, if an ath-

lete is mentally healthy, testosterone will not make him into a beast. On the other hand, if an athlete is already psychologically unbalanced, it is possible that steroids could intensify aberrant behavior.

Long-term androgen use can lead to an "abuse" or "addiction" syndrome. Characteristics include preoccupation with androgen use and difficulty in stopping use. When androgens finally are discontinued, an abstinence syndrome can develop similar to that produced by withdrawal of alcohol, opioids, and cocaine. Because of their abuse potential, most androgens are now classified under Schedule III of the Controlled Substances Act.

⠿ KEY POINTS

- Testosterone is the principal endogenous androgen.
- Important physiologic effects of androgens are pubertal transformation in males, maintenance of adult male sexual characteristics, promotion of muscle growth, and stimulation of erythropoiesis.
- The major indication for androgens is male hypogonadism.
- The major side effects of androgens are edema, virilization in females, premature epiphyseal closure in children, and liver toxicity (in people taking 17-alpha-alkylated androgens).
- Androgens are contraindicated during pregnancy.
- Large doses of androgens can increase muscle mass and strength in athletes. However, athletic use of androgens is illegal and carries significant risks.

Summary of Major Nursing Implications*

ANDROGENS

Danazol
Fluoxymesterone
Methyltestosterone
Oxandrolone
Stanozolol
Testolactone
Testosterone
Testosterone enanthate
Testosterone cypionate

Preadministration Assessment

Therapeutic Goals

Males. Treatment of hypogonadism and delayed puberty.

Females. Treatment of breast cancer and breast engorgement.

Males and Females. Treatment of anemias, hereditary angioedema, catabolic states, and osteoporosis.

Identifying High-Risk Patients

Androgens are *contraindicated* during pregnancy and for males who have breast cancer. Also, androgens are *contraindicated* for enhancing athletic performance.

Implementation: Administration

Routes

PO, IM, transdermal, SC (implantable pellets).

Administration

Oral. Advise patients to take oral androgens with food if GI upset occurs.

Transdermal. Advise patients using Testoderm to shave the scrotum before application.

Advise patients using AndroGel to wash their hands after applying the gel and to cover the site of application (so as to reduce the risk of transferring testosterone to others). Advise patients not to shower or swim for 5 to 6 hours after application (to avoid washing the drug off).

Implantable Pellets. Pellets are implanted subdermally (under local anesthesia) in the abdominal wall lateral to the umbilicus.

Ongoing Evaluation and Interventions

Minimizing Adverse Effects

Virilization. Virilization may occur in women, girls, and boys. **Inform female patients about signs of virilization**

*Patient education information is highlighted as blue text.

 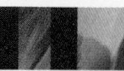

Summary of Major Nursing Implications*—cont'd

(deepening of the voice, acne, changes in body and facial hair, menstrual irregularities), and instruct them to notify the physician if these occur. Irreversible changes may be avoided if androgens are withdrawn early. In the treatment of breast carcinoma, some virilization should be tolerated.

Premature Epiphyseal Closure. Accelerated bone maturation can decrease attainable adult height. Monitor effects on epiphyses with x-rays of the hand and wrist twice yearly.

Hepatotoxicity. The *17-alpha-alkylated androgens* can cause cholestatic hepatitis, jaundice, and other liver disorders. Rarely, liver cancer develops. Obtain periodic tests of liver function. Inform patients about signs of liver dysfunction (jaundice, malaise, anorexia, fatigue, nausea), and in-struct them to notify the physician if these occur. Liver function normalizes following cessation of drug use. Avoid long-term use of 17-alpha-alkylated preparations.

Edema. Salt and water retention may result in edema. Inform patients about signs of salt and water retention (swelling of the extremities, unusual weight gain), and instruct them to notify the physician if these occur. Treatment consists of androgen withdrawal and, if necessary, use of a diuretic.

Teratogenesis. Androgens can cause masculinization of the female fetus. Rule out pregnancy prior to androgen use. Warn women against becoming pregnant while taking androgens.

*Patient education information is highlighted as blue text.

Estrogens and Progestins and Their Use in Hormone Replacement Therapy

Estrogens and progestins are hormones that promote the maturation and ongoing activity of female reproductive organs. These hormones also promote development of secondary sex characteristics in females. In addition, estrogens protect against osteoporosis. The principal endogenous estrogen is estradiol. The principal endogenous progestational hormone is progesterone. Both hormones are produced by the ovaries. During pregnancy, large amounts are also produced by the placenta.

Clinical applications of the female sex hormones fall into two major categories: contraceptive and noncontraceptive applications. In this chapter, our focus is on noncontraceptive uses; contraception is discussed in Chapter 60. The principal noncontraceptive application of estrogens and progestins is hormone replacement therapy (HRT): estrogens are given to replace estrogens that are lost following menopause; progestins are given to oppose estrogen-mediated stimulation of the endometrium.

THE MENSTRUAL CYCLE

Because much of the clinical pharmacology of the estrogens and progestins is related to their actions during the menstrual cycle, understanding the menstrual cycle is essential to understanding these hormones. Accordingly, we will begin by reviewing the menstrual cycle. The anatomic and hormonal changes that take place during the cycle are summarized in Figure 59–1. As indicated, the first half of the cycle (days 1 through 14) is called the *follicular phase;* the second half is called the *luteal phase.* One complete whole cycle typically takes 28 days.

Ovarian and Uterine Events. The menstrual cycle consists of a coordinated series of ovarian and uterine events. In the ovary, the following sequence occurs: (1) several ovarian follicles ripen; (2) one of the ripe follicles ruptures, causing ovulation; (3) the ruptured follicle evolves into a corpus luteum; and (4) if fertilization does not occur, the corpus luteum dissolves. As these ovarian events are taking place, parallel events take place in the uterus: (1) while ovarian follicles ripen, the endometrium prepares for nidation (implantation of a fertilized ovum) by increasing in thickness and vascularity; (2) following ovulation, the uterus continues its preparation by increasing secretory activity; and (3) if nidation fails to occur, the thickened endometrium breaks down, causing menstruation, and the cycle begins anew.

The Roles of Estrogens and Progesterone. The uterine changes that occur during the cycle are brought about under the influence of estrogens and progesterone produced by the ovaries. During the first half of the cycle, estrogens are secreted by the maturing ovarian follicles. As suggested by Figure 59–1, these estrogens act on the uterus to cause proliferation of the endometrium. At midcycle, one of the ovarian follicles ruptures and then evolves into a corpus luteum. For most of the second half of the cycle, estrogens and progesterone are produced by the newly formed corpus luteum. These hormones maintain the endometrium in its hypertrophied state. At the end of the cycle, the corpus luteum atrophies, causing production of estrogens and progesterone to decline. In response to the diminished supply of ovarian hormones, the endometrium breaks down.

The Role of Pituitary Hormones. Two anterior pituitary hormones—follicle-stimulating hormone (FSH) and luteinizing hormone (LH)—play central roles in regulating the menstrual cycle. During the first half of the cycle, FSH acts on the developing ovarian follicles, causing them to grow and secrete estrogens. The resultant rise in estrogen levels exerts a negative feedback influence on the pituitary, thereby suppressing further FSH release. At midcycle, LH levels rise abruptly (see Fig. 59–1). This LH surge, which is triggered by rising estrogen levels, causes one of the mature follicles to swell rapidly, burst, and release its ovum. (Why only one follicle undergoes ovulation remains a mystery.) Following ovulation, LH acts on the newly formed corpus luteum to promote secretion of estrogens and progesterone.

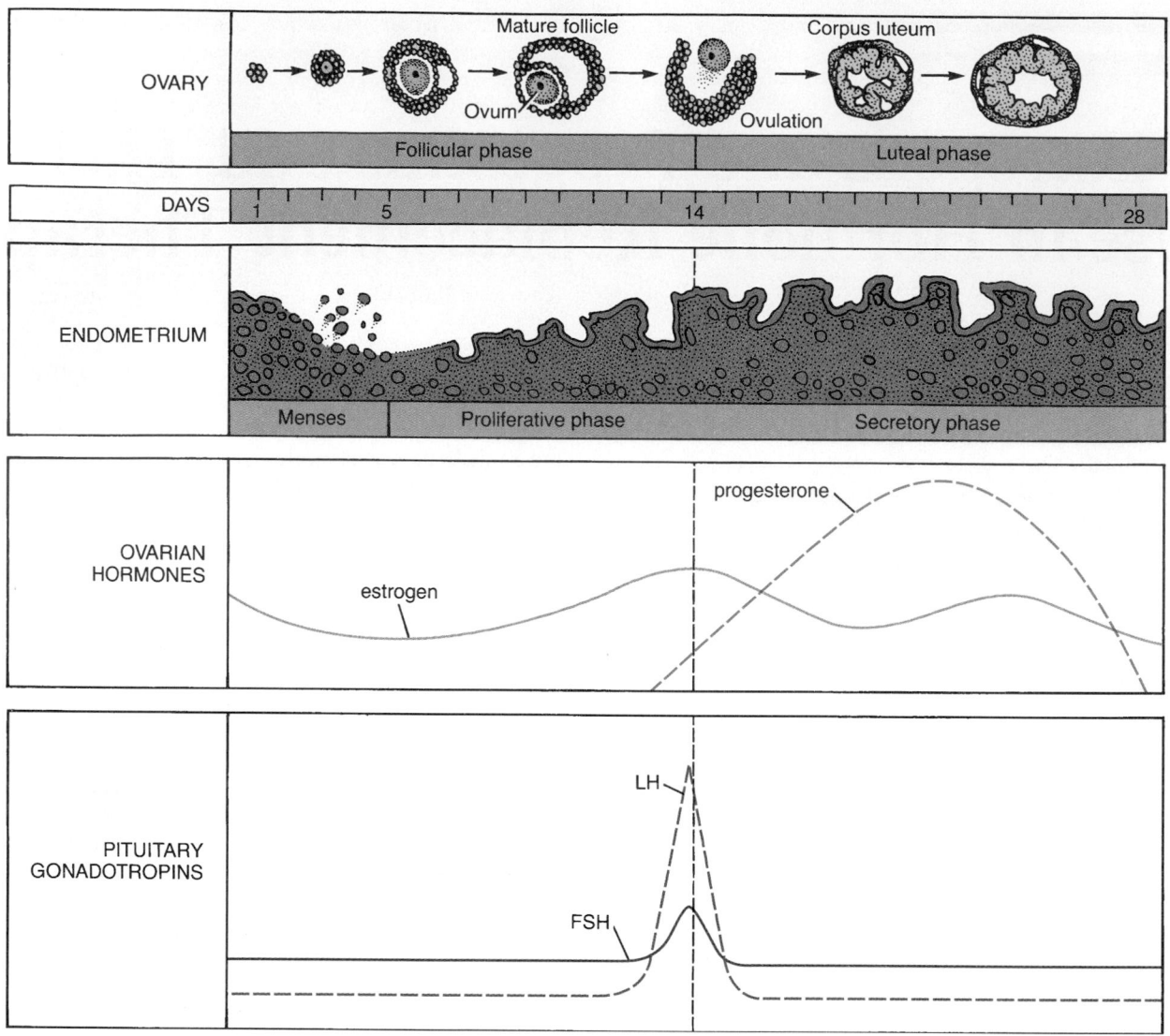

Figure 59–1 ■ **The menstrual cycle: anatomic and hormonal changes.**
(FSH = follicle-stimulating hormone, LH = luteinizing hormone.)

From the foregoing, it is clear that precisely timed alterations in the secretion of FSH and LH are responsible for coordinating the structural and secretory changes that occur throughout the menstrual cycle. The mechanisms that regulate secretion of FSH and LH are complex and incompletely understood.

ESTROGENS

Biosynthesis

Females. In premenopausal women, the ovary is the principle organ of estrogen production. During the follicular phase of the menstrual cycle, estrogens are synthesized by ovarian follicles under the direction of FSH; during the luteal phase, estrogens are synthesized by the corpus luteum under the direction of LH. The major estrogen produced by the ovaries is *estradiol*. In the periphery, some of the estradiol secreted by the ovaries is converted into *estrone* and *estriol*, hormones that are less potent than estradiol itself. Estrogens are eliminated by a combination of hepatic metabolism and urinary excretion.

During pregnancy, large quantities of estrogens are produced by the placenta. Excretion of these hormones results in high levels of estrogens in the urine. (The urine of pregnant mares is extremely rich in estrogens and serves as a commercial source of these hormones.)

Males. Estrogen production is not limited to females. In the human male, small amounts of testosterone are converted into estradiol and estrone by the testes. Enzymatic conversion of testosterone in peripheral tissues (e.g., liver, fat, skeletal muscle) results in additional estrogen production.

Physiologic and Pharmacologic Effects
Effects on Primary and Secondary Sex Characteristics of Females

Estrogens support the development and maintenance of the female reproductive tract and secondary sex characteristics. These hormones are required for the growth and maturation of the uterus, vagina, fallopian tubes, and breasts. In addition, estrogens direct development of pubic and axillary hair as well as pigmentation of the nipples and genitalia.

Estrogens have a profound influence on physiologic processes related to reproduction. During the follicular phase of the menstrual cycle, estrogens promote breast enlargement and proliferation of the vaginal and uterine epithelium, and they increase secretion from cervical glands. In addition, estrogens increase vaginal acidity (by promoting deposition of glycogen in the vaginal epithelium). At the end of the menstrual cycle, a decline in estrogen levels can bring on menstruation; however, it is the fall in progesterone levels at the end of the cycle that normally causes breakdown of the endometrium and resultant menstrual bleeding. Following menstruation, estrogens promote endometrial restoration. Although the effects of estrogens on the release of pituitary gonadotropins are not completely understood, it is clear that high levels of estrogen can suppress release of FSH. During pregnancy, estrogens stimulate uterine growth and blood flow. Also, estrogens (along with progestins) act on the breasts to promote development of the acini.

Metabolic Actions

Estrogens can affect various nonreproductive tissues. Important among these are bone, blood vessels, the heart, liver, and central nervous system (CNS).

Bone. Estrogens have a positive effect on bone mass. Under normal circumstances, bone undergoes continuous remodeling, a process in which bone mineral is resorbed and deposited in equal amounts. The principal effect of estrogens on the process is to block bone resorption, although estrogens may also promote mineral deposition. In young girls, estrogens promote the rapid growth of the long bones that occurs during puberty. In addition, they direct epiphyseal closure, and thereby bring linear growth to a halt. In postmenopausal women, estrogen replacement therapy can help maintain bone mass.

Cholesterol. Estrogens have favorable effects on cholesterol levels: levels of low-density lipoprotein (LDL) cholesterol are reduced, while levels of high-density lipoprotein (HDL) cholesterol are elevated. These beneficial effects on cholesterol metabolism result at least in part from actions in the liver. There is speculation, but no proof, that effects on cholesterol metabolism may explain the low incidence of myocardial infarction in premenopausal women.

Estrogens alter cholesterol excretion. Specifically, they increase the amount of cholesterol in bile and decrease the amount of bile acids in bile. Since bile acids are needed to keep cholesterol soluble, these effects may explain why some women taking estrogens develop cholesterol gallstones.

Clinical Pharmacology
Adverse Effects

The principal concerns with estrogen therapy are the potential for endometrial hyperplasia, endometrial cancer, breast cancer, and cardiovascular events. Other adverse effects are more of a nuisance than a concern.

Endometrial Hyperplasia and Carcinoma. Prolonged use of estrogens *alone* by postmenopausal women is associated with an increased risk of endometrial carcinoma. However, when estrogens are used in combination with a progestin, there is little or no risk of uterine cancer. Why? When used alone, estrogens act on the endometrium to cause prolif-

eration and hyperplasia. In a few cases, hyperplasia progresses to carcinoma. Progestins eliminate (or at least greatly reduce) the risk of cancer by antagonizing estrogen-mediated endometrial proliferation and by reversing hyperplasia. Accordingly, whenever estrogens are given to postmenopausal women who have an intact uterus, progestins should be given as well. If persistent or recurrent vaginal bleeding develops during the course of estrogen use, the possibility of endometrial carcinoma should be evaluated. In addition, the patient should receive an endometrial biopsy every 2 to 3 years.

Breast Cancer. The question of whether estrogens cause breast cancer has been studied intensively, but has not been fully resolved. More than 50 studies have been published. Most recently, results of the Women's Health Initiative (WHI) indicate that treatment of postmenopausal women with estrogen *plus* a progestin produces a small increase in the risk of breast cancer—but treatment with estrogen *alone* may not (see below under *Hormone Replacement Therapy*). In contrast, the Women's Contraceptive and Reproductive Experience study has shown that, when estrogen plus a progestin is used for contraception, there is *no* increase in the risk of breast cancer (see Chapter 60, Birth Control). How can we explain these contradictory results? One possibility is that risk of breast cancer is a function of age—risk being relatively high in older women and very low in younger women. In either population—old or young—the risk of breast cancer from estrogen *alone* has not been established.

Regardless of whether estrogens *cause* breast cancer, there is no question they *promote* the growth of certain cancers that have estrogen receptors. Accordingly, estrogen-dependent breast cancer must be ruled out before initiating estrogen treatment. Furthermore, because all women are at potential risk for breast cancer, and because estrogens may slightly increase that risk, women taking estrogens should be especially diligent about doing monthly breast self-exams and having a yearly breast exam by a health professional; having a periodic mammogram should also be considered.

Ovarian Cancer. In postmenopausal women, therapy with estrogen alone—but not with estrogen plus a progestin—increases the risk of ovarian cancer. Details are presented below under *Hormone Replacement Therapy.*

Adverse Effects Associated with Use During Pregnancy. Use of estrogens during pregnancy can cause cancer and developmental abnormalities. Accordingly, women who become pregnant while taking estrogens should be apprised of the risks to the fetus. *Estrogens are classified in Food and Drug Administration (FDA) Pregnancy Risk Category X: the risk of use during pregnancy clearly outweighs any potential benefit.*

Diethylstilbestrol (DES), a nonsteroidal estrogen, has caused clear cell adenocarcinoma (CCA) of the vagina in women who were exposed to this drug during fetal life (i.e., in women whose mothers took DES during pregnancy). DES was used extensively between 1948 and 1971 to decrease the risk of miscarriage, but is now contraindicated for this use. The incidence of CCA among DES-exposed daughters is about 1 in 1000—40 times higher than the incidence among daughters who were not exposed to the drug. In daughters exposed to DES, CCA usually develops between ages 15 and 27; after age 30, the chance of developing CCA is very low. Although DES is the only estrogen clearly linked to induction of vaginal cancers, other estrogens may pose a similar risk.

Use of DES during pregnancy has produced genital abnormalities (e.g., testicular hypoplasia) in males. Abnormal semen production has also occurred. There have been no reports of cancer in males following *in utero* exposure to DES.

Cardiovascular Events. Estrogen, when combined with a progestin, increases the risk of myocardial infarction, pulmonary embolism, deep vein thrombosis, and stroke. Whether estrogen alone carries the same risk has not been determined. Adverse cardiovascular effects are discussed further under *Hormone Replacement Therapy.*

Nausea and Other GI Disturbances. Nausea is the most frequent undesired response to the estrogens. Fortunately, nausea diminishes with continued use, and is rarely so severe as to necessitate treatment cessation. Nausea can be minimized by administering estrogens with food and by initiating therapy with low doses. If taken in large doses, estrogens may cause anorexia, vomiting, and diarrhea.

Other Adverse Effects. Use of estrogens during menopause produces a small increase in the risk of *gallbladder disease.* Treatment of breast cancer and bone metastases can result in severe *hypercalcemia.* Estrogens may cause *jaundice* in patients with pre-existing liver dysfunction. *CNS reactions* include headache, dizziness, and depression.

Therapeutic Uses

In this chapter, discussion is limited to the noncontraceptive uses of estrogens. Use of estrogens for contraception is discussed in Chapter 60.

HRT After Menopause. Replacement therapy in postmenopausal women is the most common noncontraceptive use of estrogens. This use is discussed separately below.

Female Hypogonadism. In the absence of estrogens, pubertal transformation will not take place. Causes of estrogen deficiency include primary ovarian failure, hypopituitarism, and bilateral oophorectomy (i.e., removal of both ovaries). In girls with estrogen insufficiency, puberty can be induced by administering exogenous estrogens. This treatment promotes breast development, maturation of the reproductive organs, and development of pubic and axillary hair. To simulate normal patterns of estrogen secretion, the regimen should consist of continuous low-dose therapy (for about a year) followed by cyclic administration of higher estrogen doses.

Acne. Estrogens, in the form of oral contraceptives, can be used to control acne. Treatment is limited to females at least 15 years old who want contraception. The use of estrogen for acne is discussed further in Chapter 101 (Drugs for the Skin).

Prostate Cancer. Growth of prostate cancer is dependent upon the presence of androgens (e.g., testosterone). Estrogens can help patients by suppressing androgen production. Estrogens reduce androgen synthesis by suppressing secretion of LH (also known as interstitial cell-stimulating hormone), the hormone required by the testes to support androgen production. Since gonadotropin-releasing hormone (GnRH) analogs (e.g., leuprolide) are also able to suppress LH secretion, but do not cause the feminizing side effects seen with estrogens, these agents have largely replaced estrogens for treatment of prostate cancer.

Routes of Administration

Oral, Intramuscular, Intravenous, Intravaginal. The principal routes of administration are *oral* and *intramuscular.* With only one exception (conjugated estrogens), preparations that are used orally are not administered IM, and vice versa. As a rule, oral formulations, because of their convenience, are preferred to parenteral formulations. In addition to oral and IM use, some estrogens may be applied *intravaginally.* One preparation—conjugated estrogens—may be administered *intravenously.*

Transdermal. Estradiol is available in transdermal patch formulations. Patches are applied to the skin of the trunk (but not the breasts), allowing estrogen to be absorbed through the skin and then directly into the bloodstream. When compared with oral formulations, the patches have two significant advantages: (1) the total dosage of estrogen is greatly reduced (because the liver is bypassed) and (2) serum levels more closely resemble those seen in healthy premenopausal women. Rates of estrogen absorption range from 37.5 to 100 μg/hr, depending on the patch employed. Trade names include Alora, Climara, Esclim, Estraderm, and Vivelle.

SELECTIVE ESTROGEN RECEPTOR MODULATORS (SERMS)

SERMs are drugs that activate estrogen receptors in some tissues and block them in others. These drugs were developed in an effort to provide the benefits of estrogen (e.g., protection against osteoporosis, maintenance of the urogenital tract, reduction of LDL cholesterol) while avoiding its drawbacks (e.g., promotion of breast cancer, uterine cancer, and thromboembolism). Three SERMs are available: tamoxifen [Nolvadex], toremifene [Fareston], and raloxifene [Evista]. None of the three offers all of the benefits of estrogen, and none avoids all of its drawbacks.

Tamoxifen was the first SERM to be widely used. By blocking estrogen receptors, tamoxifen can inhibit cell growth in the breast. As a result, the drug is used extensively to prevent and treat breast cancer. Unfortunately, blockade of estrogen receptors also produces hot flushes. By activating estrogen receptors, tamoxifen protects against osteoporosis and has a favorable effect on serum lipids. However, receptor activation also increases the risk of endometrial cancer and thromboembolism. The pharmacology of tamoxifen and toremifene (a close relative of tamoxifen) is discussed at length in Chapter 99 (Anticancer Drugs II).

Raloxifene is very similar to tamoxifen. The principal difference is that raloxifene does not activate estrogen receptors in the endometrium, and hence does not pose a risk of uterine cancer. Like tamoxifen, raloxifene protects against breast cancer and osteoporosis, promotes thromboembolism, and induces hot flushes. Currently, raloxifene is approved only for prevention and treatment of osteoporosis. However, the drug is being tested for prevention and treatment of breast cancer. Raloxifene is discussed at length in Chapter 70 (Drugs Affecting Calcium Levels and Bone Mineralization).

PROGESTINS

Progestins are compounds that have actions like those of progesterone, the principal endogenous progestational hormone. As their name implies, the progestins act prior to gestation to prepare the uterus for implantation of a fertilized ovum. In addition, progestins help maintain the uterus throughout pregnancy.

Biosynthesis

Progesterone is produced by the ovaries and placenta. Ovarian production occurs during the second half of the menstrual cycle. During this period, progesterone is synthesized by the corpus luteum, under the direction of LH from the anterior pituitary. If implantation of a fertilized ovum fails to occur, progesterone production by the corpus luteum ceases, and menstrual flow begins. However, if implantation does take place, the developing trophoblast will produce its own luteotropic hormone (chorionic gonadotropin) that will act on the corpus luteum to promote continued progesterone secretion. By the second or third month of pregnancy, the placenta begins to produce progesterone of its own (along with estrogens). After this time, ovarian progesterone is no longer needed to support gestation. Placental synthesis of progesterone and estrogens continues throughout the remainder of pregnancy.

Physiologic and Pharmacologic Effects

Effects on the Endometrium and Endocervical Glands. Progesterone secreted during the second half of the menstrual cycle converts the endometrium from a proliferative state into a secretory state. At the end of the menstrual cycle, progesterone production ceases. The resultant abrupt fall in progesterone levels is the principal stimulus for the onset of menstruation. In addition to affecting the endometrium, progesterone acts on the endocervical glands, causing their secretions to become scant and viscous. This action is opposite to that of estrogen, which promotes the flow of profuse, watery secretions.

Effects During Pregnancy. As noted, progesterone levels increase during pregnancy. These high levels are thought to have two actions that help sustain pregnancy. First, progesterone inhibits uterine contraction. Second, progesterone may suppress the maternal immune response, thereby preventing immune rejection of the fetus.

Other Effects. Pharmacologic doses of progesterone can suppress release of pituitary gonadotropins (LH and FSH). This prevents maturation of follicles and ovulation. Also, individual progestin preparations display varying degrees of estrogenic, androgenic, and anabolic activity.

Clinical Pharmacology
Adverse Effects

Teratogenic Effects. Administration of progestins in high doses during the first 4 months of pregnancy has been associated with an increased incidence of birth defects (limb reductions, heart defects, masculinization of the female fetus). Accordingly, use of progestins during early pregnancy is not recommended. Women who become pregnant while taking progestins should be apprised of the potential risk to the fetus.

Gynecologic Effects. Because of their actions on the endometrium, progestins can cause breakthrough bleeding, spotting, and amenorrhea. Other effects include breast tenderness and alteration of cervical secretions. To facilitate evaluation of potential adverse drug responses, the patient should undergo examination of the breasts and pelvic organs prior to therapy. In addition, a Papanicolaou (Pap) smear should be obtained and evaluated. Patients should be instructed to report any episodes of abnormal vaginal bleeding.

Breast Cancer. Progestins appear to increase the risk of breast cancer from estrogens (see below under *Hormone Replacement Therapy*).

Other Adverse Effects. Progestins have been associated with depression, jaundice, edema, lethargy, photosensitivity, nausea, bloating, breast tenderness, and exacerbation of acute intermittent porphyria.

Therapeutic Uses

Discussion in this chapter is limited to the noncontraceptive uses of progestins. Use of progestins for contraception is considered in Chapter 60.

Hormone Replacement Therapy. The primary noncontraceptive use of progestins is to counteract the adverse effects of estrogen on the endometrium in women undergoing HRT. This application is discussed below.

Dysfunctional Uterine Bleeding. This condition occurs when progesterone levels are insufficient to balance the stimulatory influence of estrogen on the endometrium. In the absence of sufficient progesterone, estrogen puts the endometrium in a state of continuous proliferation. Since progesterone is unavailable to induce monthly endometrial breakdown, the excessively proliferative endometrium undergoes spontaneous sloughing at irregular intervals. Irregular breakdown of the endometrium can result in periodic episodes of severe menstrual bleeding. Alternatively, chronic spotting may be produced. Dysfunctional uterine bleeding is often associated with anovulatory cycles. The disorder occurs most commonly in adolescents and in women approaching menopause.

Treatment has two objectives: the initial goal is cessation of hemorrhage; the long-term goal is to establish a regular monthly cycle. Excessive bleeding can be stopped by administering a progestin for several days. Dosing may be continued for 2 weeks for sustained suppression. When progestin administration is stopped, withdrawal bleeding takes place. Withdrawal bleeding is likely to be profuse and associated with cramping.

Cyclic therapy is employed to establish a regular monthly cycle. In this regimen, administration of an oral progestin is initiated 5 days after the onset of each menstrual period and continued for the next 20 days. This form of therapy promotes a repeating pattern of endometrial proliferation followed by endometrial breakdown and menstruation.

Amenorrhea. Progestins can induce menstrual flow in selected women who are experiencing amenorrhea. If endogenous estrogen levels are adequate, treatment with a progestin for 5 to 10 days will be followed by withdrawal bleeding when the progestin is discontinued. If estrogen levels are low, it may be necessary to induce endometrial proliferation with an estrogen prior to giving the progestin. Cyclic therapy can be used to promote regular monthly flow. This form of treatment consists of estrogen administration for 25 days coupled with progestin administration on days 15 through 25. The regimen is repeated beginning on the first day of each month.

Endometriosis. Endometriosis is a disorder in which endometrial tissue has become implanted in an abnormal location (e.g., uterine wall, ovary, extragenital sites). This condition is painful and a frequent cause of infertility and spontaneous abortion. Endometriosis can be treated surgically, or growth of the implants can be suppressed with drugs. When drug therapy is indicated, the medications employed most commonly are *danazol, nafarelin,* and *leuprolide.* All three suppress production of estrogens and progesterone, and thereby deprive implants of the hormones needed for growth.

Endometrial Carcinoma. Progestins can induce beneficial responses (palliation, tumor regression, remission) in women with metastatic endometrial carcinoma. Several months of treatment may be required for a response to occur. The progestins employed for this indication are *medroxyprogesterone acetate* (MPA) and *megestrol acetate.* MPA is given once weekly by IM injection; megestrol acetate is administered daily by mouth. In addition to its use against endometrial carcinoma, megestrol acetate may provide palliation for women with breast cancer.

Premenstrual Syndrome. In the past, progesterone was widely prescribed for premenstrual syndrome (PMS). However, it is now clear that the practice should cease. In controlled studies, progesterone was no more effective than placebo. Furthermore, there is evidence that progesterone may actually *cause* PMS symptoms. PMS is discussed at length in Box 59–1.

Preparations and Routes

Progestins may be administered orally, parenterally (IM), and topically (intravaginal, transdermal). Oral progestins include *medroxyprogesterone acetate* [Provera, Cycrin, others], *norethindrone* [Micronor, Nor-Q.D.], *norethindrone acetate* [Aygestin], and *megestrol acetate* [Megace], a micronized formulation of *progesterone* [Prometrium]. Intramuscular progestins are *medroxyprogesterone acetate* [Depo-Provera], *hydroxyprogesterone caproate* [Hylutin], and *progesterone* (in oil). Intravaginal use is limited to *progesterone* [Crinone]. Transdermal use is limited to *norethindrone,* which is available in combination with estradiol under the trade name *CombiPatch.*

Special Interest Topic

BOX 59-1 ■ PREMENSTRUAL SYNDROME

PMS consists of a constellation of psychologic and physical symptoms that develop during the luteal phase of the menstrual cycle and then resolve a few days after the onset of menses. Common psychologic symptoms include irritability, depression, mood lability, crying spells, and social withdrawal. Common physical symptoms include acne, breast tenderness, abdominal bloating, and increased appetite, especially for carbohydrates. Additional symptoms are listed in the table below. The psychologic symptoms are much more disabling than the physical symptoms. PMS is among the most common disorders in women of reproductive age.

Common Symptoms of PMS

Psychologic and Behavioral Symptoms	Physical Symptoms
• Irritability	• Acne
• Depression, sadness, or hopelessness	• Breast tenderness
• Mood lability: alternating sadness and anger	• Abdominal bloating
• Hypersensitivity to trivial events	• Ankle edema
• Loneliness and social withdrawal	• Weight gain (from water retention)
• Crying spells	• Food craving (especially carbohydrates)
• Anxiety	• Fatigue
• Difficulty concentrating	• Headache
• Decreased sense of well-being	• Backache
• Reduced efficiency or work performance	• Nausea, vomiting
• Restlessness, agitation	• Joint and muscle pain
• Tension	• Constipation or diarrhea

ETIOLOGY

Although PMS is clearly of neuroendocrine origin, the exact cause is unknown. At one time, hormonal abnormality was suspected. However, we now know that hormone levels in women who experience PMS are identical to those in women who do not. Hence, hormonal abnormality cannot be the cause. Nonetheless, because symptoms are synchronized with the menstrual cycle, it would seem that hormones are in some way involved—even if levels *are* normal. One reasonable hypothesis is that women who experience PMS are sensitive to hormonal changes in a way that other women are not. Because of this heightened sensitivity, normal hormonal changes are able to trigger PMS. The ability of selective serotonin reuptake inhibitors (SSRIs) to relieve dysphoric symptoms suggests that susceptibility to mood changes, which are the principal complaint in PMS, may result from altered serotonergic transmission in the CNS.

DIAGNOSIS

To make a diagnosis of PMS, symptoms must be *intense* and *intermittent*. That is, symptoms should be prominent in the luteal phase of the menstrual cycle, and minimal or absent in the follicular phase. Practically all women experience some PMS-like symptoms in the late luteal phase. However, in the

majority of women, symptoms are relatively mild, and hence do not constitute PMS. Only 20% to 30% of women have symptoms that are strong enough to be considered PMS. An even smaller number—3% to 5%—have symptoms that constitute *premenstrual dysphoric disorder* (PMDD), an especially severe form of PMS described in the American Psychiatric Association's *Diagnostic and Statistical Manual of Mental Disorders, Fourth Edition.*

Timing of symptoms is critical. On days 4 through 12 of the menstrual cycle, symptoms should be absent, or at least no greater than would be expected in the population at large. Symptoms should begin following ovulation (around day 14 of the cycle) and then become most intense in the fourth week of the cycle, that is, late in the luteal phase. To make a diagnosis, total symptom severity in the fourth week must be at least twice the intensity of any symptoms present in the second week. Daily charting of symptoms for at least two menstrual cycles is needed to establish whether symptoms occur in the appropriate pattern and are of sufficient intensity to permit a diagnosis of PMS (or PMDD).

When diagnosing PMS, it is essential to rule out conditions whose symptoms can intensify in the late luteal phase or menstrual phase, a phenomenon known as "menstrual magnification." Common conditions subject to menstrual magnification include depression, migraine, chronic fatigue syndrome, and irritable bowel syndrome. The differential diagnosis is relatively easy to make in that, unlike PMS, these disorders are symptomatic *throughout* the cycle—they simply can become more intense as menstruation approaches.

TREATMENT GUIDELINES

In 2000, the American College of Obstetricians and Gynecologists (ACOG) issued guidelines for the diagnosis and treatment of PMS ("Clinical Management Guidelines for Premenstrual Syndrome." *ACOG Practice Bulletin* No. 15). For women with a positive diagnosis of PMS, the guidelines recommend stepwise intervention, beginning with lifestyle changes and then progressing to drug therapy if needed.

For women with mild symptoms, lifestyle changes—including use of dietary supplements—may provide adequate relief. Measures include performing regular aerobic exercise (which can enhance mood and reduce fluid retention); getting adequate sleep (about 8 hours a night); eating foods rich in complex carbohydrates (which can enhance mood and reduce food craving); reducing salt intake (which can reduce fluid retention and bloating); and eliminating caffeine, a compound that promotes both irritability and insomnia. Three dietary supplements can reduce symptoms: *magnesium* (200 to 400 mg/day) can improve mood and reduce headache and fluid retention); *vitamin E* (400 IU/day) can reduce breast pain and perhaps other symptoms; and, as discussed below, *calcium* can reduce aches and pains, mood swings, food craving, and water retention.

If lifestyle changes fail to suppress symptoms, drug therapy may be needed. Two types of drugs are recommended: mood-altering agents and ovulation suppressants. Mood-altering agents should be tried first. Ovulation suppressants should be used only after preferred drugs have failed.

Agents that are *ineffective* should be avoided. Among these are progesterone and vitamin B_6. Progesterone has been used for years on the theory that it may produce a favorable hormonal balance. However, we now know that progesterone is no more effective than placebo, and in fact may exacerbate some symptoms (bloating, breast tenderness, emotional lability). Like progesterone, vitamin B_6 has been used widely for PMS, but proof of efficacy is lacking. Furthermore, high doses can cause peripheral neuropathy. In light of safety concerns and lack of proven efficacy, neither progesterone nor vitamin B_6 is recommended.

MOOD-ALTERING DRUGS

Selective serotonin reuptake inhibitors (SSRIs), such as fluoxetine [Prozac, Sarafem], and sertraline [Zoloft], are the most effective therapy known for the psychologic symptoms of PMS or PMDD. These drugs, which were developed as antidepressants (see Chapter 31), can significantly reduce depression, anger, irritability, tension, dysphoria, fatigue, and confusion. Success rates range from 50% to 75%. Moreover, benefits develop quickly—within 2 to 3 days, compared 2 to 4 weeks when SSRIs are used for depression. Why were SSRIs ever tried for PMS? Because the psychologic symptoms of PMS are much like those of depression. Interestingly, although SSRIs are most effective at reducing affective symptoms of PMS, they can also reduce physical symptoms, such as breast tenderness, bloating, and headache.

In clinical trials, about 15% of women discontinued treatment because of side effects. The most common are nausea, headache, insomnia, nervousness, dizziness, reduced libido, and anorgasmia. If side effects are intolerable, dosage can be reduced.

Most research on using SSRIs for PMS has been conducted with either fluoxetine or sertraline. However, other SSRIs—paroxetine [Paxil], fluvoxamine [Luvox], citalopram [Celexa], and escitalopram [Lexapro]—are probably effective too. Hence, if a patients fails to respond to fluoxetine or sertraline, a trial with a different SSRI may be merited. It should be noted that, although the SSRIs are highly effective in PMS, none of these drugs is *approved* for the disorder (although two SSRIs—fluoxetine and sertraline—*are* approved for PMDD).

With fluoxetine and sertraline, dosing may be done either (1) every day throughout the menstrual cycle or (2) just during the luteal phase, the time when symptoms are present. With the second option, dosing is begun on day 14 of the cycle and stopped on day 2 of the following cycle (i.e., the day after menstruation begins). The intermittent schedule has two obvious advantages: it's cheaper than continuous dosing and side effects are minimized. Hence, unless a woman has depression in addition to PMS, intermittent dosing is preferred. Specific dosages for fluoxetine and sertraline are as follows:

- Fluoxetine—The usual dosage is 20 mg/day, given continuously or just during the luteal phase.
- Sertraline—The usual dosage is 50 mg/day, given continuously or just during the luteal phase. Higher doses may be used if needed.

Alprazolam [Xanax], a benzodiazepine, is an alternative to SSRIs. The drug can be especially helpful when anxiety is the predominant symptom. Compared with placebo, alprazolam is superior at reducing anxiety, irritability, severe tension, and the feeling of being out of control. Unfortunately, daytime sedation is significant at the doses needed to suppress these symptoms. Alprazolam is administered only during the luteal phase. The usual dosage is 0.25 mg 4 times a day. Doses should be tapered to minimize symptoms of withdrawal.

OVULATION SUPPRESSANTS

Two classes of drugs—gonadotropin-releasing hormone (GnRH) agonists and oral contraceptives (OCs)—can suppress ovulation, and may thereby suppress both menstrual cycling and associated symptoms of PMS. According to the ACOG guidelines, ovulation suppressants are second-line drugs for PMS.

GnRH agonists (e.g., leuprolide) can reduce physical and psychologic symptoms of PMS. Treatment can relieve breast tenderness, bloating, depression, nervous tension, anxiety, and loss of control. These agents act by suppressing release of LH and FSH from the pituitary, and thereby cause levels of estrogen and progesterone to fall to postmenopausal concentrations. Unfortunately, loss of estrogen increases the risk of osteoporosis. Hence, although GnRH agonists may help reduce symptoms of PMS, serious adverse effects preclude their use for more than 6 months.

Although OCs are often prescribed for PMS, there are few data to support their efficacy. Nonetheless, these agents may be helpful for women whose symptoms are primarily physical (e.g., bloating, breast tenderness).

OTHER DRUGS

There is good evidence that **calcium** (1200 mg/day) can reduce symptoms of mild to moderate PMS. In one study, 2 to 3 months of daily calcium therapy decreased depression and mood swings by 45% (vs. 28% with placebo), generalized aches and pains by 54% (vs. a 15% *increase* with placebo), food cravings by 54% (vs. 35% with placebo), and water retention by 36% (vs. 24% with placebo). Calcium did not reduce fatigue or insomnia. These data are the first clear indication that a dietary supplement can significantly reduce symptoms of PMS. Moreover, the required dosage is low—about equal to the recommended dietary intake for preventing osteoporosis (1300 mg/day for teenagers and 1000 mg/day for women ages 19 to 40). Hence, women now have two good reasons for ensuring adequate calcium intake: alleviation of PMS and protection against osteoporosis.

Spironolactone [Aldactone], a potassium-sparing diuretic, can counteract water retention and can thereby relieve bloating and weight gain. Treatment should be reserved for women with documented weight gain, and should be limited to the luteal phase. The dosage is 100 mg/day.

Analgesics, such as ibuprofen and naproxen, have no effect on mood, but can reduce headache, dysmenorrhea, cramps, and muscle and joint pain.

HORMONE REPLACEMENT THERAPY

The term *hormone replacement therapy* (HRT) refers to giving women physiologic doses of estrogen (with or without a progestin) to compensate for the loss of estrogen that occurs during menopause. Why is estrogen lost? Because ovarian follicles, which are the primary source of estrogen, decline as women grow older. Menopause typically begins around age 50. During the initial phase, the menstrual cycle is irregular; anovulatory cycles may occur, and periods of amenorrhea may alternate with menses. Eventually, ovulation and menstruation cease entirely. Production of ovarian estrogens decreases gradually, coming to a complete stop several years after menstruation has ceased.

Loss of estrogen has multiple consequences. Prominent among these are vasomotor symptoms (manifesting as hot flushes, also known as hot flashes, and night sweats), urogenital atrophy (manifesting as vaginal dryness, itching, and burning), and accelerated bone loss (manifesting as osteoporosis and fractures). HRT can prevent or attenuate these consequences.

There are two basic regimens for HRT: (1) estrogen alone and (2) estrogen plus a progestin. The purpose of estrogen in both is to replace the estrogen that was lost because of menopause. The progestin is present for one reason only: to counterbalance estrogen-mediated stimulation of the endometrium, which can lead to cancer of the uterus. Accordingly, in women who no longer have a uterus, the progestin component is unnecessary, and hence is omitted. It should be noted that, although progestins can protect against estrogen-induced cancer of the uterus, progestins appear to *increase* the risk of estrogen-induced cancer of the breast. In addition, progestins appear to increase the risk of adverse cardiovascular events.

Over the past decade, there has been growing concern that the benefits of HRT may not outweigh the risks. Evidence from recent studies has shown that the benefits of HRT are more limited than previously believed, whereas the risks are greater than previously appreciated. Because of this new information, experts now agree that, for most women, the benefits of *long-term* HRT to *prevent chronic disorders* do not justify the risks. However, use of *short-term* HRT to *manage menopausal symptoms*

is still considered appropriate, provided the smallest effective dosage is used for the shortest time needed.

A note on nomenclature: In the discussion below, HRT that consists of *estrogen plus progestin* is abbreviated *EPT* (for estrogen-progestin therapy), and HRT that consists of *estrogen alone* is abbreviated *ET* (for estrogen therapy). These distinctions are necessary because, as we shall see, the benefits and risks of EPT and ET are not identical.

Landmark Studies: WHI and HERS

The surprising results of two recent trials—the Women's Health Initiative (WHI) and the Heart and Estrogen/progestin Replacement Study and its follow-up (HERS and HERS II)—have led to major changes in recommendations regarding HRT. Both trials were large, prospective, randomized, double-blind, placebo-controlled studies of the effects of HRT in postmenopausal women. Although these trials have limitations, they are nonetheless the most statistically valid studies on HRT to date.

The WHI was designed to assess the benefits of HRT as *primary prevention* against heart disease and other disorders in *healthy* postmenopausal women. More than 27,000 subjects were enrolled. In one arm of the study, women with an intact uterus were given either a daily placebo or daily EPT. The specific preparation used was Prempro, a combination of conjugated equine estrogens (0.625 mg) and medroxyprogesterone acetate (2.5 mg). In another arm, women who had undergone a hysterectomy received either a daily placebo or daily ET. The specific preparation used was Premarin, which contains 0.625 mg of conjugated equine estrogens. The EPT arm was terminated early (in July 2002) because the risks of treatment—cardiovascular events and invasive breast cancer—exceeded any benefits. These risks were not seen with the estrogen-only arm, which is still ongoing. Benefits and risks observed in the EPT arm of WHI are summarized in Table 59–1.

In contrast to the WHI, which was a *primary prevention* trial, HERS was designed to assess the benefits of HRT as *secondary prevention* in women with *established* coronary heart disease (CHD). The study enrolled 2763 postmenopausal women with an intact uterus. Participants received either

---

TABLE 59–1 ▪▪ Results of the Women's Health Initiative: Incidence of Benefits and Harms of Combination HRT*

Benefits/Harms	Number of Events Prevented or Caused Per Year
Benefits (Events Prevented)	
Hip fractures	5 for each 10,000 users (1 for each 2000 users)
Colon cancer	6 for each 10,000 users (1 for each 1700 users)
Harms (Events Caused)	
Myocardial infarction	7 for each 10,000 users (1 for each 1400 users)
Stroke	8 for each 10,000 users (1 for each 1250 users)
Pulmonary embolism	8 for each 10,000 users (1 for each 1250 users)
Deep vein thrombosis	10 for each 10,000 users (1 for each 1000 users)
Breast cancer (with 5 or more years of HRT use)	8 for each 10,000 users (1 for each 1250 users)
Dementia (primarily Alzheimer's disease)	23 for each 10,000 users (1 for each 434 users)

*Data on dementia are from the Women's Health Initiative Memory Study, JAMA, 289: 2651–2662, 2003. All other data are from the main Women's Health Initiative study.

placebo or daily Prempro (the same EPT regimen used in WHI). The outcome? EPT failed to protect against myocardial infarction (MI). Worse yet, during the first few years of treatment, EPT actually *increased* the risk of MI.

Benefits and Risks of HRT

Our understanding of the benefits and risks of HRT continues to evolve. Principal benefits are suppression of menopausal symptoms and prevention of osteoporosis and colorectal cancer. Known risks include CHD, stroke, thromboembolic events, breast cancer, and cholecystitis. Benefits and risks are summarized in Table 59–2.

Benefits of HRT

Replacement of estrogen offers four primary benefits: (1) suppression of vasomotor symptoms, (2) prevention of urogenital atrophy, (3) prevention of osteoporosis and related fractures, and (4) prevention of colorectal cancer. To suppress vasomotor symptoms, HRT is employed short term (a few years). To prevent urogenital atrophy, osteoporosis, and colorectal cancer, HRT must continue lifelong. Despite long-held hopes, there is no proof that HRT improves cardiovascular health.

Relief of Vasomotor Symptoms. Vasomotor symptoms (hot flashes) develop in about 70% of postmenopausal women. Episodes are characterized by sudden skin flushing, sweating, and a sensation of uncomfortable warmth. Severe episodes can cause insomnia, fatigue, and irritability. In most women, hot flashes abate within a few months to a few years; in others, they may persist for more than a decade. Vasomotor symptoms generally respond well to HRT.

Management of Urogenital Atrophy. In the absence of estrogen, urogenital degeneration is inevitable. Of all structures in the body, the urethra and vagina have the highest concentrations of estrogen receptors. Activation of these receptors maintains the functional integrity of the urethra and vaginal epithelium. Hence, when estrogen levels decline during menopause, these structures undergo degenerative change. Atrophy of the urethra results in incontinence. Atrophy of the vaginal epithelium can lead to vaginitis and decreased enjoyment of intercourse. HRT helps prevent these undesirable outcomes.

TABLE 59–2 ■ Major Benefits and Risks of HRT	
Benefits	**Risks**
• Suppression of vasomotor symptoms	• Myocardial infarction*
• Preservation of urogenital integrity	• Pulmonary embolism*
• Preservation of bone mineral density and prevention of osteoporotic fractures	• Deep vein thrombosis*
	• Stroke*
	• Breast cancer*
• Decreased risk of colorectal cancer	• Ovarian cancer†
• Possible decreased risk of Alzheimer's disease	• Uterine cancer‡
	• Cholecystitis
	• Dementia

*Risk is clearly increased by treatment with estrogen plus progestin; whether risk is increased by estrogen alone has not been established.
†Risk is increased by treatment with estrogen alone, but not by estrogen plus progestin.
‡Uterine cancer is a risk only for a woman with a uterus (obviously) and only if she uses unopposed estrogen, which should not be done (women with a uterus should always use estrogen combined with a progestin).

Prevention of Osteoporosis and Related Fractures. Osteoporosis is characterized by demineralization and weakening of the bones. Compression fractures of the vertebrae are common. In osteoporotic women, fractures of the hip and wrist can be caused by minimal trauma. Osteoporosis occurs in a majority (about 70%) of elderly white females; the incidence in males and black females is much lower. The condition develops following surgical removal of the ovaries as well as after menopause. Estrogen deficiency is the principal cause.

In postmenopausal women, HRT can reduce bone resorption and can slow development of osteoporosis. More importantly, HRT can decrease the risk of osteoporotic fractures, an effect demonstrated for the first time in the WHI. (Prior to the WHI, reduction in fracture risk was assumed, but not proved.) It should be noted that, although HRT can indeed reduce fracture risk, the *absolute* reduction is relatively small: for every 10,000 women using HRT, there would be only 5 fewer fractures per year. Like the WHI, HERS also showed a reduction in fracture risk. However, the reduction was not statistically significant. It must be stressed that HRT is primarily prophylactic: Estrogen does little to reverse bone loss that has already occurred. Furthermore, beneficial effects on bone are not permanent. Rather, they fade quickly when HRT stops. Accordingly, to maintain protection, HRT must continue lifelong.

Prevention of Colorectal Cancer. Cancer of the colon is the fourth most common cancer in the United States and the second leading cause of cancer deaths (lung cancer is first). A meta-analysis of the results of 18 observational studies indicated that, compared with women who have never used HRT, current users have a 34% decreased risk of colon cancer. However, protection appears to decline after HRT is discontinued. The WHI was the first controlled trial to report similar outcomes. A reduction in risk was also seen in HERS, although it was not large enough to be statistically significant. How might HRT confer protection? At least two mechanisms are possible: (1) reduced production of bile acids and (2) inhibited growth of colon cancer cells.

Improved Quality of Life? There is a widely held belief that HRT can improve mood and make women feel more youthful and vibrant. However, data from HERS and the WHI indicate that quality of life (QOL) benefits are very limited. In the WHI, daily EPT failed to improve energy, mood, cognition, sleep, sexual satisfaction, or any other health-related QOL parameter. In HERS, QOL benefits were seen only in women with significant vasomotor symptoms. For these women, HRT was associated with improved mental health, including a reduction in depressive symptoms—with no significant improvement or decline in energy level or physical function.

Prevention of Dementia? The impact of HRT on development of dementia is not completely known. As discussed below under *Harms of HRT,* we have good evidence that *EPT* can actually *cause* dementia. However, it remains possible that *ET* may confer *protection.* We know that, after ages 80 to 85, women appear to be at increased risk of Alzheimer's disease (AD) relative to men. Loss of protection by estrogen could explain why. How might estrogen protect against AD? In animal studies, estrogen has been shown to inhibit formation of beta-amyloid, stimulate brain cholinergic activity, induce glial cell activation, enhance synaptic plasticity, and protect against cell damage from oxidative stress. In humans, estrogen has been shown to increase blood flow and glucose metabolism in brain areas involved in memory processing and to modulate activity in brain areas affected early in AD development. Despite this plausible basis for thinking HRT might protect against AD, the association between HRT and AD remains unclear. Most of the evidence supporting possible protection is from epidemiologic studies that had methodologic flaws. However, data from a recent prospective study suggest an intriguing possibility: Yes, HRT *can* protect against AD, but only when used during the early years of menopause, the time when levels of endogenous estrogen are undergoing rapid decline; if HRT is used after this critical interval, no protection is conferred. Studies designed to confirm this possibility would be welcome. Until more is known, HRT cannot be recommended for the specific purpose of protecting against AD.

Prevention of Cardiovascular Disease—NOT. Data from HERS and HERS II indicate that, contrary to widely held beliefs, HRT does *not* protect against cardiovascular disease. Worse yet, data from the WHI indicate that, among users of HRT, the risk of cardiovascular events actually goes *up* (see *Harms of HRT* below).

Other Benefits. Postmenopausal HRT appears to have a positive effect on wound healing, tooth retention, and glycemic control. After menopause, a woman's skin becomes thinner and wounds heal more slowly. However, among women taking HRT, the rate of wound healing is close to that of premenopausal women. There is a direct correlation between duration of HRT and prevention of tooth loss: for each 4.2 years of HRT use, one additional tooth is retained. HRT greatly decreases the risk of developing type 2 diabetes and, among women who already have type 2 diabetes, HRT can improve glycemic control.

Harms of HRT

Minor Adverse Effects. Minor adverse effects are common. Nausea occurs in up to 20% of women during the first 2 to 3 months of HRT. Fluid retention may result in weight gain and breast tenderness. With cyclic regimens, menstrual bleeding occurs.

Cardiovascular Events. Over the past few years, our understanding of the cardiovascular effects of HRT has changed dramatically, owing largely to HERS and WHI. Until recently, we believed that HRT conferred significant cardioprotection. Why? First, estrogen has beneficial cardiovascular effects: It reduces levels of LDL cholesterol, raises levels of HDL cholesterol, decreases oxidation of LDL, and improves vascular endothelial function. Second, in observational studies, use of HRT was associated with a decreased incidence of CHD. Unfortunately, HERS and WHI failed to demonstrate any cardiovascular benefit for HRT—but did reveal significant cardiovascular harm.

Early results of HERS, published in 1998, raised serious doubts about the cardioprotective effects of HRT. During the first year, women taking HRT experienced 50% *more* coronary events than those taking placebo. However, over the next 3 years, women taking HRT experienced 40% *fewer* coronary events. As in other studies, HRT lowered LDL cholesterol (by 11%) and raised HDL cholesterol (by 10%). The increase in coronary events during the first year of HRT was both unexpected and disturbing. After all, HRT was supposed to protect against heart disease. The authors speculated that the initial increase in events was due to thrombogenic effects of HRT, whereas the subsequent decrease was due to antiatherogenic effects. If this theory was correct, then longer use of HRT should have revealed a net benefit. Unfortunately, in HERS II, a 2.7-year follow-up to the original HERS trial, the hoped-for net benefit failed to materialize: The incidence of coronary events in women using HRT for the longer time was no

smaller than in those taking placebo. In support of this observation, the Estrogen Replacement and Atherosclerosis Trial showed that neither ET nor EPT reduces the progression of atherosclerosis, as measured by angiography. Similarly, the Women's Estrogen for Stroke Trial demonstrated that, among women with a prior ischemic stroke, ET does not reduce the incidence of stroke recurrence.

Data from the WHI suggest that, rather than protecting against cardiovascular events, HRT actually *increases* risk—at least for women using EPT (as opposed to ET). After 5.2 years of follow-up, women using EPT experienced a higher incidence of MI, stroke, pulmonary embolism, and deep vein thrombosis (DVT) compared with women taking placebo. Fortunately, the *absolute* increase was relatively small: For every 10,000 women using EPT, there would be 7 more heart attacks each year, 8 more strokes, 8 more pulmonary emboli, and 10 more cases of DVT. Because of this increased risk, the EPT arm of the WHI was terminated early. At this time, we do not know if ET is safer than EPT. This question may be resolved when the results of the ongoing ET arm of the WHI become available.

Endometrial Cancer. Estrogens increase the risk of endometrial cancer, *but only when used alone.* When estrogens are combined with a progestin, they pose little or no risk. Accordingly, in women with an intact uterus, it is now standard practice to use EPT, rather than ET.

Breast Cancer. Observational studies have shown that HRT using EPT increases the risk of breast cancer. Furthermore, the risk climbs with increased duration of use. The WHI was the first large, randomized controlled trial to confirm these observations: Among women using EPT for 5 or more years, the risk of invasive breast cancer was 26% higher than among women taking placebo. In absolute terms, this means that, for every 10,000 women using EPT, there would be 8 more cases of breast cancer per year. Fortunately, the increase in risk appears to fall off rapidly when HRT is discontinued. As noted above, the increased risk of breast cancer was a contributing factor to the early termination of the EPT arm of the WHI. At this time, we do not know whether HRT with estrogen *alone* increases breast cancer risk. The ongoing ET arm of the WHI may answer this question.

Ovarian Cancer. In 2001, researchers reported that long-term replacement therapy with estrogen alone increases the risk of death from ovarian cancer. Specifically, among postmenopausal women using ET for 10 or more years, the mortality rate from ovarian cancer is 2.2 times the rate among nonusers. When ET is discontinued, the increased risk declines very gradually, and may still be evident after 29 years. In a separate large study, sponsored by the National Cancer Institute, researchers confirmed these results and made an additional important observation: Long-term use of estrogen *plus progestin* does *not* increase the risk of ovarian cancer. This is good news for the 8.6 million American women who use EPT—but not for the 12 million women who, because of having undergone a hysterectomy, use ET. It should be noted that ovarian cancer is relatively rare: The average woman has a 1 in 59 lifetime chance of developing the disease (compared with a 1 in 9 lifetime chance of developing breast cancer). However, even though ovarian cancer is rare, it still kills 14,000 American women each year. Women using ET should undergo regular screening for ovarian cancer—even though current methods are unable to detect early disease.

Cholecystitis. Several studies, including the Nurses' Health Study (NHS) and HERS, have shown that HRT increases the risk of cholecystitis, an inflammatory condition of the gallbladder caused by chronic gallstones. Cholecystectomy (incision of the gallbladder) is the usual remedy. In the NHS, the risk of cholecystitis depended on duration of HRT use, being highest among women using HRT for 5 or more years. In the HERS trial, the incidence of cholecystectomy among HRT users was 48% higher than among nonusers.

Dementia. Data from the Women's Health Initiative Memory Study (WHIMS), released in May 2003, indicate that *EPT increases* the risk of dementia, primarily Alzheimer's disease. WHIMS evaluated 4532 subjects from the WHI, 2229 of whom were receiving EPT and 2303 of whom were receiving placebo. After a mean follow-up of 4 years, the incidence of dementia in the EPT group was twice that in the placebo group. Fortunately, although the *relative* risk was high (a 2-fold increase over placebo), the *absolute* risk was still low: for every 10,000 women using EPT for 1 year, there would be 23 additional cases of dementia. Whether replacement therapy using *estrogen alone* promotes dementia is being studied in an ongoing arm of WHIMS.

Warnings

After reviewing the WHI results, the FDA ruled that *all* products intended for HRT, whether they contain estrogen alone or estrogen combined with a progestin, must carry strengthened warnings. Although only one estrogen-progestin product [Prempro] was studied in the WHI, until data on other products become available, all estrogen-containing products are assumed to carry similar risks. Accordingly, product labels must now have a *boxed warning* (the highest level of warning in labeling) that contains statements similar to these:

- Estrogens and progestin should not be used to prevent cardiovascular disease.
- The Women's Health Initiative (WHI) reported that postmenopausal women treated for 5 years with conjugated equine estrogens (0.625 mg/day) combined with medroxyprogesterone acetate (2.5 mg/day) experienced increased risks (compared with placebo) of myocardial infarction, stroke, pulmonary emboli, deep vein thrombosis, and invasive breast cancer.
- In the absence of comparable data, products that contain other doses of other estrogens and other progestins should be assumed to have similar risks.
- Physicians should prescribe estrogens and progestins at the lowest effective doses and for the shortest duration consistent with treatment goals and risk for the individual woman.

To further minimize risks, the new labeling advises women who use HRT to perform monthly breast self-examinations, have yearly breast exams by a healthcare provider, and undergo periodic mammograms (scheduled on the basis of the patient's age and other risk factors). In addition, healthcare providers should advise women on ways to reduce the risk of osteoporosis (e.g., taking calcium and vitamin D supplements, performing weight-bearing exercise) and heart disease (e.g., treating hypertension, maintaining a healthy weight, reducing dietary fat, avoiding smoking).

Women at high risk of complications should not use HRT. Among these are women with unusual vaginal bleeding and women who have had blood clots, breast cancer, or a stroke or MI in the past year.

Recommendations on HRT Use

Given our increased understanding of the risks and benefits of HRT, the question arises: Should *any* woman use HRT? The answer is "Yes"—provided the benefits for the individual outweigh the risks. To make this assessment, risk factors for the individual must be inventoried, and the hoped-for benefits should be clearly defined. For women with significant baseline risks (e.g., personal or family history of breast cancer, cardiovascular disease), the risk of harm from HRT goes up.

In late 2002 and early 2003, several expert sources issued revised recommendations on HRT. The recommendations below represent a composite of those offered by three groups: the North American Menopause Society, the FDA, and the third United States Preventive Services Task Force (USPSTF). These recommendations are based in large part on data from WHI and HERS. As more data become available, these recommendations are likely to change.

At this time, proof of benefits and risks for *EPT* is much stronger than the proof for *ET*. Clear benefits of EPT include preservation of bone mineral density, reduced risk of fractures, and reduced risk of colon cancer. Known harms include increased risk of breast cancer, venous thromboembolism, coronary heart disease, stroke, cholecystitis, and dementia. On the basis of this evidence, the USPSTF concluded that, when EPT is used *long term* for disease prevention, harmful effects exceed benefits for most women. Regarding ET (for women who have had a hysterectomy), the USPSTF concluded there is insufficient evidence to recommend for or against chronic use for disease prevention. The USPSTF did not address the issue of *short-term* EPT or ET to manage menopausal symptoms.

The recommendations below are based on studies using Premarin and Prempro. In the absence of data proving otherwise, we must assume that all other estrogen and estrogen-progestin products carry similar risks. Likewise, until proof is available, we cannot assume that ET is significantly safer than EPT.

General Recommendations

In order to balance benefits and risks, an individual risk profile should be compiled for every woman considering HRT. All candidates for HRT should be informed of known risks. Women with multiple risk factors should consider alternative therapies. For most women, the benefits of *long-term* HRT for disease prevention do not outweigh the risks, and hence long-term HRT should generally be avoided. Conversely, the benefits of short-term therapy (less than 4 years) to treat menopausal symptoms often *do* justify the risks. To keep risk as low as possible, HRT should be used in the lowest dosage and for the shortest time needed to accomplish treatment goals.

Use for Approved Indications

HRT has only three approved indications:

- Treatment of moderate to severe vasomotor symptoms associated with menopause

■ Treatment of moderate to severe symptoms of vulvar and vaginal atrophy associated with menopause
■ Prevention of postmenopausal osteoporosis

HRT should be restricted to achieving one or more of these goals. With the first two indications, duration of treatment is relatively short (typically 3 to 4 years), and hence the risk of harm is relatively low—except for women with established heart disease. In contrast, prevention of osteoporosis requires lifelong HRT, and hence the risk of harm is relatively high.

The only indication for long-term *progestin* therapy is protection against endometrial cancer (that could be caused by unopposed estrogen). Accordingly, use of EPT should be limited to women with an intact uterus. For women who have had a hysterectomy, estrogen alone should be used.

Treatment of Vasomotor Symptoms. HRT is the most effective treatment for vasomotor symptoms (e.g., hot flashes, night sweats), providing welcome relief for millions of women. Do the benefits of short-term therapy justify the risks? Probably, especially for women with severe symptoms and a favorable risk profile. To increase safety, the lowest effective dosage should be employed. Furthermore, because vasomotor symptoms subside over time, the need for continued HRT should be reassessed at least every 6 months. For women who chose to avoid HRT, nonhormonal alternatives can help. Among these are black cohosh (a dietary supplement), foods that contain soy products, and several prescription drugs, including clonidine [Catapres], gabapentin [Neurontin], and four antidepressants: fluoxetine [Prozac], venlafaxine [Effexor], paroxetine [Paxil], and sertraline [Zoloft].

Treatment of Symptoms of Vulvar and Vaginal Atrophy. Estrogen is the most effective treatment for reducing symptoms of menopause-related vulvar and vaginal atrophy (dryness, irritation, itching). However, because systemic estrogen carries significant risks, the FDA recommends that, if HRT is being used solely to manage vulvar and vaginal symptoms, a topical estrogen formulation should be considered. Options include vaginal creams, vaginal tablets, and an estrogen-containing vaginal ring (Table 59–3). Although long-term data are lacking, it seems likely that topical estrogen is safer than oral estrogen. Why? Because, with topical formulations, blood levels of estrogen remain low.

Prevention of Osteoporosis. HRT reduces postmenopausal bone loss, and thereby decreases the risk of osteoporosis and related fractures. However, protection is lost as soon as HRT stops. Hence, to maintain bone health, HRT must continue for life. As a result, the risk of harm is high. Accordingly, alternative treatments are preferred. In fact, labeling of HRT products now must carry the following advice: *When this prod-*

uct is being prescribed solely to prevent postmenopausal osteoporosis, approved nonestrogen treatments should be carefully considered. Furthermore, HRT should be considered only for women with significant risk of osteoporosis, and only when that risk outweighs the risks of HRT. As discussed in Chapter 70 (Drugs Affecting Calcium Levels and Bone Mineralization), effective alternatives to HRT include raloxifene [Evista], bisphosphonates (e.g., alendronate [Fosamax], calcitonin [Miacalcin]), and teriparatide [Forteo]. Of course, all women (not to mention men) should practice primary prevention of bone loss. How? By ensuring adequate intake of calcium and vitamin D, performing regular weight-bearing exercise, and avoiding smoking and excessive alcohol.

Inappropriate Uses: Attempted Prevention of Heart Disease and Dementia

Heart Disease. As noted above under *Warnings,* EPT and ET should *not* be prescribed for the express purpose of preventing heart disease. With regard to EPT, there is no evidence that it confers cardiovascular protection, whereas there *is* evidence that it promotes cardiovascular harm (MI, pulmonary embolism, DVT, and stroke). With regard to ET, long-term effects on CHD are not yet clear. In the absence of proven cardiovascular benefits, there is no rational basis for using ET to promote cardiovascular health. Finally, it should be noted that neither EPT nor ET has ever been approved for prevention of cardiovascular disease.

To reduce risk of cardiovascular events, postmenopausal women should be counseled about alternative ways to promote cardiovascular health. Among these are avoiding smoking, performing regular exercise, decreasing intake of saturated fats, and taking prescribed drugs to treat hypertension, diabetes, and high cholesterol.

Alzheimer's Disease. HRT should not be used to prevent Alzheimer's disease. There is no evidence that ET protects against dementia, and there is clear evidence that EPT can actually *cause* dementia.

Discontinuing HRT

Because the risks of HRT are greater than previously appreciated, many women are discontinuing treatment. Unfortunately, discontinuation may cause vasomotor symptoms to return, typically within 4 days of the last HRT dose. Women who had severe symptoms before initiating HRT are at highest risk of developing intolerable symptoms when they stop.

What's the best way quit? No one knows. There are two basic methods: immediate cessation and tapering slowly. However, there are no controlled studies to indicate which option

TABLE 59–3 ■ Intravaginal Estrogens for Postmenopausal Urogenital Atrophy			
Generic Name	**Trade Name**	**Formulation**	**Usual Maintenance Dosage**
Conjugated estrogens, equine	Premarin	Cream	0.5–2 gm/day*
Estradiol	Estrace	Cream	1–2 gm 1–3 times/wk
	Estring	Ring	Insert 1 ring (2 mg) every 90 days
Estradiol hemihydrate	Vagifem	Tablet	Insert 1 tablet (25 μg) twice/wk
Estropipate	Ogen	Cream	2–4 gm/day*
Dienestrol	Ortho Dienestrol	Cream	1 applicatorful 1–3 times/wk

*Administer cyclically (3 weeks on and 1 week off). For short-term use only.

might result in fewer symptoms. For women who chose to taper slowly, again there are two basic options, referred to as "dose tapering" and "day tapering." With dose tapering, dosing is done every day, but the size of the daily dose is gradually reduced. If intense symptoms return following a dosage reduction, further reductions should be delayed until symptoms improve. With day tapering, the daily dose remains unchanged, but the number of days between doses is gradually increased—starting with dosing every other day, then every third day, and so on. Regardless of which method is used—dose tapering or day tapering—only the dosage of *estrogen* should be lowered; for women on EPT, the *progestin dosage should remain unchanged.* Why? Because lowering the progestin dosage might permit estrogen to stimulate endometrial growth, thereby posing a risk of cancer.

If tapering estrogen leads to intolerable vasomotor symptoms, what can be done? One choice is to taper more slowly. Another is to substitute preparations that do not contain estrogen, but nonetheless may be able to suppress symptoms. As noted above, options include black cohosh, foods that contain soy products, and several drugs, including clonidine, gabapentin, fluoxetine, venlafaxine, paroxetine, and sertraline.

Open Questions

Despite the valuable information provided by HERS and WHI, women considering HRT could use even more information to guide their choice. Important questions that remain unanswered include the following:

- Are the benefits and risks of ET significantly different from those of EPT?
- Does ET (as opposed to EPT) have a role in primary prevention of cardiovascular disease?
- Which component of EPT—estrogen, progestin, or both—is responsible for adverse effects?
- Are Prempro and Premarin (the preparations employed in WHI and HERS) safer in lower doses? If so, are they effective in lower doses?
- Are other estrogens and progestins safer than the hormones in Prempro and Premarin? If so, are they also effective?
- Is intravaginal estrogen safer than oral estrogen (when the objective is preservation of vaginal integrity)?
- When the HRT regimen contains a progestin, which dosing schedule is safer: continuous daily progestin or sequential progestin?
- Does long-term ET protect against dementia and Alzheimer's disease?
- How much weight should women give to quality-of-life issues when deciding whether the benefits of HRT outweigh the risks?
- Does the presence of severe vasomotor symptoms tip the risk/benefit balance in favor of HRT?
- Are there genetic factors that significantly alter the risk/benefit balance of HRT?

When these questions have been answered, the risks and benefits of treatment options will be more clear, and hence

TABLE 59–4 ▪ Some Products for Hormone Replacement Therapy

Generic Name and Route	Trade Name	Usual Dosage
Estrogens		
Oral		
Conjugated estrogens, equine	Premarin	0.625 mg/day
Conjugated estrogens, synthetic	Cenestin	0.3–1.25 mg/day
Estradiol, micronized	Estrace	0.5–2 mg/day
Estropipate	Ogen, Ortho-Est	0.625 mg/day
Esterified estrogens	Estratab, Menest	0.3–1.25 mg/day
Ethinyl estradiol	Estinyl	0.02 mg/day
Transdermal		
Estradiol	Alora, Climara, Esclim, Estraderm, Vivelle	0.025–0.05 mg/day
Estrogen/Progestin Combinations		
Oral		
Conjugated estrogens, equine/ medroxyprogesterone acetate	Prempro	0.625/2.5 mg daily
Conjugated estrogens, equine/ medroxyprogesterone acetate	Premphase	*Days 1–14:* 0.625 mg estrogen (alone) daily *Days 15–28:* 0.625/5 mg estrogen/progesterone daily
Estradiol/norgestimate	Ortho-Prefest	1.0 mg estradiol every day; 0.09 mg norgestimate in a repeating cycle of 3 days on and 3 days off
Estradiol/norethindrone	Activella	1 mg/0.5 mg daily
Ethinylestradiol/norethindrone	Femhrt	5 μg/1 mg daily
Transdermal		
Estradiol/norethindrone	CombiPatch	0.05/0.14 mg daily

women will be able to chose (or reject) HRT with greater assurance than is possible today.

Drug Products for HRT
Preparations

Some drug preparations for HRT are listed in Table 59–4. The estrogens employed most often are conjugated equine estrogens [Premarin] (prepared by extraction from *preg*nant *mar*es' *urin*e), estradiol [Estrace], and transdermal estrogen [Estraderm, others]. Popular estrogen-progestin combinations include Prempro and Premphase. Topical products used to manage symptoms of vaginal atrophy are listed in Table 59–3.

Dosing Schedules

Every woman undergoing HRT receives an estrogen, and every woman with a uterus also receives a progestin (to counteract the stimulant effects of estrogen on the endometrium). Several schedules of administration may be employed. In WHI and HERS, estrogen and progestin were administered *continuously*, thereby eliminating monthly bleeding. An alternative is to give estrogen continuously but give the progestin cyclically (e.g., on calendar days 15 through 28). However, cyclic progestin has the disadvantage of promoting monthly bleeding.

⁞. KEY POINTS

- Estradiol is the principal endogenous estrogen.
- Progesterone is the principal endogenous progestational hormone.
- The first half of the 28-day menstrual cycle is called the follicular phase. The second half is called the luteal phase.
- During the follicular phase, estrogens produced by maturing ovarian follicles cause proliferation of the endometrium.
- During the luteal phase, estrogens and progesterone produced by the corpus luteum maintain the endometrium in its hypertrophied state.
- Toward the end of the menstrual cycle, progesterone levels decline, causing the hypertrophied endometrium to break down, which results in bleeding.
- In addition to their role in the menstrual cycle, estrogens are required for the growth and maturation of the uterus, vagina, fallopian tubes, and breasts. Estrogens also control development of pubic and axillary hair as well as pigmentation of the nipples and genitalia.
- Estrogens suppress bone mineral resorption, and thereby have a positive effect on bone mass.
- Estrogens raise levels of HDL cholesterol and reduce levels of LDL cholesterol. These actions partially explain the low incidence of coronary heart disease in premenopausal women.
- Nausea is the most common adverse effect of exogenous estrogens.
- Prolonged use of estrogens alone is associated with an increased risk of endometrial carcinoma. However, when estrogens are used in combination with a progestin, there is little or no risk of this cancer.

- When combined with a progestin, estrogens increase the risk of breast cancer in postmenopausal women, but apparently not in younger women. Whether estrogen alone increases risk in either population has not been established.
- Use of estrogens during pregnancy can cause vaginal cancer in female offspring and genital malformation in males. Accordingly, estrogens are contraindicated during pregnancy.
- Progestins may cause birth defects during the first 4 months of pregnancy. Hence, their use during pregnancy is not recommended.
- Because of their actions on the endometrium, exogenous progestins can cause breakthrough bleeding, spotting, and amenorrhea.
- Symptoms of menopause result from a decline in estrogen production by the ovaries.
- Two basic regimens are used for HRT: estrogen alone and estrogen combined with a progestin. The purpose of the estrogen is to replace estrogen that was lost because of menopause. The progestin is present to counteract the adverse effects that unopposed estrogen has on the endometrium. In women who no longer have a uterus, the progestin is omitted.
- The Women's Health Initiative (WHI) and the Heart and Estrogen/progestin Replacement Study (HERS)—two large, randomized, placebo-controlled trials—have given us the most statistically valid data to date on the benefits and risks of HRT.
- The principal benefits of HRT are suppression of vasomotor symptoms, prevention of urogenital atrophy, prevention of bone loss and osteoporotic fractures, and reduction of colon cancer risk. Whether HRT protects against Alzheimer's disease has not been determined.
- HRT does not protect against cardiovascular disease, and clearly should not be used with this objective in mind. To reduce cardiovascular risks, postmenopausal women should avoid smoking, perform regular exercise, decrease intake of saturated fats, and take drugs as indicated to treat hypertension, diabetes, and high cholesterol.
- The principal risks of HRT are myocardial infarction, pulmonary embolism, deep vein thrombosis, stroke, ovarian cancer, breast cancer, cholecystitis, and dementia.
- As a rule, the benefits of using HRT short term to reduce vasomotor symptoms outweigh the risks.
- The benefits of using HRT short term to manage urogenital symptoms probably outweigh the risks. However, if this is the only reason for HRT use, a topical estrogen preparation is probably safer, and hence should be considered.
- For protection against osteoporosis, HRT must be taken lifelong, and hence the risks of harm are high. Accordingly, effective alternatives are preferred. Among these are raloxifene, bisphosphonates, calcitonin, and teriparatide. To promote bone health, all women should perform regular weight-bearing exercise, ensure adequate intake of calcium and vitamin D, and avoid smoking and excessive alcohol.

- Premenstrual syndrome (PMS) consists of a constellation of psychologic and physical symptoms that develop in the luteal phase of the menstrual cycle and then resolve a few days after the onset of menses.
- Psychologic symptoms of PMS (e.g., irritability, depression, mood lability, crying spells, social withdrawal) are more disabling than physical symptoms (e.g., acne, breast tenderness, abdominal bloating, appetite disturbance).

- To make a diagnosis of PMS, symptoms must be sufficiently intense, and must be absent between days 4 and 12 of the menstrual cycle.
- Fluoxetine [Prozac] and other SSRIs are the most effective drugs known for PMS. These agents are most effective at reducing psychologic symptoms of PMS; they can also reduce physical symptoms, such as breast tenderness, bloating, and headache.

Summary of Major Nursing Implications*

ESTROGENS

Conjugated estrogens, equine
Conjugated estrogens, synthetic
Diethylstilbestrol
Estradiol
Estrone
Estropipate
Ethinyl estradiol

Preadministration Assessment

Therapeutic Goal

Estrogens are used primarily for contraception (see Chapter 60) and postmenopausal HRT, which has three approved indications: treatment of vasomotor symptoms, treatment of symptoms of vulvar and vaginal atrophy, and prevention of osteoporosis. Additional indications are female hypogonadism, prostate cancer, and dysfunctional uterine bleeding.

Baseline Data

Assessment should include a breast examination, pelvic examination, Pap smear, lipid profile, mammography, and blood pressure measurement. If the objective is HRT, menopause should be verified.

Identifying High-Risk Patients

Estrogens are *contraindicated* during pregnancy and for patients with estrogen-dependent cancers, undiagnosed abnormal vaginal bleeding, active thrombophlebitis or thromboembolic disorders, or a history of estrogen-associated thrombophlebitis, thrombosis, or thromboembolic disorders.

Implementation Administration

Routes

Oral, IM, IV, transdermal, and intravaginal.

Administration

Transdermal. Give the patient the following instructions for using the estradiol transdermal system:

Apply the transdermal patch to an area of clean, dry, intact skin on the abdomen or some other region of the trunk (but not the breasts or waistline) by pressing the patch firmly in place for 10 seconds.

If the patch falls off, reapply the same patch or, if necessary, apply a new patch.

Remove the old patch and apply a new patch once or twice weekly (depending on the product).

Rotate the application site such that the same site is not used more than once each week.

Intravaginal Creams. Instruct the patient to apply estrogen cream high into the vagina using the applicator provided.

Dosing

Schedules for HRT. Women with an intact uterus should receive EPT, whereas women who have had a hysterectomy should use ET. In both cases, dosing with estrogen is done *daily*. With EPT, the progestin component may be given *daily* or *sequentially* (days 15 through 25).

Ongoing Evaluation and Interventions

Monitoring Summary

The patient should receive a yearly follow-up breast and pelvic exam. An endometrial biopsy should be performed every 2 to 3 years.

Minimizing Adverse Effects

Nausea. Nausea is common early in treatment but diminishes with time. **Inform the patient that nausea can be reduced by taking estrogens with food.**

Endometrial Hyperplasia and Cancer. Therapy with estrogen alone during menopause increases the risk of endometrial carcinoma. Adding a progestin to the regimen eliminates (or at least greatly reduces) this risk. **Instruct the patient to notify the physician if persistent or recurrent vaginal bleeding develops so that the possibility of endometrial carcinoma can be evaluated.** Also, the patient should receive an endometrial biopsy every 2 to 3 years.

Breast Cancer. Estrogen, combined with a progestin, produces a small increase in the risk of breast cancer in postmenopausal women, but apparently not in younger women. **To minimize risk, advise patients to perform monthly breast self-exams, have yearly breast exams by a healthcare professional, and receive periodic mammograms.**

Use During Pregnancy. In utero exposure to estrogens can cause genital abnormalities in males and vaginal cancer in females. Accordingly, estrogens are *contraindicated during pregnancy.* **Inform women of child-bearing age about the potential risks to the fetus. Instruct patients to discontinue estrogens immediately if pregnancy is suspected.**

*Patient education information is highlighted as blue text.

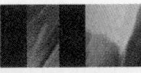

Summary of Major Nursing Implications*—cont'd

Ovarian Cancer. In postmenopausal women, replacement therapy with estrogen alone—but not with estrogen plus a progestin—increases the risk of ovarian cancer. **Advise women using ET to undergo periodic evaluation for ovarian cancer.**

Cardiovascular Events. Therapy with estrogen plus a progestin increases the risk of MI, pulmonary embolism, DVT, and stroke. Whether estrogen alone carries the same risk has not been determined. **To reduce cardiovascular risk, advise women to avoid smoking, perform regular exercise, decrease intake of saturated fats, and take appropriate drugs to treat hypertension, diabetes, and high cholesterol.**

Effects Resembling Those Caused by Oral Contraceptives. Use of estrogens for noncontraceptive purposes can produce adverse effects similar to those caused by oral contraceptives (e.g., abnormal vaginal bleeding, hypertension, benign hepatic adenoma, reduced glucose tolerance). Nursing implications regarding these effects are summarized in Chapter 60.

Minimizing Adverse Interactions

The interactions of estrogens are probably similar to those seen with oral contraceptives. Implications regarding these interactions are summarized in Chapter 60.

PROGESTINS

Hydroxyprogesterone caproate
Levonorgestrel
Medroxyprogesterone acetate
Megestrol
Norethindrone
Norgestrel
Progesterone

Preadministration Assessment

Therapeutic Goal

Progestins are used primarily for contraception (see Chapter 60) and to counteract the endometrial hyperplasia that could be caused by unopposed estrogen during HRT. Other uses include dysfunctional uterine bleeding, amenorrhea, and endometriosis.

Baseline Data

The physical examination should include breast and pelvic examinations. A Pap smear should be obtained.

Identifying High-Risk Patients

Progestins are *contraindicated* in the presence of undiagnosed abnormal vaginal bleeding, thrombophlebitis, thromboembolic disorders, severe liver disease, and carcinoma of the breast and reproductive organs. Progestins should be *avoided* during pregnancy.

Implementation: Administration

Routes

Oral, IM, transdermal.

Administration

Advise patients to take oral progestins with food if GI upset occurs.

Ongoing Evaluation and Interventions

Minimizing Adverse Effects

Teratogenic Effects. Progestins can cause birth defects (limb reductions, heart defects, masculinization of the female fetus) if taken during the first 4 months of pregnancy. **Inform women of child-bearing age about the potential risks to the fetus, and instruct them to discontinue progestins immediately if pregnancy is suspected.**

Gynecologic Effects. **Inform patients about potential side effects (breakthrough bleeding, spotting, amenorrhea, alteration of cervical secretions, breast tenderness). Instruct patients to notify the physician if abnormal vaginal bleeding occurs.**

*Patient education information is highlighted as blue text.

Birth Control

Birth control can be accomplished by interfering with the reproductive process at any step from gametogenesis to nidation (implantation of a fertilized ovum). Pharmacologic methods of contraception include oral contraceptives, levonorgestrel implants, depot medroxyprogesterone acetate, progesterone-containing intrauterine devices, and gossypol (an investigational agent that suppresses sperm production). Nonpharmacologic methods include surgical sterilization (tubal ligation, vasectomy), mechanical devices (condom, diaphragm, cervical cap), and avoiding intercourse during periods of fertility (calendar method, temperature method, cervical mucus method).

Although we have birth control methods that are safe and effective, statistics show that unwanted pregnancy is common—suggesting that available methods are not used as widely or as effectively as they could be, and that alternatives to current methods are needed. In the United States, nearly 6 of every 10 pregnancies is unplanned or unwanted. Among girls ages 15 to 17, the pregnancy rate is 1 in 10. However, although much attention is focused on teenage pregnancy, fully 80% of un-

planned pregnancies occur in women age 20 or older. Of the unplanned pregnancies that occur every year, about 1.1 million are carried to term, and another 1.4 million end in abortion.

Our principal focus in this chapter is on oral contraceptives. These agents are the second most widely used form of birth control (sterilization is first), and are among the most effective methods available. In preparing to study these agents and other forms of contraception, you should review Chapter 59, paying special attention to information on the menstrual cycle and the physiologic and pharmacologic effects of estrogens and progestins.

EFFECTIVENESS AND SAFETY OF BIRTH CONTROL METHODS

Effectiveness

The effectiveness of a birth control method can be expressed in terms of the percentage of accidental pregnancies that occur during use of the technique. Employing this criterion, Table 60–1 compares the effectiveness of the major birth control methods. As we can see, the most effective methods are Norplant, Depo-Provera, intrauterine devices (IUDs), and sterilization. Oral contraceptives (OCs) are close behind. The least reliable methods include periodic abstinence, spermicides, and the cervical cap.

Note that Table 60–1 contains two columns of figures, one labeled *optimal* and the other *typical*. The optimal figures are the pregnancy rates that are likely when a method of birth control is employed exactly as it should be (i.e., consistently and with proper technique). The *typical* figures represent pregnancy rates observed in actual practice. The higher pregnancy rates reported in the typical column are largely an indication that methods of birth control are not always used when and as they should be.

Safety

The issue of the relative safety of birth control measures is complex. Contributing to this complexity is the fact that much of our information on the adverse effects of OCs was gathered when these agents were employed in doses higher than those employed today. Newer data show that OCs, as currently prescribed, are considerably safer than indicated by older studies. An additional complication regarding the safety of birth control measures stems from the fact that the risk of mortality associated with pregnancy and delivery is greater than the risk associated with any form of birth control. Hence, a birth control measure that is inherently more safe than others, but is also less effective, may become relatively less safe when the dangers associated with a greater pregnancy rate are factored in.

TABLE 60–1 ▪■ **Effectiveness of Birth Control Methods**		
	Failure Rate* (%)	
Birth Control Method	**Typical†**	**Optimal‡**
Levonorgestrel subdermal implant [Norplant]	0.05	0.05
Surgical sterilization		
Female: tubal ligation	0.5	0.5
Male: vasectomy	0.15	0.1
Intramuscular medroxyprogesterone acetate [Depo-Provera]	0.3	0.3
Intrauterine devices		
Copper T 380A [ParaGard]	0.8	0.6
Progesterone T [Progestasert]	2	1.5
Levonorgestrel T [Mirena]	0.1	0.1
Oral contraceptives		
Combination pills	5	0.1
Progestin-only pills	5	0.5
Vaginal contraceptive ring [NuvaRing]	—	1
Condoms		
Male	14	3
Female	21	5
Diaphragm with spermicide	20	6
Cervical cap		
Parous	40	26
Nulliparous	20	9
Spermicide alone	26	6
Periodic abstinence	20	2–10
No birth control	Pregnancy rate would be 80%–85%	

*Failure rate = percentage of women who have an accidental pregnancy during first year of use.
†Typical = failure rate usually observed in actual practice.
‡Optimal = failure rate that would be expected if the birth control method were practiced exactly as it should be.

Keeping the above provisos in mind, we can make the following observations on birth control safety. Of the contraceptive methods available, OCs produce the broadest spectrum of adverse effects, ranging from nausea to menstrual irregularity to rare thromboembolic disorders. However, despite their wide variety of undesired actions, when used by nonsmoking women with normal cardiovascular function, OCs produce no greater mortality than other active forms of birth control. The lowest mortality rate is seen when barrier methods (diaphragm, condom, cervical cap) are used together with abortion (if contraceptive failure should occur). As discussed below, women who are at risk for sexually transmitted disease (STD) should not use an IUD.

SELECTING A BIRTH CONTROL METHOD

Figure 60–1 indicates the percentage of users who select particular forms of birth control. Perhaps surprisingly, the method chosen most frequently is sterilization: female sterilization (tubal ligation) plus male sterilization (vasectomy) are selected by over 42% of birth control users. OCs or condoms are chosen by most of the remaining birth control users. Diaphragms, periodic abstinence, IUDs, and other techniques account for a small fraction of birth control use.

Several factors should be considered when choosing a method of birth control. Chief among these are *effectiveness*, *safety*, and *personal preference*. As indicated in Table 60–1, the most effective methods are levonorgestrel subdermal implants [Norplant], intramuscular medroxyprogesterone acetate [Depo-Provera], sterilization, and IUDs. OCs are close behind. The remaining methods—condoms, diaphragm, cervical cap, spermicides, and periodic abstinence—must be used in a near-perfect fashion to provide any reasonable level of protection.

When factoring safety into the choice of a birth control method, several guidelines apply. OCs should be avoided by women with certain cardiovascular disorders (see below) and should be used with caution by women who smoke heavily. For women in these categories, a barrier method or an IUD is preferred to OCs. Although OCs are effective and relatively convenient, they can also cause many side effects; women who consider the benefit-to-risk ratio unfavorable should be advised about alternative contraceptive techniques. Women who are at risk for a STD (i.e., women who are not in a mutually monogamous relationship) should not use an IUD.

Personal preference is a major factor in providing the motivation needed for consistent implementation of a birth control method. Because even the best form of contraception will be ineffective if improperly practiced, the importance of personal preference cannot be stressed too much. Practitioners

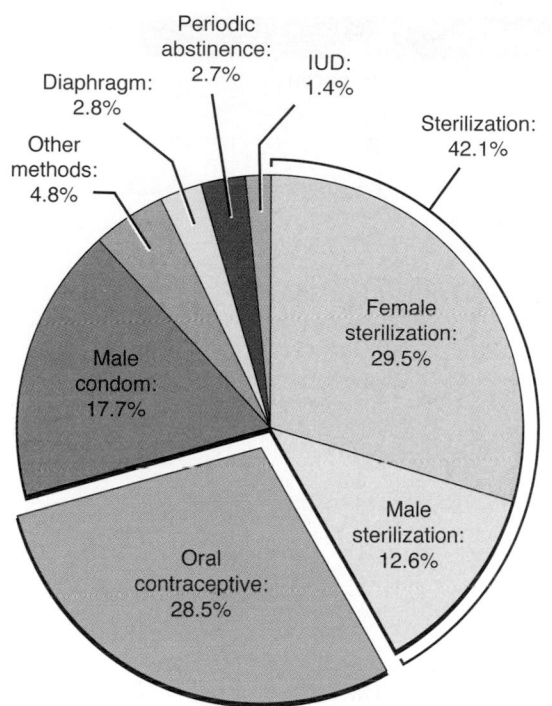

Figure 60–1 ■ Percentage use for birth control methods.
Note: the segment labeled "other methods" refers to douching, withdrawal, spermicides, IUDs, and other techniques.

should take pains to educate clients about the various contraceptive methods available so that expressions of preference can be based on understanding.

Additional factors that bear on selecting a birth control method include family planning goals, age, frequency of sexual intercourse, and the individual's capacity for compliance. If family planning goals have already been met, sterilization of either the male or female partner may be desirable. For women who engage in coitus frequently, OCs or a long-term method (e.g., Norplant, Depo-Provera, IUD) are reasonable choices. Conversely, when sexual activity is limited, use of a spermicide, condom, or diaphragm may be most appropriate. Since barrier methods combined with spermicides can offer some protection against venereal disease (as well as providing contraception), these combinations may be of special benefit to individuals who have multiple partners. If compliance is a problem (as it can be with OCs, condoms, and diaphragms), use of a long-term method (e.g., IUD, Norplant, Depo-Provera) would confer reliable protection.

ORAL CONTRACEPTIVES

Classification

There are two main categories of OCs: (1) those that contain both an estrogen and a progestin, known as *combination OCs,* and (2) those that contain only a progestin, known as "minipills" or *progestin-only OCs.* Of the two groups, combination OCs are by far the more widely used.

The combination OCs have three subgroups: *monophasic, biphasic,* and *triphasic.* In a monophasic regimen, the daily

estrogen and progestin dosage remains constant throughout the monthly cycle of use. In a biphasic regimen, the estrogen dosage remains constant, but the progestin dosage is increased during the second half of the cycle. In triphasic regimens, the monthly cycle is divided into three phases. In most triphasic regimens, the progestin dosage changes for each phase of the cycle; in two regimens, the estrogen dosage also varies.

Combination Oral Contraceptives

Since their introduction in the late 1950s, combination OCs have become one of our most widely prescribed families of drugs. As indicated in Table 60–1, these agents are nearly 100% effective, making them one of the most efficacious forms of birth control available. Not only are these drugs highly effective, they are also very safe, although minor side effects are relatively common.

Chemistry

Combination OCs consist of an estrogen plus a progestin. Only two estrogens are employed: ethinyl estradiol and mestranol, which is converted to ethinyl estradiol in the body. In contrast, several progestins are employed, norethindrone being used most often (Table 60–2).

Mechanism of Action

Combination OCs decrease fertility in several ways. Their principal effect is *inhibition of ovulation.* The precise mechanism by which inhibition occurs is unknown. In addition, OCs can promote thickening of the cervical mucus, thereby creating a barrier to the passage of sperm. Also, OCs can modify the endometrium, making it less favorable for implantation.

Adverse Effects

Combination OCs can cause a wide variety of adverse effects. However, although many types of effects may be produced, severe effects are rare. Hence, when compared with the serious risks associated with pregnancy and childbirth, the risks of OCs are low.

Because OCs are taken by women who are healthy, and because OCs represent a potential health hazard (albeit small), it is important that steps be taken to minimize risk. Accordingly, a thorough physical examination should usually be performed. This examination should include blood pressure determination, examination of the breasts and pelvic organs, and a Pap smear. These tests should be repeated at least once a year.

Thromboembolic Disorders. Combination OCs have been associated with venous and arterial thromboembolism, pulmonary embolism, myocardial infarction, and thrombotic stroke. These thrombotic disorders are caused by the *estrogen* component of combination OCs, not by the progestin. Thrombosis results at least in part from an increase in circulating levels of clotting factors. Thrombosis is not due to atherosclerosis.

In contrast to older OCs, the OCs available today carry a very low risk of thrombosis. When combination OCs first became available, they contained *high* doses of estrogens (e.g., 100 μg ethinyl estradiol). As a result, these preparations carried a significant risk of thrombotic disorders. Because today's OCs contain *low* doses of estrogens—no more than 50 μg

TABLE 60–2 ■ Composition of Oral Contraceptives

Trade Name	μg	Estrogen	mg	Progestin
Combination OCs				
Monophasic				
Loestrin 21 1/20	20	Ethinyl estradiol	1	Norethindrone
Loestrin Fe 1/20	20	Ethinyl estradiol	1	Norethindrone
Microgestin Fe 1/20	20	Ethinyl estradiol	1	Norethindrone
Alesse	20	Ethinyl estradiol	0.1	Levonorgestrel
Aviane	20	Ethinyl estradiol	0.1	Levonorgestrel
Levlite	20	Ethinyl estradiol	0.1	Levonorgestrel
Levlen	30	Ethinyl estradiol	0.15	Levonorgestrel
Levora	30	Ethinyl estradiol	0.15	Levonorgestrel
Nordette	30	Ethinyl estradiol	0.15	Levonorgestrel
Lo-Ogestrel	30	Ethinyl estradiol	0.3	Norgestrel
Lo/Ovral	30	Ethinyl estradiol	0.3	Norgestrel
Loestrin 21 1.5/30	30	Ethinyl estradiol	1.5	Norethindrone
Loestrin Fe 1.5/30	30	Ethinyl estradiol	1.5	Norethindrone
Microgestin Fe 1.5/30	30	Ethinyl estradiol	1.5	Norethindrone
Apri	30	Ethinyl estradiol	0.15	Desogestrel
Desogen	30	Ethinyl estradiol	0.15	Desogestrel
Ortho-Cept	30	Ethinyl estradiol	0.15	Desogestrel
Yasmin	30	Ethinyl estradiol	3	Drospirenone
Demulen 1/35	35	Ethinyl estradiol	1	Ethynodiol diacetate
Zovia 1/35E	35	Ethinyl estradiol	1	Ethynodiol diacetate
Ovocon-35	35	Ethinyl estradiol	0.4	Norethindrone
Brevicon	35	Ethinyl estradiol	0.5	Norethindrone
Necon 0.5/35	35	Ethinyl estradiol	0.5	Norethindrone
Nortrel 0.5/35	35	Ethinyl estradiol	0.5	Norethindrone
Modicon	35	Ethinyl estradiol	0.5	Norethindrone
Necon 1/35	35	Ethinyl estradiol	1	Norethindrone
Norinyl 1 + 35	35	Ethinyl estradiol	1	Norethindrone
Nortrel 1/35	35	Ethinyl estradiol	1	Norethindrone
Ortho-Novum 1/35	35	Ethinyl estradiol	1	Norethindrone
Ortho-Cyclen	35	Ethinyl estradiol	0.250	Norgestimate
Ogestrel	50	Ethinyl estradiol	0.5	Norgestrel
Ovral-28	50	Ethinyl estradiol	0.5	Norgestrel
Demulin 1/50	50	Ethinyl estradiol	1	Ethynodiol diacetate
Zovia 1/50E	50	Ethinyl estradiol	1	Ethynodiol diacetate
Ovocon-50	50	Ethinyl estradiol	1	Norethindrone
Necon 1/50	50	Mestranol	1	Norethindrone
Ortho-Novum 1/50	50	Mestranol	1	Norethindrone
Norinyl 1 + 50	50	Mestranol	1	Norethindrone
Biphasic				
Ortho-Novum 10/11,	35	Ethinyl estradiol	0.5	Norethindrone (phase 1)
Necon 10/11,	35	Ethinyl estradiol	1	Norethindrone (phase 2)
Janest-28				
Mircette	20	Ethinyl estradiol	0.15	Desogestrel (phase 1)
	10	Ethinyl estradiol		(phase 2)
Triphasic				
Cyclessa	25	Ethinyl estradiol	0.1	Desogestrel (phase 1)
	25	Ethinyl estradiol	0.125	Desogestrel (phase 2)
	25	Ethinyl estradiol	0.15	Desogestrel (phase 3)
Tri-Norinyl	35	Ethinyl estradiol	0.5	Norethindrone (phase 1)
	35	Ethinyl estradiol	1	Norethindrone (phase 2)
	35	Ethinyl estradiol	0.5	Norethindrone (phase 3)
Ortho-Novum 7/7/7	35	Ethinyl estradiol	0.5	Norethindrone (phase 1)
	35	Ethinyl estradiol	0.75	Norethindrone (phase 2)
	35	Ethinyl estradiol	1	Norethindrone (phase 3)
Tri-Levlen, Triphasil,	30	Ethinyl estradiol	0.05	Levonorgestrel (phase 1)
Trivora-28, Enpresse	40	Ethinyl estradiol	0.075	Levonorgestrel (phase 2)
	30	Ethinyl estradiol	0.125	Levonorgestrel (phase 3)

TABLE 60–2 ▪■ Composition of Oral Contraceptives—cont'd				
Trade Name	**µg**	**Estrogen**	**mg**	**Progestin**
Combination OCs—cont'd				
Triphasic—cont'd				
Ortho Tri-Cyclen LO	25	Ethinyl estradiol	0.18	Norgestimate (phase 1)
	25	Ethinyl estradiol	0.215	Norgestimate (phase 2)
	25	Ethinyl estradiol	0.25	Norgestimate (phase 3)
Ortho Tri-Cyclen	35	Ethinyl estradiol	0.18	Norgestimate (phase 1)
	35	Ethinyl estradiol	0.215	Norgestimate (phase 2)
	35	Ethinyl estradiol	0.25	Norgestimate (phase 3)
Estrostep 21,	20	Ethinyl estradiol	1	Norethindrone (phase 1)
Estrostep Fe	30	Ethinyl estradiol	1	Norethindrone (phase 2)
	35	Ethinyl estradiol	1	Norethindrone (phase 3)
Progestin-only OCs				
Micronor, Nor-Q.D.			0.35	Norethindrone
Orvette			0.075	Norgestrel

ethinyl estradiol, and usually less—the risk of thrombosis among users is only slightly greater than among nonusers.

The risk of thromboembolic phenomena from OCs is increased in the presence of other risk factors, especially *heavy smoking* and a *history of thromboembolism*. Additional risk factors include hypertension, cerebrovascular disease, coronary artery disease, myocardial infarction, and surgery in which postoperative thrombosis might be expected.

In the past, OCs were not recommended for women over the age of 35. Why? Because earlier studies indicated a dramatic increase in the risk of thrombosis for this group. However, more recent data show that today's low-estrogen OCs may be used up to menopause with no greater risk of thrombosis than among younger women.

Several measures can help minimize thromboembolic phenomena. First, the estrogen dose in OCs should be no greater than required for contraceptive efficacy. Second, OCs should not be prescribed for women who are heavy smokers, for women with a history of thromboembolism, or for women with other risk factors for thrombosis. Third, OCs should be discontinued at least 4 weeks prior to surgery in which postoperative thrombosis might be expected. Lastly, women should be informed about the symptoms of thrombosis and thromboembolism (e.g., leg tenderness or pain, sudden chest pain, shortness of breath, severe headache, sudden visual disturbance) and instructed to cease OC use and notify the physician if these occur.

Hypertension. The incidence of hypertension among OC users is 3 to 6 times greater than among nonusers. OCs elevate blood pressure by increasing blood levels of both angiotensin (a potent vasoconstrictor) and aldosterone (a hormone that promotes salt and water retention). The risk of hypertension increases with age and duration of OC use. Women taking OCs should undergo periodic determination of blood pressure. If hypertension develops, OCs should be discontinued. Blood pressure usually declines to pretreatment levels within a few months after OC withdrawal.

Cancer. The effects of OCs on hormone-responsive cancers—cancers of the ovaries, endometrium, cervix, and breast—have been studied intensely. Effects on three of

these cancers are clear: OCs *protect* against ovarian and endometrial cancer, and slightly *increase* the risk of cervical cancer—but only in women who test positive for the human papillomavirus.

And what about breast cancer? Until recently, the question was unresolved: some older studies found a link between OC use and breast cancer; others did not. Now, we seem to have a definitive answer: OCs do *not* increase the risk of breast cancer for most women. This conclusion is based on data from the Women's Contraceptive and Reproductive Experience (Women's CARE) study, published in 2002. This major study, involving over 9000 women, found no association between present or past use of OCs and development of breast cancer. This conclusion applied not only to study participants as a whole, but also to women in the following subgroups:

- Those who used OCs with high estrogen content
- Those who used OCs for a prolonged time
- Those who began OC use during adolescence
- Those with a first-degree relative with breast cancer

These results should reassure most OC users.

However, although this study shows that OCs do not increase risk for most women, the results of another large recent study show that OCs *do* increase risk for some women, specifically, women who have the BRCA1 gene mutation. Even without taking OCs, these women have a very high—50% to 80%—lifetime risk of breast cancer; OCs increase this risk by one-third. The same study found that OCs do *not* increase risk in women with the BRCA2 mutation.

It is important to note that, although OCs do not *cause* breast cancer, estrogens can promote the growth of *existing* breast carcinoma. Accordingly, women with this disease should not take OCs.

As discussed in Chapter 59, women who had been exposed to diethylstilbestrol (DES), a nonsteroidal estrogen, during fetal life are at increased risk of developing cervical and vaginal cancer when they mature. To minimize any possible risk to the fetus, OCs should be discontinued if contraceptive failure occurs.

Teratogenic Effects. Current data indicate that OCs can be taken during early pregnancy with no harm to the fetus. Nonetheless, when taken in very high doses, estrogens and progestins *can* cause birth defects. For example, exposure of the male fetus to DES can cause testicular hypoplasia and abnormal semen production. Accordingly, OCs should be discontinued if pregnancy occurs.

Abnormal Uterine Bleeding. By inducing endometrial regression, OCs may decrease or eliminate menstrual flow during the initial months of use. Breakthrough bleeding and spotting may occur, especially when OCs with low estrogen and progestin content are employed. If bleeding irregularities persist, the possibility of malignancy should be investigated. If two consecutive periods are missed, the client should be evaluated for pregnancy. Following discontinuation of OC use, a period of 1 to 3 months may be required before normal menstruation resumes. In extreme cases, cyclic menses may not return for up to 1 year.

Effects Related to Estrogen or Progestin Imbalance. Many of the mild side effects of OCs result from an excess or deficiency of estrogen or progestin. Effects that can result from an excess of estrogen include nausea, breast tenderness, and edema. Progestin excess can increase appetite and cause fatigue and depression. A deficiency in either hormone can cause menstrual irregularities. Side effects related to hormonal imbalance are summarized in Table 60–3. By making appropriate adjustments in the estrogen and progestin content of an OC regimen, many of these effects can be minimized.

Use in Pregnancy and Lactation. Because OCs can cause cancer in females exposed to them *in utero, OCs are contraindicated for use during pregnancy* (Food and Drug Administration [FDA] Pregnancy Risk Category X). Pregnancy should be ruled out prior to initiation of OC therapy. If pregnancy occurs during OC use, the OC should be discontinued. OCs enter breast milk and reduce milk production. Accordingly, OCs should not be taken by women who are breast-feeding.

Benign Hepatic Adenoma. Hepatic adenoma is a rare complication of OC use. Although nonmalignant, these tumors are highly vascular, and hence can be the source of severe hemorrhage if they rupture. Women using OCs should undergo periodic palpation of the liver. If a mass is detected, further tests should be performed to establish a definitive diagnosis. If hepatic adenoma is diagnosed, OCs must be discontinued; spontaneous regression of the tumor usually follows.

Multiple Births. The incidence of twin births is increased in women who become pregnant shortly after discontinuing OCs. Women who desire pregnancy, but wish to reduce the chances of multiple births, should employ an alternative form of birth control for approximately 3 months after stopping OCs.

Glucose Intolerance. Oral contraceptives can elevate plasma glucose levels. This diabetogenic effect is caused by the *progestin* in OCs. Glucose intolerance is most likely in patients who are already diabetic or have experienced gestational diabetes. Because hypoglycemic agents (e.g., insulin) can control glucose elevations induced by OCs, the presence of diabetes does not preclude OC use. Prediabetic women should be monitored for development of hyperglycemia. Glucose intolerance may occur less with OCs that contain *desogestrel* or *norgestimate* as their progestin component.

Other Adverse Effects. Rarely, OCs cause *gallbladder disease* accompanied by jaundice. This condition reverses following termination of treatment. OCs can cause a variety of *ocular lesions* (e.g., retinal vascular occlusion, retinal edema, optic neuropathy). Accordingly, OCs should be withdrawn in the event of unexplained visual disturbance. *Melanoderma* (darkening of the skin) may occur during OC use; a reduction in dosage may cause pigmentation to decrease. Progestins with androgenic actions may cause *acne, hirsutism,* and *hair loss;* these may occur less with OCs that contain *desogestrel* or *norgestimate,* rather than older progestins.

Summary of Contraindications and Precautions

Combination OCs are *contraindicated* during pregnancy and for women with the following disorders (or a history thereof): thrombophlebitis, thromboembolic disorders, cerebrovascular accident, coronary artery disease, known or suspected breast carcinoma, known or suspected estrogen-dependent neoplasm, benign or malignant liver tumors, and undiagnosed abnormal genital bleeding.

Combination OCs should be used with *caution* by women with diabetes, women who are heavy smokers (more than 15 cigarettes a day), women who have risk factors for cardiovascular disease (e.g., hypertension, obesity, hypercholesterolemia), and women anticipating elective surgery in which postoperative thrombosis might be expected.

Noncontraceptive Benefits of OCs

OCs decrease the risk of several disorders, including ovarian cancer, endometrial cancer, ovarian cysts, pelvic inflammatory disease (PID), premenstrual syndrome, fibrocystic breast

TABLE 60–3 ■ Side Effects Caused by an Excess or Deficiency in the Estrogen or Progestin Content of an Oral Contraceptive Regimen			
Estrogen		**Progestin**	
Excess	**Deficiency**	**Excess**	**Deficiency**
Nausea	Early or midcycle	Increased appetite	Late breakthrough
Breast tenderness	breakthrough	Weight gain	bleeding
Edema	bleeding	Depression	Amenorrhea
Bloating	Increased spotting	Tiredness	Hypermenorrhea
Hypertension	Hypomenorrhea	Fatigue	
Migraine headache		Hypomenorrhea	
Cervical mucorrhea		Breast regression	
Polyposis		Monilial vaginitis	
		Acne, oily scalp*	
		Hair loss*	
		Hirsutism*	

*Caused by progestins that have androgenic activity.

disease, toxic shock syndrome, anemia, and acne. In addition, OCs favorably affect menstrual symptoms: cramps are reduced, menstrual flow is smaller and of shorter duration, and menses are more predictable.

Drug Interactions

Drugs That Reduce the Effects of OCs. The effectiveness of OCs can be decreased by a variety of drugs. *Rifampin* (used for tuberculosis), *ritonavir* (used for HIV infection), *troglitazone* (used for diabetes), and several *antiepileptic drugs* (carbamazepine, phenobarbital, phenytoin, primidone, topiramate) can induce synthesis of hepatic drug-metabolizing enzymes, and can thereby accelerate OC degradation. A number of antibiotics, including *tetracyclines* and *ampicillin,* can also lower OC efficacy: By killing gut flora, these agents reduce enterohepatic recirculation of OCs, and thereby accelerate OC elimination. Women taking OCs in combination with any of the above agents should be alert for indications of reduced OC blood levels (e.g., breakthrough bleeding, spotting). If these signs appear, it may be necessary to increase OC dosage or use an alternative form of birth control.

Drugs Whose Effects Are Reduced by OCs. OCs can reduce the effects of several drugs. By increasing levels of clotting factors, OCs can decrease the effectiveness of *warfarin,* an anticoagulant. OCs can also reduce the effects of insulin and other hypoglycemic agents. Hence, when combined with OCs, warfarin and hypoglycemic agents may require increased dosage.

Drugs Whose Effects Are Increased by OCs. OCs can impair the hepatic metabolism of several agents, including *theophylline* (used for asthma) and *imipramine* (an antidepressant). Because of reduced metabolic breakdown, these drugs may accumulate to toxic levels. Accordingly, women taking these drugs in combination with OCs should be alert for signs of toxicity; a reduction in the dosage of theophylline or imipramine may be required.

Preparations

The combination OCs currently available are listed in Table 60–2. As shown, the principal estrogen in OCs is *ethinyl estradiol.* The principal progestin is *norethindrone.* The preparations in Table 60–2 are listed in order of increasing estrogen content. OCs with lower amounts of estrogen are less likely to produce serious side effects. The table also indicates which preparations belong to each of the three subgroups of combination OCs: monophasic, biphasic, and triphasic. The biphasic and triphasic preparations reflect efforts to more closely simulate ovarian production of estrogens and progestins. However, these preparations offer little if any advantage over monophasic OCs.

Yasmin. Yasmin is a new combination OC that deserves special comment. The product contains ethinyl estradiol plus *drospirenone,* a unique compound that has both progestational and antialdosterone actions. The new compound is a structural analog of spironolactone, a potassium-sparing diuretic that blocks receptors for aldosterone. Drospirenone was developed in an effort to reduce fluid retention caused by the estrogen component in combination OCs. (Estrogen promotes fluid retention by activating the renin-angiotensin-aldosterone system. Drospirenone reduces fluid retention by blocking aldosterone receptors, and thereby prevents retention of sodium and water. As a result, Yasmin may cause less bloating, weight gain, and hypertension than other combination OCs.) The principal concern with drospirenone is *hyperkalemia* secondary to renal retention of potassium. Accordingly,

the drug is inappropriate for women with conditions that predispose to hyperkalemia (e.g., renal insufficiency, adrenal insufficiency, liver disease). Furthermore, it should be used with caution in women taking other drugs that can elevate serum potassium. Important among these are angiotensin-converting enzyme inhibitors, angiotensin II receptor blockers, potassium-sparing diuretics, and potassium supplements. If women taking these drugs are given Yasmin, potassium levels should be checked during the first cycle of use.

Dosage and Administration

Dosing Schedules. Most OCs are taken in a sequence that consists of 21 days of OC use followed by 7 days on which either (1) no pill is taken, (2) an inert pill is taken, or (3) an iron-containing pill is taken. The sequence is begun on the fifth day of the menstrual cycle (i.e., 5 days after the onset of menses) and is repeated for as long as appropriate. Successive dosing cycles should commence every 28 days, regardless of whether breakthrough bleeding or spotting has occurred. Pills should be taken at the same hour every day (e.g., with a meal, at bedtime). During the first week of OC use, a backup form of birth control (e.g., condom, diaphragm) is recommended. Postpartum use of OCs can be initiated immediately after delivery, as long as breast-feeding is not intended.

Many specialists recommend taking combination OCs continuously for several months, rather than following the traditional 28-day cycle. Why? Because, with fewer interruptions of OC use, women experience fewer periods of withdrawal bleeding with its associated menstrual pain, premenstrual symptoms, headaches, and other symptoms. Prolonged use of OCs is possible because these drugs suppress endometrial thickening, and hence monthly bleeding is not required to slough off hypertrophied tissue. Importantly, when an extended cycle is used, a monophasic OC should be selected; a biphasic or triphasic formulation would be inappropriate.

Adjustments to Estrogen and Progestin Dosage. In most cases, therapy is initiated with an OC whose estrogen content is equivalent to 35 μg of estrogen or less. If this low-estrogen preparation results in signs of estrogen deficiency (e.g., spotting, breakthrough bleeding), an OC with higher estrogen content may be substituted. Conversely, if signs of estrogen excess become apparent (e.g., nausea, edema, breast discomfort), a preparation with lower estrogen content may be selected. In a similar fashion, the progestin content of the regimen can be adjusted so as to alleviate symptoms of progestin excess or deficiency. When substituting one combination OC for another, the change can be made at the beginning of any new cycle. The change will not affect contraceptive efficacy.

What to Do in the Event of Missed Dosage. The chances of ovulation (and hence pregnancy) from missing one OC dose are small. However, the risk of pregnancy becomes progressively larger with each consecutive omission. If only one dose is missed, that dose should be taken together with the next scheduled dose. If two doses are missed, two doses should be taken per day on the following 2 days. If three doses are missed, a new cycle should be initiated, starting 7 days after the last pill was taken. An additional form of birth control should be used during the first 2 weeks of the new cycle.

Progestin-Only Oral Contraceptives

Progestin-only OCs, also known as "minipills," contain a progestin (norethindrone or norgestrel) but no estrogen. Because they lack estrogen, minipills do not cause thromboembolic disorders and most of the other adverse effects associated with combination OCs. Unfortunately, although slightly safer than combination OCs, the progestin-only preparations are less effective and cause more menstrual irregularity (breakthrough bleeding, spotting, amenorrhea, inconsistent cycle length, variations in the volume and duration of monthly flow). Because of these drawbacks, minipills are considerably less popular than combination pills. Three progestin-only products are currently available (see Table 60–2).

Contraceptive effects of the minipill result largely from alteration of cervical secretions. Under the influence of progestin, cervical glands produce a thick, sticky mucus that acts as a barrier to penetration by sperm. Progestins also modify the endometrium, making it less favorable for nidation. Compared with combination OCs, minipills are weak inhibitors of ovulation, and hence this mechanism contributes little to their effects.

Unlike combination OCs, whose administration is cyclic, progestin-only OCs are taken continuously. Use is initiated on day 1 of the menstrual cycle and one pill is taken daily thereafter. Each pill should be taken at the same time each day.

The following guidelines apply in the event of missed dosage. If one pill is missed, it should be taken as soon as remembered; the next pill should be taken as scheduled. If two pills are missed, one should be taken as soon as remembered and the other should be discarded; the next pill should be taken as originally scheduled. If three pills are missed, administration should be discontinued, and use should not be resumed until menstruation occurs or until pregnancy has been ruled out. (Progestins are potentially teratogenic, and hence should be avoided if conception is suspected.)

COMBINATION CONTRACEPTIVES WITH NOVEL DELIVERY SYSTEMS

Two new combination contraceptives—a transdermal patch and a vaginal ring—have the same mechanism as combination OCs, but deliver their hormones in novel ways. Like combination OCs, both of the new contraceptives contain two hormones—an estrogen and a progestin—that undergo absorption into the systemic circulation, and then prevent pregnancy primarily by suppressing ovulation. What's new is how the hormones are delivered: with the patch, the hormones are absorbed through the skin, and with the vaginal ring, the hormones are absorbed through the vaginal mucosa. Otherwise, the pharmacology of the new contraceptives is essentially identical to that of combination OCs.

Transdermal Contraceptive Patch

On November 20, 2001, the FDA approved *Ortho Evra*, the first transdermal contraceptive patch. As noted, the new product works by the same mechanism as the combination OCs. The patch and combination OCs are equivalent with respect to contraceptive efficacy, safety, and the incidence of breakthrough bleeding and spotting. The principal difference between the two formulations lies with their dosing schedules: Whereas combination OCs must be taken every day, the patch is applied just once a week. As a result, the patch is easier to use than OCs, and hence adherence is better.

The Ortho Evra patch contains 750 μg of *ethinyl estradiol* (the estrogen found in most combination OCs) and 6 mg of *norelgestromin* (the active metabolite of norgestimate, a progestin found in some OCs). Each day, the patch releases 20 μg of ethinyl estradiol and 150 μg of norelgestromin. Following release, these hormones penetrate the skin, enter capillaries, and undergo distribution throughout the body. Plasma levels reach a plateau 2 days after the first patch is applied.

Application of the patch, which is 1.75 inches square (about the size of a matchbook), is done once a week for 3 weeks, followed by 1 week off (to permit normal menstruation). Patches are applied to the lower abdomen, buttocks, upper outer arm, or upper torso (front or back)—but not to the breasts, or to skin that is red, cut, or irritated. To enhance adhesion, the skin should be clean and dry, and free of lotions, creams, or oils.

How effective is the patch? In clinical trials, the pregnancy rate was about 1 for every 100 woman-years of patch use. However, among women who weighed 90 kg (198 lbs) or more, the pregnancy rate was significantly higher, suggesting the patch may not be appropriate for women in this weight group.

When should patch use begin? For women not currently using OCs, the first patch should be applied during the first 24 hours of the menstrual period. For women switching from OCs, the first patch should be applied on the first day of withdrawal bleeding.

In clinical trials, 4.6% of patches became partially or completely detached. When this occurs, the patch should be reattached or replaced. If the patch has been off less than 24 hours, backup contraception is unnecessary. However, if the patch has been off *more* than 24 hours, a new cycle should be started, accompanied by backup contraception during the first 7 days.

The most common adverse effects of the patch are breast discomfort, headache, local irritation, nausea, and menstrual cramps. Compared with Triphasil (a combination OC), the patch produces a higher incidence of breast discomfort (18.7% vs. 5.8%) and dysmenorrhea (13.3% vs. 9.6%). Contraindications for the patch are the same as for combination OCs, as, presumably, are drug interactions and the risk of serious adverse effects (e.g., thrombosis, embolism, hypertension).

Vaginal Contraceptive Ring

On October 3, 2001, the FDA approved *NuvaRing,* a hormonal contraceptive device designed for vaginal insertion. Just one ring is used each month. Like combination OCs, the ring contains an estrogen and a progestin. These hormones prevent pregnancy largely by suppressing ovulation. Adverse effects, drug interactions, warnings, and contraindications for the ring are the same as for combination OCs. The ring is made of transparent, flexible material and looks like a very skinny doughnut, with an overall diameter of 2.1 inches and a cross-sectional diameter of one-eighth inch. Insertion is done by the user.

The NuvaRing contains 2.7 mg of *ethinyl estradiol* and 11.7 mg of *etonogestrel* (the active metabolite of desogestrel, a progestin found in some OCs). Each day, the ring releases 15 μg of ethinyl estradiol and 120 μg of etonogestrel. Following release, these hormones penetrate the vaginal mucosa, undergo absorption into the blood, and then are distributed throughout the body. Contraception results from systemic effects—not from local effects in the vagina.

One ring is inserted once each month, left in place for 3 weeks, and then removed; a new ring is inserted 1 week later. During the ring-free week, withdrawal bleeding occurs. The new ring should be inserted on schedule, even if bleeding is still ongoing. If a ring is expelled before 3 weeks have passed, it can be washed off in warm water (not hot water) and reinserted. If the expelled ring cannot be reused, a new one should be inserted. If more than 3 hours elapse between ring expulsion and reinsertion, contraceptive effects may be diminished, and hence backup contraception should be used for 7 days.

Initiating ring use is done as follows:

- For women not currently using contraception, ring use should start any time during days 1 through 5 of the menstrual cycle, even if bleeding is ongoing; backup contraception should be used during the first 7 days.
- For women switching from combination OCs, ring use should start within 7 days of taking the last active OC; no backup contraception is needed.
- For women switching from progestin-only OCs, ring use should start on the same day the last pill is taken, which can be any day of the month; backup contraception should be used during the first 7 days.
- For women switching from Norplant, ring use should start on the same day that the implants are removed; backup contraception should be used during the first 7 days.
- For women switching from a progestin-containing IUD, ring use should start on the same day the IUD is removed; backup contraception should be used during the first 7 days.
- For women switching from IM progestin injections, ring use should start on the day of the next scheduled injection; backup contraception should be used during the first 7 days.

In clinical trials, the most common adverse effects were vaginitis, headaches, upper respiratory infection, leukorrhea, sinusitis, weight gain, and nausea. Common reasons for discontinuing ring use included foreign body sensations, coital problems, expulsion of the ring, vaginal symptoms, headache, and emotional lability. The risk of serious adverse effects—thrombosis, embolism, and hypertension—is the same as with combination OCs.

LONG-ACTING CONTRACEPTIVES

Subdermal Levonorgestrel Implants

A subdermal system [Norplant System] for delivery of levonorgestrel is available for long-term, reversible contraception. As indicated in Table 60–1, subdermal implants are one of the most effective contraceptives available. Unfortunately, implants also have a high incidence of side effects.

Description. The Norplant System consists of six tiny Silastic rubber capsules (2.4 by 34 mm), each containing 36 mg of levonorgestrel, a synthetic progestin. Under local anesthesia, the capsules are surgically implanted on the inside of the upper arm through a small incision. Levonorgestrel then diffuses slowly and continuously from the capsules, providing blood levels sufficient for contraception for up to 5 years. The capsules are removed after 5 years, and then replaced if continued contraception is desired.

Mechanism of Action. Subdermal levonorgestrel implants act much like progestin-only OCs. Cervical mucus is made thick and sticky, creating a barrier to migration of sperm. Endometrial growth is suppressed, thereby discouraging nidation. In some women, ovulation is suppressed.

Pharmacokinetics. The daily release of levonorgestrel is about 80 μg initially and declines over time. Plasma drug levels vary widely among users. The drug is slowly metabolized by the liver. Following removal of the capsules, blood levels become undetectable within 10 to 14 days.

Adverse Effects. Menstrual irregularities are common. Their incidence is as follows: prolonged bleeding or many bleeding days (28%), spotting (17%), amenorrhea (9.4%), irregular onset of bleeding (7.6%), and frequent bleeding (7%). Other common reactions include breast discharge, cervicitis, musculoskeletal pain, abdominal discomfort, leukorrhea, and vaginitis—all of which have an incidence of 5% or more. In about 6% of users, removal of the implants is difficult: some implants break during removal, some are displaced and hard to find, and some are too embedded to remove easily on the initial attempt.

Depot Medroxyprogesterone Acetate

Following a single IM injection, depot medroxyprogesterone acetate (MPA) [Depo-Provera] provides safe and effective contraception for 3 months or longer. Injections of 150 mg are repeated every 3 months to provide continuous protection. Depot MPA prevents pregnancy in three ways: (1) suppression of ovulation, (2) thickening of the cervical mucus, and (3) alteration of the endometrium such that nidation is discouraged. When injections are discontinued, an average of 12 months is required for fertility to return. However, some women remain infertile as long as 2.5 years.

Adverse effects of depot MPA are typical of those seen with other progestins. Menstrual disturbances are common; cycles become irregular at first and, after 6 to 12 months,

menstruation may cease entirely. Because the drug is used long-term, osteoporosis may be a concern. In one study, bone density was lower following 5 years of depot MPA. However, in another study, bone loss reversed after depot MPA was discontinued. Other adverse effects include abdominal bloating, headache, depression, and decreased libido. Although depot MPA has produced uterine and mammary cancers in animals, a large-scale study has shown no increase in the risk of cervical, ovarian, or breast cancer in women—and the risk of endometrial cancer is actually reduced. Depot MPA does *not* cause weight gain; women should be reassured of this fact.

Although used worldwide for contraception for many years, depot MPA was not approved for use in the United States until 1992. Approval had been withheld in large part because (1) depot MPA has caused cancer in laboratory animals and (2) when undesired effects occur with depot MPA, they are prolonged. These drawbacks are not seen with other forms of reversible contraception (e.g., combination OCs). Furthermore, it had been argued that, with the advanced healthcare system we have in the United States, the need for a long-acting, injectable contraceptive is much smaller than in many other countries. Despite these arguments, it is clear that depot MPA does have attractive features, most notably high contraceptive efficacy (see Table 60–1) and infrequent administration. With these qualities, depot MPA would seem to be a desirable form of birth control for women who are incapable of using other methods reliably or for whom other forms of contraception are contraindicated.

Depot Medroxyprogesterone Acetate plus Estradiol Cypionate

The combination of depot MPA plus estradiol, marketed as *Lunelle,* is the second injectable hormonal contraceptive approved for use in the United States—and the first injectable contraceptive to contain a progestin *plus* an estrogen. The product represents an alternative to Depo-Provera, which contains the same progestin (MPA) but lacks estrogen.

Lunelle is supplied in 0.5-ml, single-dose vials that contain 25 mg of MPA and 5 mg of estradiol cypionate. The combination is injected IM (by a healthcare professional) every 28 to 30 days. If more than 33 days have elapsed since the last dose, pregnancy should be ruled out before resuming treatment. Dosing is begun during the first 5 days of the menstrual cycle or within 2 days of discontinuing OCs. Contraceptive effects are present during the first cycle. Women who want to use the drug following pregnancy should begin treatment no sooner than 4 weeks postpartum (in the absence of breast-feeding) or 6 weeks postpartum (in the presence of breast-feeding).

Lunelle and Depo-Provera are similar in some respects and different in others. Both products have the same mechanism of action (they work primarily by suppressing ovulation) and both have high contraceptive efficacy (>99%). Also, both products are in FDA Pregnancy Risk Category X, and hence must not be used by pregnant women. In other respects, the products differ significantly. Because each dose of Lunelle contains less MPA than each dose of Depo-Provera, Lunelle must be administered more often (once a month compared with every 3 months). When treatment is discontinued, fertility returns in 2 to 4 months with Lunelle, versus about 12 months with Depo-Provera. Most women (75%) using Lunelle continue to have monthly periods, whereas, with Depo-Provera, menstruation becomes irregular and may eventually stop. Among Lunelle users, 5.7% experience some weight gain (about 4 pounds during the first year and 2 more in the second year). In contrast, weight gain does not occur with Depo-Provera. Because Depo-Provera lacks estrogen, it is preferable for women who need to avoid estrogen because they smoke or for some other reason.

Intrauterine Devices

IUDs are among the most reliable forms of reversible birth control (see Table 60–1). In addition, the IUDs available today are very safe when used by appropriate clients (see below). Worldwide, over 85 million women use these devices. However, despite their safety and efficacy, IUDs are not popular in the United States: Only 1.4% of American women who use birth control choose an IUD.

Nonuse of IUDs is largely the legacy of the Dalcon Shield, an IUD that caused miscarriages, pelvic infections, and infertility—as well as 18 deaths. The cause of these problems was a tiny string, composed of hundreds of nylon filaments and encased in a sheath. Following emplacement, the sheath rotted and thereby exposed the string, which then acted as a wick, drawing bacteria into the uterus.

With proper client selection, today's IUDs are very safe. The principal problem is pelvic inflammatory disease (PID) secondary to a sexually transmitted disease (STD). If PID occurs during the course of IUD use, the risk of infertility is about 7%. Accordingly, IUDs should be used only by women with a low risk for STDs—that is, women who are monogamous, and who are confident that their partners are monogamous too. The major side effects of IUDs are cramps. Pain and cramping are likely immediately following insertion, but are less intense in women who have had one or more children. If pregnancy occurs while an IUD is in place, there is an increased risk of ectopic pregnancy.

Three IUDs are now available: (1) the *copper T 380A* [ParaGard], (2) an *intrauterine progesterone contraceptive system* [Progestasert], and (3) a *levonorgestrel-releasing intrauterine system* [Mirena]. All three are T-shaped. ParaGard can remain in place for 10 years, Mirena for 5 years, and Progestasert for 1 year. As indicated in Table 60–1, Mirena has the lowest failure rate (0.1%), followed by ParaGard (0.6% to 0.8%), and then by Progestasert (1.5% to 2%).

How IUDs prevent conception is uncertain. ParaGard, whose active ingredient is copper, was initially thought to prevent implantation. However, later studies suggest the device causes a harmless inflammation of the endometrium, and thereby interferes with sperm motility and fertilization.

The mechanism for Progestasert differs from that of ParaGard—but is also uncertain. This IUD contains a 38-mg reservoir of progesterone. The device releases progesterone at a rate of 65 mg/day, an amount too small to elevate systemic progesterone levels. We do know that Progestasert does not inhibit ovulation. Furthermore, since models of this IUD that lack progesterone are not effective, it is clear that localized actions of progesterone are required for contraceptive effects. It has been hypothesized that the device may work by altering the endometrium to prevent implantation or by reducing the viability of sperm. To ensure that progesterone release remains adequate, a new device must be inserted annually.

Mirena has a mechanism similar to that of Progestasert. The IUD contains 52 mg of levonorgestrel in a slow-release reservoir. The rate of levonorgestrel release is 20 μg/day initially, but only 10 μg/day after 5 years. As with Progestasert, contraception results from local actions in the uterus: thickening of cervical mucus, which impedes passage of sperm; reduction of sperm survival; and changes in the endometrium that impede pregnancy. Contraceptive efficacy is high (1-year failure rate is only 0.1%) and persists for 5 years

(compared with only 1 year for Progestasert). During the first months of use, increased spotting and bleeding can occur. However, after 6 months, bleeding decreases and 20% of users experience amenorrhea. Although systemic levels of levonorgestrel remain low (150 to 200 pg/ml), progestin-related adverse effects can occur (nausea, acne, breast tenderness, headache, mood changes). According to the manufacturer, candidates for Mirena should have had at least one child and should have no history of PID and no predisposition to ectopic pregnancy. A woman's first Mirena IUD should be inserted within 7 days of the onset of menses; replacements can be inserted during any phase of the menstrual cycle. After the device is removed, 80% of women who are trying to conceive succeed within 1 year.

SPERMICIDES

Spermicides are dispensed in the form of foams, gels, creams, and suppositories. All of these preparations can be purchased without a prescription. When used alone, spermicides are only moderately effective (see Table 60–1). Combined use with a diaphragm or condom increases efficacy. As indicated in Table 60–4, spermicidal preparations employ either *nonoxynol 9* or *octoxynol 9* as their active ingredient. These agents are chemical surfactants that kill sperm by destroying their cell membrane. Adverse effects are minimal. Most studies show no relationship between spermicide use and birth defects.

Correct use of spermicides is required for contraceptive efficacy. The spermicide must be applied prior to coitus, but no more than 1 hour in advance (when used alone). Containers for foam preparations must be shaken thoroughly before each use to ensure dispersal of the spermicide. Suppositories or tablets should be inserted a minimum of 10 to 15 minutes before intercourse to allow time for dissolution. Spermicides should be reapplied each time intercourse is anticipated. Douching should be postponed for at least 6 hours following coitus.

Data from a recent trial indicate that use of nonoxynol 9 can *increase* the risk of HIV transmission. The apparent mechanism is promotion of anal and rectal lesions that facilitate HIV penetration to cells.

BARRIER DEVICES

Barrier devices—male condoms, female condoms, diaphragms, and the cervical cap—are nonpharmacologic options for birth control. Of the barrier devices available, condoms for men are by far the most commonly employed.

Condoms for Men. The condom is a thin sheath, made of latex, polyurethane, or lamb's intestine, that fits snugly over the penis, and hence traps ejaculate released during intercourse. As indicated in Figure 60–1, condoms are the fourth most common form of birth control. The typical-use failure rate is 14%.

TABLE 60–4 ■ Spermicides		
Formulation	**Active Ingredient**	**Trade Name**
Foam	Nonoxynol 9 (12.5%)	Delfen Contraceptive, Koromex
	Nonoxynol 9 (8%)	Because, Emko, Emko Pre-Fil
Jelly	Nonoxynol 9 (5%)	Ramses
	Nonoxynol 9 (3%)	Koromex, Gynol II Extra Strength Contraceptive*
Gel	Nonoxynol 9 (4%)	Conceptrol Disposable Contraceptive
	Nonoxynol 9 (3.5%)	Advantage 24*
	Nonoxynol 9 (2.2%)	K-Y Plus*
	Nonoxynol 9 (2%)	Gynol II Contraceptive,* Koromex Crystal Clear,* Shur Seal*
	Octoxynol 9 (1%)	Ortho-Gynol Contraceptive*
Cream	Octoxynol 9 (3%)	Koromex*
Suppository	Nonoxynol 9 (2.27%)	Encare
	Nonoxynol 9 (100 mg)	Semicid
	Nonoxynol 9 (150 mg)	Conceptrol Contraceptive Inserts
Vaginal Film	Nonoxynol 9 (28%)	VCF

*Intended for use only in combination with a vaginal diaphragm.

In the United States, most condoms are made of latex, which is impermeable to bacteria and viruses. Hence, in addition to protecting against pregnancy, latex condoms offer protection against STDs. There is good evidence that condom use protects against HIV (the most dangerous STD) and gonorrhea (the most easily transmitted STD); however, evidence for protection against other STDs is inconclusive. Lubricants that contain mineral oil can very rapidly decrease the barrier strength of latex—by as much as 90%—and therefore should be avoided. Allergy to latex can develop in men and women, especially with repeated exposure.

Like latex condoms, polyurethane condoms offer some protection against STDs. In addition, they are thinner than latex condoms, possibly stronger, and don't cause allergies. However, the failure rate with polyurethane is higher than with latex.

In contrast to latex and polyurethane condoms, condoms made from lamb intestine are permeable to viruses, and hence do not protect against viral STDs.

Condom for Women. The Reality female condom is a loose-fitting, tubular polyurethane pouch that has flexible rings at both ends. The ring at the closed end anchors the pouch over the cervix. The ring at the open end, which is larger than the ring at the closed end, is placed over the labia and serves as an external anchor. The Reality condom is prelubricated, available without prescription, cannot be combined with a male condom, and should be used just once and then discarded. Like male condoms, the female condom provides some protection against STDs. The failure rate with typical use is 21%.

Diaphragm. The diaphragm is a soft rubber cap with a metal spring that reinforces its rim. The device must be fitted by a healthcare provider, and the user must be taught how to insert it. When in place over the cervical os, the diaphragm blocks access of sperm to the cervix. Because the device does not fit tightly enough to completely block penetration of sperm, it must be filled with spermicidal jelly or cream before insertion. Spermicide must be reapplied externally with repeated intercourse. The diaphragm can be inserted as long as 6 hours prior to intercourse, and must remain in place for at least 6 hours after. Because of the risk of toxic shock syndrome, the diaphragm should not remain in place for more than 24 hours. With typical use, the failure rate is about 18%.

Cervical Cap. The *Prentif Cavity-Rim Cervical Cap* is a small, pliant, cup-shaped device that fits snugly over the cervix. Suction holds it in place. The device must be fitted by a healthcare provider, and the user must be taught how to insert it. Because only four sizes are available, some women cannot be fitted. Like the diaphragm, the cap is filled with spermicidal cream or jelly prior to use, and can be inserted up to 6 hours before intercourse. There is no need to apply additional spermicide with repeated intercourse. The cap should remain in place for at least 8 hours after intercourse, and probably no longer than 24 hours (although the manufacturer says it can stay in place for 48 hours). The typical-use failure rate is about 40% (for parous women) and 20% (for nulliparous women).

DRUGS FOR MEDICAL ABORTION

Mifepristone (RU 486) with Misoprostol

Mifepristone (RU 486) [Mifeprex] is a synthetic steroid that blocks receptors for progesterone and glucocorticoids. In the United States, the drug has one approved indication: termination of early intrauterine pregnancy; cotreatment with misoprostol is usually required. Investigational uses include breast cancer, ovarian cancer, meningiomas, Cushing's syndrome, uterine fibroids, and endometriosis. In addition, mifepristone is the most effective drug known for emergency contraception, although it is not used routinely for this purpose (see Box 60–1). Mifepristone has been available in Europe since 1988, but was not approved for use here until September 20, 2000.

Mifepristone, followed by misoprostol, is a safe and effective alternative to surgery for termination of early pregnancy. Together, these drugs terminate pregnancy in about 95% of women. Principal adverse effects are abdominal pain and vaginal bleeding, which are unavoidable aspects of abortion. In contrast to surgical abortion, which is generally unavailable before 8 weeks of gestation, abortion with mifepristone is performed early—within 7 weeks of conception.

Mechanism of Action. Mifepristone promotes abortion through blockade of uterine progesterone receptors. Although mifepristone also blocks receptors for glucocorticoids, this action does not contribute to abortion. In the pregnant uterus, the drug has three effects. First, blockade of progesterone receptors leads to decidual breakdown and detachment of the conceptus. Second, mifepristone promotes cervical softening and dilation. Third, through an indirect mechanism, mifepristone increases uterine production of prostaglandins and renders the myometrium more responsive to the contractile actions of these prostaglandins. All three effects lead to expulsion of the conceptus. If mifepristone alone fails to induce abortion, the patient is given misoprostol, a synthetic prostaglandin that reinforces uterine contractions induced by mifepristone. The pharmacology of misoprostol is discussed separately below.

Clinical Trials. In a study conducted in France, the abortion success rate with mifepristone-misoprostol was nearly 99%. (Success was defined as termination of pregnancy with complete expulsion of the conceptus.) All women in the study had amenorrhea for less than 50 days prior to receiving mifepristone. Dosing was done as follows: Each patient received a 600-mg oral dose of mifepristone and, if abortion had not occurred within 48 hours, each was given a 400-μg dose of oral misoprostol; a second dose of misoprostol (200 μg) was offered if abortion had not occurred by 4 hours after the first dose. Only 5.5% of the pregnancies terminated prior to dosing with misoprostol; with the addition of misoprostol (1 or 2 doses), the cumulative success rate was 98.7%. In the majority of patients (69%), abortion occurred within 4 hours of the first misoprostol dose.

In the United States, success with mifepristone-misoprostol has also been good—although not quite as good as in France. In 1999, American researchers reported that the abortion rate with mifepristone-misoprostol declined with increasing duration of gestation. Success was greatest (92%) when gestation was 49 days or less, fell to 83% during days 50 to 56 of gestation, and to 77% during days 57 to 63 of gestation. The dosages employed were the same as in the French study. Why the success rate was lower than in the French study is unknown.

There is good evidence that *intravaginal* misoprostol is more effective and better tolerated than oral misoprostol. In one study, women received 600 mg of oral mifepristone, followed by 800 μg of misoprostol, either PO or intravaginally. Following intravaginal misoprostol, 95% of conceptuses were expelled without the need for surgery, compared with only 87% following oral misoprostol. With intravaginal administration, abortion occurred within 4 hours in 93% of patients, compared with 78% of patients receiving oral misoprostol. The incidence of nausea and vomiting with intravaginal administration was significantly lower than with oral administration

Adverse Effects. Successful abortion necessarily causes abdominal pain (cramping) and bleeding. Nearly all women experience these effects. About 80% of patients experience transient cramping, beginning 1 hour after taking misoprostol; about 15% require a nonopioid analgesic for relief. Bleeding and spotting typically last 9 to 16 days. However, in some women, bleeding persists for 30 days or more. About 1% of women experience severe bleeding; treatment measures include curettage, vasoconstrictor drugs, and infusion of fluids, blood, or both. Other side effects include nausea (61%), vomiting (26%), diarrhea (20%), and headache (31%). Misoprostol (but not mifepristone) is a proven human teratogen. Hence if mifepristone-misoprostol fails to induce abortion, surgical abortion should be considered.

Mifepristone-misoprostol can rupture an ectopic pregnancy, and can thereby cause severe bleeding. At least one death from hemorrhage has occurred. Ectopic pregnancy must be ruled out before mifepristone is used.

Contraindications. Major contraindications to mifepristone-misoprostol are ectopic pregnancy, pregnancy beyond 49 days, hemorrhagic disorders, and use of anticoagulant drugs. Because mifepristone blocks receptors for glucocorticoids, it should be avoided in women with adrenal insufficiency and those on long-term glucocorticoid therapy.

Preparations, Dosage, and Administration. Mifepristone [Mifeprex] is supplied in single-dose packets containing three 200-mg tablets. The dosage is 600 mg (3 tablets) taken all at once—followed in two days by 400 μg of oral misoprostol (if mifepristone did not induce complete abortion by itself). Mifepristone is available only through qualified physicians; it is not sold in pharmacies.

FDA-Approved Protocol for Abortion. Induction of abortion with mifepristone/misoprostol requires *three visits to a qualified physician.* In order to dispense mifepristone, a physician must be qualified to determine pregnancy duration and to diagnose ectopic pregnancy. In addition, the physician must either (1) be able to perform surgical abortion (in the event mifepristone/misoprostol fails) as well as curettage (in the event of severe bleeding), or (2) have a commitment from a colleague to perform these procedures.

Day 1. Mifepristone (600 mg) is taken—but only after several conditions have been met. The physician must rule out ectopic pregnancy and must ensure that the pregnancy is indeed early (defined for this purpose as pregnancy in which no more than 49 days have elapsed since the beginning of the last menstrual period). If necessary, ultrasound should be performed

Special Interest Topic

BOX 60–1 ■ EMERGENCY CONTRACEPTION: THE SECRET'S OUT

Emergency contraception (EC) is defined as contraception that is implemented *after* intercourse. Women can use EC to prevent pregnancy following unprotected intercourse, which can result from sexual assault, contraceptive failure (e.g., broken condom), or occasional lack of forethought. Safe and effective methods of EC have been readily available for over two decades. However, most women are unaware they exist.

The data on unintended pregnancy are staggering. In the United States, nearly 50% of women ages 15 to 44 report having had at least one unintended pregnancy. Among teenagers, 88% of pregnancies are unintended. Of the 6 million pregnancies that occur each year, over half are accidental. Every year, unintended pregnancies lead to 1.4 million abortions and 1.1 million births that women did not want—at least not yet. Clearly, if EC were widely used, most abortions and unwanted births could be avoided.

Methods of EC Available in the United States

EC can be accomplished with *emergency contraceptive pills* (ECPs) or by inserting a *copper IUD*. Two types of ECPs are available: (1) pills that contain an estrogen plus a progestin (the Yuzpe regimen) and (2) pills that contain a progestin only. Mifepristone (RU 486) is more effective than either of these regimens but is not approved for EC use.

The Yuzpe regimen consists of two doses of an OC that contains an estrogen (ethinyl estradiol) plus a progestin (e.g., levonorgestrel). The first dose must be taken within 72 hours of unprotected intercourse (the sooner the better), and the second 12 hours later. Success is indicated by onset of menstrual bleeding in about 21 days. The safety and efficacy of this method was first described in 1974 by professor A. Alfred Yuzpe, a Canadian obstetrician-gynecologist.

The exact mechanism by which pregnancy is prevented has not been determined. Inhibition of ovulation is most likely. However, inhibition of fertilization or implantation may also contribute.

The Yuzpe regimen reduces the risk of pregnancy by 75%, which is better than it may seem. In the absence of ECPs, the pregnancy rate from a single act of unprotected intercourse is about 8% (i.e., 8 women in 100 would become pregnant). However, among women using the Yuzpe regimen, only 2 in 100 are likely to become pregnant—a reduction of 75%. It should be noted that ECPs are most effective when taken immediately after unprotected intercourse: the longer the delay, the greater the risk of pregnancy.

The major side effects of the Yuzpe regimen are nausea (50%) and vomiting (19%). These can be reduced by taking an antiemetic (e.g., prochlorperazine) 1 hour before the first ECP.

ECPs should not be used during pregnancy. Why? Because they won't work: These drugs cannot terminate an ongoing pregnancy. However, if the woman *is* pregnant, all available evidence indicates that ECPs will not harm the fetus.

As of 2002, there were 14 products suitable for use in the Yuzpe regimen (see table below). Only one of these—the

Preven emergency contraceptive kit—is labeled and marketed specifically for EC use. The other 13 products are ordinary combination OCs that, in sufficient dosage, can prevent pregnancy when taken after intercourse. It is completely legal to prescribe these OCs for emergency contraception, even though they are not labeled for this application. In fact, in 1997, the FDA declared these drugs safe and effective for EC use.

Emergency Contraceptive Pills*	
Trade Name	**Pills/Dose†**
Yuzpe Regimen	
Preven	2 blue pills
Alesse	5 pink pills
Aviane	5 orange pills
Levlen	4 orange pills
Levlite	5 pink pills
Levora	4 white pills
Lo-Ogestrel	4 white pills
Lo/Ovral	4 white pills
Nordette	4 orange pills
Ogestrel	2 white pills
Ovral	2 white pills
Tri-Levlen	4 yellow pills
Triphasil	4 yellow pills
Trivora	4 pink pills
Progestin Only Regimens	
Plan B	1 white pill
Ovrette	20 yellow pills

*Preven and Plan B are the only products packaged and marketed specifically for EC. All of the other products are ordinary OCs that can be used for EC when needed (color denotes which pills in multipill packs are to be taken).
†All regimens require two doses. The first dose must be taken within 72 hours of intercourse, and the second 12 hours later.

There are two **progestin-only products** suitable for EC use: *Plan B* and *Ovrette*. Plan B, like Preven, is packaged and marketed specifically for EC use. Ovrette, like most of the drugs used in the Yuzpe regimen, is an ordinary OC.

Plan B is the trade name for an ECP that contains 0.75 mg of *levonorgestrel*, a progestin. As with the Yuzpe regimen, two doses are required—the first within 72 hours of intercourse, and the second 12 hours later. The mechanism of action is the same as in the Yuzpe regimen: inhibition of ovulation, fertilization, and implantation. Plan B is more effective than the Yuzpe regimen (85% vs. 75%), and causes less nausea (23% vs. 50%) and vomiting (6% vs. 19%). Like the Yuzpe regimen, Plan B will not terminate an ongoing pregnancy—but neither will it hurt the fetus if pregnancy is present. Because of superior efficacy and tolerability, Plan B, which was introduced in 1999, seems likely to replace the Yuzpe regimen as the standard hormonal method of EC.

Special Interest Topic—cont'd

Ovrette, which contains 0.075 mg of norgestrel, is an alternative to Plan B. However, because each dose of Ovrette consists of 20 pills, Ovrette is considerably less convenient than Plan B.

Insertion of a **copper IUD** within 5 days of unprotected intercourse can prevent pregnancy in most women. The method is more than 99% effective, allowing less than 1 pregnancy for every 1000 IUD recipients. IUD insertion has the additional benefit of providing ongoing contraception for up to 10 years. Although using an IUD for EC is highly effective, the technique does have drawbacks: expense and difficulty locating a clinician to insert the IUD within 5 days.

Do ECPs Cause Abortion?

The ECPs in current use do *NOT* cause abortion (termination of pregnancy). Recall that pregnancy is defined as implantation of a fertilized egg, and that implantation occurs 7 days after ovulation. Since the available ECPs act prior to implantation of the fertilized egg (by inhibiting either ovulation, fertilization, or implantation), they cannot be considered abortifacients.

One drug—*mifepristone*—can prevent pregnancy *or* cause abortion, depending on when it is taken. If mifepristone is taken within 5 days of unprotected intercourse, it will prevent pregnancy from occurring, and hence can be considered an ECP. However, if mifepristone is taken after this time, it may terminate pregnancy that has already begun, and hence can be considered an abortifacient. When used as an ECP, mifepris-

tone is 100% effective. The drug is available in the United States, but is not approved for EC use.

How Can ECPs Be Obtained?

ECPs are readily available. Sources include private physicians, student health departments at colleges and universities, and clinics run by Planned Parenthood. In California and Washington, ECPs can be obtained directly from certified pharmacists, without seeing a physician. Women who want to locate an EC provider in their community can do so by phone or online:

- Dial *1-888-NOT-2-LATE* for information on EC methods and phone numbers of local EC providers.
- Dial *1-800-230-PLAN* to locate the nearest Planned Parenthood clinic.
- Long on to *www.plannedparenthood.org/ec/* or *ec.princeton. edu* for extensive information on EC, including a database of EC providers around the country.

It's a good idea to keep ECPs on hand "just in case." Remember, these drugs work best when taken right after intercourse. By having them on hand, delay can be avoided. Furthermore, ECPs may not be available when they're needed. For example, if unprotected intercourse takes place Friday night, it may be difficult to get ECPs before Monday night, when the window of opportunity will close. (As discussed above, ECPs must be taken within 3 days of unprotected intercourse, and EC providers may not be available over the weekend.) An ECP supply can be obtained by requesting a prescription during a routine visit to the doctor.

---

to confirm that pregnancy is intrauterine and not beyond the 49-day limit. Also, the patient must read a Medication Guide supplied by the manufacturer, and both the patient and physician must sign a Patient Agreement Form stating that the patient understands the benefits and risk of the procedure and has decided to end the pregnancy. Finally, the patient must be given clear instruction on whom to call and what to do in the event of an emergency.

Day 3. Two days after taking mifepristone, the patient returns to the physician, who performs a physical examination or ultrasound scan to determine if abortion has occurred. If abortion has not occurred, the patient takes misoprostol (400 µg).

Day 14. About 14 days after taking mifepristone, the patient returns to the physician, who confirms by physical examination or ultrasound scan that pregnancy has been terminated. If the woman is still pregnant, surgical abortion should be considered (because there is a risk of birth defects from misoprostol).

Methotrexate with Misoprostol

Methotrexate, followed by misoprostol, is a safe and effective alternative to surgical termination of early pregnancy. Methotrexate induces abortion because of its toxicity to trophoblastic tissue; misoprostol contributes by promoting uterine contraction. Abortion is accomplished by giving an intramuscular injection of methotrexate (50 mg/m²) followed in 5 days by 800 µg of intravaginal misoprostol. If abortion does not occur in 24 hours, dosing with misoprostol is repeated. In one study, 14% of patients required the second dose of misoprostol, but 96% eventually aborted. The procedure is more effective at 49 days of gestation (or less) than between 50 and 56 days of gestation. Side effects include nausea, vomiting, diarrhea, headache, dizziness, and hot flushes. Acetaminophen plus codeine is sufficient to relieve pain in most cases. The vast majority of women who have undergone the procedure said they would recommend it.

Prostaglandins: Misoprostol, Carboprost, and Dinoprostone

Prostaglandins are synthesized in all tissues of the body, where they act as local hormones. Unlike true hormones, which travel to distant sites to produce their effects, prostaglandins act on the very tissues in which they are made; degradation of prostaglandins is so rapid that these compounds rarely escape their tissue of origin intact. Although the prostaglandins produce a broad spectrum of physiologic effects, their clinical use is limited. In obstetrics, prostaglandins are indicated for induction of abortion, induction of cervical ripening, and control of postpartum hemorrhage. Use of prostaglandins for abortion is discussed here. Use for cervical ripening and control of postpartum hemorrhage is discussed in Chapter 62.

Nomenclature

Nomenclature regarding the prostaglandins can be confusing and deserves comment. Each prostaglandin has three names: a traditional name, an official generic name, and a trade name. Misoprostol, carboprost, and dinoprostone are *generic names*. For carboprost, the traditional name is *15-methyl-prostaglandin F_2 alpha* and the trade name is *Hemabate*. For *dinoprostone,* the traditional name is *prostaglandin E_2;* trade names are *Prostin E_2, Cervidil,* and *Prepidil.* For misoprostol, a synthetic *analog of prostaglandin E_1,* the trade name is *Cytotec.*

Physiologic and Pharmacologic Effects

Uterine Stimulation. Prostaglandins increase the force, frequency, and duration of uterine contractions. In the early months of pregnancy, the uterus is more responsive to prostaglandins than to oxytocin. During the second and third trimesters, prostaglandins can induce contractions of sufficient strength to cause complete evacuation of the uterus.

Like oxytocin, prostaglandins appear to have a physiologic role as promoters of uterine contraction, spontaneous labor, and delivery. Observations supporting this statement include: (1) exogenous prostaglandins can induce uterine contractions that are very similar in frequency and duration to contractions that occur spontaneously; (2) the ability of the uterus to synthesize prostaglandins increases at term; (3) the prostaglandin content of amniotic fluid, umbilical blood, and maternal blood increases at term and during labor; and (4) labor is delayed and prolonged by agents that inhibit prostaglandin synthesis.

Cervical Softening. Local application of prostaglandins produces cervical softening. This softening results from breakdown of collagen, and hence mimics the process by which natural cervical ripening occurs. Softening of the cervix is not dependent on uterine stimulation.

Therapeutic Uses

Abortion. All three prostaglandins—misoprostol, carboprost, and dinoprost—are used to induce abortion. Misoprostol (in combination with methotrexate or mifepristone [RU 486]) is used *early* in pregnancy, whereas carboprost and dinoprostone are used in the *second trimester.* With all three drugs, uterine contractions develop slowly. As a result, about 18 hours must pass before expulsion of the fetus takes place. Unlike other abortifacients, prostaglandins are not feticidal, and hence the aborted fetus may show transient signs of life. Prostaglandins are proven teratogens in animals. Accordingly, if abortion fails, it is important that pregnancy be terminated by an alternative procedure (e.g., surgery or administration of oxytocin or hypertonic saline). Following passage of the fetus and placenta, the patient should be examined for possible cervical or uterine laceration.

Control of Postpartum Hemorrhage. *Carboprost* is indicated for control of postpartum hemorrhage. The drug is reserved for bleeding that has been refractory to more conventional agents (oxytocin, ergot alkaloids). In these situations, carboprost may be lifesaving. Use of carboprost to control postpartum hemorrhage is discussed in Chapter 62.

Induction of Labor. *Misoprostol* has been used investigationally to induce labor. In one study, patients received 50 μg every 4 hours until labor occurred; both oral and vaginal administration were tried. Labor occurred sooner with vaginal administration, but side effects (fetal heart rate abnormalities) were less frequent with oral administration. Accordingly, until optimal vaginal dosing has been established, oral administration is preferred.

Cervical Ripening. *Dinoprostone* and *misoprostol* can be used to initiate ripening of the cervix prior to induction of labor. This application is discussed in Chapter 62.

Adverse Effects

Gastrointestinal Disturbances. Gastrointestinal reactions are extremely common and result from the ability of prostaglandins to stimulate smooth muscle of the alimentary canal. Vomiting and diarrhea occur in up to 60% of those treated. Nausea also occurs often. These responses can be reduced by pretreatment with antiemetic and antidiarrheal medications.

Cervical or Uterine Laceration. Intense uterine contractions can result in cervical or uterine laceration. The patient should be examined thoroughly for trauma following expulsion of the fetus and placenta.

Other Adverse Effects. Fever is common. When hyperthermia develops, it is important to distinguish between drug-induced fever and pyrexia resulting from endometritis. With dinoprostone, there is a 10% incidence of headache, shivering, and chills.

Precautions and Contraindications

Prostaglandins are *contraindicated* for women with acute pelvic inflammatory disease and active disease of the heart, lungs, kidneys, or liver. These drugs should be used with *caution* in women with a history of asthma, hypotension, hypertension, diabetes, or uterine scarring.

Preparations, Dosage, and Administration

Dinoprostone. Dinoprostone [Prepidil, Prostin E$_2$, Cervidil] is available in three formulations: (1) 20-mg vaginal suppositories, (2) 10-mg vaginal inserts, and (3) a 0.5-mg gel. Dinoprostone suppositories [Prostin E$_2$] are used for abortion. The gel [Prepidil] and vaginal inserts [Cervidil] are used for cervical ripening.

For *induction of abortion* (weeks 12 to 20), one 20-mg vaginal suppository is inserted initially, followed by one suppository every 3 to 5 hours as needed.

Carboprost Tromethamine. Carboprost tromethamine [Hemabate] is available in solution (250 μg/ml) for IM administration. For *induction of*

abortion (weeks 13 to 20), the dosage is 250 μg initially followed by 250 μg every 1.5 to 3.5 hours as needed. For *control of postpartum bleeding,* a single 250-μg dose is injected.

Misoprostol. Misoprostol [Cytotec] is available in 200- and 400-μg tablets. For induction of abortion, the drug is used in combination with mifepristone or methotrexate. Dosage and routes of administration in these combination regimens are given above.

⁘ KEY POINTS

- The most effective methods of birth control are levonorgestrel subdermal implants [Norplant], intramuscular medroxyprogesterone acetate [Depo-Provera], IUDs, and sterilization. OCs are a close second.

- Sterilization is the most common form of birth control. OCs and condoms come next.

- A long-term method of birth control (e.g., Norplant, Depo-Provera, IUD) is a good choice when compliance is a problem.

- There are two main categories of OCs: (1) combination OCs, which contain an estrogen plus a progestin, and (2) progestin-only OCs (minipills).

- The principal estrogen in combination OCs is ethinyl estradiol; the principal progestin is norethindrone.

- Combination OCs act primarily by inhibiting ovulation.

- Although combination OCs can cause a wide variety of adverse effects, serious effects are rare.

- The low-estrogen combination OCs used today pose only a minimal risk of thromboembolism—except in heavy smokers and women with a history of thromboembolic disorders.

- When used by nonsmoking women with normal cardiovascular function, OCs produce no greater mortality than other active forms of birth control.

- Combination OCs protect against ovarian and endometrial cancer, and slightly increase the risk of cervical cancer—but only in women who test positive for the human papillomavirus. Combination OCs do not seem to increase the risk of breast cancer.

- Many of the mild side effects of OCs result from an excess or deficiency of estrogen or progestin, and hence can be minimized by adjusting the estrogen and/or progestin content of the regimen.

- Because OCs may pose a small risk to a fetus, they are contraindicated during pregnancy, and should be discontinued if accidental pregnancy occurs.

- The efficacy of OCs can be reduced by drugs that induce hepatic drug-metabolizing enzymes (e.g., rifampin, phenobarbital) and by certain antibiotics (e.g., ampicillin, tetracyclines) that kill gut flora and thereby decrease enterohepatic recirculation of OCs, which in turn accelerates their excretion.

- Because they lack estrogen, progestin-only OCs are slightly safer than combination OCs—but are less effective and cause more menstrual irregularity.

- Progestin-only OCs prevent pregnancy by promoting production of thick, sticky mucus (which creates a barrier to migration of sperm) and by suppressing endometrial growth (which discourages nidation).

- Subdermal levonorgestrel implants [Norplant] are active for 5 years, and are among the most effective contraceptives available.
- Norplant has the same mechanism as progestin-only pills: production of thick, sticky mucus and alteration of the endometrium.

- Intramuscular medroxyprogesterone acetate [Depo-Provera] is active for 3 months, and is one of the most effective contraceptives available.
- Depo-Provera prevents pregnancy in three ways: it (1) suppresses ovulation, (2) thickens cervical mucus, and (3) alters the endometrium such that nidation is discouraged.

Summary of Major Nursing Implications*

COMBINATION ORAL CONTRACEPTIVES

Preadministration Assessment

Therapeutic Goal

Prevention of unwanted pregnancy.

Baseline Data

Assess for a history of hypertension, diabetes, thrombophlebitis, thromboembolic disorders, cerebrovascular disease, coronary artery disease, breast carcinoma, estrogen-dependent neoplasm, and benign or malignant liver tumors.

Identifying High-Risk Patients

Combination OCs are *contraindicated* during pregnancy and for women with the following disorders (or history thereof): thrombophlebitis, thromboembolic disorders, cerebrovascular disease, coronary artery disease, myocardial infarction, known or suspected breast carcinoma, known or suspected estrogen-dependent neoplasm, benign or malignant liver tumors, and undiagnosed abnormal genital bleeding.

Combination OCs should be used with *caution* in women with diabetes, women who smoke heavily (more than 15 cigarettes a day), women who have risk factors for cardiovascular disease (e.g., hypertension, obesity, hypercholesterolemia), and women anticipating elective surgery in which postoperative thrombosis might be expected.

Implementation: Administration

Dosing Schedule

Provide the client with the following instructions on administration:

- Initiate dosing 5 days after the onset of menstruation.
- The approved dosing sequence consists of 21 days of drug use followed by 7 days off (for the 7 "off" days, the manufacturer may provide inert tablets, iron-containing tablets, or no tablets).
- Take pills at the same time each day (e.g., with a meal, at bedtime).

Responding to Missed Doses

Provide the client with the following instructions regarding missed doses:

- If only one dose is missed, take the omitted dose together with the next scheduled dose.

- If two doses are missed, take two doses per day on the following 2 days.
- If three doses are missed, initiate a new cycle (starting 7 days after the last pill was taken) and use an additional form of contraception (e.g., condom, diaphragm) during the first 2 weeks of the new cycle.

Postpartum Use

Inform the client that OCs can be initiated immediately after delivery if breast-feeding is not intended.

Promoting Compliance

Counsel the client about the importance of taking OCs as prescribed. Encourage the client to read the package insert provided with combination OCs.

Ongoing Evaluation and Interventions

Monitoring Summary

Periodic evaluations should include pelvic and breast examinations, palpation of the liver, blood pressure determination, and a Pap smear.

Minimizing Adverse Effects

Thrombotic Disorders. Because of their estrogen content, combination OCs slightly increase the risk of thrombosis and thromboembolism. To minimize thrombosis and thromboembolism, (1) use OCs of low estrogen content, (2) avoid use of OCs by women with known risk factors for thrombotic disorders, and (3) discontinue OCs at least 4 weeks prior to elective surgeries in which postoperative thrombosis might be expected. Inform the client about symptoms of thrombosis and thromboembolism (e.g., leg tenderness or pain, sudden chest pain, shortness of breath, severe headache, sudden visual disturbance), and instruct her to notify the physician if these develop.

Hypertension. Perform periodic determinations of blood pressure. If hypertension is detected, discontinue OCs. Blood pressure usually normalizes within a few months.

Abnormal Uterine Bleeding. During initial use, combination OCs may reduce or eliminate menstrual flow; breakthrough bleeding or spotting may also occur. Menstrual irregularities may be greater with low-estrogen preparations.

Instruct the client to notify the physician if two consecutive periods are missed; the possibility of pregnancy must be evaluated.

*Patient education information is highlighted as blue text.

Summary of Major Nursing Implications*—cont'd

Instruct the client to notify the physician if bleeding irregularities persist; the possibility of malignancy must be investigated.

Inform the client that menstruation may take several months to normalize following OC withdrawal.

Effects Related to Estrogen or Progestin Imbalance. An excess or deficiency of estrogen or progestin can cause specific side effects (see Table 60–3). By adjusting the estrogen or progestin content of the OC regimen, these effects can be reduced or eliminated. Substitution of one combination OC for another can be made at the beginning of any new cycle.

Use in Pregnancy and Lactation. Using OCs during pregnancy may carry a small risk of carcinogenesis in female offspring. Accordingly, OCs are contraindicated during pregnancy. Pregnancy should be ruled out prior to OC use. Instruct the client to cease OC use if pregnancy should accidentally occur.

Inform the client that OCs enter breast milk and can reduce milk production. Instruct her not to breast-feed while taking OCs.

Benign Hepatic Adenoma. Women taking OCs should undergo periodic palpation of the liver. If a mass is detected, further tests are required for definitive diagnosis. If benign hepatoma is present, OC use must cease; regression of the tumor usually follows.

Glucose Intolerance. OCs can elevate plasma glucose levels. Advise the diabetic client to monitor blood glucose content closely; an increase in dosage of insulin or oral hypoglycemic medication may be needed. Monitor the prediabetic client for hyperglycemia.

Multiple Births. The incidence of twin births is increased when conception takes place shortly after termination of OC use. Advise the client to employ another form of birth control for 3 months after termination of OC use if she wishes to reduce the chances of multiple births.

Minimizing Adverse Interactions

Drugs That Reduce OC Levels. Levels of OCs can be reduced by drugs that induce OC metabolism (e.g., phenobarbital, phenytoin, troglitazone, rifampin, ritonavir) or accelerate OC excretion (e.g., tetracycline, ampicillin). Advise clients who are taking these agents to be alert for indications of reduced OC levels (e.g., breakthrough bleeding, spotting), and to notify the physician if these occur. An increase in OC dosage or use of an alternative method of birth control may be required.

*Patient education information is highlighted as blue text.

Drugs Whose Effects Are Reduced by OCs. OCs can reduce the effects of some drugs, including *warfarin, insulin,* and some *oral hypoglycemic agents.* When combined with OCs, these drugs may require greater than normal dosages.

Drugs Whose Effects Are Increased by OCs. OCs can increase blood levels of several drugs, including *theophylline* and *imipramine.* Women using these drugs in combination with OCs should be alert for signs of toxicity; dosage reduction for theophylline or imipramine may be required.

PROGESTIN-ONLY ORAL CONTRACEPTIVES

Preadministration Assessment

Therapeutic Goal

Prevention of unwanted pregnancy.

Identifying High-Risk Patients

Progestin-only pills are *contraindicated* during pregnancy.

Implementation: Administration

Dosing Schedule

Instruct the client to initiate OC use on day 1 of the menstrual cycle and to take one pill every day thereafter. Pills should be taken at the same time each day (e.g., with a meal or at bedtime).

Responding to Missed Doses

Provide the client with the following instructions regarding missed doses:

- If one pill is missed, take it as soon as the omission is noticed.
- If two pills are missed, take one pill as soon as the omission is noticed, discard the second pill, and take the next scheduled pill at its normal time.
- If three pills are missed, terminate OC use. Do not resume use until menstruation occurs or until pregnancy has been ruled out.

Ongoing Evaluation and Interventions

Minimizing Adverse Effects

Menstrual Irregularities. Breakthrough bleeding, spotting, amenorrhea, inconsistent cycle length, and variations in the amount and duration of monthly flow are common and unavoidable. Forewarn the client of these effects.

Drug Therapy of Infertility

INFERTILITY: CAUSES AND TREATMENT STRATEGIES
  Female Infertility
  Male Infertility
DRUGS USED TO TREAT FEMALE INFERTILITY
  Drugs for Controlled Ovarian Stimulation
  Bromocriptine
  Drugs for Endometriosis

Infertility (subfertility) is defined as a decrease in the ability to reproduce. This contrasts with sterility, which is the complete absence of reproductive ability. About 15% of couples attempting to have children experience infertility. Failure to conceive may be due to reproductive dysfunction of the male partner, the female partner, or both. When medical treatment is implemented, approximately one-half of infertile couples achieve pregnancy. To date, drug therapy of female infertility has been considerably more successful than drug therapy of male infertility.

In treating infertility, the chances of success are greatly enhanced by accurate diagnosis. A variety of diagnostic procedures may be employed, including semen analysis, determination of basal body temperature patterns, measurement of estrogen and progesterone levels, endometrial biopsy, and evaluation of fallopian tube patency. A complete medical history of both partners is essential. This history should include information on frequency and timing of coitus and use of drugs that might lower fertility.

In this chapter, we discuss the drugs employed to increase fertility in two stages. First, we discuss the underlying causes of reproductive dysfunction. Second, we discuss the fertility-promoting drugs. As preparation to study these agents, you should review the following from Chapter 59: information on the menstrual cycle and information on the biosynthesis and physiologic and pharmacologic effects of the female hormones (estrogens and progestins). Pay special attention to the roles of gonadotropin-releasing hormone (GnRH), luteinizing hormone (LH), and follicle-stimulating hormone (FSH).

INFERTILITY: CAUSES AND TREATMENT STRATEGIES

Female Infertility

Female infertility can result from disruption of any phase of the reproductive process. The most critical phases are follicular maturation, ovulation, transport of the ovum through the fallopian tubes, fertilization of the ovum, nidation (implantation), and growth and development of the conceptus. These events can take place only if the ovaries, uterus, hypothalamus, and pituitary are functioning properly. If the activity of any of these structures is disturbed, fertility can be impaired. Causes of female infertility that respond to drug therapy are discussed below.

Anovulation and Failure of Follicular Maturation

In the absence of adequate hormonal stimulation, ovarian follicles will not ripen and ovulation will not take place. Frequently, these causes of infertility can be corrected with drugs. The agents used to promote follicular maturation and/or ovulation are *clomiphene, menotropins, follitropins (e.g., urofollitropin), and human chorionic gonadotropin* (HCG). Clomiphene induces follicular maturation and ovulation by promoting release of FSH and LH from the pituitary; in some cases, induction of ovulation requires co-treatment with HCG. Menotropins and follitropins are used in conjunction with HCG: Menotropins and follitropins act directly on the ovary to promote follicular development; after follicles have matured, HCG is given to induce ovulation. Because HCG acts on mature follicles to cause ovulation, the drug is used only after follicular maturation has been induced with another agent (menotropins, a follitropin, or clomiphene). The pharmacology of clomiphene, menotropins, follitropins, and HCG is discussed below.

Unfavorable Cervical Mucus

In the periovulatory period, the cervical glands normally secrete large volumes of thin, watery mucus. These secretions, which are produced under the influence of estrogen, facilitate passage of sperm through the cervical canal. If the cervical mucus is scant or of inappropriate consistency (thick, sticky), sperm will be unable to pass through to the uterus. Production of unfavorable mucus may occur spontaneously or as a side effect of clomiphene (see below).

Cervical mucus can be restored to its proper volume and consistency by administering estrogens. Two regimens have been employed. In one, ethinyl estradiol is given beginning early in the menstrual cycle (on day 6, 7, or 8) and continued through day 12 or 13; dosages range from 20 to 80 μg/day. In the other regimen, conjugated estrogens are administered from day 5 through day 15 of the cycle; dosages range from 2.5 to 5 mg/day. When used to counteract the effects of clomiphene on the cervical mucus, estrogens are administered for 10 days beginning 1 day after the last clomiphene dose.

Hyperprolactinemia

Elevation of prolactin levels may be caused by a pituitary adenoma or by disturbed regulation of the healthy pituitary. Amenorrhea, galactorrhea, and infertility may all occur in association with excessive prolactin secretion. The mechanism by which hyperprolactinemia impairs fertility is unknown. Hyperprolactinemia can be treated with bromocriptine.

687

Luteal-Phase Defect

The term *luteal-phase defect* refers to a group of disorders in which secretion of progesterone by the corpus luteum is insufficient to maintain endometrial integrity. Dysfunction of the corpus luteum may be spontaneous or may occur secondary to hyperprolactinemia or to use of clomiphene. Luteal-phase defect can be diagnosed by making serial determinations of plasma progesterone levels or by taking a biopsy of the endometrium.

Progesterone is the preferred therapy for luteal-phase defect. This hormone will correct the defect regardless of its etiology. Only progesterone itself should be used; synthetic progestins are teratogenic and may also induce degeneration of the corpus luteum. Progesterone treatment should commence after ovulation has occurred, and should continue through the first 8 to 10 weeks of pregnancy (i.e., until the placenta has developed the capacity to make its own progestins).

Progesterone may be administered by IM injection (12.5 mg/day) or by a vaginal suppository (25 mg twice daily). Because progesterone injections are both painful and inconvenient, the suppositories are preferred.

Endometriosis

Endometriosis is a condition in which endometrial tissue has become implanted in an abnormal location (e.g., uterine wall, ovary, extragenital sites). These implants respond to hormonal stimulation in much the same fashion as the normally situated endometrium. Endometriosis is a common cause of infertility and, when pregnancies do occur, the rate of spontaneous abortion is high (about 50%).

The mechanism by which endometriosis reduces fertility is not always clear. In some cases, infertility results from ovarian or tubal adhesions that impede transport of the ovum. However, when endometriosis is mild, visible causes of infertility are frequently absent.

Endometriosis can be treated with surgery, drugs, or both. Surgery reduces symptoms of endometriosis and increases fertility. In contrast, although drugs can reduce symptoms, they do *not* enhance fertility. The drug employed most frequently is *danazol*. More recently, *nafarelin* and *leuprolide* (synthetic analogs of gonadotropin-releasing hormone) have been used. Oral contraceptives can reduce symptoms of endometriosis, but obviously won't promote fertility.

Polycystic Ovary Syndrome

Polycystic ovary syndrome (PCOS) is characterized by the presence of polycystic ovaries, anovulation, and metabolic disturbances—especially insulin resistance and hyperinsulinemia, which stimulate overproduction of androgens. The resulting androgen excess underlies anovulation. For years, *clomiphene* (with or without HCG) has been the preferred method for inducing ovulation. However, recent studies, which have focused on the metabolic changes in PCOS, indicate that insulin-sensitizing drugs can also help. Two drugs have been studied: *metformin* [Glucophage] and *troglitazone* [Rezulin]. In women with PCOS, both drugs improved insulin sensitivity, decreased blood levels of insulin and, as a result, reduced overproduction of androgens and increased rates of ovulation. Although troglitazone is no longer available (it was withdrawn because of liver toxicity), other "glitazones" (e.g.,

rosiglitazone, pioglitazone) might also work. The pharmacology of metformin and the glitazones is presented in Chapter 54 (Drugs for Diabetes Mellitus).

Male Infertility

For about 30% of couples who experience infertility, failure to conceive is due entirely to reproductive dysfunction in the male. Male infertility is due most often to decreased density or motility of sperm, or to semen of abnormal volume or quality. The most obvious manifestation of male infertility is erectile dysfunction (ED). In most cases, infertility in males is not associated with an identifiable endocrine disorder. Unfortunately, with the exception of ED, male infertility is generally unresponsive to drugs.

Hypogonadotropic Hypogonadism

A few males may be incapable of spermatogenesis because of insufficient gonadotropin secretion. In these rare cases, drug therapy may be helpful. If the gonadotropin deficiency is only partial, sperm counts can be increased using HCG (alone or in combination with menotropins). If the deficiency is severe, treatment with androgens is required (see Chapter 58). If therapy with HCG and menotropins is intended, the patient should be informed that treatment will be prolonged (3 to 4 years) and very expensive.

Erectile Dysfunction

Inability to achieve erection is the most conspicuous cause of male infertility. Sildenafil [Viagra] and other drugs for ED are discussed in Chapter 103.

Idiopathic Male Infertility

Idiopathic infertility is defined as infertility for which no cause can be identified. It is estimated that 25% to 40% of male infertility is idiopathic. Since the cause is unknown, specific drug therapy is impossible. Accordingly, treatment is empiric (trial and error). Several drugs, including androgens, clomiphene, and HCG, have been administered in hopes of improving idiopathic infertility in males. Unfortunately, success rates are low.

DRUGS USED TO TREAT FEMALE INFERTILITY

Drugs for Controlled Ovarian Stimulation

The term *controlled ovarian stimulation* refers to the use of drugs to facilitate follicular maturation and ovulation. Following ovulation, fertilization can be accomplished either naturally (through sexual intercourse) or through assisted reproduction technology (e.g., *in vitro* fertilization). Of the drugs discussed below, five are used to promote follicular maturation, two are used to stimulate ovulation, and two are used to prevent premature stimulation of ovulation by endogenous hormones (see Table 61–1).

Clomiphene

Therapeutic Use. Clomiphene [Clomid, Milophene, Serophene] is used to promote follicular maturation and ovulation in selected infertile women.

TABLE 61–1 ■ Drugs for Controlled Ovarian Stimulation

Generic Name	Trade Name	Mechanism of Action
Drugs That Promote Follicular Maturation		
Clomiphene	Clomid, Milophene, Serophene	Clomiphene blocks estrogen receptors in the hypothalamus and pituitary, and thereby causes a compensatory increase in the release of LH and FSH, which then act on the ovary to promote follicular maturation (and possibly ovulation).
Menotropins	Pergonal, Repronex	Menotropins is a 50:50 mixture of FSH and LH that acts on the ovary to promote follicular maturation. Treatment is followed by HCG to induce ovulation.
Urofollitropin Follitropin alfa Follitropin beta	Metrodin Gonal-F Follistim	These follitropins are preparations of FSH that act on the ovary to promote follicular maturation. Treatment is followed by HCG to induce ovulation.
Drugs That Stimulate Ovulation		
Human chorionic gonadotropin (HCG)	A.P.L., Chorex, Choron, Gonic, Pregnyl, Profasi	HCG is similar in structure and identical in action to LH. The drug acts on the ovary to induce ovulation.
Choriogonadotropin Alfa	Ovidrel	Choriogonadotropin is a synthetic form of LH that acts on the ovary to induce ovulation.
Drugs That Prevent Premature Ovulation		
Ganirelix Cetrorelix	Antagon Cetrotide	These drugs are GnRH antagonists that block endogenous release of LH, and thereby prevent possible premature ovulation in women receiving drugs to promote follicular maturation.

Mechanism of Fertility Promotion. Clomiphene blocks receptors for estrogen. By blocking these receptors in the hypothalamus and pituitary, clomiphene makes it appear to these structures that estrogen levels are low. In response, the pituitary increases secretion of gonadotropins (LH and FSH) and these hormones then stimulate the ovary, promoting follicular maturation and ovulation. In properly selected patients, the ovulation rate is about 90%. Because of its mechanism of action, clomiphene can induce ovulation only if the pituitary is capable of producing LH and FSH, and only if the ovaries are capable of responding. Success is impossible in women with primary failure of either the pituitary or ovaries. Accordingly, pituitary and ovarian function should be verified prior to clomiphene therapy. If treatment produces follicular maturation but ovulation fails to occur, it may be possible to induce ovulation by adding HCG to the regimen (see below). The occurrence of ovulation can be determined by three methods: (1) monitoring for an increase in basal body temperature, (2) monitoring for an increase in progesterone levels, and (3) examining a biopsy of the endometrium for evidence of secretory transformation.

Adverse Effects. Common side effects include hot flushes (similar to the vasomotor responses of menopause), nausea, abdominal discomfort, bloating, and breast engorgement. Some patients experience visual disturbances (blurred vision, visual flashes), which usually reverse following clomiphene withdrawal. Multiple births (usually twins) occur in 8% to 10% of clomiphene-facilitated pregnancies. Patients should be told of this possibility.

Excessive stimulation of the ovaries can produce *ovarian enlargement*. This reaction is most likely in women with polycystic ovaries. Hyperstimulation of the ovaries can be minimized by avoiding unnecessarily large clomiphene doses. If undue ovarian enlargement occurs, clomiphene administration should cease. The ovaries will regress to normal size following drug withdrawal.

Some actions of clomiphene may *interfere* with conception. Luteal-phase defect may be induced. This response can be corrected by giving progesterone. Because it has antiestrogenic actions, clomiphene may force the production of scant and viscous cervical mucus; estrogen therapy can render cervical secretions more hospitable to sperm.

It is recommended that clomiphene be avoided during pregnancy. Although no human fetal defects have been reported, clomiphene has produced developmental abnormalities in animals.

Preparations, Dosage, and Administration. Clomiphene [Clomid, Milophene, Serophene] is dispensed in 50-mg tablets for oral use. The initial course of treatment consists of 50 mg once daily for 5 days. If cyclic menstrual bleeding has been occurring, therapy should begin on the fifth day after the onset of menses. If menstruation has been absent, therapy can commence at any time (assuming pregnancy has been ruled out). If the first course of treatment fails to induce ovulation, a second 5-day course (using 100 mg/day) may be tried. The second course may begin as early as 30 days after the previous course. Doses may be increased in subsequent courses. However, doses above 100 mg/day are rarely needed. Once a dose that induces ovulation has been established, that dose should be used for a maximum of three cycles. If pregnancy has not occurred, further treatment is unlikely to succeed. When ovulation does occur, it is usually within 5 to 10 days after the last clomiphene dose; patients should be instructed to have coitus at least every other day during this time.

Menotropins

Menotropins [Pergonal, Repronex] (also known as human menopausal gonadotropin, or HMG) is a hormonal preparation having equal amounts of LH and FSH activity. Commercial menotropins is prepared by extraction from the urine of postmenopausal women.

Therapeutic Actions and Uses. *Anovulatory Women.*
Menotropins, in conjunction with HCG, is used to promote follicular maturation and ovulation in anovulatory patients. Menotropins acts directly on the ovaries to cause maturation of follicles. Once follicles have ripened, HCG is given to induce ovulation.

Menotropins is employed when gonadotropin secretion by the pituitary is insufficient to provide adequate ovarian stimulation. Candidates for menotropins therapy must have ovaries capable of responding to FSH and LH; menotropins is of no help in women with primary ovarian failure. Among properly selected patients, the rate of ovulation approaches 100%. It should be noted that therapy with menotropins is not cheap: A single cycle of treatment can cost between $500 and $1500 (in addition to physicians' fees and laboratory costs).

Ovulatory Women. Menotropins can be used to induce development of multiple follicles in ovulatory women participating in an *in vitro* fertilization program.

Men. Menotropins can be used to promote spermatogenesis in males with primary or secondary hypogonadotropic hypogonadism.

Adverse Effects. The most serious adverse response is *ovarian hyperstimulation syndrome,* a condition characterized by sudden enlargement of the ovaries. Mild to moderate ovarian enlargement is common, occurring in about 20% of patients. This condition is benign and resolves spontaneously upon discontinuation of drug use. Of greater concern is ovarian enlargement that occurs rapidly and that may be accompanied by ascites, pleural effusion, and considerable pain. If this manifestation of ovarian stimulation occurs, menotropins should be withdrawn and the patient hospitalized. Treatment is usually supportive (bed rest, analgesics, fluid and electrolyte replacement). If rupture of ovarian cysts occurs, surgery may be required to stop bleeding. Enlargement of the ovaries is most likely during the first 2 weeks of treatment. To ensure early detection, the patient should be examined at least every other day while taking menotropins, and for 2 weeks after termination of treatment. Ovarian stimulation can be minimized by keeping the dosage as low as possible.

In addition to causing excessive ovarian stimulation, menotropins may produce *spontaneous abortion* (in about 25% of menotropins-facilitated pregnancies) and *multiple births* (15% of pregnancies result in twins; 5% of pregnancies have three or more conceptuses).

Monitoring Therapy. Ovarian responses to menotropins must be monitored to determine timing of HCG administration and to minimize the risk of ovarian enlargement. Responses can be followed by measuring serum estrogen levels and by ultrasonography of the developing follicles. When estrogen levels rise to twice the pretreatment baseline, or when ultrasonography indicates that follicles have enlarged to 16 to 20 mm, menotropins administration should cease and HCG should be injected. However, if estrogen production is excessive (serum levels 3 to 4 times the pretreatment baseline),

HCG should be withheld, owing to the risk of ovarian hyperstimulation under these conditions. In addition, HCG should be withheld if ultrasonography indicates the presence of four or more mature follicles.

Preparations, Dosage, and Administration. Menotropins [Pergonal, Repronex] is dispensed as a powder to be reconstituted with sterile saline immediately prior to use. Ampules of menotropins contain either (1) 75 IU of FSH activity plus 75 IU of LH activity or (2) 150 IU of FSH activity plus 150 IU of LH activity. Administration is IM.

Menotropins is used sequentially with HCG: After follicular maturation has been induced with menotropins, HCG is injected to promote ovulation. For the initial cycle, the contents of one menotropins ampule is injected daily for 9 to 12 days. When estrogen measurements indicate follicular maturation has occurred, menotropins is discontinued; HCG (5000 to 10,000 USP units) is injected 24 hours after the last menotropins dose. Ovulation occurs 2 to 3 days after injecting HCG. Accordingly, patients should be instructed to have intercourse on the eve of HCG injection and on the following 2 to 3 days. If there is evidence of ovulation but conception does not take place, treatment should be repeated for two more courses using the same menotropins dosage. If treatment remains ineffective, two additional courses may be tried, using twice as much menotropins as previously. If there is still no conception, further treatment is unlikely to help.

Follitropins

Description. Three follitropins are available: *urofollitropin* [Metrodin, Fertinex, Bravelle], *follitropin alfa* [Gonal-F], and *follitropin beta* [Follistim]. All three are preparations of FSH. Urofollitropin is a highly purified preparation of FSH extracted from the urine of postmenopausal women. Follitropin alfa and follitropin beta are FSH preparations produced by recombinant DNA technology.

Use in Women. The actions, uses, and adverse effects of the follitropins are much like those of menotropins (a 50:50 mixture of FSH and LH). Like menotropins, the follitropins act directly on the ovary to stimulate follicle maturation. All three follitropins are employed to stimulate ovulation in anovulatory women, and to promote production of multiple follicles in ovulatory women participating in an *in vitro* fertilization program. For both indications, the follitropins are used sequentially with HCG: the follitropin is given first to promote follicle maturation; then HCG is given to stimulate ovulation. As with menotropins, multiple births are relatively common. The principal adverse effect of the follitropins is ovarian hyperstimulation syndrome. All of the follitropins are administered SC; follitropin beta may also be given IM.

Use in Men. Two follitropins—*follitropin alpha* and *follitropin beta*—are approved for promotion of spermatogenesis in males with primary or secondary hypogonadotropic hypogonadism.

Human Chorionic Gonadotropin

Human chorionic gonadotropin is a polypeptide hormone produced by the placenta. HCG is similar in structure and identical in action to luteinizing hormone.

Therapeutic Use. HCG is used to induce ovulation in women who are infertile because of ovulatory failure. The drug causes ovulation by simulating the midcycle LH surge. When HCG is used to promote ovulation, follicular maturation must first be induced with another agent, usually menotropins. HCG can also be used in conjunction with clomiphene when treatment with clomiphene alone has failed to promote ovulation.

Adverse Effects. The most severe adverse response to HCG is *ovarian hyperstimulation syndrome.* If this reaction occurs, hospitalization and discontinuation of HCG are indicated. HCG may also provoke *rupture of ovarian cysts* with resultant bleeding into the peritoneal cavity. *Multiple births* may be induced; the patient should be informed of this possibility. Additional adverse effects include edema, injection site pain, and central nervous system disturbances (headache, irritability, restlessness, fatigue).

Preparations, Dosage, and Administration. Commercial HCG is prepared by extraction from the urine of pregnant women. HCG is dispensed as a powder and must be reconstituted for use. Administration is by IM injection. The usual dose for induction of ovulation is 5000 to 10,000 USP units. Trade names are *A.P.L., Chorex, Choron, Gonic, Pregnyl,* and *Profasi.*

Prior to giving HCG, follicular maturation must be induced with another agent (menotropins, a follitropin, or clomiphene). When used in conjunction with menotropins or a follitropin, HCG is injected 1 day after the last menotropins/follitropin dose. When used in conjunction with clomiphene, HCG is administered 7 to 9 days after the last clomiphene dose.

Choriogonadotropin Alfa

Choriogonadotropin alfa [Ovidrel] is a form of HCG produced by recombinant DNA technology. The drug's physicochemical, immunologic, and biologic activities are equivalent to those of naturally occurring HCG, produced by extraction from the urine of pregnant women. However, unlike urine-derived HCG, which must be injected IM, choriogonadotropin alfa is injected SC. As a result, administration is more comfortable (IM injection can be painful). Choriogonadotropin alfa has two indications. First, like natural HCG, the drug is given to *trigger ovulation* in women who are infertile owing to anovulation. Second, the drug is used to *promote late follicular maturation and early luteinization* in women undergoing assisted reproductive technology (e.g., *in vitro* fertilization). For both indications, follicular maturation must first be induced with a follicle-stimulating agent (e.g., menotropins). Choriogonadotropin alfa (250 μg) is then given as a single SC injection 1 day after the last dose of the follicle-stimulating agent. Major adverse effects are the same as those of natural HCG: ovarian hyperstimulation syndrome, rupture of ovarian cysts, and multiple births.

Gonadotropin-Releasing Hormone Antagonists

Gonadotropin-releasing hormone (GnRH) antagonists are used to prevent a premature surge of endogenous LH in women undergoing controlled ovarian stimulation (with menotropins or follitropin [FSH]). As discussed above, after follicles have matured under the influence of exogenous menotropins or FSH, the patient is given an injection of HCG (LH) to cause ovulation. However, in some women, the natural midcycle LH surge occurs early, causing ovulation before her eggs have fully matured. As a result, the chances of successful conception and implantation are reduced. The GnRH antagonists prevent LH release, and thereby eliminate the chance of premature ovulation.

Two GnRH antagonists are available: *ganirelix* [Antagon] and *cetrorelix* [Cetrotide]. Both drugs block GnRH receptors, and thereby prevent GnRH from promoting the production and release of LH from the pituitary. The usual dosing schedule for both is 250 μg SC daily, beginning in the early follicular phase and continuing until the day of HCG administration. Injections are made by the patient into the upper thigh or the region around the naval.

Bromocriptine

Therapeutic Uses. Bromocriptine [Parlodel] is used to correct amenorrhea and infertility associated with excessive prolactin secretion. If galactorrhea is present, this consequence of hyperprolactinemia may also be corrected. When the source of excessive prolactin is a pituitary adenoma, bromocriptine can induce regression of the tumor, in addition to reducing prolactin secretion. Continuous treatment can suppress tumor growth for years. Bromocriptine is also used in Parkinson's disease (see Chapter 21).

Mechanism of Fertility Promotion. Bromocriptine stimulates receptors for dopamine. By stimulating dopamine receptors in the anterior pituitary, bromocriptine inhibits prolactin secretion. Reductions in prolactin levels are accompanied by normalization of the menstrual cycle and a return of fertility. The mechanism by which lowering of prolactin levels leads to a return of ovulation is unknown.

Adverse Effects. When bromocriptine is given to treat infertility, adverse effects are frequent but usually mild. Nausea occurs in 50% of patients. Headache, dizziness, fatigue, and abdominal cramps are also common. Orthostatic hypotension may occur, but is rare at the doses employed to decrease pro-

lactin secretion. Teratogenic effects have not been reported. Adverse effects can be minimized by taking bromocriptine with meals and initiating treatment at low doses.

Preparations, Dosage, and Administration. Bromocriptine mesylate [Parlodel] is dispensed in 2.5-mg tablets and 5-mg capsules. Dosing is begun at 2.5 mg once a day and then gradually increased to 2.5 mg 2 or 3 times a day. All doses should be administered with food. Normalization of the menstrual cycle may occur rapidly (within a few days) or may require up to 2 months of treatment. As soon as pregnancy is achieved, use of bromocriptine should cease. As a rule, administration should not resume until after delivery. If treatment is not reinstated, hypersecretion of prolactin is almost certain to recur within a year.

Drugs for Endometriosis
Danazol

Therapeutic Use. Danazol [Danocrine] can improve symptoms of endometriosis, but does *not* increase fertility. Treatment leads to complete regression of endometrial implants in the majority of patients. However, implants will eventually recur after treatment stops. In addition to the therapy of endometriosis, danazol has been used to treat *angioneurotic edema* and *fibrocystic breast disease.*

Mechanism of Action. Danazol acts by multiple mechanisms to induce regression of endometrial implants. First, danazol inhibits several of the enzymes required for synthesis of ovarian hormones, thereby depriving the implant of the hormonal environment it needs for maintenance. Second, danazol suppresses secretion of pituitary gonadotropins (FSH and LH), thereby further decreasing the availability of ovarian hormones. Lastly, danazol may act directly on the implant to block ovarian hormone receptors. All of these actions result in atrophy of ectopic endometrial tissue. The normal endometrium atrophies as well.

Adverse Effects and Interactions. Danazol is weakly androgenic and may induce virilization. Potential manifestations include acne, deepening of the voice, and growth of facial hair. These effects are usually reversible upon cessation of treatment. Danazol may also cause edema, and therefore should be used with caution in patients with cardiac and renal disorders. Thrombotic events have been reported, including fatal strokes. Liver impairment has also been reported, and hence liver function should be assessed before therapy and periodically thereafter. Danazol may intensify the effects of warfarin, an anticoagulant. Danazol can cause masculinization of the female fetus, and hence is contraindicated during pregnancy.

Preparations, Dosage, and Administration. Danazol [Danocrine] is dispensed in capsules (50, 100, and 200 mg) for oral administration. A dosage of 200 to 300 mg twice daily is usually effective. To ensure that danazol is not taken during pregnancy, therapy should be initiated at the time of menstruation. The usual course of treatment is 3 to 9 months.

GnRH Agonists

Nafarelin [Synarel] and leuprolide [Lupron] are synthetic agonistic analogs of GnRH. Both drugs are used to treat endometriosis. However, although these drugs reduce symptoms of endometriosis, they do not increase fertility.

Nafarelin. Mechanism of Action. Like the normal endometrium, ectopic endometrial implants are dependent on ovarian hormones. Nafarelin suppresses endometriosis by indirectly suppressing ovarian hormone production.

How does nafarelin suppress production of ovarian hormones? *Initial* doses actually increase hormone production. Why? Because nafarelin, like endogenous GnRH, acts on the pituitary to promote release of FSH and LH, which in turn act on the ovary to stimulate hormone production. However, in contrast to endogenous GnRH, which has a short half-life and is released in a *pulsatile* fashion, nafarelin has a long half-life and is administered on a continuing basis. As a result, nafarelin causes continuous stimulation of pituitary GnRH receptors. This continuous stimulation has the paradoxical effect of *suppressing* FSH and LH release, thereby depriving the ovary of the stimulation needed for hormone production.

Therapeutic Use. Nafarelin is approved for treatment of *endometriosis.* The drug is about as effective as danazol for this indication. Nafarelin reduces the area of endometriosis and improves symptoms. Because of concern about bone loss (see below), nafarelin should not be used for more than 6 months.

It must be stressed that nafarelin, like danazol, does not produce cure. Within 6 months after the drug is withdrawn, symptoms return in up to 50% of women who had previously been rendered symptom free.

Adverse Effects. Most undesired effects are secondary to estrogen deficiency. Common responses include hot flushes, vaginal dryness, decreased libido, mood changes, and headache. Nasal irritation also occurs (administration is by nasal spray). Nafarelin is teratogenic and must not be used during pregnancy.

The adverse effect of greatest concern is *bone loss*. After 3 to 6 months of treatment, bone mass and mineral content may decrease. To minimize the risk of osteoporosis, the manufacturer recommends that treatment last no more than 6 months.

Preparations, Dosage, and Administration. Nafarelin [Synarel] is dispensed in a spray for intranasal administration. (The drug cannot be given orally owing to rapid degradation by GI enzymes.) The initial dosage is 200 μg (one spray) in the morning and evening. Doses should alternate between nostrils. Treatment should begin between days 2 and 4 of the menstrual cycle.

Leuprolide. Like nafarelin, leuprolide [Lupron Depot] is a GnRH analog that can reduce symptoms of endometriosis. However, it does not improve fertility. Leuprolide has the same mechanism as nafarelin (suppression of LH and RH release with continued use) as well as the same adverse effects (hot flushes, vaginal dryness, amenorrhea, headache, depression, osteoporosis). For treatment of endometriosis, a depot formulation is used; the dosage is 3.75 mg IM once a month. In addition to endometriosis, leuprolide is indicated for advanced cancer of the prostate (see Chapter 99).

∴ KEY POINTS

■ Infertility (subfertility) is defined as a decrease in reproductive ability, whereas sterility is a complete absence of reproductive ability.

■ Infertility in a couple may result from infertility in the male partner, the female partner, or both.
■ Clomiphene is used to promote follicular maturation and ovulation.
■ Clomiphene acts by blocking estrogen receptors in the hypothalamus and pituitary, causing a compensatory increase in the release of LH and FSH, which then act on the ovary to promote follicular maturation and ovulation.
■ Menotropins is a 50:50 mixture of LH and FSH.
■ Menotropins is used sequentially with HCG: menotropins is given to promote follicular maturation, then HCG is given to promote ovulation.
■ The most serious adverse effect of menotropins is ovarian hyperstimulation syndrome, which is characterized by sudden enlargement of the ovaries.
■ HCG is given to stimulate ovulation (after another drug, such as menotropins, has been given to promote follicular maturation).
■ Like menotropins, HCG can cause ovarian hyperstimulation syndrome.
■ Bromocriptine is given to suppress excessive prolactin release.
■ Although danazol can cause regression of endometrial implants, the drug does not increase fertility.

Summary of Major Nursing Implications*

CLOMIPHENE

The implications summarized here apply only to the use of clomiphene for promoting maturation of ovarian follicles and ovulation. (Clomiphene has also been used investigationally to increase fertility in males.)

Preadministration Assessment

Therapeutic Goal

Promotion of follicular maturation and ovulation in carefully selected patients.

Baseline Data

Take a complete health and gynecologic history; a pelvic examination and an endometrial biopsy are also required. Ovarian and pituitary function must be confirmed. Pregnancy must be ruled out.

Identifying High-Risk Patients

Clomiphene is *contraindicated* during pregnancy and in women with liver disease and abnormal uterine bleeding of undetermined origin.

Implementation: Administration

Route

Oral.

Administration Schedule

If cyclic menstrual bleeding has been occurring, begin therapy 5 days after the onset of menses. If menstruation has been absent, begin at any time.

The initial course consists of 50-mg doses once daily for 5 days. If ovulation fails to occur, additional courses may be tried, each beginning no sooner than 30 days after the previous course.

Implementation: Measures to Enhance Therapeutic Effects

Timing of Coitus

Advise the couple to have coitus at least every other day during the 5- to 10-day period that follows the last clomiphene dose.

Adjunctive Use of HCG

If ovulation fails to occur under the influence of clomiphene alone, injection of HCG 7 to 9 days after the last clomiphene dose may bring success.

Ongoing Evaluation and Interventions

Evaluating Therapeutic Effects

To determine if ovulation has occurred, monitor for an increase in basal body temperature or plasma proges-

*Patient education information is highlighted as blue text.

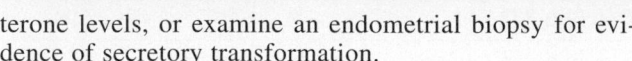

terone levels, or examine an endometrial biopsy for evidence of secretory transformation.

Minimizing Adverse Effects

Ovarian Enlargement. Instruct the patient to notify the physician if pelvic pain occurs (an indication of ovarian enlargement). If ovarian enlargement is diagnosed, clomiphene should be withdrawn, after which ovarian size usually regresses spontaneously.

Reduced Fertility. Clomiphene may cause luteal-phase defect; this response can be corrected with progesterone. Alteration of cervical mucus may occur; estrogens can be used to restore the volume and fluidity of cervical secretions.

Multiple Births. Inform the couple that multiple births (usually twins) are not uncommon in clomiphene-facilitated pregnancies.

Visual Disturbances. Forewarn the patient about possible visual disturbances (blurred vision, visual flashes), and instruct her to notify the physician if these occur. Visual aberrations usually cease following drug withdrawal.

Other Adverse Effects. Common side effects include hot flushes (similar to the vasomotor responses of menopause), nausea, abdominal discomfort, bloating, and breast engorgement. Forewarn the patient about these effects and instruct her to notify the physician if they are especially disturbing.

MENOTROPINS

The implications summarized here refer only to the use of menotropins (together with HCG) for induction of follicular maturation and ovulation. (Menotropins is also used to treat infertility in males.)

Preadministration Assessment

Therapeutic Goal

Induction of follicular maturation and ovulation (in conjunction with HCG) in carefully selected patients.

Baseline Data

A thorough gynecologic and endocrinologic evaluation should precede treatment. Ovarian function must be verified. Obtain a baseline value for serum estrogen.

Identifying High-Risk Patients

Menotropins is *contraindicated* in the presence of pregnancy, primary ovarian failure, thyroid dysfunction, adrenal dysfunction, ovarian cysts, and ovarian enlargement (other than that caused by polycystic ovary syndrome).

Implementation: Administration

Route

Intramuscular.

Administration

Reconstitute powdered menotropins with sterile saline immediately prior to injection.

Menotropins is employed sequentially with HCG. Administer menotropins for 9 to 12 days (to promote follicular maturation). Twenty-four hours after the last dose, inject HCG. Ovulation follows in 2 to 3 days.

Serum estrogen content and ultrasonography are used to assess follicular maturation; upon follicular maturation, menotropins is discontinued and HCG is injected. If estrogen production is excessive (3 to 4 times the pretreatment baseline) or if ultrasonography indicates the presence of four or more mature follicles, withhold HCG.

Implementation: Measures to Enhance Therapeutic Effects

Timing of Coitus

Advise the couple to have intercourse on the eve of HCG injection and on the following 2 to 3 days (i.e., during the probable period of ovulation).

Ongoing Evaluation and Interventions

Minimizing Adverse Effects

Ovarian Hyperstimulation Syndrome. Rapid ovarian enlargement can occur, sometimes associated with ascites, pleural effusion, and pain. If ovarian enlargement is excessive, discontinue menotropins and hospitalize the patient. Treatment is supportive (bed rest, analgesics, fluid and electrolyte replacement). If ovarian cysts rupture, surgery may be required to stop bleeding. To ensure early detection of ovarian enlargement, the patient should be examined at least every other day during menotropins use, and for 2 weeks following drug withdrawal. Because HCG can intensify ovarian stimulation, if serum estrogen levels rise to 3 to 4 times the pretreatment baseline (suggesting existing hyperstimulation of the ovaries), HCG should be withheld.

Other Adverse Effects. Forewarn the patient that treatment may result in spontaneous abortion. Inform the couple that multiple births are relatively common in menotropins-facilitated pregnancies.

HUMAN CHORIONIC GONADOTROPIN

The implications summarized here apply only to the use of HCG in the treatment of female infertility.

Preadministration Assessment

Therapeutic Goal

Induction of ovulation in women who are infertile because of anovulation. Pretreatment with menotropins, urofollitropin, or clomiphene is required.

Implementation: Administration

Route

Intramuscular.

Administration

HCG must be used in conjunction with menotropins, a follitropin, or clomiphene. When used with menotropins or a

*Patient education information is highlighted as blue text.

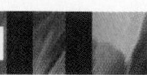

Summary of Major Nursing Implications*—cont'd

follitropin, HCG is injected 1 day after the last menotropins dose. When used with clomiphene, HCG is administered 7 to 9 days after the last clomiphene dose.

Ongoing Evaluation and Interventions

Minimizing Adverse Effects

Ovarian Hyperstimulation Syndrome. See *Minimizing Adverse Effects* for menotropins.

Multiple Births. **Inform the couple that multiple births are common in HCG-facilitated pregnancies.**

BROMOCRIPTINE

The implications summarized here refer only to the use of bromocriptine for hyperprolactinemia. They do not apply to treatment of Parkinson's disease.

Preadministration Assessment

Therapeutic Goal

Treatment of female infertility occurring secondary to hyperprolactinemia.

Identifying High-Risk Patients

Bromocriptine is *contraindicated* during pregnancy and in patients with severe ischemic heart disease or peripheral vascular disease.

Implementation: Administration

Route

Oral.

Administration

Instruct the patient to take bromocriptine with food.

Normalization of the menstrual cycle may occur within a few days or may require up to 2 months of treatment.

Bromocriptine should be withdrawn when pregnancy is achieved, and administration should not resume until after delivery.

Ongoing Evaluation and Interventions

Minimizing Adverse Effects

Nausea. **Inform the patient that nausea can be reduced by taking bromocriptine with meals.**

Other Adverse Effects. Headache, dizziness, fatigue, and abdominal cramps can be reduced by initiating therapy at low doses.

*Patient education information is highlighted as blue text.

DANAZOL

The implications summarized here refer only to the use of danazol in the treatment of endometriosis. (Danazol may also be used to treat angioneurotic edema and fibrocystic breast disease.)

Preadministration Assessment

Therapeutic Goal

Regression of ectopic endometrial implants (endometriosis). Treatment does not increase fertility.

Baseline Data

Obtain tests of liver function.

Identifying High-Risk Patients

Danazol is *contraindicated* during pregnancy and for women with undiagnosed genital bleeding or severe impairment of cardiac, renal, or hepatic function.

Implementation: Administration

Route

Oral.

Administration

Initiate therapy during menstruation. Treatment typically lasts 3 to 9 months.

Ongoing Evaluation and Interventions

Minimizing Adverse Effects

Virilization. Danazol is weakly androgenic. **Inform the patient about signs of masculinization (acne, deepening of the voice, growth of facial hair), and instruct her to notify the physician if these occur.** Virilization usually reverses following danazol withdrawal.

Use in Pregnancy. If taken during pregnancy, danazol may cause masculinization of the female fetus. **Warn the patient against becoming pregnant prior to danazol withdrawal.**

Edema. Danazol may cause edema. Use with caution in the presence of cardiac and renal disease.

Liver Dysfunction. Liver dysfunction has been reported. Liver function should be assessed prior to danazol use and periodically throughout the course of treatment.

Drugs That Affect Uterine Function

In this chapter, our principal focus is on drugs that stimulate or suppress uterine contractions. In addition, we discuss two drug used to promote cervical ripening. Drugs that stimulate uterine contraction are known as *oxytocics*. Drugs that suppress contraction are known as *tocolytics*. Oxytocic agents have three applications: (1) induction or augmentation of labor, (2) control of postpartum bleeding, and (3) induction of abortion. The tocolytic drugs have only one major use: suppression of preterm labor. Drugs that promote cervical ripening are used to soften the cervix prior to induction of labor.

UTERINE RELAXANTS (TOCOLYTICS) AND THEIR USE IN PRETERM LABOR

Premature birth, defined as birth before 37 weeks' gestation, is the leading cause of infant morbidity and neonatal mortality. In the United States, about 11% of all live births (about 440,000 annually) are premature. These preterm births account for 75% of neonatal mortality and 50% of congenital neurologic deficits. The most common complication of premature birth is *neonatal respiratory distress syndrome.* Preterm labor can be triggered by a variety of causes, the most common being intra-amniotic infection.

Because of the morbidity and mortality associated with premature birth, uterine relaxants (tocolytic drugs) are used to suppress preterm labor, and thereby delay delivery. These drugs can suppress labor briefly, but not long term. On average, delivery is postponed by only 48 hours. Hence, birth still takes place prior to term. If tocolytics don't permit pregnancy to reach term, what are they good for? The answer: Almost nothing—*if* they are used *alone*. However, when tocolytics are *combined with glucocorticoids,* which accelerate fetal lung development (see Chapter 103), the outcome is greatly improved: Infants experience less respiratory distress syndrome, intraventricular hemorrhage, and mortality.

A variety of drugs can suppress preterm labor. Intravenous *magnesium sulfate* is the current drug of choice. Other options include nifedipine (a calcium channel blocker), beta$_2$-adrenergic agonists (e.g., terbutaline), and several nonsteroidal anti-inflammatory drugs (e.g., indomethacin, naproxen). All of these drugs are equally good at suppressing labor. Accordingly, selection among them is based on severity of side effects. The efficacy, side effects, and overall risk of the major tocolytics are summarized in Table 62–1.

Magnesium Sulfate

Owing to its efficacy, safety, and low cost, magnesium sulfate is the treatment of choice for suppressing preterm labor. In 60% to 80% of cases, the drug can stop contractions for 48 to 72 hours. The underlying mechanism is inhibition of acetylcholine release at uterine neuromuscular junctions (NMJs). Arrest of labor occurs with plasma magnesium levels in the range of 4 to 7 mEq/L. At higher levels, magnesium can inhibit transmitter release at NMJs that serve skeletal muscle. As a result, if magnesium levels become excessive, the drug can cause profound muscle weakness along with respiratory arrest. Dosing consists of an initial IV bolus (4 to 6 gm), followed by IV infusion at 2 to 3 gm/hr for 48 to 72 hours. A controlled infusion pump is needed to minimize the risk of toxicity.

When plasma levels remain in the therapeutic range, magnesium is well tolerated by both the mother and fetus. Initial maternal reactions include transient hypotension, flushing, headache, dizziness, lethargy, dry mouth, and a feeling of warmth. Higher doses may cause hypothermia and paralytic ileus. Pulmonary edema, which can be fatal, is seen in 2% of patients. Pulmonary edema is managed by discontinuing magnesium and giving a diuretic to accelerate magnesium excretion. Magnesium sulfate is contraindicated in patients with myasthenia gravis (because the disease causes muscle weakness), renal failure (because magnesium is eliminated entirely by the kidneys), and hypocalcemia (because hypocalcemia intensifies magnesium-induced suppression of neurotransmitter release).

Magnesium readily crosses the placenta, and may thereby cause hypotonia (muscle weakness) and sleepiness in the newborn. Because elimination of magnesium by neonatal kidneys is slow, hypotonia may persist 3 to 4 days. During this time, mechanical assistance of ventilation may be required.

The risk of adverse effects can be reduced by monitoring (1) magnesium levels, (2) renal function (because renal impairment will cause magnesium levels to rise), (3) fluid balance (because fluid retention increases the risk of pulmonary

TABLE 62–1 ▪■ Drugs Used to Suppress Preterm Labor

| Tocolytic Drug | Efficacy | | Overall Risk | | Major Adverse Effects | |
	Short Term*	Long Term†	Maternal	Fetal	Maternal	Fetal/Neonatal
Magnesium sulfate	Good	None	Low	Low	Pulmonary edema, hypotension, muscle weakness, ileus, cardiorespiratory arrest	Neonatal hypotonia and sleepiness
Beta₂-agonists: ritodrine‡, terbutaline	Good	None	High	Low	Pulmonary edema, tachycardia, palpitations, chest pain, myocardial ischemia, hypotension, hyperglycemia	Fetal tachycardia, hypotension, ileus, hyperinsulinemia with hypoglycemia, hyperbilirubinemia, hypocalcemia
Nifedipine, a calcium channel blocker	Good	None	Low	Low	Tachycardia, hypotension, hepatotoxicity	
Indomethacin, a nonsteroidal anti-inflammatory drug	Good	None	Low	High	Nausea, gastric irritation, interstitial nephritis, prolonged postpartum bleeding	Renal failure, bronchopulmonary dysplasia, necrotizing enterocolitis, intracerebral hemorrhage, premature closure of ductus arteriosus

*Short-term efficacy is defined as the ability to delay delivery by 24 to 48 hours.
†Long-term efficacy is defined as the ability to delay labor for an extended time following successful short-term therapy.
‡No longer available.

edema), and (4) deep tendon reflexes (because loss of deep tendon reflexes is an early sign that magnesium levels are rising dangerously high).

In addition to its use in preterm labor, magnesium sulfate is the preferred drug for prevention and treatment of seizures associated with eclampsia and severe preeclampsia (see Chapter 45).

Other Uterine Relaxants
Beta₂-Adrenergic Agonists

Two beta₂-adrenergic agonists—ritodrine and terbutaline—have been used widely to suppress preterm labor. These drugs are as effective as magnesium sulfate, but pose a greater risk to the mother. Accordingly, they are now considered second-line agents. In 1998, ritodrine was voluntarily withdrawn from the market. Terbutaline is still available, but has never been approved by the Food and Drug Administration (FDA) for use in preterm labor.

Ritodrine. Ritodrine—marketed as Yutopar before being withdrawn—is classified as a beta₂-selective adrenergic agonist. By activating beta₂ receptors in the uterus, the drug relaxes uterine smooth muscle, thereby decreasing both the intensity and frequency of contractions. Ritodrine is as effective as magnesium sulfate, but poses a much greater risk to the mother. Adverse effects result from activating beta₁ receptors as well as beta₂ receptors. (Although ritodrine is classified as beta₂-selective, it also activates beta₁ receptors, albeit less readily than beta₂ receptors.) Adverse effects of greatest concern are pulmonary edema, hypotension, and hyperglycemia in the mother, and tachycardia in both the mother and fetus.

Terbutaline. Terbutaline [Brethine] is a beta₂-selective adrenergic agonist similar to ritodrine in actions and adverse effects. The drug's principal indication is asthma (see Chapter 71). In addition, terbutaline has been used to delay preterm labor, although it is not FDA approved for this use. Administration may be IV or SC for up to 48 hours.

In the past, it was common to give terbutaline by continuous SC infusion for long-term suppression of preterm labor. However, it is now clear that maintenance therapy with terbutaline is no more effective than placebo—and obviously more dangerous. Accordingly, the practice should be discouraged.

Nifedipine, a Calcium Channel Blocker

Nifedipine [Procardia, Adalat, Nifedical] can suppress preterm labor for at least 48 hours. Efficacy equals that of magnesium sulfate and ritodrine. Presumably, nifedipine stops contractions by blocking calcium entry into uterine smooth muscle. Maternal side effects, which are rare, include transient tachycardia, facial flushing, headache, dizziness, and nausea. Hypotension may occur in hypovolemic patients. There is some concern that nifedipine may also compromise uteroplacental blood flow. In animal studies, calcium channel blockers have caused acidosis, hypoxemia, and hypercapnia in the newborn. Combining nifedipine with magnesium sulfate can potentiate neuromuscular blockade. To suppress preterm labor, an initial 10-mg sublingual dose is followed at 15- to 20-minute intervals by two or three 10-mg oral doses, after which 10- or 20-mg oral doses are given every 4 to 6 hours for maintenance. The basic pharmacology of the calcium channel blockers is discussed in Chapter 43.

Indomethacin, a Nonsteroidal Anti-inflammatory Drug

Indomethacin [Indocin] is a second-line tocolytic drug generally reserved for women who are unresponsive to or intolerant of preferred agents. Indomethacin is as effective as magnesium sulfate or ritodrine, but carries a higher risk of neonatal complications. The drug suppresses labor by inhibiting synthesis of prostaglandins, local hormones that promote uterine contraction. Adverse neonatal outcomes include renal failure, bronchopulmonary dysplasia, respiratory distress syndrome, necrotizing enterocolitis, and intracerebral hemorrhage. In addition, indomethacin can cause premature closure of the ductus arteriosus. Adverse maternal effects include nausea, gastric irritation, interstitial nephritis, and increased postpartum bleeding. Tocolytic treatment is initiated with a 50- or 100-mg loading dose (usually rectal), followed by oral maintenance doses (25 to 50 mg) given every 4 to 8 hours for 2 to 3 days.

UTERINE STIMULANTS (OXYTOCICS)

There are three groups of uterine stimulants: (1) *oxytocin* (in a group by itself), (2) *ergot alkaloids,* and (3) *prostaglandins.* The principal use for oxytocin is induction of labor, and the

TABLE 62–2 ■ Clinical Uses of Uterine Stimulants

Drug Class and Generic Name	Trade Name	Clinical Use		
		Induction of Labor	Control of Postpartum Hemorrhage	Induction of Abortion
Oxytocin	Pitocin, Syntocinon	✔	✔	
Ergot alkaloids				
Ergonovine	Ergotrate		✔	
Methylergonovine	Methergine		✔	
Prostaglandins				
Carboprost	Hemabate		✔	✔
Dinoprostone*	Prostin E₂			✔
Misoprostol*	Cytotec			✔

*Dinoprostone and misoprostol are also used to promote cervical ripening, an application that is unrelated to uterine stimulation. When used for cervical ripening, dinoprostone is marketed as Cervidil or Prepidil.

principal use for ergot alkaloids is control of postpartum bleeding. The prostaglandins have three applications in obstetrics: induction of abortion, control of postpartum bleeding, and promotion of cervical ripening. Two of these uses—induction of abortion (discussed in Chapter 60) and control of postpartum bleeding—are based on the ability of prostaglandins to stimulate uterine contractions; promotion of cervical ripening is unrelated to uterine stimulation. Clinical applications of the oxytocic drugs are summarized in Table 62–2.

Oxytocin

Oxytocin [Pitocin, Syntocinon] is a peptide hormone produced by the posterior pituitary. This hormone promotes uterine contraction during parturition and stimulates the milk-ejection reflex. The primary therapeutic use of oxytocin is induction of labor near term, a procedure for which oxytocin is the agent of choice.

Physiologic and Pharmacologic Effects

Uterine Stimulation. Oxytocin can increase the force, frequency, and duration of uterine contractions. The ability of the uterus to respond to oxytocin depends on the stage of gestation: Early in pregnancy, uterine sensitivity to oxytocin is low; as pregnancy proceeds, the uterus becomes progressively more responsive; and just prior to term, a large and abrupt increase in responsiveness develops. Sensitivity increases over time because the number of oxytocin receptors on uterine smooth muscle increases throughout pregnancy. Although uterine sensitivity to oxytocin is low early in pregnancy, oxytocin can still initiate and enhance contractions at this stage. However, the doses required are much larger than those needed to stimulate the uterus at term.

Despite the profound effects of oxytocin on uterine contractility, the precise role of oxytocin in spontaneous labor and delivery has not been established. We do know that giving exogenous oxytocin can elicit contractions identical to those seen during spontaneous labor. However, we also know that parturition can take place with virtually no oxytocin present—although labor will be prolonged. Furthermore, during normal labor or during labor induced artificially (through rupture of the membranes), only modest increases in plasma oxytocin occur. From these observations we can conclude that, although oxytocin is not absolutely required for parturition, the hormone probably acts to facilitate contractions. However, it is not certain that oxytocin is responsible for *initiating* labor.

Milk Ejection. Milk is produced by glandular tissue of the breast and is later transferred, via small channels, into large sinuses within the breast. Once in these sinuses, milk is readily accessible to the suckling infant. Transfer of milk to the sinuses is brought about by the milk-ejection reflex: When the infant sucks on the breast, neuronal stimuli are sent to the posterior pituitary, causing release of oxytocin; oxytocin then causes contraction of the smooth muscle surrounding the small milk channels, thereby forcing milk into the large sinuses. In the absence of oxytocin, milk ejection does not occur.

Water Retention. Oxytocin is similar in structure to antidiuretic hormone (ADH), which acts on the kidney to decrease excretion of water. Although less potent than ADH, oxytocin can nonetheless promote renal retention of water.

Pharmacokinetics

Oxytocin is administered IV or IM. The plasma half-life is short, ranging from 12 to 17 minutes. Elimination is by hepatic metabolism and renal excretion.

Use for Induction of Labor

Rationale. Induction of labor is reserved for (1) pregnancy that has continued beyond term (i.e., beyond 42 weeks) and (2) pregnancy in which early vaginal delivery is likely to decrease morbidity and mortality for the mother or infant. Post-term pregnancy is the most common reason for induction. Reasons for *early* induction include premature rupture of the membranes, severe maternal infection, diabetes mellitus, placental insufficiency, renal insufficiency, anemia, and preeclampsia (at or near term). Labor should be induced only when continued pregnancy constitutes a greater risk to the mother and fetus than does the risk of induction itself. Induction for elective purposes (e.g., convenience of the obstetrician) is controversial.

Preinduction Preparation. Induction should not be done if the fetal lungs have not yet matured, or if the cervix is not yet ripe. Accordingly, prior to induction, if the fetal lungs are still immature, maturation should be hastened with glucocorticoids (see Chapter 103). Likewise, if the cervix is not yet ripe, ripening should be induced with dinoprostone or misoprostol (see below). Alternatively, cervical ripening can be induced mechanically (with a cervical dilator) or by membrane stripping (i.e., by separating the chorioamnionic membranes from the internal surface of the uterus).

Precautions and Contraindications. Improper use of oxytocin can be hazardous. Uterine rupture may occur, which may result in death of the mother, the infant, or both. The likelihood of trauma is especially high in the presence of cephalopelvic disproportion, fetal malpresentation, placental abnormalities, umbilical prolapse, previous uterine surgery, and fetal distress. Oxytocin is contraindicated in pregnancies with any of these characteristics. In addition, oxytocin is contraindicated in women with active genital herpes. Induction of labor in women of high parity (five or more pregnancies) carries a high risk of uterine rupture, and hence oxytocin must be used with great caution in these patients.

Adverse Effect: Water Intoxication. When administered in large doses, oxytocin exerts an antidiuretic effect. If large volumes of fluid have been administered along with oxytocin, retention of water may produce intoxication. However, at the doses employed to induce labor, water intoxication is rare.

Dosage and Administration. For induction of labor, oxytocin is administered by intravenous infusion. The flow rate must be carefully controlled with an infusion pump. Solutions should be dilute (e.g., 10 mU/ml) and infused at an initial rate of no more than 1 to 2 mU/min. The infusion rate is then gradually increased (by increments of 1 to 2 mU/min every 30 to 60 minutes) until uterine contractions resembling those of spontaneous labor have been produced (i.e., contractions every 2 to 3 minutes and lasting 45 to 60 seconds). The infusion rate should rarely exceed 10 mU/min.

During oxytocin infusion, constant monitoring is required. The mother should be monitored for blood pressure, pulse rate, and uterine contractility (frequency, duration, and intensity). The fetus should be monitored for heart rate and rhythm. In the event of significant maternal or fetal distress, the infusion should be stopped; contractions will diminish rapidly. Complications that usually require interruption of the infusion are (1) elevation of resting uterine pressure above 15 to 20 mm Hg, (2) contractions that persist for more than 1 minute, (3) contractions that occur more often than every 2 to 3 minutes, and (4) pronounced alteration in fetal heart rate or rhythm.

Additional Therapeutic Uses

Augmentation of Labor. Oxytocin may be employed if labor is dysfunctional. However, patients must be judiciously selected, and dosage must be regulated with special care. As a rule, oxytocic agents should not be used to promote labor that is already in progress, even if labor is proceeding slowly: By intensifying the force of contractions, oxytocin may cause uterine damage (laceration or rupture) or trauma to the infant.

Postpartum Use. Oxytocin can be administered IM or IV following placental delivery to control bleeding or hemorrhage and to increase uterine tone.

Abortion. Oxytocin has been employed during the second trimester to manage incomplete abortion. Intravenous infusion of 10 units at a rate of 10 to 20 mU/min is often effective in emptying the uterus. However, oxytocin is not a method of choice.

Ergot Alkaloids: Ergonovine and Methylergonovine

Ergot is a dried preparation of *Claviceps purpurea*, a fungus that grows on rye plants. The ergot alkaloids are compounds present in ergot. Ergot is capable of inducing powerful uterine contractions, a fact known to midwifes for centuries. Analysis of ergot has revealed the presence of several pharmacologically active constituents. Of these, *ergonovine* is the most effective uterine stimulant. A derivative of ergonovine—*methylergonovine*—has been synthesized and produces effects very much like those of ergonovine. Because the actions of ergonovine and methylergonovine are so similar, we will consider these agents jointly.

In obstetrics, the ergot alkaloids are used to control postpartum bleeding. However, because they carry a high risk of severe hypertension, these drugs are generally reserved for women who have not responded to safer agents: oxytocin and carboprost tromethamine.

Pharmacologic Effects

Ergot alkaloids produce their effects by stimulating a variety of receptors (adrenergic, dopaminergic, serotonergic). These drugs exert their most profound effects on uterine and vascular smooth muscle.

Effects on the Uterus. Ergot alkaloids stimulate uterine contraction. In small doses, these agents produce contractions of moderate strength that alternate with uterine relaxation of normal degree and duration. With large doses, the force and frequency of contractions are greatly increased, and the extent of uterine relaxation is reduced; sustained contraction is not uncommon. Because contractions may be prolonged, *ergot alkaloids are not employed for induction of labor.*

Vascular Effects. Ergot alkaloids can cause constriction of arterioles and veins. This ability underlies the use of two ergot alkaloids—ergotamine and dihydroergotamine—to treat migraine headache (see Chapter 29). Vasoconstriction may also contribute to control of postpartum bleeding.

Pharmacokinetics

Regardless of the route employed, ergonovine and methylergonovine act rapidly. Uterine contractions begin within 60 seconds of IV injection, and within 10 minutes of oral or IM administration. Effects persist for several hours.

Therapeutic Uses

Postpartum Use. The ergot alkaloids may be used postpartum and postabortion to increase uterine tone and decrease bleeding. The ability of these drugs to induce sustained uterine contraction makes them very effective for these purposes. Administration is usually delayed until after delivery of the placenta. The patient should be monitored for blood pressure, pulse rate, and uterine contractility. Cramping occurs as part of the therapeutic response, but may also indicate overdose. Owing to a high risk of severe hypertension, many physicians now reserve the ergot alkaloids for patients who have not responded to safer alternatives (i.e., oxytocin or carboprost tromethamine).

Augmentation of Labor. Because contractions may be both intense and prolonged, ergot alkaloids are not recommended for use during labor. If these drugs are given during labor, excessive uterine tone can cause trauma to the mother, fetus, or both. Placental blood flow may be reduced, resulting in fetal hypoxia and uterine rupture. In addition, cervical laceration may occur.

Migraine. Ergot alkaloids relieve migraine in part by constricting dilated cerebral blood vessels. The two ergot preparations employed in migraine are ergotamine and dihydroergotamine. The pharmacology of these drugs and their use in migraine are discussed in Chapter 29 (Drugs for Headache).

Adverse Effects

When ergot alkaloids are given orally or IM, significant adverse effects are rare. In contrast, IV administration frequently causes *hypertension.* This reaction can be severe and may be associated with nausea, vomiting, and headache; convulsions and even death have occurred. Accordingly, IV administration should be reserved for emergencies. Furthermore, patients with pre-existing hypertension should not be given these drugs. Caution should be exercised in patients with cardiovascular, renal, or hepatic disorders.

Contraindications

Ergot alkaloids are contraindicated for women who are pregnant, hypertensive, or hypersensitive to these drugs. The drugs are also contraindicated for induction of labor and for use in the presence of threatened or ongoing spontaneous abortion.

Preparations, Dosage, and Administration

Preparations. Ergonovine maleate [Ergotrate Maleate] and methylergonovine maleate [Methergine] are both dispensed in solution (0.2 mg/ml) for IV and IM administration. Methylergonovine is also available in 0.2-mg tablets.

Dosage and Administration. For parenteral therapy, ergonovine and methylergonovine are usually administered IM; intravenous administration is hazardous and should be reserved for emergency control of postpartum hemorrhage. Treatment is usually initiated only after passage of the placenta. Dosages for both drugs are as follows: *intramuscular* (for control of postpartum bleeding), 0.2 mg initially, repeated every 2 hours as needed; *intravenous* (for control of uterine hemorrhage), 0.2 mg infused over 60 seconds or more.

The *oral* dosage for methylergonovine (to promote involution of the uterus) is 0.2 to 0.4 mg every 6 to 8 hours for up to 1 week.

Carboprost Tromethamine
Therapeutic Use

Carboprost tromethamine [Hemabate], also known as 15-methyl prostaglandin F$_2$ alpha, is a preferred agent for controlling postpartum hemorrhage. The drug suppresses bleeding primarily by causing intense uterine contractions, and partly by causing vasoconstriction. In most cases, bleeding can be stopped with a single 250-µg IM dose. If needed, the same dose can be repeated every 15 to 90 minutes, but the cumulative dosage should not exceed 2 mg. In addition to its postpartum use, carboprost is used to induce abortion (see Chapter 60).

Adverse Effects

As with other prostaglandins, GI reactions are very common. The underlying cause is stimulation of smooth muscle of the gut. Vomiting and diarrhea occur in up to 60% of patients. Nausea is also common. Gastrointestinal reactions can be reduced by pretreatment with antiemetic and antidiarrheal medications.

Fever is common. If body temperature rises, it is important to differentiate between drug-induced fever and pyrexia resulting from endometritis.

Like other prostaglandins, carboprost causes vasoconstriction as well as constriction of the bronchi. As a result, treatment carries a risk of hypertension and impairment of respiration.

Precautions and Contraindications

Carboprost is contraindicated for women with acute pelvic inflammatory disease and active disease of the heart, lungs, kidneys, or liver. The drug should be used with caution in women with a history of asthma, hypertension, diabetes, or uterine scarring.

DRUGS USED TO PROMOTE CERVICAL RIPENING

The term *cervical ripening* refers to changes the cervix undergoes prior to normal delivery. During pregnancy, the cervix is elongated, rigid, and constricted. When ripening occurs, the cervix shortens, softens, and dilates, thereby permitting the fetus to pass through the birth canal. If induced delivery using oxytocin is attempted in the absence of ripening, maternal and fetal injury can result. Accordingly, if oxytocin is to be used before natural ripening has occurred, a ripening agent should be used first. Two drugs are employed: dinoprostone and misoprostol. Both are prostaglandins. Of the two, only dinoprostone is FDA approved for cervical ripening. However, misoprostol is also effective, and much less expensive.

Dinoprostone

Dinoprostone [Prepidil, Cervidil] is the most widely used agent for promoting cervical ripening prior to induction of labor with oxytocin. The drug is a synthetic prostaglandin identical in structure to endogenous prostaglandin E$_2$ (PGE$_2$), a compound produced by fetal membranes and by the placenta. Endogenous PGE$_2$ has two roles in the birthing process: It promotes cervical ripening, and later stimulates uterine contractions. Cervical ripening results from activation of collagenase, an enzyme that breaks down the collagen network that makes the cervix rigid. When used to promote ripening, dinoprostone shortens the duration of labor, allows a reduction in oxytocin dosage, and decreases the need for cesarean delivery. Because it can stimulate uterine contractions, dinoprostone is also used to induce abortion (see Chapter 60). For promotion of cervical ripening, dinoprostone is available in two formulations: a gel and a vaginal insert.

Dinoprostone Gel

Dinoprostone gel [Prepidil] is dispensed in single-dose, prefilled syringes that contain 0.5 mg dinoprostone/2.5 ml gel. Administration is intracervical, using the syringe and endocervical catheter (10- or 20-mm tip) supplied by the manufacturer. To prevent leakage, the patient should lie supine during administration and for at least 30 minutes after. If the desired response has not occurred within 6 hours, a second 0.5-mg dose can be given, followed 6 hours later by a third, if needed. (Most women need at least two doses, and 50% need a third.) Because dinoprostone can stimulate uterine contractions, and may thereby cause fetal distress, uterine activity and fetal heart rate should be monitored continuously. Monitoring should start before each dose and continue at least 2 hours after. Oxytocin is given 6 to 12 hours after the last dose of dinoprostone. The major adverse effect of dinoprostone is hyperstimulation of the uterus, which occurs in 1% of patients using the gel. Rarely, systemic absorption results in nausea, vomiting, diarrhea, and fever. Dinoprostone gel is unstable and must be stored refrigerated, between 2°C and 8°C. Treatment is expensive: Each 0.5-mg dose costs about $150, making the total $450 for women who require three doses.

Dinoprostone Vaginal Inserts

Dinoprostone vaginal inserts [Cervidil] consist of a pouch (containing 10 mg of the drug) to which a long tape is attached. The purpose of the tape is to permit rapid removal of the pouch. Following insertion in the posterior fornix of the vagina, the pouch releases dinoprostone slowly (0.3 mg/hr) for 12 hours. The patient should remain supine for at least 2 hours after pouch insertion. The pouch is removed when active labor occurs or when 12 hours have elapsed, whichever comes first. If oxytocin is needed, administration can begin 30 minutes after removing the pouch. As with dinoprostone gel, the major adverse effect of the insert is uterine hyperstimulation, which develops in 5% of patients (compared with only 1% of those receiving the gel). To minimize harm, uterine activity and fetal heart rate should undergo continuous monitoring while the insert is in place and for at least 15 minutes after its removal. Compared with dinoprostone gel, the inserts have two advantages. First, treatment is almost always cheaper. Second, because the inserts can be easily removed, drug delivery can be stopped as soon as (1) labor starts (thereby avoiding unnecessary drug exposure) or (2) uterine hyperstimulation develops (thereby minimizing uterine contractions and related fetal distress). The vaginal inserts are unstable and must be stored frozen, between −10°C and −20°C. The cost of one insert is about $175, compared with $150 for one dose of the gel. Nonetheless, treatment with the inserts is generally less expensive. Why? Because most women require two or three doses of the gel (total cost: $300 to $450), but only one insert (total cost: $175).

Misoprostol

Misoprostol [Cytotec] is an attractive alternative to dinoprostone for promoting cervical ripening, although misoprostol is not approved for this use. Compared with dinoprostone, misoprostol is more effective, more convenient (stores at room temperature versus refrigerated), and *much* less expensive (treatment costs about $1 versus $175 to $450). Unfortunately, misoprostol also causes a higher incidence of uterine hyperstimulation. To induce cervical ripening, a 25-μg dose (one-fourth of a 100-μg tablet) is inserted into the posterior fornix of the vagina. Dosing is repeated every 4 hours as needed. In women given misoprostol, delivery occurs faster than in those given dino-

prostone, and there is less need for oxytocin. To minimize risk from uterine hyperstimulation, fetal heart rate and uterine activity should be monitored continuously. In addition to its use for cervical ripening, misoprostol is used to induce abortion (see Chapter 60) and, primarily, to protect against peptic ulcers (see Chapter 73).

⠿ KEY POINTS

- Tocolytic drugs suppress contraction of uterine smooth muscle.
- Tocolytic drugs have only one indication: delay of preterm labor.
- Tocolytic drugs are able to delay labor for a maximum of 72 hours.
- Magnesium sulfate is the current tocolytic of choice.
- Magnesium sulfate suppresses labor by inhibiting release of acetylcholine from neurons that innervate uterine smooth muscle.
- By inhibiting transmitter release from neurons that innervate skeletal muscle, magnesium sulfate (in toxic doses) can cause profound weakness and respiratory arrest.
- About 2% of patients receiving magnesium sulfate develop pulmonary edema, which can be fatal.
- Magnesium sulfate is contraindicated in the patients with myasthenia gravis (because the disease causes muscle weakness), renal failure (because magnesium is eliminated entirely by the kidneys), and hypocalcemia (because hypocalcemia intensifies magnesium-induced suppression of neurotransmitter release).
- Oxytocic agents stimulate contraction of uterine smooth muscle.
- Oxytocics have three major applications: induction or augmentation of labor, control of postpartum bleeding, and induction of abortion.
- The principal indication for oxytocin is induction of labor, which is appropriate when (1) pregnancy has continued beyond term or (2) early vaginal delivery is likely to decrease morbidity or mortality for the mother or infant.
- Used improperly (e.g., in pregnancies with cephalopelvic disproportion), oxytocin can cause uterine rupture.
- Two oxytocic drugs—oxytocin and carboprost tromethamine—are preferred agents for controlling postpartum hemorrhage.
- Because they pose a risk of severe hypertension, ergonovine and methylergonovine are generally considered second-line drugs for controlling postpartum hemorrhage.
- Dinoprostone is a prostaglandin used to promote cervical ripening prior to inducing labor with oxytocin.

Summary of Major Nursing Implications

MAGNESIUM SULFATE

Preadministration Assessment

Therapeutic Goal

Magnesium sulfate is used to delay preterm labor up to 72 hours, thereby buying time to accelerate fetal lung maturation with glucocorticoids.

Identifying High-Risk Patients

Magnesium sulfate is *contraindicated* for women with myasthenia gravis, renal failure, or hypocalcemia.

Implementation: Administration

Route

Intravenous.

Administration

Give an initial bolus followed by continuous infusion using a controlled infusion pump.

Ongoing Evaluation and Interventions

Summary of Monitoring

Monitor magnesium levels, renal function, fluid balance, and deep tendon reflexes.

Minimizing Adverse Effects

Pulmonary Edema. Pulmonary edema develops in 2% of patients. Manage by discontinuing the magnesium infusion and giving a diuretic to accelerate magnesium excretion.

Weakness and Respiratory Arrest. Toxic doses can impair transmitter release from neurons that innervate skeletal muscle, and thereby causing profound weakness and respiratory arrest. Support respiration as needed.

Neonatal Hypotonia. Excessive magnesium can impair skeletal muscle function in the neonate. If necessary, provide mechanical support of respiration until the infant can breathe unassisted.

OXYTOCIN

The implications summarized here apply only to the use of oxytocin for induction of labor, the drug's principal use.

Preadministration Assessment

Therapeutic Goal

Oxytocin is given to initiate or improve uterine contractions. Treatment is reserved for pregnancies that have gone beyond term or for pregnancies in which early vaginal delivery is likely to decrease morbidity and mortality for the mother or infant.

Baseline Data

The history should determine parity, previous obstetric problems, stillbirths, and abortions. Full maternal and fetal status should be assessed, including the degree of cervical ripening and fetal lung maturity.

Identifying High-Risk Patients

Induction of labor is *contraindicated* in the presence of cephalopelvic disproportion, fetal malpresentation, placental abnormality, umbilical prolapse, previous major surgery to the uterus or cervix, fetal distress, and active genital herpes.

Use with *caution* in women of high parity (five or more pregnancies).

Induction should not be conducted in the absence of cervical ripening or fetal lung maturation. If indicated, promote cervical ripening mechanically or with drugs, and promote fetal lung maturation with glucocorticoids.

Implementation: Administration

Route

Intravenous.

Administration

Administer by carefully controlled infusion, using an infusion pump.

Ongoing Evaluation and Interventions

Minimizing Adverse Effects

Uterine contractions of excessive intensity, frequency, and duration can cause maternal and fetal harm. Monitor uterine contractility (frequency, duration, and intensity), maternal blood pressure, and fetal and maternal heart rate. Interrupt the infusion if any of the following occur: (1) resting intrauterine pressure rises above 15 to 20 mm Hg, (2) individual contractions persist longer than 1 minute, (3) contractions occur more often than every 2 to 3 minutes, and (4) fetal heart rate or rhythm changes significantly.

ERGOT ALKALOIDS: ERGONOVINE AND METHYLERGONOVINE

Preadministration Assessment

Therapeutic Goal

Prevention and treatment of postpartum and postabortion hemorrhage.

Identifying High-Risk Patients

Ergot alkaloids are *contraindicated* during pregnancy, for induction of labor, in women with hypertension or allergy to ergot alkaloids, and in the presence of threatened or ongoing spontaneous abortion.

Implementation: Administration

Routes

Oral and IM. Preferred.
Intravenous. Hazardous; reserve for hemorrhagic emergencies.

Administration

As a rule, administer after passage of the placenta. Perform IV injections slowly (over 60 seconds or more).

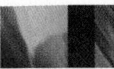 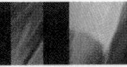

Summary of Major Nursing Implications—cont'd

Ongoing Evaluation and Interventions
Evaluating Therapeutic Effects

Monitor blood pressure, pulse rate, and uterine activity. Report sudden increases in blood pressure, excessive uterine bleeding, and insufficient uterine tone. Cramping is normal but may also indicate overdose.

Minimizing Adverse Effects

Significant adverse effects—*hypertension, nausea, vomiting, headache, convulsions,* and *death*—usually occur only with IV administration. To minimize risk, infuse slowly (over 60 seconds or more) and reserve IV administration for emergencies.

DINOPROSTONE
Preadministration Assessment
Therapeutic Goal

Dinoprostone is used to promote cervical ripening.

Identifying High-Risk Patients

Dinoprostone is *contraindicated* for women with acute pelvic inflammatory disease and active disease of the heart, lungs, kidneys, or liver. Use with *caution* in women with a history of asthma, hypotension, hypertension, diabetes, or uterine scarring.

Implementation: Administration
Routes

Vaginal insert and gel for intracervical instillation.

Ongoing Evaluation and Interventions
Evaluating Therapeutic Effects

Assess the cervix for elongation, softening, and dilation.

Minimizing Adverse Effects

GI Disturbances. Nausea, vomiting, and diarrhea can be reduced by pretreatment with antiemetic and antidiarrheal drugs.

Fever. Fever may be induced by dinoprostone or it may indicate endometritis. If fever develops, a differential diagnosis must be made.

Review of the Immune System

Life is a constant battle—and the immune system is the army that helps us prevail. This system protects us from invading organisms (viruses, bacteria, fungi, and parasites) and can destroy cancer cells before they destroy us. Unfortunately, the army does not always act in our best interest: It can attack transplanted organs and tissues and, when it runs amok, can turn on the very cells it was intended to protect.

To study the immune system, we begin with an overview. After that, we discuss the two major types of specific immune responses: antibody-mediated immunity (humoral immunity) and cell-mediated immunity.

INTRODUCTION TO THE IMMUNE SYSTEM

Our objective in this section is to establish an overview of immune system components and how they function. Much of the information introduced here is amplified later.

Natural Immunity Versus Specific Acquired Immunity

Our bodies can mount two types of immune responses, referred to as *natural immunity* (innate or native immunity) and *specific acquired immunity*. Factors that confer natural immunity include physical barriers (e.g., skin), phagocytic cells, and natural killer cells. All of these factors are present prior to exposure to a particular infectious agent and all respond nonspecifically. In contrast, specific acquired immune responses occur only after exposure to a foreign substance. The foreign substances that induce specific responses are called *antigens,* and the objective of the immune response is to destroy the antigen. With each succeeding re-exposure to a particular antigen, the specific immune response to that antigen becomes more rapid and more intense. Specific immune responses are possible because certain cells of the immune system (T lymphocytes and B lymphocytes) possess receptors that can recognize individual antigens. In this chapter, our focus is on specific acquired immunity and not on natural immunity.

Cell-Mediated Immunity Versus Antibody-Mediated (Humoral) Immunity

Specific acquired immune responses can be classified as either cell mediated or humoral. *Cell-mediated immunity* refers to immune responses in which targets are attacked directly by immune system cells—specifically, cytolytic T cells and macrophages. *Humoral immunity* refers to immune responses that are mediated by *antibodies.* (The term *humoral*—defined as "pertaining to elements dissolved in blood or body fluids"—simply connotes that antibodies are present dissolved in the blood.)

Introduction to Cells of the Immune System

Immune responses are mediated by several types of cells, some of which play a more central role than others. The major actors are the *lymphocytes* (B cells, cytolytic T cells, helper T cells), *macrophages,* and *dendritic cells.* Accessory cells include neutrophils and basophils. With the exception of some dendritic cells, all of the cells involved in the immune response arise from pluripotent stem cells in the bone marrow (Fig. 63–1) and, for at least part of their life cycle, circulate in the blood. Defining characteristics of individual immune system cells are summarized in Table 63–1.

B Lymphocytes (B Cells). B lymphocytes have the job of making *antibodies.* Hence, B cells mediate humoral immunity. As discussed below, antibody specificity is determined by the structure of highly specific receptors found on the surface of B cells. Like all other lymphocytes, B cells circulate in both the blood and the lymph. B cells are so named because in chickens, where B cells were discovered, these cells are produced in the *bursa of Fabricius,* a structure not found in mammals. In humans and other mammals, B cells are produced in the bone marrow.

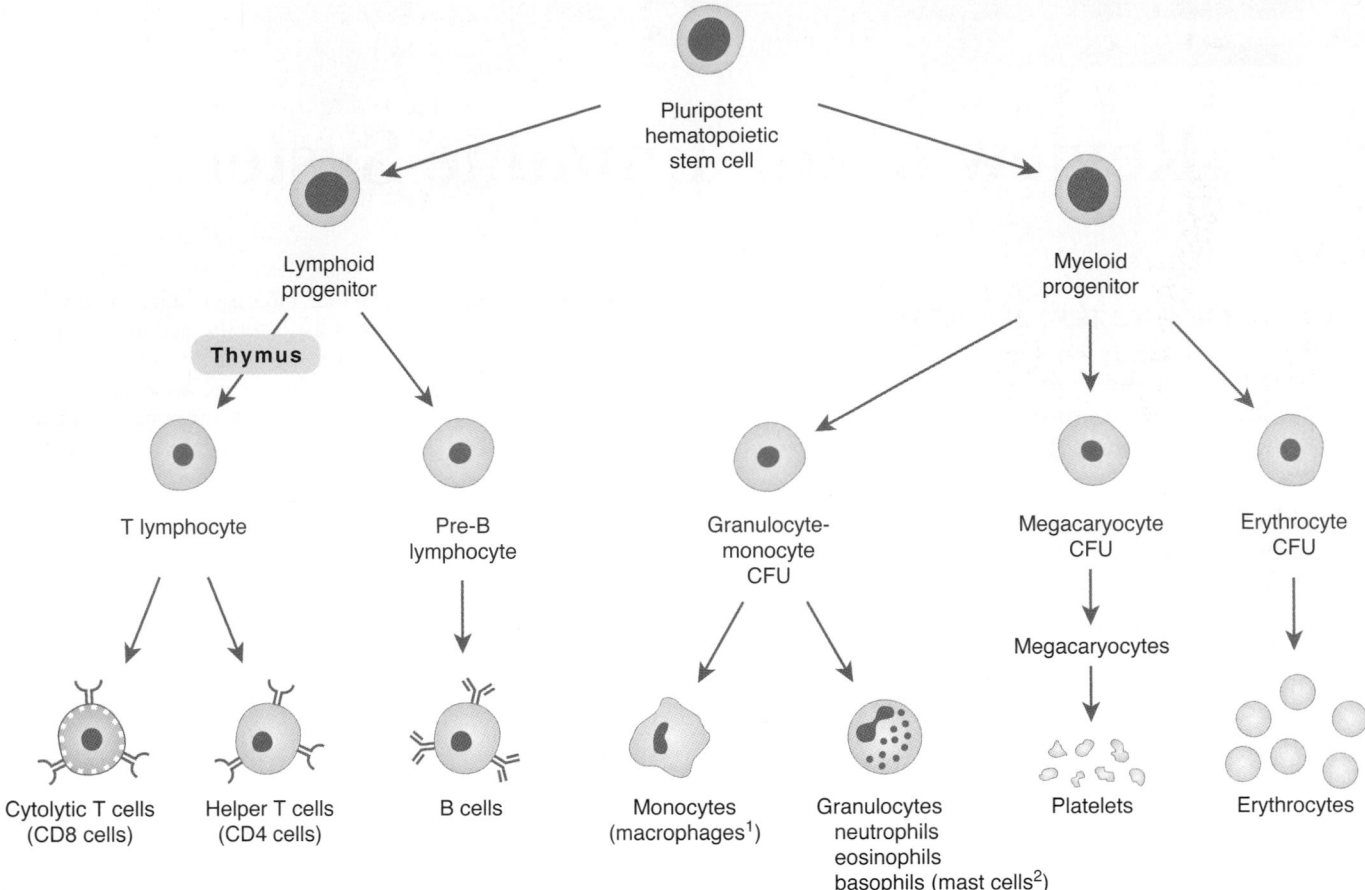

Figure 63–1 ■ **Maturation of blood cells.**
With the exception of platelets and erythrocytes, all of the mature blood cells shown participate in immune responses. However, only cells of lymphoid origin (cytolytic T cells, helper T cells, B cells) possess receptors that can recognize specific antigens. (CFU = colony forming unit.)
[1]Monocytes that have moved into tissues are called macrophages.
[2]Basophils that have moved into tissues are called mast cells.

Cytolytic T Lymphocytes (Cytolytic T Cells, CD8 Cells).
Cytolytic T cells are key players in cellular immunity. These cells do not produce antibodies. Rather, they attack and kill target cells directly. Specificity of attack is determined by the presence of antigen molecules on the surface of the target cell and specific receptors for that antigen on the surface of the T cell. Cytolytic T cells are also known as *CD8 cells* and *cytotoxic T cells*. The designation "CD8" refers to the presence of cell-surface marker molecules known as *cell differentiation complex 8*. The "T" in T cell stands for thymus, the organ in which cytolytic T cells and helper T cells mature. Like B cells, cytolytic T cells circulate in the blood and lymph.

Helper T Lymphocytes (Helper T Cells, CD4 Cells).
Helper T cells contribute to the immune response in three ways: (1) they have an essential role in antibody production by B cells, (2) they release factors that promote delayed-type hypersensitivity (DTH), and (3) they participate in the activation of cytolytic T cells. Specificity of helper T cells is achieved through highly specific cell-surface receptors that recognize individual antigens. Like other lymphocytes, helper T cells circulate in the blood and lymph. Helper T cells carry CD4 marker molecules on their surface, and hence are referred to as CD4 cells.

The term *helper* is somewhat misleading, in that it connotes a useful but dispensable role. Nothing could be further from reality. Helper T cells are not simply nice to have around, they are absolutely required for an effective immune response. The critical nature of their contribution—and the grim consequences of their absence—are manifested in people with AIDS: Helper T cells are the immune cells that HIV attacks; because of helper T-cell loss, AIDS patients are at high risk of death from opportunistic infections.

Macrophages. Macrophages begin their existence in the bone marrow, enter the blood as monocytes, and then infiltrate tissues, where they evolve into macrophages. Macrophages are present in all organs and tissues.

The primary function of macrophages is *phagocytosis* (i.e., ingestion of microbes, other foreign material, and cellular debris). In their role as phagocytes, macrophages are the principal scavengers of the body. Although their major job is phagocytosis, macrophages also have an important role in specific acquired immunity, natural immunity, and inflammation.

In specific acquired immunity, macrophages have three functions: (1) they are required for activation of T cells (both helper T cells and cytolytic T cells), (2) they are the final mediators of

TABLE 63–1 ■ Cells of the Immune System

Cell Type	Synonyms	Primary Immune-Related Actions
Major Cell Types		
B lymphocytes	B cells	• Produce antibodies
Cytolytic T lymphocytes (CTLs)	Cytolytic T cells, cytotoxic T cells, CD8 cells	• Lyse target cells
Helper T lymphocytes	Helper T cells, CD4 cells	• Promote proliferation and differentiation of B cells and CTLs • Initiate delayed-type hypersensitivity
Macrophages		• Promote proliferation and differentiation of helper T cells and CTLs by serving as antigen-presenting cells • Participate in delayed-type hypersensitivity • Phagocytize cells tagged with antibodies • Phagocytize cells in the effector stage of delayed-type hypersensitivity
Dendritic cells		• Promote proliferation of cytolytic T cells and helper T cells by serving as antigen-presenting cells
Accessory Cells		
Mast cells		• Mediate immediate hypersensitivity reactions
Basophils		• Mediate immediate hypersensitivity reactions
Neutrophils	Polymorphonuclear leukocytes	• Phagocytize foreign particles (e.g., bacteria), especially those tagged with IgG • Mediate inflammation
Eosinophils		• Attack helminths and other foreign particles that have been coated with IgE • Contribute to immediate hypersensitivity reactions

DTH, and (3) they phagocytize cells that have been tagged with antibodies. Of these three immune-related roles, activation of T cells is arguably the most critical. When performing this function, macrophages are referred to as *antigen-presenting cells* (APCs). Because antigen presentation is an absolute requirement for a specific immune response to occur (see below), we can appreciate how important macrophages are to immunity.

Dendritic Cells. Dendritic cells perform the same antigen-presenting task as macrophages. However, unlike macrophages, dendritic cells do not also serve as scavengers. Dendritic cells are found in lymph nodes and other lymphoid tissues.

Mast Cells and Basophils. These cells mediate immediate hypersensitivity reactions. Mast cells, which are derived from basophils, are concentrated in the skin and other soft tissues; basophils circulate in the blood. Both cell types release histamine, heparin, and other compounds that cause the symptoms of immediate hypersensitivity. Release of these mediators is triggered when an antigen binds to antibodies on the cell surface. The role of mast cells and basophils in allergic reactions is discussed further in Chapter 66 (Antihistamines).

Neutrophils. Neutrophils, also known as *polymorphonuclear leukocytes,* phagocytize bacteria and other foreign particles. As discussed below, neutrophils avidly devour cells that have been tagged with antibodies of the immunoglobulin G (IgG) class. Accordingly, neutrophils can be viewed as important effectors in humoral immunity. Neutrophils are also major contributors to inflammation.

Eosinophils. Eosinophils attack and destroy foreign particles that have been coated with antibodies of the IgE class.

Their usual target is helminths (parasitic worms). Eosinophils also contribute to tissue injury and inflammation associated with immediate hypersensitivity reactions.

Antibodies

Antibodies are a family of structurally related glycoproteins that mediate humoral immunity. The most characteristic feature of antibodies is their ability to recognize and bind specific antigens. Alternative names for antibodies are *immunoglobulins* and *gamma globulins.*

All antibodies are produced by B lymphocytes. Some of the antibodies that B cells produce are retained on the surface of the B cell, where they serve as the receptors whereby B cells recognize specific antigens. However, most of the antibodies that B cells produce are secreted from the cell, after which they bind to their specific antigen, thereby initiating the effector phase of humoral immunity. The process of antibody production is discussed in detail below.

All antibodies are composed of units that have the same basic structure. As shown in Figure 63–2, antibodies have four chains: two heavy chains and two light chains. Disulfide bridges connect the four chains to form a unit. Each heavy chain and each light chain has two regions, one in which the sequence of amino acids is *constant* and one in which the sequence is highly *variable.* The variable regions form the antigen-binding site.

There are five classes of antibodies, known as IgA, IgD, IgE, IgG, and IgM. All are constructed from the same basic parts described above. However, the heavy chains

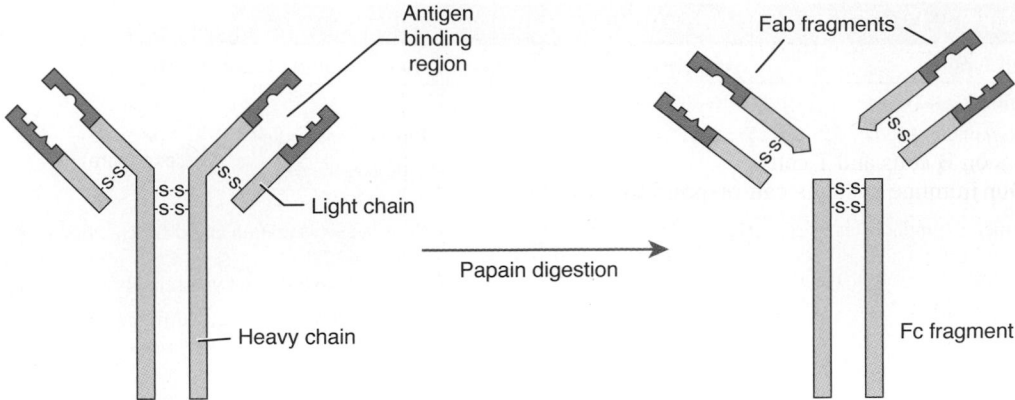

Figure 63–2 ■ Antibody structure.
The basic antibody structure depicting heavy and light chains is shown on the left. Variable regions of the heavy and light chains, which form the antigen-binding site, appear in green. As shown on the right, papain digestion of antibodies produces two types of fragments: Fab fragments, which retain the ability to bind antigen, and Fc fragments, which do not bind antigen and tend to crystallize in the test tube.

TABLE 63–2 ■ Functions of Antibody Classes	
Class	**Function**
IgA	• Located in mucous membranes of the GI tract and lungs and in many secretions, where it serves as the first line of defense against microbes entering the body via these routes • Transferred to infants via breast milk; is not absorbed from the GI tract but does protect the infant against microbes *in* the GI tract
IgD	• Found only on the surface of mature B cells, where it serves as a receptor for antigen recognition (along with IgM)
IgE	• Binds to the surface of mast cells; subsequent binding of antigen to IgE stimulates release of histamine, heparin, and other mediators from the mast cells, thereby causing symptoms of allergy (e.g., hives, hay fever) • Binds to parasitic worms, after which eosinophils bind to IgE and release compounds that lyse the worms
IgG	• Produced in copious amounts in response to antigenic stimulation, and hence is the major antibody in blood • Fixes complement and thereby promotes target-cell lysis • Binds target cells and thereby enhances phagocytosis • Transferred across the placenta to the fetal circulation, thereby providing neonatal immunity
IgM	• First class of antibody produced in response to an antigen • Fixes complement and thereby promotes target-cell lysis • Present on the surface of mature B cells, where it serves as a receptor for antigen recognition (along with IgD)

differ for each class. Primary functions of the five classes are summarized in Table 63–2.

When antibodies are subjected to digestion by papain in the laboratory, they break down into three pieces (see Fig. 63–2). Two of the pieces retain the ability to bind antigen, and hence are called *Fab fragments* (fragment, antigen binding). The third piece does not bind antigen and tends to form crystals in the test tube, and hence is called the *Fc fragment* (fragment, crystalline).

Antigens

Antigens are molecules that induce specific immune responses and, as a result, become the targets of those responses. By way of analogy, an antigen is like the child who pokes a stick in a hornet's nest, at once triggering a response and becoming its target. An antigen may trigger production of antibodies, cytotoxic T cells, or both—all of which can then attack the antigen.

Most antigens are large molecules. Because antigens are big, the antigen-binding region of the resultant antibodies cannot recognize and bind the entire antigen molecule. Rather, the antibodies recognize and bind selected small portions of the antigen, referred to as *epitopes* or *antigenic determinants*. All antigens have multiple epitopes. As a result, more than one antibody can bind the antigen.

In research and in clinical practice, we may want to generate antibodies to molecules that are too small to induce an immune response. To overcome this obstacle, we can link the small molecule to a larger molecule, usually a protein. When this is done, the small molecule is referred to as a *hapten*, and the large molecule is referred to as a *carrier*. At least some of the resultant antibodies will be selective for the hapten.

Characteristic Features of Immune Responses

Cell-mediated immunity and humoral immunity share five characteristic features: specificity, diversity, memory, time limitation, and selectivity for antigens of nonself origin (i.e., the ability to discriminate between self and nonself).

Specificity. Cell-mediated and humoral immune responses are triggered by specific antigens, and their purpose is to destroy the antigen that triggered the response. The ability to respond to a specific antigen (i.e., the ability to make subtle distinctions among related molecules) is conferred by highly specific receptors on B cells and T cells.

Diversity. Our immune systems can respond to millions of different antigenic determinants. This is possible because our immune systems have millions of clones of B and T lymphocytes—each of which is preprogrammed to recognize a different antigenic determinant. As noted, this ability to discriminate between antigens is the result of having unique cell-surface receptors.

Memory. Exposure to an antigen affects the immune system such that re-exposure produces a faster, larger, and more prolonged response than did the initial exposure (Fig. 63–3). Why does this happen? Because during the initial response, B and T lymphocytes that recognize the antigen undergo proliferation. Most of the new cells participate in the attack against the antigen. However, some of the new cells become *memory cells,* thereby increasing the pool of antigen-specific cells available to respond in the future. Hence, when the antigen is encountered again, the memory cells mobilize, and thereby accelerate and intensify the response.

Time Limitation. As indicated in Figure 63–3, immune responses don't last indefinitely. Rather they are time limited. The reasons are twofold. First, as the immune response proceeds, it greatly decreases the level of antigen that initiated the response, thereby attenuating the stimulus for continuing. Second, activated B cells and T cells only function for a short time, after which they become quiescent or die. Hence, in the absence of a continuing stimulus to generate more active B and T cells, the immune response fades.

Selectivity for Antigens of Nonself Origin. Under normal conditions, our immune systems target only foreign antigens, leaving potentially antigenic molecules on our own cells untouched. Sparing of self is possible because, as T cells develop in the thymus, cells that are able to react with antigens of self origin are eliminated. As discussed below, this discrimination between self and nonself is made possible by *major histocompatibility complex* (MHC) molecules.

When the ability to discriminate between self and nonself fails, our immune systems can attack our own cells. The result is an autoimmune disease. Diseases that result from autoimmune attack include rheumatoid arthritis, myasthenia gravis, and type 1 diabetes (insulin-dependent diabetes).

Phases of the Immune Response

Specific immune responses can be viewed as having three main phases, named the recognition phase, the activation phase, and the effector phase.

Recognition Phase. The recognition phase occurs when a mature lymphocyte encounters its matching antigen. All specific immune responses begin with antigen recognition by B cells and T cells. Antigen recognition is possible because of antigen-specific receptors on the lymphocyte surface.

Activation Phase. Antigen recognition causes the lymphocyte involved to become activated. The activated lymphocyte then undergoes proliferation and differentiation. Some of the daughter cells differentiate into cells that actively participate in

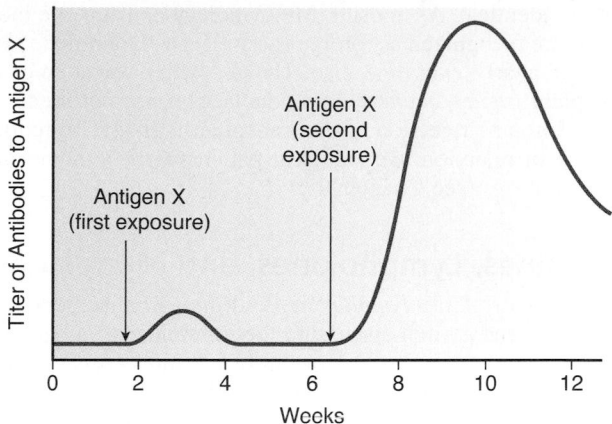

Figure 63–3 ■ Memory and time limitation of immune responses.
After the initial exposure to antigen X, antibody levels rise slowly, peak at a low level, and then decline rapidly. After the secondary exposure to antigen X, antibody levels rise more rapidly, reach a higher peak, persist longer, and then slowly decline.

the immune response, attacking the source of the antigen. Other daughter cells differentiate into memory cells, thereby preparing the host for a more intense, rapid, and prolonged response in the event of antigen re-exposure in the future.

Effector Phase. In this stage, the immune system attempts to eliminate the specific antigen that initiated the response. With cell-mediated or antibody-mediated immunity, several effector mechanisms can be involved. In cell-mediated immunity, antigen-bearing cells can be lysed by cytolytic T cells, or they can be ingested by macrophages. In antibody-mediated immunity, target cells may be primed for attack by phagocytes or by the complement system.

Major Histocompatibility Complex Molecules

The *major histocompatibility complex* is a group of *genes* that codes for *MHC molecules,* which become expressed on the surface of all cells. MHC molecules are critical to immune system function. They play a key role in the activation of helper and cytotoxic T lymphocytes; they guide cytotoxic T lymphocytes toward target cells; and they provide the basis for distinguishing between self and nonself.

There are two classes of MHC gene products, referred to as *class I MHC molecules* and *class II MHC molecules.* Class I MHC molecules are found on virtually all cells except erythrocytes; class II MHC molecules are found primarily on B cells and antigen-presenting cells (i.e., macrophages and dendritic cells). As discussed below, *class I MHC molecules* on the surface of antigen-presenting cells (APCs) help initiate immune responses by "presenting" antigen to *cytotoxic T cells.* In contrast, *class II MHC molecules* on the surface of APCs help initiate immune responses by presenting antigen to *helper T cells.*

As a rule, the sequence of amino acids in MHC molecules produced by one individual differs from the sequence of amino acids in MHC molecules produced by everyone else. That is, it is rare for two individuals to have MHC molecules that are identical. As a result, MHC molecules from one individual are recognized as foreign (nonself) by the immune systems of nearly everyone else. Hence, when we attempt to transplant organs between individuals who are not identical twins, immune rejection of the transplant is likely. To reduce the risk of rejection, we can treat patients with immunosuppressant drugs (see Chapter 65).

Cytokines, Lymphokines, and Monokines

The terms *cytokine, lymphokine,* and *monokine* are encountered frequently when discussing the immune system and can be a source of confusion. Accordingly, clarification is in order. The term *cytokine* refers to any mediator molecule (other than an antibody) released by *any* immune-system cell. A *lymphokine* is simply a cytokine released by a *lymphocyte,* and a *monokine* is simply a cytokine released by a *mononuclear phagocyte* (*monocyte* or *macrophage*). Put another way, *cytokine* is a generic term for the whole class of nonantibody mediators released by immune cells, whereas the terms *lymphokine* and *monokine* are more restrictive, referring only to nonantibody mediators released by lymphocytes and mononuclear phagocytes, respectively. Examples of cytokines and their functions are listed in Table 63–3.

TABLE 63–3 ■ Functions of Selected Cytokines	
Cytokine	**Function**
Interleukin-1	Stimulates lymphocyte progenitor cells
Interleukin-2	Stimulates proliferation and differentiation of helper T cells and cytolytic T cells
Interleukin-3	Stimulates proliferation of bone marrow lineage cells, B cells, and T cells
Interleukin-4	Activates B cells, T cells, and macrophages
Interleukin-5	Stimulates generation of eosinophils
Interleukin-6	Stimulates proliferation of bone marrow cells and plasma cells
Interleukin-7	Stimulates B cells and T cells
Interleukin-8	Attracts neutrophils, B cells, and T cells
Interleukin-9	Stimulates proliferation of mast cells
Interleukin-10	Inhibits some T cells
Interleukin-11	Enhances actions of interleukin-3
Interleukin-12	Enhances actions of interleukin-2
Interferon-alpha	Activates macrophages, cytotoxic T cells, and natural killer cells
Interferon-gamma	Activates macrophages and T cells and enhances expression of MHC molecules
Tumor necrosis factor	Kills tumor cells; promotes inflammation
Granulocyte-macrophage colony-stimulating factor	Stimulates proliferation of monocytes, macrophages, and granulocytes (neutrophils, eosinophils, basophils)

ANTIBODY-MEDIATED (HUMORAL) IMMUNITY

As noted, there are two types of immune responses: humoral immunity and cell-mediated immunity. Our objective in this section is to review humoral immunity, focusing on (1) how antibodies are produced and (2) the mechanisms by which antibodies protect us. Cell-mediated immunity is discussed in the section that follows.

Production of Antibodies

Antibody production requires the cooperative interaction of three types of cells: *B cells,* which actually make the antibodies; *helper T cells* (CD4 cells), which stimulate the B cells; and an *antigen-presenting cell* (either a macrophage or a dendritic cell), which activates the CD4 cells so that they can then help the B cells. The major steps in the process are depicted in Figure 63–4.

Overview of Antibody Production

As indicated in Figure 63–4, production of antibodies begins with binding of a specific antigen (Ag) to two types of cells: a virgin B cell and an APC. The APC may be either a macrophage or a dendritic cell. After processing the Ag, the APC is able to bind with a specific CD4 cell, thereby causing the CD4 cell to proliferate and differentiate into active CD4 cells and memory CD4 cells. The active CD4 cells then bind with processed Ag on B cells, thereby causing the B cells to proliferate and differentiate into (1) plasma cells, which manufacture the antibodies, and (2) memory B cells, which await the next Ag exposure.

Specific Cellular Events in Antibody Production

B Cells. Participation of B cells in the immune response begins with recognition and binding of a *specific antigen.* The receptor that B cells employ for antigen recognition is actually an antibody (IgD or IgM). For any given B cell, this antibody (receptor) is highly specific for just one antigenic determinant. After the antigen binds the B-cell receptor, the receptor-antigen complex is internalized and the antigen is broken down into small peptide fragments. Each fragment is then complexed with a *class II MHC molecule,* after which the *MHC II–antigen complexes* are transported to the cell surface. (In Fig. 63–4, only one such complex is shown. However, in a real cell, many such complexes, each with a different piece of the antigen, would appear on the cell surface.) The final step of B-cell activation occurs when a CD4 helper T cell recognizes and binds with an MHC II–antigen complex on the B cell. This binding causes the CD4 cell to secrete cytokines, which then stimulate the B cell to proliferate and differentiate into two types of cells: plasma cells and memory B cells. The plasma cells are the cells that make the antibodies; the memory cells serve to hasten, intensify, and prolong the immune response if antigen exposure should occur again.

Antigen-Presenting Cells. APCs are essential for activation of CD4 helper T cells. The reason is that CD4 cells cannot recognize antigen that is free in solution. Rather, they can only recognize antigen that has been complexed with an MHC II molecule.

Participation of APCs in the immune response begins with nonspecific binding of antigen to the APC (see Fig. 63–4). Next, as in B cells, the antigen is internalized and broken into fragments, which are then complexed with MHC II molecules and transported to the cell surface, where they are available for interaction with CD4 cells.

Helper T Cells (CD4 Cells). The role of CD4 cells in humoral immunity is to activate B cells. In the absence of activation by CD4 cells, B cells are unable to proliferate and produce antibodies.

Participation of CD4 cells in the immune response begins when these cells bind with an MHC II–antigen complex on the surface of an APC. Binding is mediated by a receptor on the CD4 cell that is specific for the particular antigen in the MHC II–antigen complex. (As noted, in order for the CD4 cell to recognize the antigen, the antigen must be complexed with an MHC II molecule, which is why the APC is essential for CD4 cell activation.) Upon binding with the MHC II–antigen complex, the CD4 cell releases cytokines, which then cause the CD4 cell itself to proliferate and differentiate into memory CD4 cells and activated CD4 cells. The activated CD4 cells then bind with their corresponding MHC II–antigen complexes on B cells, release cytokines, and thereby cause proliferation and differentiation of the B cells.

Antibody Effector Mechanisms

Antibodies are simply molecules with the ability to bind to other molecules. Antibodies have no special destructive powers. Hence, in order to rid the body of antigens, which is

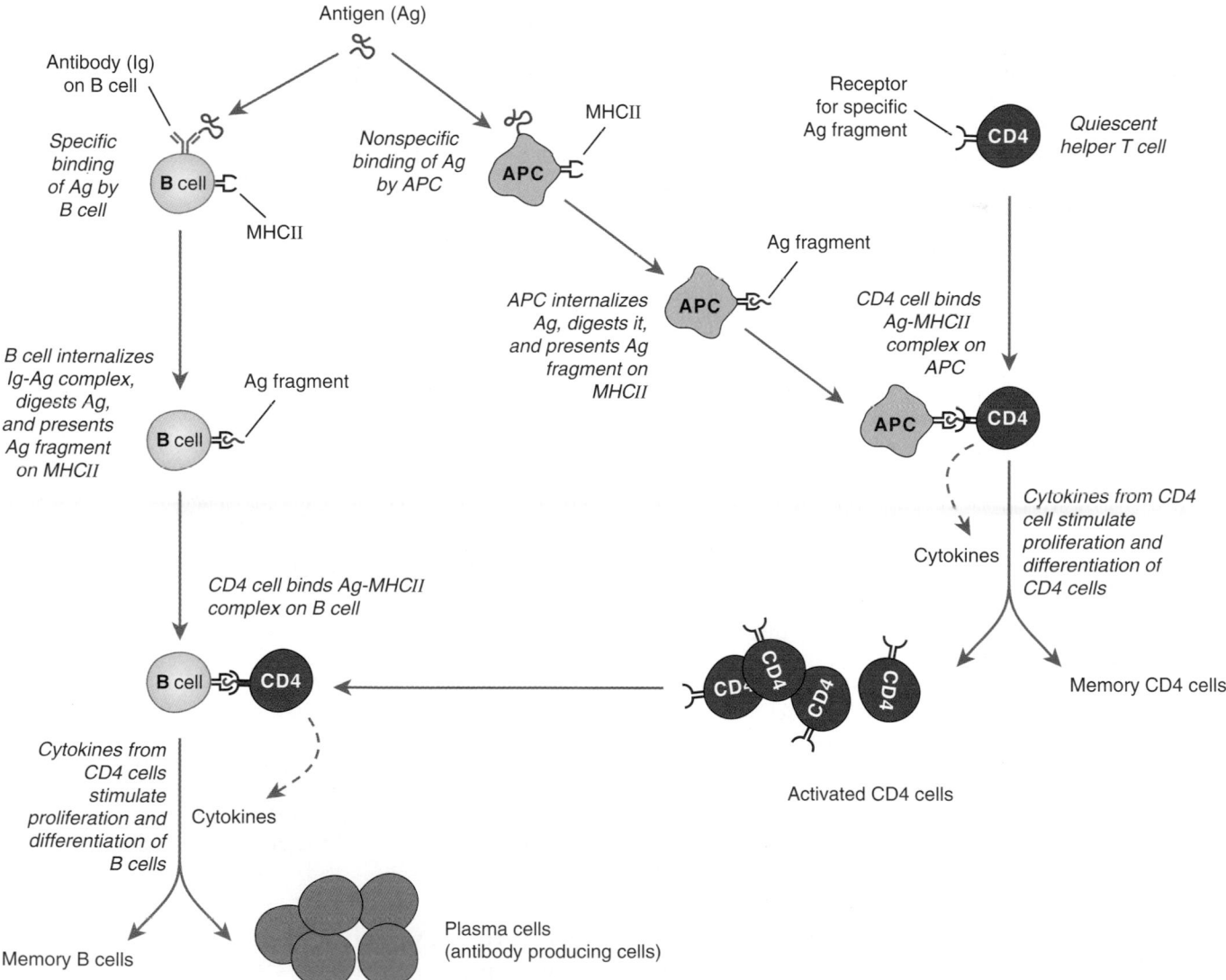

Figure 63–4 ■ Major events in antibody-mediated (humoral) immunity.
Humoral immunity requires three types of cells: B cells, APCs, and helper T cells (CD4 cells). Binding of a CD4 cell with an APC activates the CD4 cell, which then binds with a B cell and releases cytokines, which then stimulate the B cell. (Ag = antigen, APC = antigen-presenting cell [macrophage or dendritic cell], Ig = immunoglobulin [antibody], MHCII = class II MHC molecule.)

what antibodies are for, antibodies usually work in conjunction with other factors, namely, *phagocytic cells* and the *complement system*. The only antigens that antibodies can neutralize without help are bacterial toxins and viruses.

Opsonization of Bacteria

One mechanism for ridding the body of pathogenic bacteria is phagocytosis by macrophages and neutrophils. However, because of their structures, some bacteria are difficult for phagocytes to grab hold of, and hence are resistant to ingestion. Antibodies help promote phagocytosis of these bacteria by acting as *opsonins*. (An opsonin is a molecule that binds to a bacterium or other target particle and thereby promotes phagocytosis by providing a handle for phagocytes to grab on to.)

Bacterial opsonization by antibodies occurs in two steps. First, the antigen-binding region of the antibody binds with antigen on the bacterial surface, which leaves the Fc portion of the antibody projecting away from the surface. Second, phagocytes link up with the Fc portion of the antibody, which brings them in close contact with the bacterium, and hence enables them to commence phagocytosis. Phagocytes are able to bind the Fc fragment because they have high-affinity receptors for Fc on their surface. Most of the antibodies that act as opsonins belong to the IgG class.

Activation of the Complement System

The complement cascade is a complex system consisting of at least 20 serum proteins that, when activated, can cause multiple effects, including cell lysis, opsonization, degranulation of mast cells, and infiltration of phagocytes. The system may be activated in two ways, known as the *classical pathway* and the *alternative pathway*. The classical pathway is activated by *antibodies;* the alternative pathway is not. However, with both pathways, the end results are essentially the same. Consideration here is limited to the classical pathway.

The classical pathway is turned on when C1 (the first component of the complement system) encounters an antigen-antibody complex and then binds with the Fc region of the antibody. C1 will not bind with antibody that is free in solution; as a result, free antibodies cannot activate the system. Activation of the complement system triggers a cascade of reactions that amplify the response at each stage. The result is production of compounds that can injure target cells.

Lysis of target cells that have been tagged with antibodies is the most dramatic effect of the complement system. Lysis is caused by cylindrical *membrane attack complexes,* which are formed by the complement cascade. Following their insertion into the target cell membrane, the attack complexes act as pores through which fluid can enter the cell. As a result of fluid influx, the cell swells and eventually bursts.

Neutralization of Viruses and Bacterial Toxins

Neutralization of toxins and viruses is the only protective action that antibodies can perform unassisted. In order to hurt us, bacterial toxins must first bind with receptors on our cells. Likewise, in order to infect us, viruses must first bind with cell-surface receptors. By binding with antigenic determinants on toxins and viruses, antibodies make it impossible for toxins and viruses to bind with cellular receptors. As a result, these agents can no longer harm us.

CELL-MEDIATED IMMUNITY

Cell-mediated immunity has two branches, one mediated by *helper T lymphocytes* (CD4 cells) plus *macrophages,* and one mediated primarily by *cytolytic T lymphocytes* (CD8 cells). In the branch mediated by CD4 cells and macrophages, the result is called *delayed-type hypersensitivity.* In the branch mediated by CD8 cells, the result is *target-cell lysis.*

Delayed-Type Hypersensitivity

The object of delayed-type hypersensitivity (DTH) is to rid the body of bacteria that replicate primarily within macrophages (e.g., *Listeria monocytogenes, Mycobacterium tuberculosis*). For DTH to occur, two cells are needed: an *infected macrophage* and a *CD4 helper T cell.* The macrophage serves to activate the CD4 cell, which in turn activates the macrophage, thereby enabling the macrophage to kill the bacteria residing within it. Hence, the same cell (i.e., the macrophage) is both the activator of the CD4 cell and the recipient of the activated CD4 cell's help.

Activation of Helper T Cells. Activation of CD4 cells in DTH is essentially identical to the activation of CD4 cells in humoral immunity. As shown in Figure 63–5, the process begins when a macrophage becomes infected with intracellular bacteria. As in humoral immunity, the macrophage breaks down the antigen to small peptides, combines each peptide with a class II MHC molecule, and then presents the antigen–MHC II complexes on its surface. In the next step, a CD4 cell binds with an antigen–MHC II complex on the macrophage. As discussed above, selectivity of binding is determined by receptors on the CD4 cell that recognize a specific antigen fragment—but only when the fragment is bound to a class II MHC molecule. Binding of the CD4 cell with the APC causes the CD4 cell to release (1) cytokines that cause the CD4 cell itself to proliferate and differentiate into memory cells and (2) mediators of DTH, including interferon-gamma and tumor necrosis factor.

Activation of Macrophages. *Interferon-gamma,* released from the activated CD4 cell, is the major stimulus for macrophage activation. In response to interferon-gamma, macrophages increase production of lysosomes and reactive oxygen. The reactive oxygen is ultimately responsible for killing bacteria inside the macrophage. In addition to ridding macrophages of bacteria, DTH produces local inflammation.

Cytolytic T Lymphocytes

Cytolytic lymphocytes (CTLs, CD8 cells) kill other cells. Their principal job is to kill self cells that are infected with viruses, thereby halting viral replication. In addition, CTLs participate in rejection of transplants. In this chapter, discussion is limited to killing of virally infected cells.

The process by which CTLs kill other cells has two stages: activation of CTLs, followed by recognition and killing of the target cell. The overall process is depicted in Figure 63–6.

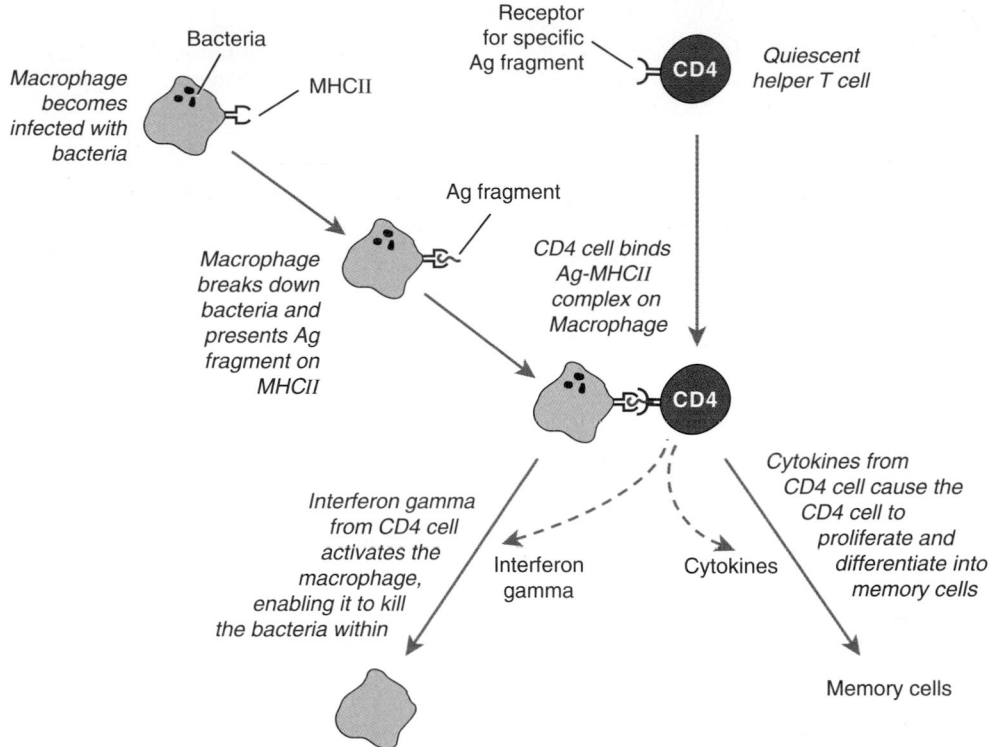

Figure 63–5 ■ Cell-mediated immunity: delayed-type hypersensitivity.
DTH requires two cells: an infected macrophage and a CD4 cell. Binding of the CD4 cell to the macrophage activates the CD4 cell, which then releases interferon-gamma and several cytokines. Interferon-gamma activates the macrophage. The cytokines cause the CD4 cell to proliferate and differentiate into memory cells. (Ag = antigen, MHCII = class II MHC molecule.)

Activation of Cytolytic T Cells. Activation of CTLs requires the participation of an *antigen-presenting cell* and a *helper T cell* (CD4 cell). The process is very similar to the activation of CD4 cells discussed above. However, there is one important difference: Whereas CD4 cells specifically recognize antigen that is bound to a *class II* MHC molecule on an APC, CTLs specifically recognize antigen that is bound to a *class I* MHC molecule on an APC.

In viral infections, activation of CTLs begins with processing of viral antigens by an APC. As shown in Figure 63–6, the APC combines the antigen with a class I MHC molecule and then presents the antigen–MHC I complex on its surface. Next, a pre-CTL binds to the antigen–MHC I complex. (Like CD4 cells, each pre-CTL has receptors that are specific for a particular antigen-MHC complex.) Linking of the pre-CTL with the APC primes the pre-CTL for the next stage of activation: stimulation by cytokines (interleukin-2, interferon-gamma, and probably others) provided by an activated CD4 cell. (Activation of the CD4 cell, which is not shown in Figure 63–6, occurs when the CD4 cell encounters an APC that has a viral antigen–MHC II complex.) In response to the cytokines released by the CD4 cell, the pre-CTL undergoes proliferation and differentiation into memory CTLs and activated CTLs.

Recognition of Virally Infected Target Cells. CTLs recognize their targets by the presence of an antigen–MHC I complex. This is the same process by which CTLs recognize

APCs. As noted earlier, virtually all cells in the body carry class I MHC molecules. (Class II molecules are limited to APCs and B cells.) Hence, when a cell is infected with a virus, viral antigens form intracellular complexes with MHC I molecules, after which the antigen–MHC I complexes are presented on the cell surface. As shown in Figure 63–6, activated CTLs recognize the antigen–MHC I complex, and hence bind with the target cell. Since only cells that are infected with the virus will bear viral antigens on their class I MHC molecules, attack by CTLs is limited to infected cells; all others are spared.

Mechanisms of Cell Kill. Binding of a CTL to its target cell causes the CTL to release mediators that kill the target. Two mechanisms of cell kill are involved: *lysis* and *apoptosis* (programmed cell death). The mediator of lysis is called *perforin,* a molecule that forms pores in the target-cell membrane; the resultant influx of fluid causes the cell to swell and then burst. (This mechanism is very similar to one by which the complement system causes cell lysis.) The mediators of apoptosis have not been identified with certainty. However, their effects are very clear. The initial effect is activation of intracellular enzymes that digest the cell's own DNA. This is followed by fragmentation of the nucleus and cell death. Only the target cell is harmed; bystander cells and the CTL itself are not touched. In fact, after releasing its mediators, the CTL disconnects from the doomed target and goes on to seek other victims.

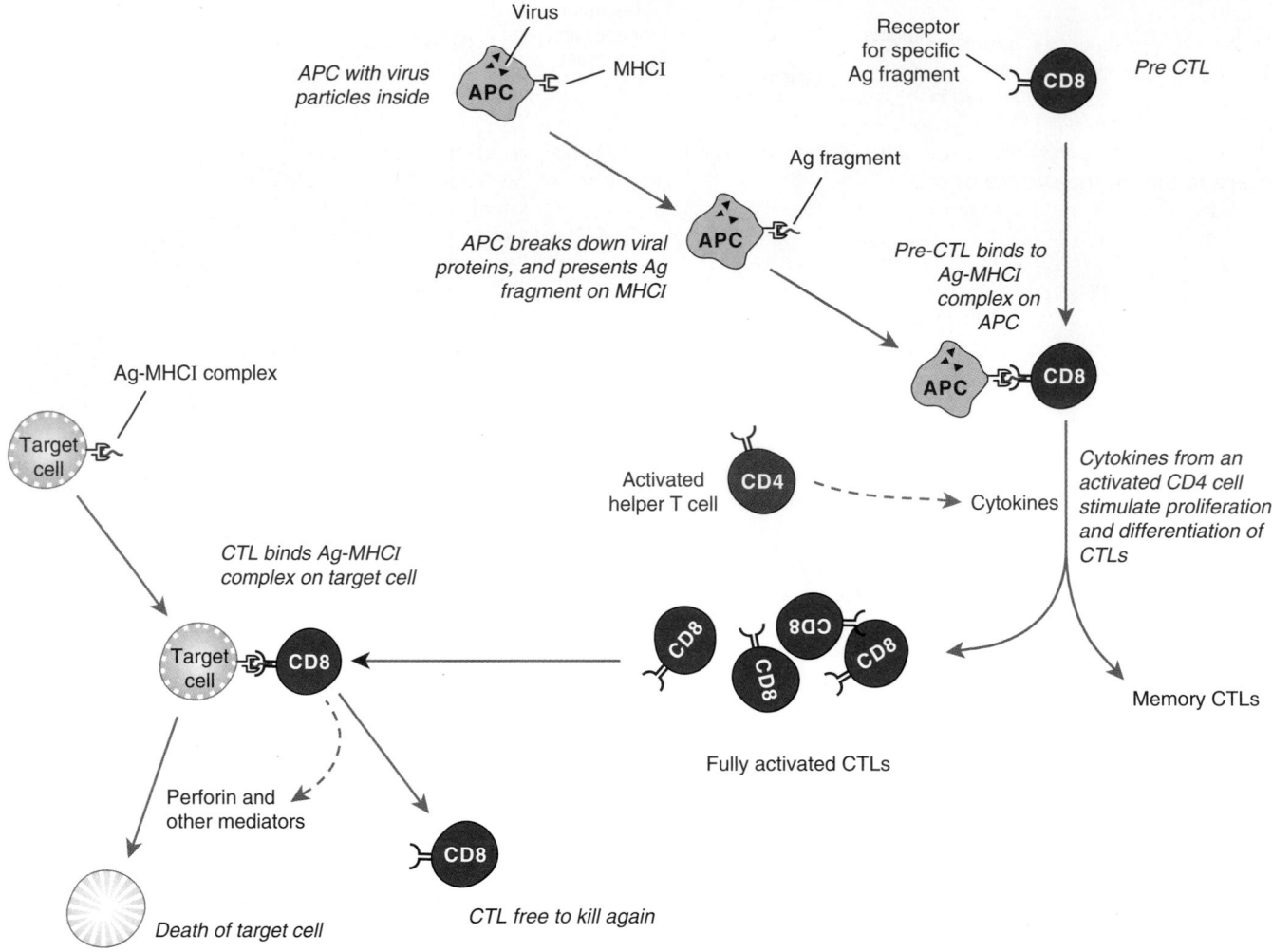

Figure 63–6 ■ Cell-mediated immunity: cytolytic T cells.
This branch of cell-mediated immunity requires three types of cells: CTLs, APCs, and CD4 cells. Binding of the CTL with the APC begins the activation of the CTL. Stimulation of the CTL by cytokines from the CD4 cell completes the activation of the CTL, which then binds with and kills its target. Activation of the CD4 cells, which is not shown, takes place essentially as depicted in Figures 63–4 and 63–5. (Ag = antigen, APC = antigen-presenting cell, CTL = cytolytic T lymphocyte, MHCI = class I MHC molecule.)

⣞ KEY POINTS

- The immune system *helps* us by attacking invading organisms (viruses, bacteria, fungi, parasites) and cancer cells. The immune system can *hurt* us by attacking transplants and our own healthy cells.
- There are two basic types of immune responses: natural immunity (native or innate immunity) and specific acquired immunity.
- There are two types of specific acquired immunity: cell-mediated immunity and humoral (antibody-mediated) immunity.
- The immune system has five major types of cells: B lymphocytes (B cells), helper T lymphocytes (CD4 cells), cytolytic T lymphocytes (CD8 cells, CTLs), macrophages, and dendritic cells.

- Only lymphocytes have receptors that can recognize specific antigens.
- B cells make antibodies.
- CTLs kill target cells directly.
- Helper T cells are essential for the activation of B cells, CTLs, and the macrophages involved in delayed type hypersensitivity (DTH).
- Macrophages have three functions in specific immunity: (1) they serve as antigen-presenting cells (APCs) in the activation of helper T cells and CTLs, (2) they are involved in DTH, and (3) they phagocytize opsonized cells in humoral immunity.
- Like macrophages, dendritic cells serve as APCs.
- An antigen is a molecule that triggers a specific immune response, and then becomes the target of that response.

- Most antigens are large molecules.
- Antibodies bind to specific, small regions of an antigen, referred to as epitopes or antigenic determinants.
- The major histocompatibility complex (MHC) is a group of genes that codes for MHC molecules, which are found on the surface of cells.
- MHC molecules have three major functions: they play a key role in the activation of helper T cells and CTLs, they guide CTLs toward target cells, and they provide the basis for distinguishing between self and nonself.
- Class II MHC molecules are found only on B cells and APCs, whereas class I MHC molecules are found on virtually all cells (including B cells and APCs).
- It is rare for two individuals to have MHC molecules that are precisely the same. As a result, MHC molecules from one individual are usually recognized as foreign (nonself) by the immune systems of everyone else.
- A cytokine is defined as any mediator molecule (other than an antibody) released by any immune-system cell.
- The most characteristic feature of antibodies is their ability to recognize specific antigens.
- Antibody production requires the cooperative interaction of three types of cells: B cells, which make the antibodies; helper T cells (CD4 cells), which stimulate the B cells; and APCs, which activate the CD4 cells so that they can then activate B cells.
- B cells have antibodies on their surface that serve as receptors for recognizing specific antigens. Binding of antigen to the receptor is the first step in B-cell activation.
- Activation of B cells is completed when a CD4 cell binds with an antigen–MHC II complex on the B cell and then releases cytokines, which then stimulate the B cell.
- In order to activate a B cell, a CD4 cell must first become activated itself. CD4 activation is initiated by binding of the CD4 cell with an antigen–MHC II complex on an APC.

- Antibodies eliminate antigens by three mechanisms: (1) direct neutralization of toxins and viruses, (2) opsonization of bacteria, and (3) activation of the complement system.
- Opsonization (coating bacteria with antibodies) helps macrophages and neutrophils hold on to bacteria, and hence facilitates phagocytosis.
- The complement system forms pores in the bacterial cell membrane, thereby promoting death by lysis.
- Cell-mediated immunity can result in delayed-type hypersensitivity (DTH) and lysis of target cells by CTLs.
- DTH involves two types of cells: an infected macrophage and a CD4 cell. The macrophage activates the CD4 cell, which then releases interferon-gamma, which in turn stimulates the macrophage, thereby enabling the macrophage to kill the bacteria inside it.
- The major role of CTLs is to kill self cells that have become infected with viruses.
- Activation of CTLs proceeds in two steps: first, the CTL binds to an APC; second, the CTL is stimulated by cytokines provided by a CD4 cell.
- Binding of CTLs with APCs differs from binding of CD4 cells with APCs in that CTLs specifically recognize antigen that is bound to a class I MHC molecule on the APC, whereas CD4 cells specifically recognize antigen that is bound to a class II MHC molecule.
- CTLs kill target cells in two ways: (1) they release perforin, which creates pores in the cell, thereby causing death by lysis; and (2) they release compounds that cause apoptosis (programmed cell death).
- Activated CTLs attack only self cells that have antigen–MHC I complexes; all other self cells, including the CTLs, are spared.
- Specific immune responses result in production of memory T cells and memory B cells. As a result, the next time an antigen is encountered, the immune response occurs faster and with greater intensity.

Childhood Immunization

The purpose of immunization is to protect against infectious diseases. As a result of widespread immunization, the incidence of several infectious diseases (diphtheria, pertussis, tetanus, measles, mumps, rubella, and *Haemophilus influenzae* type b) has been dramatically reduced, wild-type polio has been eliminated from the Western hemisphere, and smallpox has been eliminated from the planet.

Experience has shown that the most effective way to reduce vaccine-preventable diseases (VPDs) is to create a highly immune population. Accordingly, universal vaccination is a national goal. Although immunization carries some risk, the risk from failing to vaccinate is much greater.

GENERAL CONSIDERATIONS

Definitions

In order to discuss immunization, we need to use special terminology. Accordingly, we begin the chapter by defining some terms.

Vaccine. A vaccine is a preparation containing whole or fractionated microorganisms. Administration causes the recipient's immune system to manufacture antibodies directed against the microbe from which the vaccine was made. Most of the preparations discussed in this chapter are vaccines.

Killed Vaccines Versus Live Vaccines. There are two major classes of vaccines: killed and live (albeit attenuated). Killed vaccines are composed of whole, killed microbes or isolated microbial components (e.g., the polysaccharide of *H. influenzae* type b or the surface antigen of hepatitis B). In contrast, live, attenuated vaccines are composed of live microbes that have been weakened or rendered completely avirulent. Live vaccines can be dangerous in recipients who are immunocompromised. Why? Because these people are unable to mount an effective immune response, even against avirulent organisms.

Toxoid. A toxoid is a bacterial toxin that has been changed to a nontoxic form. Administration causes the recipient's immune system to manufacture antitoxins (i.e., antibodies directed against the natural bacterial toxin). Antitoxins protect against injury from toxins, but do not kill the bacteria that produce them. In this chapter, only two toxoids are considered: tetanus toxoid and diphtheria toxoid.

Vaccination. The terms *vaccination* and *vaccine* derive from vaccinia, a virus whose name in turn derives from *vacca* (Latin for cow). At one time, vaccinia virus was used as a vaccine against smallpox. (Vaccinia itself causes cowpox, a mild sickness, and in the process induces synthesis of smallpox antibodies.) Hence, when the term *vaccination* was originally coined, it had the limited meaning of giving vaccinia to generate immunity against smallpox. Today, vaccination refers broadly to administration of any vaccine or toxoid.

Immunization: Active Versus Passive. *Immunization* is a more inclusive term than *vaccination,* in that immunization refers to production of both active immunity and passive immunity, whereas vaccination refers only to production of active immunity.

Active immunity develops in response to infection or to administration of a vaccine or toxoid. In either case, the result is endogenous production of antibodies. Active immunity takes weeks or months to develop, but is long lasting. Discussion in this chapter is limited almost exclusively to active immunization.

Passive immunity is conferred by giving a patient *preformed* antibodies (immune globulins). Unlike active immunity, passive immunity protects immediately, but persists only as long as the antibodies remain in the body.

Specific Immune Globulins. These preparations contain a high concentration of antibodies directed against a specific antigen (e.g., hepatitis B virus). Administration provides immediate passive immunity. These preparations are made from donated blood and do not transmit infectious diseases.

Public Health Impact of Immunization

Widespread vaccination has had a profound impact on public health. As shown in Table 64–1, vaccination has greatly reduced the incidence of several infectious diseases (e.g., diphtheria, pertussis, tetanus). With two other diseases—polio and smallpox—results have been even more dramatic: polio is gone from the Western hemisphere, and smallpox is gone from the planet.

Despite these successes, we still have a long way to go. Nationally, more than one child in every three falls behind on his or her immunizations by the age of 2 years. In some parts of the country, more than 50% of the children are not current. The consequences of failing to vaccinate can be enormous. For example, between 1989 and 1991, a measles epidemic occurred; 55,000 cases were reported, 11,000 people were hospitalized, and more than 130 people died, half of them young children.

The Childhood Immunization Initiative, begun in 1993, is directed at preventing such epidemics in the future. The goal of the program is to eliminate all indigenous cases of diphtheria, measles, rubella, tetanus, and *H. influenzae* b infection from the United States. The program aims to achieve these goals by improving vaccine delivery systems, increasing community participation, reducing vaccine costs to parents, developing safer and simpler vaccines, and involving more federal agencies in providing vaccines to populations who otherwise might not have access to them.

From a strictly economic viewpoint, vaccination is a wonderful investment. On average, we save $14 in future health care costs for each dollar we spend on vaccination.

Adverse Effects of Immunization

Vaccines are generally very safe. Mild reactions are common, but serious events are rare. Many children experience local reactions (discomfort, swelling, and erythema at the injection site). Fever is also common. Potential severe effects include anaphylaxis (e.g., in response to measles, mumps, and rubella virus vaccine [MMR]); acute encephalopathy (caused by diphtheria and tetanus toxoids and pertussis vaccine [DTP]); and vaccine-associated paralytic poliomyelitis (VAPP) (caused by oral poliovirus vaccine [OPV]).

Immunocompromised children are at special risk from live vaccines. The reason is that, in the absence of an adequate immune response, the viruses or bacteria in these normally safe vaccines are able to multiply in profusion, thereby causing serious infection. Accordingly, live vaccines should generally be avoided in children who are severely immunosuppressed. Causes of immunosuppression include congenital immunodeficiency, HIV infection, leukemia, lymphoma, generalized malignancy, and therapy with radiation, cytotoxic anticancer drugs, and high-dose glucocorticoids.

The risk of serious adverse reactions can be minimized by observing appropriate *precautions* and *contraindications*. Table 64–2 lists contraindications that apply to all vaccines. Precautions and contraindications that apply to specific vaccines are discussed in the context of those preparations. Certain conditions, such as diarrhea and mild illness, may be inappropriately regarded as contraindications by some practitioners. As a result, vaccination may be needlessly postponed. Conditions that are often considered contraindications, although they are not, are also listed in Table 64–2.

Practitioners are required to report certain adverse events to the *Vaccine Adverse Event Reporting System* (VAERS). The information is used to help determine whether (1) a particular event that occurs after vaccination is actually caused by the vaccine, and (2) what the risk factors might be. In addition to reporting events that they are required to report, practitioners should report all other serious or unusual adverse events, regardless of whether they believe the event was caused by the vaccine. Forms for reporting adverse events can be obtained from the VAERS web site (*www.vaers.org*) or by calling 1-800-822-7967.

The *National Vaccine Injury Compensation Program* (NVICP), established by the Childhood Vaccine Injury Act of 1986, was created to provide compensation for injury or death resulting from vaccination. The program is intended as an alternative to civil litigation in that negligence need not be

TABLE 64–1 ■ Impact of Vaccination on the Incidence of Vaccine-Preventable Diseases

	Prevaccine Era: Maximum Number of Reported Cases (Year the Maximum Occurred)	Vaccine Era: Number of Reported Cases in 1998	Percentage Change in Reported Cases
Diphtheria	206,939 (1921)	1	−99.99
Pertussis	265,269 (1934)	6279	−97.6
Tetanus	1560 (1948)	34	−97.82
Measles	894,134 (1941)	89	−99.99
Mumps	152,209 (1968)	606	−99.60
Rubella	57,686 (1969)	345	−99.40
Poliomyelitis (wild)	21,269 (1952)	0	−99.99
Invasive *Haemophilus influenzae*	20,000* (1984)	54	−99.73

*Estimated because national reporting did not exist in prevaccine era.

TABLE 64–2 ■ Contraindications That Apply To All Vaccines and Conditions Often Incorrectly Regarded as Contraindications	
True Contraindications (Vaccine Should Not Be Administered)	**Not Contraindications (Vaccine May Be Administered)**
Anaphylactic reaction to a vaccine contraindicates further doses of that vaccine	Mild to moderate local reaction (soreness, erythema, swelling) following a dose of an injectable vaccine
Anaphylactic reaction to a vaccine component contraindicates use of all vaccines that contain that substance	Mild acute illness with or without low-grade fever
Moderate or severe illnesses with or without a fever	Diarrhea
	Current antimicrobial therapy
	Convalescent phase of illnesses
	Prematurity (same dosage and indications as for normal, full-term infants)
	Recent exposure to an infectious disease
	Personal or family history of either penicillin allergy or nonspecific allergies

proved. As a provision of the law, a table was created listing the vaccines covered by the program and the injuries, disabilities, illness, and conditions (including death) for which compensation may be paid. Compensation may also be paid for injuries not listed in the table, provided that (1) a listed vaccine is involved and (2) causality can be demonstrated. Injuries related to vaccines not listed in the table are not covered under the program. Additional information can be obtained by calling the NVICP automated recording at 1-800-338-2382.

Immunization Records

The National Childhood Vaccine Act of 1986 requires a permanent record of each mandated vaccination a child receives. The information should be recorded in either (1) the permanent medical record of the recipient or (2) a permanent office log or file. The following data are required:

- Date of vaccination
- Route and site of vaccination
- Vaccine type, manufacturer, lot number, and expiration date
- Name, address, and title of the person administering the vaccine

The purpose of these records is twofold. First, they help ensure the child receives appropriate vaccinations. Second, they help avoid overvaccination, and thereby reduce the risk of possible hypersensitivity reactions. To promote uniformity in record keeping, an official immunization card has been adopted by every state and the District of Columbia.

Reporting Vaccine-Preventable Diseases

Public health officials rely on healthcare providers to report cases of vaccine-preventable diseases (VPDs). Nearly all VPDs that occur in the United States are notifiable. Healthcare providers should report individual cases to their local or state health department. Each week, the state health departments make a report to the Centers for Disease Control and Prevention (CDC). The information gathered is used to (1) determine if an outbreak is occurring, (2) evaluate prevention and control strategies, and (3) evaluate the impact of national immunization policies and practices.

Childhood Immunization Schedule

Each year, the CDC's Advisory Committee on Immunization Practices (ACIP), in cooperation with the American Academy of Family Physicians and the American Academy of Pediatrics, issues revised recommendations for childhood immunization in the United States. Figure 64–1 on p. 718 shows the recommended schedule for 2003. You can find the most recent updates online at *www.cdc.gov/nip*.

TARGET DISEASES

Routine childhood vaccination is currently recommended for protection against 11 infectious diseases: diphtheria, tetanus (lockjaw), pertussis (whooping cough), measles, mumps, rubella, invasive *H. influenzae* type b, hepatitis B, polio, varicella (chickenpox), and invasive pneumococcal disease. In addition, immunization against hepatitis A is recommended for some regions. In the discussion below, certain VPDs are considered in a group (e.g., measles, mumps, rubella). The reason is that vaccination against these VPDs is usually done simultaneously using a combination vaccine.

Measles, Mumps, and Rubella

Measles. Measles is a highly contagious viral disease characterized by rash and high fever (103°F to 105°F). Infection is spread by inhalation of aerosolized sputum or by direct contact with nasal or throat secretions. Initial symptoms include fever, cough, headache, sore throat, and conjunctivitis. Three days later, rash develops. Rash begins at the hairline, spreads to the rest of the body in 36 hours, and then fades in a few days. Secondary infections can result in pneumonia and otitis media (inner ear infection). However, of the potential complications of measles, encephalitis is by far the most serious. Sequelae of encephalitis include blindness, deafness, and convulsions. Although encephalitis is rare (0.1% incidence), it carries a 10% risk of death. In the United States, measles has become very rare: In 1998, only 89 cases were reported.

Mumps. Mumps is a viral disease that primarily affects the parotid glands (the largest of the three pairs of salivary glands). Although mumps can occur in adults, it usually occurs in children ages 5 to 15. As a rule, the first symptom is swelling in one of the parotid glands. Swelling is often associated with pain and tenderness. The patients may also experience fever (100°F to 104°F). Swelling increases for 2 to 3 days and then fades entirely by day 6 or 7. Swelling in the second parotid gland often develops after swelling in the first, but may also occur simultaneously or not at all. Painful *orchitis* (inflammation of the testes) develops in about one-third of adult and adolescent males. Acute *aseptic meningitis* develops in about 10% of all patients; symptoms, which resolve completely, include dizziness, headache, and vomiting. In the United States, the incidence of reported mumps cases has declined from a high of 152,209 in 1968 to only 606 in 1998.

Rubella. Rubella, also known as German measles, is a generally mild viral infection. However, if it occurs during pregnancy, the consequences can be severe. Initial symptoms include sore throat, mild fever, and swelling in lymph nodes located behind the ears and in the back of the neck. Shortly after, a rash develops on the face and scalp, spreads rapidly to the torso and arms, and then fades in 2 or 3 days. Arthritis may also develop, mainly in women. In pregnant women, rubella can cause miscarriage, stillbirth, and congenital defects, especially if the disease occurs during the first trimester. Possible birth defects include cataracts, heart disease, mental retardation, and deafness. In the United States, the incidence of reported rubella cases peaked at 57,686 in 1969, but was only 345 in 1998.

Diphtheria, Tetanus, and Pertussis

Diphtheria. Diphtheria is a potentially fatal infection caused by *Corynebacterium diphtheriae,* a gram-positive bacillus. The bacterium colonizes the throat and nasal passages, and produces a toxin that spreads throughout the body. Initial symptoms include sore throat, fever, headache, and nausea. Colonization of the airway begins as patches of gray or dirty-yellow membrane that eventually grow together, forming a thick coating. This coating, combined with swelling, can impede swallowing and breathing; in severe cases, a tracheostomy is needed. The toxin produced by *C. diphtheriae* can damage the heart and nerves, resulting in heart failure and paralysis. Treatment of diphtheria includes administration of diphtheria antitoxin and antibiotics (e.g., erythromycin, penicillin G). In the United States, only 37 cases were reported between 1980 and 1992. However, of those infected, about 10% died, mainly children and the elderly. In 1998, only one case was reported.

Tetanus (Lockjaw). Tetanus, also known as lockjaw, is a frequently fatal disease characterized by painful spasm of all skeletal muscles. The cause is a potent endotoxin elaborated by *Clostridium tetani,* a gram-positive bacillus. Infection with *C. tetani* typically results from puncturing the skin with a nail, splinter, or other object that is contaminated with soil, street dust, or animal or human feces. The first symptom is often stiffness of the jaw, hence the name *lockjaw.* As infection progresses, the patient may experience stiff neck, difficulty swallowing, restlessness, irritability, headache, chills, fever, and convulsions. Eventually, spasm develops in muscles of the abdomen, back, neck, and face. The case fatality rate is 21%. The yearly incidence of tetanus peaked at 1560 cases in 1948, but was only 34 cases in 1998. Treatment options include tetanus antitoxin, a booster dose of tetanus toxoid, and antibiotics (e.g., penicillin G, a tetracycline).

Pertussis (Whooping Cough). Pertussis, also known as whooping cough, occurs primarily in infants and young children. The cause is *Bordetella pertussis,* a gram-negative bacillus. Initial symptoms include rhinorrhea, mild fever, and persistent cough. As infection worsens, coughing becomes more intense. The acute phase of the disease can last 4 to 6 weeks. During this time, infants experience difficulty eating, drinking, and breathing. Deaths have occurred. Complications of pertussis include pneumonia, seizures, ear infections, and, rarely, permanent neurologic injury. In the United States, reported cases dropped from a high of 265,269 in 1934 to 6279 in 1998. Worldwide, the disease afflicts about 60 million people, and kills 700,000 each year, mainly infants and young children. The drug of choice for treating pertussis is erythromycin.

Poliomyelitis

Poliomyelitis, also known as polio or infantile paralysis, is a serious disease in which the poliovirus attacks neurons of the central nervous system that control muscle movement. The result is skeletal muscle paralysis, usually in the legs; however, muscles of respiration and muscles of the arms may also be affected. In about 10% of cases, polio is fatal. The disease is caused by three different polioviruses. Paralytic polio is usually caused by type 1 poliovirus. Polio has no cure. However, proper symptomatic treatment can improve comfort and reduce or prevent some crippling effects. Vaccination against polio has eliminated the disease from the Western hemisphere, except for eight to nine cases annually caused by the vaccine itself. To prevent vaccine-induced polio, use of the live virus vaccine (oral polio vaccine) has been discontinued.

Haemophilus influenzae Type b

Haemophilus influenzae type b is a gram-negative bacterium that can cause meningitis, pneumonia, and serious throat and ear infections. The bacterium is the leading cause of serious illness in children under the age of 5 years, and the most common cause of bacterial meningitis, which has a mortality rate of 5%. Among children who survive meningitis, between 25% and 35% suffer lasting neurologic deficits. As a result of childhood vaccination, the annual incidence of infection dropped from an estimated 20,000 cases in 1984 to less than 54 in 1998. Of the cases that occurred, almost all were in unvaccinated children. Infection with *H. influenzae* can be treated successfully with antibiotics.

Varicella (Chickenpox)

Varicella (chickenpox) is a common, highly contagious, and potentially serious disease of childhood. The causative organ-

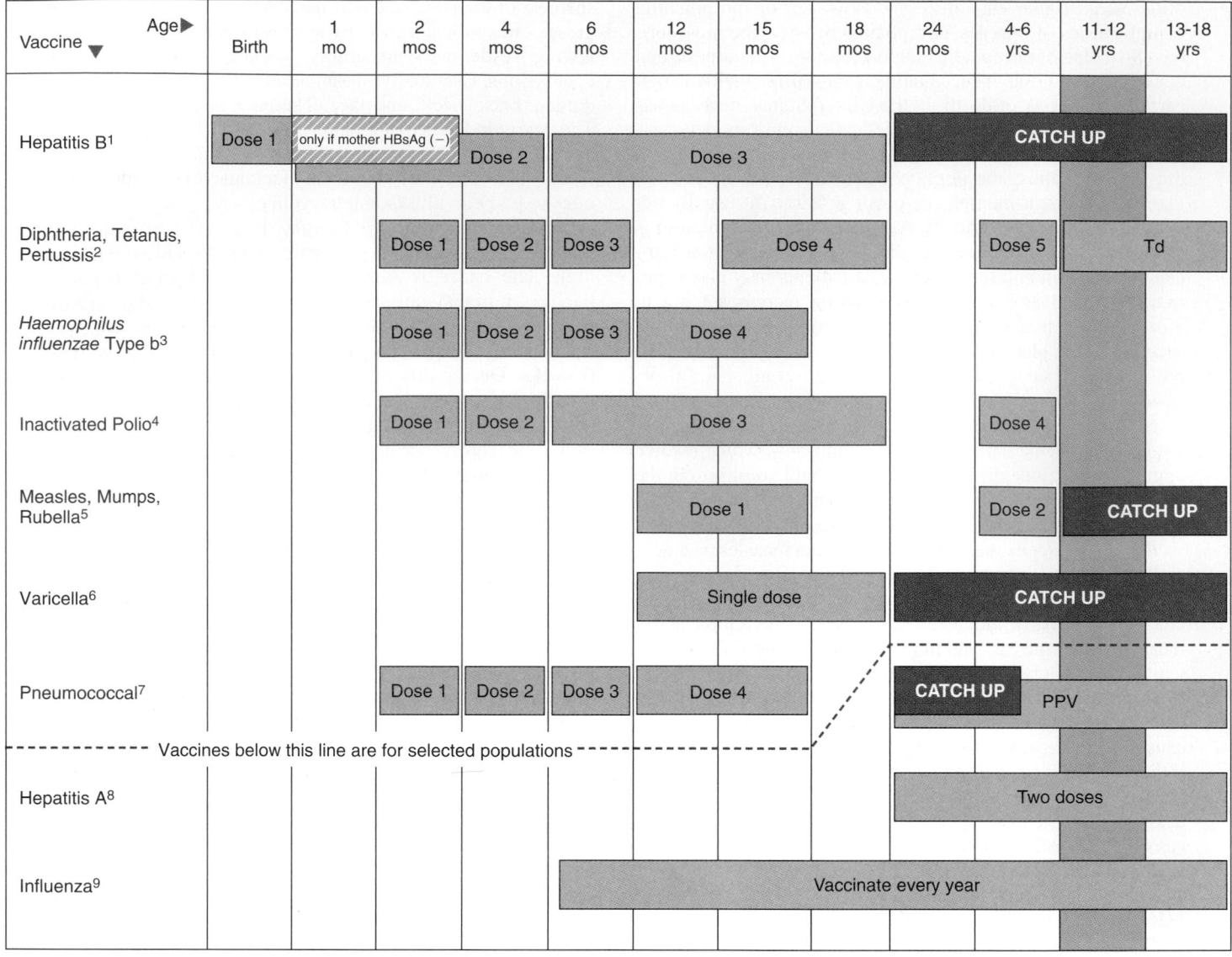

Vaccine ▼ / Age ▶	Birth	1 mo	2 mos	4 mos	6 mos	12 mos	15 mos	18 mos	24 mos	4-6 yrs	11-12 yrs	13-18 yrs
Hepatitis B[1]	Dose 1	only if mother HBsAg (−)	Dose 2		Dose 3						CATCH UP	
Diphtheria, Tetanus, Pertussis[2]			Dose 1	Dose 2	Dose 3		Dose 4			Dose 5	Td	
Haemophilus influenzae Type b[3]			Dose 1	Dose 2	Dose 3	Dose 4						
Inactivated Polio[4]			Dose 1	Dose 2	Dose 3					Dose 4		
Measles, Mumps, Rubella[5]						Dose 1				Dose 2	CATCH UP	
Varicella[6]						Single dose					CATCH UP	
Pneumococcal[7]			Dose 1	Dose 2	Dose 3	Dose 4				CATCH UP	PPV	
Hepatitis A[8]										Two doses		
Influenza[9]					Vaccinate every year							

Vaccines below this line are for selected populations

▨ = Time for preadolescent assessment

Figure 64–1 ■ Recommended childhood immunization schedule in the United States for 2003.
This immunization schedule is based on joint recommendations by the Advisory Committee on Immunization Practices (ACIP) of the Centers for Disease Control and Prevention, the American Academy of Pediatrics (AAP), and the American Academy of Family Physicians (AAFP). *Gold-colored bars* indicate recommended ages for each dose; a bar that spans more than one age bracket indicates an acceptable range of ages for that dose. *Purple bars* indicate "catch-up" vaccination. All children should undergo a preadolescent assessment between ages 11 and 12 years.

1. Hepatitis B vaccine (Hep B). The immunization schedule for infants is based on whether the mother is *hepatitis B surface antigen* (HBsAg)-*positive* or *HBsAg-negative*, that is, on whether the mother has laboratory evidence of hepatitis B infection.

All infants should receive the *first dose* of Hep B soon after birth and before hospital discharge; if the infant's mother is HBsAg-negative, the first dose may be given at any age up to 2 months. Only monovalent Hep B can be used for the birth dose. Either Hep B alone, or a combination vaccine that contains Hep B, may be used to complete the series. If a combination product is used, a total of four doses may be given. The *second dose* should be given at least 4 weeks after the first dose (and no sooner than age 6 weeks if a combination vaccine that contains *Haemophilus influenzae* type b vaccine is used). The *third dose* should be given at least 16 weeks after the first dose, and at least 8 weeks after the second dose. The *last dose* (third or fourth) should be administered after age 6 months.

Infants born to HBsAg-positive mothers should receive Hep B plus 0.5 ml hepatitis B immune globulin (HBIG), injected at separate sites, within 12 hours of birth. The second dose of Hep B is recommended at age 1 to 2 months, and the vaccination series should be completed (third or fourth dose) at age 6 months.

Continued

Figure 64–1 ▪ Continued

Infants born to mothers whose HBsAg status is unknown should receive the first dose of Hep B within 12 hours of birth. Maternal blood should be drawn at the time of delivery to determine the mother's HBsAg status; if her status is positive, the infant should receive HBIG as soon as possible, and no later than age 1 week.

Catch-up vaccination, for children who were not vaccinated during infancy, can be started at any time. Children under 11 years old should receive the standard three- or four-dose series. An optional two-dose series can be used for children 11 to 15 years old; the second dose is given 4 to 6 months after the first dose.

2. Diphtheria and tetanus toxoids and acellular pertussis vaccine (DTaP). For routine vaccination, children should receive the five-dose series as indicated. However, the fourth dose can be administered to children as young as 12 months, provided 6 months have elapsed since the third dose and the child is considered unlikely to return at age 15 to 18 months.

Tetanus and diphtheria toxoids (Td) is recommended at age 11 to 12 years if at least 5 years have elapsed since the last dose of tetanus and diphtheria toxoid–containing vaccine. Subsequent routine Td boosters are recommended every 10 years.

3. *Haemophilus influenzae* type b (Hib) conjugate vaccine. Four Hib conjugate vaccines are licensed in the United States for infant use. If PRP-OMP [PedvaxHIB, Comvax] is administered at 2 and 4 months, a dose at age 6 months is not required; otherwise, it must be given. Because clinical studies in infants have demonstrated that using some combination products may induce a lower immune response to the Hib component, DTaP/Hib combination products should not be used for primary immunization at 2, 4, or 6 months. After completing the primary series, any Hib conjugate vaccine may be used as a booster.

4. Inactivated poliovirus vaccine (IPV). Until recently, two poliovirus vaccines were available in the United States: *inactivated poliovirus vaccine* (IPV) and *oral poliovirus vaccine* (OPV). However, in 2002, OPV was withdrawn. All children should receive four doses of IPV—at ages 2 months, 4 months, 6 to 18 months, and 4 to 6 years.

5. Measles, mumps, and rubella virus vaccine (MMR). The second dose of MMR is routinely recommended at 4 to 6 years, but may be given during any visit provided that (1) at least 4 weeks have elapsed since the first dose and (2) neither dose is administered earlier than age 12 months. Children 11 to 12 years old who have not yet received the second dose should get a catch-up dose now, as should children 13 to 18 years old.

6. Varicella vaccine. Varicella vaccine is recommended at any visit at or after age 12 months for susceptible children (i.e., children who lack a reliable history of chickenpox [as judged by a healthcare provider] and who have not been immunized).

A catch-up dose is recommended for susceptible children 2 to 18 years old. Susceptible children age 13 and older should receive two doses, administered at least 4 weeks apart.

7. Pneumococcal vaccine. Two pneumococcal vaccines are available: *pneumococcal conjugate vaccine* (PCV) and *pneumococcal polysaccharide vaccine* (PPV). PCV is used for routine vaccination (doses 1 through 4 in the figure) of children ages 2 to 23 months. Catch-up vaccination with PCV is recommended for all children ages 2 to 5 years who have not already been vaccinated, giving priority to those at highest risk for serious pneumococcal disease. Children in certain high-risk groups should receive PPV in addition to PCV. See text and *MMWR* 2000;49(RR-9):1–37.

8. Hepatitis A vaccine. Routine vaccination of children is recommended only in geographic areas of high risk, and for children in certain high-risk groups. For information about your area, consult your local public health authorities or read *MMWR* 1999;48(RR-12):1–37.

Two doses are required. The first can be given at 12 months of age. The second dose should be given 6 to 12 months after the first (for Havrix) or 6 to 18 months after the first (for VAQTA).

9. Influenza vaccine. Influenza vaccine, administered annually, is now recommended for all children ages 6 to 23 months old, and for all children (over the age of 6 months) who have certain risk factors, including asthma, diabetes, heart disease, sickle cell disease, HIV infection, and use of immunosuppressive drugs (see Chapter 89 and *MMWR* 2001;50[RR-44]:1–44). The vaccine can also be given to all others wishing to obtain immunity. Dosage depends on the child's age: 0.25 ml for ages 6 to 35 months; 0.5 ml for ages 3 years and older. Children less than 9 years old who are receiving influenza vaccine for the first time should get two doses, given at least 4 weeks apart.

---

ism is varicella-zoster virus, a member of the herpesvirus group. Patients typically develop 250 to 500 maculopapular or vesicular lesions, usually on the face, scalp, or trunk. Other symptoms include fever, malaise, and loss of appetite. Among children, the most common complications are bacterial suprainfection and acute cerebellar ataxia; Reye's syndrome and encephalitis develop rarely. Among adults, the most serious common complication is varicella pneumonia. As a rule, symptoms in adults are more severe than in children: hospitalization is 10 times more likely in adults, and death is 20 times more likely. Although adults account for only 2% of varicella cases, they account for 50% of varicella-related deaths. Before varicella vaccine became available, 90% to 95% of children in the United States got chickenpox by age 11, which corresponds to 4 million cases a year.

Herpes zoster, also known as *shingles* or simply *zoster,* develops in 15% of cases years after childhood chickenpox has resolved. The cause of zoster is reactivation of varicella-zoster viruses that had been dormant within sensory nerve roots. Episodes of zoster begin with neurologic pain in the area of skin supplied by the affected nerve roots. Blister-like lesions develop within 3 to 4 days, and usually disappear 2 to 3 weeks later. However, in about 14% of patients, neurologic pain persists for a month or more—and in a few cases, pain lasts for years.

Although varicella vaccine is both safe and effective, vaccination rates remain low. Varicella vaccine became available in 1995, but only 25% of children have received it. As a result, children continue to experience unnecessary illness, hospitalization, and death.

Hepatitis B

Hepatitis B is a serious liver infection caused by the hepatitis B virus. Acute infection can cause anorexia, malaise, diarrhea, vomiting, jaundice, pain (in muscles, joints, and stomach), and death. Chronic infection can result in cirrhosis, liver cancer, and death. Each year in the United States, hepatitis B infects 150,000 people, puts 11,000 in the hospital, and kills 4000 to 5000. Worldwide, 170 million people have chronic hepatitis B, and 250,000 die from it annually.

Although hepatitis B is found in virtually all body fluids, only blood, serum-derived fluids, saliva, semen, and vaginal fluids are infectious. The most common modes of transmission are needle-stick accidents, sexual contact with an infected partner, maternal-child transmission during birth, and use of contaminated IV equipment or solutions.

Hepatitis B is discussed further in Chapter 89 (Antiviral Drugs I: Drugs for Non-HIV Viral Infections).

Hepatitis A

Hepatitis A is a serious liver infection caused by the hepatitis A virus. In the United States, hepatitis A infects between 125,000 and 200,000 people annually, and causes about 100 deaths (from acute liver failure). Symptoms of hepatitis A include fever, malaise, nausea, jaundice, anorexia, diarrhea, and stomach pain. However, not all infected persons become symptomatic. Among children less than 6 years old, only 30% develop symptoms. In contrast, symptoms are present in most older children and adults. When symptoms do occur, they develop rapidly and then usually fade in less than 2 months. However, between 10% and 15% of patients experience prolonged or relapsing disease that persists for up to 6 months. During the course of the infection, the virus undergoes replication in the liver, passage into the bile, and then excretion in the feces. As a result, the usual mode of transmission is fecal-oral in the context of close personal contact with an infected person. In addition, hepatitis A can be contracted by ingesting contaminated food or water. Blood-borne transmission is rare. Individuals at risk of infection include household and sexual contacts of infected individuals, international travelers, and people living in areas where hepatitis A is endemic (e.g., American Indian reservations, Alaskan Native villages).

Pneumococcal Infection

In the United States, *Streptococcus pneumoniae* (pneumococcus) is the leading bacterial cause of childhood meningitis, sepsis, pneumonia, and otitis media. Among children with pneumococcal meningitis, up to 50% suffer permanent brain damage or hearing loss, and about 10% die. Worldwide, pneumococcal infection ranks among the leading causes of death from infectious disease.

Each year in the United States *S. pneumoniae* causes 3000 cases of meningitis, 50,000 cases of bacteremia, 500,000 cases of pneumonia, and 7 million cases of otitis media. Among children under age 5, the pneumococcus causes 1400 cases of meningitis and 16,000 cases of bacteremia. The risk of acquiring pneumococcal infection is highest for children under the age of 2. Factors that increase risk of infection include sickle cell disease, immunodeficiency, asplenia, chronic diseases, attending a group day care center, and being a Native American, African American, Alaskan Native, or socially disadvantaged.

Influenza

Influenza is a serious infection of the respiratory tract that constitutes a major cause of morbidity and mortality around the world. Characteristics of the influenza virus and of influenza itself (mode of transmission, symptoms, time course, methods of prevention and treatment) are discussed in Chapter 89.

SPECIFIC VACCINES AND TOXOIDS

The discussion below is limited to the vaccines and toxoids used most often for childhood immunization. Also, the discussion focuses almost exclusively on immunization of children; vaccination of adults is mentioned only briefly. The major preparations used for childhood immunization are listed in Table 64–3. Their adverse effects are summarized in Table 64–4. Childhood immunization schedules for the year 2003, as recommended by the Advisory Committee on Immunization Practices (ACIP) of the Centers for Disease Control and Prevention, the American Academy of Pediatrics (AAP), and the American Academy of Family Physicians (AAFP) are summarized in Figure 64–1.

Measles, Mumps, and Rubella Virus Vaccine (MMR)

Description. Measles, mumps, and rubella vaccine (MMR), marketed under the trade name M-M-R II, is a combination product composed of three live virus vaccines. Administration induces synthesis of antibodies directed against measles, mumps, and rubella viruses. Immunization with MMR is preferred to immunization with the three vaccines separately.

Efficacy. Following a single dose of MMR, an effective response develops in 97% of vaccinees within 2 to 6 weeks.

Adverse Effects. Mild. Local soreness, erythema, and swelling may develop soon after vaccination. Within 1 to 2 weeks, some children experience glandular swelling in the cheeks and neck and under the jaw. Transient rash develops in 5% to 15% of vaccinees. Fever (103°F or higher) that persists for several days occurs in 5% to 15% of vaccinees 5 to 12 days after vaccination. MMR-induced fever poses a small risk of febrile seizures, but there is no evidence of residual seizure disorders. Within 1 to 3 weeks of the first dose, about 1% of vaccinees experience pain, stiffness, and swelling in one or more joints; these symptoms usually subside in a few days, but on rare occasions persist for a month or more. Fever, soreness, and pain can be reduced with acetaminophen or a nonaspirin nonsteroidal anti-inflammatory drug, such as ibuprofen.

Severe. Transient *thrombocytopenia* occurs rarely (0.0025% incidence). MMR-induced thrombocytopenia is generally benign, but hemorrhage has developed in a few vaccinees.

MMR may induce *anaphylactic reactions.* However, the incidence is extremely low: Only 11 certain cases have occurred in over 70 million vaccinations. Until recently, MMR-induced anaphylaxis was thought to result from allergy to eggs (the measles component of the vaccine is produced in chick embryo fibroblasts). However, new studies suggest that egg allergy is not involved. Currently, the leading suspect is a hydrolysis product of gelatin. Until more is known, authorities now recommend that MMR be used with extreme caution

TABLE 64–3 ■■ Some Vaccines and Toxoids Available in the United States

Preparation Name (Synonym)	Trade Name	Type of Preparation	Route and Site
Measles, mumps, and rubella virus vaccine (MMR)	M-M-R II	Live virus	SC, in outer aspect of upper arm
Diphtheria and tetanus toxoids and acellular pertussis vaccine (DTaP)	Tripedia, DAPTACEL Infanrix	Toxoids (diphtheria and tetanus) plus inactivated bacteria components (pertussis)	IM, in deltoid or mediolateral thigh
Diphtheria and tetanus toxoids and acellular pertussis adsorbed, hepatitis B (recombinant) and inactivated poliovirus vaccine	PEDIARIX	Toxoids (diphtheria and tetanus) plus inactivated bacteria components (pertussis) plus inactive viral antigen (hepatitis B) plus inactivated viruses (poliovirus)	IM, in deltoid or anterolateral thigh
Tetanus and diphtheria toxoids (DT [pediatric], Td [adult])	Generic only	Toxoids	IM, in deltoid or mediolateral thigh
Haemophilus influenzae type b (Hib) conjugate vaccine	HibTITER, ActHIB, PedvaxHIB	Bacterial polysaccharide conjugated to protein	IM, in midthigh or outer aspect of upper arm
Poliovirus vaccine, inactivated (IPV, Salk vaccine)	IPOL	Inactivated viruses of all three polio serotypes	SC, in anterolateral thigh
Varicella virus vaccine	Varivax	Live virus	SC, in deltoid or anterolateral thigh
Hepatitis A vaccine	Havrix, VAQTA	Inactive viral antigen	IM, in deltoid
Hepatitis B vaccine	Recombivax HB, Engerix-B	Inactive viral antigen	IM, in deltoid or anterolateral thigh
Pneumococcal conjugate vaccine	Prevnar	Bacterial polysaccharide conjugated to protein	IM, in deltoid or anterolateral thigh
Pneumococcal polysaccharide vaccine	Pneumovax 23, Pnu-Imune 23	Bacterial polysaccharide (unconjugated)	IM, in deltoid or anterolateral thigh
Influenza vaccine	FluShield, Fluzone, Fluvirin	Inactive viral antigen	IM, in deltoid or anterolateral thigh

TABLE 64–4 ■■ Adverse Effects of Some Vaccines and Toxoids

Preparation	Mild Effects	Serious Effects
Measles, mumps, and rubella virus vaccine	Local reactions; rash; fever; swollen glands in cheeks and neck and under the jaw; pain, stiffness, and swelling in joints	Anaphylaxis, thrombocytopenia
Diphtheria and tetanus toxoids and pertussis vaccine, whole-cell or acellular*	Local reactions, fever, fretfulness, drowsiness, anorexia, persistent crying	Acute encephalopathy, convulsions, shock-like state
Haemophilus influenzae type b conjugate vaccine	Local reactions, fever, crying, diarrhea, vomiting	None
Poliovirus vaccine (IPV and OPV†)	Local reactions (only from IPV)	Vaccine-associated paralytic poliomyelitis (only from OPV†)
Varicella virus vaccine	Local reactions, fever, mild varicella-like rash (local or generalized)	None
Hepatitis A vaccine	Local soreness, headache, anorexia, fatigue	Anaphylaxis
Hepatitis B vaccine	Local discomfort, fever	Anaphylaxis
Pneumococcal conjugate vaccine	Local reactions, fever	None
Influenzae vaccine	Local reactions, fever	Guillain-Barré syndrome (association not proved)

*Acellular DTP causes fewer and milder side effects than whole-cell DTP.
†OPV is no longer available.

in children with a known allergy to gelatin. The ACIP is reconsidering whether caution is still required for children with an allergy to eggs.

Precautions and Contraindications. MMR is *contraindicated* during *pregnancy* and should be used with *caution* in children with a history of (1) *thrombocytopenia* or *thrombocytopenic purpura* or (2) *anaphylactic-like reactions to gelatin, eggs,* or *neomycin* (MMR contains a small amount of this antibiotic).

MMR can be administered to children with *mild febrile illness* (e.g., upper respiratory infection with or without low-grade fever). However, for children with *moderate or severe febrile illness,* administration should be postponed until the illness has resolved.

Products that contain *immune globulins* (e.g., whole blood, serum, specific immune globulins) contain antibodies against the viruses in MMR, and therefore can inhibit the immune response to the vaccine. Accordingly, in children who have received immune globulins, vaccination with MMR should be postponed for at least 3 to 6 months.

In vaccinees who are *immunocompromised,* replication of the viruses in MMR may be much greater than normal. If the immunodeficiency is severe, death may occur. However, of the more than 200 million people who have received MMR in the United States, only 5 such deaths have been reported. Nonetheless, *children with severe immunodeficiency should NOT be given MMR.* Severe immunodeficiency may result from immunosuppressive drugs (e.g., glucocorticoids, cytotoxic anticancer drugs), certain cancers (e.g., leukemia, lymphoma, generalized malignancy), and advanced HIV infection. It is important to note, however, that if HIV infection is *asymptomatic,* MMR should be given. In these people, there is no risk of serious adverse events from MMR, whereas there *is* a risk of severe complications from measles if the disease should develop. Vaccination with MMR early in the course of HIV infection is preferred, since the immune response to vaccination diminishes as HIV infection progresses.

Route, Site, and Immunization Schedule. MMR is administered SC into the outer aspect of the upper arm. Each child should receive two vaccinations, the first between 12 and 15 months of age, and the second between 4 and 6 years. If the scheduled second dose is missed, it can be given between ages 11 and 18 years.

Diphtheria and Tetanus Toxoids and Acellular Pertussis Vaccine (DTaP)

Preparations. Vaccination against diphtheria, tetanus, and pertussis is usually done simultaneously using a combination product. Until recently, two types of products were available, one containing *whole-cell* pertussis and one containing *acellular* pertussis. The whole-cell preparation (DTwP) is composed of diphtheria toxoid, tetanus toxoid, and a whole-cell pertussis vaccine, consisting of *Bordetella pertussis* that has been inactivated or partially detoxified. The acellular preparation (DTaP) also contains diphtheria and tetanus toxoids; however, instead of whole-cell pertussis vaccine, it contains acellular pertussis vaccine. *DTaP is more effective than DTwP and causes fewer and milder side effects.* Accordingly, DTaP is recommended for routine vaccination. DTwP has been withdrawn.

Vaccination with DTaP produces antibodies directed against diphtheria and tetanus toxins and against *B. pertussis.* The preparation is available under three trade names: Tripedia, DAPTACEL, and Infanrix.

Efficacy. Immunization with DTaP reduces the risk of disease by 80% to 90%. Protection begins after the third dose and persists 4 to 6 years (against pertussis) and 10 years (against diphtheria and tetanus).

Adverse Effects. Mild. Mild reactions are common. The reactions seen most often are *low fever* (50%), *fretfulness* (50%), *drowsiness* (30%), *anorexia* (20%), and *local reactions* (pain [50%], swelling [40%], and redness [30%]). Mild reactions usually develop a few hours to 48 hours after vaccination and then resolve in 1 to 2 days. Acetaminophen or ibuprofen can be used to decrease fever and pain. Mild reactions were more likely with DTwP than with DTaP.

Moderate. Moderate reactions occur less often than mild reactions. *Persistent, inconsolable crying,* lasting 3 hours or longer, occurs in 1% of vaccinees. Crying is most likely with the first dose of DTaP and is not associated with long-term sequelae. *Fever* (105°F or higher) occurs in 0.3% of vaccinees; the pertussis component appears responsible. Approximately 0.06% of vaccinees develop *convulsions* (with or without fever). These seizures have no permanent sequelae and do not increase the risk of subsequent febrile or afebrile seizures. A *shock-like state* develops in 0.06% of vaccinees and has no lasting sequelae.

Severe: Encephalopathy. Very rarely, DTaP causes acute encephalopathy. The incidence is between zero and 10.5 episodes per million doses. Most cases occur within 3 days of vaccination. Some of the children who experience acute encephalopathy develop chronic neurologic dysfunction later in life. However, the contribution of acute encephalopathy to long-term neurologic deficits is unclear.

Precautions and Contraindications. DTaP can be administered to children with *mild febrile illness* (e.g., upper respiratory infection with or without low-grade fever). However, for children with *moderate or severe febrile illness,* administration should be postponed until the illness has resolved.

DTaP is *contraindicated* if a prior vaccination with DTaP produced (1) an immediate anaphylactic reaction or (2) encephalopathy within 7 days of vaccination.

DTaP should be administered with *caution* (if at all) if a prior vaccination with DTaP produced any of the following:

■ A shock-like state
■ Fever (105°F or higher) occurring within 48 hours of vaccination and not attributable to another identifiable cause
■ Persistent, inconsolable crying lasting 3 or more hours and occurring within 48 hours of vaccination
■ Convulsions (with or without fever) occurring within 3 days of vaccination.

Route, Site, and Immunization Schedule. DTaP is injected IM into the deltoid muscle or thigh. Most children should receive five injections, the first at 2 months, the second at 4 months, the third at 6 months, the fourth between 15 and 18 months, and the fifth between 4 and 6 years. DTaP is recommended over DTwP for all vaccinations in the series, even for children who began the series with DTwP. Children 11 to 12 years old who completed the series at least 5 years previously should receive a booster shot of tetanus plus diphtheria toxoids for adults (Td). Subsequent Td boosters are recommended every 10 years.

Poliovirus Vaccine

Preparations. Until recently, two polio vaccines were available: *oral poliovirus vaccine* (OPV, Sabin vaccine) and *inactivated poliovirus vaccine* (IPV, Salk vaccine). OPV is composed of live, attenuated viruses. In contrast, IPV is composed of *inactivated* polioviruses. As discussed below, OPV has *caused* polio in a few children, whereas IPV has not and cannot. Because the benefit/risk ratio of IPV is superior to that of OPV, IPV is clearly preferred. Accordingly, in 2002, OPV was withdrawn from the U.S. market. The trade name for IPV is IPOL; the trade name for OPV was Orimune.

Efficacy. Between 97.5% and 100% of children receiving IPV or OPV develop antibodies to poliovirus types 1, 2, and 3. Antibodies develop after two or more doses and persist for many years.

Adverse Effects of IPV. IPV is devoid of serious adverse effects. As with other injected drugs, local soreness may occur. IPV contains trace amounts of streptomycin, neomycin, and bacitracin. Children with an allergy to these drugs should be monitored.

Adverse Effects of OPV. Very rarely, OPV has caused *vaccine-associated paralytic poliomyelitis* (VAPP). The severity of VAPP is similar to that of paralytic poliomyelitis caused by the wild-type virus. In immunocompromised children, VAPP can prove fatal. The incidence of VAPP is one case for each 2.4 million doses of OPV administered, which corresponds to 1 case for each 750,000 children starting the vaccination series. In the United States, eight to nine cases of VAPP have occurred each year. Because wild-type poliovirus has been eliminated from the Western hemisphere, the risk for Americans of acquiring polio from OPV now greatly exceeds the risk of acquiring the disease from the environment. In response to this change in risk/benefit ratio, the ACIP has changed its recommendations on polio immunization: Whereas OPV had been the preferred vaccine for many years, the ACIP now recommends exclusive use of IVP.

Route, Site, and Immunization Schedule. IPV is administered SC in the anterolateral thigh. All children should receive four doses, the first at 2 months of age, the second at 4 months, the third between 6 and 18 months, and the fourth between 4 and 6 years.

Haemophilus influenzae Type b Conjugate Vaccine

Preparations. Vaccines directed against *H. influenzae* type b (Hib) are prepared by conjugating (covalently binding) a purified capsular polysaccharide (PRP) from *H. influenzae* to either (1) diphtheria toxoid, (2) tetanus toxoid, or (3) an outer membrane protein (OMP) isolated from *Neisseria meningitidis*. The reason for conjugating PRP to these other compounds is to enhance antigenicity. The vaccines made with OMP—marketed as PedvaxHIB and Comvax* and abbreviated PRP-OMP—elicit a stronger immune response than the vaccines made with diphtheria toxoid [HibTITER] or tetanus toxoid [ActHIB].

Efficacy. Immunization with Hib vaccine decreases the risk of disease by 88% to 98%. When PedvaxHIB is used,

protection begins 1 week after the first dose. However, when HibTITER or ActHIB is used, protection is delayed, beginning 1 to 2 weeks after the fourth dose. With all three vaccines, protection persists for several years.

Adverse Effects. Hib vaccine is among the safest of all vaccines. Serious adverse effects have not been reported. The few adverse effects that do occur are generally transient and mild. Between 2% and 5% of vaccinees develop local reactions (swelling, erythema, warmth, tenderness). About 1% experience fever (>101°F), crying, diarrhea, or vomiting.

Route, Site, and Immunization Schedule. Hib vaccines are administered IM into the midthigh or the outer aspect of the upper arm. Most children should receive four doses, the first at 2 months of age, the second at 4 months, the third at 6 months, and the fourth between 12 and 15 months. If PedvaxHIB is used for the first two doses, the third dose (6-month dose) can be omitted.

Varicella Virus Vaccine

Description. Varicella virus vaccine [Varivax] is composed of live, attenuated varicella viruses. Administration induces synthesis of antibodies against the virus. Varicella vaccine was developed in Japan in 1973, but was not available in the United States until March of 1995.

Efficacy. In children less than 12 years old, a single dose of varicella vaccine produces antibodies in 97% of recipients. However, in children 13 to 17 years old, only 79% develop antibodies after one dose. In Japan, testing of people who were vaccinated 20 years earlier demonstrated that antibodies were still present.

Even though most vaccinees develop antibodies to varicella viruses, not everyone with antibodies is fully protected. Complete protection against chickenpox develops in only 85% to 96% of vaccinees. However, among the 4% to 15% who get chickenpox despite vaccination, symptoms are always mild: These children develop fewer lesions (<35, compared with 250 to 500 for unvaccinated children), experience less fever, and recover more quickly. In Japan, herpes zoster (shingles) has not been observed in any adult who received varicella vaccine as a child, even if breakthrough chickenpox had occurred.

Adverse Effects. Varicella vaccine is very safe; no serious adverse events have been reported. About 25% of vaccinees experience erythema, soreness, and swelling at the injection site; 15% develop fever (>102°F); and 3% develop a mild, local varicella-like rash, consisting of just a few lesions. About 5% of healthy children develop a sparse, generalized varicella-like rash within a month of the injection; in children with leukemia, the incidence of generalized rash is much higher—about 50%.

In theory, children receiving the vaccine can transmit vaccine virus to others. However, among otherwise healthy vaccinees, such transmission has not been reported. In contrast, among leukemic children who developed a rash after vaccination, a few cases of viral transmission have occurred. To reduce the risk of transmission, vaccine recipients should temporarily avoid close contact with susceptible, high-risk individuals (e.g., neonates, pregnant women, immunocompromised people).

Precautions and Contraindications. Varicella vaccine is *contraindicated* during *pregnancy,* for individuals with cer-

*Comvax is a combination vaccine used for immunization against *H. influenzae* and hepatitis B.

tain *cancers* (e.g., leukemia, lymphomas), and for those with *hypersensitivity to neomycin or gelatin,* which are in the vaccine. In addition, the vaccine should be avoided by individuals who are *immunocompromised.* This includes those with HIV infection or congenital immunodeficiency and those taking immunosuppressive drugs.

Children receiving the vaccine should avoid *aspirin and other salicylates* for 6 weeks. This precaution is based on the theoretical risk of developing Reye's syndrome: If the child develops chickenpox (albeit a mild case) in response to the vaccine, the very small risk of developing Reye's syndrome is made somewhat larger by concurrent use of salicylates.

Route, Site, and Immunization Schedule. Varicella vaccine is administered SC into the outer aspect of the upper arm or into the anterolateral thigh. Because the vaccine wasn't available in the United States before the spring of 1995, many children missed being vaccinated at the preferred age: 12 to 18 months. Accordingly, the vaccination schedule for older children necessarily differs from that for younger children. Current recommendations are as follows:

- *Children 12 to 18 months old*—Most children in this age group should receive a single dose of vaccine. No additional doses are needed.
- *Children 19 months through 12 years old*—Children in this age group who have not been vaccinated yet and have not had chickenpox can be vaccinated now. A single dose is all that is needed. Many physicians wait until these children are 11 to 12 years old to administer this catch-up dose. However, a single vaccination can be administered at any time prior to the 13th birthday.
- *Children 13 or more years old*—Children in this age group who have not been vaccinated yet and have not had chickenpox can be given a catch-up vaccination now. Since these older children have a reduced response to the vaccine, they need two doses, administered at least 4 weeks apart.

We Need to Vaccinate More Children. Since the approval of Varivax in 1995, only 33% of eligible children have received the vaccine. Several misconceptions underlie low usage: Some people think that chickenpox is a mild disease (it's actually the leading cause of vaccine-preventable child death in the United States); some think that Varivax is not effective (vaccination prevents severe chickenpox in 100% of recipients); and some think that Varivax is not safe (serious reactions are extremely rare, and a causal relationship with Varivax has not been proved).

The major impact of failure to vaccinate will be felt when today's children grow up. Recall that chickenpox in adults is much more severe than in children: Compared with children, adults have a 10- to 20-fold increased risk of serious complications, including death. Because some children are being vaccinated, the overall incidence of chickenpox is on the decline. As a result, children who remain unvaccinated may still not get chickenpox, and hence may reach adulthood without developing antibodies to the disease. Therefore, if they do acquire the disease as adults, it is likely to be severe. The moral to this story is that vaccinating children now will not only protect them from chickenpox during childhood, it will also protect them from serious harm when they grow up.

Hepatitis B Vaccine

Preparations. Hepatitis B vaccine (Hep B) contains *hepatitis B surface antigen* (HBsAg), the primary antigenic protein in the viral envelope. Administration of Hep B promotes synthesis of specific antibodies directed against hepatitis B virus. Hep B approved for children is marketed under two trade names: Recombivax HB and Engerix-B. Recombivax is available in two formulations, both containing 10 μg of HBsAg/ml. Engerix-B is also available in two formulations, both containing 20 μg of HBsAg/ml. The HBsAg in Recombivax HB and Engerix-B is produced in yeast using recombinant DNA technology. Because these vaccines are made from a viral component, rather than from a live virus, they cannot cause disease.

In 2001, the Food and Drug Administration (FDA) approved a new vaccine directed against both hepatitis A and hepatitis B. This combination vaccine, marketed as Twinrix, is approved for adults but not for children.

Efficacy. Greater than 85% of vaccinees are protected after the second dose of Hep B, and more than 90% are protected after the third dose. Although the duration of protection has not been determined with precision, it appears to be at least 5 to 7 years.

Adverse Effects and Contraindications. Hep B is one of our safest vaccines. The most common reactions are soreness at the injection site and mild to moderate fever. Acetaminophen or ibuprofen may be used to relieve discomfort, but aspirin should be avoided. The only contraindication to Hep B is a prior anaphylactic reaction either to Hep B itself or to baker's yeast.

Route, Site, and Immunization Schedule. Hep B is injected IM. In neonates and infants, the injection is made into the anterolateral thigh. In adolescents and adults, the injection is made into the deltoid. All vaccinees should receive three doses.

The immunization schedule for *infants* is based on whether the mother is *HBsAg-positive* or *HBsAg-negative* (i.e., on whether the mother has laboratory evidence of hepatitis B infection). The following schedules for infants are recommended:

- *Infants whose mothers are HBsAg-negative*—give 5 μg of Recombivax HB or 10 μg of Engerix-B sometime between birth and 2 months of age. Give the second dose between 1 and 4 months of age (and at least 1 month after the first dose), and the third dose between 6 and 18 months of age (and at least 4 months after the first dose and at least 2 months after the second dose).
- *Infants whose mothers are HBsAg-positive*—give 5 μg of Recombivax HB or 10 μg of Engerix-B within 12 hours of birth, and give 0.5 ml of *hepatitis B immune globulin* (HBIG) at the same time but at a separate site. (The purpose of the HBIG is to provide immediate protection against hepatitis B acquired from the mother.) Give the second dose of Hep B between 1 and 2 months of age, and the third dose at 6 months of age.
- *Infants whose mothers' HBsAg status is unknown*—give 5 μg of Recombivax HB or 10 μg of Engerix-B within 12 hours of birth. Subsequent doses are based on the mother's HBsAg status, which is determined by analyzing a maternal blood sample obtained during delivery. If the mother is HBsAg-positive, the infant should be given HBIG as soon as possible—and no later than 1 week after birth.

Children and adolescents who were not vaccinated against hepatitis B during infancy may begin the three-dose series at any time. Once the first dose is given, the second is given 1 month (or more) later, and the third 4 months (or more) after the first dose and no less than 2 months after the second dose. For children 11 years and older, a new two-dose schedule can be used; the second dose is given 4 to 6 months after the first.

Hepatitis A Vaccine

Preparations. In the United States, two vaccines against hepatitis A are available: Havrix and VAQTA. Both consist of inactivated hepatitis A virus.

Efficacy. Immunization with hepatitis A vaccine decreases the risk of clinical disease by 94% to 100%. Protective levels of antibodies are seen in 94% to 100% of adults and children 1 month after the first dose, and in 100% of vaccinees 1 month after the second dose. Protection appears to be long lasting: Among vaccinated children who were followed for 7 years, no cases of hepatitis A were detected.

Who Should Be Vaccinated? At this time, routine childhood vaccination against hepatitis A is recommend only in locales where the risk of disease is high. Among these are American Indian reservations and Alaskan Native villages. Information on local risk can be obtained from local public health authorities or by reading *MMWR: Morbidity and Mortality Weekly Report,* volume 48, number RR-12, October 1, 1999.

Hepatitis A vaccine is also recommended for

- People at least 2 years old traveling to places with high rates of hepatitis A, including Central or South America, Mexico, the Caribbean islands, Africa, Asia (except Japan), and southern or eastern Europe
- People in communities that have prolonged outbreaks of hepatitis A
- Men who have sex with men
- People who use street drugs
- People with chronic liver disease
- People who receive clotting factor concentrates

Adverse Effects. Hepatitis A vaccine is extremely safe. Worldwide, over 65 million doses have been administered, while causing no serious adverse events that could be definitively linked to the vaccine.

Mild reactions are common. Soreness at the injection site occurs in about 54% of adults and 18% of children. Headache occurs in 14% of adults and 9% of children. Other mild reactions include loss of appetite and malaise. When mild reactions occur, they usually begin 3 to 5 days after vaccination and last only 1 to 2 days.

Route, Site, and Immunization Schedule. Hepatitis A vaccines should be given IM into the deltoid muscle. Two doses are required. The first can be given at 12 months of age. The second should be given 6 to 12 months after the first (for Havrix) or 6 to 18 months after the first (for VAQTA).

Pneumococcal Conjugate Vaccine

On February 12, 2000, the FDA approved a *pneumococcal conjugate vaccine* (PCV) [Prevnar] for prevention of invasive pneumococcal disease in infants and children. An unconjugated vaccine—*pneumococcal polysaccharide vaccine* (PPV) [Pneumovax 23, Pnu-Imune 23]—is also available. However, this PPV is approved only for use in adults and in high-risk children over the age of 2 years; it does not work in children younger than 2 years.

Description. PCV consists of seven pneumococcal capsular polysaccharide antigens that have been conjugated to a protein carrier—specifically, CRM_{197}, a nontoxic variant of diphtheria toxin. The protein carrier increases antigenicity, especially in infants. The seven antigens in the vaccine are from the seven serotypes of *S. pneumoniae* that cause the majority (80%) of invasive pneumococcal infections in American children under the age of 6.

Efficacy. Vaccination efficacy was evaluated in a trial that enrolled 37,868 healthy infants. Half received the vaccine, and half received a control injection. Vaccination was 100% effective in preventing invasive disease caused by the *S. pneumoniae* serotypes that the vaccine was designed to protect against. In addition, vaccination was 89% effective at preventing invasive disease caused by *all* serotypes of *S. pneumoniae*. In addition to preventing invasive pneumococcal disease, vaccination caused a modest reduction in cases of otitis media (see Chapter 102).

Adverse Effects. The pneumococcal conjugate vaccine appears to be very safe. No serious adverse effects have been reported. Mild, self-limited reactions (erythema, swelling, pain, tenderness) occur at the injection site in 10% to 20% of vaccinees. Fever (temperature over 100.3°F) develops in 21%. Irritability, drowsiness, and reduced appetite may also occur.

Who Should Be Vaccinated? The ACIP recommends vaccinating children in the following groups:

- All children under 2 years of age
- Children between ages 2 and 5 years who (1) have not already been vaccinated and (2) have conditions that put them at high risk of serious pneumococcal disease. In this group are children with sickle cell anemia, injury to the spleen, chronic heart or lung disease, or immunosuppression of any cause (e.g., diabetes, cancer, liver disease, HIV infection, use of immunosuppressive drugs). These children should receive two doses of PCV 2 months apart, followed 2 or more months later by a single dose of PPV.
- All other children between 2 and 5 years old who have not already been vaccinated, giving priority to those at highest risk (i.e., children ages 24 to 35 months, children attending day care centers, and children who are African American, Native American, or Alaskan Native). For these children, the ACIP recommends just one PCV dose.

Route, Site, and Immunization Schedule. Vaccination is done by IM injection into the anterolateral aspect of the thigh (in infants) or into the deltoid muscle of the upper arm (in toddlers and young children). The vaccine is a suspension, and hence must be shaken before use. All doses are 0.5 ml. The number of doses and their timing depend on the child's age when the first dose is given:

- *First dose at age 2 months*—four doses total; one each at ages 2, 4, and 6 months and one between ages 12 and 15 months
- *First dose between ages 7 and 11 months*—three doses total; the first two doses should be given at least 4 weeks apart, and the third should be at least 2 months after the second, but not before the child's first birthday

- *First dose between ages 12 and 23 months*—two doses total, given at least 2 months apart
- *First dose on or after age 24 months*—for children at low risk, just one dose; for children at high risk, two doses given 2 months apart, followed 2 or more months later by a single dose of PPV.

Influenza Vaccine

Annual vaccination against influenza is now recommended for all children ages 6 to 23 months, and for all children at least 6 months old who have certain risk factors, including asthma, diabetes, heart disease, sickle cell disease, HIV infection, and use of immunosuppressive drugs. Properties of the influenza vaccine (composition, efficacy, adverse effects, contraindications, preparations, dosage, route) along with a discussion of who should be vaccinated are presented in Chapter 89.

⁘ KEY POINTS

- Vaccines promote synthesis of antibodies directed against bacteria and viruses, whereas toxoids promote synthesis of antibodies directed against bacterial toxins, but not against the bacteria themselves.
- Killed vaccines are composed of whole, killed microbes or isolated microbial components, whereas live vaccines are composed of live microbes that have been weakened or rendered completely avirulent.
- Vaccination is defined as the administration of any vaccine or toxoid.
- Vaccination produces active immunity. Antibodies develop over weeks to months and then persist for years.
- Passive immunity is conferred by administering preformed antibodies (immune globulins). Protection is immediate but persists only as long as the antibodies remain in the body.
- Widespread vaccination has greatly reduced the incidence of several infectious diseases, eliminated polio from the Western hemisphere, and eliminated smallpox from the earth.
- Although vaccines are very safe, mild reactions are common, and serious reactions can occur rarely.
- Immunocompromised children are at special risk from live vaccines and should not receive them.
- Measles, mumps, and rubella virus vaccine (MMR) is a combination product composed of three live virus vaccines.
- Rarely, MMR causes thrombocytopenia and anaphylactic reactions. Until recently, anaphylactic reactions were thought to result from allergy to eggs, but we now think they result from allergy to gelatin.
- MMR is contraindicated during pregnancy and should be used with caution in children with a history of either thrombocytopenia or anaphylactic reactions to gelatin, eggs, or neomycin.

- Until recently, we had two vaccines for protection against diphtheria, tetanus, and pertussis. One (DTwP) contained whole-cell pertussis and the other (DTaP) contains acellular pertussis. DTaP is more effective than DTwP and causes fewer and milder side effects. Accordingly, DTaP is recommended for all children. DTwP is no longer available.
- Rarely, DTaP causes acute encephalopathy.
- There are two vaccines against polioviruses: oral poliovirus vaccine (OPV, Sabin vaccine) and inactivated poliovirus vaccine (IPV, Salk vaccine). OPV contains live, attenuated viruses, whereas IPV contains inactivated polioviruses.
- OPV can cause vaccine-associated paralytic poliomyelitis (VAPP); IPV does not. Because IPV is safer, it has replaced OPV for routine vaccination against polio.
- *Haemophilus influenzae* type b vaccine is one of our safest vaccines. No serious adverse events have been reported.
- Varicella virus vaccine is composed of live, attenuated varicella viruses.
- All children receiving varicella vaccine are fully protected against severe varicella (chickenpox), although some get mild disease. However, the children who get chickenpox despite vaccination develop far fewer lesions than unvaccinated children, experience less fever, and recover more quickly.
- Varicella vaccine is very safe; no serious adverse events have been reported.
- Varicella vaccine is contraindicated for pregnant women, individuals hypersensitive to neomycin or gelatin, and immunocompromised people.
- Hepatitis B vaccine (Hep B) contains hepatitis B surface antigen (HBsAg), the primary antigenic protein in the viral envelope. Administration of Hep B promotes synthesis of specific antibodies directed against hepatitis B virus.
- Hep B is one of our safest vaccines. The only contraindication is a prior anaphylactic reaction either to Hep B itself or to baker's yeast.
- Within 12 hours of birth, infants whose mothers are HBsAg-positive should be injected with Hep B and hepatitis B immune globulin (HBIG). All other infants should get their first injection of Hep B within 2 months of birth; they do not need HBIG.
- Hepatitis A vaccine is composed of inactivated hepatitis A viruses.
- Pneumococcal conjugate vaccine is the first vaccine for preventing invasive pneumococcal disease in infants and toddlers.
- Annual influenza vaccination is recommended for all children 6 to 23 months old, and for children 6 months and older who have certain risk factors, including asthma, diabetes, HIV infection, and treatment with immunosuppressive drugs.

Immunosuppressants

Immunosuppressive drugs inhibit immune responses. These agents have two principal applications: (1) prevention of organ rejection in transplant patients, and (2) treatment of autoimmune disorders (e.g., rheumatoid arthritis, systemic lupus erythematosus). At the doses required to suppress allograft rejection, almost all of these drugs are toxic. Two toxicities are of particular concern: (1) increased risk of infection and (2) increased risk of neoplasms. Furthermore, because allograft recipients must take immunosuppressants for life, the risk of toxicity continues lifelong. Sites of action of immunosuppressants are summarized in Figure 65–1.

CALCINEURIN INHIBITORS

Cyclosporine and tacrolimus are the most effective immunosuppressants available. Although cyclosporine and tacrolimus differ in structure, they share the same mechanism of action: Both drugs inhibit calcineurin, and thereby suppress production of interleukin-2 (IL-2), a compound needed for T-cell proliferation. The principal use of these drugs is prevention of organ rejection in transplant recipients. Cyclosporine was developed before tacrolimus and is used more often.

Cyclosporine

Cyclosporine [Sandimmune, Gengraf, Neoral] is a powerful immunosuppressant and the drug of choice for preventing organ rejection following allogenic transplants. Major adverse effects are nephrotoxicity and increased risk of infection.

Mechanism of Action

Cyclosporine acts on helper T lymphocytes to suppress production of IL-2, interferon-gamma, and other cytokines. The drug's primary molecular target is a protein known as *cyclophilin.* After binding to cyclophilin, cyclosporine inhibits *calcineurin,* a key enzyme in the pathway that promotes synthesis of IL-2 and other cytokines. In the absence of these compounds, proliferation of B cells and cytotoxic T cells is suppressed. In contrast to methotrexate and other cytotoxic immunosuppressants, cyclosporine does not cause bone marrow depression.

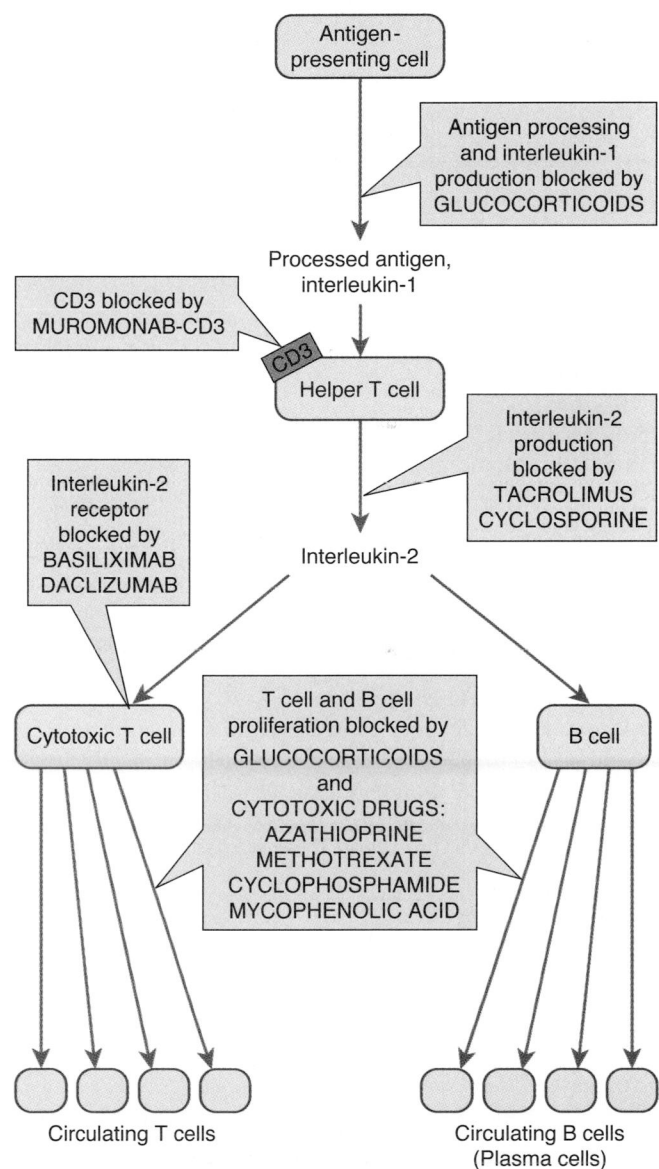

Figure 65–1 ▪ Sites of action of immunosuppressant drugs.

Therapeutic Uses

Cyclosporine is used primarily to prevent rejection of allogenic kidney, liver, and heart transplants. A glucocorticoid (prednisone) is usually given concurrently. Azathioprine, tacrolimus, or sirolimus may be given as well. In addition to its use in transplant patients, cyclosporine is used to treat autoimmune diseases, including rheumatoid arthritis, psoriasis, myasthenia gravis, and early stages of type 1 diabetes.

Pharmacokinetics

Cyclosporine may be administered orally or IV. Oral administration is preferred; IV therapy is reserved for patients who cannot take the drug orally. Absorption from the GI tract is incomplete (about 30%) and erratic. Accordingly, to avoid toxicity (from high drug levels) and organ rejection (from low drug levels), blood levels of cyclosporine should be measured periodically.

Most cyclosporine in the body is bound. In the blood, the drug is bound to red cells (60% to 70%), leukocytes (10% to 20%), and plasma lipoproteins. Outside the vascular system, the drug is bound to tissues.

Cyclosporine undergoes extensive metabolism by hepatic microsomal enzymes. Hence, drugs that increase or decrease the activity of these enzymes can have a significant impact on cyclosporine levels. Excretion of both cyclosporine and its metabolites is via the bile. Practically none of the drug appears in the urine.

Adverse Effects

The most common adverse effects are nephrotoxicity, infection, hypertension, tremor, and hirsutism. Of these, nephrotoxicity and infection are the most serious.

Nephrotoxicity. Renal damage occurs in as many as 75% of patients. Injury manifests as reduced renal blood flow and reduced glomerular filtration rate. These effects are dose dependent and usually reverse following a decrease in cyclosporine dosage.

Nephrotoxicity is evaluated by monitoring for elevated blood urea nitrogen (BUN) and serum creatinine. However, be aware that a rise in these values could also indicate rejection of a kidney transplant. Patients should be informed about the possibility of kidney damage and the importance of periodic tests for BUN and creatinine.

Infection. Cyclosporine increases the risk of infection, although less so than the cytotoxic immunosuppressants. Infectious complications occur in 74% of those treated. Patients should be warned about early signs of infection (fever, sore throat) and instructed to report these immediately.

Hepatotoxicity. Liver damage occurs in 4% to 7% of patients. Injury is evaluated by monitoring for serum bilirubin and liver transaminases. Signs of liver injury reverse rapidly with a reduction in dosage. Inform the patient about the need for periodic tests of liver function.

Lymphomas. Cyclosporine and other immunosuppressants can cause lymphoproliferative diseases. The incidence with cyclosporine alone is low. However, when cyclosporine is combined with other immunosuppressants, the risk of malignant lymphomas increases.

Other Common Adverse Effects. Hypertension, indicated by a 10% to 15% increase in blood pressure, develops in about 50% of patients; standard antihypertensive drugs can be used for treatment. *Tremor* (21% to 55%) and *hirsutism* (21% to 45%) are also common. Less frequently, patients experience *leukopenia* (6%), *gingival hyperplasia* (4%), *gynecomastia* (4%), *sinusitis* (3% to 7%), and *hyperkalemia.*

Anaphylactic Reactions. Anaphylactic reactions are rare, occurring in 1 out of 1000 patients. Signs of anaphylaxis are flushing, respiratory distress, hypotension, and tachycardia. Anaphylaxis occurs only with IV therapy—not with oral therapy. Patients should be monitored for 30 minutes after the onset of IV treatment. If anaphylaxis develops, discontinue the infusion and treat with epinephrine and oxygen.

Use in Pregnancy and Lactation. At doses 2 to 5 times those used clinically, cyclosporine is embryotoxic and fetotoxic in rats and rabbits. However, experience to date shows minimal fetal risk in humans. Nonetheless, prudence dictates avoiding the drug during pregnancy if possible. Patients taking cyclosporine should be advised to use a mechanical form of contraception (condom, diaphragm) rather than oral contraceptives. Cyclosporine is classified in Food and Drug Administration (FDA) Pregnancy Risk Category C. The drug is excreted in breast milk, and nursing should be avoided.

Drug and Food Interactions

Many interactions have been reported. However, only a few appear to have clinical significance. Important interactions are considered below.

Drugs That Can Decrease Cyclosporine Levels. Drugs that induce hepatic microsomal enzymes can accelerate metabolism of cyclosporine, causing cyclosporine levels to fall. This can result in organ rejection. Drugs known to lower cyclosporine levels include *phenytoin, phenobarbital, carbamazepine, rifampin, terbinafine,* and *trimethoprim-sulfamethoxazole.* Cyclosporine levels should be monitored and the dosage adjusted in patients taking these drugs.

Drugs That Can Increase Cyclosporine Levels. A variety of drugs can increase cyclosporine levels, thereby increasing the risk of toxicity. Drugs known to increase cyclosporine levels include *azole antifungal drugs* (e.g., ketoconazole), *macrolide antibiotics* (e.g., erythromycin), and *amphotericin B.* The mechanism is inhibition of cyclosporine metabolism. When either of these drugs is combined with cyclosporine, the dosage of cyclosporine must be reduced to prevent accumulation to toxic levels.

Some physicians administer ketoconazole concurrently with cyclosporine for the express purpose of permitting a reduction in cyclosporine dosage. By slowing metabolism of cyclosporine, ketoconazole permits cyclosporine dosage to be reduced by up to 88%, while continuing to maintain cyclosporine levels within the therapeutic range. The lowered dosage greatly reduces the cost of treatment—from about $7000 per year to about $3000 per year.

Nephrotoxic Drugs. Renal damage may be intensified by concurrent use of other nephrotoxic drugs. These include *amphotericin B, aminoglycosides,* and *nonsteroidal anti-inflammatory drugs* (NSAIDs).

Grapefruit Juice. A compound present in grapefruit juice inhibits metabolism of cyclosporine. As a result, consuming grapefruit juice can raise cyclosporine levels by 50% to 200%, thereby greatly increasing the risk of toxicity.

Preparations, Dosage, and Administration

Preparations and Storage. Cyclosporine is available under three trade names: *Sandimmune, Neoral,* and *Gengraf.* These preparations are *NOT* bioequivalent and cannot be used interchangeably. In Neoral and Gengraf, cyclosporine is present as a microemulsion. As a result, absorption from these formulations is greater than from the Sandimmune formulation. As Sandimmune, cyclosporine is available in capsules (25, 50, and 100 mg), an oral solution (100 mg/ml), and an IV solution (50 mg/ml). As Neoral or Gengraf, cyclosporine is available in capsules (25 and 100 mg) and an oral solution (100 mg/ml). To improve palatability, oral solutions can be mixed with milk, chocolate milk, or orange juice just before administration.

Dosage and Monitoring for Allograft Recipients. Dosing is complex and depends on the organ being transplanted, the formulation employed (Neoral or Gengraf vs. Sandimmune), and other immunosuppressants taken concurrently. The dosages below are representative.

Sandimmune. Oral therapy if preferred to IV therapy. The initial *oral* dose is 15 mg/kg given 4 to 24 hours prior to surgery. This dose is continued once daily for 1 to 2 weeks. Dosage is then gradually reduced to a maintenance level of 3 to 10 mg/kg/day.

For *intravenous* therapy, 1 ml of concentrate is diluted in 20 to 100 ml of 0.9% sodium chloride or 5% dextrose. The initial dose is 5 to 6 mg/kg (one-third the oral dose) infused over 2 to 6 hours. The solution should be protected from light. Because of the risk of anaphylaxis, epinephrine and oxygen must be immediately available. The patient should be switched to oral therapy as soon as possible.

Neoral and Gengraf. Dosage depends on the transplanted organ and other immunosuppressive drugs taken concurrently. Typical dosages are 9 mg/kg/day for a kidney transplant, 8 mg/kg/day for a liver transplant, and 7 mg/kg/day for a heart transplant.

Monitoring. Dosage is adjusted on the basis of nephrotoxicity and cyclosporine levels. Blood for drug levels is drawn just prior to the next dose. For patients undergoing a kidney transplant, the target trough level in *whole blood* is 100 to 200 ng/ml.

Dosage for Rheumatoid Arthritis. Rheumatoid arthritis is treated with Neoral. The initial dosage is 1.25 mg/kg twice daily. Dosage may be gradually increased to a maximum of 2 mg/kg twice daily. If there is no response by 16 weeks, cyclosporine should be discontinued.

Dosage for Psoriasis. The initial dosage is 1.25 mg/kg twice daily. This may be gradually increased to a maximum of 4 mg/kg twice daily. If the maximum dosage is not effective within 6 weeks, cyclosporine should be discontinued. If a response does occur, the dosage should be reduced to the lowest effective amount for maintenance. Continuous therapy for more than 1 year is not recommended.

Tacrolimus

Tacrolimus [Prograf], formerly known as FK506, is an alternative to cyclosporine for preventing organ transplant rejection. The drug is somewhat more effective than cyclosporine, but is also more toxic.

Therapeutic Use. At this time, systemic tacrolimus is approved only for prophylaxis of organ rejection in patients receiving liver transplants. Concurrent use of glucocorticoids is recommended. Compared with patients receiving cyclosporine, those receiving tacrolimus experience fewer episodes of acute transplant rejection, but twice as many patients discontinue the drug because of toxicity. Tacrolimus is under investigation for use in patients receiving kidney, bone marrow, heart, pancreas, and small bowel transplants. As discussed in Chapter 101, tacrolimus is also used for topical therapy of atopic dermatitis.

Mechanism of Action. Tacrolimus acts much like cyclosporine, although the two drugs are structurally dissimilar. Like cyclosporine, tacrolimus inhibits calcineurin, and thereby prevents helper T cells from producing IL-2, interferon-gamma, and other cytokines. The end result is decreased proliferation of B cells and cytotoxic T cells. Tacrolimus and cyclosporine differ only in that cyclosporine must first bind to cyclophilin in order to act, whereas tacrolimus must first bind to an intracellular protein named FKBP-12.

Pharmacokinetics. Tacrolimus may be administered orally or IV. Following oral administration, absorption is slow and incomplete; bioavailability is less than 25%. The drug is metabolized in the liver by an isozyme of cytochrome P450. Excretion is via the bile. Less than 1% is excreted unchanged in the urine. The mean plasma half-life is 8 to 9 hours.

Adverse Effects. Adverse effects are much like those of cyclosporine. As with cyclosporine, *nephrotoxicity* is the major concern; the incidence is 33% to 40%. Other common reactions include *neurotoxicity* (headache, tremor, insomnia), *GI effects* (diarrhea, nausea, vomiting), *hypertension, hyperkalemia,* and *hyperglycemia. Anaphylaxis* can occur with IV administration. Like other immunosuppressants, tacrolimus increases the risk of *infection* and *lymphomas.*

Drug and Food Interactions. Because tacrolimus is metabolized by CYP3A (i.e., the 3A isozyme of cytochrome P450), agents that inhibit CYP3A—erythromycin, ketoconazole, fluconazole, chloramphenicol, and grapefruit juice—can increase tacrolimus levels. Like tacrolimus, NSAIDs can injure the kidneys. Accordingly, NSAIDs should be avoided.

Preparations, Dosage, and Administration. Preparations. Tacrolimus [Prograf] is dispensed in capsules (0.5, 1, and 5 mg) for oral use and in solution (5 mg/ml) for IV use. For initial therapy, administration may be oral (if tolerated) or IV. For maintenance therapy, administration is oral.

Intravenous. The dosage range is 50 to 100 μg/kg/day. Administration is by continuous infusion. Treatment should begin no sooner than 6 hours after transplant surgery. Patients should switch to oral tacrolimus as soon as possible (usually 2 to 3 days after surgery).

Oral. The dosage range is 75 to 150 μg/kg every 12 hours. Oral therapy should begin 8 to 12 hours after the last IV dose. If treatment is initiated with oral therapy, the first dose should be given no sooner than 6 hours after surgery.

SIROLIMUS

Actions and Therapeutic Use. Sirolimus [Rapamune] is an immunosuppressant approved for prevention of renal transplant rejection. The drug should be used in conjunction with cyclosporine and glucocorticoids.

Sirolimus is structurally similar to tacrolimus, but works by a somewhat different mechanism. Both drugs form a complex with a regulatory protein known as FKBP-12. The ultimate result is suppression of T-cell activation and proliferation. However, there is a difference: Whereas responses to tacrolimus (as well as to cyclosporine) involve inhibition of calcineurin, responses to sirolimus do not.

Pharmacokinetics. Sirolimus is rapidly but incompletely absorbed. Food reduces the *rate* of absorption but increases the *extent.* In the blood, most of the drug is sequestered in erythrocytes. As a result, concentrations in plasma are considerably lower than in whole blood. Sirolimus undergoes extensive metabolism by CYP3A4 (i.e., the 3A4 isozyme of cytochrome P450). Excretion is via the bile. The drug's half-life is prolonged—2.5 days.

Adverse Effects. Like all other immunosuppressants, sirolimus increases the risk of *infection.* Accordingly, patients should avoid sources of contagion. In addition, for 12 months after transplant surgery, they should take medicine to prevent *Pneumocystis carinii* pneumonia, and for 3 months after transplant surgery, they should take medicine to prevent infection with cytomegalovirus.

Sirolimus *raises levels of cholesterol and triglycerides.* In clinical trials, about 50% of patients required treatment with lipid-lowering drugs. Exercise caution in patients with pre-existing hyperlipidemias.

Sirolimus, combined with cyclosporine, poses a significant risk of *renal injury.* Renal function should be monitored.

Other side effects include rash, acne, anemia, thrombocytopenia, joint pain, diarrhea, and hypokalemia. In addition, sirolimus increases the risk of lymphocele (a complication of renal transplant surgery). In contrast to cyclosporine, sirolimus is not neurotoxic, and, in contrast to tacrolimus, it is not diabetogenic.

Use in Pregnancy and Lactation. In rats, sirolimus can cause fetal death and reduced birth weight, but does not cause overt birth defects. Effects in pregnant women have not been studied systematically. At this time, sirolimus is categorized in FDA Pregnancy Risk Category C, and hence should be avoided during pregnancy. Women should initiate effective contraception before starting sirolimus, and should continue it for at least 12 weeks after stopping sirolimus. Sirolimus is excreted into breast milk, and hence women using it should not breast-feed.

Drug and Food Interactions. Levels of sirolimus can be raised or lowered by drugs that inhibit or induce CYP3A4, thereby posing a risk of toxicity or treatment failure. Drugs that *induce* CYP3A4, and thereby *decrease* sirolimus levels, include carbamazepine, phenytoin, phenobarbital, rifabutin, and rifapentine. Drugs that *inhibit* CYP3A4, and thereby *increase* sirolimus levels, include verapamil, nicardipine, azole antifungal agents (e.g., ketoconazole), macrolide antibiotics (e.g., erythromycin), and HIV-protease inhibitors (e.g., saquinavir). Because cyclosporine, tacrolimus, and sirolimus are metabolized by CYP3A4, they can compete with each other for metabolism, and can thereby raise each other's levels.

Sirolimus can reduce the immune response to all vaccines. In addition, the drug can render patients vulnerable to infection from live virus vaccines, and hence these should be avoided.

High-fat foods can increase sirolimus absorption by about 35%. To minimize variability, patients should take all doses consistently (i.e., all with food or all without food).

Grapefruit juice can inhibit the metabolism of sirolimus, causing its levels to rise. Accordingly, taking sirolimus with grapefruit juice should be avoided.

Monitoring. Routine monitoring of sirolimus blood levels is not required. However, monitoring *is* recommended for pediatric patients, patients with liver disease, and patients taking strong inducers or inhibitors of CYP3A4. Monitoring is also recommended whenever the dosage of cyclosporine (taken concurrently with sirolimus) is raised or lowered substantially.

Preparations, Dosage, and Administration. Sirolimus is available in 1-mg tablets and a 1-mg/ml oral solution. The treatment program should include cyclosporine and glucocorticoids. Sirolimus dosing should begin as soon as possible after transplant surgery. The recommended regimen consists of a 6-mg loading dose followed by 2-mg daily maintenance doses. For patients who weigh less than 40 kg (but are at least 13 years old), the loading dose is 3 mg/m² and the maintenance dosage is 1 mg/m² once a day. For all patients, maintenance doses should be taken 4 hours after taking cyclosporine, and should be taken consistently with respect to food intake (i.e., either with food or without food)—and should *not* be taken with grapefruit juice. In patients with liver impairment, maintenance doses (but not the loading dose) should be reduced by 33%.

GLUCOCORTICOIDS

Glucocorticoids (e.g., prednisone) are used widely to suppress immune responses. Immunosuppressant applications range from suppression of transplant rejection to treatment of asthma to therapy of autoimmune disorders, such as rheumatoid arthritis and systemic lupus erythematosus.

Glucocorticoids have multiple effects on elements of the immune system. They cause lysis of antigen-activated lymphocytes, suppression of lymphocyte proliferation, and sequestration of lymphocytes at extravascular locations. In addition, they reduce production of IL-2 by monocytes and lymphocytes, and they reduce the responsiveness of T lymphocytes to interleukin-1.

Immunosuppressive doses are large. For example, to prevent organ rejection, an initial dose of 0.5 to 2 mg/kg of prednisone is employed. To treat episodes of acute organ rejection, 500 to 1500 mg of IV methylprednisolone is given.

Because large doses are employed, the full range of glucocorticoid adverse effects can be expected. These include increased risk of infection, thinning of the skin, bone dissolution with resultant fractures, impaired growth in children, and suppression of the hypothalamic-pituitary-adrenal axis.

The pharmacology of glucocorticoids is discussed at length in Chapter 68 (Glucocorticoids in Nonendocrine Diseases).

CYTOTOXIC DRUGS

Cytotoxic drugs suppress immune responses by killing B and T lymphocytes that are undergoing proliferation. With the exception of mycophenolate mofetil, these drugs are nonspecific. That is, they are toxic to all proliferating cells. As a result, they can cause bone marrow depression, GI disturbances, reduced fertility, and alopecia (hair loss). Neutropenia and thrombocytopenia from bone marrow depression are of particular concern. Because of their serious adverse effects, the cytotoxic drugs are usually reserved for patients who have not responded to safer immunosuppressants (i.e., cyclosporine, tacrolimus, and glucocorticoids).

Azathioprine

Mechanism of Action. Azathioprine [Imuran] suppresses cell-mediated and humoral immune responses by inhibiting the proliferation of B and T lymphocytes. Azathioprine is a prodrug that must be converted to its active form—mercaptopurine—in the body. Mercaptopurine suppresses cell proliferation by inhibiting DNA synthesis. Hence, the drug acts selectively during the S phase of the cell cycle. As discussed in Chapter 98, mercaptopurine itself is used to treat cancer.

Therapeutic Uses. Prior to the advent of cyclosporine, azathioprine (combined with prednisone) was the principal drug employed to suppress re-

jection of renal transplants. Today, azathioprine is generally used as an adjunct to cyclosporine and glucocorticoids to help suppress transplant rejection. In addition, the drug is approved for severe refractory rheumatoid arthritis in nonpregnant adults (see Chapter 69). Azathioprine has been used investigationally to treat various autoimmune diseases, including myasthenia gravis, systemic lupus erythematosus, Crohn's disease, ulcerative colitis, and type 1 diabetes.

Adverse Effects and Interactions. Although uncommon at usual therapeutic doses, *neutropenia* and *thrombocytopenia* from bone marrow suppression can be serious concerns. Accordingly, complete blood counts should be performed at regular intervals. Azathioprine is *mutagenic* and *teratogenic* in animals, and hence should be avoided during pregnancy. Long-term therapy is associated with an increased incidence of *neoplasms*.

Allopurinol delays conversion of mercaptopurine to inactive products, and thereby increases the risk of toxicity. If allopurinol and azathioprine are used concurrently, the dose of azathioprine must be reduced by about 70%.

Preparations, Dosage, and Administration. Azathioprine [Imuran] is available in 50-mg tablets for oral administration, and as a powder to be reconstituted with sterile water for IV administration. For patients receiving a kidney transplant, therapy is initiated with a single daily dose of 3 to 5 mg/kg, usually beginning on the day of surgery. Daily maintenance doses range from 1 to 3 mg/kg. Oral administration is preferred to IV.

Cyclophosphamide

Cyclophosphamide [Cytoxan, Neosar], an anticancer drug, is discussed at length in Chapter 98. Discussion here is limited to immunosuppressant uses. Cyclophosphamide is a prodrug that is converted to its active form by the liver. The active form is an alkylating agent that cross-links DNA, leading to cell injury and death. Immunosuppressant effects result from a decrease in the number and activity of B and T lymphocytes. Toxicity to other cells produces adverse effects. These include neutropenia (from bone marrow suppression), hemorrhagic cystitis, and sterility in males and females. Cyclophosphamide has been used for its immunosuppressant actions to treat rheumatoid arthritis, systemic lupus erythematosus, and multiple sclerosis. The drug is as effective as azathioprine for suppressing rejection of renal transplants.

Methotrexate

Methotrexate [Rheumatrex, Trexall] is an anticancer drug (see Chapter 98) that is also employed for immunosuppression. As an immunosuppressant, the drug is approved for rheumatoid arthritis (see Chapter 69) and for psoriasis (see Chapter 101). Methotrexate has also been used to suppress graft-versus-host disease in bone marrow recipients. These beneficial effects result from suppression of B and T lymphocytes secondary to interference with folate metabolism. The doses employed for immunosuppression are lower than those employed to treat cancer. As a result, toxicities differ with the two applications: In cancer chemotherapy, bone marrow suppression, ulcerative stomatitis, and renal damage are primary concerns, whereas in immunosuppressive therapy, hepatic fibrosis and cirrhosis are primary concerns.

Mycophenolate Mofetil

Therapeutic Use. Mycophenolate mofetil [CellCept] is approved for prophylaxis of organ rejection in patients with allogenic heart, liver, or kidney transplants. The drug should be combined with cyclosporine and glucocorticoids.

Mechanism of Action. Following oral administration, mycophenolate mofetil is rapidly converted to mycophenolic acid (MPA), its active form. MPA then acts on B and T lymphocytes to inhibit inosine monophosphate dehydrogenase, an enzyme required for *de novo* synthesis of purines. Since these cells are uniquely dependent on *de novo* synthesis for proliferation (other cells acquire needed purines via salvage pathways), MPA causes selective inhibition of B and T lymphocyte proliferation.

Pharmacokinetics. Mycophenolate mofetil is administered orally and undergoes nearly complete absorption, followed by rapid and nearly complete hydrolysis to MPA. MPA is converted in the liver to an inactive metabolite, which is then excreted in the urine. The half-life of MPA is about 18 hours.

Adverse Effects. Major adverse effects include *diarrhea, vomiting, severe neutropenia,* and *sepsis* (primarily cytomegalovirus viremia). As with other immunosuppressive drugs, there is an *increased risk of infection and malignancies,* especially lymphomas.

Drug Interactions. Absorption of mycophenolate can be decreased by *antacids* that contain magnesium and aluminum hydroxides and by *cholestyramine,* a drug used to lower cholesterol levels. Accordingly, mycophenolate should not be given simultaneously with these drugs.

Use in Pregnancy. When given to pregnant rats in doses at or below those used clinically, mycophenolate causes fetal malformations and fetal resorption. Controlled studies in women have not been performed. Because of the serious risk of fetal toxicity, the drug should be avoided during pregnancy. Before initiating treatment, pregnancy should be ruled out. During therapy, women of child-bearing age should use *two* reliable forms of contraception.

Preparations, Dosage, and Administration. Mycophenolate mofetil [CellCept] is available in formulations for oral and IV administration. For oral use, the drug is available in 250-mg capsules, 500-mg tablets, and a 200-mg/ml suspension. For IV use, the drug is available as a lyophilized powder to be reconstituted to a 6-mg/ml solution. Intravenous administration is reserved for patients who cannot take the drug orally, and should be done by *slow infusion* (over 2 hours or longer). Dosages are as follows:

- *Kidney transplant:* 1 gm twice daily, PO or IV
- *Heart transplant:* 1.5 gm twice daily, PO or IV
- *Liver transplant:* 1 gm twice daily IV or 1.5 gm twice daily PO

Dosing should begin within 24 hours of transplant surgery. All patients who receive IV therapy initially should switch to oral therapy within 14 days. As a rule, oral dosing should be done on an empty stomach to increase drug availability.

ANTIBODIES

Antibodies directed against components of the immune system can suppress immune responses. Five preparations are considered here. Four of these—muromonab-CD3, basiliximab, daclizumab, and lymphocyte immune globulin—are used to suppress allograft rejection in transplant recipients. The fifth preparation—Rh$_o$(D) immune globulin (RhIG)—is used to prevent reactions to Rh-positive blood in Rh-negative women.

Muromonab-CD3

Actions and Uses. Muromonab-CD3 [Orthoclone OKT3] is a monoclonal antibody, developed in mice, that binds to the CD3 site on human T lymphocytes. Upon binding, the antibody blocks all T-cell functions. All T cells—both those in the circulation and those in tissues—are affected. Muromonab-CD3 is used to prevent acute allograft rejection of kidney, heart, and liver transplants. In addition, the drug is given to deplete T cells from bone marrow prior to bone marrow transplantation.

Adverse Effects. Relatively mild reactions are common. These include *fever* (73%), *chills* (59%), *dyspnea* (21%), *chest pain* (14%), and *nausea and vomiting* (12%). These effects are most intense on the first day and then rapidly subside.

In some patients, potentially fatal *anaphylactoid reactions* have occurred. Manifestations include pulmonary edema, cardiovascular collapse, and cardiac or respiratory arrest. Accordingly, patients should be monitored closely. Also, the drug should be used only in facilities with equipment and staffing for cardiopulmonary resuscitation.

Preparations, Dosage, and Administration. Muromonab-CD3 [Orthoclone OKT3] is dispensed in solution (1 mg/ml) for IV administration. The usual dosage is 5 mg/day for 10 to 14 days. Administration is by IV bolus. The preparation should be drawn through a filter before injection. Treatment is begun following diagnosis of acute transplant rejection. To minimize first-dose adverse reactions, the patient should be pretreated with an IV glucocorticoid. The wholesale cost for a course of treatment is about $7200.

Basiliximab and Daclizumab

Actions and Uses. Basiliximab [Simulect] and daclizumab [Zenapax] are monoclonal antibodies, developed in mice, that bind to the receptor for IL-2 on T lymphocytes. As a result of receptor binding, these antibodies block activation of T cells by IL-2.

Both drugs have the same indication: prophylaxis of *acute* organ rejection following a renal transplant. Both drugs must be combined with cyclosporine and a glucocorticoid. In clinical trials, these drugs helped reduce the incidence of acute organ rejection during the first 6 months after transplant surgery, but had little or no impact on graft survival after 1 year.

Adverse Effects. Basiliximab and daclizumab are generally well tolerated. The incidence and severity of adverse effects is much lower than with muromonab-CD3. In contrast to other immunosuppressants, basiliximab and daclizumab do not increase the risk of opportunistic infections. Furthermore, no cancers have been observed 1 year after treatment.

Rarely, basiliximab causes severe, acute hypersensitivity reactions, including anaphylaxis. Accordingly, medications for managing hypersensitivity should be immediately available. Patients who have experienced a severe reaction should not get the drug again.

Preparations, Dosage, and Administration. Basiliximab. Basiliximab [Simulect] is dispensed as a powder to be reconstituted for IV administration. Treatment consists of two 20-mg doses, given by either (1) IV bolus or (2) IV infusion over 20 to 30 minutes. The first dose is given within 2 hours *prior* to transplant surgery. The second dose is given 4 days later. The wholesale cost for the two doses is about $2500.

Daclizumab. Daclizumab [Zenapax] is dispensed in concentrated solution (25 mg/ml) that must be diluted in 50 ml of 0.9% saline for IV infusion. Treatment consists of five doses (1 mg/kg each) that are infused over 15 minutes. The first dose is given within 24 hours prior to transplant surgery. The next four doses are given 2, 4, 6, and 8 weeks later. The wholesale cost for a course of treatment is about $6000.

Lymphocyte Immune Globulin, Antithymocyte Globulin (Equine)

Basic Pharmacology. Lymphocyte immune globulin [Atgam] is prepared by immunizing horses with human T lymphocytes. Therapeutic effects result from a decrease in the number and activity of thymus-derived lymphocytes. Lymphocyte immune globulin is approved for preventing rejection of renal transplants. The drug is also used to suppress organ rejection following liver, bone marrow, and heart transplants. Investigational uses include myasthenia gravis and multiple sclerosis. Lymphocyte immune globulin is usually employed in combination with glucocorticoids and azathioprine. Because these other immunosuppressants are present, immune reactions to this horse-derived drug are generally mild (chills, fever, leukopenia, skin reactions). However, anaphylactic reactions can occur. Accordingly, epinephrine and facilities for respiratory support should be immediately available.

Preparations, Dosage, and Administration. Lymphocyte immune globulin is dispensed in solution (50 mg/ml) for IV administration. The concentrate should be diluted in saline solution according to the manufacturer's instructions. The infusion apparatus should have an in-line filter. The usual adult dosage is 10 to 30 mg/kg/day administered over 4 hours or longer. To minimize phlebitis, a vein with high flow should be employed. Monitor the patient for anaphylaxis.

Rh$_o$(D) Immune Globulin

Actions and Uses. Rh$_o$(D) immune globulin (RhIG) is a concentrated preparation of immune globulin that contains antibodies to Rh$_o$(D). RhIG is given to prevent development of antibodies to Rh$_o$(D) in Rh$_o$(D)-negative women following exposure to Rh$_o$(D)-positive blood. Such exposure can occur in association with a Rh$_o$(D)-positive pregnancy (as a result of the pregnancy itself, full-term delivery, spontaneous or induced abortion, or amniocentesis). RhIG acts by suppressing the immune response of Rh-negative women to Rh-positive blood cells. In many medical centers, RhIG is administered routinely at 28 weeks of gestation to all Rh$_o$(D)-negative women.

Adverse Effects, Precautions, and Contraindications. Undesired reactions are uncommon and mild. Temperature may rise slightly. RhIG is contraindicated for Rh-positive women and must not be administered to newborns.

Preparations, Dosage, and Administration. RhIG [RhoGAM, others] is dispensed in vials and prefilled syringes for IM injection. Prevention of anti–Rh$_o$(D) antibody formation is most successful if the drug is administered twice: at 28 weeks of gestation and again within 72 hours after delivery.

⸪ KEY POINTS

- Immunosuppressants are used to prevent organ rejection in transplant recipients and to treat autoimmune disorders (e.g., rheumatoid arthritis).
- Transplant recipients must take immunosuppressants for life.
- Immunosuppressants increase the risk of infection and lymphomas.

■ Cyclosporine and tacrolimus are the most effective immunosuppressants available.

■ Cyclosporine and tacrolimus are used primarily in transplant recipients.

■ Cyclosporine causes kidney injury in up to 75% of patients.

■ Renal damage from cyclosporine can be intensified by other nephrotoxic drugs, including amphotericin B, aminoglycosides, and NSAIDs.

■ Drugs that inhibit hepatic microsomal enzymes can increase cyclosporine levels, and drugs that induce these enzymes can decrease cyclosporine levels.

■ Grapefruit juice inhibits cyclosporine metabolism, and can thereby greatly increase cyclosporine levels.

■ Like cyclosporine, tacrolimus causes renal damage, and hence should not be combined with other nephrotoxic drugs.

■ Ketoconazole, fluconazole, grapefruit juice, and other agents that inhibit metabolism of tacrolimus can elevate its levels.

■ Immunosuppressant applications of glucocorticoids include suppression of transplant rejection and treatment of rheumatoid arthritis and other autoimmune disorders.

■ Prolonged use of glucocorticoids can result in osteoporosis, thinning of the skin, increased risk of infection, impaired growth in children, and adrenal insufficiency (secondary to suppression of the hypothalamic-pituitary-adrenal axis).

■ Cytotoxic immunosuppressants (e.g., azathioprine) decrease immune responses by killing B and T lymphocytes.

■ Cytotoxic immunosuppressants (except mycophenolate mofetil) injure all proliferating cells. As a result, these drugs can cause bone marrow depression (neutropenia, thrombocytopenia), GI disturbances, reduced fertility, and alopecia.

■ Immune responses can be suppressed with muromonab-CD3, basiliximab, and other antibodies directed against components of the immune system.

Summary of Major Nursing Implications*

CYCLOSPORINE

Preadministration Assessment

Therapeutic Goal

Prevention of allograft rejection.

Baseline Data

Obtain baseline data on kidney function (serum creatinine, BUN), liver function (aspartate aminotransferase, alanine aminotransferase, serum amylase, bilirubin, alkaline phosphatase), and serum potassium levels.

Identifying High-Risk Patients

Cyclosporine is *contraindicated* in the presence of hypersensitivity to cyclosporine or to its intravenous vehicle (polyoxyethylated castor oil), pregnancy, recent inoculation with live virus vaccines, and recent contact with or active infection with chickenpox or herpes zoster.

Use with *caution* in patients using potassium-sparing diuretics and in those with intestinal malabsorption, hypertension, hyperkalemia, active infection, and renal or hepatic dysfunction.

Implementation: Administration

Routes

Oral, intravenous.

Preparations

Cyclosporine is available under three trade names: Sandimmune, Neoral, and Gengraf. Sandimmune has lower bioavailability than Neoral or Gengraf, and hence is not interchangeable with them.

Patient Education for Oral Administration

Dispense the oral liquid into a glass container using the specially calibrated pipette. Mix well with diluent and drink immediately. Rinse the container with diluent and drink to ensure ingestion of the complete dose. Dry the outside of the pipette and return to its cover for storage.

To improve palatability, mix the concentrated drug solution with milk, chocolate milk, or orange juice just before administration.

Intravenous Dosage and Administration

Dilute 1 ml of concentrate in 20 to 100 ml of 0.9% sodium chloride or 5% dextrose. Protect from light. Administer the initial dose (5 to 6 mg/kg) slowly—over 2 to 6 hours. Because of the risk of anaphylactic reactions, monitor the patient closely for 30 minutes after beginning administration. Have epinephrine and oxygen available. Switch to oral therapy as soon as possible.

Dosage Adjustment

Adjust dosage on the basis of nephrotoxicity and cyclosporine levels. Draw blood for drug levels just prior to the next dose. The target trough level is 100 to 200 ng/ml in whole blood.

Ongoing Evaluation and Interventions

Evaluating Therapeutic Effects

Graft tenderness or fever may indicate rejection. In renal transplant recipients, elevated BUN and elevated serum creatinine in conjunction with low cyclosporine may indicate rejection. Therapeutic failure can be confirmed with ultrasound, a biopsy, or renal flow scan.

*Patient education information is highlighted as blue text.

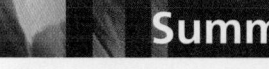

Summary of Major Nursing Implications*—cont'd

Minimizing Adverse Effects

Nephrotoxicity. Cyclosporine can cause a dose-dependent reduction in kidney function. Monitor for elevation of serum creatinine and BUN. **Inform outpatients about the importance of undergoing periodic tests of kidney function.**

Infection. Cyclosporine increases the risk of infection. **Inform patients about early signs of infection (fever, sore throat), and instruct them to report these immediately.**

Hepatotoxicity. Cyclosporine causes reversible liver damage. Monitor for elevation of serum bilirubin and liver transaminases. **Inform patients about the need for periodic tests of liver function.**

Hirsutism. Cyclosporine promotes hair growth. **Assure the patient that this effect is reversible.**

Use in Pregnancy and Lactation. Cyclosporine is embryotoxic. **Advise women of child-bearing age to use a mechanical form of contraception (diaphragm, condom) and to avoid oral contraceptives. Cyclosporine is excreted in breast milk; warn the patient against breast-feeding.**

Anaphylactic Reactions. See *Intravenous Dosage and Administration.*

Minimizing Adverse Interactions

Drugs That Can Decrease Cyclosporine Levels. *Phenytoin, phenobarbital, carbamazepine, rifampin, terbinafine,* and *trimethoprim-sulfamethoxazole* can reduce cyclosporine levels, leading to organ rejection. Monitor cyclosporine levels and increase the dosage as needed.

Drugs That Can Increase Cyclosporine Levels. *Azole antifungal drugs* (e.g., ketoconazole), *macrolide antibiotics* (e.g., erythromycin), and *amphotericin B* can elevate cyclosporine levels, thereby increasing the risk of toxicity. Monitor cyclosporine levels and reduce the dosage as needed.

Nephrotoxic Drugs. *Amphotericin B, aminoglycosides,* and *NSAIDs* increase the risk of cyclosporine-induced kidney damage. Monitor renal function.

Grapefruit Juice. Grapefruit juice inhibits cyclosporine metabolism, and can thereby increase cyclosporine levels. Toxicity may result.

*Patient education information is highlighted as blue text.

Antihistamines

Histamine is an endogenous compound found in specialized cells throughout the body. The substance plays an important role in allergic reactions and regulation of gastric acid secretion. The antihistamines, one of our most widely used families of drugs, block histamine's actions.

In order to understand the antihistamines, we must first understand histamine itself. Accordingly, the chapter begins with a discussion of histamine, emphasizing its contribution to allergic responses. After that, we discuss the antihistamines themselves.

HISTAMINE

Histamine is a locally acting substance with prominent and varied effects. In the vascular system, histamine dilates small blood vessels and increases capillary permeability. In the bronchi, histamine produces constriction. In the stomach, histamine stimulates secretion of acid. In the central nervous system (CNS), histamine acts as a neurotransmitter. Despite this impressive spectrum of actions, clinical applications for histamine itself are limited. Currently, use of histamine is restricted to diagnostic procedures. However, although its clinical utility is minimal, histamine is still of great interest because of its involvement in two common pathologic states: allergies and peptic ulcer disease.

Distribution, Synthesis, Storage, and Release

Distribution. Histamine is present in practically all tissues. Levels are especially high in the skin, lungs, and GI tract. The histamine content of plasma is relatively low.

Synthesis and Storage. Histamine is synthesized and stored in two types of cells: *mast cells* and *basophils*. Mast cells are present in the skin and other soft tissues; basophils are present in the blood. In both mast cells and basophils, histamine is stored in structures called secretory granules. (In addition to histamine, secretory granules contain other substances that, like histamine, are mediators of allergic reactions.)

Release. Release of histamine from mast cells and basophils is produced by allergic and nonallergic mechanisms.

Allergic Release. The initial requirement for allergic release of histamine is the production of antibodies of the immunoglobulin E class. These antibodies are generated in response to exposure to specific allergens (e.g., pollens, insect venoms, certain drugs). Following synthesis, the antibodies become attached to the outer surface of mast cells and basophils (Fig. 66–1). When the subject is re-exposed to the allergen, the allergen becomes bound by the antibodies. As indicated in Figure 66–1, binding of allergen to adjacent antibodies creates a bridge between those antibodies. By a mechanism that is not fully understood, this bridging process mobilizes intracellular calcium. The calcium, in turn, causes the histamine-containing storage granules to fuse with the cell membrane and disgorge their contents into the extracellular space. Note that allergic release of histamine requires *prior exposure* to the allergen; an allergic reaction cannot occur during initial contact with an allergen.

Nonallergic Release. A number of agents (certain drugs, radiocontrast media, plasma expanders) can act directly on mast cells to cause histamine release. With these agents, no prior sensitization is needed. Cell injury can also cause direct release of histamine.

Physiologic and Pharmacologic Effects

Histamine acts through two types of receptors, named H$_1$ and H$_2$. As discussed below, responses to activation of these receptors differ.

Effects of H$_1$ Stimulation

Vasodilation. Activation of H$_1$ receptors causes dilation of small blood vessels (arterioles and venules). Vasodilation is prominent in the skin of the face and upper body, causing the area to become warm and flushed. If extensive vasodilation occurs, total peripheral resistance will decline and blood pressure will fall.

Increased Capillary Permeability. Histamine$_1$ stimulation increases capillary permeability. How? By causing capillary endothelial cells to contract, which creates openings between these cells through which fluid, protein, and platelets can escape. Escape of fluid and protein into the interstitial space produces edema. If loss of intravascular fluid is substantial, blood pressure may fall.

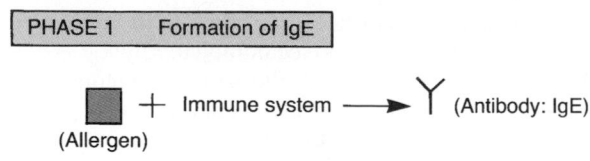

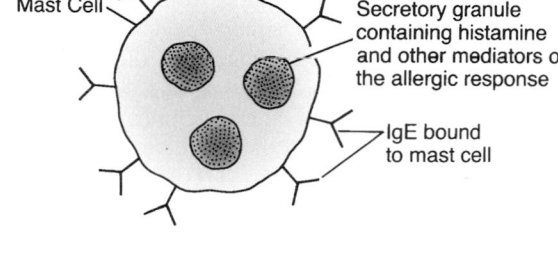

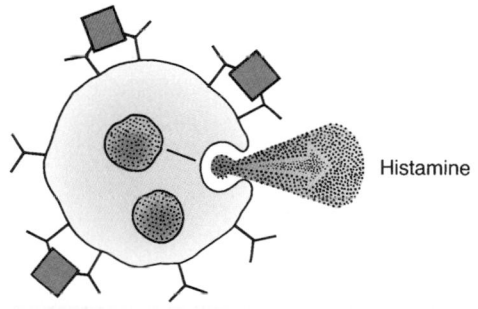

Figure 66–1 ■ Release of histamine by allergen-antibody interaction.
(IgE = immunoglobulin E.)

Bronchoconstriction. Histamine₁ stimulation causes constriction of the bronchi. If histamine is administered to an individual with asthma, severe bronchoconstriction will follow. However, although *exogenous* histamine can induce bronchial constriction, histamine is not the cause of bronchoconstriction that occurs during a spontaneous asthma attack. Consequently, antihistamines are of no use for treating asthma.

Other Effects. Stimulation of H₁ receptors located on sensory nerves produces *itching* and *pain*. Histamine₁ stimulation also promotes *secretion of mucus*. In the CNS, histamine acts as a neurotransmitter, causing *sedation* and other effects.

Effects of H₂ Stimulation

The major response to activation of H₂ receptors is *secretion of gastric acid*. Histamine acts directly on parietal cells of the stomach to promote acid release. Although acetylcholine and gastrin also help regulate acid release, histamine has a dominant role. We know this because, in the presence of H₂ blockade, acetylcholine and gastrin are unable to elicit acid secretion.

Role of Histamine in Allergic Responses

Allergic reactions are mediated by histamine and other compounds (e.g., prostaglandins, leukotrienes). The intensity of an allergic reaction is determined by which of these mediators is involved.

Mild Allergy. The symptoms of mild allergy (e.g., rhinitis, itching, localized edema) are caused largely by histamine (acting at H₁ receptors). As a result, mild allergic conditions (e.g., hay fever, acute urticaria, mild transfusion reactions) are generally responsive to antihistamine therapy.

Severe Allergic Reactions (Anaphylaxis). Severe allergic reactions manifest as *anaphylactic shock,* a syndrome characterized by bronchoconstriction, hypotension, and edema of the glottis. Although histamine is involved in anaphylaxis, it plays a minor role; other substances (e.g., leukotrienes) are the principal causative agents. Since histamine has little to do with producing anaphylaxis, it follows that antihistamines are of little help as treatment. The drug of choice for anaphylaxis is *epinephrine.* The rationale for using epinephrine is discussed in Chapter 18.

THE TWO TYPES OF ANTIHISTAMINES: H₁ ANTAGONISTS AND H₂ ANTAGONISTS

Antihistamines fall into two basic categories: H₁-receptor antagonists and H₂-receptor antagonists. The H₁ antagonists produce selective blockade of H₁ receptors. The H₂ antagonists produce selective blockade of H₂ receptors. The principal use of H₁ blockers is treatment of mild allergic disorders. The principal use of H₂ blockers is treatment of gastric and duodenal ulcers. Because H₂ antagonists do not block H₁ receptors, these drugs are of no use for treating allergies. In this chapter, our focus is on H₁ antagonists. The H₂ blockers, which are important and widely used, are discussed in Chapter 73 (Drugs for Peptic Ulcer Disease).

H₁ ANTAGONISTS I: BASIC PHARMACOLOGY

The H₁ antagonists are the classic antihistamines. These agents were in use long before H₂ blockers were developed. In fact, before H₂ blockers became available, the term *H₁ antagonist* did not exist; the drugs that we now call H₁ antagonists or H₁ blockers were simply referred to as *antihistamines.* Because of its historic use, the term *antihistamines* is still employed as a synonym for the subgroup of histamine antagonists that produce selective H₁ blockade. In this chapter, we respect tradition and continue to use the term *antihistamine* interchangeably with *H₁ blocker* and *H₁ antagonist.*

Although all H₁ antagonists available have similar antihistaminic actions, these drugs differ significantly in side effects. Because of these differences, selection of a prototype to represent the group is not feasible. Hence, rather than structuring discussion around one prototypic drug, we will discuss the H₁ antagonists collectively. Differences among individual antihistamines are addressed as appropriate.

Classification of H₁ Antagonists

The H₁ antagonists fall into two major groups: *first-generation H₁ antagonists* and *second-generation H₁ antagonists*. The principal difference between the groups is that first-generation antihistamines are highly sedating, whereas second-generation antihistamines are not.

Mechanism of Action

Histamine₁ blockers bind selectively to H₁-histaminic receptors, thereby blocking the actions of histamine at these sites. H₁ antagonists do not block H₂ receptors. Also, they do not block release of histamine from mast cells or basophils.

It should be noted that, although interaction of the classic antihistamines with *histaminic* receptors is limited to the H₁-receptor subtype, these drugs can also bind to *nonhistaminic* receptors. Of particular significance is the ability of certain antihistamines to bind to and block *muscarinic* receptors. This action underlies several important side effects.

Pharmacologic Effects

Peripheral Effects. The major effects of the H₁ antagonists can be attributed to preventing the actions of histamine at H₁ receptors. In arterioles and venules of the skin, H₁ blockers inhibit the dilator actions of histamine, and thereby reduce localized flushing. In capillary beds, the antihistamines prevent histamine-induced increases in permeability, and thereby reduce edema. By blocking the actions of histamine at sensory nerves, H₁ antagonists reduce itching and pain. Blockade of H₁ receptors in mucous membranes suppresses secretion of mucus.

Effects on the CNS. Antihistamines can cause both excitation and depression of the CNS. At *therapeutic doses,* antihistamines produce CNS *depression:* reaction time is slowed, alertness is diminished, and drowsiness is likely. These effects are more pronounced with some antihistamines than with others. With the second-generation antihistamines (e.g., fexofenadine) CNS depression is negligible.

Overdose with antihistamines can produce *CNS stimulation.* Convulsions frequently result. Very young children are especially sensitive to CNS stimulation by these drugs.

Other Pharmacologic Effects. Blockade of muscarinic cholinergic receptors by antihistamines can produce typical *anticholinergic* responses. These are discussed below under *Adverse Effects.* Several antihistamines can suppress nausea and vomiting (see below under *Motion Sickness*).

Therapeutic Uses

All of the H₁ antagonists are useful in treating allergic disorders. Some of these drugs are also indicated for other conditions (e.g., motion sickness, insomnia).

Mild Allergy. Antihistamines can reduce symptoms of mild allergies. In people with *seasonal allergic rhinitis* (also known as hay fever or rose fever), H₁ blockers can reduce sneezing, rhinorrhea, and itching of the eyes, nose, and throat. In patients with *acute urticaria,* these drugs can reduce redness, itching, and edema. The antihistamines can also reduce symptoms of *allergic conjunctivitis* and urticaria associated with *mild transfusion reactions.* In all of these conditions, benefits result from H₁-receptor blockade—not from preventing allergen-induced release of histamine from mast cells and basophils. Because mild allergic reactions may be mediated by substances in addition to histamine, antihistamines may fail to produce complete relief.

Severe Allergy. As noted, the major symptoms of anaphylaxis (hypotension, laryngeal edema, bronchospasm) are caused by mediators other than histamine. Hence, although antihistamines may be employed as adjuncts in patients with anaphylaxis, their benefits are minimal.

Motion Sickness. Some antihistamines, such as promethazine [Phenergan] and dimenhydrinate [Dramamine], are labeled for use in motion sickness. Benefits derive from blockade of H₁ receptors and muscarinic receptors in the neuronal pathway leading from the vestibular apparatus of the inner ear to the vomiting center of the medulla. Motion sickness and its treatment are discussed in Chapter 75. The antihistamines employed for motion sickness, along with their dosages, are listed in Table 75–1.

Insomnia. The ability of antihistamines to cause CNS drowsiness has been exploited in the treatment of insomnia. Practically every over-the-counter (OTC) sleep aid contains an H₁ antagonist (diphenhydramine or pyrilamine) as its active ingredient. However, although antihistamines can induce sleep when used in sufficient dosage, the doses recommended for OTC preparations are usually too small to be effective.

Common Cold. Despite their widespread presence in cold remedies, antihistamines are of practically no value against the common cold. These drugs neither prevent colds nor shorten their duration. Moreover, since histamine does not mediate symptoms of colds, H₁ blockade cannot even provide symptomatic relief. The only benefit these drugs may offer is a moderate reduction in rhinorrhea, an effect that derives from their *anticholinergic* properties, not from H₁ blockade.

Adverse Effects

All of the H₁ blockers can produce undesired effects. As a rule, these responses are more of a nuisance than a source of serious discomfort or danger. Frequently, side effects subside with continued use. Because individual antihistamines differ in their abilities to produce particular side effects (Table 66–1), adverse responses can be minimized by judicious drug selection.

Sedation. Sedation is the most common undesired effect of the antihistamines. Fortunately, tolerance to sedation often develops within a few days or weeks. If a preparation with a long half-life is being used, daytime sedation can be minimized by administering the entire daily dose at night. Patients should be advised to avoid driving and other hazardous activities if alertness is impaired. Also, patients should be warned against using alcohol and other CNS depressants. Why? Because these agents will intensify the depressant effects of the H₁ antagonist.

The second-generation antihistamines exert little or no sedative effect. These agents—azelastine, cetirizine, fexofenadine, loratadine, and desloratadine—are unable to cross the blood-brain barrier, and hence cannot alter CNS function.

For patients who experience disabling sedation with a first-generation H₁ antagonist, therapy with a second-generation (nonsedating) antihistamine is likely to help. Unfortunately, the nonsedating agents are considerably more expensive than the first-generation agents. The sedative properties of individual antihistamines are indicated in Table 66–1.

Nonsedative CNS Effects. In addition to sedation, antihistamines can cause dizziness, incoordination, confusional

TABLE 66–1 ■ Pharmacologic Effects* of H₁ Antagonists

Drug	H₁-Blocking Activity	Sedative Effects	Anticholinergic Effects
First-Generation Agents			
Alkylamines			
Chlorpheniramine	++	+	++
Dexchlorpheniramine	+++	+	++
Ethanolamines			
Clemastine	+ to ++	++	+++
Diphenhydramine	+ to ++	+++	+++
Ethylenediamines			
Tripelennamine	+ to ++	++	±
Phenothiazines			
Promethazine	+++	+++	+++
Piperidines			
Azatadine	++	++	++
Cyproheptadine	++	+	++
Phenindamine	++	†	++
Second-Generation (Nonsedating) Agents			
Azelastine	++ to +++	±	±
Cetirizine	+++	±	±
Fexofenadine	+++	±	±
Loratadine	++ to +++	±	±
Desloratadine	11 to 111	6	6

*± – low to none; + – low; ++ – moderate; +++ – high.
†May cause excitation.

states, and fatigue. The elderly are especially sensitive to these actions. In some patients, paradoxical excitation occurs, resulting in insomnia, nervousness, tremors, and even convulsions. CNS stimulation is most common in children and following overdose.

Gastrointestinal Effects. Gastrointestinal disturbances are common. Responses include nausea, vomiting, loss of appetite, and diarrhea or constipation. These reactions can be minimized by administering antihistamines with meals.

Anticholinergic Effects. The H₁ antagonists possess weak atropine-like properties. These antimuscarinic actions can produce drying of mucous membranes in the mouth, nasal passages, and throat. Cholinergic blockade may also result in urinary hesitancy, constipation, and palpitations. If dry mouth becomes distressing, discomfort can be minimized by sucking on hard (sugarless) candy and by taking frequent sips of fluid. Antihistamines should be used with caution in patients with asthma, because thickening of bronchial secretions may impair breathing. Care should also be exercised in patients with other conditions that may be exacerbated by muscarinic blockade (e.g., urinary retention, prostatic hypertrophy, hypertension). The antimuscarinic efficacy of individual H₁ blockers is indicated in Table 66–1. As you can see, the second-generation antihistamines are the least anticholinergic.

Cardiac Dysrhythmias. Potentially fatal cardiac dysrhythmias (torsades de pointes, ventricular fibrillation, others) have occurred rarely in patients taking *astemizole* [Hismanal] or *terfenadine* [Seldane], two second-generation antihistamines. These drugs promote dysrhythmias by prolonging the QT interval, but only when their levels are excessive. Because of their potential for serious harm, terfenadine and astemizole have been withdrawn from the market.

Drug Interactions

CNS Depressants. Alcohol and other CNS depressants (e.g., barbiturates, benzodiazepines, opioids) can intensify the depressant effects of H₁ antagonists. Patients should be advised against drinking alcoholic beverages. If medications with CNS-depressant properties are combined with H₁ blockers, dosage of the depressant may need to be lowered.

Use in Pregnancy and Lactation

Pregnancy. The margin of safety of antihistamines in pregnancy is unknown. There have been reports of fetal malformation, but direct involvement of H₁ antagonists has not been proved. Given the uncertainty over the safety of these drugs, it is recommended that antihistamines be used only when clearly necessary, and only when the benefits of treatment outweigh the potential risks to the fetus. Antihistamines should be avoided late in the third trimester, because newborns are particularly sensitive to the adverse actions of these drugs.

Lactation. The H₁ antagonists can be excreted in breast milk, thereby posing a risk to the nursing infant. Since infants, and especially newborns, are unusually sensitive to antihistamines, these drugs should not be used by women who are breast-feeding.

Acute Toxicity

Although the antihistamines have a large margin of safety, acute poisoning is nonetheless common, owing to the widespread availability of these drugs. CNS effects are prominent, especially anticholinergic reactions. Specific symptoms and treatment are described below.

Symptoms. The anticholinergic actions of H_1 blockers produce symptoms resembling those of atropine poisoning (dilated pupils, flushed face, hyperpyrexia, tachycardia, dry mouth, urinary retention). In children, CNS excitation is prominent, manifesting as hallucinations, incoordination, ataxia, and convulsions. In extreme cases, intoxication progresses to coma, cardiovascular collapse, and death.

Treatment. There is no specific antidote to antihistamine poisoning. Hence, treatment is directed at drug removal and managing symptoms. Emesis should be induced to expel the drug from the stomach. Following this, activated charcoal plus a cathartic is given to minimize absorption of any drug that remains in the GI tract. Convulsions should be treated with IV phenytoin. Anticonvulsants that have CNS-depressant properties must be avoided. Hyperthermia can be reduced by application of ice packs or by sponge baths.

H_1 ANTAGONISTS II: PREPARATIONS

First-Generation H_1 Antagonists

The first-generation (sedating) H_1 antagonists can be grouped into five major categories: alkylamines, ethanolamines, ethylenediamines, phenothiazines, and piperidines. As indicated in Table 66–1, these groups differ in antihistaminic efficacy and the ability to cause sedation and muscarinic blockade. Given these differences, it is often possible, through judicious drug selection, to produce effective H_1 blockade while minimizing undesired effects.

Sedation can be a significant problem. Among the first-generation agents, CNS depression is most prominent with the ethanolamines (e.g., diphenhydramine) and phenothiazines (e.g., promethazine), and least prominent with the alkylamines (e.g., chlorpheniramine). For many patients, the alkylamines can provide effective H_1 blockade while causing only a modest reduction in alertness. If sedation remains excessive with an alkylamine, a second-generation agent may be tried.

All of the H_1 blockers can be administered by mouth. In addition, some can be given parenterally or by rectal suppository. Routes and dosages for individual H_1 antagonists are summarized in Table 66–2.

Second-Generation (Nonsedating) H_1 Antagonists

Five second-generation antihistamines are available: azelastine, cetirizine, fexofenadine, loratadine, and desloratadine. Two others—astemizole [Hismanal] and terfenadine [Seldane]—were removed from the market because they posed a risk of severe dysrhythmias. The second-generation agents differ from the first-generation agents in that they do not readily cross the blood-brain barrier, and hence produce little or no sedation. Synergism with alcohol and other CNS depressants is low. Nonetheless, combined use with these drugs should be avoided. In addition to being nonsedating, the second-generation agents are largely devoid of anticholinergic actions. Unfortunately, these drugs are much more expensive than the first-generation agents. For example, they cost about 20 times more than chlorpheniramine, a representative first-generation drug. Properties of individual agents are described below.

Fexofenadine. Fexofenadine [Allegra] is approved for oral therapy of seasonal allergic rhinitis and for chronic idiopathic urticaria. Of the second-generation antihistamines now available, fexofenadine appears to offer the best combination of efficacy and safety. In clinical trials, the incidence of drowsiness and other side effects was nearly the same as with placebo.

TABLE 66–2 ■ H_1 Antagonists: Trade Names, Routes, and Dosage

Generic Name	Trade Names	Routes	Usual Adult Oral Dosage
First-Generation Agents			
Alkylamines			
Chlorpheniramine	Chlor-Trimeton, others	PO	4 mg q 4–6 h
Dexchlorpheniramine	Polaramine	PO	2 mg q 4–6 h
Ethanolamines			
Clemastine	Tavist, Antihist-1	PO	1.34 mg q 12 h
Diphenhydramine	Benadryl, others	PO, IV, IM	25–50 mg q 6–8 h
Ethylenediamines			
Tripelennamine	PBZ	PO	25–50 mg q 4–6 h
Phenothiazines			
Promethazine	Phenergan, others	PO, IV, IM, R*	12.5–25 mg q 6–24 h
Piperidines			
Azatadine	Optimine	PO	1–2 mg q 12 h
Cyproheptadine	Periactin	PO	4 mg q 6–8 h
Phenindamine	Nolahist	PO	25 mg q 4–6 h
Second-Generation (Nonsedating) Agents			
Azelastine	Astelin	Nasal spray	See text
Cetirizine†	Zyrtec	PO	See text
Fexofenadine	Allegra	PO	See text
Loratadine	Claritin, Claritin Reditabs	PO	See text
Desloratadine	Clarinex	PO	5 mg q 24 h

*R = rectal suppository.

†Cetirizine has mild sedating effects.

Fexofenadine has a plasma half-life of 14.4 hours and is excreted unchanged in the urine. The drug is available in capsules (30 mg) and tablets (30, 60, and 180 mg). The recommended dosage for adults and for children 12 years and older is 60 mg twice a day or 180 mg once a day. The dosage for children ages 6 to 11 is 30 mg twice a day. Dosage should be reduced in patients with renal impairment.

Cetirizine. Cetirizine [Zyrtec] is indicated for chronic idiopathic urticaria and for seasonal and perennial allergic rhinitis. The drug is administered orally and food delays absorption. Cetirizine is eliminated by a combination of hepatic metabolism and renal excretion, and has a half-life of 8.3 hours. Although cetirizine is generally well tolerated, it can cause drowsiness (14%), fatigue (6%), and dryness of the mouth, nose, and throat (5%). The drug is available in tablets (5 and 10 mg) and a syrup (1 mg/ml). The recommended dosage for adults and for children 6 years and older is 5 or 10 mg once a day. The dosage for children ages 2 to 5 years is 2.5 mg once a day initially, and may be increased to either 5 mg once a day or 2.5 mg twice a day. Dosage should be reduced in patients with significant hepatic or renal impairment.

Loratadine. Loratadine [Claritin] is indicated for seasonal allergic rhinitis and for chronic idiopathic urticaria. Like other second-generation antihistamines, the drug is generally well tolerated. However, in clinical trials, 8% of patients experienced drowsiness, and 12% experienced headache. Loratadine is administered orally and food delays absorption. The drug undergoes extensive hepatic metabolism and has a half-life of 8 to 28 hours. Loratadine is available in three formulations: a syrup (1 mg/ml), 10-mg standard tablets, and 10-mg rapidly disintegrating tablets [Claritin Reditabs] designed to dissolve on the tongue. The recommended dosage for adults and for children 6 years and older is 10 mg once a day. The dosage for children ages 2 to 5 years is 5 mg (of the syrup) once a day. For patients with significant hepatic or renal impairment, dosing should be done every other day.

Desloratadine. Desloratadine [Clarinex] is the major active metabolite of loratadine [Claritin]. The two drugs differ primarily in that desloratadine has a longer half-life (27 hours vs. 8.4 hours). However, although desloratadine has a longer half-life, there is no proof that its *effects* persist longer. Desloratadine has two approved uses: seasonal allergic rhinitis and chronic idiopathic urticaria. The recommended dosage for adults and for children over 12 years is 5 mg once a day. Taking higher doses offers no increase in benefits, but does increase the risk of drowsiness. For patients with liver or renal impairment, the manufacturer recommends reducing the initial dosage to 5 mg every other day. Desloratadine has no significant drug interactions and, at the recommended dosage, the incidence of adverse effects is similar to that seen with placebo. There is no indication that desloratadine prolongs the QT interval or poses a risk of dysrhythmias. About 7% of patients metabolize desloratadine very slowly, causing its effects to be more intense.

Azelastine. For two reasons, azelastine [Astelin] is unique among the second-generation agents. First, azelastine is administered by nasal spray, whereas the others are given orally. Second, in addition to blocking receptors for histamine, azelastine blocks the release of histamine and other mediators from mast cells. For patients with allergic or vasomotor rhinitis (the drug's only indications), azelastine is as effective as oral antihistamines and intranasal glucocorticoids. The recommended dosage for adults and for chil-

dren 12 years and older is 2 sprays (250 mg) per nostril twice a day. The dosage for children ages 5 to 11 is one spray per nostril twice a day. Azelastine causes mild sedation and hence should not be combined with alcohol. During clinical trials, the most common side effect was a bitter taste, which occurred in 20% of patients. Other side effects include headache (14.8%); drowsiness (11.5%); pharyngitis (3.8%); dry mouth, nose, and throat (2.8%); and nausea, vomiting, and bowel changes (2.8%).

⠿ KEY POINTS

- Histamine is synthesized and stored in mast cells and basophils.
- Histamine release may be triggered by allergic and nonallergic mechanisms.
- There are two classes of histamine receptors, called H_1 receptors and H_2 receptors.
- Activation of H_1 receptors causes vasodilation, increased capillary permeability, pain, itching, bronchoconstriction, and sedation.
- Activation of H_2 receptor causes release of gastric acid from parietal cells of the stomach.
- Histamine is an important mediator of mild allergic reactions, but is only a minor contributor to severe (anaphylactic) reactions.
- There are two major classes of histamine receptor antagonists: H_1-receptor antagonists, which are used to treat mild allergic reactions, and H_2-receptor antagonists, which are used to treat gastric and duodenal ulcers (see Chapter 73).
- Histamine$_1$-receptor antagonists relieve allergic symptoms by blocking histamine receptors on small blood vessels, capillaries, and sensory nerves. These drugs do not block release of histamine from mast cells and basophils.
- There are two major classes of H_1-receptor antagonists, known as first-generation H_1-receptor antagonists and second-generation H_1-receptor antagonists.
- First-generation H_1-receptor antagonists frequently cause sedation; second-generation agents rarely do.
- CNS depression from first-generation H_1-receptor antagonists can be intensified by alcohol and other drugs with CNS-depressant actions.

Summary of Major Nursing Implications*

H₁-RECEPTOR ANTAGONISTS

First-Generation Antihistamines

Azatadine
Brompheniramine
Chlorpheniramine
Clemastine
Cyproheptadine
Dexchlorpheniramine
Diphenhydramine
Phenindamine
Promethazine
Tripelennamine

Second-Generation Antihistamines

Azelastine
Cetirizine
Desloratadine
Fexofenadine
Loratadine

Preadministration Assessment

Therapeutic Goal

Oral Therapy. Relief of symptoms of mild to moderate allergic disorders (e.g., allergic rhinitis, allergic conjunctivitis, uncomplicated urticaria and angioedema).

*Patient education information is highlighted as blue text.

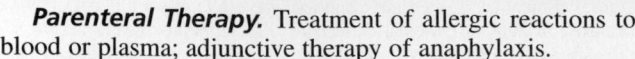

Summary of Major Nursing Implications*—cont'd

Parenteral Therapy. Treatment of allergic reactions to blood or plasma; adjunctive therapy of anaphylaxis.

Identifying High-Risk Patients

Antihistamines are *contraindicated* during the third trimester of pregnancy and for nursing mothers and newborn infants.

Exercise *caution* when treating young children, the elderly, and patients with conditions that may be aggravated by muscarinic blockade, including asthma, urinary retention, open-angle glaucoma, hypertension, and prostatic hypertrophy.

Implementation: Administration

Routes

All H_1 blockers can be administered orally. Some can also be administered parenterally, by rectal suppository, or by nasal spray (see Table 66–2).

Administration

Advise patients to take oral antihistamines with food if GI upset occurs.

Warn patients not to crush or chew enteric-coated preparations.

Ongoing Evaluation and Interventions

Minimizing Adverse Effects

Sedation. For most patients, a first-generation antihistamine in the alkylamine group (see Table 66–1) can provide effective H_1 blockade with only modest sedation. If sedation is excessive with an alkylamine, a second-generation antihistamine (e.g., fexofenadine) can be used. With long-acting antihistamines, daytime sedation can be minimized by administering the entire daily dose in the evening. **Caution the patient to avoid hazardous activities if sedation is significant.**

Anticholinergic Effects. **Advise the patient that dryness of the mouth and throat can be reduced by sucking on hard (sugarless) candy and by taking frequent sips of liquids.** Other atropine-like responses (urinary hesitancy, tachycardia, constipation) are not usually problems. Second-generation antihistamines have minimal anticholinergic effects.

Gastrointestinal Distress. **Advise the patient that GI disturbances (nausea, vomiting) can be minimized by taking antihistamines with meals.**

Minimizing Adverse Interactions

CNS Depressants. Alcohol and other CNS depressants can intensify the depressant actions of the H_1 antagonists. **Warn the patient against drinking alcohol.** Dosages of CNS depressants (e.g., barbiturates, benzodiazepines, opioids) may need to be reduced. Second-generation antihistamines have no CNS depressant effects and do not potentiate the actions of CNS depressants.

Managing Toxicity

There is no specific antidote to antihistamine overdose. Hence, treatment is directed at removing the drug and managing symptoms. To remove the drug, give an emetic and, after vomiting has occurred, give activated charcoal and a cathartic. Treat hyperthermia with ice packs or cooling sponge baths. Control convulsions with IV phenytoin.

*Patient education information is highlighted as blue text.

Cyclooxygenase Inhibitors: Nonsteroidal Anti-inflammatory Drugs and Acetaminophen

MECHANISM OF ACTION
CLASSIFICATION OF
CYCLOOXYGENASE INHIBITORS
FIRST-GENERATION NSAIDS
   Aspirin
   Other First-Generation NSAIDs
SECOND-GENERATION NSAIDS
(COX-2 INHIBITORS, COXIBS)
   Celecoxib
   Rofecoxib
   Valdecoxib
ACETAMINOPHEN

The family of cyclooxygenase inhibitors consists of aspirin and related drugs. Most of these agents can produce three useful effects: (1) suppression of inflammation, (2) relief of pain, and (3) reduction of fever. All three are produced through one central mechanism: inhibition of cyclooxygenase, the enzyme responsible for synthesis of prostaglandins and related compounds. This same mechanism underlies the principal adverse effects of these drugs: (1) gastric ulceration, (2) bleeding, and (3) renal impairment.

MECHANISM OF ACTION

All of the drugs discussed in this chapter work by inhibiting *cyclooxygenase* (COX), the enzyme that converts arachidonic acid into *prostaglandins* and related compounds (prostacyclin, thromboxane A_2 [TXA_2]). To understand the drugs that inhibit COX, we must first understand COX itself.

Cyclooxygenase is found in all tissues and helps regulate multiple processes. At sites of tissue injury, COX catalyzes the synthesis of prostaglandin E_2 (PGE_2) and prostaglandin I_2 (PGI_2, prostacyclin), which promote inflammation and sensitize receptors to painful stimuli. In the stomach, COX promotes synthesis of PGE_2 and PGI_2, which help protect the gastric mucosa. Three mechanisms are involved: reduced secretion of gastric acid, increased secretion of bicarbonate

and cytoprotective mucus, and maintenance of submucosal blood flow. In platelets, COX promotes synthesis of TXA_2, which stimulates platelet aggregation. In the kidney, COX catalyzes synthesis of PGE_2 and PGI_2, which promote vasodilation and thereby maintain renal blood flow. In the brain, COX-derived prostaglandins mediate fever and contribute to perception of pain. In the uterus, COX-derived prostaglandins help promote contractions at term. It is important to appreciate that prostaglandins, prostacyclin, and TXA_2 act *locally;* these compounds do not affect sites distant from where they were made.

Cyclooxygenase has two forms, named cyclooxygenase-1 (COX-1) and cyclooxygenase-2 (COX-2). Cyclooxygenase-1 is found in practically all tissues, where it mediates "housekeeping" chores. Important among these are protecting the gastric mucosa, supporting renal function, and promoting platelet aggregation. In contrast, COX-2 is produced mainly at sites of *tissue injury,* where it mediates inflammation and sensitizes receptors to painful stimuli. Cyclooxygenase-2 is also present in the *brain,* where it mediates fever and contributes to perception of pain. Because COX-1 mediates beneficial processes whereas COX-2 mediates harmful processes, COX-1 has been dubbed the "good COX" and COX-2 the "bad COX." Some important functions of COX-1 and COX-2 are summarized in Table 67–1.

Having established the roles of COX-1 and COX-2, we can now predict the effects of drugs that inhibit these enzymes. Inhibition of COX-1 (good COX) results largely in harmful effects:

- Gastric erosion and ulceration
- Bleeding tendencies
- Renal impairment

Inhibition of COX-1 also has one beneficial effect:

- Protection against myocardial infarction (secondary to reduced platelet aggregation)

Inhibition of COX-2 (bad COX) results in beneficial effects:

- Suppression of inflammation
- Alleviation of pain
- Reduction of fever

TABLE 67–1 ■ Cyclooxygenase-1 and Cyclooxygenase-2: Functions and Effect of Inhibition

Location	COX Isoform	COX Reaction Product	Response to COX Reaction Product	Effect of COX Inhibition
Stomach	COX-1	PGE_2, PGI_2	Gastric protection: Increased bicarbonate secretion Increased mucus production Decreased acid secretion Maintenance of submucosal blood flow	Gastric ulceration
Kidney	COX-1	PGE_2, PGI_2	Maintenance of renal function: Renal vasodilation Maintenance of renal perfusion	Renal impairment
Platelets	COX-1	TXA_2	Platelet aggregation	Bleeding tendencies Protection against MI
Injured tissue	COX-2	PGE_2	Inflammation Pain	Reduced inflammation Analgesia
Brain	COX-2	—	Fever Pain	Reduced fever Analgesia

COX-1 = cyclooxygenase-1, COX-2 = cyclooxygenase-2, PGE_2 = prostaglandin E_2, PGI_2 = prostaglandin I_2 (prostacyclin), TXA_2 = thromboxane A_2, MI = myocardial infarction.

CLASSIFICATION OF CYCLOOXYGENASE INHIBITORS

The cyclooxygenase inhibitors fall into two major categories: (1) drugs that have anti-inflammatory properties and (2) drugs that lack anti-inflammatory properties. Agents in the first group are referred to as *nonsteroidal anti-inflammatory drugs* (NSAIDs). Representative members include aspirin, ibuprofen [Motrin, Advil, others], naproxen [Naprosyn], and celecoxib [Celebrex]. The second class consists of just one drug: *acetaminophen* [Tylenol, others]. Acetaminophen can reduce pain and fever but cannot suppress inflammation.

The NSAIDs can be subdivided into two groups: (1) *first-generation NSAIDs* (conventional NSAIDs, traditional NSAIDs) and (2) *second-generation NSAIDs* (COX-2 inhibitors, coxibs). The first-generation agents inhibit COX-1 *and* COX-2. The second-generation agents inhibit COX-2 only. Because the first-generation agents inhibit both COX isoforms, they are unable to suppress pain and inflammation without posing a risk of serious side effects (gastric ulceration, bleeding, renal impairment). In contrast, because of their selectivity for COX-2, the second-generation NSAIDs are able to suppress pain and inflammation while causing fewer adverse events than the first-generation NSAIDs.

FIRST-GENERATION NSAIDS

The first-generation NSAIDs, which inhibit COX-1 and COX-2, are a large and widely used family of drugs. In the United States, more than 70 million prescriptions are written annually and more than 30 billion tablets are sold over the counter. The traditional NSAIDs are used to treat inflammatory disorders (e.g., rheumatoid arthritis, osteoarthritis, bursitis) and to alleviate mild to moderate pain, suppress fever, and relieve dysmenorrhea. Because they cannot inhibit COX-2 without inhibiting COX-1, first-generation NSAIDs cannot suppress inflammation without posing a risk of serious

harm: NSAID-induced ulcers are responsible for more than 100,000 hospitalizations and at least 16,500 deaths each year. Aspirin, the oldest member of the family, will serve as our prototype for the group.

Aspirin

Aspirin is an important drug whose effectiveness is frequently underappreciated. Given that aspirin is available without prescription, widely advertised in the media, and used somewhat casually by the general public, you may be surprised to hear that aspirin is a highly valuable and effective medication. The drug provides excellent relief of mild to moderate pain, reduces fever, protects against thrombotic disorders, and remains a drug of choice for rheumatoid arthritis and other inflammatory conditions. You may also be surprised to hear that aspirin can cause serious toxicity, especially gastric ulceration. Despite the introduction of many new NSAIDs, aspirin remains the most widely used member of the group, and is the standard against which the others must be compared.

Chemistry

Aspirin belongs to a chemical family known as *salicylates.* All members of this group are derivatives of salicylic acid (Fig. 67–1). Aspirin is produced by substituting an acetyl group onto salicylic acid. Because of this acetyl group, aspirin is commonly known as *acetylsalicylic acid,* or simply ASA.

Mechanism of Action

Aspirin is a nonselective inhibitor of cyclooxygenase. Most beneficial effects—reductions of inflammation, pain, and fever—result from inhibiting COX-2. One beneficial effect—protection against myocardial infarction (MI) and ischemic restroke—results from inhibiting COX-1. Major adverse effects—gastric ulceration, bleeding, renal impairment—also result from inhibiting COX-1.

It is important to note that aspirin is an *irreversible* inhibitor of cyclooxygenase. In contrast, all other NSAIDs are

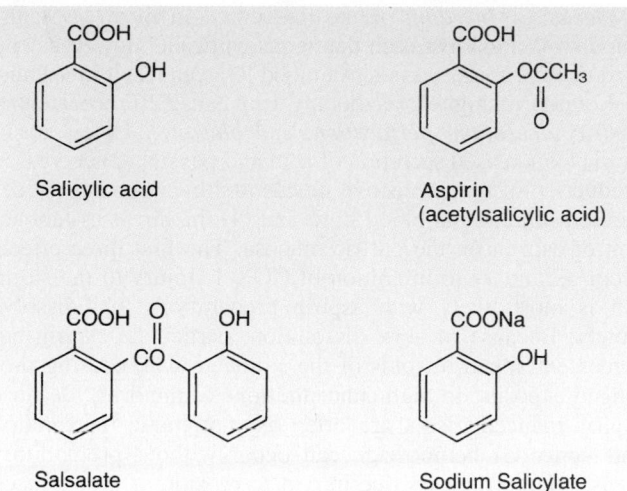

Figure 67–1 ■ Structural formulas of aspirin and related salicylates.

reversible (competitive) inhibitors. Because inhibition of cyclooxygenase by aspirin is irreversible, duration of action depends on how quickly specific tissues can synthesize new molecules of COX-1 and COX-2. With other NSAIDs, effects decline as soon as drug levels fall.

Pharmacokinetics

Absorption. Aspirin is absorbed rapidly and completely following oral administration. The principal site of absorption is the small intestine. When administered by rectal suppository, aspirin is absorbed slowly and blood levels are lower than with oral therapy.

Metabolism. Aspirin has a very short half-life (15 to 20 minutes) because of rapid conversion to *salicylic acid,* an active metabolite. The rate of inactivation of salicylic acid depends on the amount present: At low therapeutic levels, salicylic acid has a half-life of approximately 2 hours, but at high therapeutic levels, the half-life may exceed 20 hours.

Distribution. Salicylic acid is extensively bound to plasma albumin. At therapeutic levels, binding is between 80% and 90%. Aspirin undergoes distribution to all body tissues and fluids, including breast milk, fetal tissues, and the central nervous system (CNS).

Excretion. Salicylic acid and its metabolites are excreted by the kidneys. Excretion of salicylic acid is highly dependent on urinary pH. Accordingly, by raising the pH of urine from 6 to 8, we can increase the rate of excretion by a factor of 4.

Plasma Drug Levels. Low therapeutic doses of aspirin produce plasma salicylate levels in the range of 100 μg/ml. Anti-inflammatory doses produce salicylate levels of about 400 μg/ml. Signs of salicylism (toxicity) begin when plasma salicylate levels exceed 200 μg/ml. Severe toxicity occurs at levels above 400 μg/ml.

Therapeutic Uses

Suppression of Inflammation. Aspirin is an initial drug of choice for rheumatoid arthritis, osteoarthritis, and juvenile arthritis. Aspirin is also indicated for other inflammatory disorders, including rheumatic fever, tendinitis, and bursitis. The

dosages employed to suppress inflammation are considerably larger than dosages used for analgesia or reduction of fever. The use of aspirin and other NSAIDs to treat arthritis is discussed further in Chapter 69.

The precise mechanisms by which aspirin decreases inflammation have not been established. We do know that prostaglandins contribute to several, but not all, components of the inflammatory process. Hence, inhibition of COX-2 provides a partial explanation of anti-inflammatory effects. Other possible mechanisms include modulation of T-cell function, suppression of inflammatory cell infiltration, and stabilization of lysosomes.

Analgesia. Aspirin is our most widely used medication for relieving mild to moderate pain. The degree of analgesia produced depends on the type of pain. Aspirin is most active against joint pain, muscle pain, and headache. For some forms of postoperative pain, aspirin can be more effective than opioids. However, aspirin is relatively ineffective against severe pain of visceral origin. In contrast to opioid analgesics, aspirin produces neither tolerance nor physical dependence. In addition, aspirin is safer.

Aspirin relieves pain primarily through actions in the periphery. At sites of injury, prostaglandins sensitize pain receptors to mechanical and chemical stimulation. Aspirin reduces pain by inhibiting COX-2, and thereby suppresses prostaglandin production. In addition to this peripheral mechanism, aspirin has actions in the CNS that contribute to pain relief.

Reduction of Fever. Aspirin is the drug of choice for reducing temperature in febrile *adults.* However, because of the risk of Reye's syndrome (see below), *aspirin should not be used to treat fever in children.* Although aspirin readily reduces fever, it will not lower normal body temperature, nor will it lower temperature that has become elevated in response to physical activity or to a rise in environmental temperature.

How does aspirin reduce fever? Body temperature is regulated by the hypothalamus, which maintains a balance between heat production and heat loss. Fever occurs when the set point of the hypothalamus becomes elevated, causing the hypothalamus to increase heat production and decrease heat loss. Set-point elevation is triggered by local synthesis of prostaglandins in response to endogenous pyrogens (fever-promoting substances). Aspirin lowers the set point by inhibiting COX-2, and thereby inhibits pyrogen-induced synthesis of prostaglandins.

Dysmenorrhea. Aspirin can provide relief from primary dysmenorrhea. Benefits derive from inhibiting prostaglandin synthesis in uterine smooth muscle. (Prostaglandins promote uterine contraction, and hence suppression of prostaglandin synthesis relieves cramping.) Some of the newer aspirin-like drugs (e.g., ibuprofen, naproxen) are superior to aspirin for dysmenorrhea. The efficacy of the newer drugs is attributed to a greater ability to inhibit COX in the uterus.

Suppression of Platelet Aggregation. Synthesis of TXA_2 in platelets promotes aggregation. Aspirin suppresses platelet aggregation by causing *irreversible* inhibition of COX-1, the enzyme that makes TXA_2. Because platelets lack the machinery to synthesize new COX-1, the effects of a single dose persist for the life of the platelet (about 8 days).

There is a large body of evidence demonstrating that aspirin, through its antiplatelet actions, can benefit a variety of patients. Accordingly, in 1999, the Food and Drug Administration (FDA) recommended wider use of aspirin for antiplatelet effects. Professional labeling for aspirin now recommends low doses (75 to 325 mg/day) to treat men and women for the following:

- *Ischemic stroke* (to reduce the risk of death and nonfatal stroke)
- *Transient ischemic attacks* (to reduce the risk of death and nonfatal stroke)
- *Acute MI* (to reduce the risk of vascular mortality)
- *Previous MI* (to reduce the combined risk of death and nonfatal MI)
- *Chronic stable angina* (to reduce the risk of MI and sudden death)
- *Unstable angina* (to reduce the combined risk of death and nonfatal MI)
- *Angioplasty and other revascularization procedures* (in patients who have a pre-existing condition for which aspirin is already indicated)

In addition, aspirin can be used by healthy people for *primary prevention of MI*. Antiplatelet effects of aspirin are discussed further in Chapter 50.

Cancer Prevention. *Colorectal Cancer.* There is a growing body of evidence that regular use of aspirin decreases the risk of colorectal cancer. This disease kills 54,000 Americans each year and is second only to lung cancer as the leading cause of cancer deaths. Although the protective dosage of aspirin has not been determined, the minimum appears to be 2 or 3 tablets a week. Benefits are not apparent until years of use. The mechanism underlying protection may be inhibition of COX-2, which is present at high levels in colon cancer cells.

Who should take aspirin for prophylaxis? One authority recommends that people at risk for colorectal cancer take 1 aspirin tablet (325 mg) every other day (assuming there is no contraindication to using the drug). Individuals at risk include patients with inflammatory bowel disease; those with previous large-bowel cancer; those with breast, ovarian, or endometrial cancer; and those with a family history of colorectal cancer.

Other Cancers. Preliminary evidence suggests that aspirin may protect against cancers of the prostate, pancreas, and ovary. In a study involving men over the age of 60, daily use of aspirin and other NSAIDs was associated with a 50% decrease in the incidence of prostate cancer. In a study involving over 28,000 women, aspirin use was associated with a 43% decrease in the incidence of pancreatic cancer. In another study involving women, taking aspirin at least 3 times a week for at least 6 months was associated with a 40% reduction in the incidence of ovarian cancer.

Protection Against Alzheimer's Disease. There is mounting evidence that long-term use of aspirin and other NSAIDs may protect against development of Alzheimer's disease (see Chapter 22).

Adverse Effects

When administered short-term in analgesic or antipyretic (fever-reducing) doses, aspirin rarely causes serious adverse effects. However, toxicity is common when treating inflammatory disorders, which require high doses administered long term.

Gastrointestinal Effects. The most common side effects of aspirin are *gastric distress, heartburn,* and *nausea*. These reactions can be reduced by taking aspirin with food or a full glass of water.

Occult GI bleeding occurs frequently. In most cases, the amount of blood lost each day is insignificant. However, with chronic aspirin use, cumulative blood loss can result in anemia.

Long-term high-dose therapy can cause life-threatening *gastric ulceration, perforation,* and *bleeding*. Ulcers result from (1) increased secretion of acid and pepsin, (2) decreased production of cytoprotective mucus and bicarbonate, (3) decreased submucosal blood flow, and (4) the direct irritant action of aspirin on the gastric mucosa. The first three effects occur secondary to inhibition of COX-1. Injury to the stomach is most likely with aspirin preparations that dissolve slowly: Because of slow dissolution, particulate aspirin becomes entrapped in folds of the stomach wall, causing prolonged exposure to high concentrations of the drug. Because aspirin-induced ulcers are often asymptomatic, perforation and upper GI hemorrhage can occur without premonitory signs. (Hemorrhage is due in part to erosion of the stomach wall and in part to suppression of platelet aggregation.) Factors that increase the risk of ulceration include (1) advanced age, (2) a history of peptic ulcer disease, (3) previous intolerance to aspirin or other NSAIDs, (4) cigarette smoking, and (5) a history of alcoholism. Because alcohol intensifies the irritant effects of aspirin, alcohol should not be consumed.

Aspirin-induced ulcers can be managed by giving an antiulcer medication. *Histamine$_2$ (H$_2$)-receptor antagonists* (e.g., cimetidine, famotidine) and *proton pump inhibitors* (e.g., omeprazole, lansoprazole) are preferred. Drugs in both classes suppress secretion of gastric acid. The pharmacology of these agents is discussed in Chapter 73 (Drugs for Peptic Ulcer Disease).

The only drug approved for *prophylaxis* against aspirin-induced ulcers is *misoprostol* [Cytotec], a synthetic prostaglandin. Misoprostol helps prevent ulcers by (1) suppressing secretion of gastric acid, (2) promoting secretion of cytoprotective mucus and bicarbonate, and (3) maintaining normal submucosal blood flow. Because misoprostol can stimulate uterine contractions, the drug is absolutely contraindicated during pregnancy. A fixed-dose combination of misoprostol plus diclofenac (an NSAID) is available under the trade name Arthrotec. The pharmacology of misoprostol is discussed in Chapter 73.

There is evidence that infection with *Helicobacter pylori*, the bacterium that causes many ulcers (see Chapter 73), greatly increases the risk of ulcers in patients taking aspirin. In addition, there is evidence that, if the bacterium is eliminated prior to starting long-term aspirin therapy, the risk of ulcers can be significantly reduced. Accordingly, in patients at high risk for ulcers—the elderly, those with a history of ulcers, and those taking glucocorticoids or anticoagulants—it would be prudent to test for and eliminate *H. pylori* prior to initiating aspirin therapy.

Bleeding. Aspirin can promote bleeding by inhibiting platelet aggregation. After ingestion of just two aspirin tablets, bleeding time is doubled for approximately 1 week. (Recall that platelets are unable to replace aspirin-inactivated cyclooxygenase. Hence bleeding time is prolonged for the life of the platelet.) Because of its effects on platelets, *aspirin is contraindicated for patients with bleeding disorders* (e.g., hemophilia, vitamin K deficiency, hypoprothrombinemia). In order to minimize blood loss during parturition and elective surgery, aspirin should be discontinued at least 1 week prior to these procedures. However, there is no need to stop aspirin prior to *dental* surgery. Caution is needed when aspirin is used in conjunction with anticoagulants.

Renal Impairment. Aspirin can cause acute, reversible impairment of renal function, resulting in salt and water retention and edema. The risk of clinically significant effects is limited primarily to patients with additional risk factors: advanced age, pre-existing renal dysfunction, hypovolemia, hepatic cirrhosis, or heart failure. It should be noted that, although aspirin has *acute* effects on renal function, long-term use does *not* lead to chronic renal failure (although it can exacerbate pre-existing renal dysfunction). Aspirin impairs renal function by inhibiting COX-1, thereby depriving the kidney of prostaglandins needed for normal function.

Development of renal impairment is signaled by reduced urine output, weight gain despite use of diuretics, and a rapid rise in serum creatinine and blood urea nitrogen. If any of these is observed, aspirin should be withdrawn immediately. In most cases, kidney function then returns to baseline level.

The risk of renal impairment can be reduced by identifying high-risk patients and treating them with the smallest dosages possible.

Salicylism. Salicylism is a syndrome that begins to develop when aspirin levels climb just slightly above therapeutic. Overt signs include *tinnitus* (ringing in the ears), *sweating, headache,* and *dizziness.* Acid-base disturbance may also occur (see below). If salicylism develops, aspirin should be withheld until symptoms subside; therapy should then resume, but with a small reduction in dosage. In some cases, development of tinnitus can be used to adjust aspirin dosage: When tinnitus occurs, the maximum acceptable dose has been achieved. However, this guideline may be inappropriate for older patients, because they may fail to develop tinnitus even when aspirin levels become toxic.

Acid-base disturbance results from the effects of aspirin on respiration. When administered in high therapeutic doses, aspirin acts on the CNS to stimulate breathing. The resultant increase in CO_2 loss produces *respiratory alkalosis*. In response, the kidneys excrete more bicarbonate. As a result, plasma pH returns to normal and a state of *compensated respiratory alkalosis* is produced.

Reye's Syndrome. This syndrome is a rare but serious illness of childhood that has a mortality rate of 20% to 30%. Characteristic symptoms are encephalopathy and fatty liver degeneration. Epidemiologic data published in 1980 suggested a relationship between Reye's syndrome and use of aspirin by children who have influenza or chickenpox. Although a direct causal link between aspirin and Reye's syndrome was never established, the Centers for Disease Control and Prevention recommended that *aspirin (and other NSAIDs) be avoided by children and teenagers suspected of having influenza or chickenpox.* In response to this recommendation, aspirin was removed from most products intended for use by children, and use of aspirin by children declined sharply. As a result, Reye's syndrome essentially vanished: The incidence declined from a high of 555 cases in 1980 to no more than 2 cases per year between 1994 and 1997. If a child with chickenpox or influenza needs an analgesic/antipyretic, acetaminophen can be used safely.

Adverse Effects Associated with Use During Pregnancy. Aspirin poses risks to the pregnant patient and the developing fetus. Accordingly, the drug is classified in *FDA*

Pregnancy Risk Category D: there is evidence of human fetal risk, but the potential benefits from use of the drug during pregnancy may outweigh the potential for harm. The principal risks to pregnant women are (1) anemia (from GI blood loss), and (2) postpartum hemorrhage. In addition, by inhibiting prostaglandin synthesis, aspirin may suppress spontaneous uterine contractions, and may thereby prolong gestation and labor.

Aspirin crosses the placenta and may adversely affect the fetus. Since prostaglandins help keep the ductus arteriosus patent, inhibition of prostaglandin synthesis by aspirin may induce premature closure of the ductus arteriosus. Aspirin therapy has also been associated with low birth weight, stillbirth, renal toxicity, intracranial hemorrhage in preterm infants, and neonatal death.

Hypersensitivity Reactions. Hypersensitivity develops in about 0.3% of aspirin users. Reactions are most likely in adults who have certain predisposing conditions: asthma, hay fever, chronic urticaria, or nasal polyps. Hypersensitivity reactions are uncommon in children. The aspirin hypersensitivity reaction begins with profuse, watery rhinorrhea and may progress to generalized urticaria, bronchospasm, laryngeal edema, and shock. Despite its resemblance to severe anaphylaxis, this reaction is not allergic and is not mediated by the immune system. Because individuals who react to aspirin are also sensitive to most other NSAIDs, it is thought that hypersensitivity reactions are in some way related to inhibition of cyclooxygenase. However, it is not clear why the reaction is limited to those adults who have the predisposing conditions noted. As with severe anaphylactic reactions, *epinephrine* is the treatment of choice. Hypersensitivity to aspirin is a contraindication to using other drugs with aspirin-like properties.

Summary of Precautions and Contraindications

Aspirin is contraindicated in patients with *peptic ulcer disease, bleeding disorders* (e.g., hemophilia, vitamin K deficiency, hypoprothrombinemia), and *hypersensitivity to aspirin itself or other NSAIDs.* In addition, the drug should be used with extreme caution by *pregnant women* and by *children who have chickenpox or influenza.* Caution should also be exercised when treating *elderly patients, patients who smoke cigarettes,* and *patients with* H. pylori *infection, heart failure, hepatic cirrhosis, hypovolemia, renal dysfunction, asthma, hay fever, chronic urticaria, nasal polyps,* or a *history of alcoholism.* Aspirin should be withdrawn 1 week prior to elective surgery or the anticipated date of parturition.

Drug Interactions

Because of its widespread use, aspirin has been reported to interact with many other medications. However, most of these interactions have little clinical significance. Significant interactions are discussed below.

Warfarin. The most important interactions of aspirin occur with warfarin, an oral anticoagulant. Because aspirin suppresses platelet function and can decrease prothrombin production, aspirin will intensify the anticoagulant effects of warfarin. Furthermore, since aspirin can initiate gastric bleeding, augmenting anticoagulant effects can increase the risk of gastric hemorrhage. Accordingly, the combination of aspirin with warfarin must be used with great care.

Glucocorticoids. Like aspirin, glucocorticoids promote gastric ulceration. As a result, the risk of ulcers is greatly increased when these drugs are combined—as may happen when treating arthritis. To reduce the risk of gastric ulceration, patients can be given misoprostol for prophylaxis.

Alcohol. Combining alcohol with aspirin and other NSAIDs increases the risk of gastric bleeding. To alert the public to this risk, the FDA now requires that labels for aspirin include the following statement: *Alcohol Warning: If you consume three or more alcoholic drinks every day, ask your doctor whether you should take aspirin or other pain relievers/fever reducers. Aspirin [and related drugs] may cause stomach bleeding.* A similar label is required for all other NSAIDs and acetaminophen.

Ibuprofen. Data from a recent study indicate that ibuprofen (an NSAID) can reduce the antiplatelet effects of aspirin. How? By blocking access of aspirin to COX-1 in platelets. This interaction is important: In patients taking low-dose aspirin to prevent MI or ischemic stroke, ibuprofen could negate aspirin's benefits. In the same study, three other COX inhibitors—rofecoxib, diclofenac, and acetaminophen—did not antagonize the effects of aspirin. Whether other related COX inhibitors might antagonize aspirin is unknown.

Acute Poisoning

Aspirin overdose is a common cause of poisoning. Although rarely fatal in adults, aspirin poisoning may prove lethal in children. The lethal dose for adults is 20 to 25 gm. In contrast, as little as 4 gm may be sufficient to kill a child.

Signs and Symptoms. Initially, aspirin overdose produces a state of compensated respiratory alkalosis—the same state seen in mild salicylism. As poisoning progresses, respiratory excitation is replaced by respiratory depression. Acidosis, hyperthermia, sweating, and dehydration are prominent, and electrolyte imbalance is likely. Stupor and coma result from effects in the CNS. Death usually results from respiratory failure. The mechanisms that underlie these clinical manifestations are described below.

Many symptoms of aspirin overdose occur secondary to uncoupling of oxidative phosphorylation, the process by which the energy released during the oxidation of carbohydrates, fats, and proteins is used to form ATP from ADP. When oxidative phosphorylation becomes uncoupled, energy from metabolism of carbohydrates and other nutrients can no longer be transferred to ATP and stored. The consequences of this uncoupling are threefold: (1) Production of CO_2 is increased (secondary to the increased rates of metabolism that take place in futile attempts to form needed ATP). (2) There is increased production of lactic and pyruvic acids (as by-products of increased metabolism). (3) Production of heat is increased because the energy that would normally be used to make ATP is released in the form of heat. Increased heat production is responsible for hyperthermia and dehydration, two of the more serious consequences of aspirin overdosage.

The acidosis that characterizes aspirin poisoning results from multiple causes. Respiratory acidosis occurs because CO_2 production is increased and because toxic levels of salicylate act on the CNS to decrease respiration, thereby allowing even more CO_2 to accumulate. Respiratory acidosis remains uncompensated because bicarbonate stores become depleted during the initial phase of poisoning. Superimposed on respiratory acidosis is true metabolic acidosis. Metabolic acidosis results from (1) the acidity of aspirin and its metabolites, (2) increased production of lactic and pyruvic acids, and (3) accumulation of acidic products of metabolism (e.g., sulfuric and phosphoric acids) because of aspirin-induced impairment of renal excretion.

Acidosis is intensified by the following cycle: (1) Because of the pH partitioning effect, acidosis promotes penetration of salicylate into the CNS. (2) Increased entry of salicylate deepens respiratory depression. (3) Deepening of respiratory depression increases accumulation of CO_2, thereby increasing acidosis. (4) Increasing acidosis causes even more salicylate to enter the CNS, producing even further deepening of respiratory depression. This cycle continues until respiration ceases.

Treatment. Aspirin poisoning is an acute medical emergency that requires hospitalization. The immediate threats to life are respiratory depression, hyperthermia, dehydration, and acidosis. Treatment is largely symptomatic. If respiration is inadequate, mechanical ventilation should be instituted. External cooling (e.g., sponging with tepid water) can help reduce hyperthermia. Intravenous fluids are administered to correct dehydration; the composition of these fluids is determined by electrolyte and acid-base status. Slow infusion of bicarbonate is given to reverse acidosis. Several measures (induction of emesis, gastric lavage, administration of activated charcoal) can reduce further GI absorption of aspirin. Alkalinization of the urine with bicarbonate accelerates excretion of aspirin and salicylate. If necessary, hemodialysis or peritoneal dialysis can be used to remove salicylates from the body.

Formulations

Aspirin is available in several formulations, including plain and buffered tablets, enteric-coated preparations, and tablets used to produce a buffered solution. These different formulations reflect efforts to increase rates of absorption and decrease gastric irritation. For the most part, the clinical utility of the more complex formulations is no greater than that of plain aspirin tablets.

Aspirin Tablets (Plain). All brands are essentially the same with respect to analgesic efficacy, time of onset, and duration of action. Some of the less expensive tablets have greater particle size, which results in slower dissolution and prolonged contact with the gastric mucosa. These effects can augment gastric irritation. Over time, aspirin in tablets decomposes and emits an odor of vinegar (acetic acid); these tablets should be discarded.

Aspirin Tablets (Buffered). The amount of buffer in buffered aspirin tablets is too small to produce significant elevation of gastric pH. An equivalent effect on pH can be achieved by taking plain aspirin tablets with a glass of water or with food. Buffered aspirin tablets are no different from plain tablets with respect to analgesic effects and incidence of gastric distress. Buffered tablets may dissolve faster than plain tablets, resulting in a somewhat faster onset.

Buffered Aspirin Solution. A buffered aspirin solution is produced by dissolving effervescent aspirin tablets [Alka-Seltzer] in a glass of water. This solution has considerable buffering capacity due to its high content of sodium bicarbonate. Effects on gastric pH are sufficient to decrease the incidence of gastric irritation and bleeding. In addition, absorption is accelerated and peak blood levels are increased. Unfortunately, these benefits do not come without a price. The sodium content of buffered aspirin solution can be detrimental to individuals on a sodium-restricted diet. Also, absorption of bicarbonate can result in elevation of urinary pH, an effect that will accelerate aspirin excretion. Lastly, this highly buffered preparation is expensive. Because of this combination of benefits and drawbacks, the buffered aspirin solution is well suited for occasional use but is generally inappropriate for long-term therapy.

Enteric-Coated Preparations. Enteric-coated preparations dissolve in the intestine rather than the stomach, thereby reducing gastric irritation. Unfortunately, absorption from these formulations can be delayed and erratic. Patients should be advised not to crush or chew them.

Timed-Release Tablets. Timed-release tablets offer no advantage over plain aspirin tablets. Since the half-life of salicylic acid is long to begin with, and since aspirin produces irreversible inhibition of cyclooxygenase, timed-release tablets cannot increase duration of action.

Rectal Suppositories. Rectal suppositories have been employed for patients who cannot take aspirin orally. Absorption can be variable, resulting in plasma drug levels that are insufficient in some patients and excessive in others. Also, rectal irritation can occur. Because of these undesirable properties, aspirin suppositories are not generally recommended.

Dosage and Administration

Aspirin is almost always administered by mouth. Gastric irritation can be minimized by administering aspirin with a glass of water or with food. Dosage depends on the age of the patient and the condition being treated. Adult and pediatric dosages for major indications are summarized in Table 67–2.

TABLE 67–2 ■ Aspirin Dosage

Indication	Adult Dosage	Pediatric Dosage
Aches and pains; fever	325–650 mg every 4 hr	2–3 years old: 160 mg 4–5 years old: 240 mg 6–8 years old: 325 mg 9–10 years old: 405 mg 11 years old: 485 mg Over 11 years old: 650 mg *All of the above doses are administered every 4 hr*
Acute rheumatic fever	5–8 gm/day in divided doses	100 mg/kg/day (initially) then 75 mg/kg/day for 4 to 6 wk
Rheumatoid arthritis	3.6–5.4 gm/day in divided doses	90–130 mg/kg/day in divided doses at 4- to 6-hr intervals

Suppression of platelet aggregation
  Initial therapy
  Chronic therapy
	
	325 mg once a day
	80 mg once a day	

Other First-Generation NSAIDs

In attempts to produce an aspirin-like drug with fewer GI and hemorrhagic effects than aspirin, the pharmaceutical industry has produced a large number of drugs with actions very similar to those of aspirin. In the United States, over 20 NSAIDs are now available (Table 67–3). Like aspirin, all other first-generation NSAIDs are relatively nonselective inhibitors of cyclooxygenase. That is, they inhibit both COX-1 and COX-2. However, in contrast to aspirin, which causes *irreversible* inhibition of cyclooxygenase, the other traditional NSAIDs cause *reversible* inhibition. All of these drugs display anti-inflammatory, analgesic, and antipyretic properties. In addition, they all can cause gastric ulceration, bleeding, and renal impairment—although the intensity of these effects may be less with some agents. Patients who are hypersensitive to aspirin are likely to experience cross-hypersensitivity with other NSAIDs. For most NSAIDs, safety during pregnancy has not been established, and hence use by pregnant women is discouraged.

The principal indications for the nonaspirin NSAIDs are rheumatoid arthritis and osteoarthritis. In addition, certain NSAIDs are used to treat fever, bursitis, tendinitis, mild to moderate pain, and dysmenorrhea (see Table 67–3). In contrast to aspirin, the nonaspirin NSAIDs do not protect against MI.

Although individual NSAIDs differ from one another chemically, pharmacokinetically, and to some extent pharmacodynamically, all are very similar clinically: They all produce essentially equivalent antirheumatic effects and they all present an essentially equal risk of serious adverse effects (gastric ulceration, bleeding, and renal impairment). However, for reasons that are not understood, individual patients may respond better to one agent than to another. Furthermore, individual patients may tolerate one NSAID better than another. Therefore, in order to optimize therapy for each individual, therapeutic trials with more than one NSAID may be needed.

Nonacetylated Salicylates: Choline Salicylate, Magnesium Salicylate, Sodium Salicylate, and Salsalate

Similarities to Aspirin. The nonacetylated salicylates are similar to aspirin (an acetylated salicylate) in most respects. Like aspirin, these drugs inhibit COX-1 and COX-2 and are employed to treat arthritis, moderate pain, and fever. The most common adverse effects are GI disturbances. As with aspirin, these drugs should not be given to children with chickenpox or influenza owing to the possibility of precipitating Reye's syndrome.

Contrasts with Aspirin. In contrast to aspirin, the nonacetylated salicylates cause little or no suppression of platelet aggregation. Accordingly, these drugs are preferred to aspirin for use by surgical patients and patients with bleeding disorders.

Because of its sodium content, *sodium salicylate* should be avoided by patients on a sodium-restricted diet (e.g., patients with hypertension or heart failure).

Magnesium salicylate may accumulate to toxic levels in patients with chronic renal insufficiency. Accordingly, magnesium salicylate should be avoided by these people.

Salsalate is a prodrug that breaks down to release two molecules of salicylate in the alkaline environment of the small intestine. Because the stomach is not exposed to salicylate, salsalate produces less gastric irritation than aspirin.

Like salsalate, *choline salicylate* causes less gastric irritation than aspirin.

Preparations, Dosage, and Administration. *Choline salicylate* [Arthropan] is dispensed in solution (870 mg/5 ml) for oral use. The usual dosage is 870 mg every 3 to 4 hours.

Magnesium salicylate [Magan, others] is dispensed in caplets (467, 500, and 580 mg) and tablets (545 and 600 mg) for oral administration. The usual dosage is 650 mg every 4 hours or 1090 mg every 8 hours. The maximum dosage is 4800 mg/day administered in three or four doses.

Sodium salicylate (generic) is dispensed in enteric-coated tablets (325 and 650 mg) for oral use. The usual dosage is 325 to 650 mg every 4 hours.

Salsalate [Disalcid, Mono-Gesic, others] is dispensed in capsules (500 mg) and tablets (500 and 750 mg) for oral use. The usual dosage is 3000 mg/day in divided doses.

Ibuprofen

Ibuprofen [Advil, Motrin, others] is the prototype of the propionic acid derivatives. (Other members of the family are listed in Table 67–3 and discussed individually below.) Like aspirin, ibuprofen inhibits cyclooxygenase and has anti-inflammatory, analgesic, and antipyretic actions. The drug is used to treat fever, mild to moderate pain, and arthritis. In addition, ibuprofen appears superior to most other NSAIDs for relief of primary dysmenorrhea, presumably because it produces good inhibition of cyclooxygenase in uterine smooth muscle. In clinical trials, ibuprofen was highly effective at promoting closure of the ductus arteriosus in preterm infants, a condition for which indomethacin is the current treatment of choice.

Ibuprofen is generally well tolerated, and the incidence of adverse effects is low. The drug produces less gastric bleeding than aspirin and causes less inhibition of platelet aggregation. Consequently, ibuprofen is among the safer NSAIDs for use with anticoagulants.

Ibuprofen is available in four oral formulations: (1) standard tablets (100, 200, 400, 600, and 800 mg), (2) chewable tablets (50 and 100 mg), (3) a

TABLE 67–3 ■ Clinical Pharmacology of the Nonsteroidal Anti-Inflammatory Drugs

Drug	Maximum Daily Dosage (mg)	Plasma Half-Life (hr)	Major Indications*				
			Arthritis	Moderate Pain	Fever	Dysmenorrhea	Bursitis/ Tendinitis
First-Generation NSAIDs							
Salicylates							
Aspirin (many trade names)	8000	0.2–0.3	A	A	A		
Choline salicylate [Arthropan]	5200	2–30†	A	A	A		
Magnesium salicylate [Magan]	4800	2–30†	A	A	A		
Sodium salicylate (generic)	3900	2–30†	A	A	A		
Salsalate [Disalcid, Mono-Gesic]	3000	2–30†	A	A	A		
Propionic Acid Derivatives							
Fenoprofen [Nalfon]	3200	3	A	A			
Flurbiprofen [Ansaid]	300	5.7	A	I	I	I	I
Ibuprofen [Motrin, Advil, others]	3200	1.8–2	A	A	A	A	
Ketoprofen [Orudis, Oruvail]	300	2	A	A	A	A	
Naproxen [Naprosyn]	1500	12–16	A	A	A	A	A
Naproxen sodium [Anaprox, Aleve, Naprelan, others]	1375	15–17	A	A	A	A	A
Oxaprozin [Daypro]	1800	42–50	A				
Others							
Diclofenac [Voltaren, Cataflam]	200	2	A	A		A	
Diflunisal [Dolobid]	1500	11–15	A	A			
Etodolac [Lodine]	1200	7.3	A	A			I
Indomethacin [Indocin]	200	4.5	A				A
Ketorolac [Toradol]	40	5–6		A‡			
Meclofenamate (generic)	400	1.3	A	A		A	
Mefenamic acid [Ponstel]	1000	2		A		A	
Meloxicam [Mobic]	15	15–20	A				
Nabumetone [Relafen]	2000	22	A				
Piroxicam [Feldene]	20	50	A			I	
Sulindac [Clinoril]	400	7.8	A				A
Tolmetin [Tolectin]	2000	2–7	A				
Second-Generation NSAIDs (COX-2 Inhibitors)							
Celecoxib [Celebrex]	800	11	A	A		A	
Rofecoxib [Vioxx]	50	17	A	A		A	
Valdecoxib [Bextra]	40	8–11	A			A	

*A = FDA-approved indication; I = investigational use.
†Half-life increases with increasing dosage.
‡Ketorolac is approved only for *acute* pain; use should not exceed 5 days.

20-mg/ml oral suspension [Children's Advil, Children's Motrin], and (4) a 40-mg/ml oral suspension [Pediatric Advil Drops, Infant's Motrin, PediaCare Fever]. Administration with meals or milk can reduce gastric distress.

Dosages for *adults* are

- *Arthritis*—1.2 to 3.2 gm/day administered in three or four divided doses
- *Primary dysmenorrhea*—400 mg every 4 to 6 hours
- *Mild to moderate pain*—400 mg every 4 hours

Dosages for *children* are

- *Juvenile arthritis*—30 to 40 mg/kg/day in three or four divided doses
- *Fever reduction*—5 mg/kg (for temperature ≤102.5°F) or 10 mg/kg (for temperature >102.5°F). The total daily dose should not exceed 40 mg/kg.

Fenoprofen

Fenoprofen [Nalfon] belongs to the propionic acid family of NSAIDs. Like other NSAIDs, the drug inhibits synthesis of prostaglandins, thereby causing anti-inflammatory, analgesic, and antipyretic effects. Fenoprofen is indicated for arthritis and mild to moderate pain. The most common adverse effects are GI disturbances. Fenoprofen is dispensed in tablets (600 mg) and capsules (200 and 300 mg). The usual dosage for rheumatoid arthritis is 300 to 600 mg 3 or 4 times a day. The maximum daily dosage is 3.2 gm.

Flurbiprofen

Flurbiprofen [Ansaid] is chemically related to ibuprofen and the other derivatives of propionic acid. The drug is approved for arthritis and has been used investigationally for bursitis, tendinitis, moderate pain, fever, and primary dysmenorrhea. The most common adverse effects are GI disturbances (dyspepsia, nausea, diarrhea, abdominal pain). The risk of serious GI effects (ulceration, perforation, hemorrhage) may be greater than with ibuprofen. Like other NSAIDs, flurbiprofen can exacerbate renal impairment. The drug is dispensed in tablets (50 and 100 mg) for oral administration. The usual dosage for rheumatoid arthritis is 200 to 300 mg/day administered in two to four divided doses.

Ketoprofen

Ketoprofen [Orudis, Oruvail] belongs to the propionic acid family of NSAIDs. The drug inhibits synthesis of prostaglandins and has anti-inflammatory, analgesic, and antipyretic effects. Indications are rheumatoid arthritis, osteoarthritis, mild to moderate pain, and primary dysmenorrhea. The most common adverse effects are dyspepsia (11.5%), nausea, vomiting, and abdominal pain. Ketoprofen is dispensed in standard capsules (12.5, 25, 50, and 75 mg) and extended-release capsules (100, 150, and 200 mg). The usual dosage for rheumatoid arthritis is 150 to 300 mg/day administered in three or four divided doses. The dosage for moderate pain or primary dysmenorrhea is 25 to 50 mg every 6 to 8 hours.

Naproxen and Naproxen Sodium

Actions and Uses. Naproxen [Naprosyn, others] and naproxen sodium [Aleve, Anaprox, Naprelan, others] belong to the propionic acid family of NSAIDs. Because these drugs have prolonged half-lives (see Table 67–3), they can be administered less frequently than other propionic acid derivatives (e.g., ibuprofen). Naproxen and naproxen sodium are approved for arthritis, bursitis, tendinitis, primary dysmenorrhea, and mild to moderate pain. In addition, they are used investigationally to reduce fever. Like other NSAIDs, they act primarily by inhibiting cyclooxygenase.

Adverse Effects. Naproxen and naproxen sodium are among the better tolerated NSAIDs. The most common adverse effects are GI disturbances. Like other NSAIDs, these drugs can compromise renal function by decreasing renal blood flow. Bleeding time can be prolonged secondary to reversible inhibition of platelet aggregation.

Preparations, Dosage, and Administration. Naproxen is dispensed in standard tablets (250, 375, and 500 mg), delayed release enteric-coated tablets (375 and 500) as EC Naprosyn, controlled-release tablets (375 and 500 mg) as Naprelan, and as an oral suspension (25 mg/ml). The usual dosage for rheumatoid arthritis is 250 to 500 mg twice daily. The dosage for mild to moderate pain is 500 mg initially followed by 250 mg every 6 to 8 hours.

Naproxen sodium is dispensed in standard tablets (220, 275, and 550 mg), controlled-release tablets (375 and 500 mg), and gelcaps (220 mg) for oral use. The usual dosage for rheumatoid arthritis is 275 to 550 mg twice daily. The dosage for mild to moderate pain is 550 mg initially followed by 275 mg every 6 to 8 hours.

Oxaprozin

Oxaprozin [Daypro] belongs to the propionic acid family of NSAIDs. Approved uses are limited to rheumatoid arthritis and osteoarthritis. As with other NSAIDs, benefits derive from inhibiting synthesis of prostaglandins. Like other propionic acid derivatives, oxaprozin is generally well tolerated. The drug has an unusually long half-life (42 to 50 hours), and hence can be administered just once a day. Oxaprozin is available in 600-mg tablets and caplets. The dosage for arthritis is 1200 mg once a day. The maximum dosage is 1800 mg/day.

Diclofenac

Diclofenac [Voltaren, Cataflam] is approved for rheumatoid arthritis, osteoarthritis, ankylosing spondylitis, and primary dysmenorrhea. As with other NSAIDs, anti-inflammatory, analgesic, and antipyretic effects result from inhibiting cyclooxygenase. Diclofenac is well absorbed following oral administration, but undergoes extensive (40% to 50%) metabolism on its first pass through the liver. In blood, about 99.5% of the drug is protein bound, primarily to albumin. Diclofenac is metabolized by the liver and excreted in the urine.

The most common adverse effects are abdominal pain, dyspepsia, and nausea. By impairing renal function, diclofenac can cause fluid retention, which can exacerbate hypertension and heart failure. The risk of liver dysfunction is greater than with other NSAIDs. Accordingly, patients should receive periodic tests of liver function, and should be instructed to report manifestations of liver injury (e.g., jaundice, fatigue, nausea).

Diclofenac is dispensed in standard tablets (50 mg) and enteric-coated delayed-release tablets (25, 50, 75, and 100 mg) for oral administration. The dosage for rheumatoid arthritis is 150 to 200 mg/day administered in two or three divided doses. The dosage for osteoarthritis is 100 to 150 mg/day administered in two or three divided doses.

Diclofenac Plus Misoprostol [Arthrotec]

Diclofenac, in combination with misoprostol, is available under the trade name Arthrotec. Misoprostol is a prostaglandin analog that can protect against NSAID-induced ulcers. The combination product is approved for patients with rheumatoid arthritis or osteoarthritis who are at high risk for NSAID-induced gastric or duodenal ulcers. In patients with arthritis, the combination is as effective as diclofenac alone and produces significantly less GI ulceration. The most bothersome side effect is diarrhea (caused by misoprostol). Misoprostol can induce uterine contraction, and hence the product is contraindicated for use during pregnancy. Arthrotec comes in two formulations: 50 mg diclofenac plus 200 μg misoprostol and 75 mg diclofenac plus 200 μg misoprostol.

Diflunisal

Diflunisal [Dolobid] is a derivative of salicylic acid. However, unlike the salicylates, diflunisal is not converted to salicylic acid in the body. The drug is indicated for mild to moderate pain, rheumatoid arthritis, and osteoarthritis. Like other NSAIDs, the drug inhibits prostaglandin synthesis and can cause GI disturbances, suppression of platelet aggregation, and renal impairment. Diflunisal has a prolonged half-life (11 to 15 hours), which allows the drug to be administered only 2 or 3 times a day. Diflunisal is dispensed in tablets (250 and 500 mg) for oral use. For treatment of arthritis and mild to moderate pain, the initial dose is 500 to 1000 mg. Maintenance doses of 250 to 500 mg are administered every 8 to 12 hours.

Etodolac

Etodolac [Lodine] is indicated for rheumatoid arthritis, osteoarthritis, and moderate pain. The drug has been used investigationally to treat bursitis and tendinitis. Like other NSAIDs, etodolac produces many of its effects by suppressing the synthesis of prostaglandins. The drug's most common adverse effects are dyspepsia (10%), nausea, vomiting, diarrhea, and abdominal pain. Etodolac may cause less gastric ulceration and bleeding than other NSAIDs. The drug is dispensed in standard tablets (400 and 800 mg), extended-release tablets (400 mg), and capsules (200 and 300 mg). The recommended dosage for arthritis is 800 to 1200 mg/day in divided doses. The dosage for moderate pain is 200 to 400 mg every 6 to 8 hours.

Indomethacin

Actions and Uses. Indomethacin [Indocin] is an effective anti-inflammatory agent approved for arthritis, bursitis, tendinitis, and, as discussed in Chapter 69, acute gouty arthritis. In addition, the drug can be given IV to preterm infants to promote closure of the ductus arteriosus. Although indomethacin is able to reduce pain and fever, it is not routinely used for these effects (owing to its potential for toxicity).

Adverse Effects. Untoward effects are seen in 35% to 50% of patients. As a result, about 20% discontinue the drug. The most common adverse effect is severe frontal headache, which occurs in 25% to 50% of patients. Other CNS effects (dizziness, vertigo, confusion) are also common. Seizures and psychiatric changes (e.g., depression, psychosis) have occurred. Mild GI reactions (nausea, vomiting, indigestion) are experienced by 3% to 9% of users. More severe GI effects (ulceration with perforation, hemorrhage) may also develop. Hematologic reactions (neutropenia, thrombocytopenia, aplastic anemia) have occurred but are rare. Indomethacin suppresses platelet aggregation.

Precautions and Contraindications. Because of its adverse effects, indomethacin is generally contraindicated for infants and children under the age of 14, patients with peptic ulcer disease, and women who are pregnant or breast-feeding. Caution is required in patients with epilepsy and psychiatric disorders, in patients involved in hazardous activities, and in patients receiving anticoagulant therapy.

Pharmacokinetics. Indomethacin is well absorbed following oral administration and distributes to all body fluids and tissues. The drug is metabolized in the liver. Metabolites and parent drug are excreted in the urine and feces.

Preparations, Dosage, and Administration. Indomethacin [Indocin] is dispensed in standard capsules (25 and 50 mg), sustained-release capsules (75 mg), an oral suspension (5 mg/ml), and rectal suppositories (50 mg). For treatment of rheumatoid arthritis, the initial dosage is 25 mg 2 or 3 times a day. The maximum daily dosage is 200 mg. Gastrointestinal reactions can be reduced by administering indomethacin with meals. Dosages for gout are presented in Chapter 69.

Ketorolac

Actions and Uses. Ketorolac [Toradol] is a powerful analgesic with minimum anti-inflammatory actions. Pain relief is equivalent to that produced by morphine and other opioids. Although ketorolac lacks the serious adverse effects associated with opioids (respiratory depression, tolerance, dependence, abuse potential), it nonetheless has serious adverse effects of its own. Accordingly, use should be short term and restricted to managing acute pain of moderate to severe intensity. Ketorolac is not indicated for chronic pain or for treatment of minor aches and discomfort. The usual indication is postoperative pain, for which ketorolac is as effective as morphine. Therapy should begin with parenteral administration, followed by oral ketorolac, if needed. Because of the risks associated with prolonged use, treatment (parenteral plus oral) should not exceed 5 days. Like other NSAIDs, ketorolac suppresses prostaglandin synthesis. This action is thought to underlie analgesic effects.

Pharmacokinetics. Ketorolac is administered orally and parenterally (IM or IV). With parenteral administration, analgesia begins within 30 minutes, peaks in 1 to 2 hours, and persists 4 to 6 hours. The drug is eliminated by hepatic metabolism and urinary excretion. In young adults, ketorolac has a half-life of 4 to 6 hours. The half-life may be prolonged in the elderly and in patients with renal impairment.

Adverse Effects and Contraindications. Ketorolac can cause all of the adverse effects associated with other NSAIDs, including peptic ulcers, GI bleeding or perforation, prolonged bleeding time, renal impairment, hypersensitivity reactions, suppression of uterine contractions, and premature closure of the ductus arteriosus. Concurrent use with other NSAIDs increases the risk of these effects and is therefore contraindicated. Other contraindications include active peptic ulcer disease, history of peptic ulcer disease or recent GI bleeding, advanced renal impairment, confirmed or suspected intracranial bleeding, use prior to major surgery, history of NSAID hypersensitivity reactions, and use during labor and delivery.

Preparations, Dosage, and Administration. Ketorolac [Toradol] is available in 10-mg tablets for oral administration and in preloaded syringes (15 and 30 mg/ml) for parenteral administration.

Parenteral therapy can be accomplished with a single injection or with multiple injections. When a single injection is used, the IM dose is 30 or 60 mg, and the IV dose is 15 or 30 mg. When multiple injections are given, the dosage (IM or IV) is 15 or 30 mg every 6 hours. In all cases, the smaller dosage option is employed for patients over 65 years, patients with impaired kidney function, and patients who weigh less than 50 kg (110 pounds). Intravenous doses should be administered over 15 seconds or longer. Intramuscular injections should be done slowly and deep in the muscle. Treatment should not exceed 5 days.

Oral ketorolac is indicated only as a follow-up to parenteral ketorolac. Initial oral doses are based on preceding parenteral doses. The usual oral maintenance dosage is 10 mg every 4 to 6 hours. Combined oral and parenteral treatment should not exceed 5 days.

Mefenamic Acid

Mefenamic acid [Ponstel] is indicated for relief of primary dysmenorrhea and moderate pain. The principal adverse effect is diarrhea, which can be severe. Mefenamic acid is dispensed in 250-mg capsules. The dosage for primary dysmenorrhea is 500 mg initially followed by 250 mg every 6 hours. The drug should be administered with food or milk to reduce gastric distress. Duration of treatment is usually 2 to 3 days.

Meclofenamate

Meclofenamate is indicated for rheumatoid arthritis, osteoarthritis, mild to moderate pain, and dysmenorrhea. As with other NSAIDs, benefits derive from inhibiting cyclooxygenase. Therapeutic effects are no better than with other NSAIDs, but adverse GI effects are greater: 3% to 9% of patients experience nausea, vomiting, abdominal pain, and cramps; worse yet, 10% to 33% develop diarrhea. Because of this poor benefit-to-risk ratio, meclofenamate is not a drug of first choice. Meclofenamate is available in 50- and 100-mg capsules. Dosage are as follows: for arthritis, 200 to 400 mg/day in three or four divided doses; for moderate pain, 50 mg every 4 to 6 hours; and for dysmenorrhea, 100 mg 3 times a day for up to 6 days.

Nabumetone

Nabumetone [Relafen] is a prodrug that undergoes conversion to its active form (6-MNA) in the liver. In contrast to most traditional NSAIDs, 6-MNA inhibits COX-2 more than COX-1. Although nabumetone has antipyretic, analgesic, and anti-inflammatory properties, the drug is approved only for osteoarthritis and rheumatoid arthritis. Principal adverse effects are diarrhea (14%), abdominal cramps (13%), dyspepsia (12%), and nausea (3% to 9%). Nabumetone causes much less GI ulceration than other first-generation NSAIDs, probably because it preferentially inhibits COX-2. Nabumetone is dispensed in 500- and 750-mg tablets. Treatment of arthritis is begun with a single dose of 1000 mg. After this, the daily dosage is 1500 to 2000 mg administered in one or two doses. Administration with food increases the rate of absorption.

Piroxicam

Piroxicam [Feldene] has anti-inflammatory, analgesic, and antipyretic properties, but is approved only for patients with rheumatoid arthritis and osteoarthritis. The drug's most outstanding feature is its long half-life (about 50 hours). Because piroxicam is eliminated so slowly, therapeutic effects can be maintained with once-a-day dosing. In general, piroxicam is better tolerated than aspirin. Undesired effects are seen in 11% to 46% of those treated, causing between 4% and 12% to discontinue therapy. Gastrointestinal reactions are most common, occurring in about 20% of recipients. The incidence of gastric ulceration is about 1%. Like aspirin, piroxicam inhibits platelet aggregation and prolongs bleeding time. The drug is dispensed in 10- and 20-mg capsules for oral administration. The usual dosage is 20 mg once a day.

Sulindac

Sulindac [Clinoril] is a prodrug that undergoes conversion to its active form within the body. The drug is approved for rheumatoid arthritis, osteoarthritis, tendinitis, bursitis, and acute gouty arthritis. Principal adverse effects are abdominal distress, dyspepsia, nausea, vomiting, and diarrhea. Gastric ulceration is less common than with some other NSAIDs. Like other NSAIDs, sulindac causes reversible inhibition of platelet aggregation, prolongs bleeding time, and impairs renal function. The drug is dispensed in 150- and 200-mg tablets for oral administration. The usual dosage is 150 mg administered twice daily with meals. The maximum daily dosage is 400 mg.

Tolmetin

Tolmetin [Tolectin] is approved for rheumatoid arthritis and osteoarthritis. The drug has analgesic and antipyretic properties but is not employed to relieve fever or pain unrelated to inflammation. Adverse effects occur in 25% to 40% of those treated, causing between 5% and 10% to discontinue treatment. Gastrointestinal effects (nausea, vomiting, indigestion) are most common. Gastric ulceration has occurred, but less frequently than with aspirin. Nonetheless, caution should be exercised in patients with a history of peptic ulcer disease. Hypersensitivity reactions are more common than with aspirin. Effects on the CNS (headache, dizziness, anxiety, drowsiness) are less severe and less frequent than with indomethacin. Unlike most other NSAIDs, tolmetin does not augment the effects of warfarin, an oral anticoagulant. The drug is dispensed in tablets (200 and 600 mg) and capsules (400 mg). For rheumatoid arthritis, the initial dosage is 400 mg 3 times a day. The maximum daily dosage is 2 gm. Gastrointestinal distress can be minimized by administering tolmetin with food.

Meloxicam

Meloxicam [Mobic] is a new NSAID with some COX-2 selectivity. Like other NSAIDs, the drug has analgesic, anti-inflammatory, and antipyretic actions. At this time, meloxicam is indicated only for osteoarthritis. For this application, the drug is as effective as first-generation NSAIDs. Direct comparison with true COX-2 inhibitors (e.g., celecoxib) has not been made. Despite its COX-2 selectivity, meloxicam has a side effect profile like that of the first-generation NSAIDs. Gastrointestinal effects (abdominal pain, constipation, diarrhea, dyspepsia, flatulence, nausea, and vomiting) occur in 20% to 25% of patients. More serious effects—GI ulceration, bleeding, perforation, and death—have also occurred. Meloxicam does not suppress platelet aggregation. The drug has a long half-life (15 to 20 hours) and undergoes elimination in the urine (50%) and feces (50%). Meloxicam is available in 7.5- and 15-mg tablets. Because of its long half-life, the drug can be administered just once a day. The recommended daily dose for both initial and maintenance therapy is 7.5 mg. The maximum dosage is 15 mg/day. Administration may be done with or without food.

SECOND-GENERATION NSAIDS (COX-2 INHIBITORS, COXIBS)

The COX-2 inhibitors, also known as coxibs, are a new and welcome option for the treatment of chronic inflammatory disorders. Recall that traditional NSAIDs suppress pain and inflammation by inhibiting COX-2, and cause their major side effects—especially gastroduodenal ulceration—by inhibiting COX-1. In theory, NSAIDs that cause selective inhibition of COX-2 should be able to suppress pain and inflammation while posing little or no risk of serious side effects. To a significant degree, theory and reality agree: Coxibs are just as effective as traditional NSAIDs at suppressing inflammation, and they pose a lower risk of side effects. However, although coxibs are indeed safer than traditional NSAIDs, they are not as safe as had been hoped for. In particular, although the risk of serious GI complications has been reduced, it has not been eliminated: Even with coxibs, some patients develop clinically significant gastroduodenal ulceration and bleeding. Furthermore, like traditional NSAIDs, the coxibs can impair renal function, and can thereby cause hypertension and edema. In contrast to traditional NSAIDs, coxibs do not inhibit platelet aggregation, and hence do not increase the risk of bleeding.

Because the coxibs are relatively new drugs (the first one was approved in 1999), their appropriate role in therapy is not yet clear. Compared with generic versions of traditional NSAIDs, the coxibs are much more expensive. To justify this expense, we need to establish that switching a patient to a coxib will significantly decrease his or her risk of a major GI event. The data available to date suggest that, for most patients, this may not be true. Hence, until more is known, it may be best to reserve these expensive drugs for patients considered at high risk.

Celecoxib

Celecoxib [Celebrex] was the first COX-2 inhibitor to receive FDA approval and will serve as our prototype for the group. The drug can relieve symptoms of arthritis while causing less GI ulceration than traditional NSAIDs.

Mechanism of Action

Celecoxib causes selective inhibition of COX-2, the COX isoform whose products mediate inflammation and pain. At therapeutic doses, celecoxib does not inhibit COX-1, the COX isoform whose products protect the stomach, help maintain renal function, and promote platelet aggregation.

Pharmacokinetics

Celecoxib is well absorbed following oral administration. Plasma levels peak in 3 hours. Binding to plasma proteins is extensive (97%). The drug undergoes hepatic metabolism followed by renal excretion. The half-life is 11 hours.

Therapeutic Use

Celecoxib is indicated for osteoarthritis, rheumatoid arthritis, acute pain, and dysmenorrhea. In addition, the drug was recently approved for a rare genetic disorder known as familial adenomatous polyposis. For patients with arthritis, celecoxib is equal to naproxen (a conventional NSAID) at relieving joint pain, stiffness, and swelling.

It is important to note that celecoxib does *not* provide the cardiovascular benefits of aspirin. Why? Because celecoxib does not inhibit COX-1 in platelets, and hence does not suppress platelet aggregation.

Adverse Effects

In premarketing trials, celecoxib was well tolerated. The discontinuation rate owing to adverse effects was only 7.1% for celecoxib versus 6.1% for placebo. The most common complaints were *dyspepsia* (8.8% vs. 6.2% for placebo) and *abdominal pain*

(4.1% vs. 2.8% for placebo). Celecoxib does not decrease platelet aggregation and hence does not promote bleeding.

Gastroduodenal Ulceration and Bleeding. Because celecoxib does not inhibit COX-1, the isoform of COX that protects the stomach, a low incidence of gastroduodenal ulceration would be expected. Some data support this expectation; others do not. When celecoxib was first approved, conclusions about its safety were based on 6-month data from the Celecoxib Arthritis Safety Study (CLASS), which indicated that celecoxib caused less GI toxicity than conventional NSAIDs (diclofenac, naproxen, ibuprofen). However, longer term (12-month) data from the same study show *no difference* in GI toxicity between celecoxib and conventional NSAIDs. Other studies have shown that, compared with patients taking conventional NSAIDs, those taking celecoxib had a lower incidence of endoscopically detectable ulcers and a lower incidence of hospitalization for GI bleeding. What's the bottom line? Celecoxib *may* be safer than conventional NSAIDs, especially when used short term. However, more data are needed to determine just *how much* safer the drug really is.

Renal Impairment. Like conventional NSAIDs—and despite its COX-2 selectivity—celecoxib can impair renal function, thereby posing a risk to patients with hypertension, edema, heart failure, or pre-existing renal disease.

Sulfonamide Allergy. Celecoxib contains a sulfur molecule and hence can precipitate an allergic reaction in patients allergic to sulfonamides. Accordingly, the drug should be avoided by patients with sulfa allergy.

Use in Pregnancy. Celecoxib and other NSAIDs can cause premature closure of the ductus arteriosus. Accordingly, these drugs are contraindicated for use in the third trimester of pregnancy.

Drug Interactions

Warfarin. Celecoxib may increase the anticoagulant effects of warfarin, and may thereby increase the risk of bleeding. Celecoxib itself does not inhibit platelet aggregation and does not promote bleeding. However, the drug may enhance the anticoagulant effects of warfarin (perhaps by increasing warfarin levels). Celecoxib may be combined with warfarin, but effects of warfarin should be monitored closely, especially during the first few days of treatment.

Other Interactions. Information on the interactions of celecoxib with other drugs is limited. Celecoxib may decrease the diuretic effects of furosemide as well as the antihypertensive effects of angiotensin-converting enzyme inhibitors. Conversely, celecoxib may increase levels of lithium (a drug for bipolar disorder). Levels of celecoxib may be increased by fluconazole (an antifungal drug).

Preparations, Dosage, and Administration

Celecoxib [Celebrex] is available in 100-, 200-, and 400-mg capsules. Dosages are as follows:

- *Osteoarthritis*—100 mg twice daily or 200 mg once daily
- *Rheumatoid arthritis*—100 or 200 mg twice daily
- *Acute pain*—On day 1, 400 mg initially plus another 200 mg if needed; on all subsequent days, 200 mg twice daily as needed
- *Primary dysmenorrhea*—Same as for acute pain
- *Familial adenomatous polyposis*—400 mg twice daily, taken with food

Rofecoxib

Actions and Uses. Rofecoxib [Vioxx] was the second selective COX-2 inhibitor approved for use in the United States. The drug is indicated to treat patients at least 18 years old for osteoarthritis, rheumatoid arthritis, acute pain, and menstrual pain. Benefits derive from inhibiting COX-2, the isoform of cyclooxygenase whose products promote inflammation and sensitize receptors to painful stimuli. Anti-inflammatory and analgesic effects are equivalent to those of first-generation NSAIDs, but GI side effects are less common. Like celecoxib, rofecoxib does not suppress platelet aggregation and hence cannot reduce the risk of MI, stroke, and other cardiovascular disorders. Long-term efficacy and safety are not yet known.

Pharmacokinetics. Plasma levels peak 2 to 3 hours after oral administration. Food decreases the rate of absorption but not the extent. Rofecoxib is eliminated by hepatic metabolism followed by renal excretion. Plasma levels rise higher in older patients and patients with hepatic impairment. The drug's half-life is 17 hours.

Adverse Effects. The most common adverse effects are diarrhea, dyspepsia, and abdominal pain. Treatment has also been associated with headache, renal impairment, hypertension, anemia, lower extremity edema, upper respiratory tract infection, and aseptic meningitis. Like other NSAIDs, rofecoxib can affect fetal circulation near term, and hence should be avoided late in pregnancy. In contrast to celecoxib, rofecoxib does not contain a reactive sulfur molecule, and hence should be safe for patients allergic to sulfonamides.

Gastric and duodenal ulcers are less common than with traditional NSAIDs. In a 24-week trial, the incidence of ulcers was 10% with rofecoxib compared with 45% with ibuprofen. In a 12-week trial, the incidence of ulcers was 7% with placebo, 5% with 25 mg rofecoxib daily, 8% with 50 mg rofecoxib daily (twice the recommended long-term dosage), and 29% with 2.4 gm ibuprofen daily.

Warning: Possible Increased Risk of MI. In the Vioxx Gastrointestinal Outcomes Research (VIGOR) trial, patients taking *high-dose* rofecoxib (50 mg/day) experienced more MIs and other thrombotic events (e.g., unstable angina, ischemic stroke, transient ischemic attacks) than did patients taking naproxen (1000 mg/day). These data have two possible explanations: (1) high-dose rofecoxib actively promotes MI or (2) naproxen protects against MI, presumably by suppressing platelet aggregation. Although there are *theoretical* reasons as to why the second explanation is correct, *clinical* data support the first explanation. Specifically, a recent observational study found that the incidence of thrombotic events among patients taking either naproxen, celecoxib, or rofecoxib in *standard* doses (≤25 mg/day) was the same as for patients not taking NSAIDs at all—whereas the incidence among patients taking high-dose rofecoxib was significantly increased. These data suggest that (1) naproxen does not protect against thrombotic events and that (2) rofecoxib increases the risk of thrombotic events, but only if the dosage is high. Accordingly, to minimize risk, rofecoxib dosage should not exceed the recommended amount—25 mg/day—when the drug is used long term.

Drug Interactions. Information on drug interactions is limited. Rifampin (a drug for tuberculosis) decreases plasma levels of rofecoxib by 50%. Antacids decrease levels by 20%. Rofecoxib increases plasma levels of lithium (a drug for bipolar disorder) and methotrexate (a drug for arthritis and cancer); patients taking these drugs should be monitored for toxicity. Rofecoxib may increase bleeding tendencies in patients taking warfarin (an anticoagulant), but may decrease the antihypertensive effects of angiotensin-converting enzyme inhibitors.

Preparations, Dosage, and Administration. Rofecoxib [Vioxx] is available in tablets (12.5 and 25 mg) and an oral suspension (12.5 and 25 mg/ml). The initial dosage for *osteoarthritis* is 12.5 mg once daily; if needed, dosage can be increased to 25 mg once daily. The dosage for *acute pain* or *dysmenorrhea* is 50 mg once daily; there is no information on treatment for more than 5 days.

Valdecoxib

Actions and Uses. Valdecoxib [Bextra], approved November 19, 2001, is the newest coxib to hit the market. Pharmacologic effects derive from selective inhibition of COX-2; at therapeutic plasma levels, the drug does not inhibit COX-1. Currently, valdecoxib is approved for rheumatoid arthritis, osteoarthritis, and dysmenorrhea—but not for pain. Therapeutic effects are equivalent to those seen with naproxen, a conventional NSAID.

Adverse Effects. Like other coxibs, valdecoxib is generally well tolerated. The risk of gastroduodenal ulceration and bleeding appears lower than with conventional NSAIDs. Like other NSAIDs, valdecoxib can impair renal function, thereby posing a risk to patients with hypertension, edema, heart failure, or pre-existing renal disease. Valdecoxib does not suppress platelet aggregation, and hence does not pose a risk of bleeding; however, neither does it protect against MI and other thrombotic events. Whether valdecoxib may *promote* MI is unknown.

Very rarely, valdecoxib users have developed anaphylaxis and severe skin reactions, including Stevens-Johnson syndrome, exfoliative dermatitis, erythema multiforme, and toxic epidermal necrolysis. Because these allergic reactions can be life threatening, valdecoxib should be discontinued at the first sign of rash. Like celecoxib—and unlike rofecoxib—valdecoxib has a structure similar to that of the sulfonamide antibiotics. However, there is no solid evidence that valdecoxib-associated allergic reactions are due to a true sulfa allergy. Nonetheless, the drug is contraindicated for patients with known allergy to sulfa-containing drugs.

Drug Interactions. Aspirin may increase the risk of GI toxicity in patients taking valdecoxib. Conversely, valdecoxib may antagonize the antiplatelet effects of aspirin. Valdecoxib can increase plasma levels of warfarin, and can thereby increase anticoagulant effects.

Preparations, Dosage, and Administration. Valdecoxib [Bextra] is available in 10- and 20-mg tablets. Recommended dosages are 10 mg once a day (for arthritis) and 20 mg twice a day (for dysmenorrhea).

ACETAMINOPHEN

Acetaminophen [Tylenol, many others] is similar to aspirin in some respects but different in others. Acetaminophen has *analgesic* and *antipyretic* properties equivalent to those of aspirin. However, in contrast to aspirin and the other NSAIDs, *acetaminophen is devoid of clinically useful anti-inflammatory and antirheumatic actions.* In addition, acetaminophen does not suppress platelet aggregation, does not cause gastric ulceration, and does not decrease renal blood flow or cause renal impairment. Furthermore, acetaminophen overdose differs from overdose with aspirin in both manifestations and treatment. In the United States, acetaminophen is the most frequently ingested medicine.

Mechanism of Action

Differences between the effects of acetaminophen and aspirin are thought to result from selective inhibition of prostaglandin synthesis. Whereas aspirin can inhibit synthesis of prostaglandins in both the CNS and the periphery, inhibition by acetaminophen is limited to the CNS; acetaminophen has only minimal effects on prostaglandin synthesis at peripheral sites. By decreasing prostaglandin synthesis in the CNS, acetaminophen is able to reduce fever and pain. The inability of acetaminophen to inhibit prostaglandin synthesis outside the CNS may explain the absence of anti-inflammatory effects, gastric ulceration, and adverse effects on the kidneys and platelets.

Pharmacokinetics

Acetaminophen is readily absorbed following oral administration and undergoes wide distribution. Most of an administered dose is metabolized by the liver, and the metabolites are excreted in the urine. The plasma half-life of the drug is approximately 2 hours.

Acetaminophen can be metabolized by two pathways; one is major and the other is minor (Fig. 67–2). In the major pathway, acetaminophen undergoes conjugation with glucuronic acid and other compounds to form nontoxic metabolites. In the minor pathway, acetaminophen is oxidized by a P450-containing enzyme into a highly reactive and toxic compound. At therapeutic doses, practically all of the drug is converted to nontoxic compounds via the major pathway. Only a small fraction is converted into the toxic metabolite via the minor pathway. Under normal conditions, the toxic metabolite undergoes rapid conversion to a nontoxic form; glu-

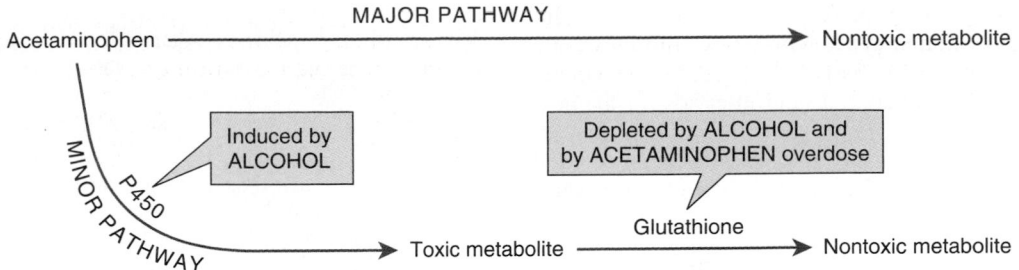

Figure 67–2 ■ **Metabolism of acetaminophen.**

tathione is required for the conversion. When an overdose of acetaminophen is taken, a larger than normal amount is processed via the minor pathway; hence, a large quantity of the toxic metabolite is produced. As the liver attempts to detoxify the metabolite, glutathione is rapidly depleted, and further detoxification stops. As a result, the toxic metabolite accumulates, causing damage to the liver (see below).

Adverse Effects

Adverse effects are extremely rare at therapeutic doses. Acetaminophen does not cause gastric ulceration or renal impairment and does not inhibit platelet aggregation. In addition, there is no evidence linking acetaminophen with Reye's syndrome. Individuals who are hypersensitive to aspirin only rarely experience cross-hypersensitivity to acetaminophen. Overdose can cause severe liver injury.

Drug Interactions

Alcohol. Regular alcohol consumption increases the risk of liver injury from acetaminophen—but only if acetaminophen dosage is excessive. Three mechanisms are involved. First, alcohol induces synthesis of the P450-containing enzyme in the minor metabolic pathway, thereby increasing production of acetaminophen's toxic metabolite (see Fig. 67–2). Second, stores of glutathione are depleted in chronic alcoholics; as a result, the liver is unable to convert the toxic metabolite to a nontoxic form (Fig. 67–2). Third, chronic alcoholics often have preexisting liver damage, which renders them less able to tolerate injury from acetaminophen.

Does alcohol increase the risk of liver damage from acetaminophen taken in *therapeutic* doses? Probably not. Although *anecdotal* reports suggest that low doses of acetaminophen can cause liver injury in alcohol users, the results of a recent randomized controlled trial indicate otherwise: In alcoholics given therapeutic doses of acetaminophen, indices of liver damage were no greater than in alcoholics given a placebo. These data suggest that, even for people who consume alcohol in large amounts, *low* (therapeutic) doses of acetaminophen are safe. Nonetheless, some authorities recommend that people who drink alcohol regularly consume no more than 2 gm of acetaminophen a day (about one-half the normal maximum).

Although therapeutic doses of acetaminophen may be safe for alcohol drinkers, high doses certainly are not. Accordingly, to alert the public to the potential risk of combining alcohol with acetaminophen, the FDA now requires that labels for acetaminophen include the following statement: *Alcohol Warning: If you consume three or more alcoholic drinks every day, ask your doctor whether you should take acetaminophen or other pain relievers/fever reducers.*

Warfarin. A recent report suggested that regular use of acetaminophen may increase the risk of bleeding in patients taking warfarin (an anticoagulant). The risk of bleeding was increased by just four acetaminophen tablets daily for 10 days. This was a surprise. After all, unlike the NSAIDs, acetaminophen does not suppress platelet aggregation, and hence should not promote bleeding. How, then, might acetaminophen cause a problem? The best guess is that acetaminophen may inhibit warfarin metabolism, which would cause warfarin levels to rise. Although this interaction has not been proved, caution is advised. If patients take more than four tablets of acetaminophen daily for several days, responses to warfarin should be monitored closely. Occasional use of acetaminophen is not a concern.

Therapeutic Uses

Acetaminophen is indicated for relief of pain and fever. Because of its lack of association with Reye's syndrome, acetaminophen is preferred to NSAIDs for use by children suspected of having chickenpox or influenza. Because it does not cause GI injury, acetaminophen is preferred to NSAIDs for patients with peptic ulcer disease. In addition, acetaminophen may be a safe alternative to aspirin for patients who have experienced aspirin hypersensitivity reactions. Because of its weak anti-inflammatory actions, acetaminophen is *not* useful for treating arthritis or rheumatic fever.

Acute Toxicity

Overdose with acetaminophen causes liver damage. The risk of liver injury is increased by fasting and by chronic consumption of alcohol.

Signs and Symptoms. The principal feature of acetaminophen overdose is *hepatic necrosis*. Severe poisoning can progress to hepatic failure, coma, and death. Early symptoms of poisoning (nausea, vomiting, diarrhea, sweating, abdominal discomfort) belie the severity of intoxication. It is not until 48 to 72 hours after drug ingestion that overt indications of hepatic injury appear.

Treatment. Liver damage can be minimized by giving *acetylcysteine* [Mucomyst], a specific antidote to acetaminophen. Acetylcysteine reduces injury by substituting for depleted glutathione in the reaction that converts the toxic metabolite of acetaminophen to its nontoxic form. Although acetylcysteine is most effective when given shortly after acetaminophen ingestion, it can still provide significant protection when administered as long as 24 hours after poisoning has occurred. Acetylcysteine is dispensed in 10% and 20% solutions, and should be diluted to 5% with water, fruit juice, or a cola beverage. The initial dose is 140 mg/kg. Additional doses of 70 mg/kg are administered at 4-hour intervals for the next 72 hours. Acetylcysteine has an extremely unpleasant odor and may induce vomiting. If vomiting interferes with oral treatment, the drug can be administered through an oroduodenal tube.

Preparations, Dosage, and Administration

Preparations. Numerous acetaminophen-containing products are on the market, including a wide assortment of fixed-dose combinations. The drug is available in rectal suppositories and multiple oral formulations (standard tablets, chewable tablets, effervescent granules, capsules, liquids, elixirs, solutions). Many products are available over the counter, and many others require a prescription. Why do I mention this plethora of products? Because it creates a significant risk of overdose: *Patients who don't carefully read the labels may well take two or more products that contain acetaminophen, thereby exceeding the safe dosage.* You should alert patients to this danger.

Dosage. The recommended dosage for adults and children over 12 years is 325 to 650 mg every 4 to 6 hours, up to a maximum of 4 gm/day. *Single* doses for younger children vary with age as follows:

- Up to 3 months—40 mg
- 4 to 11 months—80 mg
- 1 to <2 years—120 mg
- 2 to 3 years—160 mg
- 4 to 5 years—240 mg
- 6 to 8 years—320 mg
- 9 to 10 years—400 mg
- 11 to 12 years—480 mg

These doses can be given every 4 to 6 hours as needed, up to a maximum of five doses a day. For round-the-clock dosing, a 6-hour dosing interval should be used.

⁘ KEY POINTS

- Aspirin is the prototype of the first-generation (traditional) NSAIDs.
- NSAIDs have four beneficial actions: suppression of inflammation, relief of mild to moderate pain, reduction of fever, and reduction of thrombus formation (secondary to suppression of platelet aggregation).
- NSAIDs have three major adverse effects: gastric ulceration, renal impairment, and increased bleeding tendencies (secondary to suppression of platelet aggregation).
- NSAIDs produce their beneficial and adverse effects by inhibiting cyclooxygenase, an enzyme needed to form prostaglandins and related compounds from arachidonic acid.
- Cyclooxygenase has two forms: COX-1 (good COX) and COX-2 (bad COX).
- Inhibition of COX-1 can cause gastric ulceration, bleeding, and renal impairment.
- Inhibition of COX-2 reduces inflammation and pain.
- First-generation NSAIDs (e.g., aspirin, ibuprofen) inhibit COX-1 *and* COX-2.

- Second-generation NSAIDs, also known as coxibs, produce selective inhibition of COX-2, and thereby spare COX-1.
- First-generation NSAIDs cannot suppress inflammation without also posing a risk of serious adverse effects (gastric ulceration, bleeding, and renal impairment).
- By sparing COX-1, second-generation NSAIDs can suppress inflammation while causing fewer side effects than do first-generation NSAIDs.
- Aspirin causes *irreversible* inhibition of cyclooxygenase, whereas all other NSAIDs produce reversible (competitive) inhibition. As a result, the effects of aspirin persist until cells can make more cyclooxygenase, whereas the effects of all other NSAIDs decline as soon as drug levels decline.
- Because platelets are unable to synthesize new cyclooxygenase, the antiplatelet effects of a single dose of aspirin persist for the life of the platelet (about 8 days).
- Anti-inflammatory doses of aspirin are much higher than analgesic or antipyretic doses.
- Aspirin and other NSAIDs are useful drugs for rheumatoid arthritis and other chronic inflammatory conditions.
- Aspirin is a very effective analgesic. It can be as effective as opioids for some types of postoperative pain.
- The risk of NSAID-induced gastric ulcers can be reduced by (1) testing for and eliminating *H. pylori* prior to starting therapy; (2) giving misoprostol, a synthetic prostaglandin, for prophylaxis; and (3) using a coxib instead of a first-generation NSAID.
- Because of its antiplatelet actions, aspirin can protect against MI and other thrombotic events.
- Ibuprofen can antagonize the antiplatelet actions of aspirin, and can thereby decrease protection against thrombotic events.
- Because of its antiplatelet actions, aspirin should be discontinued 1 week prior to elective surgery or parturition.
- Because of its antiplatelet actions, aspirin intensifies the anticoagulant response to warfarin.
- Aspirin can impair renal function, thereby causing sodium and water retention, edema, and elevation of blood pressure. However, adverse outcomes are likely only in patients with additional risk factors: advanced age, pre-existing renal dysfunction, hypovolemia, hypertension, hepatic cirrhosis, or heart failure.
- Because of the risk of Reye's syndrome, aspirin and other NSAIDs should be avoided by children with influenza or chickenpox.
- Use of aspirin and other NSAIDs during labor and delivery can suppress spontaneous uterine contractions, induce premature closure of the ductus arteriosus, and intensify uterine bleeding.
- Although rarely fatal in adults, aspirin poisoning may prove lethal in children.
- Acetaminophen reduces pain and fever, but not inflammation.

■ Acetaminophen inhibits prostaglandin synthesis in the CNS, but not in the periphery. As a result, acetaminophen differs from the NSAIDs in four ways: it lacks anti-inflammatory actions, does not cause gastric ulceration, does not suppress platelet aggregation, and does not impair renal function.

■ Hepatic necrosis from acetaminophen overdose results from accumulation of a toxic metabolite.

■ Chronic alcohol consumption increases the risk of liver damage from acetaminophen *overdose* (but not from therapeutic doses). Two major mechanisms are in-volved: induction of cytochrome P450 (which increases production of the toxic metabolite of acetaminophen) and depletion of glutathione stores (which reduces detoxification of the metabolite).

■ Acetaminophen may increase the risk of warfarin-induced bleeding by inhibiting metabolism of warfarin.

■ Acetaminophen poisoning is treated with acetylcysteine, a drug that substitutes for depleted glutathione in the reaction that removes the toxic metabolite of acetaminophen.

Summary of Major Nursing Implications*

NONSTEROIDAL ANTI-INFLAMMATORY DRUGS

First-Generation NSAIDs

Aspirin
Choline salicylate
Diclofenac
Diflunisal
Etodolac
Fenoprofen
Flurbiprofen
Ibuprofen
Indomethacin
Ketoprofen
Ketorolac
Magnesium salicylate
Meclofenamate
Mefenamic acid
Meloxicam
Nabumetone
Naproxen
Oxaprozin
Piroxicam
Salsalate
Sodium salicylate
Sulindac
Tolmetin

Coxibs

Celecoxib
Rofecoxib
Valdecoxib

Except where noted, the nursing implications summarized below apply to aspirin and all other NSAIDs.

Preadministration Assessment

Therapeutic Goal

Major indications for the NSAIDs are inflammatory disorders (e.g., rheumatoid arthritis, osteoarthritis), mild to moderate pain, fever, primary dysmenorrhea, and preven-tion of cardiovascular disease. Applications of individual NSAIDs are summarized in Table 67–3.

Identifying High-Risk Patients

NSAIDs are *contraindicated* for patients with a history of severe NSAID hypersensitivity.

NSAIDs should be used with *extreme caution* by pregnant women and patients with peptic ulcer disease and bleeding disorders (e.g., hemophilia, vitamin K deficiency, hypoprothrombinemia) and patients taking warfarin or glucocorticoids. *Caution* is also needed when treating elderly patients and patients with heart failure, hypovolemia, hepatic cirrhosis, renal dysfunction, asthma, hay fever, chronic urticaria, nasal polyps, or a history of alcoholism or heavy cigarette smoking.

NSAIDs (especially aspirin) are *contraindicated* for children with chickenpox or influenza.

NSAIDs should be discontinued 1 week prior to elective surgery or the anticipated date of parturition.

Celecoxib and *valdecoxib*—but not rofecoxib—are contraindicated for patients with sulfa allergy.

Implementation: Administration

Routes

Oral. All NSAIDs.
Intramuscular. Ketorolac.
Rectal suppository. Aspirin and indomethacin.

Administration

Advise patients to take NSAIDs with food, milk, or a glass of water to reduce gastric upset.

Warn patients not to crush or chew enteric-coated or sustained-release formulations.

Advise patients to discard aspirin preparations that smell of vinegar.

Ongoing Evaluation and Interventions

Minimizing Adverse Effects

Gastrointestinal Effects. NSAIDs frequently cause mild GI reactions (dyspepsia, abdominal pain, nausea). To

*Patient education information is highlighted as blue text.

Summary of Major Nursing Implications*—cont'd

minimize these effects, **advise patients to take NSAIDs with food, milk, or a glass of water.**

Long-term, high-dose therapy can cause gastric ulceration, perforation, and hemorrhage. Several measures can reduce risk:

- Avoid NSAIDs in patients with a recent history of peptic ulcer disease and use NSAIDs with caution in patients with other risk factors (advanced age, previous intolerance to NSAIDs, heavy cigarette smoking, history of alcoholism)
- Test for and eliminate *H. pylori* prior to starting long-term therapy
- Give misoprostol for prophylaxis in high-risk patients—but not to patients who are pregnant (because misoprostol can stimulate uterine contractions)
- Use a coxib (instead of a traditional NSAID) in high-risk patients.
- **Warn patients not to consume alcohol.**
- **Instruct patients to notify the physician if gastric irritation is severe or persistent.**

Manage ulcers by giving an antiulcer medication (e.g., H_2-receptor antagonist, proton pump inhibitor).

Bleeding. Aspirin promotes bleeding by causing irreversible suppression of platelet aggregation. Aspirin should be discontinued 1 week prior to elective surgery or anticipated date of parturition, but need not be stopped prior to dental surgery. Exercise caution when using aspirin in conjunction with warfarin. Avoid aspirin in patients with bleeding disorders (e.g., hemophilia, vitamin K deficiency, hypoprothrombinemia).

The nonacetylated salicylates—sodium salicylate, choline salicylate, and magnesium salicylate—have minimal effects on platelet aggregation. Accordingly, these drugs are preferred for use in surgical patients and patients with bleeding disorders.

The risk of bleeding can be minimized by using a coxib instead of a traditional NSAID.

Renal Impairment. NSAIDs can cause acute renal insufficiency in elderly patients and in patients with heart failure, hypovolemia, hepatic cirrhosis, or pre-existing renal dysfunction. Keep NSAID dosages as low as possible in these patients. Monitor high-risk patients for indications of renal impairment (reduced urine output, weight gain despite diuretic therapy, rapid elevation of serum creatinine and blood urea nitrogen). Discontinue NSAIDs if these signs occur.

Hypersensitivity Reactions. These reactions are most likely in patients with asthma, hay fever, chronic urticaria, or nasal polyps. Use NSAIDs with caution in these patients. If a severe hypersensitivity reaction occurs, parenteral epinephrine is the treatment of choice. Avoid NSAIDs in patients with a history of NSAID hypersensitivity.

Salicylism. Aspirin and other salicylates can cause salicylism. **Educate patients about manifestations of salicylism (tinnitus, sweating, headache, dizziness), and advise them to notify the physician if these occur.** Aspirin should be withheld until symptoms subside, after which therapy can resume but at a slightly reduced dosage.

Reye's Syndrome. Use of NSAIDs (especially aspirin) by children with chickenpox or influenza may precipitate Reye's syndrome. Avoid NSAIDs in these patients. **Advise parents that acetaminophen can be used safely.**

Use in Pregnancy. NSAIDs can cause maternal anemia and can prolong labor and gestation. In addition, they can promote premature closure of the ductus arteriosus. NSAIDs should be avoided by expectant mothers unless the potential benefits outweigh the risks. If NSAIDs are employed during pregnancy, they should be discontinued at least 1 week before the anticipated day of delivery.

Sulfonamide Allergy. *Celecoxib* and *valdecoxib* can cause severe allergic reactions in patients with sulfa allergy, and hence must not be given to these people.

Minimizing Adverse Interactions

Warfarin. NSAIDs can increase the risk of spontaneous bleeding in patients taking warfarin. Monitor patients for signs of bleeding.

Glucocorticoids. Glucocorticoids increase the risk of gastric ulceration in patients taking NSAIDs. Prophylactic therapy with misoprostol can decrease the risk.

Alcohol. Alcohol increases the risk of gastric ulceration from NSAIDs. Exercise caution.

Aspirin-Ibuprofen Interaction. Ibuprofen can block the antiplatelet effects of aspirin. Patients taking low-dose aspirin to protect against thrombosis should avoid ibuprofen.

Managing Aspirin Toxicity

Aspirin poisoning is an acute medical emergency that requires hospitalization. Treatment is largely supportive and consists of external cooling (e.g., sponging with tepid water), infusion of fluids (to correct dehydration and electrolyte loss), infusion of bicarbonate (to reverse acidosis and promote renal excretion of salicylates), and mechanical ventilation (if respiration is severely depressed). Absorption of aspirin can be reduced by gastric lavage, induction of emesis, and giving activated charcoal. If necessary, hemodialysis or peritoneal dialysis can accelerate salicylate removal.

ACETAMINOPHEN

Preadministration Assessment

Therapeutic Goal

Acetaminophen is indicated for relief of pain and suppression of fever. The drug is preferred to NSAIDs for use in children with chickenpox or influenza, and for all patients with peptic ulcer disease.

Identifying High-Risk Patients

Use with *caution* in chronic alcoholics, patients who consume moderate amounts of alcohol daily, and patients taking warfarin.

*Patient education information is highlighted as blue text.

Summary of Major Nursing Implications*—cont'd

Implementation: Administration

Routes

Oral, rectal.

Administration

Do not exceed recommended doses.

Ongoing Evaluation and Interventions

Minimizing Adverse Effects

Acetaminophen is devoid of significant adverse effects at usual therapeutic doses, except possibly in people who consume alcohol on a regular basis.

Minimizing Adverse Interactions

Alcohol. Chronic alcohol consumption increases the risk of liver injury from *excessive* doses of acetaminophen, but probably not from *therapeutic* doses.

Warfarin. Taking acetaminophen for several days may increase the risk of bleeding in patients on warfarin. Monitor warfarin effects closely.

Managing Toxicity

Overdose can cause hepatic necrosis. Acetylcysteine is a specific antidote. Acetylcysteine has an extremely unpleasant odor and may induce vomiting. If vomiting interferes with oral administration, acetylcysteine can be administered through an oroduodenal tube.

*Patient education information is highlighted as blue text.

Glucocorticoids in Nonendocrine Diseases

The glucocorticoid drugs (e.g., cortisone, prednisone), which are also known as *corticosteroids,* are nearly identical to the glucose-regulating steroids produced by the adrenal cortex. Accordingly, we can look on the glucocorticoids as having two kinds of effects: physiologic and pharmacologic. *Physiologic* effects, such as modulation of glucose metabolism, are elicited by *low* doses of glucocorticoids. In contrast, *pharmacologic* effects (e.g., suppression of inflammation) require *high* doses.

As implied by the chapter title, glucocorticoids have both endocrine and nonendocrine applications. In low (physiologic) doses, glucocorticoids are used to treat adrenocortical insufficiency. In high (pharmacologic) doses, these agents are used to treat inflammatory disorders (e.g., asthma, rheumatoid arthritis) and certain cancers and to suppress immune responses in patients receiving organ transplants. The endocrine applications of the glucocorticoids are discussed in Chapter 57. Nonendocrine uses, which are the most common applications of these drugs, are discussed here.

Toxicity of the glucocorticoids can be severe and is determined by the pattern of drug use. Glucocorticoids are devoid of toxicity when used in physiologic doses. However, when taken in pharmacologic doses, especially for extended periods, glucocorticoids can produce an array of serious adverse effects.

All of the glucocorticoid drugs can elicit the same spectrum of therapeutic effects. Differences among individual agents pertain to time course of action and side effects. Because the similarities among these drugs are much more striking than the differences, we will forego our practice of focusing on a prototypic agent. Instead, we will discuss the glucocorticoids as a group.

REVIEW OF GLUCOCORTICOID PHYSIOLOGY

Physiologic Effects

Physiologic responses can be elicited with low doses of glucocorticoids. At higher doses, these effects are simply more intense. When glucocorticoids are used to treat nonendocrine disorders, physiologic responses occur as side effects. Physiologic effects of the glucocorticoids are discussed in depth in Chapter 57. The discussion below is a review.

Metabolic Effects. Glucocorticoids influence the metabolism of carbohydrates, proteins, and fats. The principal effect on carbohydrate metabolism is elevation of blood glucose. This is accomplished by promoting synthesis of glucose from amino acids and by reducing peripheral glucose utilization. Glucocorticoids also promote storage of glucose in the form of glycogen.

Glucocorticoids have an unfavorable impact on protein metabolism. These agents suppress synthesis of proteins from amino acids and divert amino acids for production of glucose. These actions can reduce muscle mass, decrease the protein matrix of bone, and cause thinning of the skin. Nitrogen balance becomes negative.

The most consistent effect of glucocorticoids on fat metabolism is stimulation of lipolysis (fat breakdown). Long-term, high-dose therapy can cause fat redistribution, resulting in the potbelly, "moon face," and "buffalo hump" that characterize Cushing's syndrome.

Cardiovascular Effects. Glucocorticoids are required to maintain the functional integrity of the vascular system. When levels of endogenous glucocorticoids are low, capillaries become more permeable, vasoconstriction is suppressed, and blood pressure falls. Glucocorticoids increase the number of circulating red blood cells and polymorphonuclear leukocytes. In contrasts, counts of lymphocytes, eosinophils, basophils, and monocytes decline.

Effects During Stress. At times of physiologic stress (e.g., pain, surgery, infection, trauma, hypovolemia), the adrenals secrete large quantities of glucocorticoids and epinephrine. Working together, these hormones help maintain blood pressure and plasma levels of glucose. If glucocorticoid levels are insufficient, hypotension and hypoglycemia will occur. If the stress is especially severe, glucocorticoid insufficiency can result in circulatory failure and death.

TABLE 68–1 ▪■ Glucocorticoids: Half-Lives, Relative Potencies and Equivalent Doses

Drug	Biologic Half-Life (hr)	Relative Mineralocorticoid Potency*	Relative Glucocorticoid (Anti-Inflammatory) Potency	Equivalent Anti-Inflammatory Dose (mg)†
Short Acting				
Cortisone	8–12	2	0.8	25
Hydrocortisone	8–12	2	1.0	20
Intermediate Acting				
Prednisone	18–36	1	4	5
Prednisolone	18–36	1	4	5
Methylprednisolone	18–36	0	5	4
Triamcinolone	18–36	0	5	4
Long Acting				
Betamethasone	36–54	0	20–30	0.75
Dexamethasone	36–54	0	20–30	0.75

*Relative mineralocorticoid activity (sodium and water retention; potassium depletion): 0 = very low; 1 = moderate; 2 = high.

†Approximate *oral* or *intravenous* dose needed to produce equivalent anti-inflammatory effects.

Effects on Water and Electrolytes. To varying degrees, individual glucocorticoids can exert actions like those of aldosterone, the major mineralocorticoid released by the adrenals. Accordingly, glucocorticoids can act on the kidney to promote retention of sodium and water while increasing urinary excretion of potassium. The net result is hypernatremia, hypokalemia, and edema. Fortunately, most of the glucocorticoids employed as drugs have very low mineralocorticoid activity (Table 68–1).

Respiratory System in Neonates. During labor and delivery, the adrenals of the full-term infants release a burst of glucocorticoids, which act to hasten maturation of the lungs. In the premature infant, production of glucocorticoids is low, resulting in a high incidence of respiratory distress syndrome.

Control of Synthesis and Secretion

Synthesis and release of glucocorticoids are regulated by a negative feedback loop. The principal components of the loop are the hypothalamus, anterior pituitary, and adrenal cortex (Fig. 68–1). The loop is turned on when stress or some other stimulus from the central nervous system acts on the hypothalamus to cause release of corticotropin-releasing factor (CRF). CRF then stimulates the pituitary to release adrenocorticotropic hormone (ACTH), which in turn acts on the adrenal cortex to promote synthesis and release of cortisol (the principal endogenous glucocorticoid). Cortisol has two basic effects: it (1) promotes physiologic responses and (2) acts on the hypothalamus and pituitary to suppress further release of CRF and ACTH. By inhibiting release of CRF and ACTH, cortisol suppresses its own production. As a result, this negative-feedback loop keeps glucocorticoid levels within an appropriate range. When glucocorticoids are administered chronically in large doses, the feedback loop remains continuously suppressed. As discussed later, this persistent suppression can be dangerous.

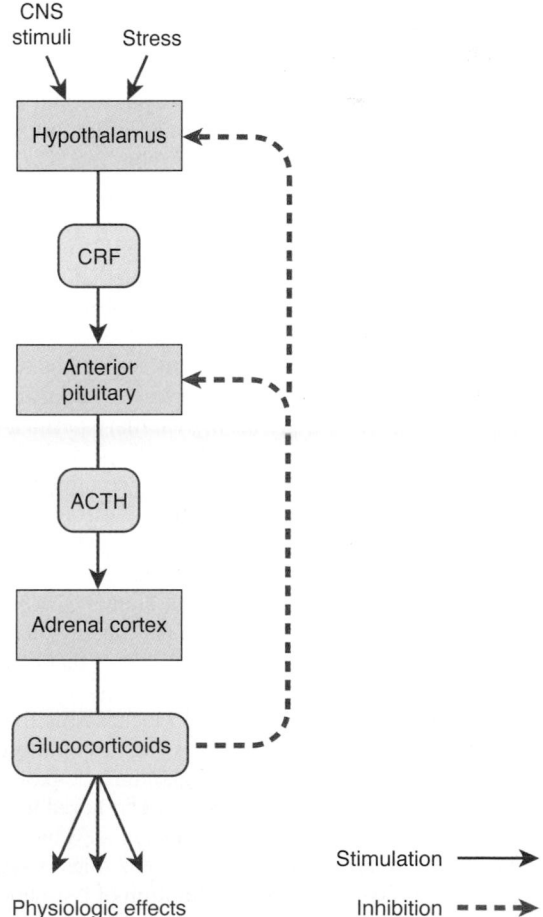

Figure 68–1 ■ Feedback regulation of glucocorticoid synthesis and secretion.
(CNS = central nervous system; CRF = corticotropin-releasing factor; ACTH = adrenocorticotropic hormone.)

PHARMACOLOGY OF THE GLUCOCORTICOIDS

Pharmacologic Actions

When administered in the high doses employed to treat nonendocrine disorders, glucocorticoids have powerful anti-inflammatory and immunosuppressive actions. These actions do not occur when glucocorticoids are given in physiologic doses. In addition to these pharmacologic effects, high-dose therapy intensifies the type of responses seen at physiologic doses.

Effects on Metabolism and Electrolytes

The effects of high-dose therapy on metabolism and electrolytes are like those seen with physiologic doses—but more intense. Hence, with high doses, glucose levels rise, protein synthesis is suppressed, and fat deposits are mobilized. As noted, most glucocorticoids have very little mineralocorticoid activity. Accordingly, these drugs do not usually induce significant sodium retention or potassium loss. However, these effects do occur in some patients and can be hazardous. In all patients, high-dose therapy can inhibit intestinal absorption of calcium. This effect is not seen when doses are physiologic.

Anti-inflammatory and Immunosuppressant Effects

The major clinical applications of the glucocorticoids stem from their ability to suppress immune responses and inflammation. Effects on the immune system and inflammation are interrelated, and hence we will consider them together.

Before discussing the actions of glucocorticoids, it will help to review the process of inflammation. The characteristic symptoms of inflammation are pain, swelling, redness, and warmth. These are initiated by chemical mediators (prostaglandins, histamine, leukotrienes) and are amplified by the actions of lymphocytes and phagocytic cells (neutrophils and macrophages). Prostaglandins and histamine promote several symptoms of inflammation—swelling, redness, and warmth—by causing vasodilation and increasing capillary permeability. Prostaglandins and histamine contribute to pain: histamine stimulates pain receptors directly; prostaglandins sensitize pain receptors to stimulation by histamine and other mediators. Neutrophils and macrophages heighten inflammation by releasing lysosomal enzymes (enzymes that cause tissue injury). Lymphocytes, which are important elements of the immune system, intensify inflammation by (1) causing direct cell injury and (2) promoting formation of antibodies that help perpetuate the inflammatory response.

Glucocorticoids act through several mechanisms to interrupt the inflammatory processes. These drugs can inhibit synthesis of chemical mediators (prostaglandins, leukotrienes, histamine) and thereby reduce swelling, warmth, redness, and pain. In addition, they suppress infiltration of phagocytes. Hence, damage from release of lysosomal enzymes is averted. Lastly, glucocorticoids suppress proliferation of lymphocytes, and thereby reduce the immune component of inflammation.

On a molecular level, most effects of glucocorticoids can be attributed to promoting the synthesis of specific regulatory proteins. Stimulation of protein synthesis is accomplished as follows: (1) glucocorticoids penetrate the cell membrane and then bind to intracellular receptors; (2) the receptor-steroid complex migrates to the cell nucleus, where it binds to chromatin in DNA; and (3) the interaction with chromatin triggers transcription of messenger RNA molecules that code for regulatory proteins, thereby increasing production of these regulatory molecules.

It is important to appreciate that the mechanisms by which glucocorticoids suppress inflammation are more diverse than the mechanisms by which nonsteroidal anti-inflammatory drugs (NSAIDs) act. As discussed in Chapter 67, NSAIDs suppress inflammation primarily by inhibiting prostaglandin production. The glucocorticoids share this mechanism and, as just discussed, act in other ways too. Because they act by multiple mechanisms, glucocorticoids have greater anti-inflammatory effects than do the NSAIDs.

Pharmacokinetics

Absorption. The rate of glucocorticoid absorption depends on route of administration and the specific glucocorticoid derivative being administered. With oral administration, absorption of all glucocorticoids is rapid and nearly complete. Following IM injection, absorption is rapid with two types of glucocorticoid esters (sodium phosphates and sodium succinates) and relatively slow with other derivatives (e.g., acetates, acetonides, tebutates). Absorption from local sites of injection (e.g., intra-articular, intrasynovial) is slower than from IM sites.

Duration of Action. Duration of action is a function of dosage, route, and drug solubility. For glucocorticoids administered orally or IV, duration of action is determined largely by biologic half-life (see Table 68–1). With IM administration, duration of action is a function of water solubility: Highly soluble preparations have a shorter duration than less soluble preparations. For locally administered glucocorticoids, duration is determined by solubility and by the specific site of administration.

Metabolism and Excretion. Glucocorticoids are metabolized primarily by the liver. As a rule, the resulting metabolites are inactive. Excretion of glucocorticoid metabolites is renal.

Therapeutic Uses in Nonendocrine Disorders

Glucocorticoids are used to treat endocrine disorders and nonendocrine disorders. Endocrine disorders (e.g., Addison's disease, acute adrenal insufficiency) can be managed with low-dose therapy and are considered in Chapter 57. Nonendocrine applications, which require much higher doses, are discussed here. Because prolonged, high-dose therapy can produce serious adverse effects, the potential benefits of treatment must be weighed carefully against the very real risks.

Rheumatoid Arthritis. Glucocorticoids are indicated for adjunctive treatment of acute exacerbations of rheumatoid arthritis. These drugs can reduce inflammation and pain, but do not alter the course of the disease. Because of the risk of serious complications, prolonged systemic use should be avoided.

When arthritis is limited to just a few joints, intra-articular injections should be employed. Local injections can be highly effective and cause less toxicity than systemic therapy. Frequently, reductions in pain and inflammation may be so dramatic as to prompt vigorous use of joints that were previously immobile. Since excessive use of diseased joints can cause injury, patients should be warned against overactivity, even though symptoms have abated.

The use of glucocorticoids in rheumatoid arthritis is discussed further in Chapter 69.

Systemic Lupus Erythematosus. Systemic lupus erythematosus (SLE) is a chronic disease similar in many ways to rheumatoid arthritis. However, in SLE, inflammation is not limited to joints; rather, it occurs throughout the body. Symptoms frequently include pleuritis, pericarditis, and nephritis. A severe episode can be fatal. Fortunately, manifestations of SLE can usually be controlled with prompt and aggressive glucocorticoid therapy.

Inflammatory Bowel Disease. Glucocorticoids are used to treat severe cases of ulcerative colitis and Crohn's disease, the two most common forms of inflammatory bowel disease. Administration may be oral, by injection, or by enema. Glucocorticoid therapy of these disorders is considered further in Chapter 75.

Miscellaneous Inflammatory Disorders. Glucocorticoids are useful in a variety of inflammatory disorders in addition to those discussed above. Conditions that respond to glucocorticoid therapy include *bursitis, tendinitis, synovitis, osteoarthritis, gouty arthritis,* and *inflammatory disorders of the eye.*

Allergic Conditions. Glucocorticoids can control symptoms of allergic reactions. Responsive conditions include hay fever (see Chapter 72), bee stings, and drug-induced allergies. Because responses to glucocorticoids are delayed, these agents have little value as acute therapy for severe allergic reactions (e.g., anaphylaxis). For life-threatening allergic reactions, epinephrine is the treatment of choice.

Asthma. Glucocorticoids are the most effective antiasthma agents available. For treatment of asthma, these drugs may be administered orally or by inhalation. Because oral therapy can be associated with serious toxicity, oral glucocorticoids should be reserved for patients who have failed to respond to safer medications (e.g., beta$_2$-adrenergic agonists, cromolyn sodium). Fortunately, adverse effects are minimal when glucocorticoids are administered by inhalation. The use of glucocorticoids in asthma is discussed at length in Chapter 71.

Dermatologic Disorders. Glucocorticoids are beneficial in a wide variety of skin diseases, including pemphigus, psoriasis, mycosis fungoides, seborrheic dermatitis, contact dermatitis, and exfoliative dermatitis. For mild disease, topical administration is usually adequate. For severe disorders, systemic therapy may be needed. It should be noted that topical glucocorticoids can be absorbed in amounts sufficient to produce systemic toxicity. Topical therapy is discussed further in Chapter 101.

Neoplasms. Glucocorticoids are used in conjunction with other anticancer agents to treat acute lymphocytic leukemia, Hodgkin's disease, and non-Hodgkin's lymphomas. Benefits derive from the direct toxicity of glucocorticoids to malignant lymphocytes. Treatment kills lymphoid cells and causes regression of lymphatic tissue. The use of glucocorticoids to treat cancers is discussed further in Chapter 99.

Suppression of Allograft Rejection. Glucocorticoids, together with other immunosuppressant agents, are used to prevent rejection of organ transplants. Treatment with glucocorticoids is initiated at the time of surgery and continued indefinitely. The use of glucocorticoids for immunosuppression is discussed further in Chapter 65.

Prevention of Respiratory Distress Syndrome in Preterm Infants. Preterm infants are at high risk of respiratory distress syndrome because their adrenals cannot produce the glucocorticoids needed for lung maturation. When preterm delivery is imminent, injecting the mother with glucocorticoids (usually dexamethasone or betamethasone) reduces the risk of respiratory distress syndrome. Steroids may also reduce the incidence of intraventricular hemorrhage and necrotizing enterocolitis (inflammation of the small intestine and colon). Antenatal use of glucocorticoids is discussed further in Chapter 103.

Adverse Effects

The adverse effects discussed below occur in response to *pharmacologic* doses of glucocorticoids. The intensity of these effects increases with dosage size and duration of treatment. These toxicities are not seen when dosage is physiologic. Furthermore, most are not seen when treatment is brief (a few days or less), even when doses are high.

Adrenal Insufficiency. Pharmacologic doses of glucocorticoids can suppress production of glucocorticoids by the adrenals, resulting in adrenal insufficiency. The mechanism, consequences, and management of adrenal insufficiency are discussed in depth later.

Osteoporosis. Osteoporosis with resultant fractures is a frequent and serious complication of glucocorticoid therapy. Most patients receiving long-term glucocorticoids have low bone mineral density; over 25% sustain osteoporotic fractures. The ribs and vertebrae are affected most. In some patients, vertebral compression fractures occur within weeks of beginning glucocorticoid use. Osteoporosis is most likely with systemic therapy. In contrast, osteoporosis is uncommon when glucocorticoids are inhaled or administered topically. Patients should be observed for signs of compression fractures (back and neck pain) and for indications of fractures in other bones.

How do glucocorticoids cause bone loss? The most important mechanism is suppression of bone formation by osteoblasts. In addition, glucocorticoids accelerate bone resorption by osteoclasts. Also, these drugs reduce intestinal absorption of calcium, causing hypocalcemia. In response to hypocalcemia, release of parathyroid hormone increases, which increases mobilization of calcium from bone.

Several measures can greatly reduce development of osteoporosis and subsequent fractures. Prior to treatment, bone mineral density of the lumbar spine should be measured. This will identify patients at highest risk and provide a baseline for evaluating bone loss during treatment. When appropriate, glucocorticoids should be administered topically or by inhalation (because less bone loss occurs with these routes than with systemic therapy). Several drugs can reduce bone loss. All patients should receive calcium and vitamin D supplements. Sodium restriction combined with a thiazide diuretic can enhance intestinal absorption of calcium and can decrease urinary excretion of calcium. There is clear evidence that a bisphosphonate (e.g., alendronate, etidronate) can prevent glucocorticoid-induced bone loss. Bisphosphonates preserve bone by inhibiting osteoclastic bone resorption. Calcitonin, which also inhibits osteoclasts, is another option. In postmenopausal women, estrogen replacement therapy (ERT) is an effective way to reduce bone loss. However, as discussed in Chapter 59, the risks of ERT may outweigh the benefits. The roles of calcium, vitamin D, bisphosphonates, calcitonin, and estrogen in the prophylaxis and treatment of osteoporosis are discussed fully in Chapter 70.

Infection. By suppressing host defenses (immune responses and phagocytic activity of neutrophils and macrophages), glucocorticoids can increase susceptibility to infection. The risk of acquiring a new infection is increased, as is the risk of reactivating a latent infection (e.g., tuberculosis). In addition, since suppression of both the immune system and neutrophils reduces inflammation and other manifestations of infection, a fulminant infection may develop without detection. Hence, not only do glucocorticoids increase susceptibility to infection, they can mask the presence of an infection as it progresses. To minimize acquisition of infection, patients should avoid close contact with individuals who have a communicable disease. If a significant infection occurs, glucocorticoids should be continued only if absolutely necessary, and then only in combination with appropriate antimicrobial or antifungal therapy.

One infection, *Pneumocystis carinii pneumonia* (PCP), occurs with alarming frequency in people receiving high doses of glucocorticoids (and not just in people with AIDS, among whom PCP is the most common opportunistic infection). Accordingly, it has been suggested that PCP prophylaxis be considered for all people taking glucocorticoids in high doses.

Glucose Intolerance. Because of their effects on glucose production and utilization, glucocorticoids can increase plasma glucose levels, thereby causing hyperglycemia and glycosuria. For patients with diabetes, these effects may necessitate an increase in insulin dosage or a reduction in caloric intake. For patients with normal pancreatic function, significant elevation of blood glucose is unlikely. However, since glucocorticoids can unmask latent diabetes, nondiabetics should undergo periodic evaluation of blood glucose levels.

Myopathy. High-dose glucocorticoid therapy can cause myopathy, manifesting as muscle weakness. The proximal muscles of the arms and legs are affected most. Damage to muscle may be sufficient to prevent ambulation. If myopathy develops, glucocorticoid dosage should be reduced. Myopathy then gradually resolves over several months.

Fluid and Electrolyte Disturbance. Because of their mineralocorticoid activity, glucocorticoids can cause sodium and water retention and potassium loss. Retention of water and sodium can cause hypertension and edema. Hypokalemia can predispose the patient to dysrhythmias and to toxicity from digitalis. Fortunately, most of the glucocorticoids in current use have very little mineralocorticoid activity (see Table 68–1). Hence, serious fluid and electrolyte disturbance is rare. The risk of fluid and electrolyte disturbance can be reduced by (1) using glucocorticoids that have low mineralocorticoid activity, (2) restricting sodium intake, and (3) taking potassium supplements or consuming potassium-rich foods (e.g., potatoes, bananas, citrus fruits). Patients should be informed about signs of fluid retention (e.g., weight gain, swelling of the lower extremities) and advised to contact the physician if these develop. Patients should also be alert for signs of hypokalemia (e.g., muscle weakness or fatigue, irregular pulses).

Growth Retardation. Glucocorticoids can suppress growth in children. Growth retardation is probably the result of reduced DNA synthesis and decreased cell division. To assess effects on growth, height and weight should be measured at regular intervals. Growth suppression can be minimized with alternate-day therapy. This dosing schedule is discussed below.

Psychologic Disturbances. Rarely, glucocorticoids have caused hallucinations, mood changes (depression, euphoria, mania), and other psychologic disturbances. These effects are related more to dosage size than to duration of treatment, and can occur within the first few days of drug use. Previous psychiatric illness does not appear to predispose patients to adverse psychologic effects of glucocorticoids. Conversely, a history of good mental health does confer immunity from psychologic disturbance.

Cataracts and Glaucoma. Cataracts are a common complication of long-term glucocorticoid therapy. Risk factors are in dispute; cataract development may be related to age, dosage, or individual susceptibility. To facilitate early detection, patients should undergo an eye examination every 6 months. Also, patients should be advised to contact the physician if vision becomes cloudy or blurred.

Oral glucocorticoids can cause open-angle glaucoma. Onset of ocular hypertension develops rapidly and reverses within 2 weeks of glucocorticoid cessation.

Peptic Ulcer Disease. Although glucocorticoids have actions that could lead to peptic ulcer disease, whether they actually cause GI ulceration is controversial. By inhibiting prostaglandin synthesis, glucocorticoids can augment secretion of gastric acid and pepsin, inhibit production of cytoprotective mucus, and reduce gastric mucosal blood flow. These actions predispose the patient to GI ulceration. Making matters worse, glucocorticoids can decrease gastric pain, thereby masking ulcer development. As a result, perforation and hemorrhage can occur without warning. The risk of ulceration is increased by concurrent use of other ulcerogenic drugs, such as aspirin and other NSAIDs. To provide early detection of ulcer formation, stools should be periodically checked for occult blood. Patients should be instructed to notify the physician if feces become black and tarry. If GI ulceration occurs, glucocorticoids should be slowly withdrawn (unless their continued use is considered essential to support life). Treatment with antiulcer medication is indicated.

Iatrogenic Cushing's Syndrome. Long-term glucocorticoid therapy can induce a cushingoid syndrome with symptoms identical to those of naturally occurring Cushing's syndrome. Prominent symptoms are hyperglycemia, glycosuria, fluid and electrolyte disturbances, osteoporosis, muscle weakness, cutaneous striations, and lowered resistance to infection. Redistribution of fat produces a potbelly, "moon face," and "buffalo hump."

Use in Pregnancy and Lactation

Pregnancy. Glucocorticoids can cross the placenta and affect the developing fetus. Animal studies indicate an increased incidence of cleft palate, spontaneous abortion, and low birth weight. No adequate studies of these effects have been done in humans. Prolonged therapy with very large doses can cause fetal adrenal hypoplasia. Therefore, when large doses have been employed, the infant should be assessed for adrenal sufficiency and given replacement therapy if indicated. Whenever glucocorticoids are to be used during pregnancy, the benefits must be carefully weighed against the potential risk to the fetus.

Lactation. Glucocorticoids enter breast milk. When physiologic doses or low pharmacologic doses are used, the concentration achieved in milk is probably too low to affect the nursing infant. However, when large pharmacologic doses are employed (e.g., doses greater than 5 mg/day of prednisone or its equivalent) the amount ingested by the infant may be sufficient to cause growth retardation and other adverse effects. Consequently, women receiving high-dose glucocorticoid therapy should be warned against breast-feeding.

Drug Interactions

Interactions Related to Potassium Loss. As noted, glucocorticoids can increase urinary loss of potassium, and can thereby induce hypokalemia. Consequently, glucocorticoids must be used with caution when combined with *digoxin* (because hypokalemia increases the risk of digoxin-induced dysrhythmias) and when combined with *thiazide diuretics* or *loop diuretics* (because these potassium-depleting diuretics will increase the risk of hypokalemia). When glucocorticoids are given together with any of the above drugs, it is advisable to monitor plasma potassium levels and be alert for signs of cardiotoxicity.

Nonsteroidal Anti-inflammatory Drugs. NSAIDs have the same effects on the gastrointestinal tract as do glucocorticoids. Accordingly, concurrent use of these agents increases the risk of ulceration.

Insulin and Oral Hypoglycemics. As noted, glucocorticoids promote hyperglycemia. To maintain glycemic control, diabetic patients may require increased doses of a glucose-lowering drug (insulin or an oral hypoglycemic agent).

Vaccines. Because of their immunosuppressant actions, glucocorticoids can decrease antibody responses to vaccines. Furthermore, if a live virus vaccine is employed, there is an increased risk of developing viral disease. Accordingly, attempts at immunization should not be made while glucocorticoids are being used.

Summary of Precautions and Contraindications

Contraindications. Glucocorticoids are contraindicated for patients with *systemic fungal infections* and for those receiving *live virus vaccines.*

Precautions. Glucocorticoids must be used with caution in *pediatric patients* and in *women who are pregnant or breast-feeding.* Caution is also required in patients with *hypertension, heart failure, renal impairment, esophagitis, gastritis, peptic ulcer disease, myasthenia gravis, diabetes mellitus, osteoporosis,* and *infections that are resistant to treatment.* In addition, caution is required during concurrent therapy with *potassium-depleting diuretics, digoxin, insulin, oral hypoglycemics,* and *NSAIDs.*

Adrenal Suppression

Development of Adrenal Suppression. Like the naturally occurring glucocorticoids (e.g., cortisol), the glucocorticoids that we administer as drugs suppress the release of CRF from the hypothalamus and ACTH from the anterior pituitary. By doing so, glucocorticoid drugs inhibit the synthesis and release of endogenous glucocorticoids by the adrenals. During long-term therapy, the pituitary loses much of its ability to manufacture ACTH and, in response to the prolonged absence of ACTH, the adrenals atrophy and lose their ability to synthesize cortisol and other glucocorticoids. As a result, when

prolonged therapy with glucocorticoids is discontinued, there is a period during which the adrenals are unable to produce glucocorticoids. The time needed for adrenal recovery is highly variable: It may be as short as 5 days or as long as a year. The extent of adrenal suppression and the time required for recovery are determined primarily by the duration of glucocorticoid use; dosage size is of secondary importance. Development of adrenal suppression can be minimized through alternate-day dosing (see below).

Adrenal Suppression and Physiologic Stress. Because of adrenal suppression, patients taking glucocorticoids long term require increased doses at times of stress. Recall that, when stress occurs, the adrenals normally secrete large amounts of glucocorticoids. If the stress is sufficiently severe (e.g., trauma, surgery), these glucocorticoids are essential for supporting life. Accordingly, *it is imperative that patients receiving long-term glucocorticoid therapy be given increased doses at times of stress* (unless the dosage is already very high). Furthermore, *once glucocorticoid use has ceased, supplemental doses are required whenever stress occurs until recovery of adrenal function is complete.* To ensure appropriate care in emergencies, patients should carry an identification card or bracelet to inform emergency personnel of their glucocorticoid needs. In addition, patients should always have an emergency supply of glucocorticoids on hand.

Glucocorticoid Withdrawal. Withdrawal of glucocorticoids should be done slowly. The withdrawal schedule is determined by the degree of adrenal suppression. A representative schedule is as follows: (1) taper the dosage to a physiologic range over 7 days; (2) switch from multiple daily doses to single doses administered each morning; (3) taper the dosage to 50% of physiologic values over the next month; and (4) monitor for production of endogenous cortisol and, when basal levels have returned to normal, cease routine steroid administration (but be prepared to give supplemental glucocorticoids at times of stress).

In addition to unmasking adrenal insufficiency, cessation of glucocorticoid use may produce a withdrawal syndrome. Symptoms include hypotension, hypoglycemia, myalgia, arthralgia, and fatigue. In patients being treated for arthritis and certain other disorders, these symptoms may be confused with return of the underlying disease. Discomfort of withdrawal can be minimized by gradual dosage reduction and by concurrent treatment with NSAIDs.

Preparations and Routes of Administration

Preparations

The glucocorticoids employed clinically include hydrocortisone (cortisol) and synthetic derivatives of this compound. Individual glucocorticoids differ from one another with respect to (1) biologic half-life, (2) mineralocorticoid potency, and (3) glucocorticoid (anti-inflammatory) potency (see Table 68–1).

The term *biologic half-life* refers to the time required for glucocorticoids to leave body tissues. In most cases, these drugs are cleared from tissues more slowly than from the blood. Hence, the biologic half-life is usually longer than the plasma half-life. When glucocorticoids are administered by mouth or by IV injection, it is the biologic half-life, and not the plasma half-life, that determines duration of action. Because of differences in their biologic half-lives, individual glucocorticoids can be classified as short acting, intermediate acting, or long acting (see Table 68–1).

Glucocorticoids with high *mineralocorticoid potency* (cortisone, hydrocortisone) can cause significant retention of sodium and water, coupled with depletion of potassium. These mineralocorticoid effects can be especially hazardous for patients with hypertension or heart failure and for patients taking digoxin. Because of the potential dangers of sodium retention and potassium loss, glucocorticoids with high mineralocorticoid activity should not be administered systemically for long periods.

The differences in *glucocorticoid potency* summarized in Table 68–1 are reflected in the doses required to produce anti-inflammatory effects (and not mineralocorticoid effects). As with other drugs, potency is a relatively unimportant characteristic. However, it is important to appreciate that, in order to produce equivalent therapeutic effects, dosages for some glucocorticoids must be much larger than for others.

Routes of Administration

Glucocorticoids can be administered *orally, parenterally* (IV, IM, SC), *topically, by local injection* (e.g., intra-articular, intralesional), and by *inhalation*. Topical application is reserved for dermatologic disorders (see Chapter 101), and inhalational therapy is reserved primarily for asthma (see Chapter 71). Since local therapy (topical application, inhalation, local injection) minimizes systemic toxicity, this form of treatment is preferred to systemic therapy (oral, parenteral). When systemic effects are needed, oral administration is preferred to parenteral. It is important to note that, even when glucocorticoids are administered for local effects, absorption can be sufficient to produce systemic effects. That is, local administration does not eliminate the risk of systemic toxicity.

Individual glucocorticoids are available as various esters (e.g., acetate, sodium phosphate, tebutate). When glucocorticoids are administered by routes other than oral or IV, the particular ester being used is a major determinant of duration of action. As indicated in Table 68–2, not all esters can be employed by all routes. Hence, when preparing to ad-

TABLE 68–2 ■ Glucocorticoid Routes of Administration*

| | Routes of Administration† | | | | | | | | |
| | Systemic | | | | Local | | | | |
Drug	PO	IM	IV	SC	IA	IB	IL	IS	ST
Betamethasone	✔								
Betamethasone sodium phosphate		✔	✔		✔		✔		✔
Betamethasone acetate/sodium phosphate		✔			✔		✔	✔	✔
Cortisone acetate	✔	✔							
Dexamethasone	✔								
Dexamethasone acetate		✔			✔		✔		✔
Dexamethasone sodium phosphate		✔	✔		✔		✔	✔	✔
Hydrocortisone	✔								
Hydrocortisone acetate					✔	✔	✔	✔	✔
Hydrocortisone cypionate	✔								
Hydrocortisone sodium phosphate		✔	✔	✔					
Hydrocortisone sodium succinate		✔	✔						
Methylprednisolone	✔								
Methylprednisolone acetate		✔			✔		✔		✔
Methylprednisolone sodium succinate		✔	✔						
Prednisolone	✔								
Prednisolone acetate		✔							
Prednisolone acetate/sodium phosphate		✔			✔	✔		✔	✔
Prednisolone sodium phosphate		✔	✔		✔		✔		✔
Prednisolone tebutate					✔		✔		✔
Prednisone	✔								
Triamcinolone	✔								
Triamcinolone acetonide		✔			✔	✔	✔		
Triamcinolone diacetate		✔			✔		✔	✔	✔
Triamcinolone hexacetonide					✔		✔		

*Topical preparations are listed in Table 99–1.
†PO = oral; IM = intramuscular; IV = intravenous; SC = subcutaneous; IA = intra-articular; IB = intrabursal; IL = intralesional; IS = intrasynovial; ST = soft tissue.

minister a glucocorticoid, you should verify that the particular ester ordered is appropriate for the intended route.

Dosage

General Guidelines for Dosing

For most patients, the objective of glucocorticoid therapy is to reduce symptoms to an acceptable level. Complete relief of symptoms is usually not an appropriate goal.

Dosages are highly individualized and, for any patient with any disease, dosage must be determined empirically (by trial and error). For patients whose disease is not an immediate threat to life, the dosage should be low initially and then increased gradually until symptoms are under control. In the event of life-threatening disease, a large initial dose should be used, and, if a response does not occur rapidly, the dose should be doubled or even tripled. When glucocorticoids are used for a prolonged period, the dosage should be reduced until the smallest effective amount has been established. Prolonged treatment with high doses should be done only if the disorder (1) is life threatening or (2) has the potential to cause permanent disability. During long-term treatment, an increase in dosage will be needed at times of stress (unless the dosage is very high to begin with). If disease status changes, appropriate adjustment of dosage must be made.

As noted, abrupt termination of long-term therapy may unmask adrenal insufficiency. To minimize the impact of adrenal insufficiency, withdrawal of glucocorticoids should be gradual. Patients must be warned against abrupt discontinuation of treatment.

Alternate-Day Therapy

In alternate-day therapy, a large dose (of an intermediate-acting glucocorticoid) is given every other morning. This dosing schedule contrasts with traditional therapy, in which multiple smaller doses are administered daily. Benefits of alternate-day therapy are (1) reduced adrenal suppression, (2) reduced risk of growth retardation, and (3) reduced toxicity overall. Adrenal insufficiency is decreased because, over the extended interval between doses, plasma glucocorticoids decline to a level that is low enough to permit some production of ACTH, thereby promoting some synthesis of cortisol by the adrenals. To allow maximal recovery of endocrine function, doses should be administered prior to 9:00 in the morning, and long-acting agents should be avoided. Early-morning administration is also helpful in that it mimics the burst of glucocorticoids normally released by the adrenals at dawn.

Unfortunately, alternate-day therapy does have one drawback: In the long interval between doses, drug levels may fall to a subtherapeutic value, thus permitting flare-up of symptoms. Symptoms are likely to be most intense late on the second day after a dose is given. If symptoms become intolerable, switching to a single daily dose may be sufficient to provide control. As with alternate-day treatment, patients taking single daily doses should administer their medicine before 9:00 AM.

⸪ KEY POINTS

- Glucocorticoids are used in low (physiologic) doses to treat endocrine disorders (see Chapter 57) and in high (pharmacologic) doses to treat nonendocrine disorders (e.g., arthritis, asthma).
- Glucocorticoids are beneficial in nonendocrine disorders primarily because of their ability to suppress inflammatory and immune responses.
- Glucocorticoids reduce inflammation by multiple mechanisms, including suppression of (1) the synthesis of inflammatory mediators (prostaglandins, leukotrienes, histamine), (2) infiltration of phagocytes, (3) release of lysosomal enzymes, and (4) proliferation of lymphocytes.
- Important nonendocrine indications for glucocorticoids include arthritis, allergic disorders, asthma, cancer, and suppression of allograft rejection.
- When used in pharmacologic doses, especially for prolonged times, glucocorticoids can cause severe adverse effects. These are not seen at physiologic doses.
- Adverse effects of the glucocorticoids include adrenal insufficiency, osteoporosis, increased vulnerability to infection, muscle wasting, thinning of the skin, fluid and electrolyte imbalance, glucose intolerance, and, possibly, peptic ulcer disease.
- By causing potassium loss, glucocorticoids can increase the risk of toxicity from digoxin, and they can exacerbate potassium loss caused by thiazide and loop diuretics.
- Concurrent use of NSAIDs with glucocorticoids increases the risk of peptic ulcer disease.
- Prolonged glucocorticoid use causes adrenal insufficiency.
- Patients with adrenal insufficiency must be given supplemental doses of glucocorticoids at times of stress (e.g., surgery, trauma). Failure to do so may be fatal!
- To minimize expression of adrenal insufficiency when glucocorticoids are discontinued, doses should be tapered very gradually.
- Following glucocorticoid withdrawal, supplemental glucocorticoids are needed at times of stress until adrenal function has fully recovered.
- Alternate-day dosing can help minimize development of adrenal insufficiency.
- Glucocorticoids should be administered before 9:00 AM. Why? Because this helps minimize adrenal insufficiency and mimics the burst of glucocorticoids released naturally by the adrenals each morning.

Summary of Major Nursing Implications*

GLUCOCORTICOIDS

The nursing implications summarized here apply to all glucocorticoids, but only to their use for *nonendocrine diseases*. Implications that apply specifically to use of glucocorticoids for *replacement therapy* are summarized in Chapter 57.

Preadministration Assessment

Therapeutic Goal

Glucocorticoids are used to suppress rejection of organ transplants, and to treat a variety of inflammatory, allergic, and neoplastic disorders. When treating inflammatory and allergic disorders, the goal is to suppress signs and symptoms to an acceptable level, not to eliminate them.

Baseline Data

Make a full assessment of the specific disorder (e.g., rheumatoid arthritis, asthma, psoriasis) to be treated. These data are used to determine the initial dosage and to guide dosage adjustments as treatment proceeds. Determine bone mineral density of the lumbar spine.

Identifying High-Risk Patients

Glucocorticoids are *contraindicated* for patients with systemic fungal infections and for individuals receiving live virus vaccines. Use glucocorticoids with *caution* in pediatric patients and in women who are pregnant or breast-feeding. In addition, exercise *caution* in patients with hypertension, open-angle glaucoma, heart failure, renal impairment, esophagitis, gastritis, peptic ulcer disease, myasthenia gravis, diabetes mellitus, osteoporosis, and infections that are resistant to treatment, and in patients receiving potassium-depleting diuretics, digoxin, insulin, oral hypoglycemics, or NSAIDs.

Implementation: Administration and Dosage

Routes and Administration

Glucocorticoids are administered orally, parenterally (IV, IM, SC), topically (to skin and mucous membranes), by inhalation, and by local injection (e.g., intra-articular, intralesional). Routes for specific preparations are summarized in Table 68–2. When getting ready to administer a glucocorticoid, verify that the preparation is appropriate for the intended route.

Dosage

Dosage is determined empirically. For patients whose disease does not threaten life, dosage should be low initially and then gradually increased until the desired response is achieved. For life-threatening disease, initial doses should be as large as needed to control symptoms. During prolonged therapy, the dosage should be reduced to the smallest effective amount. Supplemental doses are needed at times of stress (unless the dosage is very high to begin with).

Alternate-Day Therapy

Alternate-day dosing reduces adrenal suppression and other toxicities. **Instruct patients to take their medicine before 9:00 AM.**

Drug Withdrawal

Glucocorticoids must be withdrawn gradually. **Warn the patient against abrupt discontinuation of treatment.** Following termination, supplemental doses are needed during times of stress until adrenal function has recovered fully.

Ongoing Evaluation and Interventions

Evaluating Therapeutic Effects

Evaluate therapy by making periodic comparisons of current signs and symptoms with the pretreatment assessment. Dosage adjustment is based on these evaluations.

Minimizing Adverse Effects

General Measures. (1) Keep the dosage as low as possible and the duration of treatment as short as possible. (2) Use alternate-day therapy if possible. (3) When appropriate, administer glucocorticoids topically, by inhalation, or by local injection, rather than systemically.

Adrenal Insufficiency. Long-term therapy suppresses the adrenal's ability to make glucocorticoids. Increase the dosage when stress occurs (e.g., surgery, trauma, infection) unless the dosage is very high to begin with. Following termination of therapy, supplemental doses are required at times of stress until recovery of adrenal function is complete. **Advise the patient to carry identification (e.g., Medic Alert bracelet) to ensure proper dosing in emergencies. Advise the patient to always have an emergency supply of glucocorticoids on hand.** Expression of adrenal insufficiency can be reduced by withdrawing glucocorticoids gradually. Adrenal insufficiency can be minimized through alternate-day dosing and use of glucocorticoids that have an intermediate duration of action.

Osteoporosis. Glucocorticoid-induced osteoporosis predisposes the patient to fractures, especially of the ribs and vertebrae. Monitor patients for signs of compression fractures (neck or back pain) and for indications of other fractures. Evaluate status with bone densitometry. Several drugs can help prevent osteoporosis. Important among these are calcium supplements, vitamin D supplements, a thiazide diuretic (combined with salt restriction), a bisphosphonate (e.g., etidronate), and calcitonin. Estrogen replacement therapy can reduce bone loss in postmenopausal women, although the benefits may not outweigh the risks.

Infection. Glucocorticoids increase the risk of morbidity from infection. **Warn patients not to contact persons with communicable diseases. Inform patients about early signs of infection (e.g., fever, sore throat), and instruct them to notify the physician if these occur.** Treat established infections with appropriate antimicrobial drugs, and withdraw glucocorticoids unless they are absolutely required.

*Patient education information is highlighted as blue text.

Summary of Major Nursing Implications*—cont'd

Glucose Intolerance. Glucocorticoids can cause hyperglycemia and glycosuria. Diabetic patients may need to decrease their caloric intake and use higher doses of hypoglycemic medication (insulin or oral hypoglycemic).

Fluid and Electrolyte Disturbance. Glucocorticoids can cause sodium and water retention and loss of potassium. These effects can be minimized by (1) using glucocorticoids that have low mineralocorticoid activity, (2) restricting sodium intake, and (3) taking potassium supplements or consuming potassium-rich foods (e.g., bananas, citrus fruits). **Educate patients about signs and symptoms of fluid retention (e.g., weight gain, swelling of the lower extremities) and instruct them to notify the physician if these develop.**

Growth Retardation. Glucocorticoids can suppress growth in children. Evaluate growth by making periodic measurements of height and weight. Alternate-day therapy minimizes growth suppression.

Cataracts and Glaucoma. Cataracts are a common complication of long-term therapy. Open-angle glaucoma may also develop. The patient should be given an eye examination every 6 months. **Instruct the patient to notify the physician if vision becomes cloudy or blurred.**

Peptic Ulcer Disease. Glucocorticoids may increase the risk of ulcer formation and can mask ulcer symptoms. **Instruct the patient to notify the physician if feces become black and tarry.** Have stools checked periodically for occult blood. If ulcers develop, glucocorticoids should be slowly withdrawn (unless their continued use is considered essential for life), and antiulcer therapy should be instituted.

Use in Pregnancy and Lactation. Glucocorticoids can induce adrenal hypoplasia in the developing fetus. When large doses have been employed, the newborn should be assessed for adrenal insufficiency, and given replacement therapy if indicated.

During high-dose therapy, the glucocorticoid content of breast milk may become high enough to affect the nursing infant. **Warn women who are receiving high-dose therapy not to breast-feed.**

Other Adverse Effects. *Psychologic disturbances, myopathy,* and *Cushing's syndrome* can be minimized by implementing the general measures noted at the beginning of this section. There are no specific measures to prevent these complications.

Minimizing Adverse Interactions

Interactions Related to Potassium Loss. Glucocorticoid-induced potassium loss can be augmented by *potassium-depleting diuretics* (thiazides, loop diuretics) and can increase the risk of toxicity from *digoxin.* If digoxin and glucocorticoids are used concurrently, potassium levels should be monitored. Also, be alert for indications of cardiotoxicity.

Nonsteroidal Anti-inflammatory Drugs. NSAIDs can increase the risk of gastric ulceration during glucocorticoid therapy. Exercise caution when this combination is employed.

Insulin and Oral Hypoglycemics. Glucocorticoids can elevate blood levels of glucose. Diabetic patients may need to increase their dosage of insulin or oral hypoglycemic drug.

Vaccines. Glucocorticoids can decrease antibody responses to vaccines and can increase the risk of infection from live virus vaccines. Attempts at immunization should not be made while glucocorticoids are being used.

*Patient education information is highlighted as blue text.

Drug Therapy of Rheumatoid Arthritis and Gout

In this chapter we focus on the drug therapy of two inflammatory disorders: rheumatoid arthritis and gout. Some of the agents used to treat arthritis have been discussed in preceding chapters. Additional agents are introduced here.

DRUG THERAPY OF RHEUMATOID ARTHRITIS

Rheumatoid arthritis (RA) is an autoimmune, inflammatory disorder that affects about 1% of the American population. Each year, the disease results in more than 9 million physician visits and over 250,000 hospitalizations. Although RA can develop at any age, initial symptoms usually appear during the third and fourth decades. Among younger patients, the incidence of RA is 3 times greater in females than in males. However, among patients over 60, the incidence in men and women is equal. Rheumatoid arthritis follows a progressive course and can eventually cripple its victim. For some patients, drug therapy can halt the advance of the disease. However, for many others, benefits are limited to symptomatic relief.

Pathophysiology of Rheumatoid Arthritis

Onset of RA is heralded by symmetric joint stiffness and pain. Symptoms are most intense in the morning and abate as the day advances. Joints become swollen, tender, and warm. For some patients, periods of spontaneous remission occur. For others, injury progresses steadily. In addition to joint injury, RA has systemic manifestations. Among these are fever, weakness, fatigue, weight loss, thinning of the skin, scleritis (inflammation of the sclera), corneal ulcers, and nodules under the skin and periosteum (connective tissue that surrounds all bones). An especially severe manifestation is vasculitis.

The progression of joint deterioration is depicted in Figure 69–1. Inflammation begins in the synovium—the membrane that encloses the joint cavity. As inflammation intensifies, the synovial membrane thickens and begins to envelop the articular cartilage. This overgrowth is referred to as pannus. Damage to the cartilage is caused by enzymes released from the pannus and by chemicals and enzymes produced by the inflammatory process raging within the synovial space. Ultimately, the articular cartilage undergoes total destruction, resulting in direct contact between bones of the joint, followed by eventual bone fusion. After this, inflammation subsides.

Joint destruction is caused by an autoimmune process in which the immune system mounts an attack against synovial tissue. During the attack, mast cells, macrophages, and T lymphocytes produce cytokines and cytotoxins—compounds that promote inflammation and joint destruction. The cytokines of greatest importance are tumor necrosis factor, interleukin-1, interleukin-6, interferon-gamma, platelet-derived growth factor, and granulocyte-macrophage colony-stimulating factor. Why does the immune system attack joints? No one knows.

Overview of Therapy

Treatment is directed at (1) relieving symptoms (pain, inflammation, and stiffness), (2) maintaining joint function and range of motion, (3) minimizing systemic involvement, and (4) delaying disease progression. To achieve these goals, a combination of pharmacologic and nonpharmacologic measures is employed.

Nondrug Measures

Nondrug measures for managing RA include physical therapy, exercise, and surgery. Physical therapy may consist of massage, warm baths, and application of heat to the affected regions. These procedures can enhance mobility and reduce inflammation. A balanced program of rest and exercise can decrease joint stiffness and improve function. However, excessive rest or excessive exercise should be avoided: too much rest will foster stiffness, and too much activity can intensify inflammation.

Orthopedic surgery has made marked advances. For patients with severe disease of the hip or knee, total joint replacement can be performed. When joints of the hands or wrists have been damaged severely, function can be improved through removal of the diseased synovium and repair of ruptured tendons. Plastic implants can help correct deformities.

A complete program of treatment should include patient education and counseling. The patient should be informed

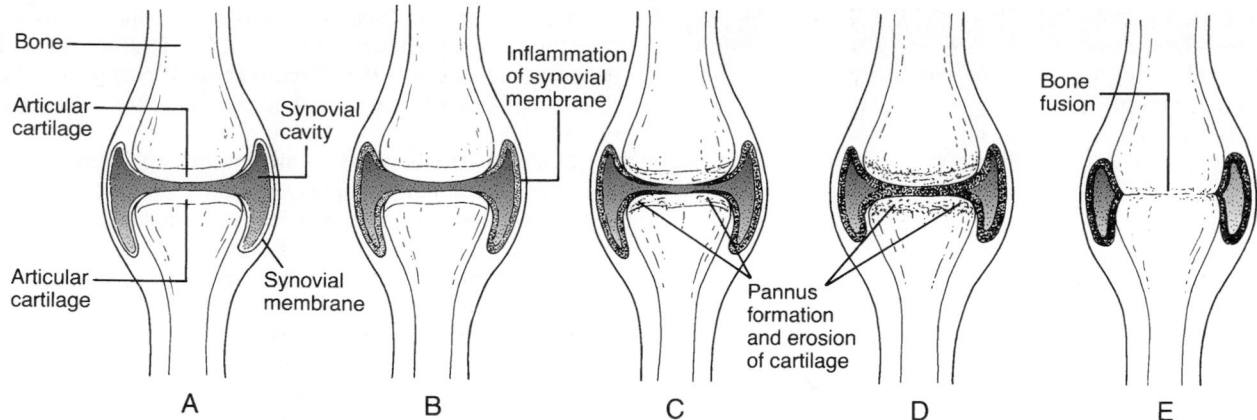

Figure 69–1 ■ Progressive joint degeneration in rheumatoid arthritis.
A, Healthy joint. *B,* Inflammation of synovial membrane. *C,* Onset of pannus formation
and cartilage erosion. *D,* Pannus formation progresses and cartilage deteriorates further.
E, Complete destruction of joint cavity together with fusion of articulating bones.

about the nature of RA, the possible consequences of joint degeneration, management measures, and the benefits and limitations of drug therapy. If loss of mobility limits function at home, on the job, or in school, consultation with a social worker, occupational therapist, or specialist in vocational rehabilitation may be appropriate.

Drug Therapy

Antiarthritic drugs can produce symptomatic relief, and, in some cases, may induce protracted remission. However, remission is rarely complete, and the disease typically advances steadily. As a result, drug therapy is chronic. Accordingly, successful treatment requires both motivation and cooperation on the part of the patient.

Classes of Antiarthritic Drugs. As indicated in Table 69–1, the antiarthritic drugs fall into three major categories: (1) *nonsteroidal anti-inflammatory drugs* (NSAIDs), (2) *disease-modifying antirheumatic drugs* (DMARDs), and (3) *glucocorticoids* (adrenal corticosteroids). These drugs differ with respect to time course of action, toxicity, and ability to slow the progression of RA.

The NSAIDs provide rapid relief of symptoms but do not prevent joint damage and do not slow disease progression. The NSAIDs are safer than DMARDs and glucocorticoids, and hence treatment requires less vigorous monitoring.

Like the NSAIDs, glucocorticoids provide rapid relief of symptoms. In addition, recent evidence indicates that glucocorticoids may be able to slow disease progression. Unfortunately, although glucocorticoids are effective drugs, with long-term use, they can cause serious toxicity. As a result, treatment is usually limited to short courses.

By definition, DMARDs are drugs that reduce joint destruction and retard disease progression. However, the onset of benefits is delayed, typically by 3 to 5 months. The DMARDs are generally more toxic than NSAIDs, and therefore close monitoring is required.

Drug Selection. Drug therapy of RA is evolving. In the past, treatment followed a simple protocol: (1) Start with an NSAID (e.g., aspirin, ibuprofen, celecoxib). (2) If symptoms can't be controlled with an NSAID, add a DMARD (e.g.,

methotrexate), and continue the NSAID until the DMARD takes effect. And (3) If necessary, provide a short course of glucocorticoid therapy while responses to the DMARD are developing, and to supplement treatment any time that symptoms "flare." Note that, in this protocol, DMARDs are used only if NSAIDs are insufficient.

Today, treatment is more aggressive. Current guidelines recommend starting a DMARD *early*—within 3 months of RA diagnosis for most new patients. The rationale is to delay joint degeneration. Recall that NSAIDs only provide symptomatic relief; they do not retard disease progression. In contrast, DMARDs may be able to arrest the disease process. Hence, by instituting DMARD therapy early (rather than waiting until joint degeneration has advanced to the point where NSAIDs can no longer control symptoms), it is possible to delay or even prevent serious joint injury. Because the effects of DMARDs take months to develop, whereas the effects of NSAIDs are immediate, an NSAID is given until the DMARD has had time to act, after which the NSAID can be withdrawn. As in the past, glucocorticoids are generally reserved for short-course management of symptom flare-ups and for control of symptoms until DMARDs take effect. If joint injury progresses despite treatment with one DMARD, another DMARD can be added or substituted.

You can find detailed information on the diagnosis and management of RA in *Guidelines for the Management of Rheumatoid Arthritis: 2002 Update,* available free at the American College of Rheumatology web site (*www.rheumatology.org/ research/guidelines*).

Pharmacology of the Drugs Used for Rheumatoid Arthritis
Nonsteroidal Anti-inflammatory Drugs

The basic pharmacology of the NSAIDs is discussed in Chapter 67. Consideration here is limited to their use in RA.

Therapeutic Role. NSAIDs are drugs of first choice for RA. These agents are both effective and fast acting. Benefits derive primarily from anti-inflammatory actions, although analgesic actions help too. Both actions result from inhibiting

TABLE 69–1 ■ Drugs for Rheumatoid Arthritis

Nonsteroidal Anti-Inflammatory Drugs (NSAIDs)

First-Generation NSAIDs
  Aspirin
  Choline salicylate [Arthropan]
  Diclofenac [Voltaren]
  Ibuprofen [Motrin, others]
  Naproxen [Naprosyn]
  Others (see Table 69–2)

Second-Generation NSAIDs (COX-2 Inhibitors)
  Celecoxib [Celebrex]
  Rofecoxib [Vioxx]
  Valdecoxib [Bextra]

Disease-Modifying Antirheumatic Drugs (DMARDs)

First-Choice DMARDs
  Methotrexate [Rheumatrex]
  Hydroxychloroquine [Plaquenil]
  Sulfasalazine [Azulfidine]

Other DMARDs
  Azathioprine [Imuran]
  Cyclosporine [Neoral]
  Gold salts
    Auranofin [Ridaura]
    Aurothioglucose [Solganal]
    Gold sodium thiomalate [Myochrysine]
  Penicillamine [Cuprimine, Depen]
  Leflunomide [Arava]
  Etanercept [Enbrel]
  Infliximab [Remicade]
  Adalimumab [Humira]
  Anakinra [Kineret]

Glucocorticoids
  Prednisone
  Prednisolone

cyclooxygenase (COX). NSAIDs only provide symptomatic relief; they do not slow the progression of RA.

NSAID Classification. As discussed in Chapter 67, there are two main classes of NSAIDs: (1) *first-generation NSAIDs,* which inhibit COX-1 *and* COX-2; and (2) *second-generation NSAIDs (coxibs),* which selectively inhibit COX-2. Anti-inflammatory and analgesic effects result from inhibiting COX-2, whereas major adverse effects—especially gastro-duodenal ulceration—result from inhibiting COX-1. Because of their selectivity, the coxibs produce less GI ulceration than the first-generation NSAIDs, while producing equal therapeutic effects.

Drug Selection. Selection of an NSAID is based largely on efficacy, safety, and cost.

Efficacy. All of the NSAIDs have essentially equal antirheumatic effects. However, for reasons that are not understood, individual patients may respond better to one NSAID than to another. Accordingly, it may be necessary to try more than one agent to achieve an optimal response.

Safety and Cost. The COX-2 inhibitors are safer than the first-generation NSAIDs, but are also more expensive. Hence, selection must balance these factors. If symptoms are controlled with a first-generation NSAID, and the drug is well tolerated, cost considerations would dictate using that drug.

However, if a first-generation NSAID produces serious gastric ulceration, then switching to a COX-2 inhibitor would be appropriate—despite the increased cost. If cost were not an issue, COX-2 inhibitors would be the first-choice NSAIDs for most all patients.

Dosage. The dosages employed for anti-inflammatory effects are considerably higher than those required for analgesia or reduction of fever. For example, treatment of RA may require 5.2 gm (16 standard tablets) of aspirin a day, compared with only 2.6 gm for aches, pain, and fever. Dosages for RA are summarized in Table 69–2.

Glucocorticoids

The glucocorticoids are powerful anti-inflammatory drugs that can relieve symptoms of severe RA, and may also retard disease progression. For patients with generalized symptoms, *oral* glucocorticoids are indicated. However, if only one or two joints are affected, *intra-articular injections* may be employed. Because long-term oral therapy can cause serious toxicity (e.g., osteoporosis, gastric ulceration, adrenal suppression), short-term therapy should be used whenever possible. Most often, these drugs are given to provide temporary relief until drugs with a slower onset of action (e.g., methotrexate, hydroxychloroquine) can provide control. Long-term therapy should be limited to patients who have failed to respond adequately to all other treatment options. The most commonly employed oral glucocorticoids are prednisone and prednisolone. For treatment of symptom flare-ups, patients may be given 10 to 20 mg/day until symptoms are controlled, followed by gradual drug withdrawal over 5 to 7 days. The pharmacology of the glucocorticoids is discussed at length in Chapter 68 (Glucocorticoids in Nonendocrine Diseases).

Methotrexate

Methotrexate [Rheumatrex, Trexall] is the most rapid-acting DMARD. Therapeutic effects may develop in 3 to 6 weeks. Many rheumatologists consider methotrexate the first-choice drug among the DMARDs, owing to its efficacy, relative safety, low cost, and extensive use in RA. Major toxicities are hepatic fibrosis, bone marrow suppression, GI ulceration, and pneumonitis. Periodic tests of liver and kidney function are mandatory, as are complete blood cell and platelet counts. Methotrexate can cause fetal death and congenital abnormalities, and therefore is contraindicated during pregnancy. For treatment of RA, the drug is administered *once a week,* either orally or by injection. The usual maintenance dosage is 7.5 to 20 mg a week. The pharmacology of methotrexate is discussed at length in Chapter 98 (Anticancer Drugs I: Cytotoxic Agents).

Hydroxychloroquine

Actions and Uses. Hydroxychloroquine [Plaquenil], a drug with antimalarial actions, is a preferred DMARD for patients with mild symptoms. By itself, the drug does not slow disease progression, but early use *can* improve long-term outcomes. Like other DMARDs, hydroxychloroquine has a delayed onset of action; full therapeutic effects take 3 to 6 months to develop. Concurrent therapy with anti-inflammatory agents (NSAIDs or glucocorticoids) is indicated during the latency period. The mechanism by which hydroxychloroquine acts is not known.

TABLE 69-2 ▪ Antiarthritic Dosages for Nonsteroidal Anti-Inflammatory Drugs

Generic Name	Trade Name	Daily Dosage
First-Generation NSAIDs		
Salicylates		
Aspirin (extended release)		800 mg qid
Choline magnesium salicylate	Trisalate	3 gm/day (in 1–3 doses)
Salsalate	Disalcid, Mono-Gesic	3.0–4.0 gm/day (in 2 or 3 doses)
Sodium salicylate		3.6–5.4 gm/day (in divided doses)
Nonsalicylates		
Diclofenac	Voltaren	150–200 mg/day (in 3 or 4 doses)
Diclofenac/Misoprostol	Arthrotec	50 mg diclofenac/200 µg misoprostol 3 or 4 times daily
Diflunisal	Dolobid	250–500 mg bid
Etodolac	Lodine	600–1200 mg/day in (2–4 doses)
Fenoprofen	Nalfon	300–600 mg tid or qid
Flurbiprofen	Ansaid	200–300 mg/day (in 2–4 doses)
Ibuprofen	Motrin, Rufen	600–800 mg tid or qid
Indomethacin	Indocin	25–50 mg tid
Ketoprofen	Orudis, Oruvail	150–300 mg (in 3 or 4 doses)
Meclofenamate	Meclomen	200–400 mg/day (in 3 or 4 doses)
Meloxicam	Mobic	7.5 mg once a day
Nabumetone	Relafen	1.5–2 gm/day (in 1 or 2 doses)
Naproxen	Naprosyn	250–500 mg bid
Naproxen sodium	Anaprox	250–500 mg bid
Oxaprozin	Daypro	1.2 gm qd
Piroxicam	Feldene	20 mg once a day
Sulindac	Clinoril	150–200 mg bid
Tolmetin	Tolectin	200–400 mg tid
Second-Generation NSAIDs (COX-2 Inhibitors)		
Celecoxib	Celebrex	100–200 mg bid
Rofecoxib	Vioxx	12.5–25 mg qd
Valdecoxib	Bextra	10 mg once a day

Toxicity. The most serious toxicity is *retinal damage.* Retinopathy may be irreversible and can produce blindness. Visual loss is directly related to dosage. Low doses may be used in long-term treatment with little risk. When dosage has been excessive, retinal damage may appear after treatment has ceased and may progress in the absence of continued drug use. Patients should receive a thorough ophthalmologic examination prior to treatment and every 6 months thereafter. Hydroxychloroquine should be discontinued at the first sign of retinal injury. Patients should be advised to contact the physician if any visual disturbance is noted.

Preparations, Dosage, and Administration. Hydroxychloroquine [Plaquenil] is dispensed in 200-mg tablets for oral administration. The initial dosage is 200 mg twice daily. Maintenance dosages range from 200 to 400 mg/day. The daily dosage should not exceed 6.4 mg/kg.

Sulfasalazine

Sulfasalazine [Azulfidine] has been used for years to treat inflammatory bowel disease (see Chapter 75) and is now used to treat RA as well. The drug can retard progression of joint deterioration, and benefits develop relatively fast, sometimes within 1 month. Gastrointestinal reactions (nausea, vomiting, diarrhea, anorexia, abdominal pain) are the most common reasons for discontinuing treatment. These reactions can be minimized by using an enteric-coated formulation and by dividing the daily dosage. Dermatologic reactions (pruritus, rash, urticaria) are also common. Fortunately, serious adverse effects—hepatitis and bone marrow suppression—are rare. To ensure early detection, periodic monitoring for hepatitis and bone marrow function (complete blood counts, platelet counts) should be performed. The initial dosage for RA is 500 mg/day, and the usual maintenance dosage is 1000 mg 2 or 3 times a day.

Etanercept

Etanercept [Enbrel] is the first member of a new class of drugs: the *tumor necrosis factor (TNF) blockers,* agents that bind to and thereby block the actions of TNF. Etanercept produces a relatively rapid reduction in symptoms and delays disease progression. There is concern that etanercept can increase the risk of serious infection.

Mechanism of Action. Etanercept suppresses inflammation by neutralizing TNF. As noted earlier, TNF is an important contributor to RA pathophysiology. In patients with RA, TNF binds to receptors on cells in the synovium, and thereby stimulates production of chemotactic factors and endothelial adhesion molecules, which in turn promote infiltration of neutrophils and macrophages. The result is inflammation and joint destruction.

How does etanercept neutralize TNF? Etanercept is a large molecule composed of two receptors for TNF linked to the Fc portion of an immunoglobulin G (IgG) molecule. The TNF receptors, which are produced through recombinant DNA technology, are identical to the TNF receptors found on human cells. Like the TNF receptors on cells, etanercept binds tightly with TNF, and thereby prevents TNF from interacting with its normal receptors.

Therapeutic Use. Etanercept is indicated for patients with moderate to severe RA. In clinical trials, etanercept was superior to methotrexate at delaying progression of joint damage, and it suppressed signs and symptoms of RA more rapidly. Among patients who had failed to respond to methotrexate, addition of etanercept for 6 months reduced symptoms in 61% of patients, compared with 27% of patients who continued taking methotrexate alone.

Pharmacokinetics. Etanercept is administered by SC injection. Plasma levels peak about 3 days after dosing. The drug is cleared from the plasma with a half-life of 115 hours (about 5 days). The mode of elimination is unknown.

Adverse Effects. Injection site reactions (itching, erythema, swelling, pain) occur in 37% of patients. Other mild but less common reactions include headache, rhinitis, dizziness, cough, and abdominal pain.

Increased risk of *serious infection* is a concern. Since TNF helps protect against infection, neutralizing TNF with etanercept may increase infection risk. During clinical trials, etanercept increased the risk of sinusitis and upper respiratory tract infections, but did *not* increase the risk of sepsis and other serious infections. However, during early postmarketing surveillance, 30 serious infections were reported, 6 of which were fatal. Because over 25,000 patients have taken etanercept, but only 30 serious infections have been reported, it is not clear that etanercept was the cause. Nonetheless, caution is advised. Accordingly, etanercept should not be given to patients with any active infection, including chronic or localized infections. Patients who develop a new infection should be monitored closely. Etanercept should be used with caution in patients with a history of recurrent infection or a condition that predisposes them to acquiring infection (e.g., advanced or poorly controlled diabetes). Prospective patients should receive a chest x-ray and tuberculin skin test to rule out tuberculosis before starting treatment.

Etanercept has been associated with rare cases of *central nervous system (CNS) demyelinating disorders* (e.g., multiple sclerosis, myelitis, optic neuritis) and *hematologic disorders,* including fatal cases of aplastic anemia. However, a causal relationship between etanercept and these disorders has not been established. Nonetheless, caution is advised, especially in patients with (1) pre-existing or recent-onset CNS demyelinating disorders or (2) a history of significant hematologic abnormalities. If patients develop signs or symptoms suggestive of blood disorders (persistent fever, bruising, bleeding, pallor), they should seek immediate medical attention. If a significant hematologic abnormality is diagnosed, discontinuing etanercept should be considered.

Drug Interactions. By neutralizing TNF, etanercept may increase the risk of acquiring or transmitting infection following immunization with a live virus vaccine. Accordingly, live virus vaccines should be avoided. Pediatric patients should be brought up to date on their vaccinations before starting the drug.

Preparations, Dosage, and Administration. Etanercept [Enbrel] is dispensed as a powder (25 mg) to be reconstituted in 1 ml of sterile bacteriostatic water (supplied by the manufacturer) for SC injection. Solutions that are discolored or cloudy or contain particles should not be used. Injections should be made immediately after reconstitution. The adult dosage is 25 mg SC twice a week. The dosage for children 4 to 17 years old is 0.4 mg/kg (up to a maximum of 25 mg) twice a week. For both adults and children, injections are made 3 to 4 days apart. Etanercept is expensive: The cost for a 12-month course of treatment is about $15,500.

Infliximab

Infliximab [Remicade] is the second TNF blocker approved for RA. Like etanercept, infliximab binds to and thereby neutralizes TNF. However, the two drugs are structurally different: whereas etanercept is composed of two TNF *receptors,* infliximab is a TNF *antibody.*

Infliximab is approved for use in combination with methotrexate to treat RA in patients who have not responded to methotrexate alone. Treatment can reduce symptoms and halt disease progression. In addition to its use in RA, infliximab is employed in Crohn's disease (see Chapter 75).

Common adverse effects include headache and infusion reactions (e.g., fever, chills, pruritus, urticaria, chest pain). In patients with heart failure, infliximab may increase the risk of hospitalization and mortality, and hence should be avoided by these patients.

Like etanercept, infliximab has immunosuppressant actions, and hence can increase the risk of serious infection, including bacterial sepsis, invasive fungal infection, and reactivation of latent tuberculosis. Accordingly, the drug should not be given to patients with chronic infections, and should be temporarily withdrawn if an acute infection develops. Patients should receive a tuberculin skin test and chest x-ray to rule out latent tuberculosis prior to treatment.

Infliximab is administered by slow IV infusion (over 2 hours or more). The dosage is 3 mg/kg at 0, 2, and 6 weeks, and every 8 weeks thereafter. Patients should also receive methotrexate (oral or SC). Infliximab is expensive: Depending on dosage and dosing schedule, treatment costs between $14,000 and $37,000 a year.

Adalimumab

Adalimumab [Humira] is the third TNF blocker approved for RA. Like infliximab, adalimumab is a monoclonal antibody that binds to and thereby neutralizes TNF. The drug is indicated for adults with moderately to severely active RA who have not responded adequately to one or more DMARDs. In these patients, adalimumab can reduce symptoms and slow progression of joint damage. The drug may be used alone or in combination with methotrexate or other DMARDs.

Adalimumab is generally well tolerated. The most common side effects are injection site reactions (rash, erythema, itching, pain, and swelling), which develop in about 20% of patients. Headache is also common (12%). Allergic reactions develop in about 1% of patients; if a serious reaction develops (e.g., anaphylaxis), the drug should be discontinued. Very rarely, adalimumab has been associated with neurologic injury; signs include numbness, tingling, dizziness, disturbed vision, and weakness in the legs. Testing in pregnant monkeys showed no evidence of fetal harm; however, there are no data on safety in pregnant women.

Like etanercept and infliximab, adalimumab has immunosuppressant actions, and hence can increase the risk of serious infection, including bacterial sepsis, invasive fungal infection, and reactivation of latent tuberculosis. Accordingly, the drug should not be given to patients with active infection. Patients who develop a new infection during treatment should be monitored closely; if the infection becomes serious, adalimumab should be discontinued. Patients should receive a tuberculin skin test and chest x-ray to rule out latent tuberculosis prior to treatment.

Adalimumab [Humira] is supplied in solution (40 mg/0.8 ml) in 1-ml prefilled syringes. Administration is by SC injection in the anterior thigh or abdomen. The injection giver—physician, patient, or caregiver—should rotate the injection site and avoid areas where the skin is tender, bruised, red, or hard. The recommended dosage is 40 mg every 2 weeks. If adalimumab is being used without methotrexate, giving it more frequently (40 mg once a week) may improve results. The drug should be stored cold—2°C to 8°C (36°F to 46°F)—and protected from light. Like etanercept and infliximab, adalimumab is expensive: For patients taking 40 mg every 2 weeks, the annual cost is about $18,000.

Leflunomide

Actions and Uses. Leflunomide [Arava] is a relatively new and powerful immunosuppressant indicated for patients with active RA. In clinical trials, the drug decreased signs and symptoms and slowed disease progression. Compared with traditional antirheumatic agents (e.g., methotrexate), leflunomide is about equally effective, but more dangerous and expensive. Accordingly, the drug should be reserved for second-line use.

Leflunomide is a prodrug that undergoes conversion to its active form—metabolite 1 (M1)—in the body. Metabolite 1 inhibits dihydroorotate dehydrogenase, a mitochondrial enzyme needed for *de novo* synthesis of pyrimidines, which in turn are needed for T-cell proliferation and antibody production. *In vitro,* the drug inhibits T-cell proliferation. In animals, it suppresses inflammation.

Pharmacokinetics. Following oral administration, leflunomide is converted to M1 by enzymes in the intestine and liver. Levels of M1 peak in 6 to 12 hours. The active form undergoes further metabolism followed by excretion in the urine and bile. The drug's half-life is 16.5 days. Because the half-life is prolonged, a series of loading doses is needed to achieve plateau level quickly.

Adverse Effects. The most common adverse effects are diarrhea (17%), respiratory infection (15%), reversible alopecia (10%), rash (10%), and nausea (9%). The drug has also been associated with much more serious reactions: pancytopenia, Stevens-Johnson syndrome, and severe hypertension.

Leflunomide is hepatotoxic. Elevation of liver enzymes occurs in about 10% of patients. In postmarketing reports, the drug has been associated with over 130 cases of severe liver injury, including 12 that were fatal. Liver function should be assessed prior to treatment and monthly thereafter. Leflunomide should be avoided in patients with liver dysfunction, hepatitis B, or hepatitis C. Patients should be informed about signs of liver injury—abdominal pain, fatigue, dark urine, and jaundice—and advised to report them immediately.

Leflunomide is carcinogenic in animals. However, the drug has not been associated with malignancy in humans.

Leflunomide and Pregnancy. *Leflunomide is contraindicated for use in pregnancy.* The drug is teratogenic and embryotoxic in animals and has been classified in Food and Drug Administration (FDA) Pregnancy Risk Category X. Women of child-bearing age must use a reliable form of contraception.

Patients who wish to become pregnant must first clear leflunomide from the body. A three-step process is used:

■ *Step 1:* Discontinue leflunomide.
■ *Step 2:* Take cholestyramine (8 gm 3 times a day) for 11 days. (Cholestyramine binds leflunomide and its metabolites in the intestine, and thereby accelerates their excretion. Without cholestyramine, safe levels might not be achieved for 2 years.)
■ *Step 3:* Verify that plasma drug levels are below 0.02 mg/L.

To minimize any risk of fetal injury, men who wish to father a child should undergo the same clearance procedure.

Drug Interactions. Leflunomide can inhibit the metabolism of certain NSAIDs (e.g., ibuprofen, diclofenac), causing their levels to rise. In addition, leflunomide can intensify liver damage from other hepatotoxic drugs (e.g., methotrexate), and hence should not be combined with such agents. Rifampin (a drug for tuberculosis) can elevate leflunomide levels by 40%. Conversely, levels of leflunomide can be rapidly decreased with cholestyramine or activated charcoal.

Preparations, Dosage, and Administration. Leflunomide [Arava] is available in tablets (10, 20, and 100 mg) for oral administration. Treatment is begun with a series of loading doses (100 mg once a day for 3 days) followed by daily maintenance doses (10 or 20 mg). Leflunomide is moderately expensive. The cost for a 12-month course of treatment is about $3000.

Anakinra

Actions and Use. Anakinra [Kineret] is the first member of a new class of DMARDs: agents that block receptors for interleukin-1 (IL-1), a proinflammatory cytokine than plays a central role in synovial inflammation and joint destruction. Structurally, anakinra is nearly identical to *human interleukin-1 receptor antagonist,* a naturally occurring compound that, like anakinra, blocks access of IL-1 to its receptors. By blocking IL-1 receptors, both compounds suppress inflammation and joint destruction.

Anakinra is approved for SC therapy of patients with moderately to severely active RA who have not responded to treatment with one or more older DMARDs (e.g., methotrexate). In clinical trials, the anakinra was superior to placebo at reducing signs and symptoms of RA and reducing disease progression. Responses to anakinra plus methotrexate were superior to those produced with methotrexate alone. Anakinra may be combined with most other DMARDs, but not with TNF blockers (etanercept, infliximab).

Pharmacokinetics. Anakinra is administered SC, yielding peak plasma levels in 3 to 7 hours. The drug is excreted in the urine, primarily as metabo-

lites. In patients with normal renal function, the terminal half-life is 4 to 6 hours. However, in patients with severe renal impairment, plasma clearance is reduced by 75%.

Adverse Effects. Injection-site reactions (pruritus, erythema, rash, pain) are common, especially during the first month of treatment. Although usually mild, these reactions can cause patients to discontinue the drug.

Like the TNF blockers, anakinra poses a risk of serious infections. In clinical trials, anakinra increased the incidence of neutropenia (8% vs. 2% with placebo) and resulting severe infections (1.8% vs. 0.6% with placebo). Anakinra should not be given to patients with active infection, and should be stopped if a serious infection develops. Because both anakinra and the TNF blockers increase infection risk, these drugs should not be combined. To detect developing neutropenia, and thereby reduce infection risk, neutrophil counts should be determined at baseline, monthly for the first 3 months of treatment, and then every 3 months through the first year of treatment.

Preparations, Dosage, and Administration. Anakinra is available in prefilled syringes that contain 100 mg of the drug in 1 ml of preservative-free solution. The recommended dosage is 100 mg/day SC. The syringes should be stored between 2°C and 8°C (36°F and 46°F) and protected from light. Treatment costs about $14,000 a year.

Gold Salts

Actions and Uses. The beneficial effects of gold in RA have been known since the 1930s. Gold can relieve pain and stiffness and, for some patients, may arrest the progression of joint degeneration. Symptomatic improvement is seen in 60% to 70% of patients; about 15% experience remission. Because the toxicity of gold can be severe, therapy is reserved for patients who have not responded adequately to other DMARDs. Therapeutic effects take 4 to 6 months to develop.

Gold preparations are available for IM and oral administration. Patients receiving IM therapy require repeated injections over a prolonged period. The oral preparation is more convenient and less toxic than the IM preparations. Unfortunately, the oral preparation is also less effective.

The exact mechanism by which gold induces remission and relieves symptoms has not been determined. Likely contributory mechanisms are suppression of lysozyme release and suppression of immune responses.

Toxicity. Gold has several toxicities that can limit its use. About 15% to 20% of patients discontinue treatment because of adverse effects. Among the most common reactions are *intense pruritus, rashes,* and *stomatitis* (lesions of the oral mucosa). *Renal toxicity,* manifested as proteinuria, occurs frequently. *Severe blood dyscrasias* (thrombocytopenia, leukopenia, agranulocytosis, aplastic anemia) have developed, but are rare. Other serious toxicities include encephalitis, hepatitis, peripheral neuritis, pulmonary infiltrates, and profound hypotension. *Oral gold causes less mucocutaneous and renal toxicity than the IM preparations, but GI reactions (diarrhea, nausea, abdominal pain) are common.

Monitoring. Frequent laboratory tests and clinical evaluations are required. At each office visit, the patient should be examined for dermatologic reactions and stomatitis. In addition, kidney and liver function must be monitored, and complete blood counts should be performed. The urine should be analyzed for protein. If signs of toxicity are detected, gold should be discontinued immediately. If the adverse reactions are mild, therapy may be resumed 2 to 3 weeks after symptoms subside. However, many rheumatologists believe that once *any* toxicity has occurred, gold should not be used again. The chances of severe toxicity can be reduced by using low initial doses.

Preparations, Dosage, and Administration. *Preparations.* Three gold preparations are available. Two of these—*aurothioglucose* [Solganal] and *gold sodium thiomalate* [Aurolate]—are administered IM. The third—*auranofin* [Ridaura]—is taken orally.

Intramuscular Dosing. On the first day, a 10-mg test dose is administered. This is followed on days 7 and 14 by 25-mg doses. After this, 50-mg doses are injected weekly until a cumulative dose of 1 gm has been given. If beneficial effects occur, therapy is continued but the dosing interval is gradually lengthened, first to 2 weeks, then to 3 weeks, and then to 1 month. In the absence of toxicity, monthly maintenance injections can be continued indefinitely.

Oral Dosing. The usual adult dosage is 6 mg/day (administered in one or two doses). If, after 6 months, the response is inadequate, dosage may be increased to 3 mg 3 times a day for an additional 3 months. If the response is still inadequate, therapy should stop.

Penicillamine

Penicillamine [Cuprimine, Depen] can relieve symptoms of RA and can retard progression of joint erosion. Unfortunately, treatment may be associated with serious toxicity, especially *bone marrow depression* and *autoimmune disorders.* Consequently, the drug is generally reserved for patients with severe disease who have failed to respond to safer DMARDs. Therapeutic effects take 3 to 6 months to develop. The initial dosage is 125 mg/day. The daily dosage can be increased by 125-mg increments every 2 to 3 months. Usual maintenance dosages range from 250 to 750 mg/day. The pharmacology of penicillamine is discussed further in Chapter 105 (Management of Poisoning).

Azathioprine

Azathioprine [Imuran] is an older DMARD that is rarely used today. Benefits derive from immunosuppressive and anti-inflammatory actions. Serious toxicities include *hepatitis* and *blood dyscrasias* (leukopenia, thrombocytopenia, anemia). To monitor for these effects, complete blood counts, platelet counts, and tests of liver function are required. Azathioprine is teratogenic in animals and should not be used during pregnancy. The drug may also pose a small risk of malignancy. For treatment of RA, the initial dosage is 1 mg/kg/day. The dosage may be gradually increased to a maximum of 2.5 mg/kg/day. As discussed in Chapter 65, azathioprine is also used to prevent rejection of kidney transplants.

Cyclosporine

Cyclosporine, an immunosuppressive drug used to prevent rejection of transplanted organs, can reduce symptoms of RA. Because it can cause kidney damage and other serious adverse effects, cyclosporine should be reserved for severe, progressive RA that has not responded to safer DMARDs. In patients with an inadequate response to methotrexate, adding cyclosporine may produce significant improvement.

Cyclosporine is available in two formulations, marketed as Sandimmune and Neoral. Only Neoral is approved for RA. The initial dosage is 1.25 mg/kg twice daily. The usual maintenance dosage is 1.25 to 2 mg/kg twice daily. If there is no response by 16 weeks, cyclosporine use should stop. Cyclosporine is discussed at length in Chapter 65.

Minocycline

Minocycline [Minocin], an antibiotic in the tetracycline family, can improve symptoms in patients with RA. The drug was originally tried because of data suggesting that RA may have an infectious origin in some patients. However, it now appears that the most likely mechanism underlying benefits is inhibition of collagenase, an enzyme that promotes joint destruction. Other potential mechanisms include inhibition of phospholipase A_2, interleukins, leukocyte infiltration, and lymphocyte proliferation.

In patients with RA, minocycline can improve morning stiffness, joint pain and tenderness, and activities of daily living. In addition, it may delay disease progression in some patients. The usual dosage is 100 mg twice daily. Increasing the dosage increases adverse effects but does not increase benefits. Symptomatic improvement develops within 12 weeks, but may not be maximal until 12 months. Adverse effects include dizziness and skin rash. Minocycline is an experimental therapy, and hence should be reserved for patients who have not responded to other DMARDs.

Protein A Column [Prosorba]

The *Prosorba* column, used in combination with plasmapheresis, decreases the titer of circulating immune complexes that promote symptoms of RA. The column contains an adsorbent compound—*protein A*—that binds to antibodies of the IgG class and to IgG-antigen complexes. When the patient's plasma is passed through the column, these antibodies and immune complexes are removed. Treatment should be reserved for patients with moderate to severe RA who have been refractory to or intolerant of methotrexate and other DMARDs.

In one clinical trial, plasmapheresis through the protein A column was done once a week for 12 weeks. Twenty weeks after the first treatment, symptoms in 32% of patients had improved by at least 20%. Benefits persisted for a mean of 37 weeks.

The most common adverse effects are transient increases in joint swelling, joint pain, and fatigue. Other common reactions include fever, chills, hypotension, nausea, abdominal pain, and headache.

Angiotensin-converting enzyme (ACE) inhibitors should be discontinued prior to treatment. Why? Because apheresis causes release of bradykinin, a compound that promotes hypotension. In the absence of ACE inhibitors, ACE rapidly converts bradykinin to an inactive form. However, if an ACE inhibitor is present, bradykinin can accumulate, thereby posing a risk of serious hypotension.

Treatment with the Prosorba column is expensive. The cost for 12 columns is about $20,400. Performing plasmapheresis adds additional expense.

DRUG THERAPY OF GOUT

Pathophysiology of Gout

Gout is a recurrent inflammatory disorder characterized by *hyperuricemia* (high blood levels of uric acid) and episodes of *severe joint pain,* typically in the large toe. Hyperuricemia can occur through two mechanisms: (1) excessive production of uric acid and (2) impaired renal excretion of uric acid. Acute attacks are precipitated by crystallization of sodium urate (the sodium salt of uric acid) in the synovial space. Deposition of urate crystals promotes inflammation by triggering a complex series of events. A key feature of the inflammatory process is infiltration of leukocytes; once inside the synovial cavity, these cells phagocytize urate crystals and then break down, causing release of destructive lysosomal enzymes. When hyperuricemia is chronic, large and gritty deposits, known as *tophi,* may form in the affected joint. Also, deposition of urate crystals in the kidney may cause renal damage. Fortunately, when gout is detected and treated early, the disease can be arrested and these chronic sequelae avoided.

In the absence of treatment, gout progresses through four stages. Stage one consists of *asymptomatic hyperuricemia.* Stage two is characterized by attacks of *acute gouty arthritis.* In stage three, symptoms subside; hence, this phase is known as the *asymptomatic intercritical period.* Stage four— *tophaceous gout*—is distinguished by development of tophi in joints.

Overview of Therapy

Five principal drugs are employed to treat gout. Two of these agents—*colchicine* and *indomethacin*—relieve inflammation. The other three—*allopurinol, probenecid,* and *sulfinpyrazone*—reduce hyperuricemia. Allopurinol reduces hyperuricemia by inhibiting uric acid formation. In contrast, probenecid and sulfinpyrazone promote uric acid excretion. Because they facilitate urate excretion, probenecid and sulfinpyrazone are called *uricosuric drugs.* In addition to the above agents, *glucocorticoids* and several *NSAIDs* may be employed.

Drug selection is based on the stage of gout being treated. During stage one—asymptomatic hyperuricemia—drugs are rarely employed; treatment is indicated only if symptoms develop or if blood levels of uric acid rise exceptionally high. Stage two—acute gouty arthritis—is treated with colchicine for the initial episode and indomethacin for subsequent attacks. Stage two may also be treated with NSAIDs and, in extreme cases, glucocorticoids. Allopurinol and the uricosuric drugs should be avoided during stage two. Treatment during stage three—the intercritical period—is variable. Some patients do well on small doses of colchicine, others respond well to antihyperuricemic agents, and still others require no treatment at all. The objective in treating stage four—chronic tophaceous gout—is to promote dissolution of tophi by lowering plasma levels of urate. Allopurinol is the preferred treatment. Drug therapy of gout is summarized in Table 69–3.

Pharmacology of the Drugs Used for Gout
Colchicine

Colchicine is an anti-inflammatory agent whose effects are specific for gout. The drug is not active against other inflammatory disorders. Colchicine is not an analgesic and does not relieve pain in conditions other than gout. The drug's principal adverse effect is GI toxicity.

Therapeutic Use. Colchicine has three distinct applications in gout. It can be used to (1) treat acute gouty attacks, (2) reduce the incidence of attacks in chronic gout, and (3) abort an impending attack.

Acute Gouty Arthritis. When taken in large doses, colchicine produces dramatic relief of acute gouty attacks. Within hours, patients whose pain had made movement impossible are able to walk. Inflammation disappears completely within 2 to 3 days. Administration may be either IV or oral. With IV administration, symptoms resolve sooner than with oral administration, and GI reactions are minimal. However, if extravasation occurs, IV colchicine can cause severe local necrosis.

Prophylaxis of Gouty Attacks. When taken during the asymptomatic intercritical period, small doses of colchicine (e.g., 0.5 to 1.0 mg/day) can decrease the frequency and intensity of acute attacks. Colchicine is also given for prophylaxis when therapy with antihyperuricemic agents is initiated. Why? Because there is a tendency for gouty episodes to increase at this time.

Abortion of an Impending Attack. During prophylactic therapy with colchicine, patients may experience prodromal signs of a developing gouty attack. If large amounts of colchicine (e.g., 0.5 mg every 2 hours) are taken immediately, the attack may be prevented. Consequently, it is recommended that patients with chronic gout always have colchicine tablets on hand.

TABLE 69–3 ■ Drug Therapy of Gout

Stage of Gout	Drug Therapy	Comments
Asymptomatic hyperuricemia	Drugs rarely indicated	
Acute gouty arthritis	Colchicine, indomethacin, and other NSAIDs	Colchicine is a drug of choice for the first episode. Indomethacin, which has fewer GI side effects, is preferred for subsequent attacks.
	Glucocorticoids	Glucocorticoids are reserved for patients who fail to respond to other agents.
Asymptomatic intercritical period	Colchicine Antihyperuricemics: Allopurinol Probenecid Sulfinpyrazone	Allopurinol is indicated if 24-hr urate excretion is high (>800 mg), indicating urate overproduction. A uricosuric agent (sulfinpyrazone, probenecid) is indicated if 24-hour urate excretion is <800 mg, indicating impaired urate excretion.
Chronic tophaceous gout	Allopurinol	The treatment objective is to decrease plasma urate below 7 mg/dl in males and 6 mg/dl in females.

Mechanism of Action. We do not fully understand the mechanisms by which colchicine relieves or prevents episodes of gout. It is clear that the drug does not influence either the production or excretion of uric acid. An important contributory action is inhibition of leukocyte infiltration; in the absence of leukocytes, there is no phagocytosis of uric acid and no subsequent release of lysosomal enzymes. Leukocyte migration is inhibited by disruption of microtubules, the structures required for cellular motility. Because microtubules are also required for cell division, colchicine is toxic to any tissue that has a large percentage of proliferating cells. Disruption of cell division underlies the GI toxicity of the drug.

Pharmacokinetics. Colchicine is readily absorbed following oral administration. At therapeutic doses, large amounts re-enter the intestine via the bile and intestinal secretions. The drug is excreted primarily in the feces.

Adverse Effects. The most characteristic signs of colchicine toxicity are *nausea, vomiting, diarrhea,* and *abdominal pain.* These responses, which occur during treatment of acute gouty attacks, result from injury to the rapidly proliferating cells of the GI epithelium. If GI symptoms develop, colchicine should be discontinued immediately, regardless of the status of joint pain. As noted, IV administration avoids most GI toxicity. Diarrhea from colchicine can be managed with opioids.

Precautions. Colchicine should be used with care in elderly and debilitated patients, and in patients with cardiac, renal, and GI diseases. Colchicine is classified in FDA Pregnancy Risk Category C (for oral use) and Category D (for IV use). Because the drug can cause fetal harm, it should be avoided during pregnancy unless the perceived benefits outweigh the potential risks to the fetus.

Preparations, Dosage, and Administration. Colchicine is dispensed in 0.6-mg oral tablets and in solution (0.5 mg/ml in 2-ml ampules) for IV use.

Oral. For an acute gouty attack, the dosage is 1.2 mg initially followed by 1.2 mg every 1 to 2 hours. Administration is repeated until pain is relieved or until signs of GI toxicity appear. The total dose should not exceed 8 mg. The usual dosage for prophylaxis is 0.6 mg/day. The dosage for aborting an impending attack is 0.6 mg every 2 hours.

Intravenous. Intravenous administration can be used to abort an acute gouty attack. In many cases, relief can be achieved with a single 2-mg injection. To minimize vascular injury, the contents of 1 ampule (1 mg) should be diluted in 20 ml of sterile 0.9% sodium chloride and then injected slowly (over 5 minutes or more). Extravasation can cause local necrosis with sloughing of skin and subcutaneous tissue. Accordingly, care must be taken to ensure that the IV line remains in place.

Indomethacin

Indomethacin [Indocin] is an NSAID used to treat acute gouty arthritis. For treatment of gout, the drug's efficacy is equivalent to that of colchicine. Like colchicine, indomethacin does not reduce hyperuricemia. Rather, it sup-

presses inflammation. In contrast to colchicine, indomethacin is devoid of acute severe GI effects. Consequently, indomethacin is considered a first-choice drug for treating acute gouty attacks. The most characteristic side effect is *severe frontal headache.* Like other NSAIDs, indomethacin can promote *gastric ulceration* and should be avoided by patients with a history of peptic ulcer disease. *Probenecid* delays excretion of indomethacin. Accordingly, if probenecid and indomethacin are used together, a reduction in indomethacin dosage may be required. For relief of acute gouty arthritis, the adult dosage is 50 mg initially followed by 25-mg doses 3 to 4 times a day. Pain is relieved rapidly (within 2 to 4 hours); swelling subsides in 3 to 5 days. After this, the dosage should be rapidly reduced, and then treatment should cease entirely. The pharmacology of indomethacin is discussed further in Chapter 67.

Allopurinol

Allopurinol [Zyloprim] is used to reduce blood levels of uric acid. The drug is indicated for primary hyperuricemia of gout and for hyperuricemia occurring secondary to cancer chemotherapy and certain blood dyscrasias (e.g., polycythemia vera, leukemia).

Mechanism of Action. Allopurinol and its major metabolite—alloxanthine—reduce uric acid levels by inhibiting uric acid production. Allopurinol and alloxanthine inhibit *xanthine oxidase,* an enzyme required for uric acid formation. As indicated in Figure 69–2, xanthine oxidase catalyzes the final two reactions that lead to formation of uric acid from DNA breakdown products.

Pharmacokinetics. Allopurinol is well absorbed following oral administration. Once absorbed, the drug undergoes rapid conversion to alloxanthine, an active metabolite. Because alloxanthine has a prolonged half-life (about 25 hours), therapeutic effects are long lasting. Consequently, allopurinol requires only once-a-day dosing.

Use in Chronic Tophaceous Gout. Allopurinol is the drug of choice for chronic tophaceous gout. By reducing production and blood levels of uric acid, the drug prevents tophus formation and promotes regression of tophi that have already formed, allowing joint function to improve. In addition, reversal of hyperuricemia decreases the risk of nephropathy that can occur from deposition of urate crystals in the kidney. During the initial months of treatment, allopurinol may *increase* the incidence of acute gouty arthritis; chances of an attack can be reduced by concurrent treatment with colchicine or indomethacin.

Use in Secondary Hyperuricemia. Hyperuricemia may occur secondary to treatment with anticancer drugs. Uric acid levels are elevated because of DNA breakdown following cell death. To minimize elevations in plasma urate levels, allopurinol should be administered prior to initiation of cancer chemotherapy. Allopurinol is also useful for treating hyperuricemia that may occur secondary to certain blood dyscrasias (e.g., polycythemia vera, myeloid metaplasia, leukemia).

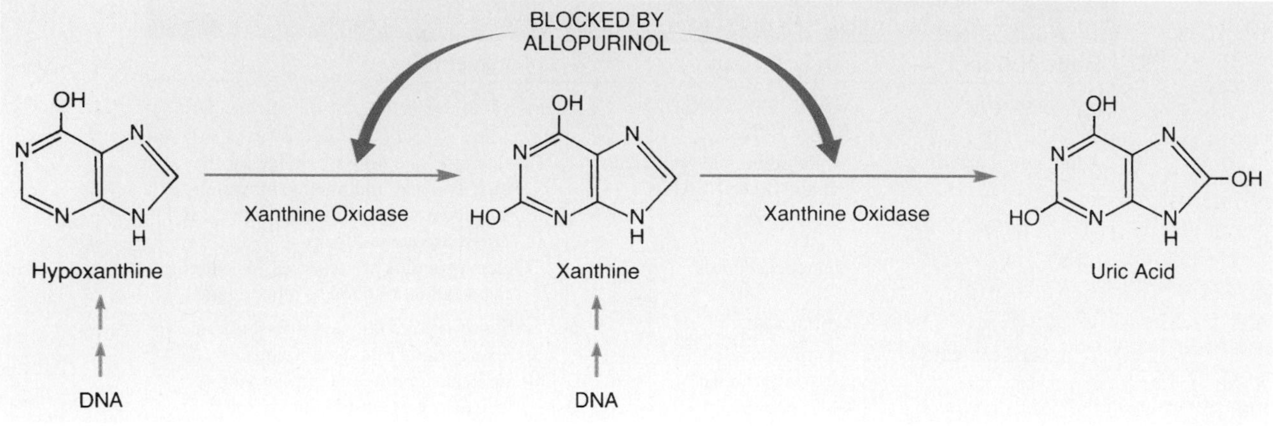

Figure 69–2 ■ **Reduction of uric acid formation by allopurinol.**

Adverse Effects. Allopurinol is generally well tolerated. The most serious toxicity is a rare but potentially fatal *hypersensitivity syndrome,* characterized by rash, fever, eosinophilia, and dysfunction of the liver and kidneys. If rash or fever develops, allopurinol should be discontinued immediately. Many patients recover spontaneously; others may require hemodialysis or glucocorticoid therapy.

Mild side effects seen occasionally include *GI reactions* (nausea, vomiting, diarrhea, abdominal discomfort) and *neurologic effects* (drowsiness, headache, metallic taste). Prolonged use (more than 3 years) may cause *cataracts;* periodic ophthalmic examinations are recommended.

Drug Interactions. Allopurinol can inhibit hepatic drug-metabolizing enzymes, thereby delaying the inactivation of other drugs. This interaction is of particular concern for patients taking *warfarin,* whose dosage should be reduced. Similarly, if allopurinol is combined with *mercaptopurine* or *azathioprine* in the treatment of cancer, dosages of mercaptopurine and azathioprine should be lowered by as much as 75%. The combination of allopurinol plus *ampicillin* is associated with a high incidence of rash; if rash develops, allopurinol should be discontinued immediately.

Preparations, Dosage, and Administration. Allopurinol [Zyloprim] is dispensed in 100- and 300-mg tablets.

For *treatment of chronic tophaceous gout,* the objective is to decrease plasma urate content to 7 mg/dl or less (in males) and 6 mg/dl or less (in females). Dosages should be individualized to achieve this goal. The usual initial dosage is 100 mg once a day. The dosage is then increased by 100-mg increments at intervals of 1 week until urate has been reduced to an acceptable level, usually at doses of 200 to 300 mg/day. To prevent renal injury, fluid intake should be sufficient to maintain a urine flow of at least 2 L/day.

For *secondary hyperuricemias in adults,* dosages range from 100 to 800 mg/day. For *children* ages 6 to 10 years who are undergoing cancer chemotherapy, the recommended dosage is 300 mg daily. The dosage for children under 6 years is 150 mg/day.

Probenecid

Actions and Uses. Probenecid (generic only) acts on renal tubules to inhibit reabsorption of uric acid. As a result, excretion of uric acid is increased and hyperuricemia is reduced. By lowering plasma urate levels, probenecid prevents formation of new tophi and facilitates regression of tophi that have already formed. The drug may exacerbate acute episodes of gout, and hence treatment should be delayed until the acute attack has been controlled. During the initial months of therapy, probenecid may induce acute attacks of gout. If an attack occurs, colchicine or indomethacin should be added to the regimen. In addition to its use in gout, probenecid may be employed to prolong the effects of penicillins and cephalosporins (by delaying their excretion by the kidneys).

Adverse Effects. Probenecid is well tolerated by most patients. Mild GI effects (nausea, vomiting, and anorexia) occur occasionally. These responses can be reduced by taking the drug with food. Hypersensitivity reactions, usually manifested as rash, develop in about 4% of patients. Renal injury may occur from deposition of urate in the kidney. The risk of kidney damage can be minimized by alkalinizing the urine and consuming 2.5 to 3 L of fluid daily during the first few days of treatment.

Drug Interactions. Aspirin and other salicylates interfere with the uricosuric action of probenecid. Accordingly, probenecid should not be used concurrently with these drugs. Probenecid inhibits the renal excretion of several drugs, including indomethacin and sulfonamides; dosages of these agents may require reduction.

Preparations, Dosage, and Administration. Probenecid is dispensed in 500-mg tablets. The initial dosage for adults is 250 mg twice daily for 1 week. The maintenance dosage is 500 mg twice daily. Administration with food decreases GI upset. Therapy should not be initiated during an acute gouty attack.

Sulfinpyrazone

Actions and Uses. Like probenecid, sulfinpyrazone [Anturane] is a uricosuric agent. The drug is used to reduce hyperuricemia in patients with *chronic* gout. Sulfinpyrazone lacks anti-inflammatory and analgesic actions and is of no benefit during an *acute* gouty attack. During the first few months of therapy, the drug may precipitate an acute gouty attack. Concurrent use of colchicine or indomethacin reduces this risk.

Adverse Effects. Gastrointestinal effects (nausea and abdominal pain) are common but rarely necessitate cessation of treatment. These reactions can be reduced by administering sulfinpyrazone with meals. Sulfinpyrazone can exacerbate GI ulcers, and hence is contraindicated in patients with active ulcers and should be used with caution in patients with a history of ulcer disease. As with probenecid, there is a risk of uric acid deposition in the kidney. This risk can be reduced by alkalinizing the urine and having the patient ingest large volumes of fluids.

Drug Interactions. *Salicylates* will counteract the uricosuric action of sulfinpyrazone, and hence should not be taken concurrently. Sulfinpyrazone can inhibit hepatic metabolism of *tolbutamide* (causing hypoglycemia) and *warfarin* (causing bleeding tendencies). If combined with sulfinpyrazone, these drugs may require a reduction in dosage.

Preparations, Dosage, and Administration. Sulfinpyrazone [Anturane] is dispensed in 100-mg tablets and 200-mg capsules. Administration with meals decreases GI side effects. The initial adult dosage is 100 to 200 mg twice daily. Maintenance dosages range from 200 to 800 mg/day in divided doses.

⁝⁚ KEY POINTS

- The objectives of RA therapy are to (1) reduce symptoms (pain, inflammation, and stiffness), (2) maintain joint function and range of motion, (3) minimize systemic involvement, and (4) delay disease progression.
- RA is treated with three classes of drugs: (1) nonsteroidal anti-inflammatory drugs (NSAIDs), (2) glucocorticoids, and (3) disease-modifying antirheumatic drugs (DMARDs).

- NSAIDs act quickly to relieve symptoms, but do not prevent joint injury and do not delay disease progression.
- Glucocorticoids act quickly and, according to recent evidence, may delay disease progression.
- DMARDs delay disease progression and reduce joint injury, but onset of effects is delayed.
- In the past, treatment of RA was initiated with NSAIDs alone; DMARDs were added only after NSAIDs could no longer control symptoms. Today's guidelines recommend initiating DMARDs within 3 months of RA diagnosis; the rationale is to delay joint degeneration and retard disease progression. During the DMARD latency period, NSAIDs (and sometimes glucocorticoids) are used to control symptoms.
- NSAIDs are much safer than glucocorticoids and most DMARDs.
- Because glucocorticoids cause serious toxicity when used long term, they are generally reserved for short-term use to (1) control symptoms while responses to DMARDs are developing or (2) supplement other drugs when symptoms flare.
- Second-generation NSAIDs (COX-2 inhibitors, coxibs) cause less GI ulceration than first-generation NSAIDs, but are more expensive.
- The doses of NSAIDs used for RA are much higher than the doses used to relieve pain or fever.
- Methotrexate, which acts relatively quickly, is considered the DMARD of first choice by many rheumatologists.
- Etanercept, a DMARD that neutralizes TNF, can prevent joint injury and delay RA progression. Unfortunately, the drug is expensive, inconvenient (owing to SC administration), and poses a risk of serious infection.
- Hydroxychloroquine can cause blindness secondary to retinal damage.

Drugs Affecting Calcium Levels and Bone Mineralization

TABLE 70–1 ▪▪ Daily Calcium Intake By Life-Stage Group		
	Calcium Intake (mg/day)	
Life-Stage Group*	Adequate Level†	Tolerable Upper Level‡
0–6 months	210	ND§
6–12 months	270	ND
1–3 years	500	2500
4–8 years	800	2500
9–18 years	1300	2500
19–50 years	1000	2500
51 years and older	1200	2500

*Values apply to males and females. For females, there is no change during pregnancy or lactation.

†Values for Adequate Intake (AI) are derived through experimental or observational data that show a mean calcium intake that appears to sustain a desired indicator of health, such as calcium retention in bone, for most members of the population group. AI values are employed for calcium because there are insufficient data to derive an Estimated Average Requirement (EAR). AI values are *not* equivalent to Recommended Dietary Allowances (RDAs).

‡The Tolerable Upper Intake level (UI) is defined as the maximum intake that is not likely to pose a risk of adverse health effects in almost all healthy individuals in a specified group. The UI is not intended to be a recommended level of intake. There is no established benefit to consuming calcium above the AI.

§ND = upper limit not determined owing to lack of data on adverse effects in this age group and concern regarding inability to handle excess calcium. To prevent excessive levels, calcium intake should be from food only.

Adapted from Food and Nutrition Board, Dietary Reference Intakes for Calcium, Phosphorus, Magnesium, Vitamin D and Fluoride. Washington, DC, National Academy Press, 1997.

It is difficult to exaggerate the biologic importance of calcium, an element critical to blood coagulation and to the functional integrity of bone, nerve, muscle, and the heart. Because these calcium-dependent processes can be seriously disrupted by alterations in calcium availability, we must maintain calcium levels within narrow limits. To regulate calcium, the body employs three factors: parathyroid hormone, vitamin D, and calcitonin. When these regulatory mechanisms fail, hypercalcemia or hypocalcemia results.

Our discussion of calcium and related drugs has four parts. First, we review calcium physiology. Second, we discuss the syndromes produced by disruption of calcium metabolism. Third, we discuss the pharmacologic agents used to treat calcium-related disorders. In the fourth, we consider osteoporosis, the most common calcium-related disorder.

CALCIUM PHYSIOLOGY

Functions and Daily Requirements

Calcium is critical to the function of the skeletal system, nervous system, muscular system, and cardiovascular system. In the skeletal system, calcium is required for the structural integrity of bone. In the nervous system, calcium helps regulate axonal excitability and transmitter release. In the muscular system, calcium participates in excitation-contraction coupling and contraction itself. In the cardio-

vascular system, calcium plays a role in myocardial contraction, vascular contraction, and coagulation of blood.

Given the widespread functions of calcium, it is important to have adequate calcium intake. Table 70–1 summarizes recommendations for calcium intake issued by the Food and Nutrition Board of the National Academy of Sciences in 1997. With the exception of children less than 4 years old, no one should consume less than 800 mg of calcium each day, and most people need 1000 mg/day or more. However, in a survey reported in 1994, Americans, on average, consume less than 800 mg/day in their diets, indicating a need to increase dietary intake or to use calcium supplements. Consuming sufficient calcium is especially important for reducing the risk of osteoporosis.

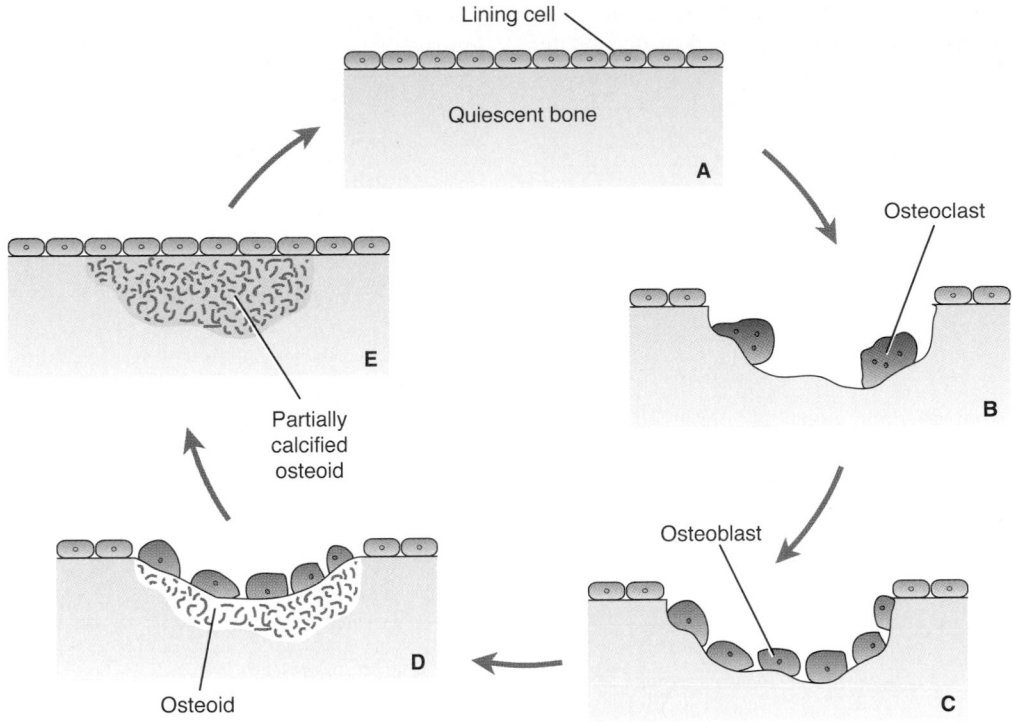

Lining cell

Quiescent bone

A

Osteoclast

B

Osteoblast

C

E

Partially
calcified
osteoid

D

Osteoid

Figure 70–1 ■ Bone remodeling cycle.
A, Quiescent bone with lining cells covering the surface. *B,* Resorption of old bone by multinucleated osteoclasts. *C,* Osteoblasts migrate to the absorption site. *D,* Osteoblasts deposit osteoid, a matrix of collagen and other proteins. *E,* Osteoid undergoes calcification.

Body Stores

Calcium in Bone. The vast majority of calcium in the body (more than 98%) is present in bone. Calcium is deposited in bone in the form of hydroxyapatite crystals. It is important to appreciate that bone—and the calcium it contains—is not static. Rather, bone undergoes continuous remodeling, a process in which old bone is resorbed, after which new bone is deposited (Fig. 70–1). The cells that resorb old bone are called *osteoclasts* and the cells that deposit new bone are called *osteoblasts*. Both cell types originate in the bone marrow. In adults, about 25% of trabecular bone (the honeycomb-like material in the center of bones) is replaced each year. In contrast, only 3% of cortical bone (the dense material that surrounds trabecular bone) is replaced annually.

Calcium in Blood. The normal value for total serum calcium is 10 mg/dl (2.5 mmol/L, 5 mEq/L). Of this total, about 50% is bound to proteins and other substances, and hence is unavailable for use. The remaining 50% is present as free, ionized calcium. It is the free calcium that participates in physiologic processes.

Absorption and Excretion

Absorption. Absorption of calcium takes place in the small intestine. Under normal conditions, about one-third of ingested calcium is absorbed. Absorption is increased by parathyroid hormone (PTH) and vitamin D (see below). In contrast, glucocorticoids decrease calcium absorption. Also, a variety of foods (e.g., spinach, whole grain cereals, bran) contain compounds that can interfere with calcium absorption.

Excretion. Calcium excretion is primarily renal. The amount lost is determined by glomerular filtration and by the extent of tubular reabsorption. Excretion can be reduced by PTH and vitamin D (see below). Conversely, excretion can be increased with loop diuretics (e.g., furosemide) and by loading with sodium. Calcitonin also augments calcium elimination (see below). In addition to renal excretion, substantial amounts of calcium can be lost through lactation.

Physiologic Regulation of Calcium Levels

Blood levels of calcium are tightly controlled. The body maintains calcium levels by adjusting the rates of three processes: (1) absorption of calcium from the intestine, (2) excretion of calcium by the kidney, and (3) resorption or deposition of calcium in bone. Regulation of these processes is under the control of three factors: *parathyroid hormone, vitamin D,* and *calcitonin.* It should be noted that preservation of plasma calcium levels takes priority over the calcium requirements of bone. Hence, if serum calcium is low, calcium will be resorbed from bone and transferred to the blood—even if resorption compromises the structural integrity of bone.

Parathyroid Hormone. PTH is released from the parathyroid glands in response to low levels of plasma calcium. The effect of PTH is to restore calcium levels to normal. PTH elevates serum calcium by three mechanisms: it (1) promotes calcium resorption from bone; (2) promotes reabsorption of calcium that had been filtered by the glomerulus; and (3) activates vitamin D, and thereby promotes absorption of calcium from the intestine. In addition to its effects on calcium, PTH reduces plasma levels of phosphate.

Vitamin D. Vitamin D is similar to PTH in two ways. First, both agents increase plasma calcium levels. Second, they increase calcium levels by the same mechanisms: (1) increasing calcium resorption from bone, (2) decreasing calcium excretion by the kidney, and (3) increasing calcium absorption from the intestine. Vitamin D differs from PTH in that vitamin D elevates plasma levels of phosphate, whereas PTH reduces phosphate levels. The actions of vitamin D are discussed further below.

Calcitonin. Calcitonin, a hormone produced by the thyroid gland, decreases plasma levels of calcium. Hence, calcitonin acts in opposition to PTH and vitamin D. Calcitonin is released from the thyroid gland when calcium levels in blood rise too high. Calcitonin lowers calcium levels by inhibiting the resorption of calcium from bone and increasing calcium excretion by the kidney. Unlike PTH and vitamin D, calcitonin does not influence calcium absorption.

CALCIUM-RELATED PATHOPHYSIOLOGY

Hypercalcemia

Clinical Presentation. Hypercalcemia is usually asymptomatic. When symptoms are present, they often involve the kidney (damage to tubules and collecting ducts, resulting in polyuria, nocturia, and polydipsia), GI tract (nausea, vomiting, and constipation), and central nervous system (lethargy and depression). Hypercalcemia may also result in dysrhythmias and deposition of calcium in soft tissues.

Causes. Hypercalcemia may arise from a variety of causes. Life-threatening elevations in plasma calcium are most often the result of cancer. Hyperparathyroidism is another common cause of severe hypercalcemia (see below). Additional causes include vitamin D intoxication, sarcoidosis, and use of thiazide diuretics.

Treatment. Calcium levels can be lowered with drugs that (1) promote urinary excretion of calcium, (2) decrease mobilization of calcium from bone, (3) decrease intestinal absorption of calcium, and (4) form complexes with free calcium in blood. For severe hypercalcemia, initial therapy consists of replacing lost fluid with IV saline, followed by diuresis using IV saline and a loop diuretic (e.g., furosemide). Other agents for lowering calcium include inorganic phosphates (which promote calcium deposition in bone and reduce calcium absorption); edetate disodium (EDTA, which binds calcium and promotes its excretion); glucocorticoids (which reduce intestinal absorption of calcium); and a group of drugs—calcitonin, bisphosphonates (e.g., pamidronate), plicamycin, inorganic phosphates, and gallium nitrate—that inhibit resorption of calcium from bone.

Hypocalcemia

Clinical Presentation and Cause. Hypocalcemia increases neuromuscular excitability. As a result, tetany, convulsions, and spasm of the pharynx and other muscles may occur. Hypocalcemia is caused most often by a deficiency of either PTH, vitamin D, or dietary calcium.

Treatment. Severe hypocalcemia is corrected by infusing an IV calcium preparation, usually calcium gluconate. Once calcium levels have been restored, an oral calcium salt (e.g., calcium citrate) can be given for maintenance. Vitamin D should be included in the regimen if there is a coexisting deficiency.

Rickets

Rickets is a disease of childhood brought on by either insufficient dietary vitamin D or limited exposure to sunlight. The disease is extremely rare in the United States. Rickets is characterized by defective bone growth and skeletal deformities. Bone abnormalities are caused as follows: (1) vitamin D deficiency results in reduced calcium absorption; (2) in response to hypocalcemia, PTH is released; (3) PTH restores serum calcium by promoting calcium resorption from bone, thereby causing bones to soften; and (4) stress on the softened bones caused by bearing weight results in deformity. Treatment consists of vitamin D replacement therapy.

Osteomalacia

Osteomalacia is the adult equivalent of rickets. Like rickets, this condition results from insufficient vitamin D. In the absence of vitamin D, mineralization of bone is impaired, resulting in back pain, bowing of the legs, fractures of the long bones, and kyphosis ("hunchback" curvature of the spine). Treatment consists of vitamin D replacement therapy.

Osteoporosis

Osteoporosis, the most common disorder of calcium metabolism, is characterized by low bone mass and increased bone fragility. Osteoporosis is discussed at length in a later section.

Paget's Disease of Bone

Clinical Presentation. Paget's disease of bone is a chronic condition seen most frequently in people over 40 years old. After osteoporosis, Paget's disease is the most common disorder of bone in the United States. The disease is characterized by increased bone resorption and replacement of the resorbed bone with abnormal bone. Increased bone turnover causes elevation in serum alkaline phosphatase (reflecting increased bone deposition) and increased urinary hydroxyproline (reflecting increased bone resorption). It is important to note that alterations in bone homeostasis do not occur evenly throughout the skeleton. Rather, alterations occur locally, most often in the pelvis, femur, spine, skull, and tibia. Although most people with Paget's disease are asymptomatic, about 10% experience bone pain and osteoarthritis; skeletal deformity may also occur. Bone weakness may lead to fractures. Neurologic complications may occur secondary to compression of the spinal cord, spinal nerves, and cranial nerves. If bone associated with hearing is affected, deafness may result.

Treatment. Asymptomatic patients are usually not treated. Mild pain can be managed with analgesics and anti-inflammatory agents. When the disease is more severe, a bisphosphonate (e.g., alendronate) is the treatment of choice. Calcitonin is an alternative. Both agents suppress bone resorption.

Hypoparathyroidism

Reductions in PTH usually result from inadvertent removal of the parathyroid glands during surgery on the thyroid gland. Lack of PTH causes hypocalcemia, which in turn may produce paresthesias, tetany, skeletal muscle spasm, laryngospasm, and convulsions. Symptoms can be relieved with calcium supplements (see *Hypocalcemia* above) and vitamin D.

Hyperparathyroidism

Clinical Presentation and Cause. Primary hyperparathyroidism usually results from parathyroid adenoma. The resulting increase in PTH secretion causes hypercalcemia and lowers serum phosphate. Hypercalcemia can cause skeletal muscle weakness, constipation (from decreased smooth muscle tone), and central nervous system (CNS) symptoms (lethargy and depression). Hypercalciuria and hyperphosphaturia are also present and may cause renal calculi. Loss of calcium and phosphate from bone may be sufficient to produce bone abnormalities.

Treatment. Primary hyperparathyroidism is usually treated by surgical resection of the parathyroid glands. If surgery is contraindicated, hypercalcemia can be managed with the drugs discussed above under *Hypercalcemia*.

DRUGS FOR DISORDERS INVOLVING CALCIUM

Calcium Salts

Calcium salts are available in oral and parenteral formulations for treatment of hypocalcemic states. The various calcium salts differ in their percentage of elemental calcium. These differences must be accounted for when determining dosage.

Oral Calcium Salts

Therapeutic Uses. Oral calcium preparations are used to treat *mild hypocalcemia.* In addition, calcium salts are taken as *dietary supplements.* People who may need supplementary calcium include children, adolescents, the elderly, postmenopausal women, and women who are pregnant or breast-feeding. As discussed in Chapter 59 (Box 59–1), calcium supplements may have the added benefit of reducing symptoms of *premenstrual syndrome*. Also, recent data indicate that calcium supplements can produce a significant, albeit moderate, reduction in recurrence of *colorectal adenomas*.

Adverse Effects. When calcium is taken chronically in high doses (3 to 4 gm/day), *hypercalcemia* can result. Hypercalcemia is most likely in patients who are also receiving large doses of vitamin D. Signs and symptoms include GI disturbances (nausea, vomiting, constipation), renal dysfunction (polyuria, nephrolithiasis), and CNS effects (lethargy, depression). In addition, hypercalcemia may cause cardiac dysrhythmias and deposition of calcium in soft tissue. Hypercalcemia can be minimized with frequent monitoring of plasma calcium content.

Drug Interactions. *Glucocorticoids* (e.g., prednisone) reduce absorption of oral calcium. Calcium reduces absorption of *tetracyclines,* and hence these agents should be administered at least 1 hour apart. Similarly, calcium reduces absorption of *thyroid hormone;* to ensure adequate thyroid hormone absorption, these agents should be administered several hours apart. *Thiazide diuretics* decrease renal calcium excretion and may thereby cause hypercalcemia.

Food Interactions. Certain foods contain substances that can suppress calcium absorption. One such substance—oxalic acid—is found in spinach, rhubarb, Swiss chard, and beets. Phytic acid, another depressant of calcium absorption, is present in bran and whole-grain cereals. Oral calcium should not be administered with these foods.

Preparations and Dosage. The calcium salts available for oral administration are listed in Table 70–2. Note that the dosage required to provide a particular amount of elemental calcium differs among preparations. Calcium carbonate, for example, has the highest percentage of calcium. Chewable tablets are preferred to standard tablets because of more consistent bioavailability. Bioavailability of *calcium citrate* appears especially good, owing to high solubility. When calcium supplements are taken, total daily calcium intake (dietary plus supplemental) should equal the values in Table 70–1. To help ensure adequate absorption, no more than 600 mg should be consumed at one time.

Parenteral Calcium Salts

Therapeutic Use. Parenteral calcium salts are given to raise calcium levels rapidly in patients with symptoms of severe hypocalcemia (i.e., hypocalcemic tetany). Three parenteral preparations are available:

calcium chloride, calcium gluconate, and *calcium gluceptate.* Intravenous calcium gluconate is the agent of choice.

Adverse Effects. *Calcium chloride* is highly irritating. Intramuscular injection may cause necrosis and sloughing; hence, this route must never be used. When the drug is administered IV, care must be taken to avoid extravasation, because local infiltration can produce severe injury. Although less irritating than calcium chloride, *calcium gluconate* can produce pain, sloughing, and abscess formation if administered IM. Overdose with any of the calcium salts can produce signs and symptoms of hypercalcemia (weakness, lethargy, nausea, vomiting, coma, and possibly death).

Drug Interactions. Parenteral calcium may cause severe bradycardia in patients taking *digoxin.* Accordingly, calcium infusions should be done slowly and cautiously in these patients. Several classes of compounds—*phosphates, carbonates, sulfates,* and *tartrates*—may cause calcium to precipitate, and hence should not be added to parenteral calcium solutions.

Dosage and Administration. All three parenteral calcium salts may be given IV; only calcium gluceptate can also be given IM. Solutions of calcium salts should be warmed to body temperature prior to administration. Intravenous injections should be done slowly (0.5 to 2 ml/min). Dosage forms and dosages are summarized in Table 70–3.

Vitamin D

The term *vitamin D* refers to two compounds: *ergocalciferol* (vitamin D_2) and *cholecalciferol* (vitamin D_3). Vitamin D_3 is the form of vitamin D produced naturally in humans when the skin is exposed to sunlight. Vitamin D_2 is a form of vitamin D that occurs in the plant kingdom. Vitamin D_2 is used as a drug and to fortify foods. Both forms of vitamin D produce nearly identical biologic effects. Therefore, rather than distinguishing between these compounds, we will use the term *vitamin D* to refer to vitamins D_2 and D_3 collectively.

Physiologic Actions

Vitamin D is an important regulator of calcium and phosphorus homeostasis. Vitamin D increases blood levels of both elements, primarily by increasing their intestinal absorption and promoting their mobilization from bone. In addition, vitamin

TABLE 70–2 ■ Oral Calcium Salts

Generic Name	Trade Names	Calcium Content	Dose Providing 500 mg Calcium
Calcium acetate	PhosLo	25%	2.0 gm
Calcium carbonate	Tums, Rolaids, others	40%	1.3 gm
Calcium citrate	Citracal	21%	2.4 gm
Calcium glubionate	Calcionate, Calciquid	6.6%	7.6 gm
Calcium gluconate*	—	9%	5.5 gm
Calcium lactate	Cal-lac	13%	3.8 gm
Tricalcium phosphate	Posture	39%	1.3 gm

*Also available in parenteral form (see Table 70–3).

TABLE 70–3 ■ Calcium Salts for Parenteral Administration

Generic Name	Dosage Form	Calcium per ml of Solution	Route	Usual Adult Dosage Range
Calcium chloride	10% solution	27 mg	IV	5–10 ml (135–270 mg Ca)
Calcium gluconate*	10% solution	9 mg	IV	5–20 ml (45–180 mg Ca)
Calcium gluceptate	22% solution	18 mg	IV IM	5–20 ml (90–360 mg Ca) 2–5 ml (36–90 mg Ca)

*Also available in an oral formulation (see Table 70–2).

D reduces renal excretion of calcium and phosphate; however, the quantitative significance of this effect is not clear. With usual doses of vitamin D, there is no net loss of calcium from bone; decalcification of bone occurs only when serum calcium concentrations cannot be maintained by increasing intestinal calcium absorption.

Sources and Daily Requirements

Vitamin D is obtained through the diet and by exposure to sunlight. In the United States, vitamin D is present as an additive in a variety of foods, including milk, other dairy products, cereals, and candy. Because of these supplements, younger Americans rarely experience nutritional vitamin D deficiency.

In 1997, the Food and Nutrition Board of the Institute of Medicine of the National Academy of Sciences issued revised guidelines for Vitamin D intake. People 50 years old or younger should consume 200 international units (IU) per day, those ages 51 through 70 should consume 400 IU/day, and people older than 70 should consume 600 IU/day.

Most older adults don't get enough vitamin D. They don't get enough sun exposure to make vitamin D, and they don't drink enough milk (the major dietary source of vitamin D) to meet daily requirements. Accordingly, older adults should use vitamin D supplements: 400 IU/day for those under 70, and 600 IU/day for those over 70. To avoid toxicity, daily intake should not exceed 800 IU.

Vitamin D Deficiency

Insufficient dietary vitamin D produces *rickets* in children and *osteomalacia* in adults. Signs and symptoms of these conditions are described above. Taking vitamin D can completely reverse the symptoms of both conditions, unless permanent deformity has already developed.

Activation of Vitamin D

In order to affect calcium and phosphate metabolism, vitamin D must first undergo activation. The extent of activation is carefully regulated, and is determined by calcium availability: When plasma calcium levels fall, activation of vitamin D is increased. The pathways for activating vitamins D_2 and D_3 are shown in Figure 70–2.

Let's begin consideration of vitamin D activation by focusing on the natural human vitamin (vitamin D_3). As shown in Figure 70–2, vitamin D_3 (cholecalciferol) is produced in the skin through the action of sunlight on provitamin D_3 (7-dehydrocholesterol). Neither provitamin D_3 nor vitamin D_3 itself possesses significant biologic activity. In the next reaction, enzymes in the liver convert cholecalciferol into calcifediol; calcifediol serves as a transport form of vitamin D_3 and possesses only slight biologic activity. In the final step of vitamin D activation, calcifediol is converted into the highly active calcitriol. This reaction occurs in the kidney and can be stimulated by (1) PTH, (2) a drop in dietary vitamin D, and (3) a fall in plasma levels of calcium.

Vitamin D_2 is activated by the same enzymes that activate vitamin D_3. As we saw with vitamin D_3, only the last compound in the series (in this case 1,25-dihydroxyergocalciferol) displays significant biologic activity.

Pharmacokinetics

Vitamin D is administered orally and absorbed from the small intestine. Bile is essential for absorption. Hence, in the absence of sufficient bile, IM administration may be required. Vitamin D is transported in the blood com-

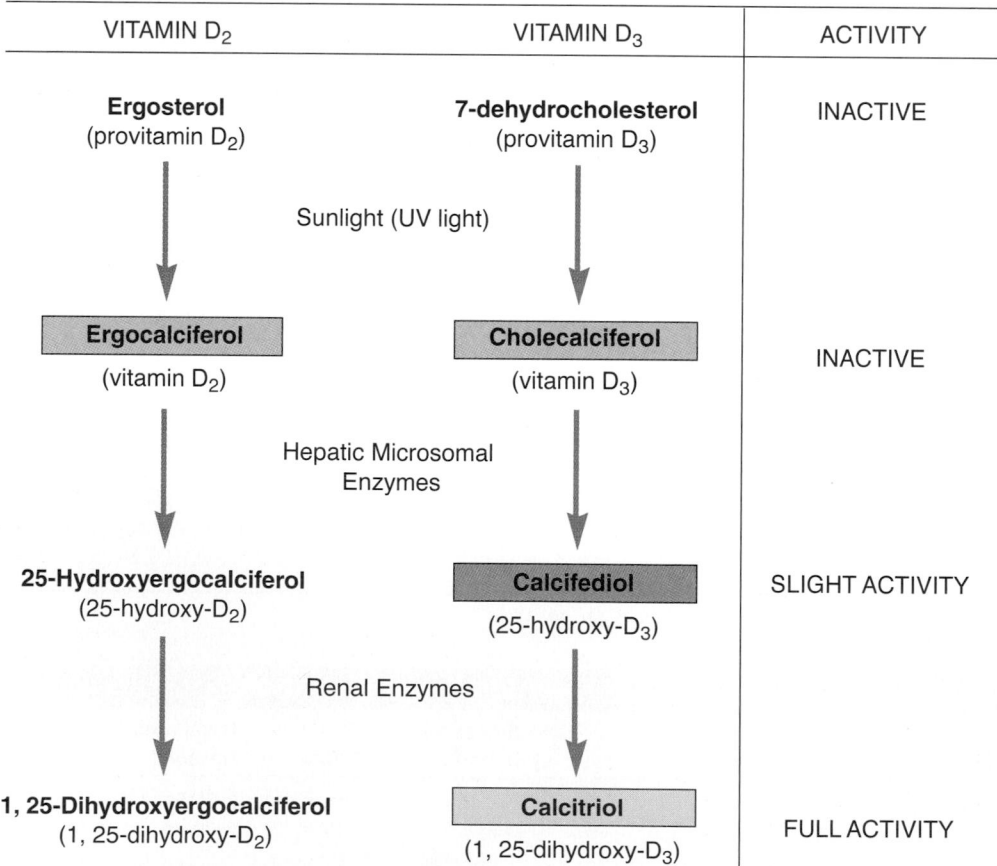

Figure 70–2 ■ Vitamin D activation.
Ergosterol is found in yeasts and fungi. 7-Dehydrocholesterol is present in the skin. (Colored boxes indicate forms of vitamin D used therapeutically.)

plexed with vitamin D–binding protein. Storage of vitamin D occurs primarily in the liver. As discussed, vitamin D undergoes metabolic activation. Reactions that occur in the liver produce the major transport form of vitamin D. A later reaction (in the kidney) produces the fully active vitamin. Excretion of vitamin D is via the bile. Very little leaves in the urine.

Viewing Vitamin D as a Hormone

Although referred to as a vitamin, vitamin D has all the characteristics of a hormone. With sufficient exposure to sunlight, the body can manufacture all the vitamin D it needs. Hence, under ideal conditions, external sources of vitamin D are probably unnecessary. Following its production in the skin, vitamin D travels to other locations (liver and kidney) for activation. Like other hormones, activated vitamin D then travels to various sites in the body (bone, intestine, and kidney) to exert regulatory actions. Also like other hormones, vitamin D undergoes feedback regulation: as plasma levels of calcium fall, activation of vitamin D increases; when plasma levels of calcium return to normal, activation of vitamin D declines.

Toxicity (Hypervitaminosis D)

Vitamin D toxicity (hypervitaminosis D) can be produced by doses of vitamin D in excess of 1000 IU/day (in infants) and 50,000 IU/day (in adults). Poisoning occurs most commonly in children; causes include accidental ingestion and excessive administration of vitamin D by parents. Doses of potentially toxic magnitude are also encountered clinically. When huge therapeutic doses are used, the margin of safety is small, and patients should be monitored closely for signs of poisoning.

Clinical Presentation. Most signs and symptoms of vitamin D toxicity occur secondary to hypercalcemia. Early responses include weakness, fatigue, nausea, vomiting, and constipation. With persistent hypercalcemia, kidney function is affected, resulting in polyuria, nocturia, and proteinuria. Calcium deposition in soft tissues can damage the heart, blood vessels, and lungs; calcium deposition in the kidneys can cause nephrolithiasis. Very large doses of vitamin D can cause decalcification of bone, resulting in osteoporosis; mobilization of bone calcium can occur despite the presence of high calcium concentrations in blood. In children, vitamin D poisoning can suppress growth for 6 months or longer.

Treatment. Treatment consists of immediate discontinuation of vitamin D, high fluid intake, and institution of a low-calcium diet. Glucocorticoids may be given to suppress calcium absorption. If hypercalcemia is severe, renal excretion of calcium can be accelerated using a combination of IV saline and furosemide (a diuretic).

Therapeutic Uses

The primary indications for vitamin D are nutritional rickets, osteomalacia, and hypoparathyroidism. Other applications include vitamin D–resistant rickets, vitamin D–dependent rickets, and renal osteodystrophy.

Preparations, Dosage, and Administration

There are seven preparations of vitamin D. Four of these—ergocalciferol, cholecalciferol, calcifediol, and calcitriol—are identical to forms of vitamin D that occur naturally. The other three—dihydrotachysterol, paricalcitol, and doxercalciferol—are synthetic derivatives of natural vitamin D. (The naturally occurring preparations are highlighted in colored boxes in Fig. 70–2.) Individual vitamin D preparations differ in their clinical applications. Indications for specific preparations are given below.

Vitamin D is usually administered by mouth. Intramuscular injections (of ergocalciferol) may also be used. Dosage is usually prescribed in international units. (One IU is equivalent to the biologic activity in 0.025 μg of vitamin D_3.) Daily dosages of vitamin D range from 400 IU (for dietary supplementation) to as high as 500,000 IU (for vitamin D–resistant rickets).

Ergocalciferol (Vitamin D₂). Ergocalciferol [Calciferol, Drisdol] is used for hypoparathyroidism, vitamin D–resistant rickets, and familial hypophosphatemia. Ergocalciferol is dispensed in capsules (50,000 IU), oral solution (8000 IU/ml), and solution for injection (500,000 IU/ml). The dosage for vitamin D–resistant rickets ranges from 12,000 to 500,000 IU daily. The dosage for hypoparathyroidism ranges from 50,000 to 200,000 IU daily (together with 4 gm of calcium lactate given 6 times/day).

Cholecalciferol (Vitamin D₃). Vitamin D_3 [Delta-D] is given as a dietary supplement and for the prophylaxis and treatment of vitamin D deficiency. Cholecalciferol is available in tablets containing 400 and 1000 IU.

Calcifediol (25-Hydroxy-D₃). Calcifediol [Calderol] is indicated for the management of metabolic bone disease and hypocalcemia in patients undergoing chronic renal dialysis. Calcifediol is available in capsules (20 and 50 μg) for oral use. The initial dosage is 300 to 350 μg/week (administered in divided doses on a daily or every-other-day schedule). For maintenance, daily doses of 50 to 100 μg are adequate for most patients.

Calcitriol (1,25-Dihydroxy-D₃). Calcitriol [Rocaltrol, Calcijex] is indicated for treatment of hypoparathyroidism and management of hypocalcemia in patients undergoing chronic renal dialysis. The drug is dispensed in capsules (0.25 and 0.5 μg), oral solution (1 μg/ml), and solution for injection (1 and 2 μg/ml). For dialysis patients, daily doses of 0.5 to 1.0 μg are usually adequate. The initial dosage for hypoparathyroidism is 0.25 μg/day.

Dihydrotachysterol. Dihydrotachysterol (DHT) is a synthetic derivative of vitamin D_2. DHT is interesting in that, unlike vitamins D_2 and D_3, it doesn't require renal enzymes for activation; metabolic conversion by the liver is all that is needed to render DHT fully active. DHT is indicated for hypoparathyroidism, postoperative tetany, and tetany of unknown cause. DHT is available in tablets (0.125, 0.2, and 0.4 mg), capsules (0.125 mg), and oral solution (0.2 mg/ml). Preparations are marketed under the trade names DHT and Hytakerol.

Doxercalciferol. Doxercalciferol [Hectorol] is indicated for prevention and treatment of secondary hyperparathyroidism in patients undergoing chronic renal dialysis. The drug is available in 2.5-μg capsules. Dosing must be carefully tailored to the patient. The recommended initial dose is 10 μg 3 times weekly administered at dialysis. Dosage may be gradually increased to a maximum of 20 μg 3 times a week.

Paricalcitol. Like doxercalciferol, paricalcitol [Zemplar] is indicated for prevention and treatment of secondary hyperparathyroidism in patients undergoing chronic renal dialysis. The drug is available in solution (5 μg/ml) for administration by IV bolus. The recommended initial dosage is 0.04 to 0.1 μg/kg given any time during dialysis—but no more frequently than every other day. Dosage may be gradually increased every 2 to 4 weeks. Doses as high as 0.24 μg/kg have been used safely.

Calcitonin-Salmon

Calcitonin-salmon [Calcimar, Miacalcin, Osteocalcin, Salmonine], a form of calcitonin derived from salmon, is similar in structure to calcitonin synthesized by the human thyroid. Salmon calcitonin produces the same metabolic effects as human calcitonin but has a longer half-life and greater milligram potency. The drug is available for administration by injection and by nasal spray. Both forms are extremely safe.

Actions

Calcitonin has two principal actions: it (1) inhibits the activity of osteoclasts, and thereby decreases bone resorption; and (2) inhibits tubular resorption of calcium, and thereby increases calcium excretion. As a result of decreasing bone turnover, calcitonin decreases alkaline phosphatase in blood and increases hydroxyproline in urine.

Therapeutic Uses

Osteoporosis. Calcitonin-salmon, administered by nasal spray, is indicated for *treatment* of established postmenopausal osteoporosis—but not for prevention. Benefits derive from suppressing bone resorption. The treatment program should include supplemental calcium and adequate intake of vitamin D. Use of calcitonin for osteoporosis is discussed further under *Osteoporosis*.

Paget's Disease of Bone. Calcitonin is helpful in moderate to severe Paget's disease and is the drug of choice for rapid relief of pain associated with this disorder. Benefits occur secondary to inhibition of osteoclasts. Neurologic symptoms caused by spinal cord compression may be reduced.

Hypercalcemia. Calcitonin can lower plasma calcium levels in patients with hypercalcemia secondary to hyperparathyroidism, vitamin D toxicity, and cancer. Levels of calcium (and phosphorus) are lowered owing to inhibition of bone resorption and increased excretion of calcium by the kidneys. Although calcitonin is effective against hypercalcemia, it is not a preferred treatment.

Adverse Effects

Calcitonin is very safe. With intranasal administration, nasal dryness and irritation are the most common complaints. Following parenteral (IM, SC) administration, about 10% of patients experience nausea, which diminishes with time. An additional 10% have inflammatory reactions at the site of injection. Flushing of the face and hands may also occur. When salmon calcitonin is taken for a year or longer, neutralizing antibodies often develop. In some patients, these antibodies bind enough calcitonin to prevent therapeutic effects.

Preparations, Dosage, and Administration

Intranasal Spray. Salmon calcitonin for intranasal use [Miacalcin] is available in a metered-dose dispenser that delivers 200 IU/activation. This formulation is approved only for *postmenopausal osteoporosis.* The dosage is 200 IU (1 spray) each day, alternating nostrils daily.

Parenteral. Salmon calcitonin for parenteral use [Calcimar, Miacalcin, Osteocalcin, Salmonine] is dispensed in 2-ml vials containing 200 IU/ml. Administration may be IM or SC. Dosages are the same for both routes. Dosages for specific indications are

- *Postmenopausal osteoporosis*—100 IU/day
- *Paget's disease of bone*—the initial dosage is 100 IU/day; the maintenance dosage is 50 IU either daily or every other day
- *Hypercalcemia*—the initial dosage is 4 IU/kg every 12 hours; the maximal dosage is 8 IU/kg every 6 hours

Bisphosphonates

Bisphosphonates are structural analogs of pyrophosphate (Fig. 70–3), a normal constituent of bone. These drugs undergo incorporation into bone, and then inhibit bone resorption by decreasing the activity of osteoclasts. Principal indications are postmenopausal osteoporosis, glucocorticoid-induced os-

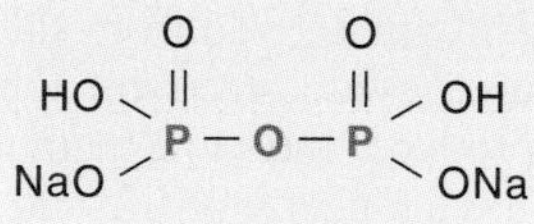

Pyrophosphate

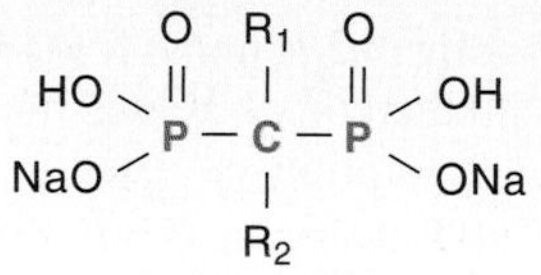

Bisphosphonate
(general structure)

Figure 70–3 ■ Structure of pyrophosphate and bisphosphonates.

teoporosis, Paget's disease of bone, and hypercalcemia of malignancy. Also, they may help prevent and treat bone metastases in patients with breast cancer (see Chapter 99). Although bisphosphonates are generally very safe, serious adverse effects can occur. All bisphosphonates are poorly absorbed from the GI tract, especially in the presence of food. At this time, six bisphosphonates are approved for use in the United States (Table 70–4). As shown in the table, these drugs differ significantly in their relative potencies.

Alendronate

Alendronate [Fosamax], a widely used bisphosphonate, will serve as our prototype for the family. The drug is approved for postmenopausal osteoporosis, male osteoporosis, glucocorticoid-induced osteoporosis, and Paget's disease of bone. Oral bioavailability is poor. Although alendronate is generally safe, esophageal ulceration has occurred in some patients.

Pharmacokinetics. Alendronate is administered orally, but bioavailability is very low (only 0.7%). If the drug is taken with solid food, essentially none is absorbed. Even coffee or orange juice can decrease absorption by 60%. Of the small fraction that undergoes absorption, about 50% is taken up rapidly by bone; the remaining 50% is excreted unchanged in the urine. Once alendronate has become incorporated into bone, it remains there for many years.

Mechanism of Action. Alendronate suppresses resorption of bone by decreasing both the number and activity of osteoclasts. Several mechanisms are involved. As osteoclasts begin to resorb alendronate-containing bone, they ingest some of the drug, which then acts on the osteoclasts to inhibit their activity. In addition to inhibiting osteoclast activity, alendronate reduces the *number* of osteoclasts by (1) acting directly to decrease their recruitment and (2) acting on osteoblasts, which then produce an inhibitor of osteoclast formation.

Therapeutic Use. Postmenopausal Osteoporosis. Alendronate is approved for both the prevention and treatment of osteoporosis in postmenopausal women. Benefits derive from decreasing bone resorption by osteoclasts. The use of alendronate for osteoporosis is discussed further under *Osteoporosis.*

Osteoporosis in Men. Alendronate is now approved for treating osteoporosis in men. When tested in men with osteoporosis, the drug increased bone mineral density (BMD), reduced vertebral fractures, and decreased loss of height.

TABLE 70–4 ■ Bisphosphonates: Relative Potencies, Routes, and Uses						
			Major Therapeutic Uses*			
Drug Name	Relative Potency	Route	Postmenopausal Osteoporosis	Paget's Disease	Hypercalcemia of Malignancy	Glucocorticoid-Induced Bone Loss
Etidronate [Didronel]	1	PO, IV	I	A	A	I
Tiludronate [Skelid]	10	PO	I	A		
Pamidronate [Aredia]	100	IV	I	A	A	I
Alendronate [Fosamax]	1000	PO	A†	A		A
Risedronate [Actonel]	1000	PO	A	A		A
Zoledronate [Zometa]	1000	IV	I		A	

*A = FDA-approved indication, I = investigational use.
†Also approved for osteoporosis in men.

Glucocorticoid-Induced Osteoporosis. Alendronate is approved for treatment of bone loss caused by long-term use of glucocorticoids (e.g., prednisone). Osteoporosis is a common complication of glucocorticoid therapy, leading to fractures in at least 50% of patients. Studies indicate that alendronate helps restore lost bone, but we don't know if it also reduces the risk of fractures. Preliminary data indicate that alendronate can help *prevent* glucocorticoid-induced loss of bone. However, the drug is not yet approved for this use.

Paget's Disease of Bone. Alendronate is a first-line drug for treating Paget's disease. Continuous daily therapy for 3 months produces a 50% decrease in serum alkaline phosphatase, indicating a substantial reduction in bone turnover. As in osteoporosis, benefits derive from inhibiting bone resorption by osteoclasts.

Adverse Effects. With the exception of causing esophagitis, alendronate is devoid of serious adverse effects. When used in the low doses employed for osteoporosis, alendronate causes no more side effects than placebo. At the higher doses employed in Paget's disease, mild GI disturbances are common.

Esophagitis, sometimes resulting in ulceration, is alendronate's most serious adverse effect. Fortunately, esophagitis is rare, occurring in only 1 of every 10,000 patients. The cause of injury is prolonged contact with the esophageal mucosa, which can occur if alendronate fails to pass completely through the esophagus. Reasons for incomplete passage include taking the drug with insufficient water, taking the drug in a supine position, lying down after taking the drug, and having a pre-existing esophageal disorder that impedes drug passage. To promote complete passage, and thereby minimize risk of esophagitis, alendronate should be administered according to recommended guidelines (see below). Patients should be instructed to discontinue alendronate and contact the physician if they experience symptoms of esophageal injury (difficulty swallowing, pain upon swallowing, or new or worsening heartburn). Because of the risk of esophagitis, alendronate is contraindicated for patients with esophageal disorders that could prevent successful swallowing and for patients who are unable to sit or stand for at least 30 minutes.

In patients with Paget's disease, alendronate can induce *hyperparathyroidism.* How? By inhibiting accelerated bone resorption, alendronate causes blood levels of calcium to fall; in response, secretion of PTH is increased. To prevent hyperparathyroidism, patients should receive calcium supplements.

Administration. Proper administration is necessary to maximize bioavailability and minimize the risk of esophagitis. To maximize bioavailability, alendronate should be taken in the morning before breakfast (i.e., on an empty stomach); no food, including orange juice or coffee, should be consumed for at least 30 minutes. To minimize the risk of esophagitis, patients should be instructed to

- Take alendronate with a full glass of water
- Remain upright (seated or standing) for at least 30 minutes and at least until completing their first meal of the day
- Avoid chewing or sucking the tablet

Preparations and Dosage. Alendronate [Fosamax] is available in tablets (5, 10, 35, 40, and 70 mg). Dosing for *osteoporosis* in women or men may be done once daily (in the morning) or once weekly (on the same morning each week). Once-weekly dosing, which is just as effective as once-daily

dosing, is possible because alendronate undergoes incorporation into bone, where it remains and acts for many weeks. Dosages are as follows:

- *Osteoporosis in postmenopausal women*—for *prevention*, 5 mg once daily or 35 mg once weekly; for *treatment*, 10 mg once daily or 70 mg once weekly
- *Osteoporosis in men*—10 mg once daily or 70 mg once weekly
- *Paget's disease*—40 mg once daily for 6 months for men or women
- *Glucocorticoid-induced osteoporosis*—5 mg once daily (for men, premenopausal women, and postmenopausal women taking estrogen replacement) or 10 mg once daily (for postmenopausal women who are not taking estrogen)

Pamidronate

Pamidronate [Aredia] is a bisphosphonate approved for IV therapy of *Paget's disease, hypercalcemia of malignancy,* and *osteolytic bone metastases.* Because of dose-related GI intolerance (e.g., mucosal erosion in the esophagus and stomach), pamidronate is not given orally.

Therapeutic Use and Dosage. Hypercalcemia of Malignancy. Many cancer cells release factors that stimulate resorption of bone by osteoclasts. The result is hypercalcemia, increased risk of fractures, and bone pain. By inhibiting osteoclast activity, pamidronate can blunt cancer-mediated bone resorption, and thereby reduce blood levels of calcium. The recommended dosage is 60 to 90 mg infused over 2 to 24 hours. Longer infusion times reduce the risk of renal injury.

Paget's Disease of Bone. Like other bisphosphonates, pamidronate can decrease bone resorption in patients with Paget's disease. The dosage is 30 mg infused slowly (over at least 4 hours) on 3 consecutive days. With this dosage, the mean duration of remission is 14 months.

Adverse Effects. Intravenous pamidronate is devoid of serious adverse effects. In some patients, the first dose causes transient flu-like symptoms. If pamidronate is not infused with sufficient fluid, venous irritation can occur. In contrast to etidronate, pamidronate does not interfere with bone mineralization. Because pamidronate inhibits accelerated bone resorption of Paget's disease, blood levels of calcium will fall, thereby triggering increased release of PTH; to prevent hyperparathyroidism, patients should receive supplemental calcium.

Etidronate

Etidronate [Didronel, Didronel IV] is approved for *Paget's disease* and *hypercalcemia of malignancy.* The drug is also used for glucocorticoid-induced and postmenopausal osteoporosis, although it is not approved for these disorders. In patients with highly active Paget's disease, etidronate can produce moderate clinical improvement. Unfortunately, when the drug is discontinued, relapse may occur rapidly. Side effects include abdominal cramps, diarrhea, nausea, and increased bone pain. In addition, etidronate causes defective mineralization of newly formed bone (osteomalacia), and can thereby increase the risk of fractures.

Preparations, Dosage, and Administration. Etidronate is available for oral and IV administration. Oral therapy is used for both Paget's disease and hypercalcemia of malignancy (HCM); IV therapy is used for hypercalcemia of malignancy only.

Oral. Etidronate [Didronel] is available in 200- and 400-mg tablets. As with all other bisphosphonates, oral bioavailability is low (less than 6%). To maximize absorption, the following should be avoided for 2 hours after taking etidronate: food, antacids high in metals (e.g., calcium, iron, magnesium, aluminum), and vitamins that contain mineral supplements.

Patients with *Paget's disease* may be given either (1) 5 to 10 mg/kg/day (for no more than 6 months), or (2) 11 to 20 mg/kg/day (for no more than 3 months). Treatment can be repeated, but not until 90 days have elapsed since completion of the prior course.

The oral dosage for *hypercalcemia of malignancy* is 20 mg/kg/day for 30 days. Oral therapy is not initiated until completion of IV therapy (see below).

Intravenous. Etidronate [Didronel IV] is dispensed in solution (300 mg/6 ml) for IV use. The appropriate dose should be diluted in 250 ml of sterile water. Administration is by slow infusion, lasting 2 hours or more. For patients with HCM, the usual dosage is 7.5 mg/kg infused once daily on 3 consecutive days. If hypercalcemia recurs, another 3-day course can be given, but at least 7 days must separate each course. Oral therapy may be initiated on the day after the last course is completed.

Tiludronate

Actions and Uses. Tiludronate [Skelid] is an oral bisphosphonate approved for *Paget's disease of bone.* In Paget's disease patients, the drug decreases abnormal bone growth and, unlike etidronate, does so without interfering with bone mineralization. Like other bisphosphonates, tiludronate undergoes incorporation into bone. When osteoclasts resorb this bone, they ingest the drug, which then inhibits further osteoclast-mediated bone resorption.

Pharmacokinetics. Tiludronate is administered by mouth and bioavailability is low (6%). Food further decreases absorption. In blood, about 90% of the drug is bound to serum proteins, mainly albumin. Tiludronate is eliminated largely unchanged in the urine.

Adverse Effects. The most common side effects are nausea (9.3%), diarrhea (9.3%), and dyspepsia (5.3%). These are usually mild and rarely require cessation of treatment. Other side effects include chest pain, edema, paresthesias, hyperparathyroidism, vomiting, and flatulence.

Preparations, Dosage, and Administration. Tiludronate [Skelid] is dispensed in 200-mg tablets. The dosage is 400 mg once a day for 3 months. Patients should be instructed to take tiludronate with a full glass of *water*. Also, they should not eat for 2 hours before or after taking the drug. Because calcium, aspirin, and antacids (containing calcium, aluminum, or magnesium) greatly reduce tiludronate absorption, these drugs should not be administered within 2 hours of administering tiludronate.

Risedronate

Actions and Uses. Risedronate [Actonel] is an oral bisphosphonate approved for *postmenopausal osteoporosis, glucocorticoid-induced osteoporosis,* and *Paget's disease of bone.* As with other bisphosphonates, benefits derive from inhibiting osteoclast-mediated resorption of bone. In postmenopausal women with osteoporosis, risedronate increases bone mineral density and reduces the risk of vertebral and nonvertebral fractures.

Pharmacokinetics. Like all other bisphosphonates, risedronate is poorly absorbed from the GI tract. Absorption is only 1% under fasting conditions, and even worse in the presence of food. Most of the absorbed drug becomes incorporated into bone. The rest is excreted unchanged in the urine. Risedronate in bone persists for months to years.

Adverse Effects. The most common adverse effects are arthralgia (32%), diarrhea (20%), headache (18%), rash (12%), nausea (10%), and a flu-like syndrome (10%). Like alendronate, risedronate poses a risk of esophagitis.

Preparations, Dosage, and Administration. Risedronate [Actonel] is available in 30-mg tablets. As with alendronate, risedronate can be taken daily or once weekly for prevention or treatment of osteoporosis. Each dose should be taken in the morning with a full glass of water, and before ingesting the first food or fluids of the day (except for water). To minimize possible adverse GI effects, patients should be upright when swallowing risedronate, and should not lie down for at least 30 minutes. Because calcium and antacids (containing calcium, aluminum, or magnesium) greatly reduce absorption, these should not be administered within 2 hours of administering risedronate. Dosages are as follows:

- *Postmenopausal osteoporosis (prevention or treatment)*—5 mg once daily or 35 mg once weekly
- *Glucocorticoid-induced osteoporosis in men or women (prevention or treatment)*—5 mg once daily
- *Paget's disease in men or women*—30 mg once daily for 2 months; if needed, a second 2-month course can be given, provided at least 2 months have elapsed since completing the first course

Zoledronate

Actions and Uses. Zoledronate [Zometa], also called zoledronic acid, is a new IV bisphosphonate approved for *hypercalcemia of malignancy* (HCM). Like other bisphosphonates, zoledronate undergoes incorporation into bone, where it remains for months or even years. When osteoclasts ingest the drug, it inhibits their activity, and thereby prevents bone resorption. In patients with HCM, inhibition of bone resorption lowers calcium levels in blood. In one clinical trial, zoledronate normalized serum calcium in 88% of patients within 10 days of a single infusion. Compared with pamidronate, another bisphosphonate used for HCM, zoledronate has three advantages. Specifically, zoledronate has a faster onset, longer duration, and, perhaps most importantly, a shorter infusion time (15 minutes vs. 2 to 4 hours), and hence is much more convenient.

Although not approved for decreasing bone resorption in *osteoporosis,* zoledronate could represent a huge therapeutic advance. In a preliminary study, a single, 15-minute infusion suppressed bone resorption for over 12 months, suggesting we might be able to manage osteoporosis with just one dose a year—compared with daily or weekly dosing with other bisphosphonates.

Adverse Effects. Adverse effects are similar to those of IV pamidronate. The most common reaction is transient fever (44%), followed by nausea (29%), constipation (26%), dyspnea (22%), abdominal pain (16%), and

bone and joint pain (12%). In addition, zoledronate can cause clinically significant reductions in serum levels of calcium, phosphorus, and magnesium. Accordingly, levels of these elements should be followed and corrected when indicated.

Zoledronate can cause dose-dependent damage to the kidney, which can progress to outright renal failure. The risk is higher at shorter infusion times. To minimize risk, dosage should be kept low (4 mg or less per infusion) and the infusion time should be 15 minutes or longer. In addition, the patient should be adequately hydrated before the infusion. To monitor for renal damage, creatinine clearance should be determined at baseline and periodically after the infusion.

Preparations, Dosage, and Administration. Zoledronate [Zometa] is dispensed as a powder (4 mg in single-use vials) that must be reconstituted with 5 ml of sterile water, and then diluted in 100 ml of 0.9% sodium chloride or 5% dextrose. The maximum recommended dose is 4 mg. All doses—maximum or smaller—must be given as a single IV infusion over *no less than 15 minutes*. If hypercalcemia does not resolve, or if it resolves and then returns, a second infusion can be given, but no sooner than 7 days after the first infusion, and only if kidney function is adequate.

Raloxifene

Raloxifene [Evista] is an important alternative to estrogen for the prevention and treatment of osteoporosis. The drug belongs to a class of agents known as *selective estrogen receptor modulators* (SERMs)—drugs that exert estrogenic effects in some tissues and antiestrogenic effects in others. Like estrogen, raloxifene preserves bone mineral density (BMD) and reduces plasma levels of cholesterol. However, in contrast to estrogen, which promotes cancer of the breast and endometrium, raloxifene may confer protection against these cancers. Tamoxifen, a SERM used to prevent and treat breast cancer, is discussed in Chapter 99.

Mechanism of Action

Raloxifene and other SERMs are structurally similar to estrogen, and hence can bind to estrogen receptors. However, unlike estrogen itself, which functions as an agonist in all tissues, SERMs function as agonists in some tissues and antagonists in others. Hence, SERMs can either mimic or block the actions of estrogen, depending on the SERM and the tissue involved. Raloxifene mimics the effects of estrogen on bone, lipid metabolism, and blood clotting, and blocks estrogen effects in the breast and endometrium.

Pharmacokinetics

Raloxifene is administered by mouth and 60% is absorbed. However, because of extensive first-pass metabolism, absolute bioavailability is below 2%. Excretion is fecal. The drug's half-life is about 28 hours.

Therapeutic Uses

Postmenopausal Osteoporosis. Like estrogen, raloxifene is used to prevent and treat osteoporosis in postmenopausal women. The drug can preserve or increase BMD, although not as effectively as estrogen. Raloxifene reduces the risk of *spinal* fractures by 55%, but does not reduce the risk of fractures at other sites. Use of raloxifene in osteoporosis is discussed further under *Osteoporosis.*

Breast Cancer. Preliminary data indicate that raloxifene protects against estrogen receptor (ER)–positive breast cancer. In animal models, raloxifene inhibits estrogen-stimulated growth of mammary cancers. In the Multiple Outcomes of Raloxifene Evaluation (MORE) trial, which enrolled 7705 postmenopausal women with osteoporosis, taking raloxifene for a median of 40 months reduced the risk of ER-positive breast cancer by 76%—but only in women with high levels of estrogen. There was no reduction in the risk of ER-negative breast cancer. Encouraged by these results, the National Cancer Institute, in 1999, funded a large 5-year trial, called the Study of Tamoxifen and Raloxifene (STAR). STAR will enroll 22,000 women at high risk of breast cancer, with the objective of comparing risk reduction induced by raloxifene or tamoxifen [Novaldex], a SERM already proved to reduce risk by 50%.

Cardiovascular Disease. Preliminary data from the MORE trial indicate that, during the first 4 years of therapy, raloxifene reduced the risk of cardiovascular events (myocardial infarction [MI], unstable angina, coronary ischemia, and stroke) by 40% in women who were at high risk for such events, but not in women who were at low risk. In contrast to estrogen, raloxifene did not increase the risk of early cardiovascular events. Although these data suggest that raloxifene might be employed to protect against cardiovascular disease, more data are needed before the drug can be recommended for this use.

Adverse Effects and Interactions

Raloxifene is generally well tolerated, although it can cause venous thromboembolism and fetal injury. Raloxifene appears devoid of significant drug-drug and drug-food interactions.

Venous Thromboembolism. Like estrogen, raloxifene increases the risk of deep vein thrombosis (DVT) and pulmonary embolism. Because inactivity promotes DVT, patients should discontinue raloxifene at least 72 hours before prolonged immobilization (e.g., postsurgical recovery, extended bed rest), and should not resume the drug until full mobility has been restored. Also, patients should minimize periods of restricted activity, as can happen when traveling (or when revising a pharmacology text). Raloxifene is contraindicated for patients with a history of venous thrombotic events.

Fetal Harm. Like estrogen, raloxifene is classified in *Food and Drug Administration (FDA) Pregnancy Risk Category X: The potential for fetal harm outweighs any possible benefits of use during pregnancy.* In animal studies, doses below those used in humans have resulted in abortion, retarded fetal development, decreased neonatal survival, and anatomic abnormalities, including hydrocephaly and uterine hypoplasia. Accordingly, raloxifene is contraindicated for use by pregnant women. Although use during pregnancy is obviously no concern for postmenopausal patients, it can be a concern for younger women taking the drug to prevent breast cancer.

Hot Flushes. In contrast to estrogen, raloxifene does not reduce hot flushes (flashes) caused by estrogen deficiency after menopause. In fact, raloxifene may *cause* hot flushes in women who were previously asymptomatic.

Comparison with Estrogen

The SERMs were developed in hopes of creating a drug with all the benefits of estrogen and none of its drawbacks. Raloxifene partly fulfills these hopes. Like estrogen, raloxifene increases BMD in postmenopausal women and reduces the risk of fractures. In contrast to estrogen, which increases the risk of breast cancer, raloxifene protects against breast cancer—but only in women with high levels of estrogen. Similarly, whereas estrogen stimulates endometrium growth, and thereby increases the risk of endometrial cancer, raloxifene does not stimulate the endometrium, and may actually protect against

cancer. Estrogen reduces plasma levels of low-density lipoprotein (LDL) cholesterol (bad cholesterol) and raises levels of high-density lipoprotein (HDL) cholesterol (good cholesterol). Like estrogen, raloxifene reduces LDL cholesterol, but does not raise HDL cholesterol. Nonetheless, raloxifene may offer superior protection against cardiovascular events. In postmenopausal women, estrogen can cause breast pain and resumption of menstruation, phenomena that are unlikely to be greeted with cheers. In contrast, raloxifene does not cause breast pain, and rarely causes menstruation to return. On the other hand, estrogen can alleviate symptoms of estrogen deficiency (e.g., hot flushes, vaginal drying and itching), whereas raloxifene cannot. Both drugs increase the risk of DVT and fetal harm. Table 70–5 summarizes the ways in which estrogen and raloxifene are alike and different.

Preparations, Dosage, and Administration

Raloxifene [Evista] is available in 60-mg tablets for oral use. The dosage for prevention or treatment of postmenopausal osteoporosis is 60 mg once a day, taken with or without food. Treatment should be accompanied by adequate intake of calcium and vitamin D.

Teriparatide

Teriparatide [Forteo] is a form of parathyroid hormone (PTH) produced by recombinant DNA technology. The drug was approved in November 2002 and is currently the only drug for osteoporosis that increases bone formation (all others decrease bone resorption). In postmenopausal women with documented osteoporosis, daily SC injections of teriparatide for 18 months increased BMD of the lumbar spine and femoral neck, and reduced the risk of vertebral fractures by 65%. Similar responses were seen in men. Teriparatide-induced increases in BMD are twice those seen with alendronate.

In clinical trials, two dosages were used: 20 µg once daily and 40 µg once daily. The larger dose produced a greater increase in vertebral BMD (13.7% vs. 9.7%), but did not produce a greater reduction in fractures. Moreover, it did produce a greater incidence of side effects. Accordingly, the smaller (20-µg) dose is recommended. With this dose, plasma levels peak about 20 minutes after SC injection, and decline to undetectable levels within 3 hours.

How does PTH affect bone? The drug has two actions: it increases bone resorption by osteoclasts, and it increases bone deposition by osteoblasts. The net effect—resorption or deposition—depends on how the drug is administered. When given by continuous IV infusion, which produces a *steady* elevation of serum PTH, the drug *decreases* BMD, primarily by accelerating calcium resorption by osteoclasts. In contrast, when given by daily SC injections, which produce *transient* elevations in serum PTH, the drug *increases* BMD, primarily by increasing bone deposition by osteoblasts.

Teriparatide is generally well tolerated. In clinical trials, adverse effects included nausea, headache, back pain, and leg cramps. In addition, serum levels of calcium, magnesium, and uric acid rose early in treatment, but then returned to normal levels within 5 weeks. Initial doses may cause orthostatic hypotension and associated dizziness. The greatest concern is bone cancer: PTH has caused a rare form of bone cancer in rats—but not in monkeys. To date, cancer has not been detected in humans. Nonetheless, teriparatide should be avoided by patients with bone metastases or a history of skeletal can-

TABLE 70–5 ▪▪ Comparison of Estrogen and Raloxifene

Drug Target	Estrogen	Raloxifene
Bone	Increases BMD and reduces fracture risk	Increases BMD (but not as much as estrogen) and reduces fracture risk
Breast	Increases risk of breast cancer; causes breast enlargement and pain	Protects against breast cancer; does *not* cause breast enlargement or pain
Endometrium	Increases risk of endometrial cancer	Does *not* promote endometrial cancer, and *may* offer protection
Plasma lipids	Lowers LDL cholesterol and raises HDL cholesterol	Lower LDL cholesterol, but does not raise HDL cholesterol
Menopausal symptoms	Alleviates menopausal symptoms (e.g,. hot flushes, vaginal dryness and itching)	Does *not* alleviate menopausal symptoms, and may actually increase hot flushes
Menstruation	Causes bleeding in 45% of postmenopausal women	Causes bleeding in 3%–5% of postmenopausal women
Blood clotting	Increases risk of DVT and pulmonary embolism	Same as estrogen
Coronary heart disease	Increases risk of MI early in therapy	No increase in MI risk early in therapy; lowers risk of MI in women with MI risk factors
Developing fetus	Contraindicated during pregnancy because of possible fetal harm	Same as estrogen

cer, and by patients at increased risk for bone cancer, including those with open epiphyses, Paget's disease of bone, or prior radiation of bone.

Preparations, Dosage, and Administration. Teriparatide [Forteo] is available in 3-ml, prefilled pen injectors that contain 750 µg of the drug. The recommended dosage is 20 µg once a day by SC injection into the anterior thigh or abdomen. Each pen can be used up to 28 days after the first injection, after which it should be discarded (even if not empty). Patients should store the pens cold—2° to 8°C (36° to 46° F)—but not frozen, and should take them out of the cold only to make an injection. Treatment costs about $20 a day—over $7000 a year.

Drugs for Hypercalcemia

Furosemide. Furosemide, a loop diuretic, promotes renal excretion of calcium. This action is useful for treating hypercalcemic emergencies. In managing such emergencies, isotonic saline (IV) must be given prior to furosemide. The dosage of furosemide for adults is 80 to 100 mg every 1 to 2 hours as needed; the infusion rate must not exceed 4 mg/min. To avoid fluid and electrolyte imbalance, urinary losses must be measured and replaced. The basic pharmacology of furosemide is discussed in Chapter 39 (Diuretics).

Glucocorticoids. Glucocorticoids reduce intestinal absorption of calcium. This action can be useful in patients with hypercalcemia. For severe hypercalcemia, parenteral glucocorticoid therapy is indicated (e.g., 100 to 500 mg hydrocortisone sodium succinate IV daily). Because glucocorticoids can produce serious adverse effects when taken chronically, the risks of long-term treatment must be carefully weighed against the benefits. The basic pharmacology of the glucocorticoids is discussed in Chapter 68 (Glucocorticoids in Nonendocrine Diseases).

Inorganic Phosphates. Phosphates reduce plasma levels of calcium and, therefore, can be used to treat hypercalcemia. Suggested mechanisms for reducing plasma calcium include (1) decreased bone resorption, (2) increased bone formation, and (3) decreased intestinal absorption of calcium (secondary to decreased renal activation of vitamin D). Intravenous use of phosphates is hazardous and limited to patients with life-threatening hypercalcemia. Oral administration is considerably safer.

Oral phosphates are given to treat mild to moderate hypercalcemia. These agents should not be given to patients with impaired kidney function or ele-

vated levels of serum phosphate. Oral phosphates should not be combined with antacids that contain aluminum, magnesium, or calcium—agents that bind phosphate and thereby prevent its absorption. Initial treatment should provide 1 to 2 gm of phosphorus/day. Doses are reduced when serum calcium levels normalize.

Edetate Disodium. EDTA is a chelating agent that binds calcium in the blood. As a result, it can rapidly reduce plasma levels of free calcium. The EDTA-calcium complex is filtered by the glomerulus but not reabsorbed by the kidney tubules, and hence renal excretion of calcium is increased. Although EDTA is highly effective at reducing hypercalcemia, this agent is also very toxic: EDTA can cause profound hypocalcemia, resulting in tetany, convulsions, dysrhythmias, and possibly death. Severe nephrotoxicity can also occur. Because of its toxicity, EDTA is used only for life-threatening hypercalcemic crisis. The usual adult dose is 40 mg/kg infused over 4 to 6 hours. The total daily dose must not exceed 3 gm.

Plicamycin. Plicamycin [Mithracin] is a cytotoxic antibiotic produced by several species of *Streptomyces*. Although used primarily for testicular cancer, plicamycin is also indicated for hypercalcemia. Plicamycin lowers plasma calcium levels by acting directly on bone to prevent calcium resorption. For management of hypercalcemia, relatively low doses are employed (e.g., 25 µg/kg/day for 3 to 4 days). Calcium-lowering effects may be visible within 1 to 2 days, and may persist from several days to 3 or more weeks. Plicamycin lowers platelet counts and reduces levels of several clotting factors; both actions result in bleeding tendencies.

Gallium Nitrate. Gallium nitrate [Ganite] is used to treat hypercalcemia of malignancy. In addition, the drug is under investigation for use in Paget's disease of bone and postmenopausal osteoporosis. Gallium reduces calcium levels by preventing bone resorption. It may also increase bone formation. Gallium is highly nephrotoxic and must not be used with other nephrotoxic drugs, such as amphotericin B and the aminoglycosides. To minimize kidney damage, the patient must be hydrated with IV fluids before treatment. Renal function must be monitored. The usual single dose is 100 to 200 mg/m². This dose is diluted in 1 L of 5% dextrose or 0.9% sodium chloride and infused over 24 hours. The dose is repeated daily for 5 days.

Bisphosphonates. Pamidronate, etidronate, and zoledronate are used for hypercalcemia of malignancy. The mechanism is suppression of bone resorption by osteoclasts. The pharmacology of these agents is discussed above.

OSTEOPOROSIS

General Considerations

Osteoporosis is a serious medical problem characterized by low bone mass and increased bone fragility. Because of bone fragility, patients are susceptible to fractures from minor traumatic events, such as coughing, rolling over in bed, or falling from a standing position. About 10 million Americans have osteoporosis—80% of them older women—and another 34 million have reduced bone mass, a risk factor for osteoporosis. Every year, osteoporosis leads to 1.5 million fractures. The most common sites are the vertebrae, forearm (distal radius), hip (femoral neck), and ribs. Vertebral fractures can result in loss of height, spinal deformity, chronic back pain, and impaired breathing. Complications from hip fractures are a significant cause of mortality: Of the 300,000 Americans who get hip fractures each year, about 50,000 die from complications.

The economic burden of osteoporosis is high. In 2001, osteoporosis was responsible for more than 1.5 million fractures, including 300,000 hip fractures, 700,000 vertebral fractures, and 250,000 wrist fractures—at an estimated direct cost (for hospitals and nursing homes) of $17 billion, or $47 million a day.

Bone Mass

In men and women, bone mass changes across the life span. Bone mass peaks in the third decade, remains stable to age 50, and then slowly declines—at a rate that is usually less than 1% a year. In addition to this slow, aging-related decline, women go through a phase of *accelerated* bone loss (2% to 3% a year) that begins after menopause and continues for several years. In both the slow and accelerated phases of decline, bone is lost because resorption of old bone outpaces deposition of new bone.

Primary Prevention: Calcium, Vitamin D, and Lifestyle

The risk of osteoporosis can be reduced by lifelong implementation of measures that can help maximize bone strength. Specifically, we need to ensure sufficient intake of calcium and vitamin D, and we need to adopt a lifestyle that promotes bone health. Calcium is needed to maximize bone growth early in life and to maintain bone integrity later in life. Vitamin D is needed to ensure calcium absorption. The amount of calcium needed for optimal bone health is indicated in Table 70–1. Note that, late in life, both men and women should take in at least 1200 mg of calcium daily. If the diet cannot provide this amount, supplements should be employed. Current recommendations for daily vitamin D intake are 200 IU prior to age 51, 400 IU from age 51 through age 70, and 600 IU thereafter. Lifestyle measures that promote bone health are

- Performing regular weight-bearing exercise (walking, jogging, dancing, racquet sports, team sports, stair climbing)
- Avoiding excessive alcohol
- Avoiding smoking

Diagnosis and Monitoring

Osteoporosis is diagnosed by measuring bone mineral density (BMD), an important predictor of fracture risk. The U.S. Preventive Services Task Force now recommends routine BMD testing for all women beginning either at age 60 (for women at increased risk for osteoporotic fractures) or at age 65 (for women who are not at increased risk).

The technique used most often to measure BMD is called *dual-energy x-ray absorptiometry* (DEXA). DEXA scans only take a few minutes, and exposure to radiation is minimal—about one-tenth that of a standard chest x-ray. Results of DEXA scans are reported in terms of *standard deviations* (SD) below mean BMD values in young adults. A BMD value that is 1 SD below the mean indicates 10% bone loss, a value that is 2 SD below the mean indicates 20% bone loss, and so forth. Using this system, the World Health Organization has defined *normal* BMD for women as being no more than 1 SD below the mean for young adults. BMD values between 1 SD below the mean and 2.5 SD below the mean define *osteopenia* (low bone mass). BMD values 2.5 SD below the mean or greater define *osteoporosis*.

Although we use BMD values to diagnose osteoporosis, it is important to note that low BMD is not the only predictor of fractures. Other important predictors are (1) a family history of osteoporotic fractures, (2) a personal history of fractures, and (3) a propensity to fall (e.g., because of parkinsonism or general frailty). Accordingly, if BMD is 2.3 SD below the mean (indicating osteopenia rather than osteoporosis), but the patient has a propensity to fall, then the patient may be at higher risk for fractures than an individual with a BMD 2.5 SD below the mean (indicating osteoporosis) but with no propensity to fall.

Although loss of bone at one site (e.g., forearm) can predict the risk of fractures at other sites (e.g., hip, spine), it is preferable to measure BMD at specific sites to predict specific risks. Accordingly, a thorough evaluation would include BMD measurements in the forearm, vertebrae, and femoral neck—the sites at which osteoporotic fractures occur most often.

Measurement of BMD is employed to monitor treatment as well as for diagnosis. If BMD stabilizes or increases, we can consider treatment a success. Conversely, if BMD continues to decline, treatment failure is indicated.

Treating Osteoporosis in Women

The objective of treatment is to reduce the occurrence of fractures. To do this, we need to maintain or increase bone strength. Two types of drugs can be used: (1) agents that decrease bone resorption and (2) agents that promote bone formation. Antiresorptive drugs—estrogen, raloxifene, bisphosphonates, and calcitonin—are used most often. These agents do a good job of preventing bone loss, but are not very good at restoring bone mass once it is gone. Accordingly, antiresorptive drugs are most beneficial when used early—before substantial loss has occurred. At this time, teriparatide [Forteo] is the only drug available that effectively promotes bone formation.

Antiresorptive Therapy

Bone resorption can be reduced with estrogen, raloxifene, bisphosphonates (e.g., alendronate), and calcitonin, all of which inhibit osteoclast activity. These antiresorptive agents can retard bone loss, but are largely unable to reverse loss that has already occurred. When these agents are used, bone density may increase slightly during the first year or two, but then levels off. With all antiresorptive drugs, success requires a sufficiency of calcium and vitamin D.

Estrogen. The basic pharmacology of estrogen as well as postmenopausal replacement therapy are discussed at length in Chapter 59. Discussion here focuses on the role of estrogen in osteoporosis. *Because of new insight into the benefits and risks of estrogen, prolonged replacement is no longer considered appropriate for most women* (see below and Chapter 59).

Estrogen acts indirectly to suppress osteoclast proliferation, and thereby maintains a brake on bone resorption. Consequently, when estrogen levels decline, either because of natural menopause or surgical removal of the ovaries, osteoclasts increase in number, causing bone resorption to increase dramatically. Estrogen replacement can restore the brake on osteoclast proliferation, and can thereby suppress bone resorption.

Estrogen replacement is approved for preventing and treating bone loss following menopause or surgical removal of the ovaries. Treatment reduces the overall risk of fractures by 24%. Estrogen replacement is most effective when initiated immediately after menopause. However, treatment begun at age 60 and even later can still offer significant protection. If estrogen is discontinued, a period of accelerated bone loss will ensue.

The standard dosage for replacement therapy is 0.625 mg/day of conjugated equine estrogens [Premarin] or its equivalent. However, less estrogen (0.3 mg/day) may be nearly as effective in osteoporosis, while causing fewer side effects (vaginal bleeding, breast tenderness, headache, nausea) and, in all probability, posing a lower risk of breast cancer.

As discussed in Chapter 59, women with an intact uterus should also receive a progestin (e.g., medroxyprogesterone) in order to minimize the risk of estrogen-induced endometrial cancer. For women without a uterus, the progestin is unnecessary.

For years, hormone replacement therapy (HRT)—estrogen with or without a progestin—had been considered the treatment of choice for preventing postmenopausal bone loss. Today, however, the benefits no longer appear to outweigh the risks. As discussed in Chapter 59, data from recent trials, including the first report from the Women's Health Initiative (WHI) and the Heart and Estrogen/progestin Replacement Study (HERS), indicate that HRT offers fewer benefits than previously thought, and carries greater risks. Yes, HRT does reduce bone loss and the risk of osteoporotic fractures. However, HRT increases the risk of breast cancer, cholecystitis, myocardial infarction, and stroke. Accordingly, in the fall of 2002, the U.S. Preventive Service Task Force recommended against using combination HRT (estrogen plus a progestin) to prevent osteoporosis or any other chronic disorder. (Using HRT short-term to manage menopausal symptoms is still considered appropriate.) Fortunately, for prevention and treatment of osteoporosis, we now have effective alternatives: raloxifene, bisphosphonates, calcitonin, and teriparatide. Women currently using HRT for osteoporosis are encouraged to consider a switch. For a more detailed discussion of the pros and cons of HRT, refer to Chapter 59.

Raloxifene. Raloxifene [Evista] is approved for prevention and treatment of postmenopausal osteoporosis. The drug reduces bone turnover, and thereby increases BMD, although not as well as estrogen. For maximal benefits, treatment must be accompanied by adequate intake of calcium and vitamin D. Raloxifene is somewhat less effective than estrogen, but is also safer, and hence is preferred. The basic pharmacology of raloxifene is discussed above.

In the MORE trial, treatment with raloxifene (60 or 120 mg once daily) for 36 months increased BMD and reduced the risk of fractures. The increase in BMD was 2.3% in the femoral neck and 2.7% in the spine. Increased BMD was associated with a reduced risk of spinal fractures: After 36 months, at least one new spinal fracture was seen in 10.1% of women taking placebo, compared with 6.6% of those taking 60 mg of raloxifene, and 5.4% of those taking 120 mg of raloxifene. This represents a 52% decrease in risk with raloxifene. However, although raloxifene reduced the risk of *spinal* fractures, it failed to reduce fractures at *nonspinal* sites (e.g., wrist, hip).

Bisphosphonates. At this time, only two bisphosphonates—alendronate and risedronate—are approved for managing osteoporosis in postmenopausal women. However, although other bisphosphonates are not approved, it is reasonable to assume they would also be effective.

Alendronate. Alendronate [Fosamax] was the first bisphosphonate approved for postmenopausal osteoporosis. The drug is safe and helps prevent fractures. Alendronate was approved initially only for *treating* existing osteoporosis, and was later approved for osteoporosis *prevention*. In both cases, benefits derive from inhibiting bone resorption by osteoclasts. To be effective, alendronate must be accompanied by adequate intake of calcium and vitamin D. The basic pharmacology of alendronate is discussed above.

When studied in osteoporotic postmenopausal women (average age 65), alendronate produced a modest increase in BMD in the hip and spine. More importantly, treatment decreased the rate of new fractures: Compared with patients taking placebo, those taking alendronate experienced 51% fewer fractures of the hip, 47% fewer fractures of the spine, and 48% fewer fractures of the wrist. Furthermore, when spinal fractures did occur, loss of height was less than in women who got spinal fractures while taking placebo. The dosage for treatment of osteoporosis is 10 mg once a day or 70 mg once a week.

When given to *prevent* osteoporosis in postmenopausal women (ages 44 to 50), alendronate produced a small increase in BMD of the spine and hip. In contrast, women taking placebo *lost* BMD at both sites. The response to alendronate was basically the same as the response to estrogen. The dosage for prevention of osteoporosis is 5 mg once a day or 35 mg once a week—half the dosage used to *treat* osteoporosis.

Risedronate. Like alendronate, risedronate [Actonel] is approved for prevention and treatment of osteoporosis in postmenopausal women. In clinical trials, the drug increased BMD and reduced the incidence of vertebral and nonvertebral fractures. The dosage for prevention or treatment is 5 mg once daily or 35 mg once weekly. As with other antiresorptive therapies, success requires adequate intake of calcium and vitamin D.

Calcitonin-Salmon Nasal Spray. Intranasal salmon calcitonin [Miacalcin] is used to treat established osteoporosis, but not to prevent osteoporosis. Benefits derive from inhibiting osteoclastic bone resorption. By doing so, the drug decreases bone loss and the risk of fractures. In women ages 68 to 72, two years of treatment with calcitonin increased BMD in the spine by 3%. In contrast, spinal BMD decreased by 1% in women taking placebo. In younger postmenopausal women (mean age 53), calcitonin increased average BMD by 2%, whereas average BMD decreased by 7% in women taking placebo. Not only is calcitonin moderately effective, it is very safe: The drug has been used for over 20 years with no long-term adverse effects. For management of osteoporosis, the dosage is one spray (200 IU) a day (into alternating nostrils daily). The basic pharmacology of calcitonin is discussed above.

Bone-Forming Therapy: Teriparatide

Teriparatide [Forteo], a recombinant form of PTH, promotes bone formation by increasing the activity of osteoblasts. In clinical trials, the drug increased BMD of the lumbar spine, femoral neck, and total body, and significantly reduced the risk of vertebral fractures. Teriparatide is the first and only drug for osteoporosis that works by increasing bone formation, rather than by decreasing bone resorption. As a rule, teriparatide should be reserved for patients at high risk of fractures. Why? Because the drug is expensive, inconvenient (it requires SC injection), and potentially dangerous (it may promote bone cancer). The pharmacology of teriparatide is discussed above.

Treating Osteoporosis in Men

In the United States, about 2 million men have aging-related osteoporosis, and another 3 million are at risk. Hip fractures occur in 80,000 American men annually, compared with 269,000 American women. Of the men who get a hip fracture, 36% will die within a year. Although rates of osteoporosis and fractures in men are significant, they are clearly much lower than rates in women. As discussed, bone mass in men peaks in the third decade, and begins progressive decline around age 50. The rate of decline in men is about equal to that in women—except that, in men, there is no counterpart to the accelerated phase of bone loss that occurs in women following menopause. If men and women lose bone mass at similar rates, why do men experience less osteoporosis? The main reason is that bones in men, at their peak, are larger and stronger than bones in women. Hence, once decline begins, male bones can tolerate more loss before fractures are likely. Factors that contribute to the risk of osteoporosis in men include low testosterone, prolonged use of glucocorticoids, white race, calcium deficiency, vitamin D deficiency, smoking, excessive alcohol consumption, and insufficient exercise.

Treatment of male osteoporosis is confounded by a paucity of research. (Osteoporosis is one of the few areas of therapeutics in which research in women has greatly exceeded research in men.) At this time, only two drugs—*alendronate* [Fosamax] and teriparatide [Forteo]—are approved for osteoporosis in men. In one clinical trial, 2 years of alendronate therapy increased BMD of the lumbar spine and hip, and significantly decreased the incidence of vertebral fractures. The recommended dosage is 10 mg once a day. (The alternative dosage—70 mg once a week—which is approved for women, is not yet approved for men, but would probably be safe and effective.) Like alendronate, teriparatide can increase BMD and reduce fracture risk. The recommended dosage is the same as in women: 20 μg SC once a day. Calcitonin has been tried in men, but proof of efficacy is lacking. If testosterone deficiency underlies osteoporosis, testosterone replacement therapy is indicated (unless the patient has testicular cancer or some other disorder that contraindicates testosterone use). All men should ensure adequate intake of calcium (1200 mg/day) and vitamin D (400 IU/day).

᛫᛫ KEY POINTS

- Calcium is critical to the function of the skeletal, nervous, muscular, and cardiovascular systems.
- More than 98% of calcium in the body is present in bone.
- Bone undergoes continuous remodeling, a process in which osteoclasts resorb old bone and osteoblasts deposit new bone.
- The body maintains calcium levels by adjusting the rates of calcium resorption from bone, calcium absorption from the intestine, and calcium excretion by the kidney. These processes are regulated by parathyroid hormone (PTH), vitamin D, and calcitonin.
- PTH elevates serum calcium by promoting resorption of calcium from bone, enhancing renal tubular resorption of calcium, and activating vitamin D, which then promotes absorption of calcium from the intestine.
- Like PTH, vitamin D increases serum calcium by increasing calcium resorption from bone, decreasing calcium excretion by the kidney, and increasing calcium absorption from the intestine.
- Calcitonin lowers calcium levels by inhibiting calcium resorption from bone and increasing calcium excretion by the kidney.
- The various calcium salts used for therapy differ widely in their percentage of calcium.
- Vitamin D is obtained through the diet and by exposure to sunlight.
- Vitamin D deficiency causes rickets in children and osteomalacia in adults.
- Calcitonin-salmon has the same metabolic effects as human calcitonin, but has a longer half-life and greater milligram potency.
- Calcitonin-salmon is used primarily for osteoporosis. Benefits derive from inhibiting bone resorption by osteoclasts.
- Calcitonin-salmon is very safe.
- Alendronate, our prototype for the bisphosphonates, has four approved indications: prevention and treatment of osteoporosis in postmenopausal women, treatment of osteoporosis in men, treatment of Paget's disease of bone in men and women, and treatment of glucocorticoid-induced osteoporosis in men and women.
- Alendronate suppresses bone resorption by decreasing both the number and activity of osteoclasts.
- Bioavailability of alendronate is very low in the absence of food, and essentially zero in the presence of food. Accordingly, nothing should be eaten for at least 30 minutes after taking the drug.
- Alendronate can cause severe esophagitis if it stays in contact with the esophageal mucosa. Accordingly, patients should take the drug with a full glass of water and then remain upright for at least 30 minutes, and at least until completing their first meal of the day.
- Raloxifene belongs to the family of SERMs, drugs that are estrogenic in some tissues and antiestrogenic in others.

- Raloxifene mimics the effects of estrogen on bone, lipid metabolism, and blood clotting, and blocks the effects of estrogen in the breast and endometrium.
- Raloxifene is indicated for the prevention and treatment of postmenopausal osteoporosis.
- Raloxifene can cause DVT and fetal harm.
- Teriparatide is the first and only drug for osteoporosis that works by increasing bone formation. (All the others decrease bone resorption.)
- Teriparatide may increase the risk of bone cancer.
- Osteoporosis is characterized by low bone mass and increased bone fragility, which renders patients vulnerable to fractures from minor trauma.
- The most common sites of osteoporotic fractures are the vertebrae, forearm (distal radius), hip (femoral neck), and ribs.
- Osteoporosis occurs mainly in the elderly. Why? Because after age 50, men and women experience aging-related bone loss that is slow but relentless. In addition, women experience several years of accelerated bone loss following menopause. In both cases, bone is lost because bone resorption by osteoclasts outpaces bone deposition by osteoblasts.
- To maximize bone strength, and thereby minimize the risk of osteoporosis, we all need to (1) ensure lifelong sufficiency of calcium and vitamin D and (2) adopt lifestyle measures that promote bone

health (regular weight-bearing exercise and avoidance of smoking and excessive alcohol).
- Osteoporosis is diagnosed by measuring BMD, which is done most commonly using dual-energy x-ray absorptiometry.
- The World Health Organization's diagnostic criterion for osteoporosis is BMD that is more than 2.5 standard deviations below the mean BMD for young adults.
- The objective of osteoporosis therapy is to reduce fractures.
- With currently available drugs, we are more able to prevent bone loss (using antiresorptive agents) than to rebuild bone that is already gone (using bone-forming agents).
- Antiresorptive drugs—estrogen, raloxifene, bisphosphonates (e.g., alendronate), and calcitonin—decrease bone loss by inhibiting the activity of osteoclasts.
- Estrogen increases BMD and reduces fracture risk.
- Until recently, estrogen was considered a treatment of choice for prevention and treatment of postmenopausal osteoporosis. Today, however, available data strongly suggest that the benefits in osteoporosis do not outweigh the risks (breast cancer, myocardial infarction, stroke, cholecystitis).
- Calcitonin is the safest drug for osteoporosis, but is less effective than estrogen or alendronate. Comparisons with raloxifene are not available.

Summary of Major Nursing Implications*

VITAMIN D

Preadministration Assessment

Therapeutic Goal

Treatment of rickets, osteomalacia, and hypoparathyroidism.

Baseline Data

The physician may order serum levels of vitamin D, calcium, phosphorus, and alkaline phosphatase as well as a 24-hour urinary calcium determination.

Assess dietary vitamin D and calcium content.

Identifying High-Risk Patients

Vitamin D is *contraindicated* in patients with hypercalcemia, hypervitaminosis D, and malabsorption syndrome. Exercise *caution* in patients taking digoxin.

Implementation: Administration

Routes

Oral, IM.

Administration

Instruct the patient to swallow oral preparations intact, without crushing or chewing.

Therapeutic responses to vitamin D require adequate calcium intake. Assess dietary calcium content and adjust to ensure calcium sufficiency.

Ongoing Evaluation and Interventions

Monitoring Summary

Monitor serum calcium, serum phosphorus, and urinary calcium.

Minimizing Adverse Interactions

Digoxin. Vitamin D–induced hypercalcemia can cause dysrhythmias in patients taking digoxin. Monitor serum calcium and make certain it remains normal.

Management of Toxicity

Large therapeutic doses may cause hypervitaminosis D, a syndrome characterized by hypercalcemia, hypercalciuria, decalcification of bone, and deposition of calcium in soft tissues. Monitor serum calcium content; levels should stay below 10 mg/dl. Monitor serum phosphorus and urinary calcium as well. If vitamin D toxicity develops, have the patient discontinue vitamin D immediately, increase fluid intake, and institute a low-calcium diet. In severe cases, calcium excretion can be accelerated with IV saline plus furosemide.

ORAL CALCIUM SALTS

Calcium acetate
Calcium carbonate
Calcium citrate

*Patient education information is highlighted as blue text.

Summary of Major Nursing Implications*—cont'd

Calcium glubionate
Calcium gluconate
Calcium lactate
Tricalcium phosphate

Preadministration Assessment

Therapeutic Goal

Treatment of mild hypocalcemia and supplementation of dietary calcium.

Baseline Data

Obtain a serum calcium level.

Identifying High-Risk Patients

Calcium salts are *contraindicated* for patients with hypercalcemia, renal calculi, and hypophosphatemia.

Implementation: Administration

Route

Oral.

Dosage

Individual calcium salts differ with respect to percentage of elemental calcium. As a result, the dose required to provide a specific amount of calcium differs among the salts. **Advise patients against switching to a different preparation.**

Administration

Advise patients to take oral calcium salts with a large glass of water; administration with or after meals promotes absorption. Advise patients to avoid taking calcium with foods that can suppress calcium absorption (e.g., spinach, Swiss chard, beets, bran, whole-grain cereals).

Ongoing Evaluation and Interventions

Minimizing Adverse Effects

Prolonged therapy can cause hypercalcemia. **Inform patients about signs of hypercalcemia (nausea, vomiting, constipation, frequent urination, lethargy, and depression), and instruct them to notify the physician if these occur.** Hypercalcemia can be minimized with frequent monitoring of serum calcium.

Minimizing Adverse Interactions

Glucocorticoids. These drugs reduce calcium absorption; increased calcium dosage may be required.

Tetracyclines. Calcium binds to tetracyclines, thereby reducing tetracycline absorption. **Instruct patients to separate administration of these agents by at least 1 hour.**

Thyroid Hormone. Calcium interferes with absorption of thyroid hormone. **Instruct patients to separate administration of these agents by several hours.**

Thiazide Diuretics. Thiazides decrease renal excretion of calcium. A reduction in calcium dosage may be needed to avoid hypercalcemia.

*Patient education information is highlighted as blue text.

PARENTERAL CALCIUM SALTS

Calcium chloride
Calcium gluceptate
Calcium gluconate

Preadministration Assessment

Therapeutic Goal

Reversal of clinical manifestations of hypocalcemia.

Baseline Data

Assess for signs and symptoms of hypocalcemia (tetany, convulsions, laryngospasm, and spasm of other muscles). Obtain measurement of serum calcium.

Identifying High-Risk Patients

Parenteral calcium is *contraindicated* for patients with hypercalcemia or ventricular fibrillation. Use with *extreme caution* in patients taking digoxin.

Implementation: Administration

Routes

Parenteral (IM, IV). All parenteral calcium salts may be given IV; only calcium gluceptate should be given IM.

Administration

Warm solutions to body temperature prior to infusion or IM injection. Perform IV injections slowly (0.5 to 2 ml/min).

Drugs that contain phosphate, carbonate, sulfate, and tartrate groups can precipitate calcium; do not mix these drugs with parenteral calcium solutions.

Calcium chloride may cause necrosis and sloughing if solutions become extravasated. Monitor the infusion closely.

Ongoing Evaluation and Interventions

Evaluating Therapeutic Effects

Evaluate the patient for reductions in tetany, muscle spasm, laryngospasm, paresthesias, and other symptoms of severe hypocalcemia.

Minimizing Adverse Effects

Hypercalcemia. Overdose can produce acute hypercalcemia, resulting in nausea, vomiting, weakness, lethargy, coma, and possibly death. Avoid hypercalcemia through careful control of dosage.

Minimizing Adverse Interactions

Digoxin. Parenteral calcium may cause severe bradycardia in patients taking digoxin. Infuse calcium slowly and cautiously in these patients.

CALCITONIN-SALMON

Preadministration Assessment

Therapeutic Goal

Treatment of postmenopausal osteoporosis, Paget's disease of bone, and hypercalcemia.

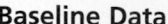

Summary of Major Nursing Implications*—cont'd

Baseline Data

The physician may order measurements of serum alkaline phosphatase, calcium, and phosphorus, as well as a 24-hour urinary hydroxyproline.

Identifying High-Risk Patients

Salmon calcitonin is *contraindicated* for patients allergic to this preparation.

Implementation: Administration

Routes

Intranasal. For osteoporosis only.
Parenteral (IM, SC). For osteoporosis, Paget's disease, and hypercalcemia.

Administration

Intranasal. Instruct patients to activate the metered-dose pump by holding the bottle upright and depressing the two white sidearms toward the bottle six times, which should produce a faint initial spray. The drug is then administered by placing the nozzle in the nostril and depressing the pump handle.

Subcutaneous. Teach patients how to inject calcitonin SC, and instruct them to rotate sites of injection.

Ongoing Evaluation and Interventions

Evaluating Therapeutic Effects

Postmenopausal Osteoporosis. Measurement of BMD should indicate retardation of bone loss (or perhaps a small increase in BMD).

Paget's Disease of Bone. Monitor for reductions in bone pain, serum alkaline phosphatase levels, and 24-hour urinary hydroxyproline value.

Hypercalcemia. Monitor for reductions in serum calcium and phosphorus levels.

ALENDRONATE (A BISPHOSPHONATE)

Preadministration Assessment

Therapeutic Goals

Alendronate is indicated for prevention and treatment of osteoporosis in postmenopausal women, treatment of osteoporosis in men, treatment of Paget's disease in men and women, and treatment of glucocorticoid-induced osteoporosis in men and women.

Baseline Data

Postmenopausal Osteoporosis. Obtain baseline values for BMD in the hip, vertebrae, and forearm.
Paget's Disease of Bone. Obtain a baseline value for serum alkaline phosphatase.

Identifying High-Risk Patients

Alendronate is *contraindicated* for patients with esophageal disorders that can impede swallowing and for patients who cannot sit or stand for at least 30 minutes.

*Patient education information is highlighted as blue text.

Implementation: Administration

Route

Oral.

Administration

Proper administration is needed to maximize absorption and minimize the risk of esophagitis. Accordingly, you should instruct patients to

- Take alendronate in the morning before breakfast.
- Take alendronate with a full glass of water.
- Avoid chewing or sucking the tablet.
- Remain upright (seated or standing) for at least 30 minutes and at least until completing breakfast.
- Postpone eating anything, including orange juice or coffee, for at least 30 minutes after taking the drug.

Ongoing Evaluation and Interventions

Evaluating Therapeutic Effects

Postmenopausal Osteoporosis. Obtain periodic determinations of BMD. If BMD increases, or at least remains constant, treatment is a success. Conversely, a significant decline in BMD indicates failure.

Paget's Disease of Bone. Obtain periodic measurements of serum alkaline phosphatase. A decline indicates that alendronate is working.

Minimizing Adverse Effects

Esophagitis. Alendronate can cause severe esophagitis, sometimes resulting in ulceration. To minimize risk, instruct patients to (1) administer the drug in accord with the guidelines described above, (2) avoid lying down after taking the drug, and (3) discontinue the drug and contact the physician if they experience symptoms of esophageal injury (difficulty swallowing, pain upon swallowing, or new or worsening heartburn). Avoid alendronate in patients with esophageal disorders that could impede swallowing and in patients who are unable to sit or stand for 30 minutes.

RALOXIFENE

Preadministration Assessment

Therapeutic Goals

Prevention and treatment of postmenopausal osteoporosis.

Baseline Data

Obtain baseline values for BMD in the hip, vertebrae, and forearm.

Identifying High-Risk Patients

Raloxifene is *contraindicated* for use by patients who are pregnant or have a history of venous thrombotic events.

Implementation: Administration

Route

Oral.

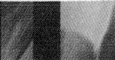

Summary of Major Nursing Implications*—cont'd

Administration

Take once daily without regard to meals.

Ongoing Evaluation and Interventions

Promoting Therapeutic Effects

Advise patients to ensure adequate intake of calcium and vitamin D.

Evaluating Therapeutic Effects

Obtain periodic determinations of BMD. If BMD increases, or at least remains constant, treatment is a success. Conversely, a significant decline in BMD indicates failure.

*Patient education information is highlighted as blue text.

Minimizing Adverse Effects

Venous Thromboembolism. Raloxifene increases the risk of DVT and pulmonary embolism. **Advise patients to discontinue raloxifene at least 72 hours prior to prolonged immobilization (e.g., postsurgical recovery, extended bed rest), and to resume treatment only after full mobility has been restored. Advise patients to avoid extended periods of restricted activity, as can happen when traveling.** Do not give raloxifene to patients with a history of venous thrombotic events.

Fetal Harm. Raloxifene can cause fetal harm, and hence must not be used during pregnancy.

ESTROGEN

Nursing implications for estrogen are summarized in Chapter 59.

Drugs for Asthma

Asthma is a common, chronic disorder that occurs in children and adults. Characteristic signs and symptoms are a sense of breathlessness and tightness in the chest, together with wheezing, dyspnea, and cough. The underlying cause is immune-mediated airway inflammation. In the year 2000, asthma attacks were reported by more than 11 million Americans, including more than 5% of children younger than 18. In 1999, asthma was the underlying cause for 2 million emergency department visits, 478,000 hospitalizations, and 4426 deaths. However, despite these statistics, with proper treatment, most asthma patients can lead full lives with no limitations.

PATHOPHYSIOLOGY OF ASTHMA

Asthma is a *chronic inflammatory* disorder of the airway. In about 50% of children with asthma and in some adults, airway inflammation results from an immune response to known allergens. In the remaining children and in most adults, the cause of airway inflammation is unknown—although as-yet unidentified allergens are suspected.

Figure 71–1 depicts the events that lead to inflammation and bronchoconstriction in patients whose asthma is caused by specific allergens. Although this model may not apply completely to all asthma patients, it nonetheless provides a basis for understanding the drugs used for treatment. The inflammatory process begins with binding of allergen molecules (e.g., house dust mite feces) to IgE antibodies on mast cells. This causes mast cells to release an assortment of mediators, including histamine, leukotrienes, prostaglandins, and interleukins. These mediators have two effects. They act immediately to cause *bronchoconstriction.* In addition, they promote infiltration and activation of inflammatory cells (eosinophils, leukocytes, macrophages). These inflammatory cells then release mediators of their own. The end result is *airway inflammation,* characterized by edema, mucus plugging, and smooth muscle hypertrophy, all of which obstruct airflow. In addition, inflammation produces a state of *bronchial hyperreactivity.* Because of this state, mild trigger factors (e.g., cold air, exercise, tobacco smoke) are able to cause intense bronchoconstriction.

From a therapeutic perspective, the important message here is that symptoms of asthma result from a combination of inflammation and bronchoconstriction. Accordingly, treatment must address both components.

OVERVIEW OF DRUGS FOR ASTHMA

The major drugs for asthma are listed in Table 71–1. As indicated, they fall into two main pharmacologic classes: anti-inflammatory agents and bronchodilators. The principal anti-inflammatory drugs are the *glucocorticoids* and *cromolyn.* The principal bronchodilators are the *beta$_2$* agonists. For chronic asthma, glucocorticoids are administered on a fixed schedule, usually by inhalation. Beta$_2$ agonists may be administered on a fixed schedule or PRN; the usual route is inhalation. Drug therapy is discussed in detail later.

ADMINISTRATION OF DRUGS BY INHALATION

Most antiasthmatic drugs can be administered by inhalation, a route with three obvious advantages: (1) therapeutic effects are enhanced (by delivering drugs directly to their site of action), (2) systemic effects are minimized, and (3) relief of acute attacks is rapid. Three types of inhalation devices are employed: metered-dose inhalers, dry-powder inhalers, and nebulizers.

Metered-Dose Inhalers

Metered-dose inhalers (MDIs) are small, hand-held, pressurized devices that deliver a measured dose of drug with each activation. Dosing is usually accomplished with 1 or

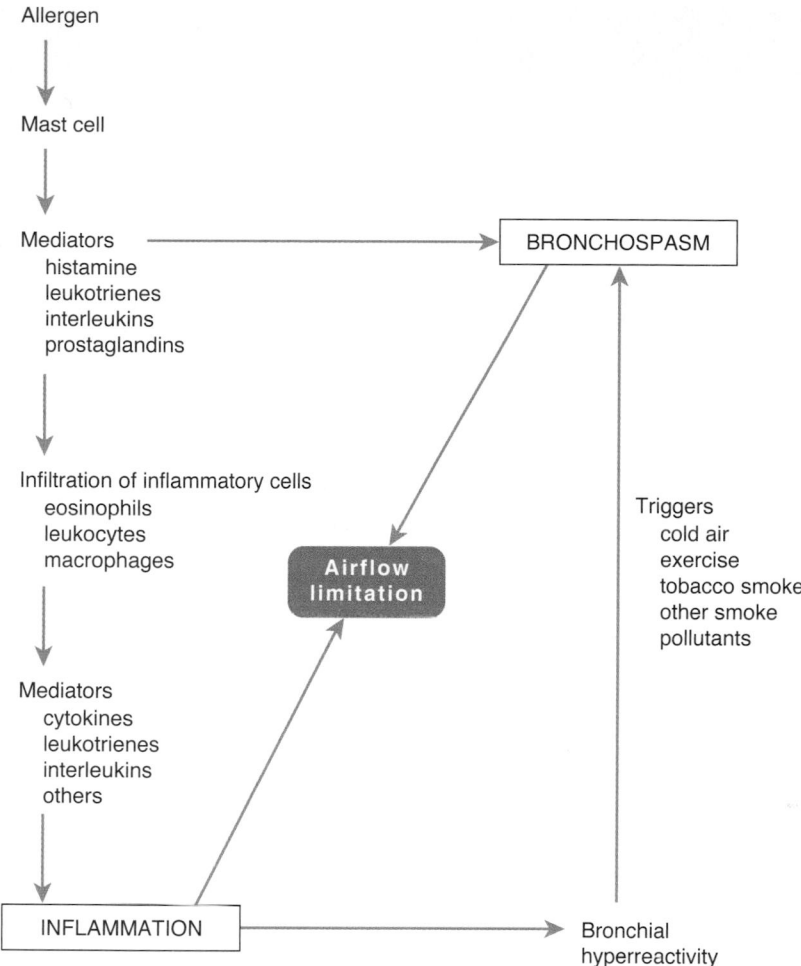

Figure 71–1 ■ Allergen-induced inflammation and bronchospasm in asthma.

2 puffs. When 2 puffs are needed, an interval of at least 1 minute should separate the first puff from the second. When using an MDI, the patient must begin to inhale prior to activating the device. Hence, hand-lung coordination is required. MDIs can be difficult to use correctly. Hence patients will need a demonstration as well as written and verbal instruction. Even with optimal use, only about 10% of the dose reaches the lungs. About 80% impacts the oropharynx and is swallowed, and the remaining 10% is left in the device or exhaled.

Several kinds of *spacers* are available for use with MDIs. All of these devices, which attach directly to the MDI, serve to increase delivery of drug to the lungs and decrease deposition of drug on the oropharyngeal mucosa (Fig. 71–2). Some spacers contain a one-way valve that activates upon inhalation, thereby obviating the need for good hand-lung coordination. Some spacers also contain an alarm whistle that sounds off when inhalation is too rapid. The ability of spacers to reduce drug deposition in the oropharynx is especially important for inhaled glucocorticoids.

MDIs in current use employ two kinds of propellants: chlorofluorocarbons (CFCs) and hydrofluoroalkane (HFA). Until recently, all MDIs employed CFCs. However, we now know that CFCs can reduce the Earth's ozone layer, and hence these propellants are being phased out. HFA does not appear to affect the ozone layer, and hence is replacing CFCs.

Dry-Powder Inhalers

Dry-powder inhalers (DPIs) are used to deliver drugs in the form of a dry, micronized powder directly to the lungs. No propellant is employed. Hence, DPIs pose no environmental risk. Unlike MDIs, DPIs are breath activated. As a result, DPIs don't require the hand-lung coordination needed with MDIs, and hence DPIs are much easier to use. Compared with MDIs, DPIs deliver more drug to the lungs (20% of the total released vs. 10%) and less to the oropharynx.

Nebulizers

A nebulizer is a small machine used to convert a drug solution into a mist. The droplets in the mist are much finer than those produced by inhalers. Inhalation of the nebulized mist can be done through a face mask or through a mouthpiece held between the teeth. Nebulizers take several minutes to deliver the same amount of drug contained in 1 puff from an inhaler. For some patients, a nebulizer may be more effective than an inhaler. Although nebulizers are usually used at home or in a hospital, these devices, which weigh under 10 pounds, are sufficiently portable for use in other locations.

BETA₂-ADRENERGIC AGONISTS

Beta₂ agonists, given by inhalation, are the most effective drugs available for relieving acute bronchospasm and preventing exercise-induced bronchospasm. In addition, long-acting formulations (given orally or by inhalation) can protect against bronchospasm over an extended time. Because of these beneficial effects, virtually all patients with asthma use these drugs. The basic pharmacology of the beta₂ agonists is presented in Chapter 17. Discussion here is limited to their use in asthma.

Mechanism of Antiasthmatic Action

The beta₂ agonists are sympathomimetic drugs that produce "selective" activation of beta₂-adrenergic receptors. By activating beta₂ receptors in smooth muscle of the lung, these drugs promote *bronchodilation,* and thereby relieve bronchospasm.

In addition, beta₂ agonists suppress histamine release in the lung and increase ciliary motility. The beta₂-selective agents have largely replaced older, less selective sympathomimetics (e.g., epinephrine, isoproterenol) for asthma therapy.

Classification by Route and Time Course

Beta₂ agonists may be administered orally or by inhalation, and their effects may be brief or prolonged. All of the oral agents are long acting. In contrast, most inhaled beta₂ agonists are short acting; only two—salmeterol and formoterol—are long acting (see Table 71–1). With the short-acting preparations, effects begin almost immediately, peak in 30 to 60 minutes, and persist for 3 to 5 hours. In contrast, effects of salmeterol and formoterol are delayed, but persist for up to 12 hours. As a result, the long-acting inhaled agents are well suited for prolonged prophylaxis, but should not be used to abort an ongoing attack.

Antiasthmatic Uses

Beta₂ agonists are employed for quick relief of an ongoing attack and for long-term control. All asthma patients inhale short-acting beta₂ agonists on a PRN basis to relieve breakthrough symptoms. Patients who experience frequent attacks may also take beta₂ agonists on a fixed schedule for long-term control; an oral preparation or a long-acting inhaled preparation (salmeterol, formoterol) may be employed. Patients subject to exercise-induced bronchospasm may inhale a short-acting beta₂ agonist immediately prior to exercise as prophylaxis against an attack. For patients undergoing an acute severe attack, a nebulized beta₂ agonist is the traditional treatment of choice; however, delivery with an MDI may be equally effective.

Adverse Effects

Inhaled Preparations. Side effects with inhaled beta₂ agonists are generally minimal. There have been reports of increased mortality associated with overuse of these drugs. However, it isn't clear whether overuse was the cause of death, or whether severe asthma, which led to increased use, was the actual cause. Systemic effects—tachycardia, angina, and tremor—are usually minimal when beta₂ agonists are inhaled, but can nonetheless occur.

Oral Preparations. The selectivity of the beta₂-adrenergic agonists is only relative, not absolute. Accordingly, when these drugs are administered orally, they are likely to produce some activation of beta₁ receptors in the heart. If dosage is excessive, stimulation of cardiac beta₁ receptors can cause *angina pectoris* and *tachydysrhythmias.* Patients should be instructed to report chest pain or changes in heart rate or rhythm.

Oral beta₂ agonists often cause *tremor* by stimulating beta₂ receptors in skeletal muscle. Tremor can be reduced by lowering the dosage. With continued drug use, tremor declines spontaneously.

Preparations, Dosage, and Administration

Seven selective beta₂ agonists are available (Table 71–2). Some are used for quick relief, some for long-term control, and some for both (depending on their route of administration).

Inhaled Preparations for Quick Relief. To provide quick relief, beta₂ agonists must be administered by inhalation. Three types of devices may be used: MDIs, DPIs, and nebulizers.

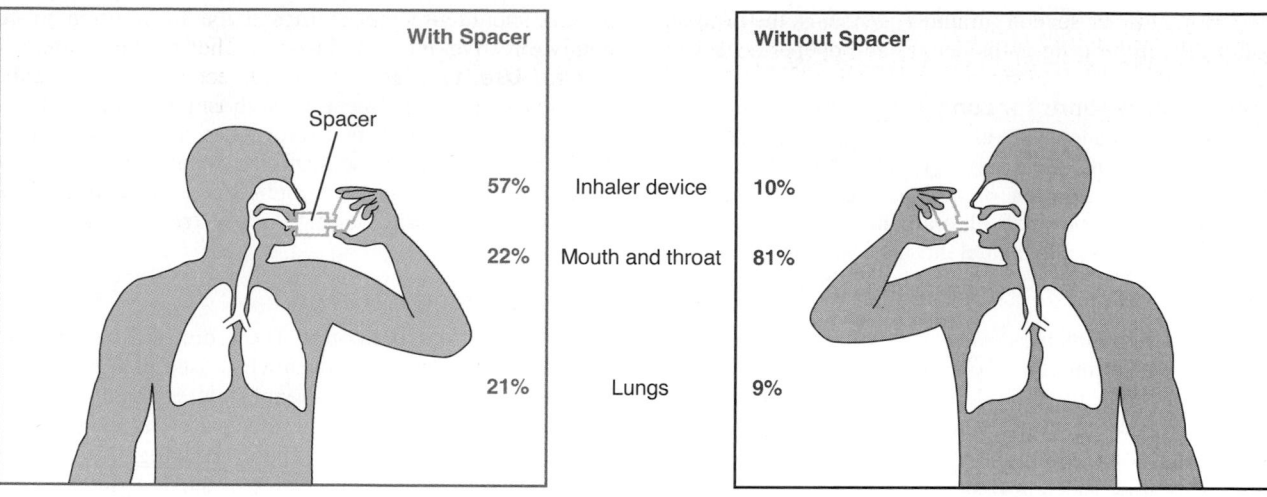

Figure 71–2 ■ Impact of a spacer device on the distribution of inhaled medication. Note that, in the presence of a spacer, more medication reaches its site of action in the lungs, and less is deposited in the mouth and throat.

TABLE 71–2 ■■ Beta₂-Adrenergic Agonists Used in Asthma

Drug [Trade Name]	Formulation	Initial Dosage	
		Adults	Children
Inhaled Agents: Short Acting			
Albuterol			
[Proventil, Proventil HFA, Ventolin, Ventolin HFA]	MDI (90 μg/puff)	2 puffs q 4–6 h PRN	2 puffs q 4–6 h PRN
[Proventil, AccuNeb]	Solution for nebulization	2.5 mg q 4–6 h PRN	0.63–2.5 mg/kg q 4–6 h PRN
Bitolterol mesylate			
[Tornalate]	Solution for nebulization	1.5–3.5 mg bid–qid PRN	1.5 mg bid–qid PRN
Levalbuterol			
[Xopenex]	Solution for nebulization	0.63 mg q 6–8 h PRN	0.63 mg q 6–8 h PRN
Pirbuterol			
[Maxair]	MDI (200 μg/puff)	2 puffs q 4–6 h PRN	2 puffs q 4–6 h PRN
[Maxair Autohaler]	BA-MDI (200 μg/puff)	2 puffs q 4–6 h PRN	2 puffs q 4–6 h PRN
Inhaled Agents: Long Acting			
Formoterol			
[Foradil Aerolizer]	DPI (12 μg/puff)	1 inhalation q 12 h	1 inhalation q 12 h
Salmeterol			
[Serevent]	MDI (21 μg/puff)	2 puffs q 12 h	2 puffs q 12 h
[Serevent Diskus]	DPI (50 μg/inhalation)	1 inhalation q 12 h	1 inhalation q 12 h
Oral Agents			
Albuterol			
[Proventil]	Tablets, syrup	2 or 4 mg tid–qid	2 mg tid–qid
Proventil Repetabs, Volmax]	Tablets (extended release)	8 mg q 12 h	4 mg q 12 h
Terbutaline			
[Brethine]	Tablets	5 mg tid	2.5 mg tid

DPI = dry-powder inhaler, MDI = metered-dose inhaler, BA-MDI = breath-activated metered-dose inhaler, HFA = hydrofluoroalkane propellant.

For drugs administered with an MDI or DPI, the usual dosing schedule is 1 or 2 puffs 3 or 4 times a day. When 2 puffs are needed, an interval of 1 minute or longer should separate puffs. During this interval, some bronchodilation develops, thereby facilitating penetration of the second puff.

For certain patients, nebulizers may be superior to inhalers. Experience has shown that some patients who have become unresponsive to a beta₂ agonist delivered with an inhaler may respond when the same drug is administered with a nebulizer. This differential effect occurs because the nebulizer delivers the dose slowly (over several minutes); hence, as the bronchi gradually dilate, the drug gains deeper and deeper access to the lungs.

Inhaled Preparations for Long-Term Control. Only two long-acting inhaled agents are available: *salmeterol* [Serevent, Serevent Diskus] and *formoterol* [Foradil Aerolizer]. Both drugs have a long duration of action, and hence are well suited for long-term control. With both, dosing is usually done every 12 hours. If supplemental bronchodilation is needed between doses, a short-acting inhaled beta$_2$ agonist should be employed.

Bronchodilation develops faster with formoterol than with salmeterol (1 to 3 minutes vs. 10 to 30 minutes). Accordingly, in addition to being used for long-term control, formoterol can be taken prior to exertion to prevent exercise-induced bronchospasm. It is important to note, however, that despite its relatively rapid onset, formoterol should *not* be used to treat an ongoing asthma attack. Rather, a short-acting inhaled beta$_2$ agonist should be taken.

Although salmeterol is usually inhaled twice daily (every 12 hours), with continuous use, more frequent dosing may be needed. Why? Because benefits seem to persist for a shorter time as the duration of treatment increases.

Oral Preparations for Long-Term Control. Two oral beta$_2$ agonists—albuterol and terbutaline—are approved for long-term control of asthma. Dosing is done 3 or 4 times a day.

GLUCOCORTICOIDS

Glucocorticoids (e.g., beclomethasone, prednisone) are the most effective antiasthma drugs available. Administration is usually by inhalation, but may also be oral or IV. Adverse reactions to inhaled glucocorticoids are generally minor, as are reactions to systemic glucocorticoids taken *acutely*. However, when *systemic* glucocorticoids are used *long term,* severe adverse effects are likely. The basic pharmacology of the glucocorticoids is presented in Chapter 68. Discussion here is limited to their use in asthma.

Mechanism of Antiasthmatic Action

Glucocorticoids reduce symptoms of asthma by *suppressing inflammation.* Specific anti-inflammatory effects include (1) decreased synthesis and release of inflammatory mediators (e.g., leukotrienes, histamine, prostaglandins); (2) decreased infiltration and activity of inflammatory cells (e.g., eosinophils, leukocytes); and (3) decreased edema of the airway mucosa (secondary to a decrease in vascular permeability). By suppressing inflammation, glucocorticoids reduce bronchial hyperreactivity. In addition to reducing inflammation, glucocorticoids decrease airway mucus production and increase the number of bronchial beta$_2$ receptors as well as their responsiveness to beta$_2$ agonists.

Use in Asthma

Glucocorticoids are used for *prophylaxis* of chronic asthma. Accordingly, administration must be done on a fixed schedule—not PRN. Because beneficial effects develop slowly, these drugs cannot be used to abort an ongoing attack.

Inhalation Use. Inhaled glucocorticoids are first-line therapy for asthma. All patients with moderate to severe asthma should use these drugs daily. In addition to being highly effective, inhaled glucocorticoids are very safe.

Oral Use. Oral glucocorticoids are reserved for patients with severe asthma. Because of their potential for toxicity, these drugs are prescribed only when symptoms cannot be controlled with safer medications (inhaled glucocorticoids, cromolyn, beta$_2$ agonists, theophylline). Because the risk of toxicity increases with duration of use, treatment should be as brief as possible.

Adverse Effects

Inhaled Glucocorticoids. These preparations are largely devoid of serious toxicity, even when used in high doses. The most serious concerns are adrenal suppression and bone loss.

The most common adverse effects are *oropharyngeal candidiasis* and *dysphonia* (hoarseness, speaking difficulty). Both effects result from local deposition of inhaled glucocorticoids. To minimize these effects, patients should (1) gargle after each administration and (2) employ a spacer device during administration, which will greatly reduce drug deposition in the oropharynx. If candidiasis develops, it can be treated with an antifungal drug.

With long-term, high-dose therapy, some *adrenal suppression* may develop, although the degree of suppression is generally low. In contrast, with prolonged use of *oral* glucocorticoids, adrenal suppression can be profound. As noted below, *patients who have been switched from oral glucocorticoids to inhaled glucocorticoids must be given supplemental oral or IV doses at times of stress.* (At times of stress, inhaled glucocorticoids can control symptoms of asthma, but cannot replace the glucocorticoids required to support life.)

Like oral glucocorticoids, inhaled glucocorticoids can promote *bone loss*—at least in premenopausal women. Fortunately, the amount of loss is much lower than that caused by oral glucocorticoids. To minimize bone loss, patients should (1) use the lowest dose possible, (2) ensure adequate intake of calcium and vitamin D, and (3) participate in weight-bearing exercise.

Glucocorticoids can *slow* growth in children and adolescents—but these drugs do *not* decrease adult height. *Short-term* studies have shown that inhaled glucocorticoids retard growth. However, we now know from *long-term* studies that adult height is not reduced. Two studies reported in the October 12, 2000, issue of the *New England Journal of Medicine* demonstrate that inhaled budesonide does indeed slow growth in children—but only temporarily. Within a year, and despite continued budesonide use, growth rate returns to normal and children eventually achieve their expected adult height. Moreover, adult height is not affected by either the duration of budesonide use or the total cumulative dose. Unfortunately, these studies focused only on *skeletal* growth, and hence we still don't know if glucocorticoids suppress growth and development of the brain, lungs, and other organs. Until more is known about how glucocorticoids affect organs, it would seem prudent to reserve these drugs for older children and for young children whose asthma is relatively severe; young children whose asthma is very mild, and hence can be treated effectively without glucocorticoids, should probably not receive these drugs.

Prolonged therapy may increase the risk of *cataracts* and *glaucoma.*

Oral Glucocorticoids. When used *acutely* (<10 days), even in very high doses, oral glucocorticoids do not cause significant adverse effects. However, prolonged therapy, even in moderate doses, can be hazardous. Potential adverse effects include *adrenal suppression, osteoporosis, hyperglycemia, peptic ulcer disease,* and, in young patients, *suppression of growth.*

Adrenal suppression is of particular concern. As discussed in Chapter 68, prolonged use of glucocorticoids can decrease the ability of the adrenal cortex to produce glucocorticoids of its own. Since high levels of glucocorticoids are required to survive severe stress (e.g., surgery, trauma, infection), and since adrenal suppression prevents production of endogenous glucocorticoids, *patients must be given increased doses of oral or IV glucocorticoids at times of stress. Failure to do so can prove fatal!* Following withdrawal of oral glucocorticoids (or transfer to inhaled glucocorticoids), several months are required for recovery of adrenocortical function. Throughout this period, all patients—*including those switched to inhaled glucocorticoids*—must be given supplemental oral or IV glucocorticoids at times of severe stress.

A complete list of contraindications to oral glucocorticoids is presented in the *Summary of Major Nursing Implications* at the end of this chapter.

Preparations, Dosage, and Administration

Inhaled Glucocorticoids. Five glucocorticoids are available for administration by inhalation (Table 71–3). Four are available in MDIs, two are available in DPIs, and one is available in suspension for nebulization. Inhaled glucocorticoids are administered on a regular schedule—not PRN. Pediatric and adult dosages are summarized in Table 71–3. In all cases, the dosage should be kept as low as possible so as to minimize bone loss, adrenal suppression, and other adverse effects.

Glucocorticoids in MDIs. As discussed earlier, two propellants—CFCs and HFA—are used in MDIs. At this time, only one glucocorticoid—beclomethasone [QVAR]—comes in an MDI that uses HFA; all other glucocorticoids come in MDIs that use CFCs. Patients using MDIs that employ CFCs should be instructed to use a *spacer device* (holding chamber) in order to (1) increase the amount of glucocorticoid delivered to the lungs (thereby increasing therapeutic effects), and (2) reduce the amount deposited in the oropharynx (thereby reducing the risk of candidiasis and dysphonia). Patients using QVAR do not need a spacer device. Why? Because the HFA propellant in QVAR produces smaller droplets than do CFCs, and hence delivery of drugs to the lungs is greatly improved. Regardless of which type of MDI is employed, penetration to the lungs can be increased by inhaling a beta$_2$ agonist 5 minutes prior to inhaling the glucocorticoid.

Nebulized Budesonide. Budesonide suspension [Pulmicort Respules] is the first inhaled glucocorticoid formulated for nebulized administration. The product is approved for maintenance therapy of persistent asthma in children 1 to 8 years old—that is, children too young to use an MDI or DPI. Improvement should begin in 2 to 8 days; maximal benefits may take 4 to 6 weeks to develop. Budesonide suspension is available in 2-ml ampules containing 250 or 500 μg of the drug. Administration is done with a jet nebulizer equipped with a mouthpiece or face mask; ultrasonic nebulizers should not be used. Administration takes 5 to 10 minutes. For children who are *not* taking an oral glucocorticoid, the initial dosage is 500 μg/day in one or two doses. For children who *are* taking an oral glucocorticoid, the initial dosage is 1000 μg/day in one or two doses. After 1 week, dosage of the oral glucocorticoid should be tapered off.

Oral Glucocorticoids. *Prednisone* and *prednisolone* are preferred glucocorticoids for oral therapy of asthma. For acute therapy, the usual adult dosage for either drug is 30 to 40 mg twice daily for 5 to 7 days.

For *long-term* treatment, *alternate-day dosing* is recommended (to minimize adrenal suppression). The *initial adult* dosage is 40 to 60 mg (of prednisone or prednisolone) administered every other morning. The *initial pediatric* dosage is 20 to 40 mg every other morning. After symptoms have been controlled for a month, dosages should be reduced by 5 to 10 mg every 2 weeks to establish the lowest dosage that can keep the patient free of symptoms. As discussed above, supplemental doses are required at times of stress.

TABLE 71–3 ■ Inhaled Glucocorticoids: Formulations and Comparable Dosages

Drug [Trade Name]	Formulation	Patient Age*	Comparable Daily Dosage (μg) Low	Medium	High
Beclomethasone dipropionate [QVAR]	MDI (40 or 80 μg/puff)	Adult	80–240	240–840	>840
		Child	80–160	160–320	>320
Budesonide [Pulmicort Turbohaler]	DPI (200 μg/inhalation)	Adult	200–600	600–1200	>1200
		Child	200–400	400–800	>800
[Pulmicort Respules]	Suspension for nebulization	Child	500	1000	2000
Flunisolide [Aerobid, Aerobid-M]	MDI (250 μg/puff)	Adult	500–1000	1000–2000	>2000
		Child	500–750	1000–1250	>1250
Fluticasone propionate [Flovent]	MDI (44, 110, or 220 μg/puff)	Adult	88–264	264–660	>600
		Child	88–176	176–440	>440
[Flovent Rotadisk, Flovent Diskus]	DPI (50, 100, or 250 μg/inhalation)	Adult	100–300	300–600	>600
		Child	100–200	200–400	>400
Triamcinolone acetonide [Azmacort]	MDI (100 μg/puff)	Adult	400–1000	1000–2000	>2000
		Child	400–800	800–1200	>1200

*Child = 12 years of age or younger.

GLUCOCORTICOID/ BETA₂-AGONIST COMBINATION

Fluticasone (an inhaled glucocorticoid) and salmeterol (a long-acting, inhaled beta₂ agonist) are available in a DPI under the trade name *Advair Diskus*. The product is indicated for maintenance therapy of asthma in adults and in children at least 12 years old. The combination should be convenient for people with step 3 or step 4 asthma who need to take both drugs anyway. Advair Diskus is available in three strengths that deliver the following doses of salmeterol/fluticasone per inhalation: 50 μg/100 μg, 50 μg/250 μg, and 50 μg/500 μg. Dosing consists of one inhalation in the morning and one in the evening. For patients who are not already taking an inhaled glucocorticoid, the starting strength should contain the lowest (100 μg) dose of fluticasone. For patients already using an inhaled glucocorticoid, the dose of fluticasone should be equivalent to the dose of the glucocorticoid already in use.

CROMOLYN

Cromolyn [Intal] is a very safe and effective drug for *prophylaxis* of asthma, but is not useful for aborting an ongoing attack. Administration is by inhalation.

Effects on the Lung

Cromolyn suppresses inflammation; it is not a bronchodilator. The drug acts in part by stabilizing the cytoplasmic membrane of mast cells, thereby preventing release of histamine and other mediators. In addition, cromolyn inhibits eosinophils, macrophages, and other inflammatory cells.

Pharmacokinetics

Cromolyn is administered by inhalation. The fraction absorbed from the lungs is small (about 8%) and produces no systemic effects. Absorbed cromolyn is excreted unchanged in the urine.

Therapeutic Uses

Chronic Asthma. Cromolyn is a first-line agent for prophylactic therapy of moderate asthma. The drug produces adequate control in 60% to 70% of patients. When administered on a fixed schedule, cromolyn reduces both the frequency and intensity of attacks. No tolerance to effects is seen with long-term use. To be of benefit, cromolyn must be administered *prior* to the onset of an attack; the drug is without benefit if taken after an episode has begun. In patients with chronic asthma, maximal effects may take several weeks to develop. Cromolyn is especially effective for prophylaxis of seasonal allergic attacks and for acute prophylaxis immediately prior to allergen exposure (e.g., when anticipating mowing the lawn). Because of cromolyn's safety and efficacy, many clinicians feel that cromolyn is the anti-inflammatory drug of first choice for childhood asthma.

Exercise-Induced Bronchospasm. Cromolyn can prevent bronchospasm in patients predisposed to exercise-induced asthma. For this use, cromolyn should be administered 15 minutes prior to anticipated exertion.

Allergic Rhinitis. Intranasal cromolyn [Nasalcrom] can relieve symptoms of allergic rhinitis. This use is discussed in Chapter 72.

Adverse Effects

Cromolyn is the safest of all antiasthma medications. Significant adverse effects occur in fewer than 1 of every 10,000 patients. Occasionally, cough or bronchospasm occurs in response to cromolyn inhalation.

Preparations, Dosage, and Administration

Cromolyn for inhalation [Intal] can be administered with two devices: (1) a power-driven nebulizer and (2) an MDI. Patients will need instruction on using these devices. With the nebulizer, the *initial* dosage for adults and children is 20 mg 4 times a day. With the MDI, the *initial* dosage for adults and children is 2 to 4 puffs (1.6 to 3.2 mg) 4 times a day. For *maintenance* therapy with either device, the lowest effective dosage should be established. For therapy of chronic asthma, cromolyn must be administered on a fixed schedule.

NEDOCROMIL

Nedocromil [Tilade] has actions and uses similar to those of cromolyn. Like cromolyn, nedocromil has anti-inflammatory and antiallergic actions that derive in part from suppressing the release of histamine and other substances from mast cells. Nedocromil is administered with an MDI. The drug is indicated for prophylactic therapy only; it cannot abort an ongoing asthma attack. Like cromolyn, nedocromil decreases the incidence and severity of attacks. The most common adverse effect is an unpleasant taste, which about 5% of patients find intolerable. Otherwise, nedocromil is generally well tolerated. The usual dosage is 2 puffs (3.5 mg) 4 times a day. Once symptoms are controlled, 2 puffs a day may suffice. Maximal effects may take several weeks to develop.

METHYLXANTHINES

We first encountered the methylxanthines (theophylline, caffeine, others) in Chapter 35 (Central Nervous System Stimulants and Attention-Deficit/Hyperactivity Disorder). As discussed in that chapter, the most prominent actions of these drugs are (1) central nervous system (CNS) excitation and (2) bronchodilation. Other actions include cardiac stimulation, vasodilation, and diuresis.

Theophylline

Theophylline is the principal methylxanthine employed in asthma. Benefits derive primarily from bronchodilation. Theophylline has a narrow therapeutic range, and hence dosage must be carefully controlled. The drug is usually administered by mouth. Theophylline is not administered by inhalation because it is not active by this route.

In the past, theophylline was a first-line drug for asthma and nearly all patients with chronic asthma took it. However, use of theophylline has declined sharply, largely because we now have safer and more effective medications (inhaled beta₂ agonists, inhaled glucocorticoids, cromolyn).

Mechanism of Action

Theophylline produces bronchodilation by relaxing smooth muscle of the bronchi. The mechanism of this effect has not been determined. Of the mechanisms that have been proposed, the most probable is blockade of receptors for adenosine.

One frequently discussed mechanism suggests that methylxanthines act by inhibiting an enzyme called phosphodiesterase, and thereby elevate intracellular levels of cyclic AMP. This mechanism was proposed based on the ability of methylxanthines, in high concentrations, to inhibit phosphodiesterase in the test tube. However, since these high concentrations are not achieved in the body, it seems unlikely that inhibition of phosphodiesterase underlies the effects of methylxanthines in humans.

Use in Asthma

Oral theophylline is used for maintenance therapy of chronic stable asthma. Although less effective than beta₂ agonists, theophylline has a longer duration of action (when administered in a sustained-release formulation). With regular use, theophylline can decrease the frequency and severity of asthma attacks. Because its effects are prolonged, theophylline may be most appropriate for patients who experience nocturnal attacks.

Intravenous theophylline has been employed in emergencies. However, the drug is no more effective than beta₂ agonists and glucocorticoids, and is clearly more dangerous.

Pharmacokinetics

Absorption. Oral theophylline is available in standard and sustained-release formulations. The standard formulations are rapidly absorbed, but produce wide fluctuations in plasma drug levels. The sustained-release preparations are absorbed more slowly and produce plasma levels that are acceptably stable. Absorption from some sustained-release preparations can be affected by food.

Metabolism. Theophylline is metabolized in the liver. Rates of metabolism are affected by multiple factors—age, disease, and drugs—and show wide individual variation. As a result, the plasma half-life of theophylline varies considerably among patients. For example, while the average half-life in nonsmoking adults is about 8 hours, the half-life can be as short as 2 hours in some adults and as long as 15 hours in others. Smoking cigarettes (one to two packs a day) accelerates metabolism and decreases the half-life of theophylline by about 50%. The *average* half-life in children is 4 hours. Metabolism is slowed in patients with certain pathologics (e.g., heart disease, liver disease, prolonged fever). Some drugs (e.g., cimetidine, fluoroquinolone antibiotics) decrease theophylline metabolism. Other drugs (e.g., phenobarbital) accelerate metabolism. Because of these variations in metabolism, individualization of dosage is essential.

Plasma Drug Levels. Safe and effective therapy requires periodic measurement of theophylline blood levels. Traditionally, dosage has been adjusted to produce theophylline levels between 10 and 20 μg/ml. However, many patients respond well at 5 μg/ml, and, as a rule, there is little benefit to increasing levels above 15 μg/ml. Hence, levels between 5 and 15 μg/ml are appropriate for most patients. At levels above 20 μg/ml, the risk of significant adverse effects is high.

Toxicity

Symptoms. Toxicity is related to theophylline levels. Adverse effects are uncommon at plasma levels below 20 μg/ml. At 20 to 25 μg/ml, relatively mild reactions occur (e.g., nausea, vomiting, diarrhea, insomnia, restlessness). Serious adverse effects are most likely at levels above 30 μg/ml. These reactions include severe dysrhythmias (e.g., ventricular fibrillation) and convulsions that can be highly resistant to treatment. Death may result from cardiorespiratory collapse.

Treatment. At the first indication of toxicity, administration of theophylline should cease. If a large amount of the drug has been ingested, ipecac can be given to induce vomiting. After this, absorption can be decreased by administering activated charcoal together with a cathartic. Ventricular dysrhythmias respond to lidocaine. Intravenous diazepam may help control seizures.

Drug Interactions

Caffeine. Caffeine is a methylxanthine with pharmacologic properties like those of theophylline (see Chapter 35). Accordingly, caffeine can intensify the adverse effects of theophylline on the CNS and heart. In addition, caffeine can compete with theophylline for drug-metabolizing enzymes, thereby causing theophylline levels to rise. Because of these interactions, individuals taking theophylline should avoid caffeine-containing beverages (e.g., coffee, many soft drinks) and other sources of caffeine.

Drugs That Reduce Theophylline Levels. Several agents—including *phenobarbital, phenytoin,* and *rifampin*—can lower theophylline levels by inducing hepatic drug-metabolizing enzymes. Concurrent use of these agents may necessitate an increase in theophylline dosage.

Drugs That Increase Theophylline Levels. Several drugs—including *cimetidine* and the *fluoroquinolone antibiotics* (e.g., ciprofloxacin)—can elevate plasma levels of theophylline, primarily by inhibiting hepatic metabolism. To avoid theophylline toxicity, the dosage of theophylline should be reduced when the drug is combined with these agents.

Oral Formulations

Oral theophylline is available in standard and sustained-release formulations. The standard formulations are rapidly absorbed, require frequent administration, and produce substantial fluctuations in plasma theophylline levels. Sus-

tained-release formulations are more convenient and can produce drug levels that are relatively stable. Accordingly, sustained-release formulations are preferred for routine therapy. Sustained-release preparations are available in 8-, 12-, and 24-hour forms.

Absorption from sustained-release formulations can be affected markedly by food. For example, absorption from one preparation—Theo-24—is accelerated in the presence of a fatty meal. In contrast, food reduces absorption from a product named Theo-Dur Sprinkle (which was recently withdrawn from the market).

Because theophylline has a narrow therapeutic range, and because sustained-release formulations contain large amounts of the drug, accelerated absorption from sustained-release formulations can produce dangerous elevations in theophylline blood levels. Because of this potential hazard, some clinicians avoid the formulations intended for once-a-day administration. These preparations pose the greatest threat because they contain the largest amount of theophylline.

Dosage and Administration

Oral. Dosage must be individualized. Traditionally, dosage has been adjusted to maintain plasma theophylline levels between 10 and 20 μg/ml. However, levels between 5 and 15 μg/ml are appropriate for most patients. To minimize chances of toxicity, doses should be low initially and then gradually increased. If a dose is missed, the following dose should not be doubled, because doing so could produce toxicity. Smokers require higher than average doses. Conversely, patients with heart disease, liver dysfunction, or prolonged fever are likely to require relatively low doses. Patients should be instructed not to chew the sustained-release formulations. Product information should be consulted for compatibility with food.

Maintenance dosages vary with the age of the patient. A typical maintenance dosage for *adults* is 200 to 300 mg 2 or 3 times a day. Guidelines for *pediatric* dosing are as follows: for children 1 to 9 years old, 22 mg/kg/day; for children 9 to 12 years old, 20 mg/kg/day; and for children 12 to 16 years old, 18 mg/kg/day. The number of daily doses depends on the duration of action of the preparation employed.

Intravenous. Intravenous theophylline is reserved for emergencies. Administration must be done slowly, since rapid injection can cause fatal cardiovascular reactions. Intravenous theophylline is incompatible with many other drugs. Accordingly, compatibility should be verified prior to mixing theophylline with other IV agents. For specific IV dosages, refer to the discussion of *aminophylline* below.

Other Methylxanthines
Aminophylline

Aminophylline [Truphylline, Phyllocontin] is a theophylline salt that is considerably more soluble than theophylline itself. In solution, each molecule of aminophylline dissociates to yield two molecules of theophylline. Hence, the pharmacologic properties of aminophylline and theophylline are identical. Aminophylline is available in formulations for oral, IV, and rectal administration. Intravenous administration is employed most often.

Administration and Dosage. Intravenous. Because of its relatively high solubility, aminophylline is the preferred form of theophylline for IV use. Infusions should be done *slowly* (no faster than 25 mg/min), because rapid injection can produce severe hypotension and death. The usual loading dose is 6 mg/kg. The maintenance infusion rate should be adjusted to provide plasma levels of theophylline that are within the therapeutic range (10 to 20 μg/ml). Aminophylline solutions are incompatible with a number of other drugs. Accordingly, compatibility must be verified before mixing aminophylline with other IV agents.

Oral. Aminophylline is available in tablets and solution for oral administration. Dosing guidelines are the same as for theophylline.

Rectal. Aminophylline is available in suppositories and solution for rectal administration. Absorption from the suppositories is erratic, and hence these preparations are not recommended. Rectal solutions provide fast and reliable dosing and are safe for occasional use. Dosages for adults and children are the same as for oral theophylline.

Oxtriphylline

Oxtriphylline [Choledyl SA] is a salt of theophylline that contains 71% theophylline by weight. The drug is administered by mouth and produces the same effects as pure theophylline. Oxtriphylline offers no therapeutic advantage over theophylline itself. The dose of oxtriphylline equivalent to 100 mg of theophylline is 156 mg.

Dyphylline

Although structurally similar to theophylline, dyphylline [Dilor, Lufyllin] is nonetheless a completely distinct compound, and is not converted to theophylline in the body. Dyphylline may be administered orally or IM. The drug has a half-life of 2 hours and is eliminated unchanged in the urine. The maximum adult oral dosage is 15 mg/kg 4 times a day. The adult IM dosage is 250 to 500 mg every 6 hours.

IPRATROPIUM

Actions and Use in Asthma. Ipratropium [Atrovent, Combivent, DuoNeb] is an atropine derivative administered by inhalation to relieve bronchospasm. The drug is approved only for bronchospasm associated with chronic obstructive pulmonary disease, but is used for asthma nonetheless. Like atropine, ipratropium is a muscarinic antagonist. By blocking muscarinic cholinergic receptors in the bronchi, ipratropium promotes *bronchodilation*. Therapeutic effects begin within 30 seconds, reach 50% of their maximum in 3 minutes, and persist about 6 hours. Ipratropium is effective against allergen-induced asthma and exercise-induced bronchospasm, but is less effective than the beta$_2$ agonists. However, because ipratropium and the beta$_2$-adrenergic agonists promote bronchodilation by different mechanisms, their beneficial effects are additive.

Adverse Effects. Systemic effects are minimal. Ipratropium is a quaternary ammonium compound, and therefore always carries a positive charge. As a result, the drug is not readily absorbed from the lungs or from the digestive tract. Hence, systemic effects are rare. The most common adverse reactions are dry mouth and irritation of the pharynx. If systemic absorption is sufficient, the drug may raise intraocular pressure in patients with glaucoma.

Preparations, Dosage, and Administration. Ipratropium is available alone [Atrovent] and in combination with albuterol [Combivent, DuoNeb].

Ipratropium by itself [Atrovent] is dispensed in an MDI that delivers 18 μg per actuation. For management of bronchospasm, the recommended adult dosage is 2 to 4 puffs 4 times a day. The pediatric dosage is 2 puffs 4 times a day.

Ipratropium plus albuterol is available in two formulations: an MDI [Combivent] and solution for nebulization [DuoNeb]. With each actuation, the Combivent MDI delivers 18 μg of ipratropium and 90 μg of albuterol; the recommended dosage is 2 inhalations 4 times a day. DuoNeb solution contains 500 μg of ipratropium and 2500 μg of albuterol in 3-ml, single-use vials; the recommended dosage is 3 ml administered 4 times a day by nebulization.

LEUKOTRIENE MODIFIERS

The leukotriene modifiers are the newest class of drugs for asthma. In fact, when they were introduced in the late 1990s, they were the first new drugs for asthma in over 20 years. All of these agents suppress the effects of leukotrienes, compounds that promote bronchoconstriction as well as eosinophil infiltration, mucus production, and airway edema. In patients with asthma, these drugs can decrease inflammation, bronchoconstriction, edema, mucus secretion, and recruitment of eosinophils and other inflammatory cells.

Currently, three leukotriene modifiers are available: zileuton, zafirlukast, and montelukast. Zileuton blocks leukotriene synthesis; zafirlukast and montelukast block leukotriene receptors. Because these drugs are relatively new, their therapeutic niche has not been firmly established.

Zileuton

Zileuton [Zyflo], an inhibitor of leukotriene synthesis, is approved for prophylactic and maintenance therapy of asthma in adults and in children 12 years of age and older. Benefits derive from inhibiting 5-lipoxygenase, the enzyme that converts arachidonic acid into leukotrienes. Symptomatic improvement can be seen within 1 to 2 hours of dosing. Because effects are not immediate, zileuton cannot be used to abort an ongoing attack.

Zileuton is given orally and undergoes rapid absorption, both in the presence and absence of food. Plasma levels peak 2 to 3 hours after dosing. Zileuton is rapidly metabolized by the liver, and the metabolites are excreted in the urine. Its plasma half-life is 2.5 hours.

Zileuton can injure the liver, as evidenced by increased plasma levels of alanine aminotransferase (ALT) activity. A few patients have developed symptomatic hepatitis, which reversed following drug withdrawal. To reduce the risk of serious liver injury, ALT activity should be monitored. The recommended schedule is once a month for 3 months, then every 2 to 3 months for the remainder of the first year, and periodically thereafter. In addition to liver injury, zileuton can cause dyspepsia. In mice taking 4 times the human dose, the drug increased the incidence of liver, kidney, and vascular tumors.

Zileuton is metabolized by cytochrome P450, and hence can compete with other drugs for metabolism, thereby increasing their levels. Combined use with theophylline can markedly increase theophylline levels. Accordingly, dosage of theophylline should be reduced. Zileuton can also increase levels of warfarin and propranolol.

Zileuton is available in 600-mg tablets. The recommended dosage is 600 mg 4 times a day. The drug may taken with or without food.

Zafirlukast

Zafirlukast [Accolate] is the first representative of a new class of anti-inflammatory agents, the *leukotriene receptor antagonists*. The drug is approved for maintenance therapy of chronic asthma in adults and children 5 years of age and older. Benefits derive in part from reduced infiltration of inflammatory cells and decreased bronchoconstriction. In clinical trials, zafirlukast produced modest symptomatic relief in patients with mild to moderate asthma. The drug is less effective than inhaled beclomethasone, a glucocorticoid.

Zafirlukast is administered orally and absorption is rapid. Food reduces absorption by 40%. Hence, the drug should be administered at least 1 hour before meals or 2 hours after. Zafirlukast undergoes hepatic metabolism followed by fecal excretion. The half-life is about 10 hours, but may be as long as 20 hours in the elderly.

Zafirlukast causes few adverse effects—although there is concern about liver injury and Churg-Strauss syndrome. The most common side effects are headache and GI disturbances, both of which are infrequent. Arthralgia and myalgia may also occur. A few patients have developed Churg-Strauss syndrome, a potentially fatal disorder characterized by weight loss, flu-like symptoms, and pulmonary vasculitis (blood vessel inflammation). However, in all cases, symptoms developed when glucocorticoids were being withdrawn, suggesting that glucocorticoid withdrawal—and not zafirlukast—may be the underlying cause.

Rarely, patients develop clinical signs of liver injury (e.g., abdominal pain, jaundice, fatigue). If these occur, zafirlukast should be discontinued, and liver function tests (especially serum ALT) should be performed immediately. If test results are consistent with liver injury, zafirlukast should not be resumed. Curiously, signs of liver injury have developed mainly in females.

Zafirlukast inhibits two isozymes of cytochrome P450, and hence can suppress metabolism of other drugs, thereby raising their levels. Concurrent use can raise serum theophylline to toxic levels. Accordingly, serum theophylline should be closely monitored, especially when zafirlukast is started or stopped. Zafirlukast can also raise levels of warfarin (an anticoagulant), and may thereby cause bleeding.

Zafirlukast is available in 10- and 20-mg tablets. The dosage for adults and children 12 years of age and older is 20 mg twice a day. The dosage for children 5 to 11 years old is 10 mg twice a day. Zafirlukast should not be administered with food.

Montelukast

Montelukast [Singulair] is a leukotriene receptor blocker indicated for maintenance therapy of asthma—but not for quick relief. The drug is approved for all patients over the age of 1 year. Maximal effects develop within 24 hours of the first dose, and are maintained with once-daily dosing in the evening. In clinical trials, montelukast decreased asthma-related nocturnal awakening, improved morning lung function, and decreased the need for a short-acting inhaled beta$_2$ agonist throughout the day. As monotherapy, montelukast is less effective than inhaled glucocorticoids. However, when combined with an inhaled glucocorticoid, montelukast can improve symptoms and may permit a reduction in glucocorticoid dosage.

Montelukast is rapidly absorbed following oral administration. Bioavailability is about 64%. Blood levels peak 3 to 4 hours after ingestion. The drug is highly bound (>99%) to plasma proteins. Montelukast undergoes extensive metabolism by hepatic P450 enzymes followed by excretion in the bile. The plasma half-life ranges from 2.7 to 5.5 hours.

Montelukast is very well tolerated. In clinical trials, adverse effects were equivalent to those of placebo. In contrast to zileuton and zafirlukast, montelukast does not seem to cause liver injury. As with zafirlukast, Churg-Strauss syndrome has occurred when glucocorticoid dosage was reduced.

Montelukast appears devoid of serious drug interactions. Unlike zileuton and zafirlukast, it does not increase levels of theophylline or warfarin. Concurrent use of phenytoin (an anticonvulsant that induces P450 enzymes) can decrease levels of montelukast.

Montelukast is available in three formulations: standard tablets (10 mg), chewable tablets (4 and 5 mg), and oral granules (4 mg/packet). The oral granules may be put directly in the mouth or may be mixed with one spoonful of either applesauce, carrots, rice, or ice cream. With all formulations, dosing is done once a day in the evening, with or without food. Dosage is based on patient age as follows:

- Age 15 years and older—one 10-mg tablet daily
- Age 6 to 14 years—one 5-mg chewable tablet daily
- Age 2 to 5 years—one 4-mg chewable tablet or 4 mg of oral granules daily
- Age 12 to 23 months—4 mg of oral granules daily

MANAGEMENT OF ASTHMA

In June 2002, the National Asthma Education and Prevention Program (NAEPP) of the National Heart, Lung, and Blood Institute introduced revised guidelines for treatment of asthma in a document titled *Expert Panel Report: Guidelines for the Diagnosis and Management of Asthma—Update on Selected Topics 2002* (EPR-Update 2002). This new report updates five sections of a more comprehensive clinical guideline titled *Expert Panel Report 2: Guidelines for the Diagnosis and Management of Asthma* (EPR-2), released in 1997. The discussion below reflects recommendations in these two guidelines.

Chronic Asthma

Therapy of chronic asthma has undergone significant change in recent years. Use of inhaled glucocorticoids and cromolyn has greatly increased, owing to increased appreciation of the role of inflammation in asthma. Conversely, use of theophylline has sharply declined: Once employed as a first-line drug for most patients, theophylline is now considered a second- or third-line agent. Inhaled, *short-acting* beta$_2$ agonists have been and remain a mainstay of treatment—and inhaled, *long-acting* beta$_2$ agonists now have a prominent role. When asthma medications are used appropriately, most patients can live normal lives, with little or no limitation of activities and few or no side effects.

Measuring Lung Function

Before considering asthma therapy, we need to address tests of lung function. Two of these are described below.

Forced expiratory volume (FEV) is the single most useful test of lung function. Unfortunately, the instrument required—a *spirometer*—is both expensive and cumbersome, and therefore not suited for use at home. To determine FEV, the patient inhales completely, and then exhales as completely and forcefully as possible into the spirometer. The spirometer measures how much air was expelled. Results are then compared to a "predicted normal value" for a healthy person of similar age, sex, height, and weight. Hence, for a patient with asthma, the FEV might be 75% of the predicted value.

Peak expiratory flow rate (PEFR) is defined as the maximal rate of airflow during expiration. To determine PEFR, the patient exhales as forcefully as possible into a *peak flowmeter,* a relatively inexpensive, handheld device. Patients should measure their peak flow every morning. If the peak flow is less than 80% of their personal best, more frequent monitoring should be done.

Classification of Chronic Asthma

As described in the EPR-2, chronic asthma has four classes of increasing severity: (1) mild intermittent, (2) mild persistent, (3) moderate persistent, and (4) severe persistent. Diagnostic criteria for these classes are summarized in Table 71–4. As shown in the table, as we progress from mild intermittent

TABLE 71–4 ■ Classification of Asthma Severity

Classification	Frequency and Duration of Symptoms*	Nighttime Symptoms	Lung Function
STEP 1: Mild Intermittent	• Symptoms <2 times a week • Asymptomatic and normal PEFR between exacerbations • Exacerbations last a few hours to a few days; intensity may vary	<2 times a month	• PEFR or FEV$_1$ ≥80% predicted • PEFR variability <20%
STEP 2: Mild Persistent	• Symptoms >2 times a week but <1 time a day • Exacerbations may affect activity	>2 times a month	• PEFR or FEV$_1$ ≥80% predicted • PEFR variability 20%–30%
STEP 3: Moderate Persistent	• Daily symptoms • Daily use of inhaled short-acting beta$_2$ agonist • Exacerbations affect activity • Exacerbations >2 times a week and may last days	>1 time a week	• PEFR or FEV$_1$ >60% and <80% of predicted • PEFR variability >30%
STEP 4: Severe Persistent	• Continual symptoms • Limited physical activity • Frequent exacerbations	Frequent	• PEFR or FEV$_1$ ≤60% predicted • PEFR variability >30%

*Patients at any level of severity can have mild, moderate, or severe exacerbations. Some patients with intermittent asthma experience severe, life-threatening exacerbations separated by long periods of normal lung function and no symptoms.
PEFR = peak expiratory flow rate, FEV$_1$ = forced expiratory volume in 1 second.
Adapted from National Asthma Education and Prevention Program. Expert Panel Report 2: Guidelines for the Diagnosis and Managment of Asthma. Bethesda, MD, National Heart, Lung, and Blood Institute, 1997.

asthma to severe persistent asthma, symptoms occur more often and last longer, exacerbations become more frequent, PEFR (or FEV) decreases to less than 60% of the predicted value, PEFR becomes more variable, and limitations on physical activity become substantial.

Drug Therapy

Drugs are employed in two ways in chronic asthma: some agents are taken to establish *long-term control* and some are taken for *quick relief* (Table 71–5). Long-term control drugs are administered daily to achieve and maintain control of persistent asthma. Anti-inflammatory drugs—especially inhaled glucocorticoids—provide the foundation for long-term control; long-acting inhaled beta$_2$ agonists are also important. Quick-relief medications are taken to promptly reverse bronchoconstriction, and thereby provide rapid relief from cough, chest tightness, and wheezing. By far the most important drugs for quick relief are the short-acting inhaled beta$_2$ agonists. With all of the drugs used for asthma, the treatment goals are to

- Prevent chronic and troublesome symptoms (e.g., coughing or breathlessness after exertion or in the night or early morning)
- Maintain normal (or near-normal) pulmonary function
- Maintain normal activity levels, including exercise
- Prevent recurrent exacerbations
- Minimize the need for emergency department visits or hospitalizations
- Provide maximum benefits with minimum adverse effects
- Meet patient and family expectations regarding asthma care

As in the EPR-2, the EPR-Update 2002 recommends *stepwise* therapy of chronic asthma (Table 71–6). The four steps of this approach correspond to the four classes of asthma severity discussed above. For patients with persistent asthma (steps 2, 3, and 4), long-term control medications provide the cornerstone of treatment; as the severity of symptoms increases, dosages are increased and additional drugs are added. For *all* patients, a quick-relief drug is taken as needed.

Stepwise therapy may be implemented in two ways. One option is to initiate treatment at the step that corresponds to the patient's asthma severity, and then gradually step up as needed. The second option, which is recommended by the Expert Panel, is to initiate treatment at a step *higher* than the patient's asthma classification, and then step down after control has been achieved. The benefit of this more aggressive approach is faster control of the underlying inflammatory process. As a result, permanent injury to the lungs *may* be reduced, thereby allowing treatment in the future with lower doses of anti-inflammatory drugs than might otherwise be required. Specific recommendations for stepwise therapy, as presented in the EPR-2 and modified in the EPR-Update 2002, are discussed below and summarized in Table 71–6.

Step 1: Mild Intermittent Asthma. Mild intermittent asthma is treated on a PRN basis; long-term control medication is not needed. The occasional acute attack is managed by inhaling a short-acting beta$_2$ agonist. If the patient needs the beta$_2$ agonist more than twice a week, moving to step 2 may be indicated.

TABLE 71–5 ■ Drugs for Asthma: Agents for Long-Term Control Versus Quick Relief

Long-Term Control Medications

Anti-inflammatory Drugs
  Glucocorticoids (inhaled or oral)
  Cromolyn and nedocromil
  Leukotriene modifiers

Bronchodilators
  Long-acting inhaled beta$_2$ agonists
  Long-acting oral beta$_2$ agonists
  Theophylline

Quick-Relief Medications

Bronchodilators
  Short-acting inhaled beta$_2$ agonists
  Ipratropium

Anti-inflammatory Drugs
  Glucocorticoids, systemic*

*Considered quick-relief drugs when used in a short burst (3 to 10 days) at the start of therapy or during a period of gradual deterioration. Glucocorticoids are not used for immediate relief of an ongoing attack.

TABLE 71–6 ■ Stepwise Approach for Managing Asthma*

Classification	Long-Term Control Drugs (Taken Daily)	Quick-Relief Drugs (PRN)
STEP 1: Mild Intermittent	• No daily medication needed	• Short-acting inhaled beta$_2$ agonist
STEP 2: Mild Persistent	• Low-dose inhaled glucocorticoids	• Same as step 1
STEP 3: Moderate Persistent	• Low-dose inhaled glucocorticoids *plus* long-acting inhaled beta$_2$ agonist **or** • Medium-dose inhaled glucocorticoids	• Same as step 1
STEP 4: Severe Persistent	• High-dose inhaled glucocorticoids *plus* long-acting inhaled beta$_2$ agonists • Oral glucocorticoids (if needed)	• Same as step 1

*This table summarizes *preferred* treatment options; additional options are discussed in the text.
Adapted from National Asthma Education and Prevention Program. Expert Panel Report: Guidelines for the Diagnosis and Management of Asthma—Update on Selected Topics 2002. Bethesda, MD, National Heart, Lung and Blood Institute, 2002.

Step 2: Mild Persistent Asthma. Mild persistent asthma requires a combination of long-term control medication plus quick-relief medication. The foundation of treatment is daily inhalation of an anti-inflammatory drug. Currently, the preferred initial drug for adults *and* children is an inhaled glucocorticoid, taken in low dosage. Second-line drugs for long-term control include cromolyn and the leukotriene receptor antagonists (e.g., zafirlukast). As in step 1, a short-acting $beta_2$ agonist is inhaled PRN to suppress breakthrough attacks. Inhaling the $beta_2$ agonist every day, or increasing its use, suggests that advancing to step 3 may be needed.

Step 3: Moderate Persistent Asthma. Moderate persistent asthma requires more intensive long-term control than does mild persistent asthma. This can be achieved by either (1) inhaling a glucocorticoid in a *medium* dosage (as compared with the low dosage used in step 1) or (2) inhaling a glucocorticoid in a *low* dosage and adding a long-acting inhaled $beta_2$ agonist (e.g., salmeterol). The second option is generally preferred. Why? Because control is often better and the risk of systemic effects from the glucocorticoid is lower. Alternatives to adding inhaled salmeterol to the low-dose glucocorticoid include (1) adding sustained-release theophylline, (2) adding a leukotriene receptor antagonist, or (3) adding a long-acting *oral* $beta_2$ agonist (e.g., sustained-release albuterol). For patients with severe, recurrent exacerbations, the preferred regimen is a *medium-dose* inhaled glucocorticoid plus a long-acting inhaled $beta_2$ agonist. As in steps 1 and 2, breakthrough episodes are managed with a short-acting inhaled $beta_2$ agonist. If the patient inhales the $beta_2$ agonist every day or increases its use, advancing to step 4 may be indicated.

Step 4: Severe Persistent Asthma. Severe chronic asthma is managed with daily inhalation of a *high-dose* glucocorticoid plus a long-acting $beta_2$ agonist. Alternatives to the inhaled $beta_2$ agonist include sustained-release theophylline or a long-acting, oral $beta_2$ agonist. If symptoms are especially severe, an *oral* glucocorticoid should be *added* to the regimen; administration may be once daily or once every other day. Breakthrough attacks are managed with a short-acting, inhaled $beta_2$ agonist.

Step-Down. Once the treatment goal has been achieved and then sustained, a reduction in drug use may be attempted. The purpose is to identify the minimal therapy required. A step-down attempt is especially important for patients who stepped up owing to seasonal allergy, but may no longer need intensified therapy after the allergy season is over.

Zone System for Monitoring Treatment

Patients can monitor their treatment using a scheme based on green, yellow, and red "zones," which are analogous to green, yellow, and red traffic lights. By using this system, patients can position themselves for early implementation of corrective measures when control begins to slip or has become dangerously inadequate. To determine which zone they are in, patients must monitor their symptoms and PEFR.

Green Zone. In this zone, patients have no symptoms and their PEFR is greater than 80% of their personal best. The green zone indicates that control is good.

Yellow Zone. In this zone, patients have some symptoms and their PEFR is 50% to 80% of their personal best. The yellow zone indicates that control is insufficient. To regain control, patients should inhale a short-acting $beta_2$ agonist. If this fails to return them to the green zone, a short course (4 days) of oral glucocorticoids may be indicated. Alternatively, the patient may need to advance to a higher step.

Red Zone. In this zone, symptoms occur at rest or interfere with activities, and the PEFR is less than 50% of the patient's personal best. The red zone indicates a medical alert. A $beta_2$ agonist should be inhaled immediately. If the PEFR remains below 50%, the patient should seek medical attention for acute severe asthma (see below).

Reducing Exposure to Allergens and Triggers

The treatment plan should include measures to control allergens and other factors that can cause airway inflammation and exacerbate symptoms. When successful, these measures can significantly reduce symptoms. Important sources of asthma-associated allergens include the house dust mite, warm-blooded pets, cockroaches, and molds. Factors that can exacerbate asthma include tobacco smoke, wood smoke, and household sprays. To the extent possible, exposure to these factors should be reduced or eliminated. For those who are reluctant to part with Fluffy (the family cat) or Ralph (the family dog), weekly washing of the critter may help. More importantly, the pet should be banned from the patient's bedroom.

The house dust mite is the most notorious cause of asthma. Allergy develops not to the microscopic mite itself, but rather to its even more microscopic feces. Measures to control or avoid dust mites and their feces include

- Encasing the patient's pillow, mattress, and box spring with covers that are impermeable to allergens
- Washing all bedding and stuffed animals weekly on the hot cycle (130°F)
- Removing carpeting or rugs from the bedroom
- Avoiding sleeping or lying on upholstered furniture
- Keeping indoor humidity below 50%

Unfortunately, even when these measure are implemented, their impact on asthma symptoms is generally small.

Acute Severe Exacerbations

Acute severe exacerbations of asthma require immediate attention. Hospitalization may be required. The goal is to relieve airway obstruction and hypoxemia, and normalize lung function as soon as possible. The foundation of treatment is repetitive inhalation of a $beta_2$ agonist, administered by nebulizer or MDI. (If the patient is unconscious or unable to generate PEFR, subcutaneous epinephrine should be given.) If there is no response to the first dose of a $beta_2$ agonist, a glucocorticoid (e.g., IV methylprednisolone or oral prednisone) should be given. Oxygen is administered to maintain oxygen saturation above 95%. As a rule, an oral glucocorticoid is taken for 1 week after discharge; addition of a high-dose inhaled glucocorticoid for 3 weeks can improve the outcome. Full recovery of lung function may take weeks.

Exercise-Induced Bronchospasm

Exercise increases airway obstruction in practically all people with chronic asthma. The cause of obstruction is bronchospasm secondary to loss of heat and/or water from the lung. Exercise-induced bronchospasm usually starts either during or immediately after exercise, peaks in 5 to 10 minutes, and resolves 20 to 30 minutes later.

With proper medication, most asthmatic patients can be as active as they wish. Indeed, many world-class athletes have asthma, including Jackie Joyner-Kersee and other Olympic gold medalists. To prevent symptoms related to exercise, patients should inhale a beta$_2$ agonist or cromolyn prophylactically. Beta$_2$ agonists should be inhaled immediately before exercise; cromolyn should be inhaled 15 minutes before exercise.

⁛ KEY POINTS

- Asthma is a chronic inflammatory disease characterized by inflammation of the airways, bronchial hyperreactivity, and bronchospasm. Allergy is often the underlying cause.
- Asthma is treated with anti-inflammatory drugs and bronchodilators.
- Most drugs for asthma are administered by inhalation, a route that increases therapeutic effects (by delivering drugs directly to their site of action), reduces systemic effects (by minimizing drug levels in blood), and facilitates rapid relief of acute attacks.
- Three devices are used for inhalation: metered-dose inhalers (MDIs), dry-powder inhalers (DPIs), and nebulizers. Patients will need instruction on their use.
- Inhaled beta$_2$ agonists are the most effective drugs available for relieving acute bronchospasm and preventing exercise-induced bronchospasm.
- Beta$_2$ agonists promote bronchodilation by activating beta$_2$ receptors in bronchial smooth muscle.
- Most inhaled beta$_2$ agonists have a rapid onset and short duration, which makes them useful for short-term prophylaxis and relief of acute attacks, but not for prolonged prophylaxis.
- Two inhaled beta$_2$ agonists—formoterol and salmeterol—have a long duration of action, and hence are indicated for prolonged prophylaxis, but not for treating acute attacks.
- Inhaled beta$_2$ agonists rarely cause systemic side effects.
- Excessive dosing with oral beta$_2$ agonists can cause tachycardia and angina by activating beta$_1$ receptors on the heart. (Selectivity is lost at high doses.)
- Glucocorticoids are the most effective antiasthma drugs available.
- Glucocorticoids reduce symptoms of asthma by suppressing inflammation. As an added bonus, glucocorticoids promote synthesis of bronchial beta$_2$ receptors, and increase their responsiveness to beta$_2$ agonists.
- Inhaled and systemic glucocorticoids are used for long-term prophylaxis of asthma—not for aborting ongoing attacks. Accordingly, they are administered on a fixed schedule—not PRN.
- Unless asthma is severe, glucocorticoids should be administered by inhalation.
- Inhaled glucocorticoids are generally very safe. Their principal side effects are oropharyngeal candidiasis and dysphonia, which can be minimized by employing a spacer device during administration and by gargling after.
- Inhaled glucocorticoids can promote bone loss. To minimize loss, dosage should be as low as possible, and patients should get regular weight-bearing exercise and should ensure adequate intake of calcium and vitamin D.
- Inhaled glucocorticoids can slow the growth rate of children, but these drugs do not reduce adult height.
- Prolonged therapy with oral glucocorticoids can cause serious adverse effects, including adrenal suppression, osteoporosis, hyperglycemia, peptic ulcer disease, and growth suppression.
- Because of adrenal suppression, patients taking oral glucocorticoids (and patients who have switched from oral glucocorticoids to inhaled glucocorticoids) must be given supplemental doses of oral or IV glucocorticoids at times of stress.
- Cromolyn is an inhaled anti-inflammatory drug used for prophylaxis of asthma.
- Cromolyn reduces inflammation primarily by preventing release of mediators from mast cells.
- For long-term prophylaxis, cromolyn is taken daily on a fixed schedule. For prophylaxis of exercise-induced bronchospasm, cromolyn is taken 15 minutes before anticipated exertion.
- Cromolyn is the safest drug for asthma. Serious adverse effects are extremely rare.
- Theophylline, a member of the methylxanthine family, relieves asthma by causing bronchodilation.
- Although theophylline was used widely in the past, it has been largely replaced by safer and more effective medications.
- There are four classes of chronic asthma: mild intermittent, mild persistent, moderate persistent, and severe persistent.
- For therapeutic purposes, asthma drugs can be classified as long-term control medications (e.g., inhaled glucocorticoids, cromolyn) and quick-relief medications (e.g., inhaled, short-acting beta$_2$ agonists).
- In the stepwise approach to asthma therapy, treatment becomes more aggressive as symptoms become more frequent and intense.
- The goals of stepwise therapy are to prevent symptoms, maintain near-normal pulmonary function, maintain normal activity, prevent recurrent exacerbations, minimize emergency room visits, minimize drug side effects, and meet patient and family expectations about treatment.
- Mild intermittent asthma is treated on a PRN basis: a short-acting beta$_2$ agonist is inhaled to abort the few acute episodes that occur.
- For mild persistent asthma, the foundation of therapy is daily inhalation of a *low-dose* glucocorticoid. A short-acting beta$_2$ agonist is inhaled PRN to suppress breakthrough attacks.
- For moderate persistent asthma, long-term control is established with either (1) a *medium-dose* inhaled glu-

cocorticoid or (2) a *low-dose* inhaled glucocorticoid plus a long-acting inhaled beta₂ agonist (e.g., salmeterol).

■ For severe persistent asthma, the foundation of therapy is a high-dose inhaled glucocorticoid plus a long-acting inhaled beta₂ agonist. An oral glucocorticoid is added if needed.

■ For acute severe exacerbations of asthma, the foundation of treatment is repetitive inhalation of a beta₂ agonist. A systemic glucocorticoid may also be needed.

■ Exercise-induced bronchospasm can be avoided by inhaling either cromolyn or a fast-acting, inhaled beta₂ agonist prior to strenuous activity.

■ By daily monitoring of symptoms and peak expiratory flow rate (PEFR), patients can poise themselves for early implementation of corrective measures when asthma control begins to slip or has become dangerously inadequate.

■ Patients should avoid allergens that can cause airway inflammation and triggers that can provoke exacerbations. Important sources of allergens are the house dust mite, warm-blooded pets, cockroaches, and molds. Important triggers are tobacco smoke, wood smoke, and household sprays.

Summary of Major Nursing Implications*

BETA₂-ADRENERGIC AGONISTS

Inhaled: Short Acting

Albuterol
Bitolterol
Levalbuterol
Pirbuterol

Inhaled: Long Acting

Formoterol
Salmeterol

Oral

Albuterol
Terbutaline

Preadministration Assessment

Therapeutic Goal

Short-acting inhaled beta₂ agonists are used PRN for prophylaxis of exercise-induced bronchospasm and to relieve ongoing asthma attacks. Oral beta₂ agonists and long-acting inhaled agents are used for maintenance therapy.

Baseline Data

Determine PEFR (or FEV) and the frequency and severity of attacks, and attempt to identify trigger factors.

Identifying High-Risk Patients

Systemic (oral, parenteral) beta₂ agonists are *contraindicated* for patients with tachydysrhythmias or tachycardia associated with digitalis toxicity. Use systemic beta₂ agonists with *caution* in patients with diabetes, hyperthyroidism, organic heart disease, hypertension, or angina pectoris.

Implementation: Administration

Routes

Usual. Inhalation.
Occasional. Oral, subcutaneous.

Administration

Inhalation. Inhaled beta₂ agonists are administered with an MDI, DPI, or nebulizer. Teach patients how to use these devices. For patients who have difficulty with hand-lung coordination, use of a spacer with a one-way valve may improve results.

Inform patients who are using MDIs or DPIs that, when 2 puffs are needed, an interval of at least 1 minute should elapse between puffs.

Warn patients against exceeding recommended dosages.

Inform patients that inhaled *formoterol* and *salmeterol* (long-acting beta₂ agonists) should be taken on a fixed schedule—not PRN.

Oral. Instruct patients to take oral beta₂ agonists on a fixed schedule—not PRN.

Instruct patients to swallow sustained-release preparations intact, without crushing or chewing.

Ongoing Evaluation and Interventions

Evaluating Therapeutic Effects

Teach patients with chronic asthma to monitor and record PEFR, symptom frequency, and symptom intensity. Teach patients to evaluate whether they are in the green, yellow, or red zone, and what the proper response to being in these zones is.

Minimizing Adverse Effects

When administered by *inhalation* at recommended doses, beta₂ agonists are generally devoid of adverse effects. Cardiac stimulation and tremors are most likely with systemic therapy.

Cardiac Stimulation. Excessive dosing with systemic beta₂ agonists can cause stimulation of beta₁ receptors on the heart, resulting in anginal pain and tachydysrhythmias. Instruct the patient to report chest pain and changes in heart rate or rhythm.

Tremor. Tremor is common with systemic beta₂ agonists, and usually subsides with continued drug use. If necessary, tremor can be reduced by lowering the dosage.

*Patient education information is highlighted as blue text.

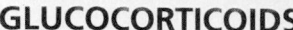

Summary of Major Nursing Implications*—cont'd

GLUCOCORTICOIDS

Inhaled

Beclomethasone
Budesonide
Flunisolide
Fluticasone
Triamcinolone

Oral

Prednisolone
Prednisone

The nursing implications summarized below refer specifically to the use of glucocorticoids in asthma. A full summary of nursing implications for glucocorticoids is presented in Chapter 68.

Preadministration Assessment

Therapeutic Goal

Glucocorticoids are used on a fixed schedule to suppress inflammation in chronic asthma. They are not used to abort an ongoing attack.

Baseline Data

Determine PEFR (or FEV) and the frequency and severity of attacks, and attempt to identify trigger factors.

Identifying High-Risk Patients

Inhaled Glucocorticoids. These preparations are *contraindicated* for patients with persistently positive sputum cultures for *Candida albicans.*

Oral Glucocorticoids. These preparations are *contraindicated* for patients with systemic fungal infections and for individuals receiving live virus vaccines. Use with *caution* in pediatric patients and in women who are pregnant or breast-feeding. In addition, exercise *caution* in patients with hypertension, heart failure, renal impairment, esophagitis, gastritis, peptic ulcer disease, myasthenia gravis, diabetes mellitus, osteoporosis, or infections that are resistant to treatment and in patients receiving potassium-depleting diuretics, digitalis glycosides, insulin, oral hypoglycemics, or nonsteroidal anti-inflammatory drugs.

Implementation: Administration

Routes

Inhalation, oral.

Administration

Inform patients that glucocorticoids are intended for preventive therapy—not for aborting an ongoing attack. Instruct patients to administer glucocorticoids on a regular schedule—not PRN.

Inhalation. Inhaled glucocorticoids are administered with an MDI, DPI, or nebulizer. Teach patients how to use these devices. **Advise patients using MDIs to employ a**

spacer device—unless they are taking budesonide [QVAR], which employs HFA as its propellant. Inform patients that delivery of glucocorticoids to the bronchial tree can be enhanced by inhaling a short-acting beta₂ agonist 5 minutes prior to inhaling the glucocorticoid.

Oral. Alternate-day therapy is recommended to minimize adrenal suppression; instruct patients to take one dose every other day in the morning. During long-term treatment, supplemental doses must be given at times of severe stress.

Ongoing Evaluation and Interventions

Evaluating Therapeutic Effects

Teach patients with chronic asthma to monitor and record PEFR, symptom frequency, and symptom intensity. Teach patients to evaluate whether they are in the green, yellow, or red zone, and what the proper response to being in these zones is.

Minimizing Adverse Effects

Inhaled Glucocorticoids. **Advise patients to gargle after each administration and to use a spacer with the MDI (except the QVAR inhaler). These measures will minimize** *dysphonia* and *oropharyngeal candidiasis.* If candidiasis develops, it can be treated with antifungal medication.

Warn patients who have been switched from long-term oral glucocorticoids to inhaled glucocorticoids that, because of *adrenal suppression,* **they must take supplemental systemic glucocorticoids at times of severe stress (e.g., trauma, surgery, infection); failure to do so can be fatal.**

To minimize *bone loss,* patients should use the lowest dose possible. Also, **advise patients to ensure adequate intake of calcium and vitamin D, and to participate in weight-bearing exercise.**

Oral Glucocorticoids. Prolonged therapy can cause *adrenal suppression* and other serious adverse effects, including *osteoporosis, hyperglycemia, peptic ulcer disease,* and *growth suppression.* These effects can be reduced with alternate-day dosing. To compensate for adrenal suppression, patients taking glucocorticoids long term must be given supplemental oral or IV glucocorticoids at times of stress (e.g., trauma, surgery, infection); failure to do so can be fatal. Additional nursing implications that apply to adverse effects of long-term glucocorticoid therapy are summarized in Chapter 68.

CROMOLYN

Preadministration Assessment

Therapeutic Goal

Cromolyn is used for acute and long-term prophylaxis of asthma. The drug will not abort an ongoing asthma attack.

Baseline Data

Determine PEFR (or FEV) and the frequency and severity of attacks, and attempt to identify trigger factors.

*Patient education information is highlighted as blue text.

Summary of Major Nursing Implications*—cont'd

Identifying High-Risk Patients

Cromolyn is *contraindicated* for the rare patient who has experienced an allergic response to cromolyn in the past.

Implementation: Administration

Route

Inhalation.

Administration

Administration Devices. Cromolyn is administered with either an MDI or a nebulizer. Instruct patients on the proper use of these devices.

Acute Prophylaxis. Instruct patients to administer cromolyn 15 minutes prior to exercise and other precipitating factors (e.g., cold, environmental agents).

Long-Term Prophylaxis. Instruct patients to administer cromolyn on a regular schedule, and inform them that full therapeutic effects may take several weeks to develop.

Ongoing Evaluation and Interventions

Evaluating Therapeutic Effects

Teach patients with chronic asthma to monitor and record PEFR, symptom frequency, and symptom intensity. Teach patients to evaluate whether they are in the green, yellow, or red zone, and what the proper response to being in these zones is.

Minimizing Adverse Effects and Interactions

Cromolyn is devoid of significant adverse effects and drug interactions.

THEOPHYLLINE

Preadministration Assessment

Therapeutic Goal

Theophylline is a bronchodilator taken on a regular schedule to decrease the intensity and frequency of moderate to severe asthma attacks.

Baseline Data

Determine PEFR (or FEV) and the frequency and severity of attacks.

Identifying High-Risk Patients

Theophylline is *contraindicated* for patients with untreated seizure disorders or peptic ulcer disease. Use with *caution* in patients with heart disease, liver or kidney dysfunction, or severe hypertension.

Implementation: Administration

Routes

Oral, intravenous.

Administration

Oral. Dosage must be individualized. Doses are low initially and then increased gradually. The dosing objective is to produce plasma theophylline levels in the therapeutic range, which for most patients is 5 to 15 μg/ml. Warn patients that, if a dose is missed, the following dose should *not* be doubled.

Instruct patients to swallow enteric-coated and sustained-release formulations intact, without crushing or chewing.

Warn patients not to switch from one sustained-release formulation to another without consulting the physician.

Consult product information regarding compatibility with food, and advise the patient accordingly.

Intravenous. Administration must be done slowly. Verify compatibility with other IV drugs prior to mixing.

Ongoing Evaluation and Interventions

Evaluating Therapeutic Effects

Monitor theophylline levels to ensure that they are in the therapeutic range (5 to 15 μg/ml for most patients).

Teach patients with chronic asthma to monitor and record PEFR, symptom frequency, and symptom intensity. Teach patients to evaluate whether they are in the green, yellow, or red zone, and what the proper response to being in these zones is.

Minimizing Adverse Effects

Mild adverse effects (e.g., nausea, vomiting, diarrhea, insomnia, restlessness) develop as plasma drug levels rise above 20 μg/ml. Severe effects (convulsions, ventricular fibrillation) can occur at drug levels above 30 μg/ml. Dosage should be adjusted to keep theophylline levels below 20 μg/ml.

Minimizing Adverse Interactions

Caffeine. Caffeine can intensify the adverse effects of theophylline on the heart and CNS and can decrease theophylline metabolism. Caution patients against consuming caffeine-containing beverages (e.g., coffee, many soft drinks) and other sources of caffeine.

Drugs That Reduce Theophylline Levels. Phenobarbital, phenytoin, rifampin, and other drugs can lower theophylline levels. In the presence of these drugs, the dosage of theophylline may need to be increased.

Drugs That Increase Theophylline Levels. Cimetidine, fluoroquinolone antibiotics, and other drugs can elevate theophylline levels. When combined with these drugs, theophylline should be used in reduced dosage.

Managing Toxicity. Theophylline overdose can cause severe dysrhythmias and convulsions. Death from cardiorespiratory collapse may occur. Manage toxicity by (1) discontinuing theophylline; (2) administering ipecac (to induce vomiting); and (3) administering activated charcoal (to decrease theophylline absorption) plus a cathartic (to accelerate fecal excretion). Give lidocaine to control ventricular dysrhythmias and IV diazepam to control seizures.

*Patient education information is highlighted as blue text.

TABLE 72–1 ▪■ **Overview of Drugs for Allergic Rhinitis**

Drug or Class	Route	Actions	Adverse Effects
Antihistamines	Oral/nasal	Block H_1 receptors and thereby decrease itching, sneezing, and rhinorrhea; do *not* reduce congestion	*Oral:* Sedation (with older agents) *Nasal:* Bitter taste
Glucocorticoids	Nasal	Prevent inflammatory response to allergens and thereby reduce all symptoms	Nasal irritation
Cromolyn	Nasal	Prevents release of inflammatory mediators from mast cells, and thereby decreases all symptoms	None
Sympathomimetics	Oral/nasal	Stimulate vascular $alpha_1$ receptors and thereby cause vasoconstriction, which reduces nasal congestion; they do *not* decrease sneezing, itching, or rhinorrhea	*Oral:* Restlessness, insomnia, increased blood pressure *Nasal:* Rebound nasal congestion
Anticholinergics	Nasal	Block nasal cholinergic receptors and thereby reduce secretions; do *not* decrease sneezing, nasal congestion, or postnasal drip	Nasal drying and irritation

TABLE 72–2 ▪■ **Some Antihistamines for Allergic Rhinitis**

Generic Name	Trade Name	Dosage
Oral Agents		
First-Generation (Sedating)		
Chlorpheniramine	Chlor-Trimeton	*Adults and children ≥12 yr:* 4 mg q 4–6 h *Children 6–12 yr:* 2 mg q 4–6 h
Diphenhydramine	Benadryl	*Adults:* 25–50 mg q 4–6 h *Children <10 kg:* 12.5–25 mg tid or qid
Second-Generation (Nonsedating)		
Cetirizine	Zyrtec	*Adults and children ≥6 yr:* 5 or 10 mg qd
Desloratadine	Clarinex	*Adults and children ≥12 yr:* 5 mg qd
Loratadine	Claritin	*Adults and children ≥6 yr:* 10 mg qd
Fexofenadine	Allegra	*Adults and children ≥12 yr:* 60 mg bid or 180 mg qd
Nasal Spray		
Azelastine*	Astelin	*Adults:* 2 sprays/nostril bid

*Azelastine is a second-generation agent.

Intranasal Glucocorticoids

The basic pharmacology of the glucocorticoids is discussed in Chapter 68. Consideration here is limited to their use in allergic rhinitis.

Actions and Uses. Intranasal glucocorticoids are the most effective drugs for treating seasonal and perennial rhinitis. With proper use, over 90% of patients respond. Because of their anti-inflammatory actions, these drugs can prevent or suppress all of the major symptoms of allergic rhinitis: congestion, rhinorrhea, sneezing, nasal itching, and erythema. In the past, intranasal steroids were reserved for patients whose symptoms could not be controlled with more conventional drugs (sympathomimetics, antihistamines, intranasal cromolyn). However, because of their proven safety and superior efficacy, glucocorticoids have now joined the H_1 antagonists as a first-line therapy. Seven agents are available: *beclomethasone, budesonide, dexamethasone, flunisolide, fluticasone, mometasone,* and *triamcinolone.* All are equally effective.

Adverse Effects. Adverse effects are mild. The most common are drying of the nasal mucosa and a burning or itching sensation. These effects are caused by the vehicle employed for administration and not by the steroids themselves. Preparations that employ an *aqueous* vehicle (Table 72–3) are much less irritating than preparations that use a nonaqueous vehicle (Freon, alcohol, polyethylene glycol). Systemic effects, including adrenocortical suppression, may occur. However, these responses are rare at recommended doses.

Dosage and Administration. Intranasal glucocorticoids are administered using a metered-spray device. Full doses are given initially (see Table 72–3). Once symptoms have been controlled, the dosage should be reduced to the lowest effective amount. For patients with seasonal allergic rhinitis, *maximal* effects may require a week or more to develop. However, an initial response can be seen within hours. For patients with perennial rhinitis, maximal responses may take 2 to 3 weeks to develop. If nasal passages are blocked, they should be cleared with a topical decongestant prior to glucocorticoid administration.

TABLE 72–3 ▪■ Some Glucocorticoid Nasal Sprays for Allergic Rhinitis

Drug	Trade Name	Vehicle	Dose/Spray (µg)	Patient Age (yr)	Initial Dosage (Sprays/Nostril)
Beclomethasone	Beconase, Vancenase Pockethaler	Nonaqueous	42	6–11	1 tid
				≥12	1 bid–qid
	Beconase AQ, Vancenase AQ	Aqueous	42	6–11	1 bid
				≥12	1 or 2 bid
	Beconase AQ 84 µg	Aqueous	84	6–11	1 qd
				≥12	1 or 2 qd
Budesonide	Rhinocort	Nonaqueous	32	≥6	4 qd
	Rhinocort Aqua	Aqueous	32	≥6	1 qd
Flunisolide	Nasalide, Nasarel	Aqueous	25	6–13	1 tid or 2 bid
				≥14	2 bid
Fluticasone	Flonase	Aqueous	50	4–11	1 qd
				≥12	2 qd
Mometasone	Nasonex	Aqueous	50	3–11	1 qd
				≥12	2 qd
Triamcinolone	Nasacort	Nonaqueous	55	≥6	2 qd
	Nasacort AQ	Aqueous	55	6–11	1 qd
				≥12	2 qd
	TriNasal	Aqueous	50	≥6	2 qd

Intranasal Cromolyn Sodium

The basic pharmacology of cromolyn sodium is discussed in Chapter 71 (Drugs for Asthma). Consideration here is limited to the use of cromolyn for allergic rhinitis.

Actions and Uses. Intranasal cromolyn is used to both prevent and treat allergic rhinitis. The drug is very safe and very effective. Cromolyn reduces symptoms by suppressing release of histamine and other inflammatory mediators from mast cells. For patients with seasonal allergic rhinitis, cromolyn is as effective as antihistamines but less effective than intranasal glucocorticoids. Like the antihistamines, cromolyn is most effective when taken prior to onset of symptoms. Beneficial effects may take a week or two to develop; patients should be informed of this delay. Adverse reactions are minimal—less than with any other drug for allergic rhinitis.

Dosage and Administration. Intranasal cromolyn sodium [Nasalcrom] is administered with a metered-spray device. The usual dosage for adults and children over the age of 6 years is one spray (5.2 mg) per nostril 3 to 6 times a day. If nasal congestion is present, a topical decongestant should be used prior to administering cromolyn. Like the antihistamines, cromolyn should be administered on a regular schedule throughout the allergy season.

Sympathomimetics (Decongestants)
Actions and Uses

Sympathomimetics (e.g., phenylephrine) reduce nasal congestion. How? By stimulating alpha$_1$-adrenergic receptors on nasal blood vessels, which causes vasoconstriction, which in turn causes shrinkage of swollen membranes followed by nasal drainage. With *topical* administration, vasoconstriction is both rapid and intense. With *oral* administration, responses are delayed, moderate, and prolonged.

In patients with allergic rhinitis, sympathomimetics only relieve stuffiness. They do not reduce rhinorrhea, sneezing, or itching. In addition to their use in allergic rhinitis, sympathomimetics can reduce congestion associated with sinusitis and colds.

Adverse Effects

Rebound Congestion. Rebound congestion develops when *topical* agents are used more than a few days. With prolonged use, as the effects of each application wear off, congestion becomes progressively more severe. To overcome this rebound congestion, the patient must use progressively larger and more frequent doses. Hence, once established, rebound congestion can lead to a cycle of escalating congestion and increased drug use. The cycle can be broken by abrupt decongestant withdrawal. However, this tactic can be extremely uncomfortable. A less drastic approach is to discontinue drug use in one nostril at a time. Rebound congestion can be minimized by limiting use of topical agents to 3 to 5 days. Accordingly, topical sympathomimetics are inappropriate for individuals with chronic rhinitis.

Central Nervous System Stimulation. Central nervous system (CNS) excitation is the most common adverse effect of the *oral* sympathomimetics. Symptoms include restlessness, irritability, anxiety, and insomnia. These responses are unlikely with topical agents.

Cardiovascular Effects. By stimulating alpha$_1$-adrenergic receptors on systemic blood vessels, sympathomimetics can cause widespread vasoconstriction. For most patients, effects on systemic vessels are inconsequential. However, for individuals with hypertension or coronary artery disease, widespread vasoconstriction can be hazardous. Generalized vasoconstriction is most likely with *oral* agents. However, if taken in excess, even the topical agents can cause significant systemic vasoconstriction.

Hemorrhagic Stroke. On November 6, 2000, the Food and Drug Administration (FDA) ordered that *phenylpropanola-*

mine, an alpha-adrenergic agonist, be removed from the market because it was shown to cause subarachnoid and intracerebral hemorrhage in women (but not in men). Although the risk of stroke is small, the FDA ruled that the risk was not justified by the relatively benign disorders for which phenylpropanolamine was used. (In addition to its use as a nasal decongestant, phenylpropanolamine had been used widely as an over-the-counter weight loss aid.) We do not know if other alpha agonists (e.g., phenylephrine, ephedrine, pseudoephedrine) also pose a risk of hemorrhagic stroke.

Abuse. By causing CNS stimulation, sympathomimetics can produce subjective effects similar to those of amphetamine. As a result, these drugs are subject to abuse. Among the sympathomimetics employed as decongestants, abuse is most common with *pseudoephedrine* and *ephedrine.* Although these drugs are available without prescription and are not regulated under the Controlled Substances Act, pharmacies are beginning to keep them behind the counter, so as to hamper inappropriate use.

Factors in Topical Administration

General Considerations. Because of the risk of rebound congestion, topical sympathomimetics should be used for no more than 5 consecutive days. To avoid systemic effects, doses should not exceed those recommended by the manufacturer. The applicator should be cleansed after each use to prevent contamination.

Drops. Drops should be administered with the patient in a lateral, head-low position. This causes the drops to spread slowly over the nasal mucosa, thereby promoting beneficial effects while reducing the amount that is swallowed. Because the number of drops can be precisely controlled, drops allow better control of dosage than do sprays. Accordingly, since young children are particularly susceptible to toxicity, drops are preferred to sprays for these patients.

Sprays. Sprays deliver the decongestant in a fine mist. Although convenient, sprays are less effective than an equal volume of properly instilled drops.

Summary of Contrasts Between Oral and Topical Agents

Oral and topical sympathomimetics differ in several important respects: (1) Topical agents act faster than the oral agents and are usually more effective. (2) Oral agents act longer than topical preparations. (3) Systemic effects (vasoconstriction, CNS stimulation) occur primarily with oral agents; topical agents elicit these responses only when dosage is excessive. (4) Rebound congestion is common with prolonged use of topical agents, but is rare with oral agents.

Preparations and Dosage

Properties of Individual Decongestants. Phenylephrine is one of the most widely used nasal decongestants. The drug is administered topically (by itself) and orally (as a component of combination preparations). *Ephedrine* causes a high incidence of CNS stimulation. CNS effects are much lower with *pseudoephedrine,* a stereoisomer of ephedrine. *Naphazoline,* one of the newer topical agents, can cause severe rebound congestion. As noted above, *phenylpropanolamine* poses a risk of hemorrhagic stroke and has been withdrawn from the market. Prior to its removal, phenylpropanolamine was one of our most widely used oral decongestants.

Dosage and Administration. Dosages and routes of administration for the sympathomimetics are summarized in Table 72–4.

Sympathomimetic-Antihistamine Combinations

Some patients require combined therapy with a sympathomimetic and an antihistamine. Although antihistamines alone are a first-line treatment, they do not relieve nasal congestion, and hence may be inadequate for some patients. For these patients, addition of a sympathomimetic may be indicated. This can be accomplished in two ways: by giving the antihistamine and sympathomimetic separately, or by using a combination product. Some popular antihistamine-sympathomimetic combinations are listed in Table 72–5.

Ipratropium, an Anticholinergic Agent

Ipratropium bromide [Atrovent] is an anticholinergic agent similar to atropine. The drug is indicated for allergic rhinitis, asthma, and the common cold. For treatment of allergic rhinitis, ipratropium is administered as a 0.03% nasal spray. Blockade of cholinergic receptors inhibits glandular secretions, and thereby decreases rhinorrhea. The drug does not decrease sneezing, nasal congestion, or postnasal drip. At the doses used for allergic rhinitis, side effects are minimal, the most common being nasal drying and irritation. Ipratropium does not readily cross membranes (it's a quaternary ammonium compound), and hence systemic effects are absent. The recommended dosage for rhinitis in patients 12 years and older is 2 sprays (42 µg) per nostril 2 or 3 times a day. Use of ipratropium for asthma is discussed in Chapter 71.

Omalizumab

Omalizumab is a monoclonal antibody directed against IgE, an immunoglobulin that plays a central role in the allergic release of inflammatory mediators from mast cells and basophils. In patients with ragweed-induced seasonal allergic rhinitis, omalizumab can greatly decrease nasal symptoms. In one study, patients received a 300-mg SC dose just prior to ragweed season, followed by additional 300-mg SC doses every 3 to 4 weeks during the season. The result? Omalizumab decreased serum levels of IgE by 95%, and prevented practically all symptoms of rhinitis. At this time, omalizumab is investigational, and hence not available for general use.

DRUGS FOR COUGH

Cough is a complex reflex involving the CNS, the peripheral nervous system, and the muscles of respiration. The cough reflex can be initiated by irritation of the bronchial mucosa as well as by stimuli arising at sites distant from the respiratory tract. Cough is often beneficial, serving to remove foreign matter and excess secretions from the bronchial tree. Productive cough is characteristic of chronic lung disease (e.g., emphysema, asthma, bronchitis) and should not be suppressed. Not all cough, however, is useful; cough frequently serves only to deprive us of comfort or sleep. Under these conditions, antitussive medication is appropriate. The most common use of cough medicines is suppression of nonproductive cough associated with the common cold and other upper respiratory infections.

Antitussives

Antitussives are drugs that suppress cough. Some of these agents act within the CNS; others act peripherally. The antitussives fall into two major groups: (1) opioid anti-

TABLE 72–4 ■ Sympathomimetics Used for Nasal Decongestion

Decongestant	Mode of Use	Dosing Interval	Dosage Size*
Ephedrine [Pretz-D]	Spray	q 4 or more h	≥12 yr: 2 or 3 sprays (0.25%) 6–11 yr: 1 or 2 sprays (0.25%)
Epinephrine [Adrenalin]	Drops	q 4–6 hr	≥6 yr: 1–2 drops (0.1%) <6 yr: Not recommended
Naphazoline [Privine]	Drops	q 6 or more h	≥6 yr: 1 or 2 drops (0.05%) <6 yr: Not recommended
	Spray	q 6 or more h	≥6 yr: 1 or 2 sprays (0.05%) <6 yr: Not recommended
Oxymetazoline [Afrin 12-Hour, Neo-Synephrine 12-Hour]	Spray	q 10–12 h	≥6 yr: 2–3 sprays (0.05%) <6 yr: Not recommended
Phenylephrine [Neo-Synephrine]	Drops	q 4 or more h	≥6 yr: 2–3 drops (0.25%–1%) <6 yr: 2–3 drops (0.125%)
	Spray	q 4 or more h	≥12 yr: 2–3 sprays (0.25%–1%) 6–12 yr: 2–3 sprays (0.25%) <6 yr: Not recommended
	Oral	q 4 h	≥12 yr: 10–20 mg 6–12 yr: 10 mg <6 yr: 1 ml (0.25% drops)
Pseudoephedrine [Sudafed]	Oral	q 4–6 h	≥12 yr: 60 mg 6–12 yr: 30 mg <6 yr: 15 mg
	Oral SR†	q 12 h	≥12 yr: 120 mg <12 yr: Not recommended
	Oral CR‡	q 24 h	≥12 yr: 240 mg <12 yr: Not recommended
Tetrahydrozoline [Tyzine]	Drops	q 3 or more h	≥6 yr: 2–4 drops (0.1%) 2–6 yr: 2–3 drops (0.05%)
	Spray	q 3 or more h	≥6 yr: 3–4 sprays (0.1%) <6 yr: Not recommended
Xylometazoline [Natru-Vent, Otrivin]	Drops	q 8–10 h	≥12 yr: 2–3 drops (0.1%) 2–12 yr: 2–3 drops (0.05%)
	Spray	q 8–10	≥12 yr: 1–3 sprays (0.1%) 2–12 yr: 1 spray (0.05%)

*For drops and sprays, dosage listed is applied to *each* nostril; numbers in parentheses indicate concentration of solution employed.
†SR = sustained release.
‡CR = controlled release.

TABLE 72–5 ■ Some Antihistamine-Sympathomimetic Combinations

Antihistamine/Sympathomimetic	Trade Name	Dosage
Acrivastine/pseudoephedrine	Semprex-D Capsules	8 mg/60 mg qid
Chlorpheniramine/pseudoephedrine	Allarest Maximum Strength Tablets	4 mg/60 mg q 4–6 h
Loratadine/pseudoephedrine	Claritin-D 12 Hour Tablets	5 mg/120 mg q 12 h
Fexofenadine/pseudoephedrine	Allegra-D Tablets	60 mg/120 mg bid
Triprolidine/pseudoephedrine	Actifed Cold & Allergy Tablets	2.5 mg/60 mg q 4–6 h

tussives and (2) nonopioid antitussives. Interestingly, although the major antitussives—codeine, dextromethorphan, and diphenhydramine—are clearly effective against chronic nonproductive cough and experimentally induced cough, there is no good evidence that these drugs can suppress cough associated with the common cold.

Opioid Antitussives

All of the opioid analgesics have the ability to suppress cough. The two opioids used most frequently for cough suppression are *codeine* and *hydrocodone*. Both agents act in the CNS to elevate cough threshold. Hydrocodone is somewhat more potent than codeine and carries a greater liability for abuse. The basic pharmacology of the opioids is discussed in Chapter 27.

Codeine. Codeine is the most effective cough suppressant available. The drug is active orally and can decrease both the frequency and intensity of cough. Doses are low, about one-tenth those needed to relieve pain. At these doses, the risk of physical dependence is small.

Like all other opioids, codeine can suppress respiration. Accordingly, the drug should be employed with caution in patients with reduced respiratory reserve. In the event of overdose, respiratory depression may prove fatal; an opioid antagonist (e.g., naloxone) should be used to reverse toxicity.

When dispensed by itself, codeine has a significant potential for abuse, and is classified under Schedule II of the Controlled Substances Act. However, the abuse potential of the antitussive mixtures that contain codeine is low. Accordingly, these mixtures are classified under Schedule V.

For treatment of cough, the adult dosage is 10 to 20 mg orally, 4 to 6 times a day. Codeine is rarely recommended for children.

Nonopioid Antitussives

Dextromethorphan. Dextromethorphan is the most effective nonopioid cough medicine. Except when used for severe acute cough, this drug works as well as codeine. Like the opioids, dextromethorphan acts in the CNS. Although dextromethorphan is a derivative of the opioids, it does not produce euphoria or physical dependence, and lacks any potential for abuse. At therapeutic doses, it does not depress respiration. Adverse effects are mild and rare. Dextromethorphan is the active ingredient in most nonprescription antitussive preparations. The usual adult dosage is 10 to 30 mg every 4 to 8 hours.

In the past, dextromethorphan was considered devoid of analgesic actions; however, it now appears the drug *can* reduce pain. The mechanism is blockade of receptors for *N*-methyl-D-aspartate (NMDA) in the brain and spinal cord. In contrast, opioids relieve pain primarily through activation of mu receptors. Although dextromethorphan has minimal analgesic effects when used alone, it can enhance analgesic effects of the opioids. For example, we can double the analgesic response to 30 mg of morphine by combining morphine with 30 mg of dextromethorphan.

Other Nonopioid Antitussives. Diphenhydramine is an antihistamine with the ability to suppress cough. The mechanism of antitussive action is unclear. Like other antihistamines, diphenhydramine has sedative and anticholinergic properties. Cough suppression is achieved only at doses that produce prominent sedation. The usual adult dosage is 25 mg every 4 hours.

Benzonatate [Tessalon] is a structural analog of tetracaine, a local anesthetic. The drug is believed to suppress cough by decreasing the sensitivity of respiratory tract stretch receptors (components of the cough-reflex pathway); CNS mechanisms may also be involved. Adverse effects are usually mild (e.g., sedation, dizziness, constipation). Benzonatate is dispensed in capsules for oral administration. The capsules should be swallowed intact, since chewing will anesthetize the mouth and pharynx. The usual adult dosage is 100 mg 3 times a day. The drug should not be given to infants because anesthesia of the mouth may impair swallowing.

Expectorants and Mucolytics

Expectorants. An expectorant is a drug that renders cough more productive by stimulating the flow of respiratory tract secretions. A variety of compounds (e.g., terpin hydrate, ammonium chloride, iodide products) have been promoted for their supposed expectorant actions. However, in almost all cases, efficacy is doubtful. One agent, *guaifenesin* (glyceryl guaiacolate), may be an exception to this rule. However, for this drug to be effective, doses higher than those normally employed may be needed.

Mucolytics. A mucolytic is a drug that reacts directly with mucus to make it more watery. This action should help make cough more productive. Two preparations—*hypertonic saline* and *acetylcysteine*—are employed for their mucolytic actions. Both are administered by inhalation. Unfortunately, both can trigger bronchospasm. Because of its sulfur content, acetylcysteine [Mucomyst] has the additional drawback of smelling like rotten eggs.

COLD REMEDIES: COMBINATION PREPARATIONS

The common cold is an acute upper respiratory infection of viral origin. Causative agents include rhinoviruses, adenoviruses, respiratory syncytial virus, and parainfluenza virus. Characteristic symptoms are rhinorrhea, nasal congestion, cough, sneezing, sore throat, hoarseness, headache, malaise, and myalgia; fever is common in children but rare in adults. Colds are self-limited and usually benign. Persistence or worsening of symptoms suggests development of a secondary bacterial infection.

There is no cure for the cold, and hence treatment is purely symptomatic. Because colds are caused by viruses, there is no justification for the routine use of antibacterial drugs. Antibiotics are appropriate only if a bacterial infection arises. There is no evidence that vitamin C can prevent or cure colds. Benefits of zinc lozenges are unclear (see Box 72–1).

Because no single drug can relieve all of the symptoms of a cold, the pharmaceutical industry has formulated a vast number of cold remedies that contain mixtures of ingredients. These combination cold remedies should be reserved for patients with multiple symptoms. In addition, the combination chosen should contain only those agents that are appropriate for the symptoms to be treated. Patients who require relief from just a single symptom (e.g., rhinitis, cough, or headache) are best treated with a single-entity preparation.

Combination cold remedies frequently contain two or more of the following: (1) a nasal decongestant, (2) an antitussive, (3) an analgesic, (4) an antihistamine, and (5) caffeine. The purpose of the first three agents is self-evident. In contrast, the roles of antihistamines and caffeine require explanation. Since histamine has nothing to do with the symptoms of a cold, antihistamines are not present to counteract the actions of histamine. Rather, because of their anticholinergic actions, antihistamines are included to suppress secretion of mucus. Caffeine is added to offset the sedative effects of the antihistamine.

Although they can be convenient, combination cold remedies do have disadvantages. As with all fixed-dose combinations, there is the chance that a dosage (e.g., one capsule or one tablet) that produces therapeutic levels of one ingredient may produce levels of other ingredients that are either excessive or subtherapeutic. In addition, the combination may contain ingredients for which the patient has no need. Furthermore, under FDA regulations, a brand-name product can be reformulated and then sold under the same name. Hence, without carefully reading the label, the consumer has no assurance that the brand name product purchased this year contains the same amounts of the same drugs that were present in last year's version of that combination product.

Special Interest Topic

BOX 72–1 ■ ZINC FOR KIDS WITH COLDS?

In an effort to develop a cure for the common cold, researchers have been studying zinc. Results of 10 studies in adults have been mixed: in 5 studies, zinc reduced symptoms; in 5 others, zinc didn't help. Only one study has been done in children. The result? Zinc had no beneficial effect. However, until more research is done, a final conclusion cannot be drawn.

A theoretical basis for how zinc might work has not been firmly established. The predominant theory suggests that zinc blocks viral binding to cells of the nasal epithelium, and thereby suppresses infection. This theory is based on the observation that zinc can prevent rhinovirus (the most common cause of colds) from binding to epithelial cells grown in culture. However, there is no clear proof that zinc can block the adhesion of other cold viruses (e.g., adenoviruses, respiratory syncytial virus, parainfluenza virus). Hence, experimental support for the reduced-adhesion theory is limited. Alternative theories posit that zinc may inhibit viral replication, boost immune function, enhance cytoprotection, or suppress cold-related inflammatory responses.

Having shown that zinc can benefit adults with colds, Dr. Michael Macknin of the Cleveland Clinic wanted to see if zinc would also benefit children. Accordingly, he and his team studied responses in 249 students in grades 1 through 12 from two school districts in the eastern suburbs of Cleveland, Ohio. The objective was to determine if zinc could shorten the duration of cold symptoms (cough, headache, hoarseness, muscle ache, nasal congestion, nasal drainage, scratchy throat, sore throat, sneezing). Treatment was begun within 24 hours of the onset of symptoms and consisted of either placebo (cherry-flavored lozenges) or 10-mg zinc gluconate glycine lozenges (also cherry flavored) administered 5 or 6 times a day. The outcome? The time to resolution of symptoms was unaffected by zinc. Not only did zinc fail to accelerate recovery, it produced annoying side effects: bad taste in the mouth (60% vs. 38% for placebo); nausea (29% vs. 16%); diarrhea (11% vs. 4%); and mouth, tongue, or throat discomfort (37% vs. 24%).

Should we conclude from these results that zinc is unable to benefit children with colds? No. Other interpretations are possible:

- Benefits may be related to zinc in the diet. Zinc is a normal micronutrient. If the children in this study had adequate zinc in their diets, it may be that little or no benefit would be seen by giving additional zinc. Conversely, if the study had been done in a region where children are zinc deficient, beneficial effects might have been observed.
- The dosage may have been inadequate. In one successful study in adults, the dosage was 23.7 mg 8 times a day—for a total of 190 mg each day. In the children's study, the daily dosage was only 50 to 60 mg—less than one-third of the dosage used in adults. Since the mechanism by which zinc acts is unknown, it is impossible to predict how much is actually needed. Hence, perhaps a higher dosage would have worked.
- The causative viruses may have been insensitive. We know that zinc can block adhesion of *rhinoviruses* to nasal epithelial cells (at least in culture), but may not block adhesion of other cold viruses. If blockade of viral binding really is the mechanism by which zinc acts, treatment would fail if the causative viruses were not sensitive. Since causative agents may be different in different locales or at different times of the year, perhaps the outcome would have been successful if the study had been done in a different place or at a different time.
- The zinc may have been inactivated. In the successful studies done with adults, zinc was formulated in lemon-lime lozenges—not the cherry-flavored lozenges employed in the children's study. It may be that, somehow, the cherry flavoring inactivated the zinc.

At this time, it would be premature to dismiss zinc as a useful medication. More research is needed. Unanswered questions include:

- How does zinc work?
- Which cold viruses are sensitive?
- What dosage is most effective?
- What formulation is most effective?
- Are benefits limited to children who are zinc deficient?

When these questions have been answered, we will be able to draw a more firm conclusion about the utility of zinc as a cold remedy for kids.

⁙ KEY POINTS

- Allergic rhinitis is the most common allergic disorder.
- Allergic rhinitis is treated primarily with antihistamines, intranasal glucocorticoids, intranasal cromolyn sodium, and sympathomimetics (decongestants).
- Antihistamines (H_1-receptor antagonists) are first-line drugs for allergic rhinitis. They relieve rhinorrhea, sneezing, and itching, but not congestion.
- Sedation is a common side effect of the first-generation antihistamines but not the second-generation antihistamines.
- Intranasal glucocorticoids are the most effective drugs for allergic rhinitis. These first-line agents relieve rhinorrhea, congestion, itching, and sneezing.
- Intranasal cromolyn sodium provides effective treatment of allergic rhinitis, but only when taken prophylactically. Benefits take a week or so to develop.
- Intranasal cromolyn has no significant adverse effects.
- Sympathomimetics decrease nasal congestion by activating alpha$_1$-adrenergic receptors on blood vessels, which causes vasoconstriction and thereby shrinks swollen nasal membranes.
- *Topical* sympathomimetics decrease nasal congestion rapidly and produce minimal systemic effects, but cause rebound congestion when used for more than a few days.
- *Oral* sympathomimetics decrease nasal congestion slowly and produce CNS stimulation, but do *not* cause rebound congestion, and hence are suited for long-term use.
- Codeine, a member of the opioid family of drugs, is the most effective cough suppressant available. Doses are only one-tenth those used for analgesia.
- Dextromethorphan is the most effective nonopioid cough suppressant available.
- There is not good evidence that codeine, dextromethorphan, or any other cough medicine can suppress cough associated with the common cold.

CHAPTER

73

Drugs for Peptic Ulcer Disease

The term *peptic ulcer disease* (PUD) refers to a group of upper GI disorders characterized by varying degrees of erosion of the gut wall. Severe ulcers can be complicated by hemorrhage and perforation. Although peptic ulcers can develop in any region exposed to acid and pepsin, ulceration is most common in the lesser curvature of the stomach and in the duodenum. PUD is a very common disorder that affects about 10% of Americans at some time in their lives. About 4.5 million Americans get ulcers each year. Until recently, PUD was considered a chronic, relapsing disorder of unknown cause and with no known cure; therapy promoted healing but did not prevent ulcer recurrence. However, we now know that most cases of PUD are caused by infection with *Helicobacter pylori,* and that eradication of this bacterium not only promotes healing, but greatly reduces the chance of recurrence.

PATHOGENESIS OF PEPTIC ULCERS

Peptic ulcers develop when there is an imbalance between mucosal defensive factors and aggressive factors (Fig. 73–1). The major defensive factors are mucus and bicarbonate. The major aggressive factors are *H. pylori,* nonsteroidal anti-inflammatory drugs (NSAIDs), gastric acid, and pepsin.

Defensive Factors

Defensive factors serve the physiologic role of protecting the stomach and duodenum from self-digestion. When defenses are intact, generation of ulcers is unlikely. Conversely, when defenses are compromised, aggressive factors are able to cause injury. Two important agents that can weaken defenses are *H. pylori* and NSAIDs.

Mucus. Mucus is secreted continuously by cells of the GI mucosa, forming a barrier that protects underlying cells from attack by acid and pepsin.

Bicarbonate. Bicarbonate is secreted by epithelial cells of the stomach and duodenum. Most bicarbonate remains trapped in the mucus layer, where it serves to neutralize any hydrogen ions that penetrate the mucus. Bicarbonate produced by the pancreas is secreted into the lumen of the duodenum, where it neutralizes acid delivered from the stomach.

Blood Flow. Sufficient blood flow to cells of the GI mucosa is essential for maintaining mucosal integrity. If submucosal blood flow is reduced, the resultant local ischemia can lead to cell injury, thereby increasing vulnerability to attack by acid and pepsin.

Prostaglandins. Prostaglandins play an important role in maintaining defenses. These compounds stimulate secretion of mucus and bicarbonate, and they promote vasodilation, which helps maintain submucosal blood flow. Prostaglandins provide additional protection by suppressing secretion of gastric acid.

Aggressive Factors

Helicobacter pylori. *Helicobacter pylori* is a gram-negative bacillus that can colonize the stomach and duodenum. By taking up residence in the space between epithelial cells and the mucus barrier that protects them, this organism manages to escape destruction by acid and pepsin. Once established, *H. pylori* can remain in the GI tract for decades. Although about half of the world's population is infected with *H. pylori,* the vast majority of infected people never develop symptomatic PUD.

Why do we think *H. pylori* causes PUD? First, between 60% and 75% of patients with PUD have *H. pylori* infection. (Several years ago, the prevalence was even higher—about 90%). Second, duodenal ulcers are much more common among

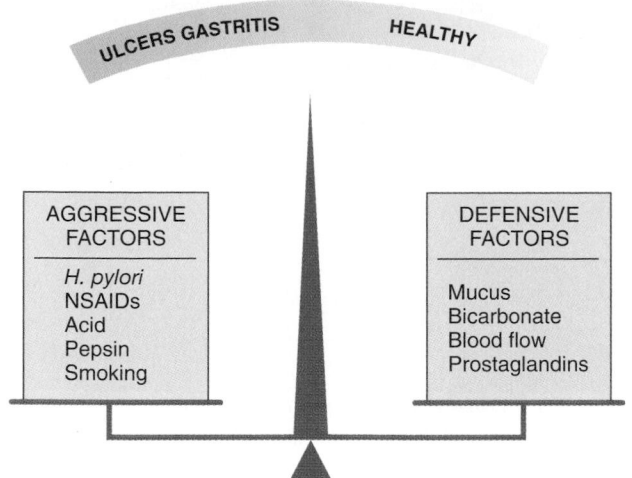

Figure 73–1 ■ **The relationship of mucosal defenses and aggressive factors to health and peptic ulcer disease.** When aggressive factors outweigh mucosal defenses, gastritis and peptic ulcers result. (NSAIDs = nonsteroidal anti-inflammatory drugs.)

people with *H. pylori* infection than among people who are not infected. Third, eradication of the bacterium promotes ulcer healing. Fourth, eradication of the bacterium minimizes ulcer recurrence. (One-year recurrence rates approach 80% when *H. pylori* remains present, compared with only 10% when the organism has been eliminated.)

Although the mechanism by which *H. pylori* promotes ulcers has not been firmly established, likely possibilities are enzymatic degradation of the protective mucus layer, elaboration of a cytotoxin that injures mucosal cells, and infiltration of neutrophils and other inflammatory cells in response to the bacterium's presence. Also, *H. pylori* produces *urease*, an enzyme that forms carbon dioxide and ammonia from urea in gastric juice; the carbon dioxide and ammonia are potentially toxic to the gastric mucosa. In addition to its role in PUD, *H. pylori* is strongly associated with development of gastric cancer.

Nonsteroidal Anti-inflammatory Drugs. NSAIDs are the underlying cause of many gastric ulcers and some duodenal ulcers. As discussed in Chapter 67, aspirin and other NSAIDs inhibit the biosynthesis of prostaglandins. By doing so, these drugs can decrease submucosal blood flow, suppress secretion of mucus and bicarbonate, and promote secretion of gastric acid. Furthermore, NSAIDs can irritate the mucosa directly. NSAID-induced ulcers are most likely with long-term, high-dose therapy.

Gastric Acid. Gastric acid is an absolute requirement for peptic ulcer formation: in the absence of acid, no ulcer will form. Acid causes ulcers by (1) injuring cells of the GI mucosa and (2) activating pepsin, a proteolytic enzyme. In most cases, acid hypersecretion, by itself, is insufficient to generate ulcers. In fact, in most patients with gastric ulcers, acid secretion is normal or reduced, and among patients with duodenal ulcers, only one-third produce excessive amounts of acid. From these observations, we can conclude that, in the majority of patients with peptic ulcers, factors in addition to acid must be involved.

Zollinger-Ellison syndrome is the primary disorder in which hypersecretion of acid alone appears to be the sole cause of ulcer generation. The underlying cause of this syndrome is a tumor that secretes gastrin, a hormone that stimulates gastric acid release. In response to high levels of gastrin, gastric acid is produced in huge quantities—quantities that are sufficient to overwhelm mucosal defenses. Zollinger-Ellison syndrome is a rare disorder that accounts for about 0.1% of duodenal ulcers.

Pepsin. Pepsin is a proteolytic enzyme present in gastric juice. Like gastric acid, pepsin can injure unprotected cells of the gastric and duodenal mucosa.

Smoking. Smoking delays ulcer healing and increases the risk of recurrence. Possible mechanisms include reduction of the beneficial effects of antiulcer medications, reduced secretion of bicarbonate, and accelerated gastric emptying, which would deliver more acid to the duodenum.

Summary

Infection with *H. pylori* is now recognized as the most common cause of gastric and duodenal ulcers. However, among people whose PUD can be ascribed to *H. pylori,* additional factors must be involved. We know this because more than 50% of the population harbors *H. pylori,* but only 10% develop ulcers. Factors that may increase the risk of PUD in people infected with *H. pylori* include smoking, increased acid secretion, and reduced bicarbonate production. Following infection with *H. pylori,* the second most common cause of gastric ulcers is NSAIDs. Hypersecretion of acid underlies a few cases of PUD that are not caused by *H. pylori* or NSAIDs.

OVERVIEW OF TREATMENT
Drug Therapy

The goal of drug therapy is to (1) alleviate symptoms; (2) promote healing; (3) prevent complications (hemorrhage, perforation, obstruction); and (4) prevent recurrences. With the exception of antibiotics, antiulcer drugs do not alter the disease process; rather, they simply create conditions conducive to healing. Since nonantibiotic therapies do not cure ulcers, the relapse rate following their discontinuation is high. In contrast, the relapse rate following antibiotic therapy is low.

Classes of Antiulcer Drugs

As shown in Table 73–1, the antiulcer drugs fall into five major classes:

- Antibiotics
- Antisecretory agents (histamine$_2$-receptor antagonists, proton pump inhibitors)
- Mucosal protectants
- Antisecretory agents that enhance mucosal defenses
- Antacids

From this classification, we can see that drugs act in three basic ways to promote ulcer healing. First, drugs can eradicate *H. pylori;* antibiotics do this. Second, drugs can reduce gastric acidity; antisecretory agents, misoprostol, and antacids do this. Third, drugs can enhance mucosal defenses; sucralfate and misoprostol do this.

TABLE 73–1 ■ Classification of Antiulcer Drugs

Class	Drugs	Mechanism of Action
Antibiotics	Amoxicillin [Amoxil] Bismuth [Pepto-Bismol] Clarithromycin [Biaxin] Metronidazole [Flagyl] Tetracycline [Achromycin V]	Eradication of *H. pylori*
Antisecretory Agents		
H₂ receptor antagonists	Cimetidine [Tagamet] Famotidine [Pepcid] Nizatidine [Axid] Ranitidine [Zantac] Esomeprazole [Nexium]	Suppression of acid secretion by blocking H₂ receptors on parietal cells
Proton pump inhibitors	Lansoprazole [Prevacid] Omeprazole [Prilosec] Pantoprazole [Protonix] Rabeprazole [Aciphex]	Suppression of acid secretion by inhibiting H⁺, K⁺-ATPase, the enzyme that makes gastric acid
Muscarinic antagonists	Pirenzepine [Gastrozepine]	Suppression of acid secretion by blocking muscarinic cholinergic receptors (on parietal cells?)
Mucosal Protectant	Sucralfate [Carafate]	Forms a barrier over the ulcer crater that protects against acid and pepsin
Antisecretory Agent That Enhances Mucosal Defenses	Misoprostol [Cytotec]	Protects against NSAID-induced ulcers by stimulating secretion of mucus and bicarbonate, maintaining submucosal blood flow, and suppressing secretion of gastric acid
Antacids	Aluminum hydroxide Calcium carbonate Magnesium hydroxide	React with gastric acid to form neutral salts

Drug Selection

Helicobacter pylori–*Associated Ulcers.* In 1994, a National Institutes of Health Consensus Development Conference recommended that all patients with gastric or duodenal ulcers and documented *H. pylori* infection be treated with antibiotics. This recommendation applies to patients with newly diagnosed PUD, recurrent PUD, and PUD in which use of NSAIDs is a contributing factor. To hasten healing and relieve symptoms, an antisecretory agent should be given along with the antibiotics. By eliminating *H. pylori,* antibiotics can cure PUD, and thereby prevent recurrence. Diagnosis of *H. pylori* infection and specific antibiotic regimens are discussed below under *Antibacterial Drugs.*

NSAID-Induced Ulcers. *Prophylaxis.* For patients with risk factors for ulcer development (e.g., age over 60, history of ulcers, high-dose NSAID therapy), prophylactic therapy is indicated. At this time, only one drug—*misoprostol*—is approved for prophylaxis of NSAID-induced ulcers. However, a recent study indicates that omeprazole (a proton pump inhibitor) is just as effective and better tolerated. Antacids, sucralfate, and histamine₂-receptor blockers are not recommended.

Treatment. NSAID-induced ulcers can be treated with any ulcer medication. However, histamine₂-receptor blockers and proton pump inhibitors are preferred. If possible, the offending NSAID should be discontinued to accelerate healing. If the NSAID cannot be discontinued, a proton pump inhibitor is the best choice to promoting healing.

Evaluation

We can evaluate ulcer healing by monitoring for relief of pain and by radiologic or endoscopic examination of the ulcer site. Unfortunately, evaluation is seldom straightforward. Why? Because cessation of pain and disappearance of the ulcer rarely coincide: In most cases, pain subsides prior to complete healing. However, the converse may also be true: Pain may persist even though endoscopic or radiologic examination reveals healing is complete.

Eradication of *H. pylori* can be determined with several methods, including a breath test, serologic tests, and microscopic observation of a stained biopsy sample. These methods are discussed below under *Tests for Helicobacter pylori.*

A Note About the Effects of Drugs on Pepsin

Pepsin is a proteolytic enzyme that can contribute to ulcer formation. This enzyme promotes ulcers by breaking down protein in the gut wall.

Like most enzymes, pepsin is sensitive to alterations in pH. As pH rises from 1.3 (the usual pH of the stomach) to 2, peptic activity increases by a factor of 4. As pH goes even higher, peptic activity begins to decline. At a pH of 5, peptic activity drops below baseline rates. When pH exceeds 6 to 7, pepsin undergoes irreversible inactivation.

Because the activity of pepsin is pH dependent, drugs that elevate gastric pH (e.g., antacids, histamine₂ antagonists) can cause peptic activity to increase, thereby enhancing pepsin's destructive effects. For example, treatment that produces a 99% reduction in gastric acidity will cause pH to rise from a base level of 1.3 up to 3.3. At pH 3.3, peptic activity will be significantly increased. To avoid activation of pepsin, drugs that reduce acidity should be administered in doses sufficient to raise gastric pH above 5.

Nondrug Therapy

Optimal antiulcer therapy requires implementation of nondrug measures in addition to drug therapy.

Diet. Despite commonly held beliefs, diet plays a minor role in ulcer management. The traditional "ulcer diet," consisting of bland foods together with milk or cream, does not accelerate healing. Furthermore, there is no convincing evidence that caffeine-containing beverages (coffee, tea, colas) promote ulcer formation or interfere with recovery. A change in *eating pattern* may be beneficial: Consumption of five or six small meals a day, rather than three larger ones, can reduce fluctuations in intragastric pH, and may thereby facilitate healing.

Other Nondrug Measures. *Smoking* is associated with an increased incidence of ulcers and also retards recovery. Accordingly, cigarettes should be avoided. Because of their ulcerogenic actions, *aspirin and other NSAIDs* should be avoided by patients with PUD. The exception to this rule is use of aspirin to prevent cardiovascular disease; in the low doses employed, aspirin is not a significant factor in PUD. There are no hard data indicating that *alcohol* contributes to PUD. However, if the patient notes a temporal relationship between alcohol consumption and exacerbation of symptoms, then alcohol use should stop. Many people feel that reduction of *stress and anxiety* may encourage ulcer healing; however, there is no good evidence that this is true.

ANTIBACTERIAL DRUGS

As noted, antibacterial drugs should be given to all patients with gastric or duodenal ulcers and confirmed infection with *H. pylori*. At this time, antibiotics are not recommended for asymptomatic individuals who test positive for *H. pylori*.

Tests for *Helicobacter pylori*

Several tests for *H. pylori* are available. Some are invasive; some are not. The invasive tests require an endoscopically obtained biopsy sample, which can be evaluated in three ways: (1) staining and viewing under a microscope to see if *H. pylori* is present; (2) assaying for the presence of urease (a marker enzyme for *H. pylori*); and (3) culturing and then assaying for the presence of *H. pylori*. Three types of noninvasive tests are available: breath, serologic, and stool tests. In the breath test, patients are given radiolabeled urea. If *H. pylori* is present, the urea is converted to carbon dioxide and ammonia; radiolabeled carbon dioxide can then be detected in the breath. In the serologic test, blood samples are evaluated for antibodies to *H. pylori*. In the stool test, fecal samples are evaluated for the presence of *H. pylori* antigens.

Antibiotics Employed

The antibiotics employed most often are clarithromycin, amoxicillin, bismuth, metronidazole, and tetracycline. None is effective alone. Furthermore, if these drugs *are* used alone, the risk of developing resistance is increased.

Bismuth. Bismuth compounds act topically to disrupt the cell wall of *H. pylori,* thereby causing lysis and death.

Bismuth may also inhibit urease activity and may prevent *H. pylori* from adhering to the gastric surface.

Bismuth can impart a harmless black coloration to the tongue and stool. Patients should be forewarned. Stool discoloration may confound interpretation of gastric bleeding. Long-term therapy may carry a risk of neurologic injury.

In the United States, bismuth is available by itself as bismuth subsalicylate [Pepto-Bismol, others], and in a complex with ranitidine (ranitidine bismuth citrate), marketed under the trade name Tritec. In Europe the drug is available as bismuth subcitrate [De-Nol].

Clarithromycin. Clarithromycin [Biaxin] suppresses growth of *H. pylori* by inhibiting protein synthesis. Treatment is highly effective. The rate of resistance is about 10%. The most common side effects are nausea, diarrhea, and distortion of taste. The basic pharmacology of clarithromycin is presented in Chapter 82.

Amoxicillin. *Helicobacter pylori* is highly sensitive to amoxicillin. The rate of resistance is about 3%. Amoxicillin kills bacteria by disrupting the cell wall. Antibacterial activity is highest at neutral pH, and hence can be enhanced by reducing gastric acidity with an antisecretory agent (e.g., omeprazole). The most common side effect is diarrhea. The basic pharmacology of amoxicillin is discussed in Chapter 80.

Tetracycline. Tetracycline, an inhibitor of bacterial protein synthesis, is highly active against *H. pylori*. Resistance is rare (<1%). Because tetracycline can stain developing teeth, it should not be used by pregnant women or young children. The pharmacology of tetracycline is discussed in Chapter 82.

Metronidazole. Metronidazole [Flagyl] is very effective against sensitive strains of *H. pylori*. Unfortunately, 54% of strains are now resistant. The most common side effects are nausea and headache. A disulfiram-like reaction can occur if metronidazole is used with alcohol. Accordingly, alcohol should be avoided. Metronidazole should not be taken during pregnancy. The basic pharmacology of metronidazole is discussed in Chapter 95.

Antibiotic Regimens

In 1998, the American College of Gastroenterology issued updated guidelines for managing *H. pylori* infection. To minimize emergence of resistance, the guidelines recommend using at least two antibiotics—and preferably three. As a rule, an antisecretory agent (histamin$_2$-receptor antagonist or proton pump inhibitor) should be included as well. Eradication rates are consistently higher with a 14-day course of treatment than with a shorter course. Some highly effective regimens are summarized in Table 73–2.

For several reasons, compliance with antibiotic therapy can be difficult. First, antibiotic regimens are complex, requiring the patient to ingest as many as 12 pills a day. Second, side effects—especially nausea and diarrhea—are common. Third, treatment is somewhat expensive (about $200). However, it costs much less to eradicate *H. pylori* with antibiotics than it does to treat ulcers over and over again with traditional antiulcer drugs, which merely promote healing without eliminating the cause.

TABLE 73–2 ▪■ Some Regimens for Helicobacter pylori

Drugs	Duration
Antisecretory Agent Plus Three Antibiotics	
Lansoprazole (30 mg qd) Metronidazole (500 mg tid) Tetracycline (500 mg qid) Bismuth subsalicylate (525 mg qid)	14 days
Famotidine (40 mg qd) Metronidazole (250 mg qid) Tetracycline (500 mg qid) Bismuth subsalicylate (525 mg qid)	14 days
Antisecretory Agent Plus Two Antibiotics	
Omeprazole (20 mg bid) Clarithromycin (500 mg bid) Amoxicillin (1 gm bid)	14 days
Lansoprazole (30 mg bid)* Clarithromycin (500 mg bid) Amoxicillin (1 gm bid)	10 or 14 days
Ranitidine bismuth citrate (400 mg bid) Clarithromycin (500 mg bid) Amoxicillin (1 gm bid)	14 days

*Lansoprazole, clarithromycin, and amoxicillin are available as a package under the trade name *Prevpac.*

HISTAMINE₂-RECEPTOR ANTAGONISTS

The histamine$_2$-receptor antagonists (H$_2$RAs) are drugs of first choice for treating gastric and duodenal ulcers. These agents promote ulcer healing by suppressing secretion of gastric acid. Four H$_2$RAs are available: cimetidine, ranitidine, famotidine, and nizatidine. All four are equally effective. Serious side effects are uncommon.

Cimetidine

Cimetidine [Tagamet] was the first H$_2$RA available and will serve as our prototype for the family. At one time, cimetidine was the most frequently prescribed drug in the United States.

Mechanism of Action

As discussed in Chapter 66, histamine acts through two types of receptors, named H$_1$ and H$_2$. Activation of H$_1$ receptors produces symptoms of allergy. In contrast, activation of H$_2$ receptors, which are located on parietal cells of the stomach (Fig. 73–2), promotes secretion of gastric acid. By blocking H$_2$ receptors, cimetidine reduces both the volume of gastric juice and its hydrogen ion concentration. Cimetidine suppresses basal acid secretion and secretion stimulated by gastrin and acetylcholine. Because cimetidine produces selective blockade of H$_2$ receptors, the drug does not reduce symptoms of allergy.

Pharmacokinetics

Cimetidine may be given orally, IM, or IV. Comparable blood levels are achieved with all three routes. When the drug is taken orally, food decreases the rate of absorption but not the extent. Hence, if cimetidine is taken with meals, absorption will be slowed and beneficial effects prolonged. Cimetidine crosses the blood-brain barrier—albeit with difficulty—and central nervous system (CNS) side effects can occur. Although some hepatic metabolism takes place, most of each dose is eliminated intact in the urine. The drug's half-life is relatively short (about 2 hours), but increases in patients with renal impairment. Accordingly, dosage should be reduced in these patients.

Therapeutic Uses

Gastric and Duodenal Ulcers. Cimetidine promotes healing of gastric and duodenal ulcers. To heal duodenal ulcers, 4 to 6 weeks of therapy are generally required. To heal gastric ulcers, 8 to 12 weeks may be needed. Long-term therapy with low doses may be given as prophylaxis against recurrence of gastric and duodenal ulcers.

Gastroesophageal Reflux Disease (GERD). Reflux esophagitis is an inflammatory condition caused by reflux of gastric contents back into the esophagus. Cimetidine is a drug of choice for relieving symptoms. However, cimetidine does little to hasten healing.

Zollinger-Ellison Syndrome. This syndrome is characterized by hypersecretion of gastric acid and development of peptic ulcers. The underlying cause is secretion of gastrin from a gastrin-producing tumor. Cimetidine can promote healing of ulcers in patients with Zollinger-Ellison syndrome, but only if high doses are employed. These high doses may cause significant adverse effects.

Aspiration Pneumonitis. Anesthesia suppresses the glottal reflex, permitting aspiration of gastric acid. When acid is aspirated, pulmonary injury develops within seconds and can be fatal. Surgical patients at high risk for this disorder include obese patients and women undergoing obstetric procedures. Cimetidine is a drug of choice for preventing aspiration pneumonitis. Gastric acidity can be reduced substantially by administering cimetidine 60 to 90 minutes prior to anesthesia.

Heartburn, Acid Indigestion, and Sour Stomach. Cimetidine is now available over the counter to treat these common acid-related symptoms.

Adverse Effects

The incidence of side effects is low. Furthermore, the effects that do occur are usually benign.

Antiandrogenic Effects. Cimetidine binds to androgen receptors, producing receptor blockade. This action may result in *gynecomastia, reduced libido,* and *impotence.* These effects reverse following termination of treatment.

CNS Effects. Effects on the CNS are most likely in elderly patients who have renal or hepatic impairment. Possible reactions include *confusion, hallucinations, CNS depression* (lethargy, somnolence), and *CNS excitation* (restlessness, seizures).

Other Adverse Effects. When administered by IV bolus, cimetidine can cause hypotension and dysrhythmias. These reactions are rare and do not occur with oral therapy. By reducing gastric acidity, cimetidine may permit growth of *Candida* in the stomach. Hematologic effects (neutropenia, leukopenia, thrombocytopenia) occur rarely. Minor side effects include headache, dizziness, myalgia, nausea, diarrhea, constipation, rash, and pruritus.

Drug Interactions

Interactions Related to Inhibition of Drug Metabolism. Cimetidine inhibits hepatic drug-metabolizing enzymes, and hence can cause levels of many other drugs to rise. Agents

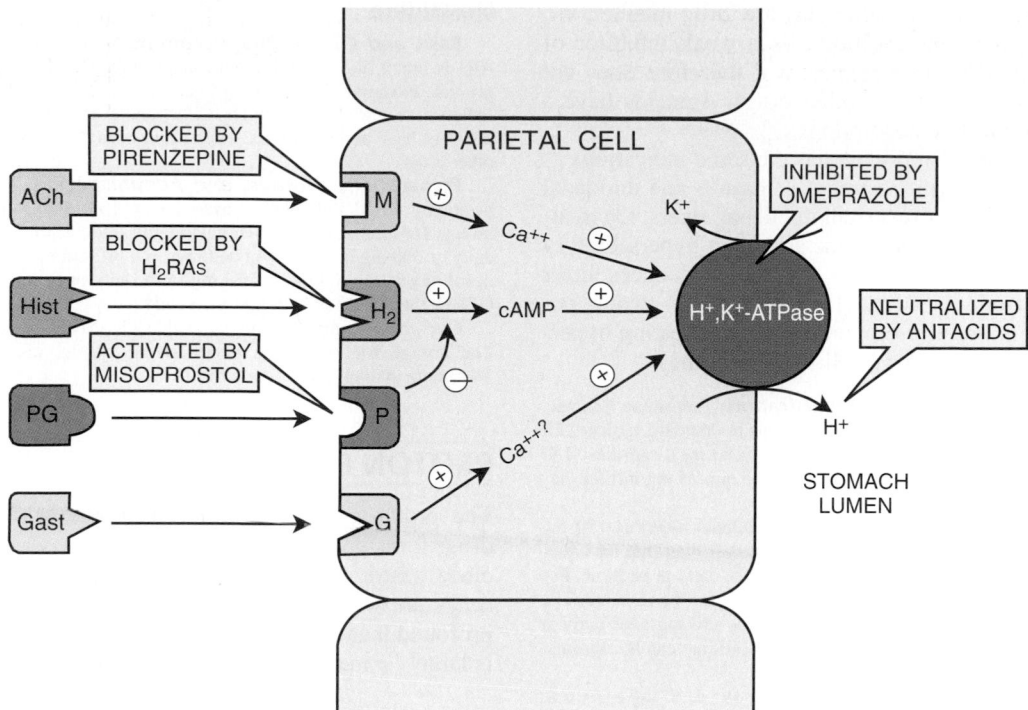

Figure 73–2 ■ **A model of the regulation of gastric acid secretion showing the actions of antisecretory drugs and antacids.**
Production of gastric acid is stimulated by three endogenous compounds: (1) acetylcholine (ACh) acting at muscarinic (M) receptors; (2) histamine (Hist) acting at histamine$_2$ (H$_2$) receptors; and (3) gastrin (Gast) acting at gastrin (G) receptors. As indicated, all three compounds act through intracellular messengers—either calcium (Ca^{++}) or cyclic AMP (cAMP)—to increase the activity of H$^+$,K$^+$-ATPase, the enzyme that actually produces gastric acid. Prostaglandins (PG) decrease acid production, perhaps by suppressing production of intracellular cAMP. The actions of histamine$_2$-receptor antagonists (H$_2$RAs), other antisecretory drugs, and antacids are indicated. (P = prostaglandin receptor.)

of particular concern are *warfarin, phenytoin, theophylline,* and *lidocaine,* all of which have a narrow margin of safety. If these agents are used concurrently with cimetidine, their dosages should be reduced.

Antacids. Antacids can decrease absorption of cimetidine. Accordingly, cimetidine and antacids should be administered at least 1 hour apart.

Preparations, Dosage, and Administration

Oral. Cimetidine [Tagamet] is available in tablets (100, 200, 300, 400, and 800 mg) and an oral solution (300 mg/5 ml). For treatment of duodenal and gastric ulcers, the drug may be given once daily (800 mg at bedtime), twice daily (400 mg each dose), or 4 times a day (300 mg with meals and at bedtime). In patients with renal impairment, dosage should be lowered to 300 mg every 12 hours. For prophylaxis against recurrence of ulcers, a single 400-mg dose at bedtime may be employed. Patients with Zollinger-Ellison syndrome require high doses, but not more than 2.4 gm/day.

Parenteral. Parenteral cimetidine is reserved for patients with hypersecretory conditions (e.g., Zollinger-Ellison syndrome) and ulcers that have failed to respond to oral therapy. The usual dosage (IM or IV) is 300 mg every 6 to 8 hours. Intramuscular injections are made with a concentrated solution (300 mg/2 ml). For IV administration, two concentrations may be employed: (1) 300 mg may be diluted in 20 ml and injected slowly (over 2 minutes), or (2) 300 mg may be diluted in 100 ml and infused over 15 minutes.

Ranitidine

Ranitidine [Zantac] shares many of the properties of cimetidine. However, although similar to cimetidine, ranitidine does differ in three important respects: ranitidine is more potent than cimetidine, produces fewer adverse effects, and causes fewer drug interactions.

Actions. Like cimetidine, ranitidine suppresses secretion of gastric acid by blocking H$_2$ receptors on parietal cells. The drug does not block H$_1$ receptors, and hence does not reduce symptoms of allergy.

Pharmacokinetics. Ranitidine can be administered PO, IM, or IV. Oral bioavailability is about 50%. In contrast to cimetidine, ranitidine is absorbed at the same rate in the presence or absence of food. The ability of ranitidine to enter the CNS is even less than that of cimetidine. Elimination is by hepatic metabolism and renal excretion. Accumulation will occur in patients with renal impairment unless the dosage is reduced. The drug's half-life is 2 to 3 hours.

Adverse Effects. Significant side effects are uncommon. Because ranitidine penetrates the blood-brain barrier poorly, CNS effects are rare. In contrast to cimetidine, ranitidine does not bind to androgen receptors, and hence does not cause antiandrogenic effects (e.g., gynecomastia, impotence).

Drug Interactions. Ranitidine has few drug interactions. In contrast to cimetidine, ranitidine is a weak inhibitor of hepatic drug-metabolizing enzymes, and therefore does not greatly depress metabolism of other drugs. Antacids have a small effect on ranitidine absorption.

Therapeutic Uses. Ranitidine has the same indications as cimetidine: (1) short-term treatment of gastric and duodenal ulcers, (2) prophylaxis of recurrent duodenal ulcers, (3) treatment of Zollinger-Ellison syndrome and other hypersecretory states, and (4) treatment of GERD. Because it produces fewer side effects than cimetidine, and because of its greater potency, ranitidine is preferred to cimetidine for treating hypersecretory states (e.g., Zollinger-Ellison syndrome).

Preparations, Dosage, and Administration. Ranitidine [Zantac, Zantac EFFERdose, Zantac GELdose] is available in standard tablets (75, 150, and 300 mg), effervescent tablets or granules (150 mg), capsules (150 and 300 mg), a syrup (15 mg/ml), and in solution (0.5 and 25 mg/ml) for parenteral use.

Oral. The usual adult dosage for gastric or duodenal ulcers is 150 mg twice a day. (Note that this dosage is considerably lower than that for cimetidine.) Alternatively, a 300-mg dose can be given once daily at bedtime. For patients with Zollinger-Ellison syndrome, higher doses may be required. The dosage for preventing recurrence of duodenal ulcers is 150 mg once daily at bedtime. Since absorption is not affected by food, ranitidine can be administered without regard to meals.

Parenteral. The usual parenteral dosage (IM or IV) is 50 mg every 6 to 8 hours. Intramuscular doses can be injected without dilution. For IV injection, the preparation should be diluted to a volume of 20 ml and administered slowly (over 5 or more minutes). For IV infusion, the drug should be diluted in 100 ml and administered over 15 to 20 minutes.

Ranitidine Bismuth Citrate

Ranitidine bismuth citrate [Tritec] is a compound that dissociates into ranitidine and bismuth in stomach acid. The drug is indicated only for duodenal ulcers associated with *H. pylori* infection, and must be used in combination with clarithromycin—never alone. The role of ranitidine is to suppress secretion of gastric acid. The role of bismuth is to help kill *H. pylori*. Ranitidine bismuth citrate is dispensed in 400-mg tablets. The recommended dosage is 400 mg twice daily for 4 weeks, combined with clarithromycin (500 mg tid) for the first 2 weeks. Dosage should be reduced in patients with significant renal impairment. The drug may be taken with or without food.

Famotidine

Basic and Clinical Pharmacology. Famotidine [Pepcid, Pepcid AC, Pepcid RPD] is very similar to ranitidine. The drug is approved for treatment and prevention of duodenal ulcers, treatment of gastric ulcers, treatment of GERD, and treatment of hypersecretory states (e.g., Zollinger-Ellison syndrome). An over-the-counter formulation is approved for heartburn, acid indigestion, and sour stomach. Like ranitidine, famotidine does not bind to androgen receptors, and hence does not have antiandrogenic effects. Famotidine does not inhibit hepatic drug-metabolizing enzymes, and hence does not suppress the metabolism of other drugs.

Preparations, Dosage, and Administration. Prescription-strength famotidine [Pepcid] is available in standard tablets (20 and 40 mg), orally disintegrating tablets (20 and 40 mg), powder for oral suspension (40 mg/5 ml when reconstituted), and solution (0.4 and 10 mg/ml) for IV use. For treatment of duodenal and gastric ulcers, the dosage is 20 mg twice daily or 40 mg once daily at bedtime. For preventing recurrence of duodenal ulcers, the dosage is 20 mg once daily at bedtime. For treatment of GERD, the dosage is 20 to 40 mg twice daily. For treatment of hypersecretory states, the initial dosage is 20 mg every 6 hours; severe cases may require up to 160 mg every 6 hours. All doses should be reduced in patients with moderate to severe renal impairment.

Over-the-counter famotidine [Pepcid AC] is available in three 10-mg formulations: standard tablets, chewable tablets, and gelcaps. Indications are prevention and relief of heartburn, acid indigestion, and sour stomach. For prevention of symptoms, the drug is taken 1 hour before eating. The dosage for prevention or relief is 10 mg, taken with a glass of water. As with prescription-strength famotidine, dosages should be reduced in patients with moderate to severe renal impairment.

Nizatidine

Basic and Clinical Pharmacology. Nizatidine [Axid Pulvules, Axid AR] is much like ranitidine and famotidine. The drug is used to treat and prevent duodenal ulcers and to treat gastric ulcers, GERD, heartburn, acid indigestion, and sour stomach. Like ranitidine and famotidine, nizatidine does not have antiandrogenic effects and does not inhibit the metabolism of other drugs.

Preparations, Dosage, and Administration. Prescription-strength nizatidine [Axid Pulvules] is available in 150- and 300-mg capsules. The dosage for treatment of active gastric and duodenal ulcers is 150 mg twice daily or 300 mg once daily at bedtime. For preventing the recurrence of duodenal ulcers, the dosage is 150 mg once daily at bedtime. For treatment of GERD, the dosage is 150 mg twice daily.

Over-the-counter nizatidine [Axid AR] is available in 75-mg capsules. The dosage for preventing heartburn is 75 mg, taken any time in the 30-minute interval preceding a meal.

PROTON PUMP INHIBITORS

The proton pump inhibitors (PPIs) are the most effective drugs for suppressing secretion of gastric acid. Indications include gastric and duodenal ulcers and GERD. All of these drugs are well tolerated. Similarities among them are more profound than their differences. Hence, selection among them is largely a matter of cost and prescriber preference.

Omeprazole

Omeprazole [Prilosec] was the first PPI available and will serve as our prototype for the group. The drug is a powerful suppressant of acid secretion. Effects are superior to those of the H_2RAs. Side effects from short-term therapy are minimal.

Mechanism of Action. Omeprazole is a prodrug that undergoes conversion to its active form within parietal cells of the stomach. The active form causes irreversible inhibition of H^+,K^+-ATPase—the enzyme that generates gastric acid (see Fig. 73–2). Because it blocks the final common pathway of gastric acid production, omeprazole can inhibit basal and stimulated acid release. A single 30-mg oral dose reduces production of gastric acid by 97% within 2 hours. Because inhibition of the ATPase is irreversible, effects persist until new enzyme is synthesized. Partial recovery of acid production occurs 3 to 5 days after termination of treatment. Full recovery may take weeks.

Pharmacokinetics. Administration is oral. Because the drug is acid labile, it is dispensed in capsules that contain protective enteric-coated granules. The capsule dissolves in the stomach, but the granules don't dissolve until they reach the relatively alkaline environment of the duodenum, and hence they protect the drug from destruction by stomach acid. About 50% of each dose reaches the systemic circulation. The drug undergoes hepatic metabolism followed by renal excretion. The plasma half-life is short (about 1 hour). However, since omeprazole acts by irreversible enzyme inhibition, its effects persist long after the drug has been cleared from the body.

Therapeutic Use. Omeprazole is approved for short-term therapy of duodenal ulcers, gastric ulcers, and GERD, and for long-term therapy of hypersecretory conditions (e.g., Zollinger-Ellison syndrome). Except for therapy of hypersecretory states, treatment should be limited to 4 to 8 weeks.

In clinical trials, duodenal ulcers healed faster with omeprazole (40 mg/day) than with conventional doses of H_2RAs. However, by the end of 8 weeks, the success rate was equivalent with both treatments. Patients who fail to respond to H₂RAs can often benefit from omeprazole. The 6-month relapse rate following discontinuation of omeprazole is equivalent to that seen with H₂RAs.

Adverse Effects. Effects seen with short-term therapy are generally inconsequential. Like the H₂RAs, omeprazole can cause headache, diarrhea, nausea, and vomiting. The incidence of these effects is less than 1%.

With long-term therapy, there may be a risk of cancer. Gastric carcinoid tumors have developed in rats given omeprazole daily for 2 years. These tumors are related to hypersecretion of gastrin, which occurs in response to omeprazole-induced suppression of gastric acidity. Gastrin has a trophic effect on cells of the gastric epithelium; hyperplasia of these cells may precede development of gastric carcinoid tumors. However, omeprazole has been on the market for several years now, and no gastric tumors have been attributed to the drug.

Preparations, Dosage, and Administration. Omeprazole [Prilosec] is dispensed in delayed-release capsules (10, 20, and 40 mg) for oral use. For treatment of active duodenal ulcer and GERD, the usual dosage is 20 mg once a day for 4 to 8 weeks. For treatment of Zollinger-Ellison syndrome and other hypersecretory states, doses up to 120 mg 3 times a day may be needed.

Lansoprazole

Lansoprazole [Prevacid] is very similar to omeprazole. Both drugs cause prolonged inhibition of H⁺,K⁺-ATPase. Hence, suppression of acid secretion is sustained. Like omeprazole, lansoprazole is well tolerated. The most common adverse effects are diarrhea, abdominal pain, and nausea. Lansoprazole is available in two oral formulations: (1) delayed-release capsules (15 and 30 mg) and (2) enteric-coated granules (15 and 30 mg/packet) that form a suspension when mixed with water (2 tablespoons). The dosage for duodenal ulcers (prevention and treatment) and GERD is 15 mg once daily. The dosage for erosive gastritis and active gastric ulcers is 30 mg once daily. For hypersecretory states, the initial dosage is 60 mg/day; for severe cases, up to 90 mg twice daily may be needed. All doses should be taken before a meal.

Rabeprazole

Rabeprazole [Aciphex] is much like omeprazole and lansoprazole in actions, uses, and adverse effects. The drug is approved for duodenal ulcers, GERD, and hypersecretory states, such as Zollinger-Ellison syndrome. Like other PPIs, rabeprazole suppresses acid secretion by inhibiting H⁺,K⁺-ATPase in parietal cells. However, in contrast to omeprazole, the drug causes *reversible* inhibition of H⁺,K⁺-ATPase, and hence its effects are less long lasting. In addition to suppressing acid secretion, rabeprazole has antibacterial activity. As a result, it may help other antibacterial drugs eradicate *H. pylori*. The most common adverse effects are diarrhea, headache, dizziness, malaise, nausea, and rash. Although rabeprazole is metabolized by cytochrome P450 enzymes, it does not appear to influence the metabolism of other drugs. However, it can increase digoxin levels by 20%. Accordingly, levels of digoxin should be monitored. Rabeprazole is available in 20-mg delayed-release, enteric-coated tablets. The dosage for GERD and duodenal ulcers is 20 mg once daily. The initial dosage for hypersecretory states is 60 mg once daily; for severe cases, 60 mg twice daily may be needed. Although rabeprazole is not approved for treating gastric ulcers, 20 to 40 mg once daily has been effective.

Pantoprazole

Pantoprazole [Protonix, Protonix I.V.] is similar to omeprazole and the other PPIs, but with one important exception: pantoprazole is the only PPI that can be given IV (as well as PO). Indications are duodenal ulcers, gastric ulcers, GERD, and hypersecretory states. Like other PPIs, pantoprazole is well tolerated. With oral therapy, the most common adverse effects are diarrhea (1.5%), headache (1.3%), and dizziness (0.7%). And with IV therapy, the most common adverse effects are diarrhea, headache, nausea, dyspepsia, and injection site reactions, including thrombophlebitis and abscess. Pantoprazole does not affect cytochrome P450 enzymes, and hence does not affect the metabolism of other drugs. Pantoprazole is available in delayed-release tablets (20 and 40 mg) for oral use, and as a powder (40 mg/vial) to be re-

constituted for IV use. Infusions are done over 15 minutes, and a filter *must* be used to remove precipitates. The usual dosage, either PO or IV, is 40 mg/day.

Esomeprazole

Esomeprazole [Nexium] is nearly identical to omeprazole [Prilosec], our prototype for the PPI family. Structurally, esomeprazole is the *S*-isomer of omeprazole, which is a mixture of *S*- and *R*-isomers. The *S*-isomer (esomeprazole) is metabolized more slowly than the *R*-isomer, and hence esomeprazole achieves higher blood levels than omeprazole, and its effects last somewhat longer. Otherwise the two drugs are essentially the same. The most common adverse effects are headache and diarrhea. In addition, esomeprazole may cause nausea, flatulence, abdominal pain, and dry mouth. Approved indications are erosive esophagitis, GERD, and duodenal ulcers associated with *H. pylori* infection. Esomeprazole is dispensed in 20- and 40-mg delayed-release capsules. For treatment of erosive gastritis, the usual dosage is 20 or 40 mg once daily, taken at least 1 hour before a meal, for 4 to 8 weeks. For treatment of GERD, the usual dosage is 20 mg once daily for 4 to 8 weeks. And for treatment of duodenal ulcers associated with *H. pylori*, the recommended regimen is 10 days of triple therapy, consisting of esomeprazole (40 mg once daily), amoxicillin (1000 mg twice daily), and clarithromycin (500 mg twice daily). The goal is to eradicate *H. pylori*.

OTHER ANTIULCER DRUGS

Sucralfate

Sucralfate [Carafate] is an effective antiulcer medication notable for its minimal side effects and lack of significant drug interactions. The drug promotes ulcer healing by creating a protective barrier against acid and pepsin. Sucralfate has no acid-neutralizing capacity and does not decrease acid secretion.

Mechanism of Antiulcer Action. Sucralfate is a complex substance composed of sulfated sucrose and aluminum hydroxide. Under mildly acidic conditions (pH <4), sucralfate undergoes polymerization and cross-linking reactions. The resultant product is a viscid and very sticky gel that adheres to the ulcer crater, creating a barrier to back-diffusion of hydrogen ions, pepsin, and bile salts. Attachment to the ulcer appears to last up to 6 hours.

Pharmacokinetics. Sucralfate is administered orally, and systemic absorption is minimal (3% to 5%). About 90% of each dose is eliminated in the feces.

Therapeutic Uses. Sucralfate is approved for acute and maintenance therapy of duodenal ulcers. Rates of healing are comparable to those achieved with cimetidine. Controlled trials indicate that sucralfate can also promote healing of gastric ulcers.

Adverse Effects. Sucralfate has no known serious adverse effects. The most significant side effect is constipation, which occurs in only 2% of patients. Because sucralfate is not absorbed, systemic effects are absent.

Drug Interactions. Interactions with other drugs are minimal. By raising gastric pH above 4, antacids may interfere with sucralfate's effects. This interaction can be minimized by administering these drugs at least 30 minutes apart.

Sucralfate may impede the absorption of some drugs, including phenytoin, theophylline, digoxin, warfarin, and fluoroquinolone antibiotics (e.g., ciprofloxacin, norfloxacin). These interactions can be minimized by administering sucralfate at least 2 hours apart from these other drugs.

Preparations, Dosage, and Administration. Sucralfate [Carafate] is dispensed in 1-gm tablets and a suspension (1 gm/10 ml) for oral administration. The drug should be taken on an empty stomach. The recommended adult dosage is 1 gm 4 times a day, administered 1 hour before meals and at bedtime. However, a dosing schedule of 2 gm twice a day appears equally effective. Treatment should continue for 4 to 8 weeks.

Sucralfate tablets are large and difficult to swallow, especially by the elderly. The oral suspension is much easier to ingest.

Misoprostol

Therapeutic Use. Misoprostol [Cytotec] is an analog of prostaglandin E_1. In the United States, the drug is approved only for *preventing gastric ulcers caused by long-term therapy with NSAIDs*. In other countries, misoprostol is also used to treat peptic ulcers unrelated to NSAIDs. In addition to its use in PUD, misoprostol, in combination with mifepristone (RU-486), can be used for abortion (see Chapter 60). The drug is also used to promote cervical ripening (see Chapter 62).

Mechanism of Action. In normal individuals, prostaglandins help protect the stomach by (1) suppressing secretion of gastric acid, (2) promoting secretion of bicarbonate and cytoprotective mucus, and (3) maintaining submucosal blood flow (by promoting vasodilation). As discussed in Chapter 67, aspirin and other NSAIDs cause gastric ulcers in part by inhibiting prostaglandin biosynthesis. Misoprostol prevents NSAID-induced ulcers by serving as a replacement for endogenous prostaglandins.

Adverse Effects. The most common reactions are dose-related *diarrhea* (13% to 40%) and abdominal pain (7% to 20%). Some women experience spotting and dysmenorrhea.

Misoprostol is contraindicated for use during pregnancy. The drug is classified in Food and Drug Administration Pregnancy Risk Category X: the risk of use by pregnant women clearly outweighs any possible benefits. Prostaglandins stimulate uterine contractions. Administration during pregnancy has caused partial or complete expulsion of the developing fetus. If women of child-bearing age are to use misoprostol, they must (1) be able to comply with birth control measures, (2) be given oral and written warnings about the dangers of misoprostol, (3) have a negative serum pregnancy test result within 2 weeks prior to beginning therapy, and (4) begin therapy only on the second or third day of the next normal menstrual cycle.

Preparations, Dosage, and Administration. Misoprostol [Cytotec] is dispensed in 100- and 200-μg tablets for oral administration. The usual dosage is 200 μg 4 times a day administered with meals and at bedtime. Patients who cannot tolerate this dosage may try 100 μg 4 times a day.

Antacids

Antacids are alkaline compounds that neutralize stomach acid. The principal indications for these drugs are PUD and GERD.

Beneficial Actions

Antacids react with gastric acid to produce neutral salts or salts of low acidity. By neutralizing acid, these drugs decrease destruction of the gut wall. In addition, if acid neutralization is sufficient to elevate gastric pH above 5, activity of pepsin declines as well. In addition to neutralizing acid and inactivating pepsin, antacids may be able to enhance mucosal protection by stimulating production of prostaglandins. Antacids do not coat the ulcer crater to protect it from acid and pepsin. With the exception of sodium bicarbonate, antacids are poorly absorbed, and therefore do not alter systemic pH.

Therapeutic Uses

Peptic Ulcer Disease. The primary indication for antacids is PUD. Rates of healing are equivalent to those achieved with H2RAs. At one time, antacids were the mainstay of antiulcer therapy. However, these drugs have been largely replaced by newer medications (H2RAs, PPIs, sucralfate) that are equally effective, more convenient to administer, and cause fewer side effects.

Other Uses. Antacids are administered prior to anesthesia to prevent aspiration pneumonitis. In addition, these drugs can provide prophylaxis against stress-induced ulcers. For patients with GERD, antacids can produce symptomatic relief, but they do not accelerate healing. Although these drugs are used widely by the general public to relieve functional symptoms (dyspepsia, heartburn, acid indigestion), there are no controlled studies that demonstrate efficacy in these conditions.

Potency, Dosage, and Formulations

Potency. Antacid potency is expressed in terms of acid-neutralizing capacity (ANC). ANC is defined as the number of milliequivalents of hydrochloric acid that can be neutralized by a given weight or volume of antacid. Individual antacids differ widely in ANC. The ANC of commonly used proprietary preparations is listed in Table 73–3.

Dosage. The objective of peptic ulcer therapy is to promote healing, and not simply to relieve pain. Consequently, antacids should be taken on a regular schedule, not just in response to discomfort. In the usual dosing schedule, antacids are administered 7 times a day: 1 and 3 hours after each meal and at bedtime.

Dosage recommendations should be based on ANC and not on weight or volume of antacid. The ANC of a single dose usually ranges from 20 to 80 mEq. Single doses for gastric ulcers are relatively low (20 to 40 mEq), whereas single doses for duodenal ulcers are higher (40 to 80 mEq). Frequent administration of even larger doses (120 mEq) may be required if ulceration is especially severe.

To provide maximum benefits, treatment should elevate gastric pH above 5. At this pH there is inhibition of pepsin's activity in addition to nearly complete (greater than 99.9%) neutralization of acid.

Antacids are inconvenient and unpleasant to ingest, making compliance difficult to achieve—especially in the absence of pain. Patients should be encouraged to take their medication as prescribed, even after symptoms are gone.

Formulations. Antacids are available in tablets and liquid formulations. Antacid tablets should be chewed thoroughly and followed with a glass of water or milk. Liquid preparations should be shaken before dispensing. As a rule, liquids (suspensions) are more effective than tablets.

Adverse Effects

Constipation and Diarrhea. Most antacids affect the bowel. Some (e.g., aluminum hydroxide) promote constipation, whereas others (e.g., magnesium hydroxide) promote diarrhea. Effects on the bowel can be minimized by combining an antacid that promotes constipation with one that promotes diarrhea. Patients should be taught to adjust the dosage of one agent or the other to normalize bowel function.

Sodium Loading. Some antacid preparations contain substantial amounts of sodium (see Table 73–3). Because sodium excess can exacerbate hypertension and heart failure, patients with these disorders should avoid preparations that have a high sodium content.

Drug Interactions

By raising gastric pH, antacids can influence the dissolution and absorption of many other drugs, including *cimetidine* and *ranitidine*. These interactions can be minimized by allowing 1 hour between administration of antacids and administration of other drugs.

Antacids can interfere with the actions of sucralfate, a locally acting antiulcer medication. To minimize this interaction, these drugs should be administered 1 hour apart.

If absorbed in substantial amounts, antacids can alkalinize the urine. Elevation of urinary pH can accelerate excretion of acidic drugs and delay excretion of basic drugs.

Antacid Families

There are four major groups of antacids: (1) aluminum compounds, (2) magnesium compounds, (3) calcium compounds, and (4) sodium compounds. Individual agents that belong to these groups are listed in Table 73–4. Representative members of these groups are discussed below.

TABLE 73–3 ▪ Composition and Acid-Neutralizing Capacity of Commonly Used Over-the-Counter Antacid Suspensions

Product	Acid Neutralizing Capacity (mEq/5 ml)	Active Ingredients (mg/5 ml)				Sodium (mg/5 ml)
		Al(OH)₃	Mg(OH)₂	Simethicone	Magaldrate	
AlternaGEL	16	600				<2.5
Aludrox	12	307	103			2.3
Amphojel	10	320				2.3
Kudrox DS	25	565	180			<15
Maalox	15	225	200			1.4
Maalox TC	27	600	300			0.8
Milk of Magnesia	14		390			0.1
Mylagen II	24	400	400	40		1.3
Mylanta DS	25	400	400	40		1.1
Riopan	15				540	<0.1
Riopan Plus	15			40	540	<0.1
Riopan Plus DS	30			40	1080	0.3

DS = double strength, TC = therapeutic concentrate.

Representative Antacids

Antacids differ from one another with respect to ANC, onset and duration of action, effects on the bowel, systemic effects, and special applications. In this section, we discuss the two most commonly used antacids—magnesium hydroxide and aluminum hydroxide—and two less commonly used drugs—calcium carbonate and sodium bicarbonate. The distinguishing properties of these agents are summarized in Table 73–5.

Magnesium Hydroxide. This antacid is rapid acting, has high ANC, and produces effects of long duration. These properties make magnesium hydroxide an antacid of choice. The liquid formulation of magnesium hydroxide is often referred to as milk of magnesia.

The most prominent adverse effect is diarrhea, which results from retention of water in the intestinal lumen. To compensate for this effect, magnesium hydroxide is usually administered in combination with aluminum hydroxide, an antacid that promotes constipation. However, if the dose of magnesium hydroxide is sufficiently high, no amount of aluminum hydroxide will prevent diarrhea. Since stimulation of the bowel can be hazardous for patients with intestinal obstruction or appendicitis, magnesium hydroxide should be avoided in patients with undiagnosed abdominal pain. Because of its effect on the bowel, magnesium hydroxide is frequently employed as a laxative (see Chapter 74). In patients with renal impairment, magnesium may accumulate to high levels, causing signs of toxicity (e.g., CNS depression).

Aluminum Hydroxide. This drug has relatively low ANC and is slow acting, but produces effects of long duration. Although rarely used alone, this compound is widely used in combination with magnesium hydroxide (see Table 73–3). Aluminum hydroxide preparations contain significant amounts of sodium; appropriate caution should be exercised. The most common adverse effect is constipation.

Aluminum hydroxide adsorbs a variety of compounds. Binding of certain drugs (e.g., tetracyclines, warfarin, digoxin) may reduce their effects. Aluminum hydroxide has a high affinity for phosphate. By binding with phosphate, the drug can reduce phosphate absorption, and can thereby cause hypophosphatemia. Aluminum hydroxide can also bind to pepsin, which may facilitate ulcer healing.

Calcium Carbonate. Calcium carbonate, like magnesium hydroxide, is rapid acting, has high ANC, and produces effects of long duration. Because of these properties, calcium carbonate was once considered the ideal antacid. However, because of concerns about acid rebound (stimulation of acid secretion), use of calcium carbonate has declined. The principal adverse effect is constipation. This can be overcome by using the drug in combination with a magnesium-containing antacid (e.g., magnesium hydroxide). Calcium carbonate releases carbon dioxide in the stomach, and can thereby cause eructation (belching) and flatulence. Rarely, systemic absorption is sufficient to produce the milk-alkali syndrome, a condition characterized by hypercalcemia, meta-

TABLE 73–4 ▪ Classification of Antacids

Aluminum Compounds
Aluminum hydroxide
Aluminum carbonate
Aluminum phosphate
Dihydroxyaluminum sodium carbonate

Magnesium Compounds
Magnesium hydroxide (milk of magnesia)
Magnesium oxide

Calcium Compounds
Calcium carbonate

Sodium Compounds
Sodium bicarbonate

Other
Magaldrate (a complex of magnesium and aluminum compounds)

bolic alkalosis, soft tissue calcification, and impaired renal function. The palatability of calcium carbonate is low, and this can detract from compliance.

Sodium Bicarbonate. Although capable of neutralizing gastric acid, sodium bicarbonate is unfit for treating ulcers. This agent has a rapid onset but its effects are short lasting. Like calcium carbonate, sodium bicarbonate liberates carbon dioxide, thereby increasing intra-abdominal pressure and promoting eructation and flatulence. Absorption of sodium can exacerbate hypertension and heart failure. In patients with renal impairment, sodium bicarbonate can cause systemic alkalosis. (Other antacids rarely alter systemic pH.) Because of its brief duration, high sodium content, and capacity for causing alkalosis, sodium bicarbonate is inappropriate for treating PUD. The drug *is* useful, however, for treating acidosis and elevating urinary pH to promote excretion of acidic drugs following overdose.

Anticholinergics

Atropine and other classic muscarinic antagonists have a very limited role in treating PUD. Why? Because the doses required to inhibit acid secretion are so high that they produce muscarinic blockade throughout the body. Hence,

TABLE 73–5 ▪■ Representative Antacids: Summary of Distinguishing Properties

Antacid	Effect on the Bowel		Effect on Systemic pH	Comments
	Constipation	Diarrhea		
Aluminum hydroxide	Yes	No	None	Can cause hypophosphatemia; can treat hyperphosphatemia
Magnesium hydroxide	No	Yes	None	Can cause Mg toxicity (CNS depression) in patients with renal impairment
Calcium carbonate	Yes	No	None	May cause acid rebound or milk-alkali syndrome; releases CO_2
Sodium bicarbonate	No	No	Increase	Not used routinely to treat ulcers; used to treat acidosis and to alkalanize urine; high risk of sodium loading; releases CO_2

when used to treat ulcers, these drugs cause a high incidence of anticholinergic side effects, such as dry mouth, constipation, urinary retention, and disturbance of vision.

Pirenzepine. Pirenzepine [Gastrozepine] is a unique muscarinic antagonist available for treatment of PUD. In contrast to the classic anticholinergic drugs, pirenzepine produces "selective" blockade of the muscarinic receptors that regulate gastric acid secretion (see Fig. 73–2). As a result, the drug can inhibit acid secretion without causing pronounced anticholinergic side effects. For treatment of duodenal ulcers, pirenzepine (50 mg 2 to 3 times/day) is about equal to cimetidine (1 gm/day).

Following oral administration, about 20% to 30% of the drug is absorbed. Very little crosses the blood-brain barrier. About 80% is excreted unchanged in the urine. The drug's half-life is approximately 10 hours.

The most common side effect is dry mouth. In addition, pirenzepine can cause constipation, visual disturbances, nausea, vomiting, and diarrhea.

⁘ KEY POINTS

- The term *peptic ulcer disease* (PUD) refers to a group of upper GI disorders characterized by varying degrees of erosion of the gut wall.
- PUD develops when aggressive factors (*H. pylori*, NSAIDs, acid, pepsin) outweigh defensive factors (mucus, bicarbonate, submucosal blood flow, prostaglandins).
- Gastric acid is an absolute requirement for ulcer formation. In the absence of acid, no ulcer will form.
- The major underlying cause of PUD is infection with *H. pylori*. The second most common cause is use of NSAIDs.
- The goal of PUD therapy is to alleviate symptoms, promote healing, prevent complications (hemorrhage, perforation, obstruction), and prevent recurrences.
- The major drugs for treating ulcers are antibiotics, antisecretory agents (H2RAs, PPIs), and sucralfate, a mucosal protectant.

- With the exception of antibiotics, antiulcer drugs do not alter the disease process; rather, they simply create conditions conducive to healing. Since non-antibiotic therapies do not cure ulcers, the relapse rate following discontinuation is high. In contrast, the relapse rate following successful antibiotic therapy is low.
- All patients with gastric or duodenal ulcers and confirmed infection with *H. pylori* should be treated with antibiotics, preferably in combination with an antisecretory agent.
- The antibiotics employed most often are clarithromycin, tetracycline, amoxicillin, bismuth, and metronidazole.
- To avoid resistance and increase efficacy, at least two antibiotics should be used.
- Cimetidine and other H2RAs suppress secretion of gastric acid by blocking histamine2 receptors on parietal cells of the stomach.
- Cimetidine inhibits hepatic drug-metabolizing enzymes, and can thereby cause levels of other drugs to rise.
- In contrast to cimetidine, ranitidine has little effect on drug metabolism.
- Proton pump inhibitors (e.g., omeprazole, lansoprazole) suppress acid secretion by inhibiting gastric H^+,K^+-ATPase, the enzyme that makes gastric acid. PPIs are the most effective inhibitors of acid secretion.
- Sucralfate promotes ulcer healing by creating a protective barrier against acid and pepsin.
- Misoprostol, an analog of prostaglandin E_1, is used to prevent gastric ulcers caused by NSAIDs.
- Misoprostol stimulates uterine contraction and hence is contraindicated during pregnancy.

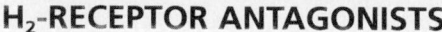

Summary of Major Nursing Implications*

H₂-RECEPTOR ANTAGONISTS

Cimetidine
Famotidine
Nizatidine
Ranitidine

Preadministration Assessment

Therapeutic Goal

The objective in treating PUD is to relieve pain, promote healing, prevent ulcer recurrence, and prevent complications.

Baseline Data

Diagnosis requires radiographic or endoscopic visualization of the ulcer and testing for *H. pylori* infection.

Identifying High-Risk Patients

Use H₂RAs with *caution* in patients with renal or hepatic dysfunction.

Implementation: Administration

Routes

Cimetidine and Ranitidine. Oral, IM, and IV.
Famotidine. Oral and IV.
Nizatidine. Oral only.

Administration

Oral. Inform patients that H₂RAs may be taken without regard to meals.

Dosing may be done once daily at bedtime, twice daily, or 4 times a day. Make sure the patient knows which dosing schedule has been prescribed.

Intramuscular. *Cimetidine and ranitidine:* Use concentrated solutions for IM injections.

Intravenous. *Cimetidine, famotidine, and ranitidine:* For IV injection, dilute in a small volume (e.g., 20 ml) and inject slowly (over 5 or more minutes). For IV infusion, dilute in a large volume (100 ml) and infuse over 15 to 20 minutes.

Implementation: Measures to Enhance Therapeutic Effects

Advise patients to avoid cigarettes and ulcerogenic over-the-counter drugs (aspirin and other NSAIDs). Advise patients to stop drinking alcohol if drinking exacerbates ulcer symptoms. Inform patients that five or six small meals per day may be preferable to three larger ones. Advise patients that reducing stress may accelerate ulcer healing.

Ongoing Evaluation and Interventions

Evaluating Therapeutic Effects

Ulcer Healing. Monitor for relief of pain. Radiologic or endoscopic examination of the ulcer site may also be employed. Monitor gastric pH; treatment should increase pH to 5 or above. Educate patients about signs of GI bleeding (e.g., black, tarry stools, "coffee-grounds" vomitus), and instruct them to notify the physician if these are observed.

*Patient education information is highlighted as blue text.

Helicobacter pylori. If *H. pylori* was present at the onset of treatment, it may be useful to determine if the infection was eradicated.

Minimizing Adverse Effects

Antiandrogenic Effects. *Cimetidine* can cause gynecomastia, reduced libido, and impotence. These effects reverse after drug withdrawal.

CNS Effects. *Cimetidine* can cause confusion, hallucinations, lethargy, somnolence, restlessness, and seizures. These responses are most likely in elderly patients who have renal or hepatic impairment. Inform patients about possible CNS effects and instruct them to notify the physician if these occur. CNS effects are less likely with ranitidine, famotidine, and nizatidine.

Minimizing Adverse Interactions

Interactions Secondary to Inhibition of Drug Metabolism. *Cimetidine* inhibits hepatic drug-metabolizing enzymes and can thereby increase levels of other drugs. Drugs of particular concern are *warfarin, phenytoin, theophylline,* and *lidocaine.* Dosages of these drugs may need to be reduced.

Ranitidine inhibits drug metabolism, but to a lesser degree than cimetidine. Famotidine and nizatidine do not inhibit drug metabolism.

Antacids. Antacids can decrease absorption of *cimetidine* and *ranitidine.* At least 1 hour should separate administration of antacids and these drugs.

ANTACIDS

Aluminum hydroxide
Calcium carbonate
Magnesium hydroxide
Sodium bicarbonate

Preadministration Assessment

Therapeutic Goal and Baseline Data

See nursing implications for H₂RAs above.

Identifying High-Risk Patients

Use all antacids with *caution* in patients with hypertension or heart failure. Use *magnesium-containing antacids* with *caution* in patients with renal insufficiency.

Implementation: Administration

Route

Oral.

Administration

Instruct patients to administer antacids 7 times a day: 1 and 3 hours after meals and at bedtime.

Instruct patients to take their medication on a regular schedule even after pain has subsided—because relief of pain does not necessarily indicate healing.

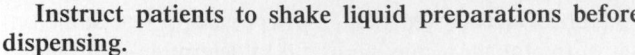

Summary of Major Nursing Implications*—cont'd

Instruct patients to shake liquid preparations before dispensing.

Instruct patients to chew antacid tablets thoroughly and to follow administration with a glass of water or milk.

Ongoing Evaluation and Interventions

Evaluating Therapeutic Effects

See nursing implications for H$_2$RAs above.

Minimizing Adverse Effects

Constipation and Diarrhea. To minimize disruption of bowel function, a constipating antacid (aluminum hydroxide, calcium carbonate) is combined with a laxative antacid (magnesium hydroxide). **Teach patients to adjust the dosage of the constipating agent and laxative agent as needed to normalize bowel function.**

*Patient education information is highlighted as blue text.

Sodium Loading. Sodium in antacids can exacerbate hypertension and heart failure. Patients with these disorders should use a low-sodium preparation.

Minimizing Adverse Interactions

Interactions Caused by Elevation of Gastric pH. By raising gastric pH, antacids can reduce the availability of other drugs, including cimetidine and ranitidine, and can decrease the antiulcer effects of sucralfate. To minimize these interactions, **instruct patients to allow 1 hour or more between antacid administration and administration of other drugs.**

Aluminum Hydroxide. This antacid can bind to a variety of drugs (e.g., tetracyclines, warfarin, digoxin), thereby decreasing their availability. Increased doses of these agents may be needed.

Laxatives

Laxatives are used to ease or stimulate defecation. These agents can soften the stool, increase stool volume, hasten fecal passage through the intestine, and facilitate evacuation from the rectum. When properly employed, laxatives are valuable medications. However, these agents are also subject to widespread abuse. Misuse of laxatives is largely the result of misconceptions about what constitutes normal bowel function.

Before we talk about laxatives, we need to distinguish between two terms: *laxative effect* and *catharsis*. The term *laxative effect* refers to production of a soft formed stool over a period of 1 or more days. In contrast, the term *catharsis* refers to a prompt, fluid evacuation of the bowel. Hence, a laxative effect is leisurely and relatively mild, whereas catharsis is fast and intense.

GENERAL CONSIDERATIONS

Function of the Colon

The principal function of the colon is to absorb water and electrolytes. Absorption of nutrients is minimal. Normally, about 1500 ml of fluid enters the colon each day, and approximately 90% gets absorbed. When colon function is healthy, the extent of fluid absorption is such that the resulting stool is soft (but formed) and capable of elimination without strain. However, when fluid absorption is excessive, as can happen when transport through the intestine is delayed, the resultant stool is dehydrated and hard. Conversely, if insufficient fluid is absorbed, watery stools result.

Frequency of bowel evacuation varies widely among individuals. For some people, bowel movements occur 2 or 3 times a day. For others, elimination may occur only 2 times a week. Because of this wide individual variation, we can't define a normal frequency for bowel movements. That is, although a daily bowel movement may be normal for many people, it may be abnormal for many others.

Dietary Fiber

Proper function of the bowel is highly dependent on dietary fiber—the component of vegetable matter that escapes digestion in the stomach and small intestine. Fiber facilitates colonic function in two ways: (1) it can absorb water, thereby softening the feces and increasing their mass; and (2) it can be digested by colonic bacteria, whose subsequent growth increases fecal mass. The best source of fiber is bran. Fiber can also be obtained from fruits and vegetables. Ingestion of 20 to 60 gm of fiber a day should optimize intestinal function.

Constipation

Constipation is determined primarily by stool *consistency* (degree of hardness); alterations in the *frequency* of bowel movements are of secondary importance. Hence, if the interval between bowel movements becomes prolonged, but the stool remains soft and hydrated, a diagnosis of constipation would be improper. Conversely, if bowel movements occur with regularity, but the feces are hard and dry, we would consider constipation to be present—despite the regular and frequent passage of stool.

The principal cause of constipation is poor diet—specifically, a diet deficient in fiber and fluid. Certain drugs (e.g., opioids, anticholinergics, some antacids) may also cause constipation.

In most cases, constipation can be readily corrected. Stools will become softer and more easily passed within days of increasing fiber and fluid in the diet. Mild exercise, especially after meals, also helps improve function of the bowel. If necessary, a laxative may be employed—but only briefly and only as an adjunct to diet and exercise.

Indications for Laxative Use

Laxatives can be highly beneficial when employed for valid indications. By softening the stool, laxatives can reduce the painful elimination that can be associated with episiotomy and with hemorrhoids and other anorectal lesions. In patients with cardiovascular diseases (e.g., aneurysm, myocardial infarction, disease of the cerebral or cardiac vasculature), softening of the stool decreases the amount of straining needed to defecate, thereby avoiding dangerous elevation of blood pressure. In geriatric patients, laxatives can help compensate for loss of tone in abdominal and perineal muscle. As an adjunct to anthelmintic therapy, laxatives can be used for (1) obtaining a fresh stool sample for diagnosis; (2) emptying the bowel prior to treatment (so as to increase parasitic exposure to anthelmintic medication); and (3) facilitating export of dead parasites following anthelmintic use. Additional applications include (1) emptying of the bowel prior to surgery and diagnostic procedures (e.g., radiologic examination, proctosigmoidoscopy);

TABLE 74–1 ■ Classification of Laxatives by Pharmacologic Category

Class and Agent	Site of Action	Mechanism of Action
Bulk-Forming Laxatives		
Methylcellulose	Small and large intestine	Absorb water, thereby softening and enlarging the fecal mass; fecal swelling promotes peristalsis
Psyllium		
Polycarbophil		
Surfactant Laxatives		
Docusate sodium	Small and large intestine	Surfactant action softens stool by facilitating penetration of water; also cause secretion of water and electrolytes into intestine
Docusate calcium		
Docusate potassium		
Stimulant Laxatives		
Bisacodyl	Colon	(1) Stimulate peristalsis and (2) soften feces by increasing secretion of water and electrolytes into the intestine and decreasing water and electrolyte absorption
Senna		
Castor oil	Small intestine	
Osmotic Laxatives		
Magnesium hydroxide	Small and large intestine	Osmotic action retains water and thereby softens the feces; fecal swelling promotes peristalsis
Magnesium sulfate		
Magnesium citrate		
Magnesium phosphate		
Polyethylene glycol		
Miscellaneous Laxatives		
Mineral oil	Colon	Lubricates and reduces water absorption
Glycerin suppository	Colon	Lubricates and causes reflex rectal contraction
Lactulose	Colon	Similar to osmotic laxatives
Polyethylene glycol–electrolyte solution	Small and large intestine	Similar to osmotic laxatives

(2) modification of the effluent from an ileostomy or colostomy; (3) prevention of fecal impaction in bedridden patients; (4) removal of ingested poisons; and (5) correction of constipation associated with pregnancy and certain drugs.

Contraindications to Laxative Use

Laxatives are contraindicated for individuals with certain disorders of the bowel. Specifically, laxatives must be avoided by individuals experiencing abdominal pain, nausea, cramps, or other symptoms of appendicitis, regional enteritis, diverticulitis, and ulcerative colitis. Laxatives are also contraindicated for patients with acute surgical abdomen. In addition, laxatives should not be used in the presence of fecal impaction or obstruction of the bowel; under these conditions, increased peristalsis may cause bowel perforation. Lastly, laxatives should not be employed habitually for the treatment of constipation. Reasons why are discussed below under *Laxative Abuse.*

Laxative Classification Schemes

Traditionally, laxatives have been classified according to general *mechanism of action.* This scheme has four major categories: (1) bulk-forming laxatives, (2) surfactant laxatives, (3) stimulant laxatives, and (4) osmotic laxatives. Drugs representing these classes are listed in Table 74–1.

From a clinical perspective, it can be helpful to classify laxatives according to *therapeutic effect* (time of onset and impact on stool consistency). When these properties are considered, most laxatives fall into one of three groups (labeled I,

II, and III in this chapter). Group I agents act rapidly (within 2 to 6 hours) to impart a watery consistency to the stool. Laxatives in group I are especially useful when preparing the bowel for diagnostic procedures or surgery. Group II agents have an intermediate latency (6 to 12 hours) and produce a stool that is semifluid. Group II agents are the ones most frequently abused by the general public. Group III laxatives act slowly (in 1 to 3 days) to produce a soft but formed stool. Uses for this group include treating constipation and preventing straining at stool. Representative members of groups I, II, and III are listed in Table 74–2.

BASIC PHARMACOLOGY OF LAXATIVES

Bulk-Forming Laxatives

The bulk-forming laxatives (e.g., methylcellulose, psyllium) have actions and effects much like those of dietary fiber. These agents consist of natural or semisynthetic polysaccharides and celluloses derived from grains and other plant material. With regard to clinical response, the bulk-forming agents belong to category III: These drugs produce a soft, formed stool 1 to 3 days after the onset of treatment.

Mechanism of Action. The effects of bulk-forming agents on bowel function are identical to those of dietary fiber. Following ingestion, these agents, which are nondigestible and nonabsorbable, swell in water to form a viscous solution or gel, thereby softening the fecal mass and increasing its bulk. Fecal volume may be further enlarged by growth

TABLE 74–2 ▪▪ Classification of Laxatives by Therapeutic Response

Group I: Produce Watery Stool in 2–6 Hr	Group II: Produce Semifluid Stool in 6–12 Hr	Group III: Produce Soft Stool in 1–3 Days
Osmotic laxatives (in high doses) 　Magnesium salts 　Sodium salts	Osmotic laxatives (in low doses) 　Magnesium salts 　Sodium salts 　Polyethylene glycol	Bulk-forming laxatives 　Methylcellulose 　Psyllium 　Polycarbophil
Castor oil	Stimulant laxatives (except castor oil)	Surfactant laxatives 　Docusalt salts
Polyethylene glycol–electrolyte 　solution	Bisacodyl, oral* 　Senna	Lactulose

*Bisacodyl suppositories act in 15 minutes.

of colonic bacteria, which can utilize these materials as nutrients. Transit through the intestine is hastened because swelling of the fecal mass stretches the intestinal wall, thereby stimulating peristalsis.

Indications. Bulk-forming laxatives are preferred agents for temporary treatment of constipation. Also, these drugs are widely used in patients with diverticulosis and irritable bowel syndrome. In addition, by altering fecal consistency, these agents can provide symptomatic relief of diarrhea and can reduce discomfort and inconvenience for patients with an ileostomy or colostomy.

Adverse Effects. Untoward effects are minimal. Because the bulk-forming agents are not absorbed, systemic reactions are rare. *Esophageal obstruction* can occur if these agents are swallowed in the absence of sufficient fluid. Accordingly, bulk-forming laxatives should be administered with a full glass of water or juice. If their passage through the intestine is arrested, the bulk-forming agents may produce *intestinal obstruction* or *impaction.* Accordingly, these agents should be avoided if there is narrowing of the intestinal lumen.

Preparations, Dosage, and Administration. *Psyllium* (prepared from *Plantago* seed), *methylcellulose,* and *polycarbophil* are the principal bulk-forming laxatives. All three preparations should be administered with a full glass of water or juice. Dosages for psyllium and methylcellulose are presented in Table 74–3.

Surfactant Laxatives

Actions. The surfactants (e.g., docusate sodium) are group III laxatives: These agents produce a soft stool several days after the onset of treatment. Surfactants alter stool consistency by lowering surface tension, which facilitates penetration of water into the feces. The surfactants may also act on the intestinal wall to (1) inhibit fluid absorption and (2) stimulate secretion of water and electrolytes into the intestinal lumen. In this respect, surfactants resemble the stimulant laxatives (see below).

Preparations, Dosage, and Administration. The surfactant family consists of two *docusate salts:* docusate sodium and docusate calcium. The dosage for docusate sodium [Colace, others], the prototype surfactant, is presented in Table 74–3. Administration of surfactants should be accompanied by a full glass of water.

Stimulant Laxatives

The stimulant laxatives (e.g., bisacodyl, castor oil) have two effects on the bowel. First, they stimulate intestinal motility—hence their name. Second, they increase the amount of water and electrolytes within the intestinal lumen. How? By increasing the secretion of water and ions into the intestine, and reducing water and electrolyte absorption. Most stimulant laxatives act on the colon, producing a semifluid stool within 6 to 12 hours.

Stimulant laxatives are widely used—and abused—by the general public, and are of concern for this reason. They have few legitimate applications. Properties of individual agents are discussed below.

Bisacodyl. Bisacodyl [Correctol, Dulcolax, Feen-a-mint, others] is unique among the stimulant laxatives in that it can be administered by rectal suppository as well as by mouth. *Oral* bisacodyl acts within 6 to 12 hours. Hence, tablets may be given at bedtime to produce a response the following morning. Bisacodyl *suppositories* act rapidly (in 15 to 60 minutes). Dosages for bisacodyl are presented in Table 74–3.

Bisacodyl tablets are enteric coated to prevent gastric irritation. Accordingly, patients should be advised to swallow them intact, without chewing or crushing. Because milk and antacids accelerate dissolution of the enteric coating, the tablets should be administered no sooner than 1 hour after ingesting these substances.

Bisacodyl suppositories may cause a burning sensation and, with continued use, proctitis may develop. Accordingly, long-term use should be discouraged.

Anthraquinones: Senna and Cascara Sagrada. Anthraquinone compounds are the active ingredients in *senna* and *cascara sagrada,* which are laxatives derived from plants. The actions and applications of these laxatives are similar to those of bisacodyl and phenolphthalein. The anthraquinones act on the colon to produce a soft or semifluid stool in 6 to 12 hours. Systemic absorption followed by renal secretion may be sufficient to impart a harmless yellowish-brown or pink color to the urine; patients should be forewarned of this effect. Dosages for senna are presented in Table 74–3. Because of concerns about carcinogenicity, products containing cascara sagrada have been removed from the market.

Castor Oil. Castor oil is the only stimulant laxative that acts on the *small intestine.* As a result, the drug acts quickly (in 2 to 6 hours) to produce a watery stool. Hence, unlike

TABLE 74–3 ▪■ Representative Laxatives: Trade Names, Dosage Forms, and Dosages

Class and Generic Name	Trade Names	Dosage Forms	Dosage and Administration
Bulk-Forming			
Methylcellulose	Citrucel	Powder	*Powder:* 1 heaping tbsp in 8 oz cold water 1–3 times a day
Psyllium	Metamucil, others	Granules, powder, effervescent powder, wafer	*Adults:* 1 rounded tsp (or 1 packet) mixed with water or other fluid, taken 1–3 times daily *Children over 6 yr:* 1/3 to 1/2 adult dose
Surfactant			
Docusate sodium	Colace, Ex-Lax, Modane Soft, Phillips' Liqui-Gels, others	Capsules, tablets, syrup, liquid	*Adults and children over 12 yr:* 50–500 mg/day *Children 6–12 yr:* 40–120 mg/day (All doses taken with a full glass of water)
Stimulant			
Bisacodyl	Correctol, Dulcolax, Feen-a-mint, others	Tablets, suppositories	*Adults:* 10–15 mg (tablets) or 10-mg suppository once daily *Children:* 5-mg tablet or 5-mg suppository once daily
Senna	Ex-Lax, Senokot, others	Tablets	*Adults:* 2 tablets once or twice a day *Children 6–12 yr:* 1 tablet once or twice a day
Osmotic			
Magnesium hydroxide (milk of magnesia)		Liquid	*Low dose:* 15–30 ml *High dose:* 30–60 ml
Polyethylene glycol	MiraLax	Powder	*Adults:* 17 gm (dissolved in 8 oz of water once a day)
Other			
Mineral oil		Liquid	*Adults:* 45 ml PO twice a day *Children:* 5–20 ml PO at bedtime

other stimulant laxatives, which are all group II agents, castor oil belongs to group I. Use of castor oil is limited to situations in which rapid and thorough evacuation of the bowel is desired (e.g., preparation for radiologic procedures). The drug is far too powerful for routine treatment of constipation. Because of its relatively prompt action, castor oil should not be administered at bedtime. The drug has an unpleasant taste that can be improved by chilling and mixing with fruit juice.

Phenolphthalein. Phenolphthalein is similar in structure and actions to bisacodyl. This agent acts on the colon to produce a semifluid stool in 6 to 8 hours. Because phenolphthalein undergoes enterohepatic recirculation, effects may persist for 3 to 4 days. The drug can impart a harmless pink tint to the urine; patients should be forewarned of this effect.

Recent data indicate that phenolphthalein can cause *cancer*. Mice given 30 to 100 times the daily human dose for 6 months to 2 years developed a variety of tumors. Genetic damage was also observed. Although there is no evidence that phenolphthalein causes cancer in humans, a Food and Drug Administration advisory panel has recommended banning the drug from over-the-counter (OTC) sales. In response to this recommendation, makers of brand-name laxatives that once contained phenolphthalein have replaced the drug with other stimulant agents. For example, Ex-Lax now contains senna, while Feen-a-mint and Correctol now contain bisacodyl.

Osmotic Laxatives
Laxative Salts

Actions and Uses. The laxative salts (e.g., magnesium hydroxide, sodium phosphate) are poorly absorbed salts whose osmotic action draws water into the intestinal lumen. Accumulation of water causes the fecal mass to soften and swell; swelling, in turn, stretches the intestinal wall and thereby stimulates peristalsis. When administered in low doses, the osmotic laxatives produce a soft or semifluid stool in 6 to 12 hours. In high doses, these agents act rapidly (in 2 to 6 hours) to cause a fluid evacuation of the bowel. High-dose therapy is employed to empty the bowel in preparation for diagnostic and surgical procedures. High doses are also employed to purge the bowel of ingested poisons, and to evacuate dead parasites following anthelmintic therapy.

Preparations. The osmotic laxatives include *magnesium salts* (magnesium hydroxide, magnesium citrate, and magnesium sulfate), *sodium salts* (sodium phosphate and sodium biphosphate), and *potassium salts* (potassium bitartrate and potassium phosphate). Dosages for magnesium hydroxide solution (also known as milk of magnesia) are presented in Table 74–3.

Adverse Effects. Osmotic laxatives can cause substantial loss of water. To avoid dehydration, treatment should be accompanied by augmented intake of fluids. Although the osmotic laxatives are poorly and slowly absorbed, some absorption does take place. In patients with renal dysfunction, magnesium and potassium can accumulate to toxic levels. Accordingly, osmotic laxatives that contain these elements are contraindicated in patients with kidney disease. Sodium absorption can cause fluid retention, which in turn can exacerbate heart failure, hypertension, and edema. Accordingly, sodium-containing laxatives are contraindicated for patients with these disorders.

Polyethylene Glycol

Polyethylene glycol [MiraLax] is an osmotic laxative indicated for occasional constipation. Like the laxative salts, this nonabsorbable compound retains water in the intestinal lumen, causing the fecal mass to soften and swell. The most common adverse effects are nausea, abdominal bloating, cramping, and flatulence. High doses may cause diarrhea. The recommended dosage is 17 gm, dissolved in 8 ounces of water, taken once a day. Bowel movement may not occur for another 2 to 4 days.

Miscellaneous Laxatives

Mineral Oil. Mineral oil is a mixture of indigestible and poorly absorbed hydrocarbons. Laxative action is produced by lubrication. Mineral oil is especially useful when administered by enema to treat fecal impaction.

Mineral oil can produce a variety of adverse effects. Aspiration of oil droplets can cause lipid pneumonia. Anal leakage can cause pruritus and soiling. Systemic absorption can produce deposition of mineral oil in the liver. Excessive dosing can decrease the absorption of fat-soluble vitamins.

Lactulose. Lactulose is a semisynthetic disaccharide composed of galactose and fructose. Lactulose is poorly absorbed and cannot be digested by intestinal enzymes. In the colon, resident bacteria metabolize lactulose to lactic, formic, and acetic acids. These acids exert a mild osmotic action, producing a soft, formed stool in 1 to 3 days. Although lactulose can relieve constipation, this agent is more expensive than therapeutically equivalent agents (bulk-forming laxatives) and also causes unpleasant side effects (flatulence and cramping are common). Accordingly, lactulose should be reserved for patients who do not respond adequately to bulk-forming laxatives.

In addition to its laxative action, lactulose can enhance intestinal excretion of ammonia. This property has been exploited to lower blood ammonia content in patients with portal hypertension and hepatic encephalopathy occurring secondary to chronic liver disease.

Glycerin Suppository. Glycerin is an osmotic agent that softens and lubricates inspissated feces. The drug may also stimulate rectal contraction. Evacuation occurs about 30 minutes after suppository insertion. Glycerin suppositories have been useful for re-establishing normal bowel function following termination of chronic laxative use.

Polyethylene Glycol–Electrolyte Solutions. These bowel-cleansing solutions [CoLyte, GoLYTELY, others] contain a mixture of polyethylene glycol (a nonabsorbable osmotic agent) together with potassium chloride, sodium chloride, sodium sulfate, and sodium bicarbonate. The mixture is isosmotic with body fluids, and its composition is such that water and electrolytes are neither absorbed from nor secreted into the intestinal lumen. Hence, water is not lost and electrolyte balance is preserved. As a result, polyethylene glycol–electrolyte solutions can be used safely in patients who are dehydrated and in those who are especially sensitive to alterations in electrolyte levels (e.g., patients with renal impairment or cardiovascular disease). These preparations are indicated primarily for cleansing the bowel prior to diagnostic procedures. The volume of administration is huge (about 4 L). Patients must ingest 250 to 300 ml every 10 minutes for 2 to 3 hours. Bowel movements commence about 1 hour after initiation of treatment.

LAXATIVE ABUSE

Causes. Many people believe that a daily and bountiful bowel movement is a requisite of good health, and that any deviation from this pattern merits correction. Such misconceptions are reinforced by aggressive marketing of OTC laxative preparations. Not infrequently, the combination of tradition supported by advertising has led to habitual self-prescribing of laxatives by people for whom these agents are not indicated.

Laxatives can help perpetuate their own use. Strong laxatives can purge the entire bowel. When such overemptying occurs, spontaneous evacuation will be impossible until bowel content has been replenished, which may take 2 to 5 days. During this time, the laxative user, having experienced no movement of the bowel, often becomes convinced that constipation has returned. In response, he or she takes yet another dose of laxative, thereby purging the bowel once more. In this manner, a vicious cycle of repeated laxative use and purging becomes established.

Consequences. Chronic exposure to laxatives can diminish defecatory reflexes, leading to further reliance on laxatives. Laxative abuse may also cause more serious pathologic changes, including electrolyte imbalance, dehydration, and colitis.

Treatment. The first step in breaking the laxative habit is abrupt cessation of laxative use. Following drug withdrawal, bowel movements will be absent for several days; the patient should be informed of this fact. Any misconceptions that the patient has regarding bowel function should be corrected: The patient should be taught that a once-daily bowel movement may not be normal for him or her and that stool *quality* is more important than frequency or quantity. Instruction on bowel training (heeding the defecatory reflex, establishing a consistent time for bowel movements) should be provided. Increased consumption of fiber (bran, fruits, vegetables) should be stressed. The patient should be encouraged to exercise daily, especially after meals. Finally, the patient should be advised that, if a laxative must be used, it should be used only briefly and in the smallest effective dosage. Agents that produce catharsis must be avoided.

⠿ KEY POINTS

■ Laxatives are given to promote defecation.
■ Constipation is determined primarily by stool consistency, not by frequency or volume of bowel movements.
■ Legitimate indications for laxatives include cardiovascular disorders, episiotomy, hemorrhoids, emptying the bowel before surgery and diagnostic procedures, ileostomy or colostomy, prevention of fecal impaction in bedridden patients, and constipation associated with pregnancy.
■ Like dietary fiber, bulk-forming laxatives swell in water to form a viscous solution or gel, thereby softening the feces and increasing fecal mass. Increased mass stretches the bowel wall, thereby promoting peristalsis.

■ Administer bulk-forming laxatives with fluid to avoid esophageal obstruction.
■ Patients receiving osmotic laxatives must increase fluid intake to avoid dehydration.
■ Because of their relatively rapid onset, group I laxatives (castor oil, high-dose osmotic agents) should not be given at bedtime.
■ Laxatives—especially the stimulant type—are commonly misused (abused) by the public. To reduce abuse, educate clients about normal bowel function and about alternatives to laxatives (diet high in fiber and fluids, exercise, establishing regular bowel habits).

Summary of Major Nursing Implications*

LAXATIVES

Implications That Apply to All Laxatives

Identifying High-Risk Patients

Laxatives are *contraindicated* for individuals with abdominal pain, nausea, cramps, and other symptoms of appendicitis, regional enteritis, diverticulitis, and ulcerative colitis. Laxatives are also *contraindicated* for patients with acute surgical abdomen, fecal impaction, and obstruction of the bowel.

Reducing Laxative Abuse

Patient education is a key factor in reducing laxative abuse. Educate the patient about normal bowel function (to correct misconceptions), and provide instruction on establishing good bowel habits (heeding the defecatory reflex, establishing a consistent time for bowel movements). Advise the patient to exercise (especially after meals) and to increase consumption of fiber (bran, fruits, vegetables). Inform the patient that laxatives should be used only when clearly necessary and then only briefly in the lowest effective dosage. Warn the patient against using cathartics.

Implications That Apply to Specific Laxatives

Bulk-Forming Laxatives: Psyllium, Methylcellulose, and Polycarbophil

Instruct the patient to take bulk-forming agents with a full glass of water or juice to prevent esophageal obstruction.

Bulk-forming laxatives are contraindicated for individuals with narrowing of the intestinal lumen, a condition that increases the risk of intestinal obstruction and impaction.

Surfactants: Docusate Salts

Instruct the patient to take surfactant agents with a full glass of water.

Stimulant Laxatives

Stimulant agents are the laxatives most commonly abused by the general public. Discourage the patient from inappropriate use of these drugs.

Bisacodyl. Administered PO and by rectal suppository. Instruct the patient to take oral bisacodyl no sooner than 1 hour after ingestion of milk or antacids. Instruct the patient to swallow tablets intact, without crushing or chewing.

Suppositories may cause a burning sensation; forewarn the patient. Warn the patient that prolonged use of bisacodyl suppositories can cause proctitis.

Senna. Forewarn the patient that senna can impart a harmless yellowish-brown or pink color to the urine.

Castor Oil. Castor oil acts rapidly (in 2 to 6 hours); do not administer at bedtime. Advise the patient not to take castor oil late at night. Warn the patient that castor oil is a powerful laxative and should not be used to treat routine constipation. Administer in chilled fruit juice to improve palatability.

Osmotic Laxatives: Magnesium Salts, Sodium Salts, and Potassium Salts

Effects are dose dependent. Low doses produce a soft or semifluid stool in 6 to 12 hours. Higher doses cause watery evacuation of the bowel in 2 to 6 hours.

To prevent dehydration, increase fluid intake during treatment.

Magnesium salts and *potassium salts* are contraindicated for patients with *renal dysfunction*.

Sodium salts are contraindicated for patients with *heart failure, hypertension,* or *edema*.

*Patient education information is highlighted as blue text.

Other Gastrointestinal Drugs

In this chapter we discuss an assortment of GI drugs whose indications range from emesis to colitis to gallstones. Four groups are emphasized: (1) antiemetics, (2) antidiarrheals, (3) drugs for irritable bowel syndrome, and (4) drugs for inflammatory bowel disease.

ANTIEMETICS

Antiemetics are given to suppress vomiting. We begin the discussion by reviewing the emetic response. Next we discuss the major antiemetic classes. And then we finish by considering the most important application of these drugs: management of chemotherapy-induced emesis.

The Emetic Response

Emesis is a complex reflex brought about by activation of the vomiting center, a nucleus of neurons located in the medulla oblongata. Some stimuli activate the vomiting center directly; others act indirectly (Fig. 75–1). Direct-acting stimuli include signals from the cerebral cortex (anticipation or fear), signals from sensory organs (upsetting sights, noxious odors, or pain), and signals from the vestibular apparatus of the inner ear. Indirect-acting stimuli first activate the chemoreceptor trigger zone (CTZ), which in turn activates the vomiting center. Activation of the CTZ occurs in two ways: (1) by signals from the stomach and small intestine (traveling along vagal afferents);

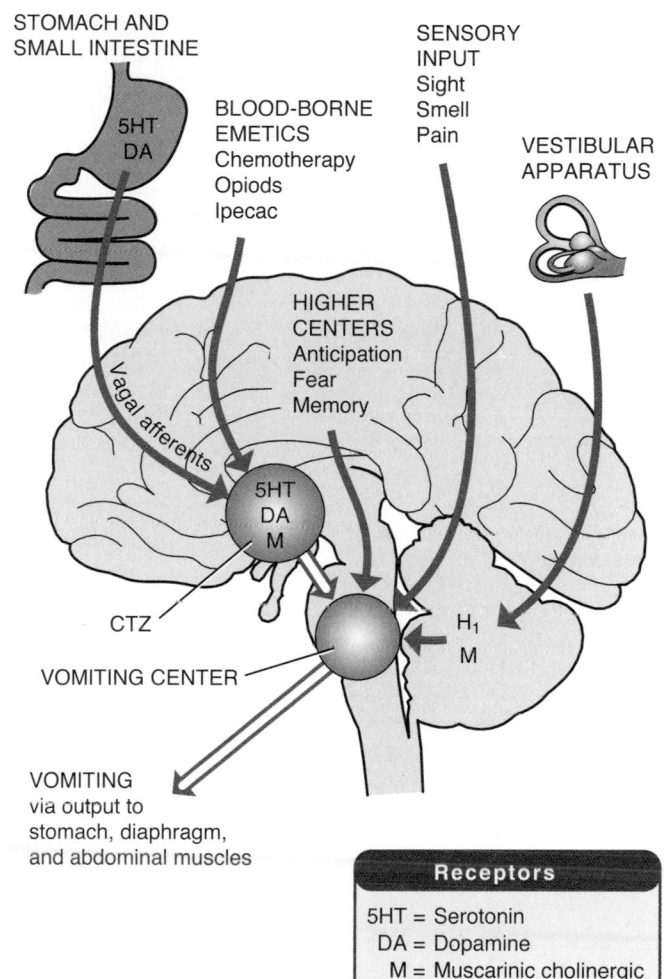

Figure 75–1 ■ The emetic response: stimuli, pathways, and receptors. CTZ = chemoreceptor trigger zone.

and (2) by the direct action of emetogenic compounds (e.g., anticancer drugs, opioids, ipecac) that are carried to the CTZ in the blood. Once activated, the vomiting center signals the stomach, diaphragm, and abdominal muscles; the resulting coordinated response expels gastric contents.

Several types of receptors are involved in the vomiting response. Important among these are receptors for serotonin, dopamine, acetylcholine, and histamine (see Fig. 75–1). Many antiemetics, including ondansetron [Zofran], prochlorperazine [Compazine], and dimenhydrinate [Dramamine], act by blocking one or more of these receptors.

Antiemetic Drugs

Several types of antiemetics are available. Their classes, trade names, and dosages are summarized in Table 75–1. Uses and mechanisms are summarized in Table 75–2. Properties of the principal classes are discussed below.

Serotonin Receptor Antagonists

The serotonin receptor antagonists are the most effective drugs available for suppressing nausea and vomiting caused by cisplatin and other highly emetogenic anticancer drugs. These agents are also used to suppress nausea and vomiting

TABLE 75–1 ■ Antiemetics

Class and Generic Name	Trade Name	Adult Dosage
Serotonin Antagonists		
Ondansetron	Zofran	See Table 75–3
Granisetron	Kytril	See Table 75–3
Dolasetron	Anzemet	See text
Dopamine Antagonists		
Phenothiazines		
Chlorpromazine	Thorazine	10–25 mg (PO, IM, IV) q 4–6 h PRN
Perphenazine	Trilafon	8–30 mg/day in divided doses (PO, IM, IV)
Prochlorperazine	Compazine	5–10 mg (PO, IM, IV) 3–4 times a day PRN
Promethazine	Phenergan	12.5–25 mg (PO, IM, IV) q 4–6 h
Thiethylperazine	Torecan	10 mg (PO) 3 times a day
Butyrophenones		
Haloperidol	Haldol	1–5 mg (PO, IM, IV) q 12 h PRN
Droperidol	Inapsine	2.5–5 mg (IM, IV) q 4–6 h PRN
Others		
Metoclopramide*	Reglan	See Table 75–3
Domperidone	Motilium	15 mg (IV), then 7.5 mg q 2 h × 7
Anticholinergics		
Antihistamines		
Buclizine	Bucladin-S	50 mg (PO) q 4–6 h
Cyclizine	Marezine	50 mg (PO, IM) q 4–6 h PRN
Dimenhydrinate	Dramamine	50–100 mg (PO, IM, IV) q 4–6 h PRN
Diphenhydramine	Benadryl	10–50 mg (PO, IM, IV) q 4–6 h PRN
Hydroxyzine	Vistaril, Atarax	25–100 mg (PO, IM) q 6 h PRN
Meclizine	Bonine, Antivert	25–50 mg (PO) q 24 h PRN
Others		
Scopolamine	Transderm Scōp	0.5 mg (transdermal) q 72 h PRN
Glucocorticoids		
Dexamethasone	Decadron	10–20 mg (IV) before chemotherapy, then 4–8 mg
Methylprednisolone	Solu-Medrol	2 doses of 125–500 mg (IV) 6 hr apart before chemotherapy
Cannabinoids		
Dronabinol	Marinol	5–7.5 mg/m^2 (PO) q 24 h PRN
Nabilone	Cesamet	1–2 mg (PO) 3–4 times a day PRN
Benzodiazepines		
Lorazepam	Ativan	1.0–1.5 mg (IV) before chemotherapy
Diazepam	Valium	2–5 mg (PO) q 3 h
Miscellaneous		
Diphenidol	Vontrol	25–50 mg (PO) q 4 h PRN
Benzquinamide	Emete-Con	25–50 mg (IM, IV) q 3–4 h PRN
Phosphorated carbohydrate solution	Emetrol	15–30 ml (PO) q 1–3 h PRN

*Also blocks serotonin receptors.

associated with radiation therapy and anesthesia. At this time, three serotonin antagonists are in use: ondansetron, granisetron, and dolasetron.

Ondansetron. Ondansetron [Zofran] was the first serotonin receptor antagonist approved for suppressing chemotherapy-induced emesis. The drug acts by blocking type 3 serotonin receptors (5-HT$_3$ receptors*) located in the CTZ and on afferent vagal neurons in the upper GI tract. Ondansetron, which is very effective by itself, is even more effective when combined with dexamethasone. The drug's most common side effects are headache, diarrhea, and dizziness. Since ondansetron does not block dopamine receptors, it does not cause the extrapyramidal effects (e.g., akathisia, acute dystonia) seen with antiemetic phenothiazines. As discussed in Chapter 37, ondansetron is being used investigationally to facilitate abstinence in people with early-onset alcoholism.

Administration is intravenous or oral. The initial IV dose is 0.15 mg/kg infused slowly (over 15 minutes) beginning 30 minutes before chemotherapy; this dose is repeated 4 and 8 hours later. Alternatively, ondansetron can be given as a single 32-mg IV dose. The usual oral dosage is 8 mg 3 times a day.

Granisetron. Like ondansetron, granisetron [Kytril] suppresses emesis by blocking 5-HT$_3$ receptors on afferent vagal neurons and in the CTZ. The drug is approved for suppressing nausea and vomiting associated with cancer chemotherapy, radiation therapy, and surgery. Principal adverse effects are headache (responsive to acetaminophen), weakness, tiredness, and either diarrhea or constipation. Administration is oral or IV. The recommended dosage for chemotherapy patients is 10 μg/kg IV infused over 5 minutes, starting 30 minutes before chemotherapy. The dosage for patients undergoing radiation therapy is 2 mg (tablets or oral solution) once daily given within 1 hour of radiation treatment. The dosage for prevention of postoperative nausea and vomiting is 1 mg IV injected slowly (over 30 seconds) either prior to induction of anesthesia or just before reversing anesthesia.

Dolasetron. Dolasetron [Anzemet] is approved for suppressing nausea and vomiting caused by emetogenic chemotherapy. Administration is oral or IV. The usual IV dosage for adults and children is 1.8 mg/kg administered 30 minutes before chemotherapy.

Dolasetron has been used on an investigational basis to suppress nausea and vomiting associated with radiation therapy and anesthesia. The IV dosage for adults undergoing radiation therapy is 40 mg or 0.3 mg/kg. The IV dosage for prevention of postoperative nausea and vomiting in adults is 12.5 mg administered 15 minutes before termination of anesthesia.

Dopamine Antagonists

Phenothiazines. The phenothiazines (e.g., prochlorperazine) suppress emesis by blocking dopamine$_2$ receptors in the CTZ. These drugs can reduce emesis associated with surgery, cancer chemotherapy, and toxins. Side effects include extrapyramidal reactions, anticholinergic effects, hypotension, and sedation. The basic pharmacology of the phenothiazines is discussed in Chapter 30 (Antipsychotic Agents and Their Use in Schizophrenia).

Butyrophenones. Two butyrophenones—*haloperidol* [Haldol] and *droperidol* [Inapsine]—are used as antiemetics. Like the phenothiazines, the butyrophenones suppress emesis by blocking dopamine$_2$ receptors in the CTZ. The butyrophenones are useful for postoperative nausea and vomiting, and for emesis caused by cancer chemotherapy, radiation therapy, and toxins. Potential side effects are similar to those of the phenothiazines: extrapyramidal reactions, sedation, and hypotension. In addition, droperidol may pose a risk of fatal dysrhythmias owing to prolongation of the QT interval. Accordingly, patients receiving the drug should undergo electrocardiographic monitoring. The pharmacology of the butyrophenones is discussed in Chapter 30.

Metoclopramide. Metoclopramide [Reglan] suppresses emesis through blockade of dopamine receptors in the CTZ. The drug can suppress postoperative nausea and vomiting as well as emesis caused by anticancer drugs, opioids, toxins, and radiation therapy. The pharmacology of metoclopramide is discussed below under *Prokinetic Agents*.

Glucocorticoids

Two glucocorticoids—*methylprednisolone* [Solu-Medrol, others] and *dexamethasone* [Decadron, others]—are commonly used to suppress emesis caused by cancer chemotherapy (even though they are not approved by the Food and Drug Adminis-

*Serotonin is also known as 5-hydroxytryptamine, 5-HT. Hence, the abbreviation 5-HT$_3$ for type 3 serotonin receptors.

TABLE 75–2 ■ Antiemetics: Uses and Mechanism of Action

Class	Prototype	Antiemetic Use	Mechanism of Antiemetic Action
Serotonin antagonists	Ondansetron [Zofran]	Chemotherapy, radiation, postoperative	Blocks serotonin receptors on vagal afferents and in the CTZ
Dopamine antagonists	Prochlorperazine [Compazine]	Chemotherapy, postoperative, general	Blocks dopamine receptors in the CTZ
Glucocorticoids	Dexamethasone [Decadron]	Chemotherapy	Unknown
Cannabinoids	Dronabinol [Marinol]	Chemotherapy	Unknown
Anticholinergics	Scopolamine [Transderm Scōp]	Motion sickness	Blocks muscarinic receptors in the pathway from the inner ear to the vomiting center
Antihistamines	Dimenhydrinate [Dramamine]	Motion sickness	Blocks H$_1$ receptors and muscarinic receptors in the pathway from the inner ear to the vomiting center

tration [FDA] for this application). These drugs are effective alone and in combination with other antiemetics. The mechanism by which glucocorticoids suppress emesis is unknown. Both dexamethasone and methylprednisolone are administered IV. Because antiemetic use is intermittent and short term, serious side effects are absent. The pharmacology of the glucocorticoids is discussed in Chapter 68.

Dronabinol: A Cannabinoid

Dronabinol [Marinol], also known as delta-9-tetrahydrocannabinol or THC, belongs to the cannabinoid family of drugs. At this time, dronabinol is the only cannabinoid available for medical use. A second cannabinoid—*nabilone* [Cesamet]—has been withdrawn from the market. Dronabinol is the principal psychoactive agent in marijuana (*Cannabis sativa*). The basic pharmacology of the cannabinoids is discussed in Chapter 38.

Therapeutic Uses. Dronabinol is approved for suppressing nausea and vomiting associated with cancer chemotherapy. The mechanism underlying benefits is unknown. Dronabinol is also approved for stimulating appetite in patients with AIDS. The goal is to reduce AIDS-induced anorexia and prevent or reverse weight loss.

Adverse Effects. In theory, dronabinol can produce subjective effects identical to those elicited by smoking marijuana. Potential unpleasant effects include temporal disintegration, dissociation, depersonalization, and dysphoria. Because of these effects, dronabinol is contraindicated for patients with psychiatric disorders. In addition to its subjective effects, dronabinol can cause tachycardia and hypotension, and therefore must be used with caution in patients with cardiovascular diseases.

Abuse Potential. Because it can mimic the subjective effects of marijuana, dronabinol has some potential for abuse. When first approved for medical use, the drug was classified under Schedule II of the Controlled Substances Act—a classification reserved for drugs with a high abuse potential. However, in 1998, the manufacturer petitioned the Drug Enforcement Agency (DEA) to reclassify dronabinol under Schedule III. Two arguments for the reduced classification were offered: (1) because of its slow onset, dronabinol does not produce the same "high" produced by smoking marijuana, and (2) there is little or no interest in dronabinol on the street. Apparently, the DEA agreed: Dronabinol is now classified under Schedule III.

Preparations, Dosage, and Administration. Dronabinol [Marinol] is dispensed in capsules (2.5, 5, and 10 mg) for oral use. To *prevent emesis,* the dosage is 5 to 7.5 mg/m² every 2 hours as needed. To *stimulate appetite* in patients with AIDS, the recommended initial dosage is 2.5 mg twice daily, before lunch and supper. If this dosage is intolerable, 2.5 mg once daily may be tried. The maximum recommended daily dosage is 20 mg in divided doses.

Benzodiazepines

Lorazepam [Ativan] is used in combination regimens to suppress nausea and vomiting caused by cancer chemotherapy. The drug has three principal benefits: sedation, suppression of anticipatory emesis, and production of anterograde amnesia. In addition, lorazepam may help control extrapyramidal reactions caused by phenothiazine antiemetics. The basic pharmacology of lorazepam and other benzodiazepines is discussed in Chapter 33.

Management of Chemotherapy-Induced Emesis

Many anticancer drugs cause severe nausea and vomiting. These reactions can be so intense that patients may discontinue chemotherapy rather than endure further discomfort. Fortunately, nausea and vomiting can be minimized with the antiemetics available today.

Chemotherapy is associated with three types of emesis: (1) anticipatory, (2) acute, and (3) delayed. *Anticipatory emesis* occurs before anticancer drugs are actually given; it is triggered by the memory of severe nausea and vomiting from a previous round of chemotherapy. *Acute emesis* happens shortly (1 to 2 hours) after receiving chemotherapy. In contrast, *delayed emesis* develops a day or more after drug administration.

Antiemetics are more effective at *preventing* emesis than at *suppressing* emesis that has already begun. For prevention, antiemetics are administered orally or parenterally. To suppress ongoing emesis, oral therapy won't work, and hence parenteral administration is required.

For patients taking highly emetogenic drugs, antiemetic combinations are more effective than single-drug therapy. A serotonin receptor antagonist (e.g., ondansetron) plus dexamethasone is the current treatment of choice. Lorazepam may be added to reduce anxiety and anticipatory emesis, and to provide amnesia. The superior efficacy of combination therapy suggests that anticancer drugs may induce emesis by multiple mechanisms. Three representative combination regimens are shown in Table 75–3.

DRUGS FOR MOTION SICKNESS

Motion sickness can be caused by sea, air, automobile, and space travel. Symptoms are nausea, vomiting, pallor, and cold sweats. The drugs used to treat motion sickness are most effective when given prophylactically, rather than after symptoms have begun.

Scopolamine

Scopolamine, a muscarinic antagonist, is the most effective drug for prophylaxis and treatment of motion sickness. Benefits derive from suppressing nerve traffic in the neuronal pathway that connects the vestibular apparatus of the inner ear to the vomiting center (see Fig. 75–1). The most common side effects are dry mouth, blurred vision, and drowsiness. More severe but less common effects are urinary retention, constipation, and disorientation.

Scopolamine is available for oral, subcutaneous, and transdermal administration. The transdermal system [Transderm-Scōp], an adhesive patch that contains scopolamine, is applied behind the ear. Anticholinergic side effects with transdermal administration may be less intense than with oral or subcutaneous administration.

Antihistamines

The antihistamines used most often for motion sickness are *dimenhydrinate* [Dramamine], *meclizine* [Antivert], and *cyclizine* [Marezine]. Because these drugs block receptors for acetylcholine in addition to receptors for histamine, they appear in Table 75–1 as a subclass under *Anticholinergics.* Sup-

TABLE 75–3 ■ Antiemetic Combinations for Patients Receiving Highly Emetogenic Anticancer Drugs

Regimen	Dosage
Combination 1	
Ondansetron	32 mg IV once *or* 0.15 mg/kg IV q 4 h for 3 doses
Dexamethasone	10–20 mg IV once
Lorazepam*	1.0–1.5 mg IV once, or more
Combination 2	
Granisetron	10 μg/kg IV once *or* 1 mg IV once
Dexamethasone	10–20 mg IV once
Lorazepam*	1.0–1.5 mg IV once, or more
Combination 3	
Metoclopramide	3 mg/kg IV q 2–4 h for 3 doses
Dexamethasone	10–20 mg IV once
Lorazepam	1.0–1.5 mg IV once, or more
Diphenhydramine	25–50 mg IV q 4–6 h

*Lorazepam is optional.

pression of motion sickness is thought to result from blockade of histaminergic (H_1) and cholinergic (muscarinic) receptors in the neuronal pathway that leads from the inner ear to the vomiting center (see Fig. 75–1). The most important side effect of the antihistamines is sedation. In addition, these drugs can cause typical anticholinergic effects, including dry mouth, blurred vision, and urinary retention. Unfortunately, sedation limits their utility. For treatment of motion sickness, the antihistamines are less effective than scopolamine.

ANTIDIARRHEAL AGENTS

Diarrhea is characterized by stools of excessive volume and fluidity, and by increased frequency of defecation. Diarrhea is a symptom of GI disease and not a disease per se. Causes include infection, maldigestion, inflammation, and functional disorders of the bowel (e.g., irritable bowel syndrome). The most serious complications of diarrhea are dehydration and depletion of electrolytes. Management is directed at the following: (1) diagnosis and treatment of the underlying disease, (2) replacement of lost water and salts, (3) relief of cramping, and (4) reducing the passage of unformed stools.

Antidiarrheal drugs fall into two major groups: (1) specific antidiarrheal drugs and (2) nonspecific antidiarrheal drugs. The specific agents are drugs that treat the underlying cause of diarrhea. Included in this group are anti-infective drugs and drugs used to correct malabsorption syndromes. Nonspecific antidiarrheals are agents that act on or within the bowel to provide symptomatic relief; these drugs do not influence the actual cause of diarrhea.

Nonspecific Antidiarrheal Agents
Opioids

Opioids are our most effective antidiarrheal agents. By activating opioid receptors in the GI tract, these drugs decrease intestinal motility, and thereby slow intestinal transit, which allows more time for absorption of fluid and electrolytes. In addition, activation of opioid receptors decreases secretion of fluid into the small intestine and increases absorption of fluid and salt. The net effect is to present the large intestine with less water. As a result, the fluidity and volume of stools are reduced, as is the frequency of defecation.

At the doses employed to relieve diarrhea, subjective effects and dependence do not occur. However, excessive doses can elicit typical morphine-like subjective effects. If severe overdose occurs, it should be treated with naloxone. In patients with inflammatory bowel disease, opioids may cause toxic megacolon.

Several opioid preparations—diphenoxylate, difenoxin, loperamide, paregoric, and opium tincture—are approved for diarrhea. Of these, diphenoxylate [Lomotil, others] and loperamide [Imodium, others] are the most frequently employed. Pharmacologic properties of these agents are discussed below. Dosages for diarrhea are summarized in Table 75–4.

Diphenoxylate. Diphenoxylate is an opioid whose only indication is diarrhea. The drug is insoluble in water, and hence cannot be abused by parenteral routes. When taken orally in antidiarrheal doses, diphenoxylate has no significant effect on the central nervous system. However, if taken in high doses, the drug can elicit typical morphine-like subjective responses.

Diphenoxylate is dispensed only in combination with atropine. The combination, whose most common trade name is *Lomotil,* is available in tablets and an oral liquid. Each tablet or 5 ml of liquid contains 2.5 mg of diphenoxylate and 25 μg of atropine sulfate. The atropine is present to discourage diphenoxylate abuse: Doses of the combination that are sufficiently high to produce euphoria from the diphenoxylate would produce unpleasant side effects from the correspondingly high dose of atropine. Accordingly, the combination has a very low potential for abuse and is classified under Schedule V of the Controlled Substances Act.

Loperamide. Loperamide [Imodium, others] is a structural analog of meperidine. The drug is employed to treat diarrhea and to reduce the volume of discharge from ileostomies. Benefits result from suppressing bowel motility and from suppressing fluid secretion into the intestinal lumen. The drug is poorly absorbed and does not readily cross the blood-

TABLE 75-4 ■ Opioids Used to Treat Diarrhea

Generic Name	Trade Name	CSA* Schedule	Antidiarrheal Dosage
Diphenoxylate (plus atropine)†	Lomotil, Lonox, Logen, Lomanate	V	*Adults:* 5 mg, 4 times/day *Children (initial dosage):* Age 2–5 years—1 mg, 4 times/day Age 5–8 years—1–2 mg, 4 times/day Age 8–12 years—1–2 mg, 4 times/day
Difenoxin (plus atropine)†	Motofen	IV	*Adults:* 2 mg initially, then 1 mg after each loose stool
Loperamide	Imodium, Kaopectate II Caplets, Pepto Diarrhea Control	NR‡	*Adults (initial dose):* 4 mg *Children (initial dosage):* Age 2–5 years—1 mg, 3 times/day Age 5–8 years—2 mg, 2 times/day Age 8–12 years—2 mg, 3 times/day
Paregoric (camphorated tincture of opium; contains 0.4 mg morphine/ml)		III	*Adults:* 5–10 ml, 1–4 times/day *Children:* 0.25–0.5 ml/kg, 1–4 times/day
Opium tincture (opioid content equivalent to 10 mg morphine/ml)		II	0.6 ml 4 times/day

*Controlled Substances Act
†Diphenoxylate and difenoxin are dispensed only in combination with atropine. The atropine dose is subtherapeutic and is present to discourage abuse.
‡Not regulated under the CSA.

brain barrier. Very large oral doses fail to elicit morphine-like subjective effects. Loperamide has little or no potential for abuse, and is not regulated under the Controlled Substances Act. The drug is dispensed in 2-mg capsules, 2-mg tablets, and in two liquid formulations (0.2 and 1 mg/ml).

Difenoxin. Difenoxin is the major active metabolite of diphenoxylate. Like diphenoxylate, difenoxin can elicit morphine-like subjective effects if taken in high doses. To discourage excessive dosing, difenoxin, like diphenoxylate, is dispensed only in combination with atropine. The trade name for the combination is *Motofen.* Because its abuse potential is somewhat greater than that of diphenoxylate plus atropine, Motofen is classified as a Schedule IV preparation.

Paregoric. Paregoric (camphorated tincture of opium) is a dilute solution of opium, containing morphine (0.4 mg/ml) as its main active ingredient. The primary indication for paregoric is diarrhea, although the preparation is also approved for the same indications as morphine. Antidiarrheal doses cause neither euphoria nor analgesia. Very high doses can cause typical morphine-like responses. Paregoric has a moderate potential for abuse and is classified as a Schedule III preparation.

Opium Tincture. Opium tincture is an alcohol-based solution that contains 10% opium by weight. The principal active ingredient—morphine—is present at 10 mg/ml. The primary indication for opium tincture is diarrhea. In addition, the preparation (after dilution) may be given to suppress symptoms of withdrawal in opioid-dependent neonates. When administered in antidiarrheal doses, opium tincture does not produce analgesia or euphoria. However, high doses can cause typical opioid agonist effects. Opium tincture has a high potential for abuse and is classified under Schedule II.

Other Nonspecific Antidiarrheals

Bulk-Forming Agents. Paradoxically, methylcellulose, polycarbophil, and other bulk-forming laxatives are useful in the management of diarrhea. Benefits derive from giving the stool a more firm, less watery consistency. Stool volume is not decreased. The bulk-forming laxatives are discussed in Chapter 74.

Anticholinergic Antispasmodics. Muscarinic antagonists (e.g., atropine) can relieve cramping associated with diarrhea, but do not alter fecal consistency or volume. Because of undesirable side effects (e.g., blurred vision, photophobia, dry mouth, urinary retention, tachycardia), anticholinergic drugs are of limited use. The pharmacology of the muscarinic blockers is discussed in Chapter 14.

Management of Infectious Diarrhea

General Considerations. Infectious diarrhea may be produced by enteric infection with a variety of bacteria and protozoa. These infections are usually self-limited. Mild diarrhea can be managed with nonspecific antidiarrheals. However, in many cases, no treatment is required at all. Antibiotics should be administered only when clearly indicated. Indiscriminate use of antibiotics is undesirable in that it can promote emergence of antibiotic-resistant organisms, and can produce an asymptomatic carrier state by killing most, but not all, of the infectious agents. Conditions that *do* merit antibiotic treatment include severe infections with *Salmonella, Shigella, Campylobacter,* or *Clostridium.*

Traveler's Diarrhea. Tourists are often plagued by infectious diarrhea. This condition is known variously as Montezuma's revenge, the Aztec two-step, or Rangoon runs. In most cases, the causative organism is *Escherichia coli.* As a rule, treatment is unnecessary: Infection with *E. coli* is self-limited and will run its course in a few days. However, if symptoms are especially severe, treatment with one of the fluoroquinolone antibiotics—*ciprofloxacin* (500 mg bid), *levofloxacin* (500 mg once daily), *ofloxacin* (300 mg bid), or *norfloxacin* (400 mg bid)—is indicated. *Azithromycin* [Zithromax] is preferred for children (10 mg/kg on day 1 and 5 mg/kg on days 2 and 3) and for pregnant women (1000 mg once or 500 mg once daily for 3 days). For milder symptoms, relief can be achieved with *loperamide,* a nonspecific antidiarrheal. However, by slowing peristalsis, loperamide may delay export of the offending organism, and may thereby prolong the infection.

Prophylaxis is possible with *ciprofloxacin, ofloxacin,* or *norfloxacin.* However, because these drugs can cause serious side effects, prophylaxis is not generally recommended. The risk of traveler's diarrhea can be greatly reduced by avoiding local drinking water and by carefully washing foods.

DRUGS FOR IRRITABLE BOWEL SYNDROME

Irritable bowel syndrome (IBS) is the most common disorder of the GI tract, affecting an estimated 20% of Americans—about 54 million people. The incidence in women is 3 times higher than in men. IBS is responsible for 12% of all visits to primary care physicians, and 28% of all visits to gastroenterologists. The direct medical costs are estimated at $8 billion a year; the indirect costs are much higher—about $25 billion a year. IBS is second only to the common cold as the leading cause of days missed from work.

What is IBS? A GI disorder characterized by crampy abdominal pain—sometimes severe—occurring in association with diarrhea, constipation, or both. Formally, IBS is defined by the presence, for at least 12 weeks in the past year, of abdominal pain or discomfort that cannot be explained by structural or chemical abnormalities and that has at least two of the following features:

- Pain is relieved by defecation.
- Onset of pain occurred in association with development of diarrhea or constipation.
- Onset of pain occurred in association with a change in stool consistency (to loose, watery, or pellet-like).

IBS has three major forms, characterized by either

- Abdominal pain in association with diarrhea (diarrhea-predominant IBS)
- Abdominal pain in association with constipation (constipation-predominant IBS)
- Abdominal pain in association with alternating episodes of diarrhea and constipation.

What causes IBS? No one knows. Despite extensive research, no underlying pathophysiologic mechanism has been identified. What we do know is that the bowel appears hypersensitive and hyper-responsive. As a result, mild stimuli that would have no effect on most people can trigger an intense response. In addition, we know that symptoms can be triggered by stress, depression, and dietary factors, including caffeine, alcohol, fried foods, fatty foods, gas-generating vegetables (beans, broccoli, cabbage), and too much sorbitol, a sweetener found in chewing gum and some diet products. Recent evidence suggests that excessive bacterial colonization of the small intestine may be involved. Overproduction of gastric acid has also been implicated.

Fortunately, many people achieve significant relief with treatment. Nondrug measures and drug therapy are employed. Patients should keep a log to identify foods and stressors that trigger symptoms. Because large meals stretch and stimulate the bowel, switching to smaller, more frequent meals may help. Increasing dietary fluid and fiber may reduce constipation.

Two groups of drugs are used for treatment: nonspecific drugs and drugs specific for IBS. Both groups are discussed below.

Nonspecific Drugs

Four groups of drugs—*antispasmodics* (e.g., hyoscyamine, dicyclomine), *bulk-forming agents* (e.g., psyllium, polycarbophil), *antidiarrheals* (e.g., loperamide), and *tricyclic antide-pressants* (TCAs)—have been employed for years to provide symptomatic relief of IBS. However, a recent report from the American College of Gastroenterology (ACG) concluded that, for most of these agents, there is no good proof of clinical benefits. Specifically, after reviewing available data, the authors concluded that loperamide and the bulk-forming agents are no better than placebo at relieving global symptoms of IBS. In contrast, they concluded there is good evidence that TCAs can reduce abdominal pain, and that this benefit is unrelated to relief of depression. Regarding antispasmodic agents, they concluded that the available evidence is insufficient to make a recommendation for or against their use.

Two recent studies suggest that, for some patients, symptoms of IBS can be relieved with *antibiotics* or with *acid suppressants*. In one study, the authors observed that many patients with IBS have excessive bacteria in the small intestine. When these people were treated with antibiotics, bacterial colonization was reduced, and so were symptoms of IBS. In the other study, researchers evaluated the impact of drugs that suppress production of stomach acid in patients who routinely experienced exacerbation of symptoms after eating. Two kinds of acid suppressants were used: proton pump inhibitors (lansoprazole or omeprazole) and histamine$_2$-receptor blockers (famotidine or ranitidine). In all cases, patients experienced a significant reduction of postprandial urgency and other symptoms. Benefits developed quickly (within days) and reversed when the drugs were stopped.

IBS-Specific Drugs

In this section we discuss two new drugs: alosetron and tegaserod. These are the only drugs approved by the FDA for IBS. The ACG report concluded that both drugs are beneficial.

Alosetron

Alosetron [Lotronex] is a potentially dangerous drug approved for diarrhea-predominant IBS in *women*. Safety and efficacy in men have not been demonstrated. Alosetron was first approved on February 9, 2000, and then, in response to reports of severe GI toxicity and several deaths, was withdrawn on November 28, 2000, less than 10 months after being introduced. However, on June 7, 2002, alosetron was *reapproved* by the FDA, marking the first time the agency has allowed a drug back on the market after it had been pulled for safety reasons. To reduce risk, physicians, patients, and pharmacists must adhere to a strict risk-management program (see below).

Indications. At this time, alosetron is approved only for treating women with severe, diarrhea-predominant IBS that has lasted for 6 months or more and has not responded to conventional treatment. Diarrhea-predominant IBS is considered severe if the patient experiences one or more of the following: (1) frequent and severe abdominal pain or discomfort, (2) frequent bowel urgency or fecal incontinence, and (3) disability or restriction of daily activities because of IBS. Less than 5% of IBS cases qualify as severe.

Mechanism of Action and Clinical Effects. Alosetron causes selective blockade of type 3 serotonin receptors (5-HT$_3$ receptors), which are found primarily on neurons that innervate the viscera. In patients with diarrhea-predominant IBS, alosetron can decrease abdominal pain, increase colonic transit time, reduce intestinal secretions, and increase absorption of water and sodium. As a result, the drug can increase stool firmness and decrease both fecal urgency and frequency. Presumably, all of these effects result from 5-HT$_3$ blockade. Symptoms decline 1 to 4 weeks after starting the drug, and recur 1 week after treatment stops.

Pharmacokinetics. Alosetron is administered orally, and absorption is rapid but incomplete (50% to 60%). Bioavailability is decreased by food. Plasma levels peak about 1 hour after ingestion. Alosetron undergoes extensive metabolism by hepatic cytochrome P450 enzymes, followed by excretion primarily in the urine. The half-life is 1.5 hours.

Drug Interactions. Alosetron has no known adverse interactions with other drugs. It does not interact with theophylline, oral contraceptives, cisapride, ibuprofen, alprazolam, amitriptyline, fluoxetine, or hydrocodone combined with acetaminophen. Because alosetron is metabolized by P450 enzymes, drugs that induce these enzymes (e.g., carbamazepine, phenobarbital) may decrease alosetron levels.

Adverse Effects and Contraindications. Although alosetron is generally well tolerated, it *can* cause severe adverse effects. Deaths have occurred. The most common problem is constipation (29%), which can be complicated by impaction, bowel obstruction, and perforation. In addition, alosetron can cause ischemic colitis (intestinal damage secondary to reduced blood flow). Ischemic colitis and complications of constipation have led to hospitalization, blood transfusion, surgery, and death. As of March 8, 2002, 84 cases of ischemic colitis had been reported, of which three were fatal. Because of its potential for GI toxicity, alosetron is *contraindicated* for patients with ongoing constipation or with history of

- Chronic constipation, severe constipation, or sequelae from constipation
- Intestinal obstruction or stricture, toxic megacolon, or GI perforation or adhesions
- Ischemic colitis, impaired intestinal circulation, thrombophlebitis, or hypercoagulable state
- Crohn's disease or ulcerative colitis
- Diverticulitis

Risk Management Program. To ensure the best possible benefit-to-risk ratio, the manufacturer and the FDA have established a risk management program that involves active participation of the patient, physician, and pharmacist. The program emphasizes that

- Alosetron can cause potentially fatal GI toxicity.
- Only physicians enrolled in the program can write prescriptions for the drug.
- Alosetron is indicated only for women with severe, chronic diarrhea-dependent IBS that has not responded to conventional therapy.
- Treatment should be discontinued immediately if constipation or signs of ischemic colitis develop.

Each enrolled physician must attest that he or she

- Is qualified to diagnose and treat IBS
- Is qualified to diagnose and manage ischemic colitis
- Is qualified to diagnose and manage constipation and complication of constipation
- Understands the risks and benefits of alosetron for diarrhea-predominant IBS

- Agrees to educate the patient about risks and benefits of alosetron, will confirm that each patient has signed a Patient-Physician Agreement, and will give each patient a copy of that agreement and a copy of an alosetron Medication Guide
- Will report serious adverse events to the manufacturer or the FDA
- Will place a qualification sticker on all prescriptions for alosetron (Pharmacists must not fill prescriptions that lack the sticker.)

Each patient must sign a Patient-Physician Agreement indicating that she

- Has been informed about and understands the severity of potential risks of alosetron treatment and understands the balance between risks and benefits
- Agrees to treatment with alosetron
- Will not take alosetron if she is constipated, and will immediately discontinue alosetron and contact the physician if she becomes constipated or develops signs of ischemic colitis
- Will stop taking alosetron and call the physician if the drug does not control IBS symptoms after 4 weeks

Preparations, Dosage, and Administration. Alosetron [Lotronex] is available in 1-mg tablets. Currently, the recommended initial dosage is 1 mg once a day—one-half the dosage recommended when alosetron was first approved. If, after 4 weeks, the dosage is well tolerated but inadequate, it can be increased to 1 mg twice a day. If, after 4 weeks at the higher dosage, treatment is still inadequate, the drug is not likely to help and hence should be stopped.

Patients who develop constipation or signs of ischemic colitis (rectal bleeding, bloody diarrhea, new or worsening abdominal pain) should immediately inform the physician and discontinue the drug. Those with ischemic colitis should never use alosetron again. Those with constipation may resume treatment, but only after constipation has resolved, and only on the advice of the physician. If constipation does not resolve, the physician should be seen for evaluation.

Tegaserod

Actions and Uses. Tegaserod [Zelnorm] is a serotonin analog approved for short-term therapy of constipation-predominant IBS in women. Long-term efficacy and safety have not been determined. At this time, the drug is not approved for use in men.

Tegaserod is a partial agonist at type 4 serotonin receptors (5-HT$_4$ receptors), which are found on neurons that innervate the viscera. By activating these receptors, the drug can decrease visceral sensation and increase GI motility and secretions. As a result, tegaserod can reduce bloating, constipation, and abdominal pain. Unfortunately, benefits are modest and may take a month to develop. Nonetheless, because treatment options for constipation-predominant IBS are limited, the drug is a welcome addition.

Pharmacokinetics. Tegaserod is rapidly absorbed but bioavailability is low (about 10% in the absence of food and only 5% in the presence of food). In the blood, the drug is highly bound to plasma proteins. Tegaserod undergoes metabolism to inactive products followed by excretion in the bile.

Adverse Effects and Drug Interactions. Tegaserod is generally well tolerated. In clinical trials, the most common adverse effect was *diarrhea* (9% vs. 4% in patients taking placebo). Most cases occurred during the first week of treatment and resolved despite continued drug use. Furthermore, most patients who experienced diarrhea had only one episode. Patients with ongoing diarrhea, and those who experience frequent diarrhea, should not take the drug. Tegaserod appears devoid of adverse interactions with other drugs.

Contraindications. Tegaserod is contraindicated for patients with severe renal impairment, moderate or severe hepatic impairment, a history of bowel obstruction, symptomatic gallbladder disease, abdominal adhesions, or sphincter of Oddi dysfunction.

Contrasts with Alosetron. Although tegaserod and alosetron are both used for IBS, the drugs differ with regard to mechanism of action, pharmacologic effects, indications, and adverse effects. Specifically:

- Whereas tegaserod is a partial *agonist* at *5-HT₄* receptors, alosetron is an *antagonist* at $5\text{-}HT_3$ receptors.
- Whereas tegaserod *increases* intestinal motility and secretions, alosetron *decreases* motility and secretions.
- Whereas tegaserod is used for *constipation*-predominant IBS, alosetron is used for *diarrhea*-predominant IBS.
- Whereas tegaserod can cause *diarrhea,* alosetron can cause *constipation* and *ischemic colitis.*
- Tegaserod is much safer than alosetron, and hence there are no restrictions on tegaserod use.

Preparations, Dosage, and Administration. Tegaserod [Zelnorm] is available in 2- and 6-mg tablets for oral administration. The recommended dosage is 6 mg twice daily (taken at least 30 minutes before meals) for 4 to 6 weeks. If there is a favorable response, treatment may continue for another 4 to 6 weeks.

DRUGS FOR INFLAMMATORY BOWEL DISEASE

Inflammatory bowel disease (IBD) has two forms: *Crohn's disease* and *ulcerative colitis.* Crohn's disease is characterized by transmural inflammation. The disease usually affects the terminal ileum, but can also affect any other part of the GI tract. Ulcerative colitis is characterized by inflammation of the mucosa and submucosa of the colon and rectum. Both diseases produce abdominal cramps and diarrhea. Ulcerative colitis may cause rectal bleeding as well. About 15% of patients with ulcerative colitis eventually have an attack severe enough to require hospitalization for IV glucocorticoid therapy, which produces remission in 60% of patients; the re-

maining 40% usually require total colectomy. In the United States, IBD afflicts about 1 million people. Drug therapy of IBD is summarized in Table 75–5.

Three classes of medications are employed: *aminosalicylates* (e.g., sulfasalazine), *glucocorticoids* (e.g., hydrocortisone), and *immunomodulators* (e.g., azathioprine). None is curative; at best, these drugs may control the disease process. Patients frequently require therapy with more than one agent.

Aminosalicylates

Aminosalicylates are used to treat mild or moderate ulcerative colitis and Crohn's disease, and to maintain remission after symptoms have subsided. Four aminosalicylates are available: sulfasalazine, mesalamine, olsalazine, and balsalazide.

Sulfasalazine. Sulfasalazine [Azulfidine] belongs to the same chemical family as the sulfonamide antibiotics. However, although similar to the sulfonamides, sulfasalazine is not employed to treat infections; rather, the drug is approved only for IBD. In addition, the drug has been used on an investigational basis to treat rheumatoid arthritis (see Chapter 69).

Actions. Sulfasalazine is metabolized by intestinal bacteria into two compounds: 5-aminosalicylic acid (5-ASA) and sulfapyridine. 5-ASA is the component responsible for reducing inflammation; sulfapyridine is responsible for adverse effects. Possible mechanisms by which 5-ASA reduces inflammation include suppression of prostaglandin synthesis and suppression of the migration of inflammatory cells into the affected region.

Therapeutic Uses. Sulfasalazine is most effective against acute episodes of mild to moderate ulcerative colitis. Responses are less satisfactory when symptoms are severe. Sulfasalazine can also benefit patients with Crohn's disease.

Adverse Effects. Nausea, fever, rash, and arthralgia are common. Hematologic disorders (e.g., agranulocytosis, hemolytic anemia, macrocytic anemia) may also occur. Accordingly, complete blood counts should be obtained periodically. Sulfasalazine appears safe for use during pregnancy and lactation.

TABLE 75–5 ■ Therapeutic Options for Inflammatory Bowel Disease			
	Disease Form		
Disease Intensity	**Ulcerative Colitis (Distal Only)**	**Ulcerative Colitis (Extensive)**	**Crohn's Disease**
Mild	Aminosalicylate: PO or rectal Glucocorticoid: rectal	Aminosalicylate: PO	Aminosalicylate: PO Metronidazole: PO Budesonide: PO Ciprofloxacin: PO
Moderate	Same as mild	Same as mild	Glucocorticoid: PO Azathioprine: PO Mercaptopurine: PO
Severe	Glucocorticoid: PO or rectal Glucocorticoid: IV	Glucocorticoid: PO or IV Cyclosporine: IV	Glucocorticoid: PO or IV Methotrexate: IV or SC Infliximab: IV
Refractory	Glucocorticoid: PO or IV Azathioprine: PO Mercaptopurine: PO	Glucocorticoid: PO or IV Azathioprine: PO Mercaptopurine: PO	Infliximab: IV
Remission	Aminosalicylate: PO or rectal Azathioprine: PO Mercaptopurine: PO	Aminosalicylate: PO Azathioprine: PO Mercaptopurine: PO	Mesalamine: PO Azathioprine: PO Mercaptopurine: PO Metronidazole: PO

Preparations, Dosage, and Administration. Sulfasalazine [Azulfidine] is available in 500-mg tablets (standard and delayed release) for oral administration. The initial adult dosage is 500 mg/day. Maintenance dosages range from 2 to 4 gm/day in divided doses.

Mesalamine. Mesalamine [Asacol, Pentasa, Rowasa] is the generic name for 5-ASA, the active component in sulfasalazine. The drug is used for acute treatment of mild to moderate IBD and for maintenance therapy. Mesalamine can be administered by retention enema, by rectal suppository, and by mouth (in tablets and capsules that dissolve when they reach the terminal ileum). Adverse effects are less than with sulfasalazine. The most common side effects of *oral* therapy are headache and GI upset. The adult dosage for oral mesalamine is 800 mg 3 times a day (for Asacol tablets) or 1 gm 4 times a day (for Pentasa capsules). The 500-mg rectal suppositories [Rowasa] are administered twice daily. The retention enema [Rowasa] is administered once daily (4 gm in 60 ml).

Olsalazine. Olsalazine [Dipentum] is a dimer composed of two molecules of 5-ASA, the active component of sulfasalazine. Olsalazine is approved for maintenance therapy of ulcerative colitis in patients unable to tolerate sulfasalazine. The drug's most common adverse effect is watery diarrhea, which occurs in 17% of patients. Other adverse effects include abdominal pain, cramps, acne, rash, and joint pain. Olsalazine is dispensed in 250-mg tablets for oral administration. The adult dosage is 500 mg twice daily with food.

Balsalazide. Balsalazide [Colazal] is an aminosalicylate indicated for mildly to moderately active ulcerative colitis. As with sulfasalazine, colonic bacteria act on balsalazide to release 5-ASA, the active portion of the molecule. Practically all of the drug remains in the intestine; less than 1% is absorbed. As a result, balsalazide is well tolerated. The most common adverse effects are headache (8%), abdominal pain (6%), and diarrhea and nausea (5%). Balsalazide is available in 750-mg capsules for oral administration. The recommended dosage is 3 capsules 3 times a day for 8 to 12 weeks. This dosage delivers 2.4 gm of free 5-ASA to the colon daily.

Glucocorticoids

The basic pharmacology of the glucocorticoids is presented in Chapters 57 and 68; discussion here is limited to their use in IBD. Glucocorticoids (e.g., dexamethasone, budesonide) can relieve symptoms of ulcerative colitis and Crohn's disease. Benefits derive from anti-inflammatory actions. Glucocorticoids are indicated primarily for induction of remission, and not for long-term maintenance. Administration may be oral, IV, or rectal. Prolonged use of glucocorticoids can cause severe adverse effects, including adrenal suppression, osteoporosis, increased susceptibility to infection, and a cushingoid syndrome.

Oral *budesonide* [Entocort EC] was recently approved for treating mild to moderate Crohn's disease that involves the ileum and ascending colon. Entocort EC capsules are formulated to release budesonide when it reaches the ileum and ascending colon. As a result, high local concentrations are produced. Systemic effects are lower than with other glucocorticoids because absorbed budesonide undergoes extensive first-pass metabolism.

Immunomodulators

Immunosuppressants—azathioprine, mercaptopurine, cyclosporine, methotrexate, and infliximab—are used for long-term therapy of selected patients with ulcerative colitis and Crohn's disease. Clinical experience is greatest with azathioprine and mercaptopurine.

Azathioprine and Mercaptopurine. These drugs are discussed together because one is the active form of the other. That is, azathioprine itself is inactive; once in the body, azathioprine is converted to mercaptopurine, a compound with pharmacologic activity.

Although not approved for IBD, azathioprine [Imuran] and mercaptopurine [Purinethol] have been employed with suc-

cess to induce and maintain remission in both ulcerative colitis and Crohn's disease. Because onset of effects may be delayed for up to 6 months, these agents cannot be used for acute monotherapy. Furthermore, because these drugs are more toxic than aminosalicylates or glucocorticoids, they are generally reserved for patients who have not responded to traditional therapy. Major adverse effects are pancreatitis and neutropenia (secondary to bone marrow suppression). At the doses used for IBD, these drugs are neither carcinogenic nor teratogenic. The basic pharmacology of azathioprine and mercaptopurine is discussed in Chapters 65 and 98, respectively.

Cyclosporine. Cyclosporine [Sandimmune, Neoral] is a stronger immunosuppressant than azathioprine or mercaptopurine, and acts faster too. When used for IBD, the drug is generally reserved for patients with acute, severe ulcerative colitis or Crohn's disease that has not responded to glucocorticoids. For these patients, continuous IV infusion can rapidly induce remission. In addition to IV administration, the drug has been administered orally in low doses to maintain remission, but results have been inconsistent. Cyclosporine is a toxic compound that can cause renal impairment, neurotoxicity, and generalized suppression of the immune system. The basic pharmacology of cyclosporine is discussed in Chapter 65.

Infliximab. Infliximab [Remicade] is a new and unique drug for Crohn's disease. This highly effective agent is a monoclonal antibody that binds with and thereby inactivates *tumor necrosis factor-alpha,* a key immunoinflammatory modulator. In clinical trials, infliximab reduced symptoms in 65% of patients with moderate to severe Crohn's disease and produced clinical remission in 33%. Effects of a single infusion may last a year.

During clinical trials, 5% of patients dropped out because of adverse effects. Infections (21%) and infusion reactions (16%) were most common. Infusion reactions seen most often were fever, chills, pruritus, urticaria, and cardiopulmonary reactions (chest pain, hypotension, hypertension, dyspnea).

Infliximab is dispensed as a powder to be reconstituted for IV infusion. For patients with moderate to severe Crohn's disease, treatment consists of a single 5-mg/kg infusion. Patients with fistulizing Crohn's disease get three infusions: an initial infusion of 5 mg/kg, followed by two more 5-mg/kg infusions 2 weeks and 6 weeks after the first one.

Methotrexate. In patients with Crohn's disease, methotrexate can promote short-term remission, and thereby reduce the need for glucocorticoids. Because the doses employed are low (25 mg once a week), the toxicity associated with high-dose therapy in cancer patients is avoided. The basic pharmacology of methotrexate is discussed in Chapter 98.

Other Drugs

Nicotine. There is observational and experimental evidence that nicotine can help protect against ulcerative colitis. It is well known that ulcerative colitis occurs mainly in *nonsmokers.* Furthermore, the disease frequently develops soon after smoking cessation, and resumption of smoking can help reduce symptoms. These observations in smokers have been reinforced by controlled experiments, which have shown that transdermal nicotine (nicotine patches) and a nicotine enema can reduce symptoms in patients with mild to moderate ulcerative colitis. However, until more information is available, nicotine cannot be recommended for routine treatment.

Metronidazole. In patients with mild or moderate Crohn's disease, metronidazole [Flagyl, Protostat] is as effective as sulfasalazine. The dosages employed—up to 750 mg 3 times a day—are high. Furthermore, because relapse is likely if metronidazole is discontinued, long-term therapy is required. Unfortunately prolonged use of high-dose metronidazole poses a risk of peripheral neuropathy. Although metronidazole can help patients with Crohn's disease, benefits are minimal in those with ulcerative colitis.

PROKINETIC AGENTS

Prokinetic drugs increase the tone and motility of the GI tract. Indications include gastroesophageal reflux disease, chemotherapy-induced nausea and vomiting, and diabetic gastroparesis. At this time, metoclopramide is the only prokinetic agent available in the United States. Another prokinetic agent—*cisapride* [Propulsid]—was withdrawn on July 14, 2000, owing to a significant risk of severe cardiac dysrhythmias (see the fourth edition of this text).

Metoclopramide

Actions. Metoclopramide [Reglan, others] has two beneficial actions: (1) it suppresses emesis (by blocking receptors for dopamine and serotonin in the CTZ); and (2) it increases upper GI motility (by enhancing the actions of acetylcholine).

Therapeutic Uses. Metoclopramide is a valuable drug for suppressing nausea and vomiting caused by highly emetogenic anticancer agents (e.g., cisplatin, dacarbazine). In addition, metoclopramide is given to suppress postoperative emesis as well as emesis caused by radiation therapy, toxins, and opioids. Other applications include relief of diabetic gastroparesis and suppression of gastroesophageal reflux.

Adverse Effects. With high-dose therapy, sedation and diarrhea are common. Like other dopamine antagonists, metoclopramide may cause extrapyramidal reactions, especially in children. These reactions can often be controlled with parenteral diphenhydramine (a drug with prominent anticholinergic actions). Because of its ability to increase gastric and intestinal motility, metoclopramide is contraindicated in patients with obstruction, hemorrhage, or perforation of the GI tract.

Preparations, Dosage, and Administration. Metoclopramide [Reglan, others] is available in four formulations: tablets (5 and 10 mg), syrup (1 mg/ml), concentrated oral solution (10 mg/ml), and solution for injection (5 mg/ml). Oral preparations are used for diabetic gastroparesis and gastroesophageal reflux.

For prophylaxis of chemotherapy-induced emesis, treatment is IV. Dosing is begun 30 minutes prior to chemotherapy. The initial dose is 1 to 2 mg/kg infused over 15 minutes or more. Additional doses of 1 to 2 mg/kg are administered 2, 4, 7, 10, and 13 hours after the first dose.

PANCREATIC ENZYMES

The pancreas produces four digestive enzymes: *lipase, amylase, chymotrypsin,* and *trypsin.* These enzymes are secreted into the duodenum, where they help digest fats, carbohydrates, and proteins. To protect these enzymes from stomach acid and pepsin, the pancreas secretes bicarbonate. The bicarbonate neutralizes acid in the duodenum, and the resulting elevation in pH inactivates pepsin.

Deficiency of pancreatic enzymes can compromise digestion, especially the digestion of fats. Fatty stools are characteristic of the deficiency. When availability of pancreatic enzymes is reduced, replacement therapy is needed. Causes of deficiency include pancreatectomy, cystic fibrosis, pancreatitis, and obstruction of the pancreatic duct.

Pancreatic enzymes are available as two basic preparations: *pancreatin* and *pancrelipase.* Pancreatin is made from hog or beef pancreas. Pancrelipase is made from hog pancreas. Pancrelipase has enzyme activity far greater than that of pancreatin. As a result, pancrelipase is the preferred preparation. Trade names for pancrelipase include *Viokase, Lipram, Pancrease MT,* and *Pancrecarb MS.*

Both pancreatin and pancrelipase are available in capsules that contain enteric-coated microspheres. The microsphere-containing preparations are preferred to conventional formulations (tablets, capsules) because the conventional formulations frequently fail to dissolve within the appropriate region of the intestine (i.e., the duodenum and upper jejunum).

Antacids and histamine₂-receptor blockers may be employed as adjuvants to pancreatic enzyme therapy. Their purpose is to reduce gastric pH, thereby protecting the enzymes from inactivation. However, these adjuvants are beneficial only when secretion of gastric acid is excessive.

Adverse reactions to pancreatic enzymes are rare. Allergic reactions occur occasionally. Large doses can cause diarrhea, nausea, and cramping.

Dosage is adjusted on an individual basis. Determining factors include the extent of enzyme deficiency, dietary fat content, and enzyme activity of the preparation selected. The efficacy of therapy can be evaluated by measuring the reduction in 24-hour fat excretion. Pancreatic enzymes should be taken with every meal and snack.

DRUGS USED TO DISSOLVE GALLSTONES

The gallbladder serves as a repository for bile, a fluid composed of cholesterol, bile acids, and other substances. Following its production in the liver, bile may be secreted directly into the small intestine or it may be transferred to the gallbladder, where it is concentrated and stored.

Bile has two principal functions: (1) it aids in the digestion of fats, and (2) it serves as the only medium by which cholesterol is excreted from the body. The acids present in bile facilitate the absorption of fats. In addition, bile acids help solubilize cholesterol.

Cholelithiasis—development of gallstones—is the most common form of gallbladder disease. Most stones are formed from cholesterol. Stones made of cholesterol alone cannot be detected with x-rays, and hence are said to be *radiolucent.* In contrast, stones that contain calcium (in addition to cholesterol) are *radiopaque* (i.e., they absorb x-rays and therefore can be seen in a radiograph). Risk factors for cholelithiasis include obesity and high blood levels of cholesterol.

For many people, gallstones can be present for years without causing symptoms. When symptoms do develop, they can be much like those of indigestion (bloating, abdominal discomfort, gassiness). If a stone should lodge in the bile duct, severe pain and jaundice may result.

Cholelithiasis may be treated by cholecystectomy (surgical removal of the gallbladder) or with drugs. As a rule, when intervention is required, cholecystectomy is the preferred modality. In asymptomatic patients, more conservative measures (weight loss and reduced fat intake) may be indicated. Medications employed to dissolve gallstones are discussed below.

Chenodiol (Chenodeoxycholic Acid)

Actions. Chenodiol [Chenix] is a naturally occurring bile acid that reduces hepatic production of cholesterol. Reduced cholesterol production lowers the cholesterol content of bile, which in turn facilitates the gradual dissolution of cholesterol gallstones. Chenodiol may also increase the amount of bile acid in bile, an effect that may enhance cholesterol solubility. It should be noted that chenodiol is useful only for dissolving radiolucent stones. Radiopaque stones (stones with significant calcium content) are not affected.

Therapeutic Use. Chenodiol is given to promote dissolution of cholesterol gallstones, but only in carefully selected patients. Success is most likely in women who have low cholesterol levels, stones of small size, and the ability to tolerate high doses of the drug. Complete disappearance of stones occurs in only 20% to 40% of patients. Therapy is usually prolonged; 2 years is common.

Adverse Effects. Diarrhea occurs in 30% to 40% of patients; dosage reduction will decrease this response. Of much greater concern, chenodiol can damage the liver. Hence, patients must have periodic tests of liver function. Because of its hepatotoxic effects, chenodiol is contraindicated for patients with pre-existing liver disease. Chenodiol is also contraindicated during pregnancy (FDA Pregnancy Risk Category X).

Ursodiol (Ursodeoxycholic Acid)

Ursodiol [Actigall] is an analog of chenodiol. Like chenodiol, ursodiol reduces the cholesterol content of bile, thereby facilitating the gradual dissolution of cholesterol gallstones. In contrast to chenodiol, ursodiol does not increase production of bile acids. Like chenodiol, ursodiol promotes dissolution of *radiolucent* gallstones but not radiopaque gallstones. Ursodiol is indicated for dissolution of cholesterol gallstones in carefully selected patients.

Ursodiol is well tolerated. Significant adverse effects are rare. The drug is classified in FDA Pregnancy Risk Category B.

Ursodiol is dispensed in 300-mg capsules for oral administration. The usual adult dosage is 4 to 5 mg/kg twice daily (1 capsule in the morning and 1 in the evening). Treatment lasts for months.

Monooctanoin

Monooctanoin [Moctanin] is a semisynthetic vegetable oil that can dissolve *cholesterol* gallstones; extended direct contact with the gallstones is required. The only use for monooctanoin is removal of stones that remain in the common bile duct following cholecystectomy. Administration is by continuous perfusion through a catheter placed directly in the common bile duct. Duration of perfusion is usually 2 to 10 days. Complete dissolution of stones occurs in approximately one-third of patients. Partial dissolution occurs in about 30% more. The most common side effects are GI disturbances (abdominal pain, nausea, vomiting).

ANORECTAL PREPARATIONS

Anorectal preparations can provide symptomatic relief from the discomfort of hemorrhoids and other anorectal disorders. The composition of these preparations varies widely. *Local anesthetics* (e.g., benzocaine, dibucaine) and *hydrocortisone* (a glucocorticoid) are common ingredients. Hydrocortisone suppresses inflammation, itching, and swelling. Local anesthetics reduce itching and pain. Anorectal preparations may also contain *emollients* (e.g., mineral oil, lanolin), whose lubricant properties reduce irritation, and *astringents* (e.g., bismuth subgallate, witch hazel, zinc oxide), which serve to reduce irritation and inflammation. Anorectal preparations are available in multiple formulations: suppositories, creams, ointments, foams, tissues, and pads.

⁙ KEY POINTS

- Emesis results from activation of the vomiting center, which receives its principal stimulatory input from the chemoreceptor trigger zone (CTZ), cerebral cortex, and inner ear.
- Serotonin antagonists, such as ondansetron [Zofran], are the most effective antiemetics available.
- To suppress chemotherapy-induced emesis, a combination of drugs is more effective than monotherapy. The current combination of choice is a serotonin antagonist (e.g., ondansetron) plus a glucocorticoid (e.g., dexamethasone), with or without lorazepam (a benzodiazepine).
- For management of chemotherapy-related emesis, antiemetics are more effective when given before chemotherapy (to prevent emesis) than when given after chemotherapy (in an effort to stop ongoing emesis).
- Opioids (e.g., diphenoxylate) are the most effective antidiarrheal agents available.
- Traveler's diarrhea can be treated with loperamide, a nonspecific antidiarrheal drug; with a fluoroquinolone antibiotic (e.g., ciprofloxacin); or with azithromycin (for children and pregnant women).
- Irritable bowel syndrome (IBS) is the most common disorder of the GI tract.
- Only two drugs—alosetron and tegaserod—are approved by the FDA for treating IBS.
- Alosetron is approved for treating diarrhea-predominant IBS in women. Benefits derive from blocking 5-HT₃ receptors on neurons that innervate the viscera.
- Alosetron can cause ischemic colitis and severe constipation. Colitis and complications of constipation have lead to hospitalization, blood transfusion, surgery, and death.
- Inflammatory bowel disease (ulcerative colitis, Crohn's disease) is treated with aminosalicylates (e.g., sulfasalazine, mesalamine), glucocorticoids (e.g., dexamethasone, budesonide), and immunomodulators (e.g., azathioprine, mercaptopurine, infliximab).
- Metoclopramide, a prokinetic agent, has two beneficial actions: it increases upper GI motility and suppresses emesis.

Vitamins

Vitamins have the following defining characteristics: (1) they are *organic compounds,* (2) they are required in *minute amounts* for growth and maintenance of health, and (3) they do not serve as sources of energy (in contrast to fats, carbohydrates, and proteins), but rather are *essential for energy transformation and regulation of metabolic processes.* Several vitamins are inactive in their native form and must be converted into active compounds in the body.

GENERAL CONSIDERATIONS

Dietary Reference Intakes

Reference values on vitamin intake are established by the *Food and Nutrition Board of the Institute of Medicine of the National Academy of Sciences.* The purpose is to provide a standard for good nutrition. In a 1998 report—*Dietary Reference Intakes for Thiamin, Riboflavin, Niacin, Vitamin B_6, Folate, Vitamin B_{12}, Pantothenic Acid, Biotin, and Choline*—the Food and Nutrition Board defined four reference values: *Recommended Dietary Allowance* (RDA), *Adequate Intake* (AI), *Tolerable Upper Intake Level* (UL), and *Estimated Average Requirement* (EAR). Collectively, these four values are referred to as *Dietary Reference Intakes* (DRIs).

Recommended Dietary Allowance. The RDA is the average daily dietary intake sufficient to meet the nutrient requirements of nearly all (97% to 98%) healthy individuals. RDAs are based on extensive experimental data. Because

RDAs represent *average* daily intakes, low intake on one day can be compensated for by high intake on another. RDAs change as we grow older. In addition, they often differ for males and females, and typically increase for women who become pregnant or breast-feed. You should appreciate that RDAs apply only to individuals in good health. Vitamin requirements can be increased by illness, and therefore published RDA values may not be appropriate for sick people. RDAs are revised periodically as new information becomes available. Table 76–1 summarizes when the most recent revisions were made.

Until recently, nutrition experts believed that, for most people, diet alone could be relied on to provide RDAs of all vitamins. Hence, dietary supplements were considered generally unnecessary. Now, however, expert opinion has changed. Nutrition experts now agree that, for two vitamins—folic acid and vitamin B_{12}—supplements are clearly required. Specifically, they recommend supplements of folic acid for all women of child-bearing age and supplements of vitamin B_{12} for all people over age 50. In addition, to prevent chronic illnesses caused by subclinical vitamin deficiency, supplements for all other vitamins may be appropriate too.

Adequate Intake. The AI is an *estimate* of the average daily intake required to meet nutritional needs. AIs are employed when experimental evidence is not strong enough to establish an RDA. AIs are set with the expectation that they will meet the needs of all individuals. However, because AIs are only estimates, there is no guarantee they will be adequate.

Tolerable Upper Intake Level. The UL is the highest average daily intake that can be consumed by nearly everyone without a significant risk of adverse effects. Please note that the UL is not a *recommended* upper limit for intake. It is simply an index of safety. There is no known benefit to exceeding the RDA.

Estimated Average Requirement. The EAR is the level of intake that will meet nutrition requirements for 50% of the healthy individuals in any life-stage or gender group. By definition, the EAR will be insufficient for the other 50%. The EAR for a vitamin is based on extensive experimental data, and serves as the basis for establishing an RDA. If there is not enough information to establish an EAR, no RDA can be set. Instead, an AI is assigned, using the limited data on hand.

Classification of Vitamins

The vitamins are divided into two major groups: *fat-soluble vitamins* and *water-soluble vitamins.* In the fat-soluble group are vitamins A, D, E, and K. The water-soluble group consists of vitamin C and members of the vitamin B complex (thiamin, riboflavin, niacin, pyridoxine, pantothenic acid, biotin, folic acid, and cyanocobalamin). As a rule, water-soluble vi-

TABLE 76–1 ▪■ Where to Find Food and Nutrition Board Updates for Specific Vitamins*

Vitamin	Publication	Date
Vitamin D	Dietary Reference Intakes for Calcium, Phosphorous, Magnesium, Vitamin D, and Fluoride	1997
Biotin, folate, niacin, pantothenic acid, riboflavin, thiamin, and vitamins B_6 and B_{12}	Dietary Reference Intakes for Thiamin, Riboflavin, Niacin, Vitamin B_6, Folate, Vitamin B_{12}, Pantothenic Acid, Biotin, and Choline	1998
Vitamins C and E	Dietary Reference Intakes for Vitamin C, Vitamin E, Selenium, and Carotenoids	2000
Vitamins A and K	Dietary Reference Intakes for Vitamin A, Vitamin K, Arsenic, Boron, Chromium, Copper, Iodine, Iron, Manganese, Molybdenum, Nickel, Silicon, Vanadium, and Zinc	2002

*All publications are from the Food and Nutrition Board, Institute of Medicine, and published by the National Academy Press, Washington, DC.

tamins undergo minimal storage in the body. Hence, frequent ingestion is needed to replenish supplies. In contrast, fat-soluble vitamins can be stored in massive amounts, which is good news and bad news. The good news is that extensive storage minimizes the risk of deficiency. The bad news is that extensive storage greatly increases the potential for toxicity if intake is excessive.

FAT-SOLUBLE VITAMINS
Vitamin A (Retinol)

Actions. Vitamin A, also known as retinol, has multiple functions. In the eyes, vitamin A plays an important role in adaptation to dim light. The vitamin also has a role in embryogenesis, spermatogenesis, immunity, growth, and maintaining the structural and functional integrity of the skin and mucous membranes.

Sources. Requirements for vitamin A can be met by (1) consuming foods that contain *preformed vitamin A* (retinol) and (2) consuming foods that contain *provitamin A carotenoids* (beta-carotene, alpha-carotene, beta-cryptoxanthin), which are converted to retinol by cells of the intestinal mucosa. Preformed vitamin A is present only in foods of animal origin. Good sources are dairy products, meat, fish oil, and fish. Provitamin A carotenoids are found in darkly colored, carotene-rich fruits and vegetables. Especially rich sources are carrots, cantaloupe, mangoes, spinach, tomatoes, pumpkins, and sweet potatoes.

Units. The unit employed to measure vitamin A activity is called the *retinol activity equivalent* (RAE). By definition, 1 RAE equals 1 μg of retinol, 12 μg of beta-carotene, 24 μg of alpha-carotene, or 24 μg of beta-cryptoxanthin. Why are the RAEs for the provitamin A carotenoids 12 to 24 times higher than the RAE for retinol? Because dietary carotenoids are poorly absorbed and incompletely converted into retinol. Hence, to produce the nutritional effect of retinol, we need to ingest much higher amounts of the carotenoids. In the past, vitamin A activity was measured in international units (IU). One IU is equal to 0.3 RAEs.

Requirements. RDAs for vitamin A were revised in 2002. The new RDAs are slightly lower than the old ones, which were established in 1989. The new RDA for adult males is 900 RAEs, and the RDA for adult females is 700 RAEs. RDAs for individuals in other life-stage groups are shown in Table 76–2.

Pharmacokinetics. Under normal conditions, dietary vitamin A is readily absorbed and then stored in the liver. As a rule, liver reserves of vitamin A are large and will last for months if intake of retinol ceases. Normal plasma levels for retinol range between 30 and 70 μg/dl. In the absence of vitamin A intake, levels are maintained through mobilization of liver reserves. As liver stores approach depletion, plasma levels begin to decline. Signs and symptoms of deficiency appear when plasma levels fall below 20 μg/dl.

Deficiency. Because vitamin A is needed for dark adaptation, night blindness is often the first indication of deficiency. With time, vitamin A deficiency may lead to *xerophthalmia* (a dry, thickened condition of the conjunctiva) and *keratomalacia* (degeneration of the cornea with keratinization of the corneal epithelium). When vitamin A deficiency is severe, blindness may occur. In addition to effects on the eye, deficiency can produce skin lesions and dysfunction of mucous membranes.

Toxicity. In high doses, vitamin A can cause birth defects, liver injury, and bone-related disorders. To reduce risk, the Food and Nutrition Board has set 3000 μg/day as the UL for vitamin A.

Vitamin A is highly *teratogenic.* Excessive intake during pregnancy can cause malformation of the heart, skull, and other structures of cranial–neural crest origin. Risk is highest among women taking vitamin A supplements. Pregnant women should definitely not exceed the UL for vitamin A, and should probably not exceed the RDA.

Excessive doses of vitamin A can cause a toxic state, referred to as *hypervitaminosis A.* Chronic intoxication affects multiple organ systems, especially the liver. Symptoms are diverse and may include vomiting, jaundice, hepatosplenomegaly, skin changes, hypomenorrhea, and elevation of intracranial pressure. Most symptoms disappear following vitamin A withdrawal.

Vitamin A excess can damage bone. In infants and young children, vitamin A can cause bulging of the skull at sites where bone has not yet formed. In adult females, too much vitamin A can increase the risk of hip fracture—apparently by blocking the ability of vitamin D to enhance calcium absorption.

Therapeutic Uses. The only indication for vitamin A is prevention or correction of vitamin A deficiency. Contrary to earlier hopes, it is now clear that vitamin A, in the form of beta-carotene supplements, does not decrease the risk of cancer or cardiovascular disease. In fact, in a study comparing placebo with dietary supplements (beta-carotene plus vitamin A), subjects taking the supplements had a significantly *increased* risk of lung cancer and overall mortality. As discussed in Chapter 101, certain derivatives of vitamin A (e.g., isotretinoin, etretinate) are used to treat acne and other dermatologic disorders.

Preparations, Dosage, and Administration. Vitamin A (retinol) is available in the form of drops, tablets, and capsules for oral administration and in solution for IM injection. Oral administration is generally preferred. To *prevent* deficiency, dietary plus medicinal vitamin A should add up to the RDA (see Table 76–2). To *treat* deficiency, doses up to 100 times the RDA may be required.

Vitamin D

Vitamin D plays a critical role in the regulation of calcium and phosphorus metabolism. In children, deficiency causes *rickets*. In adults, deficiency causes *osteomalacia*. Excessive amounts of vitamin D are toxic. Symptoms result primarily from hypercalcemia. The pharmacology and physiology of vitamin D are discussed at length in Chapter 70. Values for adequate intake are summarized in Table 76–2. At this time, RDAs are not available.

Vitamin E (Alpha-Tocopherol)

Vitamin E (alpha-tocopherol) is essential to the health of many animal species, but has no clearly established role in human nutrition. Unlike other vitamins, vitamin E has no known role in metabolism. Deficiency, which is rare, can result in neurologic deficits.

Vitamin E helps maintain health primarily through antioxidant actions. Specifically, the vitamin helps protect against peroxidation of lipids. A large body of evidence suggests that large doses of vitamin E may protect against chronic diseases. However, definitive proof of such protection is lacking (see Box 76–1).

Forms of Vitamin E. Vitamin E exists in a variety of forms (e.g., alpha-tocopherol, beta-tocopherol, alpha-tocotrienol), each of which has multiple stereoisomers. However, only four stereoisomers are found in blood, all of them variants of *alpha-tocopherol*. These isomers are designated *RRR-*, *RRS-*, *RSR-*, and *RSS*-alpha-tocopherol. Of the four, only *RRR-alpha-tocopherol* occurs naturally in foods. However, all four can be found in fortified foods and dietary supplements. Why are other forms of vitamin E absent from the blood? Because they are unable to bind to *alpha-tocopherol transfer protein* (alpha-TTP), the hepatic protein required for secretion of vitamin E from the liver and subsequent transport throughout the body.

Sources. Most dietary vitamin E comes from vegetable oils (e.g., corn oil, olive oil, cottonseed oil, safflower oil, canola oil). The vitamin is also found in nuts, wheat germ, whole-grain products, and mustard greens.

Requirements. RDAs for vitamin E were revised in 2000 (see Table 76–2). The new RDAs are higher than the RDAs set in 1989. For men and women, the new RDA is 15 mg/day. RDAs increase for women who are breast-feeding, but not for those who are pregnant.

Deficiency. Vitamin E deficiency is rare. In the United States, deficiency is limited primarily to people with an inborn deficiency of alpha-TTP and to those who have fat malabsorption syndromes, and hence are unable to absorb fat-soluble vitamins. Symptoms of deficiency include ataxia, sensory neuropathy, areflexia, and muscle hypertrophy.

Adverse Effects. Excessive vitamin E may increase the risk of *bleeding*. In animals, vitamin E can suppress coagulation, increase prothrombin time, and cause hemorrhage—but only at very high doses (e.g., 500 mg/kg/ day). Furthermore, vitamin E–induced bleeding can be counteracted by vitamin K, which promotes synthesis of clotting factors. Data on the hemorrhagic

effects of vitamin E in humans are inconsistent. Individuals who are vitamin K deficient may be at some risk. To protect against possible bleeding, the Food and Nutrition Board has set the adult UL for vitamin E at 1000 mg/day.

Vitamin K

Action. Vitamin K is required for synthesis of prothrombin and three other clotting factors (factors VII, IX, and X). All of these vitamin K–dependent factors are needed for coagulation of blood.

Forms and Sources of Vitamin K. Vitamin K occurs in nature in two forms: (1) vitamin K_1, or phytonadione (phylloquinone); and (2) vitamin K_2. Phytonadione is present in a wide variety of foods. Vitamin K_2 is synthesized by the normal flora of the gut. Two other forms—vitamin K_4 (menadiol) and vitamin K_3 (menadione)—are produced synthetically. At this time, phytonadione is the only form of vitamin K available for therapeutic use.

Requirements. Human requirements for vitamin K have not been precisely defined. In 2002, the Food and Nutrition Board set the AI for adult males at 120 μg, and the AI for adult females at 90 μg. AIs for other life-stage groups are shown in Table 76–2. For most individuals, vitamin K requirements are readily met through dietary sources and through vitamin K synthesized by intestinal bacteria. Since bacterial colonization of the gut is not complete until several days after birth, levels of vitamin K may be low during the immediate postnatal period.

Pharmacokinetics. Intestinal absorption of the natural forms of vitamin K (phytonadione and vitamin K_2) is adequate only in the presence of bile salts. Menadione and menadiol do not require bile salts for absorption. Following absorption, vitamin K is concentrated in the liver. Metabolism and secretion occur rapidly. Very little storage occurs.

Deficiency. Vitamin K deficiency produces bleeding tendencies. If the deficiency is severe, spontaneous hemorrhage may occur. In newborns, intracranial hemorrhage is of particular concern.

An important cause of deficiency is reduced absorption. Since the natural forms of vitamin K require bile salts for their uptake, any condition that decreases availability of these salts (e.g., obstructive jaundice) can lead to deficiency. Malabsorption syndromes (sprue, celiac disease, cystic fibrosis of the pancreas) can also decrease vitamin K uptake. Other potential causes of impaired absorption are ulcerative colitis, regional enteritis, and surgical resection of the intestine.

Disruption of intestinal flora may result in deficiency by eliminating vitamin K–synthesizing bacteria. Hence, deficiency may occur secondary to use of antibiotics. In infants, diarrhea may cause bacterial losses sufficient to result in deficiency.

The normal infant is born vitamin K deficient. Consequently, in order to rapidly elevate prothrombin levels, and thereby reduce the risk of neonatal hemorrhage, it is recommended that all infants receive a single injection of phytonadione (vitamin K_1) immediately after delivery.

As discussed in Chapter 50, the anticoagulant warfarin acts as an antagonist of vitamin K, and thereby decreases synthesis of vitamin K–dependent clotting factors. As a result, warfarin produces a state functionally equivalent to vitamin K deficiency. If the dosage of warfarin is excessive, hemorrhage can occur secondary to lack of prothrombin.

Adverse Effects. Severe Hypersensitivity Reactions. *Intravenous* administration of phytonadione can cause serious reactions (shock, respiratory arrest, cardiac arrest) that resemble anaphylaxis or hypersensitivity reactions. Death has oc-

TABLE 76-2 ■ Recommended Vitamin Intakes for Individuals

Life Stage Group	Vitamin A (µg)[a]	Vitamin C (mg)	Vitamin D (µg)[b,c]	Vitamin E (mg)[d]	Vitamin K (µg)	Thiamin (mg)	Riboflavin (mg)	Niacin (mg)[e]	Vitamin B6 (mg)	Folate (µg)[f]	Vitamin B12 (µg)	Pantothenic Acid (mg)	Biotin (µg)
Infants													
0–6 mo	400*	40*	5*	4*	2.0*	0.2*	0.3*	2*	0.1*	65*	0.4*	1.7*	5*
7–12 mo	500*	50*	5*	5*	2.5*	0.3*	0.4*	4*	0.3*	80*	0.5*	1.8*	6*
Children													
1–3 yr	300	15	5*	6	30*	0.5	0.5	6	0.5	150	0.9	2*	8*
4–8 yr	400	25	5*	7	55*	0.6	0.6	8	0.6	200	1.2	3*	12*
Males													
9–13 yr	600	45	5*	11	60*	0.9	0.9	12	1.0	300	1.8	4*	20*
14–18 yr	900	75	5*	15	75*	1.2	1.3	16	1.3	400	2.4	5*	25*
19–30 yr	900	90	5*	15	120*	1.2	1.3	16	1.3	400	2.4	5*	30*
31–50 yr	900	90	5*	15	120*	1.2	1.3	16	1.3	400	2.4	5*	30*
51–70 yr	900	90	10*	15	120*	1.2	1.3	16	1.7	400	2.4[i]	5*	30*
>70 yr	900	90	15*	15	120*	1.2	1.3	16	1.7	400	2.4[i]	5*	30*
Females													
9–13 yr	600	45	5*	11	60*	0.9	0.9	12	1.0	300	1.8	4*	20*
14–18 yr	700	65	5*	15	75*	1.0	1.0	14	1.2	400[g]	2.4	5*	25*
19–30 yr	700	75	5*	15	90*	1.1	1.1	14	1.3	400[g]	2.4	5*	30*
31–50 yr	700	75	5*	15	90*	1.1	1.1	14	1.3	400[g]	2.4	5*	30*
51–70 yr	700	75	10*	15	90*	1.1	1.1	14	1.5	400	2.4[i]	5*	30*
>70 yr	700	75	15*	15	90*	1.1	1.1	14	1.5	400	2.4[i]	5*	30*
Pregnancy													
≤18 yr	750	80	5*	15	75*	1.4	1.4	18	1.9	600[h]	2.6	6*	30*
19–30 yr	770	85	5*	15	90*	1.4	1.4	18	1.9	600[h]	2.6	6*	30*
31–50 yr	770	85	5*	15	90*	1.4	1.4	18	1.9	600[h]	2.6	6*	30*
Lactation													
≤18 yr	1200	115	5*	19	75*	1.4	1.6	17	2.0	500	2.8	7*	35*
19–30 yr	1300	120	5*	19	90*	1.4	1.6	17	2.0	500	2.8	7*	35*
31–50 yr	1300	120	5*	19	90*	1.4	1.6	17	2.0	500	2.8	7*	35*

Recommended Vitamin Intake Per Day

NOTE: This table presents Recommended Dietary Allowances (RDAs) in **bold type** and Adequate Intakes (AIs) in ordinary type followed by an asterisk (*). RDAs and AIs may both be used as goals for individual intake. RDAs are set to meet the needs of almost all (97% to 98%) individuals in a group. For healthy breast-fed infants, the AI is the mean intake. The AI for other life stage and gender groups is believed to cover needs of all individuals in the group, but lack of data or uncertainty in the data prevent being able to specify with confidence the percentage of individuals covered by this intake.

[a] As retinol activity equivalents (RAEs). 1 RAE = 1 μg retinol, 12 μg beta-carotene, 24 μg alpha-carotene, or 24 μg beta-cryptoxanthin. To calculate RAEs from retinol equivalents (REs) of provitamin A carotenoids in foods, divide the REs by 2. For preformed vitamin A in foods or supplements and for provitamin A carotenoids in supplements, 1 RE = 1 RAE.

[b] As cholecalciferol. 1 μg cholecalciferol = 40 IU vitamin D.

[c] In the absence of adequate exposure to sunlight

[d] As alpha-tocopherol. Alpha-tocopherol includes RRR-alpha-tocopherol, the only form of alpha-tocopherol that occurs naturally in foods, and the 2R-stereoisomeric forms of alpha-tocopherol (RRR-, RSR-, RRS-, and RSS-alpha-tocopherol) that occur in fortified foods and supplements. It does not include the 2S-stereoisomeric forms of alpha-tocopherol (SRR-, SSR-, SRS-, and SSS-alpha-tocopherol), also found in fortified foods and supplements.

[e] As niacin equivalents (NE). 1 mg of niacin = 60 mg of tryptophan; 0–6 months = preformed niacin (not NE).

[f] As dietary folate equivalents (DFE). 1 DFE = 1 μg food folate = 0.6 μg of folic acid from fortified food or as a supplement consumed with food = 0.5 μg of a supplement taken on an empty stomach.

[g] In view of evidence linking folate deficiency with neural tube defects in the fetus, it is recommended that all women capable of becoming pregnant consume 400 μg from supplements or fortified foods in addition to intake of food folate from a varied diet.

[h] It is assumed that women will continue consuming 400 μg from supplements or fortified food until their pregnancy is confirmed and they enter prenatal care, which ordinarily occurs after the end of the periconceptional period—the critical time for formation of the neural tube.

[i] Because 10% to 30% of older people may malabsorb food-bound B_{12}, it is advisable for those older than 50 years to meet their RDA mainly by consuming foods fortified with B_{12} or by consuming a supplement containing B_{12}.

Data from a summary table in Food and Nutrition Board, Institute of Medicine. Dietary Reference Intakes for Vitamin A, Vitamin K, Arsenic, Boron, Chromium, Copper, Iodine, Iron, Manganese, Molybdenum, Nickel, Silicon, Vanadium, and Zinc. Washington, DC, National Academy Press, 2002:770–771. However, except for the information on vitamins A and K, all of the information in this table was first released in the earlier publications listed in Table 76–1.

Special Interest Topic

BOX 76-1 ■ LOSING HOPE FOR ANTIOXIDANTS

On April 10, 2000, the National Academy of Sciences issued a report stating there is no conclusive evidence that megadoses of dietary antioxidants can protect against cancer, heart disease, Alzheimer's disease, or any other chronic disorder. Furthermore, they noted that excessive doses can cause harm. Accordingly, they recommended limiting intake of antioxidants to amounts that will prevent nutritional deficiency, and recommended avoiding doses that are potentially harmful. The report, titled *Dietary Reference Intakes for Vitamin C, Vitamin E, Selenium, and Carotenoids,* is available from the National Academy Press.

Dietary antioxidants are defined as substances present in food that can significantly decrease cellular and tissue injury caused by highly reactive forms of oxygen and nitrogen, known as "free radicals." These free radicals, which are normal by-products of metabolism, readily react with other molecules. The result is tissue injury known as "oxidative stress." Antioxidants help reduce oxidative stress by neutralizing free radicals before they can cause harm. There is no question that dietary antioxidants can decrease injury. However, the available data are insufficient to prove that taking large doses reduces the risk of chronic disease.

Which dietary constituents function as antioxidants? There is good evidence that three agents—*selenium, vitamin C,* and *vitamin E*—exert significant antioxidant actions. Data for *beta-carotene* (a precursor of vitamin A) are less clear: Although beta-carotene has antioxidant activity *in vitro,* convincing evidence of *in vivo* antioxidant activity is lacking.

How might antioxidants protect against chronic disease? By reducing oxidative damage to DNA, they could reduce the risk of cancer. By reducing oxidation of LDL cholesterol, a critical step in the formation of atherosclerotic plaque, they could protect against heart disease. Reducing oxidation of other biologic molecules could explain protection against other diseases.

Researchers have been studying the clinical effects of antioxidants for more than a decade. Unfortunately, although initial findings were encouraging, recent studies indicate that benefits are less extensive than originally suspected.

When evaluating antioxidants for clinical effects, scientists have conducted two kinds of studies: *observational studies* and *randomized controlled trials* (RCTs). Observational studies are based on patient histories (e.g., what did patients eat and what was their medical status). In contrast, RCTs are rigorous, prospective studies in which patients are randomly assigned to either an experimental group or a placebo group; conclusions are based on differences between the two. The results of RCTs are much more reliable than are the results of observational studies.

Nearly all of the early studies on antioxidants were observational. These studies indicated that daily consumption of vegetables rich in antioxidants is associated with a reduced risk of heart disease and several types of cancer. The problem is, these results have more than one interpretation. Yes, they may mean that antioxidant vitamins protected against heart disease and cancer. However, they may also mean that protection was conferred by some other aspect of the diet (e.g., high

fiber content and/or low content of cholesterol and saturated fat). Or, perhaps diet had nothing to with it: Maybe protection resulted from a generally healthy lifestyle, and not from a healthy diet. Hence, although observational studies suggest that antioxidants may protect against heart disease and cancer, they certainly don't prove it.

To establish definitive proof of cardiovascular benefits, scientists conducted large RCTs. The outcomes were unexpected and discouraging. Two studies on vitamin E are especially noteworthy. Results of the most definitive RCT to date—the *Heart Outcomes Prevention Evaluation (HOPE) Study*—were reported in the January 20, 2000, issue of the *New England Journal of Medicine.* The HOPE Study enrolled 9541 patients ages 55 and older, of whom 80% had cardiovascular disease and 40% had diabetes. Half the patients were given 400 IU of vitamin E daily, and half received a placebo. In addition, the patients were randomly assigned to receive either ramipril (an angiotensin-converting enzyme inhibitor) or a second placebo. After 4.5 years, the results were conclusive: Ramipril provided clear protection against cardiovascular events, whereas vitamin E provided none. In August 1999, an Italian group reported similar results in the British journal *Lancet.* This study, known as the *GISSI-Prevenzione* trial, involved 11,000 patients who had suffered myocardial infarction (MI). Half were randomly assigned treatment with vitamin E (300 IU daily) and half were given placebo. After 3.5 years, the incidence of nonfatal MI and death from coronary heart disease was the same for both groups, indicating no benefit from vitamin E. Results of other RCTs support the results of these two.

Do the HOPE study and other RCTs tell us that antioxidants confer virtually no protection against cardiovascular disease? At this time, we don't know enough to say for sure. Before we can answer the question, we need to investigate the following:

- *Prolonged treatment*—RCTs to date were conducted for a relatively short time (3.5 to 4.5 years). Perhaps giving vitamin E for a longer time would reveal benefits. However, the Physician's Health Study argues against this possibility: 12 years of treatment with beta-carotene (a suspected antioxidant) offered no benefit.
- *Effect in healthy subjects*—RCTs to date have been conducted on people with pre-existing heart disease. Perhaps antioxidants can *prevent* heart disease in healthy subjects, even if they can't reverse it in sick ones.
- *Combination vitamin therapy*—RCTs to date evaluated monotherapy with vitamin E. Perhaps benefits would be revealed if vitamin E were combined with other antioxidants, as occurs when we eat vitamin-containing foods.

Even if vitamin E and other antioxidants prove devoid of cardiovascular benefits, the story doesn't end there. These agents may still offer protection against other disorders. Possibilities under investigation include cataracts, macular degeneration, and Alzheimer's disease. Results of ongoing RCTs should provide further insight.

curred. Consequently, phytonadione should not be administered IV unless other routes are not feasible, and then only if the potential benefits clearly outweigh the risks.

Hyperbilirubinemia. When administered *parenterally* to newborns, vitamin K derivatives can elevate plasma levels of bilirubin, thereby posing a risk of *kernicterus.* The incidence of hyperbilirubinemia is greater among premature infants than full-term infants. Although all forms of vitamin K can elevate bilirubin levels, the risk is higher with menadione and menadiol than with phytonadione.

Therapeutic Uses and Dosage. Vitamin K has two major applications: (1) correction or prevention of hypoprothrombinemia and bleeding caused by vitamin K deficiency, and (2) control of hemorrhage caused by overdose with oral anticoagulants.

Vitamin K Deficiency. As discussed, vitamin K deficiency can result from impaired vitamin absorption and from insufficient synthesis of the vitamin by intestinal flora. Rarely, deficiency results from inadequate diet. For children and adults, the usual dosage for correction of vitamin K deficiency ranges between 5 and 15 mg/day.

As noted above, infants are born vitamin K deficient. To prevent hemorrhagic disease in neonates, it is recommended that all newborns be given an injection of phytonadione (0.5 to 1 mg) immediately after delivery.

Warfarin Overdose. Vitamin K reverses hypoprothrombinemia and bleeding caused by excessive dosing with warfarin, an oral anticoagulant. Bleeding is controlled within hours of vitamin K administration (see Chapter 50 for dosage).

Preparations and Routes of Administration. *Phytonadione* (vitamin K_1) is available in 5-mg tablets, marketed as Mephyton, and in parenteral formulations, marketed as AquaMEPHYTON. Parenteral phytonadione may be administered IM, SC, and IV. However, since IV administration is dangerous, this route should be used only when other routes are not feasible, and only if the perceived benefits outweigh the substantial risks.

WATER-SOLUBLE VITAMINS

The group of water-soluble vitamins consists of vitamin C and members of the vitamin B complex (thiamin, riboflavin, niacin, pyridoxine, pantothenic acid, biotin, folic acid, and cyanocobalamin). The B vitamins differ widely from one another in both structure and function. They are grouped together because they were first isolated from the same sources (yeast and liver). Vitamin C is not found in the same foods as the B vitamins, and hence is classified by itself. DRIs for the B vitamins were revised in 1998. DRIs for vitamin C were revised in 2000.

Two compounds—*pangamic acid* and *laetrile*—have been falsely promoted as B vitamins. Pangamic acid has been marketed as "vitamin B_{15}" and laetrile as "vitamin B_{17}." There is no proof these compounds act as vitamins or have any other role in human nutrition.

Vitamin C (Ascorbic Acid)

Actions. Vitamin C participates in multiple biochemical reactions. These include synthesis of adrenal steroids, conversion of folic acid to folinic acid, and regulation of the respiratory cycle in mitochondria. At the tissue level, vitamin C is required for production of collagen and other compounds that comprise the intercellular matrix that binds cells together. In addition, vitamin C has antioxidant activity (see Box 76–1) and facilitates GI absorption of iron.

Sources. The main dietary sources of ascorbic acid are citrus fruits and juices, tomatoes, potatoes, strawberries, melons, and broccoli. Orange juice and lemon juice are especially rich sources.

Requirements. The RDAs for vitamin C were revised in 2000 (see Table 76–2). The new RDAs are higher than those set in 1989. As in the past, RDAs increase for women who are pregnant or breast-feeding. For smokers, the RDA is increased by 35 mg/day.

Deficiency. Deficiency of vitamin C can lead to *scurvy,* a disease that is rare in the United States. Symptoms include faulty bone and tooth development, loosening of the teeth, gingivitis, bleeding gums, poor wound healing, hemorrhage into muscles and joints, and ecchymoses (skin discoloration caused by leakage of blood into subcutaneous tissues). Many of these symptoms result from disruption of the intercellular matrix of capillaries and other tissues.

Adverse Effects. Excessive doses can cause nausea, abdominal cramps, and diarrhea. The mechanism is direct irritation of the intestinal mucosa. To protect against GI disturbances, the Food and Nutrition Board has set 2 gm/day as the adult UL for vitamin C.

Therapeutic Use. The only established indication for vitamin C is prevention and treatment of scurvy. For severe, acute deficiency, parenteral administration is recommended. The usual adult dosage is 0.3 to 1 gm/day.

Vitamin C has been advocated for therapy of many conditions unrelated to deficiency, including cancers, asthma, osteoporosis, and the common cold. Claims of efficacy for several of these conditions have been definitively disproved. Other claims remain unproved. Studies have shown that large doses do not reduce the incidence of colds, although the intensity or duration of illness may be reduced slightly. Research has failed to show any benefit of vitamin C therapy for patients with advanced cancer, atherosclerosis, or schizophrenia. Vitamin C does not promote healing of wounds.

Preparations and Routes of Administration. Vitamin C is available in formulations for oral and parenteral administration. Oral products include tablets (ranging from 25 to 1500 mg), timed-release capsules (500 mg), and syrups (20 and 100 mg/ml). For parenteral use, vitamin C is available as ascorbic acid, sodium ascorbate, and calcium ascorbate. Administration may be SC, IM, or IV.

Niacin (Nicotinic Acid)

Niacin has a role as both a vitamin and a medicine. In its medicinal role, niacin is used to reduce cholesterol levels; the doses required are much higher than those used to correct or prevent nutritional deficiency. Discussion in this chapter focuses on niacin as a vitamin. Use of nicotinic acid to reduce cholesterol levels is discussed in Chapter 48.

Physiologic Actions. Before it can exert physiologic effects, niacin must first be converted into either nicotinamide-adenine dinucleotide (NAD) or nicotinamide-adenine dinucleotide phosphate (NADP). NAD and NADP then act as coenzymes in oxidation-reduction reactions essential for cellular respiration.

Sources. Nicotinic acid (or its nutritional equivalent, nicotinamide) is present in many foods of plant and animal origin. Particularly rich sources are liver, chicken, yeast, peanuts, cereal bran, and cereal germ.

In humans, the amino acid tryptophan can be converted to nicotinic acid. Hence, proteins can be a source of the vitamin. About 60 mg of dietary tryptophan is required to produce 1 mg of nicotinic acid.

Requirements. RDAs for nicotinic acid are stated as niacin equivalents (NEs). By definition, 1 NE is equal to 1 mg of niacin (nicotinic acid) or 60 mg of tryptophan. New RDAs for niacin were established in 1998 (see Table 76–2). These are slightly lower than the RDAs set in 1989.

Deficiency. The syndrome caused by niacin deficiency is called *pellagra,* a term that is a condensation of the Italian words *pelle agra,* meaning "rough skin." As suggested by this name, a prominent symptom of pellagra is dermatitis, characterized by scaling and cracking of the skin in areas exposed to the sun. Other symptoms involve the GI tract (abdominal pain, diarrhea, soreness of the tongue and mouth) and central nervous system (irritability, insomnia, memory loss, anxiety, dementia). All symptoms are readily reversed with niacin replacement therapy.

Adverse Effects. Nicotinic acid has very low toxicity. Small doses are completely devoid of adverse effects. When taken in large doses, nicotinic acid can cause vasodilation with resultant *flushing, dizziness,* and *nausea.* Using flushing as an index of excess niacin consumption, the Food and Nutrition Board has set 50 mg as the adult UL for this vitamin. Toxicity associated with high-dose therapy is discussed in Chapter 48.

Nicotinamide, a compound that can substitute for nicotinic acid in the treatment of pellagra, is not a vasodilator, and hence does not produce the adverse effects associated with large doses of nicotinic acid. Accordingly, nicotinamide is often preferred to nicotinic acid for treating pellagra, which requires high doses of the vitamin.

Therapeutic Uses. In its capacity as a vitamin, nicotinic acid is indicated only for the prevention or treatment of niacin deficiency. As noted, if given in large doses, nicotinic acid may also be used to lower cholesterol levels (see Chapter 48).

Preparations, Dosage, and Administration. *Nicotinic acid* (niacin) is available in tablets (20 to 500 mg), in capsules (125 to 500 mg), and as an elixir (10 mg/ml) for oral use. Dosages for mild deficiency range from 10 to 20 mg/day. For treatment of pellagra, daily doses may be as high as 500 mg. Dosages for hyperlipidemia are given in Chapter 48.

Nicotinamide (niacinamide) is dispensed in 100- and 500-mg tablets for oral use. For treatment or prevention of pellagra, dosages range from 150 to 500 mg/day. Unlike nicotinic acid, nicotinamide has no effect on plasma lipoproteins, and hence is not used to treat hyperlipidemias.

Riboflavin (Vitamin B₂)

Actions. Riboflavin participates in numerous enzymatic reactions. However, in order to exert physiologic effects, the vitamin must first be converted into one of two active forms: flavin adenine dinucleotide (FAD) or flavin mononucleotide (FMN). In the form of FAD or FMN, riboflavin acts as a coenzyme for multiple oxidative reactions.

Sources and Requirements. In the United States, most dietary riboflavin comes from milk, bread products, and fortified cereals. Organ meats are also rich in the vitamin. New RDAs for riboflavin were established in 1998 (see Table 76–2). These are somewhat lower than the RDAs set in 1989.

Toxicity. Riboflavin appears devoid of toxicity to humans. When large doses are administered, the excess is rapidly excreted in the urine. Because large doses are harmless, no UL has been set.

Use in Riboflavin Deficiency. Riboflavin is indicated only for prevention and correction of riboflavin deficiency, which usually occurs in conjunction with deficiency of other B vitamins. In its early state, riboflavin deficiency manifests as sore throat and angular stomatitis (cracks in the skin at the corners of the mouth). Symptoms that may appear later include cheilosis

(painful cracks in the lips), glossitis (inflammation of the tongue), vascularization of the cornea, and itchy dermatitis of the scrotum or vulva. Oral riboflavin is used for treatment. The dosage is 10 to 15 mg/day.

Use in Migraine Headache. As discussed in Chapter 29, riboflavin can help prevent migraine headaches. The daily dosage is 400 mg—much higher than the dosage for riboflavin deficiency.

Thiamin (Vitamin B₁)

Actions and Requirements. The active form of thiamin (thiamin pyrophosphate) is an essential coenzyme for carbohydrate metabolism. Thiamin requirements are related to caloric intake, and are greatest when carbohydrates are the primary source of calories. For maintenance of good health, thiamin consumption should be at least 0.3 mg/1000 kcal in the diet. The 1998 revised RDAs for thiamin appear in Table 76–2. As indicated, thiamin requirements increase significantly during pregnancy and lactation. Compared with the RDAs set in 1989, the new RDAs are largely unchanged for women, and somewhat reduced for men.

Sources. In the United States, the principal dietary sources of thiamin are enriched, fortified, or whole-grain products, especially breads and ready-to-eat cereals. The richest source of the natural vitamin is pork.

Deficiency. Severe thiamin deficiency produces *beriberi,* a disorder having two distinct forms: *wet beriberi* and *dry beriberi. Wet beriberi* is so named because its primary symptom is fluid accumulation in the legs. Cardiovascular complications (palpitations, electrocardiogram abnormalities, high-output heart failure) are common and may progress rapidly to circulatory collapse and death. *Dry beriberi* is characterized by neurologic and motor deficits (e.g., anesthesia of the feet, ataxic gait, footdrop, wrist drop); edema and cardiovascular symptoms are absent. Wet beriberi responds rapidly and dramatically to replacement therapy. In contrast, recovery from dry beriberi can be very slow.

In the United States, thiamin deficiency occurs most commonly among alcoholics. In this population, deficiency manifests as *Wernicke-Korsakoff syndrome* rather than frank beriberi. This syndrome is a serious disorder of the central nervous system, having neurologic and psychologic manifestations. Symptoms include nystagmus, diplopia, ataxia, and an inability to remember the recent past. Failure to correct the thiamin deficit may result in irreversible damage to the brain. Accordingly, if Wernicke-Korsakoff syndrome is suspected, parenteral thiamin should be administered immediately.

Adverse Effects. When taken orally, thiamin is devoid of adverse effects. Accordingly, no UL for the vitamin has been established.

Therapeutic Use. The only indication for thiamin is treatment and prevention of thiamin deficiency.

Preparations, Dosage, and Administration. Thiamin is dispensed in standard tablets (50, 100, and 250 mg) and enteric-coated tablets (20 mg) for oral use and in solution (100 mg/ml) for IM or IV administration. For mild deficiency, oral thiamin is preferred. Parenteral administration is reserved for severe deficiency states (wet or dry beriberi, Wernicke-Korsakoff syndrome). The dosage for beriberi is 50 to 100 mg IM daily for 1 to 2 weeks, followed by 2.5 to 10 mg PO daily until recovery is complete.

Pyridoxine (Vitamin B₆)

Actions. Pyridoxine functions as a coenzyme in the metabolism of amino acids and proteins. However, before it can influence biologic processes, pyridoxine must first be converted to its active form: pyridoxal phosphate.

Requirements. RDAs for pyridoxine were revised in 1998 (see Table 76–2). For most people, and especially the young, the new RDAs are considerably lower than the RDAs set in 1989. As before, RDAs increase significantly for women who are pregnant or breast-feeding.

Sources. In the United States, the principal dietary sources of pyridoxine are fortified, ready-to-eat cereals; meat, fish, and poultry; white potatoes and other starchy vegetables; and noncitrus fruits. Especially rich sources are organ meats (e.g., beef liver) and cereals or soy-based products that have been highly fortified.

Deficiency. Pyridoxine deficiency may result from poor diet, use of isoniazid, and inborn errors of metabolism. Symptoms include seborrheic dermatitis, microcytic anemia, peripheral neuritis, convulsions, depression, and confusion.

In the United States, dietary deficiency of vitamin B_6 is rare, except among alcoholics. Within the alcoholic population, vitamin B_6 deficiency has an incidence of about 20% to 30%, and occurs in combination with deficiency of other B vitamins.

Isoniazid (a drug for tuberculosis) prevents conversion of vitamin B_6 to its active form, and may thereby induce symptoms of deficiency (peripheral neuritis). Patients who are predisposed to this neuropathy (e.g., alcoholics, diabetics) should receive daily pyridoxine supplements.

Inborn errors of metabolism can prevent efficient utilization of vitamin B_6, resulting in greatly increased pyridoxine requirements. Among infants, symptoms include irritability, convulsions, and anemia. Unless treatment with vitamin B_6 is initiated early, permanent retardation may result.

Adverse Effects. At low doses, pyridoxine is devoid of adverse effects. However, if extremely large doses are taken, neurologic injury may result. Symptoms include ataxia and numbness of the feet and hands. To minimize risk, adults should not consume more than 100 mg/day, the UL for this vitamin.

Drug Interactions. Vitamin B_6 interferes with the utilization of levodopa, a drug for Parkinson's disease. Accordingly, patients receiving levodopa should be advised against taking this vitamin.

Therapeutic Uses. Pyridoxine is indicated for prevention and treatment of all vitamin B_6 deficiency states (dietary deficiency, isoniazid-induced deficiency, pyridoxine dependency syndrome).

Preparations, Dosage, and Administration. Pyridoxine is dispensed in tablets (25 to 500 mg) for oral use and in solution (100 mg/ml) for IM or IV administration. To correct dietary deficiency, the dosage is 10 to 20 mg/day for 3 weeks followed by 1.5 to 2.5 mg/day for maintenance. To treat deficiency induced by isoniazid, the dosage is 50 to 200 mg/day. To protect against isoniazid-induced deficiency, the dosage is 25 to 50 mg/day. Pyridoxine dependency syndrome may require initial doses up to 600 mg/day followed by 25 to 50 mg/day for life.

Cyanocobalamin (Vitamin B_{12}) and Folic Acid

Cyanocobalamin (vitamin B_{12}) and folic acid (folacin) are essential factors in the synthesis of DNA. Deficiency of either vitamin manifests as megaloblastic anemia. Cyanocobalamin deficiency produces neurologic damage as well. Because deficiency presents as anemia, folic acid and cyanocobalamin are discussed at length in Chapter 52 (Drugs for Deficiency Anemias).

RDAs and ULs. Revised RDAs for vitamin B_{12} and folate were published in 1998 (see Table 76–2). The new adult RDA for B_{12} (2.4 µg) is about 20% higher than the RDA established in 1989, and the new adult RDA for folic acid (400 µg) is 100% higher than the old one. Because adults over age 50 often have difficulty absorbing dietary vitamin B_{12}, they should ingest at least 2.4 µg daily in the form of a supplement. A UL of 1000 µg/day has been set for folic acid. Because of insufficient data, no UL has been set for B_{12}.

Food Folate Versus Synthetic Folate. The form of folate that occurs naturally (food folate) has a different chemical structure than synthetic folate (pteroylglutamic acid). Synthetic folate is more stable than food folate, and has greater bioavailability. In the presence of food, the bioavailability of synthetic folate is at least 85%. In contrast, bioavailability of food folate is less than 50%.

To increase folate in the American diet, the Food and Drug Administration issued the following order: Beginning January 1, 1998, all enriched grain products (e.g., enriched bread, pasta, flour, breakfast cereal, grits, rice) must be fortified with synthetic folate—specifically, 140 µg/100 gm of grain. As a result of grain fortification, the incidence of folic acid deficiency in the United States has declined dramatically.

Folic Acid Deficiency and Fetal Development. Deficiency of folic acid during pregnancy can impair development of the central nervous system, resulting in *neural tube defects* (NTDs): *anencephaly* and *spina bifida*. Anencephaly (failure of the brain to develop) is uniformly fatal. Spina bifida, a condition characterized by defective development of the bony encasement of the spinal cord, can result in nerve damage, paralysis, and other complications. The time of vulnerability for NTDs is days 21 through 28 after conception. Hence, the damage can occur before a woman recognizes her pregnancy by missing a period. Because NTDs occur very early in pregnancy, it is essential that adequate levels of folic acid be present *when pregnancy begins;* women cannot wait until pregnancy is confirmed before establishing adequate intake. To ensure sufficient folate at the onset of pregnancy, the U.S. Public Health Service recommends that *all women who may become pregnant consume 400 µg of supplemental folic acid each day*—in addition to the folates they get from food. Since pregnancy can occur despite birth control measures, this recommendation applies even to women who don't intend to become pregnant.

Folic Acid and Colorectal Cancer. Data from the Nurse's Health Study suggest that folate protects against colorectal cancer, the third most common cancer in the United States. In this study, women who took a vitamin supplement containing 400 µg of folate every day for 15 or more years reduced their risk of colon cancer by 75%. Although the mechanism of protection is unknown, it may relate to the role of folate in DNA synthesis and repair: Researchers speculate that insufficient folate may predispose to cancer-causing genetic changes, whereas maintaining adequate folate may reduce the incidence of these changes.

Folic Acid, Homocysteine, and Atherosclerosis. Folic acid reduces blood levels of homocysteine, a suspected factor in atherosclerosis. The roles of folic acid and homocysteine in atherosclerosis are discussed in Chapter 48.

Pantothenic Acid

Pantothenic acid is an essential component of two biologically important molecules: *coenzyme A* and *acyl carrier protein*. Coenzyme A is an essential factor in multiple biochemical processes, including gluconeogenesis, intermediary metabolism of carbohydrates, and biosynthesis of steroid hormones, porphyrins, and acetylcholine. Acyl carrier protein is required for synthesis of fatty acids. Pantothenic acid is present in virtually all foods. As a result, spontaneous deficiency has not been reported. There are insufficient data to establish RDAs for pantothenic acid. However, the Food and Nutrition Board *has* assigned AIs (see Table 76–2). There are no reports of toxicity from pantothenic acid. Accordingly, no UL has been set. Pantothenic acid is available in single-ingredient tablets and in multivitamin preparations. However, because deficiency does not occur, there is no reason to take supplements.

Biotin

Biotin is an essential cofactor for several reactions involved in the metabolism of carbohydrates and fats. The vitamin is found in a wide variety of foods, although the exact amount in most foods has not been determined. In addition to being available in foods, biotin is synthesized by intestinal bacteria. Biotin deficiency is extremely rare. In fact, in order to determine the effects of deficiency, scientists had to induce it experimentally. When this was done, subjects experienced dermatitis, conjunctivitis, hair loss, muscle pain, peripheral paresthesias, and psychologic effects (lethargy, hallucinations, depression). At this time, the data are insufficient to establish RDAs for biotin. However, as with pantothenic acid, the Food and Nutrition Board *has* assigned AIs (see Table 76–2). Biotin appears devoid of toxicity: Subjects given large doses experienced no adverse effects. Accordingly, no UL has been set.

⬛ KEY POINTS

- Vitamins can be defined as organic compounds, required in minute amounts, that promote growth and maintenance of health by participating in energy transformation and regulation of metabolic processes.
- Recommended Dietary Allowances (RDAs) for vitamins, which are set by the Food and Nutrition Board of the National Academy of Sciences, represent the average daily dietary intake sufficient to meet the nutrient requirements of nearly all (97% to 98%) healthy individuals in a particular life-stage or gender group.
- The Tolerable Upper Intake Limit (UL) for a vitamin is the highest average daily intake that can be consumed by nearly everyone without a significant risk of adverse effects. The UL is simply an index of safety—not a recommendation to exceed the RDA.
- Until recently, nutrition experts believed that diet alone could supply the RDAs of most vitamins, with two important exceptions: vitamin B_{12} (for adults over age 50) and folic acid (for women of child-bearing age). Today, however, experts suggest it would be prudent for *all* adults to take daily supplements of *all* vitamins, not just vitamin B_{12} and folic acid. The objective is to reduce the risk of chronic illnesses caused, in part, by chronic, subclinical vitamin deficiency.

- Vitamins are divided into two major groups: fat-soluble vitamins (A, D, E, and K) and water-soluble vitamins (vitamin C and members of the vitamin B complex).
- Vitamin A deficiency can cause night blindness, xerophthalmia (a dry, thickened condition of the conjunctiva), and keratomalacia (degeneration of the cornea with keratinization of the corneal epithelium).
- Too much vitamin A can cause birth defects, liver injury, and bone abnormalities. Accordingly, vitamin A intake should not exceed the UL, set at 3000 μg/day.
- Vitamin D plays a critical role in the regulation of calcium and phosphorus metabolism.
- In children, vitamin D deficiency causes rickets. In adults, deficiency causes osteomalacia.
- Vitamin K is required for synthesis of prothrombin and other clotting factors.
- Vitamin K deficiency causes bleeding tendencies. Severe deficiency can cause spontaneous hemorrhage.
- Vitamin K is used to treat vitamin K deficiency (including neonatal deficiency) and overdose with warfarin (an anticoagulant).
- Vitamin C deficiency can cause scurvy.
- Niacin (nicotinic acid) is both a vitamin and a drug.
- When niacin is used as a drug (to reduce cholesterol levels), doses are much higher than when niacin is used to prevent or correct deficiency.
- Niacin deficiency results in pellagra.
- Severe thiamin deficiency produces beriberi.
- In the United States, thiamin deficiency occurs most commonly among alcoholics. In this population, deficiency manifests as Wernicke-Korsakoff syndrome rather than beriberi.
- Pyridoxine (vitamin B_6) deficiency can cause peripheral neuritis and other symptoms.
- Isoniazid, a drug for tuberculosis, prevents conversion of pyridoxine to its active form, and can thereby induce deficiency.
- Folic acid deficiency during early pregnancy can cause neural tube defects (anencephaly and spina bifida). To ensure folic acid sufficiency at the start of pregnancy, all women with the potential for becoming pregnant should consume 400 μg of folic acid every day.
- At this time, there are no convincing data that large doses of antioxidants (e.g., vitamin C, vitamin E) reduce the risk of cancer, heart disease, or any other chronic disorder.

Enteral and Parenteral Nutrition

Good nutrition is required to maintain health and permit healing during illness. As a rule, required nutrients—amino acids, carbohydrates, fats, vitamins, and minerals—can be obtained simply by ingesting appropriate foods. However, this is not always the case; circumstances frequently arise in which nutritional needs cannot be fulfilled by eating. Under these conditions, nutritional support is required. Specific indications for nutritional support include (1) malnutrition; (2) coma; (3) bowel obstruction; (4) cancer chemotherapy (because of associated nausea and vomiting); and (5) trauma, major burns, and severe infection (because these disorders cause a hypermetabolic state). Nutritional support is also given to permit bowel rest for patients with inflammatory bowel disease and for those recovering from bowel surgery.

There are two major categories of nutritional support: *enteral* (via the GI tract) and *parenteral* (intravenous). *Enteral* nutritional therapy is indicated for (1) patients who have a healthy digestive tract but are unable or unwilling to eat sufficient food, and (2) patients who have a digestive or absorptive disorder that cannot be overcome by diet modification. *Parenteral* nutritional support is indicated when nutrition cannot be maintained by eating or by enteral therapy.

ENTERAL NUTRITIONAL THERAPY

Enteral nutritional therapy is defined formally as provision of nutrients by way of the GI tract. However, in everyday practice, enteral nutrition is taken to mean feeding by tube. In the discussion below, we limit consideration to tube feeding.

Enteral therapy is indicated for two groups of patients: (1) those with a healthy digestive tract but who cannot or will not ingest sufficient food (e.g., anorectic patients, patients with an impaired ability to chew or swallow); and (2) those with a digestive or absorptive disorder that cannot be compensated for by modification of diet. Depending on patient status, enteral therapy may be used as a supplement to oral feeding or to meet all nutritional needs. Contraindications to enteral therapy include total bowel obstruction, uncontrollable vomiting, paralytic ileus, and severe malabsorption.

Modes of Delivery
Tube Placement

For *short-term* therapy, a *nasogastric* tube is commonly used. When intragastric administration is contraindicated (e.g., poor gastric motility, no gag reflex) or when the risk of aspiration is high, a *nasoduodenal* or *nasojejunal* tube may be employed.

For *long-term* therapy (more than 1 to 3 months), feeding tubes may be surgically implanted directly into the esophagus, stomach, or jejunum.

Schedule of Administration

Enteral nutritional support may be administered by four schedules: continuous infusion, cyclic infusion, intermittent infusion, and bolus administration. With *continuous infusion,* the total daily feeding is delivered at a constant rate over 24 hours. With *cyclic infusion,* the total daily feeding is delivered at a constant rate over several hours (rather than over 24 hours). With *intermittent infusion,* the total daily feeding is divided into three to six separate feedings that last 30 to 60 minutes each. *Bolus administration* is like intermittent infusion, except that the individual feedings last only a few minutes, rather than 30 to 60 minutes.

Method of Administration

Enteral nutrition may be administered (1) by syringe, (2) by gravity using a drip chamber, and (3) by enteral pump. Use of a *syringe,* which is the least expensive method of delivery, is appropriate only for bolus administration or for short infusions. *Gravity feeding with a drip chamber* costs somewhat more than syringe administration, but is clearly easier for infusions that last for 30 minutes or more. When a drip chamber is employed, the rate of delivery must be adjusted manually when the patient changes position (e.g., sits up, stands, lies down). Use of an *enteral infusion pump* is the most expensive form of administration, but is also the most consistent. Furthermore, for administering infusion solutions that are too viscous to flow by gravity, a pump is the only instrument that will work.

Components of an Enteral Nutritional Regimen

Amino Acids. All patients require an adequate supply of amino acids in order to conserve or rebuild lean body mass. Enteral solutions provide amino acids in various forms: intact proteins, hydrolyzed proteins, and free amino acids.

Specialized products are available to meet the unique amino acid needs of patients with renal failure, severe hepatic dysfunction, and other disorders. However, since proof of benefits for these formulas is generally lacking, their use is somewhat controversial.

Carbohydrates. Carbohydrates—in the form of dextrose, sucrose, lactose, starch, dextrin, and glucose oligosaccharides—are the primary source of calories in most enteral regimens. The simple sugars (dextrose, sucrose, and lactose) are absorbed more readily than complex carbohydrates (e.g., dextrin, starch). Hence, for patients with limited absorptive capacity, the simple sugars may be preferred. Because of their high osmolality, simple sugars can retain water in the intestinal lumen and can thereby promote diarrhea. Lactose intolerance (an inability to digest and absorb lactose) is common. Accordingly, most formulations are lactose free.

Fats. Fats serve as a source of calories and are required to prevent and correct essential fatty acid deficiency. Most enteral formulations contain a high percentage of fat (in the form of polyunsaturated fats). However, the fat content of some formulas is quite low. The fats employed most frequently are corn oil, soybean oil, and safflower oil.

Other Components. Enteral formulations should provide required *electrolytes, vitamins,* and *trace elements.* As a rule, enteral fluids do not contain sufficient water to maintain adequate hydration, and hence supplemental water is often needed. Many oral formulations contain flavoring agents; the patient should be consulted regarding taste preference.

Complications of Treatment

The most dangerous complication of enteral therapy is *aspiration pneumonitis,* a condition that can be fatal. To reduce the risk of aspiration, the upper body should be elevated (by raising the head of the bed to a 30-degree angle) during the infusion and for at least 1 hour after. High-risk patients (e.g., those prone to vomiting and those who lack a gag reflex) must not be given bolus feeding. For these people, feeding should be done by slow drip, and then only if the tip of the feeding tube has been placed into the duodenum or jejunum. If these tube placements are not possible, enteral therapy should be replaced with parenteral nutritional support.

About 10% of patients who are fed through a nasogastric tube experience adverse effects (e.g., diarrhea, vomiting, insufficient gastric emptying, GI bleeding). These can be minimized by initiating therapy at a slow rate using a dilute nutrient solution. As the patient adjusts to therapy, the infusion rate and nutrient concentration can be increased.

Enteral therapy may be associated with metabolic disturbances (e.g., hyperglycemia, fluid and electrolyte imbalance, fatty acid deficiency). Monitoring serum glucose and electrolyte levels will help minimize metabolic disorders.

PARENTERAL NUTRITIONAL THERAPY

Routes of Administration

Parenteral nutritional therapy may be administered through a *peripheral vein* or a *central venous catheter* (which delivers nutrient solution directly into the superior vena cava). Peripheral infusion is indicated only for *short-term* therapy with relatively dilute nutrient solutions. If therapy is to be *prolonged* (i.e., lasting more than 10 to 12 days) or if *strongly hypertonic* solutions are to be given, central administration is required.

Components of a Parenteral Nutritional Regimen

The core component of a parenteral nutritional regimen is a mixture of amino acids. Dextrose, fats, vitamins, and minerals are added as required.

Amino Acids

Nutritional Role. Amino acids serve two purposes: they (1) foster conservation of existing lean body mass and (2) promote wound healing and restoration of lean body mass. For healthy adults, the recommended dietary allowance (RDA) for amino acids is 0.9 gm/kg. The RDA for healthy infants and children ranges from 1.4 to 2.2 gm/kg. RDA values increase significantly in patients with malnutrition, trauma, burns, or infection.

Complications of Therapy. Blood urea nitrogen (BUN) may rise to dangerous levels, especially in patients with kidney dysfunction. If elevation of BUN exceeds normal limits, amino acid administration should be re-evaluated. In patients with liver disease, amino acid infusion may result in hepatic coma owing to accumulation of nitrogenous compounds. Caution must be exercised in patients with cirrhosis, viral hepatitis, or cancer of the liver.

Formulations. Amino acid solutions are available in general and specialized formulations. The general formulations consist of essential and nonessential amino acids; total amino acid concentrations range from 3.0% to 11.4%. Some mixtures also contain electrolytes. The general formulations will satisfy the nutritional requirements of most patients. Specialized products have been formulated to meet the unique needs of certain patients—specifically, patients in a state of high metabolic stress and patients experiencing liver failure or severe renal impairment. Special formulations are also available for pediatric patients.

Administration. The route of administration depends on the amino acid concentration. Solutions whose amino acid content exceeds 4% are very hypertonic and, as a result, will cause phlebitis if administered peripherally. Accordingly, these concentrated solutions must be administered through a central venous catheter. Solutions composed of less than 4% amino acids may be administered peripherally.

Dextrose

Nutritional Role. In order to utilize amino acids for conservation and synthesis of protein, the body requires a source of nonprotein calories. Dextrose (*d*-glucose) can provide these calories. For the average adult, daily requirements range from 25 to 35 kcal/kg, including those from protein.

Complications of Therapy. *Glucose intolerance* (hyperglycemia, glycosuria, osmotic diuresis) can occur. This response is most likely during the first few days of treatment. Glucose intolerance can be minimized by initiating therapy with low doses, followed by gradual dosage elevation. This progressive dosing permits the body to produce the extra amounts of insulin needed to process the abnormal glucose load. Glucose content of blood and urine should be measured every 6 hours until glucose tolerance has been demonstrated (usually within 2 to 3 days). If tolerance fails to develop, insulin can be added to the infusion mixture to control hyperglycemia. This IV insulin can be supplemented with SC insulin as needed. Special care must be exercised with diabetic patients.

Hypertonic solutions of dextrose may cause *thrombosis* if administered into a peripheral vein. Consequently, solutions in excess of 10% dextrose should be infused into a central venous catheter.

Because insulin levels are elevated during dextrose therapy, and because insulin promotes cellular uptake of potassium, infusion of dextrose may be accompanied by *hypokalemia*. Hypokalemia can be avoided by monitoring plasma potassium content and giving potassium as required.

If dextrose is abruptly discontinued, *hypoglycemia* may develop (because of continued release of endogenous insulin). Accordingly, dextrose should be withdrawn slowly: When infusion of hypertonic dextrose is stopped, infusion of 10% dextrose should be instituted and maintained for 1 to 2 hours.

Administration. Depending on their concentrations, dextrose solutions may be administered through a peripheral vein or centrally. Hypertonic solutions (i.e., solutions containing more than 10% dextrose) can be administered safely only through a central venous catheter. More dilute solutions may be given by peripheral infusion. Dextrose solutions may be mixed with amino acid solutions prior to administration.

Fat

Nutritional Role. Intravenous fat emulsions can serve two functions: (1) they can prevent or reverse essential fatty acid deficiency (EFAD) and (2) they can serve as a source of nonprotein calories. When the objective of treatment is avoidance or reversal of EFAD, fat emulsions are given in relatively small amounts (3% to 8% of total caloric intake). Much larger doses (up to 60% of total caloric intake) are used when fats are intended as a source of energy. When fats are administered for their caloric content, dextrose dosage must be reduced to keep total caloric intake constant.

Most fat emulsions are prepared from soybean oil. The principal components of these emulsions are linoleic, oleic, palmitic, linolenic, and stearic acids.

Complications of Therapy. Although fat emulsions are generally very safe, *death has occurred following administration to preterm infants.* Autopsy findings indicate fat accumulation within the blood vessels of the lungs. Intravenous fats should be administered slowly to preterm infants, and then only if the potential benefits clearly outweigh the risks.

The most common adverse effect of fat infusion is *hyperlipidemia*. This is especially likely in patients whose capacity to metabolize fats is impaired. Hyperlipidemia may also occur in patients with normal fat-metabolizing capacity if administration is too rapid or if too much dextrose is administered concurrently. Blood should be monitored for fat content to ensure that lipemia clears between infusions.

Administration. Fat emulsions are isotonic with plasma, and hence may be administered safely through a peripheral vein. Central administration may be performed as well. Some preparations may be mixed with amino acid and dextrose solutions. Others must be administered separately. Fat emulsions may be infused in the same vein as dextrose–amino acid

solutions. When this is done, the Y-connector through which the fat will flow should be placed *below* any in-line filter that may be present. This placement is needed because particles in fat emulsions are too large to pass through bacterial and particulate filters. Infusion of fat emulsion should be slow (0.5 to 1 ml/min) for the first 15 to 30 minutes. In the absence of adverse reactions (e.g., dyspnea, cyanosis, allergic responses), the infusion rate may then be increased.

Electrolytes, Vitamins, and Trace Elements

In addition to amino acids, carbohydrates, and fats, patients receiving parenteral nutrition must be supplied with vitamins, electrolytes (sodium, potassium, calcium, magnesium, phosphate), and trace elements (copper, chromium, iodine, manganese, molybdenum, selenium, zinc). These nutrients should be incorporated into the regimen from the onset of treatment. The pharmacology of electrolytes and vitamins is discussed in Chapters 40 and 76, respectively.

Preparation of Parenteral Nutrient Solutions

Parenteral nutrient solutions are prepared by mixing hypertonic dextrose with an amino acid solution. Vitamins, minerals, and electrolytes are added as indicated. Although a fat emulsion may also be added to this mixture, the usual practice is to administer fats separately. To prevent bacterial contamination, parenteral solutions should be prepared aseptically under a laminar-flow hood. Solutions should be stored under refrigeration and administered within 24 hours. Preparations that have become cloudy or darkened should be discarded. Drugs should not be added to solutions unless compatibility has been established.

Monitoring Treatment

Nutritional therapy is assessed through bedside examination, determination of blood and urine chemistries, and daily monitoring of weight, intake, and output. Weight measurement provides the best overall index of the efficacy of treatment. However, although weight gain can be a measure of success, be aware that large increases in weight (greater than 0.5 kg/day) may indicate excessive fluid retention. This possibility should be evaluated.

Blood and urine chemistries should be determined prior to treatment and throughout the period of nutritional support. Serum should be measured frequently for BUN, electrolytes, and glucose. To assess the response to treatment, albumin, cholesterol, and triglycerides should be measured weekly. Prothrombin time, platelet counts, and serum osmolarity should also be determined weekly. Blood for laboratory tests should *not* be drawn from the vein being used to infuse nutrients.

Complications of Treatment

The principal complications of parenteral nutritional therapy are infection and metabolic disturbances. Mechanical complications related to the catheter may also occur.

Infection. Patients receiving parenteral nutritional support are at constant risk of infection. This risk can be minimized by employing aseptic technique during catheter insertion and during preparation and administration of solutions. Risk of infection can be further reduced by using a central venous catheter that has been impregnated with antiseptics (chlorhexidine plus silver sulfadiazine). Use of a 0.22-micron filter can provide partial protection. A filter can hold back bacteria in the feeding solution, but cannot hold back bacterial endotoxins. Also, the filter can only retain bacteria that have entered the line at a site above the filter.

In the event of fever, sepsis should be suspected. To assess for sepsis, blood for culture should be drawn from the tip of the IV line as well as from a separate venous site. If temperature remains elevated and no cause can be found, the catheter and nutrient solution should be replaced and the tip of the catheter should be cultured for bacterial contamination. If the fever does not drop rapidly, antibiotic therapy should be instituted.

Metabolic Disturbances. The principal metabolic complications of parenteral nutritional therapy have been discussed. These include hyperglycemia, hypoglycemia, hyperlipidemia, and elevation of BUN. In addition, the patient may experience overhydration, dehydration, acid-base imbalance, electrolyte imbalance, and deficiencies in trace elements and vitamins.

Catheter-Related Complications. Infusion into a peripheral vein may produce phlebitis at or near the site of catheter insertion. If this occurs, the catheter should be moved. The risk of phlebitis can be reduced by selecting a large peripheral vein and by infusing the nutrient solution slowly. Other catheter-related complications include pneumothorax (caused by insertion of a central catheter) and central venous thrombosis.

⠿ KEY POINTS

- Enteral nutritional therapy can be defined as nutritional support administered via tube into the GI tract.
- For short-term therapy, enteral feeding tubes are inserted through the nose; for long-term therapy, tubes are surgically implanted directly into the esophagus, stomach, or jejunum.
- Enteral nutritional solutions may be delivered to the feeding tube with (1) a syringe; (2) a gravity method (employing a drip chamber or rate controller); or (3) an enteral infusion pump.
- The major complication of enteral nutritional therapy is aspiration pneumonitis.
- Parenteral nutrition is administered via a central venous catheter (for long-term therapy or for hypertonic feeding solutions) or a peripheral vein (for short-term therapy or for dilute feeding solutions).
- With parenteral nutritional therapy, glucose intolerance may occur during the first few days (until the pancreas increases insulin release).
- The fat component of peripheral nutritional solutions can cause death in premature infants.
- Parenteral nutritional therapy poses a significant risk of infection.
- Enteral and parenteral nutritional solutions consist of amino acids, carbohydrates, fats, electrolytes, vitamins, and trace elements.

Drugs for Obesity

Obesity is a public health epidemic. In the United States, nearly two-thirds (64.5%) of adults and 15.5% of teens are overweight or obese—and the numbers continue to climb. Excessive body fat increases the risk of morbidity from hypertension, heart disease, stroke, type 2 diabetes, gallbladder disease, osteoarthritis, sleep apnea, and certain cancers. Among women, obesity also increases the risk of menstrual irregularities, amenorrhea, and polycystic ovary syndrome; during pregnancy, obesity increases the risk of morbidity and mortality for both the mother and child. Obesity-related disorders kill about 300,000 Americans a year, making obesity second only to smoking as the leading cause of preventable death.

Obesity is now viewed as a chronic disease, much like hypertension and diabetes. Despite intensive research, the underlying cause remains incompletely understood. Contributing factors include genetics, metabolism, and appetite regulation, along with environmental, psychosocial, and cultural factors. Although obese people can lose weight, the tendency to regain weight cannot be eliminated. Put another way, obesity cannot yet be cured. Accordingly, for most patients, lifelong management is indicated.

In 1998, the National Heart, Lung, and Blood Institute (NHLBI) in cooperation with the National Institute of Diabetes and Digestive and Kidney Diseases, released the first federal clinical guidelines on obesity, titled *Clinical Guidelines on the Identification, Evaluation, and Treatment of Overweight and Obesity in Adults: Evidence Report.* Two years later, the NHLBI, in cooperation with the North American Association for the Study of Obesity, released a companion document—*The Practical Guide: Identification, Evaluation, and Treatment of Overweight and Obesity in Adults*—to give clinicians specific tools to help their patients lose weight

and keep it off. Much of our discussion is based on these two documents. The first is available online at *www.nhlbi.nih.gov/ guidelines/obesity/ob_gdlns.htm,* and the second at *www.nhlbi. nih.gov/guidelines/obesity/practgde.htm.*

ASSESSMENT OF OBESITY-RELATED HEALTH RISK

Health risk is determined by (1) the degree of obesity (as reflected in the body mass index), (2) the pattern of fat distribution (as reflected in the waist circumference measurement), and (3) the presence of obesity-related diseases and/or cardiovascular risk factors. Accordingly, all three factors must be assessed when establishing a treatment plan.

Body Mass Index. The body mass index (BMI), which is derived from the patient's weight and height, is a simple way to estimate body fat content. Studies indicate a close correlation between BMI and total body fat. The BMI is calculated by dividing a patient's weight (in kilograms) by the square of the patient's height (in meters). Hence, BMI is expressed in units of kg/m^2. BMI can also be calculated using the patient's weight in *pounds* and height in *inches* (Fig. 78–1). According to the federal guidelines, a BMI of 30 or higher indicates obesity. Individuals with a BMI of 25 to 29.9 are considered overweight, but not obese. There is good evidence that the risk of cardiovascular disease and other disorders rises significantly when the BMI exceeds 25. When the BMI exceeds 30, there is an increased risk of death. These specific associations between BMI and health risk do not apply to growing children, women who are pregnant or lactating, and competitive athletes or body builders, who are heavy because of muscle mass rather than excess fat. Table 78–1 summarizes weight classifications based on BMI.

Waist Circumference. Waist circumference (WC) is an indicator of *abdominal* fat content, an independent risk factor for obesity-related diseases. Accumulation of fat in the upper body, and especially within the abdominal cavity, poses a greater risk to health than does accumulation of fat in the lower body (hips and thighs). People with too much abdominal fat are at increased risk of insulin resistance, diabetes, hypertension, coronary atherosclerosis, and ischemic stroke. Fat distribution can be estimated simply by looking in the mirror: an apple shape indicates too much abdominal fat, whereas a pear shape indicates fat on the hips and thighs. Measurement of WC provides a quantitative estimate of abdominal fat. A WC exceeding 40 inches (102 cm) in men or 35 inches (88 cm) in women signifies an increased health risk—but only for people with a BMI between 25 and 34.9 (see Table 78–1).

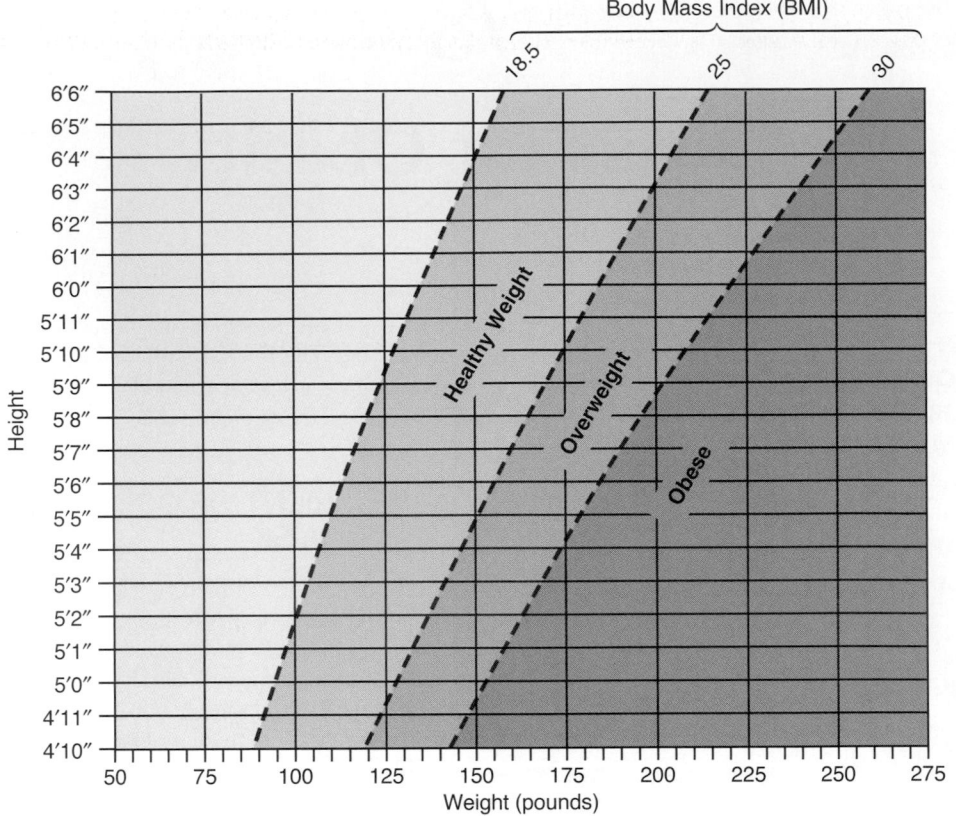

Body Mass Index (BMI)

Directions: Find your weight on the bottom of the graph. Go straight up from that point until you come to the line that matches your height. Then look to find your weight group.

- **Healthy Weight:** BMI from 18.5 to 24.9
- **Overweight:** BMI from 25 to 29.9
- **Obese:** BMI 30 or higher

Figure 78–1 ■ **Weight classification based on Body Mass Index (BMI).**

Risk Status. Overall obesity-related health risk is determined by BMI, WC, and the presence of obesity-related diseases and cardiovascular risk factors. Certain obesity-related diseases—established coronary heart disease, other atherosclerotic diseases, type 2 diabetes, and sleep apnea—confer a very high risk for complications and mortality. Other obesity-related diseases—gynecologic abnormalities, osteoarthritis, gallstones, and stress incontinence—confer less risk. Cardiovascular risk factors—smoking, hypertension, high levels of low-density lipoprotein (LDL) cholesterol, low levels of high-density lipoprotein (HDL) cholesterol, high fasting glucose, family history of premature coronary heart disease, physical inactivity, and advancing age—confer a high risk when three or more of these factors are present.

Not surprisingly, health risk rises as BMI gets larger (see Table 78–1). In addition, the risk is increased by the presence of an excessive WC. The risk is further increased by obesity-related diseases and cardiovascular risk factors. In the absence of an excessive WC and other risk factors, health risk is minimal with a BMI below 25, and relatively low with a BMI below 30. Conversely, a BMI of 30 or more indicates significant risk. In the presence of an excessive WC, health risk is high for all individuals with a BMI above 25.

OVERVIEW OF OBESITY TREATMENT

The strategy for losing weight is simple: take in fewer calories per day than are burned. Of course, implementation is tough. The key components of a weight loss program are diet and exercise. Drugs and other measures are employed only as adjuncts.

Who Should be Treated?

Accordingly to the federal guidelines, weight loss therapy is indicated for people with

- A BMI of 30 or more
- A BMI of 25 to 25.9 *plus* two risk factors
- A WC greater than 40 inches (in men) or greater than 35 inches (in women) *plus* two risk factors

Benefits of Treatment

It is well established that obesity increases morbidity and mortality. It is also well established that weight reduction reduces morbidity, and probably mortality. In overweight and obese people, weight reduction confers the following proven benefits:

- Reduction of high blood pressure in patients with hypertension

TABLE 78–1 ⁝■ Disease Risk Based on BMI and WC

BMI (kg/m²)	Weight Class	Obesity Class	Disease Risk* Nonexcessive WC†	Disease Risk* Excessive WC‡
<18.5	Underweight	—	—	—
18.5–24.9	Normal	—	—	—
25.0–29.9	Overweight	—	Increased	High
30.0–34.9	Obesity	I	High	Very high
35.0–39.9	Obesity	II	Very high	Very high
40 or more	Extreme obesity	III	Extremely high	Extremely high

*Risk for hypertension, cardiovascular disease, and type 2 diabetes, relative to individuals of normal weight.
†Nonexcessive WC = waist circumference of 40 inches or less for men, and 35 inches or less for women.
‡Excessive WC = waist circumference above 40 inches for men, and above 35 inches for women.
Adapted from National Institutes of Health, National Heart, Lung and Blood Institute, Obesity Education Initiative. Clinical Guidelines on the Identification, Evaluation, and Treatment of Overweight and Obesity in Adults, Bethesda, MD, National Institutes of Health, 1998.

- Improvement of blood lipid status (elevation of HDL cholesterol and reduction of LDL cholesterol, total cholesterol, and triglycerides)
- Reduction of elevated blood glucose in patients with type 2 diabetes.

To date, no prospective trials have been conducted to determine if weight loss actually reduces mortality. However, given that weight loss reduces risk factors for cardiovascular disease and diabetes, it seems likely that it also reduces mortality.

Treatment Goal

The goal of treatment is to promote and maintain weight loss. The initial objective is to reduce weight by 10% over 6 months. For patients with a BMI of 27 to 35, this can usually be achieved by reducing energy intake by 300 to 500 kcal/day, which should allow a loss of 0.5 to 1 pound a week—or 13 to 26 pounds in 6 months. More severely obese people (BMI above 35) require greater caloric restriction (500 to 1000 kcal/day) to lose 10% of their weight in 6 months. After 6 months, the goal for all patients is to prevent lost weight from returning. This can be accomplished by a combination of diet, physical activity, and behavioral therapy. If appropriate, additional weight reduction can be attempted.

Treatment Modalities

Weight loss can be accomplished with five treatment modalities: diet therapy, physical activity, behavior therapy, drug therapy, and surgery. For any individual, the treatment mode is determined by the degree of obesity and personal preference.

Diet Therapy. A reduced-calorie diet is central to any weight loss program. As noted, the only way to lose weight is to take in fewer calories than we burn. Depending on the individual, the caloric deficit should range from 300 to 1000 kcal/day. Because fats contain more calories than either carbohydrates or proteins (on an ounce-for-ounce basis), reducing dietary fat is the most practical way to reduce caloric intake. Accordingly, no more than 30% of total calories should come from fat. Also, when reducing fat intake, patients should focus on saturated fats, which elevate LDL cholesterol. As a rule, the desired caloric deficit cannot be achieved by decreasing fat intake alone; carbohydrate intake must be decreased too.

Exercise. Physical activity should be a component of all weight loss and weight maintenance programs. Exercise makes a modest contribution to weight loss by increasing energy expenditure. In addition, exercise can help reduce abdominal fat, increase cardiorespiratory fitness, and maintain weight loss once loss has occurred. Initially, patients should try to perform 30 to 45 minutes of moderate exercise 3 to 5 days a week. The long-range goal is to exercise 30 minutes or more on most (preferably all) days of the week.

Behavior Modification. Behavior therapy is directed at modifying eating and exercise habits. As such, behavior therapy can strengthen a program of diet and exercise. In the absence of continuing behavior therapy, most patients regain lost weight when treatment stops. Techniques of behavior therapy include self-monitoring of eating and exercise habits, stress management (because stress can trigger eating), and stimulus control (limiting exposure to stimuli that promote eating). There is no evidence that any one of these techniques is superior to others.

Drug Therapy. Drugs can be used as an adjunct to diet and exercise—but only for people at increased health risk, and only after a 6-month program of diet and exercise has failed. Drugs should never be used alone. Rather, they should be part of a comprehensive weight reduction program—one that includes exercise, behavior modification, and a reduced-calorie diet.

Candidates for drug therapy should be at increased health risk owing to excessive body fat. Specifically, drugs should be reserved for patients whose BMI is 30 or greater (in the absence of additional risk factors), or 27 or greater (in the presence of additional risk factors). Drugs are not appropriate for patients whose BMI is relatively low.

Benefits of drugs are usually modest. Weight loss attributable to drugs generally ranges between 4.4 and 22 pounds, although some people lose significantly more. As a rule, the majority of weight loss occurs during the first 6 months of treatment.

Expert opinion regarding duration of therapy has changed. In the past, drug use was limited to a few months. Today, however, long-term treatment is recommended. Why? Because we now know that, when drugs are discontinued, most patients regain lost weight. This is similar to the return of high blood pressure when antihypertensive drugs are withdrawn. Accordingly, when treatment has been effective and well tolerated, it should continue indefinitely. At this time, only two drugs—sibutramine and orlistat—are approved for long-term use, and hence are preferred to all other agents.

Not everyone responds to drugs, and hence regular assessment is required. Patients should lose at least 4 pounds during the first 4 weeks of drug treatment. If this initial response is absent, further drug use should be questioned. For patients who *do* respond, ongoing assessment must show that (1) the drug is effective at *maintaining* weight loss weight, and that (2) serious adverse effects are absent. Otherwise, drug therapy should cease.

In theory, drugs can promote weight loss in three ways: They can suppress appetite, reduce absorption of nutrients, or increase metabolic rate. With one exception—orlistat—all of the drugs currently approved for obesity work by suppressing appetite. Orlistat works by reducing absorption of fat. None of the available drugs increases metabolic rate.

Surgery. Surgical procedures can produce substantial weight loss. However, they are indicated only for severely obese patients—that is, people with a BMI of 40 or more (in the absence of comorbidity) or 35 or more (in the presence of comorbidity). Furthermore, surgery should be reserved for patients who have failed to respond to less invasive therapies and who are at high risk for obesity-related morbidity or mortality. The two most widely used procedures are gastric resection (vertical banded gastroplasty) and gastric bypass (Roux-en-Y). Unlike surgeries used in the past, which were designed to reduce nutrient absorption, these procedures are designed to reduce food consumption. Surgery is highly effective: In 6 months to a year, patients can loose between 110 pounds and 220 pounds. Furthermore, benefits are sustained.

WEIGHT-LOSS DRUGS I: DRUGS APPROVED FOR LONG-TERM THERAPY

At this time, sibutramine and orlistat are the only antiobesity drugs approved for long-term use. Sibutramine promotes weight loss by suppressing appetite, and orlistat decreases absorption of fats. Because management of obesity requires prolonged treatment, these two drugs are preferred to all others.

Sibutramine, an Appetite Suppressant
Actions and Use

Sibutramine [Meridia], in combination with a reduced-calorie diet, is indicated for promoting and maintaining weight loss in obese people. Candidates should have a BMI of 30 or greater (in the absence of other risk factors), or 27 or greater (in the presence of other risk factors, such as hypertension, diabetes, or hyperlipidemia). Sibutramine promotes weight loss by *suppressing appetite,* and possibly by increasing metabolic rate. The underlying mechanism is blockade of serotonin (5-hydroxytryptamine [5-HT]) and norepinephrine (NE) reuptake, which increases availability of these transmitters at synapses in the brain. Like other drugs that increase concentrations of 5-HT and/or NE, sibutramine has antidepressant actions.

In clinical trials, sibutramine was moderately effective. In one 6-month trial, subjects taking sibutramine (5, 10, 15, or 20 mg/day) lost 6.8, 9.7, 11.7, and 12.8 pounds, respectively, compared with 2.0 pounds for subjects taking placebo. In a 12-month trial, subjects taking sibutramine (10 or 15 mg/day) lost 10 pounds and 14 pounds, respectively, compared with 3.5 pounds for those taking placebo. As a rule, early responders to sibutramine—that is, those who lost at least 4 pounds during the first 4 weeks of treatment—do better than late responders. The safety and efficacy of sibutramine beyond 1 year of use has not been studied.

Pharmacokinetics

Sibutramine is well absorbed following oral administration. On its first pass through the liver, the drug is rapidly converted into two active metabolites by the 3A4 isozyme of cytochrome P450 (CYP3A4). Concentrations of the metabolites peak in 3 to 4 hours, and decline with half-lives of 14 to 16 hours. The metabolites undergo enzymatic inactivation followed by excretion in the urine.

Adverse Effects

The most common adverse effects are headache (30%), dry mouth (17%), constipation (11.5%), and central nervous system (CNS) stimulation, manifested as insomnia (10.7%), nervousness (5.2%), and anxiety (4.5%). Unlike two other serotonergic drugs—fenfluramine and dexfenfluramine (see below)—sibutramine has not been associated with valvular heart disease or primary pulmonary hypertension. Sibutramine has a low potential for abuse, and hence is classified under Schedule IV of the Controlled Substances Act (CSA).

Sibutramine can *elevate blood pressure.* For most patients, the increase is small, only 1 to 3 mm Hg. However, in a few patients, a substantial increase has occurred. Accordingly, blood pressure should be measured before treatment and periodically thereafter. Sibutramine should be avoided in patients with uncontrolled hypertension or with a history of coronary artery disease, heart failure, dysrhythmias, or stroke.

Sibutramine can *increase heart rate.* For most patients, the increase is small, only 4 to 5 beats/min. Rarely, patients develop tachycardia (heart rate above 100 beats/min).

Drug Interactions

Serotonergic Agents. Combining sibutramine with another serotonergic drug may cause *serotonin syndrome,* a potentially fatal reaction characterized by incoordination, myoclonus, hyperreflexia, tremor, fever, sweating, and mental changes (e.g., agitation, anxiety, hallucinations). Accordingly, sibutramine should not be used with other drugs that enhance serotonergic transmission. Among these are *selective serotonin reuptake inhibitors* (e.g., fluoxetine [Prozac]), *serotonin agonists taken for migraine* (e.g., sumatriptan [Imitrex]), and *lithium.* Certain opioids—including meperidine [Demerol], fentanyl [Sublimaze], and pentazocine [Talwin]—also increase the risk of serotonin syndrome, and hence should be avoided.

Monoamine Oxidase Inhibitors. By blocking reuptake of norepinephrine, sibutramine can increase the risk of hypertensive crisis in patients taking monoamine oxidase inhibitors (MAOIs). Accordingly, MAOIs should be withdrawn at least 2 weeks before starting sibutramine, and sibutramine should be discontinued at least 2 weeks before staring an MAOI.

Sympathomimetics. Because sibutramine can elevate blood pressure, it should be used cautiously with other drugs that raise blood pressure. Among these are ephedrine and pseudoephedrine—drugs that are commonly found in over-the-counter (OTC) remedies for colds, allergies, and nasal congestion. Amphetamines should also be avoided.

Cytochrome P450 3A4 Inhibitors. In theory, drugs such as ketoconazole and erythromycin, which inhibit CYP3A4, could slow the metabolism of sibutramine, and thereby alter its effects. However, in actual practice, this interaction appears insignificant.

Preparations, Dosage, and Administration

Sibutramine [Meridia] is available in 5-, 10-, and 15-mg capsules for oral use. The recommended initial dosage is 10 mg once a day, administered in the morning to minimize insomnia. For patients who fail to lose at least 4 pounds in the first 4 weeks, the clinician should consider either increasing the dosage to 15 mg daily or discontinuing treatment. Dosages above 15 mg/day should be avoided.

Although sibutramine is usually taken continuously, a recent study found that intermittent dosing is just as effective. In this study, patients took sibutramine on a repeating cycle consisting of once-daily dosing for 12 weeks followed by 6 weeks off.

Orlistat, a Lipase Inhibitor

Actions and Use. Orlistat [Xenical] is a novel drug for promoting and maintaining weight loss. Unlike most other weight-loss drugs, which act in the brain to curb appetite, orlistat acts in the GI tract to reduce absorption of fat. Specifically, the drug acts in the stomach and small intestine to inhibit gastric and pancreatic lipases, enzymes that break down triglycerides into monoglycerides and free fatty acids. If triglycerides are not broken down, they can't be absorbed. In patients taking orlistat, absorption of dietary fat is reduced by about 30%. Like sibutramine, orlistat should be reserved for patients with a BMI of at least 30—or 27 in the presence of other risk factors (e.g., diabetes, hypertension, hyperlipidemia). Patients must adopt a reduced-calorie diet in which 30% of calories come from fat.

In clinical trials, orlistat produced modest but sustained benefits. When taken for 2 years, the drug enhanced weight loss, reduced regain of lost weight, and improved some obesity-related risk factors. Patients treated for 2 years lost an average of 19 pounds, compared with 12 pounds for those taking placebo. In addition, treatment reduced total and LDL cholesterol, raised HDL cholesterol, reduced fasting blood glucose, and lowered systolic and diastolic blood pressure. Safety and efficacy beyond 2 years of treatment have not been evaluated.

Adverse Effects and Interactions. Orlistat undergoes minimal (<1%) absorption, and hence systemic effects are absent. In contrast, GI effects are common. Patients frequently experience oily spotting (27%), flatulence with discharge (24%), fecal urgency (22%), fatty or oily stools (20%), oily evacuation (12%), increased defecation (11%), and fecal incontinence (8%). All of these result directly from effects on dietary fats, and all can be minimized by reducing fat intake. For many patients, these unpleasant effects provide strong motivation for adhering to a low-fat diet, and hence may be viewed as beneficial as well as adverse. Recent data indicate that daily doses of psyllium [Metamucil, others], a bulk-forming laxative, can greatly reduce the GI effects of orlistat. The underlying mechanism is absorption of dietary fat.

By reducing fat absorption, orlistat can reduce absorption of fat-soluble vitamins (vitamins A, D, E, and K). To avoid deficiency, patients should take a daily multivitamin supplement. Administration should be done 2 hours before or 2 hours after taking orlistat.

Vitamin K deficiency can intensify the effects of warfarin, an anticoagulant. In patients taking warfarin, anticoagulant effects should be monitored closely.

Orlistat is contraindicated for patients with malabsorption syndrome or cholestasis.

Preparations, Dosage, and Administration. Orlistat is available in 120-mg capsules. The dosage is 120 mg 3 times a day. Each dose should be administered during a major meal or up to 1 hour after. There is no benefit to exceeding three daily doses. Orlistat dosing can be omitted if a meal is missed, or if a meal has little or no fat.

WEIGHT-LOSS DRUGS II: MISCELLANEOUS AGENTS

In this section, we consider one group of drugs—appetite suppressants—and two individual agents: metformin and leptin. None of these drugs is approved for long-term therapy of obesity. In fact, most of them are not approved for obesity therapy at all, be it long-term *or* short-term.

Appetite Suppressants

The family of appetite suppressants consists of sibutramine (discussed above) along with the sympathomimetics and other drugs discussed here. Sibutramine is the only appetite suppressant approved for long-term therapy, and hence is preferred to the drugs below.

Sympathomimetic Amines

The sympathomimetic amines act primarily by increasing availability of NE at receptors in the brain. The result is a decrease in appetite. These drugs are approved for short-term use only (3 months or less). The sympathomimetics fall into two major groups: amphetamines and nonamphetamines. The amphetamines have a higher abuse potential than the nonamphetamines. Accordingly, nonamphetamines are preferred. All of these drugs can increase heart rate and blood pressure, and hence must be used with caution in patients with cardiovascular disease. In addition, all are CNS stimulants, and hence can interfere with sleep.

Nonamphetamines. At this time, only four nonamphetamine sympathomimetics are available: *benzphetamine, diethylpropion, phendimetrazine,* and *phentermine*. All four require a prescription. Trade names and dosages are summarized in Table 78–2.

All nonamphetamines are CNS stimulants. Consequently, like the amphetamines, they can increase alertness, decrease fatigue, and induce nervousness and insomnia. Because they can interfere with sleep, these drugs should be administered no later than 4:00 PM. Upon discontinuation of treatment, fatigue and depression may replace CNS stimulation.

Like the amphetamines, most of the nonamphetamines have effects in the periphery as well as the CNS. Peripheral effects of greatest concern are tachycardia, anginal pain, and hypertension. Accordingly, these drugs should be used with caution in patients with cardiovascular disease.

Although the risk of abuse with the nonamphetamine anorexiants is lower than with the amphetamines, abuse can nonetheless occur. As indicted in Table 78–2, all of these drugs are regulated by the CSA, under Schedule III or Schedule IV. To reduce the risk of abuse, an attempt should be made to identify abuse-prone patients prior to treatment.

Tolerance is common and may be seen in 6 to 12 weeks. Tolerance to the anorexiant effects of one agent produces cross-tolerance to the others. If tolerance develops, the appropriate response is to discontinue the drug rather than increase the dosage.

For two reasons, these drugs are not recommended for use during pregnancy. First, they are not very effective during pregnancy; hence there is little point in taking them. Second, *in utero* exposure to these agents poses an increased risk of cleft palate and congenital heart defects.

Phenylpropanolamine. Phenylpropanolamine (PPA) is a nonamphetamine sympathomimetic agent that, until recently, was widely available in OTC cold remedies and weight-loss products. The drug is effective for both applications, and had been considered safe. However, data from a new study—*Phenylpropanolamine and Risk of Hemorrhagic Stroke: Final Report of the Hemorrhagic Stroke Project*—indicate that systemic therapy with PPA significantly increases the risk of hemorrhagic stroke in women (but not in men). On the basis of this information, the Food and Drug Administration (FDA) concluded that the benefits from using PPA for nasal decongestion or weight loss do not justify exposing users to the risk of stroke—even though

TABLE 78–2 ■ Sympathomimetic Appetite Suppressants			
Generic Name	**Trade Name**	**Adult Dosage**	**CSA* Schedule**
Benzphetamine	Didrex	25–50 mg 1–3 times a day	III
Diethylpropion	Tenuate, Tepanil	25 mg tid 1 hr before meals *or*, for sustained-release pills, 75 mg once a day in midmorning	IV
Phendimetrazine	Bontril, Plegine, Prelu-2, X-Trozine	35 mg bid or tid 1 hr before meals *or*, for sustained-release pills, 105 mg qd before breakfast	III
Phentermine	Adipex-P, Ionamin, Fastin, others	8 mg tid 30 min before meals *or* 15–37.5 mg qd before breakfast	IV

*CSA = Controlled Substances Act.

that risk is very small. Accordingly, on November 6, 2000, the FDA ordered manufacturers to remove PPA from all *OTC* cold remedies and weight-loss products. (Removal of PPA from prescription products is under review.) For people with colds, there are many OTC alternatives to PPA. In contrast, for people trying to lose weight, there is no OTC alternative to PPA: All other weight-loss drugs require a prescription. At this time, we do not know if other sympathomimetics, which share the same mechanism as PPA, also pose a risk of stroke.

Amphetamines. Because of their ability to suppress appetite, the amphetamines have been employed as adjunctive aids in programs for weight loss. However, because of their high abuse potential, and because they offer no advantages over less dangerous drugs, amphetamines are not recommended—nor are they approved by the FDA for either short-term or long-term therapy of obesity.

Bupropion

Bupropion [Wellbutrin, Zyban] is under investigation for use in obesity. The drug is currently approved for depression (see Chapter 31) and as an aid to smoking cessation (see Chapter 38). Like sibutramine, bupropion blocks reuptake of NE and 5-HT, and thereby reduces appetite. In a small trial, 31 women on a reduced-calorie diet were treated with bupropion or placebo. Their average weight before treatment was 222 pounds. After 8 weeks, the 18 women who took bupropion lost, on average, 6.2% of their body weight (13.8 pounds), compared with 1.5% (3.5 pounds) for the 13 women who took placebo. We don't know if benefits of treatment will be sustained. The basic pharmacology of bupropion is discussed in Chapter 31.

Dexfenfluramine and Fenfluramine

Dexfenfluramine and fenfluramine—two highly effective appetite suppressants—can damage valves of the heart. Accordingly, on September 15, 1997, they were voluntarily withdrawn from the market. Although these drugs are no longer available, they are discussed here because some former users remain at risk of complications.

Dexfenfluramine. Dexfenfluramine [Redux] hit the market in 1996, and became an instant success. At the time, it was the only drug approved for long-term therapy of obesity, and millions took it. Unfortunately, a serious side effect—valvular heart disease—soon became apparent. As a result, dexfenfluramine was withdrawn—only 16 months after its debut.

In 1997, physicians at the Mayo Clinic reported that dexfenfluramine can cause valvular heart disease. Echocardiographic examination of patients taking the drug indicated a 30% incidence of regurgitation involving the mitral, aortic, and/or tricuspid valves. Although most patients with valve injury were asymptomatic, some displayed symptoms of heart failure (dyspnea, fatigue, edema). A few required surgery to correct valve leakage.

Subsequent studies confirmed that dexfenfluramine can damage the heart. However, these studies also indicated that valve damage is less common and less severe than originally suspected. Furthermore, there is evidence that, in some patients, the damage can heal—at least in part. Clinically significant valve damage is most likely with long-term, high-dose treatment. Injury is unlikely with short-term treatment (<3 months). Altogether, the data indicate that, although the risk of valve damage is real, clinically significant damage is uncommon, and serious problems are rare.

What should former users of dexfenfluramine do? (1) All patients should undergo clinical evaluation for signs and symptoms of heart disease. (2) Echocardiography is recommended for all patients with clinical evidence of valvular disease (e.g., heart murmur), to ascertain the extent of injury. In addition, echocardiography should be considered for all patients who took the drug in high doses or for more than 3 months. (3) Regardless of cardiac signs and symptoms, echocardiography should be considered for all patients anticipating dental and surgical procedures that can cause transient bacteremia. Why? Because, in patients with valvular heart disease, bacteremia can lead to bacterial endocarditis. Hence, it is important to know whether or not valvular disease exists. If valve damage is confirmed, the patient should receive prophylactic antibiotic therapy prior to the dental or surgical procedure.

Fenfluramine. Fenfluramine [Pondimin] is a racemic mixture of *d*-fenfluramine (dexfenfluramine) and *l*-fenfluramine. Only the *d*-isomer is active. Accordingly, the pharmacologic profile of fenfluramine is nearly identical to that of dexfenfluramine. Like dexfenfluramine, fenfluramine carries a risk of valvular heart disease, and hence has been withdrawn from the market. Patient follow-up is the same as for dexfenfluramine (see above). Prior to being withdrawn, fenfluramine was frequently prescribed in combination with phentermine (see below).

Fenfluramine Plus Phentermine (Fen-Phen)

Prior to 1997, when fenfluramine was withdrawn from the market, it was common practice to treat patients with a combination of fenfluramine (a serotonergic agent) and phentermine (a sympathomimetic agent)—although the combination, commonly known as "fen-phen," was never approved by the FDA. (Phentermine and other sympathomimetics are discussed above.) In theory, fen-phen has two potential benefits. First, since fenfluramine and phentermine act by different mechanisms, the combination might suppress appetite while allowing both drugs to be given in reduced dosages, thereby decreasing side effects. Second, since fenfluramine and phentermine have opposing effects on arousal (fenfluramine causes drowsiness whereas phentermine causes stimulation), combined therapy might neutralize both effects. As discussed above, fenfluramine has caused valvular heart disease, and hence is no longer available. In contrast, phentermine does not injure the heart, and hence is still on the market. Some clinicians are now prescribing "phen-pro"—a combination of phentermine with fluoxetine [Prozac]. Like fenfluramine, fluoxetine increases the concentration of serotonin at brain synapses.

Metformin

Metformin [Glucophage], a drug approved for type 2 diabetes, is under investigation as an aid to weight loss in nondiabetic adults and children. In a study involving overweight nondiabetic women, subjects who combined metformin with a low-calorie diet lost 20 to 30 pounds in 12 months. Although the mechanism underlying weight loss is unknown, a likely possibility is increased insulin sensitivity and reduced insulin levels. (Overweight people often have elevated insulin levels, which increase appetite and promote fat storage, and thereby oppose attempts to lose weight.) The most common side effect of metformin is diarrhea. The most serious side effect is lactic acidosis, which develops most often in patients with heart failure, renal insufficiency, pulmonary dysfunction, or liver disease. Accordingly, metformin is contraindicated for these people. The basic pharmacology of metformin is discussed in Chapter 54.

TABLE 78–3 ▪ Calorie-Free Sugar Substitutes

Generic Name	Trade Name	Relative Sweetness*	Heat Stability	Comments
Saccharin	Sweet 'N Low	300	Good	Bitter aftertaste. High doses cause bladder cancer in rats, but there is no evidence of cancer in humans. OK for cooking.
Aspartame	NutraSweet, Equal	180	Poor	No aftertaste. Made of two amino acids: aspartate and phenylalanine. Phenylalanine makes it dangerous for phenylketonurics. Because of poor heat stability, it is not good for cooking.
Sucralose	Splenda	600	Very good	No aftertaste. The only low-calorie sweetener derived from sucrose. Very heat stable, and hence excellent for cooking.
Acesulfame	Sunett, Sweet One	200	Good	No aftertaste. Derived from acetoacetic acid. OK for cooking.
Neotame		8000	Good	No aftertaste. OK for cooking.

*Intensity of sweetness relative to sucrose (e.g., saccharin is 300 times sweeter than sucrose).

Leptin

In 1994, Jeffrey Friedman of Rockefeller University announced the discovery of leptin, a hormone the helps regulate appetite and energy metabolism. In addition, leptin participates in sexual development. The name *leptin* derives from *leptos,* the Greek word for thin. Mice and humans that lack the gene for leptin are obese. For this reason, leptin is also known as the *antiobesity hormone.*

The physiology of leptin is only partly understood. The hormone is released by adipocytes (fat cells) when they fill with fat. Leptin then acts in the hypothalamus to reduce appetite, increase physical activity, and increase fat metabolism. These actions serve to halt further fat accumulation. Hence, the leptin system behaves like a typical feedback loop: When fat storage climbs too high, leptin is released and suppresses further storage; when fat storage falls too low, leptin release is suppressed, allowing more fat to accumulate. The evolutionary purpose of this system is unknown, although there are two obvious possibilities: it may serve to protect against storing too much fat, or it may serve to ensure storage of sufficient fat.

Genetic deficiency of leptin causes extreme obesity. Congenital deficiency is characterized by hyperphagia (overeating), excessive weight gain early in life, and severe obesity. In addition, sexual development is delayed. In 1999, researchers from England described the effects of leptin deficiency and leptin replacement therapy in a young girl. The child had a normal weight at birth, but began gaining excessive weight after 4 months. She was constantly hungry (despite hyperphagia), demanded food continuously, and expressed great discontent when food was denied. By age 6, she weighed 125 pounds and needed leg liposuction to improve mobility. By age 9, she weighed 208 pounds. At that time, she began daily SC injections of leptin. Within a week, her appetite subsided. After 1 year, she had lost 36 pounds, almost all of it fat. Interestingly, she also showed signs of early puberty. (As noted, leptin stimulates sexual development.) This was the first report that leptin replacement is effective in a leptin-deficient person.

Unlike the girl just described, the vast majority of obese people have no problem making leptin. In fact, their leptin levels are usually *high*—not low, as might be expected. High levels suggest leptin resistance. Possible causes include failure to produce enough leptin receptors or production of receptors that are faulty.

Leptin is now undergoing trials in obese people. Reports to date indicate the drug is safe but only moderately effective. One study enrolled 73 subjects who weighed an average of 200 pounds. Every day, subjects gave themselves an SC injection of leptin or placebo. After 6 months, leptin users had lost 15 pounds—all of it fat—compared with 3 pounds for those injecting placebo. The principal adverse effect was local discomfort (redness, itching, and swelling) at the injection site. Among subjects using the highest leptin doses, local discomfort led one-third to discontinue treatment.

CALORIE-SAVING FOODS

Sugar Substitutes
Calorie-Free Sweeteners

Five non-nutritive sweeteners are available: *saccharin* [Sweet 'N Low], *aspartame* [NutraSweet, Equal], *sucralose* [Splenda], *acesulfame* [Sunett], and *neotame* (no trade name yet). Their calorie content is negligible. As indicated in Table 78–3, all five are much sweeter than sucrose (table sugar), when compared on an ounce-for-ounce basis. With the exception of aspartame, which is unstable at high heat, all can be used for cooking. These sweeteners are present in literally thousands of commercial food products, including soft drinks, alcoholic beverages, canned goods, baked goods, candies, and various deserts. For people trying to lose pounds or keep them off, switching to foods made with these sweeteners may help.

Calorie-free sweeteners have been used extensively for years, and have proved very safe. At very high doses, saccharin can cause bladder cancer in rats. However, at the doses consumed in the diet, there is no evidence that it causes cancer in humans. Aspartame contains phenylalanine, and hence can be harmful to people with phenylketonuria. All of these sweeteners are safe for people with diabetes. There is no evidence to support rumors that aspartame contributes to multiple sclerosis, systemic lupus erythematosus, Alzheimer's disease, and other disorders.

Tagatose, A Reduced-Calorie Sweetener

Tagatose is a naturally occurring sugar with properties much like those of sucrose—but with only 38% of the calories. Tagatose tastes like sucrose and, unlike saccharin, has no bitter aftertaste. When used for cooking and baking, tagatose behaves the same as sucrose. Tagatose received FDA approval in October 2001.

Olestra, a Fat Substitute

Olestra [Olean] is a nonabsorbable, calorie-free fat substitute used to make potato chips, corn chips, crackers, and other snack foods. Olestra cannot be broken down by pancreatic enzymes, and hence cannot be absorbed. As a result, it provides no dietary fat or calories.

Olestra is very well tolerated. Two randomized, double-blind trials failed to support anecdotal reports of olestra-induced GI symptoms. In one trial, subjects were given a large bag of potato chips—fried in olestra or a traditional fat—to eat while watching a movie. Later, 563 subjects were interviewed. The result? Olestra produced virtually no increase in gas, diarrhea, or abdominal cramping—although the participants did rate the olestra chips as less tasty (5.6 vs. 6.4 on a 9-point scale). In the second study, 3181 subjects ate traditional potato chips or olestra potato chips over 6 weeks. Again, olestra caused no increase in GI symptoms (heartburn, nausea, vomiting, gas, bloating, cramping, frequency of bowel movements, or loose stools).

Olestra can reduce the absorption of fat-soluble vitamins (A, D, E, and K). When these vitamins are ingested at the same time as olestra, they can dissolve in the olestra, and then pass through the intestine without being absorbed. To compensate for this action, snack foods made with olestra are fortified with fat-soluble vitamins. Hence, there is no risk of vitamin deficiency.

⁙ KEY POINTS

- Obesity increases the risk of morbidity and mortality.
- Obesity is a chronic disease that requires lifelong treatment.
- The body mass index (BMI) is a measure of body fat content.
- A BMI of 25 to 29.9 indicates overweight, and a BMI of 30 or more indicates obesity.
- Waist circumference (WC) is an index of abdominal fat. Accumulation of abdominal fat poses a greater risk to health than accumulation of fat in the hips and thighs.
- Obesity-related health risk is determined by the degree of obesity, excessive abdominal fat, and the presence of obesity-related diseases (e.g., type 2 diabetes, sleep apnea) and cardiovascular risk factors (e.g., smoking, hypertension, high LDL cholesterol).
- Weight reduction reduces morbidity and probably mortality.
- Weight reduction can be accomplished with diet therapy, physical activity, behavior therapy, drug therapy, and surgery.
- Antiobesity drugs should be used only as adjuncts to a comprehensive weight-loss program that includes exercise, behavior modification, and a reduced-calorie diet.
- Antiobesity drugs are indicated for patients with a BMI of 30 or more (in the absence of other risk factors) or 27 or more (in the presence of other risk factors).
- Most patients regain lost weight when antiobesity drugs are discontinued. Hence, to remain effective, these drugs must be taken indefinitely.
- Only two drugs—sibutramine and orlistat—are approved for long-term therapy of obesity.
- Sibutramine promotes weight loss by suppressing appetite. The underlying mechanism is blockade of NE and 5-HT reuptake.
- Sibutramine can elevate blood pressure and heart rate, and hence must be used with caution in patients with hypertension or a history of dysrhythmias.
- Sibutramine poses a risk of serotonin syndrome, and hence must not be combined with other serotonergic drugs. Among these are selective serotonin reuptake inhibitors (e.g., fluoxetine [Prozac]), serotonin agonists used for migraine (e.g., sumatriptan [Imitrex]), and lithium.
- By blocking reuptake of norepinephrine, sibutramine can increase the risk of hypertensive crisis in patients taking MAOIs. At least 2 weeks should separate use of these drugs.
- Orlistat promotes weight loss by decreasing absorption of dietary fat. The underlying mechanism is inhibition of gastric and pancreatic lipases.
- Orlistat frequently causes GI symptoms (oily spotting, fecal urgency, oily stools, and fecal incontinence). These symptoms, which are a direct result of reduced fat absorption, can be minimized by reducing fat intake, and by taking the bulk-forming laxative psyllium [Metamucil, others].
- Orlistat can reduce absorption of fat-soluble vitamins (vitamins A, D, E, and K). To avoid deficiency, patients should take a daily multivitamin supplement.

Basic Principles of Antimicrobial Therapy

SELECTIVE TOXICITY
CLASSIFICATION OF ANTIMICROBIAL DRUGS
ACQUIRED RESISTANCE TO
ANTIMICROBIAL DRUGS
SELECTION OF ANTIBIOTICS
HOST FACTORS THAT MODIFY DRUG CHOICE,
ROUTE OF ADMINISTRATION, OR DOSAGE
DOSAGE SIZE AND DURATION OF TREATMENT
THERAPY WITH ANTIBIOTIC COMBINATIONS
PROPHYLACTIC USE OF ANTIMICROBIAL DRUGS
MISUSES OF ANTIMICROBIAL DRUGS
MONITORING ANTIMICROBIAL THERAPY

With this chapter we begin our study of drugs used to treat infectious diseases. These drugs, which are given to about 30% of all hospitalized patients, constitute one of our most widely used families of medicines.

Modern antimicrobial agents had their debut in the 1930s and 1940s, and have greatly reduced morbidity and mortality from infection. As newer drugs are introduced, our ability to fight infections increases even more. However, despite impressive advances, continued progress is needed: There are organisms that respond poorly to available drugs; there are effective drugs whose use is limited by toxicity; and there is, because of evolving microbial resistance, the constant threat that currently effective antibiotics will be rendered useless.

In this introductory chapter, our discussion focuses on two principal themes. The first is microbial susceptibility to drugs, with special emphasis on microbial drug resistance. The second theme addresses how to use antimicrobial agents properly. This discussion includes criteria for drug selection, host factors that modify drug use, use of antimicrobial combinations, and use of antimicrobial agents for prophylaxis.

Before addressing our major topics, we should clarify three terms: *chemotherapy, antibiotic,* and *antimicrobial agent.* Although we often think of *chemotherapy* as the use of drugs to kill or suppress cancer cells, this term was first defined as *the use of chemicals against invading organisms* (e.g., bacteria, viruses, fungi). Today, the word is applied to both the treatment of cancer and the treatment of infection. Hence, not only do we speak of cancer chemotherapy, we also speak of chemotherapy of infectious diseases.

It has become common practice to use the terms *antibiotic* and *antimicrobial drug* interchangeably. We will follow that practice. However, you should be aware that the formal definitions of these words are not identical. Strictly speaking, an *antibiotic* is a chemical that is produced by one microorganism and has the ability to harm other microbes. Under this definition, only those compounds that are actually made by microorganisms qualify as antibiotics. Drugs such as the sulfonamides, which are produced in the laboratory, would not be considered antibiotics under the strict definition. In contrast, an *antimicrobial drug* is defined as any agent, natural or synthetic, that has the ability to kill or suppress microorganisms. Under this definition, no distinction is made between compounds produced by microbes and those made by chemists. From the perspective of therapeutics, there is no benefit to distinguishing between drugs made by microorganisms and drugs made by chemists. Hence, the current practice is to use the terms *antibiotic* and *antimicrobial drug* as synonyms.

SELECTIVE TOXICITY

What Is Selective Toxicity?

The term *selective toxicity* is defined as the ability of a drug to injure a target cell or target organism without injuring other cells or organisms that are in intimate contact with the target. As applied to antimicrobial drugs, selective toxicity indicates the ability of an antibiotic to kill or suppress infecting microbes without causing injury to the host. Selective toxicity is the property that makes antibiotics valuable. If it weren't for their selective toxicity—that is, if antibiotics were as harmful to the host as they are to infecting organisms—these drugs would have no therapeutic utility.

How Is Selective Toxicity Achieved?

How is it that a drug can be highly toxic to microbes but benign to cells of the host? The answer lies with differences in the cellular chemistry of mammals and microbes. There are biochemical processes that are critical to microbial well-being that do not take place in mammalian cells. Hence, drugs that selectively interfere with these unique microbial processes can cause serious injury to microorganisms while leaving mammalian cells intact.

Disruption of the Bacterial Cell Wall. Unlike mammalian cells, bacteria are encased in a rigid cell wall. The protoplasm within this wall has a high concentration of solutes, making osmotic pressure within the bacterium high. If it were not for the cell wall, bacteria would absorb water, swell, and then burst. Several families of drugs (penicillins, cephalosporins, others) act to weaken the cell wall and thereby promote bacterial lysis. Because mammalian cells have no cell wall, drugs directed at this structure do not affect the host.

Inhibition of an Enzyme Unique to Bacteria. The sulfonamides exemplify drugs whose selective toxicity derives from inhibition of an enzyme that is essential for bacterial growth but is not present in cells of the host. The enzyme that the sulfonamides inhibit is needed by bacteria for production of folic acid, a compound required by all cells—mammalian and bacterial—for synthesis of essential molecules (DNA, RNA, proteins). The folic acid used by mammalian cells is acquired directly from dietary sources. In contrast, bacteria lack the ability to take up folic acid from their environment. Hence, to meet their needs, bacteria first take up *para*-aminobenzoic acid (PABA), a precursor of folic acid, and then use the PABA to form folic acid. The sulfonamide drugs suppress bacterial growth by inhibiting an enzyme required to synthesize folic acid from PABA. Since mammalian cells do not synthesize folic acid, toxicity of sulfonamides is selective for microbes.

Disruption of Bacterial Protein Synthesis. In bacteria as in mammalian cells, synthesis of proteins employs cellular components called ribosomes. However, although both cell types employ ribosomes, bacteria have ribosomes that differ in structure from those of mammalian cells. Because of this difference, it is possible for drugs to disrupt the function of bacterial ribosomes while having little or no effect on ribosomes of the host. By doing so, drugs can alter protein synthesis in bacteria while leaving mammalian protein synthesis untouched. Hence, once again we see that biochemical differences between microbes and host cells can be exploited to produce selectively toxic effects.

CLASSIFICATION OF ANTIMICROBIAL DRUGS

Various schemes are employed to classify antimicrobial drugs. The two schemes most suited to our objectives are considered below.

Classification by Susceptible Organism

Antibiotics differ widely in their antimicrobial activity. Some agents, called *narrow-spectrum antibiotics,* are active against only a few species of microorganisms. In contrast, *broad-spectrum antibiotics* are active against a wide variety of microbes. As discussed below, *narrow-spectrum drugs are generally preferred to broad-spectrum drugs.* Because of differences in antimicrobial spectra, not all drugs are appropriate for all patients: If therapy is to succeed, we must choose an antibiotic that is active against the specific organism responsible for the infection to be treated.

Table 79–1 classifies the major antimicrobial drugs according to susceptible organisms. The table shows three major groups: *antibacterial drugs, antifungal drugs,* and *antiviral drugs.* In addition, the table subdivides the antibacterial drugs into narrow-spectrum and broad-spectrum agents, and indicates the principal classes of bacteria against which these drugs are active.

Classification by Mechanism of Action

The antimicrobial drugs fall into seven major groups based on mechanisms of action. This classification is summarized in Table 79–2. Properties of the seven major classes are discussed briefly below.

- *Drugs that inhibit bacterial cell wall synthesis or activate enzymes that disrupt the cell wall.* These drugs (e.g., penicillins, cephalosporins) weaken the cell wall and thereby promote bacterial lysis and death.
- *Drugs that increase cell membrane permeability.* Drugs in this group (e.g., amphotericin B) increase the permeability of cell membranes, causing leakage of intracellular material.
- *Drugs that cause lethal inhibition of bacterial protein synthesis.* The aminoglycosides (e.g., gentamicin) are the only drugs in this group. We do not know why inhibition of protein synthesis by these agents results in cell death.

TABLE 79–1 ▪■ Classification of Antimicrobial Drugs by Susceptible Organisms*
Antibacterial Drugs
Narrow Spectrum
Gram-positive cocci and gram-positive bacilli
Penicillin G and V
Penicillinase-resistant penicillins: methicillin, nafcillin
Vancomycin
Erythromycin
Clindamycin
Gram-negative aerobes
Aminoglycosides: gentamicin, others
Cephalosporins (first and second generations)
Mycobacterium tuberculosis
Isoniazid
Rifampin
Ethambutol
Pyrazinamide
Broad Spectrum
Gram-positive cocci and gram-negative bacilli
Broad-spectrum penicillins: ampicillin, others
Extended-spectrum penicillins: carbenicillin, others
Cephalosporins (third generation)
Tetracyclines
Imipenem, meropenem
Trimethoprim
Sulfonamides: sulfisoxazole, sulfamethoxazole, others
Fluoroquinolones: ciprofloxacin, norfloxacin, others
Antiviral Drugs
Acyclovir
Azidothymidine
Zidovudine
Amantadine
Saquinavir
Antifungal Drugs
Amphotericin B
Ketoconazole
Itraconazole

*The classification in this table is simplified. Table 79–4 presents a more comprehensive list of microorganisms and the drugs active against them.

- *Drugs that cause nonlethal inhibition of protein synthesis.* Like the aminoglycosides, these drugs (e.g., tetracyclines) inhibit bacterial protein synthesis. However, in contrast to the aminoglycosides, these agents only slow microbial growth; they do not kill bacteria at clinically achievable concentrations.
- *Drugs that inhibit bacterial synthesis of nucleic acids.* These drugs inhibit synthesis of DNA or RNA by binding directly to nucleic acids or by interacting with enzymes required for nucleic acid synthesis. Members of this group include rifampin and the fluoroquinolones (e.g., ciprofloxacin).
- *Antimetabolites.* These drugs disrupt specific biochemical reactions. The result is either a decrease in the synthesis of essential cell constituents or synthesis of nonfunctional analogs of normal metabolites. Examples of antimetabolites include trimethoprim and the sulfonamides.
- *Inhibitors of viral enzymes.* Two classes of drugs, protease inhibitors and nucleoside analogs, inhibit enzymes necessary for viral replication and infectivity. Examples are zidovudine, acyclovir, and saquinavir.

When considering the *antibacterial* drugs, it is useful to distinguish between agents that are *bactericidal* and agents that are *bacteriostatic*. *Bactericidal* drugs are directly lethal to bacteria at clinically achievable concentrations. In contrast, *bacteriostatic* drugs can slow microbial growth but do not cause cell death. When a bacteriostatic drug is used, elimination of bacteria must ultimately be accomplished by host defenses (i.e., the immune system working in concert with phagocytic cells).

TABLE 79–2 ■ Classification of Antimicrobial Drugs by Mechanism of Action	
Drug Class	**Representative Antibiotics**
Inhibitors of cell wall synthesis	Penicillins Cephalosporins Imipenem Vancomycin
Drugs that disrupt the cell membrane	Amphotericin B Ketoconazole
Bactericidal inhibitors of protein synthesis	Aminoglycosides
Bacteriostatic inhibitors of protein synthesis	Clindamycin Erythromycin Linezolid Tetracyclines
Drugs that interfere with synthesis of bacterial DNA and RNA	Fluoroquinolones Rifampin
Antimetabolites	Flucytosine Sulfonamides Trimethoprim
Drugs that inhibit viral enzymes	Acyclovir Zidovudine Saquinavir Indinavir
Inhibitor of mycolic acid synthesis	Isoniazid

ACQUIRED RESISTANCE TO ANTIMICROBIAL DRUGS

Over time, an organism that had once been highly responsive to an antibiotic may become less susceptible, or it may lose sensitivity to the drug entirely. In some cases, resistance to several drugs develops. Acquired resistance is of great concern in that it can render currently effective drugs useless, thereby creating a clinical crisis and a constant need for new antimicrobial agents. Organisms for which drug resistance is now a serious clinical problem include *Enterococcus faecalis, Enterococcus faecium, Staphylococcus aureus, Staphylococcus epidermidis, Streptococcus pneumoniae,* and *Klebsiella pneumoniae* (Table 79–3).

TABLE 79–3 ■ Drugs for Some Highly Resistant Bacteria		
Bacterium	**Resistant To**	**Preferred Treatment**
Enterococcus faecalis Beta-lactamase negative Beta-lactamase producing	Vancomycin + streptomycin or gentamicin Penicillin	Penicillin G or ampicillin Vancomycin, ampicillin-sulbactam
Enterococcus faecium	Vancomycin, streptomycin, gentamicin Vancomycin, streptomycin, gentamicin, penicillin G, ampicillin	Penicillin G or ampicillin Linezolid, quinupristin-dalfopristin
Staphylococcus aureus	Methicillin Methicillin, vancomycin	Vancomycin Possibly: linezolid, quinupristin-dalfopristin, very high doses of vancomycin
Staphylococcus epidermidis	Methicillin Methicillin, vancomycin, and other glycopeptides	Vancomycin Quinupristin-dalfopristin
Streptococcus pneumoniae	Penicillin G (MIC >0.1 to ≤1.0 µg/ml) Penicillin G (MIC ≥2.0 µg/ml) Penicillin G, erythromycin, tetracycline, chloramphenicol, TMP-SMZ	Ceftriaxone, cefotaxime Vancomycin ± rifampin Vancomycin ± rifampin
Klebsiella pneumoniae	Ceftazidime, third-generation cephalosporins	Imipenem-cilastatin, meropenem, a fluoroquinolone

MIC = minimum inhibitory concentration, TMP-SMZ = trimethoprim-sulfamethoxazole.

In the discussion that follows, we examine the mechanisms by which microbial drug resistance is acquired and the measures by which emergence of resistance can be delayed. As you read this section, keep in mind that it is the *microbe* that becomes drug resistant, *not the patient.*

Mechanisms of Microbial Drug Resistance

Microbes become drug resistant because of alterations in their function or structure. Four such alterations are described below. All of these alterations are ultimately the result of inheritable changes in microbial DNA.

- *Microbes may elaborate drug-metabolizing enzymes.* For example, many bacteria are now resistant to penicillin G because of increased production of penicillinase, an enzyme that converts penicillin into an inactive product. Through production of enzymes, some microorganisms are able to inactivate several different kinds of antibiotics.
- *Microbes may cease active uptake of certain drugs.* Because the site of action of many antibiotics is intracellular, reduced drug uptake will produce resistance. This mechanism is responsible for some cases of resistance to tetracyclines.
- *Microbial drug receptors may undergo change, resulting in decreased antibiotic binding and action.* For example, some bacteria are now resistant to streptomycin because of structural changes in bacterial ribosomes, the sites at which streptomycin acts to inhibit protein synthesis.
- *Microbes may synthesize compounds that antagonize drug actions.* For example, by acquiring the ability to synthesize increased quantities of PABA, some bacteria have developed resistance to sulfonamides.

Mechanisms by Which Resistance Is Acquired

The alterations in structure and function discussed above are brought about by changes in the microbial genome. These genetic changes may result from spontaneous mutation or by acquisition of DNA from an external source. One important mechanism by which bacteria obtain external DNA is conjugation with other bacteria.

Spontaneous Mutation. Spontaneous mutations produce random changes in a microbe's DNA. The result is a gradual increase in resistance. Low-level resistance develops first. With additional mutations, resistance becomes increasingly great. As a rule, spontaneous mutations confer resistance *to only one drug.* Development of multiple drug resistance would require multiple mutations, a phenomenon that is rare.

Conjugation. Conjugation is a process by which extrachromosomal DNA is transferred from one bacterium to another. In order to transfer resistance by conjugation, the donor organism must possess two unique DNA segments, one that codes for the mechanisms of drug resistance and one that codes for the "sexual" apparatus required for DNA transfer. Together, these two DNA segments constitute an *R factor* (resistance factor).

Conjugation takes place primarily among *gram-negative* bacteria. Genetic material may be transferred between members of the same species or between members of different species. Because transfer of R factors is not species specific, it is possible for pathogenic bacteria to acquire R factors from the normal flora of the body. Because R factors are becoming common in normal flora, the possibility of transferring resistance from normal flora to pathogens is a serious clinical concern.

In contrast to spontaneous mutation, conjugation frequently results in *multiple drug resistance.* This can be achieved, for example, by transferring DNA that codes for several different drug-metabolizing enzymes. Hence, in a single event, a drug-sensitive bacterium can become highly drug resistant.

Relationships Between Antibiotic Use and the Emergence of Drug-Resistant Microbes

Use of antibiotics promotes the emergence of drug-resistant microbes. Please note, however, that although antibiotics promote drug resistance, these agents are not mutagenic and do not directly cause the genetic changes that underlie reduced drug sensitivity. Spontaneous mutation and conjugation are random events whose incidence is independent of drug use. Drugs simply serve to make conditions favorable for overgrowth of those microbes that have already acquired mechanisms for drug resistance.

How Do Antibiotics Promote Resistance? To answer this question, we need to recall two aspects of microbial ecology: (1) microbes secrete compounds that are toxic to other microbes, and (2) microbes within a given ecologic niche (e.g., large intestine, urogenital tract, skin) compete with one another for available nutrients. Under drug-free conditions, the various microbes in a given niche keep one another in check. Furthermore, if none of these organisms is drug resistant, introduction of antibiotics will be equally detrimental to all members of the population, and therefore will not promote the growth of any individual. However, *if a drug-resistant organism is present, antibiotics will create selection pressure favoring the growth of that microbe.* How? By killing off the sensitive organisms, the drug will eliminate toxins produced by those microbes, and thereby facilitate survival of the microbe that is drug resistant. Also, elimination of sensitive organisms will remove competition for available nutrients, thereby making conditions even more favorable for the drug-resistant microbe to flourish. Hence, although drug resistance is of no benefit to an organism when there are no antibiotics present, when antibiotics are introduced, they create selection pressure favoring overgrowth of those microbes that are resistant.

Which Antibiotics Promote Resistance? *All* antimicrobial drugs promote the emergence of drug-resistant organisms. However, some agents are more likely to promote resistance than others. Because broad-spectrum antibiotics kill off more competing organisms than do narrow-spectrum drugs, emergence of resistance is facilitated most by the broad-spectrum agents.

Does the Amount of Antibiotic Use Influence the Emergence of Resistance? You bet! The more that antibiotics are used, the faster drug-resistant organisms will emerge. Not only do antibiotics promote emergence of resistant pathogens, they also promote overgrowth of normal flora that possess mechanisms for resistance. Because drug use can increase resistance in normal flora, and because normal flora can transfer resistance to pathogens, every effort should be made to avoid use of antibiotics by individuals who don't actually need them (i.e., individuals who don't have a treatable infection). Because all use of antibiotics will further the emergence of resistance, there can be no excuse for casual or indiscriminate dispensing of antimicrobial drugs.

Because hospitals are sites of intensive antibiotic use, resident organisms can be extremely drug resistant. As a result, *nosocomial infections* (defined as infections acquired in hospitals) are among the most difficult to treat.

Suprainfection

Suprainfection is simply a special example of the emergence of drug resistance. A suprainfection is defined as a *new* infection that appears during the course of treatment for a primary infection. New infections develop when antibiotics eliminate the inhibitory influence of normal flora, thereby allowing a second infectious agent to flourish. Because broad-spectrum antibiotics kill off more normal flora than do narrow-spectrum drugs, suprainfections are more likely in patients receiving broad-spectrum agents. Because suprainfections are caused by drug-resistant microbes, these infections are often difficult to treat. It should be noted that, in most texts, suprainfections are referred to as *superinfections;* this name may have been chosen to reflect the difficulties of treatment.

Delaying the Emergence of Resistance

In the Spring of 2002, the Centers for Disease Control and Prevention (CDC) launched its Campaign to Prevent Antimicrobial Resistance. The campaign is directed primarily at hospitals, which are major breeding grounds for resistant pathogens. As shown in Figure 79–1, the campaign consists of 12 action steps that fall under four major headings:

- Prevent infection
- Diagnose and treat infection effectively
- Use antimicrobials wisely
- Prevent transmission

The 12 steps are discussed briefly below. You can get more information online at *www.cdc.gov/drugresistance.*

Because the CDC campaign is limited to antibiotic use by humans, there is a major cause of resistance that it doesn't address: Feeding thousands of tons of antibiotics to livestock to promote growth. This important and contentious topic is discussed in Box 79–1.

Step 1. Vaccinate. By preventing infection, vaccination reduces the need to use antimicrobial drugs, and thereby helps prevent emergence of resistance. Accordingly, the CDC recommends predischarge vaccination of all at-risk patients, especially against two respiratory infections: influenza and pneumococcal pneumonia. In addition, all healthcare personnel who have patient-care duties should receive a flu shot annually.

Step 2. Get the catheters out. Catheters and other invasive devises are the leading exogenous cause of nosocomial infections. Infections can occur in association with IV catheters, arterial catheters, urinary tract catheters, endotracheal tubes, and other devices. Every year, an estimated 250,000 Americans develop bacteremia related to use of central venous catheters alone; the cost of treatment ranges between $35,000 and $56,000 *per patient.* To help prevent these infections, catheters should be used only when essential for patient care, and should be removed as soon as they are no longer needed.

Step 3. Target the pathogen. Proper antimicrobial therapy requires that we choose drugs that are active against the causative organism. To do so, we must determine both the

identity and drug sensitivity of the pathogen. This important issue is discussed fully under the heading *Selection of Antibiotics* below.

Step 4. Access the experts. Not surprisingly, input from an infectious disease expert can improve patient outcomes, decrease treatment costs, and shorten the time to discharge. Expert assistance can be especially helpful in (1) patients with serious infections, (2) patients receiving complex antimicrobial regimens, (3) patients who fail to respond as expected, and (4) patients with complicated underlying illnesses.

Step 5. Practice antimicrobial control. To facilitate antimicrobial control, institutions are encouraged to implement procedures and programs that can help clinicians use antimicrobial drugs more wisely. Perhaps the most effective option is to implement a computerized support system designed to help clinicians select antimicrobial regimens. Other effective measures include use of standardized antimicrobial order forms, providing interactive education for prescribers, giving individual prescribers critical feedback on their choices, and establishing a multidisciplinary system to evaluate drug utilization.

Step 6. Use local data. Drug susceptibility of microbes varies over time and according to locale, patient population, and hospital unit. To facilitate drug selection, institutions often compile data on drug susceptibility into an "antibiogram," which provides an overview of common local pathogens and

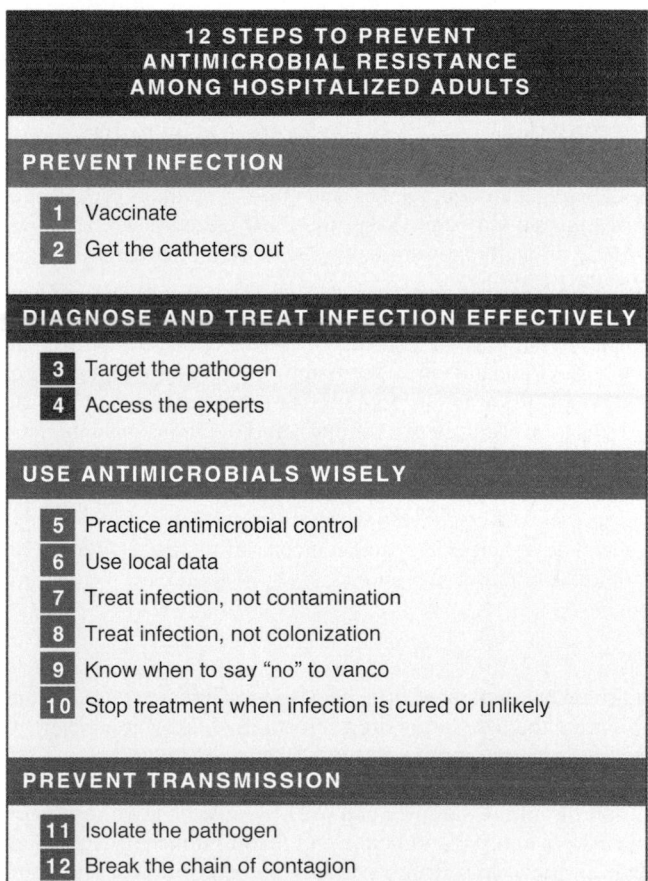

12 STEPS TO PREVENT ANTIMICROBIAL RESISTANCE AMONG HOSPITALIZED ADULTS

PREVENT INFECTION

1. Vaccinate
2. Get the catheters out

DIAGNOSE AND TREAT INFECTION EFFECTIVELY

3. Target the pathogen
4. Access the experts

USE ANTIMICROBIALS WISELY

5. Practice antimicrobial control
6. Use local data
7. Treat infection, not contamination
8. Treat infection, not colonization
9. Know when to say "no" to vanco
10. Stop treatment when infection is cured or unlikely

PREVENT TRANSMISSION

11. Isolate the pathogen
12. Break the chain of contagion

Figure 79–1 ■ Pocket card from the CDC's Campaign to Prevent Antimicrobial Resistance.

Special Interest Topic

BOX 79–1 ■ ANTIBIOTICS IN ANIMAL FEED: HASTENING ANTIBIOTIC ARMAGEDDON

Drug-resistant infection resulting from use of antibiotics in agriculture is a global public health concern. Antibiotics are employed extensively in the livestock and poultry industries. Not surprisingly, this practice has created a large reservoir of drug-resistant bacteria, some of which now infect humans. In addition to being a direct detriment to health, these infections pose an even larger threat: passage of resistance genes to normal intestinal flora, and then from normal flora to other human pathogens.

The amount of antibiotics given to food animals is staggering. According to estimates made by the Union for Concerned Scientists, of the 14,800 tons of antibiotics produced in the United States each year, nearly 90% (13,300 tons) goes to animals. Even more surprisingly, of the antibiotics that animals receive, only 7.5% (1000 tons) is given to treat infection. The vast majority—12,300 tons—is mixed with feed to promote growth. Both uses encourage the emergence of resistance.

Of the two agricultural uses—growth promotion and treatment of infection—growth promotion is by far the more controversial. Few authorities would argue that we should not give animals antibiotics to treat infection. In contrast, there are strong arguments against giving these drugs to promote growth. The doses employed for growth promotion are much lower than those used for infection, and hence are *more* likely to encourage emergence of resistance. Moreover, since growth can be promoted by other means, giving antibiotics for this purpose is unnecessary.

Which antibiotics are employed in agriculture? Essentially all of the antibiotics used in humans are also used in animals—including fluoroquinolones and third-generation cephalosporins, agents that are among the most effective we have. Because all antibiotics are being used, we are hastening the day when all will be useless.

The story of virginiamycin and Synercid illustrates the potentially serious consequences of giving antibiotics to farm animals. Virginiamycin is a mixture of two streptogramins. For 30 years, the drug has been used to promote animal growth. In 1999, a mixture of two similar streptogramins—quinupristin and dalfopristin, sold as Synercid—was approved for medical use in the United States. Synercid is an extremely important drug because it can kill vancomycin-resistant *Enterococcus faecium,* a dangerous pathogenic strain that is resistant to all other antibiotics. Unfortunately, agricultural use of virginiamycin is likely to shorten Synercid's useful life: A study of chickens that were fed virginiamycin indicates that 50% of the birds carried Synercid-resistant *E. faecium.* Sooner or later, these birds will pass these resistant pathogens on to humans—if they haven't already.

How can we reduce agriculture-related resistance? Clearly, if we want to delay emergence of resistance, and thereby extend the useful life of our antibiotics, we must limit agricultural use of these drugs. To this end, the World Health Organization has recommended that all antibiotics used by humans be banned from use to promote growth in animals. Fifteen countries in the European Union have banned four widely used antibiotics, including virginiamycin, from use as growth promoters. In Denmark, use of antibiotics in animal feed has stopped entirely—with no apparent detriment to either animal health or the incomes of producers. Furthermore, within a few years after these drugs were discontinued, rates of antibiotic resistance among farm animals dropped dramatically. For example, resistance to avoparcin dropped from 73% to 5% in less than 5 years.

In the United States, public health and agriculture officials have discussed and debated the issue for nearly 25 years, but no legislation has been enacted. A major stumbling block has been the inability to quantify the problem. That is, although there is universal agreement that giving antibiotics to animals represents a threat to public health, we lack sufficient data to determine just how big the threat is. Hopefully, our government will take appropriate action before the threat has grown too large to overcome.

Although restrictions are not yet in place, they may be forthcoming: In September 2002, the Food and Drug Administration proposed a draft "guidance" on antibiotic use in animals. If adopted, the guidance would require manufacturers of agricultural antibiotics to assess the ability of new drugs to promote emergence of pathogens resistant to antibiotics used in humans; drugs that did so could be kept off the market. In addition, the guidance proposes to review the impact of drugs already in use. Important among these are virginiamycin, penicillins, fluoroquinolones, tetracyclines, and third-generation cephalosporins.

Note: Use of antibiotics by vegetable and fruit growers is just as widespread as in animal husbandry, and probably just as detrimental to public health—but that's another story.

---

their current pattern of drug sensitivity. Clinicians use the antibiogram to guide initial drug selection while awaiting patient-specific data on drug susceptibility from the microbiology lab.

Step 7. Treat infection, not contamination. Contamination of culture samples can lead to false-positive results on bacteriologic tests, and hence can lead to unneeded treatment with antimicrobial drugs. Studies indicate, in fact, that contamination is a major cause of unnecessary antimicrobial use. To decrease contamination, clinicians should simply use approved procedures to obtain and process all culture samples.

For example, to prevent contamination when drawing blood, clinicians can decontaminate the skin with tincture of iodine.

Step 8. Treat infection, not colonization. A small, localized colony of bacteria does not constitute an infection. However, for two reasons, colonization is a concern. First, in patients who do *not* have an active infection, treatment because of colonization would be an unnecessary use of antibiotics. Second, in patients who *do* have an active infection, wrongly attributing the infection to colonizing bacteria could lead to treatment with drugs that are inactive against the real cause. To avoid both problems, it is essential that we differentiate between bacteria that are simply colonizing a region and those that are causing an actual infection.

Step 9. Know when to say "no" to vanco. Vanco (i.e., vancomycin) is a drug of last resort against several important pathogens, including methicillin-resistant *Staphylococcus aureus* (MRSA) and multidrug-resistant *Streptococcus pneumoniae*. To delay emergence of vancomycin-resistant organisms, we must use the drug only when clearly necessary. Guidelines from the CDC spell out situations in which using vancomycin is deemed appropriate and situations in which using the drug should be discouraged.

Step 10. Stop treatment when infection is cured or unlikely. Common sense dictates that we administer antibiotics only when they are actually needed: If the patient doesn't have an infection, we shouldn't use these drugs. When an infection has been cured, antibiotics should be discontinued. Similarly, if antibiotics were started before culture results were available, and if the culture comes back negative, then the antibiotics should be stopped.

Step 11. Isolate the pathogen. By using standard infection control procedures, such as proper containment and disposal of contagious body fluids, we can isolate the pathogen, and can thereby reduce the risk of transferring resistant organisms from one patient to another.

Step 12. Break the chain of contagion. This step could also be titled *Wash your hands!* All too often, bacteria are transferred from patient to patient on the hands of physicians, nurses, and other hospital workers. Fortunately, this transfer can be stopped by following a simple rule: Wash your hands before and after touching any patient. Unfortunately, at least 50% of the time, clinicians fail to do so.

SELECTION OF ANTIBIOTICS

When treating infection, the therapeutic objective is to produce maximal antimicrobial effects while causing minimal harm to the host. To achieve this goal, we must select the most appropriate antibiotic for the individual patient. When choosing an antibiotic, three principal factors must be considered: (1) the identity of the infecting organism, (2) drug sensitivity of the infecting organism, and (3) host factors, such as the site of infection and the status of host defenses.

For any given infection, several drugs may be effective. However, for most infections, there is usually one drug that is superior to the alternatives (Table 79–4). This drug of first choice may be preferred for several reasons, such as greater efficacy, lower toxicity, or more narrow spectrum. Whenever possible, the drug of first choice should be employed. Alternative agents should be used only when the first-choice drug is inappropriate. Conditions that might rule out a first-choice agent include (1) allergy to the drug of choice, (2) inability of the drug of choice to penetrate to the site of infection, and (3) unusual susceptibility of the patient to toxicity of the first-choice drug.

Empiric Therapy Prior to Completion of Laboratory Tests

Optimal antimicrobial therapy requires identification of the infecting organism and determination of its drug sensitivity. However, when the patient has a severe infection, it may be necessary to begin treatment before test results are available. Under these conditions, drug selection must be based on clinical evaluation and knowledge of which microbes are most likely to cause infection at a particular site. If necessary, a broad-spectrum agent can be used for initial treatment. Once the identity and drug sensitivity of the infecting organism have been determined, we can switch to a more selective antibiotic. When conditions demand that we start therapy in the absence of laboratory data, it is essential that samples of exudates and body fluids be obtained for culture *prior to initiation of treatment;* if antibiotics are present at the time of sampling, these agents can suppress microbial growth in culture, and can thereby confound identification.

Identifying the Infecting Organism

The first rule of antimicrobial therapy is to *match the drug with the bug.* Hence, whenever possible, the infecting organism should be identified prior to initiation of therapy. If treatment is begun in the absence of a definitive diagnosis, positive identification should be established as soon as possible, since this will permit adjustment of the regimen to better conform with the drug sensitivity of the infecting organism.

The quickest, simplest, and most versatile technique for identifying microorganisms is microscopic examination of a *gram-stained preparation.* Samples for examination can be obtained from pus, sputum, urine, blood, and other body fluids. The most useful samples are direct aspirates from the site of infection.

In some cases, only a small number of infecting organisms will be present. Under these conditions, positive identification may require that the microbes be grown out in culture. As stressed above, material for culture should be obtained prior to initiating treatment. Furthermore, the samples should be taken in a fashion that minimizes contamination with normal body flora. Also, the samples should not be exposed to low temperature, antiseptics, or oxygen.

Determining Drug Susceptibility

Because of the emergence of drug-resistant organisms, testing for drug sensitivity is common. However, sensitivity testing is not always needed. Rather, testing is indicated only when the infecting organism is one in which resistance is likely. Hence, for microbes such as the group A streptococci, which have remained highly susceptible to penicillin G, sensitivity testing is unnecessary. In contrast, when resistance is common, as it is with *Staph. aureus* and the gram-negative bacilli, tests for drug sensitivity should be performed.

Disk-Diffusion Test. The most widely used method for assessing drug sensitivity is the disk-diffusion test, also known as the Kirby-Bauer test. This test is performed by inoculating an agar plate with the infecting organism and then placing on that plate several small disks, each of which is impregnated with a different antibiotic. Because of diffusion, an antibiotic-containing zone becomes established around each disk. As the bacteria proliferate, growth will be inhibited around the disks that contain an antibiotic to which the bacteria are sensitive. The degree of drug sensitivity is proportional to the size of the bacteria-free zone. Hence, by measuring the diameter of these zones, we can determine the drugs to which the organism is more susceptible, as well as those to which it is highly resistant.

TABLE 79–4 ▪■ Antibacterial Drugs of Choice

Organism	Drug of First Choice	Some Alternative Drugs
Gram-Positive Cocci		
*Enterococcus**		
Endocarditis and other severe infections	Penicillin G *or* ampicillin with gentamicin or streptomycin	Vancomycin with gentamicin or streptomycin, quinupristin-dalfopristin, linezolid
Uncomplicated urinary tract infection	Ampicillin *or* amoxicillin	Nitrofurantoin, a fluoroquinolone; fosfomycin
Staphylococcus aureus or *epidermidis**		
Penicillinase producing	A penicillinase-resistant penicillin	A cephalosporin, vancomycin, amoxicillin–clavulanic acid
Methicillin resistant	Vancomycin	Linezolid, quinupristin-dalfopristin, trimethoprim-sulfamethoxazole, a fluoroquinolone
Streptococcus pyogenes (group A) and groups C and G	Penicillin G or V	Clindamycin, vancomycin, erythromycin
Streptococcus, group B	Penicillin G or ampicillin	A cephalosporin, vancomycin, erythromycin
Streptococcus viridans group	Penicillin G with or without gentamicin	A cephalosporin, vancomycin
Streptococcus bovis	Penicillin G	A cephalosporin, vancomycin
Streptococcus, anaerobic	Penicillin G	Clindamycin, a cephalosporin, vancomycin
*Streptococcus pneumoniae** (pneumococcus)	Penicillin G	Ceftriaxone, cefotaxime
Gram-Negative Cocci		
Neisseria gonorrhoeae (gonococcus)	Ceftriaxone or cefixime or ciprofloxacin or ofloxacin	Cefotaxime, penicillin G
Neisseria meningitidis (meningococcus)	Penicillin G	Cefotaxime, chloramphenicol, a fluoroquinolone
Gram-Positive Bacilli		
Bacillus anthracis (anthrax)	Ciprofloxacin	Amoxacillin, doxycycline
Clostridium difficile	Metronidazole	Vancomycin (PO)
Clostridium perfringens	Penicillin G, clindamycin	Metronidazole, chloramphenicol, imipenem, meropenem
Clostridium tetani	Metronidazole	A tetracycline, penicillin G
Corynebacterium diphtheriae	Erythromycin	Penicillin G
Listeria monocytogenes	Ampicillin with or without gentamicin	Trimethoprim-sulfamethoxazole
Enteric Gram-Negative Bacilli		
Bacteroides	Metronidazole or clindamycin	Imipenem or meropenem, amoxicillin–clavulanic acid, ticarcillin–clavulanic acid, gatifloxacin
Campylobacter jejuni	Erythromycin or azithromycin	A fluoroquinolone, gentamicin, a tetracycline
Escherichia coli	Cefotaxime, ceftizoxime, cefepime, ceftriaxone	Ampicillin with or without gentamicin, ticarcillin–clavulanic acid, trimethoprim–sulfamethoxazole, imipenem or meropenem
Enterobacter	Imipenem or meropenem	Trimethoprim-sulfamethoxazole, gentamicin, ciprofloxacin, cefotaxime
Helicobacter pylori	Tetracycline plus metronidazole plus bismuth subsalicylate	Tetracycline plus clarithromycin plus bismuth subsalicylate
*Klebsiella pneumoniae**	Cefotaxime, ceftizoxime	Imipenem or meropenem, gentamicin, tobramycin, amikacin
Proteus, indole positive (including *Providencia rettgeri* and *Morganella morganii*)	Cefotaxime, ceftizoxime, ceftriaxone, cefepime, or ceftazidime	Imipenem or meropenem, gentamicin, a fluoroquinolone, trimethoprim–sulfamethoxazole
Proteus mirabilis	Ampicillin	A cephalosporin, ticarcillin, trimethoprim–sulfamethoxazole, imepenem or meropenem
Salmonella typhi	Ceftriaxone or a fluoroquinolone	Trimethoprim–sulfamethoxazole, ampicillin, amoxicillin, chloramphenicol, azithromycin
Other *Salmonella*	Ceftriaxone or cefotaxime or a fluoroquinolone	Trimethoprim–sulfamethoxazole, chloramphenicol, ampicillin, amoxicillin
Serratia	Imipenem or meropenem	Gentamicin, amikacin, cefotaxime, a fluoroquinolone, trimethoprim–sulfamethoxazole, aztreonam

*Drugs for highly resistant strains are listed in Table 79–3.

TABLE 79–4 ▪ Antibacterial Drugs of Choice *(continued)*

Organism	Drug of First Choice	Some Alternative Drugs
Enteric Gram-Negative Bacilli—cont'd		
Shigella	A fluoroquinolone	Trimethoprim–sulfamethoxazole, ampicillin, ceftriaxone, azithromycin
Yersinia enterocolitica	Trimethroprim-sulfamethoxazole	A fluoroquinolone, gentamicin, tobramycin, cefotaxime
Other Gram-Negative Bacilli		
Acinetobacter	Imipenem or meropenem	Trimethoprim-sulfamethoxazole, tobramycin, gentamicin, ticarcillin, doxycycline
Bordetella pertussis (whooping cough)	Erythromycin	Trimethoprim-sulfamethoxazole, azithromycin, clarithromycin
Brucella (brucellosis)	A tetracycline plus rifampin	A tetracycline plus gentamicin, trimethoprim-sulfamethoxazole with or without gentamicin, chloramphenicol with or without streptomycin
Calymmatobacterium granulomatis	Trimethoprim-sulfamethoxazole	Doxycycline or ciprofloxacin
Francisella tularensis (tularemia)	Streptomycin	Gentamicin, a tetracycline, chloramphenicol, ciprofloxacin
Gardnerella vaginalis	Metronidazole (PO)	Topical clindamycin or metronidazole, clindamycin (PO)
Haemophilus ducreyi (chancroid)	Azithromycin or ceftriaxone	Ciprofloxacin or erythromycin
Haemophilus influenzae		
Meningitis, epiglottitis, arthritis, and other serious infections	Cefotaxime or ceftriaxone	Cefuroxime, chloramphenicol, meropenem
Upper respiratory infection and bronchitis	Trimethoprim-sulfamethoxazole	Cefuroxime, amoxicillin–clavulanic acid, a fluoroquinolone
Legionella species	Azithromycin, a fluoroquinolone with or without rifampin	Doxycycline with or without rifampin, trimethoprim-sulfamethoxazole, erythromycin
Pasteurella multocida	Penicillin G	A tetracycline, a cephalosporin, amoxicillin–clavulonic acid
Pseudomonas aeruginosa		
Urinary tract infection	Ciprofloxacin	Levofloxacin, piperacillin, ceftazidime, imipenem, carbenicillin, ticarcillin, gentamicin, meropenem
Other infections	Ticarcillin, mezlocillin or piperacillin plus tobramycin, gentamicin, or amikacin	Ceftazidime, gentamicin or amikacin, imipenem, meropenem, aztreonam, ciprofloxacin
Spirillum minus (rat bite fever)	Penicillin G	A tetracycline, streptomycin
Streptobacillus moniliformis (rat bite fever)	Penicillin G	A tetracycline, streptomycin
Vibrio cholerae (cholera)	A tetracycline	Trimethoprim-sulfamethoxazole, a fluoroquinolone
Yersinia pestis (plague)	Streptomycin with or without a tetracycline	Chloramphenicol, gentamicin, trimethoprim-sulfamethoxazole
Mycobacteria		
Mycobacterium tuberculosis	Isoniazid plus rifampin plus pyrazinamide with or without ethambutol or streptomycin	A fluoroquinolone, cycloserine, ethionamide, kanamycin, capreomycin, ciprofloxacin, *para*-aminosalicylic acid
Mycobacterium leprae (leprosy)	Dapsone plus rifampin with or without clofazimine	Minocycline, ofloxacin, sparfloxacin, clarithromycin
Mycobacterium avium complex	Clarithromycin or azithromycin plus ethambutol ± rifabutin	Ciprofloxacin, amikacin
Actinomycetes		
Actinomycetes israelii	Penicillin G	A tetracycline, erythromycin, clindamycin
Nocardia	Trimethoprim-sulfamethoxazole	Sulfisoxazole, imipenem or meropenem, amikacin, a tetracycline, linezolid
Chlamydiae		
Chlamydia psittaci	A tetracycline	Chloramphenicol
Chlamydia trachomatis		
Trachoma	Azithromycin	Doxycycline
Inclusion conjunctivitis	Erythromycin	A sulfonamide
Pneumonia	Erythromycin	A sulfonamide
Urethritis, cervicitis	Doxycycline or azithromycin	Erythromycin, ofloxacin, amoxicillin
Lymphogranuloma venereum	Doxycycline	Erythromycin

Continued

TABLE 79–4 ▪ Antibacterial Drugs of Choice (continued)

Organism	Drug of First Choice	Some Alternative Drugs
Mycoplasma		
Mycoplasma pneumoniae	Erythromycin, clarithromycin, azithromycin, or a tetracycline	A fluoroquinolone
Ureaplasma urealyticum	Erythromycin	A tetracycline, clarithromycin, azithromycin, ofloxacin
Rickettsia		
Rocky Mountain spotted fever, endemic typhus (murine), trench fever, typhus, scrub typhus, Q fever	Doxycycline	Chloramphenicol, a fluoroquinolone, rifampin
Spirochetes		
Borrelia burgdorferi (Lyme disease)	Doxycycline or amoxicillin	Ceftriaxone, cefotaxime, penicillin G, azithromycin, clarithromycin
Borrelia recurrentis (relapsing fever)	A tetracycline	Penicillin G
Leptospira	Penicillin G	A tetracycline
Treponema pallidum (syphilis)	Penicillin G	A tetracycline, ceftriaxone
Treponema pertenue (yaws)	Penicillin G	A tetracycline

Broth Dilution Procedure. In this procedure, bacteria are grown in a series of tubes containing different concentrations of an antibiotic. The advantage of this method over the disk-diffusion test is that it provides a more precise measure of drug sensitivity. By using the broth dilution procedure, we can establish close estimates of two clinically useful values: (1) the *minimum inhibitory concentration* (MIC), defined as the lowest concentration of antibiotic that produces complete inhibition of bacterial growth (but does not *kill* bacteria); and (2) the *minimum bactericidal concentration* (MBC), defined as the lowest concentration of drug that produces a 99.9% decline in the number of bacterial colonies (indicating bacterial kill). Because of the quantitative information provided, broth dilution procedures are especially useful for guiding therapy of infections that are unusually difficult to treat.

HOST FACTORS THAT MODIFY DRUG CHOICE, ROUTE OF ADMINISTRATION, OR DOSAGE

In addition to matching the drug with the bug and determining the drug sensitivity of an infecting organism, we must consider host factors when prescribing an antimicrobial drug. Two host factors—host defenses and the site of infection—are unique to the selection of antibiotics. Other host factors, such as age, pregnancy, and previous drug reactions, are the same factors that must be considered when choosing any other drug.

Host Defenses

Host defenses consist primarily of the immune system and phagocytic cells (macrophages, neutrophils). Without the contribution of these defenses, successful antimicrobial therapy would be rare. In most cases, the drugs we use to treat infection do not produce cure on their own. Rather, they work in concert with host defense systems to subdue infection. Accordingly, the usual objective of antibiotic treatment is not outright kill of infecting organisms. Rather, the goal is to suppress microbial growth to the point at which the balance is tipped in favor of the host. Underscoring the critical role of host defenses is the grim fact that people whose defenses are impaired, such as those with AIDS and those undergoing cancer chemotherapy, frequently die from infections that drugs alone are unable to control. When treating the immunocompromised host, our only hope lies with drugs that are rapidly bactericidal, and even these may prove inadequate.

Site of Infection

To be effective, an antibiotic must be present at the site of infection in a concentration greater than the MIC. At some sites, drug penetration may be hampered, making it difficult to achieve the MIC. For example, drug access can be impeded in meningitis (because of the blood-brain barrier), endocarditis (because bacterial vegetations in the heart are difficult to penetrate), and infected abscesses (because of poor vascularity and the presence of pus and other material). When treating meningitis, two approaches may be used to achieve the MIC: (1) we can select a drug that can readily cross the blood-brain barrier, and (2) we can inject an antibiotic directly into the subarachnoid space. When pus and other fluids hinder drug access, surgical drainage is indicated.

Foreign materials (e.g., cardiac pacemakers, prosthetic joints and heart valves, synthetic vascular shunts) present a special local problem. Phagocytes react to these objects and attempt to destroy them. Because of this behavior, the phagocytes are less able to attack bacteria, thereby allowing microbes to flourish. When attempts are made to treat these infections, relapse and failure are common. In many cases, the infection can be eliminated only by removing the foreign material.

Other Host Factors

Age. Infants and the elderly are highly vulnerable to drug toxicity. In the elderly, heightened drug sensitivity is due in large part to reduced rates of drug metabolism and drug excretion, which can result in accumulation of antibiotics to toxic levels.

Multiple factors contribute to antibiotic sensitivity in infants. Because of poorly developed kidney and liver function, neonates eliminate drugs slowly. To avoid drug accumulation, many antibiotics must be used in low dosage. The very young are also subject to special toxicities. For example, use of sulfonamides in newborns can produce kernicterus, a severe neurologic disorder caused by displacement of bilirubin from plasma proteins (see Chapter 84). The tetracyclines provide another example of toxicity unique to the young: These antibiotics bind to developing teeth, causing discoloration.

Pregnancy and Lactation. Antimicrobial drugs can cross the placenta, posing a risk to the developing fetus. For example, when gentamicin is used during pregnancy, irreversible hearing loss may result. Also, tetracyclines can stain immature teeth.

Antibiotic use during pregnancy may pose a risk to the expectant mother. It has been shown, for example, that during pregnancy there is an increased incidence of toxicity from tetracycline, characterized by hepatic necrosis, pancreatitis, renal damage, and, in extreme cases, death.

Antibiotics can enter breast milk, possibly affecting the nursing infant. Sulfonamides, for example, can reach levels in milk that are sufficient to cause kernicterus in nursing newborns. As a general guideline, antibiotics and all other drugs should be avoided by women who are breast-feeding.

Previous Allergic Reaction. Severe allergic reactions are more common with the penicillins than with any other family of drugs. As a rule, patients with a history of allergy to the penicillins should not receive them again. The exception to this rule is treatment of a life-threatening infection for which no suitable alternative is available. In addition to the penicillins, other antibiotics (sulfonamides, trimethoprim, erythromycin) are associated with a high incidence of allergic responses. However, severe reactions to these agents are rare.

Genetic Factors. As with other drugs, responses to antibiotics can be influenced by the patient's genetic heritage. For example, some antibiotics (e.g., sulfonamides, nalidixic acid) can cause hemolysis in patients who, because of their genetic makeup, have red blood cells that are deficient in glucose-6-phosphate dehydrogenase. Clearly, people with this deficiency should not be given antibiotics that are likely to induce red cell lysis.

Genetic factors can also affect rates of metabolism. For example, hepatic inactivation of isoniazid is rapid in some people and slow in others. If the dosage is not adjusted accordingly, isoniazid may accumulate to toxic levels in the slow metabolizers, but may fail to achieve therapeutic levels in the rapid metabolizers.

DOSAGE SIZE AND DURATION OF TREATMENT

Successful therapy requires that the antibiotic be present at the site of infection in an effective concentration for a sufficient time. Dosages should be adjusted to produce drug concentrations that are equal to or greater than the MIC for the infection being treated. Drug levels 4 to 8 times the MIC are often desirable.

Duration of therapy depends on a number of variables, including the status of host defenses, the site of the infection, and the identity of the infecting organism. *It is imperative that antibiotics not be discontinued prematurely.* Accordingly, *patients should be instructed to take their medication for the en-*

tire prescribed course, even though symptoms may subside before the full course has been completed. Early withdrawal is a common cause of recurrent infection, and the organisms responsible for relapse are likely to be more drug resistant than those present when therapy began.

THERAPY WITH ANTIBIOTIC COMBINATIONS

Therapy with a combination of antimicrobial agents is indicated only in specific situations. Under these well-defined conditions, use of multiple drugs may be life saving. However, it should be stressed that, although antibiotic combinations do have a valuable therapeutic role, routine use of two or more antibiotics should be discouraged. When an infection is caused by a single, identified microbe, treatment with just one drug is usually most appropriate.

Antimicrobial Effects of Antibiotic Combinations

When two antibiotics are used together, the result may be *additive, potentiative,* or, in certain cases, *antagonistic.* An *additive* response is one in which the antimicrobial effect of the combination is equal to the sum of the effects of the two drugs alone. A *potentiative* interaction (also called a *synergistic* interaction) is one in which the effect of the combination is greater than the sum of the effects of the individual agents. A classic example of potentiation is produced by trimethoprim plus sulfamethoxazole, drugs that inhibit sequential steps in the synthesis of tetrahydrofolic acid (see Chapter 84).

In certain cases, a combination of two antibiotics may be *less* effective than one of the agents by itself. Such reduced responses indicate *antagonism* between the drugs. Antagonism is most likely when a *bacteriostatic* agent (e.g., tetracycline) is combined with a *bactericidal* drug (e.g., penicillin). Antagonism occurs because bactericidal drugs are usually effective only against organisms that are actively growing. Hence, when bacterial growth has been suppressed by a bacteriostatic drug, the effects of a bactericidal agent can be reduced. If host defenses are intact, antagonism between two antibiotics may have little clinical significance. However, if host defenses are compromised, the consequences of antagonism can be dire.

Indications for Antibiotic Combinations

Initial Therapy of Severe Infection. The most common indication for use of multiple antibiotics is initial therapy of severe infection of unknown etiology, especially in the neutropenic host. Until the infecting organism has been identified, wide antimicrobial coverage is indicated. Just how broad the coverage should be depends on the clinician's skill in narrowing the field of potential causative organisms. Once the identity of the infecting microbe is known, drug selection can be adjusted accordingly. As discussed above, samples for culture should be obtained before drug therapy is initiated.

Mixed Infections. An infection may be caused by more than one microbe. Multiple infecting organisms are common in brain abscesses, pelvic infections, and infections resulting from perforation of abdominal organs. When the infecting microbes differ from one another in drug susceptibility, treatment with more than one antibiotic is required.

Prevention of Resistance. Although use of multiple antibiotics is usually associated with *promoting* drug resistance, there is one disease—tuberculosis—in which drug combinations are employed for the specific purpose of *suppressing* the emergence of resistant bacteria. Just why tuberculosis differs from other infections in this regard is discussed in Chapter 86.

Decreased Toxicity. In some situations, an antibiotic combination can reduce toxicity to the host. For example, by combining flucytosine with amphotericin B in the treatment of fungal meningitis, the dosage of amphotericin B can be reduced, thereby decreasing the risk of amphotericin-induced damage to the kidneys.

Enhanced Antibacterial Action. In specific infections, a combination of antibiotics can have greater antibacterial action than a single agent. This is true of the combined use of penicillin plus an aminoglycoside in the treatment of enterococcal endocarditis. Penicillin acts to weaken the bacterial cell wall; the aminoglycoside acts to suppress protein synthesis. The combination has enhanced antibacterial action because, by weakening the cell wall, penicillin facilitates penetration of the aminoglycoside to its intracellular site of action.

Disadvantages of Antibiotic Combinations

Use of multiple antibiotics has several drawbacks, including (1) increased risk of toxic and allergic reactions, (2) possible antagonism of antimicrobial effects, (3) increased risk of suprainfection, (4) selection of drug-resistant bacteria, and (5) increased cost. Accordingly, antimicrobial combinations should be employed only when clearly indicated.

PROPHYLACTIC USE OF ANTIMICROBIAL DRUGS

Estimates indicate that between 30% and 50% of the antibiotics used in the United States are administered for prophylaxis. That is, these agents are given to prevent infection rather than to treat an established infection. Much of the prophylactic use of antibiotics is uncalled for. However, in certain situations, antimicrobial prophylaxis is both appropriate and effective. Whenever prophylaxis is attempted, the benefits must be weighed against the risks of toxicity, allergic reactions, suprainfection, and selection of drug-resistant organisms. Generally approved indications for prophylaxis are discussed below.

Surgery. Prophylactic use of antibiotics can decrease the incidence of infection in certain kinds of surgery. Procedures in which prophylactic efficacy has been documented include cardiac surgery, peripheral vascular surgery, orthopedic surgery, and surgery on the GI tract (stomach, duodenum, colon, rectum, and appendix). Prophylaxis is also beneficial for women undergoing a hysterectomy or an emergency cesarean section. In "dirty" surgery (operations performed on perforated abdominal organs, compound fractures, or lacerations from animal bites), the risk of infection is nearly 100%. For these operations, use of antibiotics is considered *treatment,* not prophylaxis. When antibiotics are given for prophylaxis, they should be administered before surgery has begun. If the procedure is unusually long, readministration during surgery may be indicated. As a rule, postoperative antibiotics are unnecessary. For most operations, a first-generation cephalosporin (e.g., cefazolin) will suffice.

Bacterial Endocarditis. Individuals with congenital or valvular heart disease and those with prosthetic heart valves are unusually susceptible to bacterial endocarditis. For these people, endocarditis can develop following surgery, dental procedures, and other procedures that may dislodge bacteria into the bloodstream. Hence, prior to undergoing such procedures, these patients should receive prophylactic antimicrobial medication.

Neutropenia. Severe neutropenia puts individuals at high risk of infection. There is some evidence that the incidence of bacterial infection may be reduced through antibiotic prophylaxis. However, prophylaxis may increase the risk of infection with fungi: By killing normal flora, whose presence helps suppress fungal growth, antibiotics can encourage fungal invasion.

Other Indications for Antimicrobial Prophylaxis. For young women with recurrent urinary tract infection, prophylaxis with trimethoprim-sulfamethoxazole may be helpful. Amantadine (an antiviral agent) may be employed for prophylaxis against type A influenza. For individuals who have had severe rheumatic endocarditis, lifelong prophylaxis with penicillin may be needed. Antimicrobial prophylaxis is indicated following exposure to organisms responsible for sexually transmitted diseases (e.g., syphilis, gonorrhea).

MISUSES OF ANTIMICROBIAL DRUGS

Throughout this chapter, we have focused on the proper use of antimicrobial medications. In this section, we consider important ways in which these drugs are misused. The data in Table 79–5 illustrate how common these misuses can be.

Attempted Treatment of Untreatable Infection. The majority of viral infections—including mumps, chickenpox, and the common cold—do not respond to currently available drugs. Hence, when drug therapy of these disorders is attempted, patients are exposed to all the risks of drug use without receiving any benefits.

Treatment of Fever of Unknown Origin. Although fever can be a sign of infection, it can also signify other diseases, including hepatitis, arthritis, and cancer. Unless the cause of a fever is a proven infection, antibiotics should not be employed. Why? Because (1) if the fever is *not* due to an infection, antibiotics would not only be inappropriate, they would expose the patient to unnecessary toxicity and delay correct diagnosis of the fever's cause; and (2) if the fever *is* caused by infection, antibiotics could hamper later attempts to identify the infecting organism.

The only situation in which fever, by itself, constitutes a legitimate indication for antibiotic use is when fever occurs in the severely immunocompromised host. Since fever may indicate infection, and since infection can be lethal to the immunocompromised patient, these patients should be

TABLE 79–5 ■ Examples of Inappropriate Antibiotic Prescriptions

Type of Infection	Prescriptions per Year	Percent Inappropriate	Comment
Common cold	18 million	100	Antibiotics are ineffective against the common cold
Bronchitis	16 million	80	Antibiotics are ineffective against bronchitis, except in a few infections or in patients with chronic severe lung disease
Sore throat	13 million	50	Antibiotics should be used only in patients with confirmed strep infection
Sinusitis	13 million	50	In the absence of facial pain or swelling, antibiotics should be withheld for about 10 days to see if symptoms improve without drugs

given antibiotics when fever occurs—even if fever is the only indication that an infection may be present.

Improper Dosage. Like all other medications, antibiotics must be used in appropriate dosage. If the dosage is too low, the patient will be exposed to a risk of adverse effects without benefit of antibacterial effects. If the dosage is too high, the risks of suprainfection and adverse effects become unnecessarily high.

Treatment in the Absence of Adequate Bacteriologic Information. As stressed earlier, proper antimicrobial therapy requires information on the identity and drug sensitivity of the infecting organism. Except in life-threatening situations, therapy should not be undertaken in the absence of bacteriologic information. This important guideline is often ignored.

Omission of Surgical Drainage. Antibiotics may have limited efficacy in the presence of foreign material, necrotic tissue, or pus. Hence, when appropriate, surgical drainage and cleansing should be performed to promote antimicrobial effects.

MONITORING ANTIMICROBIAL THERAPY

Antimicrobial therapy is assessed by monitoring clinical responses and laboratory results. The frequency of monitoring is directly proportional to the severity of infection. Important clinical indicators of success are reduction of fever and resolution of signs and symptoms related to the affected organ system (e.g., improvement of breath sounds in patients with pneumonia).

Various laboratory tests are used to monitor treatment. Serum drug levels may be monitored for two reasons: to ensure that levels are sufficient for antimicrobial effects and to avoid toxicity from excessive levels. Success of therapy is indicated by the disappearance of infectious organisms from post-treatment cultures. Cultures may become sterile within hours of the onset of treatment (as may happen with urinary tract infections), or they may not become sterile for weeks (as may happen with tuberculosis).

⁞■ KEY POINTS

- In antimicrobial therapy, the term *selective toxicity* refers to the ability of a drug to injure invading microbes without injuring cells of the host.
- Narrow-spectrum antibiotics are active against only a few microorganisms, whereas broad-spectrum antibiotics are active against a wide array of microbes.
- Bactericidal drugs kill bacteria, whereas bacteriostatic drugs only suppress growth.
- Emergence of microbial resistance to drugs is a major concern in antimicrobial therapy.
- An important method by which bacteria acquire resistance is conjugation, a process in which DNA coding for drug resistance is transferred from one bacterium to another.
- Antibiotics do not cause the genetic changes that underlie resistance. Rather, antibiotics promote emergence of drug-resistant organisms by creating selection pressures that favor them.
- Broad-spectrum antibiotics promote the emergence of resistance more than do narrow-spectrum antibiotics.
- In the hospital, we can delay the emergence of antibiotic resistance in four basic ways: preventing infection, diagnosing and treating infection effectively, using antimicrobial drugs wisely, and preventing patient-to-patient transmission.
- Use of antibiotics to promote growth in livestock is a major force for promoting emergence of resistance.
- Effective antimicrobial therapy requires that we determine both the identity and drug sensitivity of the infecting organism.
- The minimum inhibitory concentration (MIC) of an antibiotic is defined as the lowest concentration needed to completely suppress bacterial growth.
- The minimum bactericidal concentration (MBC) is defined as the concentration that decreases the number of bacterial colonies by 99.9%.

- Host defenses—the immune system and phagocytic cells—are essential to the success of antimicrobial therapy.
- Patients should complete the prescribed course of antibiotic treatment, even though symptoms may abate before the full course is over.
- Although combinations of antibiotics should generally be avoided, they are appropriate in several situations, including (1) initial treatment of severe infections, (2) infection with more than one organism, (3) treatment of tuberculosis, and (4) treatment of an infection in which combination therapy can greatly enhance antibacterial effects.

- Appropriate indications for prophylactic antimicrobial treatment include (1) certain surgeries, (2) neutropenia, (3) recurrent urinary tract infections, and (4) patients at risk of bacterial endocarditis (e.g., those with prosthetic heart valves or congenital heart disease).
- Important misuses of antibiotics include (1) treatment of untreatable infections (e.g., the common cold and most other viral infections); (2) treatment of fever of unknown origin (except in the immunocompromised host); (3) treatment in the absence of adequate bacteriologic information; and (4) treatment in the absence of appropriate surgical drainage.

Drugs That Weaken the Bacterial Cell Wall I: Penicillins

INTRODUCTION TO THE PENICILLINS

The penicillins are practically ideal antibiotics. They are active against a variety of bacteria and their direct toxicity is low. Allergic reactions are the principal adverse effect. Owing to their safety and efficacy, the penicillins are widely prescribed.

Because they have a beta-lactam ring in their structure (Fig. 80–1), the penicillins are known as *beta-lactam antibiotics*. The beta-lactam family also includes the cephalosporins, aztreonam, imipenem, meropenem, and ertapenem (see Chapter 81). All of the beta-lactam antibiotics share the same mechanism of action: disruption of the bacterial cell wall.

Mechanism of Action

To understand the actions of the penicillins, we must first understand the structure and function of the bacterial cell wall. The cell wall is a rigid, permeable, mesh-like structure that lies outside the cytoplasmic membrane. Inside the cytoplasmic membrane, osmotic pressure is very high, creating a strong tendency for bacteria to take up water and swell. If it were not for the rigid cell wall, which prevents bacteria from expanding, water would be absorbed to such an extent that they would eventually burst.

The penicillins weaken the cell wall, causing the bacteria to take up excessive amounts of water and then rupture. As a result, the penicillins are generally *bactericidal*. For reasons that are not fully understood, penicillins are lethal only to bacteria undergoing active growth and division.

Penicillins weaken the cell wall by two actions: (1) *inhibition of transpeptidases* and (2) *disinhibition (activation) of autolysins*. Transpeptidases are enzymes critical to cell wall synthesis. Specifically, they catalyze the formation of crossbridges between the peptidoglycan polymer strands that form the cell wall; these bridges give the cell wall its strength (Fig. 80–2). Autolysins are bacterial enzymes that cleave bonds in the cell wall. Bacteria employ these enzymes to break down segments of the cell wall to permit growth and division. By simultaneously inhibiting transpeptidases and activating autolysins, the penicillins (1) disrupt synthesis of the cell wall and (2) promote its active destruction. These combined actions result in cell lysis and death.

The molecular targets of the penicillins (transpeptidases, autolysins, other bacterial enzymes) are known collectively as *penicillin-binding proteins* (PBPs). These molecules are called PBPs because penicillins must bind to them to produce antibacterial effects. More than eight different PBPs have been identified. The PBPs that are most important in mediating the bactericidal actions of the penicillins are named PBP1 and PBP3. As indicated in Figure 80–3, PBPs are located on the outer surface of the cytoplasmic membrane.

Since mammalian cells lack a cell wall, and since penicillins act specifically on enzymes that affect cell wall integrity, the penicillins have virtually no *direct* effects on cells of the host. As a result, the penicillins are among our safest antibiotics.

Mechanisms of Bacterial Resistance

Bacterial resistance to penicillins is determined primarily by two factors: (1) inability of penicillins to reach their targets (PBPs) and (2) inactivation of penicillins by bacterial enzymes.

The Gram-Negative Cell Envelope

All bacteria are surrounded by a cell envelope. However, the cell envelope of gram-negative organisms differs from that of gram-positive organisms. Because of this difference, most penicillins are ineffective against gram-negative bacteria.

887

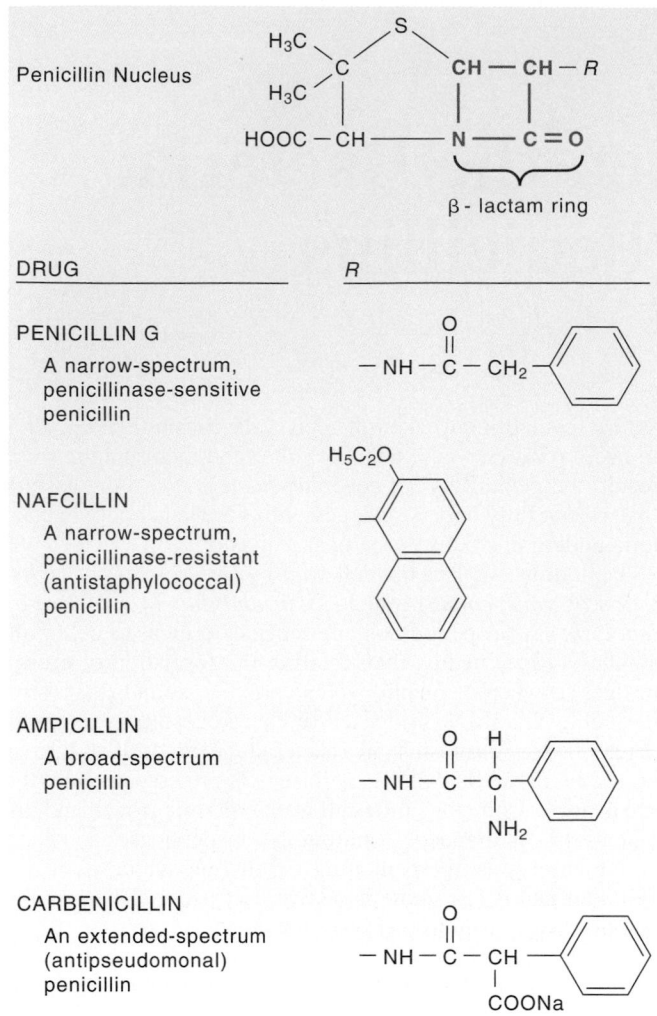

Figure 80–1 ■ **Structural formulas of representative penicillins.**
The unique structure of individual penicillins is determined by the side chain coupled to the penicillin nucleus at the position labeled R. This side chain influences acid stability, pharmacokinetic properties, penicillinase resistance, and ability to bind specific penicillin-binding proteins.

As indicated in Figure 80–3, the cell envelope of *gram-positive* bacteria has only two layers: the cytoplasmic membrane plus a relatively thick cell wall. Despite its thickness, the cell wall can be readily penetrated by penicillins, giving them easy access to PBPs on the cytoplasmic membrane. As a result, penicillins are generally very active against gram-positive organisms.

The *gram-negative* cell envelope has three layers: the cytoplasmic membrane, a relatively thin cell wall, and an additional *outer membrane* (Fig. 80–3). Like the gram-positive cell wall, the gram-negative cell wall can be easily penetrated by penicillins. The outer membrane, however, is difficult to penetrate: Only those penicillins that can pass through the small pores in the outer membrane are able to cross and reach PBPs on the cytoplasmic membrane. Since most peni-

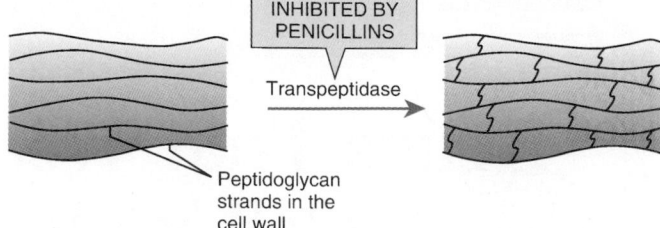

Figure 80–2 ■ **Inhibition of transpeptidase by penicillins.**
The bacterial cell wall is composed of long strands of a peptidoglycan polymer. As depicted, transpeptidase enzymes create cross-bridges between the peptidoglycan strands, giving the cell wall its strength. By inhibiting transpeptidases, penicillins prevent cross-bridge synthesis and thereby weaken the cell wall.

cillins cannot pass through the outer membrane, most penicillins are inactive against gram-negative organisms.

Penicillinases (Beta-Lactamases)

Beta-lactamases are enzymes that cleave the beta-lactam ring, and thereby render penicillins and other beta-lactam antibiotics inactive (Fig. 80–4). Bacteria produce a variety of beta-lactamases; some are specific for penicillins, some are specific for other beta-lactam antibiotics (e.g., cephalosporins), and some act on several kinds of beta-lactam antibiotics. Those beta-lactamases that act selectively on penicillins are referred to as *penicillinases*.

Penicillinases are synthesized by gram-positive and gram-negative bacteria. Gram-positive organisms produce large amounts of these enzymes, and then export them into the surrounding medium. In contrast, gram-negative bacteria produce penicillinases in relatively small amounts, and, rather than exporting them to the environment, secrete them into the periplasmic space (see Fig. 80–3).

The genes that code for synthesis of beta-lactamases are located on plasmids (extrachromosomal DNA) and chromosomes. The genes found on plasmids may be transferred from one bacterium to another, thereby promoting the spread of penicillin resistance.

Transfer of resistance is of special importance with *Staphylococcus aureus*. When penicillin was first introduced in the early 1940s, all strains of *S. aureus* were sensitive to the drug. However, by 1960, as many as 80% of *S. aureus* isolates in hospitals displayed penicillin resistance. Fortunately, a penicillin derivative (methicillin) that has resistance to the actions of beta-lactamases was introduced at this time. To date, no known strains of *S. aureus* produce beta-lactamases capable of inactivating methicillin or related penicillinase-resistant penicillins (although some strains of this organism are resistant to these drugs for other reasons).

Chemistry

All of the penicillins are derived from a common nucleus: 6-aminopenicillanic acid. As shown in Figure 80–1, this nucleus contains a beta-lactam ring joined to a second ring. The beta-lactam ring is essential for antibacterial actions. Properties of individual penicillins are determined by additions

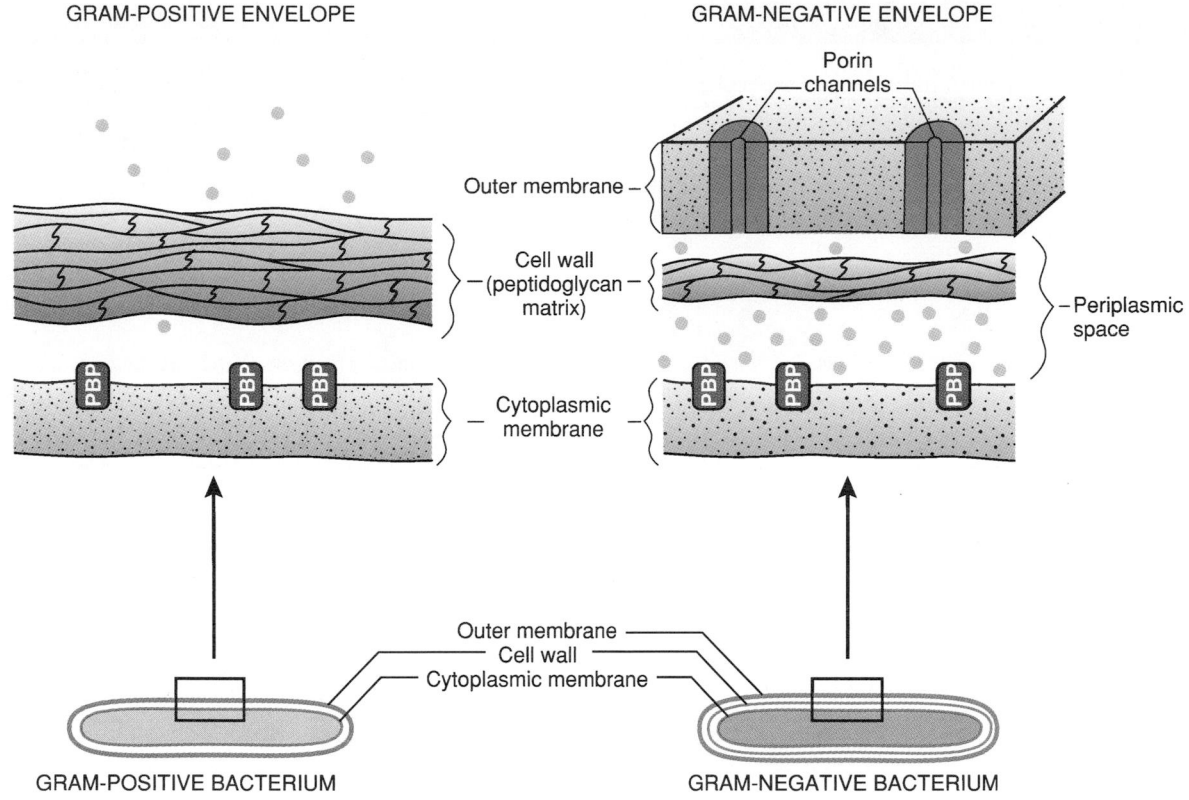

GRAM-POSITIVE ENVELOPE

GRAM-NEGATIVE ENVELOPE

Figure 80–3 ■ The bacterial cell envelope.
Note that the gram-negative cell envelope has an outer membrane, whereas the gram-positive envelope does not. The outer membrane of the gram-negative cell envelope prevents certain penicillins from reaching their target molecules. (PBP = penicillin-binding protein [transpeptidases and other penicillin target molecules]; • = beta-lactamases.)

made to the basic nucleus, primarily at the site labeled R. These modifications determine (1) affinity for PBPs, (2) resistance to penicillinases, (3) ability to penetrate the gram-negative cell envelope, (4) resistance to stomach acid, and (5) pharmacokinetic properties.

Classification

The most useful classification of penicillins is based on antimicrobial spectrum. When classified according to spectrum, the penicillins fall into four major groups: (1) narrow-spectrum penicillins that are penicillinase sensitive, (2) narrow-spectrum penicillins that are penicillinase resistant (antistaphylococcal penicillins), (3) broad-spectrum penicillins (aminopenicillins), and (4) extended-spectrum penicillins (antipseudomonal penicillins). The individual agents that belong to these groups, together with their principal target organisms, are listed in Table 80–1.

PROPERTIES OF INDIVIDUAL PENICILLINS

Penicillin G

Penicillin G (benzylpenicillin) was the first penicillin available and is the prototype for the penicillin family. This agent is often referred to simply as *penicillin*. Penicillin G

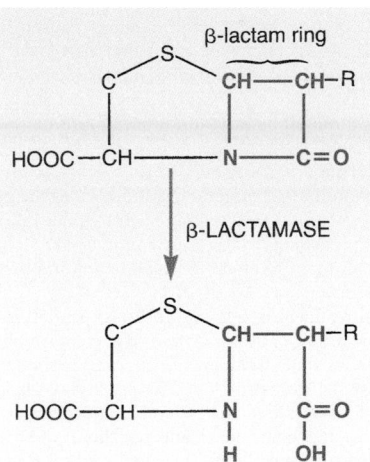

Figure 80–4 ■ The effect of beta-lactamase on the penicillin nucleus.

is bactericidal to a number of gram-positive bacteria as well as to some gram-negative bacteria. Despite the introduction of newer antibiotics, penicillin G remains a drug of choice for many infections. The structure of penicillin G is shown in Figure 80–1.

TABLE 80–1 ■ Classification of the Penicillins

Penicillin Class	Drug	Clinically Useful Antimicrobial Spectrum
Narrow-spectrum penicillinase sensitive	Penicillin G Penicillin V	*Streptococcus* species, *Neisseria* species, many anaerobes, spirochetes, others
Narrow-spectrum penicillins: penicillinase resistant (antistaphylococcal penicillins)	Nafcillin Oxacillin Cloxacillin Dicloxacillin	*Staphylococcus aureus*
Broad-spectrum penicillins (aminopenicillins)	Ampicillin Amoxicillin Bacampicillin	*Haemophilus influenzae, Escherichia coli, Proteus mirabilis,* enterococci, *Neisseria gonorrhoeae*
Extended-spectrum penicillins (antipseudomonal penicillins)	Carbenicillin indanyl Ticarcillin Mezlocillin Piperacillin	Same as broad-spectrum penicillins plus *Pseudomonas aeruginosa, Enterobacter* species, *Proteus* (indole positive), *Bacteroides fragilis,* many *Klebsiella*

Antimicrobial Spectrum

Penicillin G is active against most *gram-positive bacteria* (except penicillinase-producing staphylococci), gram-negative cocci (*Neisseria meningitidis* and non–penicillinase-producing strains of *Neisseria gonorrhoeae*), anaerobic bacteria, and spirochetes (including *Treponema pallidum*). With few exceptions, gram-negative bacilli are resistant. Although many organisms respond to penicillin G, the drug is considered a narrow-spectrum agent (as compared with other members of the penicillin family).

Therapeutic Uses

Penicillin G is a drug of first choice for infections caused by sensitive gram-positive cocci. Important among these infections are pneumonia and meningitis caused by *Streptococcus pneumoniae* (pneumococcus), pharyngitis caused by *Streptococcus pyogenes,* and infectious endocarditis caused by *Streptococcus viridans.* Penicillin is also the preferred drug for use against those few strains of *S. aureus* that do not produce penicillinase.

Penicillin is a preferred agent for infections caused by several gram-positive bacilli. These infections are gas gangrene (caused by *Clostridium perfringens*), tetanus (caused by *Clostridium tetani*), and anthrax (caused by *Bacillus anthracis*).

Penicillin is the drug of first choice for meningitis caused by *N. meningitidis* (meningococcus).

Although once the drug of choice for gonorrhea (caused by *N. gonorrhoeae*), penicillin has been replaced by ceftriaxone as the primary treatment for this infection. Penicillin is now limited to treating infections caused by non–penicillinase-producing strains of *N. gonorrhoeae.*

Penicillin is the drug of choice for syphilis, an infection caused by the spirochete *T. pallidum.*

In addition to treatment of active infections, penicillin G has important *prophylactic* applications. The drug is used to prevent syphilis in sexual partners of individuals known to have this infection. Benzathine penicillin G (administered monthly for life) is employed for prophylaxis against recurrent attacks of rheumatic fever; treatment is recommended for patients with a history of recurrent rheumatic fever and for those with clear evidence of rheumatic heart disease. Penicillin is also employed for *prophylaxis of bacterial endocarditis;* candidates for therapy include individuals with (1) prosthetic heart valves, (2) most congenital heart diseases, (3) acquired valvular heart disease, (4) mitral valve prolapse, and (5) previous history of bacterial endocarditis. For prevention of endocarditis, penicillin is administered prior to dental procedures and other procedures that are likely to produce temporary bacteremia.

Pharmacokinetics

Absorption. Penicillin G is available as three different salts: (1) *potassium* penicillin G, (2) *procaine* penicillin G, and (3) *benzathine* penicillin G. These salts differ with respect to route of administration and time course of action. With all three preparations, the salt dissociates to release penicillin G, the active form of these preparations.

Oral. Oral administration is obsolete. Penicillin G is unstable in acid, and the majority of an oral dose is destroyed in the stomach.

Intramuscular. All forms of penicillin may be administered IM. However, it is important to note that the different salts are absorbed at very different rates. As indicated in Figure 80–5, absorption of *potassium* penicillin G is rapid; peak blood levels are achieved about 15 minutes after injection. In contrast, the *procaine* and *benzathine* salts are absorbed slowly. Because of their delayed absorption, these salts are referred to as *repository* forms of penicillin. When benzathine penicillin is injected IM, penicillin G is absorbed into the blood for weeks, but serum levels remain very low (see Fig. 80–5). Consequently, this preparation is useful only against highly sensitive organisms (e.g., *T. pallidum,* the bacterium that causes syphilis).

Intravenous. When high blood levels are needed rapidly, penicillin can be administered IV. Only the potassium salt should be given by this route. Procaine and benzathine salts must never be administered IV.

Distribution. Penicillin distributes well to most tissues and body fluids. In the *absence* of inflammation, penetration of the meninges and into fluids of joints and the eye is poor. However, in the *presence* of inflammation, entry into cerebrospinal fluid, joints, and the eye is enhanced, permitting treatment of infections caused by susceptible organisms.

Elimination. Penicillin is eliminated by the kidneys, primarily as the unchanged drug. Renal excretion of penicillin is accomplished mainly (90%) by active tubular secretion; the remaining 10% results from glomerular filtration. In older children and adults, the half-life of penicillin is very short (about 30 minutes). Kidney dysfunction causes the half-life to increase dramatically, and may necessitate a reduction in dosage. In patients at high risk of toxicity (those with renal impairment, the acutely ill, the elderly, the very young), kidney function should be monitored.

Renal excretion of penicillin can be delayed with *probenecid,* a compound that competes with penicillin for active tubular transport. In the past, when penicillin was both scarce and expensive, probenecid was employed

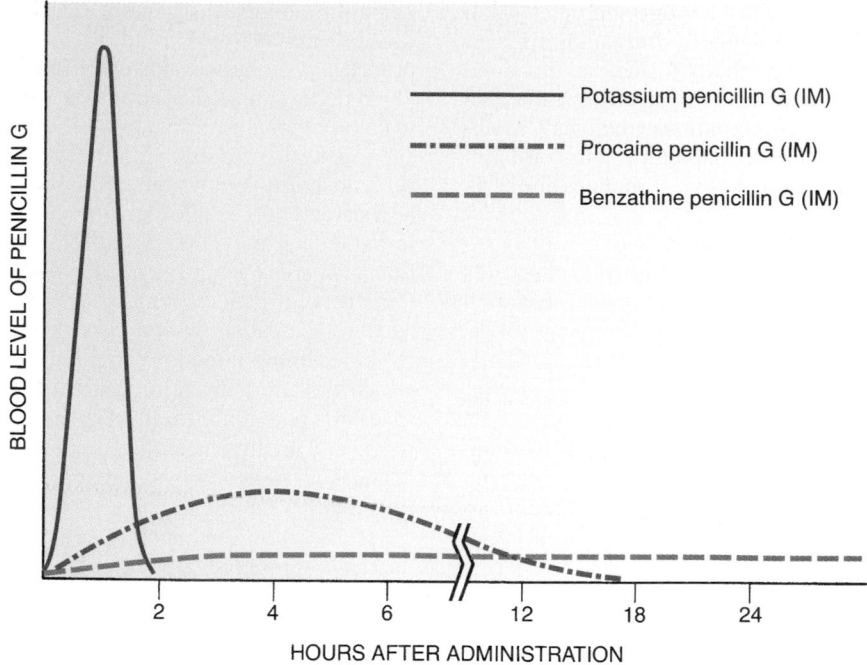

Figure 80–5 ▪ **Penicillin G blood levels following the administration of oral and intramuscular formulations of penicillin G.** (Adapted from Pratt WB, Fekety R. The Antimicrobial Drugs. New York, Oxford University Press, 1986.)

routinely to prolong the effects of the drug. However, since penicillin is now available in abundance at low cost, concurrent use of probenecid is rarely indicated.

Side Effects and Toxicities

Penicillin G is the least toxic of all antibiotics, and is among the safest of all medications. *Allergic reactions,* the principal concern with penicillin, are discussed separately below. In addition to allergic reactions, penicillin G may cause *pain at sites of IM injection,* prolonged (but reversible) *sensory and motor dysfunction* following accidental injection into a peripheral nerve, and *neurotoxicity* (seizures, confusion, hallucinations) if blood levels are allowed to rise too high. Inadvertent *intra-arterial* injection can produce severe reactions (gangrene, necrosis, sloughing of tissue) and must be avoided.

Certain adverse effects may be caused by compounds coadministered with penicillin. For example, the procaine component of procaine penicillin G may cause bizarre behavioral effects when procaine penicillin is given in large doses. When large IV doses of potassium penicillin G are administered rapidly, hyperkalemia can result, possibly causing dysrhythmias and even cardiac arrest.

Penicillin Allergy

General Considerations. *Penicillins are the most common cause of drug allergy.* Between 1% and 10% of patients who receive penicillins experience an allergic response. Reactions range in severity from minor rash to life-threatening anaphylaxis. As with most allergic reactions, there is no direct relationship between the size of the dose and the intensity of the allergic response. Although prior exposure to penicillins is required for an allergic reaction, responses may occur in the absence of prior penicillin use. How can this be? Because patients may have been exposed to penicillins produced by fungi or to penicillins present in foods of animal origin.

Because of cross-sensitivity, patients allergic to one penicillin should be considered allergic to all penicillins. In addition, about 5% to 10% of individuals allergic to penicillins display cross-sensitivity to *cephalosporins*. If at all possible, patients with penicillin allergy should not be treated with any member of the penicillin family; cephalosporins may be used cautiously in some patients.

Individuals allergic to penicillin should be encouraged to wear a Medic Alert bracelet or some other form of identification to alert healthcare personnel to their condition.

Types of Allergic Reactions. Penicillin reactions are classified as *immediate, accelerated,* and *late*. Immediate reactions occur 2 to 30 minutes after drug administration; accelerated reactions occur within 1 to 72 hours; and late reactions take days or even weeks to develop.

Anaphylaxis (laryngeal edema, bronchoconstriction, severe hypotension) is an immediate hypersensitivity reaction, and is the reaction of greatest concern. Anaphylactic reactions occur more frequently with penicillins than with any other drugs. Fortunately, even with penicillins, the incidence of anaphylaxis is only about 0.02%. However, when these reactions do occur, the risk of mortality is high (about 10%). The primary treatment for anaphylaxis is *epinephrine* (SC, IM, or IV) plus respiratory support. To ensure prompt treatment if anaphylaxis should develop, patients should remain in the physician's office for at least 30 minutes after drug injection (i.e., until the risk of an anaphylactic reaction has passed).

Development of Penicillin Allergy. Before discussing penicillin allergy further, we need to review development of allergy to small molecules as a class. Drugs and other small molecules are unable to induce antibody formation directly. Therefore, in order to promote antibody formation, the small molecule must first bond covalently to a larger molecule (usually a protein). In these combinations, the small molecule is referred to as a *hapten.* The hapten-protein combination constitutes the complete *antigen* that stimulates antibody formation.

The hapten involved in development of penicillin antibodies is rarely intact penicillin itself. Rather, compounds formed from the degradation of penicillin are the actual haptens. As a result, most "penicillin antibodies" are not directed at penicillin itself. Rather, they are directed at various penicillin degradation products.

Skin Tests for Penicillin Allergy. Allergy to penicillin can decrease over time. Hence, an intense allergic reaction in the past does not necessarily mean that an intense reaction will occur again. In patients with a history of penicillin allergy, skin tests can be employed to assess the current risk of a severe reaction. These tests are performed by injecting a tiny amount of allergen intradermally and observing for an allergic response.

Two reagents can be employed to assess penicillin allergy. One of these, *benzylpenicilloyl-polylysine* [Pre-Pen], tests primarily for *delayed* hypersensitivity. This reagent is referred to as a *major antigenic determinant,* a term indicating that the antibodies for which this reagent tests are relatively common. Benzylpenicilloyl-polylysine is a large polymeric molecule that is poorly absorbed. Hence, even in patients with severe penicillin allergy, a skin test with this compound carries little risk of a systemic reaction.

The second skin test reagent, known as the *minor determinant mixture* (MDM), detects antibodies that mediate *immediate* allergic responses (e.g., anaphylaxis). The term *minor* indicates that the antibodies being tested for are relatively uncommon and not that the allergic response mediated by these antibodies is of minor significance. It is important to note that skin testing with MDM can be dangerous: In patients with severe penicillin allergy, the skin test itself can precipitate an anaphylactic reaction. Accordingly, the test should be performed only if epinephrine and facilities for respiratory support are immediately available.

For two reasons, penicillin itself is rarely employed for skin tests. First, skin testing with penicillin can elicit an anaphylactic reaction in highly sensitized individuals. Second, use of penicillin can produce a false-negative result. This second point is paradoxical and requires explanation. Recall that most antibodies that mediate penicillin allergy are directed against degradation products of penicillin, and not against penicillin itself. Nonetheless, intact penicillin is able to bind to the active site of these antibodies—but that binding will not trigger an immune response. As a result, when small amounts of degradation products are formed following intradermal injection of penicillin, the presence of large amounts of intact penicillin can compete with those products for antibody-binding sites, thereby preventing the degradation products from triggering an allergic reaction.

Management of Patients with a History of Penicillin Allergy. All patients who are candidates for penicillin therapy should be asked if they have experienced an allergic reaction to penicillin. For patients who indicate a history of

penicillin allergy, the general rule is to avoid penicillins entirely. If the allergy is mild, a *cephalosporin* is often an appropriate alternative. However, if there is a history of anaphylaxis or some other severe allergic reaction, it is prudent to avoid cephalosporins as well (because there is a 5% to 10% risk of cross-sensitivity to cephalosporins). When a cephalosporin is indicated, an oral cephalosporin is preferred to a parenteral cephalosporin—because the risk of severe allergic responses is lower with oral therapy. For many infections, *vancomycin* and *erythromycin* are effective and safe alternatives for patients with penicillin allergy.

Rarely, a patient with a history of anaphylaxis may have a life-threatening infection (e.g., enterococcal endocarditis) for which the alternatives to penicillins are ineffective. In these cases, the potential benefits of penicillin therapy outweigh the risks, and treatment should be instituted. To minimize the chances of an anaphylactic reaction, penicillin should be administered according to a desensitization schedule. In this procedure, an initial small dose is followed at 60-minute intervals by progressively larger doses until the full therapeutic dose has been achieved. It should be noted that the desensitization procedure is not without risk. Accordingly, epinephrine and facilities for respiratory support should be immediately available.

Drug Interactions

Aminoglycosides. For some infections, penicillins are used in combination with an aminoglycoside (e.g., gentamicin). By weakening the cell wall, the penicillin facilitates access of the aminoglycoside to its intracellular site of action, thereby increasing bactericidal effects. Unfortunately, when penicillins are present in high concentrations, they interact chemically with aminoglycosides to cause inactivation of the aminoglycoside. Accordingly, *penicillins and aminoglycosides should not be mixed in the same IV solution.* Rather, these drugs should be administered separately. Once a penicillin has been diluted in body fluids, the potential for inactivation of aminoglycosides is minimal.

Probenecid. As noted in the discussion of penicillin elimination, probenecid can delay renal excretion of penicillin, thereby prolonging antibacterial effects.

Bacteriostatic Antibiotics. Since penicillins are most effective against actively growing bacteria, concurrent use of a bacteriostatic antibiotic (e.g., tetracycline) could, in theory, reduce the bactericidal effects of the penicillin. However, the clinical significance of such interactions is not known. Moreover, there are infections for which combined therapy with a bacteriostatic agent and a penicillin is indicated. When such combined chemotherapy is employed, the penicillin should be administered a few hours before the bacteriostatic drug to minimize any reduction of penicillin's effects.

Preparations, Dosage, and Administration

Preparations and Routes of Administration. Penicillin G is available as three different salts (potassium, procaine, and benzathine). These salts differ with respect to routes of administration: *potassium* penicillin G [Pfizerpen] is administered IM, IV, and by local infusion (e.g., intrapleural); and *benzathine* penicillin G [Bicillin L-A, Permapen], *procaine* penicillin G [Wycillin], and a combination product [Bicillin C-R], composed of benzathine penicillin G plus procaine penicillin G, are all administered IM. Check to ensure that the penicillin salt to be administered is appropriate for the intended route.

Dosage. Dosage of penicillin G is prescribed in units (1 unit equals 0.6 mg). Dosage ranges are summarized in Table 80–2. For any particular patient, the specific dosage will depend on the type and severity of infection. The dosage should be reduced in patients with severe renal impairment.

TABLE 80–2 ■ Dosages for Penicillin

Generic Name	Trade Name	Route	Dosing Interval (hr)	Total Daily Dosage[a] Adults	Children
Narrow-Spectrum Penicillins: Penicillinase-Sensitive					
Penicillin G	Bicillin L-A, Permapen, Pfizerpen, Wycillin	IM, IV	4	1.2–2.4 million units[b]	100,000–250,000 units/kg[b]
Penicillin V	Beepen-VK, Veetids, Pen-Vee K	PO	4–6	0.5–2 gm	25–50 mg/kg
Narrow-Spectrum Penicillins: Penicillinase-Resistant (Antistaphylococcal Penicillins)					
Nafcillin	Nallpen, Unipen	PO	6	2–4 gm	50–100 mg/kg
		IM, IV	4–6	2–9 gm	100–200 mg/kg
Oxacillin	Bactocill	PO	6	2–4 gm	50–100 mg/kg
		IM, IV	4–6	2–12 gm	100–200 mg/kg
Cloxacillin	Cloxapen	PO	6	2–4 gm	50–100 mg/kg
Dicloxacillin	Dycill, Dynapen, Pathocil	PO	6	1–2 gm	12.5–25 mg/kg
Broad-Spectrum Penicillins (Aminopenicillins)					
Ampicillin	Marcillin, Omnipen, Principen, Totacillin	PO	6–8	2–4 gm	50–100 mg/kg
		IM, IV	6–8	2–12 gm	10–200 mg/kg
Ampicillin-sulbactam	Unasyn	IM, IV	6	4–8 gm[c]	—
Amoxicillin	Amoxil, Trimox, Wymox	PO	8	0.75–1.5 gm	20–40 mg/kg
Amoxicillin-clavulanate	Augmentin	PO	8	250–500 mg[d]	20–40 mg/kg[d]
	Augmentin ES-600	PO	12	—	90 mg/kg
	Augmentin XR	PO	12	4000 mg	—
Bacampicillin	Spectrobid	PO	12	0.8–1.6 gm	25–50 mg/kg
Extended-Spectrum Penicillins (Antipseudomonal Penicillins)					
Carbenicillin indanyl	Geocillin	PO	4–6	1.5–3 gm	—
		IM	6	4–8 gm	50–200 mg/kg
		IV	4–6	30–40 gm	100–600 mg/kg
Ticarcillin	Ticar	IM	6	4 gm	50–100 mg/kg
		IV	4–6	200–300 mg/kg	200–300 mg/kg
Ticarcillin-clavulanate	Timentin	IV	4–6	200–300 mg/kg[e]	—
Mezlocillin	Mezlin	IM	6	4–8 gm	—
		IV	4–6	6–18 gm	300 mg/kg
Piperacillin	Pipracil	IM	6–12	6–8 gm	—
		IV	4–6	12–24 gm	200–300 mg/kg
Piperacillin-tazobactam	Zosyn	IV	6	12 gm[f]	—

[a]Doses vary widely, depending upon the type and severity of infection; doses and dosing intervals presented here may not be appropriate for all patients.
[b]10,000 units = 6 mg.
[c]Dose based on ampicillin content.
[d]Dose based on amoxicillin content.
[e]Dose based on ticarcillin content.
[f]Dose based on piperacillin content.

Administration. Solutions for parenteral administration should be prepared according to the manufacturer's instructions. During IM administration, take care to avoid inadvertent injection into an artery or peripheral nerve.

Penicillin V

Penicillin V, also known as penicillin VK, is similar to penicillin G in most respects. These drugs differ primarily in their acid stability: penicillin V is stable in stomach acid, whereas penicillin G is not. Because of its stability in stomach acid, penicillin V has replaced penicillin G for oral therapy. Penicillin V may be taken with meals. Dosages are summarized in Table 80–2. Trade names are Beepen-VK, Pen-Vee K, and Veetids.

Penicillinase-Resistant Penicillins (Antistaphylococcal Penicillins)

By altering the penicillin side chain, pharmaceutical chemists have created a group of penicillins that are highly resistant to inactivation by beta-lactamases. In the United States, four such drugs are currently available: *nafcillin, oxacillin, cloxacillin,* and *dicloxacillin.* (A fifth drug—*methicillin*—is no longer on the market.) These agents have a very narrow antimicrobial spectrum and are used only against penicillinase-producing strains of staphylococcus (*S. aureus* and *Staph. epidermidis*). Since most strains of staphylococci produce penicillinase, the penicillinase-resistant penicillins are drugs of choice for the majority of staphylococcal infections. It should be noted that these agents should not be used against infections caused by non–penicillinase-producing staphylococci, since they are less active than penicillin G against those bacteria.

An increasing clinical problem is the emergence of staphylococcal strains referred to as *methicillin resistant,* a term used to indicate *lack of susceptibility to methicillin (an obsolete penicillinase-resistant penicillin) and all other penicillinase-resistant penicillins.* Resistance appears to result from production of altered PBPs to which the penicillinase-resistant penicillins are unable to bind. Currently, vancomycin (alone or combined with rifampin) is the treatment of choice for infections caused by methicillin-resistant staphylococci.

Nafcillin

Nafcillin [Nallpen, Unipen] is usually administered IM or IV. Although the drug is available in a formulation for oral use, absorption from the GI tract is incomplete and erratic; consequently, oral administration is not recommended. Dosages are summarized in Table 80–2.

Oxacillin, Cloxacillin, and Dicloxacillin

These three drugs are similar in structure and pharmacokinetic properties. All three are acid stable and available for oral administration; oxacillin may also be administered parenterally (IM and IV). Oral administration of all three may be done with meals. Dosages and trade names are summarized in Table 80–2.

Methicillin

Methicillin, the oldest penicillinase-resistant penicillin, is no longer available in the United States. In addition to causing allergic reactions typical of all penicillins, methicillin may produce interstitial nephritis, an adverse effect that is usually reversible but sometimes progresses to complete renal failure.

Broad-Spectrum Penicillins (Aminopenicillins)

The family of broad-spectrum penicillins consists of *ampicillin, amoxicillin,* and *bacampicillin.* These drugs have the same antimicrobial spectrum as penicillin G, *plus* increased activity against certain gram-negative bacilli, including *Haemophilus influenzae, Escherichia coli, Salmonella,* and *Shigella.* This broadened spectrum is due in large part to an increased ability to penetrate the gram-negative cell envelope. All of the broad-spectrum penicillins are readily inactivated by beta-lactamases. Hence, these drugs are ineffective against most infections caused by *S. aureus.*

Properties of individual broad-spectrum penicillins are discussed below. Dosages are summarized in Table 80–2.

Ampicillin

Ampicillin was the first broad-spectrum penicillin available for clinical use. The agent is a preferred or alternative drug for infections caused by *Streptococcus faecalis, Proteus mirabilis, E. coli, Salmonella, Shigella,* and *H. influenzae.* The drug's most common side effects are rash and diarrhea; both reactions occur more frequently with ampicillin than with any other penicillin. Administration may be parenteral or oral. It should be noted, however, that for oral therapy, amoxicillin is preferred (see below). Trade names for ampicillin are Marcillin, Omnipen, Principen, and Totacillin. Routes and usual dosages are summarized in Table 80–2. Dosages must be reduced in patients with renal impairment. As discussed below, ampicillin is also available in a fixed-dose combination with sulbactam, an inhibitor of bacterial beta-lactamases. The combination is marketed as Unasyn.

Amoxicillin

Amoxicillin is similar to ampicillin in structure and actions. The drugs differ primarily in acid stability, amoxicillin being the more acid resistant. Hence, when the two are administered orally in equivalent doses, blood levels of amoxicillin are greater than those of ampicillin. Accordingly, when oral therapy is indicated, amoxicillin is preferred. Amoxicillin produces less diarrhea than ampicillin, perhaps because less amoxicillin remains unabsorbed in the intestine. Trade names are Amoxil, Trimox, and Wymox. As discussed below, amoxicillin is also available in fixed-dose combinations with clavulanic acid, an inhibitor of bacterial beta-lactamases. The combination is marketed as Augmentin. Amoxicillin, by itself, is one of our most frequently prescribed antibiotics.

Bacampicillin

Bacampicillin [Spectrobid] is a prodrug form of ampicillin. Once in the body, bacampicillin is rapidly converted to ampicillin, its active form. Bacampicillin is acid stable and administration is oral. The drug may be taken with meals. Because of its resistance to acid, bacampicillin produces blood levels of ampicillin that are 2 times greater than those achieved with equivalent oral doses of ampicillin itself. Despite this difference, bacampicillin offers no clinical advantage over ampicillin or amoxicillin, and is usually more expensive.

Extended-Spectrum Penicillins (Antipseudomonal Penicillins)

The family of extended-spectrum penicillins consists of four drugs: *ticarcillin, carbenicillin indanyl, mezlocillin,* and *piperacillin.* The antimicrobial spectrum of these drugs includes organisms that are susceptible to the aminopenicillins plus *Pseudomonas aeruginosa, Enterobacter* species, *Proteus* (indole positive), *Bacteroides fragilis,* and many *Klebsiella.* All of the extended-spectrum penicillins are susceptible to beta-lactamases, and hence are ineffective against most strains of *S. aureus.*

The extended-spectrum penicillins are used primarily for infections with *P. aeruginosa.* These infections often occur in the immunocompromised host and can be very difficult to eradicate. To increase killing of *Pseudomonas,* an antipseudomonal aminoglycoside (gentamicin, tobramycin, amikacin, netilmicin) is almost always added to the regimen. When these combinations are employed, the penicillin and the aminoglycoside should not be mixed in the same IV solution. Why? Because high concentrations of penicillins can inactivate aminoglycosides.

Properties of individual extended-spectrum penicillins are discussed below. Dosages are summarized in Table 80–2.

Ticarcillin

Antimicrobial Spectrum and Therapeutic Use. Ticarcillin [Ticar] has one of the broadest antimicrobial spectra of all penicillins. However, like other extended-spectrum penicillins, the drug is susceptible to destruction by penicillinase.

The primary indication for ticarcillin is infection caused by *P. aeruginosa.* When used against *Pseudomonas,* ticarcillin is usually combined with an aminoglycoside.

Adverse Effects. In addition to promoting the allergic reactions typical of all penicillins, ticarcillin can cause unique effects. Since the drug is administered as the *disodium salt,* and since large IV doses are often required, symptoms of *sodium overload* (e.g., congestive heart failure) may develop. Also, ticarcillin interferes with platelet function and can thereby promote *bleeding.*

Preparations and Administration. Ticarcillin [Ticar] is unstable in acid, and hence must be given parenterally (IM or IV). When ticarcillin is used in combination with an aminoglycoside, the two drugs should be administered separately.

As discussed later in the chapter, ticarcillin is available in a fixed-dose combination with clavulanic acid, a beta-lactamase inhibitor. The combination [Timentin] is administered intravenously.

Dosages for patients with normal kidney function are summarized in Table 80–2. Dosages must be reduced in patients with renal impairment.

Carbenicillin Indanyl

Carbenicillin indanyl [Geocillin] is acid stable and administered orally. Once absorbed, the drug is converted to carbenicillin, its active form. Excretion is renal, and the drug becomes concentrated in urine. Carbenicillin indanyl is indicated only for urinary tract infections caused by *P. aeruginosa* or by indole-positive *Proteus*. Drug levels at sites outside the urinary tract are too low for clinically significant antibacterial effects. Oral carbenicillin should not be taken with meals.

Mezlocillin and Piperacillin

Mezlocillin [Mezlin] and piperacillin [Pipracil] have broad antimicrobial spectra. However, like other extended-spectrum penicillins, these drugs are penicillinase sensitive. Both are highly active against *P. aeruginosa*, their principal target. Like ticarcillin, mezlocillin and piperacillin can cause bleeding secondary to disruption of platelet function. Both drugs are acid labile and must be administered parenterally (IM or IV). The risk of sodium overload with IV mezlocillin or IV piperacillin is much less than with IV ticarcillin. When these drugs are used in combination with an aminoglycoside, they should not be mixed in the same IV solution. Dosages of mezlocillin and piperacillin for patients with normal kidney function are shown in Table 80–2. Dosages for both drugs should be reduced in patients with renal impairment. As discussed below, piperacillin is also available in a fixed-dose combination with tazobactam, a beta-lactamase inhibitor. The combination is marketed as Zosyn.

Penicillins Combined with a Beta-Lactamase Inhibitor

As their name indicates, beta-lactamase inhibitors are drugs that inhibit bacterial beta-lactamases. By combining a beta-lactamase inhibitor with a penicillinase-sensitive penicillin, we can extend the antimicrobial spectrum of the penicillin. In the United States, three beta-lactamase inhibitors are used: *clavulanic acid, tazobactam,* and *sulbactam*. These drugs are not available alone. Rather, they are available only in fixed-dose combinations with a penicillin. Four such combination products are in use now:

- Ampicillin + sulbactam = [Unasyn]
- Amoxicillin + clavulanic acid = [Augmentin]
- Ticarcillin + clavulanic acid = [Timentin]
- Piperacillin + tazobactam = [Zosyn]

Because beta-lactamase inhibitors have minimal toxicity, any adverse effects that occur with the combination products are due to the penicillin. Routes of administration and dosages are summarized in Table 80–2.

.˙. KEY POINTS

- Penicillins weaken the bacterial cell wall, causing lysis and death.
- Some bacteria resist penicillins by producing penicillinases (beta-lactamases), enzymes that inactivate penicillins.
- Gram-negative bacteria are resistant to most penicillins because most penicillins are unable to penetrate the gram-negative cell envelope.
- Penicillins are the safest antibiotics available.
- The principal adverse effect of penicillins is allergic reactions, which can range in intensity from rash to life-threatening anaphylaxis.
- Patients allergic to one penicillin should be considered cross-allergic to all other penicillins. In addition, they have a 5% to 10% chance of cross-allergy to cephalosporins.
- Vancomycin and erythromycin are safe and effective alternatives to penicillins for patients with penicillin allergy.
- Penicillins are normally eliminated rapidly by the kidney, but can accumulate to harmful levels if renal function is severely impaired.
- The principal differences among the penicillins relate to antibacterial spectrum, stability in stomach acid, and duration of action.
- Penicillin G has a narrow antibacterial spectrum and is unstable in stomach acid.
- Benzathine penicillin G is released very slowly following IM injection, and thereby produces prolonged antibacterial effects.
- The penicillinase-resistant penicillins (e.g., nafcillin) are used primarily against penicillinase-producing strains of *Staph. aureus*.
- In contrast to penicillin G, the broad-spectrum penicillins, such as ampicillin and amoxicillin, have useful activity against gram-negative bacilli.
- Extended-spectrum penicillins, such as ticarcillin, are useful against *P. aeruginosa*.
- Beta-lactamase inhibitors, such as clavulanic acid, are combined with certain penicillins to increase their activity against beta-lactamase–producing bacteria.
- Penicillins should not be combined with aminoglycosides (e.g., gentamicin) in the same IV solution.

Summary of Major Nursing Implications*

PENICILLINS

Amoxicillin
Ampicillin
Bacampicillin
Carbenicillin
Cloxacillin
Dicloxacillin
Mezlocillin
Nafcillin
Oxacillin

Penicillin G
Penicillin V
Piperacillin
Ticarcillin

Except where indicated otherwise, the implications summarized below apply to all members of the penicillin family.

Preadministration Assessment

Therapeutic Goal

Treatment of infections caused by sensitive bacteria.

*Patient education information is highlighted as blue text.

Summary of Major Nursing Implications*—cont'd

Baseline Data

The physician may order tests to identify the infecting organism and its drug sensitivity. Take samples for microbiologic culture prior to starting treatment.

In patients with a history of penicillin allergy, a skin test may be performed to determine current allergic status.

Identifying High-Risk Patients

Penicillins are *contraindicated* for patients with a history of severe allergic reactions to penicillins, cephalosporins, or imipenem.

Implementation: Administration

Routes

Penicillins are administered orally, IM, and IV. Routes for individual agents are summarized in Table 80–2. Before giving a penicillin, check to ensure that the preparation is appropriate for the intended route.

Dosage

Doses for penicillin G are prescribed in units (1 unit equals 0.6 mg). Doses for all other penicillins are prescribed by weight.

Dosages for individual penicillins are summarized in Table 80–2.

Administration

During IM injection, aspirate to avoid injection into an artery. Take care to avoid injection into a nerve.

Instruct the patient to take oral penicillins with a full glass of water 1 hour before meals or 2 hours after. *Penicillin V, amoxicillin, amoxicillin-clavulanate,* and *bacampicillin* may be taken with meals.

Instruct the patient to complete the prescribed course of treatment, even though symptoms may abate before the full course is over.

Ongoing Evaluation and Interventions

Evaluating Therapeutic Effects

Monitor the patient for indications of antimicrobial effects (e.g., reduction in fever, pain, or inflammation; improved appetite or sense of well-being).

Monitoring Kidney Function

Renal impairment can cause penicillins to accumulate to toxic levels, and hence monitoring kidney function can help avoid injury. Measurement of intake and output is of particular value in patients with kidney disease, in acutely ill patients, and in the very old and very young. Notify the physician if a significant change in intake-output ratio develops.

*Patient education information is highlighted as blue text.

Minimizing Adverse Effects

Allergic Reactions. Penicillin allergy is common. Rarely, life-threatening anaphylaxis occurs. Interview the patient for a history of penicillin allergy.

For patients with prior allergic responses, a skin test may be ordered to assess current allergy status. Exercise caution: The skin test itself can cause a severe reaction. When skin tests are performed, epinephrine and facilities for respiratory support should be immediately available.

Advise the patient with penicillin allergy to wear some form of identification (e.g., Medic Alert bracelet) to alert emergency healthcare personnel.

Instruct outpatients to report any signs of an allergic response (e.g., skin rash, itching, hives).

Whenever a parenteral penicillin is used, keep the patient under observation for at least 30 minutes. If anaphylaxis occurs, treatment consists of *epinephrine* (SC, IM, or IV) plus respiratory support.

As a rule, patients with a history of penicillin allergy should not receive penicillins again. If previous reactions have been mild, a cephalosporin (preferably oral) may be an appropriate alternative. However, if severe immediate reactions have occurred, cephalosporins should be avoided too.

Rarely, a patient with a history of anaphylaxis nonetheless requires penicillin. To minimize the risk of a severe reaction, administer penicillin according to a desensitization schedule. Be aware, however, that the procedure does not guarantee that anaphylaxis will not occur. Accordingly, have epinephrine and facilities for respiratory support immediately available.

Sodium Loading. High IV doses of *carbenicillin* or *ticarcillin* can produce sodium overload. Exercise caution in patients under sodium restriction (e.g., cardiac patients, those with hypertension). Monitor electrolytes and cardiac status.

Hyperkalemia. High doses of IV *potassium penicillin G* may cause hyperkalemia, possibly resulting in dysrhythmias or cardiac arrest. Monitor electrolyte and cardiac status.

Effects Resulting from Incorrect Injection. Take care to avoid intra-arterial injection or injection into peripheral nerves, because serious injury can result.

Minimizing Adverse Interactions

Aminoglycosides. When present in high concentration, penicillins can inactivate aminoglycosides (e.g., gentamicin). Do not mix penicillins and aminoglycosides in the same IV solution.

Bacteriostatic Antibiotics. Suppression of bacterial growth with a bacteriostatic agent can, in theory, decrease the effectiveness of penicillins. When a bacteriostatic drug is combined with a penicillin, administer the penicillin a few hours before the bacteriostatic drug.

Drugs That Weaken the Bacterial Cell Wall II: Cephalosporins, Carbapenems, Aztreonam, Vancomycin, Teicoplanin, and Fosfomycin

CEPHALOSPORINS
CARBAPENEMS
  Imipenem
  Meropenem
  Ertapenem
OTHER INHIBITORS OF CELL WALL SYNTHESIS
  Aztreonam
  Vancomycin
  Teicoplanin
  Fosfomycin

Like the penicillins, the drugs discussed in this chapter are inhibitors of cell wall synthesis. By disrupting the cell wall, these drugs produce bacterial lysis and death. Most of the chapter focuses on the cephalosporins, our most widely used antibacterial drugs. With only three exceptions—vancomycin, teicoplanin, and fosfomycin—the drugs addressed in this chapter belong to the beta-lactam family.

CEPHALOSPORINS

The cephalosporins are beta-lactam antibiotics similar in structure and actions to the penicillins. These drugs are bactericidal, often resistant to beta-lactamases, and active against a broad spectrum of pathogens. Their toxicity is low. Because of these attributes, the cephalosporins are popular therapeutic agents and constitute our most widely used group of antibiotics. Hospitals in the United States spend more money on cephalosporins than on all other antibiotics combined.

Chemistry

All cephalosporins are derived from the same nucleus. As shown in Figure 81–1, this nucleus contains a *beta-lactam ring* fused to a second ring. The beta-lactam ring is required for antibacterial activity. Unique properties of individual cephalosporins are determined by additions made to the nucleus at the sites labeled R_1 and R_2. Structures of four representative cephalosporins are shown.

Mechanism of Action

The cephalosporins are bactericidal drugs with a mechanism of action like that of the penicillins. These agents bind to penicillin-binding proteins (PBPs) and thereby (1) disrupt cell wall synthesis and (2) activate autolysins (enzymes that cleave bonds in the cell wall). The resultant damage to the cell wall causes death by lysis. Like the penicillins, cephalosporins are most effective against cells undergoing active growth and division.

Resistance

The principal cause of cephalosporin resistance is production of beta-lactamases, enzymes that cleave the beta-lactam ring of cephalosporins, and thereby render them inactive. The beta-lactamases that act on cephalosporins are sometimes referred to as *cephalosporinases*. Some of the beta-lactamases that act on cephalosporins can also cleave the beta-lactam ring of penicillins.

Not all cephalosporins are equally susceptible to beta-lactamases. Most *first-generation* cephalosporins are destroyed by beta-lactamases; *second-generation* cephalosporins are less sensitive to destruction; and *third-* and *fourth-generation* cephalosporins are highly resistant to destruction.

In some cases, bacterial resistance results from production of altered PBPs that have a low affinity for cephalosporins. Methicillin-resistant staphylococci produce these unusual PBPs and are resistant to cephalosporins as a result.

Classification and Antimicrobial Spectra

The cephalosporins can be grouped into four "generations" based on the order of their introduction to clinical use. The generations differ significantly with respect to antimicrobial spectrum and susceptibility to beta-lactamases. In general, *as we progress from first-generation agents to fourth-generation agents, there is (1) increasing activity against gram-negative bacteria and anaerobes, (2) increasing resistance to destruction by beta-lactamases, and (3) increasing ability to reach the cerebrospinal fluid (CSF).* These differences are summarized in Table 81–1.

897

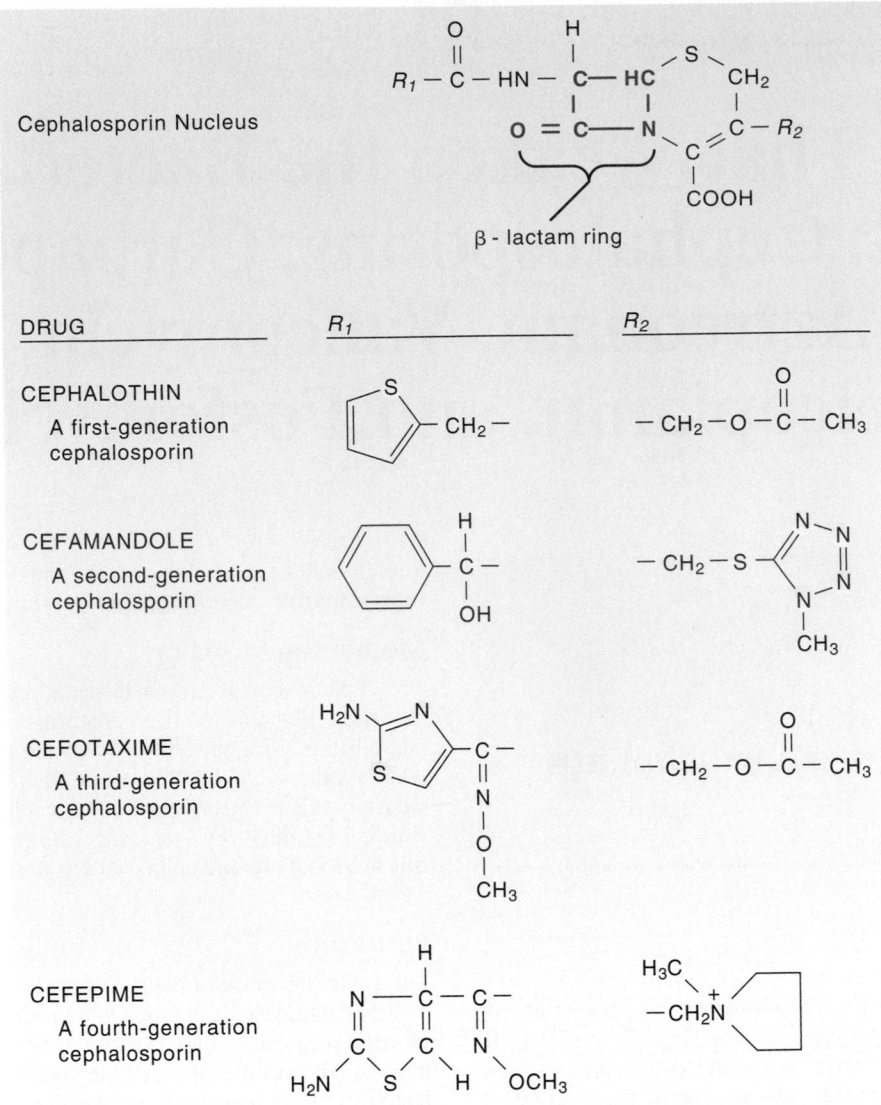

FIGURE 81–1 ▪ Structural formulas of representative cephalosporins.
The unique structure and pharmacologic properties of individual cephalosporins are determined by additions made to the cephalosporin nucleus at the positions labeled R_1 and R_2.

TABLE 81–1 ▪▪ Major Differences Between Cephalosporin Generations

Class	Activity Against Gram-Negative Bacteria	Resistance to Beta-Lactamases	Distribution to Cerebrospinal Fluid
First generation (e.g., cephalothin)	Low	Low	Poor
Second generation (e.g., cefamandole)	Higher	Higher	Poor
Third generation (e.g., cefotaxime)	Higher	Higher	Good
Fourth generation (e.g., cefepime)	Highest	Highest	Good

TABLE 81-2 ::■ Pharmacokinetic Properties of the Cephalosporins

Class	Drug	Routes of Administration	Major Route of Elimination	Half-life (hr)	
				Normal Renal Function	Severe Renal Impairment
First generation	Cefadroxil	PO	Renal	1.2–1.3	20–25
	Cefazolin	IM, IV	Renal	1.5–2.2	24–50
	Cephalexin	PO	Renal	0.4–1.0	10–20
	Cephapirin	IM, IV	Renal	0.3–0.7	2.4
	Cephradine	PO, IM, IV	Renal	0.8–2.0	8–15
Second generation	Cefaclor	PO	Renal	0.6–0.9	2–3
	Cefmetazole	IV	Renal	1.2	—
	Cefonicid	IM, IV	Renal	3.5–4.9	17–56
	Cefotetan	IM, IV	Renal	3.0–4.5	13–35
	Cefoxitin	IM, IV	Renal	0.7–1.0	13–22
	Cefprozil	PO	Renal	1.3	5–6
	Cefuroxime	PO, IM, IV	Renal	1.0–1.9	15–22
	Loracarbef	PO	Renal	1	32
Third generation	Cefdinir	PO	Renal	1.7	16
	Cefditoren	PO	Renal	1.6	—
	Cefixime	PO	Renal	3–4	11.5
	Cefoperazone	IM, IV	Biliary	1.7–2.6	2.2
	Cefotaxime	IM, IV	Renal	0.9–1.4	3–11
	Cefpodoxime	PO	Renal	2–3	9.8
	Ceftazidime	IM, IV	Renal	1.9–2.0	—
	Ceftibuten	PO	Renal	2	Increased
	Ceftizoxime	IM, IV	Renal	1.1–2.3	30
	Ceftriaxone	IM, IV	Hepatic	5.8–8.7	15.7
Fourth generation	Cefepime	IM, IV	Renal	2	Increased

First Generation. First-generation cephalosporins, represented by cephalothin, are highly active against gram-positive bacteria. These drugs are the most active of all cephalosporins against staphylococci and nonenterococcal streptococci. However, those staphylococci that are resistant to methicillin-like drugs are also resistant to first-generation cephalosporins (and to most other cephalosporins as well). The first-generation agents have only modest activity against gram-negative bacteria and do not reach effective concentrations in CSF.

Second Generation. Second-generation cephalosporins (e.g., cefamandole) have enhanced activity against gram-negative bacteria. The increase is due to a combination of factors: (1) increased affinity for PBPs of gram-negative bacteria, (2) increased ability to penetrate the gram-negative cell envelope, and (3) increased resistance to beta-lactamases produced by gram-negative organisms. However, none of the second-generation agents is active against *Pseudomonas aeruginosa*. These drugs do not reach effective concentrations in CSF.

Third Generation. Third-generation cephalosporins (e.g., cefotaxime) have a broad spectrum of antimicrobial activity. Because of increased resistance to beta-lactamases, these agents are considerably more active against gram-negative aerobes than are the first- and second-generation drugs. Some third-generation cephalosporins (e.g., ceftazidime) have important activity against *P. aeruginosa*. Others (e.g., cefixime) lack such activity. In contrast to first- and second-generation cephalosporins, the third-generation agents are able to reach clinically effective concentrations in CSF.

Fourth Generation. Cefepime, the only fourth-generation cephalosporin, is highly resistant to beta-lactamases and has a very broad antibacterial spectrum. Activity against *P. aeruginosa* is equal to that of ceftazidime. Penetration to the CSF is good.

Pharmacokinetics

Absorption. Because of poor absorption from the GI tract, *many cephalosporins must be administered parenterally* (IM or IV). Of the 24 cephalosporins used in the United States, only 12 can be administered by mouth (Table 81–2).

Of these, only two (cephradine and cefuroxime) can be administered orally *and* by injection.

Distribution. Cephalosporins distribute well to most body fluids and tissues. Therapeutic concentrations are achieved in pleural, pericardial, and peritoneal fluids. Concentrations in ocular fluids are generally low. Penetration to the CSF by first- and second-generation drugs is unreliable, and hence these drugs should not be used for bacterial meningitis. In contrast, CSF levels achieved with third- and fourth-generation drugs are generally sufficient for bactericidal effects.

Elimination. Practically all cephalosporins are eliminated by the *kidney;* excretion is by a combination of glomerular filtration and active tubular secretion. Probenecid can decrease tubular secretion of some cephalosporins, thereby prolonging their effects. In patients with renal insufficiency, dosages of most cephalosporins must be reduced (to prevent accumulation to toxic levels).

Two cephalosporins—*cefoperazone* and *ceftriaxone*—are eliminated largely by nonrenal routes. Consequently, there is no need to reduce their dosage in patients with renal impairment.

Adverse Effects

The cephalosporins are generally well tolerated and constitute one of our safest groups of antimicrobial drugs. Serious adverse effects are rare.

Allergic Reactions. Hypersensitivity reactions are the most frequent adverse effects. Maculopapular rash that develops several days after the onset of treatment is most common. Severe, immediate reactions (e.g., bronchospasm, anaphylaxis) are rare. If, during the course of treatment, signs of allergy appear (e.g., urticaria, rash, hypotension, difficulty in breathing), the cephalosporin should be discontinued immediately. Anaphylaxis is treated with respiratory support and parenteral epinephrine. Patients with a history of cephalosporin allergy should not be given these drugs.

Because of structural similarities between penicillins and cephalosporins, patients allergic to one type of drug may experience cross-reactivity with the other. In clinical practice, the incidence of cross-reactivity has been low: Only 5% to 10% of penicillin-allergic patients experience an allergic reaction if given a cephalosporin. For patients with mild penicillin allergy, cephalosporins can be used with minimal concern about allergic responses. However, because of the potential for fatal anaphylaxis, *cephalosporins should not be given to patients with a history of severe allergic reactions to penicillins.*

Bleeding. Three cephalosporins—*cefmetazole, cefoperazone,* and *cefotetan*—cause bleeding tendencies. The mechanism is reduction of prothrombin levels through interference with vitamin K metabolism.

Several measures can reduce the risk of hemorrhage. During prolonged treatment, patients should be monitored for prothrombin time, bleeding time, or both. Parenteral vitamin K can correct an abnormal prothrombin time. Patients should be observed for signs of bleeding, and, if bleeding develops, the cephalosporin should be withdrawn. Caution should be exercised during concurrent use of anticoagulants or thrombolytic agents. Because of their antiplatelet effects, aspirin and other nonsteroidal anti-inflammatory drugs should be used with care. Caution should be exercised in patients with a history of bleeding disorders.

Thrombophlebitis. Thrombophlebitis may develop during IV infusion. This reaction can be minimized by rotating the infusion site and by administering cephalosporins slowly and in dilute solution. Patients should be observed for phlebitis. If the reaction develops, the infusion site should be changed.

Other Adverse Effects. Cephalosporins may cause *pain at sites of IM injection;* patients should be forewarned of this possibility. Rarely, cephalosporins may be the cause of *antibiotic-associated pseudomembranous colitis* due to overgrowth with *Clostridium difficile.* If this suprainfection develops, the cephalosporin should be discontinued and, if necessary, oral vancomycin or metronidazole should be given. Cephalothin may cause *nephrotoxicity.*

With one cephalosporin—*cefditoren*—there are two unique concerns. First, the drug contains a milk protein (sodium caseinate), and hence should be avoided by patients with *milk-protein hypersensitivity* (as opposed to lactose intolerance). Second, cefditoren is excreted in combination with carnitine, and can cause *carnitine loss.* Accordingly, the drug is contraindicated for patients with existing carnitine deficiency or conditions that predispose them to carnitine deficiency.

Drug Interactions

Probenecid. Probenecid delays renal excretion of some cephalosporins and can thereby prolong their effects. This is the same interaction that occurs between probenecid and the penicillins.

Alcohol. Three cephalosporins—*cefmetazole, cefoperazone,* and *cefotetan*—induce a state of alcohol intolerance. If a patient receiving these drugs were to ingest alcohol, a disulfiram-like reaction could occur. (As discussed in Chapter 37, the disulfiram effect is brought on by accumulation of acetaldehyde and can be extremely dangerous.) Accordingly, patients taking these cephalosporins must not consume alcohol in any form.

Drugs That Promote Bleeding. As noted, three cephalosporins—*cefmetazole, cefoperazone,* and *cefotetan*—promote bleeding. Caution should be exercised if these drugs are used in combination with other drugs that also promote bleeding (anticoagulants, thrombolytics, nonsteroidal anti-inflammatory drugs and other antiplatelet drugs).

Therapeutic Uses

The therapeutic role of the cephalosporins is continually evolving as new agents are introduced and more experience is gained with older agents. Only general recommendations are considered here.

The cephalosporins are broad-spectrum, bactericidal drugs with a high therapeutic index. These agents have been employed widely and successfully against a variety of infections. Cephalosporins can be useful alternatives for patients with mild penicillin allergy.

The four generations of cephalosporins differ significantly in their applications. *The first- and second-generation cephalosporins are rarely drugs of choice for active infections.* In most cases, equally effective and less expensive alternatives are available. In contrast, *the third-generation agents have qualities that make them the preferred therapy for several infections.* The role of *fourth-generation agents* is yet to be established.

First-Generation Cephalosporins. When a cephalosporin is indicated for a *gram-positive infection,* a first-generation drug should be used; these agents are the most active of the cephalosporins against gram-positive organisms and are less expensive than other cephalosporins. First-generation agents are frequently employed as alternatives to penicillins to treat infections caused by staphylococci or streptococci (except enterococci) in patients with penicillin allergy. However, it is important to note that cephalosporins should be given only to patients with a history of *mild* penicillin allergy—not to those who have experienced a severe, immediate hypersensitivity reaction.

The first-generation agents have been employed widely for *prophylaxis against infection in surgical patients.* First-generation agents are preferred to second- or third-generation cephalosporins for surgical prophylaxis because they are as effective as the newer drugs, less expensive, and have a less broad antimicrobial spectrum.

Second-Generation Cephalosporins. Specific indications for second-generation cephalosporins are limited. *Cefuroxime,* a prototype for the group, has been used with success against pneumonia caused by *Haemophilus influenzae, Klebsiella,* pneumococci, and staphylococci. Oral cefuroxime is useful for otitis, sinusitis, and respiratory tract infections. *Cefoxitin* is useful for abdominal and pelvic infections.

Third-Generation Cephalosporins. Because they are highly active against gram-negative organisms, and because they penetrate to the CSF, third-generation cephalosporins are drugs of choice for meningitis caused by enteric, gram-negative bacilli. *Ceftazidime* is of special utility for treating meningitis caused by *P. aeruginosa. Nosocomial infections* caused by gram-negative bacilli, which are often resistant to first- and second-generation cephalosporins and most other commonly used antibiotics, are appropriate indications for the third-generation drugs. Two third-generation agents—*ceftriaxone* and *cefotaxime*—are drugs of choice for infections caused by *Neisseria gonorrhoeae* (gonorrhea), *H. influenzae, Proteus, Salmonella, Klebsiella,* and *Serratia.*

The third-generation cephalosporins should not be used routinely. Rather, they should be given only when conditions demand, because in this way emergence of organisms resistant to them will be delayed.

Drug Selection

Twenty-four cephalosporins are currently employed in the United States, and selection among them can be a challenge. Within each generation, the similarities among cephalosporins are more pronounced than the differences. Hence, aside from cost, there is frequently no rational basis for choosing one drug over another. However, there *are* some differences between cephalosporins, and these differences may render one agent preferable to another for treating a specific infection in a specific host. The differences that do exist can be grouped into three main categories: (1) antimicrobial spectrum, (2) adverse effects, and (3) pharmacokinetics (e.g., route of administration, penetration to the CSF, time course, mode of elimination). Drug selection based on consideration of these differences is discussed below.

Antimicrobial Spectrum. A prime rule of antimicrobial therapy is to match the drug with the bug: The drug should be active against known or suspected pathogens, but its spectrum should be no broader than required. When a cephalosporin is appropriate, we should select from among those drugs known to have good activity against the causative pathogen. The third- and fourth-generation agents, with their very broad antimicrobial spectra, should be avoided in situations where a narrower spectrum, first- or second-generation drug would suffice.

For some infections, one cephalosporin may be decidedly more effective than all others, and should be selected on this basis. For example, *ceftazidime* (a third-generation drug) is the most effective of all cephalosporins against *P. aeruginosa* and is clearly the preferred cephalosporin for treating infections caused by this microbe.

Adverse Effects. Although most cephalosporins produce the same spectrum of adverse effects, a few agents can cause unique reactions. In particular, three cephalosporins—*cefmetazole, cefoperazone,* and *cefotetan*—produce bleeding tendencies and intolerance to alcohol. When an equally effective alternative is available, it would be prudent to avoid these drugs.

Pharmacokinetics. Four pharmacokinetic properties are of interest: (1) route of administration, (2) duration of action, (3) distribution to CSF, and (4) route of elimination. The relationship of these properties to drug selection is discussed below.

Route of Administration. Twelve cephalosporins can be administered orally. These drugs may be preferred for treating mild to moderate infections in patients who can't tolerate parenteral agents.

Duration of Action. In patients with normal renal function, the half-lives of the cephalosporins range from about 30 minutes to 9 hours (see Table 81–2). Because they require fewer administrations per day, drugs with a long half-life are frequently preferred to those with a short half-life. The drugs with the longest half-lives in each generation are as follows: first generation, *cefazolin* (1.5 to 2 hours); second generation, *cefonicid* (4.5 hours); and third generation, *ceftriaxone* (6 to 9 hours).

Distribution to CSF. Only the third- and fourth-generation agents produce CSF levels sufficient for bactericidal effects. Hence, for treatment of meningitis caused by susceptible organisms, these drugs are preferred over first- and second-generation cephalosporins. One third-generation drug—*cefoperazone*—is notable for its *inability* to achieve therapeutic concentrations in the CSF.

Route of Elimination. Most cephalosporins are eliminated by the kidneys and, if dosage is not carefully adjusted, may accumulate to toxic levels in patients with kidney dysfunction. Only two agents—*cefoperazone* and *ceftriaxone*—are eliminated in significant amounts by nonrenal routes, and hence can be used with relative safety in patients with renal impairment.

Dosage and Administration

Routes of Administration. Many cephalosporins cannot be absorbed from the GI tract and must therefore be administered parenterally (IM or IV). As shown in Table 81–2, only 12 cephalosporins can be given orally. Two drugs—*cephradine* and *cefuroxime*—can be administered both orally and by injection.

Dosage. Dosages are summarized in Table 81–3. For most cephalosporins (*cefoperazone* and *ceftriaxone* excepted), the dosage should be reduced in patients with significant renal impairment.

TABLE 81–3 ■ Cephalosporin Dosages

Drug	Trade Name	Route	Dosing Interval (hr)	Total Daily Dosage* Adults (gm)	Total Daily Dosage* Children (mg/kg)
First Generation					
Cefadroxil	Duricef	PO	12, 24	1–2	30
Cefazolin	Ancef, Kefzol, Zolicef	IM, IV	6, 8	2–12	80–160
Cephalexin	Biocef, Keflex, Keftab	PO	6	1–4	25–50
Cephapirin	Cefadyl	IM, IV	4, 6	2–12	40–80
Cephradine	Velosef	IM, IV	4, 6	2–12	50–100
		PO	6	1–4	25–50
Second Generation					
Cefaclor	Ceclor, Ceclor CD	PO	8	0.75–1.5	20–40
Cefmetazole	Zefazone	IV	6, 12	4–8	—
Cefonicid	Monocid	IM, IV	24	0.5–2	—
Cefotetan	Cefotan	IM, IV	12	2–6	—
Cefoxitin	Mefoxin	IM, IV	4, 8	3–12	80–160
Cefprozil	Cefzil	PO	12, 24	0.5–1	30
Cefuroxime	Ceftin, Kefurox, Zinacef	IM, IV	8	2.25–9	50–100
		PO	12	0.5–1	250–500
Loracarbef	Lorabid	PO	12, 24	0.5–1	30
Third Generation					
Cefdinir	Omnicef	PO	12, 24	0.6	14
Cefditoren	Spectracef	PO	12	0.4–0.8	—
Cefixime	Suprax	PO	24	0.4	8
Cefoperazone	Cefobid	IM, IV	6, 8	2–12	100–150
Cefotaxime	Claforan	IM, IV	4, 8	2–12	100–200
Cefpodoxime	Vantin	PO	12	0.2–0.4	10
Ceftazidime	Ceptaz, Fortaz, Tazidime, Tazicef	IM, IV	8, 12	0.5–6	90–150
Ceftibuten	Cedax	PO	24	0.4	9
Ceftizoxime	Cefizox	IM, IV	6, 12	2–12	150–200
Ceftriaxone	Rocephin	IM, IV	12, 24	1–4	50–100
Fourth Generation					
Cefepime	Maxipime	IM, IV	12	1–2	—

*With the exceptions of cefoperazone and ceftriaxone, cephalosporins require a reduction of dosage for patients with severe renal impairment.

Administration. Oral. If oral cephalosporins produce nausea, administration with food can reduce the response. Oral suspensions should be stored under refrigeration.

Intramuscular. Intramuscular injections should be made deep into a large muscle. Intramuscular injection of cephalosporins is frequently painful; the patient should be forewarned. The injection site should be checked for induration, tenderness, and redness, and the physician should be informed if these occur.

Intravenous. For IV therapy, cephalosporins may be administered by three techniques: (1) bolus injection, (2) slow injection (over 3 to 5 minutes), and (3) continuous infusion. The physician's order should state which method to use. If there is uncertainty as to method of administration, clarification should be requested. Solutions for parenteral administration should be prepared according to the manufacturer's recommendations.

CARBAPENEMS

Carbapenems are beta-lactam antibiotics that have very broad antimicrobial spectrums. At this time three carbapenems are available: imipenem, meropenem, and ertapenem. All three are administered parenterally.

Imipenem

Imipenem [Primaxin], a beta-lactam antibiotic (Fig 81–2), has the broadest antimicrobial spectrum of any drug. Because of its broad spectrum, imipenem may be of special use for treating mixed infections in which anaerobes, *Staphylococcus aureus,* and gram-negative bacilli may all be involved. Imipenem is dispensed in fixed-dose combinations with cilastatin, a compound that inhibits destruction of imipenem by renal enzymes.

Mechanism of Action. Imipenem binds to two PBPs (PBP1 and PBP2), causing weakening of the bacterial cell wall with subsequent lysis and death. Antimicrobial effects are enhanced by the drug's resistance to practically all beta-lactamases, and by its ability to penetrate the gram-negative cell envelope.

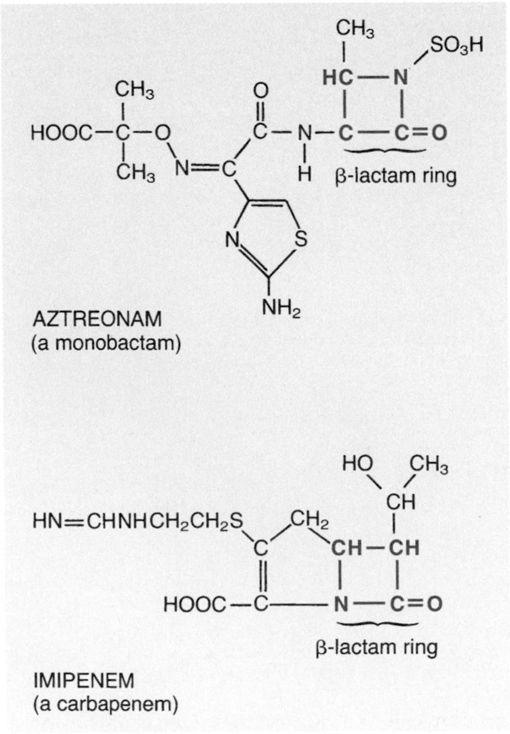

Antimicrobial Spectrum. Imipenem is active against most bacterial pathogens, including organisms resistant to other antibiotics. The drug is highly active against gram-positive cocci and most gram-negative cocci and bacilli. In addition, imipenem is the most effective beta-lactam antibiotic for use against anaerobic bacteria.

Pharmacokinetics. Imipenem is not absorbed from the GI tract and hence must be given parenterally (IV or IM). The drug is well distributed to body fluids and tissues. Imipenem penetrates the meninges to produce therapeutic concentrations in CSF.

Elimination is primarily renal. When employed alone, imipenem is inactivated by an enzyme (dipeptidase) present in the kidney. As a result, drug levels in urine are low. To increase urinary concentrations, imipenem is administered in combination with *cilastatin,* a dipeptidase inhibitor. When the combination is used, about 70% of imipenem is excreted unchanged in the urine. The elimination half-life is about 1 hour.

Adverse Effects. Imipenem is generally well tolerated. *Gastrointestinal effects* (nausea, vomiting, diarrhea) are most common. *Hypersensitivity reactions* (rashes, pruritus, drug fever) have occurred, and patients allergic to other beta-lactam antibiotics may be cross-allergic with imipenem. *Suprainfections* with bacteria or fungi develop in about 4% of patients. Rarely, *seizures* have occurred.

Therapeutic Use. Because of its broad spectrum and low toxicity, imipenem has been used widely. The drug has proved effective for serious infections caused by gram-positive cocci, gram-negative cocci, gram-negative bacilli, and anaerobic bacteria. This broad antimicrobial spectrum gives imipenem special utility for chemotherapy of mixed infections (e.g., simultaneous infection with aerobic and anaerobic bacteria). When imipenem has been given alone to treat infection with *P. aeruginosa,* resistant organisms have emerged. Consequently, imipenem should be combined with another antipseudomonal drug for use against this microbe.

Preparations, Dosage, and Administration. Imipenem is dispensed in 1:1 fixed-dose combinations with cilastatin. The combination products are marketed under the trade name Primaxin. Two formulations are available: Primaxin I.V. and Primaxin I.M., for intravenous and intramuscular use, respectively. These products are dispensed in powdered form and must be reconstituted in accord with the manufacturer's instructions. The usual adult dosage (based on imipenem content) is 250 to 500 mg every 6 hours. Dosage should be reduced in patients with renal impairment.

Meropenem

Actions and Uses. Meropenem [Merrem IV] is a beta-lactam antibiotic similar in structure and actions to imipenem. Meropenem is active against most clinically important gram-positive and gram-negative aerobes and anaerobes. Approved indications are (1) bacterial meningitis in children age 3 months or older and (2) complicated intra-abdominal infections in children and adults. Meropenem may prove especially useful for nosocomial infections caused by organisms resistant to other antibiotics.

Pharmacokinetics. Meropenem is administered IV and distributes to all body fluids and tissues. The drug has a plasma half-life of 1 hour and is eliminated primarily unchanged in the urine. In contrast to imipenem, meropenem is not degraded by renal dipeptidases, and hence is not combined with cilastatin.

Adverse Effects. Like other beta-lactam antibiotics, meropenem is generally well tolerated. Principal adverse effects are rashes, diarrhea, nausea,

FIGURE 81–2 ■ **Miscellaneous beta-lactam antibiotics.**

and vomiting. As with imipenem, seizures occur rarely. The risk of seizures is highest in patients with CNS disorders (e.g., brain lesions, history of seizures) and bacterial meningitis.

Preparations, Dosage, and Administration. Meropenem [Merrem IV] is dispensed in powdered form to be reconstituted for IV administration. Depending on the volume employed, the drug may be (1) infused over 15 to 30 minutes or (2) injected as a bolus over 3 to 5 minutes. The dosage for adults is 1 gm every 8 hours. The dosage for pediatric patients is 20 mg/kg every 8 hours (for intra-abdominal infections) and 40 mg/kg every 8 hours (for bacterial meningitis). Adult and pediatric dosages must be reduced for patients with significant renal impairment (creatinine clearance <50 ml/min).

Ertapenem

Actions and Uses. Ertapenem [Invanz] is the newest member of the carbapenem family. Like penicillins and cephalosporins, carbapenems weaken the bacterial cell wall, and thereby cause cell lysis and death. Like other carbapenems, ertapenem is highly resistant to beta-lactamases, and hence has a very broad antimicrobial spectrum—but less broad than that of imipenem or meropenem. Ertapenem is active against most gram-positive bacteria and most anaerobes. However, in contrast to imipenem and meropenem, the drug has little or no activity against *P. aeruginosa* or *Acinetobacter* species. In addition, ertapenem has minimal activity to pneumococci that are highly resistant to penicillin, and has no activity against methicillin-resistant staphylococci, *Enterococcus faecium*, *Enterococcus faecalis*, or atypical respiratory tract pathogens, including *Chlamydia* species, *Legionella* species, and *Mycoplasma pneumoniae*. Ertapenem is indicated for parenteral therapy of acute pelvic infections, community-acquired pneumonia, and complicated infections of the urinary tract, abdomen, and skin and skin structures.

Pharmacokinetics. Ertapenem may be administered by IM injection or IV infusion. Absorption following IM injection is complete. In the blood, ertapenem is highly bound to plasma proteins. The drug undergoes some hydrolysis of the beta-lactam ring prior to excretion in the urine (80%) and feces (10%). Its half life is approximately 4 hours (compared with only 1 hour for imipenem or meropenem).

Adverse Effects. Like other carbapenems, ertapenem is generally well tolerated. In clinical trials, the most common adverse effects were diarrhea (10.3%), nausea (8%), infused-vein complications (7.1%), headache (5.6%), vomiting (3.7%), and edema (3.4%). In addition, CNS effects (agitation, confusion, disorientation, decreased mental acuity, somnolence, stupor) were reported in 5.1% of patients. Like imipenem and meropenem, ertapenem can cause seizures—but the incidence is relatively low (0.5%).

Preparations, Dosage, and Administration. Ertapenem [Invanz] is available as a powder to be reconstituted for IM or IV administration. For IV therapy, the drug is infused over 30 minutes, and should not be mixed with other drugs or with diluents that contain dextrose. The recommended dosage (IM or IV) is 1 gm once daily (for patients with good kidney function) or 500 mg once daily (for patients with significant renal impairment). The duration of treatment is 3 to 14 days, depending on the infection being treated.

OTHER INHIBITORS OF CELL WALL SYNTHESIS

Aztreonam

Chemistry. Aztreonam [Azactam] belongs to a new class of beta-lactam antibiotics known as *monobactams*. These agents contain a beta-lactam ring, but the ring is not fused with a second ring. The structure of aztreonam is shown in Figure 81–2.

Mechanism of Action. Aztreonam binds to PBP3. Hence, like most beta-lactam antibiotics, the drug inhibits bacterial cell wall synthesis, ultimately causing the cell to rupture and die. The drug does not bind to PBPs produced by anaerobes or gram-positive bacteria.

Antimicrobial Spectrum and Therapeutic Use. Aztreonam has a narrow antimicrobial spectrum: The drug is active only against gram-negative aerobic bacteria. Susceptible organisms include *Neisseria* species, *H. influenzae*, *P. aeruginosa*, and Enterobacteriaceae (e.g., *Escherichia coli*, *Klebsiella*, *Proteus*, *Serratia*, *Salmonella*, *Shigella*). Aztreonam is highly resistant to beta-lactamases, and therefore is active against many gram-negative aerobes that produce these enzymes. The drug is not active against gram-positive bacteria and anaerobes.

Pharmacokinetics. Aztreonam is not absorbed from the GI tract and hence must be administered parenterally (IM or IV). Once in the blood-

stream, the drug distributes widely to most body fluids and tissues. Therapeutic concentrations can be achieved in the CSF. Aztreonam is eliminated by the kidneys, primarily as the unchanged drug.

Adverse Effects. Aztreonam is generally well tolerated. Adverse effects are like those of other beta-lactam antibiotics. The most common side effects are pain and thrombophlebitis at sites of injection. Because aztreonam differs greatly in structure from penicillins and cephalosporins, there is little cross-allergenicity between these drugs. Hence, it appears that aztreonam is safe for patients with allergies to other beta-lactam antibiotics.

Preparations, Dosage, and Administration. Aztreonam [Azactam] is dispensed in powdered form to be reconstituted for IM or IV administration. The usual adult dosage is 1 to 2 gm every 8 to 12 hours. Dosage should be reduced in patients with kidney dysfunction.

Vancomycin

Vancomycin [Vancocin, Vancoled] is a potentially toxic drug used only for serious infections. Principal indications are antibiotic-associated pseudomembranous colitis (caused by *C. difficile*), infection with methicillin-resistant *S. aureus*, and treatment of serious infections with susceptible organisms in patients allergic to penicillins. Unlike most other drugs discussed in this chapter, vancomycin does not contain a beta-lactam ring.

Mechanism of Action. Like the beta-lactam antibiotics, vancomycin inhibits cell wall synthesis and thereby promotes bacterial lysis and death. However, in contrast to the beta-lactam antibiotics, vancomycin does not interact with PBPs. Instead, vancomycin disrupts the cell wall by binding to molecules that serve as precursors for cell wall biosynthesis.

Antimicrobial Spectrum. Vancomycin is active only against gram-positive bacteria. The drug is especially active against *Staph. aureus* and *Staphylococcus epidermidis*, including strains of both species that are methicillin resistant. Other susceptible organisms include streptococci and *C. difficile*.

Pharmacokinetics. Absorption from the GI tract is poor. Hence, for most infections, vancomycin is given parenterally (by slow IV infusion). Oral administration is employed only for infections of the intestine.

Vancomycin is well distributed to most body fluids and tissues. Although the drug enters the CSF, levels may be insufficient to treat meningitis. Hence, if meningeal infection fails to respond to IV therapy, concurrent intrathecal administration may be required.

Vancomycin is eliminated unchanged by the kidneys. In patients with renal impairment, dosage must be reduced.

Therapeutic Use. Vancomycin should be reserved for treatment of serious infections. This agent is the drug of choice for infections caused by methicillin-resistant *Staph. aureus* or *Staph. epidermidis;* most strains of these bacteria remain vancomycin sensitive. The drug is also employed as an alternative to penicillins and cephalosporins to treat severe infections (e.g., staphylococcal and streptococcal endocarditis) in patients allergic to the beta-lactam antibiotics.

Until recently, oral vancomycin was considered the treatment of choice for antibiotic-associated pseudomembranous colitis caused by suprainfection with *C. difficile*. However, to delay emergence of resistance to vancomycin, metronidazole is now tried first. Vancomycin is used only in severely ill patients who have not responded to metronidazole.

Adverse Effects. The most serious adverse effect is *ototoxicity*. Although hearing impairment is often reversible, permanent impairment can occur. Ototoxicity is most likely when plasma levels of vancomycin exceed 30 μg/ml. The risk of hearing loss is increased by high dosage, prolonged treatment, renal impairment, and concurrent use of other ototoxic drugs (e.g., aminoglycosides, ethacrynic acid).

Rapid infusion of vancomycin can cause a variety of disturbing effects, including rashes, flushing, tachycardia, and hypotension. These effects, which are thought to result from release of histamine, can be avoided by infusing vancomycin slowly (over 60 minutes or more).

Thrombophlebitis is common. The reaction can be minimized by administering vancomycin in dilute solution and by changing the infusion site frequently.

Patients allergic to penicillins do not show cross-reactivity with vancomycin. Accordingly, vancomycin is an alternative to penicillins in patients allergic to them.

Preparations, Dosage, and Administration. For treatment of *systemic infection,* vancomycin is administered by intermittent infusion over 60 minutes or more. The usual adult dosage is 2 gm/day administered in divided doses at 6- or 12-hour intervals. The dosage for children is 44 mg/kg/day administered in divided doses at 6- or 12-hour intervals. In patients with renal impairment, dosages must be reduced. Serum drug levels should be monitored to ensure that dosage is appropriate. Blood for measuring peak drug levels should be drawn 1.5 to 2.5 hours after completing the IV infusion. Peak levels of 30 to 40 µg/ml are generally acceptable.

For treatment of *antibiotic-associated pseudomembranous colitis,* vancomycin is given orally. The adult dosage is 125 to 500 mg every 6 hours. The dosage for children is 11 mg/kg every 6 hours. Because vancomycin is not absorbed from the GI tract, there is no need to decrease oral doses in patients with renal impairment.

Teicoplanin

Chemistry and Actions. Teicoplanin [Targocid] is an investigational drug similar in structure and actions to vancomycin. Both drugs disrupt cell wall synthesis to cause lysis and death, and both are active only against gram-positive bacteria. Sensitive organisms include methicillin-resistant *Staph. aureus,* enterococci, and *C. difficile.* Like vancomycin—and unlike the other drugs discussed in the chapter—teicoplanin does not have a beta-lactam ring.

Pharmacokinetics. The kinetics of teicoplanin are much like those of vancomycin—except that teicoplanin can be administered IM as well as IV. Neither drug is absorbed from the GI tract, so oral administration is reserved for infections of the intestine. Following parenteral administration, teicoplanin is well distributed to tissues and most body fluids, but not to CSF. Teicoplanin has a long half-life (up to 100 hours) and is eliminated intact by the kidneys.

Therapeutic Use. Teicoplanin has been used with success against an array of infections, but its therapeutic niche is yet to be established. Potential applications include osteomyelitis and endocarditis caused by methicillin-resistant staphylococci, streptococci, and enterococci. Combining the drug with gentamicin can increase bactericidal actions.

Teicoplanin represents a safe and effective alternative to vancomycin, and offers several advantages. These are (1) the option of IM administration, (2) shorter infusion time with IV administration (30 vs. 60 minutes), (3) once-a-day dosing, and (4) the absence of serious adverse effects, including infusion-related reactions.

Adverse Effects. Teicoplanin is largely devoid of adverse effects. In contrast to vancomycin, teicoplanin does not promote histamine release, and hence does not cause infusion-related reactions (flushing, tachycardia, hypotension). Ototoxicity may occur but is rare. Not surprisingly, patients allergic to beta-lactam antibiotics are *not* cross-allergic to teicoplanin.

Dosage and Administration. Teicoplanin may be given parenterally or orally. Parenteral administration is done by IM injection, IV injection, or 30-minute IV infusion. For parenteral therapy, the usual adult dosage is 6 mg/kg initially followed by 3 mg/kg every 24 hours. Dosage should be reduced in patients with renal impairment. As noted, oral therapy is used only for intestinal infections.

Fosfomycin

Fosfomycin [Monurol] is a new bactericidal agent approved for single-dose therapy of uncomplicated urinary tract infections (i.e., acute cystitis) caused by *E. coli* or *Streptococcus faecalis.* The drug kills bacteria by disrupting synthesis of the peptidoglycan polymer strands that compose the cell wall. (As discussed in Chapter 80, penicillins kill bacteria in part by preventing cross-linking of peptidoglycan strands.)

The most common adverse effects are diarrhea (10.4%), headache (10.3%), vaginitis (7.6%), and nausea (5.2%). Fosfomycin may also cause abdominal pain, rhinitis, drowsiness, dizziness, and rash.

Fosfomycin is dispensed as a water-soluble powder in single-dose, 3-gm packets. The drug may be taken with or without food. Symptoms of cystitis should improve in 2 to 3 days. If symptoms fail to improve, additional doses will not help—but will increase the risk of side effects.

⸪ KEY POINTS

■ Cephalosporins are beta-lactam antibiotics that weaken the bacterial cell wall, causing lysis and death.
■ The major cause of cephalosporin resistance is production of beta-lactamases.
■ Cephalosporins can be grouped into four "generations." As we progress from first- to fourth-generation drugs, there is (1) increasing activity against gram-negative bacteria, (2) increasing resistance to destruction by beta-lactamases, and (3) increasing ability to reach the CSF.
■ Many cephalosporins must be administered parenterally; only 12 of the 24 available in the United States can be administered orally.
■ Except for cefoperazone and ceftriaxone, all cephalosporins are eliminated by the kidneys, and therefore must be given in reduced dosage to patients with renal impairment.
■ The most common adverse effects of cephalosporins are allergic reactions. Patients allergic to penicillins have a 5% to 10% risk of cross-reactivity with cephalosporins.
■ Three cephalosporins—cefmetazole, cefoperazone, and cefotetan—cause bleeding tendencies and disulfiram-like reactions.
■ Imipenem, a beta-lactam antibiotic, has the broadest antimicrobial spectrum of any drug.
■ Vancomycin is an important but potentially toxic drug generally reserved for (1) antibiotic-associated pseudomembranous colitis (caused by *C. difficile*), (2) infections with methicillin-resistant *Staph. aureus,* and (3) serious infections by susceptible organisms in patients allergic to penicillins.

Summary of Major Nursing Implications*

CEPHALOSPORINS

Cefaclor
Cefadroxil
Cefazolin
Cefdinir
Cefditoren
Cefepime
Cefixime

Cefmetazole
Cefonicid
Cefoperazone
Cefotaxime
Cefotetan
Cefoxitin
Cefpodoxime
Cefprozil

*Patient education information is highlighted as blue text.

Summary of Major Nursing Implications*—cont'd

Ceftazidime
Ceftibuten
Ceftizoxime
Ceftriaxone
Cefuroxime
Cephalexin
Cephapirin
Cephradine
Loracarbef

Except where indicated, the implications summarized below apply to all members of the cephalosporin family.

Preadministration Assessment

Therapeutic Goal

Treatment of infections caused by susceptible organisms.

Baseline Data

The physician may order tests to determine the identity and drug sensitivity of the infecting organism. Take samples for culture prior to initiating treatment.

Identifying High-Risk Patients

Cephalosporins are *contraindicated* for patients with a history of allergic reactions to cephalosporins or severe allergic reactions to penicillins.

Implementation: Administration

Routes

More than half of all cephalosporins are administered parenterally (IM or IV). Twelve are administered orally. Two—*cephradine* and *cefuroxime*—are administered orally *and* parenterally. Routes for individual cephalosporins are given in Table 81–3.

Dosage

Dosages are summarized in Table 81–3. Dosages for all cephalosporins—except *cefoperazone* and *ceftriaxone*—should be reduced in patients with significant renal impairment.

Administration

Oral. Advise the patient to take oral cephalosporins with food if gastric upset occurs. Instruct the patient to refrigerate oral suspensions.

Instruct the patient to complete the prescribed course of therapy even though symptoms may abate before the full course is over.

Intramuscular. Make IM injections deep into a large muscle. **These injections are frequently painful; forewarn the patient.** Check the injection site for induration, tenderness, and redness; notify the physician if these occur.

Intravenous. Techniques for IV administration are bolus injection, slow injection (over 3 to 5 minutes), and continuous infusion. The physician's order should specify which method to use; request clarification if the order is unclear.

Ongoing Evaluation and Interventions

Evaluating Therapeutic Effects

Monitor for indications of antimicrobial effects (e.g., reduction in fever, pain, or inflammation; improved appetite or sense of well-being).

Minimizing Adverse Effects

Allergic Reactions. Hypersensitivity reactions are relatively common. Rarely, life-threatening anaphylaxis occurs. Avoid cephalosporins in patients with a history of cephalosporin allergy or severe penicillin allergy. If penicillin allergy is *mild,* cephalosporins can be used with relative safety. **Instruct the patient to report any signs of allergy (e.g., skin rash, itching, hives).** If anaphylaxis occurs, administer parenteral epinephrine and provide respiratory support.

Bleeding. Cefmetazole, cefoperazone, and *cefotetan* can promote bleeding. Monitor prothrombin time, bleeding time, or both. Parenteral vitamin K can correct abnormal prothrombin time. Observe patients for signs of bleeding and, if bleeding develops, discontinue the drug. Exercise caution in patients with a history of bleeding disorders and in patients receiving drugs that can interfere with hemostasis (anticoagulants; thrombolytics; antiplatelet drugs, including aspirin and other nonsteroidal anti-inflammatory drugs).

Thrombophlebitis. Intravenous cephalosporins may cause thrombophlebitis. To minimize this reaction, rotate the injection site and inject cephalosporins slowly and in dilute solution. Observe the patient for phlebitis; change the infusion site if phlebitis develops.

Antibiotic-Associated Pseudomembranous Colitis (AAPMC). AAPMC may develop, especially with use of broad-spectrum cephalosporins. Notify the physician if diarrhea occurs (a possible indication of colitis). If AAPMC is diagnosed, discontinue the cephalosporin. Oral vancomycin or metronidazole may be needed.

Milk-Protein Hypersensitivity. Cefditoren tablets contain sodium caseinate, a milk protein. Do not give cefditoren to patients with milk-protein allergy. (The drug is safe in patients with lactose intolerance.)

Carnitine Deficiency. Cefditoren is excreted in combination with carnitine, and can thereby lower carnitine levels. Do not give cefditoren to patients with pre-existing carnitine deficiency or with conditions that predispose to carnitine deficiency.

Minimizing Adverse Interactions

Alcohol. Cefmetazole, cefoperazone, and *cefotetan* can cause alcohol intolerance. A serious disulfiram-like reaction may occur if alcohol is consumed. **Inform patients about alcohol intolerance and warn them not to drink alcoholic beverages.**

Drugs That Promote Bleeding. Drugs that interfere with hemostasis—anticoagulants, thrombolytics, and antiplatelet drugs (including aspirin and other nonsteroidal anti-inflammatory drugs)—can intensify bleeding tendencies caused by *cefmetazole, cefoperazone,* and *cefotetan.* Do not combine these drugs.

*Patient education information is highlighted as blue text.

Bacteriostatic Inhibitors of Protein Synthesis: Tetracyclines, Macrolides, Clindamycin, Chloramphenicol, Linezolid, Dalfopristin/Quinupristin, and Spectinomycin

TETRACYCLINES

MACROLIDES

   Erythromycin

   Other Macrolides

OTHER BACTERIOSTATIC INHIBITORS
OF PROTEIN SYNTHESIS

   Clindamycin

   Chloramphenicol

   Linezolid

   Dalfopristin/Quinupristin

   Spectinomycin

All of the drugs discussed in this chapter inhibit bacterial protein synthesis. Unlike the aminoglycosides, whose effects on protein synthesis produce microbial death, the drugs considered here are usually bacteriostatic. That is, these agents suppress bacterial growth and replication but do not produce outright kill. In general, the drugs presented here are second-line agents, primarily because of emerging resistance or toxicity.

TETRACYCLINES

The tetracyclines are *broad-spectrum* antibiotics. Six members of the family are available for systemic therapy in the United States. All six—tetracycline, oxytetracycline, demeclocycline, methacycline, doxycycline, and minocycline—are similar in structure, antimicrobial actions, and adverse effects. Principal differences among the tetracyclines are pharmacokinetic. Because the similarities among these drugs are more pronounced than their differences, we will discuss the tetracyclines as a group, rather than focusing on a prototype. Unique properties of individual tetracyclines are indicated as appropriate.

Mechanism of Action

The tetracyclines suppress bacterial growth by inhibiting protein synthesis. They do so by binding to the 30S ribosomal subunit, thereby inhibiting binding of transfer RNA to the messenger RNA–ribosome complex. As a result, addition of amino acids to the growing peptide chain is prevented. At the concentrations achieved clinically, the tetracyclines are bacteriostatic.

Selective toxicity of the tetracyclines is determined in large part by the relative inability of these drugs to cross mammalian cell membranes. In order to influence protein synthesis, tetracyclines must first gain access to the cell interior. Entry into bacteria is accomplished by way of an energy-dependent transport system. Mammalian cells lack this transport system, and therefore do not actively accumulate the drug. Consequently, although tetracyclines are inherently capable of inhibiting protein synthesis in mammalian cells, drug levels within host cells remain too low to be harmful.

Microbial Resistance

Bacterial resistance to the tetracyclines results from reduced drug accumulation, increased drug inactivation, and decreased access of drug to ribosomes (owing to the presence of ribosome protection proteins). Regarding reduced accumulation, two mechanisms are involved: (1) decreased uptake and (2) acquisition of the ability to actively extrude tetracyclines.

Antimicrobial Spectrum

The tetracyclines are broad-spectrum antibiotics. These drugs are active against a wide variety of gram-positive and gram-negative bacteria. Sensitive organisms include *Rickettsia*, spirochetes, *Brucella*, *Chlamydia*, *Mycoplasma*, *Helicobacter pylori*, *Borrelia burgdorferi*, *Bacillus anthracis*, and *Vibrio cholerae*.

Therapeutic Uses

   Treatment of Infectious Diseases. Extensive use of tetracyclines has resulted in increasing bacterial resistance. Because of microbial resistance, and because antibiotics with greater selectivity and less toxicity are now available, use of tetracyclines has declined. Today, tetracyclines are rarely drugs of first choice. Disorders for which tetracyclines *are* considered first-line drugs include (1) rickettsial diseases (e.g., Rocky Mountain spotted fever, typhus fever, Q fever); (2) infections caused by *Chlamydia trachomatis* (trachoma, lymphogranuloma venereum, urethritis, cervicitis); (3) brucellosis; (4) cholera; (5) pneumonia caused by *Mycoplasma pneumoniae;* (6) Lyme disease; (7) anthrax; and (8) gastric infection with *H. pylori.*

Treatment of Acne. Tetracyclines are used topically and orally for severe acne vulgaris. Beneficial effects derive from suppressing the growth and metabolic activity of *Propionibacterium acnes,* causing the organism to reduce secretion of inflammatory chemicals. Oral doses of tetracyclines employed in acne are relatively low. As a result, adverse effects are minimal. Treatment of acne is discussed further in Chapter 101 (Drugs for the Skin).

Peptic Ulcer Disease. *Helicobacter pylori,* a bacterium that lives in the stomach, is a major contributing factor to peptic ulcer disease. Tetracyclines, in combination with metronidazole and bismuth subsalicylate, are a treatment of choice for eradicating this organism. The role of *H. pylori* in ulcer formation is discussed in Chapter 73 (Drugs for Peptic Ulcer Disease).

Periodontal Disease. Three tetracyclines—*doxycycline, minocycline,* and *tetracycline*—are used for periodontal disease. Doxycycline is taken orally, whereas minocycline and tetracycline are applied topically. Benefits of oral doxycycline [Periostat] result from inhibiting collagenase (an enzyme that destroys connective tissue in the gums) and not from killing bacteria. The small doses employed—20 mg twice daily—are too low to exert antibacterial effects.

Topical tetracycline [Actisite] and minocycline [Arestin] are employed as adjuncts to scaling and root planing. The objective is to reduce pocket depth and bleeding in adults with periodontitis. With both drugs, benefits derive from suppressing bacterial growth. Topical tetracycline is available as a polymer thread impregnated with the drug. The thread is packed into periodontal pockets, where it releases tetracycline slowly for 10 days, after which the thread is removed. Topical minocycline is available as a powder composed of "microspheres" that contain the drug. Like topical tetracycline, the minocycline powder is applied directly into periodontal pockets.

Rheumatoid Arthritis. *Minocycline* can reduce symptoms in patients with rheumatoid arthritis, suggesting a possible infectious component to the disease.

Pharmacokinetics

Individual tetracyclines differ significantly in their pharmacokinetic properties. Of particular significance are differences in half-life and route of elimination. Also of clinical importance are differences in the extent to which food decreases absorption. The pharmacokinetic properties of individual tetracyclines are summarized in Table 82–1.

Duration of Action. The tetracyclines can be divided into three groups: short acting, intermediate acting, and long acting (see Table 82–1). These differences are related to differences in lipid solubility: The short-acting tetracyclines (tetracycline, oxytetracycline) have relatively low lipid solubility, whereas the long-acting agents (doxycycline, minocycline) have relatively high lipid solubility.

Absorption. All of the tetracyclines are orally effective, although the extent of absorption differs among individual agents (see Table 82–1). Absorption of the short-acting and intermediate-acting tetracyclines is reduced in the presence of food. In contrast, food does not reduce absorption of the long-acting agents.

The tetracyclines form insoluble chelates with calcium, iron, magnesium, aluminum, and zinc. Formation of chelates decreases absorption. Accordingly, *tetracyclines should not be administered together with* (1) *calcium supplements,* (2) *milk products* (because they contain calcium), (3) *iron supplements,* (4) *magnesium-containing laxatives,* and (5) *most antacids* (because they contain magnesium, aluminum, or both).

Distribution. Tetracyclines are widely distributed to most tissues and body fluids. However, penetration to the cerebrospinal fluid (CSF) is poor, and levels achieved in the CSF are inadequate for treating meningeal infections. Tetracyclines readily cross the placenta and enter the fetal circulation.

Elimination. Tetracyclines are eliminated by the kidneys and liver. All tetracyclines are excreted by the liver into the bile. After the bile enters the intestine, most tetracyclines are reabsorbed.

Ultimate elimination of short-acting and intermediate-acting tetracyclines is in the urine, largely as the unchanged drug (see Table 82–1). Because these agents undergo renal excretion, they can accumulate to toxic levels if the kidneys fail. Consequently, *short-acting and intermediate-acting tetracyclines should not be administered to patients with renal failure.*

Long-acting tetracyclines are eliminated by the liver, primarily as metabolites. Because these agents are excreted by

			Percent of Oral	Effect of	Principal	Half-life	
		Lipid	Dose	Food on	Route of	Normal	Anuric
Class	Drug	Solubility	Absorbed	Absorption	Elimination	(hr)	(hr)
Short Acting	Tetracycline	Low	76	Decrease	Renal	8	57–108*
	Oxytetracycline	Low	58	Decrease	Renal	9	47–66*
Intermediate Acting	Demeclocycline	Moderate	66	Decrease	Renal	12	40–60*
	Methacycline	Moderate	58	Decrease	Renal	14	44*
Long Acting	Doxycycline	High	93	No change	Hepatic	18	12–22
	Minocycline	High	95	No change	Hepatic	16	11–23

TABLE 82–1 ■ Pharmacokinetic Properties of the Tetracyclines

*Because of greatly prolonged half-life and potential for accumulation to toxic levels, this drug should not be employed in patients with kidney dysfunction.

the liver, their half-lives are unaffected by kidney dysfunction. Accordingly, *the long-acting agents are drugs of choice for tetracycline-responsive infections in patients with renal impairment.*

Adverse Effects

Gastrointestinal Irritation. Tetracyclines irritate the GI tract. As a result, oral therapy is frequently associated with epigastric burning, cramps, nausea, vomiting, and diarrhea. These reactions can be reduced by giving tetracyclines with meals—although food may decrease absorption. Occasionally, tetracyclines cause esophageal ulceration. This can be minimized by avoiding administration at bedtime. Because diarrhea may result from suprainfection of the bowel (in addition to nonspecific irritation), it is important that the cause of diarrhea be determined.

Effects on Bones and Teeth. Tetracyclines bind to calcium in developing teeth, resulting in yellow or brown discoloration; hypoplasia of the enamel may also occur. The intensity of tooth discoloration is related to the total cumulative dose: Staining is darker with prolonged and repeated treatment. When taken after the fourth month of gestation, tetracyclines can cause staining of *deciduous* teeth. However, use of these drugs during pregnancy will not affect the *permanent* teeth. Discoloration of permanent teeth occurs when tetracyclines are taken by patients ages 4 months to 8 years, the interval during which tooth enamel is being formed. Accordingly, these drugs should be avoided by children under the age of 8 years. The risk of tooth discoloration with *doxycycline* and *oxytetracycline* may be less than with other tetracyclines.

Tetracyclines can suppress long-bone growth in premature infants. This effect is reversible upon discontinuation of treatment.

Suprainfection. As discussed in Chapter 79, a suprainfection is an overgrowth with drug-resistant microbes. This overgrowth occurs secondary to suppression of drug-sensitive organisms. Because the tetracyclines are broad-spectrum agents, and therefore can decrease viability of a wide variety of microbes, the risk of suprainfection is greater than with antibiotics that have a more narrow spectrum.

Suprainfection of the bowel with staphylococci or with *Clostridium difficile* produces severe diarrhea and can be life threatening. The infection caused by *C. difficile* is known as *antibiotic-associated pseudomembranous colitis* (AAPMC). Patients should be instructed to notify the physician if significant diarrhea occurs so that the possibility of bacterial suprainfection can be evaluated. If a diagnosis of suprainfection with staphylococci or *C. difficile* is made, tetracyclines should be discontinued immediately. Treatment consists of oral *vancomycin* or *metronidazole* plus vigorous fluid and electrolyte replacement.

Overgrowth with fungi (commonly *Candida albicans*) may occur in the mouth, pharynx, vagina, and bowel. Symptoms include vaginal or anal itching; inflammatory lesions of the anogenital region; and a black, furry appearance of the tongue. Suprainfection with *Candida* can be managed by discontinuing tetracycline use. When this is not possible, antifungal therapy is indicated.

Hepatotoxicity. Tetracyclines can cause fatty infiltration of the liver. Hepatotoxicity manifests clinically as lethargy and jaundice. Rarely, the condition progresses to massive liver failure. Liver damage is most likely when tetracyclines are administered intravenously in high doses (greater than 2 gm/day). Pregnant and postpartum women with kidney disease are at particularly high risk.

Renal Toxicity. Tetracyclines may exacerbate renal impairment in patients with pre-existing kidney disease. Because most tetracyclines are excreted by the kidneys, these agents should not be given to patients with renal impairment. Exceptions to this rule are *doxycycline* and perhaps *minocycline;* since these two agents are eliminated primarily by the liver, decreased kidney function does not cause them to accumulate.

Photosensitivity. All of the tetracyclines can increase the sensitivity of the skin to ultraviolet light. The most common result is exaggerated sunburn. Advise patients to avoid prolonged exposure to sunlight, wear protective clothing, and apply a sunscreen to exposed skin.

Other Adverse Effects. *Vestibular toxicity,* manifesting as dizziness, lightheadedness, and unsteadiness, has occurred with *minocycline.* Rarely, tetracyclines have produced *pseudotumor cerebri* (a benign elevation in intracranial pressure). In a few patients, *demeclocycline* has produced *nephrogenic diabetes insipidus,* a syndrome characterized by thirst, increased frequency of urination, and unusual weakness or tiredness. Because of their irritant properties, tetracyclines can cause *pain at sites of IM injection and thrombophlebitis when administered intravenously.*

Drug and Food Interactions

As noted, tetracyclines can form nonabsorbable chelates with certain metal ions (calcium, iron, magnesium, aluminum, zinc). Substances that contain these ions include *milk products, calcium supplements, iron supplements, magnesium-containing laxatives,* and *most antacids.* If a tetracycline is administered with these agents, its absorption will be decreased. To minimize interference with absorption, tetracyclines should be *administered at least 2 hours before or 2 hours after ingestion of chelating agents.*

Dosage and Administration

Administration. For systemic therapy, tetracyclines may be administered orally, intravenously, and by IM injection. Oral administration is preferred, and all tetracyclines are available in oral formulations. As a rule, oral tetracyclines should be taken on an empty stomach (1 hour before or 2 hours after meals) and with a full glass of water. An interval of at least 2 hours should separate administration of oral tetracyclines and ingestion of products capable of chelating these drugs (e.g., milk, calcium or iron supplements, antacids). Several tetracyclines can be given intravenously (Table 82–2), but this route should be employed only when oral therapy cannot be tolerated or has proved inadequate. Intramuscular injection is extremely painful and used only rarely.

In addition to their systemic use, two agents—tetracycline and minocycline—are available in formulations for topical therapy of periodontal disease.

Dosage. Dosage is determined by the nature and intensity of the infection being treated. Typical systemic doses for adults and children over the age of 8 years are summarized in Table 82–2.

Summary of Major Precautions

With the exceptions of doxycycline and minocycline, the tetracyclines are eliminated primarily in the urine, and will accumulate to toxic levels in the presence of kidney dis-

TABLE 82–2 ▪ Tetracyclines: Routes of Administration, Dosing Interval, and Dosage

Class	Drug	Trade Names	Route	Usual Dosing Interval (hr)	Total Daily Dose Adult (mg)	Total Daily Dose Pediatric (mg/kg)[a]
Short Acting	Tetracycline	Panmycin, Sumycin, Tetracap, Tetracyn, Tetralan	PO	6	1000–2000	25–50
			IV[b]	12	500–1000	10–20
			IM[c]	12	300	15–25
	Oxytetracycline	Terramycin, Uri-Tet	PO	6	1000–2000	25–50
			IM[c]	12	300	15–25
Intermediate Acting	Demeclocycline	Declomycin	PO	12	600	6–12
	Methacycline	Rondomycin	PO	12	600	6–12
Long Acting	Doxycycline	Vibramycin, others	PO	24	100[d]	2.2[e]
			IV[b]	24	100–200[f]	2.2–4.4[g]
	Minocycline	Minocin, Dynacin, Vectrin	PO	12	200[h]	4[i]
			IV[b]	12	200[h]	4[i]

[a]Doses presented are for children over the age of 8 years; use in children below this age may cause permanent staining of teeth.
[b]The intravenous route is used only if oral therapy cannot be tolerated or is inadequate.
[c]Intramuscular injection is extremely painful and used only rarely.
[d]First-day regimen is 100 mg initially followed by 100 mg 12 hours later.
[e]First-day regimen is 2.2 mg/kg initially followed by 2.2 mg/kg 12 hours later.
[f]First-day regimen is 200 mg in one or two slow infusions (1 to 4 hours).
[g]First-day regimen is 4.4 mg/kg in one or two slow infusions (1 to 4 hours).
[h]First-day regimen is 200 mg initially followed by 100 mg 12 hours later.
[i]First-day regimen is 4 mg/kg initially followed by 2 mg/kg 12 hours later.

ease. Accordingly, most tetracyclines should not be administered to patients with renal failure.

Tetracyclines can cause discoloration of deciduous and permanent teeth. Tooth discoloration can be avoided by withholding these drugs from pregnant women and from children under the age of 8 years.

Diarrhea may indicate a potentially life-threatening suprainfection of the bowel. Advise patients to notify the physician if diarrhea occurs.

High-dose IV therapy has been associated with severe liver damage, particularly in pregnant and postpartum women who have kidney disease. As a rule, these women should not receive tetracyclines.

Summary of Unique Properties of Individual Tetracyclines

Tetracycline. Tetracycline hydrochloride [Sumycin, others] is the least expensive and most widely used member of the tetracycline family. When employed systemically, the drug has the indications, pharmacokinetics, adverse effects, and drug interactions described for the tetracyclines as a group. Like most tetracyclines, tetracycline hydrochloride should not be administered with food, and is contraindicated for patients with kidney dysfunction. This agent and all other tetracyclines should not be given to pregnant women or to children under the age of 8 years.

In addition to its systemic use, tetracycline is available in a topical formulation [Actisite] for treatment of periodontal disease in adults.

Oxytetracycline. Oxytetracycline [Terramycin, Uri-Tet] is a short-acting agent similar to tetracycline in most respects. The principal difference between these drugs is cost: Brand-name preparations of oxytetracycline are more expensive than brand name preparations of tetracycline.

Demeclocycline. Demeclocycline [Declomycin] shares the actions, indications, and adverse effects described above for the tetracyclines as a group. Because of its intermediate duration of action, demeclocycline can be administered at dosing intervals that are longer than those used for tetracycline.

Demeclocycline is unique among the tetracyclines in its ability to stimulate urine flow. This side effect can lead to excessive urination, thirst, and tiredness. Interestingly, because of its effect on renal function, demeclocy-

cline has been employed therapeutically to promote urine production in patients suffering from the syndrome of inappropriate (excessive) secretion of antidiuretic hormone.

Methacycline. Methacycline [Rondomycin] shares the actions, indications, and adverse effects described above for the tetracyclines as a group. Like demeclocycline, methacycline is an intermediate-acting agent, and hence administration can be less frequent than with tetracycline.

Doxycycline. Doxycycline [Vibramycin, others] is a long-acting agent that shares the actions and adverse effects described above for the tetracyclines as a group. Because of its extended half-life, doxycycline can be administered once daily. Absorption of oral doxycycline is greater than that of tetracycline, and is not diminished by food or milk, and hence the drug may be administered with meals. Doxycycline is eliminated primarily by nonrenal mechanisms. As a result, this agent is safe for patients with renal failure. Doxycycline is a first-line drug for Lyme disease, anthrax, chlamydial infections (urethritis, cervicitis, lymphogranuloma venereum), and sexually acquired proctitis (in combination with ceftriaxone). A low-dose oral formulation [Periostat] is used for periodontal disease.

Minocycline. Minocycline [Minocin] is a long-acting agent similar in most respects to doxycycline. Like doxycycline, minocycline can be taken with food. Minocycline is safe for patients with kidney disease. The drug is unique among the tetracyclines in that it can damage the vestibular system, causing unsteadiness, lightheadedness, and dizziness. This toxicity limits the use of the drug. Minocycline is expensive; treatment costs significantly more than with tetracycline. In addition to fighting systemic infection, minocycline can reduce symptoms of arthritis (see Chapter 69). Also, the drug is available in a topical formulation [Arestin] for treatment of periodontal disease.

MACROLIDES

The macrolides are broad-spectrum antibiotics that act by inhibiting bacterial protein synthesis. These drugs are called macrolides because they are big molecules. Erythromycin is the oldest member of the family. The newer members—azithromycin, clarithromycin, dirithromycin, and troleandomycin—are derivatives of erythromycin.

Erythromycin

Erythromycin has a relatively broad spectrum of antimicrobial action and is a preferred or alternative treatment for a number of infections. The drug is one of our safest antibiotics and will serve as our prototype for the macrolide family.

Mechanism of Action

Antibacterial effects result from inhibition of protein synthesis: Erythromycin binds to the 50S ribosomal subunit and thereby blocks addition of new amino acids to the growing peptide chain. Erythromycin is usually bacteriostatic, but can be bactericidal against highly susceptible organisms or when present in high concentration. The drug is selectively toxic to bacteria because ribosomes in the cytoplasm of mammalian cells do not bind the drug. Also, in contrast to chloramphenicol (see below), erythromycin cannot cross the mitochondrial membrane, and therefore does not inhibit protein synthesis in host mitochondria.

Antimicrobial Spectrum

Erythromycin has an antibacterial spectrum similar to that of penicillin. The drug is active against most gram-positive bacteria as well as some gram-negative bacteria. Bacterial sensitivity is determined in large part by the ability of erythromycin to gain access to the cell interior.

Therapeutic Uses

Erythromycin is a commonly used antimicrobial agent. *This drug is the treatment of first choice for several infections and may be used as an alternative to penicillin G in patients allergic to penicillins.*

Erythromycin is a preferred treatment for pneumonia caused by *Legionella pneumophila* (legionnaires' disease).

Erythromycin is considered the drug of first choice for individuals infected with *Bordetella pertussis,* the causative agent of *whooping cough.* Since symptoms are caused by a toxin produced by *B. pertussis,* erythromycin does little to alter the course of the disease. However, by eliminating *B. pertussis* from the nasopharynx, treatment does lower infectivity.

Corynebacterium diphtheriae is highly sensitive to erythromycin. Accordingly, erythromycin is the treatment of choice for *acute diphtheria* and eliminating the diphtheria carrier state.

Several infections respond equally well to erythromycin and to tetracyclines. Both agents are drugs of first choice for certain chlamydial infections (urethritis, cervicitis) and for pneumonia caused by *M. pneumoniae.*

Erythromycin may be employed as an alternative to penicillin G in patients with penicillin allergy. The drug is used most frequently as a substitute for penicillin to treat respiratory tract infections caused by *Streptococcus pneumoniae* and by group A *Streptococcus pyogenes.* Erythromycin can also be employed as an alternative to penicillin for preventing recurrences of rheumatic fever and bacterial endocarditis.

Pharmacokinetics

Absorption and Bioavailability. Erythromycin for oral administration is available in four forms: *erythromycin base* and three derivatives of the base, *erythromycin estolate, erythromycin stearate,* and *erythromycin ethylsuccinate.* The base is unstable in stomach acid, and absorption can be variable; the derivatives were synthesized to improve bioavailability. Bioavailability has also been enhanced by use of acid-resistant coatings, which protect erythromycin while in the stomach and then dissolve in the duodenum, thereby permitting absorption of erythromycin from the small intestine. As a rule, *food decreases the absorption of erythromycin base and erythromycin stearate,* whereas absorption of the estolate and ethylsuccinate forms is not affected. Only erythromycin base is biologically active; the derivatives must be converted to the base (either in the intestine or following absorption) in order to work. When used properly (i.e., when dosage is correct and the effects of food are accounted for), all of the oral erythromycins produce equivalent therapeutic effects.

In addition to its oral forms, erythromycin is available as *erythromycin lactobionate* and *erythromycin gluceptate* for IV use. These IV preparations produce plasma drug levels that are higher than those achieved with oral therapy.

Distribution. Erythromycin is readily distributed to most tissues and body fluids. Penetration to the CSF, however, is poor. Erythromycin crosses the placenta, but adverse effects on the fetus have not been observed.

Elimination. Erythromycin is eliminated primarily by hepatic mechanisms. The drug is concentrated in the liver and then excreted in the bile. A small amount (10% to 15%) is excreted unchanged in the urine. Because elimination is primarily hepatic, dosage reduction is unnecessary in patients with renal dysfunction.

Adverse Effects

Erythromycin is generally free of serious toxicity and is one of the safest antibiotics available. The toxicity of principal concern is occasional liver injury from *erythromycin estolate.*

Gastrointestinal Effects. Gastrointestinal disturbances (epigastric pain, nausea, vomiting, diarrhea) are the most common adverse effects. These can be reduced by administering erythromycin with meals. However, this should be done only when using those forms of erythromycin whose absorption is unaffected by food (erythromycin estolate, erythromycin ethylsuccinate, certain enteric-coated formulations of erythromycin base). Patients who experience persistent or severe GI reactions should notify the physician.

Liver Injury. The drug's most serious toxicity is *cholestatic hepatitis.* This reaction occurs almost exclusively in adults, and is caused by *erythromycin estolate* and not by other forms of the drug. Symptoms include nausea, vomiting, abdominal pain, jaundice, and elevations in plasma levels of bilirubin and liver transaminases. Hepatic injury usually develops 10 to 20 days after initiation of treatment. However, the reaction can occur in a few hours if erythromycin is administered to patients who experienced hepatotoxicity in the past. Because of its ability to injure the liver, erythromycin estolate should be avoided by patients with pre-existing liver disease. Patients should be instructed to report signs of liver injury (e.g., severe abdominal pain, yellow discoloration of the skin or eyes, darkened urine, pale stools). Symptoms reverse following drug withdrawal.

Other Adverse Effects. By killing off sensitive gut flora, erythromycin can promote *suprainfection of the bowel. Thrombophlebitis* can occur with IV administration; this reaction can be minimized by infusing the drug slowly in dilute solution. Rarely, erythromycin causes *torsades de pointes,* a ventricular dysrhythmia. *Transient hearing loss* occurs rarely with high-dose therapy.

A recent report indicates that erythromycin may cause *hypertrophic pyloric stenosis in infants,* especially those under 2 weeks of age.

Drug Interactions

Erythromycin can increase the plasma levels and half-lives of several drugs, thereby posing a risk of toxicity. Erythromycin raises drug levels by inhibiting hepatic drug-metabolizing enzymes that employ cytochrome P450. Elevation of drug levels is a particular concern with *astemizole* and *terfenadine,* two nonsedating antihistamines that can cause fatal dysrhythmias when present in excessive amounts.* Accordingly, erythromycin should never be combined with these drugs. Elevated levels are also a concern with *theophylline* (used to treat asthma), *carbamazepine* (an anticonvulsant), and *warfarin* (an anticoagulant); when these agents are combined with erythromycin, the patient should be monitored closely for signs of toxicity.

Erythromycin prevents binding of *chloramphenicol* and *clindamycin* to bacterial ribosomes, thereby antagonizing the effects of these antibiotics. Accordingly, concurrent use of erythromycin with these two drugs is not recommended.

Preparations, Dosage, and Administration

Preparations. Erythromycin is available in formulations for oral and IV administration. All preparations have the same antimicrobial spectrum and indications. Adverse effects are also similar, except that cholestatic hepatitis occurs only with erythromycin estolate.

Oral Dosage and Administration. Oral erythromycins should be administered on an empty stomach and with a full glass of water. If necessary, some preparations (erythromycin estolate, erythromycin ethylsuccinate, certain enteric-coated preparations of erythromycin base) can be administered with food to decrease GI reactions. The usual *adult* dosage for *erythromycin base, estolate,* and *stearate* is 250 to 500 mg every 6 hours; the adult dosage for *erythromycin ethylsuccinate* is 400 to 800 mg every 6 hours. The usual *pediatric* dosage for all oral erythromycins is 7.5 to 12.5 mg/kg every 6 hours.

Trade names for oral erythromycins include E-Mycin, E-base, Ery-Tab, PCE Dispertab, and Erythromycin Filmtabs (for erythromycin base); Ilosone (for erythromycin estolate); and E.E.S. and EryPed (for erythromycin ethylsuccinate). Erythromycin stearate is available only as a generic product.

Intravenous Dosage and Administration. Intravenous administration is reserved for severe infections and used only rarely. Continuous infusion is preferred to intermittent administration. Only *erythromycin lactobionate* [Erythrocin] and *erythromycin gluceptate* [Ilotycin Gluceptate] are given IV. The usual *adult* dosage is 1 to 4 gm daily. The usual *pediatric* dosage is 15 to 50 mg/kg/day. Erythromycin should be infused slowly and in dilute solution to minimize the risk of thrombophlebitis. For instruction on preparation and storage of IV solutions, consult the manufacturer's literature.

Other Macrolides

All of the macrolides are similar to erythromycin with respect to mechanism of action, antimicrobial spectrum, and resistance. Major differences among these drugs are kinetic.

Clarithromycin

Actions and Therapeutic Uses. Like erythromycin, clarithromycin [Biaxin, Biaxin XL] binds the 50S subunit of bacterial ribosomes, causing inhibition of protein synthesis. The drug is approved for respiratory tract infections, uncomplicated infections of the skin and skin structures, and prevention of disseminated *Mycobacterium avium* complex infections in patients with advanced HIV infection. It is also used for *H. pylori* infection and as a substitute for penicillin G in penicillin-allergic patients.

Pharmacokinetics. Clarithromycin is available in three oral formulations: standard tablets, extended-release tablets, and granules. The standard tablets and granules are well absorbed, regardless of the presence of food. In contrast, the extended-release tablets are absorbed poorly if food is present. Following absorption, clarithromycin is widely distributed and readily penetrates cells. Elimination is by hepatic metabolism and renal excretion. A reduction in dosage may be needed for patients with severe renal dysfunction.

Adverse Effects and Interactions. Clarithromycin is well tolerated and does not produce the intense nausea seen with erythromycin. The most common reactions (3%) have been diarrhea, nausea, and distorted taste—all described as mild to moderate. In clinical trials, only 3% of patients withdrew because of side effects, compared with 20% of those taking erythromycin. High doses of clarithromycin have caused fetal abnormalities in laboratory animals; possible effects on the human fetus are unknown.

Like erythromycin, clarithromycin can inhibit hepatic metabolism of other drugs, and can thereby elevate their levels. Because of the risk of fatal dysrhythmias, clarithromycin must not be combined with *terfenadine* or *astemizole,* which are no longer sold in the United States. Like erythromycin, clarithromycin can elevate levels of *warfarin, carbamazepine,* and *theophylline;* dosages of these drugs may need to be reduced.

Preparations, Dosage, and Administration. Clarithromycin is available in standard tablets (250 and 500 mg), sold as Biaxin; extended-release tablets (500 mg), sold as Biaxin XL; and granules for oral suspension (25 and 50 mg/ml), sold as Biaxin. With the standard tablets and granules, the recommended dosage is 250 or 500 mg every 12 hours for 7 to 14 days; the exact dosage size and duration depend on the infection being treated. With the extended-release tablets, the recommended dosage is 500 mg once a day for 7 to 14 days. The standard tablets and granules may be taken without regard to meals, but the extended-release tablets should be taken with food.

Azithromycin

Actions and Therapeutic Uses. Like erythromycin, azithromycin [Zithromax] binds the 50S subunit of bacterial ribosomes, causing inhibition of protein synthesis. The drug is used for respiratory tract infections, chancroid, otitis media, uncomplicated infections of the skin and skin structures, and infections caused by *C. trachomatis,* for which it is a drug of choice. It may also be used as a substitute for penicillin G in penicillin-allergic patients. Like clarithromycin, azithromycin is under investigation for treatment of disseminated *M. avium* complex infections and other infections associated with AIDS.

Pharmacokinetics. Absorption of azithromycin is reduced by 50% in the presence of food. Accordingly, the drug should not be administered with meals. Following absorption, azithromycin is widely distributed to tissues and becomes concentrated in cells. The drug is eliminated in the bile, as both metabolites and parent drug.

Adverse Effects and Interactions. Like clarithromycin, azithromycin is well tolerated and does not produce the intense nausea seen with erythromycin. The most common reactions have been diarrhea (5%) and nausea and abdominal pain (3%). In one clinical trial, only 0.7% of patients withdrew because of drug-induced side effects. Aluminum- and magnesium-containing antacids reduce the rate (but not the extent) of azithromycin absorption. In contrast to erythromycin and clarithromycin, azithromycin does not inhibit the metabolism of other drugs, and hence can be used safely with terfenadine and astemizole.

Preparations, Dosage, and Administration. Oral. Azithromycin [Zithromax] is dispensed in two oral formulations: tablets (250 and 600 mg) and a suspension (20 and 40 mg/ml). The usual dosing schedule is 500 mg once on the first day, followed by 250 mg once daily on the following 4 days. The drug should be taken 1 hour before meals or 2 hours after. It must not be taken with food or with aluminum- or magnesium-containing antacids.

Intravenous. Azithromycin is dispensed as powder (500 mg) to be reconstituted for IV infusion. The usual dosage is 500 mg infused slowly (over 60 minutes or more) on 2 or more days. Intravenous therapy is followed by oral therapy. A complete course of treatment takes 7 days.

Dirithromycin

Actions and Therapeutic Uses. Dirithromycin [Dynabac] is similar to erythromycin with respect to mechanism of action, antimicrobial spectrum, and clinical effects. Approved indications include bronchitis caused by *S. pneumoniae* (but not by *Haemophilus influenzae*); community-acquired pneumonia caused by pneumococci, *M. pneumoniae,* or *L. pneumophila;* and skin and soft tissue infections caused by *Staphylococcus aureus.*

Pharmacokinetics. Following oral administration, dirithromycin is absorbed from the GI tract and converted by nonenzymatic hydrolysis into

---

*Because they can cause fatal dysrhythmias, terfenadine and astemizole are no longer available in the United States.

erythromycylamine, an active metabolite. The drug reaches high concentrations in tissues, although serum concentrations may be low. Dirithromycin and its metabolite are eliminated slowly in the bile, with a half-life of about 40 hours. Because of this extended half-life, once-daily dosing is sufficient.

Adverse Effects and Interactions. As with erythromycin, nausea and abdominal pain are common; the reported incidence is about 10%, but the actual incidence may be higher. In contrast to erythromycin and clarithromycin, dirithromycin does not inhibit the metabolism of other drugs, and hence appears safe for patients taking terfenadine or astemizole.

Preparations, Dosage, and Administration. Dirithromycin [Dynabac] is dispensed in 250-mg enteric-coated tablets for oral use. The usual dosage is 500 mg once daily for 7 to 14 days. Dirithromycin should be taken with meals or within 1 hour after eating. Food does not reduce absorption.

Troleandomycin

Troleandomycin [Tao] is the newest member of the macrolide family. Like other macrolides, the drug suppresses bacterial growth by inhibiting protein synthesis. At this time, troleandomycin has only two approved indications: pneumococcal pneumonia and upper respiratory tract infections caused by group A beta-hemolytic streptococci. Some patients have developed jaundice while taking the drug. Accordingly, liver function should be monitored. Troleandomycin inhibits cytochrome P450, and hence can suppress metabolism of other drugs, causing their levels to rise. Troleandomycin is available in 250-mg tablets for oral administration. The usual adult dosage is 250 to 500 mg 4 times a day for 10 days.

OTHER BACTERIOSTATIC INHIBITORS OF PROTEIN SYNTHESIS

Clindamycin

Clindamycin [Cleocin] can promote severe *antibiotic-associated pseudomembranous colitis,* a condition that can be fatal. Because of the risk of colitis, indications for clindamycin are limited. Currently, the drug is indicated only for certain anaerobic infections located outside the central nervous system (CNS).

Mechanism of Action

Clindamycin binds to the 50S subunit of bacterial ribosomes and thereby inhibits protein synthesis. The ribosomal site at which clindamycin binds overlaps the binding sites for erythromycin and chloramphenicol. As a result, these agents may antagonize each other's effects. Accordingly, there are no indications for concurrent use of clindamycin with these other antibiotics.

Antimicrobial Spectrum

Clindamycin is active against most anaerobic bacteria (gram positive and gram negative) and most gram-positive aerobes. Gram-negative aerobes are generally resistant. Susceptible anaerobes include *Bacteroides fragilis, Fusobacterium, Clostridium perfringens,* and anaerobic streptococci. Clindamycin is usually bacteriostatic. However, bactericidal effects may occur if the target organism is especially sensitive. Resistance can be a significant problem with *B. fragilis.*

Therapeutic Use

Because of its efficacy against gram-positive cocci, clindamycin was once used widely as an alternative to penicillin. However, following the discovery that clindamycin can promote AAPMC (see below), use of the drug has declined. Today, clindamycin is employed primarily for anaerobic infections outside the CNS (the drug does not cross the blood-brain barrier). Clindamycin is a preferred drug for abdominal and pelvic infections caused by *B. fragilis.* In addition, it can be used as a substitute for penicillin G to treat severe infections with other anaerobes (e.g., *C. perfringens, Fusobacterium nucleatum,* anaerobic streptococci).

Pharmacokinetics

Absorption and Distribution. Clindamycin may be administered orally, IM, and IV. Absorption from the GI tract is nearly complete and is not affected by food. The drug is widely distributed to most body fluids and tissues, including synovial fluid and bone. Penetration to the CSF is poor.

Elimination. Clindamycin undergoes hepatic metabolism to active and inactive products. These metabolites are excreted in the urine and bile. About 10% of the drug is eliminated unchanged by the kidneys. In normal individuals, the half-life is approximately 3 hours, and is increased only slightly in patients with substantial reductions in liver or kidney function. Hence, dosage need not be reduced. However, the drug may accumulate to toxic levels in the presence of *combined* renal and hepatic disease. Under these conditions, a reduction in dosage is indicated.

Adverse Effects

Antibiotic-Associated Pseudomembranous Colitis. AAPMC is the most severe toxicity associated with clindamycin. The cause is suprainfection of the bowel with *C. difficile,* an anaerobic gram-positive bacillus. AAPMC is characterized by profuse, watery diarrhea (10 to 20 stools per day), abdominal pain, fever, and leukocytosis. Stools often contain mucus and blood. Symptoms usually begin during the first week of treatment, but may also develop as long as 4 to 6 weeks after clindamycin withdrawal. Left untreated, the condition can be fatal. AAPMC occurs with parenteral and oral therapy. Because of the risk of colitis, patients should be instructed to report significant diarrhea (more than five watery stools per day). If suprainfection with *C. difficile* is diagnosed, clindamycin should be discontinued and the patient should be given oral vancomycin or metronidazole, which are drugs of choice for eliminating *C. difficile* from the bowel. Diarrhea usually ceases 3 to 5 days after starting vancomycin. Vigorous replacement therapy with fluids and electrolytes is usually indicated. Drugs that decrease bowel motility (e.g., opioids, anticholinergics) may worsen symptoms and should not be used.

Other Adverse Effects. Diarrhea (unrelated to AAPMC) is relatively common. *Hypersensitivity reactions* (especially rashes) occur frequently. *Hepatotoxicity* and *blood dyscrasias* (agranulocytosis, leukopenia, thrombocytopenia) develop rarely. Rapid IV administration can cause *electrocardiographic changes, hypotension,* and *cardiac arrest.*

Preparations, Dosage, and Administration

Preparations. Clindamycin is available as *clindamycin hydrochloride* and *clindamycin palmitate* for oral use and as *clindamycin phosphate* for IM or IV use. Clindamycin hydrochloride [Cleocin] is dispensed in capsules (75, 150, and 300 mg). Clindamycin palmitate [Cleocin Pediatric] is dispensed as flavored granules, which are reconstituted with fluid to make an oral solution containing 15 mg of clindamycin per milliliter. Clindamycin phosphate [Cleocin Phosphate] is dispensed in solution (150 mg/ml).

Oral Dosage and Administration. For *clindamycin hydrochloride,* the adult dosage ranges from 150 to 450 mg every 6 hours; the pediatric dosage ranges from 8 to 20 mg/kg daily in three or four divided doses. For *clindamycin palmitate,* adult and pediatric dosages range from 8 to 25 mg/kg/day administered in three or four divided doses. Oral clindamycin should be taken with a full glass of water. The drug may be administered with meals.

Parenteral Dosage and Administration. For parenteral (IM or IV) therapy, *clindamycin phosphate* is employed. Intramuscular and IV dosages are the same. The usual adult dosage is 0.6 to 3.6 gm/day administered in three or four divided doses. The usual pediatric dosage is 15 to 40 mg/kg/day in three or four divided doses.

Chloramphenicol

Chloramphenicol [Chloromycetin] is a broad-spectrum antibiotic with the potential for causing *fatal aplastic anemia* and other blood dyscrasias. Because of the risk of severe blood disorders, use of chloramphenicol is limited to serious infections for which less toxic drugs are ineffective.

Mechanism of Action

Chloramphenicol inhibits bacterial protein synthesis. The drug binds reversibly to the 50S subunit of bacterial ribosomes and thereby prevents addition of new amino acids to the growing peptide chain. Chloramphenicol is usually bacteriostatic, but can be bactericidal against highly susceptible organisms or when its concentration is high.

Since most protein synthesis in mammalian cells is carried out in the cytoplasm employing ribosomes that are insensitive to chloramphenicol, toxic effects of chloramphenicol are restricted largely to bacteria. However, because the ribosomes of mammalian *mitochondria* are very similar to the ribosomes of bacteria, chloramphenicol can decrease mitochondrial protein synthesis in the host. This action may underlie certain adverse effects (e.g., dose-dependent bone marrow depression, gray syndrome in infants).

Antimicrobial Spectrum

Chloramphenicol is active against a broad spectrum of bacteria. A large number of gram-positive and gram-negative aerobic organisms are sensitive. Among these are *Salmonella typhi, H. influenzae, Neisseria meningitidis,* and *S. pneumoniae.* Most anaerobic bacteria (e.g., *B. fragilis*) are also susceptible. In addition, chloramphenicol is active against rickettsiae, chlamydiae, mycoplasmas, and treponemes.

Resistance

Resistance among gram-negative bacteria results from acquisition of an R factor that codes for acetyltransferase, an enzyme that inactivates chloramphenicol. This same R factor also codes for resistance to tetracyclines, and frequently confers resistance to penicillins too.

Pharmacokinetics

Chloramphenicol is available in two forms: *chloramphenicol base,* which is administered PO, and *chloramphenicol succinate,* which is administered IV. Chloramphenicol base is active when administered. In contrast, chloramphenicol succinate is a prodrug that must be hydrolyzed to free chloramphenicol before it can act.

Availability of Active Drug. Chloramphenicol base is absorbed rapidly following oral administration, and bioavailability is high (between 75% and 90%). In contrast, when the drug is administered IV as chloramphenicol succinate, conversion to the active form (free chloramphenicol) is variable and incomplete. Production of active drug is especially erratic in newborns, infants, and young children.

Distribution. Chloramphenicol is highly lipid soluble and widely distributed to body tissues and fluids. Therapeutic concentrations are readily achieved in the CSF, and drug levels in the brain may be as much as 9 times those in plasma. As a result, chloramphenicol is of special value for treating meningitis and brain abscesses caused by susceptible bacteria. The drug crosses the placenta and is secreted in breast milk.

Metabolism and Excretion. Chloramphenicol is eliminated primarily by hepatic metabolism. Inactive metabolites are excreted in the urine. In patients with liver dysfunction, the drug's half-life is prolonged and accumulation can occur. Accordingly, dosage should be reduced in patients with liver disease. Because the kidneys serve only to excrete inactive metabolites, there is no need for dosage reduction in patients with renal dysfunction. In neonates, hepatic metabolism is not fully developed and hence the half-life of chloramphenicol is prolonged.

Monitoring Chloramphenicol Serum Levels. Because chloramphenicol has a low therapeutic index, and because serum levels of the drug can vary substantially among patients, monitoring of drug levels is frequently indicated. Monitoring is especially important for neonates, infants, and young children—because chloramphenicol levels in these patients can be highly variable. Monitoring is also important for patients with liver disease and those receiving certain drugs (e.g., phenytoin, phenobarbital, rifampin) that can alter the rate of chloramphenicol metabolism. For most infections, effective therapy is achieved with peak serum drug levels of 10 to 20 $\mu g/ml$ and trough levels of 5 to 10 $\mu g/ml$. The risk of dose-dependent bone marrow depression is significantly increased when peak levels rise above 25 $\mu g/ml$.

Therapeutic Use

Initially, chloramphenicol was employed widely. However, use was sharply restricted when its ability to cause fatal aplastic anemia became evident. Today, chloramphenicol is indicated only for life-threatening infections for which safer drugs are ineffective or contraindicated.

Chloramphenicol is a drug of choice for acute typhoid fever caused by sensitive strains of *S. typhi.* However, it is not recommended for routine therapy of the typhoid carrier state.

Chloramphenicol is lethal to *H. influenzae,* an organism that can infect the meninges and other sites. At one time, chloramphenicol plus ampicillin was considered the regimen of choice for initial therapy of meningitis caused by this microbe. However, third-generation cephalosporins, which readily penetrate the meninges, are now preferred.

Adverse Effects

The most important adverse effects are gray syndrome and toxicities related to the blood. Because of these toxicities, indications for chloramphenicol are limited.

Gray Syndrome. Gray syndrome is a potentially fatal toxicity observed most commonly in newborns. Initial symptoms are vomiting, abdominal distention, cyanosis, and gray discoloration of the skin. These may be followed by vasomotor collapse and death. The syndrome results from accumulation of chloramphenicol to high levels. Newborns are especially vulnerable to gray syndrome because (1) hepatic function is insufficient to detoxify chloramphenicol and (2) renal function is insufficient to excrete active drug. Although gray syndrome is usually observed in neonates, it can occur in older children and adults if dosage is excessive. If drug use is discontinued immediately when early symptoms appear, the syndrome is usually reversible. The risk of gray syndrome in infants can be reduced by using low doses and by monitoring chloramphenicol levels in serum.

Reversible Bone Marrow Depression. Chloramphenicol can produce dose-related depression of the bone marrow, resulting in anemia, and sometimes leukopenia and thrombocytopenia. Marrow depression is a toxic reaction to chloramphenicol and occurs most commonly when plasma drug levels exceed 25 $\mu g/ml$. The cause of bone marrow depression appears to be inhibition of protein synthesis in host mitochondria. To promote early detection of bone marrow depression, complete blood counts should be performed prior to therapy and every 2 days thereafter. Advise patients to notify the physician if signs of blood disorders develop (e.g., sore throat, fever, unusual bleeding or bruising). Chloramphenicol should be withdrawn if evidence of bone marrow depression is detected. Depression of bone marrow usually reverses within 1 to 3 weeks following drug withdrawal. The anemia associated with toxic bone marrow depression is not related to aplastic anemia (discussed next).

Aplastic Anemia. Rarely, chloramphenicol produces aplastic anemia, a condition characterized by pancytopenia and bone marrow aplasia. The reaction is usually fatal. Aplastic anemia develops in 1 of 35,000 patients, and is not related to dosage. As a rule, the reaction develops weeks or months after termination of treatment. Aplastic anemia can occur with oral, IV, or even topical (ophthalmic) use of the drug. The mechanism underlying aplastic anemia has not been determined, but toxicity may result from a genetic predisposition. Unfortunately, aplastic anemia cannot be predicted by monitoring the blood.

Other Adverse Effects. *Gastrointestinal effects* (vomiting, diarrhea, glossitis) occur occasionally. *Herxheimer reactions* have occurred during treatment of typhoid fever. *Neurologic effects* (peripheral neuropathy, optic neuritis, confusion, delirium) develop rarely, usually in association with prolonged treatment. Other rare toxicities include *suprainfection of the bowel, allergic reactions,* and *fever.*

Drug Interactions

Chloramphenicol can inhibit hepatic drug-metabolizing enzymes, thereby prolonging the half-lives of certain drugs. Agents whose metabolism may be affected include *phenytoin* (an anticonvulsant), *warfarin* (an anticoagulant), and two oral hypoglycemics: *tolbutamide* and *chlorpropamide.* If any of these drugs are taken concurrently with chloramphenicol, their dosages should be reduced (to avoid accumulation to toxic levels).

Preparations, Dosage, and Administration

General Considerations Regarding Route of Administration and Dosage. For treatment of systemic infections, chloramphenicol may be administered PO or IV. For initial therapy of serious infections, IV administration is generally preferred; oral therapy may be substituted later if conditions warrant.

As a rule, the dosing objective is to produce peak chloramphenicol plasma levels that range between 10 and 20 μg/ml. This can be accomplished by monitoring serum levels of the drug. Monitoring is especially important in newborns, in patients with liver disease, and in patients receiving drugs that can alter chloramphenicol disposition (e.g., phenytoin).

Preparations. For *oral* therapy, chloramphenicol is available in 250-mg capsules as *chloramphenicol base.* For *intravenous* therapy, chloramphenicol is available in powdered form as *chloramphenicol sodium succinate* [Chloromycetin Sodium Succinate], which must be reconstituted to a 100-mg/ml solution.

Dosage and Administration. Recommended dosages for oral and IV administration are the same. As a rule, oral doses should be taken on an empty stomach at least 1 hour before meals or 2 hours after. If gastric upset occurs, discomfort may be reduced by taking chloramphenicol with food. The usual dosage for adults and children is 12.5 to 25 mg/kg every 6 hours. For infants 7 days old or younger, the usual dosage is 25 mg/kg once a day. For infants more than 7 days old, the recommended dosage is 25 mg/kg every 12 hours. Dosage should be reduced for patients with liver dysfunction.

Linezolid

Linezolid [Zyvox] is the first member of a new class of antibiotics, the *oxazolidinones*. The drug is important because it has activity against multidrug-resistant gram-positive pathogens, including vancomycin-resistant enterococci (VRE) and methicillin-resistant *Staphylococcus aureus* (MRSA). To delay the emergence of resistance, linezolid should generally be reserved for infections caused by VRE or MRSA, even though it has additional approved uses.

Mechanism, Resistance, and Antimicrobial Spectrum

Linezolid is a bacteriostatic inhibitor of protein synthesis. The drug binds to the 23S portion of the 50S ribosomal subunit, and thereby blocks formation of the initiation complex. No other antibiotic works quite this way. As a result, cross-resistance with other agents is unlikely. In clinical trials, development of resistance to linezolid was rare, and occurred only in association with prolonged treatment of VRE infections and the presence of a prosthetic implant or undrained abscess.

Linezolid is active primarily against aerobic and facultative gram-positive bacteria. Susceptible pathogens include *Enterococcus faecium* (vancomycin-sensitive and vancomycin-resistant strains), *Enterococcus faecalis* (vancomycin-resistant strains), *Staph. aureus* (methicillin-sensitive and methicillin-resistant strains), *Staphylococcus epidermidis* (including methicillin-resistant strains), and *S. pneumoniae* (penicillin-sensitive and penicillin-resistant strains). Linezolid is not active against gram-negative bacteria, because these organisms readily export the drug.

Pharmacokinetics

Oral linezolid is rapidly and completely absorbed. Food decreases the rate of absorption but not the extent. The drug is eliminated by hepatic metabolism and renal excretion. Its half-life is about 5 hours.

Adverse Effects

Linezolid is generally well tolerated. The most common side effects are diarrhea (5.3%), nausea (3.5%), and headache (2.7%). Linezolid oral suspension contains phenylalanine, and hence must not be used by people with phenylketonuria.

Linezolid can cause reversible *myelosuppression,* manifesting as anemia, leukopenia, thrombocytopenia, or even pancytopenia. Risk is related to duration of use. Complete blood counts should be done weekly. Special caution is needed in patients with pre-existing myelosuppression, those taking other myelosuppressive drugs, and those receiving linezolid for more than 2 weeks. If existing myelosuppression worsens or new myelosuppression develops, discontinuing linezolid should be considered.

Drug Interactions

Linezolid is a weak inhibitor of monoamine oxidase (MAO), and hence poses a risk of hypertensive crisis. As discussed in Chapter 31, MAO inhibitors can cause severe hypertension if they are combined with *indirect-acting sympathomimetics* (e.g., ephedrine, pseudoephedrine, methylphenidate, cocaine) or with foods that contain large amounts of *tyramine.* Accordingly, patients using linezolid should be warned to avoid these agents.

In theory, combining linezolid with a *selective serotonin reuptake inhibitor* (e.g., fluoxetine [Prozac]) can increase the risk of serotonin syndrome (because inhibition of MAO increases the serotonin content of CNS neurons). However, serotonin syndrome has not been observed.

Preparations, Dosage, and Administration

Linezolid is available in three formulations: (1) 400- and 600-mg *tablets,* (2) a powder for reconstitution to a 20-mg/ml *oral suspension,* and (3) a 2-mg/ml *intravenous solution* supplied in 100-, 200-, and 300-ml bags. Oral linezolid can be taken with or without food. Intravenous linezolid is infused over 30 to 120 minutes, and should not be combined with additives or other drugs. Dosages for specific infections are as follows:

- *VRE infections*—600 mg PO or IV every 12 hours for 14 to 28 days
- *Pneumonia (nosocomial or community acquired)*—600 mg PO or IV every 12 hours for 10 to 14 days
- *Complicated skin and skin structure infections (including MRSA infections)*—same as for pneumonia
- *Uncomplicated skin and skin structure infections*—400 mg PO every 12 hours for 10 to 14 days

Dalfopristin/Quinupristin

Dalfopristin and quinupristin are the first members of a new class of antibiotics known as *streptogramins.* The two drugs are available in a fixed-dose combination (70 parts dalfopristin/30 parts quinupristin) under the trade name *Synercid.*

Mechanism of Action. Dalfopristin and quinupristin inhibit bacterial protein synthesis. When used separately, dalfopristin and quinupristin are bacteriostatic. However, in combination they are bactericidal.

Therapeutic Use. The principal indication for dalfopristin/quinupristin is vancomycin-resistant *E. faecium.* (The drugs are not active against *E. faecalis.*) To delay emergence of resistance, dalfopristin/quinupristin should be reserved for infections that have not responded to vancomycin. Other indications include MRSA, methicillin-resistant *Staph. epidermidis,* and drug-resistant *S. pneumoniae.* Dalfopristin/quinupristin is safe for patients who are allergic to penicillins and cephalosporins.

Adverse Effects. *Hepatotoxicity* is the major concern. Blood should be tested for liver enzymes and bilirubin at least twice during the first week of therapy and once weekly thereafter. Other adverse effects include irritation at the infusion site, joint and muscle pain, rash, pruritus, vomiting, and diarrhea.

Drug Interactions. Dalfopristin and quinupristin inhibit hepatic drug-metabolizing enzymes, specifically CYP3A4 (a form of cytochrome P450). Accordingly, the combination is likely to inhibit the metabolism of many other drugs, including cyclosporine, tacrolimus, and cisapride.

Preparations, Dosage, and Administration. Dalfopristin/quinupristin [Synercid] is dispensed as a powder in 500-mg vials to be reconstituted for IV administration. The usual dosage is 7.5 mg/kg infused slowly (over 1 hour) 2 or 3 times a day. To minimize venous irritation, flush the vein with 0.5% dextrose after the infusion. If irritation occurs despite flushing, the drug may be infused through a central venous catheter. Because dalfopristin and quinupristin are eliminated by hepatic metabolism, dosage should be reduced in patients with liver impairment.

Spectinomycin

Mechanism of Action and Antimicrobial Spectrum. Spectinomycin [Trobicin] binds to the 30S ribosomal subunit and thereby suppresses bacterial protein synthesis. The drug is active against a number of gram-negative bacteria. Resistance develops frequently.

Therapeutic Use. Because resistant organisms emerge rapidly, use of spectinomycin is limited. The principal indication for the drug is anogenital *gonorrhea* in patients who cannot tolerate preferred drugs (e.g., ceftriaxone, cefixime).

Pharmacokinetics. Spectinomycin is administered only by IM injection; the drug is not absorbed from the GI tract and hence cannot be used orally. Most of each dose is excreted unchanged in the urine. The plasma half-life is approximately 2 hours.

Adverse Effects. Spectinomycin is generally well tolerated. Adverse effects seen occasionally include soreness at the site of injection, dizziness, nausea, urticaria, pruritus, chills, fever, and insomnia.

Preparations, Dosage, and Administration. Spectinomycin [Trobicin] is dispensed as a sterile powder together with sufficient diluent to produce a 400-mg/ml solution. For treatment of uncomplicated gonorrhea of the rectum or genitalia, the usual adult dose is 2 gm administered as a single IM (intragluteal) injection. For children weighing less than 45 kg, a single injection of 40 mg/kg is given. For disseminated gonococcal infection, the adult dosage is 2 gm twice a day for 3 days.

⠿ KEY POINTS

- Tetracyclines are broad-spectrum, bacteriostatic antibiotics that act by inhibiting bacterial protein synthesis.
- Tetracyclines are first-choice drugs for only a few infections. These include infections caused by *C. trachomatis,* rickettsia (e.g., Rocky Mountain spotted fever), *H. pylori* (i.e., peptic ulcer disease), *Bacillus anthracis* (anthrax), *Borrelia burgdorferi* (Lyme disease) and *M. pneumoniae.*
- Tetracyclines form insoluble chelates with calcium, iron, magnesium, aluminum, and zinc. Accordingly, these drugs must not be administered with calcium supplements, milk products, iron supplements, magnesium-containing laxatives, and most antacids.
- Except for doxycycline and minocycline, tetracyclines should not be given to patients with renal failure.
- Except for doxycycline and minocycline, tetracyclines should not be administered with food.
- Tetracyclines can stain developing teeth, and therefore should not be given to pregnant women or children under 8 years old.
- Because they are broad-spectrum antibiotics, tetracyclines can cause suprainfections—especially antibiotic-associated pseudomembranous colitis (AAPMC) and overgrowth of the mouth, pharynx, vagina, or bowel with *C. albicans.*
- High doses of tetracyclines can cause severe liver damage, especially in pregnant and postpartum women who have kidney impairment.
- Erythromycin, the prototype of the macrolide antibiotics, is a bacteriostatic drug that inhibits bacterial protein synthesis.
- Erythromycin has an antimicrobial spectrum similar to that of penicillin G, and hence can be used in place of penicillin G in patients with penicillin allergy.
- Although erythromycin is generally very safe, one form of the drug—erythromycin estolate—can cause serious liver injury.
- Clindamycin causes a high incidence of AAPMC, and hence has limited uses.
- Chloramphenicol can cause fatal aplastic anemia and other serious blood dyscrasias. As a result, the drug should be used only when clearly indicated.
- Linezolid is important because it can suppress multidrug-resistant gram-positive pathogens, including vancomycin-resistant enterococci (VRE) and methicillin-resistant *Staph. aureus* (MRSA).

Summary of Major Nursing Implications*

TETRACYCLINES

Demeclocycline
Doxycycline
Methacycline
Minocycline
Oxytetracycline
Tetracycline

Except where stated otherwise, the implications summarized below pertain to all members of the tetracycline family.

Preadministration Assessment

Therapeutic Goal

Treatment of tetracycline-sensitive infections, acne, and periodontal disease.

Identifying High-Risk Patients

Tetracyclines should not be used during pregnancy or by children under the age of 8 years. Except for *doxycycline* and *minocycline,* tetracyclines must be used with great *caution* in patients with significant renal impairment.

Implementation: Administration

Routes

Systemic. *All* tetracyclines are used systemically. For specific routes (PO, IM, or IV) applicable to individual agents, see Table 82–2.

Topical. Tetracycline and *minocycline* are used topically to treat periodontal disease.

Administration

Oral. **Advise patients to take oral tetracyclines on an empty stomach (1 hour before meals or 2 hours after) and with a full glass of water.** *Doxycycline* and *minocycline* may be taken with food.

Absorption of tetracyclines will be reduced by certain chelating agents: *milk products, calcium supplements, iron*

---

*Patient education information is highlighted as blue text.

Summary of Major Nursing Implications*—cont'd

supplements, magnesium-containing laxatives, and *most antacids.* **Instruct the patient to allow at least 2 hours between ingestion of tetracyclines and these chelators.**

Instruct the patient to complete the prescribed course of treatment, even though symptoms may abate before the full course is over.

Parenteral. Intravenous administration is performed only when oral administration is ineffective or cannot be tolerated. *Intramuscular* injection is painful and used only rarely.

Ongoing Evaluation and Interventions
Minimizing Adverse Effects

Gastrointestinal Irritation. **Inform patients that GI distress (epigastric burning, cramps, nausea, vomiting, diarrhea) can be reduced by taking tetracyclines with meals.**

Effects on Teeth. Tetracyclines can discolor developing teeth. To prevent this effect, avoid use of tetracyclines by pregnant women and by children under the age of 8 years.

Suprainfection. Tetracyclines can promote bacterial suprainfection of the bowel, resulting in severe diarrhea. **Instruct patients to notify the physician if significant diarrhea develops.** If suprainfection is diagnosed, discontinue tetracyclines immediately; treatment consists of (1) oral vancomycin or metronidazole, plus (2) vigorous fluid and electrolyte replacement therapy.

Fungal overgrowth may occur in the mouth, pharynx, vagina, and bowel. **Inform patients about symptoms of fungal infection (vaginal or anal itching; inflammatory lesions of the anogenital region; black, furry appearance of the tongue), and advise them to notify the physician if these occur.** Suprainfection caused by *Candida* can be managed by discontinuing the tetracycline or by giving an antifungal drug.

Hepatotoxicity. Tetracyclines can cause fatty infiltration of the liver, resulting in jaundice and, rarely, massive liver failure. The risk of liver injury can be reduced by (1) avoiding high-dose IV therapy and (2) withholding tetracyclines from pregnant and postpartum women who have kidney disease.

Renal Toxicity. Tetracyclines can exacerbate pre-existing renal impairment. With the exception of *doxycycline* and perhaps *minocycline,* tetracyclines should not be used by patients with kidney disease.

Photosensitivity. Tetracyclines can increase the sensitivity of the skin to ultraviolet light, thereby increasing the risk of sunburn. **Advise patients to avoid prolonged exposure to sunlight, wear protective clothing, and apply a sunscreen to exposed skin.**

ERYTHROMYCIN

The implications summarized below pertain to all forms of erythromycin, except where noted otherwise.

Preadministration Assessment
Therapeutic Goal

Erythromycin is indicated for legionnaires' disease, whooping cough, diphtheria, chancroid, chlamydial infections, and other infections caused by erythromycin-sensitive organisms. The drug is also used as a substitute for penicillin G in penicillin-allergic patients.

Identifying High-Risk Patients

All erythromycins are contraindicated in patients taking astemizole or terfenadine, two antihistamines no longer available in the United States. *Erythromycin estolate* is *contraindicated* for patients with liver disease.

Implementation: Administration
Routes

Oral. Erythromycin base, erythromycin estolate, erythromycin ethylsuccinate, and erythromycin stearate.

Intravenous. Erythromycin lactobionate, erythromycin glucceptate.

Administration

Oral. **Advise the patient to take oral preparations on an empty stomach (1 hour before meals or 2 hours after) and with a full glass of water. However, if GI upset occurs, administration may be done with meals.**

Inform patients using erythromycin estolate, erythromycin ethylsuccinate, and enteric-coated formulations of erythromycin base that they make take these drugs without regard to meals.

Instruct patients to complete the prescribed course of treatment, even though symptoms may abate before the full course is over.

Intravenous. Administer by slow infusion and in dilute solution to minimize thrombophlebitis.

Ongoing Evaluation and Interventions
Minimizing Adverse Effects

Gastrointestinal Effects. Gastrointestinal disturbances (epigastric pain, nausea, vomiting, diarrhea) can be reduced by administering erythromycin with meals. **Advise patients to notify the physician if GI reactions are severe or persistent.**

Liver Injury. Erythromycin estolate may cause cholestatic hepatitis. **Inform patients about signs of liver injury (e.g., severe abdominal pain, yellow discoloration of skin or eyes, darkened urine, pale stools), and advise them to notify the physician if these develop.** If cholestatic hepatitis occurs, erythromycin estolate should be withdrawn. Do not give erythromycin estolate to patients with liver dysfunction.

Minimizing Adverse Interactions

Erythromycin can increase the half-lives and plasma levels of several drugs. Raising levels of *astemizole* or *terfenadine* can cause fatal dysrhythmias, and hence these drugs must never be combined with erythromycin. When erythromycin is combined with *theophylline, carbamazepine,* or *warfarin,* patients should be monitored closely for toxicity.

Erythromycin can antagonize the antibacterial actions of *clindamycin* and *chloramphenicol.* Concurrent use of erythromycin with these agents is not recommended.

---

*Patient education information is highlighted as blue text.

Summary of Major Nursing Implications*—cont'd

CLINDAMYCIN

Preadministration Assessment

Therapeutic Goal

Treatment of anaerobic infections outside the CNS.

Implementation: Administration

Routes

Oral, IM, IV.

Administration

Instruct patients to take oral clindamycin with a full glass of water.

Instruct patients to complete the prescribed course of treatment, even though symptoms may abate before the full course is over.

Ongoing Evaluation and Interventions

Minimizing Adverse Effects

Antibiotic-Associated Pseudomembranous Colitis. Clindamycin can promote AAPMC, a potentially fatal suprainfection. Prominent symptoms are profuse watery diarrhea, abdominal pain, fever, and leukocytosis. Stools often contain mucus and blood. **Instruct the patient to report significant diarrhea (more than five watery stools per day).** If AAPMC is diagnosed, discontinue clindamycin. Treat with oral vancomycin or metronidazole and vigorous replacement of fluids and electrolytes. Drugs that decrease bowel motility (e.g., opioids, anticholinergics) may worsen symptoms and should be avoided.

CHLORAMPHENICOL

Preadministration Assessment

Therapeutic Goal

Treatment of life-threatening infections for which safer drugs are ineffective or contraindicated.

Baseline Data

Obtain blood cell counts.

Identifying High-Risk Patients

Chloramphenicol is *contraindicated* for patients with a history of toxic reactions to chloramphenicol. The drug should be used with *caution* in patients with liver disease and during pregnancy and lactation.

Implementation: Administration

Routes

Oral, IV. Dosage is the same for both routes.

*Patient education information is highlighted as blue text.

Administration

Instruct patients to take chloramphenicol on an empty stomach at least 1 hour before meals or 2 hours after. If GI upset occurs, the drug may be taken with meals.

Instruct the patient to complete the prescribed course of treatment, even though symptoms may abate before the full course is over.

Ongoing Evaluation and Interventions

Monitoring Drug Levels

Knowledge of plasma drug levels is especially valuable in patients with liver disease, the young (newborns, infants, young children), and patients receiving drugs that can alter chloramphenicol disposition (e.g., phenobarbital, phenytoin, rifampin). The dosage is adjusted to produce peak plasma levels of 10 to 20 $\mu g/ml$ and trough levels of 5 to 10 $\mu g/ml$.

Minimizing Adverse Effects

Gray Syndrome. The gray syndrome usually occurs in newborns. Manifestations include vomiting, abdominal distention, cyanosis, and gray discoloration of the skin; vasomotor collapse and death can occur. Observe the patient for symptoms and terminate therapy if they occur. The risk of gray syndrome can be reduced by giving appropriately low doses and monitoring chloramphenicol levels.

Reversible Bone Marrow Depression. Chloramphenicol can produce reversible, dose-related depression of bone marrow, manifesting as anemia, leukopenia, and thrombocytopenia. Blood cell counts should be obtained prior to therapy and every 2 days thereafter. **Inform patients about early signs of hematologic toxicity (e.g., sore throat, fever, unusual bleeding or bruising), and instruct them to notify the physician if these occur.** If bone marrow depression is diagnosed, chloramphenicol should be withdrawn immediately. The risk of bone marrow depression can be minimized by keeping peak plasma drug levels below 25 $\mu g/ml$.

Aplastic Anemia. Very rarely, chloramphenicol causes aplastic anemia, a condition with a high mortality rate. The risk of aplastic anemia can be minimized by using chloramphenicol only when clearly indicated.

Minimizing Adverse Interactions

Chloramphenicol can prolong the half-lives of a variety of drugs, including *phenytoin, warfarin,* and some *oral hypoglycemics.* If these drugs are combined with chloramphenicol, their dosages should be reduced.

Aminoglycosides: Bactericidal Inhibitors of Protein Synthesis

The aminoglycosides are narrow-spectrum antibiotics, used primarily against aerobic gram-negative bacilli. These drugs disrupt protein synthesis, resulting in rapid bacterial death. The aminoglycosides can cause serious injury to the inner ear and kidney. Because of these toxicities, indications for the aminoglycosides are limited. All of the aminoglycosides carry multiple positive charges. As a result, these drugs are not absorbed from the GI tract, and hence must be administered parenterally to treat systemic infections. In the United States, eight aminoglycosides are approved for clinical use. The agents employed most commonly are gentamicin, tobramycin, and amikacin.

BASIC PHARMACOLOGY OF THE AMINOGLYCOSIDES

Chemistry

The aminoglycosides are composed of two or more amino sugars connected by a glycoside linkage, hence the family name. At physiologic pH, these drugs are highly polar polycations (i.e., they carry several positive charges), and therefore cannot readily cross membranes. As a result, aminoglycosides are not absorbed from the GI tract, do not enter the cerebrospinal fluid, and are rapidly excreted by the kidneys. Structural formulas for the three major aminoglycosides are shown in Figure 83–1.

Mechanism of Action

The aminoglycosides disrupt bacterial protein synthesis. As indicated in Figure 83–2, these drugs bind to the 30S ribosomal subunit, and thereby cause (1) inhibition of protein synthesis, (2) premature termination of protein synthesis, and (3) production of abnormal proteins (secondary to misreading of the genetic code).

The aminoglycosides are *bactericidal.* Cell kill is concentration dependent. Hence, the higher the concentration, the more rapidly the infection will clear. Of note, bactericidal activity persists for several hours *after* serum levels have dropped below the minimal bactericidal concentration, a phenomenon known as the *postantibiotic effect.*

Bacterial kill appears to result from production of abnormal proteins rather than from simple inhibition of protein synthesis. Studies suggest that abnormal proteins become inserted in the bacterial cell membrane, causing it to leak. The resultant loss of cell contents causes death. Inhibition of protein synthesis per se does not seem the likely cause of bacterial death. This statement is based on the observation that complete blockade of protein synthesis by other antibiotics (e.g., tetracyclines, chloramphenicol) is usually bacteriostatic—not bactericidal.

Microbial Resistance

The principal cause for bacterial resistance is production of enzymes that can inactivate aminoglycosides. Among gram-negative bacteria, the genetic information needed to synthesize these enzymes is acquired by transfer of R factors. To date, more than 20 different aminoglycoside-inactivating enzymes have been identified. Since each of the aminoglycosides can be modified by more than one of these enzymes, and since each enzyme can act on more than one aminoglycoside, patterns of bacterial resistance can be complex.

Of all the aminoglycosides, *amikacin* is least susceptible to inactivation by bacterial enzymes. As a result, resistance to amikacin is uncommon. To minimize emergence of bacteria resistant to amikacin, the drug should be reserved for infections that are unresponsive to other aminoglycosides.

Antimicrobial Spectrum

Bactericidal effects of the aminoglycosides are limited almost exclusively to *aerobic gram-negative bacilli.* Sensitive organisms include *Escherichia coli, Klebsiella pneumoniae, Serratia marcescens, Proteus mirabilis,* and *Pseudomonas aeruginosa.* Aminoglycosides are inactive against most gram-positive bacteria.

Aminoglycosides *cannot kill anaerobes.* To produce antibacterial effects, aminoglycosides must be transported across the bacterial cell membrane, a process that is oxygen dependent. Since, by definition, anaerobic organisms live in the absence of oxygen, these microbes cannot take up aminoglycosides, and hence are resistant. For the same reason, aminoglycosides are inactive against facultative bacteria when these organisms are living under anaerobic conditions.

Therapeutic Use

Parenteral Therapy. The principal use for parenteral aminoglycosides is treatment of *serious infections due to aerobic gram-negative bacilli.* Primary target organisms are

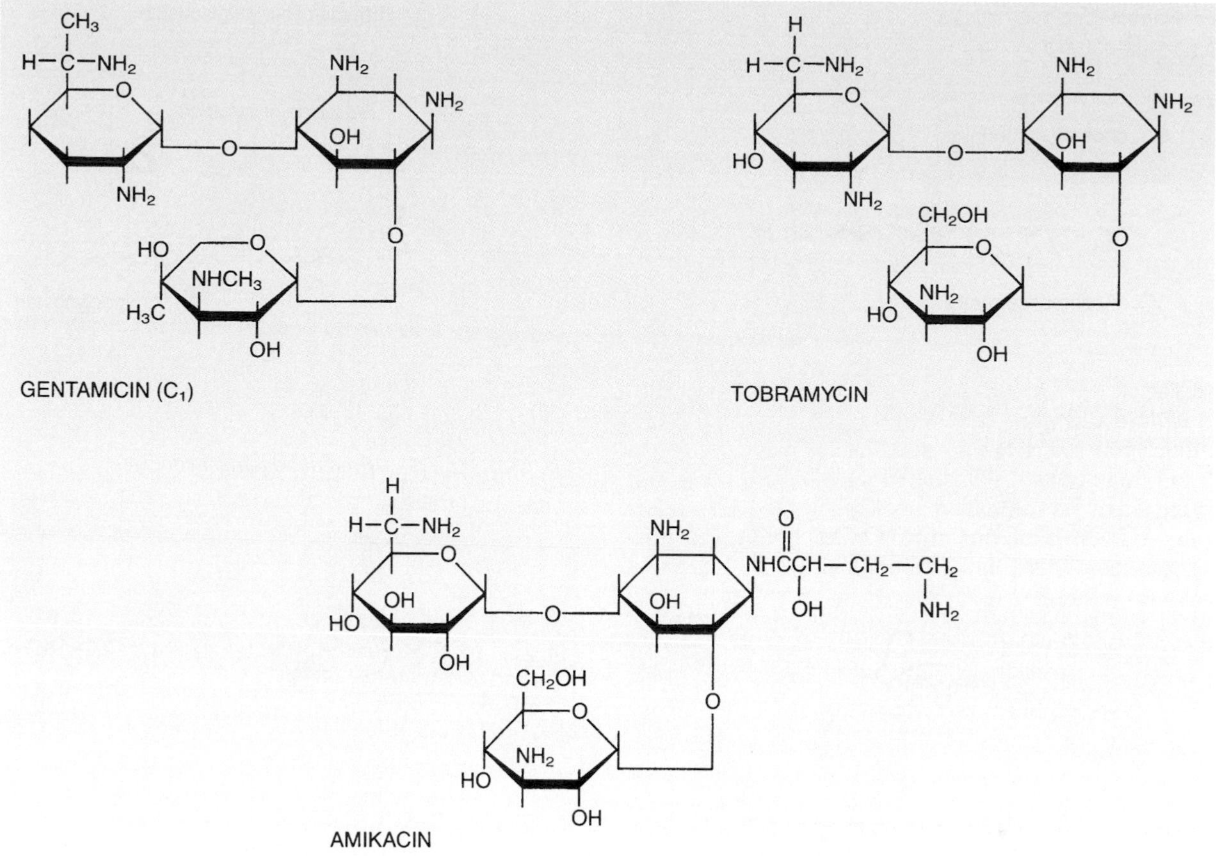

Figure 83–1 ■ **Structural formulas of the major aminoglycosides.**

P. aeruginosa and the Enterobacteriaceae (e.g., *E. coli, Klebsiella, Serratia, P. mirabilis*).

The aminoglycosides used most commonly for parenteral therapy are gentamicin, tobramycin, and amikacin. Selection among the three depends in large part on patterns of resistance in a given community or hospital. In settings where resistance to aminoglycosides is uncommon, either gentamicin or tobramycin is usually preferred. Of the two, gentamicin is less costly and may be selected on this basis. Organisms resistant to both gentamicin and tobramycin are usually sensitive to amikacin. Accordingly, in settings where resistance to gentamicin and tobramycin is common, amikacin may be preferred for initial therapy.

Oral Therapy. Aminoglycosides are not absorbed from the GI tract, and hence oral therapy is used only for local effects within the intestine. In patients anticipating elective colorectal surgery, oral aminoglycosides have been given prophylactically to suppress bacterial growth in the bowel. One aminoglycoside—paromomycin—is used to treat intestinal amebiasis and tapeworm infestation.

Topical Therapy. *Neomycin* is available in formulations for application to the eyes, ears, and skin. Topical preparations of *gentamicin* and *tobramycin* are used to treat conjunctivitis caused by susceptible gram-negative bacilli. Until recently, *gentamicin* was also available in a formulation for application to the skin. However, this product has been withdrawn.

Pharmacokinetics

All of the aminoglycosides have similar pharmacokinetic profiles. Pharmacokinetic properties of the principal aminoglycosides are summarized in Table 83–1.

Absorption. Because they are polycations, the aminoglycosides cross membranes poorly. As a result, very little (about 1%) of an oral dose is absorbed. Hence, for treatment of systemic infections, aminoglycosides must be given parenterally

(IM or IV). Absorption following application to the intact skin is minimal. However, when used for wound irrigation, aminoglycosides may be absorbed in amounts sufficient to produce systemic toxicity.

Distribution. Distribution of aminoglycosides is limited largely to extracellular fluid. Entry into the cerebrospinal fluid is insufficient to treat meningitis in adults. Aminoglycosides bind tightly to renal tissue, achieving levels in the kidney up to 50 times higher than levels in serum. These high levels are responsible for nephrotoxicity (see below). Aminoglycosides penetrate readily to the perilymph and endolymph of the inner ear, and can thereby cause ototoxicity (see below). Aminoglycosides can cross the placenta and may have toxic effects on the fetus.

Elimination. The aminoglycosides are eliminated primarily by the kidney. These drugs are not metabolized. In patients with normal renal function, the half-lives of the aminoglycosides range from 2 to 3 hours. However, because elimination is almost exclusively renal, half-lives increase dramatically in patients with renal impairment (see Table 83–1). *Accordingly, to avoid serious toxicity, we must reduce dosage size or increase the dosing interval in patients with kidney disease.*

Interpatient Variation. Different patients receiving the same aminoglycoside dosage (in milligrams per kilogram of body weight) can achieve widely different serum levels of drug. This interpatient variation is caused by several factors, including age, percent body fat, and pathophysiology (e.g.,

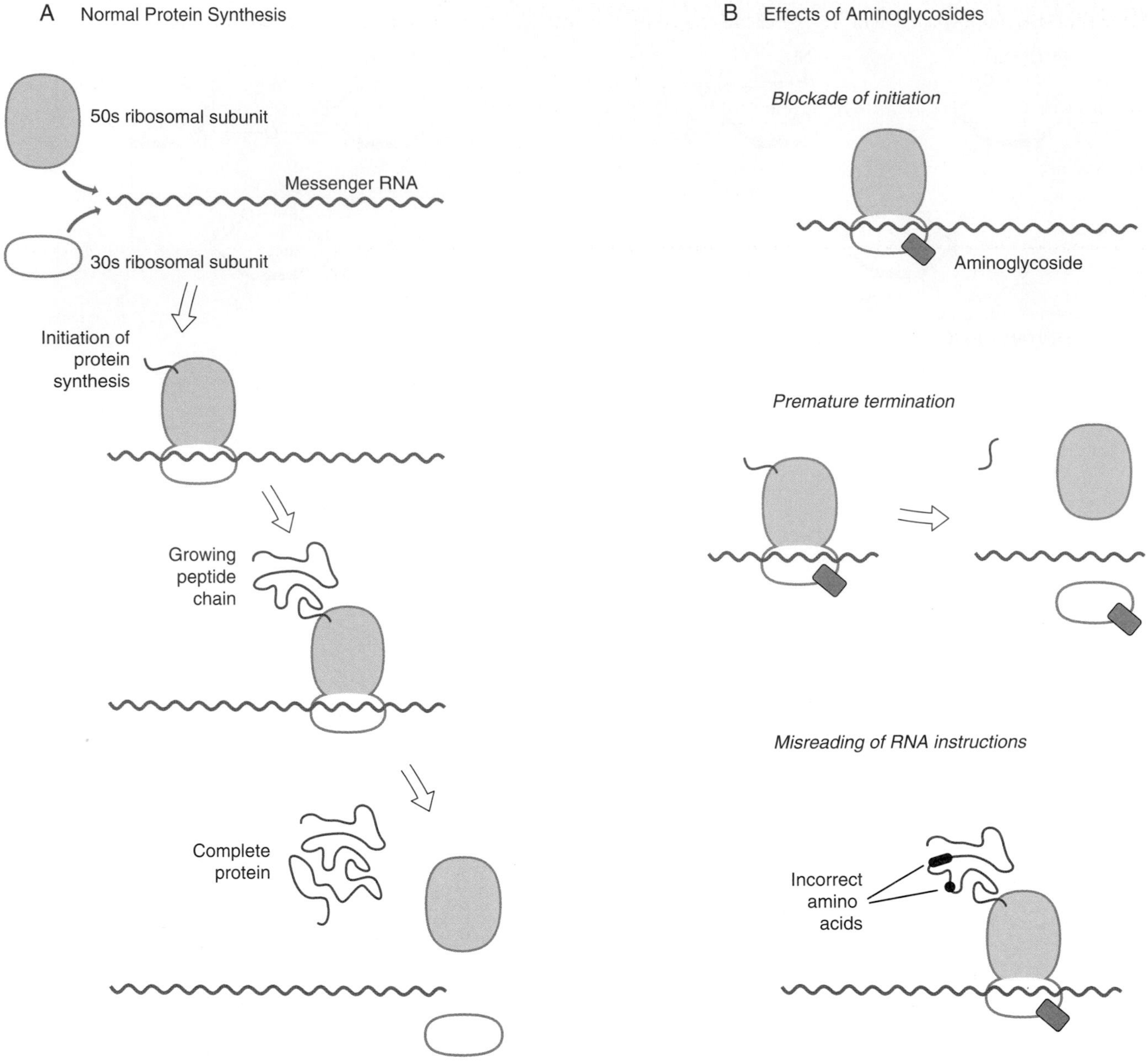

A Normal Protein Synthesis

B Effects of Aminoglycosides

Figure 83–2 ■ Mechanism of action of aminoglycosides.
A, Protein synthesis begins with binding of the 50S and 30S ribosomal subunits to messenger RNA (mRNA), followed by attachment of the first amino acid of the new protein to the 50S subunit. As the ribosome moves down the mRNA strand, additional amino acids are added to the growing peptide chain. When the new protein is complete, it separates from the ribosome and the ribosomal subunits separate from the mRNA. *B,* Aminoglycosides bind to the 30S ribosomal subunit and can thereby (1) block initiation, (2) terminate synthesis before the new protein is complete, and (3) cause misreading of the genetic code, which causes synthesis of faulty proteins.

kidney dysfunction, fever, edema, dehydration). Because of variability among patients, aminoglycoside dosage must be individualized. As dramatic evidence of this need, in one clinical study it was observed that, in order to produce equivalent serum drug levels, the doses required ranged from as little as 0.5 mg/kg in one patient to a high of 25.8 mg/kg in another—a difference of more than 50-fold.

Adverse Effects

The aminoglycosides can produce serious toxicity, especially to the inner ear and kidney. The inner ear and kidney are vulnerable because aminoglycosides become concentrated within cells of these structures.

Ototoxicity. All aminoglycosides can accumulate within the inner ear, causing cellular injury that can impair both

TABLE 83–1 ■ Dosages and Pharmacokinetics of Systemic Aminoglycosides

Generic Name	Trade Name	Total Daily Dosage (mg/kg)[a,b]		Half-Life in Adults (hr)		Therapeutic (Peak) Level[c,d] (μg/ml)	Safe Trough Level[e,f] (μg/ml)
		Adults	Children	Normal	Anuric		
Amikacin	Amikin	15	15	2–3	24–60	15–30	<5–10
Gentamicin	Garamycin	3–5	6–7.5	2	24–60	4–10	<1–2
Tobramycin	Nebcin	3–5	6–7.5	2–2.5	24–60	4–10	<1–2
Netilmicin	Netromycin	4–6.5	5.5–8	2–2.7	40	4–10	<1–2

[a]The total daily dose may be administered as one large dose each day, or as two or three divided doses given at equally spaced intervals around the clock.

[b]Because of interpatient variability, standard doses cannot be relied upon to produce appropriate serum drug levels, and hence dosage should be adjusted on the basis of serum drug measurements.

[c]Measured 30 minutes after IM injection or a 30-minute IV infusion.

[d]The peak values presented refer to levels obtained when the total daily dosage is given in *divided* doses, rather than as a single large daily dose.

[e]Measured just prior to the next dose.

[f]To minimize ototoxicity, drug levels should drop *below* the listed values between doses.

hearing and balance. Impairment of *hearing* is caused by damage to sensory hair cells in the *cochlea; disruption of balance* is caused by damage to sensory hair cells of the *vestibular apparatus.*

The risk of ototoxicity is related primarily to excessive *trough levels** of drug—rather than to excessive *peak* levels. Why? Because, when trough levels remain persistently elevated, aminoglycosides are unable to diffuse out of inner ear cells, and hence the cells are exposed to the drug continuously for an extended time. It is this prolonged exposure, rather than brief exposure to high levels, that underlies cellular injury. In addition to high trough levels, the risk of ototoxicity is increased by (1) renal impairment (which can cause accumulation of aminoglycosides), (2) concurrent use of ethacrynic acid (a drug that has ototoxic properties of its own), and (3) administration of aminoglycosides in excessive doses or for more than 10 days.

Patients should be monitored for ototoxicity. The first sign of impending *cochlear* damage is high-pitched tinnitus (ringing in the ears). As injury to cochlear hair cells proceeds, hearing in the high-frequency range begins to decline. Loss of low-frequency hearing develops with continued drug use. Since the initial decline in high-frequency hearing is subtle, audiometric testing is needed to detect it. The first sign of impending *vestibular* damage is headache, which may last for 1 or 2 days. After that, nausea, unsteadiness, dizziness, and vertigo begin to appear. Patients should be informed about the symptoms of vestibular and cochlear damage and instructed to report them.

Ototoxicity is largely irreversible. Accordingly, if permanent injury is to be avoided, aminoglycosides should be withdrawn at the first sign of damage (i.e., tinnitus, persistent headache, or both).

The risk of ototoxicity can be minimized in several ways. Dosages should be adjusted so that trough serum drug levels do not exceed recommended values. (Aminoglycosides diffuse out of the endolymph and perilymph during the trough time, thereby decreasing exposure of sensory hair cells to these drugs.) Special care should be taken to ensure safe trough levels in patients with kidney dysfunction. When possible, amino-

glycosides should be used for no more than 10 days. Concurrent use of ethacrynic acid should be avoided.

Nephrotoxicity. Aminoglycosides can injure cells of the proximal renal tubules. These drugs are taken up by tubular cells and achieve high intracellular concentrations. The risk of injury is related primarily to the total cumulative dose, and partly to excessive trough levels. Aminoglycoside-induced nephrotoxicity usually manifests as *acute* tubular necrosis. Prominent symptoms are proteinuria, casts in the urine, production of dilute urine, and elevations in serum creatinine and blood urea nitrogen (BUN). Serum creatinine and BUN should be monitored. The risk of nephrotoxicity is especially high in the elderly, in patients with pre-existing kidney disease, and in patients receiving other nephrotoxic drugs (e.g., amphotericin B, cephalothin). Fortunately, cells of the proximal tubule readily regenerate. As a result, injury to the kidney reverses following cessation of aminoglycoside use. The most significant consequence of renal damage is accumulation of aminoglycosides themselves, which can lead to ototoxicity.

Nephrotoxicity correlates with the *total cumulative dose* of aminoglycosides. High *peak levels* do *not* seem to increase toxicity.

Neuromuscular Blockade. Aminoglycosides can inhibit neuromuscular transmission, causing flaccid paralysis and potentially fatal depression of respiration. Most episodes of neuromuscular blockade have occurred following intraperitoneal or intrapleural instillation of aminoglycosides. However, neuromuscular blockade has also occurred following IV, IM, and oral administration. The risk of paralysis is increased by concurrent use of neuromuscular blocking agents and general anesthetics. Myasthenia gravis is an additional risk. Neuromuscular blockade can be reversed with calcium; IV infusion of a calcium salt (e.g., calcium gluconate) is the treatment of choice. Because of increased physician awareness, aminoglycoside-induced neuromuscular blockade is now rare.

Other Adverse Effects. Hypersensitivity reactions (e.g., rash, pruritus, urticaria) occur occasionally. Blood dyscrasias (neutropenia, agranulocytosis, aplastic anemia) are rare. *Streptomycin* has been associated with neurologic disorders (optic nerve dysfunction, peripheral neuritis, paresthesias of the face and hands). Oral neomycin has caused suprainfection of the bowel and intestinal malabsorption. Topical neomycin can cause contact dermatitis.

Drug Interactions

Penicillins. Penicillins and aminoglycosides are frequently employed in combination to enhance bacterial kill. The combination is effective because penicillins disrupt the cell wall,

---

*The trough serum level is defined as the lowest level between doses, and occurs just prior to administering the next dose.

and thereby facilitate access of aminoglycosides to their site of action. Unfortunately, when present in high concentrations, penicillins can inactivate aminoglycosides by direct chemical interaction. Therefore, *penicillins and aminoglycosides should not be mixed together in the same IV solution.* (Inactivation is not likely to occur once the drugs are in the body, because drug concentrations are usually too low for significant chemical interaction.)

Ototoxic Drugs. The risk of injury to the inner ear is significantly increased by concurrent use of *ethacrynic acid,* a loop diuretic that has ototoxic actions of its own. The combination of aminoglycosides with two other loop diuretics—furosemide and bumetanide—appears to cause no more ototoxicity than aminoglycosides alone.

Nephrotoxic Drugs. The risk of renal damage is increased by concurrent therapy with other nephrotoxic agents. Additive or potentiative nephrotoxicity has been observed with *amphotericin B, cephalosporins, polymyxins,* and *vancomycin.*

Skeletal Muscle Relaxants. Aminoglycosides can intensify neuromuscular blockade induced by tubocurarine, pancuronium, and other skeletal muscle relaxants. If aminoglycosides are used with these agents, caution must be exercised to avoid respiratory arrest.

Dosing Schedules

Systemic aminoglycosides may be administered in the form of one large dose each day, or as two or three divided doses. Traditionally, these drugs have been administered in divided doses, given at equally spaced intervals around the clock (e.g., every 8 hours). Today, however, it is common practice to administer the total daily dose all at once, rather than dividing it up. Multiple studies have shown that once-daily doses are just as effective as divided doses, and are at least as safe, if not safer. Because once-daily dosing is both safe and effective, and because it's easier and cheaper than giving divided doses, once-daily dosing has become the preferred dosing schedule. Keep in mind, however, that this schedule is not appropriate for some patients, including neonates and women who are pregnant.

How can it be that giving one large daily dose is just as safe and effective as giving divided doses? The answer lies in the hypothetical data plotted in Figure 83–3. As indicated, when we give one large dose (15 mg) once a day, we achieve a very high peak plasma level—much higher than when we give the same daily total in the form of 3 smaller doses (5 mg) every 8 hours. Because of this high peak concentration, and because aminoglycosides exhibit a postantibiotic effect (see *Mechanism of Action* above), bacterial kill using a single daily dose is just as great as when we use divided doses—even though, with once-daily dosing, plasma drug levels are subtherapeutic for a prolonged time between doses. This prolonged period of low drug levels also explains why once-daily dosing is very safe: Because levels are low for a long time, aminoglycosides are able to wash out from vulnerable cells, thereby reducing injury. In contrast, when we use divided doses, the time during which drug levels are low enough to permit washout is quite short, and hence the risk of toxicity is high.

Monitoring Serum Drug Levels

Monitoring serum drug levels provides the best basis for adjusting aminoglycoside dosage. To produce bacterial kill, peak levels must be sufficiently high. To minimize ototoxicity, trough levels must be sufficiently low. (Recall that, when trough levels remain too high, aminoglycosides can't diffuse out of inner ear cells, and hence injury results.) Therapeutic levels and trough levels for the major systemic aminoglycosides are listed in Table 83–1.

How monitoring is done depends on the dosing schedule employed (i.e., once-daily dosing or use of divided doses). When once-daily dosing is employed, we only need to measure trough levels. As a rule, there is no need to measure peak levels. Why? Because, when the entire daily dose is given at once, high peak levels are guaranteed. (They're typically 3 to 4 times those achieved with divided doses.) In contrast, when divided doses are employed, we need to measure both the peak and the trough.

When drawing blood samples for aminoglycoside levels, timing is important. Samples for *peak* levels should be taken 30 minutes after giving an IM injection or after completing a 30-minute IV infusion. Sampling for *trough* levels depends on the dosing schedule employed. For patients receiving *divided doses,* trough samples should be taken just prior to the next dose. For patients receiving *once-daily doses,* two samples are usually drawn (e.g., 2 and 12 hours after dosing). The trough level is then determined by extrapolation from these values.

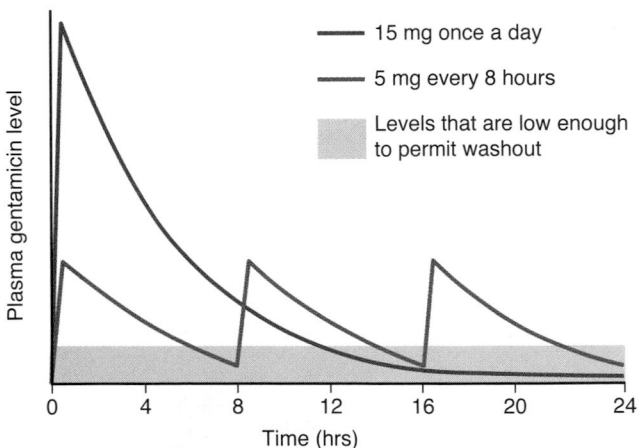

Figure 83–3 ■ **Plasma gentamicin levels produced with once-daily doses versus divided doses.**
The curves depict plasma levels of gentamicin produced with (1) a single large dose administered once a day versus (2) the same daily total given as three smaller doses spaced 8 hours apart. Plasma levels with both regimens are high enough to produce good bactericidal effects. The *shaded area* indicates levels that are low enough to permit washout of the drug from vulnerable cells in the inner ear. Note that, with once-daily dosing, levels are in the washout range for over 12 hours, versus only 6 hours when divided doses are used. As a result, ototoxicity is lower with the once-a-day schedule.

PROPERTIES OF INDIVIDUAL AMINOGLYCOSIDES

Gentamicin

Therapeutic Use. Gentamicin [Garamycin] is used to treat serious infections caused by aerobic gram-negative bacilli. Primary targets are *Pseudomonas aeruginosa* and the

Enterobacteriaceae (e.g., *E. coli, Klebsiella, Serratia, Proteus mirabilis*). In hospitals where resistance is not a problem, gentamicin is often the preferred aminoglycoside for use against these bacteria. The principal advantage of gentamicin over the other major aminoglycosides (tobramycin and amikacin) is low cost. Unfortunately, resistance to gentamicin is increasing, and cross-resistance to tobramycin is common. For infections that are resistant to gentamicin and tobramycin, amikacin is usually effective. In addition to its use against gram-negative bacilli, gentamicin can be combined with ampicillin or penicillin to treat enterococcal endocarditis.

Adverse Effects and Interactions. Like all other aminoglycosides, gentamicin is toxic to the kidney and inner ear. Caution must be exercised when combining gentamicin with other nephrotoxic or ototoxic drugs. Gentamicin is inactivated by penicillins and should not be mixed with these drugs in the same IV solution.

Preparations, Dosage, and Administration. *Intravenous and Intramuscular.* Gentamicin sulfate [Garamycin] is dispensed in solution (10 and 40 mg/ml) for IM and IV administration. The dosage for both routes is the same. For adults, the traditional dosing scheme consists of a loading dose (2 mg/kg) followed by doses of 1 to 1.7 mg/kg every 8 hours—for a total of 3 to 5.1 mg/kg/day. When once-daily dosing is employed, the loading dose is followed by doses of 5.1 mg/kg every 24 hours. For children, the traditional maintenance dosage is 2 to 2.5 mg/kg every 8 hours. In patients with renal impairment, the total daily dosage should be reduced. Duration of treatment is usually 7 to 10 days.

Because of substantial interpatient variation, it is desirable to monitor serum drug levels and to adjust dosage accordingly. Peak levels should range between 4 and 10 μg/ml (for traditional dosing) or between 16 and 24 μg/ml (for once-daily dosing). The trough should not exceed 2 μg/ml.

For IV administration, gentamicin should be diluted in either Sodium Chloride for Injection or 5% dextrose and infused over 30 minutes or longer. The drug should not be mixed with penicillins in the same IV solution.

Intrathecal. Intrathecal therapy is done with a 2-mg/ml solution devoid of preservatives. The usual dosage for children under 3 months old is 1 to 2 mg once daily. The usual dosage for adults is 4 to 8 mg once daily. For all patients, treatment should continue for 1 day after samples of cerebrospinal fluid become negative for the infecting organism.

Tobramycin

Uses, Adverse Effects, and Interactions. Tobramycin [Nebcin, TOBI] is similar to gentamicin regarding uses, adverse effects, and interactions. The drug is more active than gentamicin against *Pseudomonas aeruginosa*, but less active against enterococci and *Serratia*. Inhaled tobramycin is used for patients with cystic fibrosis (see Chapter 103). Like all other aminoglycosides, tobramycin can injure the inner ear and kidney. If possible, concurrent therapy with other ototoxic or nephrotoxic drugs should be avoided.

Preparations, Dosage, and Administration. *Intravenous and Intramuscular.* Tobramycin sulfate [Nebcin] is dispensed in solution (10 and 40 mg/ml) and as a powder (30 mg/ml after reconstitution) for IM and IV administration. Dosages and serum levels are the same as those given for gentamicin. Ideally, dosages should be individualized to produce peak and trough levels within the ranges indicated in Table 83–1. In patients with renal impairment, the total daily dosage should be reduced. For IV administration, the drug should be diluted in either 0.9% Sodium Chloride for Injection or 5% dextrose and infused over 30 minutes or more. Tobramycin should not be mixed with penicillins in the same IV solution. Duration of treatment is usually 7 to 10 days.

Nebulization. For patients with *cystic fibrosis*, tobramycin [TOBI] is available in solution (300 mg/5 ml) for use in a nebulizer. The dosage is 300 mg twice daily administered in a repeating cycle consisting of 28 days of drug use followed by 28 days off. Cystic fibrosis is discussed in Chapter 103.

Amikacin

Uses, Adverse Effects, and Interactions. Amikacin [Amikin] has two outstanding features: (1) of all the aminoglycosides, amikacin has the broadest spectrum of action against gram-negative bacilli; and (2) of all the aminoglycosides, amikacin is the least vulnerable to inactivation by bacterial enzymes. Because most aminoglycoside-inactivating enzymes do not affect amikacin, the incidence of bacterial resistance to this agent is lower than with other aminoglycosides. As a result, amikacin is often effective against bacteria that are resistant to the other major aminoglycosides (gentamicin and tobramycin). In hospitals where resistance to gentamicin and tobramycin is common, amikacin is the preferred agent for initial treatment of infections caused by aerobic gram-negative bacilli. However, in settings where resistance to the other aminoglycosides is infrequent, amikacin should be reserved for infections of proven aminoglycoside resistance. Why? Because this practice will delay emergence of organisms resistant to amikacin. Like all other aminoglycosides, amikacin is toxic to the kidney and inner ear. Caution should be exercised if amikacin is used in combination with other ototoxic or nephrotoxic drugs.

Preparations, Dosage, and Administration. Amikacin sulfate [Amikin] is available in solution (50 and 250 mg/ml) for parenteral IM and IV administration. For IV use, amikacin should be diluted in sodium chloride or 5% dextrose for injection; infusion time should be 30 to 60 minutes in adults and 1 to 2 hours in infants. The recommended dosage for adults and children is 15 mg/kg/day administered either (a) as a single daily dose or (b) in equally divided doses at 8- or 12-hour intervals. In patients with renal impairment, dosage should be reduced or the dosing interval increased. Dosage adjustments should be based on measurements of serum drug levels. As a rule, duration of treatment should not exceed 10 days.

Other Aminoglycosides
Netilmicin

Netilmicin [Netromycin] has an antibacterial spectrum similar to that of gentamicin. Netilmicin has some resistance to the bacterial enzymes that inactivate gentamicin and tobramycin. However, netilmicin is more vulnerable to inactivation than amikacin. Like other aminoglycosides, netilmicin is ototoxic and nephrotoxic, although ototoxicity may be less than with other aminoglycosides. Administration is IM or IV. The recommended dosage for adults is 1.3 to 2.2 mg/kg every 8 hours. The dosage for children is 1.8 to 2.7 mg/kg every 8 hours. Duration of treatment ranges from 7 to 14 days.

Neomycin

Neomycin is more ototoxic and nephrotoxic than any other aminoglycoside. Because of this toxicity, neomycin is not used parenterally. Instead, the drug is employed for topical treatment of infections of the eye, ear, and skin. The drug is also administered orally to suppress bowel flora prior to surgery of the intestine. Because aminoglycosides are not absorbed from the GI tract, oral administration constitutes a local (nonsystemic) use of the drug. Oral neomycin can cause suprainfection of the bowel as well as an intestinal malabsorption syndrome.

Kanamycin

Kanamycin [Kantrex] is an older aminoglycoside to which bacterial resistance is common. The drug is still active against some gram-negative bacilli, but *Serratia* and *Pseudomonas aeruginosa* are resistant. Because of resistance, systemic use of the drug has sharply declined; gentamicin, tobramycin, and amikacin are preferred. Like neomycin, kanamycin is employed to suppress bacterial flora of the bowel prior to elective colorectal surgery. Kanamycin is dispensed in capsules for oral use and in solution for IM and IV use.

Streptomycin

Streptomycin, discovered in 1943, was the first aminoglycoside drug. Although once employed widely, streptomycin has been largely replaced by safer or more effective medications. As discussed in Chapter 86, streptomycin can be used in combination with other drugs to treat tuberculosis, but newer and safer agents (rifampin, isoniazid, ethambutol) are generally preferred. Streptomycin is also indicated for several uncommon infections (plague, tularemia, glanders, brucellosis). When combined with ampicillin or penicillin G, streptomycin may be used for enterococcal endocarditis.

Paromomycin

Paromomycin [Humatin] is an aminoglycoside employed only for local effects within the intestine. The drug is administered orally to treat intestinal amebiasis and tapeworm infestations. The dosage for both indications is 8 to 12 mg/kg 3 times daily for 5 to 10 days. Principal adverse effects are nausea, cramps, and diarrhea. Paromomycin is dispensed in 250-mg capsules.

KEY POINTS

- Aminoglycosides are narrow-spectrum antibiotics, used primarily against aerobic gram-negative bacilli.
- Aminoglycosides disrupt protein synthesis and cause rapid bacterial death.
- Aminoglycosides are highly polar polycations. As a result, they are not absorbed from the GI tract, do not cross the blood-brain barrier, and are excreted rapidly by the kidney.
- Aminoglycosides can cause irreversible injury to sensory cells of the inner ear, resulting in hearing loss and disturbance of balance.
- The risk of ototoxicity is related primarily to persistently elevated trough drug levels, rather than to excessive peak levels.
- Aminoglycosides are nephrotoxic, but renal injury is usually reversible.
- The risk of nephrotoxicity is related primarily to the total cumulative dose, and only partly to elevated trough levels.
- Because the same aminoglycoside dose can produce very different plasma levels in different patients, monitoring of serum levels is common. *Peak* levels must be high enough to cause bacterial kill; *trough* levels must be low enough to minimize toxicity.

Summary of Major Nursing Implications*

AMINOGLYCOSIDES

Amikacin
Gentamicin
Kanamycin
Neomycin
Netilmicin
Paromomycin
Tobramycin

Except where noted, the implications summarized below apply to all aminoglycosides.

Preadministration Assessment

Therapeutic Goal

Parenteral Therapy. Treatment of serious infections caused by gram-negative aerobic bacilli.

Oral Therapy. Suppression of bowel flora prior to elective colorectal surgery.

Topical Therapy. Treatment of local infections of the eyes, ears, and skin.

Identifying High-Risk Patients

Aminoglycosides must be used with *caution* in patients with renal impairment, pre-existing hearing impairment, and myasthenia gravis, and in patients receiving ototoxic drugs (especially ethacrynic acid), nephrotoxic drugs (e.g., amphotericin B, cephalosporins, vancomycin), and neuromuscular blocking agents.

Implementation: Administration

Routes

Intramuscular and Intravenous. Gentamicin, tobramycin, amikacin, netilmicin, kanamycin.

Oral. Neomycin, kanamycin, paromomycin.
Topical. Neomycin, gentamicin, tobramycin.

Administration

Aminoglycosides must be given parenterally (IV, IM) to treat systemic infections. Intravenous infusions should be done slowly (over 30 minutes or more). Do not mix aminoglycosides and penicillins in the same IV solution.

When possible, adjust the dosage on the basis of plasma drug levels. Draw blood samples for measurement of peak levels 1 hour after IM injection and 30 minutes after completion of an IV infusion. Draw samples for trough levels just prior to the next dose.

In patients with renal dysfunction, the dosage should be reduced or the dosing interval increased.

Dosing Schedule

Aminoglycosides may be given as one large dose each day, or in 2 or 3 divided doses administered at equally spaced intervals around the clock.

Ongoing Evaluation and Interventions

Monitoring Summary

Monitor aminoglycoside levels (peaks and troughs), inner ear function (hearing and balance), creatinine clearance, BUN, and urine output.

Minimizing Adverse Effects

Ototoxicity. Aminoglycosides can damage the inner ear, causing irreversible impairment of hearing and balance. Monitor for ototoxicity; use audiometry in high-risk patients. **Instruct patients to report symptoms of ototoxicity**

*Patient education information is highlighted as blue text.

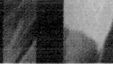

Summary of Major Nursing Implications*—cont'd

(tinnitus, high-frequency hearing loss, persistent headache, nausea, unsteadiness, dizziness, vertigo). If ototoxicity is detected, aminoglycosides should be withdrawn.

Nephrotoxicity. Aminoglycosides can cause reversible acute tubular necrosis. To evaluate renal injury, monitor serum creatinine and BUN. If oliguria or anuria develops, withhold the aminoglycoside and notify the physician.

Neuromuscular Blockade. Aminoglycosides can inhibit neuromuscular transmission, causing potentially fatal respiratory depression. Carefully observe patients with myasthenia gravis and patients receiving skeletal muscle relaxants or general anesthetics. Aminoglycoside-induced neuromuscular blockade can be reversed with IV calcium gluconate.

Minimizing Adverse Interactions

Penicillins. Aminoglycosides can be inactivated by high concentrations of penicillins. Never mix penicillins and aminoglycosides in the same IV solution.

Ototoxic and Nephrotoxic Drugs. Exercise caution when using aminoglycosides in combination with other nephrotoxic or ototoxic drugs. Increased nephrotoxicity has been observed with *amphotericin B, cephalosporins, polymyxins,* and *vancomycin.* The risk of ototoxicity is increased by *ethacrynic acid.*

Skeletal Muscle Relaxants. Aminoglycosides can intensify neuromuscular blockade induced by tubocurarine, pancuronium, and other skeletal muscle relaxants. When aminoglycosides are used concurrently with these agents, exercise caution to avoid respiratory arrest.

*Patient education information is highlighted as blue text.

Sulfonamides and Trimethoprim

The sulfonamides and trimethoprim are broad-spectrum antimicrobial drugs that have closely related mechanisms of action: They all disrupt the synthesis of tetrahydrofolic acid. In approaching these drugs, we begin with the sulfonamides, followed by trimethoprim, and then conclude with trimethoprim-sulfamethoxazole, an important fixed-dose combination product.

SULFONAMIDES

The sulfonamides were the first drugs available for systemic treatment of bacterial infections. The introduction and subsequent widespread use of these drugs produced a sharp decline in morbidity and mortality from susceptible infections. Until the penicillins became generally available, sulfonamides remained the mainstay of antibacterial chemotherapy. With the advent of newer antimicrobial drugs, use of sulfonamides has greatly declined. However, the sulfonamides still have an important therapeutic role, primarily in the treatment of urinary tract infections. With the introduction of trimethoprim-sulfamethoxazole in the 1970s, indications for the sulfonamides have expanded.

Basic Pharmacology

Similarities among the sulfonamides are more striking than the differences. Accordingly, rather than focusing on a representative prototype, we will discuss the sulfonamides as a group.

Chemistry

The general structural formula for the sulfonamides is shown in Figure 84–1. As you can see, sulfonamides are structural analogs of *para-aminobenzoic acid* (PABA). The antimicrobial actions of sulfonamides are based on this structural similarity.

Individual sulfonamides vary greatly with respect to solubility in water. Older sulfonamides had low solubility; as a result, these agents often crystallized out in the urine, causing

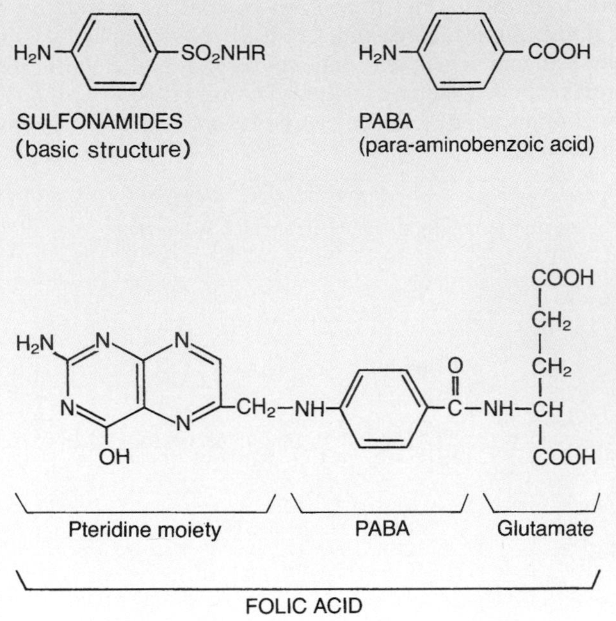

Figure 84–1 ■ **Structural relationships among sulfonamides, PABA, and folic acid.**

injury to the kidneys. The sulfonamides in current use have relatively high water solubility, and hence the risk of renal damage is low.

Mechanism of Action

Sulfonamides suppress bacterial growth by inhibiting synthesis of *folic acid* (folate), a compound required by all cells for biosynthesis of DNA, RNA, and proteins. The steps in folate synthesis are shown in Figure 84–2. As indicated, sulfonamides block the step in which PABA is combined with pteridine to form dihydropteroic acid. Because of their structural similarity to PABA, sulfonamides act as competitive inhibitors of this reaction. Sulfonamides are usually bacteriostatic. Hence, host defenses are essential for complete elimination of an infection.

If all cells require folate, why don't sulfonamides harm humans? To answer this question, we need to understand how bacteria and mammalian cells acquire folic acid. Bacteria are unable to take up folate from their environment, and hence must synthesize folic acid from precursors. It is this process that sulfonamides disrupt. In contrast to bacteria, mammalian cells do not manufacture their own folate. Rather, they simply take up folic acid obtained from the diet, using a specialized

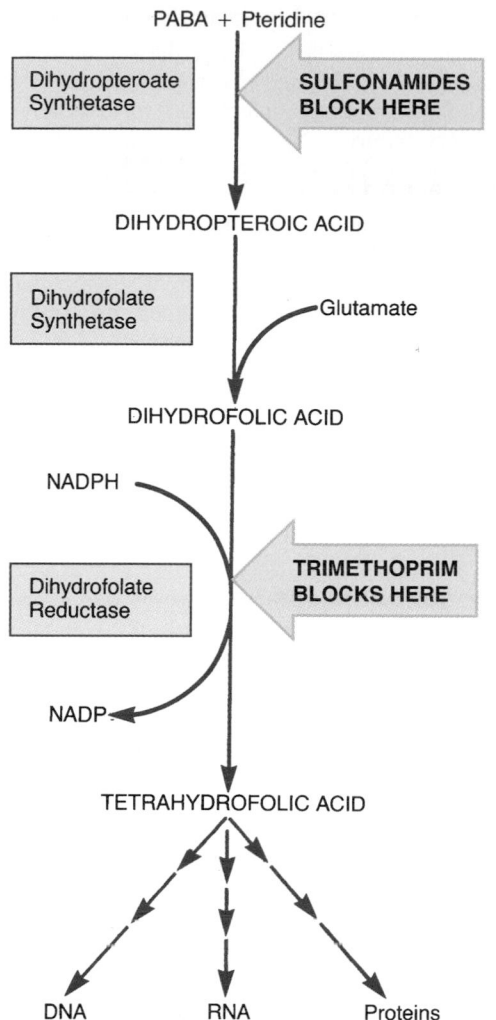

Figure 84–2 ▪ Sites of action of sulfonamides and trimethoprim.
Sulfonamides and trimethoprim inhibit sequential steps in the synthesis of tetrahydrofolic acid (FAH₄). In the absence of FAH₄, bacteria are unable to synthesize DNA, RNA, and proteins.

transport system for uptake. Because mammalian cells use preformed folic acid rather than synthesizing it, sulfonamides are harmless to us.

Microbial Resistance

Many bacterial species have developed resistance to sulfonamides, thereby decreasing the utility of these drugs. Resistance is especially high among gonococci, meningococci, staphylococci, streptococci, and shigellae. Resistance may be acquired by spontaneous mutation or by transfer of R factors. Principal mechanisms of resistance are (1) synthesis of PABA in amounts sufficient to overcome sulfonamide-mediated inhibition of dihydropteroate synthetase, (2) alteration in the structure of dihydropteroate synthetase such that binding and inhibition by sulfonamides is reduced, and (3) reduced sulfonamide uptake.

Antimicrobial Spectrum

The sulfonamides are active against a broad spectrum of microbes. Susceptible organisms include gram-positive cocci, gram-negative bacilli, actinomycetes (e.g., *Nocardia*), chlamydiae (e.g., *Chlamydia trachomatis*), and some protozoa (e.g., *Toxoplasma,* plasmodia).

Therapeutic Uses

Although the sulfonamides were once employed widely, their applications are now limited. Sulfonamide use has declined for two reasons: (1) introduction of bactericidal antibiotics that have less toxicity than do the sulfonamides, and (2) development of bacterial resistance to sulfonamides. Today, urinary tract infection is the principal indication for sulfonamides.

Urinary Tract Infections. Sulfonamides are often preferred drugs for acute infections of the urinary tract. About 90% of these infections are due to *Escherichia coli,* a bacterium that is usually sulfonamide sensitive. Of the sulfonamides available, *sulfisoxazole* is generally favored. This drug has high solubility in urine, achieves effective concentrations within the urinary tract, and is less expensive than other sulfonamides. When infection is recurrent, or when urinary tract obstruction is present, treatment with a sulfonamide alone may not be sufficient. Treatment of urinary tract infections is discussed further in Chapter 85.

Other Uses. Sulfonamides are useful drugs for nocardiosis (infection with *Nocardia asteroides*). In addition, sulfonamides are alternatives to doxycycline and erythromycin for infections caused by *C. trachomatis* (trachoma, inclusion conjunctivitis, urethritis, lymphogranuloma venereum). Sulfonamides are used in conjunction with pyrimethamine to treat two protozoal infections: toxoplasmosis and malaria caused by chloroquine-resistant *Plasmodium falciparum*. Topical sulfonamides are used to treat superficial infections of the eye and to prevent bacterial colonization in burn patients.

One sulfonamide preparation—sulfasalazine—is used to treat *ulcerative colitis*. However, benefits in this disorder do not result from suppression of microbial growth. Treatment of ulcerative colitis is considered in Chapter 75.

Pharmacokinetics

Absorption. Sulfonamides are well absorbed following oral administration. When applied topically to the skin or mucous membranes, sulfonamides may be absorbed in amounts sufficient to cause systemic effects.

Distribution. Sulfonamides are well distributed to all tissues. Concentrations in pleural, peritoneal, ocular, and similar body fluids may be as much as 80% of the concentration in blood. Sulfonamides readily cross the placenta, and levels achieved in the fetus are sufficient to produce both antimicrobial effects and toxicity.

Metabolism. Sulfonamides are metabolized in the liver; the principal reaction is acetylation. Acetylated derivatives of sulfonamides lack antimicrobial activity, but are just as toxic as the parent compounds. Acetylation may decrease sulfonamide solubility, thereby increasing the risk of renal damage from crystal formation.

Excretion. Sulfonamides are excreted primarily by the kidneys. Hence, the rate of renal excretion is the principal determinant of sulfonamide half-life.

Adverse Effects

Sulfonamides can cause multiple adverse effects. Prominent among these are hypersensitivity reactions, blood dyscrasias, and kernicterus, which occurs in newborn infants. Renal damage from crystalluria was a problem with older sulfonamides but is of minimal concern with the drugs available today.

Hypersensitivity Reactions. Sulfonamides can induce a variety of hypersensitivity reactions. Mild reactions—rash, drug fever, and photosensitivity—are relatively common. To minimize photosensitivity reactions, patients should avoid prolonged exposure to sunlight, wear protective clothing, and apply a sunscreen to exposed skin.

Hypersensitivity reactions are especially frequent with topical sulfonamides. As a result, these preparations are no longer employed routinely. Rather, they are reserved for ophthalmic infections, burns, and vaginitis caused by *Gardnerella vaginalis* or *Candida albicans*.

The most severe hypersensitivity response to sulfonamides is *Stevens-Johnson syndrome,* a rare reaction that has a mortality rate of about 25%. Symptoms include widespread lesions of the skin and mucous membranes, together with fever, malaise, and toxemia. The reaction is most likely with long-acting sulfonamides, agents that have been banned in the United States. Shorter acting sulfonamides may also induce the syndrome, but the incidence is low. To minimize the risk of severe reactions, sulfonamides should be discontinued immediately if skin rash of any sort is observed. In addition, sulfonamides should not be given to patients with a history of hypersensitivity to the sulfonamides or to chemically related drugs, including thiazide diuretics, loop diuretics, and sulfonylurea-type oral hypoglycemics (e.g., tolbutamide).

Hematologic Effects. Sulfonamides can cause *hemolytic anemia* in patients whose red blood cells have a genetically determined deficiency in glucose-6-phosphate dehydrogenase (G-6-PD). This inherited trait is most common among African Americans and people of Mediterranean origin. Rarely, hemolysis occurs in the absence of G-6-PD deficiency. Red cell lysis can produce fever, pallor, and jaundice; patients should be observed for these signs. In addition to hemolytic anemia, sulfonamides can cause agranulocytosis, leukopenia, thrombocytopenia, and, very rarely, aplastic anemia. When sulfonamides are used for a long time, periodic blood tests should be obtained.

Kernicterus. Kernicterus is a disorder in newborns caused by deposition of bilirubin in the brain. Bilirubin is neurotoxic and can cause severe neurologic deficits and even death. Under normal conditions, infants are not vulnerable to kernicterus because any bilirubin present in their blood is tightly bound to plasma proteins, and therefore is not free to enter the central nervous system (CNS). Sulfonamides promote kernicterus by displacing bilirubin from plasma proteins. Since the blood-brain barrier of infants is poorly developed, the newly freed bilirubin has easy access to sites within the brain. *Because of the risk of kernicterus, sulfonamides should not be administered to infants under the age of 2 months. In addition, sulfonamides should not be given to pregnant women near term or to mothers who are breast-feeding.*

Renal Damage from Crystalluria. Because of their low solubility, older sulfonamides tended to come out of solution in the urine, forming crystalline aggregates in the kidneys, ureters, and bladder. These aggregates caused irritation and obstruction, sometimes resulting in anuria and even death. Renal damage is uncommon with today's sulfonamides (because their solubility is relatively high). To minimize the risk of renal damage, adults should maintain a daily urine output of 1200 ml. This can be accomplished by consuming 8 to 10 glasses of water each day. Since the solubility of sulfonamides is highest at elevated pH, alkalinization of the urine (e.g., with sodium bicarbonate) can further decrease the chances of crystalluria.

Drug Interactions

Sulfonamides can intensify the effects of warfarin, phenytoin, and sulfonylurea-type oral hypoglycemics (e.g., tolbutamide). The principal mechanism is inhibition of hepatic metabolism. When combined with sulfonamides, these drugs may require a reduction in dosage to prevent toxicity.

Sulfonamide Preparations

The sulfonamides fall into two major categories: (1) systemic sulfonamides and (2) sulfonamides used for local effects. The sulfonamides employed for systemic therapy are more widely used.

Systemic Sulfonamides

The systemic sulfonamides can be subdivided based on duration of action. As indicated in Table 84–1, two groups are available in the United States: (1) short-acting agents and (2) intermediate-acting agents. Long-acting sulfonamides produce a high incidence of Stevens-Johnson syndrome and have been withdrawn from the American market. The short-acting sulfonamides are used primarily to treat infections of the urinary tract. Except where noted below, the adverse effects and drug interactions of individual sulfonamides are the same as those discussed above. Dosages and trade names for systemic sulfonamides are summarized in Table 84–1.

Sulfisoxazole. Sulfisoxazole, a short-acting sulfonamide, can be considered the prototype of the sulfonamide family. This drug is the preferred sulfonamide for urinary tract infections. Sulfisoxazole is just as effective as other sulfonamides and less expensive. Moreover, because of its high water solubility, sulfisoxazole poses a minimal risk of crystalluria. Since high plasma concentrations of sulfisoxazole can be achieved, the drug is useful against a variety of systemic infections (e.g., nocardiosis, melioidosis, chancroid). Sulfisoxazole may be administered orally or by injection (IV, SC, IM). Oral administration is preferred.

Sulfamethoxazole. Sulfamethoxazole [Gantanol] is the only intermediate-acting sulfonamide available. Indications for the drug are the same as for sulfisoxazole. Because of its prolonged duration of action, sulfamethoxazole can be administered less frequently than the short-acting sulfonamides.

TABLE 84–1 ▪ Systemic Sulfonamides			
Class*	Generic Name	Trade Name	Usual Adult Oral Maintenance Dosage
Short Acting	Sulfisoxazole	—	1 gm every 4–6 hr
	Sulfadiazine	—	1 gm every 4–6 hr
	Sulfamethizole	Thiosulfil Forte	0.5–1 gm every 6 hr
Intermediate Acting	Sulfamethoxazole	Gantanol	1 gm every 12 hr

*Long-acting sulfonamides (e.g., sulfamethoxypyridazine, sulfameter) are no longer available in the United States.

This drug has lower water solubility than sulfisoxazole, and hence presents a greater risk of injury to the kidneys. The risk of renal damage can be minimized by maintaining adequate hydration. Sulfamethoxazole is employed primarily in fixed-dose combination with trimethoprim. This combination is discussed later in the chapter. Administration is oral.

Sulfadiazine. Sulfadiazine is a short-acting sulfonamide. The drug is less soluble than other short-acting agents. Hence, if renal damage is to be avoided, high urine flow must be maintained. Sulfadiazine crosses the blood-brain barrier with ease, and therefore is the best sulfonamide for prophylaxis of meningitis. When combined with pyrimethamine, sulfadiazine is useful against toxoplasmosis. The drug is dispensed in tablets for oral administration.

Sulfamethizole. Sulfamethizole [Thiosulfil Forte] is a short-acting sulfonamide. The drug is used only for urinary tract infections. Sulfamethizole is dispensed in tablets for oral administration.

Topical Sulfonamides

Topical sulfonamides have been associated with a high incidence of hypersensitivity reactions and are not used routinely. The preparations discussed below have proven utility and a relatively low incidence of hypersensitivity.

Sulfacetamide. Sulfacetamide is widely used for superficial infections of the eye (e.g., conjunctivitis, corneal ulcer). The drug may cause blurred vision, sensitivity to bright light, headache, brow ache, and local irritation. Hypersensitivity is rare, but severe reactions have occurred. Accordingly, sulfacetamide should not be used by patients with a history of hypersensitivity to sulfonamides, sulfonylureas, or thiazide or loop diuretics. Sulfacetamide is available in solution and ointment formulations for local application to the eye. Trade names include Isopto Cetamide and Sodium Sulamyd.

Silver Sulfadiazine and Mafenide. Both of these sulfonamides are employed to prevent bacterial colonization in patients with second- and third-degree burns. Mafenide acts by the same mechanism as other sulfonamides. In contrast, antibacterial effects of silver sulfadiazine are due primarily to release of free silver—and not to the sulfonamide portion of the molecule. Local application of mafenide is frequently painful. In contrast, application of silver sulfadiazine is usually pain free. Following topical application, both agents can be absorbed in amounts sufficient to produce systemic effects. Mafenide, but not silver sulfadiazine, is metabolized to a compound that can suppress renal excretion of acid, thereby causing acidosis. Accordingly, patients receiving mafenide should be monitored for acid-base status. If acidosis becomes severe, mafenide should be discontinued for 1 to 2 days. Mafenide is marketed under the trade name Sulfamylon. Trade names for silver sulfadiazine are Silvadene, Thermazene, and SSD Cream.

TRIMETHOPRIM

Like the sulfonamides, trimethoprim [Proloprim, Trimpex] suppresses production of tetrahydrofolic acid. Trimethoprim is active against a broad spectrum of microbes.

Mechanism of Action

As indicated in Figure 84–2, trimethoprim *inhibits dihydrofolate reductase,* the enzyme that converts dihydrofolic acid to its active form: tetrahydrofolic acid. Hence, like the sulfonamides, trimethoprim suppresses bacterial synthesis of DNA, RNA, and proteins. Depending on conditions at the site of infection, trimethoprim may be bactericidal or bacteriostatic.

Although mammalian cells also contain dihydrofolate reductase, trimethoprim is selectively toxic to bacteria. Why? Because bacterial dihydrofolate reductase differs in structure from mammalian dihydrofolate reductase. As a result, trimethoprim inhibits the bacterial enzyme at concentrations about 40,000 times lower than those required to inhibit the mammalian enzyme. This differential sensitivity allows suppression of bacterial growth with doses that have essentially no effect on the host.

Microbial Resistance

Bacteria acquire resistance to trimethoprim by three mechanisms: (1) synthesis of increased amounts of dihydrofolate reductase, (2) production of an altered dihydrofolate reductase that has a low affinity for trimethoprim, and (3) reduced cellular permeability to trimethoprim. Resistance has resulted from spontaneous mutation and from transfer of R factors. In the United States, bacterial resistance is uncommon.

Antimicrobial Spectrum

Trimethoprim is active against many gram-positive bacilli and some gram-negative bacilli (e.g., *Corynebacterium diphtheriae, Listeria monocytogenes*). Most aerobic gram-negative bacilli of clinical importance are also sensitive, including *E. coli, Klebsiella, Proteus mirabilis, Serratia marcescens, Salmonella, Shigella,* and *Haemophilus influenzae.* In addition, trimethoprim is active against some pathogenic protozoa (e.g., *Pneumocystis carinii, Toxoplasma gondii,* and the protozoa responsible for malaria).

Therapeutic Uses

Trimethoprim is approved only for initial therapy of acute, uncomplicated urinary tract infections due to susceptible organisms (e.g., *E. coli, P. mirabilis, Enterobacter* species, and *Staphylococcus saprophyticus*). When combined with sulfamethoxazole, trimethoprim has considerably more applications; these are discussed later in the chapter.

Pharmacokinetics

Trimethoprim is absorbed rapidly and completely from the GI tract. The drug is quite lipid soluble, and therefore undergoes wide distribution to body fluids and tissues. Trimethoprim readily crosses the placenta. Most of an administered dose is excreted unchanged by the kidneys. Hence, in the presence of renal dysfunction, the half-life of trimethoprim is prolonged. The concentration of trimethoprim achieved in urine is considerably higher than the concurrent concentration in blood.

Adverse Effects

Trimethoprim is generally well tolerated. The most frequent adverse effects are itching and rash. Gastrointestinal reactions (e.g., epigastric distress, nausea, vomiting, glossitis, stomatitis) occur occasionally.

Hematologic Effects. Since mammalian dihydrofolate reductase is relatively insensitive to trimethoprim, toxicities related to suppression of tetrahydrofolate production are rare. These rare effects—*megaloblastic anemia, thrombocytopenia,* and *neutropenia*—occur only in individuals with pre-existing folic acid deficiency. Accordingly, caution should be exercised when administering trimethoprim to patients in whom folate deficiency might be likely (e.g., alcoholics, pregnant women, debilitated patients). If early signs of bone marrow suppression occur (e.g., sore throat, fever, pallor), complete blood counts should be performed. If a significant reduction in blood cell counts is observed, trimethoprim should be discontinued. Administration of folinic acid (leucovorin) will restore normal hematopoiesis.

Use in Pregnancy and Lactation. Large doses of trimethoprim have caused fetal malformations in animals. To date, no developmental abnormalities have been observed in humans. However, since trimethoprim readily crosses the placenta, prudence dictates avoiding routine use of the drug during pregnancy. The risk of exacerbating pregnancy-related folate deficiency is an additional reason not to use the drug at this time.

Trimethoprim is excreted in breast milk and may interfere with folic acid utilization by the nursing infant. The drug should be administered with caution to women who are breast-feeding.

Preparations, Dosage, and Administration

Trimethoprim [Proloprim, Trimpex] is dispensed in 100- and 200-mg tablets for oral use. For urinary tract infections, the usual dosage is 100 mg every 12 hours or 200 mg every 24 hours. Duration of treatment is 10 days. Dosage should be reduced in patients with renal dysfunction.

TRIMETHOPRIM-SULFAMETHOXAZOLE

Trimethoprim (TMP) and sulfamethoxazole (SMZ) are marketed together in a fixed-dose combination product. This combination (TMP-SMZ) is a powerful antimicrobial preparation whose components act in concert to inhibit sequential steps in tetrahydrofolic acid synthesis. Trade names for TMP-SMZ are Bactrim, Cotrim, and Septra. In many countries the combination is known generically as *co-trimoxazole*.

Mechanism of Action

The antimicrobial effects of TMP-SMZ result from inhibiting consecutive steps in the synthesis of tetrahydrofolic acid: SMZ acts first to inhibit incorporation of PABA into folic acid; TMP then inhibits dihydrofolate reductase, the enzyme that converts dihydrofolic acid into tetrahydrofolate (see Fig. 84–2). As a result, the ability of the target organism to produce nucleic acids and proteins is greatly suppressed. By inhibiting two reactions required for synthesis of tetrahydrofolate, TMP and SMZ potentiate each other's effects. That is, the antimicrobial effect of the combination is more powerful than the sum of the effects of TMP alone plus SMZ alone. TMP-SMZ is selectively toxic to microbes because (1) mammalian cells use preformed folic acid, and therefore are not affected by SMZ; and (2) dihydrofolate reductases of mammalian cells are relatively insensitive to inhibition by TMP.

Microbial Resistance

Resistance to the combination of TMP plus SMZ is less than to either drug alone. This is logical in that the chances of an organism acquiring resistance to both drugs are less than its chances of developing resistance to just one or the other. Specific mechanisms of resistance to sulfonamides and TMP are presented earlier in the chapter.

Antimicrobial Spectrum

TMP-SMZ is active against a wide range of gram-positive and gram-negative bacteria. This should be no surprise since TMP and SMZ by themselves are broad-spectrum antimicrobial drugs. Most urinary tract pathogens are susceptible. Specific bacteria against which TMP-SMZ is consistently effective include *E. coli, P. mirabilis, Salmonella typhi, Shigella* species, *Vibrio cholerae, H. influenzae,* and *Yersinia pestis.* TMP-SMZ is also active against *Nocardia* and certain protozoa (*P. carinii* and *Plasmodium* species).

Therapeutic Uses

TMP-SMZ is a preferred or alternative medication for a variety of infectious diseases. The combination is especially valuable for urinary tract infections, otitis media, bronchitis, shigellosis, and pneumonia and other infections caused by *P. carinii.*

Urinary Tract Infection. TMP-SMZ is indicated for chemotherapy of uncomplicated urinary tract infection caused by susceptible strains of *E. coli, Klebsiella, Entero-*

bacter, P. mirabilis, Proteus vulgaris, and *Morganella morganii.* The combination is particularly useful for chronic and recurrent infections.

Pneumocystis carinii Infections. TMP-SMZ is the treatment of choice for pneumonia and other infections caused by *P. carinii,* an opportunistic organism that thrives in immunocompromised hosts (e.g., cancer patients, organ transplant recipients, individuals with AIDS). When given to AIDS patients, TMP-SMZ produces a high incidence of adverse effects.

Gastrointestinal Infections. TMP-SMZ is a drug of choice for infections caused by several gram-negative bacilli, including *Yersinia enterocolitica, Aeromonas,* and *Calymmatobacterium granulomatis.* In addition, the combination is a preferred treatment for shigellosis caused by susceptible strains of *Shigella flexneri* and *S. sonnei.*

Other Infections. TMP-SMZ can be used for otitis media and acute exacerbations of chronic bronchitis when these infections are due to susceptible strains of *H. influenzae* or *Streptococcus pneumoniae.* The preparation is also useful against urethritis and pharyngeal infection caused by penicillinase-producing *Neisseria gonorrhoeae.* Other infections that can be treated with TMP-SMZ include whooping cough, nocardiosis, brucellosis, melioidosis, and chancroid.

Pharmacokinetics

Absorption and Distribution. TMP-SMZ may be administered orally or by IV infusion. Both components of TMP-SMZ are well distributed throughout the body. Therapeutic concentrations are achieved in tissues and body fluids (e.g., vaginal secretions, cerebrospinal fluid, pleural effusions, bile, aqueous humor). Both TMP and SMZ readily cross the placenta, and both enter breast milk.

Plasma Drug Levels. Optimal antibacterial effects are produced when the ratio of TMP to SMZ is 1:20. To achieve this ratio in plasma, TMP and SMZ must be administered in a ratio of 1:5. Hence, standard tablets contain 80 mg of TMP and 400 mg of SMZ. Because the plasma half-lives of TMP and SMZ are similar (10 hours for TMP and 11 hours for SMZ), levels of both drugs decline in parallel, and the 1:20 ratio is maintained as the drugs undergo elimination.

Elimination. Both TMP and SMZ are excreted primarily by the kidneys. About 70% of urinary SMZ is present as inactive metabolites. In contrast, TMP undergoes little hepatic metabolism prior to excretion. Both agents are concentrated in the urine. Hence, levels of active drug are higher in the urine than in plasma, despite some conversion to inactive products.

Adverse Effects

TMP-SMZ is generally well tolerated; toxicity from routine use is rare. The most common adverse effects are nausea, vomiting, and rash. However, although infrequent, all of the serious toxicities associated with sulfonamides can occur with TMP-SMZ. That is, the combination can cause hypersensitivity reactions (including Stevens-Johnson syndrome), blood dyscrasias (hemolytic anemia, agranulocytosis, leukopenia, thrombocytopenia, aplastic anemia), kernicterus, and renal damage. Primarily because of its TMP component, TMP-SMZ can induce megaloblastic anemia, but only in patients who are folate deficient. TMP-SMZ may also cause adverse CNS effects (headache, depression, hallucinations). Hyperkalemia is a potential complication of TMP-SMZ therapy, especially when the dosage is high. Patients suffering from AIDS are unusually susceptible to TMP-SMZ toxicity. In this group, the incidence of adverse effects (rash, recurrent fever, leukopenia) is about 55%.

Several measures can reduce the incidence and severity of adverse effects. Crystalluria can be avoided by maintaining adequate hydration. Periodic blood tests permit early detection of hematologic disorders. To avoid kernicterus, TMP-SMZ should be withheld from pregnant women near term, nursing mothers, and infants under the age of 2 months. The risk of megaloblastic anemia can be reduced by withholding sulfonamides from individuals likely to be folate deficient (e.g., debilitated patients, pregnant women, alcoholics). Hypersensitivity reactions can be minimized by avoiding TMP-SMZ in patients with a history of hypersensitivity to sulfonamides or to chemically related drugs, including thiazide diuretics, loop diuretics, and sulfonylurea-type oral hypoglycemics.

Drug Interactions

Interactions of TMP-SMZ with other drugs are due primarily to the presence of SMZ. Hence, like sulfonamides used alone, SMZ in the combination can intensify the effects of warfarin, phenytoin, and sulfonylurea-type oral hypoglycemics (e.g., tolbutamide). Accordingly, when these drugs are combined with TMP-SMZ, a reduction in their dosage may be needed.

Preparations, Dosage, and Administration

Preparations. Trimethoprim-sulfamethoxazole [Bactrim, Cotrim, Septra] is dispensed in tablets and a suspension for oral use, and in solution for IV infusion. The ratio of TMP to SMZ in all preparations is 1:5. Two strengths of tablets are available: *standard tablets* contain 80 mg TMP and 400 mg SMZ; *double-strength tablets* contain 160 mg TMP and 800 mg SMZ. Each milliliter of the *oral suspension* contains 8 mg TMP and 40 mg SMZ. Each milliliter of the *IV infusion solution* contains 16 mg TMP and 80 mg SMZ.

Oral Dosing. For management of most infections, the usual *adult* dosage is 160 mg TMP plus 800 mg SMZ administered every 12 hours for 10 to 14 days. To treat shigellosis or traveler's diarrhea, the same dose is administered every 12 hours for 5 days. In the presence of renal impairment (creatinine clearance 15 to 30 ml/min), the dosage should be reduced by 50%. If creatinine clearance is below 15 ml/min, TMP-SMZ should not be used.

To treat urinary tract infections and acute otitis media in *children,* the usual dosage is 4 mg/kg TMP plus 20 mg/kg SMZ administered every 12 hours for 10 days. The same dose, administered every 12 hours for 5 days, is used to treat shigellosis. As in adults, the dosage should be reduced in patients with renal dysfunction.

For prophylaxis of *P. carinii* pneumonia in patients with AIDS, the usual dosage is 160 mg TMP plus 800 mg SMZ once daily.

Intravenous Dosing. Intravenous TMP-SMZ is used for severe infections. The following dosages are for adults and children, and are based on the TMP component of TMP-SMZ. For urinary tract infection or shigellosis, the total daily dose is 8 to 10 mg/kg. This total dose is administered in two to four divided doses given at equally spaced intervals. Duration of treatment is 14 days for urinary tract infection and 5 days for shigellosis. For treatment of *P. carinii* pneumonia, the total daily dose is 15 to 20 mg/kg. This dose is administered in three or four divided doses given at equally spaced intervals. Duration of treatment is 2 weeks or less. Dosage for all indications should be reduced in patients with renal impairment.

⊷ KEY POINTS

- The sulfonamides and trimethoprim act by inhibiting bacterial synthesis of folic acid.
- Sulfonamides are used primarily to treat urinary tract infections.
- The principal adverse effects of sulfonamides are (1) hypersensitivity reactions, ranging from rash and photosensitivity to Stevens-Johnson syndrome; (2) hemolytic anemia; (3) kernicterus; and (4) renal damage.
- The combination product TMP-SMZ inhibits sequential steps in bacterial folic acid synthesis, and therefore is much more powerful than TMP or SMZ alone.
- TMP-SMZ is a preferred drug for treating urinary tract infections and is the drug of choice for *P. carinii* infections in patients with AIDS and other immunodeficiency states.
- The principal adverse effects of TMP-SMZ are like those caused by sulfonamides (i.e., hypersensitivity reactions, hemolytic anemia, kernicterus, and renal injury).

Summary of Major Nursing Implications*

SULFONAMIDES (SYSTEMIC)

Sulfadiazine
Sulfamethizole
Sulfamethoxazole
Sulfisoxazole

The nursing implications summarized here apply to systemic sulfonamides. Implications specific to topical sulfonamides are not summarized.

Preadministration Assessment

Therapeutic Goal

Sulfonamides are used primarily for urinary tract infections caused by *E. coli* and other susceptible organisms.

Identifying High-Risk Patients

Sulfonamides are *contraindicated* during pregnancy and lactation, for infants under the age of 2 months, and for patients with a history of hypersensitivity to sulfonamides and chemically related drugs, including thiazide diuretics, loop diuretics, and sulfonylurea-type oral hypoglycemics. Exercise *caution* in patients with renal impairment.

Implementation: Administration

Routes

All systemic sulfonamides can be administered orally. *Sulfisoxazole* can also be administered parenterally (IV, SC, IM).

Administration

Instruct patients to complete the prescribed course of treatment, even though symptoms may abate before the full course is over.

Advise patients to take oral sulfonamides on an empty stomach and with a full glass of water.

Administer IV *sulfisoxazole* by slow injection or IV drip.

Ongoing Evaluation and Interventions

Minimizing Adverse Effects

Hypersensitivity Reactions. Sulfonamides can induce severe hypersensitivity reactions (e.g., Stevens-Johnson syndrome). Do not give sulfonamides to patients with a history of hypersensitivity to sulfonamides or to chemically related drugs, including sulfonylureas, thiazide diuretics, and loop

*Patient education information is highlighted as blue text.

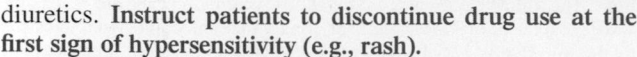

Summary of Major Nursing Implications*—cont'd

diuretics. **Instruct patients to discontinue drug use at the first sign of hypersensitivity (e.g., rash).**

Photosensitivity. Photosensitivity reactions may occur. **Advise the patient to avoid prolonged exposure to sunlight, wear protective clothing, and apply a sunscreen to exposed skin.**

Hematologic Effects. Sulfonamides can cause hemolytic anemia and other blood dyscrasias (agranulocytosis, leukopenia, thrombocytopenia, aplastic anemia). Observe patients for signs of hemolysis (fever, pallor, jaundice). When sulfonamide therapy is prolonged, periodic blood cell counts should be made.

Kernicterus. Sulfonamides can cause kernicterus in newborns. Do not give these drugs to pregnant women near term, nursing mothers, or infants under the age of 2 months.

Renal Damage. Deposition of sulfonamide crystals can injure the kidney. To minimize crystalluria, maintain hydration sufficient to produce a daily urine flow of 1200 ml in adults. Alkalinization of urine (e.g., with sodium bicarbonate) can also help. **Advise outpatients to consume 8 to 10 glasses of water per day.**

Minimizing Adverse Interactions

Sulfonamides can intensify the effects of *warfarin, phenytoin,* and *sulfonylurea-type oral hypoglycemics* (e.g., tolbutamide). When combined with sulfonamides, these drugs may require a reduction in dosage.

TRIMETHOPRIM

Preadministration Assessment

Therapeutic Goal

Initial treatment of uncomplicated urinary tract infections caused by *E. coli* and other susceptible organisms.

Identifying High-Risk Patients

Trimethoprim is *contraindicated* in patients with folate deficiency (manifested as megaloblastic anemia). When possible, the drug should be avoided during pregnancy and lactation.

Implementation: Administration

Route

Oral.

Dosage and Administration

Instruct patients to complete the prescribed course of treatment, even though symptoms may abate before the full course is over.

Reduce the dosage in patients with renal dysfunction.

Ongoing Evaluation and Interventions

Minimizing Adverse Effects

Hematologic Effects. Trimethoprim can cause blood dyscrasias (megaloblastic anemia, thrombocytopenia, neutropenia) by exacerbating pre-existing folic acid deficiency. Avoid trimethoprim when folate deficiency is likely (e.g., in alcoholics, pregnant women, debilitated patients). **Inform**

patients about early signs of blood disorders (e.g., sore throat, fever, pallor), and instruct them to notify the physician if these occur. Complete blood counts should be performed. If a significant reduction in counts is observed, discontinue trimethoprim. Normal hematopoiesis can be restored with folinic acid (leucovorin).

Use in Pregnancy and Lactation. Trimethoprim should be avoided during pregnancy and lactation. The drug can exacerbate folate deficiency in pregnant women and cause folate deficiency in the nursing infant whose mother is taking trimethoprim.

TRIMETHOPRIM-SULFAMETHOXAZOLE

Preadministration Assessment

Therapeutic Goal

Indications include urinary tract infections caused by *E. coli* and other susceptible organisms, shigellosis, and infections caused by *P. carinii.*

Identifying High-Risk Patients

TMP-SMZ is *contraindicated* during pregnancy and lactation, for infants under the age of 2 months, in patients with folate deficiency (manifested as megaloblastic anemia), and for patients with a history of hypersensitivity to sulfonamides and chemically related drugs, including thiazide diuretics, loop diuretics, and sulfonylurea-type oral hypoglycemics.

Implementation: Administration

Routes

Oral; IV (for severe infections).

Dosage

Adjustment. In patients with renal impairment (creatinine clearance of 15 to 30 ml/min), decrease dosage by 50%. If creatinine clearance falls below 15 ml/min, discontinue drug use.

Administration

Instruct the patient to complete the prescribed course of treatment, even though symptoms may abate before the full course is over.

Ongoing Evaluation and Interventions

Minimizing Adverse Effects

Although serious adverse reactions are rare, TMP-SMZ can nonetheless cause all of the toxicities associated with sulfonamides and trimethoprim used alone. Hence, the nursing implications summarized above regarding adverse effects of the sulfonamides alone and trimethoprim alone also apply to the combination of TMP-SMZ.

Minimizing Adverse Interactions

TMP-SMZ has the same drug interactions as sulfonamides used alone. That is, TMP-SMZ can increase the effects of *warfarin, phenytoin,* and *sulfonylurea-type oral hypoglycemics.* When combined with TMP-SMZ, these drugs may require a reduction in dosage.

*Patient education information is highlighted as blue text.

Drug Therapy of Urinary Tract Infections

Urinary tract infections (UTIs) are the most common infections encountered today. In the United States, UTIs account for over 7 million visits to physicians annually. Among sexually active young women, 25% to 35% have at least one UTI a year. Among elderly women in nursing homes, between 30% and 50% have bacteriuria at any given time. UTIs occur much less frequently in males than in females, but are more likely to be associated with complications (e.g., septicemia, pyelonephritis).

Infections may be limited to bacterial colonization of the urine, or bacteria may invade tissues of the urinary tract. When bacteria invade tissues, characteristic inflammatory syndromes result: *urethritis* (inflammation of the urethra), *cystitis* (inflammation of the urinary bladder), *pyelonephritis* (inflammation of the kidney and its pelvis), and *prostatitis* (inflammation of the prostate).

UTIs may be classified according to their location—in either the lower urinary tract (bladder and urethra) or the upper urinary tract (kidney). Within this classification scheme, *cystitis* and *urethritis* are considered *lower tract infections,* whereas *pyelonephritis* is considered an *upper tract infection.*

UTIs are referred to as being *complicated* or *uncomplicated. Complicated* UTIs occur in males and females and are associated with some predisposing factor, such as calculi (stones), prostatic hypertrophy, an indwelling catheter, or an impediment to the flow of urine (e.g., physical obstruction). *Uncomplicated* UTIs occur primarily in women of child-bearing age and are not associated with any particular predisposing factor.

Several classes of antibiotics are used to treat UTIs. Among these are sulfonamides, trimethoprim, penicillins, aminoglycosides, cephalosporins, fluoroquinolones, and the urinary tract antiseptics: nitrofurantoin, methenamine, nalidixic acid, and cinoxacin. With the exception of the urinary tract antiseptics, all of these drugs are discussed at length in other chapters. The basic pharmacology of the urinary tract antiseptics is presented here.

ORGANISMS THAT CAUSE URINARY TRACT INFECTIONS

The bacteria that cause UTIs differ between community-acquired infections and hospital-acquired (nosocomial) infections. The majority (>80%) of uncomplicated, community-acquired UTIs are caused by *Escherichia coli.* Rarely, other gram-negative bacilli—*Klebsiella pneumoniae, Enterobacter, Proteus, Providencia,* and *Pseudomonas*—are the cause. Gram-positive cocci, especially *Staphylococcus saprophyticus,* account for 10% to 15% of community-acquired infections. Hospital-acquired UTIs are frequently caused by *Klebsiella, Proteus, Enterobacter, Pseudomonas,* staphylococci, and enterococci; *E. coli* is responsible for less than 50% of nosocomial infections. Although most UTIs involve only one organism, infection with multiple organisms may occur, especially in patients with an indwelling urinary catheter, renal stones, or chronic renal abscesses.

SPECIFIC URINARY TRACT INFECTIONS AND THEIR TREATMENT

In this section, we consider the characteristics and treatment of the major UTIs: acute cystitis, acute urethral syndrome, acute pyelonephritis, acute bacterial prostatitis, and recurrent UTIs. Most of these infections can be treated with oral therapy at home. The principal exception is severe pyelonephritis, which requires IV therapy in a hospital. Drugs and dosages for outpatient therapy in women are summarized in Table 85–1.

Acute Cystitis

Acute cystitis is a lower urinary tract infection that occurs most often in women of child-bearing age. Clinical manifestations are dysuria, urinary urgency, urinary frequency, suprapubic discomfort, pyuria, and bacteriuria (more than 100,000 bacteria per milliliter of urine). It is important to note that many women

TABLE 85–1 ■ Regimens for Oral Therapy of Urinary Tract Infections in Women

Drug	Dose	Duration
Acute Cystitis		
First-Line Drugs		
Trimethoprim/sulfamethoxazole	160/800 mg bid	3–7 days
Trimethoprim	100 mg bid	3–7 days
Nitrofurantoin	50–100 mg qid	7 days
Fosfomycin	3 gm once	1 day
Second-Line Drugs		
Norfloxacin	400 mg bid	3 days
Ciprofloxacin	250 mg bid	3 days
Ofloxacin	400 mg bid	3 days
Levofloxacin	400 qd	3 days
Amoxicillin (with clavulanic acid)	500 mg tid	3–7 days
Cephalexin	500 mg qd	7 days
Cefixime	400 mg qd	7 days
Acute Pyelonephritis		
First-Line Drugs		
Trimethoprim/sulfamethoxazole	160/800 bid	14 days
Trimethoprim	100 mg bid	14 days
Norfloxacin	400 mg bid	14 days
Ciprofloxacin	250–500 mg bid	14 days
Ofloxacin	400 mg bid	14 days
Second-Line Drugs		
Amoxicillin (with clavulanic acid)	500 mg tid	14 days
Cephalexin	500 mg qid	14 days
Cefotaxime	1 mg tid	14 days
Ceftriaxone	1–2 mg qd	14 days
Complicated Urinary Tract Infections		
Trimethoprim/sulfamethoxazole	160/800 mg bid	7–14 days
Norfloxacin	400 mg bid	7–14 days
Ciprofloxacin	250–500 mg bid	7–14 days
Ofloxacin	400 mg bid	7–14 days
Levofloxacin	400 mg bid	7–14 days
Amoxicillin (with clavulanic acid)	500 mg tid	7–14 days
Cephalexin	500 mg tid	7–14 days
Prophylaxis of Recurrent Infection		
Trimethoprim/sulfamethoxazole	40/200 mg* qhs 3 times/wk	6 months
Trimethoprim	100 mg qhs	6 months
Nitrofurantoin	50–100 mg qhs	6 months
Norfloxacin	200 mg qhs	6 months
Cephalexin	250 mg qhs	6 months
Cefaclor	250 mg qhs	6 months

*One-half of a single-strength tablet.

(30% or more) with symptoms of acute cystitis also have asymptomatic upper urinary tract infection (subclinical pyelonephritis). In uncomplicated, community-acquired cystitis, the principal causative organisms are *E. coli* (80%), *S. saprophyticus* (11%), and *Streptococcus faecalis*.

For community-acquired infections, three types of oral therapy can be employed; (1) single-dose therapy, (2) short-course therapy (3 days), and (3) conventional therapy (7 days). *Single-dose* therapy and *short-course* therapy are recommended only for uncomplicated, community-acquired infections in women who are not pregnant and whose symptoms began less than 7 days before starting treatment. Short-course therapy is more effective than single-dose therapy and is generally preferred. Advantages of short-course therapy over conventional therapy are lower cost, greater compliance, fewer side effects, and less potential for promoting emergence of bacterial resistance. *Conventional* therapy is indicated for all patients who do not meet the criteria for short-course therapy. These patients include males, children, pregnant women, and women with suspected upper tract involvement.

As indicated in Table 85–1, a variety of drugs can be used for treatment. Trimethoprim/sulfamethoxazole and trimethoprim alone are traditional agents of first choice. In communities where resistance to these drugs exceeds 20%, the fluoroquinolones (e.g., norfloxacin, ofloxacin) are good alternatives. When compliance is a concern, fosfomycin, which requires just one dose, is an attractive choice. As a rule, beta-lactam antibiotics (e.g., amoxicillin; cephalexin and other cephalosporins) should be avoided. Why? Because these drugs are less effective than the alternatives, and are not as well tolerated.

Acute Pyelonephritis

Acute pyelonephritis is an infection of the kidneys. This disorder is common in young children, the elderly, and women of child-bearing age. Clinical manifestations include fever, chills, severe flank pain, dysuria, urinary frequency, urinary urgency, pyuria, and, usually, bacteriuria (more than 100,000 bacteria per milliliter of urine). *Escherichia coli* is the causative organism in 90% of initial, community-acquired infections.

Mild to moderate infection can be treated at home with oral antibiotics. Options include trimethoprim-sulfamethoxazole, ciprofloxacin, norfloxacin, ofloxacin, and amoxicillin-clavulanate. Treatment should last 14 days. Some regimens for oral therapy are shown in Table 85–1.

Severe pyelonephritis requires hospitalization and IV antibiotics. Several options are available, including ciprofloxacin, ceftriaxone, ceftazidime, ampicillin plus gentamicin, and ampicillin-sulbactam. Once the infection has been controlled with IV antibiotics, therapy with oral antibiotics should be instituted.

Complicated Urinary Tract Infections

Complicated UTIs occur in males and females who have a structural or functional abnormality of the urinary tract that predisposes them to developing infection. Among these predisposing factors are prostatic hypertrophy, renal calculi (stones), nephrocalcinosis, renal or bladder tumors, ureteric stricture, or an indwelling urethral catheter. Symptoms of complicated UTIs can range from mild to severe. Some patients even develop systemic illness, manifesting as fever, bacteremia, and septic shock.

The microbiology of complicated UTIs is less predictable than the microbiology of uncomplicated UTIs. Although *E. coli* is a common pathogen, it is by no means the only one. Others possibilities include *Klebsiella, Proteus, Pseudomonas, Staphylococcus aureus, Enterobacter* species, *Serratia* species, and even *Candida* species. Accordingly, if treatment is to succeed, we must determine the identity and drug sensitivity of causative organism. To do so, urine for microbiologic testing should be obtained *before* giving any antibiotics. If symptoms of the UTI are relatively mild, treatment should wait until test results are available. However, if symptoms are severe, immediate treatment with a broad-spectrum antibiotic can be instituted. Some options are presented in Table 85–1. Once test results are known, a drug specific to the pathogen can be substituted. Duration of treatment ranges from 7 days (for patients with cystitis) to 14 days (for patients with pyelonephritis or systemic involvement).

Recurrent Urinary Tract Infection

Recurrent UTI results from *relapse* or from *reinfection*. *Relapse* is caused by recolonization with the same organism responsible for the initial infection. In contrast, *reinfection* is caused by colonization with a new organism.

Reinfection. More than 80% of recurrent UTIs in females are due to reinfection. These usually involve the lower urinary tract and may be related to sexual intercourse or use of a contraceptive diaphragm. If reinfections are *infrequent* (only one or two a year), each episode should be treated as a separate infection. Single-dose or short-course therapy can be used.

When reinfections are *frequent* (three or more a year), long-term prophylaxis may be indicated. Prophylaxis can be achieved with low daily doses of several agents, including trimethoprim (100 mg), nitrofurantoin (50 or 100 mg), or trimethoprim/sulfamethoxazole (160 mg/800 mg). Prophylaxis should continue for at least 6 months. During this time, periodic urine cultures should be obtained. If a symptomatic episode occurs, standard therapy for acute cystitis should be given. If reinfection is associated with sexual intercourse, the risk can be decreased by voiding after intercourse and by single-dose prophylaxis (e.g., trimethoprim/sulfamethoxazole [160 mg/800 mg] taken after intercourse).

Relapse. Recolonization with the original infecting organism accounts for 20% of recurrent UTIs. Symptoms that reappear shortly after completion of a course of therapy suggest either a structural abnormality of the urinary tract, involvement of the kidneys, or chronic bacterial prostatitis (the most common cause of recurrent UTI in males). If obstruction of the urinary tract is present, it should be corrected surgically. If renal calculi are the cause of relapse, they should be removed.

Drug therapy is progressive. When relapse occurs in women after short-course therapy, a 2-week course of therapy should be tried. If this fails, an additional 4 to 6 weeks of therapy should be tried. If this too is unsuccessful, long-term therapy (6 months) may be indicated. Drugs employed for long-term therapy of relapse include trimethoprim-sulfamethoxazole, norfloxacin, and cephalexin.

Acute Bacterial Prostatitis

Acute bacterial prostatitis is defined as inflammation of the prostate caused by local bacterial infection. Clinical manifestations include high fever, chills, malaise, myalgia, localized pain, and various urinary tract symptoms (dysuria, nocturia, urinary urgency, urinary frequency, urinary retention). In most cases (80%), *E. coli* is the causative organism. Infection is frequently associated with an indwelling urethral catheter, urethral instrumentation, or transurethral prostatic resection. However, in many patients the infection has no obvious cause. Bacterial prostatitis responds well to antimicrobial therapy. For oral therapy, the fluoroquinolones (e.g., ciprofloxacin, norfloxacin) are preferred. Dosages are the same as for acute cystis (see Table 85–1). For parenteral therapy, aminoglycosides (e.g., gentamicin, amikacin) are employed.

URINARY TRACT ANTISEPTICS

The urinary tract antiseptics are drugs whose use is limited to treatment of UTIs. The major urinary tract antiseptics are nitrofurantoin, methenamine, nalidixic acid, and cinoxacin. All four drugs become concentrated in the urine, and are active against the common urinary tract pathogens. These drugs do not achieve effective antibacterial concentrations in blood or tissues, and hence cannot be used for infections at sites outside the urinary tract. As a rule, the urinary tract antiseptics are second-choice drugs for treatment or prophylaxis of UTIs.

Nitrofurantoin

Nitrofurantoin [Furadantin, Macrodantin, Macrobid] is a broad-spectrum antimicrobial drug. The agent is bacteriostatic in low concentrations and bactericidal in high concentrations. Therapeutic levels are achieved only in urine. Hence the drug is useful only against infections of the urinary tract. Nitrofurantoin can cause serious adverse effects.

Nitrofurantoin injures bacteria by causing damage to DNA. However, in order to damage DNA, the drug must first be converted to a reactive form. Nitrofurantoin is selectively toxic to bacteria because, unlike mammalian cells, bacteria possess relatively high levels of the enzyme that activates the drug.

Antimicrobial Spectrum

Nitrofurantoin is active against a large number of gram-positive and gram-negative bacteria. Susceptible organisms include staphylococci, streptococci, *Neisseria, Bacteroides,* and most strains of *E. coli.* These sensitive bacteria rarely acquire resistance. Organisms that are frequently insensitive include *Proteus, Pseudomonas, Enterobacter,* and *Klebsiella.*

Therapeutic Use

Nitrofurantoin is indicated for acute infections of the lower urinary tract caused by susceptible organisms. In addition, nitrofurantoin can be used for prophylaxis of recurrent lower UTI. The drug is not recommended for infections of the upper urinary tract.

Pharmacokinetics

Absorption and Distribution. Nitrofurantoin is available in two oral formulations: *macrocrystalline* and *microcrystalline.* The macrocrystalline preparation is absorbed relatively slowly and produces less GI distress than does the microcrystalline form. Both formulations produce equivalent therapeutic effects. Nitrofurantoin is distributed to tissues, but only in small amounts. Therapeutic concentrations are achieved only in urine.

Metabolism and Excretion. About two-thirds of each dose undergoes metabolic degradation, primarily in the liver; the remaining one-third is excreted intact in the urine. Nitrofurantoin achieves a urinary concentration of about 200 μg/ml (compared with less than 2 μg/ml in plasma). The drug imparts a harmless brown color to the urine; patients should be forewarned of this effect.

For two reasons, the drug should not be administered to individuals with kidney impairment, defined here as creatinine clearance less than 40 ml/min. First, in the absence of good renal function, levels of nitrofurantoin in the urine are too low to be effective. Second, renal dysfunction reduces nitrofurantoin excretion, causing plasma levels of the drug to rise, thereby presenting a risk of systemic toxicity.

Adverse Effects

Gastrointestinal Effects. The most frequent adverse reactions are GI disturbances (e.g., anorexia, nausea, vomiting, diarrhea). These can be minimized by administering nitrofurantoin with milk or with meals, by reducing the dosage, and by using the macrocrystalline formulation.

Pulmonary Reactions. Nitrofurantoin can induce two kinds of pulmonary reactions: acute and subacute. Acute reactions, which are most common, are manifested by dyspnea, chest pain, chills, fever, cough, and alveolar infiltrates. These symptoms resolve 2 to 4 days after discontinuing the drug. Acute pulmonary responses are thought to be hypersensitivity reactions. Patients with a history of these responses should not receive nitrofurantoin again. Subacute reactions are rare and occur during prolonged treatment. Symptoms (e.g., dyspnea, cough, malaise) usually regress over weeks to months following nitrofurantoin withdrawal. However, in some patients, permanent lung damage may occur.

Hematologic Effects. Nitrofurantoin can cause a variety of hematologic reactions, including agranulocytosis, leukopenia, thrombocytopenia, and megaloblastic anemia. In addition, hemolytic anemia may occur in infants and in patients whose red blood cells have an inherited deficiency in glucose-6-phosphate dehydrogenase. Because of the potential for hemolytic anemia in newborns, nitrofurantoin is contraindicated for pregnant women near term and for infants under the age of 1 month.

Peripheral Neuropathy. Damage to sensory and motor nerves is a serious concern. Demyelinization and nerve degeneration can occur and may be irreversible. Early symptoms include muscle weakness, tingling sensations, and numbness. Patients should be informed about these symptoms and instructed to report them. Neuropathy is most likely in patients with renal impairment and in those taking nitrofurantoin chronically.

Other Adverse Effects. Nitrofurantoin can cause multiple neurologic effects (e.g., headache, vertigo, drowsiness, nystagmus); all are readily reversible. Hepatotoxicity (cholestatic jaundice, chronic hepatitis, hepatocellular damage) occurs rarely.

Preparations, Dosage, and Administration

Preparations. Microcrystalline nitrofurantoin [Furadantin] is dispensed in a 5-mg/ml oral suspension. Macrocrystalline nitrofurantoin [Macrodantin, Macrobid] is dispensed in 25-, 50-, and 100-mg capsules.

Dosage and Administration. For *treatment of acute UTI,* the adult dosage is 50 mg 3 to 4 times a day; the pediatric dosage is 5 to 7 mg/kg/day administered in four divided doses. For *prophylaxis of recurrent UTI,* low doses are employed (e.g., 50 to 100 mg at bedtime for adults and 1 mg/kg/day in one or two doses for children). Nitrofurantoin can be administered with meals or with milk to reduce GI distress.

Methenamine
Mechanism of Action

Under acidic conditions, methenamine [Mandelamine, Hiprex, Urex] decomposes into ammonia and formaldehyde. The formaldehyde denatures bacterial proteins, causing cell death. For formaldehyde to be released, the urine must be acidic (pH 5.5 or less). Since formaldehyde is not formed at physiologic systemic pH, methenamine is devoid of systemic toxicity.

Antimicrobial Spectrum

Virtually all bacteria are susceptible to formaldehyde; resistance does not exist. Certain bacteria (e.g., *Proteus* species) can elevate urinary pH (by splitting urea to form ammonia). Since formaldehyde is not released under alkaline conditions, infections with these urea-splitting organisms are often unresponsive.

Therapeutic Uses

Methenamine is used for *chronic* UTI, but is *not* recommended for *acute* infection. The drug can suppress recurrent UTI in females, but trimethoprim-sulfamethoxazole is preferred. Methenamine is not active against infections of the upper urinary tract—because there is insufficient time for formaldehyde to form as the drug traverses the kidney. Methenamine does not prevent UTIs associated with catheters.

Pharmacokinetics

Absorption and Distribution. Methenamine is rapidly absorbed after oral administration. However, approximately 30% of each dose may be converted to ammonia and formaldehyde in the acidic environment of the stomach. This can be minimized by using enteric-coated preparations. The drug is distributed throughout total body water.

Excretion. Methenamine is eliminated by the kidneys. Within the urinary tract, about 20% of the drug decomposes to form formaldehyde. Levels of formaldehyde are highest in the bladder. Since formaldehyde generation takes place slowly, and since transit time through the kidney is brief, formaldehyde levels in the kidney remain subtherapeutic. Ingestion of large amounts of fluid reduces antibacterial effects by diluting methenamine and raising urinary pH. Poorly metabolized acids (e.g., hippuric acid, mandelic acid, ascorbic acid) have been administered with methenamine in attempts to acidify the urine, and thereby increase formaldehyde formation. However, there is no evidence that these acids enhance therapeutic effects.

Adverse Effects and Precautions

Methenamine is relatively safe and generally well tolerated. Gastric distress occurs occasionally, probably from formaldehyde release in the stomach. Use of enteric-coated preparations may reduce this response. Chronic high-dose therapy can cause bladder irritation, manifested as dysuria, frequent voiding, urinary urgency, proteinuria, and hematuria. Since decomposition of methenamine generates ammonia (in addition to formaldehyde), the drug is contraindicated for patients with liver dysfunction. Methenamine salts (methenamine mandelate, methenamine hippurate) should not be used by patients with renal impairment, since crystalluria may be caused by precipitation of the mandelate or hippurate moiety.

Drug Interactions

Urinary Alkalinizers. Drugs that elevate urinary pH (e.g., acetazolamide, sodium bicarbonate) inhibit formaldehyde production, and can thereby reduce the antibacterial effects. Patients taking methenamine should not be given alkalinizing agents.

Sulfonamides. Methenamine should not be combined with sulfonamides: Formaldehyde forms an insoluble complex with sulfonamides, thereby posing a risk of urinary tract injury from crystalluria.

Preparations, Dosage, and Administration

Methenamine is available as two salts: methenamine mandelate and methenamine hippurate.

Methenamine mandelate [Mandelamine] is dispensed in enteric-coated tablets (0.5 and 1 gm) and a suspension (0.1 gm/ml) for oral use. The usual adult dosage is 1 gm 4 times a day. The dosage for children 6 to 12 years old is 0.5 gm 4 times a day. For children under the age of 6, the dosage is 18 mg/kg 4 times a day.

Methenamine hippurate [Hiprex, Urex] is dispensed in 1-gm oral tablets. The dosage for adults and for children over the age of 12 years is 1 gm twice a day. For children ages 6 to 12 years, the dosage is 500 mg to 1 gm twice a day.

Nalidixic Acid

Mechanism of Action

Nalidixic acid [NegGram], a chemical relative of the fluoroquinolones, inhibits replication of bacterial DNA, thereby causing DNA degradation and cell death. The precise target of nalidixic acid is *DNA gyrase,* the bacterial enzyme that converts closed circular DNA into a supercoiled configuration. If supercoiling does not occur, DNA replication cannot take place.

Microbial Resistance

Resistant bacteria often emerge during treatment. Two mechanisms have been described: (1) production of an altered DNA gyrase that has reduced sensitivity to nalidixic acid and (2) reduced bacterial uptake of nalidixic acid. Cross-resistance with cinoxacin is common. A frequent factor in resistance is use of suboptimal doses. (Low levels of nalidixic acid favor overgrowth with drug-resistant organisms.) Fortunately, resistance to nalidixic acid is not carried on R factors, and therefore is not transferable.

Antimicrobial Spectrum

Nalidixic acid is active against most gram-negative urinary tract pathogens, including *E. coli, Klebsiella, Enterobacter,* and *Proteus* species. *Pseudomonas aeruginosa* is resistant, as are most gram-positive aerobic cocci. .

Therapeutic Uses

Nalidixic acid is approved only for UTIs. The drug has been used to control acute infection and to prevent recurrent UTI. However, for both applications, other drugs are preferred. Nalidixic acid is not useful against infections outside the urinary tract.

Pharmacokinetics

Nalidixic acid is well absorbed from the GI tract, and then undergoes rapid hepatic metabolism. Only one metabolite—hydroxynalidixic acid—has antibacterial actions. Nalidixic acid and its metabolites are excreted in the urine. The concentration of active drug in urine is about 10 times greater than in plasma. Therapeutic levels are achieved in urine even in patients with moderate to severe renal impairment. Drug concentrations outside the urinary tract are too low for antibacterial effects.

Adverse Effects

Although nalidixic acid can cause multiple untoward effects, the incidence of severe reactions is low. The most common effects are GI disturbances (nausea, vomiting, abdominal discomfort), visual disturbances (blurred vision, diplopia, poor accommodation, photophobia, altered color perception), and rash. Patients who experience reduced visual acuity should exercise appropriate caution (e.g., when driving). Photosensitivity reactions can occur. Accordingly, patients should be advised to avoid excessive exposure to sunlight, wear protective clothing, and apply a sunscreen to exposed skin. Convulsions have occurred on occasion, making nalidixic acid inappropriate for individuals with a history of convulsive disorders. Nalidixic acid may produce intracranial hypertension in pediatric patients, and hence the drug should not be administered to children under the age of 3 months. Blood dyscrasias (thrombocytopenia, leukopenia, hemolytic anemia) and jaundice are rare. Nonetheless, when nalidixic acid is used for more than 2 weeks, blood cell counts and liver function tests should be performed.

Drug Interactions

Nalidixic acid can intensify the effects of warfarin (by displacing the anticoagulant from binding sites on plasma proteins). Accordingly, when warfarin is combined with nalidixic acid, a reduction in warfarin dosage may be needed.

Preparations, Dosage, and Administration

Nalidixic acid [NegGram] is dispensed in tablets (250 mg, 500 mg, 1 gm) and in suspension (50 mg/ml) for oral use. The adult dosage is 1 gm 4 times a day for 1 or 2 weeks. For children under the age of 12 years, the dosage is 55 mg/kg/day in four divided doses. Nalidixic acid should not be given to children less than 3 months old.

Cinoxacin

Cinoxacin [Cinobac] is a close chemical relative of nalidixic acid. Both drugs have the same mechanism of action, antimicrobial spectrum, and indications. Furthermore, organisms that are resistant to nalidixic acid are often resistant to cinoxacin. As with other urinary tract antiseptics, therapeutic levels of cinoxacin are achieved only in the urine. Adverse effects are like those of nalidixic acid, but their incidence is relatively low. Cinoxacin is excreted by the kidneys, primarily unchanged. The drug is dispensed in 250- and 500-mg capsules for oral use. The usual adult dosage is 1 gm/day administered in two or four divided doses. Dosage should be reduced in patients with renal impairment—because failure to do so could result in accumulation of cinoxacin to toxic levels.

⠂⠂ KEY POINTS

- *Escherichia coli* is the most common cause of uncomplicated, community-acquired UTIs.
- Except for pyelonephritis, most UTIs can be treated with oral therapy at home.
- Trimethoprim-sulfamethoxazole is frequently the treatment of choice for oral therapy of UTIs.
- Many drugs, including penicillins, cephalosporins, and fluoroquinolones, may be used for parenteral therapy of UTIs.
- Prophylaxis of recurrent UTI can be achieved with daily low doses of oral antibiotics (e.g., trimethoprim-sulfamethoxazole).
- The urinary tract antiseptics—nitrofurantoin, methenamine, nalidixic acid, and cinoxacin—are second-choice drugs for treating UTIs.

Antimycobacterial Agents: Drugs for Tuberculosis, Leprosy, and *Mycobacterium avium* Complex Infection

Our topic for this chapter is infections caused by three mycobacteria: *Mycobacterium tuberculosis, Mycobacterium leprae,* and *Mycobacterium avium.* The mycobacteria are slow-growing microbes, and the infections they cause require prolonged treatment. Because therapy is prolonged, drug toxicity and poor patient compliance are significant clinical problems. In addition, prolonged treatment promotes the emergence of drug-resistant microbes.

TUBERCULOSIS I: CLINICAL CONSIDERATIONS

Tuberculosis is a global epidemic. Worldwide, approximately 2 billion people are infected—nearly one-third of the Earth's population. Each year, tuberculosis kills 2 to 3 million people—more than any other infectious disease, more than AIDS and

malaria combined. Although new cases in the United States continue to decline (down from 20,673 in 1992 to 16,377 in 2000), in the rest of the world, new cases are increasing. The current estimate is 8 million new cases a year. Of these, the vast majority (95%) occur in developing countries. There are two reasons for the resurgence of tuberculosis: AIDS and the emergence of multidrug-resistant mycobacteria.

Pathogenesis

Tuberculosis is caused by *Mycobacterium tuberculosis,* an organism also known as the tubercle bacillus. Infections may be limited to the lungs or may become disseminated. In most cases, the bacteria are quiescent, and the infected individual has no symptoms. However, when the disease is active, morbidity can be significant. In the United States, approximately 10 million people harbor tubercle bacilli. However, only a small fraction have symptomatic disease.

Primary Infection

Infection with *M. tuberculosis* is transmitted from person to person by inhaling infected sputum that has been aerosolized, usually by coughing or sneezing. As a result, initial infection is in the lung. Once in the lung, tubercle bacilli are taken up by phagocytic cells (macrophages and neutrophils). At first, the bacilli are resistant to the destructive activity of phagocytes and multiply freely within them. Infection can spread from the lungs to other organs via the lymphatic and circulatory systems.

In most cases, immunity to *M. tuberculosis* develops within a few weeks, and the infection is brought under complete control. The immune system facilitates control by increasing the ability of phagocytes to suppress multiplication of tubercle bacilli. Because of this rapid response by the immune system, most individuals (90%) with primary infection never develop clinical or radiologic evidence of disease. However, even though symptoms are absent and the progression of infection is halted, the infected individual is likely to harbor tubercle bacilli lifelong (unless drugs are given to eliminate quiescent bacilli). Hence, in the absence of treatment, there is always some risk that latent infection may become active.

If the immune system fails to control the primary infection, clinical disease (tuberculosis) develops. The result is necrosis and cavitation of lung tissue. Lung tissue may also become caseous (cheese-like in appearance). Because phagocytes do not function at sites of necrosis, cellular immunity is unable to suppress the active infection. In the absence of treatment, tissue destruction progresses, and death may result.

Reactivation

The term *reactivation* refers to renewed multiplication of tubercle bacilli that had been dormant following control of a primary infection. Until recently, it was assumed that most new cases of symptomatic tuberculosis resulted from reactivation of an old (latent) infection. However, we now know that, among some groups, reactivation may be responsible for only 60% of new infections—the remaining 40% result from recent person-to-person transmission.

Diagnosis and Treatment of Active Tuberculosis

The availability of modern chemotherapeutic agents has dramatically altered the treatment of tuberculosis. Whereas patients once faced lengthy hospitalization, therapy can now be performed on an outpatient basis for most patients. Prolonged bed rest is not required, nor is it recommended. To reduce emergence of resistance, treatment is always done with two or more drugs. In addition, direct observation of drug administration is now considered standard care.

The goal of treatment is to eliminate symptoms and prevent relapse. To accomplish this, treatment must kill tubercle bacilli that are actively dividing as well as those that are "resting." Success is indicated by an absence of observable mycobacteria in sputum and by the failure of sputum cultures to yield colonies of *M. tuberculosis*.

Diagnosis

Diagnostic testing is indicated for (1) individuals with clinical manifestations that suggest tuberculosis and (2) individuals with a positive tuberculin skin test (see below under *Diagnosis and Treatment of Latent Tuberculosis*) who are at high risk of developing active disease. A definitive diagnosis is made with a chest radiograph and microbiologic evaluation of sputum. A chest radiograph should be ordered for all persons suspected of active infection.

Sputum is evaluated in two ways: (1) by microscopic examination of sputum smears and (2) by culturing sputum samples. Microscopic examination cannot provide a definitive diagnosis. Why? Because direct observation cannot distinguish between *M. tuberculosis* and other mycobacteria. Furthermore, microscopic examination is much less sensitive than culturing. Accordingly, sputum cultures are required for definitive diagnosis. Because *M. tuberculosis* grows very slowly, results of sputum cultures are often delayed by as long as 3 to 6 weeks. However, with newer culturing techniques, results can be obtained in less than 1 week. In addition to providing positive identification of *M. tuberculosis*, cultures are necessary to determine drug sensitivity.

Drug Resistance

Drug resistance is a major impediment to successful therapy. Some infecting bacilli are inherently resistant; others develop resistance over the course of treatment. Some bacilli are re-

sistant to just one drug; others are resistant to multiple drugs. Infection with a resistant organism may be acquired in two ways: (1) through contact with someone who harbors resistant bacteria, and (2) through repeated ineffectual courses of therapy (see below).

Multidrug resistance is a recent and ominous development. Resistance to isoniazid and rifampin—two mainstays of therapy—is of particular concern. Infection with multidrug-resistant organisms greatly increases the risk of death, especially among patients with AIDS. In addition, multidrug resistance is expensive: The cost of treating one case of resistant tuberculosis is about $180,000, compared with $12,000 per case for nonresistant tuberculosis.

The incidence of drug resistance is increasing. Thirty years ago, primary resistance to isoniazid occurred in less than 2% of patients; today the incidence is 9%. The incidence of multidrug resistance varies among communities. Nationwide, the average is 1 of every 10 patients. The highest incidence of multidrug resistance is found in New York City, where fully two-thirds of all cases occur.

The principal cause underlying the emergence of resistance is inadequate drug therapy. Treatment may be too short; dosage may be too low; patient compliance may be erratic; and, perhaps most importantly, the regimen may contain too few drugs (see below).

The Prime Directive: Always Treat Tuberculosis with Two or More Drugs

Antituberculosis regimens must always contain two or more drugs to which the infecting organism is sensitive. To understand why this is so, we need to begin with five facts:

- Resistance in *M. tuberculosis* occurs because of spontaneous mutations.
- Each mutational event confers resistance to only one drug.
- Mutations conferring resistance to a single drug occur in about 1 of every 100 million (10^8) bacteria.
- The bacterial burden in active tuberculosis is well above 10^8 organisms but far below 10^{16}.
- *M. tuberculosis* grows slowly, hence treatment is prolonged.

Now, let's assume we initiate therapy with a single drug, and that all bacteria in our patient are sensitive at the start of treatment. What will happen? Over time, at least one of the more than 10^8 bacteria in our patient will mutate to a resistant form. Hence, as we proceed with treatment, we will kill all sensitive bacteria, but the descendants of the newly resistant bacterium will continue to flourish, thereby causing treatment failure. In contrast, if we initiate therapy with *two* drugs, treatment will succeed. Why? Because failure would require that at least one bacterium undergo *two* resistance-conferring mutations, one for each drug. Since two such mutations occur in only 1 of every 10^{16} bacteria (10^{16} is the product of the probabilities for each mutation), and since the total bacterial load is much less than 10^{16}, the chances of the two events occurring in one of the bacteria in our patient are nil.

Not only do drug combinations decrease the risk of resistance, combination therapy can reduce the incidence of relapse. Because some drugs (e.g., isoniazid, rifampin) are especially effective against actively dividing bacilli, whereas other drugs (e.g., pyrazinamide) are most active against intracellular (quiescent) bacilli, by using certain combinations of antituberculosis agents, we can increase the chances of killing all tubercle bacilli present, whether they are actively multiplying or dormant. Hence, the risk of relapse is lowered.

In Chapter 79 (Basic Principles of Antimicrobial Therapy), we noted that treatment with multiple antibiotics broadens the spectrum of antimicrobial coverage, thereby increasing the risk of suprainfection. This is not the case with multiple drug therapy of tuberculosis. The major drugs used against *M. tuberculosis* are *selective* for this organism. As a result, these drugs, even when used in combination, do not kill off other microorganisms, and therefore do not create the conditions that lead to suprainfection.

In summary, because treatment is prolonged, there is a high risk that drug-resistant bacilli will emerge if only one antituberculosis agent is employed. Because the chances of a bacterium developing resistance to two drugs are very low, treatment with two or more drugs minimizes the risk of drug resistance. Accordingly, when treating tuberculosis, we must always use two or more drugs to which the organism is sensitive.

Determining Drug Sensitivity

Because resistance to one or more antituberculosis drugs is common, and because many patterns of resistance are possible, it is essential that we determine drug sensitivity in isolates from each patient at the onset of treatment. Unfortunately, sensitivity tests often take several weeks to complete. Until test results are available, drug selection must be empiric, based on patterns of drug resistance in the community and the immunocompetence of the patient. However, once test results are available, the regimen should be adjusted accordingly. In the event of treatment failure, sensitivity tests should be repeated.

Treatment Regimens

A variety of regimens are employed for active tuberculosis. Drug selection is based largely on the susceptibility of the infecting organism and the immunocompetence of the host. Therapy is usually initiated with a *four-drug* regimen; isoniazid and rifampin are almost always included. In the event of suspected or proved resistance, more drugs are added; the total may be as high as seven. Representative regimens are shown in Table 86–1 and discussed below.

Treatment can be divided into two phases. The goal of the initial phase (induction phase) is to eliminate actively dividing extracellular tubercle bacilli, and thereby render the sputum noninfectious. The goal of the second phase (continuation phase) is to eliminate intracellular "persisters."

Drug-Sensitive Tubercle Bacilli. If the infecting organism is not resistant to isoniazid or rifampin, treatment can be relatively simple. The regimen employed most frequently is summarized in Table 86–1. As indicated, the induction phase, which lasts 2 months, consists of daily therapy with four drugs: *isoniazid, rifampin, pyrazinamide,* and *ethambutol*. The continuation phase, which lasts 4 months, consists of daily or biweekly therapy with just two drugs: *isoniazid* and *rifampin*. Note that the entire course of treatment is prolonged, making compliance a significant problem.

Multidrug-Resistant Tubercle Bacilli. Multidrug resistance is defined as resistance to at least isoniazid and rifampin. Treatment requires at least three drugs to which the organism is sensitive, and should continue for 12 to 24 months after sputum conversion. Initial therapy may consist of five, six, or even seven drugs. Hence, an initial regimen might include (1) isoniazid; (2) rifampin; (3) pyrazinamide; (4) ethambutol; (5) kanamycin, amikacin, or capreomycin; (6) ciprofloxacin or ofloxacin; and (7) cycloserine, ethionamide, or *para*-aminosalicylic acid.

TABLE 86–1 ■ Representative Antituberculosis Regimens

Drug Resistance	HIV-Negative Patients*	HIV-Positive Patients*	Interaction with Drugs for HIV Infection
None	*Induction Phase:* IRPE for 2 months *Continuation Phase:* IR for 4 months	*Induction Phase:* IRPE for 2 months *Continuation Phase:* IR for 4–7 months OR	Protease inhibitors and NNRTIs cannot be used with rifampin.
		Induction Phase: IPE + rifabutin for 2 months *Continuation Phase:* I + rifabutin for 4–7 months	Rifabutin can be used with two protease inhibitors (indinavir, nelfinavir) but not with saquinavir, ritonavir, or NNRTIs.
Isoniazid resistance	RPE for 6 months	RPE for 6–9 months OR PE + rifabutin for 6–9 months	Protease inhibitors and NNRTIs cannot be used with rifampin. Rifabutin can be used with indinavir and nelfinavir but not with saquinavir, ritonavir, or NNRTIs.
Rifampin resistance	IPE for 18–24 months	IPE for 18–24 months OR *Induction Phase:* IPSE for 2 months *Continuation Phase:* IPS for 7–10 months	All drugs for HIV infection can be used. All drugs for HIV infection can be used.

*Drugs used in these regimens: E = ethambutol, I = isoniazid, P = pyrazinamide, R = rifampin, S = streptomycin.
NNRTI = non-nucleoside reverse transcriptase inhibitor.

Therapy in Patients with HIV Infection. Between 2% and 20% of patients with HIV infection develop active tuberculosis. Because of their reduced ability to fight infection, these patients require more aggressive therapy than do immunocompetent patients. As a rule, treatment should last several months longer than in HIV-negative patients.

Drug interactions are a big problem. Two important drugs for tuberculosis—rifampin and rifabutin—can accelerate the metabolism of antiretroviral drugs (i.e., drugs used to fight HIV), and can thereby decrease their effects. Specifically, rifampin and rifabutin can decrease the effects of (1) protease inhibitors (the most effective drugs we have against HIV) and (2) non-nucleoside reverse transcriptase inhibitors (NNRTIs). Accordingly, it is best to avoid combining rifampin and rifabutin with these agents. Unfortunately, this means that patients will be denied optimal treatment for one of their infections. That is, if they take rifampin or rifabutin to treat tuberculosis, they will be unable to take protease inhibitors or NNRTIs for HIV. Conversely, if they take protease inhibitors and NNRTIs to treat HIV, they will be unable to take rifampin or rifabutin for tuberculosis. This dilemma does not have an easy solution.

Duration of Treatment

The ideal duration of treatment has not been established. For patients with drug-sensitive tuberculosis, the minimum duration is 6 months. For patients with multidrug-resistant infection, and for patients with HIV or AIDS, treatment may last as long as 24 months after sputum cultures have become negative.

Directly Observed Therapy

In directly observed therapy (DOT), administration of each dose is done in the presence of an observer, usually a representative of the health department. DOT is now considered the standard of care for tuberculosis. Recall that patients with tuberculosis must take multiple drugs every day for 6 months or more, making compliance a very real problem. The purpose of DOT is to ensure compliance, which, in turn, will accelerate bacterial kill, decrease the risk of disease transmission, and decrease the risk of drug resistance. In addition, DOT permits ongoing evaluation of both the response to treatment and adverse drug effects.

Evaluating Treatment

Three modes are employed to evaluate therapy: bacteriologic evaluation of sputum, clinical evaluation, and chest radiographs.

In patients with positive pretreatment sputum tests, sputum should be evaluated every 2 to 4 weeks initially, and then monthly after sputum cultures become negative. With proper drug selection and good compliance, sputum cultures become negative in over 90% of patients after 3 months of treatment.

Treatment failures should be evaluated for drug resistance and patient compliance. In the absence of demonstrated drug resistance, treatment with the same regimen should continue, using direct observation of drug administration to ensure that medication is being taken as prescribed. In patients with drug-resistant tuberculosis, *two* effective drugs should be added to the regimen.

In patients with negative pretreatment sputum tests, treatment is monitored by chest radiographs and clinical evaluation.

In most patients, clinical manifestations (e.g., fever, malaise, anorexia, cough) should decrease markedly within 2 weeks. The radiograph should show improvement within 3 months.

After completing therapy, patients should be examined every 3 to 6 months for signs and symptoms of relapse.

Diagnosis and Treatment of Latent Tuberculosis

Because latent tuberculosis can progress to active tuberculosis, the condition can pose a threat both to the infected individual and to society. Accordingly, testing and treatment are clearly desirable—but not for everyone: Because treatment of latent tuberculosis is prolonged and carries a risk of drug toxicity, testing and treatment should be limited to people who really need it. In 2000, the American Thoracic Society and the Centers for Disease Control issued revised guidelines—"Targeted Tuberculin Testing and Treatment of Latent Tuberculosis Infection"—that specify who should be tested, who should be treated, and what drugs should be used. The discussion below reflects the new recommendations.

Targeted Tuberculin Skin Testing

How Do We Test for Latent Tuberculosis? The tuberculin skin test is the primary tool used to identify individuals with latent tuberculosis. The test is performed by giving an intradermal injection of a preparation know as *purified protein derivative (PPD)*, an antigen derived from *M. tuberculosis*. If the individual has an intact immune system and has been exposed to *M. tuberculosis* in the past, the PPD will elicit a local immune response. The test is read 48 to 72 hours after the injection. A positive reaction is indicated by a region of induration (hardness) around the injection site.

Who Should Be Tested? Testing should be limited to people who are at high risk of either (1) having acquired the infection recently or (2) progression from latent tuberculosis to active tuberculosis. Included in this group are people with HIV infection, people receiving immunosuppressive drugs, recent contacts of tuberculosis patients, and people with high-risk medical conditions, such as diabetes mellitus, silicosis, or chronic renal failure. A complete list of candidates for testing is given in Table 86–2. Routine testing of low-risk individuals is not recommended.

Interpreting the Results: Who Should Be Treated? The decision to treat latent tuberculosis is based on the risk category of the individual and the size of the region of induration produced by the tuberculin test (Table 86–3). For individuals at high risk, treatment is recommended if the region of induration is relatively small (5 mm or larger). For individuals at moderate risk, treatment is indicated when the region of induration is larger (10 mm or more). And for individuals at low risk (who should not be routinely tested), the region must be larger still (15 mm or more) to justify treatment.

Treatment of Latent Tuberculosis

Isoniazid has been the treatment of choice for latent tuberculosis for over 30 years, and remains so today. The drug is effective, relatively safe, and inexpensive. However, isoniazid does have two drawbacks. First, to be effective, treatment must continue a long time—at least 6 months and preferably 9 months. Second, isoniazid poses a risk of liver damage. Be-

TABLE 86–2 ■ Candidates for Targeted Tuberculin Skin Testing

Individuals at High Risk of Recent Tuberculosis Infection

Contacts of tuberculosis patients

Residents and staff of high-risk congregate settings:
- Prisons and jails
- Nursing homes
- Hospitals and other healthcare facilities
- Homeless shelters
- Residential facilities for patients with AIDS

Persons who, in the last 5 years, immigrated from a country where tuberculosis is prevalent

Staff of mycobacteriology laboratories

Children and adolescents exposed to high-risk adults

Children under the age of 4 years

Individuals at High Risk of Progression from Latent to Active Tuberculosis

HIV-infected persons

Intravenous drug abusers

Patients taking immunosuppressive drugs for 1 month or more

Patients with a chest radiograph indicating fibrotic changes consistent with prior tuberculosis

Patients with other high-risk medical conditions, including
- Diabetes mellitus
- Chronic renal failure
- Silicosis
- Leukemia or lymphoma
- Clinical conditions associated with substantial weight loss, including postgastrectomy state, intestinal bypass surgery, chronic peptic ulcer disease, chronic malabsorption syndromes, and carcinomas of the oropharynx and upper GI tract that inhibit adequate nutritional intake

cause of these problems, alternative regimens have been developed (Table 86–4). Unfortunately, although the alternative regimens are of shorter duration, they still pose a risk of liver damage.

Before starting treatment for latent tuberculosis, active tuberculosis must be ruled out. Why? Because latent tuberculosis is treated with just one (or two) drugs, and hence, if active tuberculosis were present, treatment would promote emergence of resistant bacilli. To exclude active disease, the patient should undergo a physical examination and chest radiography; if indicated, bacteriologic studies may also be done.

Isoniazid. Isoniazid is the preferred drug for treating latent tuberculosis in all patients, including those who are HIV positive. Ideally, treatment should continue for 9 months. Treatment for 6 months is an option, but is not as reliable. Two dosing schedules can be used: daily or twice weekly. When twice-weekly dosing is selected, each dose should be administered under direct observation of a healthcare provider (to ensure compliance).

Isoniazid is hepatotoxic. To reduce the risk of liver injury, liver function should be evaluated at the beginning of therapy and every 4 weeks thereafter. If hepatotoxicity develops, isoniazid should be withdrawn.

Short-Course Therapy: Rifampin Plus Pyrazinamide. Two months of daily therapy with rifampin plus pyrazinamide is as effective as 9 months of daily isoniazid. However, although this regimen has the advantage of being short, it is more expensive than isoniazid, and the risk of liver injury is greater (both rifampin and pyrazinamide are hepatotoxic). To reduce the risk of liver injury, patients should be evaluated every 2 weeks, compared with every 4 weeks for those taking isoniazid. As with isoniazid therapy, dosing may

TABLE 86–3 ■ Tuberculin Test Results That Are Considered Positive—and Hence Justify Treatment—in Patients at Low, Moderate, and High Risk of Latent Tuberculosis

Risk Category	Who Is In the Risk Category?	Test Result Considered Positive
High	HIV-positive people Recent contacts of patients with tuberculosis People with fibrotic changes on their chest radiograph consistent with prior tuberculosis People taking immunosuppressive drugs for more than 1 month	≥5 mm of induration
Moderate	Recent immigrants from countries with a high prevalence of tuberculosis Intravenous drug abusers Residents and staff of high-risk congregate settings (e.g., prisons, nursing homes, hospitals, homeless shelters) Mycobacteriology laboratory personnel Persons with high-risk medical conditions (e.g., diabetes mellitus, chronic renal failure, silicosis, leukemia, lymphoma) Children and adolescents exposed to high-risk adults Children under 4 years old	≥10 mm of induration
Low	Persons with no risk factors for tuberculosis	≥15 mm of induration

TABLE 86–4 ■ Options for Treating Latent Tuberculosis Infection

Drugs	Duration (months)	Dosing Schedule	Adult Dosage	Recommendation* HIV⁻	Recommendation* HIV⁺
Isoniazid	9	Daily	5 mg/kg (max 300 mg)	A	A
		Twice weekly†	15 mg/kg (max 900 mg)	B	B
Isoniazid	6	Daily	5 mg/kg (max 300 mg)	B	C
		Twice weekly†	15 mg/kg (max 900 mg)	B	C
Rifampin *and* pyrazinamide	2	Daily	10 mg/kg (max 600 mg) *and* 15–20 mg/kg (max 2 gm)	B	A
	2–3	Twice weekly†	10 mg/kg (max 600 mg) *and* 50 mg/kg (max 4 gm)	C	C
Rifampin	4	Daily	10 mg/kg (max 600 mg)	B	B

*A = preferred treatment; B = acceptable alternative to A; C = offer when A and B cannot be given.
†Twice-weekly dosing should be administered by directly observed therapy.
Data from Centers for Disease Control and Prevention. Targeted tuberculin testing and treatment of latent tuberculosis infection. MMWR Morb Mortal Wkly Rep 2000;49(RR-6):1–54.

be done daily or twice a week; twice-weekly dosing should be done under direct observation of a healthcare provider.

Short-Course Therapy: Rifampin Alone. Four months of daily therapy with rifampin alone is an alternative for patients who cannot take isoniazid or pyrazinamide. Dosing should be done daily. Twice-weekly dosing is not an option.

TUBERCULOSIS II: PHARMACOLOGY OF INDIVIDUAL ANTITUBERCULOSIS DRUGS

Based on their clinical utility, the antituberculosis drugs can be divided into two groups: first-line drugs and second-line drugs. The first-line drugs are *isoniazid, rifampin, rifapentine, rifabutin, pyrazinamide, ethambutol,* and *streptomycin.* Of these, isoniazid and rifampin are the most important. The second-line drugs—*para-aminosalicylic acid, kanamycin, amikacin, capreomycin, ethionamide, cycloserine, ciprofloxacin,* and *ofloxacin*—are generally less effective and more toxic than the primary drugs. The second-line agents are used in combination with the primary drugs to treat disseminated tuberculosis and tuberculosis caused by organisms resistant to first-line drugs. Adverse effects and routes of administration of the antituberculosis drugs are summarized in Table 86–5.

Isoniazid

Isoniazid is the primary agent for treatment and prophylaxis of tuberculosis. This drug is superior to alternative drugs with regard to efficacy, toxicity, ease of use, patient acceptance, and affordability. With the exception of patients who cannot tolerate the drug, isoniazid should be taken by all individuals infected with isoniazid-sensitive strains of *M. tuberculosis.*

Antimicrobial Spectrum and Mechanism of Action

Isoniazid is highly selective for mycobacteria. The drug can kill tubercle bacilli at concentrations 10,000 times lower than those needed to affect gram-positive and gram-negative bacte-ria. Isoniazid is bactericidal to mycobacteria that are actively dividing, but is only bacteriostatic to "resting" organisms.

Although the mechanism by which isoniazid acts is not known with certainty, available data suggest the drug suppresses bacterial growth by inhibiting synthesis of mycolic acid, a component of the mycobacterial cell wall. Since mycolic acid is not produced by other bacteria or by cells of the host, this mechanism would explain why isoniazid is so selective for mycobacteria.

Resistance

Tubercle bacilli can develop resistance to isoniazid during treatment. Acquired resistance results from spontaneous mutation—not from transfer of R factors. The precise mechanism underlying resistance has not been established. Emergence of resistance can be decreased through multiple-drug therapy. Organisms resistant to isoniazid are cross-resistant to ethionamide, but not to other drugs used for tuberculosis.

Pharmacokinetics

Absorption and Distribution. Isoniazid is administered orally and IM. Absorption is good with both routes. Once in the blood, isoniazid is widely distributed to tissues and body fluids. Concentrations in cerebrospinal fluid (CSF) are about 20% of those in plasma.

Metabolism. Isoniazid is inactivated in the liver, primarily by *acetylation.* The ability to acetylate isoniazid is genetically determined: about 50% of people in the United States are *rapid* acetylators and the other 50% are *slow* acetylators. The drug's half-life is about 1 hour in rapid acetylators and 3 hours in slow acetylators. It is important to note that differences in rates of acetylation generally have little impact on the *efficacy* of isoniazid, provided patients are taking the drug daily. However, *nonhepatic toxicities* may be more likely in slow acetylators, because drug accumulation is greater in these patients.

Excretion. Isoniazid is excreted in the urine, primarily as inactive metabolites. In patients who are slow acetylators and who also have renal insufficiency, the drug may accumulate to toxic levels.

Therapeutic Use

Isoniazid is indicated only for treating active and latent tuberculosis. When used for latent tuberculosis, the drug is administered alone. When used for active tuberculosis, it must be taken in combination with at least one other antituberculosis agent (e.g., rifampin).

TABLE 86–5 ■ Antituberculosis Drugs: Routes and Major Adverse Effects

Drug	Route	Major Adverse Effects
First-Line Drugs		
Isoniazid	PO, IM	Hepatotoxicity, peripheral neuritis
Rifampin	PO, IV	Hepatotoxicity
Rifapentine	PO	Hepatotoxicity
Rifabutin	PO	Hepatotoxicity
Pyrazinamide	PO	Hepatotoxicity
Ethambutol	PO	Optic neuritis
Streptomycin	IM	Eighth nerve damage, nephrotoxicity
Second-Line Drugs		
Capreomycin	IM	Eighth nerve damage, nephrotoxicity
Kanamycin	IM, IV	Eighth nerve damage, nephrotoxicity
Amikacin	IM, IV	Eighth nerve damage, nephrotoxicity
Cycloserine	PO	Psychoses, seizure, rash
Ethionamide	PO	GI intolerance, hepatotoxicity
Ciprofloxacin	PO	GI intolerance
Ofloxacin	PO	GI intolerance
p-Aminosalicylic acid	PO	GI intolerance

Adverse Effects

Peripheral Neuropathy. Dose-related peripheral neuropathy is the drug's most common adverse effect. Principal symptoms are symmetric paresthesias (tingling, numbness, burning, pain) of the hands and feet. Clumsiness, unsteadiness, and muscle aches may also develop. Peripheral neuropathy results from isoniazid-induced deficiency in pyridoxine (vitamin B_6). If peripheral neuropathy develops, it can be reversed by administering pyridoxine (50 to 200 mg daily). In patients predisposed to neuropathy (e.g., alcoholics, diabetics), small doses of pyridoxine (6 to 50 mg/day) can be administered with isoniazid as prophylaxis against peripheral neuritis. This practice reduces the risk of neuropathy from 20% down to less than 1%.

Hepatotoxicity. Isoniazid can cause hepatocellular injury and multilobular necrosis. Deaths have occurred. Liver injury is thought to result from production of a toxic isoniazid metabolite. The greatest risk factor for liver damage is advancing age: The incidence of hepatotoxicity is nil in patients under 20 years; 1.2% in those ages 35 to 49, 2.3% in those ages 50 to 64, and 8% in those over 65. Patients should be informed about signs of hepatitis (anorexia, malaise, fatigue, nausea, yellowing of the skin or eyes) and instructed to notify the physician if these develop. Patients should also undergo monthly evaluation for these signs. Some clinicians perform monthly determinations of serum aspartate transaminase (AST) activity, because elevation of AST activity is indicative of liver injury. However, because AST levels may rise and then return to normal, despite continued isoniazid use, increases in AST may not be predictive of clinical hepatitis. It is recommended that isoniazid be withdrawn if signs of hepatitis develop or if AST activity rises to a level 3 times greater than the pretreatment baseline. Caution should be exercised when giving isoniazid to alcoholics and individuals with pre-existing disorders of the liver.

Other Adverse Effects. A variety of *central nervous system (CNS) effects* can occur, including optic neuritis, seizures, dizziness, ataxia, and psychologic disturbances (depression, agitation, impairment of memory, hallucinations, toxic psychosis). *Anemia* may result from isoniazid-induced deficiency in pyridoxine. *GI distress, dry mouth,* and *urinary retention* occur on occasion. *Allergy* to isoniazid can produce fever, rashes, and a syndrome resembling lupus erythematosus.

Drug Interactions

Phenytoin. Isoniazid can interfere with the metabolism of phenytoin, thereby causing the anticonvulsant to accumulate to toxic levels. Signs of phenytoin excess include ataxia and incoordination. Plasma levels of phenytoin should be monitored, and phenytoin dosage should be reduced as appropriate. Dosage of isoniazid should not be changed.

Alcohol, Rifampin, and Pyrazinamide. Daily ingestion of alcohol or concurrent therapy with rifampin or pyrazinamide increases the risk of hepatotoxicity. Patients should be encouraged to reduce or eliminate consumption of alcohol.

Preparations, Dosage, and Administration

Preparations. Isoniazid [Nydrazid] is dispensed in tablets (100 and 300 mg) and a syrup (10 mg/ml) for oral use, and in solution (100 mg/ml in 10-ml vials) for IM injection. Isoniazid is also available in fixed-dose combinations: capsules, sold as *Rifamate,* contain 150 mg of isoniazid and 300 mg of rifampin; and tablets, sold as *Rifater,* contain 50 mg of isoniazid, 120 mg of rifampin, and 300 mg of pyrazinamide.

Oral Dosage. For treatment of *active tuberculosis,* the adult dosage is 5 mg/kg/day or 15 mg/kg twice a week. The pediatric dosage for active tuberculosis is 10 to 20 mg/kg/day or 20 to 40 mg/kg twice a week. For treatment of *latent tuberculosis,* the adult dosage is 300 mg/day and the pediatric dosage is 10 mg/kg/day.

Intramuscular Dosage. Parenteral therapy is administered in critical situations when oral treatment is not possible. The dosage is 300 mg daily.

Rifampin

Rifampin [Rifadin, Rimactane] is equal to isoniazid in importance as an antituberculosis drug. Prior to the appearance of resistant tubercle bacilli, the combination of rifampin plus isoniazid was the most frequently prescribed regimen for uncomplicated pulmonary tuberculosis. Rifampin is a powerful inducer of cytochrome P450 enzymes, and hence can decrease the levels of many other drugs.

Antimicrobial Spectrum

Rifampin is a broad-spectrum antibiotic. The drug is active against most gram-positive bacteria as well as many gram-negative organisms. The drug is bactericidal to *M. tuberculosis* and *M. leprae*. Other bacteria that are highly sensitive include *Neisseria meningitidis, Haemophilus influenzae, Staphylococcus aureus,* and *Legionella* species.

Mechanism of Action and Bacterial Resistance

Rifampin inhibits bacterial DNA-dependent RNA polymerase, and thereby suppresses RNA synthesis and, consequently, protein synthesis. The results are bactericidal. Because mammalian RNA polymerases are not affected by the drug, rifampin is selectively toxic to microbes. Bacterial resistance to rifampin results from production of an altered form of RNA polymerase.

Pharmacokinetics

Absorption and Distribution. Rifampin is well absorbed if taken on an empty stomach. However, if the drug is taken with or shortly after a meal, both the rate and extent of absorption can be significantly reduced. Rifampin is distributed widely to tissues and body fluids, including the CSF. The drug is lipid soluble, and hence has ready access to intracellular bacteria.

Elimination. Rifampin is eliminated primarily by hepatic metabolism. Only about 20% of the drug leaves in the urine. Rifampin induces hepatic drug-metabolizing enzymes, including those responsible for its own inactivation. As a result, the rate at which rifampin is metabolized increases over the first weeks of therapy, causing the half-life of the drug to decrease—from an initial value of about 4 hours down to 2 hours at the end of 2 weeks.

Therapeutic Use

Tuberculosis. Rifampin is one of our most effective antituberculosis drugs. This agent is bactericidal to tubercle bacilli at extracellular and intracellular sites. Rifampin is a drug of choice for treating pulmonary tuberculosis and disseminated disease. Because resistance can develop rapidly when rifampin is employed alone, the drug is always employed in combination with at least one other antituberculosis agent. Despite the capacity of rifampin to produce a variety of adverse effects, toxicity rarely requires discontinuation of treatment.

Leprosy. Rifampin is bactericidal to *M. leprae* and has become an important agent for the treatment of leprosy (see below under *Drugs for Leprosy [Hansen's Disease]*).

Meningococcus Carriers. Rifampin is highly active against *Neisseria meningitidis* and is indicated for short-term therapy to eliminate this bacterium from the nasopharynx of asymptomatic carriers. Because resistant organisms emerge rapidly, rifampin should not be used to treat active meningococcal disease.

Adverse Effects

Rifampin is generally well tolerated. When employed at recommended dosages, the drug rarely causes significant toxicity. The most common adverse effect of concern is hepatitis.

Hepatotoxicity. Rifampin is toxic to the liver and may cause jaundice and even hepatitis. Asymptomatic elevation of liver enzymes occurs in about 14% of patients. However, the incidence of overt hepatitis is less than 1%. Hepatotoxicity is most likely in alcoholics and patients with pre-existing liver disease. These individuals should be monitored closely for signs of liver dysfunction. Tests of liver function (serum transaminase levels) should be made prior to treatment and every 2 to 4 weeks thereafter. Patients should be informed about signs of hepatitis (jaundice, anorexia, malaise, fatigue, nausea) and instructed to notify the physician if these develop.

Discoloration of Body Fluids. Rifampin frequently imparts a red-orange color to urine, sweat, saliva, and tears. Patients should be forewarned of this harmless effect. Permanent staining of soft contact lenses has occurred on occasion; the patient should consult an ophthalmologist regarding the advisability of contact lens use.

Other Adverse Effects. *Gastrointestinal disturbances* (anorexia, nausea, abdominal discomfort) and *cutaneous reactions* (flushing, itching, rash) occur occasionally. Rarely, intermittent high-dose therapy has produced a *flu-like syndrome,* characterized by fever, chills, muscle aches, headache, and dizziness. This reaction appears to have an immunologic basis. In some patients, high-dose therapy has been associated with *shortness of breath, hemolytic anemia, shock,* and *acute renal failure*.

Drug Interactions

Accelerated Metabolism of Other Drugs. Because rifampin induces cytochrome P450 enzymes, it can hasten the metabolism of many drugs, thereby reducing their effects. This interaction is of special concern with *oral contraceptives, warfarin* (an anticoagulant), and certain drugs for HIV infection: *protease inhibitors* and *NNRTIs*. Because of this potential interaction, protease inhibitors and NNRTIs should not be used with rifampin. Women taking oral contraceptives should consider a nonhormonal form of birth control. The dosage of warfarin may need to be increased.

Isoniazid and Pyrazinamide. Rifampin, isoniazid, and pyrazinamide are all hepatotoxic. Hence, when these drugs are used in combination, as they often are, the risk of liver injury is greater than when they are used alone.

Preparations, Dosage, and Administration

Preparations. Rifampin [Rifadin, Rimactane] is dispensed in capsules (150 and 300 mg) for oral administration. Oral rifampin is also available in two fixed-dose combinations: capsules, sold as *Rifamate,* contain 300 mg of rifampin and 150 mg of isoniazid; and tablets, sold as *Rifater,* contain 120 mg of rifampin, 50 mg of isoniazid, and 300 mg of pyrazinamide.

Rifampin [Rifadin] is available in powdered form to be reconstituted for IV infusion.

Oral Dosage and Administration. For treatment of tuberculosis, the usual adult dosage is 600 mg or 10 mg/kg daily. The pediatric dosage is 10 to 20 mg/kg/day. Rifampin is administered as a single daily dose 1 hour before meals or 2 hours after. Because rifampin is eliminated by hepatic metabolism, patients with liver impairment require a reduction in dosage. No change in dosage is needed in patients with kidney disease.

Intravenous Administration. Dissolve 600 mg of powdered rifampin in 10 ml of Sterile Water for Injection to make a concentrated solution (60 mg/ml). Dilute an appropriate dose of the concentrate in 500 ml of 5% dextrose and infuse over 3 hours.

Rifapentine

Rifapentine [Priftin] is a long-acting analog of rifampin. Both drugs have the same mechanism of action, adverse effects, and drug interactions. The principal difference between them is their dosing schedules: Whereas rifampin must be taken every day, rifapentine is taken just twice a week. Rifapentine is the first new drug for tuberculosis in over 25 years.

Actions and Uses. Rifapentine is indicated only for pulmonary tuberculosis. At therapeutic doses, the drug is lethal to *M. tuberculosis*. The mechanism underlying cell kill is inhibition of DNA-dependent RNA polymerase. To minimize emergence of resistance, rifapentine must always be combined with at least one other antituberculosis drug.

Pharmacokinetics. Rifapentine is well absorbed from the GI tract, especially in the presence of food. Plasma levels peak 5 to 6 hours after administration. In the liver, rifapentine undergoes conversion to 25-desacetyl rifapentine, an active metabolite. Excretion is primarily (70%) in the feces. Rifapentine and its metabolite have the same half-life—about 13 hours.

Adverse Effects. Rifapentine is well tolerated at recommended doses. Like rifampin, the drug imparts a red-orange color to urine, sweat, saliva, and tears. Permanent staining of contact lenses can occur.

Hepatotoxicity is the principal concern. In clinical trials, serum transaminase levels increased in 5% of patients. However, overt hepatitis occurred in only one patient. Because of the risk of hepatotoxicity, liver function tests (bilirubin, serum transaminases) should be performed at baseline and monthly thereafter. Patients should be informed about signs of hepatitis (jaundice, anorexia, malaise, fatigue, nausea) and instructed to notify the physician if these develop.

Drug Interactions. Like rifampin, rifapentine is a powerful inducer of cytochrome P450 drug-metabolizing enzymes. As a result, it can decrease the levels of other drugs. Important among these are *protease inhibitors* and *NNRTIs* (used for HIV infection), *oral contraceptives,* and *warfarin* (an anticoagulant).

Preparation, Dosage, and Administration. Rifapentine [Priftin] is available in 150-mg tablets for oral use. For the first 2 months, the dosage is 600 mg twice a week (with at least 3 days between doses). For the next 4 months, the dosage is 600 mg once a week. Like all other drugs for tuberculosis, rifapentine must always be combined with at least one other antituberculosis agent.

Rifabutin

Actions and Use. Rifabutin [Mycobutin] is a close chemical relative of rifampin. Like rifampin, rifabutin inhibits mycobacterial DNA-dependent RNA polymerase, and thereby suppresses protein synthesis. The drug is approved for prevention of disseminated *M. avium* complex (MAC) disease in patients with advanced HIV infection (CD4 lymphocyte counts below 200 cells/mm^3). In addition to this approved application, rifabutin is used to treat active MAC disease and tuberculosis in patients with HIV infection.

Pharmacokinetics. Rifabutin is administered orally. Absorption is unaffected by food. Peak plasma levels are reached in 2 to 3 hours. The drug is widely distributed and achieves high concentrations in the lungs. Rifabutin is metabolized in the liver and excreted in the urine, bile, and feces. Its half-life is 45 hours.

Adverse Effects. Rifabutin is generally well tolerated. The most common side effects are rash (4%), GI disturbances (3%), and neutropenia (2%). Like rifampin, rifabutin can impart a harmless red-orange color to urine, sweat, saliva, and tears; soft contact lenses may be permanently stained. Rifabutin poses a risk of uveitis, and hence should be discontinued if ocular pain or blurred vision develops. Other adverse effects include myositis, hepatitis, arthralgia, chest pain with dyspnea, and a flu-like syndrome.

Drug Interactions. Like rifampin, rifabutin *induces cytochrome P450 enzymes,* although not as strongly. By increasing enzyme activity, rifabutin can decrease blood levels of other drugs, especially *oral contraceptives, protease inhibitors,* and *NNRTIs.* In patients being treated for HIV infection, rifabutin can be combined with two protease inhibitors—indinavir and nelfinavir—but not with saquinavir, ritonavir, or NNRTIs. Women using oral contraceptives should be advised to use a nonhormonal method of birth control.

Preparations, Dosage, and Administration. Rifabutin [Mycobutin] is dispensed in 150-mg capsules for oral administration. The usual dosage is 300 mg once a day. To reduce GI upset, an alternative dosing schedule of 150 mg twice daily may be used.

Pyrazinamide
Antimicrobial Activity and Therapeutic Use

Pyrazinamide is bactericidal to *M. tuberculosis.* The mechanism of antibacterial action is unknown. Currently, the combination of pyrazinamide with rifampin, isoniazid, and ethambutol is a preferred regimen for initial therapy of active tuberculosis caused by nonresistant bacteria. In addition, pyrazinamide, in combination with rifampin, is used for short-course therapy of latent tuberculosis.

Pharmacokinetics

Pyrazinamide is well absorbed following oral administration and is widely distributed to tissues and body fluids. In the liver, the drug is converted to pyrazinoic acid, an active metabolite, and then to 5-hydroxypyrazinoic acid, which is inactive. Excretion is renal, primarily as inactive metabolites.

Adverse Effects and Interactions

Hepatotoxicity. Liver injury is the principal adverse effect. High-dose therapy has caused hepatitis, and, rarely, fatal hepatic necrosis. Fortunately, these reactions are relatively uncommon with the low-dose, short-term therapy employed today. The earliest manifestations of liver damage are elevations in serum levels of transaminases (aspartate aminotransferase [AST] and alanine aminotransferase [ALT]). Levels of these enzymes should be measured prior to treatment and every 2 weeks thereafter. Patients should be informed about signs of hepatitis (e.g., malaise, anorexia, nausea, vomiting, yellowish discoloration of the skin and eyes) and instructed to notify the physician if these develop. Pyrazinamide should be discontinued if significant injury to the liver occurs. The drug should not be used by patients with pre-existing liver dysfunction.

The risk of liver injury is increased by concurrent therapy with isoniazid or rifampin, both of which are hepatotoxic. Pyrazinamide plus rifampin should not be used by patients with pre-existing liver disease or by those with previous hepatotoxicity from isoniazid.

Other Adverse Effects. Pyrazinamide and its metabolites can inhibit renal excretion of uric acid, thereby causing *hyperuricemia;* although usually asymptomatic, pyrazinamide-induced hyperuricemia has resulted in *gouty arthritis* rarely. Additional adverse effects include *arthralgia, GI disturbances* (nausea, vomiting, diarrhea), *rashes,* and *photosensitivity.*

Preparations, Dosage, and Administration

Pyrazinamide is dispensed in 500-mg tablets for oral administration. The usual dosage for adults and children is 15 to 30 mg/kg once a day. The maximum daily dosage should not exceed 2 gm. Pyrazinamide is also available in a fixed-dose combination with isoniazid and rifampin, sold under the trade name *Rifater.*

Ethambutol
Antimicrobial Action

Ethambutol [Myambutol] is active only against mycobacteria; nearly all strains of *M. tuberculosis* are sensitive. The drug is bacteriostatic, not bactericidal. Ethambutol is usually active against tubercle bacilli that are resistant to isoniazid and rifampin. Although we know that ethambutol can suppress incorporation of mycolic acid in the cell wall, the precise mechanism by which the drug suppresses bacterial growth has not been established.

Therapeutic Use

Ethambutol is an important antituberculosis drug. This agent is employed for initial treatment of tuberculosis and for treating patients who have received therapy previously. Like other drugs for tuberculosis, ethambutol is always employed as part of a multidrug regimen.

Pharmacokinetics

Ethambutol is readily absorbed following oral administration. The drug is widely distributed to most tissues and body fluids; levels in CSF, however, remain low. Ethambutol undergoes little hepatic metabolism and is excreted primarily in the urine. In patients with normal kidney function, the drug's half-life is 3 to 4 hours; the half-life increases to 8 hours in patients with renal impairment.

Adverse Effects

Ethambutol is generally well tolerated. The only significant adverse effect is optic neuritis.

Optic Neuritis. Ethambutol can produce dose-related optic neuritis, resulting in blurred vision, constriction of the visual field, and disturbance of color discrimination. The mechanism underlying these effects is unknown. Symptoms usually resolve upon discontinuation of treatment. However, for some patients, visual disturbance may persist. Color discrimination and visual acuity should be assessed prior to treatment and monthly thereafter. Patients should be advised to report any alteration in vision. If ocular toxicity develops, ethambutol should be withdrawn immediately. Because visual changes can be difficult to monitor in pediatric patients, ethambutol is not recommended for children less than 8 years old.

Other Adverse Effects. Ethambutol can produce *allergic reactions* (dermatitis, pruritus), *GI upset*, and *confusion*. The drug inhibits renal excretion of uric acid, causing *asymptomatic hyperuricemia* in about 50% of patients; occasionally, elevation of uric acid levels results in *acute gouty arthritis*. Rare adverse effects include *peripheral neuropathy, renal damage*, and *thrombocytopenia*.

Preparations, Dosage, and Administration

Ethambutol [Myambutol] is dispensed in 100- and 400-mg tablets for oral administration. For initial therapy of tuberculosis, the usual dosage for adults and children is 15 to 25 mg/kg once a day. For re-treatment therapy, the usual dosage is 25 mg/kg/day for the first 60 days and 15 mg/kg/day thereafter. Ethambutol may be taken with food if GI upset occurs.

Streptomycin

Streptomycin, an aminoglycoside antibiotic, was our first effective antituberculosis drug. The basic pharmacology of streptomycin and the other aminoglycosides is discussed in Chapter 83. Consideration here is limited to treatment of tuberculosis.

Antibacterial Activity. Streptomycin is bactericidal to tubercle bacilli *in vitro;* however, the drug has relatively low sterilizing activity *in vivo.* This discrepancy is explained by the inability of streptomycin to penetrate mammalian cells; because tubercle bacilli are frequently present at intracellular sites, many escape exposure to the drug.

Adverse Effects. The most characteristic toxicity is *injury to the eighth cranial nerve, resulting in hearing loss and disturbance of balance.* However, when the drug is prescribed properly, effects on auditory and vestibular function are rare. The risk of eighth nerve toxicity is increased by advanced age and kidney dysfunction. Tests of hearing and balance should be performed periodically during the course of treatment. Special care should be taken to adjust the dosage in patients with renal impairment. Additional adverse effects include *nephrotoxicity, facial paresthesias*, and *rash.*

Therapeutic Status, Dosage, and Administration. Streptomycin must be administered by IM injection. Because it cannot be used orally, and because of its potential for eighth nerve toxicity, streptomycin is considerably less attractive than the newer antituberculosis drugs (rifampin, isoniazid, pyrazinamide, ethambutol) for initial treatment. Accordingly, use of this once-popular agent has declined sharply. Today, streptomycin is employed primarily in three-drug regimens for chemotherapy of severe mycobacterial infection. The usual adult dosage is 15 mg/kg/day. The recommended dosage for children is 20 to 40 mg/kg/day.

Second-Line Antituberculosis Drugs

The group of second-line antituberculosis drugs consists of *para-aminosalicylic acid (PAS), kanamycin, capreomycin, ethionamide, cycloserine, ofloxacin,* and *ciprofloxacin.* In general, these drugs are less effective and more toxic than the first-line drugs. As a result, their principal indication is tuberculosis caused by organisms that have proved resistant to first-line agents. In addition, second-line drugs are used to treat severe pulmonary tuberculosis as well as disseminated (extrapulmonary) infection. The second-line drugs are always employed in conjunction with a major antituberculosis drug. Principal toxicities are summarized in Table 86-5.

*Para-*Aminosalicylic Acid

Actions and Uses. PAS is similar in structure and actions to the sulfonamides. Like the sulfonamides, PAS exerts its antibacterial effects by inhibiting synthesis of folic acid. However, in contrast to the sulfonamides, which are broad-spectrum antibiotics, PAS is active only against mycobacteria. In the United States, PAS has been employed primarily as a substitute for ethambutol in pediatric patients. The drug is always used in combination with other antituberculosis agents.

Pharmacokinetics. PAS is administered orally and is well absorbed from the GI tract. The drug is distributed widely to most tissues and body fluids, although levels in CSF remain low. PAS undergoes extensive hepatic metabolism. Metabolites and parent drug are excreted in the urine.

Adverse Effects. PAS is poorly tolerated by adults; children accept the drug somewhat better. The most frequent adverse effects are GI disturbances (nausea, vomiting, diarrhea). Because PAS is administered in large doses as a sodium salt, substantial sodium loading may occur. Additional adverse effects are allergic reactions, hepatotoxicity, and goiter.

Preparations, Dosage, and Administration. Aminosalicylate sodium [Sodium P.A.S.] is dispensed in 500-mg tablets for oral administration. Tablets that are discolored (brown, purple) should not be used. The drug loses its effectiveness if exposed to sunlight, extreme heat, or moisture. Accordingly, it should not be stored in kitchen or bathroom cabinets. If stomach upset occurs, PAS may be administered with food. The daily dosage for adults is 14 to 16 gm in two or three divided doses. The daily dosage for children is 275 to 420 mg/kg in three to four divided doses.

Ethionamide

Actions and Uses. Ethionamide [Trecator-SC], a relative of isoniazid, is active against mycobacteria, but less so than isoniazid. Ethionamide is administered with other antituberculosis drugs to treat tuberculosis that is resistant to first-line agents. Gastrointestinal disturbances limit patient acceptance. Ethionamide is the least well tolerated of all antituberculosis agents, and hence should be used only when there are no alternatives.

Pharmacokinetics. Ethionamide is readily absorbed following oral administration. The drug is widely distributed to tissues and body fluids, including the CSF. Ethionamide undergoes extensive metabolism and is excreted in the urine, primarily as metabolites.

Adverse Effects. Gastrointestinal effects (anorexia, nausea, vomiting, diarrhea, metallic taste) occur often; intolerance of these effects frequently leads to discontinuation. Ethionamide is toxic to the liver. Hepatotoxicity is assessed by measuring serum transaminases (AST, ALT) prior to treatment and periodically thereafter. Additional adverse effects include peripheral neuropathy, CNS effects (convulsions, mental disturbance), and allergic reactions.

Preparations, Dosage, and Administration. Ethionamide [Trecator-SC] is dispensed in 250-mg tablets for oral administration. The usual adult dosage is 0.5 to 1 gm/day in divided doses. The recommended pediatric dosage is 15 to 20 mg/kg/day (maximum of 1 gm).

Cycloserine

Actions and Uses. Cycloserine [Seromycin Pulvules] is an antibiotic produced by a species of *Streptomyces.* The drug is bacteriostatic and acts by inhibiting cell wall synthesis. Cycloserine is used for tuberculosis resistant to first-line drugs.

Pharmacokinetics. Cycloserine is rapidly absorbed following oral administration. The drug is widely distributed to tissues and body fluids, including the CSF. Elimination is by hepatic metabolism and renal excretion; about 50% of the drug leaves the body unchanged in the urine. Cycloserine may accumulate to toxic levels in patients with renal impairment.

Adverse Effects. CNS effects occur frequently and can be severe. Possible reactions include anxiety, depression, confusion, hallucinations, paranoia, hyperreflexia, and seizures. Psychotic episodes occur in approximately 10% of patients; symptoms usually subside within 2 weeks following drug withdrawal. Pyridoxine may prevent neurotoxic effects. Other adverse effects include peripheral neuropathy, hepatotoxicity, and folate deficiency. To minimize the risk of adverse effects, serum concentrations of cycloserine should be measured regularly; peak concentrations, measured 2 hours after dosing, should be 25 to 35 µg/ml.

Preparations, Dosage, and Administration. Cycloserine [Seromycin Pulvules] is dispensed in 250-mg capsules for oral administration. The initial dosage for adults is 250 mg twice daily for 2 weeks; the maintenance dosage is 500 mg to 1 gm daily in divided doses. The dosage for children is 10 to 20 mg/kg/day.

Capreomycin

Capreomycin [Capastat Sulfate] is an antibiotic derived from a species of *Streptomyces*. Antibacterial effects probably result from inhibiting protein synthesis. The drug is bacteriostatic to *M. tuberculosis*. Capreomycin is used only for tuberculosis resistant to primary agents. The drug's principal toxicity is renal damage, and hence it should not be taken by patients with kidney disease. Capreomycin may also cause eighth nerve damage, resulting in hearing loss, tinnitus, and disturbance of balance. Administration is by deep IM injection (the drug is not absorbed from the GI tract, and therefore cannot be administered PO). The usual adult dosage is 1 gm/day for 60 to 120 days, followed by 1-gm doses 2 to 3 times a week. The pediatric dosage is 15 mg/kg/day (up to a maximum of 1 gm).

Kanamycin and Amikacin

Kanamycin [Kantrex, others] and amikacin [Amikin] are aminoglycoside antibiotics that have good activity against *M. tuberculosis*. Like streptomycin and other aminoglycosides, kanamycin and amikacin are nephrotoxic and may damage the eighth cranial nerve. Neither drug is absorbed from the GI tract, and hence administration is parenteral (IM or IV). The adult dosage for both drugs is 15 mg/kg/day; the pediatric dosage is 15 to 30 mg/kg/day. The pharmacology of kanamycin, amikacin, and the other aminoglycosides is discussed in Chapter 83.

Ofloxacin and Ciprofloxacin

Ofloxacin [Floxin] and ciprofloxacin [Cipro] are fluoroquinolone antibiotics indicated for a wide variety of bacterial infections (see Chapter 87). Both drugs have good activity against *M. tuberculosis*. As therapy for tuberculosis, these agents are reserved for infection caused by multidrug-resistant organisms. Both agents are generally well tolerated, although GI disturbances are relatively common. Tendon rupture occurs rarely. The adult dosage for ofloxacin is 600 to 800 mg daily, given in one or two doses. The adult dosage for ciprofloxacin is 500 to 750 mg twice a day. Neither drug is recommended for children.

DRUGS FOR LEPROSY (HANSEN'S DISEASE)

Leprosy is a chronic infectious disease caused by *M. leprae*, an acid-fast bacillus. The disease was first described by G. A. Hansen in 1873. Left untreated, leprosy can cause grotesque disfiguration. Fortunately, with the drugs available today, most patients can be cured. As a result, the worldwide incidence of leprosy has declined dramatically—from an estimated 12 million cases in the mid-1980s to only 738,284 registered cases in 2000. In the United States, only 91 new cases were reported in 2000, and these occurred primarily among immigrants from endemic areas (e.g., India, Brazil, Indonesia).

Infection with *M. leprae* affects the skin, peripheral nerves, and mucous membranes of the upper respiratory tract. Characteristic features are (1) skin lesions with local loss of sensation, (2) thickening of peripheral nerves, and (3) acid-fast bacilli in smears from skin lesions.

Leprosy is divided into two main classes: (1) paucibacillary (PB) leprosy and (2) multibacillary (MB) leprosy. Classification is based on clinical manifestations and the presence of *M. leprae* in skin smears. If skin smears are negative, the diagnosis is PB leprosy. Conversely, if any smear is positive, the diagnosis is MB leprosy. In many places, microbiologic analysis of skin smears is either unavailable or unreliable. Hence, in these places, classification must be based on clinical findings alone. In this case, if the patient has one to five skin lesions, the diagnosis is PB leprosy; if the patient has six or more skin lesions, the diagnosis is MB leprosy. The distinction between PB leprosy and MB leprosy is important because treatment differs for the two forms.

Overview of Treatment

As with tuberculosis, the cornerstone of treatment is multidrug therapy. If just one drug is used, resistance will occur. Most regimens include *rifampin,* the most effective drug for killing *M. leprae*. For patients with *MB leprosy,* the World Health Organization (WHO) recommends 12 months of treatment with three drugs: rifampin, dapsone, and clofazimine. For patients with *PB leprosy,* WHO recommends 6 months of treatment with two drugs: rifampin and dapsone. For patients with *single-lesion PB leprosy* (i.e., PB leprosy with just one skin lesion), WHO recommends a single dose of the "ROM" regimen: rifampin, ofloxacin, and minocycline. With all three regimens, the relapse rate is very low (about 0.1%). Accordingly, all three are considered curative. Specific dosages for these regimens are summarized in Table 86–6.

Pharmacology of Individual Antileprosy Drugs
Rifampin

The basic pharmacology of rifampin [Rifadin, Rimactane] is discussed above under *Tuberculosis II: Pharmacology of Individual Antituberculosis Drugs*. Discussion here is limited to its use in leprosy.

Rifampin is by far our most effective agent for treating leprosy. In fact, the drug is more effective than any *combination* of other agents. A single dose kills more than 99.9% of viable *M. leprae*. After three monthly doses, less than 0.001% of the initial *M. leprae* population remains. Because of its powerful bactericidal actions, rifampin is a key component of standard antileprosy regimens.

The dosage currently recommended by WHO is 600 mg *once a month*. In the past, rifampin was administered daily. However, we now know that monthly administration is just as effective as daily administration. Moreover, monthly administration is much less expensive and minimizes adverse effects, including hepatotoxicity. Resistance can occur if rifampin is used alone. Accordingly, the drug is always combined with other antileprosy agents (e.g., dapsone plus clofazimine).

Dapsone

Actions and Uses. Dapsone is weakly bactericidal to *M. leprae*. The drug is safe, inexpensive, and moderately effective. Dapsone is chemically related to the sulfonamides and shares their mechanism of action: inhibition of folic acid synthesis. Although once employed alone to treat leprosy, dapsone is now employed in combination with other antileprosy drugs, usually rifampin and clofazimine.

Pharmacokinetics. Dapsone is absorbed rapidly and nearly completely from the GI tract. Once in the blood, the drug is widely distributed to tissues and body fluids. Dapsone undergoes hepatic metabolism followed by excretion in the urine. Its average half-life is 28 hours.

Adverse Effects. Dapsone is generally well tolerated. The drug has been taken for years without significant untoward effects. The most common adverse effects are GI disturbances, headache, rash, and a syndrome that resembles mononucleosis. Hemolytic anemia occurs occasionally; severe reactions are usually limited to patients with profound glucose-6-phosphate dehydrogenase deficiency. Rare reactions include agranulocytosis, exfoliative dermatitis, and hepatitis.

Preparations, Dosage, and Administration. Dapsone is dispensed in 25- and 100-mg tablets for oral administration. The usual dosage for adults is 100 mg/day. The dosage for children is 1 mg/kg/day. To prevent emergence of resistance, dapsone is always combined with another antileprosy drug (e.g., rifampin, clofazimine).

Clofazimine

Actions and Uses. Clofazimine [Lamprene] is slowly bactericidal to *M. leprae*. Its mechanism of action is unknown. To prevent emergence of resistance, clofazimine is always combined with another antileprosy drug (e.g., rifampin, dapsone). In addition to its antibacterial action, clofazimine has anti-inflammatory actions.

Pharmacokinetics. Clofazimine is administered orally and undergoes partial absorption. Absorbed drug is retained in fatty tissue and the skin. Because of tissue retention, the half-life of clofazimine is extremely long—about 70 days.

Adverse Effects. Clofazimine is very safe. Dangerous reactions are rare. GI symptoms (nausea, vomiting, cramping, diarrhea) are common but mild. The drug frequently imparts a harmless red color to feces, urine, sweat, tears, and saliva. Deposition of clofazimine in the small intestine produces the most serious effects: intestinal obstruction, pain, and bleeding.

Clofazimine causes reversible reddish-black discoloration of the skin in most patients. Pigmentation begins 4 to 8 weeks after the onset of treatment, and generally clears within 12 months of drug cessation. Because it can darken the skin, patients with light-colored skin often find clofazimine unacceptable.

Preparations, Dosage, and Administration. Clofazimine [Lamprene] is dispensed in 50- and 100-mg capsules for oral use. The usual adult dosage is 50 mg daily.

The ROM Regimen

The ROM regimen (rifampin, ofloxacin, minocycline) is indicated for patients with single-lesion PB leprosy. Treatment consists of one-time dosing with rifampin (600 mg), ofloxacin (400 mg), and minocycline (100 mg). Ofloxacin [Floxin], a fluoroquinolone antibiotic, is discussed in Chapter 87. Minocycline [Minocin], a member of the tetracycline family, is discussed in Chapter 82.

TABLE 86–6 ■ Regimens for Leprosy Recommended by the World Health Organization

Multibacillary Leprosy

Rifampin	600 mg once a month, supervised
Dapsone	100 mg daily, self-administered
Clofazimine	300 mg once a month, supervised
	50 mg daily, self-administered
Duration	12 months

Paucibacillary Leprosy

Rifampin	600 mg once a month, supervised
Dapsone	100 mg daily, self-administered
Duration	6 months

Single-Lesion Paucibacillary Leprosy

Rifampin	600 mg, once
Ofloxacin	400 mg, once
Minocycline	100 mg, once

Rifampin-Resistant Leprosy

First 6 months

Clofazimine	50 mg daily
Ofloxacin	400 mg daily
Minocycline	100 mg daily

Next 6 months

Clofazimine	50 mg daily
Ofloxacin	400 mg daily
or	
Clofazimine	50 mg daily
Minocycline	100 mg daily

DRUGS FOR *MYCOBACTERIUM AVIUM* COMPLEX INFECTION

Mycobacterium avium complex (MAC) consists of two nearly indistinguishable organisms: *M. avium* and *M. intracellulare*. Colonization with MAC begins in the lungs or GI tract, but then may spread to the blood, bone marrow, liver, spleen, lymph nodes, brain, kidneys, and skin. Disseminated infection is common in patients with HIV infection; the incidence at autopsy is 50%. In patients without HIV infection, symptomatic MAC infection is usually limited to the lungs. Signs and symptoms of disseminated MAC infection include fever, night sweats, weight loss, lethargy, anemia, and abnormal liver function tests.

Drug therapy is done for prophylaxis and for treatment of active infection. The preferred agents for *prophylaxis* of disseminated infection are *azithromycin* and *clarithromycin*. Regimens for treating *active infection* should include either *azithromycin* or *clarithromycin*, plus at least one other drug—usually *ethambutol*. Additional drugs may be added as needed; options include rifabutin, rifampin, ciprofloxacin, clofazimine, and amikacin.

Macrolide Antibiotics: Azithromycin and Clarithromycin. The basic pharmacology of azithromycin [Zithromax] and clarithromycin [Biaxin] is discussed in Chapter 82. Consideration here is limited to their use against MAC.

Azithromycin and clarithromycin are drugs of choice for prophylaxis and treatment of MAC infection. All patients with active disease should receive one of these drugs. To prevent emergence of resistance, azithromycin or clarithromycin should be combined with at least one other agent; ethambutol is recommended. The most common side effects of the macrolides are GI disturbances (nausea, diarrhea, vomiting, abdominal pain). For patients with MAC infection, the dosage of azithromycin is 500 daily; the dosage for clarithromycin is 500 to 2000 mg twice daily.

Ethambutol. Ethambutol is combined with either azithromycin or clarithromycin to treat disseminated MAC infection. The toxicity of greatest concern is optic neuritis. The dosage for MAC disease is 15 to 25 mg/kg/day. The basic pharmacology of ethambutol is discussed above.

Other Agents. If a macrolide plus ethambutol is insufficient to control disseminated MAC infection, one or more of the following may be added: *rifabutin* (450 to 600 mg/day), *rifampin* (600 mg/day), *ciprofloxacin* (750 mg twice daily), *clofazimine* (100 to 300 mg/day), and *amikacin* (7.5 to 15 mg/kg/day). All of these drugs are administered orally, except amikacin, which is administered IM or IV.

⁂ KEY POINTS

- Most people infected with *M. tuberculosis* remain asymptomatic, although they will harbor dormant bacteria for life (in the absence of drug therapy).
- Symptomatic tuberculosis can result from reactivation of an old infection or from recent person-to-person transmission of a new infection.
- Drug resistance, and especially multidrug resistance, is a serious impediment to successful therapy of tuberculosis.
- The principal cause of drug resistance in tuberculosis is inadequate drug therapy, which kills sensitive bacteria while allowing resistant mutants to flourish.
- To prevent emergence of resistance, tuberculosis must always be treated with at least two drugs to which the infecting organism is sensitive. Accordingly, isolates from all patients must be tested for resistance.
- Therapy of tuberculosis is prolonged, lasting from a minimum of 6 months to 2 years or even longer.
- The principal first-line drugs for tuberculosis are isoniazid, rifampin, pyrazinamide, ethambutol, and streptomycin.
- For initial therapy of active tuberculosis, patients may be given four drugs: isoniazid, rifampin, pyrazinamide, and ethambutol.
- Initial therapy of multidrug-resistant tuberculosis may require up to seven drugs.
- Tuberculosis in HIV-positive patients can be treated with the same regimens used for HIV-negative patients, although the duration of treatment is longer.
- Three methods are employed to evaluate tuberculosis therapy: bacteriologic evaluation of sputum, clinical evaluation, and chest radiographs.
- Isoniazid can cause peripheral neuropathy by depleting pyridoxine (vitamin B_6). Peripheral neuropathy can be reversed or prevented with pyridoxine supplements.
- Isoniazid can injure the liver. The greatest risk factor is advancing age.
- Rifampin induces drug-metabolizing enzymes, and can thereby increase the metabolism of other drugs; important among these are oral contraceptives, warfarin, and drugs for HIV infection (protease inhibitors, NNRTIs).
- Like isoniazid, rifampin and pyrazinamide are hepatotoxic. Accordingly, when these three drugs are combined, as they often are, the risk of liver injury can be significant.
- Ethambutol can cause optic neuritis.
- The *tuberculin skin test*—used to identify people with latent tuberculosis—is performed by giving an intradermal injection of PPD (purified protein derivative) and then measuring the zone of induration (hardness) at the site 48 to 72 hours later.
- Isoniazid, taken daily for 9 months, is the preferred treatment for latent tuberculosis.

Summary of Major Nursing Implications*

The nursing implications summarized below are limited to the drug therapy of tuberculosis.

IMPLICATIONS THAT APPLY TO ALL ANTITUBERCULOSIS DRUGS

Promoting Compliance

Treatment of active tuberculosis is prolonged and demands concurrent use of two or more drugs; as a result, compliance can be a significant problem. **To promote compliance, educate the patient about the rationale for multidrug therapy and the need for long-term treatment. Encourage patients to take their medication exactly as prescribed, and to continue treatment until the infection has resolved.** In many locales, directly observed administration is employed to ensure compliance.

Evaluating Treatment

Success is indicated by (1) reductions in fever, malaise, anorexia, cough, and other clinical manifestations of tuberculosis (usually within weeks); (2) radiographic evidence of improvement (usually in 3 months); and (3) an absence of *M. tuberculosis* in sputum cultures (usually after 3 to 6 months).

ISONIAZID

In addition to the implications summarized below, see above for implications on *promoting compliance* and *evaluating treatment* that apply to all antituberculosis drugs.

Preadministration Assessment

Therapeutic Goal

Treatment of active or latent infection with *M. tuberculosis.*

Baseline Data

Obtain a chest radiograph, microbiologic tests of sputum, and baseline tests of liver function.

Identifying High-Risk Patients

Isoniazid is *contraindicated* for patients with acute liver disease or a history of isoniazid-induced hepatotoxicity. Use with *caution* in alcoholics, diabetic patients, patients with vitamin B_6 deficiency, patients over the age of 50, and patients who are taking phenytoin, rifampin, or pyrazinamide.

Implementation: Administration

Routes

Oral, IM.

Administration

Advise patients to take isoniazid on an empty stomach, either 1 hour before meals or 2 hours after. Advise patients to take the drug with meals if GI upset occurs.

Ongoing Evaluation and Interventions

Minimizing Adverse Effects

Peripheral Neuropathy. Inform patients about symptoms of peripheral neuropathy (tingling, numbness, burn-ing, or pain in the hands or feet), and instruct them to notify the physician if these occur. Peripheral neuritis can be reversed with small daily doses of pyridoxine (vitamin B_6). In patients at high risk of neuropathy (e.g., alcoholics, diabetics), give pyridoxine prophylactically.

Hepatotoxicity. Isoniazid can cause hepatocellular damage and multilobular hepatic necrosis. **Inform patients about signs of hepatitis (jaundice, anorexia, malaise, fatigue, nausea), and instruct them to notify the physician if these develop.** Evaluate patients monthly for signs of hepatitis. Monthly determinations of AST activity may be ordered. If clinical signs of hepatitis appear, or if AST activity exceeds 3 times the pretreatment baseline, isoniazid should be withdrawn. Daily ingestion of alcohol increases the risk of liver injury; **urge the patient to minimize or eliminate alcohol consumption.**

Minimizing Adverse Interactions

Phenytoin. Isoniazid can suppress the metabolism of phenytoin, thereby causing phenytoin levels to rise. Plasma phenytoin should be monitored. If necessary, phenytoin dosage should be reduced.

RIFAMPIN

In addition to the implications summarized below, see above for implications on *promoting compliance* and *evaluating treatment* that apply to all antituberculosis drugs.

Preadministration Assessment

Therapeutic Goal

Treatment of active tuberculosis or leprosy.

Baseline Data

Obtain a chest radiograph, microbiologic tests of sputum, and baseline tests of liver function.

Identifying High-Risk Patients

Rifampin is *contraindicated* for patients taking protease inhibitors or NNRTIs. Use with *caution* in alcoholics, patients with liver disease, and patients using *warfarin.*

Implementation: Administration

Routes

Oral, IV.

Dosage

Reduce the dosage in patients with liver dysfunction.

Administration

Instruct the patient to take oral rifampin once a day, either 1 hour before a meal or 2 hours after.

Administer IV rifampin by slow infusion (over 3 hours).

Ongoing Evaluation and Interventions

Minimizing Adverse Effects

Hepatotoxicity. Rifampin may cause jaundice or hepatitis. **Inform patients about signs of liver dysfunction**

*Patient education information is highlighted as blue text.

Summary of Major Nursing Implications*—cont'd

(anorexia, darkened urine, pale stools, yellow discoloration of eyes or skin) and instruct them to notify the physician if these develop. Monitor patients for signs of liver dysfunction. Tests of liver function should be made prior to treatment and every 2 to 4 weeks thereafter.

Discoloration of Body Fluids. Forewarn patients that rifampin may impart a harmless red-orange color to urine, sweat, saliva, and tears. Warn patients that soft contact lenses may undergo permanent staining; advise them to consult an ophthalmologist about continued use of these lenses.

Minimizing Adverse Interactions

Accelerated Metabolism of Other Drugs. Rifampin can accelerate the metabolism of many drugs, thereby reducing their effects. This action is of particular concern with *oral contraceptives, warfarin, protease inhibitors,* and *NNRTIs.* Advise women taking oral contraceptives to use a nonhormonal form of birth control. Monitor warfarin effects and increase dosage as needed. Do not combine protease inhibitors and NNRTIs with rifampin.

Pyrazinamide and Isoniazid. These hepatotoxic antituberculosis drugs can increase the risk of liver injury when used with rifampin.

PYRAZINAMIDE

In addition to the implications summarized below, see above for implications on *promoting compliance* and *evaluating treatment* that apply to all antituberculosis drugs.

Preadministration Assessment

Therapeutic Goal

Treatment of active and latent tuberculosis.

Baseline Data

Obtain a chest radiograph, microbiologic tests of sputum, and baseline tests of liver function.

Identifying High-Risk Patients

Pyrazinamide is *contraindicated* for patients with severe liver dysfunction or acute gout. Use with *caution* in alcoholics.

Implementation: Administration

Route

Oral.

Administration

Usually administered once a day.

*Patient education information is highlighted as blue text.

Ongoing Evaluation and Interventions

Minimizing Adverse Effects

Hepatotoxicity. Inform patients about symptoms of hepatitis (malaise, anorexia, nausea, vomiting, yellowish discoloration of the skin and eyes), and instruct them to notify the physician if these develop. Levels of AST and ALT should be measured prior to treatment and every 2 weeks thereafter. If severe liver injury occurs, pyrazinamide should be withdrawn. The risk of liver injury is increased by concurrent therapy with isoniazid and rifampin, both of which are hepatotoxic.

ETHAMBUTOL

In addition to the implications summarized below, see above for implications on *promoting compliance* and *evaluating treatment* that apply to all antituberculosis drugs.

Preadministration Assessment

Therapeutic Goal

Treatment of active tuberculosis.

Baseline Data

Obtain a chest radiograph, microbiologic tests of sputum, and baseline vision tests.

Identifying High-Risk Patients

Ethambutol is *contraindicated* for patients with optic neuritis.

Implementation: Administration

Route

Oral.

Administration

Usually administered once a day. **Advise patients to take ethambutol with food if GI upset occurs.**

Ongoing Evaluation and Interventions

Minimizing Adverse Effects

Optic Neuritis. Ethambutol can cause dose-related optic neuritis. Symptoms include blurred vision, altered color discrimination, and constriction of visual fields. Baseline vision tests are required. **Instruct patients to report any alteration in vision (e.g., blurring of vision, reduced color discrimination).** If ocular toxicity develops, ethambutol should be withdrawn at once.

Miscellaneous Antibacterial Drugs: Fluoroquinolones, Metronidazole, Rifampin, Bacitracin, and Polymyxins

FLUOROQUINOLONES

The fluoroquinolones are close chemical relatives of nalidixic acid, a narrow-spectrum antibiotic used only for urinary tract infections (UTIs). However, in contrast to nalidixic acid, the fluoroquinolones have broad antimicrobial spectra and multiple applications. Side effects are generally mild, and resistance develops slowly.

Ciprofloxacin

Ciprofloxacin [Cipro] was among the first fluoroquinolones available and will serve as our prototype for the family. The drug can be administered orally and is active against a broad spectrum of bacterial pathogens. Ciprofloxacin has been used as an alternative to parenteral antibiotics for treatment of several serious infections. Because it can be administered by mouth, the drug allows easy treatment on an outpatient basis rather than requiring hospitalization for parenteral antibacterial therapy.

Mechanism of Action

Like nalidixic acid, ciprofloxacin *inhibits bacterial DNA gyrase,* an enzyme that converts closed circular DNA into a supercoiled configuration. In the absence of supercoiling, DNA replication cannot take place. The drug is rapidly bactericidal. However, the precise mechanism of cell death is not understood. Since the mammalian equivalent of DNA gyrase is relatively insensitive to fluoroquinolones, cells of the host are not affected.

Antimicrobial Spectrum

Ciprofloxacin is active against a broad spectrum of bacteria, including most aerobic gram-negative bacteria and some gram-positive bacteria. Most urinary tract pathogens, including *Escherichia coli* and *Klebsiella,* are sensitive.

The drug is also highly active against most bacteria that cause enteritis (e.g., *Salmonella, Shigella, Campylobacter jejuni, E. coli*). Other sensitive organisms include *Bacillus anthracis, Pseudomonas aeruginosa, Haemophilus influenzae,* gonococci, meningococci, and many streptococci. Activity against anaerobes is fair to poor. *Clostridium difficile* is resistant.

Bacterial Resistance

Resistance to fluoroquinolones has developed during treatment of infections with *Staphylococcus aureus, Serratia marcescens, C. jejuni,* and *P. aeruginosa.* Two mechanisms appear responsible: (1) alterations in DNA gyrase and (2) reduced ability of ciprofloxacin to cross bacterial membranes. There have been no reports of transfer of resistance via R factors.

Pharmacokinetics

Ciprofloxacin may be administered orally or IV. Following oral administration, the drug is rapidly but incompletely absorbed. High concentrations are achieved in urine, stool, bile, saliva, bone, and prostate tissue. Drug levels in cerebrospinal fluid remain low. Ciprofloxacin has a plasma half-life of about 4 hours. Elimination is by hepatic metabolism and renal excretion.

Therapeutic Uses

Ciprofloxacin is approved for a wide variety of infections. These include infections of the respiratory tract, urinary tract, GI tract, bones, joints, skin, and soft tissues. Also, ciprofloxacin is a preferred drug for preventing anthrax in people who have inhaled anthrax spores. Because it is active against a variety of pathogens and can be given orally, ciprofloxacin represents an alternative to parenteral treatment for many serious infections. The drug is not useful against infections caused by anaerobes.

Adverse Effects

Ciprofloxacin can induce a variety of mild adverse effects, including GI reactions (nausea, vomiting, diarrhea, abdominal pain) and central nervous system (CNS) effects (dizziness, headache, restlessness, confusion). *Candida* infections of the pharynx and vagina may develop as a result of treatment. Very rarely, seizures have occurred.

Rarely, ciprofloxacin and other fluoroquinolones have caused *tendon rupture*—usually of the Achilles tendon. When given to immature animals, fluoroquinolones disrupt the extracellular matrix of cartilage. A similar mechanism may underlie tendon rupture in humans. Since tendon injury is reversible if diagnosed early, fluoroquinolones should be discontinued at the first sign of tendon pain or inflammation. In addition, the patient should refrain from exercise until tendinitis has been ruled out. Because of the risk of tendon rupture, ciprofloxacin is not recommended for children under 18 years of age. Although there are no controlled studies on the use of ciprofloxacin during pregnancy or lactation, available information indicates that such use poses little or no risk of tendon damage to either the fetus or nursing infant.

Drug and Food Interactions

Cationic Compounds. Absorption of ciprofloxacin can be reduced by compounds that contain cations. Among these are (1) aluminum- or magnesium-containing antacids, (2) iron salts, (3) zinc salts, (4) sucralfate, and (5) milk and other dairy products, which contain calcium ions. These cationic agents should be administered at least 6 hours before or 2 hours after ciprofloxacin.

Theophylline. Ciprofloxacin can increase plasma levels of the asthma drug theophylline. Theophylline levels should be monitored and the dosage adjusted accordingly.

Warfarin. Ciprofloxacin can elevate levels of warfarin. Prothrombin time should be monitored and the dosage of warfarin reduced as appropriate.

Preparations, Dosage, and Administration

Preparations. Ciprofloxacin is available for oral and IV administration. For oral therapy, ciprofloxacin [Cipro] is dispensed in tablets (100, 250, 500, and 750 mg) and suspension (5 and 10 gm/100 ml). For IV therapy, ciprofloxacin [Cipro I.V.] is dispensed in solution (10 mg/ml).

Dosage and Administration. Oral. The dosage for urinary tract infections is 250 or 500 mg 2 times a day, usually for 7 to 14 days. For other infections, dosages range from 500 to 750 mg 2 times a day. Dosage should be reduced for patients with renal impairment. Dosages for anthrax prevention are presented below.

Intravenous. Intravenous dosages range from 200 to 400 mg every 12 hours. Infusions should be done slowly (over 60 minutes). Dosage for anthrax prevention is presented below.

Inhalational Anthrax. Ciprofloxacin is used to reduce the incidence of anthrax, or prevent the progression of anthrax, in people who have inhaled *B. anthracis* spores. The dosage for adults is 500 mg PO (or 400 mg IV) every 12 hours for 60 days. The dosage for children is 15 mg/kg PO (or 10 mg/kg IV) every 12 hours for 60 days (with the proviso that individual oral doses not exceed 500 mg, and individual IV doses not exceed 400 mg).

Other Fluoroquinolones
Ofloxacin

Basic Pharmacology. Ofloxacin [Floxin] is similar to ciprofloxacin in mechanism of action, antimicrobial spectrum, therapeutic applications, and adverse effects. Like ciprofloxacin, the drug may be administered orally or IV. In the absence of food, bioavailability of oral ofloxacin is 90%; food greatly reduces availability. Ofloxacin is widely distributed to tissues and excreted in the urine. Like ciprofloxacin, ofloxacin can cause a variety of mild adverse effects, including nausea, vomiting, headache, and dizziness. In addition, ofloxacin may intensify sensitivity to sunlight, thereby increasing the risk of severe sunburn. Like other fluoroquinolones, ofloxacin poses a risk of tendon rupture and should not be used by children under 18 years of age, and should generally be avoided by women who are pregnant or breast-feeding. Ofloxacin elevates plasma levels of warfarin, but, in contrast to ciprofloxacin, has little effect on levels of theophylline. Absorption of oral ofloxacin is reduced by cationic substances (milk, milk products, sucralfate, iron and zinc salts, and magnesium- and aluminum-containing antacids).

Preparations, Dosage, and Administration. Ofloxacin is available in tablets (200, 300, and 400 mg) for oral administration and in solution (4 and 40 mg/ml) for slow IV infusion; concentrated solutions must be diluted prior to administration. The usual oral dosage is 200 to 400 mg every 12 hours; duration of treatment may last 1 day to 6 weeks. Dosage should be reduced in patients with renal impairment. Oral ofloxacin may be taken with or without food.

Lomefloxacin

Actions, Uses, and Pharmacokinetics. Lomefloxacin [Maxaquin] is similar to ciprofloxacin with regard to mechanism and antimicrobial spectrum. Approved indications are limited to UTIs and to acute bronchitis caused by *H. influenzae* or *Moraxella catarrhalis*. Administration is oral and bioavailability is high (98%), even in the presence of food. The drug is widely distributed to tissues and eliminated by the kidney. Lomefloxacin has a prolonged half-life that permits once-a-day dosing.

Adverse Effects. Photosensitivity reactions (e.g., sunburn, blistering) can be moderate to severe. These can occur following exposure to direct sunlight, indirect sunlight, and sunlamps—even if a sunscreen has been applied. Patients should be warned about phototoxicity and advised to avoid sunlight and sunlamps. Lomefloxacin should be withdrawn at the first sign of a phototoxic reaction (e.g., burning sensation, redness, rash).

Like ciprofloxacin, lomefloxacin can cause various mild adverse effects, including nausea, vomiting, headache, and dizziness. Like other fluoroquinolones, lomefloxacin poses a risk of tendon rupture and therefore should not be used by children under the age of 18 or, generally, by women who are pregnant or breast-feeding.

Drug and Food Interactions. Absorption of lomefloxacin is reduced by magnesium- and aluminum-containing antacids, iron and zinc salts, sucralfate, and milk products. In contrast to ciprofloxacin, lomefloxacin does not elevate plasma levels of theophylline.

Preparations, Dosage, and Administration. Lomefloxacin is available in 400-mg tablets for oral administration. The drug may be taken without regard to meals. The usual dosage is 400 mg once a day for 10 to 14 days. Dosage should be reduced in patients with renal impairment.

Sparfloxacin

Actions and Uses. Sparfloxacin [Zagam] is an oral fluoroquinolone approved for once-daily treatment of community-acquired pneumonia (CAP) and acute bacterial exacerbations of chronic bronchitis. The drug is active against virtually all common respiratory tract pathogens, including drug-resistant strains of *Streptococcus pneumoniae,* a major cause of CAP.

Adverse Effects. Sparfloxacin is generally well tolerated. However, like lomefloxacin, the drug can promote serious *photosensitivity reactions.* Accordingly, patients should avoid exposure to direct sunlight, indirect sunlight, and sunlamps. Sparfloxacin can prolong the cardiac QT interval, thereby posing a risk of *dysrhythmias.* Accordingly, the drug should be avoided by patients with pre-existing QT prolongation and by patients taking drugs that can prolong the QT interval (e.g., quinidine, sotalol, astemizole). Additional side effects include tendinitis, GI disturbances (nausea, diarrhea, abdominal discomfort), headache, dizziness, and insomnia.

Drug Interactions. As with other fluoroquinolones, absorption of sparfloxacin is reduced by cations (e.g., magnesium- and aluminum-containing antacids, zinc and iron salts, milk products, sucralfate). In contrast to some other fluoroquinolones, sparfloxacin does not elevate levels of theophylline.

Preparations, Dosage, and Administration. Sparfloxacin is available in 200-mg tablets for oral use. The dosage is 400 mg on day 1, followed by 200 mg once a day on days 2 through 10.

Trovafloxacin and Alatrofloxacin

Trovafloxacin [Trovan] and its prodrug form, alatrofloxacin [Trovan IV], were introduced in 1998. The drugs are active against more bacterial pathogens than any other fluoroquinolones. Unfortunately, within a year of their introduction, reports of drug-induced liver dysfunction began to appear, including several cases of fatal liver failure. Symptomatic pancreatitis has also been reported. Because of these serious adverse effects, these drugs should be reserved for patients with life-threatening infections that cannot be treated with safer agents.

Description, Actions, and Uses. Trovafloxacin is a highly active fluoroquinolone antibiotic. Alatrofloxacin is a prodrug that undergoes conversion to its active form—trovafloxacin—within the body. When these drugs were first introduced, they were approved for a wide assortment of bacterial infections, including nosocomial and community-acquired pneumonia; acute bacterial exacerbations of chronic bronchitis; acute sinusitis; gynecologic and pelvic infections; complicated and uncomplicated infections of the skin and skin structures; urethral, cervical, and rectal gonorrhea; and pelvic inflammatory disease. However, because of hepatotoxicity, the Food and Drug Administration has recommended that their use be limited to a few life-threatening conditions: nosocomial and community-acquired pneumonia, serious abdominal infections, serious gynecologic and pelvic infections, and complicated infections of skin and soft tissues.

Adverse Effects. Hepatotoxicity is the effect of greatest concern. Trovafloxacin and alatrofloxacin can cause liver enzyme abnormalities, symptomatic hepatitis, and acute hepatic necrosis. Deaths have occurred. Clinicians should monitor liver function tests and they should monitor patients for clinical signs of liver dysfunction (fatigue, loss of appetite, jaundice, dark urine).

The drugs may also cause *pancreatitis*. Clinicians should monitor tests of pancreatic function and should monitor patients for clinical signs of pancreatitis.

The most common adverse effects include dizziness, headache, nausea, vomiting, diarrhea, vaginitis, pruritus, and rash. Like other fluoroquinolones, trovafloxacin and alatrofloxacin may pose a risk of tendinitis and tendon rupture, and hence should be avoided by children and, generally, by women who are pregnant or nursing. In contrast to some of the newer fluoroquinolones, these drugs do not prolong the QT interval and they cause little or no photosensitivity.

Drug Interactions. As with other fluoroquinolones, cationic substances (e.g., zinc and iron salts, aluminum- and magnesium-containing antacids, milk products, sucralfate) can decrease the absorption of trovafloxacin. Interestingly, absorption can also be decreased by IV morphine. In contrast to some other fluoroquinolones, these drugs do not increase blood levels of theophylline.

Preparations, Dosage, and Administration. *Trovafloxacin* [Trovan] is available in tablets (100 and 200 mg) for oral administration. *Alatrofloxacin* [Trovan IV] is available in solution (5 mg/ml) for IV administration. Dosing with either preparation is done just once a day. For some infections (e.g., nosocomial pneumonia, gynecologic and pelvic infections), treatment is begun with an initial IV dose of alatrofloxacin, followed by daily oral doses of trovafloxacin. Other infections (e.g., acute exacerbations of bacterial bronchitis) are treated just with oral trovafloxacin. The dosage range for alatrofloxacin is 200 to 300 mg/day. The dosage range for trovafloxacin is 100 to 200 mg/day. Because of concerns about liver damage, treatment duration should not exceed 14 days.

Moxifloxacin

Basic Pharmacology. Moxifloxacin [Avelox] is a broad-spectrum fluoroquinolone indicated for oral therapy of respiratory tract infections (community-acquired pneumonia [CAP], acute sinusitis, acute exacerbations of chronic bronchitis) as well as skin and skin structure infections. Administration is oral or IV. The drug is well absorbed from the GI tract, undergoes wide distribution, and is eliminated by hepatic metabolism and renal excretion. Side effects are generally mild, the most common being nausea, vomiting, diarrhea, stomach pain, dizziness, and altered sense of taste. Like other fluoroquinolones, moxifloxacin can cause tendon rupture, and hence should generally be avoided by children under 18 years old and by women who are pregnant or breast-feeding. The drug does not cause photosensitivity and does not increase levels of warfarin or digoxin. However, it does prolong the QT interval, and hence poses a risk of dysrhythmias. Accordingly, moxifloxacin should not be given to patients taking prodysrhythmic drugs or to those with hypokalemia or pre-existing QT prolongation.

Preparations, Dosage, and Administration. Moxifloxacin [Avelox] is available in 400-mg tablets and in solution for IV infusion. Oral and IV dosages are the same. The dosage for sinusitis and pneumonia is 400 mg once a day for 10 days; the dosage for bronchitis is 400 mg once a day for 5 days. Oral dosing may be done without regard to meals. However, because absorption can be reduced by cationic substances (e.g., milk, sucralfate, iron and zinc salts, magnesium- or aluminum-containing antacids), moxifloxacin should be administered at least 4 hours before or 8 hours after these agents.

Gatifloxacin

Actions and Uses. Gatifloxacin [Tequin] is a broad-spectrum fluoroquinolone with activity against gram-positive, gram-negative, and anaerobic bacteria. The drug is approved for *respiratory tract infections* (CAP, acute bacterial exacerbations of chronic bronchitis, acute sinusitis), *urinary tract infections,* and *gonorrhea.* Gatifloxacin is very active against CAP caused by penicillin-resistant *S. pneumoniae,* but is not yet approved for this infection.

Pharmacokinetics. Gatifloxacin is given PO or IV. Oral gatifloxacin is well absorbed, both in the presence and absence of food. Most of each dose (70%) is excreted unchanged in the urine.

Adverse Effects and Interactions. The most common adverse effects are nausea, vomiting, diarrhea, stomach pain, headache, and dizziness. Like other fluoroquinolones, gatifloxacin poses a risk of tendon rupture, and hence should generally be avoided by children under 18 years old and by women who are pregnant or breast-feeding. In contrast to sparfloxacin and lomefloxacin, gatifloxacin does not cause photosensitivity.

Although gatifloxacin can prolong the QT interval, clinically significant prolongation has not been observed. Hence, the risk of dysrhythmias seems low. Nonetheless, package labeling warns against using the drug in patients with hypokalemia or pre-existing QT prolongation, or by those taking drugs known to prolong the QT interval or promote dysrhythmias (e.g., quinidine, procainamide, amiodarone, sotalol).

As with other fluoroquinolones, absorption of gatifloxacin can be reduced by cationic substances (e.g., milk, sucralfate, iron and zinc salts, magnesium- or aluminum-containing antacids). Accordingly, oral gatifloxacin should be administered at least 4 hours before or 4 hours after these agents.

Gatifloxacin may increase levels of warfarin and digoxin. Elevation of warfarin can cause bleeding; elevation of digoxin can cause dysrhythmias. Caution with both drugs is advised.

Preparations, Dosage, and Administration. Gatifloxacin [Tequin] is available in tablets (200 and 400 mg) and solution for IV infusion (2 and 10 mg/ml). Infusions are done over 60 minutes. The usual dosage is 400 mg once a day (or 200 mg once a day for patients with significant renal impairment). The duration of treatment depends on the infection. For example, CAP is treated for 7 to 14 days, whereas gonorrhea is treated with just one dose.

Norfloxacin

Norfloxacin [Noroxin] is a fluoroquinolone antibiotic with an antimicrobial spectrum like that of ciprofloxacin. The drug is used orally and labeled only for UTIs.

Pharmacokinetics. Norfloxacin undergoes rapid but incomplete absorption following oral administration. The drug is widely distributed to body tissues and fluids. Excretion is primarily renal, and high concentrations are achieved in the urine. About 30% of the drug is eliminated in the bile and feces. In patients with normal kidney function, the half-life is approximately 4 hours; this value doubles in patients with renal impairment.

Therapeutic Uses. Urinary Tract Infections. Norfloxacin was originally approved only for UTIs. The drug has proved effective against UTIs caused by *P. aeruginosa* and other gram-negative bacteria that can display multiple drug resistance.

Other Uses. Norfloxacin is now approved for prostatitis caused by *E. coli,* and for uncomplicated urethral and cervical gonorrhea. In addition to these labeled uses, norfloxacin is employed to treat bacterial gastroenteritis (caused by *E. coli, Shigella, Salmonella,* and other pathogens).

Adverse Effects. Norfloxacin is generally well tolerated. Gastrointestinal effects (nausea, vomiting, anorexia) have been most frequent. The drug has produced a variety of CNS reactions, including headache, dizziness, drowsiness, lightheadedness, depression, and disturbance of vision. Skin rash develops occasionally. Like ciprofloxacin, norfloxacin poses a risk of tendon rupture. Accordingly, norfloxacin is not recommended for children under 18 years of age or for women who are pregnant or breast-feeding.

Drug and Food Interactions. Norfloxacin shares the same interactions as ciprofloxacin. Absorption is suppressed by cationic agents, including milk products, aluminum- and magnesium-containing antacids, iron and zinc salts, and sucralfate. The drug can elevate levels of theophylline and intensify effects of warfarin.

Preparations, Dosage, and Administration. Norfloxacin [Noroxin] is dispensed in 400-mg tablets for oral administration. The drug should be taken on an empty stomach with a full glass of water. For uncomplicated UTIs, the usual dosage is 400 mg twice daily for 3 days. Prolonged treatment (10 days to 3 weeks) is employed for patients with complicated infections of the urinary tract. Dosage should be reduced in the presence of kidney dysfunction.

Levofloxacin

Levofloxacin [Levaquin] is approved for UTIs, respiratory tract infections (acute maxillary sinusitis, CAP, acute bacterial exacerbations of chronic bronchitis), and complicated skin and skin structure infections. In addition, in 2000, levofloxacin became the first drug approved for treating penicillin-resistant pneumococcal CAP. Susceptible pathogens include *S. pneumoniae* (also known as pneumococcus), *H. influenzae, S. aureus, Enterococcus faecalis, Streptococcus pyogenes,* and *Proteus mirabilis.* Administration is oral or IV. Absorption of oral levofloxacin is reduced by cationic substances (e.g., magnesium- and aluminum-containing antacids, zinc and iron salts, sucralfate, milk and milk products) but not by most foods. The usual dosage is 500 mg once a day for 7 to 14 days. In patients with renal impairment, the dosage is 500 mg every 48 hours.

Enoxacin

Basic Pharmacology. Enoxacin [Penetrex] is similar to ciprofloxacin in mechanism of action and adverse effects. The drug's antimicrobial spectrum is narrower than that of ciprofloxacin. Approved indications are limited to UTIs and to uncomplicated urethral and cervical gonorrhea. Administration is oral and bioavailability is high (90%); food reduces availability. The drug is widely distributed to tissues and eliminated by the kidney. Like ciprofloxacin, enoxacin can cause a variety of mild adverse effects, including nausea, vomiting, headache, and dizziness. Serious reactions are rare. Like other fluoroquinolones, enoxacin poses a risk of tendon rupture, and therefore should generally be avoided by children under the age of 18 and by women who are pregnant or breast-feeding. Absorption of enoxacin is reduced by magnesium- and aluminum-containing antacids, iron and zinc salts, milk products, and sucralfate. Like ciprofloxacin, enoxacin can elevate plasma levels of theophylline and warfarin.

Preparations, Dosage, and Administration. Enoxacin is available in tablets (200 and 400 mg) for oral administration. The drug should be taken 1 hour before meals or 2 hours after. The dosage for UTIs is 200 or 400 mg every 12 hours for 7 to 14 days. The dosage for uncomplicated gonorrhea is 400 mg once. Doses should be reduced in patients with renal impairment.

ADDITIONAL ANTIBACTERIAL DRUGS

Metronidazole

Metronidazole [Flagyl, Protostat] is used for protozoal infections and infections caused by obligate anaerobic bacteria. The basic pharmacology of metronidazole is discussed in Chapter 95, as is the drug's use against protozoal infections. Consideration here is limited to antibacterial applications.

Mechanism of Antibacterial Action. Metronidazole is lethal to anaerobic organisms only. To exert bactericidal effects, metronidazole must first be taken up by cells and then converted into its active form; only anaerobes can perform the conversion. The active form of metronidazole interacts with DNA to cause strand breakage and loss of helical structure, effects that result in inhibition of nucleic acid synthesis and, ultimately, cell death. Since aerobic bacteria are unable to activate metronidazole, they are insensitive to the drug.

Antibacterial Spectrum. Metronidazole is active against obligate anaerobes only. Sensitive bacterial pathogens include *Bacteroides fragilis* (and other *Bacteroides* species), *C. difficile* (and other *Clostridium* species), *Fusobacterium* species, *Gardnerella vaginalis*, *Peptococcus* species, and *Peptostreptococcus* species.

Therapeutic Uses. Metronidazole is active against a variety of anaerobic bacterial infections, including infections of the CNS, abdominal organs, bones and joints, skin and soft tissues, and genitourinary tract. Frequently, such infections also involve aerobic bacteria, and hence therapy must include a drug active against them. Metronidazole is employed for prophylaxis in surgical procedures associated with a high risk of infection by anaerobes (e.g., colorectal surgery, abdominal surgery, vaginal surgery). In addition, the drug is used in combination with a tetracycline and bismuth subsalicylate to eradicate *Helicobacter pylori* in people with peptic ulcer disease. Development of resistance to metronidazole is rare.

Preparations, Dosage, and Administration. For initial treatment of serious bacterial infections, metronidazole is administered by IV infusion. Under appropriate conditions, the patient may switch to oral therapy.

Intravenous Formulations. Metronidazole is available in two formulations—powder and solution—for IV use. The powdered form [Flagyl IV] is dispensed in 500-mg vials and must be reconstituted prior to use (see below). The IV solution [Flagyl I.V. RTU] contains 5 mg of metronidazole per milliliter and is ready to use.

Preparation of Powdered Metronidazole for IV Infusion. The powder is readied for infusion in three steps: (1) reconstitution, (2) dilution in IV solution, and (3) neutralization. These steps must be performed in the order given. The powder is reconstituted using 4.4 ml of any of the following liquids: Sterile Water for Injection, Bacteriostatic Water for Injection, 0.9% Sodium Chloride Injection, or Bacteriostatic 0.9% Sodium Chloride Injection. The resulting concentrated solution contains approximately 100 mg of metronidazole per milliliter. This solution is then diluted to a concentration of 8 mg/ml (or less) using any of the following IV solutions: 0.9% Sodium Chloride Injection, 5% Dextrose Injection, or Lactated Ringer's Injection. Neutralization of the diluted solution is accomplished by adding 5 mEq of sodium bicarbonate injection for each 500 mg of metronidazole present; this procedure should elevate pH to a value between 6.0 and 7.0. Neutralized solutions should not be refrigerated, because cooling may cause metronidazole to precipitate.

Intravenous Dosage and Administration. Infusions must be done slowly (over a 1-hour interval). Therapy of anaerobic infections in adults is initiated with a loading dose of 15 mg/kg. After this, maintenance doses of 7.5 mg/kg are administered every 6 to 8 hours. Duration of treatment is usually 1 to 2 weeks. Patients who have kidney dysfunction and are receiving prolonged treatment may need a reduced dosage to avoid accumulation of the drug to toxic levels.

Oral Preparations and Dosage. Metronidazole [Flagyl, Flagyl ER, Flagyl 375] is dispensed in capsules (375 mg), standard tablets (250 and 500 mg), and extended-release tablets (750 mg) for oral administration. The adult dosage for anaerobic infections is 7.5 mg/kg every 6 hours. For bacterial vaginosis in adults, a dosage of 750 mg (extended-release formulation) once daily for 7 days is effective. Pseudomembranous colitis caused by *C. difficile* is treated with 500 mg 3 times a day for 7 to 15 days.

Rifampin

Rifampin [Rifadin, Rimactane] is a broad-spectrum antibacterial drug employed primarily for tuberculosis (see Chapter 86). However, the drug is also used against several nontuberculous infections. Rifampin is useful for treating *asymptomatic carriers of Neisseria meningitidis,* but is not given to treat active meningococcal infection. Unlabeled uses include treatment of leprosy, gram-negative bacteremia in infancy, and infections caused by *Staphylococcus epidermidis* and *S. aureus* (e.g., endocarditis, osteomyelitis, prostatitis). Rifampin has also been employed for prophylaxis of meningitis due to *H. influenzae*. Because resistance can develop rapidly, established bacterial infections should not be treated with rifampin alone. The basic pharmacology of rifampin and its use in tuberculosis are presented in Chapter 86.

Bacitracin

Bacitracin is a polypeptide antibiotic produced by a strain of *Bacillus subtilis*. The drug is almost always employed topically. Because systemic administration can cause serious toxicity, and because superior systemic agents are available, bacitracin is no longer used for systemic infections.

Mechanism of Action and Antimicrobial Spectrum. Bacitracin inhibits synthesis of the bacterial cell wall, thereby causing cell lysis and death. The drug is active against most gram-positive bacteria, including staphylococci, streptococci, and *C. difficile*. *Neisseria* species and *H. influenzae* are also susceptible, but most other gram-negative bacteria are resistant. Acquisition of resistance by sensitive organisms is uncommon.

Adverse Effects. Rarely, topical bacitracin causes local hypersensitivity reactions. Parenteral (IM) administration can produce severe nephrotoxicity.

Therapeutic Uses. Bacitracin is used for topical treatment of bacterial infections. The drug is very active against staphylococci and group A streptococci, the pathogens that cause most acute infections of the skin. Because of this activity, bacitracin has been marketed in a variety of topical preparations for treatment of skin infections. Many of these preparations contain additional antibiotics, usually polymyxin B, neomycin, or both.

Polymyxin B

Polymyxin B is a bactericidal drug employed primarily for local effects. Because of serious systemic toxicity, parenteral administration is rare.

Antibacterial Spectrum and Mechanism of Action. Polymyxin B is bactericidal to a broad spectrum of aerobic, gram-negative bacilli. Gram-positive bacteria and most anaerobes are resistant.

Bactericidal effects result from binding of polymyxin B to the bacterial cell membrane, an action that disrupts membrane structure and thereby increases membrane permeability. The increase in permeability leads to inhibition of cellular respiration and cell death. The resistance displayed by gram-positive bacteria has been attributed to the thick gram-positive cell wall, a structure that may block access of polymyxin B to the cell membrane.

Therapeutic Uses. Polymyxin B is used primarily for topical treatment of the eyes, ears, and skin. Preparations designed for application to the skin frequently contain other antibiotics, such as bacitracin and neomycin. In addition to its topical uses, polymyxin B (together with neomycin) has been employed as a bladder irrigant to prevent infection in patients with indwelling catheters.

Parenteral use is extremely limited; polymyxin B is not a drug of choice for any systemic infection. The primary indication for parenteral polymyxin B is serious infection caused by *P. aeruginosa*. Polymyxin may be given when preferred drugs have been ineffective or intolerable.

Adverse Effects. The major adverse effects associated with parenteral therapy are neurotoxicity and nephrotoxicity. Both occur frequently and limit the systemic use of the drug. Polymyxin B is not absorbed when applied topically, and hence topical use does not cause systemic effects. Rarely, topical polymyxin B produces hypersensitivity.

⁙ KEY POINTS

- Fluoroquinolones are broad-spectrum antibiotics with a wide variety of clinical applications.
- Patients who might otherwise require hospitalization for parenteral antibacterial therapy can often be treated as outpatients with oral ciprofloxacin.
- Fluoroquinolones act by inhibiting bacterial DNA gyrase.
- Because fluoroquinolones can cause tendon rupture, they should be discontinued at the first sign of tendon pain or inflammation. Also, the patient should not exercise until tendinitis has been ruled out.
- Absorption of fluoroquinolones can be reduced by cationic substances, including milk products (calcium), aluminum- and magnesium-containing antacids, iron and zinc salts, and sucralfate.
- In addition to its use against protozoa, metronidazole is used against infections caused by obligate anaerobic bacteria (e.g., *B. fragilis, C. difficile*).

Antifungal Agents

The antifungal agents fall into two major groups: drugs for *systemic mycoses* (i.e., systemic fungal infections) and drugs for *superficial mycoses*. Some drugs are used for both. Systemic infections occur much less frequently than superficial infections, but are considerably more dangerous. Accordingly, therapy of systemic mycoses is our primary focus.

DRUGS FOR SYSTEMIC MYCOSES

Systemic mycoses can be subdivided into two categories: (1) opportunistic infections and (2) nonopportunistic infections. The opportunistic mycoses—*candidiasis, aspergillosis, cryptococcosis,* and *mucormycosis*—are seen primarily in debilitated or immunocompromised hosts. In contrast, nonopportunistic infections can occur in any host. These latter mycoses, which are relatively uncommon, include *sporotrichosis, blastomycosis, histoplasmosis,* and *coccidioidomycosis*. Treating systemic mycoses can be difficult: These infections often resist treatment and hence may require prolonged therapy with drugs that frequently prove toxic.

Amphotericin B

Amphotericin B [Fungizone, Abelcet, Amphotec, AmBisome] is an important but dangerous drug. This agent is active against a broad spectrum of pathogenic fungi and is a drug of choice for most systemic mycoses (see Table 88–1). Unfortunately, amphotericin B is highly toxic: To varying degrees, infusion re-

actions and renal damage occur in all patients. Because of its potential for harm, amphotericin B should be employed only against infections that are progressive and potentially fatal.

Amphotericin B is available in four formulations: a conventional formulation (amphotericin B deoxycholate) and three lipid-based formulations. The lipid-based formulations are as effective as the conventional formulation and cause less toxicity. For treatment of systemic mycoses, all formulations are given by IV infusion. Administration is performed daily or every other day for several months.

Chemistry

Amphotericin B belongs to a group of drugs known as *polyene antibiotics,* so named because their structures contain a series of conjugated double bonds. Nystatin, another antifungal drug, is also in this family.

Mechanism of Action

Amphotericin B binds to components of the fungal cell membrane, thereby increasing permeability. The resultant leakage of intracellular cations (especially potassium) reduces viability. Depending on the concentration of amphotericin B and the susceptibility of the fungus, the drug may be fungicidal or fungistatic.

The component of the fungal membrane to which amphotericin B binds is *ergosterol,* a member of the *sterol* family of compounds. Hence, for a cell to be susceptible, its cytoplasmic membrane must contain sterols. Since bacterial membranes lack sterols, bacteria are not affected.

Much of the toxicity of amphotericin is attributable to the presence of sterols (principally cholesterol) in mammalian cell membranes. By binding to cholesterol in mammalian membranes, amphotericin is thought to affect host cells in much the same way it affects fungi. Fortunately, there is some selective toxicity for fungi: Amphotericin binds more strongly to ergosterol (the major sterol in fungal membranes) than it does to cholesterol (the major sterol in mammalian cell membranes).

Microbial Susceptibility and Resistance

Amphotericin B is active against a broad spectrum of fungi. Some protozoa (e.g., *Leishmania braziliensis*) are also susceptible. As noted, bacteria are resistant.

Emergence of resistant fungi during amphotericin therapy is extremely rare. On occasion, resistance has been observed during long-term treatment. In all cases of resistance, the fungi had membranes whose ergosterol content was reduced or absent.

Therapeutic Uses

Amphotericin B is a drug of choice for most systemic mycoses (see Table 88–1). Prior to the availability of this agent, systemic fungal infections usually proved fatal. Treatment is pro-

TABLE 88–1 ■ Drugs of Choice for Systemic Mycoses

Infection	Causative Organism	Drugs of Choice	Alternative Drugs
Aspergillosis	*Aspergillus* species	Amphotericin B	Itraconazole, voriconazole, caspofungin
Blastomycosis	*Blastomyces dermatitidis*	Amphotericin B *or* itraconazole	Ketoconazole, fluconazole
Candidiasis	*Candida* species	Amphotericin B *or* fluconazole, either one ± flucytosine	
Coccidioidomycosis	*Coccidioides immitis*	Amphotericin B *or* fluconazole	Itraconazole, ketoconazole
Cryptococcosis Chronic suppression	*Cryptococcus neoformans*	Amphotericin B ± flucytosine Fluconazole	Itraconazole Amphotericin B
Histoplasmosis Chronic suppression	*Histoplasma capsulatum*	Amphotericin B *or* itraconazole Itraconazole	Ketoconazole, fluconazole Amphotericin B
Mucormycosis	*Mucor*	Amphotericin B	No dependable alternative
Paracoccidioidomycosis	*Paracoccidioides brasiliensis*	Amphotericin B *or* itraconazole	Ketoconazole
Sporotrichosis	*Sporothrix schenckii*	Amphotericin B *or* itraconazole	Fluconazole

longed; 6 to 8 weeks is common. In some cases, treatment may last for 3 or 4 months. In addition to its antifungal applications, amphotericin B is a drug of choice for leishmaniasis (see Chapter 95).

Pharmacokinetics

Absorption and Distribution. Absorption of amphotericin B from the GI tract is poor, and oral therapy of systemic infection is not effective. Hence, for treatment of deep mycoses, the drug must be administered IV. In the body, most amphotericin is bound to sterol-containing membranes of various tissues. Levels about half those in plasma are achieved in aqueous humor and in peritoneal, pleural, and joint fluids. The drug does not readily penetrate to the cerebrospinal fluid (CSF).

Metabolism and Excretion. Little is known about the elimination of amphotericin B. We do not know whether the drug is metabolized or how the majority of the drug is removed from the body. Renal excretion of unchanged amphotericin is minimal. Accordingly, there is no need to reduce the dosage in patients with pre-existing renal impairment. Complete elimination of amphotericin takes a long time; the drug has been detected in tissues more than a year after cessation of treatment.

Adverse Effects

Amphotericin can cause a variety of serious adverse effects. Patients should be under close supervision, preferably in a hospital.

Infusion Reactions. Intravenous amphotericin frequently produces fever, chills, rigors, nausea, and headache. These reactions are caused by release of proinflammatory cytokines (tumor necrosis factor, interleukin-1, interleukin-6) from monocytes and macrophages. Symptoms begin 1 to 3 hours after starting the infusion and persist about 1 hour. Mild reactions can be reduced by pretreatment with diphenhydramine plus either aspirin or acetaminophen. Intravenous meperidine or dantrolene can be given if rigors occur. If other measures fail, hydrocortisone (a glucocorticoid) can be used to decrease fever and chills. However, since glucocorticoids can reduce the patient's ability to fight infection, routine use of hydrocortisone should be avoided. The intensity of infusion reactions is less with the lipid-based formulations of amphotericin than with the conventional formulation.

Infusion of amphotericin produces a high incidence of phlebitis. This can be minimized by changing peripheral venous sites often, administering amphotericin through a large central vein, and pretreatment with heparin.

Nephrotoxicity. Amphotericin exerts direct toxicity on cells of the kidney. Renal impairment occurs in practically all patients. The extent of kidney damage is related to the total dose administered over the full course of treatment. In most cases, renal function returns to normal following cessation of drug use. However, if the total dose exceeds 4 gm, residual impairment is likely. Kidney damage can be minimized by infusing 1 L of saline on the days of amphotericin administration. Other nephrotoxic drugs (e.g., aminoglycosides, cyclosporine) should be avoided. To evaluate renal injury, tests of kidney function should be performed weekly; intake and output should be monitored. If plasma creatinine content rises above 3.5 mg/dl, amphotericin dosage should be reduced. The degree of renal damage is less with the lipid-based formulations than with the conventional amphotericin.

Hypokalemia. Damage to the kidneys often causes hypokalemia. Potassium supplements may be needed to correct the problem. Patients should undergo frequent determinations of potassium levels and serum creatinine content.

Effects Associated with Intrathecal Injection. Intrathecal administration may cause nausea, vomiting, headache, and pain in the back, legs, and abdomen. Rare reactions include visual disturbances, impairment of hearing, and paresthesias (tingling, numbness, or pain in the hands and feet).

Other Adverse Effects. Infusion of amphotericin may be associated with delirium, hypotension, hypertension, wheezing, and hypoxia. Bone marrow depression has occurred, resulting in normocytic, normochromic anemia; for evaluation, hematocrit determinations should be performed. Rarely, amphotericin has caused rash, convulsions, anaphylaxis, dysrhythmias, acute liver failure, and nephrogenic diabetes insipidus.

Drug Interactions

Nephrotoxic Drugs. Use of amphotericin with other nephrotoxic drugs (e.g., aminoglycosides, cyclosporine) increases the risk of injury to the kidneys. Accordingly, these combinations should be avoided if at all possible.

Flucytosine. Amphotericin potentiates the antifungal actions of flucytosine, apparently by enhancing entry of flucytosine into fungal cells. Because of this potentiative interaction, the combination of flucytosine with a relatively low dose of amphotericin can produce antifungal effects equivalent to those of a high dose of amphotericin alone. By allowing a reduction in amphotericin dosage, the combination decreases the risk of amphotericin-induced toxicity.

Preparations, Dosage, and Administration

Preparations. Amphotericin B is available in a conventional formulation—*amphotericin B deoxycholate* [Fungizone Intravenous]—and three lipid-based formulations: *liposomal amphotericin B* [AmBisome], *amphotericin B cholesteryl sulfate complex* [Amphotec], and *amphotericin B lipid complex* [Abelcet]. The lipid-based formulations cause less nephrotoxicity and fewer infusion reactions than the conventional formulation. However, the newer formulations are considerably more expensive. As a rule, the lipid-based formulations are reserved for patients who are refractory to or intolerant of conventional therapy.

Routes. For treatment of systemic mycoses, amphotericin B is almost always administered by IV infusion. Infusions should be performed slowly (over 2 to 4 hours) to minimize phlebitis and cardiovascular reactions. Alternate-day dosing can reduce adverse effects. For most patients, several months of therapy are required. Because amphotericin B does not readily enter the CSF, intrathecal injection is used for fungal meningitis.

Intravenous Dosage and Administration. Fungal Infections. Dosage is individualized based on the severity of the disease and the patient's ability to tolerate treatment. Optimal dosage has not been established. A small (1-mg) test dose is often infused to assess patient reaction. After this, therapy is initiated with a dosage of 0.25 mg/kg/day. Maintenance dosages range from 1.5 to 6.0 mg/kg/day, depending on the severity of the infection and the form of amphotericin being used. Dosage should be reduced in patients with renal impairment. The infusion solution should be checked periodically for a precipitate and, if a precipitate is seen, administration should be discontinued immediately. Because the treatment period is prolonged, the administration site should be rotated; this will reduce the risk of phlebitis and help ensure continued availability of a suitable vein.

Leishmaniasis. Leishmaniasis can be treated with *amphotericin B deoxycholate* [Fungizone Intravenous] or *liposomal amphotericin B* [AmBisome]. When Fungizone is used, the dosage is 0.5 to 1 mg/kg daily every other day for up to 8 weeks. When AmBisome is used, the dosage is 3 mg/kg on days 1, 2, 3, 4, 5, 14, and 21.

Ketoconazole

Ketoconazole [Nizoral] belongs to the *azole* family of antifungal agents, for which it can be considered the prototype. Other family members are fluconazole, itraconazole, miconazole, clotrimazole, econazole, and voriconazole. All are active against a broad spectrum of fungi. Some are used for systemic mycoses, some for superficial mycoses, and some for both.

Ketoconazole is an oral alternative to amphotericin B for treating less severe systemic mycoses. The drug is safer than amphotericin B and has the additional advantage of being used orally. The adverse effect of greatest concern is liver injury. Ketoconazole and other azoles inhibit cytochrome P450–dependent drug-metabolizing enzymes, and can thereby cause levels of other drugs to rise. Toxicity can result.

Mechanism of Action

Ketoconazole inhibits the synthesis of *ergosterol,* an essential component of the fungal cytoplasmic membrane. This results in increased membrane permeability and leakage of cellular components. Accumulation of ergosterol precursors may also contribute to antifungal actions. Ketoconazole suppresses ergosterol synthesis by inhibiting fungal cytochrome P450–dependent enzymes. Ketoconazole is fungistatic at low concentrations and fungicidal at high concentrations.

Antifungal Spectrum

Most of the fungi that cause systemic mycoses are susceptible. Ketoconazole is also active against the fungi that cause superficial infections (dermatophytes and *Candida* species). Emergence of resistance is rare.

Therapeutic Uses

Ketoconazole is an alternative to amphotericin B for treatment of systemic mycoses. The drug is much less toxic than amphotericin and only somewhat less effective. Specific indications are listed in Table 88–1. Responses to ketoconazole are slow. Accordingly, the drug is less useful for severe, acute infections than for long-term suppression of chronic mycoses. Ketoconazole is also a valuable drug for treating superficial mycoses; these applications are considered later in the chapter.

Pharmacokinetics

Absorption. Ketoconazole is a weak base and hence requires an acidic environment for dissolution and absorption. Oral ketoconazole is well absorbed from the GI tract, provided that gastric acid levels are normal. In patients with achlorhydria (absence of gastric acid), absorption is low. Drugs that reduce gastric acidity (e.g., antacids, histamine$_2$ [H$_2$] blocking agents, proton pump inhibitors) decrease ketoconazole absorption.

Distribution. Most ketoconazole in the blood is bound to plasma proteins. The drug crosses the blood-brain barrier poorly and concentrations in CSF remain low. In contrast, high levels of ketoconazole are achieved in the skin, making oral ketoconazole useful against superficial mycoses.

Elimination. Ketoconazole is eliminated by hepatic metabolism. Its half-life is approximately 3 hours. In the presence of liver dysfunction, the half-life can be substantially prolonged. Because elimination is hepatic, renal impairment does not influence the intensity or duration of effects. Hence, no dosage adjustment is needed in patients with kidney disease.

Adverse Effects

Ketoconazole is generally well tolerated. The most common adverse reactions—nausea and vomiting—can be reduced by giving the drug with food. The most serious effects involve the liver.

Hepatotoxicity. Effects of ketoconazole on the liver are rare but potentially severe. Fatal hepatic necrosis has occurred. Liver function should be evaluated prior to treatment and at least monthly thereafter. Ketoconazole should be discontinued at the first sign of liver injury. The drug should be employed with caution in patients with a history of hepatic disease. Patients should be advised to notify the physician if they experience symptoms suggesting liver dysfunction (e.g., unusual fatigue, anorexia, nausea, vomiting, jaundice, dark urine, pale stools).

Effects on Sex Hormones. Just as ketoconazole inhibits steroid synthesis in fungi, the drug can inhibit steroid synthesis in humans. In males, inhibition of testosterone synthesis has caused gynecomastia, decreased libido, and reduced potency; reversible sterility has occurred with high doses. In females, reduction of estradiol synthesis has caused menstrual irregularities.

Other Adverse Effects. Ketoconazole can produce a variety of relatively mild adverse effects, including rash, itching, dizziness, fever, chills, constipation, diarrhea, photophobia, and headache. Rarely, ketoconazole has caused anaphylaxis, severe epigastric pain, and altered function of the adrenals.

Drug Interactions

Drugs That Raise Gastric pH. Drugs that decrease gastric acidity—antacids, H$_2$ antagonists, proton pump inhibitors, anticholinergic drugs—can greatly reduce ketoconazole absorption. Accordingly, these agents should be administered no sooner than 2 hours after ingestion of ketoconazole. (Since proton pump inhibitors have a prolonged duration of action, patients using these drugs may have insufficient stomach acid for ketoconazole absorption, regardless of when the proton pump inhibitor is given.)

Inhibition of Hepatic Drug-Metabolizing Enzymes.
Ketoconazole and other azole antifungal drugs inhibit cytochrome P450–dependent drug-metabolizing enzymes, and can thereby increase levels of several other drugs (see Table 88–2). The most important of these are *terfenadine** [Seldane], *astemizole** [Hismanal], and *cisapride†* [Propulsid]. When present at excessive levels, all three can cause potentially fatal cardiac dysrhythmias. Accordingly, concurrent use of these agents with ketoconazole is contraindicated.

Rifampin. Rifampin reduces plasma levels of ketoconazole, apparently by enhancing hepatic metabolism. If these drugs are used concurrently, ketoconazole dosage should be increased—and even then it may be impossible to achieve therapeutic levels.

Preparations, Dosage, and Administration

Ketoconazole [Nizoral] is dispensed in 200-mg tablets for oral administration. The recommended adult dosage is 200 mg once a day. For chemotherapy of severe infection, daily doses of 400 to 800 mg may be required. The dosage for children over 2 years old 3.3 to 6.6 mg/kg/day in a single dose. Duration of treatment is 6 months or longer. Since an acidic environment is needed for ketoconazole absorption, patients with achlorhydria should dissolve the tablets in 4 ml of 0.2 N hydrochloric acid; the solution should be sipped through a plastic or glass straw to avoid damaging the teeth.

Itraconazole

Actions and Uses. Itraconazole [Sporanox], a member of the azole family, is active against a broad spectrum of fungal pathogens. Like ketoconazole, the drug inhibits cytochrome P450, and thereby inhibits synthesis of ergosterol, an essential component of the fungal cytoplasmic membrane. Approved indications are *blastomycosis* (pulmonary and extrapulmonary), *histoplasmosis, aspergillosis, onychomycosis,* and oral and esophageal *candidiasis.* However, because of its broad antifungal spectrum, the drug has been used for other systemic fungal infections (*coccidioidomycosis, cryptococcosis, paracoccidioidomycosis, sporotrichosis*) and for superficial fungal infections.

---

*Terfenadine and astemizole are no longer available in the United States.
†In 2000, cisapride was voluntarily withdrawn from the U.S. market, and is now available only through an investigational limited-access program.

Pharmacokinetics. Itraconazole may be administered PO (in capsules or suspension) or by IV infusion. Food increases absorption of itraconazole *capsules,* but decreases absorption of itraconazole oral *suspension.* Once absorbed, the drug is widely distributed to lipophilic tissues. Concentrations in aqueous fluids (e.g., saliva, CSF) are negligible. The drug undergoes extensive hepatic metabolism. About 40% of each dose is excreted in the urine as inactive metabolites.

Adverse Effects. Itraconazole is well tolerated in usual doses. Gastrointestinal reactions (nausea, vomiting, diarrhea) are most common, occurring in about 10% of patients. Other common reactions include rash (8.6%), headache (3.8%), abdominal pain (3.3%), and edema (3.5%). Intravenous administration may produce vein disorders (e.g., irritation, swelling, hardness, pain). In addition to these relatively benign effects, itraconazole (PO or IV) may cause two potentially serious effects: cardiac suppression and liver injury.

Cardiac Suppression. Itraconazole has negative inotropic actions that can cause a transient decrease in ventricular ejection fraction. Cardiac function returns to normal by 12 hours after dosing. Because of its negative inotropic actions, itraconazole should not be used for *superficial* fungal infections (dermatomycoses, onychomycosis) in patients with heart failure, a history of heart failure, or other indications of ventricular dysfunction. The drug may still be used to treat *serious* fungal infections in patients with heart failure, but only with careful monitoring, and only if the benefits clearly outweigh the risks. If signs and symptoms of heart failure worsen, discontinuation of itraconazole should be considered.

Liver Injury. As of March 2001, the Food and Drug Administration (FDA) had received 24 reports of liver failure, including 11 deaths, in patients taking itraconazole. Although a causal link has not been established, caution is nonetheless advised. Patients should be informed about signs of liver dysfunction (persistent nausea, anorexia, fatigue, vomiting, right upper abdominal pain, jaundice, dark urine or stools) and, if they appear, should seek medical attention immediately.

Drug Interactions. Like other azole antifungal drugs, itraconazole inhibits cytochrome P450–dependent drug metabolizing enzymes. As a result, itraconazole can elevate plasma levels of several drugs, including cyclosporine, digoxin, warfarin, terfenadine, astemizole, cisapride, and sulfonylurea-type oral hypoglycemics. In patients taking cyclosporine or digoxin, levels of these drugs should be monitored; in patients taking sulfonylureas, levels of blood glucose should be monitored; and in patients taking warfarin, prothrombin time should be monitored. Because the combination of itraconazole with astemizole, terfenadine, or cisapride can result in potentially fatal cardiac dysrhythmias, itraconazole should not be used with these drugs.

Levels of itraconazole can be lowered by drugs that increase its metabolism or reduce its absorption. Drugs that accelerate itraconazole metabolism include phenytoin, isoniazid, and rifampin. Drugs that reduce itraconazole absorption (by decreasing gastric acidity) include antacids, H₂-receptor blockers (e.g., cimetidine), and proton pump inhibitors (e.g., omeprazole). If itraconazole is combined with any of these agents, its dosage may need to be increased.

TABLE 88–2 ■ Drugs Whose Levels Can be Increased by Azole Antifungal Drugs		
Target Drug	**Class**	**Consequence of Excessive Level**
Astemizole [Hismanal]*	Antihistamine	Fatal dysrhythmias
Terfenadine [Seldane]*	Antihistamine	Fatal dysrhythmias
Cisapride [Propulsid]†	Prokinetic agent	Fatal dysrhythmias
Warfarin [Coumadin]	Anticoagulant	Bleeding
Sulfonylureas	Oral hypoglycemic	Hypoglycemia
Phenytoin [Dilantin]	Antiseizure drug	CNS toxicity
Cyclosporine [Sandimmune]	Immunosuppressant	Increased nephrotoxicity
Tacrolimus [Prograf]	Immunosuppressant	Increased nephrotoxicity
Lovastatin [Mevacor]	Antihyperlipidemic	Rhabdomyolysis
Simvastatin [Zocor]	Antihyperlipidemic	Rhabdomyolysis

*No longer available in the United States.
†In 2000, cisapride was voluntarily withdrawn from the U.S. market, and is now available only through an investigational limited-access program.

Preparations, Dosage, and Administration. Oral. Itraconazole [Sporanox] for oral use is dispensed in suspension (10 mg/ml) and capsules (100 mg). The capsules should be taken with food to increase absorption. The recommended dosage is 200 mg once a day. If needed, the dosage may be increased to 200 mg twice a day.

Intravenous. Itraconazole [Sporanox] for IV use is supplied in a kit that contains a 25-ml ampule of itraconazole (10 mg/ml) and a 50-ml bag of 0.9% saline. The two solutions are combined to produce a 75-ml itraconazole solution (3.33 mg/ml). A single dose consists of 200 mg (60 ml) infused over 60 minutes. The recommended dosing schedule is 200 mg twice a day for four doses, followed by 200 mg once a day for up to 14 days, after which the patient should be switched to oral itraconazole (200 mg once a day).

Fluconazole

Actions and Uses. Fluconazole [Diflucan] belongs to the azole group of antifungal agents. The drug has the same mechanism of action as ketoconazole: inhibition of cytochrome P450–dependent synthesis of ergosterol, with resultant damage to the cytoplasmic membrane and accumulation of ergosterol precursors. The drug is primarily fungistatic. Fluconazole is used to treat blastomycosis; histoplasmosis; meningitis caused by *Cryptococcus neoformans* and *Coccidioides immitis;* and vaginal, oropharyngeal, esophageal, and disseminated *Candida* infections. In addition to its antifungal applications, fluconazole is used investigationally for leishmaniasis (see Chapter 95).

Pharmacokinetics. Fluconazole is well absorbed (90%) following oral administration. The drug is widely distributed to tissues and body fluids, including the CSF. Most of each dose is eliminated unchanged in the urine. Fluconazole has a half-life of 30 hours, making once-a-day dosing sufficient.

Adverse Effects. Fluconazole is less toxic than ketoconazole and is generally well tolerated. The most common reactions are nausea (3.7%), headache (1.9%), rash (1.8%), vomiting (1.7%), abdominal pain (1.7%), and diarrhea (1.5%). Rarely, treatment has been associated with hepatic necrosis, Stevens-Johnson syndrome, and anaphylaxis. Fluconazole is teratogenic in animals and may be in humans; appropriate caution should be exercised.

Drug Interactions. Like other azole antifungal drugs, fluconazole can inhibit cytochrome P450–dependent drug-metabolizing enzymes, and can thereby increase levels of other drugs, including warfarin, phenytoin, cyclosporine, zidovudine, rifabutin, and sulfonylureas (oral hypoglycemics).

Preparations, Dosage, and Administration. Fluconazole [Diflucan] is dispensed in solution (2 mg/ml) for IV infusion, and in tablets (50, 100, 150, and 200 mg) and suspension (10 and 40 mg/ml) for oral use. Because oral absorption is rapid and nearly complete, oral and IV dosages are the same. For treatment of *oropharyngeal and esophageal candidiasis,* the usual dosage is 200 mg on the first day, followed by 100 mg once daily thereafter. For treatment of *systemic candidiasis* and *cryptococcal meningitis,* the usual dosage is 400 mg on the first day, followed by 200 mg once daily thereafter. Duration of treatment ranges from 3 weeks to more than 3 months, depending on the infection being treated.

Miconazole

Miconazole [Monistat i.v.], like ketoconazole, belongs to the azole family of compounds. The antifungal actions of both drugs are similar. Miconazole is employed primarily for topical treatment of superficial mycoses (see below). Because of toxicity, miconazole is rarely employed for systemic infections. When used for systemic therapy, the drug must be given IV. Administration by this route is associated with a high incidence of adverse effects, including phlebitis, thrombocytosis, nausea, vomiting, pruritus, rash, and fever. Miconazole increases levels of warfarin, and hence warfarin dosage must be reduced. Miconazole can antagonize the effects of amphotericin B in the treatment of candidiasis.

Miconazole for IV use is dispensed as a 10-mg/ml solution in 20-ml ampules. The drug is diluted in 0.9% saline plus 5% dextrose and infused slowly (over 30 to 60 minutes). The daily dosage for adults is 0.2 to 3.6 gm administered in three or four divided doses at equally spaced intervals. Duration of treatment is 2 to 20 weeks.

Voriconazole

Actions and Uses. Voriconazole [Vfend], a member of the azole family, is an important new drug for treating life-threatening fungal infections. Like other azoles, voriconazole inhibits cytochrome P450–dependent enzymes, and thereby suppresses synthesis of ergosterol, a critical component of the fungal cytoplasmic membrane. As a result, voriconazole is active

against a broad spectrum of fungal pathogens, including *Aspergillus* species, *Candida* species, *Scedosporium* species, *Fusarium* species, *Histoplasma capsulatum, Blastomyces dermatitidis,* and *C. neoformans.* At this time, voriconazole is approved only for (1) primary therapy of invasive aspergillosis, and (2) infections caused by *Scedosporium apiospermum* or *Fusarium* species in patients unresponsive to or intolerant of other drugs.

Compared with amphotericin B, the current first-choice drug for invasive aspergillosis, voriconazole is equally effective and poses a much lower risk of kidney damage. However, the new drug does have its own set of adverse effects, including hepatotoxicity, visual disturbances, hypersensitivity reactions, hallucinations, and fetal injury. In addition, like other azoles, voriconazole can interact with many drugs.

Pharmacokinetics. Voriconazole may be administered IV or PO. With oral administration, bioavailability is high (96%), but can be reduced by food. Plasma levels peak 2 hours after ingestion. The drug's half-life is dose dependent, and can range from 6 hours up to 24 hours. Voriconazole undergoes extensive metabolism by hepatic P450 enzymes.

Adverse Effects. The most common adverse effects are visual disturbances, fever, rash, nausea, vomiting, diarrhea, headache, sepsis, peripheral edema, abdominal pain, and respiratory disorders. During clinical trials, the effects that most often led to discontinuing treatment were liver damage, visual disturbances, and rash.

Hepatotoxicity. Voriconazole can cause hepatitis, cholestasis, and fulminant hepatic failure. Fortunately, these events are both uncommon and generally reversible. To monitor for injury, liver function tests should be obtained before treatment and periodically thereafter.

Visual Disturbances. Reversible, dose-related visual disturbances develop in 30% of patients. Symptoms include reduced visual acuity, increased brightness, altered color perception, and photophobia. As a rule, these begin within 30 minutes of dosing and then greatly diminish over the next 30 minutes. Owing to the risk of photophobia and blurred vision, patients should be warned against driving at night.

Hypersensitivity Reactions. Voriconazole may cause dermatologic reactions, ranging from rash to life-threatening Stevens-Johnson syndrome. During infusion, anaphylactoid reactions have occurred, manifesting with tachycardia, chest tightness, dyspnea, faintness, flushing, fever, and sweating. If these symptoms develop, the infusion should be stopped.

Teratogenicity. Voriconazole is teratogenic in rats and can cause fetal harm in humans. The drug is classified in FDA Pregnancy Risk Category D, and hence should not be used during pregnancy unless the potential benefits are deemed to outweigh the risk to the fetus. Women taking the drug should use effective contraception.

Drug Interactions. Voriconazole can interact with many other drugs. Several mechanisms are involved. Voriconazole is both a substrate for and inhibitor of hepatic P450 enzymes. As a result, drugs that inhibit P450 can raise voriconazole levels, and drugs that induce P450 can lower voriconazole levels. On the other hand, because voriconazole itself can inhibit P450, voriconazole can raise levels of other drugs. Therefore

- To ensure that voriconazole levels are adequate, voriconazole should not be combined with powerful P450 inducers, including rifampin, rifabutin, carbamazepine, and phenobarbital.
- To avoid excessive voriconazole levels, voriconazole should not be combined with powerful P450 inhibitors.
- To avoid toxicity from accumulation of other drugs, voriconazole should not be combined with some agents that are P450 substrates, including astemizole, terfenadine, cisapride, pimozide, and sirolimus.

Preparations, Dosage, and Administration. Voriconazole [Vfend] is available in 200-mg single-use vials for IV infusion, and in tablets (50 and 200 mg) for oral therapy. Treatment is initiated with IV voriconazole and later can be switched to oral voriconazole as appropriate.

Intravenous therapy consists of two loading doses (6 mg/kg each given 12 hours apart) followed by maintenance doses of 4 mg/kg every 12 hours. All IV doses should be infused slowly, over 1 to 2 hours (maximum rate is 3 mg/kg/hr). If the response is inadequate, maintenance doses can be increased by 50%. Patients with *mild to moderate* hepatic cirrhosis should receive the standard two loading doses, but maintenance doses should be halved. (There are no data on dosing in patients with *severe* cirrhosis.) Patients with significant renal impairment (creatinine clearance <50 ml/min), should use *oral* voriconazole, not IV voriconazole. Why? Because, in the absence of adequate kidney function, the solubilizing agent (not voriconazole itself) in the IV formulation can accumulate to dangerous levels.

After receiving their IV loading doses, patients who can tolerate oral therapy may be switched to voriconazole tablets. The usual dosage is 200 mg every 12 hours (for patients over 40 kg) and 100 mg every 12 hours (for patients under 40 kg). If the response is inadequate, doses can be increased by 50%. Oral dosing should be done 1 hour before meals or 1 hour after.

Flucytosine

Flucytosine [Ancobon] is employed for serious infections caused by *Candida* species and *C. neoformans*. Because development of resistance is common, flucytosine is almost always used in combination with amphotericin B. Caution must be exercised in patients with renal impairment and hematologic disorders.

Mechanism of Action. The antifungal effects of flucytosine derive from disruption of DNA and RNA synthesis. Flucytosine is taken up by fungal cells and converted to 5-fluorouracil, its active form. The enzyme responsible for this conversion is cytosine deaminase. Fungi that lack cytosine deaminase are not susceptible to the drug. Since mammalian cells lack cytosine deaminase, flucytosine has relatively low toxicity to the host.

Fungal Resistance. Development of resistance to flucytosine during therapy is common and constitutes a serious clinical problem. Several mechanisms of resistance have been described, including (1) a reduction in fungal cytosine permease, the enzyme required for uptake of flucytosine; and (2) loss of cytosine deaminase, the enzyme required to convert flucytosine to its active form.

Antifungal Spectrum and Therapeutic Uses. Flucytosine has a narrow antifungal spectrum. Fungicidal activity is highest against *Candida* species and *C. neoformans*. Most other fungi are resistant. Because of this narrow spectrum, flucytosine is indicated only for candidiasis and cryptococcosis. For treatment of serious infections (e.g., cryptococcal meningitis, systemic candidiasis), flucytosine should be combined with amphotericin B. This combination offers two advantages over flucytosine alone: (1) antifungal activity is enhanced and (2) emergence of resistant fungi is reduced.

Pharmacokinetics. Flucytosine is readily absorbed from the GI tract and is well distributed throughout the body. The drug has good access to the central nervous system; levels in CSF are about 80% of those in plasma. Flucytosine is eliminated by the kidneys, principally as the unchanged drug. Its half-life is about 4 hours in patients with normal renal function. However, in patients with renal insufficiency, the half-life is greatly prolonged. Accordingly, dosages must be reduced in these patients.

Adverse Effects. *Hematologic Effects.* Bone marrow depression is the most serious complication of treatment. Marrow depression usually manifests as reversible neutropenia or thrombocytopenia. Rarely, fatal agranulocytosis develops. Platelet and leukocyte counts should be determined weekly. Adverse hematologic effects are most likely when plasma levels of flucytosine exceed 100 mg/ml. Accordingly, the dosage should be adjusted to keep drug levels below this value. Flucytosine should be used with caution in patients with pre-existing bone marrow suppression.

Hepatotoxicity. Mild and reversible liver dysfunction occurs frequently, but severe hepatic injury is rare. Liver function should be monitored by making weekly determinations of serum transaminase and alkaline phosphatase levels.

Drug Interactions. Flucytosine is often combined with *amphotericin B*. As noted, this combination offers several advantages. However, the combination can also be detrimental. Since amphotericin B is nephrotoxic, and since flucytosine is eliminated by the kidneys, amphotericin B–induced kidney damage may suppress flucytosine excretion, and may thereby promote flucytosine toxicity. Therefore, *it is important to monitor renal function and flucytosine levels when amphotericin B and flucytosine are employed concurrently.*

Like ketoconazole, flucytosine inhibits hepatic drug-metabolizing enzymes, and can thereby raise levels of several other drugs. With at least four drugs—*cisapride, pimozide, dofetilide,* and *quinidine*—elevated levels can lead to potentially fatal cardiac dysrhythmias. Accordingly, flucytosine must not be combined with these drugs.

Preparations, Dosage, and Administration. Flucytosine [Ancobon] is dispensed in 250- and 500-mg capsules for oral administration. The usual dosage for patients with normal kidney function is 50 to 150 mg/kg/day administered in divided doses at 6-hour intervals. At this dosage, some patients must ingest 10 or more capsules 4 times a day. Dosages must be reduced for patients with renal insufficiency. Nausea and vomiting associated with drug administration can be decreased by taking flucytosine capsules over a 15-minute interval.

Caspofungin

Actions and Use. Caspofungin [Cancidas] is the first representative of a new class of antifungal agents, the *echinocandins*. These drugs inhibit the synthesis of beta-1,3-D-glucan, an essential component of the fungal cell wall. Caspofungin is approved only for invasive aspergillosis in patients unresponsive to or intolerant of traditional agents (e.g., amphotericin B, itraconazole). Caspofungin is also active against *Candida* species, but is not yet approved for candidal infections.

Pharmacokinetics. Caspofungin is not absorbed from the GI tract, and hence must be given parenterally (by IV infusion). In the blood, most (97%) of the drug is protein bound. Caspofungin is cleared from the blood with a half-life of 9 to 11 hours. The principal mechanism of plasma clearance is redistribution to tissues, not metabolism or excretion. Over time, the drug undergoes gradual metabolism followed by excretion in the urine and feces.

Adverse Effects. Caspofungin is generally well tolerated. The most common adverse effects are fever (3.6% to 26%) and phlebitis at the injection site (11.3% to 15.7%). Less common reactions include headache (6% to 11.3%), rash (4.6%), nausea (2.5% to 6%), and vomiting (1.2% to 3.1%). In addition, caspofungin can cause effects that appear to be mediated by histamine release. Among these are rash, facial flushing, pruritus, and a sense of warmth. One case of anaphylaxis has been reported.

Use in Pregnancy. Caspofungin is embryotoxic in rats and rabbits. To date, there are no adequate data on effects in pregnant women. Currently, the drug is classified in FDA Pregnancy Risk Category C, and hence should be avoided during pregnancy unless the potential benefits outweigh the potential risks to the fetus.

Drug Interactions. *Drugs that induce cytochrome P450* may decrease levels of caspofungin. Powerful inducers include efavirenz [Sustiva], nelfinavir [Viracept], rifampin [Rifadin], carbamazepine [Tegretol], and phenytoin [Dilantin]. Patients taking these drugs with caspofungin may need to increase caspofungin dosage.

Caspofungin can decrease levels of *tacrolimus* [Prograf], an immunosuppressant. If these drugs are taken concurrently, levels of tacrolimus should be monitored and dosage increased as necessary.

Combining caspofungin with *cyclosporine* [Sandimmune] increases the risk of liver injury, as evidenced by a transient elevation in plasma levels of liver enzyme. Accordingly, the combination should generally be avoided.

Preparations, Dosage, and Administration. Caspofungin [Cancidas] is dispensed as a powder (50 and 70 mg) to be reconstituted in sterile saline for IV infusion. Treatment consists of a 70-mg loading dose followed by daily maintenance doses of 50 mg each. All doses should be infused slowly (over 1 hour). Duration of treatment depends on the severity of the infection and the clinical response. For patients with *moderate* liver impairment, maintenance doses should be reduced to 35 mg. There are no data on dosage for patients with *severe* liver impairment.

DRUGS FOR SUPERFICIAL MYCOSES

The superficial mycoses are caused by two groups of organisms: (1) *Candida* species and (2) dermatophytes (species of *Epidermophyton, Trichophyton,* and *Microsporum*). *Candida* infections usually occur in mucous membranes and moist skin; chronic infections may involve the scalp, skin, and nails. Dermatophytoses are generally confined to the skin, hair, and nails. Superficial infections with dermatophytes are more common than superficial infections with *Candida*.

Overview of Drug Therapy

Superficial mycoses can be treated with a variety of topical and oral drugs. For mild to moderate infections, topical agents are generally preferred. Specific indications for the drugs used against superficial mycoses are summarized in Tables 88–3 and 88–4. Some of these drugs are also used for systemic infections.

Dermatophytic Infections (Ringworm)

Dermatophytic infections are commonly referred to as ringworm (because of characteristic ring-shaped lesions). There are four principal dermatophytic infections, defined by their location: *tinea pedis* (ringworm of the foot, or "athlete's

TABLE 88-3 ■ Drugs for Superficial Fungal Infections*

Drug	Route	Ringworm†	Candida Infection Skin	Candida Infection Mouth	Onychomycosis‡
Azoles					
Clotrimazole	Topical	✔	✔	✔	
Econazole	Topical	✔	✔		
Fluconazole	Oral			✔	✔
Itraconazole	Oral	✔			✔
Ketoconazole	Oral	✔		✔	✔
	Topical	✔	✔		
Miconazole	Topical	✔	✔		
Oxiconazole	Topical	✔			
Sulconazole	Topical	✔			
Allylamines					
Butenafine	Topical	✔			
Naftifine	Topical	✔			
Terbinafine	Oral				✔
	Topical	✔			
Others					
Amphotericin B	Topical		✔		
Ciclopirox	Topical	✔	✔		✔
Griseofulvin	Oral	✔			✔
Haloprogin	Topical	✔			
Nystatin	Topical		✔	✔	
Tolnaftate	Topical	✔			
Undecylenate	Topical	✔			

*Vulvovaginal candidiasis is addressed in Table 88–4.
†*Ringworm* is a popular term for dermatophytic infections, including tinea pedis (ringworm of the foot, "athlete's foot"), tinea cruris (ringworm of the groin, "jock itch"), and tinea corporis (ringworm of the body).
‡*Onychomycosis* is a clinical term for fungal infection of the toenails and fingernails.

foot"), *tinea corporis* (ringworm of the body), *tinea cruris* (ringworm of the groin, or "jock itch"), and *tinea capitis* (ringworm of the scalp).

Tinea Pedis. Tinea pedis, the most common fungal infection, generally responds well to topical therapy. Available agents are listed in Table 88–3. Patients should be advised to wear absorbent cotton socks, change their shoes often, and dry their feet after bathing.

Tinea Corporis. Tinea corporis usually responds to a topical azole or allylamine (see Table 88–3). Treatment should continue for at least 1 week after symptoms have cleared. Severe infection may require a systemic antifungal agent (e.g., griseofulvin).

Tinea Cruris. Tinea cruris responds well to topical therapy. Treatment should continue for at least 1 week after symptoms have abated. If the infection is severely inflamed, a systemic antifungal drug (e.g., clotrimazole) may be needed; topical or systemic glucocorticoids may be needed as well.

Tinea Capitis. Tinea capitis is difficult to treat. Topical drugs are not likely to work. Oral griseofulvin, taken for 6 to 8 weeks, is considered standard therapy. However, recent data indicate that oral terbinafine, taken for only 2 to 4 weeks, may be more effective.

Candidiasis

Vulvovaginal Candidiasis. Vulvovaginal candidiasis is very common, occurring in 75% of women at least once. Most cases are caused by *Candida albicans,* although a few are caused by other *Candida* species. Predisposing factors include pregnancy, obesity, diabetes, debilitation, HIV infection, and use of certain drugs, including oral contraceptives, systemic glucocorticoids, anticancer agents, immunosuppressants, and systemic antibiotics. In the past, most regimens required daily application of a topical drug for 1 to 2 weeks. However, with the medications available today, just 1 to 3 days of topical therapy can be curative. Most recently, *oral* fluconazole has been employed; a single 150-mg dose can be curative—but causes more side effects (headache, rash, GI disturbance) than topical agents. The drugs available for vulvovaginal candidiasis are summarized in Table 88–4. All appear equally effective. Hence, selection among them is largely a matter of patient preference. The longer regimens have no demonstrated advantage over the shorter ones.

Oral Candidiasis. Oral candidiasis, also known as *thrush,* is seen often. Topical agents—*nystatin, clotrimazole,* and *amphotericin B*—are generally effective. In the immunocom-

TABLE 88–4 ■ Drugs for Vulvovaginal Candidiasis

Generic Name	Trade Name	Formulation	Dosage
Oral Preparation			
Fluconazole	Diflucan	150-mg oral tablet	1 tablet once
Topical Preparations			
Butoconazole	Femstat 3	2% vaginal cream	5 gm at hs × 3 days
	Mycelex-3	2% vaginal cream	5 gm at hs × 3 days
	Gynazole 1	2% vaginal cream, SR*	5 gm once
Clotrimazole	Gyne-Lotrimin-3	200 mg vaginal tablet	1 tablet at hs × 3 days
	Gyne-Lotrimin-7	100-mg vaginal tablet	1 tablet at hs × 7 days
		1% vaginal cream	5 gm at hs × 7 days
	Mycelex-7	100-mg vaginal tablet	1 tablet at hs × 7 days
		1% vaginal cream	5 gm at hs × 7 days
	Mycelex-G	500-mg vaginal tablet	1 tablet at hs once
Miconazole	Femizol-M	2% vaginal cream	5 gm at hs × 7 days
	Monistat 3	200-mg vaginal suppository	1 suppository at hs × 3 days
		4% vaginal cream	5 gm at hs × 3 days
	Monistat 7	100-mg vaginal suppository	1 suppository at hs × 7 days
		2% vaginal cream	5 gm at hs × 7 days
Terconazole	Terazol 3	80-mg vaginal suppository	1 suppository at hs × 3 days
		0.8% vaginal cream	5 gm at hs × 3 days
	Terazol 7	0.4% vaginal cream	5 gm at hs × 7 days
Tioconazole	Monistat 1	6.5% vaginal ointment	4.6 gm at hs once
	Vagistat-1	6.5% vaginal ointment	4.6 gm at hs once
Nystatin	Mycostatin	100,000-U vaginal tablet	1 tablet at hs × 14 days

*SR = sustained-release formulation.

promised host, systemic therapy with oral *fluconazole* or *ketoconazole* is usually required.

Onychomycosis (Fungal Infection of the Nails)

Fungal infection of the nails, known as onychomycosis, is difficult to eradicate and requires prolonged therapy. Infections may be caused by dermatophytes or by *Candida* species. Because onychomycosis is largely a cosmetic concern, treatment is usually optional.

Onychomycosis may be treated with oral antifungal drugs or with topical ciclopirox. Success rates with oral therapy are quite low. Success rates with topical therapy are even lower.

Oral Therapy. The drugs used most often are *terbinafine* [Lamisil] and *itraconazole* [Sporanox]. Both agents are active against *Candida* species as well as dermatophytes. Once in the body, these antifungal drugs become incorporated into keratin as the nails grow. Some drugs also diffuse into the nails from the tissue below. Side effects include GI reactions (e.g., nausea, vomiting, abdominal pain), headache, and skin reactions (e.g., itching, rash). Treatment generally lasts 3 to 6 months. Unfortunately, even with this prolonged therapy, the cure rate is relatively low (less than 50%).

Topical Therapy. *Ciclopirox* [Penlac Nail Lacquer] is the first topical treatment for onychomycosis. In contrast to oral terbinafine or itraconazole, which are active against *Candida* species and several dermatophytes, topical ciclopirox is active only against one dermatophyte—*Trichophyton rubrum*—and has no activity against *Candida*. Ciclopirox is applied once a day to the nails and immediately adjacent skin. New coats are applied over old ones. Once a week, all coats are removed with alcohol. Side effects are minimal and localized. Unfor-

tunately, despite prolonged use (up to 48 weeks), ciclopirox confers only modest benefits: Complete cure occurs in less than 12% of patients and, even when complete cure *does* occur, the recurrence rate is high—about 40%. Compared with oral therapy, topical ciclopirox is safer and cheaper, but also less effective.

Use of ciclopirox for superficial fungal infections of the *skin* is discussed below.

Azoles: Clotrimazole, Ketoconazole, Others

Ten members of the azole family are used for superficial mycoses (see Tables 88–3 and 88–4). The usual route is topical. Three of the azoles—fluconazole, miconazole, and ketoconazole—are used for systemic mycoses in addition to superficial mycoses.

The azoles are active against a broad spectrum of pathogenic fungi, including dermatophytes and *Candida* species. Antifungal effects result from inhibiting the biosynthesis of ergosterol, an essential component of the fungal cytoplasmic membrane.

Clotrimazole

Therapeutic Uses. Topical clotrimazole is a drug of choice for dermatophytic infections and candidiasis of the skin, mouth, and vagina.

Adverse Effects. When applied to the skin, clotrimazole can cause stinging, erythema (redness), edema, urticaria, pruritus, and peeling. However, the incidence of these reactions is low. Intravaginal administration occasionally causes burning sensations and lower abdominal cramps. The oral formulation can cause GI distress.

Preparations, Dosage, and Administration. Clotrimazole is available as an oral troche, a cream or tablet for intravaginal use, and in three formulations for application to the skin (cream, lotion, solution). For fungal infections of the skin, the drug is applied twice daily for 2 to 4 weeks. For vulvovaginal candidiasis, several dosing schedules have been employed, including (1) intravaginal insertion of one 200-mg tablet nightly for 7 days, (2) intravaginal insertion of one 500-mg tablet once at bedtime, and (3) intravaginal application of 5 gm of 1% cream once a day for 1 week. Trade names include Gyne-Lotrimin and Mycelex.

Ketoconazole

Ketoconazole [Nizoral] is approved for oral and topical therapy of superficial mycoses. Oral ketoconazole provides effective treatment of dermatophytic infections as well as candidiasis of the skin, mouth, and vagina. However, because of the toxicity associated with oral use, this route should be reserved for infections that have failed to respond to topical agents (e.g., clotrimazole, miconazole). Ketoconazole is available in cream and shampoo formulations for topical therapy of dermatophytic infections and for candidiasis of the skin. The basic pharmacology of ketoconazole is discussed above under *Drugs for Systemic Mycoses*.

Miconazole

Therapeutic Uses. Miconazole [Micatin, Monistat-Derm, Monistat 3, Monistat 7, others] is an azole antifungal drug available for topical and systemic administration. Topical miconazole is a drug of choice for dermatophytic infections as well as for cutaneous and vaginal candidiasis. Systemic use is discussed above.

Adverse Effects. Adverse effects of topical miconazole are generally mild. Intravaginal administration causes burning, itching, and irritation in about 7% of patients. When applied to the skin, miconazole occasionally causes irritation, burning, and maceration. Topical application is not associated with systemic toxicity.

Drug Interactions. *Intravaginal miconazole can intensify the anticoagulant effects of warfarin.* One woman using the combination reported bruising, bleeding gums, and a nosebleed. We have long known that *systemic* miconazole can inhibit metabolism of warfarin, thereby causing warfarin levels to rise. Apparently, intravaginal miconazole can be absorbed in amounts sufficient to do the same thing. Because of this interaction, women taking warfarin should not use intravaginal miconazole. If the drugs must be used concurrently, anticoagulation should be monitored closely and warfarin dosage reduced as indicated.

Preparations, Dosage, and Administration. Miconazole is available in cream, liquid, and powder formulations for application to the skin, and in cream and suppository formulations for intravaginal application. Cutaneous mycoses are treated with twice-daily applications for 2 to 4 weeks. For vaginal candidiasis, 2% miconazole cream or a 100-mg suppository is administered nightly for 1 week. Alternatively, a 4% vaginal cream or a 200-mg suppository can be administered nightly for 3 days.

Fluconazole

Fluconazole [Diflucan] can be used for *oral* therapy of vulvovaginal candidiasis, oropharyngeal candidiasis, and onychomycosis. The dosage for vulvovaginal candidiasis is 150 mg once. The dosage for oropharyngeal candidiasis is 200 mg on day 1 followed by 100 mg daily for 2 weeks. The dosage for onychomycosis is 100 mg daily for 3 to 12 weeks. The basic pharmacology of fluconazole is discussed above under *Drugs for Systemic Mycoses*.

Newer Azole Drugs

Econazole. Econazole [Spectazole] is available for topical application only. The drug is indicated for ringworm infections and superficial candidiasis. Local adverse effects (burning, erythema, stinging, itching) occur in about 3% of patients. Less than 1% of topical econazole is absorbed, and systemic toxicity has not been reported. Econazole, dispensed in a 1% cream, is applied twice daily for 2 to 4 weeks.

Oxiconazole and Sulconazole. Oxiconazole [Oxistat] and sulconazole [Exelderm] are broad-spectrum antifungal drugs. Both are approved for topical treatment of tinea infections. Local adverse effects (itching, burning, irritation, erythema) occur in less than 3% of patients. Neither drug is absorbed to a significant degree, and systemic toxicity has not been reported. Oxiconazole is dispensed as a cream and lotion, and sulconazole is dispensed as a cream and solution. Both drugs are applied once daily for 2 to 4 weeks.

Butoconazole, Terconazole, and Tioconazole. These azole drugs are approved only for topical treatment of vulvovaginal candidiasis. All three are fungicidal. Local adverse effects (burning, itching) occur in 2% to 6% of patients. Absorption following intravaginal administration is low, and systemic reactions are rare (except for headache from terconazole). Because of a small risk of fetal injury, these drugs are not recommended for use during the first trimester of pregnancy. Trade names, formulations, and dosages are presented in Table 88–4.

Griseofulvin

Griseofulvin is administered orally for treatment of superficial mycoses. The drug is inactive against organisms that cause systemic fungal infections.

Mechanism of Action. Following absorption, griseofulvin is deposited in the keratin precursor cells of skin, hair, and nails. Because griseofulvin is present, newly formed keratin is resistant to fungal invasion. Hence, as infected keratin is shed, it is replaced by fungus-free tissue.

Griseofulvin kills fungi by inhibiting fungal mitosis. It does so by binding to components of microtubules, the structures that form the mitotic spindle. Because griseofulvin acts by disrupting mitosis, the drug only affects fungi that are actively growing.

Pharmacokinetics. Griseofulvin is administered orally. Absorption can be enhanced by taking the drug with a fatty meal. As noted, griseofulvin is deposited in the keratin precursor cells of skin, hair, and nails. Elimination is by hepatic metabolism and renal excretion.

Therapeutic Uses. Griseofulvin is employed orally to treat dermatophytic infections of the skin, hair, and nails. The drug is not active against *Candida* species, nor is it useful for treating systemic mycoses. Dermatophytic infections of the skin respond relatively quickly (in 3 to 8 weeks). However, infections of the palms may require 2 to 3 months of treatment, and a year or more may be needed to eliminate infections of the toenails.

Adverse Effects. Most untoward effects are not serious. Transient headache is common, occurring in about 15% of patients. Other mild reactions include rash, insomnia, tiredness, and GI effects (nausea, vomiting, diarrhea). Griseofulvin may cause hepatotoxicity and photosensitivity in patients with porphyria. The drug is contraindicated for individuals with a history of porphyria or hepatocellular disease.

Drug Interactions. Griseofulvin induces hepatic drug-metabolizing enzymes and can thereby decrease the effects of *warfarin*. When this combination is used, the dosage of warfarin may need to be increased.

Preparations, Dosage, and Administration. Griseofulvin is prepared in two particle sizes: microsized and ultramicrosized. The microcrystalline form [Fulvicin-U/F, Grifulvin V, Grisactin] is dispensed in tablets (250 and 500 mg), capsules (250 mg), and a suspension (25 mg/ml). The ultramicrocrystalline form [Fulvicin P/G, Grisactin Ultra, Gris-PEG] is dispensed in tablets (125, 165, 250, and 330 mg).

Dosage depends to some degree upon the formulation (microsized or ultramicrosized). With microsized formulations, the usual adult dosage is 500 mg to 1 gm/day, and the usual pediatric dosage is 11 mg/kg/day. The ultramicrosized particles are better absorbed than the microsized particles. As a result, doses of ultramicrocrystalline griseofulvin are about 30% lower than doses of microcrystalline griseofulvin.

Polyene Antibiotics
Amphotericin B

Amphotericin B [Fungizone] is a broad-spectrum antifungal drug available for IV and topical use. As discussed above, intravenous amphotericin B is a drug of choice for most systemic mycoses. In contrast, topical amphotericin is limited to treatment of *candidiasis of the skin*. The drug is not used for vaginal candidiasis, and is ineffective against dermatophytic infections. Adverse effects (burning, itching, erythema) from topical application occur occasionally. Absorption following topical application is minimal, and does not result in systemic toxicity. Topical amphotericin B is dispensed as a cream, lotion, and ointment. The drug is applied 2 to 4 times each day. Duration of treatment is 1 to 4 weeks.

Nystatin

Actions, Uses, and Adverse Effects. Nystatin is a polyene antibiotic. Use is limited to candidiasis. This agent is the drug of choice for chemotherapy of intestinal candidiasis, and is also employed to treat candidal infections of the skin, mouth, esophagus, and vagina. Nystatin can be administered orally and topically. There is no significant absorption from either route. Oral nystatin occasionally causes GI disturbance (nausea, vomiting, diarrhea). Topical application may produce local irritation.

Preparations, Dosage, and Administration. For oral administration, nystatin is dispensed as a suspension and in tablets and lozenges; dosages range from 100,000 to 1 million units 3 to 4 times a day. Vaginal tablets are employed for vaginal candidiasis; the usual dosage is 100,000 units once a day for 2 weeks. Nystatin is dispensed as a cream, ointment, and powder to treat candidiasis of the skin. The cream and ointment formulations are applied twice daily; the powder is applied 3 times daily. Trade names for nystatin include Mycostatin, Nilstat, and Nystex.

Allylamines
Naftifine

Naftifine [Naftin] is the first representative of a new class of antifungal drugs, the allylamines. Although approved only for topical treatment of dermatophytic infections, naftifine is active against a broad spectrum of pathogenic fungi. The drug acts by inhibiting squalene epoxidase, and thereby inhibits synthesis of ergosterol, a key component of the fungal cell membrane. The most common adverse effects are burning and stinging. Absorption following topical administration is low (about 6%). Systemic effects have not been reported. Naftifine is dispensed in two formulations: 1% cream and 1% gel. The cream is applied once daily; the gel is applied twice daily. The usual duration of treatment is 4 weeks.

Terbinafine

Actions and Uses. Terbinafine [Lamisil] belongs to the same chemical family as naftifine and has the same mechanism of action: inhibition of squalene epoxidase with resultant inhibition of ergosterol synthesis. The drug is highly active against dermatophytes, and less active against *Candida* species. Terbinafine is available in topical and oral formulations. Topical therapy is used for ringworm infections (e.g., tinea corporis, tinea cruris, tinea pedis). Oral therapy is used for onychomycosis (fungal infection of the nails).

Adverse Effects. Adverse effects with *topical* terbinafine are minimal. The discussion that follows applies to *oral* therapy. The most common side effects are headache, diarrhea, dyspepsia, and abdominal pain. Oral terbinafine may also cause skin reactions and disturbance of taste. Of much greater concern, terbinafine may pose a risk of *liver failure:* As of April 2001, the FDA had received 16 reports of liver failure—including 11 deaths and 2 liver transplantations—in patients taking oral terbinafine. Although a causal link has not been established, caution is nonetheless advised. Baseline tests for serum alanine and aspartate transaminases (ALT and AST) are recommended. In addition, patients should be informed about signs of liver dysfunction (persistent nausea, anorexia, fatigue, vomiting, jaundice, right upper abdominal pain, dark urine or stools) and, if they appear, should discontinue terbinafine immediately and undergo evaluation of liver function. Terbinafine is not recommended for patients with pre-existing liver disease.

Preparations, Dosage, and Administration. Terbinafine for oral therapy is available in 250-mg tablets. The dosage for nail infections is 250 mg/day for 6 to 12 weeks. Terbinafine for topical therapy is available in two formulations: 1% cream and 1% gel. Topical therapy typically lasts 1 to 2 weeks.

Butenafine

Butenafine [Mentax] is chemically similar to naftifine and terbinafine, although the drug is not a true allylamine. However, it does have the same mechanism of action: inhibition of squalene epoxidase with resultant inhibi-

tion of ergosterol synthesis. Butenafine is indicated for topical therapy of tinea pedis (athlete's foot), tinea corporis (ringworm), tinea cruris (jock itch), and tinea versicolor. Absorption is minimal and systemic side effects have not been reported. Local reactions include burning, stinging, erythema, irritation, and itching. Butenafine 1% cream is applied once daily for 2 to 4 weeks.

Other Drugs for Superficial Mycoses
Tolnaftate

Tolnaftate is employed topically to treat a variety of superficial mycoses. The drug is active against dermatophytes, but not against *Candida* species. The mechanism of antifungal action is unknown. Adverse effects (sensitization, irritation) are extremely rare. Tolnaftate is available in several formulations. Creams, gels, and solutions are most effective; powders are used adjunctively. The drug is applied twice daily for 2 to 4 weeks. Trade names include Aftate, Tinactin, and Ting.

Haloprogin

Haloprogin [Halotex] is a topical antifungal agent that is active against dermatophytes and *Candida* species. The drug's primary indication is tinea pedis (athlete's foot). Principal side effects are irritation, burning sensations, and peeling of skin. Haloprogin is dispensed as a cream and in solution. Treatment consists of twice-daily application for 2 to 3 weeks.

Undecylenic Acid

Undecylenic acid [Desenex, Cruex, Fungoid AF] is a topical agent used to treat superficial mycoses. The drug is active against dermatophytes but not *Candida* species. Its major indication is tinea pedis (athlete's foot). However, other drugs (tolnaftate, haloprogin, the azoles) are more effective.

Ciclopirox

Ciclopirox is a broad-spectrum, topical antifungal drug. Benefits derive from chelating iron and aluminum present in metal-dependent enzymes that protect fungi from peroxides. Ciclopirox is used for infections of the skin (discussed here) and for infections of the fingernails and toenails (discussed above under *Onychomycosis*). The formulations used for skin infections are marketed under the trade name *Loprox.* The formulation used for nail infections is marketed as *Penlac Nail Lacquer.*

When applied to the skin, ciclopirox is active against dermatophytes and *Candida* species. The drug is effective against superficial candidiasis and tinea pedis, tinea cruris, and tinea corporis. Ciclopirox penetrates the epidermis to the dermis, but systemic absorption is minimal, and hence no significant systemic accumulation occurs. There is no toxicity from local application. For treatment of skin infections, ciclopirox is available in cream and lotion formulations. Treatment consists of twice-daily application for 2 to 4 weeks.

⁙ KEY POINTS

- Amphotericin B is a drug of choice for most systemic mycoses—despite its potential for serious harm.
- Amphotericin B binds to ergosterol in the fungal cell membrane, thereby making the membrane more permeable. The resultant leakage of intracellular cations reduces viability.
- Much of the toxicity of amphotericin B results from binding to cholesterol in host cell membranes.
- Because oral absorption of amphotericin B is poor, the drug must be administered IV to treat systemic mycoses.
- Amphotericin B infusion frequently causes fever, chills, rigors, nausea, and headache. Pretreatment with diphenhydramine plus an analgesic (aspirin or acetaminophen) can reduce mild symptoms. A glucocorticoid can be used for severe reactions. Meperidine or dantrolene can reduce rigors.
- Amphotericin B causes renal injury in most patients. Kidney damage can be minimized by infusing 1 L of saline on the day of amphotericin use.

- If possible, amphotericin B should not be combined with other nephrotoxic drugs (e.g., aminoglycosides, cyclosporine).
- Ketoconazole, the prototype of the azole family of antifungal agents, is active against a broad spectrum of fungi.
- Ketoconazole inhibits cytochrome P450–dependent synthesis of ergosterol, an essential component of the fungal cell membrane. As a result, cell membrane permeability increases, causing cellular components to leak out.
- Ketoconazole is an alternative to IV amphotericin for many fungal infections. Advantages are less toxicity and oral usability.
- Ketoconazole requires an acidic environment for dissolution and absorption. Accordingly, antacids, H$_2$ blocking agents, proton pump inhibitors, and other drugs that reduce gastric acidity will decrease ketoconazole absorption.

- Ketoconazole is hepatotoxic. Liver function must be monitored.
- Ketoconazole inhibits cytochrome P450–dependent drug metabolism, and can thereby cause levels of many drugs to rise. Increased levels of terfenadine, astemizole, and cisapride can lead to fatal dysrhythmias. Accordingly, concurrent use of ketoconazole with these drugs is contraindicated.
- Topical clotrimazole, a member of the azole family of antifungals, is a drug of choice for many superficial mycoses caused by dermatophytes and *Candida* species.
- Onychomycosis (fungal infection of the fingernails and toenails) is difficult to treat and requires prolonged therapy. Preferred agents for treatment are terbinafine and itraconazole.
- Vulvovaginal candidiasis can be treated with a single oral dose of fluconazole or with short-term topical therapy (e.g., one 500-mg vaginal tablet of clotrimazole).

Summary of Major Nursing Implications*

The implications summarized below pertain only to use of antifungal drugs against *systemic* mycoses.

AMPHOTERICIN B

Preadministration Assessment

Therapeutic Goal

Treatment of progressive and potentially fatal systemic fungal infections. Flucytosine may be given to enhance therapeutic effects.

Identifying High-Risk Patients

When used as it should be (i.e., for life-threatening infections), amphotericin has no contraindications.

Implementation: Administration

Routes

Intravenous, intrathecal.

Intravenous Administration

Use aseptic technique when preparing infusion solutions. Infuse slowly (over 2 to 4 hours). Check the solution periodically for a precipitate and, if one forms, discontinue the infusion immediately. Therapy lasts several months; rotate the infusion site to reduce phlebitis and ensure availability of a usable vein. Dosage must be individualized. Alternate-day dosing may be ordered to reduce adverse effects.

Ongoing Evaluation and Interventions

Minimizing Adverse Effects

General Considerations. Amphotericin B can produce serious adverse effects. The patient should be under close supervision, preferably in a hospital.

Infusion Reactions. Infused amphotericin can cause fever, chills, rigors, nausea, and headache. Pretreatment with diphenhydramine plus aspirin or acetaminophen can minimize these reactions. Give meperidine or dantrolene if rigors develop. If other measures fail, give hydrocortisone to suppress symptoms. Rotate the infusion site and pretreat with heparin to minimize phlebitis. Infusion reactions can be reduced by using a lipid-based formulation of amphotericin B instead of the conventional formulation.

Nephrotoxicity. Almost all patients experience renal impairment. Monitor and record intake and output. Kidney function should be tested weekly; if plasma creatinine content rises above 3.5 mg/dl, amphotericin dosage should be reduced. The risk of renal damage can be decreased by infusing 1 L of saline on the day of amphotericin administration, avoiding other nephrotoxic drugs (e.g., aminoglycosides, cyclosporine), and using a lipid-based formulation instead of conventional amphotericin.

Hypokalemia. Renal injury may cause hypokalemia. Serum potassium should be measured frequently. Correct hypokalemia with potassium supplements.

Hematologic Effects. Normocytic, normochromic anemia has occurred secondary to amphotericin-induced suppression of bone marrow. Hematocrit determinations should be performed to monitor for this anemia.

Minimizing Adverse Interactions

Nephrotoxic Drugs. Unless clearly required, amphotericin should not be combined with other nephrotoxic drugs, such as the aminoglycosides and cyclosporine.

*Patient education information is highlighted as blue text.

Summary of Major Nursing Implications*—cont'd

KETOCONAZOLE

Preadministration Assessment

Therapeutic Goal

Treatment of systemic and superficial mycoses. Because of its slow onset, ketoconazole is best suited for long-term therapy of chronic fungal infections.

Baseline Data

Obtain baseline tests of liver function.

Identifying High-Risk Patients

Ketoconazole is *contraindicated* for patients taking terfenadine, astemizole, or cisapride. Use with *caution* in patients with liver disease.

Implementation: Administration

Route

Oral.

Administration

Advise patients to take ketoconazole with food to minimize nausea and vomiting.

An acidic environment is needed for absorption. Instruct patients with achlorhydria to dissolve ketoconazole tablets in 4 ml of 0.2 N HCl and to sip this solution through a glass or plastic straw (to protect the teeth), and to follow drug administration with a glass of water.

Ongoing Evaluation and Interventions

Minimizing Adverse Effects

Hepatotoxicity. Hepatotoxicity is rare but potentially serious; fatal hepatic necrosis has occurred. Tests of liver function should be obtained prior to treatment and at intervals of 1 month or less thereafter. At the first indication of liver injury, ketoconazole should be withdrawn. **Inform patients about symptoms of liver dysfunction (e.g., unusual fatigue, anorexia, nausea, vomiting, jaundice, dark urine, pale stools), and advise them to notify the physician if these occur.**

Minimizing Adverse Interactions

Drugs That Raise Gastric pH. Antacids, H_2 antagonists, anticholinergic drugs, and proton pump inhibitors can reduce ketoconazole absorption. These drugs should be administered no sooner than 2 hours after ingestion of ketoconazole. (Because proton pump inhibitors have a prolonged duration of action, patients using these agents may have insufficient stomach acid for ketoconazole absorption, regardless of when the proton pump inhibitor is administered.)

Terfenadine, Astemizole, and Cisapride. Concurrent use of these drugs with ketoconazole is contraindicated because of the risk of potentially fatal dysrhythmias.

Rifampin. Rifampin reduces plasma levels of ketoconazole. Ketoconazole dosage should be increased if these drugs are used concurrently.

FLUCYTOSINE

Preadministration Assessment

Therapeutic Goal

Treatment of serious infections caused by *Candida* species and *Cryptococcus neoformans*. Flucytosine is usually combined with amphotericin B.

Baseline Data

Obtain baseline tests of renal function, hematologic status, and serum electrolytes.

Identifying High-Risk Patients

Use with *extreme caution* in patients with kidney disease or bone marrow depression.

Implementation: Administration

Route

Oral.

Dosage and Administration

Treatment may require ingestion of 10 or more capsules 4 times a day. **Advise patients to take capsules a few at a time over a 15-minute interval to minimize nausea and vomiting.** Dosage must be reduced in patients with renal impairment.

Ongoing Evaluation and Interventions

Monitoring Summary

Obtain weekly tests of liver function (serum transaminase and alkaline phosphatase levels) and hematologic status (leukocyte counts). In patients receiving amphotericin B concurrently, and in those with pre-existing renal impairment, monitor kidney function and flucytosine levels.

Minimizing Adverse Effects

Hematologic Effects. Flucytosine-induced bone marrow depression can cause neutropenia, thrombocytopenia, and fatal agranulocytosis. The risk of these effects can be minimized by adjusting the dosage to keep plasma flucytosine levels below 100 mg/ml. Obtain weekly leukocyte counts to monitor hematologic effects.

Hepatotoxicity. Mild and reversible liver dysfunction occurs frequently; severe hepatic damage is rare. Obtain weekly determinations of serum transaminase and alkaline phosphatase levels to evaluate liver function.

Minimizing Adverse Interactions

Amphotericin B. Kidney damage from amphotericin B may decrease flucytosine excretion, thereby increasing toxicity secondary to flucytosine accumulation. When these drugs are combined, renal function and flucytosine levels must be monitored.

*Patient education information is highlighted as blue text.

Antiviral Agents I: Drugs for Non-HIV Viral Infections

PURINE NUCLEOSIDE ANALOGS (DNA POLYMERASE INHIBITORS)
Acyclovir
Valacyclovir
Ganciclovir
Valganciclovir
Famciclovir
Cidofovir
Penciclovir
DRUGS FOR HEPATITIS B AND HEPATITIS C
Interferon Alfa
Ribavirin (Oral)
Lamivudine
Adefovir
DRUGS FOR INFLUENZA
Influenza Vaccines
First-Generation Drugs:
Amantadine and Rimantadine
Second-Generation Drugs:
Neuraminidase Inhibitors
OPHTHALMIC ANTIVIRAL DRUGS
Trifluridine
Vidarabine
Idoxuridine
OTHER ANTIVIRAL DRUGS
Foscarnet
Ribavirin (Inhaled)
Palivizumab
Fomivirsen
Docosanol Cream

Antiviral drugs are discussed in this chapter and the one that follows. In this chapter, we consider drugs used to treat infections caused by viruses other than HIV. In Chapter 90, we consider drugs used against HIV infection. Although several new antiviral drugs have been introduced in the last decade, our ability to treat viral infections remains limited. Compared with the dramatic advances made in antibacterial therapy over the past half-century, efforts to develop safe and effective antiviral drugs have been much less successful. A major reason for this lack of success resides in the process of viral replica-tion: Viruses are obligate intracellular parasites that use the biochemical machinery of host cells to reproduce. Because the viral growth cycle employs host-cell enzymes and sub-strates, it is difficult to suppress viral replication without do-ing significant harm to the host. The antiviral drugs used clin-ically act by suppressing biochemical processes unique to viral reproduction. As our knowledge of viral molecular biol-ogy advances, additional virus-specific processes will surely be discovered, thereby giving us new targets against which to direct drugs.

At this time, 22 drugs are available in the United States for treating non-HIV viral infections. These drugs are active against a narrow spectrum of viruses, and hence their utility is limited to a few types of infections. Three drugs are used to treat viral infections of the eye. The rest are used against sys-temic infections. Drugs of first choice for systemic infections are listed in Table 89–1.

PURINE NUCLEOSIDE ANALOGS (DNA POLYMERASE INHIBITORS)

Acyclovir

Acyclovir [Zovirax] is the agent of first choice for most in-fections caused by herpes simplex viruses and varicella-zoster virus. The drug can be administered topically, orally, and in-travenously. Serious side effects are uncommon.

Antiviral Spectrum

Acyclovir is active only against members of the herpesvirus family, a group that includes *herpes simplex viruses* (HSVs), *varicella-zoster virus* (VZV), and *cytomegalovirus* (CMV). Of these, HSVs are most sensitive, VZV is moderately sensi-tive, and most strains of CMV are resistant.

Mechanism of Action

Acyclovir inhibits viral replication by suppressing synthesis of viral DNA. To exert antiviral effects, acyclovir must first un-dergo activation. The critical step in activation is conversion of acyclovir to acyclo-GMP by *thymidine kinase*. Once formed, acyclo-GMP is converted to acyclo-GTP, the compound di-rectly responsible for inhibiting DNA synthesis. Acyclo-GTP suppresses DNA synthesis by (1) inhibiting viral DNA poly-merase and (2) becoming incorporated into the growing strand of viral DNA, which blocks further strand growth.

The selectivity of acyclovir is based in large part on the ability of certain viruses to activate the drug. HSVs are espe-cially sensitive to acyclovir because the drug is a much better

TABLE 89–1 ■ Drugs of Choice for Non-HIV Viral Infections

Virus and Infection	Drugs of Choice
Herpes Simplex Virus	
Orolabial herpes in immunocompetent host	Penciclovir
Genital herpes	Acyclovir *or* famciclovir *or* valacyclovir
Encephalitis	Acyclovir
Mucocutaneous disease in the immunocompromised host	Acyclovir
Neonatal	Acyclovir
Acyclovir-resistant	Foscarnet
Keratoconjunctivitis	Trifluridine
Varicella-Zoster Virus	
Varicella (chickenpox)	Acyclovir
Herpes zoster (shingles)	Acyclovir *or* famciclovir *or* valacyclovir
Varicellaor zoster in the immunocompromised host	Acyclovir
Acyclovir-resistent	Foscarnet
Cytomegalovirus	
Retinitis	Ganciclovir *or* valganciclovir *or* foscarnet *or* cidofovir *or* fomivirsen
Influenza A Virus	
Respiratory tract infection	Amantadine *or* rimantadine
Influenza A and B Virus	Zanamivir *or* oseltamivir
Respiratory Syncytial Virus	Ribavirin
Hepatitis B Virus	
Chronic hepatitis	Interferon alfa, lamivudine
Hepatitis C Virus	
Chronic hepatitis	Interferon alfa *plus* ribavirin

substrate for thymidine kinase produced by HSV than it is for mammalian thymidine kinase. Hence, formation of acyclo-GMP, the limiting step in the activation of acyclovir, occurs almost exclusively in cells infected with HSV. Cytomegalovirus is inherently resistant to the drug because acyclovir is a poor substrate for the form of thymidine kinase produced by this virus.

Resistance

Herpesviruses develop resistance to acyclovir by three mechanisms: (1) decreased production of thymidine kinase, (2) alteration of thymidine kinase such that it no longer converts acyclovir to acyclo-GMP, and (3) alteration of viral DNA polymerase such that it is less sensitive to inhibition. Of these mechanisms, thymidine kinase deficiency is by far the most common. Resistance is rare in immunocompetent patients, but many cases have been reported in transplant patients and patients with AIDS. Lesions caused by resistant HSVs can be extensive and severe, progressing despite continued acyclovir therapy. Acyclovir-resistant HSVs and VZV usually respond to IV foscarnet.

Therapeutic Uses

Herpes Simplex Genitalis. Most genital herpes infections are caused by *type 2 HSV* (HSV-2). For patients with *initial* infection, *topical* acyclovir reduces the duration of viral shedding, but does not accelerate healing. Topical acyclovir is not effective for *recurrent* genital infections. *Oral* acyclovir is superior to topical therapy for initial genital infections and for recurrent infections. For patients with initial infection, oral therapy decreases formation of additional lesions and decreases the duration and severity of the initial episode. For patients with recurrent herpes genitalis, continuous oral therapy reduces the frequency at which lesions appear. When initial genital infection is especially severe, *intravenous* acyclovir may be indicated. Patients with primary or recurrent herpes genitalis should be informed that, although acyclovir can decrease symptoms, the drug does not eliminate the virus and does not produce cure. Patients should be advised to avoid all sexual contact when lesions are present, and should use a condom even when lesions are absent.

Mucocutaneous Herpes Simplex Infections. Herpes infections of the face and oropharynx are usually caused by HSV-2. For immunocompetent patients, *oral* acyclovir can be used to treat primary infections of the gums and mouth. Oral acyclovir can also be taken *prophylactically* to prevent episodes of *recurrent* herpes labialis (fever blisters). However, there is no truly effective treatment for active herpes labialis. Mucocutaneous herpes infections can be especially severe in immunocompromised patients. For these people, *intravenous* acyclovir is the treatment of choice.

Varicella-Zoster Infections. High doses of *oral* acyclovir are effective for herpes zoster (shingles) in older adults. Oral therapy is also effective for varicella (chickenpox) in children, adolescents, and adults, provided that dosing is begun early (within 24 hours of rash onset). *Intravenous* acyclovir is the treatment of choice for varicella-zoster infection in the immunocompromised host.

Pharmacokinetics

Acyclovir may be administered topically, orally, or intravenously. Oral bioavailability is low, ranging from 15% to 30%. No significant absorption occurs with topical use. Once in the blood, acyclovir is distributed widely to body fluids and tissues. Levels achieved in cerebrospinal fluid are 50% of those in plasma. Elimination is renal, primarily as the unchanged drug. In patients with normal kidney function, acyclovir has a half-life of 2.5 hours. The half-life is prolonged by renal impairment, reaching 20 hours in anuric patients. Accordingly, dosages should be reduced in patients with kidney disease.

Adverse Effects

Intravenous Therapy. Intravenous acyclovir is generally well tolerated. The most common reactions are *phlebitis* and *inflammation* at the site of infusion. Reversible *nephrotoxicity,* manifested as elevations in serum creatinine and blood urea nitrogen, occurs in some patients. The cause of nephrotoxicity is deposition of acyclovir in renal tubules. The risk of renal injury is increased by dehydration and by use of other nephrotoxic drugs. Kidney damage can be minimized by infusing acyclovir slowly (over 1 hour) and by ensuring adequate hydration during the infusion and for 2 hours after.

Oral and Topical Therapy. Oral acyclovir is devoid of serious adverse effects. Renal impairment has not been reported. The most common reactions to oral therapy are nausea, vomiting, diarrhea, headache, and vertigo. Topical acyclovir frequently causes transient burning or stinging sensations; systemic reactions do not occur.

Preparations, Dosage, and Administration

Topical. Acyclovir [Zovirax] is dispensed as a 5% ointment for topical use. This formulation is indicated for initial episodes of herpes genitalis and for mild mucocutaneous herpes simplex infections in the immunocompromised host. The drug is applied 6 times a day at 3-hour intervals for 7 days. Patients should be advised to apply the drug with a finger cot or rubber glove to avoid viral transfer to other body sites and other people.

Oral. Oral acyclovir [Zovirax] is available in capsules (200 mg), tablets (400 and 800 mg), and a suspension (200 mg/5 ml). Dosages for patients with normal kidney function are given below. Dosages must be reduced for patients with renal impairment.

- For *initial episodes of herpes genitalis,* the usual dosage is 400 mg 3 times a day for 7 to 10 days.
- For *episodic recurrences of herpes genitalis,* the usual dosage is 400 mg 3 times a day for 5 days.
- For *long-term suppressive therapy of recurrent genital infections,* the usual dosage is 400 mg twice daily for up to 12 months.
- For *acute therapy of herpes zoster,* the dosage is 800 mg 5 times a day (at 4-hour intervals) for 7 to 10 days.
- For *varicella* (chickenpox), the dosage is 20 mg/kg (but no more than 800 mg) 4 times a day for 5 days. Treatment should begin at the earliest sign of rash.

Intravenous. Acyclovir [Zovirax] is dispensed as a powder (500 mg/10-ml vial, 1000 mg/20-ml vial) to be reconstituted for IV administration. The drug is administered by slow IV infusion (over 1 hour or more). It must not be given by IV bolus or by IM or SC injection. To minimize the risk of renal damage, hydrate the patient during the infusion and for 2 hours after. Dosages for patients with normal kidney function are given below. Dosages should be reduced for patients with renal impairment.

- For *mucocutaneous herpes simplex infection in the immunocompromised host,* the adult dosage is 5 mg/kg infused every 8 hours for 7 days. The dosage for children under 12 years is 250 mg/m² infused every 8 hours for 7 days.
- For *varicella-zoster infection in the immunocompromised host,* the adult dosage is 10 mg/kg infused every 8 hours for 7 days. The dosage for children under 12 years is 500 mg/m² infused every 8 hours for 7 days.
- For *severe episodes of herpes genitalis in the immunocompetent host,* the adult dosage is 5 to 10 mg/kg infused every 8 hours for 5 to 7 days (or until symptoms resolve). The dosage for children under 12 years is 250 mg/m² infused every 8 hours for 5 days.

Valacyclovir

Actions and Uses. Valacyclovir [Valtrex], a prodrug form of acyclovir, has three approved indications: (1) herpes zoster (shingles) in the immunocompetent host, (2) herpes simplex genitalis, and (3) herpes labialis (cold sores). In all three infections, benefits depend on conversion of valacyclovir to acyclovir, its active form. In a clinical trial in patients with *herpes zoster,* valacyclovir (1000 mg 3 times a day for 7 or 14 days) was somewhat more effective than acyclovir (800 mg 5 times a day for 7 days) in reducing the duration of pain and the duration of postherpetic neuralgia. In clinical trials in patients with initial or recurrent *herpes genitalis,* valacyclovir (1000 mg twice a day) and acyclovir (200 mg 5 times a day) produced similar results.

In patients receiving immunosuppressive drugs following a kidney transplant, prophylaxis with valacyclovir (2 gm 4 times a day for 90 days) can reduce the risk of CMV disease, a major complication of transplant surgery.

Pharmacokinetics. After oral administration, valacyclovir undergoes rapid absorption followed by rapid and essentially complete conversion to acyclovir. When acyclovir itself is given orally, bioavailability is only 15% to 30%. In contrast, when valacyclovir is given orally, the effective bioavailability of acyclovir is greatly increased—to about 55%. Hence, valacyclovir represents a more efficient way of getting acyclovir into the body. Following conversion of valacyclovir to acyclovir, the kinetics are the same as if acyclovir itself had been given.

Adverse Effects. In some immunocompromised patients, valacyclovir has produced a syndrome known as *thrombotic thrombocytopenic purpura/hemolytic uremic syndrome* (TTP/HUS). This syndrome, which is potentially fatal, has not occurred in immunocompetent patients. Valacyclovir is not approved for use in immunocompromised hosts. Aside from causing TTP/HUS, valacyclovir is generally well tolerated, producing the same side effects seen with oral acyclovir (e.g., nausea, vomiting, diarrhea, headache, vertigo).

Preparations, Dosage, and Administration. Valacyclovir [Valtrex] is available in 500- and 1000-mg capsules for oral use. The drug may be taken without regard to meals. In patients with renal impairment, dosages should be reduced.

For patients with *herpes zoster,* the recommended dosage is 1000 mg 3 times a day for 7 days. Therapy should begin as soon as possible after onset of symptoms.

For patients with *herpes simplex genitalis,* the dosage is 1 gm twice daily for 10 days (for initial episode), 500 mg twice daily for 3 days (for episodic recurrences), and 500 to 1000 mg once daily (for long-term suppression).

For patients with *herpes labialis* (cold sores) the dosage is 2 gm twice, taken 12 hours apart. Dosing should begin as soon as possible after onset of symptoms.

Ganciclovir

Ganciclovir [Cytovene, Vitrasert] is a synthetic antiviral agent with activity against herpesviruses, including CMV. Because the drug can cause serious adverse effects, especially granulocytopenia and thrombocytopenia, use should be restricted to prevention and treatment of CMV infection in the immunocompromised host.

Mechanism of Action. Ganciclovir is converted to its active form, ganciclovir triphosphate, inside infected cells. As ganciclovir triphosphate, it suppresses replication of viral DNA by (1) inhibiting viral DNA polymerase and (2) undergoing incorporation into the growing DNA chain, which causes premature chain termination.

Pharmacokinetics. Bioavailability of oral ganciclovir is low: only 5% (under fasting conditions) and 9% (when taken with food). Once in the blood, the drug is widely distributed to body fluids and tissues. Ganciclovir is excreted unchanged in the urine. In patients with normal renal function, the half-life is about 3 hours. In patients with renal impairment, the half-life is prolonged. Accordingly, dosages should be reduced in patients with kidney disease.

Therapeutic Use. Ganciclovir has two approved indications: (1) treatment of CMV retinitis in immunocompromised patients, including those with AIDS; and (2) prevention of CMV infection in transplant patients considered at risk. In patients with AIDS, CMV retinitis has an incidence of 15% to 40%. Although most AIDS patients respond initially, the relapse rate is high. Accordingly, for most patients, maintenance therapy should continue indefinitely. The risk of relapse is higher with oral ganciclovir than with IV ganciclovir. Since viral resistance can develop during treatment, this possibility should be considered if the patient responds poorly.

Adverse Effects. Granulocytopenia and Thrombocytopenia. The adverse effect of greatest concern is bone marrow suppression, which can result in granulocytopenia (40%) and thrombocytopenia (20%). These hematologic responses can be exacerbated by concurrent therapy with zidovudine. Conversely, granulocytopenia can be reduced with granulocyte colony-stimulating factors (see Chapter 53). Because of the risk of adverse hematologic effects, blood cell counts must be monitored. Treatment should be interrupted if the absolute neutrophil count falls below 500/mm³ or if the platelet count falls below 25,000/mm³. Cell counts usually begin to recover within 3 to 5 days. Ganciclovir should be used with caution in patients with pre-existing cytopenias, in those with a history of cytopenic reactions to other drugs, and in those taking other bone marrow suppressants (e.g., zidovudine, trimetrexate).

Reproductive Toxicity. Ganciclovir is teratogenic and embryotoxic in laboratory animals and probably in humans. Women should be advised to avoid pregnancy during therapy and for 90 days after ending treatment. At doses equivalent to those used therapeutically, ganciclovir inhibits spermatogenesis in mice; sterility is reversible with low doses and irreversible with high doses. Female infertility may also occur. Patients should be forewarned of these effects.

Other Adverse Effects. Incidental effects include nausea, fever, rash, anemia, liver dysfunction, and confusion and other central nervous system (CNS) symptoms.

Preparations, Dosage, and Administration. Intravenous. Ganciclovir [Cytovene] is available as a powder to be reconstituted for IV infusion. Solutions are alkaline and must be infused into a freely flowing vein to avoid local injury. For treatment of CMV retinitis, the *initial dosage* for adults with normal renal function is 5 mg/kg (infused over 1 hour) every 12 hours for 14 to 21 days. Two *maintenance dosages* can be used: (1) 5 mg/kg infused over 1 hour once every day or (2) 6 mg/kg infused over 1 hour once a day, 5 days each week. Dosages must be reduced for patients with renal impairment. Since many patients with AIDS must continue maintenance therapy for life, they need a permanent IV line and equipment for home infusion. Adequate hydration must be maintained in all patients to ensure renal excretion of ganciclovir.

Oral. Oral ganciclovir [Cytovene] is indicated for maintenance therapy in patients with CMV retinitis. The dosage is 1000 mg 3 times daily with food.

Intraocular. The ganciclovir intraocular implant [Vitrasert] is indicated for CMV retinitis in patients with AIDS. Surgical implantation, which takes about 1 hour, is performed under local anesthesia on an outpatient basis. Vision is usually blurred for 2 to 4 weeks after the procedure. The implant must be replaced every 5 to 8 months. Clinical trials indicate that CMV retinitis progresses more slowly in patients who receive intraocular ganciclovir compared with those on IV ganciclovir.

Valganciclovir

Basic and Clinical Pharmacology. Valganciclovir [Valcyte] is a prodrug version of ganciclovir [Cytovene] with greater oral bioavailability (60% vs. 9%). Like ganciclovir, valganciclovir is indicated for CMV retinitis. Following absorption from the GI tract, valganciclovir is rapidly metabolized to ganciclovir, its active form—and eventually undergoes excretion as unchanged ganciclovir in the urine. When compared with *intravenous* ganciclovir in patients with active CMV retinitis, oral valganciclovir was just as effective—and much more convenient. Recently, valganciclovir was shown to reduce transmission of genital herpes (see Chapter 91).

Adverse effects are the same as with ganciclovir. The principal concern is blood dyscrasias—granulocytopenia (27%), anemia (26%), and thrombocytopenia (6%)—secondary to bone marrow suppression. In addition, valganciclovir frequently causes diarrhea (41%), nausea (30%), vomiting (21%), fever (31%), and headache (22%). Valganciclovir is presumed to pose the same risks of mutagenesis, aspermatogenesis, and carcinogenesis as ganciclovir.

Preparations, Dosage, and Administration. Valganciclovir [Valcyte] is available in 450-mg tablets for oral use. The dosage for *induction* (treatment of active CMV retinitis) is 900 mg (2 tablets) twice daily for 21 days. The dosage for *maintenance* is 900 mg once daily. All doses should be taken with food to enhance bioavailability. Dosage must be reduced for patients with renal impairment.

Because valganciclovir has the potential for mutagenesis and carcinogenesis, it should be handled carefully. Tablets should be ingested intact, without crushing or chewing. Direct contact with broken tablets should be avoided. If contact does occur, the area should be washed with soap and water. When handling or disposing of the drug, healthcare workers should follow the same guidelines established for cytotoxic anticancer drugs.

Famciclovir

Famciclovir [Famvir] is a prodrug used to treat acute herpes zoster and genital herpes infection. Benefits are equivalent to those of acyclovir. Adverse effects are minimal.

Pharmacokinetics. Famciclovir undergoes rapid absorption from the GI tract followed by enzymatic conversion to *penciclovir,* its active form. Food decreases the rate of famciclovir absorption but not the extent. As a result, the amount of penciclovir produced is the same whether famciclovir is taken with or without food. Penciclovir is excreted in the urine, largely unchanged. The plasma half-life of penciclovir is about 2.5 hours. However, the half-life of penciclovir within cells is much longer. In patients with renal impairment, the plasma half-life of penciclovir is prolonged.

Mechanism of Action and Antiviral Spectrum. Penciclovir undergoes intracellular conversion to penciclovir triphosphate, a compound that inhibits viral DNA polymerase, and thereby prevents replication of viral DNA. Under clinical conditions, formation of penciclovir triphosphate requires viral thymidine kinase. As a result, inhibition of DNA synthesis is limited to cells that are infected, leaving the vast majority of host cells unharmed. *In vitro,* penciclovir is active against type 1 HSV (HSV-1), HSV-2, and VZV.

Therapeutic Use. Famciclovir is approved for treatment of acute herpes zoster (shingles) and herpes simplex genitalis. In patients with herpes zoster, the drug can decrease the time to full crusting from 7 days down to 5 days. Famciclovir does not decrease the *incidence* of postherpetic neuralgia, but can decrease the *duration* (from 112 days down to 61 days). In a trial comparing famciclovir with acyclovir, both drugs had equivalent effects against herpes zoster.

In patients with genital herpes simplex infection, famciclovir is active against the first episode and recurrent episodes. In addition, it can be used for long-term suppression.

Adverse Effects. Famciclovir is very well tolerated. In clinical trials, the incidence of side effects was the same as in patients taking a placebo. Safety for use during pregnancy or breast-feeding and in children under the age of 18 has not been established.

Preparations, Dosage, and Administration. Preparations. Famciclovir [Famvir] is dispensed in tablets (125, 250, and 500 mg) for oral administration. Famciclovir can be taken without regard to meals.

Acute Herpes Zoster. The recommended dosage is 500 mg every 8 hours for 7 days. Treatment should start no later than 72 hours after onset of symptoms. In patients with renal impairment, the interval between doses should be increased to 12 hours or 24 hours, depending on the degree of impairment.

Herpes Simplex Genitalis. For initial episodes, the dosage is 250 mg 3 times a day for 5 to 10 days. For episodic recurrence, the dosage is 125 mg twice a day for 5 days. For long-term suppression, the dosage is 250 mg twice daily.

Cidofovir

Cidofovir [Vistide] is an IV drug with just one indication: CMV retinitis in patients with AIDS. Alternative drugs for this infection are foscarnet, which is given IV, and ganciclovir, which may be administered IV, PO, or by ocular insert. Compared with IV foscarnet or IV ganciclovir, cidofovir has the distinct advantage of needing fewer infusions: Whereas foscarnet and ganciclovir must be infused daily, cidofovir is infused just once a week or every other week. The major adverse effect of the drug is kidney damage.

Mechanism of Action. Once inside cells, cidofovir is converted to cidofovir diphosphate, its active form. As the diphosphate, cidofovir causes selective inhibition of viral DNA polymerase, and thereby inhibits viral DNA synthesis. Intracellular concentrations of cidofovir diphosphate are too low to inhibit human DNA polymerases. Hence, host cells are spared.

Antiviral Spectrum and Therapeutic Use. Cidofovir is active against herpesviruses, including CMV, HSV-1, HSV-2, and VZV. At this time, the drug is approved only for CMV retinitis in patients with AIDS. Whether cidofovir is active against CMV infections in other patients or at other sites (e.g., GI tract, lungs) is unknown. In clinical trials in patients with AIDS and established CMV retinitis, cidofovir significantly delayed progression of retinitis.

Pharmacokinetics. Cidofovir is administered by IV infusion and is excreted by the kidneys. Probenecid competes with cidofovir for renal tubular secretion, and thereby delays elimination. Cidofovir has a prolonged *intracellular* half-life (17 to 65 hours), and therefore long intervals can separate doses. In contrast, IV foscarnet and ganciclovir must be infused daily.

Adverse Effects. The principal adverse effect is *kidney damage*. To reduce the risk of renal injury, all patients must receive probenecid and IV hydration therapy with each cidofovir infusion. Also, they should be monitored for signs of kidney damage (proteinuria, elevation of serum creatinine). If injury is detected, cidofovir should be withheld or the dosage reduced, depending on the degree of damage. Cidofovir is contraindicated for patients taking other drugs that can injure the kidney.

In addition to kidney damage, cidofovir can cause *granulocytopenia*, and hence neutrophil counts should be monitored.

In animal studies, cidofovir was carcinogenic and teratogenic, and caused hypospermia.

Preparations, Dosage, and Administration. Cidofovir [Vistide] is dispensed in solution (75 mg/ml) in 5-ml ampules. To reduce the risk of renal injury, cidofovir infusions must be accompanied by IV hydration therapy and PO probenecid.

Each cidofovir dose—for induction or maintenance—consists of 5 mg/kg infused IV over 1 hour. For induction, two doses are given 1 week apart. For maintenance, one dose is given every 2 weeks. The size of each dose must be reduced for patients with renal impairment. If impairment is severe, cidofovir should be withheld.

Oral probenecid must accompany each infusion. The dosage is 2 gm given 3 hours before the infusion, 1 gm given 1 hour after the infusion, and 1 gm more given 8 hours after that. Ingesting food before each dose can decrease probenecid-induced nausea and vomiting. An antiemetic may also be used.

Hydration is accomplished by infusing 1 L of 0.9% saline solution over 1 to 2 hours immediately before infusing cidofovir. For patients who can tolerate it, 1 L more can be infused over 1 to 3 hours, beginning when the cidofovir infusion begins or as soon as it is over.

Penciclovir

Penciclovir [Denavir] is a topical drug indicated for recurrent herpes labialis (cold sores) in immunocompetent adults. The drug suppresses viral replication by inhibiting DNA polymerase, the enzyme that makes DNA. Penciclovir is dispensed in a 1% cream to be applied every 2 hours (except when sleeping) for 4 days. In clinical trials, benefits were modest: The average duration of pain and time to healing was decreased by just half a day, from 5 days down to 4.5 days. The only common adverse effect is mild local erythema.

DRUGS FOR HEPATITIS B AND HEPATITIS C

Viral hepatitis is the most common liver disorder. Millions of Americans are affected. Viral hepatitis can be caused by six different hepatitis viruses, labeled A, B, C, D, E, and G. All six can cause *acute* hepatitis, but only B, C, and D also cause *chronic* hepatitis. Acute hepatitis lasts for 6 months or less and is characterized by liver inflammation, jaundice, and elevation of serum alanine aminotransferase (ALT) activity. In most cases, acute hepatitis resolves spontaneously, and hence intervention is generally unnecessary. In contrast, chronic hepatitis can lead to cirrhosis, hepatocellular carcinoma, and life-threatening liver failure, and hence treatment should be considered.

Most cases (90%) of chronic hepatitis are caused by either hepatitis B virus (HBV) or hepatitis C virus (HCV). Accordingly, our discussion focuses on hepatitis B and hepatitis C. About 1.5% of Americans are infected with HBV or HCV—5 times more than the number infected with HIV. Comparisons between hepatitis A, B, and C are summarized in Table 89–2.

Hepatitis B Infection. In the United States, about 1.25 million people have chronic hepatitis B. Transmission is primarily through exchange of blood or semen. Between 45% and 60% of exposed adults develop acute hepatitis. Of these, about 11,000 require hospitalization for deep fatigue, muscle pain, and jaundice. In adults, acute infection leads to viral clearance by the immune system. Hence, only 3% to 5% of infected adults develop chronic infection. The best strategy against HBV is prevention: All children should receive HBV vaccine before entering school (see Chapter 64). Three drugs are used for treatment: *interferon alfa* [PEG-Intron, others], *lamivudine* [Epivir HBV], and *adefovir* [Hepsera]. With all three, rates of long-term remission are relatively low (about 30%).

Hepatitis C Infection. About 2.7 million Americans have chronic hepatitis C. As with hepatitis B, transmission occurs largely through exchange of blood or semen. Among those exposed to HCV, 75% to 85% develop infection. However, most people with chronic hepatitis C have no symptoms, although they can transmit HCV to others. Chronic HCV infec-

TABLE 89–2 ■ Characteristics of Hepatitis A, Hepatitis B, and Hepatitis C			
Point of Comparison	**Hepatitis A**	**Hepatitis B**	**Hepatitis C**
Causative agent	Hepatitis A virus	Hepatitis B virus	Hepatitis C virus
Infections that become chronic	None	3%–5%	>70%
Acute infections each year in the U.S.	179,000	185,000	38,000
U.S. residents with chronic infection	None	1.25 million	2.7 million
Annual deaths in the U.S. from chronic infection	None	6000	8000–10,000
People worldwide with chronic infection	None	350 million	170 million
Method of prevention	Hepatitis A vaccine	Hepatitis B vaccine	None available
Preferred treatment	None	Interferon alfa *or* lamivudine	Interferon alfa *plus* ribavirin

tion undergoes slow progression, and, in some people, eventually causes liver failure, cancer, and death. In fact, chronic hepatitis C is the leading reason for liver transplants, and kills 8000 to 10,000 Americans each year. Currently, treatment is recommended only for patients with HCV viremia, persistent elevation of ALT, and evidence of hepatic fibrosis and inflammation upon liver biopsy. The most effective treatment for hepatitis C is *pegylated interferon alfa combined with ribavirin*. There is no vaccine for hepatitis C.

It is important to note that not all hepatitis C viruses are the same. There are 6 genotypes of HCV, and more than 50 subtypes. In the United States, 75% of HCV infections are caused by HCV genotype 1, which, unfortunately, is less responsive to treatment than other HCV genotypes.

Interferon Alfa

Human interferons are naturally occurring compounds with complex antiviral, immunomodulatory, and antineoplastic actions. The interferon family has three major classes, designated alpha, beta, and gamma. All of the interferons used for hepatitis belong to the alpha class (Table 89–3). In the discussion below, these compounds are referred to collectively as *interferon alfa*. None of these agents can be used orally, and hence administration is parenteral—usually SC. Commercial production is by recombinant DNA technology.

Mechanism of Action. Interferon alfa has multiple effects on the viral replication cycle. After binding to receptors on host cell membranes, the drug blocks viral entry into cells, synthesis of viral messenger RNA and viral proteins, and viral assembly and release.

Standard Versus Long-Acting Interferons. The alfa interferons can be divided into two groups—standard and long acting—based on their time course of action (see Table 89–3). The standard preparations have short half-lives, and hence must be administered frequently—at least *3 times a week*. In contrast, the long-acting preparations are administered less frequently—just *once a week*—making them much more convenient. In addition, with the long-acting preparations, blood levels remain high between doses, and hence clinical responses are superior.

How are long-acting interferons made? By conjugating a standard interferon (e.g., interferon alfa-2a) with polyethylene glycol (PEG), in a process known as *pegylation*. Therapeutic effects of the pegylated product are due solely to its interferon component. The PEG component serves only to delay elimination. At this time, two long-acting interferons are available: *pegylated interferon (peg-interferon) alfa-2a* [Pegasys] and *peg-interferon alfa-2b* [PEG-Intron]. Because of their convenience and superior efficacy, these products are generally preferred to the standard interferons.

Effects in Chronic Hepatitis B. In patients with chronic hepatitis B, parenteral interferon alfa-2b (4 months of either 5 million IU/day or 10 million IU 3 times a week) reduces serum ALT and improves liver histology in about 40% of recipients. Remissions have been prolonged.

Effects in Chronic Hepatitis C. In patients with chronic hepatitis C, responses are equally modest with all forms of interferon alfa. After 12 months of treatment (e.g., with 3 million IU of interferon alfacon-1 three times a week), serum ALT normalizes in 40% to 50% of patients, and serum levels of HCV RNA (a marker for HCV in blood) become undetectable in 30% to 40%. Unfortunately, about half of these people relapse when treatment is stopped; sustained responses are maintained in only 5% to 15% of patients. As discussed below, combining interferon alfa with ribavirin can improve response rates.

Adverse Effects. All formulations of interferon alfa produce the same spectrum of adverse effects. However, the incidence is higher with the long-acting preparations.

The most common side effect is a *flu-like syndrome* characterized by fever, fatigue, myalgia, headache, and chills. The incidence is about 50%. Fortunately, symptoms tend to diminish with continued therapy. Some symptoms (fever, headache, myalgia) can be reduced with acetaminophen.

Interferon alfa frequently causes *neuropsychiatric effects*—especially *depression*. Suicidal ideation and outright suicide have occurred. The risk of depression is increased by large doses and by prolonged treatment. The mechanism underlying depression is unknown. In many patients, depression responds to antidepressant drugs (e.g., paroxetine). If depression persists, a reduction in dosage or cessation of treatment is indicated.

		Dosage	
Generic Name	**Trade Name**	**Chronic Hepatitis B**	**Chronic Hepatitis C**
Standard Alfa Interferons			
Interferon alfa-2a	Roferon-A	—	3 million IU SC 3 times/wk
Interferon alfa-2b	Intron A	5 million IU/day SC *or* 10 million IU SC 3 times/wk	3 million IU SC 3 times/wk
Interferon alfacon-1	Infergen	—	9 µg SC 3 times/wk
Long-Acting Alfa Interferons			
Pegylated interferon alfa-2a	Pegasys	—	180 µg SC once/wk
Pegylated interferon alfa-2b	PEG-Intron	—	*Monotherapy:* 1 µg/kg SC once/wk *With ribavirin:* 1.5 µg/kg SC once/wk

TABLE 89–3 ■ Interferon Alfa Preparations: Dosages for Chronic Hepatitis

Prolonged or high-dose therapy can cause fatigue, hair loss, thyroid dysfunction, heart damage, and bone marrow depression, manifesting as neutropenia and thrombocytopenia.

Other adverse effects include alopecia and GI effects: nausea, diarrhea, anorexia, and vomiting. Injection-site reactions (inflammation, bruising, itching, irritation) are common, especially with the long-acting agents.

Ribavirin (Oral)

Actions and Therapeutic Use. Oral ribavirin [Rebetol, Copegus], combined with SC interferon alfa, is the treatment of choice for chronic hepatitis C. When used alone against HCV, ribavirin is not effective: Treatment produces a transient normalization of serum ALT, but does not reduce serum HCV RNA. Combining ribavirin with interferon alfa greatly improves response rates. The drug was originally approved for combined use with standard interferon alfa. However, combined use with pegylated interferon alfa is more effective, and hence is now preferred. Ribavirin has a broad spectrum of antiviral activity, but its mechanism of action remains unclear.

In addition to its use against HCV, ribavirin is available as an aerosol for treating children infected with respiratory syncytial virus. This use is discussed below under *Ribavirin (Inhaled)*.

Clinical Trials. The objective of hepatitis C therapy is to elicit a sustained virologic response (SVR), defined as loss of detectable serum HCV RNA that persists for at least 6 months after treatment. By this criterion, treatment with ribavirin plus standard interferon alfa for 24 to 48 weeks produces a SVR in 30% to 40% of previously untreated patients. In recent trials using pegylated interferon alfa, response rates were even higher. For example, in one trial, the response rate was 68% with peg-interferon alfa plus ribavirin versus only 51% with standard interferon alfa plus ribavirin.

Adverse Effects. Although ribavirin and interferon alfa are generally well tolerated, both drugs can cause significant adverse effects. As discussed above, interferon alfa frequently causes *flu-like symptoms,* and occasionally causes *severe depression.*

The principal concerns with ribavirin are *hemolytic anemia* and *birth defects.* Because anemia can develop rapidly, blood counts should made before treatment, 2 weeks and 4 weeks into treatment, and periodically thereafter. In laboratory animals, ribavirin is teratogenic and embryolethal when taken by females, and causes sperm abnormalities when taken by males. Accordingly, *ribavirin is classified in Food and Drug Administration (FDA) Pregnancy Risk Category X, and therefore is contraindicated for use during pregnancy.* Before initiating treatment, pregnancy must be ruled out. During treatment, pregnancy must be avoided—both by females taking ribavirin, and by female partners of men taking ribavirin. To avoid pregnancy, couples should use *two* reliable forms of birth control during treatment and for 6 months after.

Preparations, Dosage, and Administration. For treatment of chronic hepatitis C, ribavirin *must be combined with interferon alfa;* the drug is not effective when used alone. Ribavirin is approved specifically for combined use with interferon alfa-2b; however, combined use with a pegylated interferon is now preferred. Duration of therapy is prolonged, typically 24 to 48 weeks.

Preparations. Ribavirin is available (1) in 200-mg *capsules,* marketed as *Rebetol;* (2) in 200-mg *tablets,* marketed as *Copegus;* and (3) in a kit, marketed as *Rebetron,* that contains ribavirin capsules plus interferon alfa-2b [Intron A].

Dosage for Ribavirin Capsules (Rebetol). Rebetol is administered PO, and dosage depends on the patient's weight. For patients weighing 75 kg or less, the dosage is 1000 mg/day (400 mg in the morning and 600 mg in the evening). For patients weighing more than 75 kg, the dosage is 1200 mg/day (600 mg in the morning and 600 mg in the evening).

Dosage for Ribavirin Tablets (Copegus). Copegus is administered PO with food. Dosage depends on (1) patient weight and (2) the strain (genotype) of the hepatitis C virus.

For Genotype 1 or 4. For patients weighing 75 kg or less, the dosage is 1000 mg/day (400 mg in the morning and 600 mg in the evening). For patients weighing more than 75 kg, the dosage is 1200 mg/day (600 mg in the morning and 600 mg in the evening).

For Genotype 2 or 3. For all patients, regardless of weight, the dosage is 800 mg/day (400 mg in the morning and 400 mg in the evening).

Interferon Alfa Dosage. Dosage of interferon alfa depends on the specific preparation employed. Dosages for two examples—interferon alfa-2b [Intron A] and peg-interferon alfa-2b [PEG-Intron]—are as follows: 3 million IU SC 3 times a week (for interferon alfa-2b) and 1.5 μg/kg SC once a week (for peg-interferon alfa-2b).

Lamivudine

Lamivudine [Epivir HBV] is a nucleoside analog approved for treating infections caused by HIV or HBV. The drug was originally developed to treat HIV infection, and was later proved effective against HBV. Formulations and dosages for treating HIV and HBV infections differ, and hence must not be thought of as interchangeable. The basic pharmacology of lamivudine is discussed in Chapter 90. Discussion here is limited to treatment of HBV.

Lamivudine suppresses HBV replication by inhibiting viral DNA synthesis. The process begins with intracellular conversion of lamivudine to lamivudine triphosphate, its active form. As the triphosphate, lamivudine undergoes incorporation into the growing DNA chain, and thereby causes premature chain termination.

Lamivudine offers at least some benefit to most patients. In one clinical trial, 52 weeks of daily lamivudine normalized serum ALT in 72% of patients, and reduced liver inflammation and fibrosis in 56%. How long these benefits are maintained is unknown. Also, emergence of resistance is a concern: Resistant isolates appear in 14% of patients after 1 year of continuous treatment, and in 38% after 2 years.

At the dosage employed to treat hepatitis B, side effects are minimal. In clinical trials, the incidence of most side effects was no greater than with placebo. *Lactic acidosis* is a rare but dangerous complication. If lactic acidosis occurs, lamivudine should be discontinued.

For treatment of HBV, lamivudine [Epivir HBV] is formulated in 100-mg tablets and a 5-mg/ml oral solution. The dosage is 100 mg once a day (compared with 150 mg twice a day for HIV). Since lamivudine is eliminated primarily by renal excretion, dosage must be reduced in patients with renal impairment.

Adefovir

Actions and Therapeutic Use. Adefovir [Hepsera] is a new drug for chronic hepatitis B. It was approved on September 20, 2002, for treating adults with chronic hepatitis B who have evidence of active viral replication along with persistently elevated serum aminotransferases or histologic evidence of active disease. Adefovir was originally developed to fight HIV infection, but was not approved owing to a high incidence of nephrotoxicity at the doses required. The doses used for hepatitis B are much lower, and hence the risk of renal injury is lower too.

Adefovir was approved for chronic hepatitis B on the basis of two randomized, placebo-controlled trials, both lasting for 48 weeks. In one trial, significant improvement was seen in 53% of those taking adefovir, compared with only 25% of those taking placebo. Results of the second trial were similar: improvement was seen in 64% of those taking adefovir, compared with 35% of those taking placebo.

Adefovir is a purine nucleoside analog with a mechanism similar to that of acyclovir. Both drugs inhibit viral DNA synthesis, and both must be converted to their active form within the body. Activation of adefovir is mediated by cellular kinases—enzymes that convert the drug into adefovir diphosphate, a compound with two actions: (1) it directly inhibits viral DNA polymerase (by competing with deoxyadenosine triphosphate, a natural substrate for the enzyme) and (2) it undergoes incorporation into the growing strand of viral DNA, and thereby causes premature strand termination. Host cells are spared because adefovir diphosphate is a poor inhibitor of human DNA polymerase.

Pharmacokinetics. Adefovir is administered orally. Bioavailability is about 60%, both in the presence and absence of food. Plasma levels peak about 2 hours after dosing. Elimination is renal, as a result of glomerular filtration and active tubular secretion. In patients with normal kidney function, the drug's half-life is 7.5 hours. In patients with renal impairment, the half-life is significantly increased.

Adverse Effects. *Nephrotoxicity* is the principal concern. Increased serum creatinine, a sign of kidney damage, was seen in 4% of patients who received 48 weeks of therapy, and in 9% of patients who received 96 weeks of therapy. To reduce risk, kidney function should be assessed at baseline and periodically thereafter, paying special attention to patients at high risk (i.e., patients with pre-existing renal impairment and those taking nephrotoxic drugs [e.g., cyclosporine, tacrolimus, aminoglycosides, vancomycin, aspirin and other nonsteroidal anti-inflammatory drugs]).

When adefovir is discontinued, patients may experience *acute exacerbation of hepatitis B*. In clinical trials, serum ALT levels rose dramatically in 25% of patients when treatment was stopped. Hepatic function should be assessed periodically following adefovir withdrawal.

Drug Interactions. Drugs that are eliminated by active tubular secretion can complete with adefovir for renal excretion. As a result, if one of these agents were to be combined with adefovir, excretion of adefovir, the other drug, or both could be decreased, causing their plasma levels to rise.

Precautions. Because adefovir is related to the nucleoside analogs used against HIV, there is a concern that, if the patient were infected with HIV, giving adefovir in the low doses used against HBV could allow emergence of HIV viruses resistant to nucleoside analogs. Accordingly, HIV infection should be ruled out before adefovir is used.

The nucleoside analogs used to treat HIV infection can cause lactic acidosis and severe hepatomegaly. Hence, there is concern that adefovir can cause these effects too. If the patient develops clinical or laboratory findings that suggest lactic acidosis or pronounced hepatotoxicity, adefovir should be withdrawn.

Preparations, Dosage, and Administration. Adefovir [Hepsera] is available in 10-mg tablets. For patients with good kidney function, the dosage is 10 mg once a day, taken with or without food. For patients with impaired kidney function, as indicated by reduced creatinine clearance (CrCl), the dosing *interval* should be increased. Adjusted dosages are as follows:

- CrCl 20 to 49 ml/min—10 mg every 48 hours
- CrCl 10 to 19 ml/min—10 mg every 72 hours
- Patients on hemodialysis—10 mg once a week, taken after dialysis

DRUGS FOR INFLUENZA

Influenza is a serious respiratory tract infection that constitutes a major cause of morbidity and mortality worldwide. During the 1918–1919 global pandemic, influenza killed 21 million people, including more than 500,000 Americans. In the United States today, complications of influenza (e.g., bronchitis, pneumonia) cause up to 300,000 hospitalizations and 20,000 deaths each year. The cost of influenza is huge: Direct and indirect expenses total between $3 billion and $5 billion annually.

Influenza is caused by influenza viruses, of which there are two major types: *influenza A* and *influenza B*. Type A influenza viruses cause far more infections than type B influenza viruses. The influenza viruses are highly variable and undergo constant evolution. Because of this ongoing evolution, the World Health Organization (WHO) has established a global network of laboratories to monitor the emergence and spread of new variants.

Influenza is a highly contagious infection spread via aerosolized droplets produced by coughing or sneezing. The virus enters the body through mucous membranes of the nose, mouth, or eyes. Viral replication takes place in the respiratory tract. Symptoms begin 2 to 4 days after exposure, and last 5 to 6 days. Influenza is characterized by fever, cough, chills, sore throat, headache, and myalgia (muscle pain). For typical patients, infection results in 5 to 6 days of restricted activity, 3 to 4 days of bed disability, and 3 days of absence from work or school. In the United States, the influenza "season" begins in November and extends through March or April.

Influenza is managed by vaccination and with drugs. Vaccination is the primary management strategy; drug therapy is secondary. The drugs for influenza fall into two groups: first-generation agents (e.g., amantadine) and second-generation agents (e.g., oseltamivir). The first-generation drugs are active against influenza A only, whereas the second-generation drugs are active against influenza A *and* influenza B.

Influenza Vaccines

Annual vaccination is the best protection against influenza. Because influenza viruses are constantly evolving, influenza vaccines must continuously change too. Each year, manufacturers produce a new vaccine directed against the three strains of influenza virus deemed most likely to cause disease during the upcoming flu season. Identification of the three strains is done jointly by the Centers for Disease Control and Prevention, the FDA, and the WHO. At this time, all influenza vaccines are given by IM injection. However, an intranasal formulation is in development.

Intramuscular Vaccine

Description. Influenza vaccines for IM injection are composed of *inactivated* influenza viruses. As noted, these vaccines contain three viral strains, and are reformulated each year.

Efficacy. Protection begins 1 to 2 weeks after vaccination and generally lasts 6 months or longer. However, among elderly vaccinees, protection may be lost in 4 months or even less. Intramuscular vaccination is 70% to 90% effective in healthy young adults, but only 30% to 40% effective among elderly residents of nursing homes. Efficacy in very young children has not been fully studied.

Adverse Effects. Adverse effects of vaccination are uncommon, except for possible soreness at the injection site. People who have not been vaccinated previously may experience fever, myalgia, and malaise lasting 1 or 2 days.

Influenza vaccination may carry a very small risk of Guillain-Barré syndrome (GBS), a severe, paralytic illness. In 1976, swine flu vaccine was associated with GBS. However, there has been no clear link between GBS and influenza vaccines used since then. If there *is* a risk, it is very small, estimated at 1 to 2 cases per million vaccinees—much smaller than the risk posed by severe influenza.

Precautions and Contraindications. People with acute febrile illness should defer vaccination until symptoms abate. Minor illnesses (e.g., common cold), with or without fever, do not preclude vaccination.

Influenza vaccines are contraindicated for persons with hypersensitivity to eggs. Why? Because the vaccines are produced from viruses grown in eggs, and hence may contain trace amounts of egg proteins. Individuals suspected of egg hypersensitivity should undergo a skin test before receiving the vaccine. If the test is positive, the vaccine should be withheld.

Who Should Be Vaccinated? The Advisory Committee on Immunization Practices (ACIP) *recommends* vaccinating all individuals 6 months of age and older who are *at risk for getting a serious case of influenza or influenza complications.* Physicians, nurses, family members, and all others making close contact with at-risk individuals should be vaccinated too. Individuals considered at risk include the following:

- All children 6 to 23 months old
- All children 6 months to 18 years old receiving long-term therapy with aspirin (because they are at risk of developing Reye's syndrome if they get influenza)
- All individuals 6 months and older who have long-term health problems, including heart disease, kidney disease, asthma, diabetes, or anemia
- All individuals 6 months and older who have a weakened immune system (e.g., owing to HIV infection or therapy with immunosuppressive drugs)
- All individuals 50 years and older
- All residents of nursing homes and other facilities where persons with chronic medical conditions live.
- Women who will be in the second or third trimester of pregnancy during the flu season
  In addition, ACIP *encourages* annual vaccination for
- Household members and other close contacts of infants less than 6 months of age
- People who provide essential community services
- People living in dormitories or other crowded conditions (to prevent outbreaks of influenza)
- Anyone who wants to reduce his or her chance of catching influenza

Preparations, Dosage, and Administration. IM influenza vaccines are available under three trade names: FluShield, Fluzone, and Fluvirin. FluShield and Fluzone are approved for all individuals 6 months of age or older. Fluvirin is approved only for individuals at least 4 years old. Because the influenza virus evolves rapidly, all three products are reformulated annually. Accordingly, to maintain protection, revaccination is required each year.

Vaccination is done by IM injection into the anterolateral aspect of the thigh (for infants and young children) or into the deltoid muscle (for older children, adolescents, and adults).

Dosage is a function of age and vaccination history. Most recipients require just one injection. However, children under 9 years old who have not been vaccinated before require two, administered at least 4 weeks apart. The dosage size is 0.5 ml for all recipients over the age of 3 years, and 0.25 ml for recipients 6 months to 35 months of age.

When should influenza vaccine be administered? The best time is in October or November. However, December is not too late.

Intranasal Vaccine

An intranasal influenza vaccine [FluMist] is in development. Unlike the IM vaccine, which contains *inactivated* influenza viruses, the intranasal formulation contains *live, attenuated* influenza viruses. Inhalation of the vaccine appears to stimulate formation of antibodies locally in the nose, a major port of entry for influenza viruses. Testing in adults and children suggests that the intranasal vaccine is about as effective as the IM vaccine. Of 1070 children who received the new vaccine, only 14 (1%) developed influenza, compared with 95 out of 533 (18%) who inhaled a placebo. In addition, vaccination prevented influenza-related otitis media (middle ear infection). The only side effects of the vaccine are rhinorrhea (runny nose) and sore throat.

First-Generation Drugs: Amantadine and Rimantadine

Prior to 1999, amantadine and rimantadine were the only drugs available to treat influenza. These agents have moderate activity against influenza A, and none against influenza B. With amantadine, adverse CNS effects are common, and with both drugs, resistance can develop rapidly.

Amantadine

Amantadine [Symmetrel] is employed for prophylaxis and treatment of infections caused by type A influenza virus. As discussed in Chapter 21, the drug is also used to treat Parkinson's disease.

Mechanism of Antiviral Action. Just how amantadine suppresses viral growth is not completely understood. The drug can prevent penetration of influenza A virus into host cells and can inhibit viral uncoating. In addition, it inhibits an early step in replication of viral components.

Therapeutic Use. Antiviral applications of amantadine are limited to prophylaxis and treatment of respiratory tract infections caused by type A influenza virus strains. The drug is not active against type B influenza. Prophylaxis should be instituted only in the presence of a documented influenza A epidemic. Candidates for prophylaxis include (1) individuals at high risk of developing complications from influenza (e.g., elderly patients and those with cardiopulmonary disease) and (2) healthcare workers and family members who have extensive contact with patients at risk. Prophylaxis is continued until the epidemic abates (usually in 5 to 6 weeks). It should be noted that immunization against influenza A is preferred to prophylaxis with amantadine. Since amantadine does not impede the immune response to influenza A vaccine, individuals at risk can be vaccinated while receiving amantadine for prophylaxis. Amantadine can be discontinued 2 weeks after vaccination. For treatment of active influenza A infection, amantadine is most effective when therapy is instituted early (within 48 hours of the onset of symptoms).

Pharmacokinetics. Amantadine is well absorbed following oral administration and is distributed widely to body fluids and tissues. The drug crosses the blood-brain barrier and placenta. It also appears in saliva, nasal secretions, and breast milk. Amantadine is not metabolized. Excretion is renal. In patients with renal impairment, amantadine will accumulate to high levels if the dosage is not reduced.

Adverse Effects. Amantadine is generally well tolerated at the doses employed for prophylaxis and treatment of influenza.

CNS Effects. CNS effects occur in 10% to 30% of patients. Reactions include dizziness, nervousness, insomnia, and difficulty concentrating. Individuals involved in hazardous activities should exercise appropriate caution. More serious CNS effects (depression, hallucinations, seizures) have occurred. Accordingly, care should be exercised in patients with a history of epilepsy or psychosis.

Cardiovascular Effects. Rarely, amantadine has caused congestive heart failure (CHF). The drug should be used with caution in patients with CHF or peripheral edema. Patients should be instructed to contact their physician if they experience shortness of breath or swelling of the extremities.

Orthostatic hypotension has occurred. Patients should be advised to move slowly when assuming an upright position. Also, they should be advised to sit or lie down if dizziness or lightheadedness occurs.

Use in Pregnancy and Lactation. Amantadine is teratogenic and embryotoxic in rats. Adequate studies during human pregnancy have not been performed. The drug crosses the placenta and is classified in FDA Pregnancy Risk Category C. It should be avoided by pregnant women unless the benefits of treatment are deemed to outweigh the potential risks to the fetus. Amantadine is secreted in breast milk and should not be used by nursing mothers.

Drug Interactions. Amantadine can intensify the peripheral and CNS effects of anticholinergic drugs. When amantadine has been combined with anticholinergic drugs, psychotic reactions resembling those associated with atropine poisoning have occurred. These responses can be reduced by lowering the dosage of either amantadine or the anticholinergic agent.

Preparations, Dosage, and Administration. Amantadine [Symmetrel] is dispensed in a syrup (10 mg/ml) and in 100-mg tablets and capsules. For treatment or prophylaxis of influenza A, the dosage for patients older than 9 years is 100 mg twice daily. For children ages 1 to 9 years, the dosage is 4.4 to 8.8 mg/kg/day in two or three divided doses. The dosage must be reduced in patients with kidney dysfunction. Prophylactic administration should commence prior to anticipated viral exposure and should continue for as long as the influenza A epidemic lasts. For treatment of active influenza A infection, therapy should begin within 48 hours of the onset of symptoms and should continue for 4 to 5 days.

Rimantadine

Rimantadine [Flumadine] is very similar to amantadine in structure, actions, and uses. Like amantadine, rimantadine is indicated only for prophylaxis and treatment of influenza A virus infections. Administration is oral and bioavailability appears to be greater than 90%. In contrast to amantadine, which is not metabolized, rimantadine undergoes extensive metabolism prior to excretion in the urine. Primary adverse effects are nervousness, lightheadedness, difficulty in concentration, sleep disturbances, and fatigue. However, these occur less frequently than with amantadine (3% vs. up to 30%). The *adult* dosage for *treatment* or *prophylaxis* is 100 mg twice a day; the duration of therapy is 5 days for treatment of active infection and up to 6 weeks for prophylaxis. The dosage for *prophylaxis* in *children* is 5 mg/kg/day. Rimantadine is not approved for treating active infection in children. Rimantadine is available in 100-mg capsules and a 10-mg/ml syrup.

Second-Generation Drugs: Neuraminidase Inhibitors

The neuraminidase inhibitors—oseltamivir and zanamivir—are relatively new drugs for the prevention and treatment of influenza. Both agents were introduced in 1999. In contrast to amantadine and rimantadine, which suppress only influenza A, the neuraminidase inhibitors suppress influenza A *and* influenza B. Neuraminidase inhibitors cost more than amantadine, but are more effective, better tolerated, and pose a lower risk of resistance. As with the first-generation agents, these drugs should not be viewed as an alternative to vaccination.

Oseltamivir

Therapeutic Effects. Oseltamivir [Tamiflu] is an oral drug approved for prevention and treatment of influenza. When used for treatment, dosing must begin early—no later than 2 days after symptom onset, and preferably much sooner. Why? Because benefits decline greatly when treatment is delayed: When treatment is started within 12 hours of symptom onset, symptom duration is reduced by more than 3 days; when started within 24 hours, symptom duration is reduced by less than 2 days; and when started with 36 hours, symptom duration is reduced by only 29 hours. In addition to reducing the duration of symptoms, oseltamivir can reduce the severity of symptoms as well as the incidence of complications (sinusitis, bronchitis). Unfortunately, treatment is expensive (about $60 for a 5-day course). Furthermore, in the real world, patients may be unable to obtain and fill a prescription soon enough to be of significant benefit.

Oseltamivir has been studied for its ability to *prevent* influenza in residents of nursing homes, in family members of someone with the flu, and in the community at large. When used in nursing homes, most of whose residents had been vaccinated, oseltamivir decreased the incidence of influenza from 4.4% down to 0.4%. When used to protect family members, the drug decreased the incidence of influenza from 12% down to 1%. And when given to unvaccinated individuals during a community outbreak of influenza, it reduced the incidence of infection from 4.8% down to 1.2%.

Mechanism of Action. Antiviral effects derive from inhibiting neuraminidase, a viral enzyme required for replication. As a result of neuraminidase inhibition, newly formed viral particles are unable to bud off from the cytoplasmic membrane of infected host cells. Hence, viral spread is stopped. Oseltamivir is active against all strains of influenza A and influenza B. Emergence of resistance over the course of treatment is rare.

Pharmacokinetics. Oseltamivir is well absorbed following oral administration. In the liver, the drug undergoes conversion to oseltamivir carboxylate, its active form. Bioavailability of the carboxylate is 80%. Plasma levels of active drug peak in 2.5 to 6 hours. The plasma half-life is 6 to 10 hours. The drug is eliminated in the urine, primarily as the carboxylate form.

Adverse Effects and Interactions. Oseltamivir is generally well tolerated. The most common side effects are nausea (9.9%) and vomiting (9.4%). Nausea can be reduced by giving the drug with food. No interactions with other drugs have been reported.

Preparations, Dosage, and Administration. Oseltamivir [Tamiflu] is available in 75-mg tablets and as a powder to be reconstituted to a 12-mg/ml oral suspension. The drug may be administered without regard to meals, although taking it with food can reduce nausea.

For *treatment* of influenza, the dosage for *adults and for children* ≥13 years old is 75 mg twice daily for 5 days, beginning no later the 2 days after the onset of symptoms. Dosage should be reduced to 75 mg once daily in patients with significant renal impairment. The dosage for *children* ≥1 year old is based on body weight as follows: ≤33 lbs, 30 mg bid; 33 to 51 lbs, 45 mg bid; 51 to 88 lbs, 60 mg bid; and >88 lbs, 75 mg bid.

For *prevention* of influenza in adults and children ≥13 years old, the dosage is 75 mg once a day—one half the dosage used for treatment. Candidates for prophylactic therapy include family members of someone with flu and residents of nursing homes. To protect family members, dosing should begin within 48 hours of exposure and should continue for 7 days. To protect residents of nursing homes or high-risk members of the community at large, dosing can be done continuously for up to 42 days.

Zanamivir

Actions and Uses. Zanamivir [Relenza], administered by oral inhalation, is approved for treating uncomplicated influenza infection in patients at least 12 years old who have been symptomatic for no more than 2 days. At this time, the drug is not approved for flu prevention; however, studies indicate that it *does* confer protection. As with oseltamivir, benefits derive from inhibiting viral neuraminidase, an enzyme required for viral replication. Like oseltamivir, zanamivir is well tolerated, although benefits appear to be limited.

Clinical Trials. Zanamivir is moderately effective at shortening the duration of influenza symptoms. In Phase III clinical trials, improvement in symptoms was defined as (1) the absence of fever and (2) mild or no headache, myalgia, cough, or sore throat. In patients taking zanamivir (10 mg twice daily for 5 days, beginning no later than 36 hours after the onset of symptoms) the average duration of symptoms was 5 days, compared with 6.5 days for patients taking placebo. In addition, zanamivir reduced the incidence of complications (sinusitis, bronchitis) requiring antibacterial drugs.

Zanamivir can provide prophylaxis against influenza, although it is not approved for this use. In a 4-week trial conducted during the influenza season, once-daily treatment with 10 mg of inhaled zanamivir was 84% effective at preventing febrile illness.

Pharmacokinetics. Zanamivir is formulated as a dry powder for oral inhalation. The drug is poorly absorbed from the GI tract, and hence cannot be administered by mouth. Most (70% to 90%) of an inhaled dose is deposited in the oropharynx and throat. About 10% to 20% reaches the tracheobronchial tree and lungs. Between 4% and 17% of each dose undergoes absorption into the systemic circulation. Zanamivir has a plasma half-life of 2.5 to 5 hours and is eliminated unchanged in the urine. No metabolites have been detected.

Adverse Effects and Interactions. In patients with healthy lung function, adverse effects are rare. Because zanamivir is administered as an inhaled powder, patients may experience cough or throat irritation. Zanamivir is devoid of drug interactions.

In patients with pre-existing lung disorders (e.g., asthma, chronic obstructive pulmonary disease), zanamivir may cause severe bronchospasm and respiratory decline. Some patients have required immediate treatment or hospitalization. Deaths have occurred—however, given the impact of flu itself on lung function, it's not clear that zanamivir was responsible.

Nonetheless, owing to the potential risk, zanamivir is not generally recommended for patients with underlying airway disease.

Preparations, Dosage, and Administration. Zanamivir [Relenza] is dispensed in blister packs that contain 5 mg of powdered drug. Administration is by oral inhalation using the *Diskhaler* provided by the manufacturer. The dosage is 10 mg (two 5-mg inhalations) twice daily for 5 days. Each 10-mg dose should be separated by 12 hours. However, on the first day of treatment, less separation (as little as 2 hours) is permitted if the first dose cannot be taken early enough in the day to allow 12 hours between doses. Patients who are using an inhaled bronchodilator (e.g., albuterol) should administer the bronchodilator before inhaling zanamivir.

OPHTHALMIC ANTIVIRAL DRUGS

Trifluridine

Trifluridine [Viroptic] is indicated only for topical treatment of ocular infections caused by HSV-1 and HSV-2. The drug is given to treat acute keratoconjunctivitis and recurrent epithelial keratitis. Antiviral actions result from inhibiting DNA synthesis. The most common side effects are localized burning and stinging. Edema of the eyelid occurs in about 3% of patients. Systemic absorption is minimal following topical administration. Hence, the drug is devoid of systemic toxicity. Trifluridine is dispensed in a 1% ophthalmic solution. Treatment consists of placing 1 drop on the cornea every 2 hours (while the patient is awake) for a maximum of 9 drops/day. Once re-epithelialization of the cornea has occurred, the dosage is reduced to 5 drops/day administered one drop every 4 hours. Treatment continues for 7 days.

Vidarabine

Like trifluridine, topical vidarabine [Vira-A] is indicated for acute keratoconjunctivitis and recurrent epithelial keratitis caused by HSV-1 and HSV-2. Antiviral effects result from inhibition of viral DNA polymerase and from premature termination of the growing viral DNA chain. The most frequent side effects are burning sensations, photophobia, and lacrimation. Absorption of topical vidarabine is insignificant, and systemic toxicity has not been reported. Vidarabine is available in a 3% ointment for application to the eye. About one-half inch of ointment is administered into the lower conjunctival sac five times a day at 3-hour intervals. As a rule, treatment lasts for no more than 3 weeks.

Idoxuridine

Idoxuridine [Herplex] was the first effective antiviral drug for use in humans. Antiviral effects result from incorporation of a metabolite of idoxuridine into viral DNA. Idoxuridine is indicated only for keratitis caused by HSV-1; the drug is inactive against HSV-2. Because vidarabine and trifluridine are more effective and less toxic than idoxuridine, these newer agents have largely replaced idoxuridine for treating herpes simplex keratitis. Side effects of idoxuridine include inflammation, itching, photophobia, edema of the eyelid, lacrimal duct occlusion, and punctate defects in the corneal epithelium. Topical application has not been associated with systemic toxicity. Idoxuridine is dispensed in a 0.5% ointment and a 0.1% solution.

OTHER ANTIVIRAL DRUGS

Foscarnet

Foscarnet [Foscavir] is an IV drug active against all known herpesviruses, including CMV, HSV-1, HSV-2, and VZV. Compared with ganciclovir, foscarnet is more difficult to administer, less well tolerated, and much more expensive (the cost to the pharmacy is about $20,000 a year). The major adverse effect is renal injury.

Mechanism of Action. Foscarnet, an analog of pyrophosphate, inhibits viral DNA polymerases and reverse transcriptases, and thereby inhibits synthesis of viral nucleic acids. At the concentrations achieved clinically, the drug does not inhibit host DNA replication. Unlike many other antiviral drugs, which must undergo conversion to an active form, foscarnet is active as administered.

Therapeutic Use. Foscarnet has two approved indications: (1) CMV retinitis in patients with AIDS and (2) acyclovir-resistant mucocutaneous HSV infection in the immunocompromised host. CMV retinitis resistant to ganciclovir may respond to foscarnet.

Pharmacokinetics. Foscarnet has low oral bioavailability and must be administered IV. The drug is poorly soluble in water and does not penetrate cells easily. As a result, it must be given in large doses with large volumes of fluid. Between 10% and 28% of each dose is deposited in bone; the remainder is excreted unchanged in the urine. Because foscarnet is eliminated by the kidneys, dosages must be reduced in patients with renal impairment. The plasma half-life is 3 to 5 hours.

Adverse Effects and Interactions. Foscarnet is generally less well tolerated than ganciclovir. However, unlike ganciclovir, foscarnet does not cause granulocytopenia or thrombocytopenia.

Nephrotoxicity. Renal injury, as evidenced by a rise in serum creatinine concentration, is the most common dose-limiting toxicity. Most patients develop some degree of renal impairment. Renal injury occurs most often during the second week of therapy. The risk of nephrotoxicity is increased by concurrent use of other nephrotoxic drugs, including amphotericin B, aminoglycosides (e.g., gentamicin), and pentamidine. Prehydration with IV saline may reduce the risk of renal injury. Renal function (creatinine clearance) should be monitored closely and the dosage should be reduced if renal impairment develops.

Electrolyte and Mineral Imbalances. Foscarnet frequently causes hypocalcemia, hypokalemia, hypomagnesemia, and hypo- or hyperphosphatemia. Ionized serum calcium may be reduced despite normal levels of total serum calcium. Patients should be informed about symptoms of low ionized calcium (e.g., paresthesias, numbness in the extremities, perioral tingling) and instructed to report these. Severe hypocalcemia can result in dysrhythmias, tetany, and seizures. Serum levels of calcium, magnesium, potassium, and phosphorus should be measured frequently. Special caution is required in patients with pre-existing electrolyte, cardiac, or neurologic abnormalities. The risk of hypocalcemia is increased by concurrent use of pentamidine.

Other Adverse Effects. Common reactions include fever (65%), nausea (47%), anemia (33%), diarrhea (30%), vomiting (26%), and headache (26%). In addition, foscarnet can cause fatigue, tremor, irritability, genital ulceration, abnormal liver function tests, neutropenia, and seizures.

Preparations, Dosage, and Administration. Foscarnet [Foscavir] is dispensed in solution (24 mg/ml) for IV infusion. An infusion pump is essential to reduce the risk of accidental overdose. Infusions may be administered through a central venous line or a peripheral vein. When a central line is used, a concentrated (24 mg/ml) solution may be given. When a peripheral vein is used, the solution should be diluted to 12 mg/ml. For patients with normal kidney function, the *initial* dosage is 60 mg/kg (for CMV infection) or 40 mg/kg (for HSV infection) infused over 1 hour (or longer) every 8 hours for 2 to 3 weeks. The *maintenance* dosage (for CMV or HSV infection) is 90 to 120 mg/kg infused over 2 hours once daily. All dosages must be reduced for patients with renal impairment.

Ribavirin (Inhaled)

Ribavirin, a broad-spectrum antiviral drug, is available in two formulations: aerosol and oral. The aerosol formulation, marketed as Virazole, is used for infection with respiratory syncytial virus (RSV). The oral formulation, marketed as Rebetol, is used to treat chronic hepatitis C. Discussion here focuses on treatment of RSV. Use of ribavirin against hepatitis C is discussed above.

Antiviral Actions. Ribavirin [Virazole] is virustatic. The drug is active against RSV, HCV, influenza virus (types A and B), and HSV. Although several biochemical actions of the drug have been described, it is not known which (if any) is responsible for antiviral effects.

Use in RSV Infection. Ribavirin is labeled only for severe viral pneumonia caused by RSV in carefully selected, hospitalized infants and young children. Unfortunately, benefits of treatment are usually minimal—and the cost is high (over $1300/day). Ribavirin should not be used for mild RSV infections.

Pharmacokinetics. For treatment of RSV, ribavirin is administered by oral inhalation. The drug is absorbed from the lungs and achieves high concentrations in respiratory tract secretions and erythrocytes. Concentrations in plasma remain low. The drug is metabolized to active and inactive products. Excretion is via the urine (30% to 55%) and feces (15%). Ribavirin that is sequestered in erythrocytes remains in the body for weeks.

Adverse Effects. Inhalation of ribavirin produces little or no systemic toxicity. However, although generally safe, inhaled ribavirin does pose a hazard to infants undergoing mechanical assistance of ventilation: The drug can precipitate in the respiratory apparatus, thereby interfering with safe and effective respiratory support. Consequently, ribavirin should not be administered to infants who need respiratory assistance. In some infants and in adults who have asthma or chronic obstructive lung disease, ribavirin has caused deterioration of pulmonary function. Accordingly, respiratory function should be carefully monitored. If deterioration occurs, ribavirin should be discontinued. When administered systemically (PO or IV), ribavirin frequently causes anemia. This has not been reported with inhalational therapy.

Use in Pregnancy. Ribavirin is *contraindicated for use during pregnancy.* Although studies in primates indicate no effect on the developing fetus, ribavirin has proved either teratogenic or embryolethal in nearly all other species tested. No studies in humans have been performed. *Ribavirin is classified under FDA Pregnancy Risk Category X:* The risk of use during pregnancy clearly outweighs any potential benefits. Because of the risk of significant drug exposure, pregnant women should not directly care for patients undergoing ribavirin aerosol therapy.

Preparations, Dosage, and Administration. For treatment of RSV, ribavirin [Virazole] is dispensed as a powder (6 gm/100-ml vial) to be reconstituted for aerosol administration. According to the manufacturer, only one device—the Viratek Small Particle Aerosol Generator (SPAG) model SPAG-2—should be employed for ribavirin administration. The SPAG-2 is used to deliver ribavirin to an infant oxygen hood. Treatment is given 12 to 18 hours a day for no less than 3 days and no more than 1 week. The drug should not be administered to patients who require ventilatory assistance. To reconstitute powdered ribavirin, dissolve 6 gm of the drug in Sterile Water for Injection or Inhalation, transfer this concentrated solution to the SPAG-2 reservoir, and dilute to a final volume of 300 ml using Sterile Water for Injection or Inhalation. The final concentration of ribavirin is 20 mg/ml. This solution is aerosolized and inhaled by the patient.

Palivizumab

Actions, Uses, and Adverse Effects. Palivizumab [Synagis] is a monoclonal antibody indicated for preventing RSV infection in premature infants and in young children with chronic lung diseases. The antibody binds to a surface protein on RSV and thereby prevents replication. In clinical trials, the rate of hospitalization was 1.8% for premature infants treated with palivizumab, compared with 8.1% for those receiving placebo. In young children with chronic lung disease, the hospitalization rate was 7.9% for those receiving the antibody, versus 12.8% for those receiving placebo. Except for a possible increase in aminotransferase activity (suggesting liver injury), palivizumab is devoid of adverse effects.

Preparations, Dosage, and Administration. Palivizumab [Synagis] is dispensed as a lyophilized powder (100 mg) to be dissolved in 1 ml of sterile water at least 20 minutes before use (to allow time for the solution to clarify). The dosage is 15 mg/kg once a month, injected IM into the anterolateral aspect of the thigh. Dosing should commence before the RSV season (November through April in the United States) and continue until the season ends. The cost for a full season of treatment is about $7000. However, although this seems high, it could save more than $50,000 by avoiding hospitalization.

Fomivirsen

Clinical Pharmacology. Fomivirsen [Vitravene] is a unique drug approved for treating CMV retinitis in HIV-infected patients who are intolerant of or unresponsive to other drugs. Administration is by direct injection into the vitreous humor (following application of a topical anesthetic and antimicrobial drugs). The dosage is 0.05 ml (0.33 mg) on days 1 and 14, and every 4 weeks thereafter. Enzymes within the eye degrade fomivirsen to inactive mononucleotide fragments over a span of 7 to 10 days. The most common adverse effect is ocular inflammation, which develops in 25% of patients. Inflammation can be suppressed with topical glucocorticoids. Other common reactions include vision changes and elevated intraocular pressure.

Mechanism of Action. Fomivirsen is the first representative of a new class of drugs, known as "antisense" agents. Antisense drugs consist of a single strand of DNA designed to bind to specific molecules of messenger RNA and thereby block synthesis of disease-causing proteins. Benefits of fomivirsen derive from blocking production of viral proteins required by CMV for replication.

Docosanol Cream

Docosanol [Abreva] is a topical preparation indicated for recurrent herpes labialis (cold sores, fever blisters). The drug is available over the counter as a 10% cream. Application is done 5 times a day, beginning at the first sign of recurrence. Benefits are modest. In one clinical trial, treatment reduced the time to healing from 4.8 days down to 4.1 days—about the same response we see with penciclovir. Docosanol cream appears devoid of adverse effects.

Docosanol has a broad antiviral spectrum and a unique mechanism of action. Unlike penciclovir, which inhibits viral DNA synthesis (and thereby suppresses replication), docosanol blocks viral entry into host cells. The drug does not kill viruses and does not prevent them from binding to cells. As a result, viable virions can remain attached to the cell surface for a long time. Because docosanol does not affect processes of replication, it is unlikely to promote resistance.

⠂⠆ KEY POINTS

- Because viruses use host-cell enzymes and substrates to reproduce, it is difficult to suppress viral reproduction without also harming cells of the host.
- Acyclovir is the drug of choice for most infections caused by herpes simplex viruses and varicella-zoster virus.
- Following conversion to its active form, acyclovir suppresses viral reproduction by inhibiting viral DNA polymerase and by causing premature termination of viral DNA strand growth. Because the active form of acyclovir is not a good inhibitor of human DNA polymerase, cells of the host are spared.
- In patients with genital herpes infections, oral acyclovir can decrease the duration and severity of the initial episode and the frequency of lesion recurrence.
- Although acyclovir reduces symptoms of genital herpes, the drug does not produce cure (i.e., it does not eliminate the virus) and does not prevent transmission to sexual partners.
- Acyclovir is eliminated unchanged by the kidneys. Accordingly, dosage must be reduced in patients with renal impairment.
- Intravenous acyclovir can injure the kidneys. Renal damage can be minimized by infusing acyclovir slowly and by ensuring adequate hydration during and after the infusion.
- Ganciclovir is the drug of choice for prophylaxis and treatment of CMV infection in immunocompromised patients, including those with AIDS.
- Ganciclovir does not cure CMV retinitis in patients with AIDS, and hence, in most cases, treatment must continue for life.
- Like acyclovir, ganciclovir becomes activated within infected cells, after which it inhibits viral DNA polymerase and causes premature termination of viral DNA strand growth.
- Like acyclovir, ganciclovir is excreted unchanged in the urine. Hence, dosage must be reduced in patients with renal impairment.
- The major adverse effects of ganciclovir are granulocytopenia and thrombocytopenia.
- Chronic hepatitis is caused primarily by HBV and HCV.
- Hepatitis B can be prevented by vaccination. There is no vaccine for hepatitis C.
- Hepatitis B can be treated with interferon alfa, lamivudine, or adefovir.

- The treatment of choice for chronic hepatitis C is interferon alfa plus ribavirin.
- The principal adverse effects of interferon alfa are a flu-like syndrome and severe depression.
- Ribavirin is teratogenic and embryolethal, and can cause sperm abnormalities. Accordingly, the drug is contraindicated for use during pregnancy. Pregnancy must be avoided by women taking ribavirin, and by female partners of men taking the drug.

- Vaccination is the best way to prevent influenza. Because influenza viruses evolve rapidly, influenza vaccines must be reformulated each year, and persons wanting protection must receive the new vaccine each year.
- Amantadine is used for prophylaxis and treatment of influenza A infections, but not influenza B infections.
- In contrast to amantadine, the neuraminidase inhibitors—zanamivir and oseltamivir—are active against influenza A *and* influenza B.

Summary of Major Nursing Implications*

ACYCLOVIR

Preadministration Assessment

Therapeutic Goal

Treatment of infections caused by herpes simplex viruses and varicella-zoster virus.

Identifying High-Risk Patients

Use with *caution* in patients with dehydration or renal impairment and in those taking other nephrotoxic drugs.

Implementation: Administration

Routes

Topical, oral, IV.

Dosage

Oral and IV dosages must be reduced in patients with renal impairment.

Administration

Topical. Advise patients to apply the drug with a finger cot or rubber glove to avoid viral transfer to other body sites or people.

Oral. Dosages vary widely for different indications.

Intravenous. Give by slow IV infusion (over 1 hour or more). Never administer by IV bolus.

Implementation: Measures to Enhance Therapeutic Effects

Inform patients with herpes simplex genitalis that acyclovir only decreases symptoms; it does not eliminate the virus and does not produce cure. Advise patients to cleanse the affected area with soap and water 3 to 4 times a day, drying thoroughly after each wash. Advise patients to avoid all sexual contact while lesions are present, and to use a condom even when lesions are absent.

Ongoing Evaluation and Interventions

Evaluating Therapeutic Effects

Observe for decreased clinical manifestations of herpes simplex and varicella-zoster infection. Virologic testing may also be performed.

Minimizing Adverse Effects

Nephrotoxicity. Intravenous acyclovir can precipitate in renal tubules, causing reversible kidney damage. To minimize risk, infuse acyclovir slowly and ensure adequate hydration during the infusion and for 2 hours after. Exercise caution in patients with pre-existing renal impairment and in those who are dehydrated or taking other nephrotoxic drugs.

GANCICLOVIR

Preadministration Assessment

Therapeutic Goal

Treatment and prevention of CMV infection in immunocompromised patients, including those with AIDS and those taking immunosuppressive drugs following organ transplantation.

Baseline Data

Obtain a complete blood count and platelet count.

Identifying High-Risk Patients

Ganciclovir is *contraindicated* during pregnancy and for patients with neutrophil counts below $500/mm^3$ or platelet counts below $25,000/mm^3$. Use with *caution* in patients taking zidovudine or nephrotoxic drugs (e.g., amphotericin B, cyclosporine) and in patients with a history of cytopenic reactions to other drugs.

Implementation: Administration

Routes

Oral, IV, intraocular.

Dosage

Oral and IV dosages must be reduced in patients with renal impairment. AIDS patients with CMV retinitis must take ganciclovir for life.

Administration

Intravenous. Give by slow IV infusion (over 1 hour or more). Ensure adequate hydration to promote renal excretion.

*Patient education information is highlighted as blue text.

Summary of Major Nursing Implications*—cont'd

Oral. Administer with food.

Intraocular Implants. Surgical implants are replaced every 5 to 8 months.

Ongoing Evaluation and Interventions

Minimizing Adverse Effects

Granulocytopenia and Thrombocytopenia. Ganciclovir suppresses bone marrow function when given IV or PO. Obtain complete blood counts and platelet counts frequently. Discontinue ganciclovir if the neutrophil count falls below 500/mm³ or the platelet count falls below 25,000/mm³. The risk of granulocytopenia can be reduced by giving granulocyte colony-stimulating factors. The risk of granulocytopenia is increased by concurrent therapy with zidovudine (a drug for AIDS).

Reproductive Toxicity. In animals, ganciclovir is teratogenic and embryotoxic and suppresses spermatogenesis. **Warn female patients against becoming pregnant. Inform males about possible sterility.**

*Patient education information is highlighted as blue text.

Antiviral Agents II: Drugs for HIV Infection and Related Opportunistic Infections

In this chapter we discuss drug therapy of infection with the *human immunodeficiency virus* (HIV), the microbe that causes *acquired immunodeficiency syndrome* (AIDS). HIV promotes immunodeficiency by killing CD4 T lymphocytes (CD4 T cells), which are key components of the immune system (see Chapter 63). As a result of HIV-induced immunodeficiency, patients are at risk of opportunistic infections and certain neoplasms.

It is important to appreciate that HIV infection is not synonymous with AIDS, which develops years after HIV infection is acquired. The definition of AIDS, established by the Centers for Disease Control and Prevention (CDC) in 1993, is a syndrome in which the individual is HIV positive and has either (1) CD4 T-cell counts below 200 cells/μl or (2) an AIDS-defining illness. Included in the CDC's long list of AIDS-defining illnesses are *Pneumocystis carinii* pneumonia, cytomegalovirus retinitis, disseminated histoplasmosis, tuberculosis, and Kaposi's sarcoma.

Since being identified as a new disease in 1981, AIDS has become a global epidemic. In the United States, between 850,000 and 950,000 people are now infected, and more than 460,000 have died. Worldwide, an estimated 42 million are infected and, in 2002 alone, approximately 3.1 million died, including 610,000 children under the age of 15. The economic cost of AIDS is staggering—estimated at over $15 billion for prevention and treatment. The personal and societal costs are incalculable.

Therapy of HIV infection has made dramatic advances. Today, standard treatment consists of three or four drugs, in regimens known as *highly active antiretroviral therapy* (HAART). Because of HAART, we can decrease plasma HIV to levels that are undetectable with current technology, and can thereby delay or reverse loss of immune function, preserve health, and prolong life. In the United States, HAART has reduced annually AIDS-related deaths by 70%—from a peak of 51,670 in 1995 to 15,603 in 2001. However, these benefits have not come without a price: HAART is complex and expensive, poses a risk of toxicity and serious drug interactions, and must continue lifelong. Accordingly, if treatment is to succeed, patients must be both highly motivated and well informed about all aspects of the treatment program.

HAART cannot cure HIV infection. Although treatment can greatly reduce HIV levels—often rendering the virus undetectable—discontinuation has always been followed by a rebound in HIV replication. Because HAART does not eliminate HIV, patients continue to be infectious and must be warned to avoid behaviors that can transmit the virus to others.

Understanding this chapter requires a basic understanding of the immune system. Accordingly, you may find it helpful to read Chapter 63 (Review of the Immune System) before proceeding.

PATHOPHYSIOLOGY

Characteristics of HIV

HIV is a *retrovirus*. Like all other viruses, retroviruses lack the machinery needed for self-replication, and hence are obligate intracellular parasites. However, in contrast to other viruses, retroviruses have positive-sense single-stranded RNA as their genetic material. Accordingly, in order to replicate, retroviruses must first transcribe their RNA into DNA. The enzyme employed for this process is viral *RNA-dependent DNA polymerase,* commonly known as *reverse transcriptase.* (The enzyme is called reverse transcriptase to distinguish it from DNA-dependent RNA polymerase, the host enzyme that transcribes DNA into RNA, which is the usual ["forward"] transcription process.) The name *retrovirus* is derived from the first two letters of *reverse* and *transcriptase.*

There are two types of HIV, referred to as HIV-1 and HIV-2. HIV-1 is found worldwide, whereas HIV-2 is found mainly in West Africa. Although HIV-1 and HIV-2 differ with respect to genetic makeup and antigenicity, they both cause similar disease syndromes. Not all drugs that are effective against HIV-1 are effective against HIV-2.

Target Cells

The principal cells attacked by HIV are *CD4 T cells* (helper T lymphocytes). As discussed in Chapter 63, these cells are essential components of the immune system. They are required for production of antibodies by B lymphocytes and for activation of cytolytic T lymphocytes. Accordingly, as HIV kills CD4 T cells, the immune system undergoes progressive decline. As a result, infected individuals become increasingly vulnerable to opportunistic infections, the major cause of death among people with AIDS. HIV targets CD4 T cells because the CD4 proteins on the surface of these cells provide points of attachment for HIV (see below). Without such a receptor, HIV would be unable to connect with and penetrate these cells. Once HIV has infected a CD4 T cell, the cell dies in about 1.25 days. It is important to appreciate that only a few percent of CD4 T cells circulate in the blood; the vast majority reside in lymph nodes and other lymphoid tissues.

In addition to infecting CD4 T cells, HIV infects *macrophages* and *microglial cells* (the central nervous system [CNS] counterparts of macrophages), both of which carry CD4 proteins. Since macrophages and microglial cells are resistant to destruction by HIV, they can survive despite being infected. As a result, they serve as a reservoir of HIV during chronic infection.

Structure of HIV

The structure of HIV is very simple. As shown in Figure 90–1, the HIV *virion* (i.e., the entire virus particle) consists of *nucleic acid* (RNA) surrounded by *core proteins,* which in turn are surrounded by a *capsid* (protein shell),

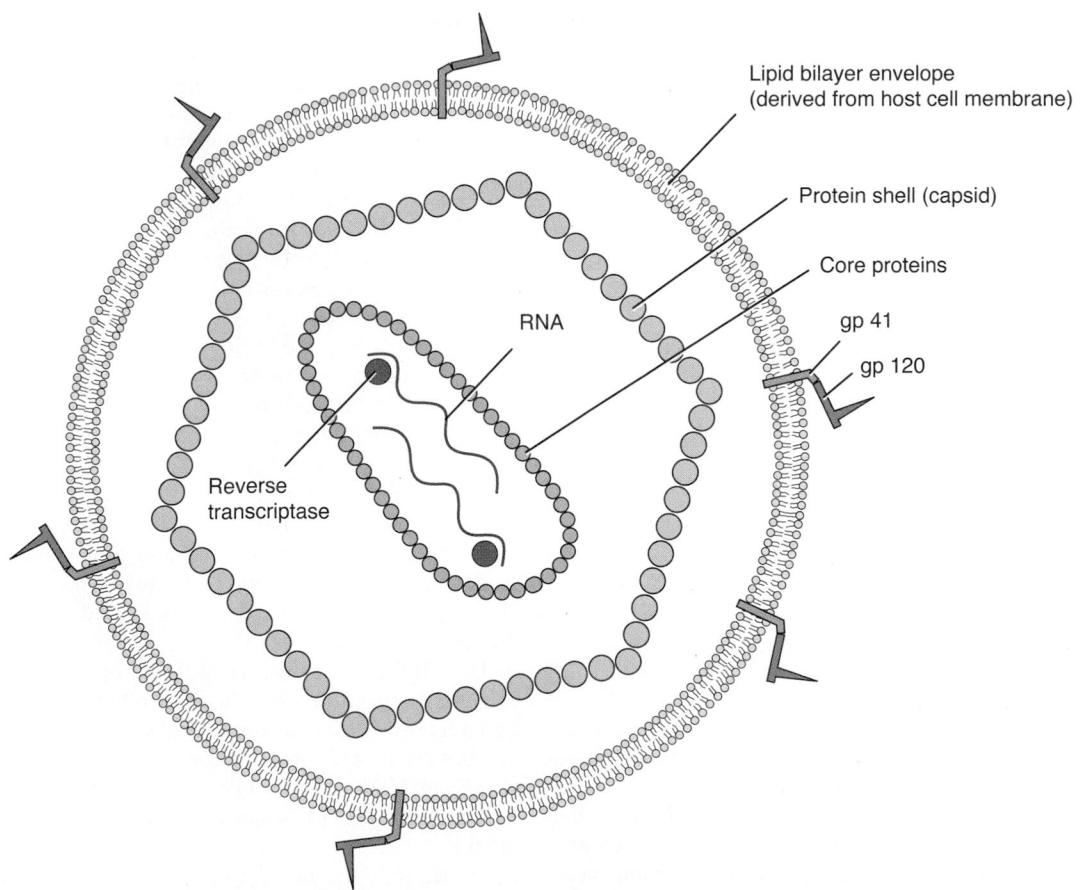

Lipid bilayer envelope
(derived from host cell membrane)

Protein shell (capsid)

Core proteins

gp 41

gp 120

RNA

Reverse
transcriptase

Figure 90–1 ■ **Structure of the human immunodeficiency virus.**
Note that HIV has two single strands of RNA, and that each strand is associated with a molecule of reverse transcriptase. (gp 41 = glycoprotein 41, gp 120 = glycoprotein 120.)

which in turn is surrounded by a *lipid bilayer envelope* (derived from the membrane of the host cell).

The central core contains two separate but identical single strands of RNA, each with its own molecule of *reverse transcriptase* attached. The RNA serves as the template for DNA synthesis.

The outer envelope of HIV contains *glycoproteins* that are needed for attachment to host cells. Each glycoprotein consists of two subunits, known as *gp41* and *gp120*. The smaller protein (gp41) is embedded in the lipid bilayer of the viral envelope; the larger protein (gp120) is connected firmly to gp41. (The numbers 41 and 120 simply indicate the mass of these glycoproteins in thousands of daltons.)

Replication Cycle of HIV

The replication cycle of HIV is depicted in Figure 90–2. The numbers below correspond to the steps in the figure.

- *Step 1*—The cycle begins with attachment of HIV to the host cell. The primary connection takes place between *gp120* on the HIV envelope and a *CD4* protein on the host cell membrane. Several other host proteins act in concert with CD4 to tighten the bond with HIV. Two of these co-receptors—known as CCR5 and CXCR4—are of particular importance.
- *Step 2*—The lipid bilayer envelope of HIV fuses with the lipid bilayer of the host cell membrane. Fusion is followed by release of HIV RNA into the host cell. In 2003, the first HIV fusion inhibitor became available for general use.
- *Step 3*—HIV RNA is transcribed into single-stranded DNA by HIV *reverse transcriptase*. Ten of the antiretroviral drugs in current use inhibit this enzyme.
- *Step 4*—Reverse transcriptase converts the single strand of HIV DNA into double-stranded HIV DNA.
- *Step 5*—Double-stranded HIV DNA becomes integrated into the host's DNA, under the direction of a viral enzyme known (aptly) as integrase. Although integrase could be a good target for drugs, such agents have proved difficult to develop.
- *Step 6*—HIV DNA undergoes transcription into RNA. Some of the resulting RNA becomes the genome for daughter HIV virions (step 6a). The rest of the RNA is messenger RNA that codes HIV proteins (step 6b).
- *Step 7*—Messenger RNA is translated into HIV glycoproteins (step 7a) and HIV enzymes and structural proteins (step 7b).
- *Step 8*—The components of HIV migrate to the cell surface and assemble into a new virus. Prior to virus assembly, HIV glycoproteins become incorporated into the host cell membrane (step 8a). In steps 8b and 8c, the other components of the virion migrate to the cell surface, where they undergo assembly into the new virus.
- *Step 9*—The newly formed virus buds off from the host cell. As indicated, the outer envelope of the virion is derived from the cell membrane of the host.
- *Step 10*—In this step, which occurs either during or immediately after budding off, HIV undergoes final maturation under the influence of protease, an enzyme that cleaves certain large polyproteins into their smaller, functional forms. If protease fails to cleave these proteins, HIV will remain immature and noninfectious. HIV protease is the target of several important drugs.

Replication Rate

HIV replicates rapidly during *all* stages of the infection. During the initial phase of infection, replication is massive. This is because (1) the population of CD4 cells is still large, thereby providing a large viral breeding ground, and (2) the host has not yet mounted an immune response against HIV, hence replication can proceed unopposed. As a result of massive replication, plasma levels of HIV can exceed 10 million virions/ml. During this stage of high viral load, patients often experience an *acute retroviral syndrome* (see below).

Over the next few months, as the immune system begins to attack HIV, plasma levels of HIV undergo a sharp decline and then level off. A typical steady-state level is between 1000 and 100,000 virions/ml. Please note, however, that steady state numbers can be deceptive. The plasma half-life of HIV is only 6 hours; that is, every 6 hours, half of the HIV virions in plasma are lost. Accordingly, in order to maintain the steady-state levels typically seen during chronic HIV infection, the actual rate of *replication* is between 1 and 10 *billion* virions/day. Despite this high rate of ongoing replication, infected individuals may remain asymptomatic for about 10 years, after which symptoms of advanced HIV disease appear.

Mutation and Drug Resistance

HIV mutates rapidly. Why? Because HIV reverse transcriptase is an error-prone enzyme. Hence, whenever it transcribes HIV RNA into single-stranded DNA and then into double-stranded DNA, there is a high probability of introducing base-pair errors. In fact, according to one estimate, up to 10 incorrect bases may be incorporated into HIV DNA during each round of replication. Because of these errors, HIV can rapidly mutate from a drug-sensitive into a drug-resistant form. The probability of developing resistance in the individual patient is directly related to the total viral load. Hence, the more virions the patient harbors, the greater the likelihood that at least one will become resistant. To minimize the emergence of resistance, patients should be treated with a combination of antiretroviral drugs. This is the same strategy we employ to prevent emergence of resistance when treating tuberculosis (see Chapter 86).

Transmission of HIV

HIV is transmitted sexually and by other means. The virus is present in all body fluids of infected individuals. Transmission can be via intimate contact with semen, vaginal secretions, and blood. The disease can be transmitted by sexual contact, transfusion, sharing IV needles, and accidental needle sticks. In addition, it can be transmitted to the fetus by an infected mother, usually during the perinatal period. Initially, HIV infection was limited largely to homosexual males, injection drug users, and hemophiliacs. However, the disease can now be found routinely in the population at large. The risk of contracting HIV can be greatly reduced by using condoms and by screening blood supplies for HIV.

Clinical Course of HIV Infection

HIV infection follows a triphasic clinical course. During the initial phase, HIV undergoes massive replication, causing blood levels of HIV to rise very high. As a result, between

50% and 90% of patients experience a flu-like *acute retroviral syndrome*. Signs and symptoms include fever, lymphadenopathy, pharyngitis, rash, myalgia, and headache (Table 90–1). Soon, however, the immune system mounts a counterattack, causing HIV levels to fall. As a result, symptoms of the acute syndrome fade. Very often, the acute retroviral syndrome is perceived as influenza, and hence goes unrecognized for what it really is.

The middle phase of HIV infection is characterized by prolonged *clinical latency*. Blood levels of HIV remain relatively

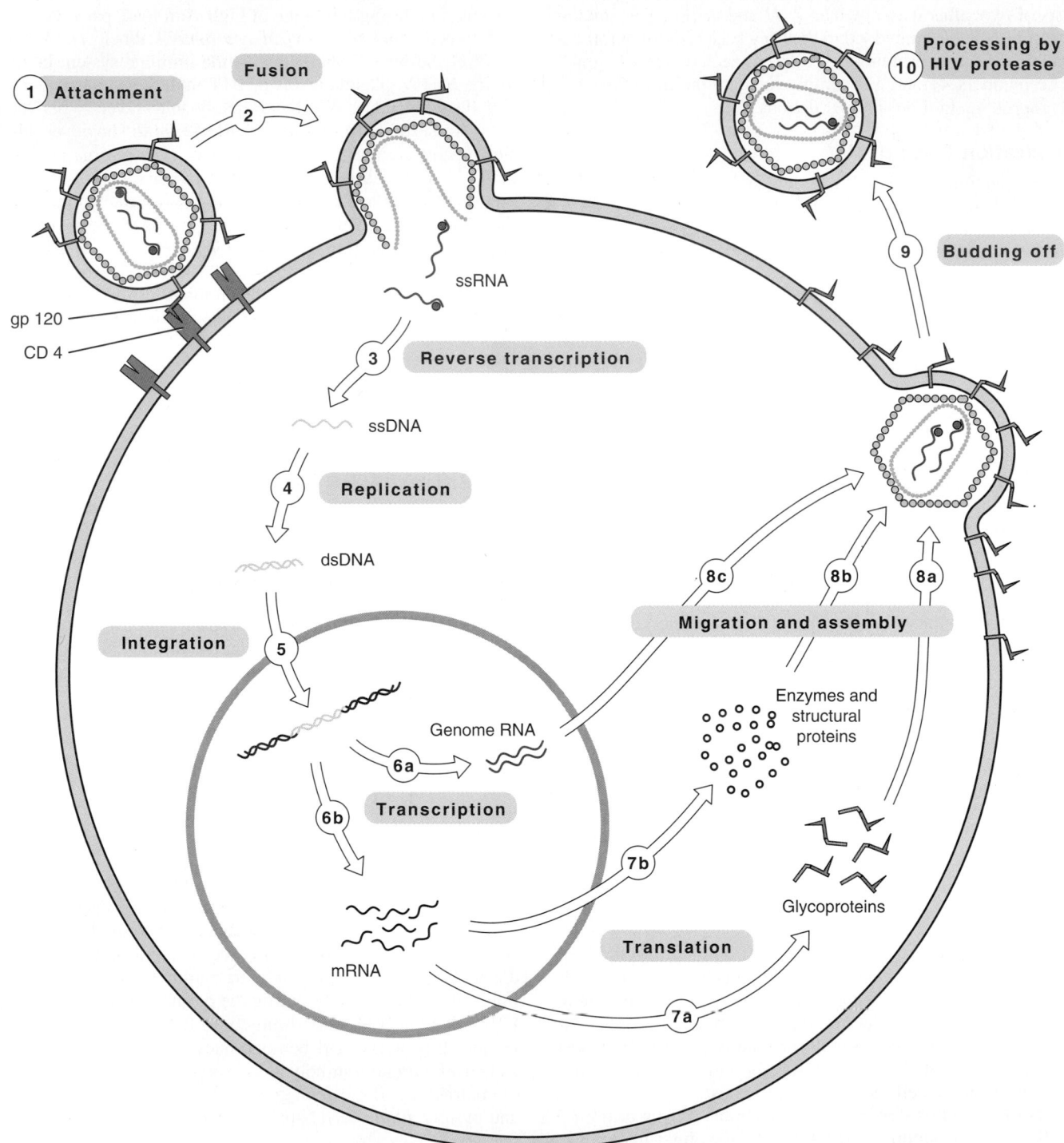

Figure 90–2 ■ Replication cycle of the human immunodeficiency virus.
See text for description of events. (gp 120 = glycoprotein 120; ssRNA = single-stranded RNA, ssDNA = single-stranded DNA, dsDNA = double-stranded DNA, mRNA = messenger RNA.)

low, and most patients are asymptomatic. However, as noted above, HIV continues to replicate despite apparent dormancy. Because of persistent HIV replication, CD4 T cells undergo progressive decline. The average duration of clinical latency is 10 years. The late phase is when AIDS occurs.

During the late phase of HIV infection, CD4 T cells drop below a critical level (200 cells/μl), rendering the patient highly vulnerable to opportunistic infections and certain neoplasms (e.g., Kaposi's sarcoma). The late phase is when AIDS occurs.

Many patients with HIV infection experience neurologic complications. Both the peripheral and central nervous systems may be involved. *Peripheral neuropathies* affect 20% to 40% of patients and may develop at any time in the course of HIV infection. In contrast, *CNS complications* usually occur late in the disease. Symptoms of CNS injury include decreased cognition, reduced concentration, memory loss, mental slowness, and motor complaints (e.g., ataxia, tremors). Neuronal injury may be the direct result of HIV infection, or may develop secondary to an opportunistic infection in the CNS.

CLASSIFICATION OF ANTIRETROVIRAL DRUGS

At this time, we have three types of antiretroviral drugs: *HIV fusion inhibitors, reverse transcriptase inhibitors, and protease inhibitors.* The reverse transcriptase inhibitors are subdivided into (1) agents that are structural analogs of nucleosides, referred to as *nucleoside reverse transcriptase inhibitors* (NRTIs), and (2) agents that are not analogs of nucleosides, referred to as *non-nucleoside reverse transcriptase inhibitors* (NNRTIs). Drugs that belong to these classes are listed in Table 90–2. All antiretroviral drugs are administered orally, and one (zidovudine) may also be given IV.

TABLE 90–1 ■ Acute Retroviral Syndrome: Associated Signs and Symptoms

- Fever (96%)
- Lymphadenopathy (74%)
- Pharyngitis (70%)
- Rash and mucocutaneous ulceration (70%)
  - Erythematous maculopapular rash with lesions on face and trunk and sometimes extremities, including palms and soles
  - Mucocutaneous ulceration involving mouth, esophagus, or genitals
- Myalgia or arthralgia (54%)
- Diarrhea (32%)
- Headache (32%)
- Nausea and vomiting (27%)
- Hepatosplenomegaly (14%)
- Weight loss (13%)
- Thrush (12%)
- Neurologic symptoms (12%)
  - Meningoencephalitis or aseptic meningitis
  - Peripheral neuropathy or radiculopathy
  - Facial palsy
  - Guillain-Barré neuritis
  - Brachial neuritis
  - Cognitive impairment or psychosis

TABLE 90–2 ■ Classification of Antiretroviral Drugs

Generic Name	Trade Name	Chemical Name/Abbreviation
Nucleoside Reverse Transcriptase Inhibitors		
Abacavir	Ziagen	ABC
Didanosine	Videx	Dideoxyinosine, ddI
Lamivudine	Epivir	3TC
Stavudine	Zerit	d4T
Tenofovir	Viread	PMPA
Zalcitabine	Hivid	Dideoxycytidine, ddC
Zidovudine	Retrovir	Azidothymidine, AZT, ZDV
Zidovudine + lamivudine	Combivir	
Non-nucleoside Reverse Transcriptase Inhibitors		
Delavirdine	Rescriptor	
Efavirenz	Sustiva	
Nevirapine	Viramune	
Protease Inhibitors		
Amprenavir	Agenerase	
Indinavir	Crixivan	
Nelfinavir	Viracept	
Ritonavir	Norvir	
Saquinavir		
Hard gel capsule	Invirase	
Soft gel capsule	Fortovase	
Lopinavir + ritonavir	Kaletra	
Fusion Inhibitor		
Enfuvirtide	Fuzeon	T-20

NUCLEOSIDE REVERSE TRANSCRIPTASE INHIBITORS

The nucleoside reverse transcriptase inhibitors (NRTIs) were the first drugs used against HIV infection and remain mainstays of treatment. As their name suggests, the NRTIs are chemical relatives of naturally occurring nucleosides, the building blocks of DNA. Antiretroviral effects derive from suppressing synthesis of viral DNA by reverse transcriptase. To be effective, all of the NRTIs must first undergo intracellular conversion to their active (triphosphate) forms. The NRTIs have few drug interactions, and most can be taken without regard to meals. Rarely, these agents cause a potentially fatal syndrome characterized by lactic acidosis and hepatomegaly with steatosis; pregnant women taking two NRTIs may be at increased risk. At this time, seven NRTIs are approved for general use. Major properties are summarized in Table 90–3.

Zidovudine

Zidovudine [Retrovir] was the first NRTI available and will serve as our prototype for the group. The drug is an analog of thymidine, a naturally occurring nucleoside. When employed in combination with other antiretroviral drugs, zidovudine can decrease viral load, increase CD4 T-cell counts, delay onset of disease symptoms, and reduce symptom severity. The drug's principal dose-limiting toxicities are *severe anemia* and *neutropenia*. Abbreviations for this agent are ZDV (for zidovudine) and AZT (for azidothymidine, its original name).

Mechanism of Antiviral Action

Zidovudine inhibits HIV replication by suppressing synthesis of viral DNA. To do this, zidovudine must first undergo intracellular conversion to its active form, zidovudine triphosphate (ZTP). As ZTP, the drug acts as a substrate for reverse transcriptase. However, when ZTP becomes incorporated into the growing DNA strand, it prevents reverse transcriptase from adding more bases; hence, further growth of the strand is blocked. In addition to causing premature strand termination, ZTP competes with natural nucleoside triphosphates for binding to the active site of reverse transcriptase; the result is competitive inhibition of the enzyme.

Therapeutic Use

Zidovudine is indicated for HIV infection. This agent penetrates to the CNS better than most other antiretroviral drugs, and hence can be especially valuable for relieving cognitive symptoms. Because monotherapy with any antiretroviral drug can rapidly lead to resistance, zidovudine should always be combined with at least one other antiretroviral agent. The role of zidovudine and other agents in the management of HIV infection is discussed at length later in the chapter.

Pharmacokinetics

Zidovudine is readily absorbed following oral administration and distributes to all body tissues, including the CNS. After entering the blood, some of the drug is taken up by cells and converted to ZTP, the active form. The remainder undergoes rapid hepatic conversion to an inactive metabolite. Both zidovudine and its inactive metabolite are eliminated by renal excretion. The *plasma* half-life of the drug is 1.1 hours, and the *intracellular* half-life is 3 hours.

Adverse Effects

Anemia and Neutropenia. Severe anemia and neutropenia are the principal toxic effects. Multiple transfusions may be required. The risk of hematologic toxicity is increased by high-dose therapy, advanced HIV infection, deficiencies in vitamin B_{12} and folic acid, and concurrent use of drugs that are myelosuppressive, nephrotoxic, or directly toxic to circulating blood cells. Anemia and neutropenia generally resolve following zidovudine withdrawal.

Hematologic status (hemoglobin concentration and neutrophil counts) should be determined before treatment and at least every 4 weeks thereafter. Hemoglobin levels may fall significantly within 2 to 4 weeks; neutrophil counts may not fall until after week 6. For patients who develop severe anemia (hemoglobin <5 gm/dl or down 25% from baseline) or severe neutropenia (neutrophil count <750 cells/μl or down 50% from baseline), zidovudine should be interrupted until there is evidence of bone marrow recovery. If neutropenia and anemia are less severe, a reduction in dosage may be sufficient. Transfusions may permit some patients to continue drug use.

Granulocyte colony-stimulating factors may be given to reverse zidovudine-induced neutropenia. Also, if erythropoietin levels are not already elevated, *epoetin alfa* (recombinant erythropoietin) can be given to reduce transfusion requirements in patients with anemia. Granulocyte colony-stimulating factors and epoetin alfa are discussed in Chapter 53.

Lactic Acidosis. Rarely, zidovudine causes a syndrome of lactic acidosis with severe hepatomegaly (liver enlargement) and hepatic steatosis (fatty degeneration of the liver). Symptoms include nausea, vomiting, abdominal pain, malaise, fatigue, anorexia, and hyperventilation (blowing off carbon dioxide can reduce acidosis). Left untreated, the syndrome can be fatal. Diagnosis is based on lactic acid measurement in *arterial* blood. If clinically significant lactic acidosis is present, zidovudine should be discontinued. Lactic acidosis is believed to result from toxicity to mitochondria.

Combining NRTIs during pregnancy may increase the risk of lactic acidosis. At least three fatal cases have occurred in pregnant women who were taking the NRTIs didanosine and stavudine. Because lactic acidosis is a potential side effect of *all* NRTIs, it may be prudent to avoid combining any of these drugs during pregnancy.

Other Adverse Effects. *Gastrointestinal effects* (anorexia, nausea, vomiting, diarrhea, abdominal pain, stomach upset) occur on occasion. Possible *CNS reactions* include headache, insomnia, confusion, anxiety, nervousness, and seizures. *Myopathy* (damage to muscle fibers) may also occur.

Drug Interactions

Drugs that are myelosuppressive, nephrotoxic, or directly toxic to circulating blood cells can increase the risk of zidovudine-induced hematologic toxicity. Notable among these is *ganciclovir,* an antiviral agent used to treat cytomegalovirus retinitis, a common infection in patients with AIDS. Other drugs of concern include *dapsone, pentamidine, pyrimethamine, trimethoprim-sulfamethoxazole, amphotericin B, flucytosine, vincristine, vinblastine,* and *doxorubicin.*

Preparations, Dosage, and Administration

Preparations. Zidovudine [Retrovir] is available in capsules (100 mg), tablets (300 mg), and a syrup (10 mg/ml) for oral therapy and in solution (10 mg/ml) for IV use. The drug is also available in combination with

TABLE 90–3 ■ Properties of Nucleoside Reverse Transcriptase Inhibitors

	Zidovudine (AZT, ZDV)	Didanosine (ddI)	Zalcitabine (ddC)	Stavudine (d4T)	Lamivudine (3TC)	Abacavir (ABC)	Tenofovir (PMPA)
Trade Name	Retrovir	Videx, Videx EC†	Hivid	Zerit, Zerit XR‡	Epivir	Ziagen	Viread
Formulations	Capsules: 100 mg Tablets: 300 mg Syrup: 10 mg/ml IV soln: 10 mg/ml	Tablets: 25, 50, 100, 150, 200 mg EC capsules: 125, 200, 250, 400 mg Powder for PO soln: 125, 200, 250, 400 mg	Tablets: 0.375, 0.75 mg	Capsules: 15, 20, 30, 40 mg Capsules, XR: 37.5, 50, 75, 100 mg PO soln: 1 mg/ml	Tablets: 150, 300 mg PO soln: 10 mg/ml	Tablets: 300 mg PO soln: 20 mg/ml	Tablets: 300 mg
Dosage	200 mg tid *or* 300 mg bid	*Tablets* >60 kg: 200 mg bid *or* 400 mg qd <60 kg: 125 mg bid *or* 250 mg qd *EC capsules* >60 kg: 400 mg qd <60 kg: 250 mg qd *PO solution* >60 kg: 250 mg bid <60 kg: 167 mg bid	0.75 mg tid	*Capsules, PO soln* >60 kg: 40 mg bid <60 kg: 30 mg bid *XR capsules* >60 kg: 100 mg qd <60 kg: 75 mg qd	*Adults:* 150 mg bid *or* 300 mg qd *Children:* 4 mg/kg bid (max 150 mg bid)	300 mg bid	300 mg once a day
Impact of Food	Take without regard to meals	Take 30 min before meals or 2 hr after	Take without regard to meals	Take without regard to meals	Take without regard to meals	Take without regard to meals—but alcohol increases levels by 41%	Take with a meal to enhance absorption
Bioavailability	60%	30%–40%	85%	86%	86%	83%	39% (with food)
Serum Half-life	1.1 hr	1.6 hr	1.2 hr	1.0 hr	3–6 hr	1.5 hr	17 hr
Intracellular Half-life	3 hr	25–40 hr	3 hr	3.5 hr	12 hr	3.3 hr	10–50 hr
Elimination	Hepatic metabolism followed by renal excretion	Partial metabolism followed by renal excretion	Partial metabolism followed by renal excretion	Partial metabolism followed by renal excretion	Renal excretion (unchanged)	Metabolized by alcohol dehydrogenase, then excreted in the urine	Renal excretion
Adverse Events	• Lactic acidosis* • Bone marrow depression: anemia, neutropenia • GI intolerance • Headache • Insomnia • Myopathy	• Lactic acidosis* • Pancreatitis • Peripheral neuropathy • GI: nausea, diarrhea	• Lactic acidosis* • Peripheral neuropathy • Stomatitis	• Lactic acidosis* • Pancreatitis • Peripheral neuropathy	• Lactic acidosis*	• Lactic acidosis* • Potentially fatal hypersensitivity reactions (fever, rash, nausea, vomiting, fatigue, abdominal pain, respiratory symptoms)	• Lactic acidosis* • Asthenia • Headache • Diarrhea • Nausea • Vomiting • Flatulence

*Lactic acidosis with steatosis is a rare but potentially fatal toxicity associated with *all* NRTIs.

†EC = enteric coated.

‡XR = extended release.

Adapted from *Guidelines for the Use of Antiretroviral Agents in HIV-Infected Adults and Adolescents*, prepared by the Panel on Clinical Practices for Treatment of HIV Infection convened by the DHHS and the Henry J. Kaiser Family Foundation, February 4, 2002.

lamivudine under the trade name Combivir, and in combination with lamivudine and abacavir under the trade name Trizivir.

Oral Therapy. The recommended dosage is 300 mg twice a day or 200 mg 3 times a day. The dosage for treating CNS effects (cognitive slowing, motor slowing, dementia) is 1200 mg/day (i.e., twice the normal dosage).

Hematologic monitoring should be done every 2 weeks. If severe anemia or severe neutropenia develops, treatment should be interrupted until there is evidence of bone marrow recovery. If anemia or neutropenia is mild, a reduction in dosage may be sufficient.

Intravenous Therapy. Intravenous zidovudine is indicated for adults with AIDS who have a history of cytologically confirmed *Pneumocystis carinii* pneumonia or a CD4 T-cell count below 200 cells/μl. The IV dosage is 1 to 2 mg/kg (infused over 1 hour) every 4 hours around the clock. Rapid infusion and bolus injection must be avoided. Intravenous therapy should be stopped as soon as oral therapy is appropriate.

Intravenous solutions are prepared by withdrawing the calculated dose from the stock vial and diluting it to 4 mg/ml (or less) in 5% dextrose for injection. The solution should not be mixed with biologic or colloidal fluids (e.g., blood products, protein solutions) and should be administered within 8 hours (if held at room temperature) or within 24 hours (if held under refrigeration).

Other NRTIs
Didanosine

Actions and Uses. Didanosine [Videx, Videx EC], also known as dideoxyinosine (ddI), is an analog of inosine, a naturally occurring nucleoside. The drug is taken up by host cells, where it undergoes conversion to its active form, dideoxyadenosine triphosphate (ddATP). Like the active form of zidovudine, ddATP suppresses viral replication primarily by causing premature termination of the growing DNA strand. In addition, it competes with natural nucleoside triphosphates for binding to the active center of reverse transcriptase, and thereby further suppresses DNA synthesis. In clinical trials, didanosine increased CD4 T-cell counts, decreased viremia, and reduced symptoms in patients with AIDS.

Didanosine is approved only for HIV infection. Because monotherapy with any antiretroviral drug can rapidly lead to resistance, the regimen should always include at least one other antiretroviral agent.

Pharmacokinetics. Didanosine is administered orally and bioavailability is low (about 35%). Absorption is greatly reduced by food and gastric acidity. To decrease gastric acidity, and thereby enhance absorption, older formulations of didanosine [Videx] contain buffering agents; newer formulations [Videx EC] are protected by an enteric coating. Didanosine crosses the blood-brain barrier poorly; levels in cerebrospinal fluid are only 20% of those in plasma. Much of the drug (35% to 60%) is excreted unchanged in the urine. The plasma half-life in patients with normal renal function is 1.6 hours, but is 3 times longer in patients with renal failure. The intracellular half-life is 25 to 40 hours.

Adverse Effects. Pancreatitis. Pancreatitis, which can be fatal, is the major dose-limiting toxicity. The incidence is 3% to 17%. Patients should be monitored for indications of developing pancreatitis (increased serum amylase in association with increased serum triglycerides; decreased serum calcium; and nausea, vomiting, or abdominal pain). If evolving pancreatitis is diagnosed, didanosine should be withdrawn. The risk of pancreatitis is increased by a history of pancreatitis or alcoholism and by use of IV pentamidine. Caution should be exercised in such patients.

Lactic Acidosis. Like all other NRTIs, didanosine can cause lactic acidosis. Fatal lactic acidosis has developed in at least three pregnant women taking didanosine plus stavudine. Accordingly, the manufacturer warns against combining these drugs during pregnancy, unless resistance to all other antiretrovirals leaves no option. Because lactic acidosis is a potential side effect of *all* NRTIs, it may be prudent to avoid combining didanosine with any of these drugs during pregnancy.

Other Adverse Effects. Additional adverse effects include diarrhea (28%), peripheral neuropathy (20%), chills or fever (12%), and rash or pruritus (9%). In contrast to zidovudine, didanosine causes minimal bone marrow suppression.

Drug Interactions. For treatment of HIV infection, didanosine is combined with stavudine or zidovudine plus a protease inhibitor or efavirenz (an NNRTI). Because of overlapping toxicities, the combination of didanosine and zalcitabine should be avoided. Buffered didanosine formulations can interfere with the absorption of drugs that require gastric acidity, including delavirdine and indinavir. Ribavirin can increase levels of didanosine, and may thereby pose a risk of toxicity. Accordingly, the combination should be used with caution.

Preparations, Dosage, and Administration. Didanosine is available in three formulations: buffered chewable tablets [Videx], enteric-coated capsules [Videx EC], and a buffered powder for oral solution [Videx].

All Formulations. Because absorption is greatly reduced by food, didanosine should be administered on an empty stomach, either 30 minutes before meals or 2 hours after. Because didanosine is eliminated by the kidneys, dosage must be reduced in patients with renal impairment.

Buffered Chewable Tablets. Didanosine tablets [Videx] are available in five strengths: 25, 50, 100, 150, and 200 mg. Instruct patients to either (1) chew the tablets thoroughly, or (2) manually crush them or disperse them in at least 1 ounce of water. Dosage is based on body weight. For adults over 60 kg, the dosage is 400 mg once daily or 200 mg twice daily. For adults under 60 kg, the dosage is 250 mg once daily or 125 mg twice daily. To ensure adequate buffering of gastric acid, patients must take two tablets (of appropriate size) for each dose.

Enteric-Coated Capsules. Didanosine enteric-coated capsules [Videx EC] are available in four strengths: 125, 200, 250, and 400 mg. Dosage is 400 mg once daily (for patients >60 kg) and 250 mg once daily (for patients <60 kg). In contrast to the buffered tablets, which must be crushed or chewed, the enteric-coated capsules must be swallowed whole.

Buffered Powder for Oral Solution. Didanosine powder for oral solution is available in single-dose packets (100, 167, and 250 mg) and in bottles (2 and 4 gm) for pediatric use. Instruct patients using the single-dose packets to (1) pour the contents of one packet into 4 ounces of water (not fruit juice or any other acid-containing beverage); (2) stir the mixture until the drug dissolves (about 2 to 3 minutes); and (3) drink the solution immediately. Dosage is 250 mg bid (for patients >60 kg) or 167 mg bid (for patients <60 kg).

Zalcitabine

Actions and Uses. Zalcitabine [Hivid], also known as dideoxycytidine (ddC), is an analog of cytidine, a naturally occurring nucleoside. Zalcitabine is a prodrug that undergoes conversion to its active form (ddC triphosphate) within host cells. The active form inhibits viral DNA synthesis by (1) causing premature termination of the growing DNA strand and (2) competing with natural nucleoside triphosphates for binding to reverse transcriptase. Toxicity of zalcitabine results in part from inhibiting mitochondrial DNA polymerase in host cells.

Zalcitabine is the least potent NRTI and hence infrequently used. Like all other drugs for HIV, zalcitabine should combined with at least one other antiretroviral agent to reduce the risk of resistance.

Pharmacokinetics. Zalcitabine is administered orally and bioavailability is 85%. Food delays absorption and reduces the amount absorbed by 14%. The drug crosses the blood-brain barrier poorly; levels in cerebrospinal fluid are only 20% of those in blood. Elimination is primarily by renal excretion; hepatic metabolism is minimal. The plasma half-life is 1.2 hours, and the intracellular half-life is 3 hours.

Adverse Effects. *Peripheral neuropathy,* which develops in 10% to 30% of patients, manifests initially as numbness and burning sensations in the extremities. These symptoms may progress to sharp shooting pain and severe continuous burning if the drug is not withdrawn. Pain of severe neuropathy requires opioid analgesics for control. Patients should be informed about early symptoms of neuropathy and instructed to report them immediately. Neuropathy reverses slowly if zalcitabine is withdrawn early, but may become irreversible if the drug is continued.

Pancreatitis from zalcitabine is uncommon (<1% incidence), but can be fatal. Patients should be monitored for indications of impending pancreatitis (rising serum amylase in association with rising serum triglycerides, decreasing serum calcium, and nausea, vomiting, or abdominal pain). If evolving pancreatitis is diagnosed, zalcitabine should be withdrawn. Caution is required in patients with a history of pancreatitis or alcoholism and in those receiving IV pentamidine.

Severe *stomatitis* (oral ulcers) occurred in 3% of patients in two clinical trials. In other trials, the incidence was even higher—but the severity was lower.

Like all other NRTIs, zalcitabine poses a small risk of potentially fatal *lactic acidosis.* Combining NRTIs may increase the risk of lactic acidosis in pregnant women, and hence should be avoided when feasible.

Drug Interactions. Like zalcitabine, *didanosine* and *stavudine* both cause peripheral neuropathy. Accordingly, zalcitabine should not be combined with these drugs. *Didanosine, alcohol,* and *IV pentamidine* increase the risk of pancreatitis.

Preparations, Dosage, and Administration. Zalcitabine [Hivid] is available in tablets (0.375 and 0.75 mg) for oral administration. The recommended dosage is 0.75 mg every 8 hours.

Stavudine

Actions and Uses. Stavudine [Zerit, Zerit XR], also known as didehydrodeoxythymidine (d4T), is an analog of thymidine, a naturally occurring nucleoside. Following uptake by cells, stavudine is converted to its active form, stavudine triphosphate. The active drug then suppresses HIV replication by (1) causing premature termination of the growing DNA strand and (2) competing with natural nucleoside triphosphates for binding to reverse transcriptase.

Stavudine is an effective drug for HIV infection. Like all other drugs used against HIV, stavudine should be combined with at least one other antiretroviral agent to decrease the risk of resistance.

Pharmacokinetics. Stavudine is administered orally and bioavailability is high (86%). Food has little or no effect on absorption. Penetration to the CNS is good. Elimination is by a combination of hepatic metabolism and renal excretion. The plasma half-life is 1 hour, and the intracellular half-life is 3.5 hours.

Adverse Effects. Peripheral Neuropathy. Like didanosine and zalcitabine, stavudine can cause peripheral neuropathy. In clinical trials, neuropathy developed in 15% to 21% of patients. Patients should be informed about early symptoms of neuropathy (numbness, tingling, or pain in hands and feet) and instructed to report them immediately. Neuropathy may resolve if the drug is withdrawn. If symptoms resolve completely, resumption of treatment may be considered, but the dosage should be reduced.

Pancreatitis. Stavudine can cause pancreatitis. Although the incidence is low (1%), pancreatitis can be fatal. Patients should be monitored for indications of pancreatitis, and, if evolving pancreatitis is diagnosed, stavudine should be withdrawn.

Lactic Acidosis. Like all other NRTIs, stavudine can cause lactic acidosis. In fact, the incidence with stavudine may be higher than with all other NRTIs. As noted above, fatal lactic acidosis has developed in at least three *pregnant women* taking stavudine plus didanosine. Accordingly, the manufacturer warns against combining these drugs during pregnancy, unless resistance to all other antiretrovirals leaves no option. Because lactic acidosis is a potential side effect of *all* NRTIs, it may be prudent to avoid combining stavudine with any NRTI during pregnancy.

Drug Interactions. Like stavudine, *didanosine* and *zalcitabine* both can cause peripheral neuropathy. Accordingly, any combination of these agents should be used with caution.

Preparations, Dosage, and Administration. Stavudine is available in standard capsules (15, 20, 30, and 40 mg) sold as Zerit, extended-release capsules (37.5, 50, 75, and 100 mg) sold as Zerit XR, and a powder (1 mg/ml) for making an oral solution. Dosage for the standard capsules and oral solution is 40 mg twice a day (for patients >60 kg) or 30 mg twice a day (for patients <60 kg). Dosage for the extended-release capsules is 100 mg once a day (for patients >60 kg) or 75 mg once a day (for patients <60 kg). Stavudine may be administered with or without food.

Lamivudine

Actions and Uses. Lamivudine [Epivir], also known as dideoxy-3′-thiacytidine (3TC), is an analog of cytidine, a naturally occurring nucleoside. Following uptake by cells, the drug is converted to its active form, lamivudine triphosphate, which then suppresses HIV replication by (1) causing premature termination of the growing DNA strand and (2) competing with natural nucleoside triphosphates for binding to reverse transcriptase.

Lamivudine is approved for HIV infection and also for hepatitis B. (The formulation used for hepatitis is marketed as Epivir HBV [see Chapter 89]). Like all other drugs used against HIV, lamivudine should be combined with at least one other antiretroviral agent, so as to decrease the risk of resistance.

Pharmacokinetics. Lamivudine is administered orally and bioavailability is high (86%). Food slows the rate of absorption but does not decrease the extent. The drug is eliminated intact in the urine. The plasma half-life is 3 to 6 hours, and the intracellular half-life is 12 hours.

Adverse Effects. Of all the NRTIs, lamivudine is the best tolerated. Side effects are minimal. Some patients experience insomnia and headache, but these effects usually fade in a few weeks.

Like all other NRTIs, lamivudine poses a small risk of potentially fatal lactic acidosis. Combining NRTIs may increase the risk of lactic acidosis in pregnant women, and hence should be avoided when feasible.

Preparations, Dosage, and Administration. For treatment of HIV, lamivudine [Epivir] is available in tablets (150 and 300 mg) and an oral solution (10 mg/ml). The drug is also available in combination with zidovudine under the trade name Combivir, and in combination with abacavir and zidovudine under the trade name Trizivir. The dosage for adults is 300 mg/day, administered as 150 mg twice daily or 300 mg once daily. The dosage for children ages 3 months to 16 years is 4 mg/kg twice daily (up to a maximum of 150 mg twice daily). In patients with renal impairment, dosage should be reduced. Lamivudine may be administered with or without food.

Abacavir

Actions and Uses. Abacavir [Ziagen], also known as ABC, is an analog of guanine, a naturally occurring pyrimidine. The drug is taken up by host cells, where it undergoes conversion to its active form, carbovir triphosphate, an analog of deoxyguanosine triphosphate. Carbovir triphosphate suppresses viral replication by causing premature termination of the growing DNA strand and by competing with natural nucleoside triphosphates for binding to the active center of reverse transcriptase.

Abacavir is approved only for HIV infection. Because monotherapy with any antiretroviral drug can rapidly lead to resistance, abacavir should always be combined with at least one other antiretroviral agent.

Pharmacokinetics. Abacavir is administered orally and bioavailability is high (83%). Absorption is not affected by food. Penetration to cerebrospinal fluid is good. The drug is converted to inactive metabolites by *alcohol dehydrogenase*. Metabolites are excreted in the urine. The plasma half-life is 1.5 hours, and the intracellular half-life is 3.3 hours.

Adverse Effects. Hypersensitivity Reactions. Hypersensitivity reactions occur in 5% of patients. These reactions, which usually develop during the first 6 weeks of treatment, can be severe and even fatal. Symptoms include fever, rash (typically maculopapular or urticarial), myalgia, arthralgia, and GI disturbances (nausea, vomiting, diarrhea, abdominal pain). A severe reaction can result in liver failure, renal failure, anaphylaxis, and death. If a hypersensitivity reaction occurs, abacavir should be withdrawn and never used again.

Recent observations indicate that abacavir hypersensitivity reactions can manifest initially as *respiratory symptoms* (e.g., pharyngitis, dyspnea, cough). Because abacavir hypersensitivity can rapidly prove fatal, early recognition is critical. Accordingly, if respiratory symptoms develop, abacavir hypersensitivity should be suspected, even though alternative diagnoses (e.g., pneumonia, bronchitis, pharyngitis, flu-like illness) are possible. If a clear differentiation between acute respiratory illness and abacavir hypersensitivity cannot be made, abacavir should be withdrawn and never used again.

Other Adverse Effects. Abacavir can cause *nausea* (47%), *nausea with vomiting* (16%), *diarrhea* (12%), *reduced appetite* (11%), and *sleep disturbances* (7%). Like all other NRTIs, abacavir poses a small risk of potentially fatal *lactic acidosis.* Combining NRTIs may increase the risk of lactic acidosis in pregnant women, and hence should be avoided when feasible.

Drug Interactions. Alcohol can compete with abacavir for metabolism by alcohol dehydrogenase, and can thereby increase abacavir levels substantially (about 40%). The clinical significance of this interaction is unclear. Nonetheless, it would seem prudent to minimize alcohol consumption.

Significant interactions with drugs other than alcohol have not been reported.

Preparations, Dosage, and Administration. Abacavir [Ziagen] is available in 300-mg tablets and a 20-mg/ml oral solution. The adult dosage is 300 mg twice daily. The pediatric dosage is 8 mg/kg twice daily, but should not exceed 300 mg twice daily.

Tenofovir Disoproxil Fumarate

Mechanism of Action. Tenofovir disoproxil fumarate [Viread] is a nucleo*tide* reverse transcriptase inhibitor—not a nucleo*side* reverse transcriptase inhibitor. The drug is discussed in this section because nucleotides and nucleosides are very similar (a nucleotide is simply a nucleoside with a phosphate group added) and hence have similar effects on reverse transcriptase. Once inside cells, tenofovir disoproxil fumarate undergoes conversion to tenofovir, and then to tenofovir diphosphate, its active form. Like the NRTIs, tenofovir diphosphate inhibits viral DNA synthesis in two ways: it competes with the natural substrate (in this case, deoxyadenosine triphosphate) for binding to reverse transcriptase and, after being incorporated into the growing DNA chain, it causes premature chain termination. Toxicity results in part from inhibiting mitochondrial DNA polymerase.

Therapeutic Use. Tenofovir is indicated only for treatment of HIV infection. To delay emergence of resistance, the regimen should always include other antiretroviral drugs.

Pharmacokinetics. Tenofovir is administered orally, and bioavailability is low (25% in the absence of food and 39% in the presence of food). Blood levels peak about 1 hour after administration. Binding to plasma proteins is low. Tenofovir is eliminated primarily by the kidneys; both glomerular filtration and active tubular secretion are involved. Because elimination is renal, tenofovir can accumulate to dangerous levels if kidney function is impaired. Tenofovir has a prolonged half-life—17 hours in plasma and 10 to 50 hours within cells—and hence can be administered just once a day.

Adverse Effects. Tenofovir is generally well tolerated. The most common reactions are mild to moderate *GI effects*: nausea (11%), diarrhea (9%), vomiting (5%), and flatulence (4%). *Asthenia* (8%) and *headache* (6%) may also occur.

Like other NRTIs, tenofovir poses a small risk of potentially fatal *lactic acidosis*. Combining NRTIs may increase the risk of lactic acidosis in pregnant women, and hence should be avoided when feasible.

Drug Interactions. Tenofovir has little or no effect on the metabolism of other drugs. However, combining tenofovir with another drug that undergoes active tubular secretion could lead to the accumulation of tenofovir, the other drug, or both. Through a mechanism that has not been determined, tenofovir can raise plasma levels of didanosine. Accordingly, patients using the combination should be monitored for long-term didanosine toxicity.

Preparations, Dosage, and Administration. Tenofovir [Viread] is available in 300-mg tablets for oral use. The recommended dosage is 300 mg once a day, taken with a meal to enhance bioavailability. If the patient is also taking didanosine, tenofovir should be administered 2 hours before didanosine or 1 hour after. Patients with significant renal impairment (creatinine clearance <60 ml/min) should not use the drug.

Abacavir plus Zidovudine plus Lamivudine

Description and Dosage. Abacavir, lamivudine, and zidovudine are available in a single tablet under the trade name *Trizivir*. The amount of each drug in the combination is the same as in their individual formulations: abacavir, 300 mg; lamivudine, 150 mg; and zidovudine, 300 mg. Dosing is done twice a day—the same schedule employed when the drugs are taken separately. The only benefit of the combination is that patients can now take just one pill twice a day, instead of three. Dosing may be done with or without food. Because dosage of each component cannot be adjusted separately, the product should not be used by patients with renal or hepatic impairment.

Adverse Effects. Abacavir can cause potentially fatal *hypersensitivity reactions.* Early manifestations include fever, rash, fatigue, GI symptoms, and respiratory symptoms. If these develop, treatment should be interrupted while an evaluation is conducted. If hypersensitivity cannot be ruled out, the drug should be discontinued permanently.

Zidovudine can cause *anemia* and *neutropenia.* Hematologic status should be closely monitored.

All NRTIs can cause *lactic acidosis.* Death from this disorder has resulted when two NRTIs—didanosine and stavudine—were combined during pregnancy. Accordingly, it would seem prudent to avoid Trizivir in pregnant women.

Lamivudine Plus Zidovudine

Lamivudine (150 mg) and zidovudine (300 mg) are available in a single tablet under the trade name *Combivir.* The dosage for adults and for children at least 12 years old is 1 tablet twice a day, taken without regard to meals. Because the dosage of each component cannot be adjusted separately, the product should not be used by patients with renal or hepatic impairment. Principal adverse effects are anemia and neutropenia (caused by zidovudine) and lactic acidosis (caused by both drugs).

NON-NUCLEOSIDE REVERSE TRANSCRIPTASE INHIBITORS

The non-nucleoside reverse transcriptase inhibitors (NNRTIs) differ from the NRTIs in structure and mechanism of action. As their name suggests, the NNRTIs are not structurally related to naturally occurring nucleosides—and, in contrast to the NRTIs, which inhibit synthesis of HIV DNA primarily by causing premature termination of the growing DNA strand, the NNRTIs bind to the active center of reverse transcriptase, and thereby cause direct inhibition. In addition, whereas NRTIs must undergo intracellular conversion to their active forms, the NNRTIs are active as administered. At this time, three NNRTIs are available: nevirapine [Viramune], delavirdine [Rescriptor], and efavirenz [Sustiva]. The principal adverse effect of these drugs is rash, which can be severe. Pharmacologic properties of the NNRTIs are summarized in Table 90-4.

Nevirapine

Mechanism of Action. Nevirapine [Viramune] binds directly to HIV reverse transcriptase and thereby disrupts the active center of the enzyme. As a result, enzyme activity is suppressed. Nevirapine only inhibits reverse transcriptase of HIV-1; it does not inhibit reverse transcriptase of HIV-2. In addition, nevirapine does not inhibit human DNA polymerase, and hence is harmless to us.

Pharmacokinetics. Nevirapine is well absorbed (>90%) following oral administration, both in the presence and absence of food. The drug is very lipid soluble, and hence can cross both the placenta and blood-brain barrier and can enter breast milk with ease. Concentrations achieved in cerebrospinal fluid are about 45% of those in plasma. Elimination results from hepatic metabolism followed by excretion in the urine (80%) and feces.

Resistance. Resistance to nevirapine develops rapidly if the drug is used alone. Accordingly, nevirapine should always be combined with other antiretroviral drugs.

Therapeutic Use. Nevirapine is approved only for treating infection with HIV-1; the drug is not active against HIV-2. To reduce the risk of resistance, nevirapine should never be used alone. Rather it should always be combined with at least one other antiretroviral drug, and preferably with two.

Adverse Effects. Rash. The most common adverse effect is rash, which usually occurs early in therapy and can be severe or even life threatening. For most patients, the rash is benign and, if needed, can be managed with an antihistamine or topical glucocorticoid. However, if the patient experiences severe rash or rash associated with fever, blistering, oral lesions, conjunctivitis, muscle pain, or joint pain, nevirapine should be withdrawn. Why? Because these symptoms may indicate development of *erythema multiforme* or *Stevens-Johnson syndrome.* Rash can be minimized by using a low dosage initially and then increasing the dosage if rash does not occur.

Hepatotoxicity. Nevirapine can cause severe hepatotoxicity, including fulminant and cholestatic hepatitis, hepatic necrosis, and hepatic failure. Death has occurred. The risk is highest during the first 12 weeks of treatment, and is increased by a history of chronic hepatitis B or hepatitis C. Liver function tests should be done at baseline, prior to dosage escalation, 2 weeks after dosage escalation, and whenever patients have symptoms (fatigue, malaise, anorexia, nausea) suggesting an early stage of liver damage. If hepatotoxicity is diagnosed, nevirapine should be withdrawn as soon as possible.

Drug Interactions. Nevirapine induces the activity of hepatic cytochrome P450 drug-metabolizing enzymes, and can thereby increase the metabolism of other drugs, causing their levels to decline. The ability to decrease levels of *protease inhibitors, oral contraceptives,* and *methadone* is of particular concern.

TABLE 90–4 ▪ Properties of Non-Nucleoside Reverse Transcriptase Inhibitors

	Nevirapine	Delavirdine	Efavirenz
Trade Name	Viramune	Rescriptor	Sustiva
Formulations	Tablets: 200 mg PO suspension: 10 mg/ml	Tablets: 100, 200 mg	Capsules: 50, 100, 200 mg Tablets: 600 mg
Impact of Food	Take without regard to meals	Take without regard to meals	Don't take with or after a high-fat meal (levels will increase by 50%)
Dosage	200 mg once a day for 14 days, then 200 mg twice a day	400 mg tid (mix four 100-mg tabs in 3 or more ounces of water to produce a slurry)	600 mg at bedtime
Bioavailability	>90%	85%	Data not available
Serum Half-life	25–30 hr	5.8 hr	40–55 hr
Elimination	Metabolized by P450, followed by excretion in urine (80%) and feces (10%)	Metabolized by P450, followed by excretion in urine (51%) and feces (44%)	Metabolized by P450, followed by excretion in the urine (14%–34%) and feces (16%–61%)
Adverse Events	• Rash* • Increased transaminase levels • Hepatitis	• Rash* • Increased transaminase levels • Headache	• Rash* • Increased transaminase levels • CNS symptoms† • Teratogenic in monkeys
Drug Interactions	• *Induces* P450 and may thereby *decrease* levels of other drugs; effects on protease inhibitors, oral contraceptives, and methadone are of particular concern • Rifampin also induces P450, and may thereby decrease levels of nevirapine. The combination is not recommended.	• *Inhibits* P450 and may thereby *increase* levels of other drugs • Because of P450 inhibition, the following drugs are *contraindicated:* astemizole,‡ terfenadine,‡ midazolam, triazolam, simvastatin, lovastatin, and cisapride‡ • Because of P450 inhibition, the following drugs should be used with *caution:* indinavir, saquinavir, clarithromycin, dapsone, ergot alkaloids, dihydropyridine calcium channel blockers, quinidine, warfarin, and sildenafil [Viagra] • Antacids, histamine$_2$-receptor blockers (e.g., cimetidine), proton pump inhibitors (e.g., omeprazole), and buffered formulations of didanosine can decrease absorption of delavirdine • Rifampin and rifabutin induce P450 and can thereby reduce levels of delavirdine substantially (80% to 96%). Don't use delavirdine with these drugs	• Efavirenz can compete with other drugs for metabolism by P450, thereby causing them to accumulate to toxic levels. Accordingly, efavirenz should not be combined with astemizole,‡ terfenadine,‡ cisapride,‡ midazolam, triazolam, or ergot alkaloids • Efavirenz induces P450, and can thereby decrease levels of saquinavir and indinavir. Don't combine with saquinavir. Increase indinavir dosage. • Combining efavirenz with ritonavir increases levels of both drugs; toxicity can result

*Rarely, rash evolves into Stevens-Johnson syndrome, which can be fatal.
†CNS symptoms, including dizziness, somnolence, insomnia, abnormal dreams, abnormal thinking, confusion, impaired concentration, amnesia, agitation, depersonalization, hallucinations, and euphoria, occur in about 50% of patients.
‡No longer available in the United States.

Like nevirapine, *rifampin* can induce P450, and can thereby significantly reduce nevirapine levels. Accordingly, the combination is not recommended.

St. John's wort—an herbal supplement taken for depression—may reduce levels of nevirapine and other NNRTIs. The principal mechanism is accelerated metabolism secondary to induction of P450 (see Chapter 31).

Preparations, Dosage, and Administration. Nevirapine [Viramune] is available in 200-mg tablets and a 10-mg/ml oral suspension. Dosages are as follows:

- *Adults*—Start with 200 mg once a day for 14 days and then, if no rash develops, use 200 mg twice a day thereafter.

- *Children 8 years and older*—Start with 4 mg/kg once a day for 14 days and then, if no rash develops, use 4 mg/kg twice a day thereafter.
- *Children 2 months to 8 years*—Start with 4 mg/kg once a day for 14 days and then, if no rash develops, use 7 mg/kg (but not more than 400 mg total) twice a day thereafter.

Other NNRTIs
Efavirenz

Efavirenz [Sustiva] is the only NNRTI deemed a preferred agent for treating HIV. The drug is effective and, because of its long half-life, can be administered once a day. Its principal drawbacks are teratogenicity and transient adverse CNS effects.

Mechanism of Action. Like other NNRTIs, efavirenz binds directly to HIV reverse transcriptase, causing noncompetitive inhibition of the enzyme. Efavirenz is selective for HIV-1. It does not affect HIV-2, and does not inhibit human DNA polymerase.

Therapeutic Use. At this time, efavirenz is the only NNRTI recommended as first-line therapy for HIV infection. In clinical trials, the combination of efavirenz plus two NRTIs (zidovudine and lamivudine) was at least as effective as indinavir (a protease inhibitor) combined with the same two NRTIs. Furthermore, the efavirenz-based regimen was better tolerated.

Pharmacokinetics. Efavirenz is administered orally and can be taken with or without food—but not with a high-fat meal, which can increase absorption by 50%. Plasma levels peak 3 to 5 hours after dosing. In the blood, efavirenz is highly (>99%) protein bound. The drug crosses the blood-brain barrier and can reduce HIV levels in the CNS. Efavirenz undergoes metabolism by P450, followed by excretion in the urine and feces. The drug has a long half-life (40 to 55 hours), and hence can be taken just once a day.

Adverse Effects. *CNS symptoms* occur in over 50% of patients. The most common are dizziness, insomnia, impaired consciousness, drowsiness, vivid dreams, and nightmares. Delusions, hallucinations, and severe acute depression may also occur, primarily in patients with a history of mental illness or drug abuse. Patients who experience these severe reactions should discontinue the drug. CNS symptoms are prominent at the onset of treatment, but generally resolve within 2 to 4 weeks, despite continuous drug use.

As with other NNRTIs, *rash* is common. In clinical trials, rash developed in 27% of adults and 40% of children. The median time to rash onset was 11 days, and the median duration was 14 days. Rash can range in severity from mild (erythema, pruritus) to moderate (diffuse maculopapular rash, dry desquamation) to severe (vesiculation, moist desquamation, ulceration). Very rarely, patients develop Stevens-Johnson syndrome, which can be fatal. If severe rash occurs, efavirenz should be withdrawn. Rash may respond to antihistamines and topical glucocorticoids.

Efavirenz is *teratogenic*. In monkeys, doses equivalent to those used in humans produced a high incidence of fetal malformation. Women using the drug must avoid getting pregnant. A barrier method of birth control (e.g., condom) should be used in conjunction with a hormonal method (e.g., oral contraceptive). Pregnancy must be ruled out before efavirenz is used.

Like other NNRTIs, efavirenz may pose a risk of *liver damage*. Liver enzymes should be monitored, especially in patients with hepatitis B or C.

Drug Interactions. Efavirenz can compete with other drugs for metabolism by P450, thereby causing them to accumulate, possibly to dangerous levels. To avoid harm, efavirenz should not be combined with astemizole, terfenadine, and cisapride (all no longer available in the United States) or with midazolam, triazolam, dihydroergotamine, or ergotamine.

Efavirenz *induces P450,* and can thereby accelerate its own metabolism and the metabolism of certain other drugs. Increased metabolism of two protease inhibitors—saquinavir and indinavir—is of particular concern. If efavirenz is combined with indinavir, the dosage of indinavir should be increased. Combined use with saquinavir, a drug with low bioavailability, should be avoided.

Combining efavirenz with ritonavir (a protease inhibitor) can increase levels of both drugs. Toxicity may result.

Preparations, Dosage, and Administration. Efavirenz [Sustiva] is available in 600-mg tablets and in 50-, 100-, and 200-mg capsules. The adult dosage is 600 mg once daily. To reduce the impact of CNS effects, dosing should be done at bedtime for the first few weeks. Efavirenz may be taken with or without food—but not with high-fat meals, which increase absorption.

Delavirdine

Actions, Resistance, and Use. Delavirdine [Rescriptor] is similar to nevirapine in actions and uses. Like nevirapine, delavirdine is a nonnucleoside that acts directly to inhibit reverse transcriptase, thereby suppressing HIV replication. Because resistant forms of HIV rapidly emerge when delavirdine is used alone, the drug should always be combined with at least one other antiretroviral agent. Like nevirapine, delavirdine is active only against HIV-1.

Adverse Effects. Like nevirapine, delavirdine causes potentially serious *rash*. In clinical trials, rash developed in up to 50% of patients; erythema multiforme and Stevens-Johnson syndrome have been reported. If severe rash develops, the drug should be withdrawn. Other common side effects include headache, fatigue, GI intolerance (nausea, vomiting, diarrhea), and elevation of liver enzymes.

Drug Interactions. In contrast to nevirapine, which induces cytochrome P450, delavirdine *inhibits* cytochrome P450. As a result, levels of drugs taken concurrently may rise. To avoid toxicity from excessive drug levels, patients taking delavirdine should not take astemizole, terfenadine, or cisapride (all no longer available in the United States), or alprazolam, midazolam, triazolam, lovastatin, or simvastatin. Other drugs whose levels may be increased include indinavir, saquinavir, clarithromycin, dapsone, warfarin, quinidine, ergot alkaloids, sildenafil [Viagra], and the dihydropyridine-type calcium channel blockers; all of these agents should be used with caution.

Drugs that induce P450 (e.g., rifampin, rifabutin, phenytoin, phenobarbital, carbamazepine) may decrease levels of delavirdine, and may thereby reduce its efficacy.

Drugs that reduce gastric acidity—antacids, histamine$_2$-receptor antagonists, proton pump inhibitors, and buffered didanosine formulations—can decrease absorption of delavirdine.

Preparations, Dosage, and Administration. Delavirdine [Rescriptor] is available in 100- and 200-mg tablets for oral use. The recommended dosage is 400 mg 3 times a day, taken with or without food. Patients who are unable to swallow tablets whole can mix 4 of the 100-mg tablets with water (at least 3 ounces) and swallow the resulting suspension. Acidity enhances absorption. Accordingly, patients with achlorhydria (lack of stomach acid) should administer delavirdine with an acidic beverage (e.g., orange juice, cranberry juice).

PROTEASE INHIBITORS

The protease inhibitors are the most effective antiretroviral drugs available. When used in combination with reverse transcriptase inhibitors, they can reduce viral load to a level that is undetectable with current assays.

In early clinical trials, protease inhibitors were generally well tolerated, although they did cause GI disturbances. However, widespread use of these drugs has revealed additional side effects: fat redistribution, hyperglycemia and diabetes, reduced bone mineral density, increased bleeding in hemophiliacs, and elevation of triglyceride and transaminase levels.

All of the protease inhibitors can inhibit cytochrome P450, and can thereby increase levels of other drugs. Because of this mechanism and others, protease inhibitors are subject to a bewildering array of drug interactions.

As with other antiretroviral drugs, HIV resistance can be a significant problem. Mutant strains of HIV that are resistant to one protease inhibitor are likely to be cross-resistant with other protease inhibitors. In contrast, since protease inhibitors do not share the same mechanism as the reverse transcriptase inhibitors or fusion inhibitors, cross-resistance between protease inhibitors and these other antiretroviral drugs does not occur. To reduce the risk of resistance, protease inhibitors should never be used alone; rather, they should always be combined with at least one reverse transcriptase inhibitor, and preferably two.

Five protease inhibitors are now approved for general use. Studies comparing these drugs have not been conducted. Accordingly, selection among them cannot be based on relative efficacy. Until data on relative efficacy are available, drug selection can be based on side effect profiles, drug interactions, and patient acceptance. The major properties of the protease inhibitors are summarized in Table 90–5.

Group Properties
Adverse Effects

Hyperglycemia/Diabetes. Protease inhibitors have been associated with hyperglycemia, new-onset diabetes, abrupt exacerbation of existing diabetes, and diabetic ketoacidosis. Onset typically occurs after 2 months of drug use, but can also develop much earlier. Hyperglycemia can be managed with insulin and oral hypoglycemics (e.g., metformin). Because of the possible risk of diabetes, patients should be instructed to report signs of the disease, such as polydipsia (increased fluid intake), polyphagia (increased food intake), and polyuria. In patients with existing diabetes, blood glucose should be monitored closely. In others, blood glucose should be measured at baseline, every 3 to 4 months during the first year of treatment, and less frequently thereafter. Although withdrawing protease inhibitors may restore normal glucose metabolism, discontinuation is not recommended.

Fat Redistribution. Use of protease inhibitors has been associated with redistribution of body fat, sometimes referred to as *lipodystrophy syndrome* or *pseudo-Cushing's syndrome.* Fat accumulates in the abdomen ("protease paunch"), in the breasts of men and women, and between the shoulder blades ("buffalo hump"). Fat is lost from the face, arms, buttocks, and legs. Leg and arm veins become prominent. Muscle mass and strength are unaffected. The underlying mechanism has not been determined. Although these fat changes resemble those of Cushing's syndrome, which is caused by excessive cortisol, elevated cortisol has not been observed. Health risks of the syndrome are unknown, although it can be psychologically distressing. Drug withdrawal may cause symptoms to resolve, but is not recommended.

Hyperlipidemia. All protease inhibitors can elevate plasma levels of cholesterol and triglycerides. These effects may occur with or without redistribution of fat. Elevation of cholesterol can lead to atherosclerosis and associated cardiovascular events. Elevation of triglycerides can lead to pancreatitis. Changes in plasma lipids can be detected by monitoring lipid levels every 3 to 4 months. Potential interventions for hyperlipidemia include diet, exercise, and lipid-lowering drugs. However, benefits of these interventions have not been established. If lipid-lowering drugs are employed, lovastatin and simvastatin should be avoided. Why? Because inhibition of P450 by protease inhibitors can cause lovastatin and simvastatin to accumulate to dangerous levels.

Increased Bleeding in Hemophiliacs. Protease inhibitors may increase the risk of bleeding in patients with hemophilia. Bleeding typically occurs in the joints and soft tissues, where danger is low. However, serious bleeds in the brain and GI tract have also occurred. The mean time to increased bleeding is 22 days after the onset of treatment. Patients may need to increase their dosage of coagulation factors.

Reduced Bone Mineral Density. Protease inhibitors can accelerate bone loss. In some patients, loss is severe enough to meet the definition of osteoporosis. In a study conducted at Washington University, involving 122 patients on HAART, 21% of those taking protease inhibitors had osteoporosis. In an Australian study involving 74 patients taking protease inhibitors, 28% of patients had low bone mineral density and 10% had osteoporosis. To help protect against bone loss, patients should ensure adequate intake of calcium and vitamin D. If significant bone loss develops, bisphosphonates, raloxifene, calcitonin, or teriparatide may be indicated (see Chapter 70, Drugs That Affect Calcium Levels and Bone Mineralization).

Elevation of Serum Transaminases. Protease inhibitors can increase serum levels of transaminases, indicating injury to the liver. Exercise caution in patients with chronic liver disease (e.g., hepatitis B or C, cirrhosis). Serum transaminases should be measured before treatment and periodically thereafter.

Drug Interactions

All protease inhibitors are metabolized by cytochrome P450 enzymes, and all protease inhibitors can inhibit cytochrome P450 enzymes. As a result, protease inhibitors can interact with drugs that inhibit or induce P450 enzymes, and with drugs that are substrates for P450 enzymes. Drug interactions of the protease inhibitors are summarized in Table 90–6.

P450 Inhibitors. Agents that inhibit P450 can retard metabolism of the protease inhibitors, thereby increasing their levels. Important inhibitors include *ketoconazole* (an antifungal drug), *clarithromycin* (an antibacterial drug), and *grapefruit juice.* If inhibition of metabolism is substantial, dosage of the protease inhibitor should be reduced.

P450 Inducers. Drugs that induce P450 can accelerate the metabolism of protease inhibitors, and can thereby reduce their levels. Important inducers include *rifampin* and *rifabutin* (used for mycobacterial infections) and three anti-seizure drugs: *phenobarbital, phenytoin,* and *carbamazepine.* If induction of P450 is substantial, loss of therapeutic effects can result. For example, when rifampin is combined with indinavir (a protease inhibitor), total body content of indinavir is reduced by 92%. Similar reductions occur with other protease inhibitors. Accordingly, combined use of rifampin and protease inhibitors should be avoided.

P450 Substrates. By inhibiting P450, protease inhibitors can slow the metabolism of other drugs, thereby causing their levels to rise. Serious toxicity can result. To avoid toxicity, protease inhibitors should not be combined with the following P450 substrates: *astemizole* and *terfenadine* (nonsedating antihistamines; no longer available in the United States), *cisapride* (a drug for heartburn; no longer available in the United States), *triazolam* and *midazolam* (benzodiazepine sedative-hypnotics), *ergotamine* and *dihydroergotamine* (drugs that promote vasoconstriction and relieve migraine), and *lovastatin* and *simvastatin* (drugs that lower cholesterol).

TABLE 90–5 ■■ Properties of Protease Inhibitors (PIs)

	Indinavir	Ritonavir	Saquinavir (HGC)*
Trade Name	Crixivan	Norvir	Invirase
Formulations	Caps: 100, 200, 333, 400 mg	Caps: 100 mg PO soln: 600 mg/7.5 ml	Hard-gel caps: 200 mg
Dosage	800 mg q 8 h Separate dosing with buffered didanosine by 1 hr	600 mg q 12 h Separate dosing with buffered didanosine by 2 hr	400 mg bid, *and only in combination with ritonavir*
Impact of Food	Food decreases levels by 77%. Take 1 hr before meals or 2 hr after; may take with skim milk or a low-fat meal.	Food increases levels by 15%. Take with food, if possible, to improve tolerability.	No food effect when taken with ritonavir
Storage	Room temperature	Refrigerate capsules. Do *not* refrigerate oral solution.	Room temperature
Bioavailability	65%	Adequate	Low (4%) and erratic
Plasma Half-life	1.5–2 hr	3–5 hr	1–2 hr
Adverse Effects Common to All PIs	• Fat redistribution • Hyperlipidema • Hyperglycemia—PIs may exacerbate hyperglycemia in patients with existing diabetes, and may cause new-onset diabetes • Possible increased risk of bleeding in patients with hemophilia • Bone loss • Elevation of serum transaminases		
Adverse Effects of Individual PIs	• GI: nausea • Nephrolithiasis • Miscellaneous: headache, asthenia, blurred vision, dizziness, rash, metallic taste, thrombocytopenia	• GI: nausea, vomiting, diarrhea • Paresthesias (circumoral and peripheral) • Asthenia • Taste perversion	• GI: nausea, diarrhea • Headache
Drug Interactions	*See* Table 90–6		

*HCG = hard gelatin capsule, SGC = soft gelatin capsule.

The interaction of protease inhibitors with *sildenafil* [Viagra] can intensify and prolong sildenafil's effects, with possibly dangerous results. Sildenafil dosage should not exceed 25 mg in 48 hours.

Protease Inhibitor Combinations. By inhibiting P450, one protease inhibitor can increase levels of another protease inhibitor. As discussed below, the combination of ritonavir with saquinavir [Invirase] is employed for the specific purpose of ensuring that saquinavir levels will be therapeutic. Likewise, the only purpose of ritonavir in the fixed-dose combination product that contains ritonavir plus lopinavir (marketed as Kaletra) is to ensure adequate blood levels of lopinavir.

Herb Interactions

St. John's Wort. St. John's wort, an herbal supplement taken for depression, can decrease levels of all protease inhibitors. The principal mechanism is accelerated metabolism owing to induction of P450 (see Box 31–2, Chapter 31). To avoid loss of efficacy, patients using protease inhibitors must not use St. John's wort.

Garlic. Garlic supplements can decrease levels of saquinavir, and probably levels other protease inhibitors. Scientists at the National Institutes of Health reported that garlic supplements can produce a dramatic (50%) decrease in blood levels of saquinavir. Not only is this effect profound, it persists: 10 days after stopping garlic intake, saquinavir levels remained 30% to 40% below baseline. These observations are significant. Why? Because many patients with HIV infection take garlic supplements on the belief (albeit unfounded) that garlic can suppress HIV replication and stimulate immune function. Although we don't know how garlic lowers saquinavir levels, induction of P450 is suspected. If this is correct, garlic supplements are likely to reduce levels of other drugs, including other protease inhibitors and NNRTIs. Accordingly, it would seem prudent for patients taking protease inhibitors or NNRTIs to avoid garlic supplements. The small amount of garlic in *prepared* foods is probably no concern.

Saquinavir

Saquinavir [Invirase, Fortovase] was the first protease inhibitor to receive Food and Drug Administration (FDA) approval and will serve as our prototype for the group. In the test tube, the drug appears more potent than other protease inhibitors.

Saquinavir is available in two formulations: hard gelatin capsules [Invirase] and soft gelatin capsules [Fortovase]. The hard-gel formulation was released first and has lower bioavailability than the soft-gel formulation. Now that the soft-gel formulation is available, the hard-gel formulation is

Saquinavir (SGS)*	Nelfinavir	Amprenavir	Lopinavir + Ritonavir
Fortovase	Viracept	Agenerase	Kaletra
Soft-gel caps: 200 mg	Tablets: 250, 625 mg PO powder: 50 mg	Capsules: 50, 150 mg PO soln: 15 mg/ml Note: Capsules and solution are not interchangeable on a mg-for-mg basis	Caps: 133.3 mg lopinavir + 33.3 mg ritonavir PO soln: 80 mg/ml lopinavir + 20 mg/ml ritonavir
1200 mg tid	750 tid or 1250 mg bid	*Adults:* 1200 mg bid using capsules; PO soln. not recommended *Children:* see text	400 mg lopinavir + 100 mg ritonavir bid
Food increases levels 6-fold. Take with a large meal.	Food increases levels 2-to 3-fold. Take with a meal or a snack.	High-fat meals decrease absorption. May take with or without food, but not with a high-fat meal.	Moderate-fat meal increases absorption from capsules and solution by 48% and 80%, respectively. Take with food.
Can store at room temperature up to 3 mo; refrigerate for long-term storage	Room temperature	Room temperature	Can store at room temperature up to 2 mo; refrigerate for long-term storage
Greater than with HCG saquinavir	20%–80%	Not determined	Not determined
1–2 hr	3.5–5 hr	7.1–10 hr	5–6 hr
• GI: Nausea, diarrhea, abdominal pain, dyspepsia • Headache	• GI: diarrhea	• GI: nausea, vomiting, diarrhea • Rash • Oral paresthesias • Propylene glycol toxicity (with the oral solution)	• GI: nausea, vomiting, diarrhea • Weakness/tiredness

being phased out. However, Invirase will continue to be available, under a limited distribution program, to patients who were using it prior to release of Fortovase.

Soft-Gel Formulation

Saquinavir in soft gelatin capsules [Fortovase] was approved by the FDA on November 10, 1997. This preparation is more effective than saquinavir in hard gelatin capsules, in part because of greater bioavailability, and in part because the approved dosage is higher.

Mechanism of Action. To understand the effects of saquinavir and the other protease inhibitors, we must first understand the function of HIV protease. As noted above, protease catalyzes the final step in HIV maturation. When the various enzymes and structural proteins of HIV are synthesized, they are not produced as separate entities; rather, they are strung together in large polyproteins. The role of protease is to cleave bonds in the polyproteins, thereby freeing the individual enzymes and structural proteins. Once these components have been freed, HIV can complete its maturation.

Protease inhibitors bind to the active site of HIV protease and thereby prevent the enzyme from cleaving HIV polyproteins. As a result, the structural proteins and enzymes of HIV are unable to function, and hence the virus remains immature and noninfectious.

Pharmacokinetics. Fortovase is administered orally. Bioavailability is about 3 times greater than with the Invirase formulation. Food increases levels sixfold. Saquinavir undergoes metabolism by P450 enzymes, followed by excretion in the feces. The drug's plasma half-life is 1 to 2 hours.

Therapeutic Use. Saquinavir is approved only for HIV infection. To reduce emergence of resistance, it should always be combined with at least one inhibitor of reverse transcriptase.

Adverse Effects. Saquinavir is generally well tolerated. The most common side effects are GI reactions: nausea, diarrhea, dyspepsia, and abdominal pain. As discussed above, saquinavir and all other protease inhibitors may pose a risk of hyperglycemia, new-onset diabetes, exacerbation of existing diabetes, fat redistribution, hyperlipidemia, bone loss, elevation of transaminase levels, and increased bleeding in patients with hemophilia.

Drug and Food Interactions. As discussed above, agents that *inhibit* P450 (e.g., ketoconazole, clarithromycin, grapefruit juice) can raise levels of saquinavir and all other protease inhibitors. Conversely, agents that *induce* P450

TABLE 90–6 ▪▪ Drug Interactions of Protease Inhibitors (PIs)

	Indinavir [Crixivan]	Ritonavir [Norvir]	Saquinavir [Invirase, Fortovase]
Interactions Shared by All PIs	• All PIs inhibit P450 (ritonavir inhibits the most) and hence can cause other drugs to accumulate to dangerous levels. Accordingly, *patients must not take the following drugs:* astemizole,* terfenadine,* cisapride,* triazolam, midazolam, ergotamine, dihydroergotamine, lovastatin, and simvastatin. • By inhibiting P450, PIs can increase levels of sildenafil [Viagra]; sildenafil dosage should not exceed 25 mg/48 hr. • St. John's wort induces P450 and thereby decreases levels of protease inhibitors. Combined use of *St. John's wort and protease inhibitors must be avoided.* • Certain antiseizure drugs—phenobarbital, phenytoin, and carbamazepine—induce P450, and may thereby decrease levels of PIs substantially.		
Interactions of Individual PIs	• Rifampin reduces indinavir levels by 89%; avoid the combination • Indinavir increases rifabutin levels 2-fold; reduce rifabutin dosage • Ketoconazole increases indinavir levels by 68%; reduce indinavir dosage • Buffered formulations of didanosine reduce indinavir absorption; take at least 1 hr apart	• Because of P450 inhibition, *patients must avoid the following drugs* (in addition to those listed above for all PIs): amiodarone bepridil, bupropion, clorazepate, clozapine, diazepam, encainide, estazolam, flecainide, flurazepam, meperidine, piroxicam, propoxyphene, propafenone, quinidine, and zolpidem • Ritonavir decreases levels of ethinyl estradiol found in oral contraceptives; use a different method of birth control • Ritonavir increases levels of rifabutin (4-fold), ketoconazole (3-fold), clarithromycin (77%), and desipramine (145%); reduce dosages of these drugs • Buffered formulations of didanosine reduce ritonavir absorption; take at least 2 hr apart	• Rifampin and rifabutin reduce levels of saquinavir; don't use these drugs • Saquinavir levels increased by ritonavir, ketoconazole, clarithromycin, and grapefruit juice

*No longer available in the United States.

(e.g., rifampin, rifabutin, phenobarbital, St. John's wort) can reduce levels of saquinavir and all other protease inhibitors.

Because saquinavir and other protease inhibitors cause inhibition of P450, these agents can raise levels of other drugs. To avoid toxicity from excessive levels, certain drugs—astemizole, terfenadine, and cisapride (all no longer available in the United States), as well as triazolam, midazolam, bepridil, ergot alkaloids, simvastatin, and lovastatin—must not be combined with saquinavir or any other protease inhibitor.

Preparations, Storage, Dosage, and Administration. Saquinavir (as Fortovase) is available in 200-mg soft gelatin capsules. Fortovase can be stored at room temperature for 3 months. For more prolonged storage, refrigeration is required. The recommended dosage is 1200 mg (6 capsules) every 8 hours. To improve absorption, the drug should taken with food.

Hard-Gel Formulation

Saquinavir in hard gelatin capsules [Invirase] received FDA approval in December 1995. The pharmacologic properties of Invirase are identical to those of Fortovase (saquinavir in soft gelatin capsules), with one important difference: The bioavailability of saquinavir in Invirase is only 4%—much lower than the bioavailability of saquinavir in Fortovase. Low bioavailability appears to result from poor absorption and extensive first-pass metabolism. Invirase is recommended for use *only in combination with ritonavir,* a protease inhibitor that causes profound inhibition of P450, and thereby greatly increases Invirase levels. The recommended dosage of Invirase (in combination with ritonavir) is 400 mg twice a day. Although Invirase is being phased out, it will remain available to patients who began using it prior to the release of Fortovase.

Other Protease Inhibitors
Indinavir

Actions and Use. Indinavir [Crixivan] inhibits HIV protease and thereby prevents the cleavage of large HIV polyproteins into their smaller, functional forms. As a result, HIV particles remain immature and noninfec-

tious. Indinavir is approved only for treatment of HIV infection. To reduce the risk of resistance, indinavir should be combined with at least one inhibitor of reverse transcriptase.

Pharmacokinetics. When administered on an empty stomach, indinavir has moderate (30%) bioavailability. Administration with a meal high in fat, protein, or calories can decrease absorption by 70%. Indinavir undergoes metabolism by hepatic P450 followed by excretion in the feces (83%) and urine (19%). The drug's plasma half-life is 1.5 to 2 hours. In patients with liver dysfunction, indinavir levels may increase and the half-life may be prolonged.

Adverse Effects. Indinavir is generally well tolerated. The major adverse effect of note is *nephrolithiasis* (kidney stones), manifested by flank pain with or without hematuria. As a rule, indinavir-induced nephrolithiasis does not compromise kidney function, and resolves following hydration and interruption of indinavir for 1 to 3 days. To decrease the risk of nephrolithiasis, patients should consume at least 48 ounces (1.5 L) of water daily. Like other protease inhibitors, indinavir may pose a risk of hyperglycemia, new-onset diabetes, exacerbation of existing diabetes, fat redistribution, hyperlipidemia, bone loss, elevation of transaminase levels, and increased bleeding in patients with hemophilia. Other side effects include GI intolerance, headache, asthenia (weakness), blurred vision, dizziness, rash, metallic taste, and thrombocytopenia.

Drug Interactions. Indinavir *inhibits cytochrome P450,* and can thereby decrease the metabolism of other drugs. As a result, drugs may accumulate to dangerous or even life-threatening levels. Agents that can produce serious toxicity because of this interaction include *astemizole, terfenadine,* and *cisapride* (no longer available in the United States), as well as *triazolam, midazolam, ergot alkaloids, simvastatin,* and *lovastatin.* Accordingly, patients taking indinavir must not be given these drugs.

Buffered formulations of didanosine can decrease absorption of indinavir. The mechanism is reduction of acidity. Let me explain. Didanosine and indinavir differ in their acidity requirements: whereas indinavir needs acidity for absorption, acidity decreases absorption of didanosine. Because acidity decreases absorption of didanosine, some formulations contain a buffering agent to neutralize gastric acid (other formulations are enteric coated). Hence, if buffered didanosine and indinavir are administered together, the buffering agent in didanosine will reduce absorption of indinavir. To prevent this interaction, indinavir and buffered didanosine should be administered at least 1 hour apart.

Nelfinavir [Viracept]	Amprenavir [Agenerase]	Lopinavir + Ritonavir [Kaletra]
• Rifampin reduces nelfinavir levels by 82%; avoid the combination • Rifabutin reduces nelfinavir levels by 32%; increase nelfinavir dosage • Nelfinavir decreases levels of ethinyl estradiol and norethindrone found in oral contraceptives; use a different method of birth control • Nelfinavir increases levels of ketoconazole	• Rifampin reduces amprenavir levels by 90%; avoid the combination • Amprenavir increases rifabutin levels 193%; reduce rifabutin dosage • Amprenavir may reduce efficacy of oral contraceptives; use a different method of birth control • Disulfiram and metronidazole increase the risk of toxicity from propylene glycol in amprenavir oral solution; avoid these drugs • Don't take within 1 hr of antacids or buffered didanosine	• Because of P450 inhibition, *patients must avoid the following drugs* (in addition to those listed above for all PIs): flecainide, propafenone, ergonovine, methylergonavine, and pimozide • Rifampin, efavirenz, and nevirapine greatly reduce levels of lopinavir, and hence should be avoided • Because of P450 inhibition, dosages of the following drugs must be *greatly reduced:* clarithromycin, ketoconazole, itraconazole, and rifabutin • Lopinavir/ritonavir decreases levels of ethinyl estradiol found in oral contraceptives: use a different form of birth control • Lopinavir/ritonavir decreases methadone availability by 53%; monitor methadone efficacy and increase dose as needed. • Owing to its alcohol content, the PO solution of lopinavir/ritonavir should not be combined with disulfiram or metronidazole

Rifampin, rifabutin, and *St. John's wort* can induce cytochrome P450. As a result, these agents can accelerate metabolism of indinavir, thereby decreasing its levels. In contrast, levels of indinavir can be increased by *ketoconazole,* a drug that inhibits P450.

Preparations, Dosage, Administration, and Storage. Indinavir [Crixivan] is available in capsules (100, 200, 333, and 400 mg) for oral administration. The recommended dosage is 800 mg every 8 hours. To maximize absorption, administer the drug either (1) with water but on an empty stomach (i.e., 1 hour before a meal or 2 hours after) or (2) with skim milk, coffee, tea, or a low-fat meal (e.g., corn flakes with skim milk and sugar). Do not administer with a large meal. If the regimen includes buffered didanosine, indinavir and didanosine should be administered at least 1 hour apart.

Indinavir should be stored at room temperature and protected from moisture, which can degrade the drug. To protect indinavir from moisture, store tightly sealed in the vesicant-containing package supplied by the manufacturer.

Ritonavir

Actions and Uses. Ritonavir [Norvir] inhibits HIV protease, and thereby prevents maturation of HIV. The drug is active against both HIV-1 and HIV-2. Ritonavir is approved for treatment of HIV infection in adults and children. To reduce emergence of resistance, ritonavir should always be combined with at least one reverse transcriptase inhibitor. Because of its ability to inhibit P450, ritonavir is often combined with other protease inhibitors to delay their degradation.

Pharmacokinetics. Ritonavir is well absorbed following administration in capsules or oral solution. Food increases absorption of ritonavir in capsules by 15%. Dilution of the oral solution in chocolate milk, Ensure, or Advera has no impact on absorption, but does improve its taste (which is otherwise unpleasant). Ritonavir undergoes metabolism by the hepatic P450 system, followed by excretion in the feces (84%) and urine (11%). The drug's plasma half-life is 3 to 5 hours.

Adverse Effects. Adverse effects are common during the initial weeks of therapy and then tend to fade. The effects seen most often are nausea (25%), diarrhea (16%), vomiting (14%), muscle weakness (12%), altered taste (8%), and paresthesias (tingling or numbness) around the mouth and in the extremities. These effects can be reduced by initiating therapy at a low dosage and then gradually titrating up to the maintenance dosage. Like other protease inhibitors, ritonavir may pose a risk of hyperglycemia, new-onset diabetes, exacerbation of existing diabetes, fat redistribution, hyperlipidemia, bone loss, elevation of transaminase levels, and increased bleeding in patients with hemophilia.

Drug Interactions. Ritonavir is a *powerful inhibitor of P450 drug-metabolizing enzymes,* and can thereby decrease the metabolism of other drugs, causing their levels to rise. Because drug accumulation can result in serious adverse effects, ritonavir is contraindicated for use with a large number of agents, including terfenadine and astemizole (no longer available in the United States), which can cause fatal dysrhythmias when present at excessive levels. A complete list of contraindicated drugs is given in Table 90–6.

Although ritonavir inhibits P450, it appears to *induce* other drug-metabolizing enzymes, and can thereby *decrease* levels of certain drugs. Among these are *ethinyl estradiol* (a component of many oral contraceptives), *zidovudine, clarithromycin, sulfamethoxazole,* and *theophylline.* Care must be taken to ensure that concentrations of these drugs do not fall to subtherapeutic levels.

Ritonavir is used concurrently with the soft-gel formulation of *saquinavir* [Invirase] to increase saquinavir levels, and is coformulated with *lopinavir* to increase lopinavir levels. In both cases, benefits derive from inhibiting P450.

St. John's wort induces cytochrome P450, and can thereby decrease levels of ritonavir. Accordingly, the combination should be avoided.

Preparations, Dosage, Administration, and Storage. Preparations. Ritonavir [Norvir] is available in 100-mg capsules and an oral solution (600 mg/7.5 ml). In addition, the drug is available in a fixed-dose combination with lopinavir under the trade name Kaletra (see below).

Dosage and Administration. The maintenance dosage for adults is 600 mg every 12 hours. The maintenance dosage for children is 400 mg/m^2 every 12 hours. Adverse effects can be minimized by starting therapy with a low dosage and then titrating up to the maintenance dosage. If possible, ritonavir should be administered with food. Palatability of the oral solution can be improved by mixing it with chocolate milk, Ensure, or Advera within 1 hour of administration. Ritonavir should be stored refrigerated (2°C to 8°C; 36°F to 46°F) and protected from light.

Nelfinavir

Actions and Uses. Nelfinavir [Viracept] inhibits HIV protease, and thereby prevents maturation of HIV. The drug is approved for treatment of HIV infection in adults and in children as young as 2 years old. To reduce emergence of resistance, nelfinavir should always be combined with at least one reverse transcriptase inhibitor.

Pharmacokinetics. Nelfinavir is administered orally, and food increases absorption greatly (two- to threefold). In blood, more than 98% of the drug is protein bound. Nelfinavir undergoes extensive hepatic metabolism followed by excretion in the feces. Only 1% of the drug is excreted in the urine. The plasma half-life of nelfinavir is 3.5 to 5 hours.

Adverse Effects. *Diarrhea* can be dose limiting. During clinical trials, 20% to 32% of patients developed moderate to severe diarrhea. In most cases, diarrhea can be managed with an over-the-counter antidiarrheal drug (e.g., loperamide).

Like other protease inhibitors, nelfinavir may pose a risk of hyperglycemia, new-onset diabetes, exacerbation of existing diabetes, fat redistribution, hyperlipidemia, bone loss, elevation of transaminase levels, and increased bleeding in patients with hemophilia.

Drug Interactions. Like all other protease inhibitors, nelfinavir *inhibits P450,* and can thereby decrease the metabolism of other drugs, causing their levels to rise. Accumulation of several drugs, including *astemizole and cisapride* (no longer available in the United States), *midazolam,* and *ergot alkaloids,* can result in serious adverse effects. Accordingly, these agents are contraindicated for patients taking nelfinavir.

Like ritonavir, nelfinavir can *decrease* levels of *ethinyl estradiol* and *norethindrone,* a combination found in many oral contraceptives. Women taking oral contraceptives should be advised to use an alternative or additional form of contraception.

Rifampin, rifabutin, and *St. John's wort* induce hepatic drug-metabolizing enzymes, and can thereby decrease levels of nelfinavir. Accordingly, patients receiving nelfinavir should avoid these agents.

Preparations, Dosage, and Administration. Nelfinavir [Viracept] is available in tablets (250 and 625 mg) and a powder (50 mg/g) for oral administration. The powder should be mixed with a small amount of water, milk, formula, soy formula, soy milk, or dietary supplement; it should *not* be mixed with acidic foods or juices (e.g., applesauce, apple juice, orange juice) because the resulting combination may have a bitter taste. The recommended adult dosage is 750 mg every 8 hours or 1250 mg every 12 hours. The pediatric dosage is 20 to 30 mg/kg every 8 hours. Nelfinavir should be administered with food to enhance absorption.

Amprenavir

Actions and Use. Amprenavir [Agenerase] inhibits HIV protease, and thereby prevents maturation of HIV. The drug is approved for use in combination with other antiretroviral agents for treating HIV-infected adults and children over 4 years old.

Pharmacokinetics. Amprenavir is rapidly absorbed following oral administration. High-fat meals reduce absorption and should be avoided. Otherwise, food has no effect on drug levels. Amprenavir has a relatively long half-life (7.1 to 10 hours), which permits dosing just 2 times a day. The drug undergoes metabolism by hepatic P450 followed by excretion in the urine (14%) and feces (75%).

Amprenavir is available in two formulations: capsules and oral solution. Bioavailability with the oral solution is lower than with the capsules. Accordingly, dosage must be increased when using the solution.

Adverse Effects. The most common adverse effects are nausea (73%), vomiting (29%), perioral paresthesias (26%), rash (25%), mood disorders (15%), and altered taste (10%). Rash is generally mild or moderate, and does not preclude continuing therapy. Rarely, severe rash develops, including potentially fatal Stevens-Johnson syndrome. Like other protease inhibitors, amprenavir may pose a risk of hyperglycemia, new-onset diabetes, exacerbation of existing diabetes, fat redistribution, hyperlipidemia, bone loss, elevation of transaminase levels, and increased bleeding in patients with hemophilia.

Amprenavir *oral solution* contains a large amount of *propylene glycol,* which can be toxic. Under normal conditions, propylene glycol is converted to a harmless metabolite by alcohol dehydrogenase. However, in patients who cannot metabolize the compound fast enough, propylene glycol can accumulate to toxic levels, causing stupor, seizures, tachycardia, hyperosmolality, lactic acidosis, renal toxicity, and hemolysis. Because of the risk of propylene glycol accumulation, *amprenavir oral solution is contraindicated for pregnant women, children under 4 years old, patients with renal or hepatic failure, and patients taking disulfiram or metronidazole.* Alcohol consumption may also pose a risk.

Amprenavir is a chemical relative of the sulfonamide antibiotics. At this time, we do not know if people with sulfonamide hypersensitivity will also experience hypersensitivity to amprenavir. Until more is known, amprenavir should be avoided in patients with a history of sulfonamide reactions.

Drug Interactions. Like all other protease inhibitors, amprenavir *inhibits P450,* and can thereby cause other drugs to accumulate to dangerous levels. Accordingly, patients must not be given the following agents: astemizole, terfenadine, and cisapride (no longer available in the United States) or triazolam, midazolam, bepridil, ergot alkaloids, simvastatin, and lovastatin.

Rifampin reduces amprenavir levels by 90%. The combination should be avoided.

St. John's wort induces P450, and can thereby reduce amprenavir levels. The combination should be avoided.

Like ritonavir and nelfinavir, amprenavir may reduce the efficacy of *oral contraceptives.* An alternative form of contraception should be used.

To enhance stability, amprenavir formulations contain a large amount of *vitamin E*—much more than the recommended daily allowance. Accordingly, patients should be warned against taking vitamin E supplements.

Patients taking amprenavir oral solution must not take metronidazole or disulfiram, and probably should avoid alcohol.

Preparations, Dosage, and Administration. Amprenavir [Agenerase] is available in capsules (50 and 150 mg) and an oral solution (15 mg/ml). Dosages for the capsules and oral solution are not interchangeable. At least 1 hour should separate administration of amprenavir and administration of antacids or buffered formulations of didanosine.

Because propylene glycol in the oral solution can be harmful, this formulation should be reserved for patients who cannot swallow amprenavir capsules, and cannot use a different protease inhibitor. The oral solution is contraindicated for pregnant women, children under 4 years old, patients with renal or hepatic failure, and patients taking disulfiram or metronidazole.

Adult Dosage. The adult dosage is 1200 mg (eight 150-mg capsules) twice daily. The oral solution is not generally recommended.

Pediatric Dosage: Capsules. For children 13 to 16 years old who weigh more than 50 kg, the dosage is 1200 mg twice daily. For children 13 to 16 years old who weigh less than 50 kg, and for children 4 to 12 years old, the dosage is 20 mg/kg twice daily or 15 mg/kg 3 times a day—up to a maximum of 2400 mg/day.

Pediatric Dosage: Oral Solution. For children 13 to 16 years old who weigh less than 50 kg, and for children 4 to 12 years old, the dosage is 22.5 mg/kg twice daily or 17 mg/kg 3 times a day—up to a maximum of 2800 mg/day.

Lopinavir plus Ritonavir

Description and Use. Lopinavir and ritonavir are available in a fixed-dose combination under the trade name Kaletra. The combination is approved for HIV infection in adults and in children over 6 months old. Lopinavir is a new protease inhibitor available only in this combination. Ritonavir is an older protease inhibitor that is often combined with other protease inhibitors (e.g., saquinavir, indinavir) to boost their effects; the mechanism is inhibition of P450. The ritonavir in Kaletra raises lopinavir levels substantially, and thereby greatly enhances antiviral actions. The amount of ritonavir, although large enough to inhibit P450, is too small to exert significant antiretroviral effects. Hence, therapeutic responses to the combination are due solely to lopinavir. In clinical trials, lopinavir/ritonavir was as effective as older antiretroviral drugs, and even worked against some HIV strains that had become resistant to other protease inhibitors.

Pharmacokinetics. Pharmacokinetics of ritonavir are discussed above, and hence discussion here is limited to lopinavir. Lopinavir is administered orally and absorption is enhanced by food. In blood, the drug is highly (99%) bound to plasma proteins. Lopinavir undergoes extensive metabolism by the CYP3A4 isozyme, followed by excretion in the urine (10%) and feces (83%). The drug's half-life is 5 to 6 hours.

Two observations tell us that antiretroviral effects of lopinavir/ritonavir are due entirely to lopinavir. First, when patients take lopinavir/ritonavir, steady-state levels of lopinavir are 15- to 20-fold *higher* than those of ritonavir. Second, in the test tube, the concentration of lopinavir required to suppress HIV replication is 10-fold *lower* than that of ritonavir. Therefore, since lopinavir achieves much higher concentrations than ritonavir, and yet works at much lower concentrations than ritonavir, it is clear that virtually all of the antiviral effects of the combination are due to lopinavir.

Adverse Effects. Lopinavir/ritonavir is generally well tolerated. The most common adverse effects are diarrhea (13.8%), nausea (6.4%), headache (2.5%), and weakness or tiredness (3.4%). Like other protease inhibitors, lopinavir/ritonavir poses a risk of hyperglycemia, new-onset diabetes, exacerbation of existing diabetes, fat maldistribution, hyperlipidemia, bone loss, elevation of transaminases, and increased bleeding in patients with hemophilia. Rash may occur in children.

Drug Interactions. Lopinavir/ritonavir *inhibits* two drug-metabolizing enzymes—CYP3A4 and CYP2D6—and can thereby cause drugs that are substrates for these enzymes to accumulate. Serious toxicity can result. To avoid toxicity, certain drugs must be used in greatly reduced dosage, and others must not be used at all. Drugs that require a large reduction in dosage include clarithromycin, ketoconazole, itraconazole, rifabutin, and sildenafil [Viagra]. Drugs that must be avoided entirely include astemizole, terfenadine, and cisapride (no longer available in the United States), as well as flecainide, propafenone, dihydroergotamine, ergonovine, ergotamine, methylergonovine, pimozide, midazolam, triazolam, lovastatin, and simvastatin.

Paradoxically, lopinavir/ritonavir can *induce* metabolism of some drugs, including methadone and ethinyl estradiol, a component of many oral contraceptives. Methadone efficacy should be monitored and dosage increased as needed. Women using ethinyl estradiol–based oral contraceptives should switch to an alternative form of birth control.

Agents that induce CYP3A4 can accelerate metabolism of lopinavir/ritonavir, and can thereby decrease antiretroviral effects. Known inducers include rifampin, efavirenz, nevirapine, phenobarbital, phenytoin, carbamazepine, and St. John's wort. Concurrent use of these agents should be avoided.

Because of its alcohol content (see below), the oral solution of lopinavir/ritonavir should not be combined with disulfiram [Antabuse] or metronidazole. Why? Because, both drugs will cause accumulation of acetaldehyde, a toxic metabolite of alcohol.

Preparations, Dosage, and Administration. Lopinavir/ritonavir [Kaletra] is available in soft gelatin capsules (133.3 mg lopinavir/33.3 mg ritonavir) and an oral solution (80 mg lopinavir/20 mg ritonavir per milliliter) prepared in 42% alcohol. The *adult dosage* is 400 mg/100 mg (3 capsules or 5 ml of oral solution) twice daily with meals. *Pediatric dosages* are based on body weight: For children weighing 7 to 14.9 kg, the dosage is 12/3 mg/kg bid; for children weighing 15 to 40 kg, the dosage is 10/2.5 mg/kg bid; and for children weighing more than 40 kg, the dosage is the same as for adults.

ENFUVIRTIDE, AN HIV FUSION INHIBITOR

Enfuvirtide [Fuzeon], widely known as T-20, is the first representative of a new class of antiretroviral drugs: the HIV fusion inhibitors. Unlike all other drugs for HIV, which inhibit essential viral enzymes—either reverse transcriptase or protease—the new drug blocks entry of HIV into CD4 T cells. Unfortunately, although enfuvirtide is effective, it is also inconvenient (treatment requires twice daily SC injections) and very expensive (treatment costs about $20,000 a year). Furthermore, injection-site reactions occur in nearly all patients. Significant interactions with other drugs have not been observed. Enfuvirtide received FDA approval on March 13, 2003.

Chemistry

Enfuvirtide is a synthetic peptide that contains 36 amino acids. Its molecular weight is 4492. Synthesis of enfuvirtide is complex: 106 steps are involved, compared with 8 to 12 steps for traditional antiretroviral drugs. As a result, the new drug is expensive to make, which largely explains its high cost.

Mechanism of Action

Enfuvirtide prevents the HIV envelope from fusing with the cell membrane of CD4 cells (step 2 in Fig. 90–2), and thereby blocks viral entry and replication. Fusion inhibition results from binding of enfuvirtide to gp41, a subunit of the glycoproteins embedded in the HIV envelope (see Fig. 90–1). As a result of enfuvirtide binding, the glycoprotein becomes rigid, and hence cannot undergo the configurational change needed to permit fusion of HIV with the cell membrane.

Resistance

Resistance to enfuvirtide has developed in cultured cells and in patients. The cause is a structural change in gp41. In clinical trials, reductions in drug susceptibility have ranged from 4- to 422-fold. Fortunately, the HIV mutations that confer resistance to enfuvirtide do not confer cross-resistance to NRTIs, NNRTIs, or protease inhibitors. Conversely, resistance to NRTIs, NNRTIs, or protease inhibitors does not confer cross-resistance to enfuvirtide.

The rate at which resistance develops depends on the efficacy of the drugs used concurrently. When the patient's other antiretroviral drugs are still effective, resistance to enfuvirtide develops relatively slowly. However, if there is significant resistance to the other drugs, then resistance to enfuvirtide will develop rapidly.

Pharmacokinetics

Enfuvirtide is administered SC, and plasma levels peak in 3 to 12 hours. Bioavailability is about 84%, regardless of the site of injection (upper arm, thigh, abdomen). In the blood, enfuvirtide is 92% protein bound, mainly to albumin. Because enfuvirtide is a peptide, it is presumed to undergo breakdown to its constituent amino acids—although studies to identify specific metabolic pathways have not been conducted. The drug's elimination half-life is 3.8 hours.

Therapeutic Use

Enfuvirtide is reserved for treating HIV-1 infection that has become resistant to other antiretroviral agents. Specifically, the drug is indicated for HIV-1 infection in adults and in children 6 years of age and older who are treatment-experienced and who have evidence of HIV replication despite ongoing antiretroviral therapy. To delay emergence of resistance, enfuvirtide should always be combined with other antiretroviral drugs.

In clinical trials, enfuvirtide was given to patients with measurable plasma HIV RNA despite use of an optimized antiretroviral regimen (OAR). The result? Compared with patients receiving the OAR alone, those receiving the OAR plus enfuvirtide showed a significant reduction in plasma HIV RNA and an increase in circulating CD4 T cells. Benefits were sustained for at least 24 weeks. At this time, we do not know if enfuvirtide prolongs survival or reduces the occurrence of opportunistic infections.

Adverse Effects

Injection-Site Reactions. In clinical trials, injection-site reactions (ISRs) developed in 98% of patients, usually within the first week of treatment. Principal manifestations are pain and tenderness (95%), erythema and induration (89%), nodules or cysts (76%), pruritus (62%), and ecchymosis (small hemorrhagic spots; 48%). Although generally mild to moderate, symptoms can also be severe. In 17% of patients, individual ISRs persisted more than 7 days. Because ISRs are both common and long lasting, 23% of patients had six or more ongoing ISRs at any given time. The intensity of ISRs can be reduced by rotating the injection site, avoiding sites with an active ISR, and avoiding unnecessarily deep injections. If a severe ISR occurs, or if local infection develops, patients should seek immediate medical attention.

Pneumonia. Enfuvirtide appears to increase the risk of bacterial pneumonia. Patients should be informed about signs of pneumonia (cough, fever, breathing difficulties), and instructed to report them immediately. Enfuvirtide should be used with caution in patients who have pneumonia risk factors: low initial CD4 cell counts, high initial viral load, IV drug use, smoking, and a history of lung disease.

Hypersensitivity Reactions. Because enfuvirtide is a foreign peptide, it can trigger hypersensitivity reactions. Typical symptoms, which may occur individually and in combination, are rash, fever, nausea, vomiting, chills, rigors, hypotension, and elevated serum transaminases. Enfuvirtide has also been associated with respiratory distress, glomerulonephritis, Guillain-Barré syndrome, and primary immune complex reaction, all of which may be immune mediated. If a systemic hypersensitivity reaction occurs, enfuvirtide should be discontinued immediately and never used again.

Effects During Pregnancy and Lactation. In animal studies, enfuvirtide failed to cause fetal harm. Studies in pregnant humans have not been conducted. Until more is known, the drug should be used during pregnancy only if clearly indicated. Enfuvirtide is classified in FDA Pregnancy Risk Category B.

Women with HIV infection should not breast-feed their infants, owing to the risk of HIV transmission. Whether enfuvirtide enters breast milk is unknown.

Drug Interactions

Enfuvirtide appears devoid of significant drug interactions. There are no interactions with other antiretroviral drugs that would require a dosage adjustment for either enfuvirtide or the other agent.

Availability

Because enfuvirtide is hard to make, the supply is limited. Production should be sufficient for 12,000 to 15,000 patients by December 2003, and up to 39,000 patients by 2005. Unfortunately, this is well below the need in the United States, let alone the need worldwide. Until the supply is much larger, enfuvirtide will be dispensed on a first-come, first-served basis. However, once a patient has started treatment, there is a program to ensure that his or her supply will be uninterrupted. To obtain the drug, patients must enroll in the Fuzeon Progressive Distribution Program established by the manufacturer. Details are available online at *www.fuzeon.com* and by phone at 1-866-694-6670.

Preparations, Dosage, Administration, and Storage

Preparation and Storage. Enfuvirtide [Fuzeon] is dispensed in single-use vials that contain 108 mg of powdered drug, which must be reconstituted to a 90-mg/ml solution by adding 1.1 ml of sterile water for injection. The solution can be used immediately or stored cold (2°C to 8°C; 36°F to 46°F) for up to 24 hours. Before injection, stored solutions should be brought to room temperature and inspected to ensure they are still clear, colorless, and free of bubbles and particulate matter. Undissolved enfuvirtide can be stored at room temperature.

Dosage and Administration. The dosage for *adults* is 90 mg (1 ml) injected SC twice a day. The dosage for *children ages 6 through 12 years* is 2 mg/kg (but not more than 90 mg total) injected SC twice a day. Injections are made into the upper arm, anterior thigh, or abdomen (but not the navel), using aseptic technique to avoid infection. The site should be moved for each injection. Injections should not be made into tissue that is scarred or bruised, or into sites where there is an ongoing reaction to a previous dose.

MANAGEMENT OF HIV INFECTION

Management of HIV infection has changed dramatically in recent years. Most patients now take multiple antiretroviral drugs—typically a protease inhibitor plus two NRTIs.

These highly effective regimens can reduce plasma HIV to undetectable levels. As a result, CD4 T-cell counts return toward normal, thereby restoring some immune function, which in turn may permit the patient to discontinue drugs for some opportunistic infections. However, despite these advances, treatment cannot cure HIV. In all cases, discontinuation of antiretroviral drugs has led to a rebound in plasma HIV.

Therapy of HIV disease is complex. Patients take three or four different drugs for HIV itself, and may take additional drugs for opportunistic infections. As a result, the potential for adverse effects and drug interactions is large. Also, among the drugs used for HIV, resistance is a common complication. Furthermore, the pill burden and adverse effects make adherence difficult. Because of these complexities, management is best done by a clinician with extensive experience in treating HIV disease.

Guidelines for treatment of HIV infection are published by two groups: (1) the International AIDS Society (IAS) and (2) the Department of Health and Human Services (DHHS) in conjunction with the Henry J. Kaiser Foundation. Both sets of guidelines are updated periodically, and both contain similar recommendations. Updated IAS guidelines were published in the July 10, 2002, issue of *JAMA*. Updated DHHS guidelines were released on February 4, 2002. The discussion that follows is based largely on DHHS guidelines for treating older patients, titled *Guidelines for the Use of Antiretroviral Agents in HIV-Infected Adults and Adolescents.* This document is available online at *aidsinfo.nih.gov,* along with companion guidelines for treating pediatric and pregnant patients.

Diagnosis

We can diagnose HIV infection with several tests. Some tests detect antibodies to HIV, some detect HIV RNA, and some detect HIV proteins. Tests that detect HIV antibodies and HIV RNA are used most often.

Antibodies to HIV are measured with two tests: an *enzyme-linked immunosorbent assay* (ELISA) and a *Western blot.* ELISAs measure the entire population of HIV antibodies in blood. In contrast, the Western blot measures individual antibody classes. To be considered positive, the Western blot must detect antibodies against at least two of the following three proteins: p24 (a core protein of HIV), and gp41 and gp120/161 (HIV proteins needed for attachment to CD4 T cells). At most testing centers in the United States, an ELISA is used as the primary screen for HIV infection. If the ELISA is positive, a Western blot is performed to confirm the diagnosis.

Measurement of HIV RNA detects the presence of HIV in blood. Tests for HIV RNA are discussed below under *Laboratory Monitoring.*

The test chosen to diagnose HIV infection depends on how long the infection has been present. Antibodies to HIV cannot be detected until several weeks after infection is acquired. Hence, during this time, an ELISA or Western blot cannot be used for diagnosis. Instead, diagnosis can be accomplished by measuring plasma HIV RNA. If the test for HIV RNA is positive, it should be confirmed with an ELISA and Western blot 2 to 4 months later.

Laboratory Monitoring

The principal laboratory tests employed to monitor HIV infection and guide therapy are *plasma HIV RNA* (viral load) *assays* and *CD4 T-cell counts*. In some cases, *drug resistance assays* are also performed. Measurement of viral load indicates the magnitude of HIV replication and predicts the rate of CD4 T-cell destruction. In contrast, CD4 T-cell counts indicate how much damage the immune system has already suffered.

Viral Load (Plasma HIV RNA)

Treatment of HIV infection is guided primarily by monitoring viral load, which is determined by measuring HIV RNA in plasma. The source of the RNA is intact HIV virions (virus particles), each of which has two copies of HIV RNA. Guidelines regarding when to measure HIV RNA are summarized in Table 90–7.

The principal tests employed to measure HIV RNA are (1) the reverse transcriptase–polymerase chain reaction (RT-PCR) assay and (2) the branched-chain DNA amplification (bDNA) assay. With both tests, results are expressed as either (1) the number of copies of HIV RNA per milliliter or (2) the log of the number of copies of HIV RNA per milliliter. It is important to note, however, that values obtained using the RT-PCR assay may be as much as twofold higher than values obtained using the bDNA assay. Accordingly, in order to interpret test results, the clinician must know which test was employed. Also, to obtain reliable test results, it is essential that blood for HIV RNA determinations be collected and preserved according to recommended procedures.

Given that the vast majority of HIV in the body is present in lymphoid tissues rather than in the blood, you might ask whether measurement of HIV RNA in *plasma* is a true reflection of the *total body* load of HIV. The answer is "Yes." Why?

Because, when HIV in lymphoid tissues replicates, many of the new virions are released into the blood. As a result, levels of HIV in blood parallel levels of HIV in lymphoid tissues. Accordingly, measurement of HIV RNA in blood gives an accurate picture of the total HIV load.

Plasma HIV RNA is the best measurement available for predicting clinical outcome. If HIV RNA is high (e.g., 100,000 copies/ml), the prognosis is poor. Conversely, if HIV RNA is low (e.g., 500 copies/ml), the risk of disease progression and death is greatly reduced. Accordingly, the goal of therapy is to decrease plasma HIV RNA as much as possible—preferably to a level that is undetectable with current assays (i.e., below 50 copies/ml of plasma). It is important to appreciate, however, that even when plasma HIV RNA is below the current limits of detection, the patient may still be able to transmit HIV to others—although the risk of transmission is greatly reduced.

When patients are treated with HAART, levels of HIV RNA should decline to 10% of baseline within 2 to 8 weeks. After 16 to 20 weeks of treatment, plasma HIV RNA should reach its minimum. With optimal therapy, the minimum should be undetectable (less than 50 copies/ml).

CD4 T-Cell Counts

Before assays for HIV RNA were available, CD4 T-cell counts were the primary laboratory test for monitoring therapy. Although CD4 T-cell counts remain important, they lack the predictive power of viral load measurements. However, CD4 T-cell counts can still tell us how much damage HIV has already caused. By knowing the extent of immunodeficiency, we can assess the risk of opportunistic infection, and hence can initiate timely prophylactic therapy.

As antiretroviral therapy takes effect, CD4 T-cell counts will begin to rise, indicating some return of immune function.

TABLE 90–7 ■ Times When Plasma HIV RNA Should Be Measured

When to Measure Plasma HIV RNA	Information Obtained	Use of the Information
When a patient presents with a syndrome consistent with acute HIV infection	Establishes presence of HIV when HIV antibody test is negative or indeterminate	Diagnosis of HIV infection
Following initial diagnosis of HIV infection	Establishes baseline viral load	Decision to start or defer therapy
Every 3–4 months in patients with diagnosed HIV infection but who are not on antiretroviral therapy	Extent to which viral load has increased	Decision to initiate therapy
2–8 weeks after starting antiretroviral therapy	Initial assessment of drug efficacy	Decision to continue or change therapy
3–4 months after starting antiretroviral therapy	Maximal effect of therapy	Decision to continue or change therapy
Every 3–4 months in patients on antiretroviral therapy	Durability of drug effects	Decision to continue or change therapy
When a clinical event or a decline in CD4 T cells occurs	Establishes whether the clinical event or decline in CD4 T cells occurred in association with an increase in viral load	Decision to initiate, continue, or change therapy

Adapted from Guidelines for the Use of Antiretroviral Agents in HIV-Infected Adults and Adolescents, prepared by the Panel on Clinical Practices for Treatment of HIV Infection convened by the DHHS and the Henry J. Kaiser Family Foundation, February 4, 2002.

With HAART, increases of 100 to 250 cells/μl have been observed. Although restoration of CD4 T-cell counts may not produce *complete* immunocompetence, it is often sufficient to permit discontinuation of prophylactic therapy against some opportunistic infections.

Measurement of CD4 T cells should be done when HIV infection is diagnosed and every 3 to 6 months thereafter. A healthy range for CD4 T cells is 800 to 1200 cells/μl. A 30% reduction is considered significant. Among people with HIV infection, a CD4 T-cell count above 500 cells/μl is considered relatively high. In contrast, a count below 50 cells/μl indicates very advanced HIV disease.

HIV Drug Resistance

Resistance is a significant concern in HIV therapy. In most cases, resistance emerges over the course of treatment as a result of noncompliance with the prescribed regimen. Rarely, resistance results from primary infection with a drug-resistant HIV variant. Resistance tests can be used to guide drug selection, especially when changing a regimen that has failed.

Two types of resistance assays are employed: *phenotypic assays* and *genotypic assays*. Phenotypic assays measure the ability of HIV to grow in the presence of increasing concentrations of antiretroviral drugs. (The ability to grow in high concentrations indicates resistance.) Genotypic assays are designed to detect resistance-conferring mutations in HIV genes that code for the targets that drugs attack (i.e., reverse transcriptase and protease). Unfortunately, assays for resistance have multiple drawbacks: they are expensive ($400 to $1000); turnaround time is slow (2 to 4 weeks); sensitivity is low; phenotypic assays can produce false-negative results; and genotypic assays are difficult to interpret. Furthermore, evidence showing that resistance testing improves clinical outcome is scant. There are no prospective data showing that one type of assay (genotypic or phenotypic) is superior to the other.

When should resistance be tested? At this time, resistance testing is recommended primarily in cases of treatment failure. Testing helps determine the role of resistance in treatment failure and helps guide the selection of replacement drugs. Resistance testing can be considered for patients with acute HIV infection who have not yet been treated. In this case, the objective is to determine if the primary infection was caused by a resistant variant.

Treatment of Adult Patients

As discussed above, HIV disease has three phases, an initial acute phase, followed by a prolonged asymptomatic phase, followed by a late symptomatic phase during which AIDS occurs. In the discussion below, we consider drug therapy for each phase separately. However, to facilitate discussion, the phases are discussed in reverse sequence. That is, we discuss symptomatic HIV disease first, then asymptomatic HIV disease, and then acute HIV disease. For patients with symptomatic or acute HIV disease, the benefits of treatment clearly outweigh the risks; hence, immediate and aggressive treatment is recommended. In contrast, for patients with asymptomatic HIV disease, the benefits of immediate treatment may not outweigh the risks; hence, in some cases, it

may be appropriate to delay treatment. During all phases of HIV disease, treatment has four basic goals:

- Maximal and durable suppression of viral load
- Restoration or preservation of immune function
- Improved quality of life
- Reduction of HIV-related morbidity and mortality.

Symptomatic HIV Disease

All patients with symptomatic (advanced) HIV disease should receive maximally effective antiretroviral therapy. The virologic goal is to produce maximal and sustained suppression of HIV replication, as evidenced by reduction of plasma HIV RNA to an undetectable level. The treatments employed are referred to as HAART (highly active antiretroviral therapy).

HAART regimens contain *three or four drugs*. Regimens that contain only two drugs are not generally recommended, and monotherapy should always be avoided, except possibly during pregnancy.

Recommended regimens are summarized in Table 90–8. As indicated, nearly all regimens contain drugs from *two different classes* (e.g., two NRTIs combined with a protease inhibitor, or two NRTIs combined with an NNRTI). By using drugs from different classes, we can attack HIV in two different ways (e.g., inhibition of reverse transcriptase and protease), and can thereby enhance antiviral effects.

In addition to enhancing antiviral effects, *use of multiple drugs reduces the risk of resistance.* Why? Because the probability that HIV will undergo a mutation that confers simultaneous resistance to three or four drugs is much smaller than the probability of undergoing a mutation that confers resistance to just one drug. For example, if our patient is taking three drugs—nelfinavir, zidovudine, and lamivudine—and a virion mutates to a form that is resistant to nelfinavir, the other two drugs—zidovudine and lamivudine—will still be effective against the resistant virion, and hence suppression of replication will be sustained. On the other hand, if our patient were only taking nelfinavir, then treatment would obviously fail. Because of concerns about resistance, when a patient who began treatment with monotherapy is switched to multidrug therapy, we should employ drugs that (1) the patient has not used before and (2) are not cross-resistant with drugs the patient has used before.

Most regimens employ drugs from only one or two of the three available classes of antiretroviral agents. Because at least one class of antiretroviral drugs is *not* used, these regimens are considered *class-sparing.* For example, a regimen that employed protease inhibitors and NRTIs would spare the use of NNRTIs. A major benefit of class-sparing regimens is that they postpone development of resistance to the unused class of drugs, and thereby ensure that the unused class will be effective for the patient in the future. The major advantages and disadvantages of class-sparing regimens are summarized in Table 90–9.

Plasma HIV RNA should be monitored to assess the impact of treatment. With HAART, plasma HIV RNA should show a 10-fold decrease by 8 weeks, and should be undetectable (i.e., less than 50 copies/μl) by 4 to 6 months.

HAART cannot cure HIV. Why? Because some HIV remains dormant in memory CD4 T cells, and hence escapes harm. In all cases, discontinuation of HAART has led to a

TABLE 90–8 ■ Regimens for Initial Therapy of Established HIV Infection

Strongly Recommended Regimens

Recommended regimens consist of 3 or 4 drugs: one entry from the left column (PIs and NNRTIs) and one entry from the right column (NRTI pairs). These regimens can produce a sustained reduction in plasma HIV RNA, a sustained increase in CD4 T-cell counts, and a favorable clinical outcome (i.e., delayed progression to AIDS and death).

Protease Inhibitors
- Indinavir
- Nelfinavir
- Ritonavir* + saquinavir (SCG or HGC)
- Ritonavir* + lopinavir
- Ritonavir* + indinavir

NNRTI
- Efavirenz

NRTI Pairs
- Stavudine + didanosine
- Stavudine + lamivudine
- Zidovudine + didanosine
- Zidovudine + lamivudine
- Didanosine + lamivudine

Recommended Alternatives

The alternative regimens consist of 3 or 4 drugs: one entry from the left column (PIs, NNRTI, and NRTIs) and one entry from the right column (NRTI pair).

Protease Inhibitors
- Amprenavir
- Ritonavir
- Saquinavir (SGC)
- Nelfinavir + saquinavir (SGC)

NNRTI
- Delavirdine

NRTIs
- Abacavir
- Nevirapine

NRTI Pair
- Zidovudine + zalcitabine

HGC = hard gel capsule formulation [Invirase], NNRTI = non-nucleoside reverse transcriptase inhibitor, NRTI = nucleoside reverse transcriptase inhibitor, PI = protease inhibitor, SGC = soft gel capsule formulation [Fortovase].
*The purpose of ritonavir in these combinations is to inhibit metabolism of the other PI by P450.

rise in HIV RNA. Accordingly, patients must understand that reducing HIV RNA to undetectable levels does not mean that HIV has been eradicated, and does not mean they have been cured. It only means that the amount of HIV in plasma is too low to measure. Patients with undetectable HIV RNA should be told that they are still infectious, and hence must avoid behaviors that can transmit HIV to others. Because patients still harbor HIV, treatment should continue indefinitely.

A combination of factors—complex regimens, adverse effects, and drug-drug and drug-food interactions—make safe and effective HAART difficult. The following examples illustrate the extent of the problem.

- *Complexity of the regimen*—A typical regimen might include nelfinavir, zidovudine, and didanosine. The dosage for nelfinavir is 750 mg (3 tablets) taken every 8 hours with food; the dosage for zidovudine is 200 mg (2 capsules) taken every 8 hours without regard to meals; and the dosage for didanosine is 200 mg (1 tablet) taken twice daily, 1 hour before meals or 2 hours after—for a total of 17 tablets or capsules a day. In addition to these antiretroviral drugs, the patient may be taking medications to treat or prevent opportunistic infections, along with medication to promote appetite.

- *Adverse effects*—In the regimen described above, the patient is at risk of multiple adverse effects. Nelfinavir can cause diarrhea, fat redistribution, hyperglycemia, hyperlipidemia, and bone resorption; zidovudine can cause neutropenia and anemia; and didanosine can cause pancreatitis and peripheral neuropathy. Drugs for opportunistic infections will increase the potential for side effects. To decrease the risk of serious injury, drugs with overlapping toxicities should be avoided.

- *Drug-drug interactions*—The potential for significant drug interactions is huge. Nelfinavir inhibits cytochrome P450, and can thereby suppress metabolism of many other drugs, causing their levels to rise. Didanosine (buffered formulations) can reduce absorption of indinavir, unless the drugs are administered 2 hours apart. Drugs that depress bone marrow function can increase the risk of anemia and neutropenia from zidovudine. One such bone-marrow depressant—ganciclovir—is encountered often because of its use against cytomegalovirus retinitis, a common opportunistic infection in people with AIDS.

- *Drug-food interactions*—Food decreases absorption of didanosine, hence the drug should be taken on an empty stomach. In contrast, food enhances absorption of nelfinavir, hence the drug should be administered with meals. Since patients with AIDS are frequently anorectic, administration with meals may be problematic.

TABLE 90–9 ■ Comparison of Class-Sparing Regimens

	PI-Based Regimens (NNRTI Sparing)	NNRTI-Based Regimens (PI Sparing)	NRTI-Based Regimens (NNRTI and PI Sparing)
Composition	1 or 2 PIs + 2 NRTIs	1 NNRTI + 2 NRTIs	3 NRTIs
Potential Advantages	Clinical, virologic, and immunologic efficacy well documented Benefits may continue despite viral breakthrough Resistance requires multiple mutations Targets two steps of HIV replication cycle (protease and reverse transcriptase)	Easier to use and adhere to than PI-based regimens Avoids PI-induced side effects Causes fewer drug interactions than PIs	Easier to use and adhere to than PI-based regimens Avoids PI-induced and NNRTI-induced side effects Resistance to 1 NRTI does not confer cross-resistance to all other NRTIs Drug interactions are more manageable than with PIs
Potential Disadvantages	Complex, and hence adherence is difficult Long-term use may cause lipodystrophy, hyperlipidemia, insulin resistance, and osteoporosis PIs inhibit cytochrome P450, and hence may cause other drugs to accumulate to toxic levels	Clinical efficacy relative to PI-based regimens is unknown A single mutation can cause resistance	Clinical efficacy relative to PI-based regimens is unknown Long-term virologic efficacy may be suboptimal in patients with a high baseline viral load
Impact on Future Options	Preserves NNRTIs for later use Resistance to 1 PI can produce cross-resistance to other PIs	Preserves PIs for later use Resistance to 1 NNRTI usually causes cross-resistance to all other NNRTIs	Preserves PIs and NNRTIs for later use Resistance to 1 NRTI causes only limited cross-resistance to other NRTIs

NNRTI = non-nucleoside reverse transcriptase inhibitor, NRTI = nucleoside reverse transcriptase inhibitor, PI = protease inhibitor.

Because of these multiple difficulties, extensive patient education is essential. Accordingly, patients should be counseled about the importance of strict adherence to the regimen, timing of dosing with regard to meals, and potential adverse effects and interactions. Measures to promote adherence are discussed below.

Chronic Asymptomatic HIV Disease

Making the decision to treat during the chronic asymptomatic phase of HIV disease is more difficult than during the symptomatic phase. Why? Because we lack strong clinical data to guide the decision. For patients in the symptomatic phase, we have solid evidence that the benefits of treatment outweigh the risks, and hence all patients should be given the option of treatment. However, for most patients in the asymptomatic phase, we simply don't know if the benefits will outweigh the risks, and hence the optimal time to initiate therapy is uncertain. Given this lack of certainty, patients and their physicians must weigh multiple factors when deciding whether to initiate HAART. Specifically, they must consider the potential benefits and risks of treatment, as well as factors unique to each patient, especially viral load and the existing degree of immunodeficiency. Table 90–10 summarizes these factors.

Early intervention offers several benefits, the most obvious being reduction of viral load. As a result, progression of immunodeficiency is slowed, progression to AIDS is delayed, life may be prolonged, and the risk of transmitting HIV is reduced. In addition, suppression of replication decreases the rate of HIV mutation, and can thereby decrease production of drug-resistant mutants. Finally, when therapy is begun while the patient is still relatively healthy, the patient will be better able to tolerate drug toxicity.

Unfortunately, early intervention does have drawbacks. Drug therapy *will* decrease quality of life by (1) exposing an otherwise symptom-free person to adverse effects and (2) creating the need to rigidly follow a complex regimen. In addition, neither the long-term efficacy nor the long-term toxicity of current drugs is fully known. Hence, the patient is facing a potential risk of losing benefits as well as experiencing adverse effects of which we are currently unaware. Finally, although it is true that decreasing viral load and replication will decrease spontaneous production of resistant mutants, if resistant mutants *are* produced, the presence of drugs will create selection pressure favoring their emergence. Hence, it is possible that drug therapy will allow resistance to develop sooner than it would have in the absence of drugs. This is especially true if the patient fails to adhere to the regimen. Furthermore, if resistance does develop, drug options for future therapy will be limited, and the risk of transmitting resistance will be increased.

In addition to balancing benefits versus risks, factors unique to the patient must be considered before initiating therapy. Obviously, the patient must want treatment. Also, the patient must be prepared to adhere to a demanding dosing schedule. Finally, the patient's HIV status must be considered. Specifically, we must consider (1) the degree of immunodeficiency, as evidenced by CD4 T-cell counts, and (2) the risk of disease progression, as evidenced by plasma HIV RNA level.

Current recommendations for treatment are summarized in Table 90–11. As indicated, *treatment should be offered to all patients with very low CD4 T-cell counts (<200 cells/μl) and to most patients with moderately low counts (200 to 350 cells/μl), regardless of HIV RNA counts. For patients with* a high viral load (>55,000 copies of HIV RNA/ml, as measured by RT-PCR assay or the current bDNA assay [version 3.0]) but with reasonable immunologic status (>350 CD4 T cells/µl) experts disagree about what to do: some would recommend immediate treatment, whereas others would defer it. For patients at even lower risk (>350 CD4 T cells/µl and <55,000 copies of HIV RNA/ml), postponing treatment is probably safe: In the absence of treatment, the 3-year risk of developing AIDS is less than 15%. In all cases, when treatment is deferred, immunologic status (CD4 T-cell counts) should be assessed frequently (every 3 to 4 months).

If the patient and physician do agree to initiate treatment, the goal is the same as with symptomatic patients: reduction of HIV RNA to levels that are undetectable with sensitive assays. As with symptomatic patients, the preferred regimens consist of three or four drugs (see Table 90–8).

Acute HIV Disease

All patients with primary acute HIV disease should receive maximally effective antiretroviral therapy. As with symptomatic HIV disease, the preferred regimens consists of three or four drugs (see Table 90–8).

Early and aggressive intervention offers multiple potential benefits. Of greatest interest is the possibility of eradicating HIV before it gets firmly established, although eradication has not yet been demonstrated. However, even if we can't clear HIV from the body, early treatment still offers the following benefits:

- By suppressing the initial burst of viral replication, treatment may decrease the extent to which HIV disseminates throughout the body.
- By reducing viral load, treatment can preserve immune system function, and may also slow the progression of HIV disease.

TABLE 90–10 ■■ Factors to Consider When Deciding to Initiate Antiretroviral Therapy During the Asymptomatic Phase of HIV Disease

Potential Benefits

- Reduction of viral load
- Control of viral replication decreases rate of mutation, and can thereby decrease production of drug-resistant mutants
- Prevention of progressive immunodeficiency; potential preservation of a normal immune system
- Delayed progression to AIDS and prolongation of life
- Treatment while the patient is still healthy allows better tolerance of drug side effects
- Possible decreased risk of transmission (owing to decreased viral load)

Potential Risks

- Reduction in quality of life owing to adverse drug effects and the constraints imposed by a complex dosing schedule
- Exposure of HIV to antiretroviral drugs can lead to earlier emergence of drug-resistant mutants
- If resistance develops, drug options for future therapy will be limited
- If resistance develops, the risk of transmitting resistant mutants will be increased
- Long-term toxicity of certain antiretroviral drugs is not yet known
- Long-term efficacy of current antiretroviral therapies is not yet known

Factors Unique to the Patient

- Willingness to start therapy
- Likelihood of adhering to the regimen
- Degree of immunodeficiency, as indicated by CD4 T-cell count
- Risk of disease progression, as indicated by plasma HIV RNA

TABLE 90–11 ■■ Treatment Recommendations for Asymptomatic Patients With Chronic HIV-1 Infection

CD4 T-Cell Count (cells/µl)	Plasma HIV RNA (copies/ml)	Treatment Recommendation
<200	Any count	Start treatment
200–350	Any count	Treatment should generally be offered, although controversy exists.
>350	>55,000 (by bDNA or RT-PCR)*	*Aggressive Approach:* Some experts would recommend starting treatment, recognizing that the 3-year risk of developing AIDS in untreated patients is >30%. *Conservative Approach:* Some experts would defer therapy and monitor CD4 T-cell counts more frequently.
>350	<55,000 (by bDNA or RT-PCR)*	Many experts would defer therapy and monitor CD4 T-cell counts more frequently, recognizing that the 3-year risk of developing AIDS in untreated patients is <15%.

*With the branched-chain DNA (bDNA) assay in current use (version 3.0), RNA counts are close to those measured with the reverse transcriptase–polymerase chain reaction (RT-PCR) assay, except when the count is relatively low (<1500 copies/ml), in which case, counts measured with the bDNA assay are significantly lower than those measured with the RT-PCR assay. With older versions of the bDNA assay, RNA counts were half those measured with the RT-PCR assay, regardless of whether the RNA concentration was low or high.

Adapted from *Guidelines for the Use of Antiretroviral Agents HIV-infected Adults and Adolescents,* prepared by the Panel on Clinical Practices for Treatment of HIV Infection convened by the DHHS and the Henry J. Kaiser Family foundation, February 4, 2002.

- By reducing viral load and the rate of replication, treatment can decrease the rate of mutation, and hence can decrease the risk that a drug-resistant virion will emerge.
- By reducing viral load, treatment can decrease the severity of acute illness, and can reduce the risk of viral transmission.

As with asymptomatic HIV disease, treatment of acute HIV infection does have potential drawbacks. Among these are

- Reduction in quality of life because of drug toxicity and the constraints imposed by a complex dosing schedule
- Possible blunting of the early immune response to HIV because of reduced viral presence
- Emergence of drug-resistant HIV if treatment fails

Nonetheless, given the potential benefits of treatment, these drawbacks do not comprise a compelling reason to postpone therapy.

Changing the Regimen

There are three basic reasons for changing antiretroviral therapy: treatment failure, treatment with a suboptimal regimen, and drug toxicity. Guidelines for altering the regimen under these three conditions are discussed below. Unfortunately, options for changing the regimen are limited: There are only four classes of antiretroviral drugs, with a total of 17 members among them.

Treatment Failure. Treatment failure is arguably the most compelling reason for changing the regimen. Failure is indicated if

- Plasma HIV RNA fails to drop by 10-fold within the first 8 weeks of treatment
- Plasma HIV RNA fails to drop to undetectable levels within the first 4 to 6 months of treatment
- Plasma HIV RNA rebounds after falling to an undetectable level
- CD4 T-cell counts continue to drop despite antiretroviral treatment
- Clinical disease progresses despite antiretroviral treatment

Of these five signs of failure, the first three are the most meaningful, in that they represent a direct measurement of antiretroviral efficacy.

When treatment failure occurs, the reason must be determined. Possibilities include patient nonadherence, poor drug absorption, accelerated drug metabolism owing to drug interactions, and viral resistance. If nonadherence is the cause, several measures may help (see below). If poor absorption is the cause, changing the timing of administration with respect to meals or increasing the dosage may help. If accelerated metabolism is the cause, increasing the dosage may help; alternatively, it may be appropriate to substitute a different drug for the one that is causing metabolism to increase.

When failure is the result of resistance, the preferred response is to change *all* drugs in the regimen. This makes sense in that failure means that HIV is replicating despite current treatment, indicating the presence of at least one HIV strain that is resistant to all drugs in the regimen. If we were to add or change just one drug, resistance would quickly develop to that agent, and failure would recur. The risk of renewed resistance is substantially lower if we change at least two drugs,

and even lower if we change three. When we change the regimen, the new drugs should be agents that (1) the patient has not taken previously and (2) are not cross-resistant with drugs the patient has taken before. Ideally, selection of replacement drugs would be guided by resistance testing.

Unfortunately, some patients are already resistant to nearly all available drugs, and hence their options are limited. In such cases, it is rational to continue with the current regimen, which may at least provide partial suppression. To date, there is limited experience with regimens that consist of either two protease inhibitors or a protease inhibitor plus an NNRTI. Nonetheless, for patients who have no other choice, these combinations are potential options. Because cross-resistance is common between ritonavir and indinavir (two protease inhibitors), these drugs should not be substituted for each other. Similarly, because cross-resistance is common among *all* NNRTIs, changing among drugs in this family should be avoided.

One drug—*enfuvirtide*—may be especially valuable for managing treatment failure. As discussed above, enfuvirtide is the first representative of a new class of antiretroviral agents, the HIV fusion inhibitors. Because enfuvirtide is different from all other antiretroviral drugs, cross-resistance between enfuvirtide and the other agents does not exist. Furthermore, because enfuvirtide is new, patients are unlikely to harbor HIV strains resistant to it.

Treatment with a Suboptimal Regimen. Suboptimal therapy is indicated by a failure to suppress plasma HIV RNA to an undetectable level. In addition to this laboratory definition of suboptimal, treatment with a single NRTI is always considered suboptimal, and treatment with two NRTIs is generally considered suboptimal. For patients taking either a single NRTI or two NRTIs, substituting two new NRTIs plus a protease inhibitor would be appropriate. Note that the new drugs *replace* the old drugs; they are not taken in addition to the old ones.

Drug Toxicity. If a patient experiences toxicity typical of a particular drug in the regimen, that drug should be withdrawn and replaced with a drug that is (1) from the same class and (2) of equal efficacy. For example, if a patient taking zidovudine were to develop anemia and neutropenia, zidovudine should be discontinued and replaced with another NRTI (e.g., stavudine). Note that, when toxicity is the reason for altering the regimen, changing just one drug is proper, whereas when resistance or suboptimal treatment is the reason, *all* of the drugs should be changed.

Promoting Patient Adherence

In order to achieve treatment goals and delay emergence of resistance, strict adherence to the prescribed regimen is critical. Unfortunately, several factors—duration of treatment, complexity of the regimen, adverse drug effects, drug-drug interactions, and drug-food interactions—make adhering to antiretroviral therapy unusually hard. The DHHS guidelines identify factors that predict *poor* adherence (e.g., poor clinician-patient relationship, active use of alcohol or street drugs, depression and other mental illnesses) as well as factors that predict *good* adherence (e.g., availability of emotional and practical support, ability to fit dosing into the daily routine, appreciation that poor adherence will cause treatment failure). Strategies for promoting adherence are summarized below.

Patient- and Medication-Related Strategies

- Thoroughly educate the patient, using multiple sessions, about the goals of therapy and the importance of adherence.
- Ensure that the patient is motivated to take medication *before* the first prescription is written.
- Negotiate a treatment plan that the patient understands and will commit to.
- Devise a regimen that minimizes both pill burden and dosing frequency, and that integrates the dosing schedule with meals and the patient's daily routine.
- Inform the patient about side effects; anticipate side effects and treat them.
- Avoid adverse drug interactions.
- Recruit family and friends to support the treatment plan.
- Provide mechanical aids to adherence, including a written schedule, pictures of prescribed drugs, daily or weekly pill boxes, alarm clock, and pager.
- Organize an adherence support group, or add adherence issues to the agenda of an existing group.
- Consider a practice "pill trial" substituting jelly beans for the real thing.

Clinician- and Health Team–Related Strategies

- Establish trust.
- Serve as educator and information resource.
- Provide ongoing support and monitoring.
- Be available between scheduled visits for questions or problems; provide access via pager when away (including on vacation and at conferences).
- Monitor adherence and, when it's low, intensify management (i.e., schedule more frequent visits, recruit family and friends, deploy other team members, provide referral to mental health or chemical dependence services).
- Utilize the health team for all patients, and especially for difficult patients and those with special needs (e.g., provide peer educators for adolescents or injection drug users).
- Consider the impact of new diagnoses (e.g., depression, liver disease, wasting, recurrent chemical dependency) on adherence, and include adherence intervention in management.
- Utilize all concerned people—pharmacists, peer educators, volunteers, case managers, drug counselors, physician's assistants, and all nurses, including nurse practitioners and research nurses—to reinforce the adherence message.
- Educate the support team about antiretroviral therapy and adherence.

Treatment of Pregnant Patients
Basic Principles

In general, *management of HIV infection in pregnant women should follow the same guidelines for managing HIV infection in nonpregnant adults.* Accordingly, HAART is recommended for all pregnant women whose clinical, immunologic, or virologic status indicates that treatment is needed—and should be strongly considered for *any* woman, regardless of clinical or immunologic status, if her plasma HIV RNA is above 1000 copies/ml.

When treating HIV infection in pregnant women, the goal is to balance the benefits of treatment (reducing viral load, thereby promoting the health of the mother and decreasing the risk of HIV transmission to the fetus) against the risks of treatment (causing teratogenic harm to the fetus). As a rule, the benefits of treatment outweigh the risks. Accordingly, the primary determinants of therapy are the clinical, virologic, and immunologic status of the mother; pregnancy is a secondary consideration. Nonetheless, pregnancy should not be ignored. Because the risk of teratogenesis is greatest during the first 10 to 12 weeks of pregnancy, it might be appropriate to interrupt therapy until the first trimester is over, especially if maternal risk is low (i.e., CD4 T-cell count exceeds 350 cells/μl and plasma HIV RNA is below 1000 copies/ml). The drawback, of course, is that viral load will increase, and may thereby intensify HIV disease in the mother and enhance transmission to the fetus. Accordingly, many experts recommend continuation of maximally effective treatment even during the first trimester. If the mother *does* decide to interrupt treatment, *all* antiretroviral drugs should be stopped. (This is necessary because continuing treatment with just one or two drugs would increase the risk of resistance, and would thereby render those drugs ineffective for current or future use by the patient.) When treatment resumes, the full regimen should be reinstituted.

Drug selection is problematic in that information on pharmacokinetics and safety during pregnancy is limited. Two drugs—*delavirdine* and *efavirenz*—pose a definite risk of fetal harm and should be avoided. All of the *protease inhibitors* increase the risk of gestational diabetes, and hence blood sugar should be monitored closely.

Reducing Perinatal HIV Transmission

Most mother-to-child transmission of HIV occurs during the perinatal period, and primarily during delivery itself. Among American children, perinatal transmission accounts for nearly all new HIV infections. In the absence of antiretroviral drugs, the rate of perinatal transmission in the United States is 25%. A high viral load increases risk. The risk of transmission can be reduced by giving antiretroviral drugs to the mother during gestation and labor, and to the infant for several weeks postpartum. Delivery by cesarean section may reduce the risk even further.

Preferred Approach: Initiating Antiretroviral Therapy Early. The best way to reduce the risk of transmission is to minimize maternal viral load with HAART. Treatment should begin early in pregnancy and the regimen should contain *zidovudine,* the preferred drug for preventing perinatal HIV transmission.

Zidovudine treatment has three parts, consisting of (1) oral zidovudine beginning after week 14 of gestation and continuing until delivery, (2) IV zidovudine during labor and delivery, and (3) oral (or IV) zidovudine given to the infant for 6 weeks postpartum. This regimen is founded on results of the Pediatric AIDS Clinical Trials Group Protocol 076. Dosing details are summarized in Table 90–12. To date, zidovudine has not been associated with birth defects, impaired cognition, developmental abnormalities, or malignancies among children exposed to the drug *in utero.* However, long-term effects are unknown.

Initiating Antiretroviral Therapy During Labor. Some HIV-positive women do not receive antiretroviral therapy during pregnancy, either by choice or from ignorance of their HIV status. In these cases, treatment begun during labor can still reduce the risk of transmission. Several effective regimens are available:

- Oral *nevirapine* for both the mother and infant
- Intravenous *zidovudine* for the mother and oral (or IV) *zidovudine* for the infant (similar to the second and third parts of the three-part zidovudine regimen described above)

TABLE 90–12 ■ Three-Part Zidovudine Regimen for Reducing Perinatal Transmission of HIV*		
Time of Administration	**Zidovudine Recipient**	**Dosage**
Antepartum	Mother	300 mg PO twice a day or 200 mg 3 times a day, initiated between weeks 14 and 34 of gestation and continued until day of delivery
Intrapartum	Mother	2 mg/kg infused IV over 1 hr, then 1 mg/kg/hr by continuous infusion until delivery
Postpartum	Infant	2 mg/kg zidovudine syrup every 6 hr for 6 weeks, beginning 6 to 12 hr postpartum (For infants who cannot tolerate oral medication, give 1.5 mg/kg IV zidovudine every 6 hr.)†

*Based on results of the Pediatric AIDS Clinical Trials Group Protocol 076.
†For infants <35 weeks gestation at birth, dosing is done every 12 hours initially, rather than every 6 hours. Later, dosing is changed to every 8 hours (after 2 weeks for infants >30 weeks gestation at birth, or after 4 weeks for infants <30 weeks gestation at birth).

- Oral *nevirapine* for both the mother and infant (as above), combined with *zidovudine* for both the mother and infant (as above)
- Oral *zidovudine* plus oral *lamivudine* for both the mother and infant

Details of these regimens are summarized in Table 90–13.

The *nevirapine-alone* regimen is of special interest. It is simple (just one oral dose for mother and infant), inexpensive (about $4), and administration can be directly observed by a clinician. Simplicity and low cost make the regimen especially attractive for use in countries where health care resources are limited.

Initiating Antiretroviral Therapy Postpartum. If an HIV-positive mother did not receive antiretroviral therapy during pregnancy or labor, treatment of the infant soon after delivery can confer some protection. Only one regimen is recommended: the 6-week postpartum component of the three-part zidovudine regimen. Treatment should be initiated as soon as possible after delivery, preferably within 6 to 12 hours. In one study, the risk of transmission was reduced from 26.6% in the absence of zidovudine to only 9.3% when zidovudine was initiated within 48 hours of delivery. Some clinicians may choose to combine zidovudine with other antiretroviral drugs, especially if zidovudine resistance is known or suspected. The guidelines recommend testing the infant early for HIV so that, if zidovudine failed to prevent infection, long-term treatment can be started when the infection is still at an early stage.

Mitochondrial Toxicity from NRTIs

NRTIs can disrupt synthesis of mitochondrial DNA, and can thereby impair mitochondrial function. The major clinical consequence is *lactic acidosis associated with hepatic steatosis.* Mitochondrial injury may also manifest as neuropathy, myopathy, cardiomyopathy, and pancreatitis. Among the NRTIs, zalcitabine is the most potent inhibitor of mitochondrial DNA synthesis, followed in turn by didanosine, stavudine, zidovudine lamivudine, abacavir, and tenofovir.

As discussed above, zidovudine (and other NRTIs) can cause a syndrome characterized by lactic acidosis and hepatic steatosis (fatty degeneration of the liver). Some pregnant women taking didanosine plus stavudine have died. Clinicians and patients should be alert for signs and symptoms of lactic acidosis/hepatic steatosis (nausea, vomiting, abdominal pain, malaise, fatigue, anorexia, and hyperventilation). If these develop, a thorough evaluation should be conducted. During the third trimester, measurement of electrolytes and hepatic enzymes should be done more frequently.

Some infants with *in utero* exposure to NRTIs have developed symptoms suggestive of mitochondrial damage. Two infants (exposed to zidovudine plus lamivudine) died of severe neurologic disease. However, an association between NRTIs and these deaths has not been firmly established. Moreover, available data suggest that, even if *in utero* exposure to NRTIs does pose a risk to the infant, the risk is extremely low—and must be compared with the known benefit of using an NRTI (usually zidovudine) during pregnancy.

Preconception Counseling and Care

In women with HIV infection, as in all other women, preconception interventions are directed at optimizing maternal and fetal health. We need to identify risk factors for adverse maternal and fetal outcomes; we need to stabilize existing medical conditions prior to conception; and we need to provide education and counseling targeted at needs of the individual. Specific recommendations for HIV-infected women include the following:

- Selection of effective contraceptive methods to reduce the risk of unintended pregnancy
- Education and counseling about potential effects of both HIV infection and antiretroviral therapy on pregnancy course and outcomes
- Education and counseling regarding perinatal HIV transmission risk and strategies to reduce that risk
- Initiation or modification of antiretroviral therapy prior to conception in order to
  - Avoid fetotoxic agents (e.g., efavirenz, delavirdine)
  - Choose agents known to reduce perinatal HIV transmission
  - Attain maximal and stable suppression of maternal viral load
  - Evaluate and manage side effects that can harm the fetus or mother (e.g., hyperglycemia, anemia, hepatotoxicity)
- Evaluation for opportunistic infections and initiation of appropriate prophylaxis
- Immunization (e.g., for influenza, hepatitis B) as indicated
- Optimization of maternal nutritional status
- Implementation of standard recommendations for preconceptional evaluation and management (e.g., assessment of

TABLE 90–13 ▪▪ Intrapartum/Postpartum Regimens for Preventing Perinatal HIV Transmission in the Absence of Antiretroviral Therapy During Pregnancy

Regimen	Recipient	Dosage
Nevirapine	Mother	200 mg PO at the onset of labor
	Infant	2 mg/kg PO 48–72 hr postpartum (If the mother was dosed less than 1 hr before delivery, the infant gets 2 oral doses, one immediately after delivery and one 48–72 hr later.)
Zidovudine	Mother	2 mg/kg by IV bolus, then 1 mg/kg/hr by continuous IV infusion until delivery
	Infant	2 mg/kg PO q 6 h for 6 weeks
Nevirapine + zidovudine	Mother and infant	Dosages are the same as when using nevirapine and zidovudine alone
Zidovudine + lamivudine	Mother	Zidovudine: 600 mg PO at the onset of labor, then 300 mg PO q 3 h until delivery Lamivudine: 150 mg PO at the onset of labor, then 150 mg PO q 12 h until delivery
	Infant	Zidovudine: 4 mg/kg PO q 12 h for 7 days Lamivudine: 3 mg/kg PO q 12 h for 7 days

reproductive history and family genetic history; starting folic acid supplementation; screening for infectious disease, including sexually transmitted diseases)

▪ Screening for maternal psychologic disorders and substance abuse
▪ Planning for perinatal consultation if desired or indicated

Treatment of Adolescent Patients

The same principles that guide antiretroviral therapy in adults also apply to adolescents. Most studies on HIV replication and antiretroviral therapy have been conducted in adults. However, it is unlikely that HIV behaves any differently in adolescents or that the fundamentals of antiretroviral therapy differ either. In fact, the few studies that have been conducted indicate that the virology of HIV is the same in adolescents and adults, suggesting that optimal antiretroviral therapy should be similar. Accordingly, like adults, adolescents should be treated with a combination of antiretroviral drugs that produces lasting suppression of plasma HIV RNA to levels that cannot be detected by current assays.

At this time, information on the pharmacokinetics of antiretroviral drugs in adolescents is limited. As a result, dosages for some drugs have not been determined. Hence, if these agents were to be used, the resulting plasma levels might be too low to be effective or too high to be safe. Therefore, to ensure maximal efficacy and minimal harm, children should be treated only with drugs for which pediatric dosages have been established.

Treatment of Infants and Young Children

Pediatric HIV infection is common and increasing in poor countries, but rare and declining in the United States. Worldwide in 2002, an estimated 3.2 million children under the age of 15 were with living with HIV/AIDS, 730,000 became

newly infected, and 610,000 died from HIV-related causes. In stark contrast, only 101 new pediatric cases were reported in the United States in 2001, down from 954 new cases in 1992. As a rule, most HIV infected children acquired the virus through mother-to-child transmission.

In young children, the course of HIV infection is accelerated. Whereas adults generally remain symptom free for a decade or more, many children develop symptoms by their first birthday. Death usually ensues by age 5—even with antiretroviral therapy. Why do young children succumb so soon? Primarily because their immune systems are immature, and hence less able to fend off the virus. Because immune function is limited, levels of HIV RNA climb higher in toddlers than in adults, and then decline at a much slower rate.

Like older patients, young patients should be treated with a combination of highly active antiretroviral drugs. Three regimens are strongly recommended:

▪ A highly active protease inhibitor (nelfinavir or ritonavir) plus two NRTIs (e.g., zidovudine plus didanosine)
▪ Efavirenz (an NNRTI) plus two NRTIs
▪ Efavirenz plus nelfinavir (a protease inhibitor) plus one NRTI

Recommended alternatives include

▪ Nevirapine (an NNRTI) plus two NRTIs
▪ Three NRTIs: abacavir plus zidovudine plus lamivudine
▪ Lopinavir/ritonavir (a protease inhibitors) plus two NRTIs
▪ Indinavir (a protease inhibitor) plus two NRTIs

Unfortunately, therapy in young patients is confounded by limited information on dosing, pharmacokinetics, and safety, and by the limited availability of pediatric formulations. The information we do have on dosage, formulations, monitoring, and other aspects of therapy can be found in two documents—*Guidelines for the Use of Antiretroviral Agents in Pediatric HIV Infection* and its supplement, *Pediatric Antiretroviral*

Drug Information—prepared by the Working Group on Antiretroviral Therapy and Medical Management of HIV-Infected Children, convened by the National Pediatric and Family HIV Resource Center, the Health Resources and Services Administration, and the National Institutes of Health (NIH). Both documents, which undergo periodic updates, are available online at *aidsinfo.nih.gov.*

Postexposure Prophylaxis

One-time exposure to HIV carries a very small, but nonetheless real, risk of infection. Sources of exposure include unprotected vaginal or anal intercourse, receptive oral intercourse, sharing a contaminated needle, or an accidental needle stick. Risk is especially high following exposure to a large quantity of infected blood or blood with a high virus titer, and following deep percutaneous penetration with a needle recently removed from the bloodstream of an infected person.

The risk of developing HIV disease after a single exposure can be reduced—but not eliminated—with prophylactic drugs. Prophylaxis should be initiated as soon as possible after HIV exposure—preferably within 1 or 2 hours—and should continue 4 weeks. The basic regimen recommended by the U.S. Public Health Service consists of two NRTIs. The following pairs may be used:

- *Lamivudine* plus *zidovudine*
- *Lamivudine* plus *stavudine*
- *Didanosine* plus *stavudine*

Selection among the three pairs is based on suspected resistance to one or both drugs in any pair. If the exposure poses a high risk of transmission, or if drug resistance is *certain,* a third drug should be added to the basic regimen. Preferred options are

- *Indinavir* (a protease inhibitor)
- *Nelfinavir* (a protease inhibitor)
- *Abacavir* (an NRTI)
- *Efavirenz* (an NNRTI)

Prophylactic therapy is based on the premise that early treatment may prevent initial cellular infection and local propagation of HIV, thereby allowing host immune defenses to eliminate the virus before it can become established. All patients should undergo testing for antibodies against HIV, preferably at 6 weeks, 12 weeks, and 6 months after exposure.

Additional information on postexposure prophylaxis, including dosages for the drugs noted above, can be found in *Updated U.S. Public Health Service Guidelines for the Management of Occupational Exposures to HBV, HCV, and HIV and Recommendations for Postexposure Prophylaxis,* last revised on June 29, 2001. This document is available online at *aidsinfo.nih.gov.*

PROPHYLAXIS AND TREATMENT OF OPPORTUNISTIC INFECTIONS

Individuals with advanced HIV disease are vulnerable to infections caused by opportunistic organisms (i.e., organisms that rarely cause serious disease, except when host defenses are compromised). Vulnerability to opportunistic infections (OIs) is caused by immunodeficiency resulting from loss of CD4 T cells. The risk of OIs is greatest in patients with fewer than 200 CD4 T cells/μl. Because of the risk of OIs, patients with low CD4 counts must take antibiotics as prophylaxis. Prior to the advent of HAART, prophylaxis was required lifelong.

Since the introduction of HAART, the incidence of new OIs has declined dramatically. For example, the incidences of cytomegalovirus retinitis and disseminated mycobacterial infection have fallen by as much as 75% to 80%. In many patients with low CD4 T-cell counts, HAART has caused CD4 counts to rise, thereby restoring some immunocompetence and permitting withdrawal of prophylaxis drugs. Unfortunately, HAART cannot help all patients. In the discussion below, we consider prophylaxis and treatment of OIs in these people. Additional details on the management of OIs can be found in *Guidelines for Preventing Opportunistic Infections Among HIV-Infected Persons—2002.* This document, developed jointly by the U.S. Public Health Service and the Infectious Diseases Society of America, is available online at *www.cdc.gov/mmwr/preview/mmwrhtml/rr5108a1.htm.*

Pneumocystis carinii Pneumonia

Before the use of HAART and prophylactic drugs, *Pneumocystis carinii* pneumonia (PCP) was the leading cause of death among people with AIDS. At one time, PCP developed in 60% to 80% of HIV-infected people, and killed about 20%. Following control of an initial bout of PCP, the rate of recurrence was 60% within the first year. In patients receiving HAART, PCP is rare, and prophylaxis is often unnecessary.

Clinical manifestations of PCP are generally nonspecific. Early symptoms include fever, cough, dyspnea, chest discomfort, pallor, and cyanosis. In advanced infection, lung morphology is altered. Left untreated, PCP has a mortality rate of 90%.

Treatment of Active PCP. The treatment of choice for PCP is *trimethoprim plus sulfamethoxazole* (TMP-SMZ), marketed as Bactrim, Cotrim, and Septra. TMP-SMZ is effective in 90% of patients. Nothing works better. As a rule, clinical improvement is seen in 4 to 8 days. For patients who are severely immunocompromised, IV *pentamidine* [Pentam 300] may be preferred. Alternatives to TMP-SMZ or pentamidine include *atovaquone* [Mepron], *trimethoprim plus dapsone, trimetrexate plus leucovorin,* and *primaquine plus clindamycin.* All of these regimens are less effective than TMP-SMZ or pentamidine, but may be better tolerated. Atovaquone is noteworthy for its cost ($11,627 wholesale for a year's supply). Dosages are summarized in Table 90–14.

Prophylaxis of PCP. Prophylactic therapy is recommended for all patients with a CD4 T-cell count below 200 cells/μl. If HAART raises CD4 counts above 200 cells/μl, prophylaxis can be discontinued a few months later.

The preferred medication for prophylaxis is *trimethoprim plus sulfamethoxazole,* given as 1 double-strength tablet each day. For patients who cannot tolerate TMP-SMZ, *aerosolized pentamidine* [NebuPent] may be used instead. Unfortunately, although aerosolized pentamidine is better tolerated than TMP-SMZ, it is less effective. Dosages for TMP-SMZ, pentamidine, and other drugs for prophylaxis are summarized in Table 90–14.

TABLE 90–14 ■■ Drugs for *Pneumocystis Carinii* Pneumonia

Drugs	Dosage	
	Adults and Adolescents	**Infants and Young Children**
Treatment of Active Infection		
Drugs of Choice		
Trimethoprim + sulfamethoxazole	TMP: 15 mg/kg/day in 3 or 4 divided doses SMZ: 75 mg/kg day in 3 or 4 divided doses Administer both drugs together, PO or IV, for 14 to 21 days	Same as adult
Alternatives		
Pentamidine (IV)	3 to 4 mg/kg IV qd for 14 to 21 days	Same as adult
Trimetrexate + leucovorin	TMX: 45 mg/m^2 IV qd for 21 days LEU: 20 mg/m^2 PO or IV q 6 h for 24 days	
Trimethoprim + dapsone	TMP: 5 mg/kg PO tid for 21 days DAP: 100 mg PO qd for 21 days	
Atovaquone	750 mg bid PO for 21 days	
Primaquine + clindamycin	PRM: 30 mg base PO qd for 21 days CLN: 600 mg IV q 8 h for 21 days *or* 300 to 450 mg PO q 6 h for 21 days	
Prophylaxis (Primary or Secondary)		
Drugs of Choice		
Trimethoprim + sulfamethoxazole	1 single-strength tablet* PO qd *or* 1 double-strength tablet* PO qd	TMP: 75 mg/m^2 PO bid SMZ: 375 mg/m^2 PO bid Administer both drugs together on 3 consecutive days each week
Alternatives		
Pentamidine (inhaled)	300 mg inhaled once a month	5 years and older: Same as adult
Atovaquone	750 mg PO bid	4–24 months: 45 mg/kg PO qd 1–3 months and >24 months: 30 mg/kg PO qd
Dapsone	50 mg PO bid *or* 100 mg PO qd	2 mg/kg (max of 100 mg) PO qd *or* 4 mg/kg (max of 200 mg) PO once a week
Dapsone + pyrimethamine + leucovorin	Either (1) DAP 50 mg PO qd + PYR 50 mg PO q 7 d + LEU 25 mg PO q 7 d *or* (2) DAP 200 mg PO + PYR 75 mg PO + LEU 25 mg PO, all taken q 7 d	

*Single-strength tablet = 80 mg TMP plus 400 mg SMZ; double-strength tablet = 160 mg TMP + 800 mg SMZ.

Cytomegalovirus Retinitis

Cytomegalovirus (CMV) retinitis is the leading cause of vision loss in people with AIDS. Prior to availability of HAART, the incidence of CMV retinitis was about 40%. Individuals with CD4 T-cell counts below 50 cells/μl are most vulnerable. Left untreated, CMV retinitis invariably leads to retinal necrosis and loss of vision.

Drug therapy of CMV retinitis proceeds in two stages: induction followed by maintenance. The induction phase reduces CMV load and greatly slows the rate of disease progression. However, induction does not eliminate CMV. Accordingly, maintenance therapy is given to reduce the risk of relapse. Before HAART was available, maintenance therapy was required lifelong. However, when HAART is able to restore sufficient immune function (by raising CD4 T-cell counts above 100 to 150 cells/μl for 3 to 6 months), maintenance therapy can be discontinued.

CMV retinitis can be treated with five agents: ganciclovir, cidofovir, foscarnet, fomivirsen, and valganciclovir. The basic pharmacology of these drugs is discussed in Chapter 89. Three agents—ganciclovir, foscarnet, and cidofovir—may be given intravenously. In addition, ganciclovir may be given orally, by intraocular implant, and by direct injection into the eye. Fomivirsen is administered only by injection into the eye. Valganciclovir is administered only by mouth.

Maintenance therapy is expensive. Current *wholesale* prices for a year's supply are $13,093 for IV ganciclovir, $17,794 for PO ganciclovir, $6500 to $10,000 for ganciclovir intraocular implants, $20,904 for IV cidofovir, $21,582 for PO valganciclovir, $12,000 for intraocular fomivirsen, and between $27,770 and $37,027 for IV foscarnet!

Ganciclovir. Ganciclovir [Cytovene, Vitrasert] is the drug of choice for CMV retinitis. For induction, IV administration is traditional, although intraocular implants or direct intraocular injections may also be used. For maintenance, intraocular implants or daily IV infusions via a central venous catheter are preferred. The implants are more effective than the infusions and cause fewer side effects. To reduce the risk of systemic CMV infection, patients with ocular implants can also take oral ganciclovir. Dose-limiting toxicities of IV ganciclovir are neutropenia and thrombocytopenia secondary to bone marrow depression. In addition, there is a risk of infection in the central venous catheter.

Foscarnet. Foscarnet [Foscavir] is less well tolerated than ganciclovir and much more expensive. As a rule, the drug is administered by IV infusion—twice daily for induction and once daily for maintenance. To receive infusions daily, patients require an indwelling central venous catheter, and hence face a risk of catheter infection. Dose-limiting toxicities are nephrotoxicity, electrolyte imbalance (especially hypocalcemia), genital ulceration, and fluid overload.

Cidofovir. Cidofovir [Vistide] is a relatively new IV drug for CMV retinitis. This agent has a longer effective half-life than ganciclovir or foscarnet, and hence can be administered less often. Specifically, whereas ganciclovir and foscarnet must be infused daily for maintenance therapy, cidofovir is infused just once every 2 weeks. Because cidofovir infusions are infrequent, patients do not require an indwelling central catheter, and hence do not face a risk of catheter infection. The major dose-limiting toxicities of cidofovir are kidney damage and neutropenia. To reduce the risk of kidney injury, all patients must be given probenecid and IV hydration therapy with each infusion.

Fomivirsen. Fomivirsen [Vitravene], a relatively new drug, has a unique mechanism of action: "antisense" binding to viral RNA, with subsequent inhibition of viral protein synthesis. Administration is by intravitreal injection, which must be repeated monthly. Ocular inflammation develops in about 25% of patients, and can be suppressed with glucocorticoids.

Valganciclovir. Valganciclovir [Valcyte] is a prodrug version of ganciclovir, but has greater oral bioavailability. Adverse effects are the same as those of ganciclovir. The principal concern is blood dyscrasia—granulocytopenia, anemia, and thrombocytopenia—secondary to bone marrow suppression.

Mycobacterium tuberculosis and Mycobacterium avium Complex

Mycobacterium tuberculosis and *Mycobacterium avium* complex (MAC) are slow-growing microbes that require prolonged drug exposure to be eradicated. Because therapy is prolonged, emergence of resistance is a significant concern. To reduce the risk of resistance, these infections are always treated with multiple drugs—just like HIV itself. Mycobacterial infections and their treatment are discussed at length in Chapter 86. A brief summary of treatment is presented here.

Mycobacterium tuberculosis. Between 2% and 20% of people with AIDS become infected with *M. tuberculosis*. If the infection is caused by drug-sensitive mycobacteria, treatment is relatively simple. In one protocol, treatment is initiated with a four-drug regimen—*isoniazid, rifabutin, pyrazinamide, and ethambutol*—and then switched to a two-drug regimen—*isoniazid plus rifabutin*—2 months later. Treatment should last for at least 9 months, and for at least 3 months after sputum tests for *M. tuberculosis* become negative. Treatment of drug-resistant infections can be very difficult, sometimes requiring as many as seven drugs. Specific regimens for drug-sensitive and drug-resistant tuberculosis are summarized in Table 86–1.

HIV-infected patients with a positive tuberculin skin test should take prophylactic drugs to prevent active *M. tuberculosis* infection. The preferred regimen consists of *isoniazid* for 9 months.

Mycobacterium avium Complex. MAC consists of two nearly identical microbes: *Mycobacterium avium* and *Mycobacterium intracellulare*. Infection with MAC begins in the lungs or GI tract, but may later disseminate to the blood, bone marrow, liver, spleen, lymph nodes, brain, kidneys, and skin.

Among people with AIDS, disseminated infection is common, being present in 50% at autopsy. Signs and symptoms of disseminated MAC infection include fever, night sweats, weight loss, lethargy, anemia, and abnormal liver function tests.

Primary prophylaxis against MAC is indicated for patients with fewer than 50 CD4 T cells/μl. Either *azithromycin* or *clarithromycin* should be used. If HAART produces a 3-month increase in CD4 counts to 100 cells/μl or more, prophylaxis can be discontinued.

If disseminated infection develops, the preferred treatment is *clarithromycin* plus *ethambutol,* with or without *rifabutin.* If needed, azithromycin can be substituted for clarithromycin. In the absence of immune recovery, treatment should continue lifelong. However, if the patient (1) has been treated for at least 12 months and is free of MAC symptoms, and (2) has had a 6-month sustained CD4 elevation (to >100 cells/μl) following HAART, then drugs for MAC may be discontinued.

Toxoplasma Encephalitis

Toxoplasma gondii is a protozoan of the Sporozoa class. In the immunocompetent host, infection with *T. gondii* is generally benign. However, in the immunocompromised host, infection can be lethal. Among patients with AIDS, toxoplasmosis usually manifests as *encephalitis* (inflammation of the brain or brainstem). Symptoms include fever, headache, seizures, aphasia (loss of speech), lethargy, confusion, dementia, focal neurologic deficits, and progression to coma. *Toxoplasma* encephalitis is most likely late in HIV disease, usually after CD4 T-cell counts fall below 100 cells/μl. In the United States, the incidence of *Toxoplasma* encephalitis among AIDS patients is 3% to 10%, making this the most common opportunistic infection of the CNS in these people.

Patients who are seropositive for *T. gondii* and have low CD4 T-cell counts (below 100 cells/μl) should take drugs to prevent active infection. The preferred regimen is 1 double-strength tablet of TMP-SMZ daily (the same regimen used to prevent PCP). Prophylaxis can be discontinued if HAART produces a 3-month sustained increase in CD4 T cells (to >200 cells/μl).

If active infection develops, the treatment of choice is *pyrimethamine plus sulfadiazine.* The sulfadiazine component can cause rash and crystalluria. For patients who cannot tolerate sulfadiazine, *pyrimethamine plus clindamycin* is an alternative.

Once toxoplasmosis has been controlled, lifelong suppressive therapy is needed to reduce the risk of relapse. The preferred regimen is *pyrimethamine plus sulfadiazine plus leucovorin. Pyrimethamine plus clindamycin* is an alternative. Recent data indicate that prophylaxis can be discontinued in patients who (1) have remained free of encephalitis symptoms and (2) have had a 6-month sustained increase in CD4 T-cell counts (to >200 cells/μl) following HAART.

Cryptococcal Meningitis

Cryptococcus neoformans is a fungus that infects 9% to 13% of patients with AIDS. In 80% of these patients, cryptococcosis manifests as meningitis (inflammation of the meninges). The most common symptoms are fever and headache. Other symptoms include nausea, vomiting, photophobia, and altered mental status. Cryptococcal meningitis typically occurs late in HIV disease, usually after CD4 T-cell counts fall below 100 cells/μl. In addition to infecting the meninges, *C. neoformans* can infect the blood, lungs, skin, and prostate.

The treatment of choice for cryptococcal meningitis is *amphotericin B plus flucytosine* infused daily for 2 weeks or longer. The major adverse effect of amphotericin is kidney damage, whereas the major concern with flucytosine is bone marrow depression (neutropenia, thrombocytopenia). Compared with amphotericin B alone, the combination of amphotericin plus flucytosine decreases rates of treatment failure and relapse. However, mortality rates with both treatments are similar. Because bone-marrow depression is a significant concern for patients with AIDS, those taking flucytosine should be monitored closely.

After the initial infection has been controlled, patients should continue maintenance therapy indefinitely. The treatment of choice is oral *fluconazole* daily. In the absence of maintenance therapy, patients are at increased risk of relapse and death. However, limited experience suggests that discontinuing maintenance therapy may be reasonable in patients who (1) have no signs or symptoms of cryptococcosis and (2) have developed a 6-month sustained increase in CD4 T-cell counts to 100 to 200 cells/μl following HAART.

The pharmacology of amphotericin B, flucytosine, and fluconazole is discussed at length in Chapter 88.

Varicella-Zoster Virus Infection

Varicella-zoster virus (VZV) can cause *chickenpox* and *herpes zoster,* also known as *shingles* or simply *zoster.* Among adults with AIDS, VZV infection usually manifests as shingles, which results from reactivation of latent VZV infection. The preferred treatment for shingles is high-dose *oral acyclovir* (800 mg 5 times daily for 7 to 10 days). *Oral famciclovir* and *IV foscarnet* are alternatives. For patients with disseminated VZV infection, the preferred treatment is *IV acyclovir* (10 mg/kg every 8 hours for 1 to 2 weeks); IV foscarnet is an alternative. The pharmacology of acyclovir, famciclovir, and foscarnet is discussed at length in Chapter 89.

Herpes Simplex Virus Infection

Infection with herpes simplex virus (HSV) is common among patients with HIV disease. Lesions may occur at multiple sites, including the lips, tongue, oral cavity, genitals, and perianal region. In patients with advanced HIV disease, HSV may infect the esophagus, colon, lungs, eyes, and CNS. For infection at all sites, *acyclovir* is the drug of choice. Administration may be oral or IV. Responses usually occur within 3 to 10 days. Duration of treatment ranges from 7 to 21 days. For patients with acyclovir-resistant HSV, *IV foscarnet* or *IV cidofovir* can be used. Patients with who experience frequent or severe recurrences can take oral acyclovir or *famciclovir* for prophylaxis.

Candidiasis

HIV-infected patients frequently develop infection with *Candida* species, usually *Candida albicans*. The most common sites are the oropharynx and esophagus. Up to 75% of patients experience oral candidiasis (thrush), which often responds to topical therapy, such as "swishing and swallowing" a *nystatin suspension* or sucking *miconazole troches*. Systemic therapy with an oral azole—*fluconazole, ketoconazole,*

or *itraconazole*—is an alternative. Oral azoles are more convenient than topical therapy and probably more effective. However, they are also more expensive. Prophylaxis of recurrent oral candidiasis is not always needed. However, if recurrence is frequent or severe, chronic intermittent therapy with an oral azole may be considered.

For esophageal candidiasis, systemic therapy is required. Options include oral *ketoconazole,* oral *fluconazole,* and IV *amphotericin B.* All patients with a documented history of esophageal candidiasis should be considered for chronic suppressive therapy with oral *fluconazole.*

HIV VACCINES

Development of an HIV vaccine is critical to controlling the AIDS epidemic worldwide. Although HIV infection can now be managed with HAART, treatment is expensive, complex, and potentially dangerous, and must continue lifelong. Furthermore, HAART is largely unavailable in developing countries, where most AIDS cases occur. Accordingly, vaccine development has been assigned high priority. At the NIH, funding for research on HIV vaccines was increased to about $350 million for fiscal 2002, more than 3 times the funding level for 1995.

Obstacles to Vaccine Development

Making a safe and effective vaccine against HIV has proved exceedingly and unexpectedly difficult. Obstacles include the wide global variation in HIV strains, lack of information on natural immunity to HIV, multiple modes of HIV transmission, and lack of an ideal animal model for studying vaccine effects. Also, scientists are concerned that the vaccine may need to (1) *prevent* HIV infection, rather than minimize it, and may need to (2) stimulate cell-mediated immunity in addition to humoral immunity. These two concerns are discussed below.

Vaccines don't prevent infection—they only attenuate it. By priming the immune system, vaccines reduce microbial replication and accelerate microbial kill. As a result, infection doesn't spread as far as it would in an unvaccinated person and doesn't injure as many cells. Unfortunately, HIV is different from all other microbes: It kills the very cells that are meant to attack it and that vaccination is meant to stimulate. Given the nature of HIV, we must ask, "Will a vaccine that permits HIV to infect even a small number of immune cells be able to contain the infection—or will HIV eventually break through?" The answer is unknown.

Vaccines elicit two kinds of immune responses: *humoral immunity* (production of antibodies) and *cell-mediated immunity* (activation of cytotoxic T lymphocytes, also known as killer T cells). Most authorities agree that, to be effective, an HIV vaccine should elicit both types of responses. Why? The answer is simple: We already know that HIV-positive people produce billions of antibodies against HIV, and yet the infection progresses relentlessly; hence, a vaccine that only stimulates humoral immunity would seem likely to fail. Unfortunately, although it's relatively easy to make a safe vaccine that stimulates humoral immunity, it's much harder to make a safe vaccine that stimulates cellular immunity. Why? Because the best way to stimulate cellular immunity is with a *live-virus* vaccine—that is, a vaccine made from HIV that has been attenuated by removing some of its genes, but has not been killed. The problem is that live-virus vaccines pose a risk of infection—a risk that is unacceptable with HIV. The potential danger of this approach was underscored when monkeys were given a simian version of such a vaccine and subsequently developed simian AIDS, presumably from the vaccine itself.

Current Status of Vaccine Development

HIV vaccines are undergoing intensive study. Nearly 60 vaccines have been evaluated in clinical trials, which enrolled more than 10,000 HIV-negative volunteers.

To date, only one vaccine—AIDSVAX—has undergone a Phase III trial. AIDSVAX is a bivalent vaccine composed of gp120 proteins, which are found in the outer envelope of HIV. The vaccine activates the antibody-producing arm of the immune system, but does not activate killer T cells. The Phase III trial enrolled 5095 HIV-negative men and 308 HIV-negative women, all considered at high risk of acquiring HIV. One third of participants received placebo, and two-thirds were injected with vaccine. The result? HIV infection developed in 5.8% of placebo recipients and 5.7% of those given the vaccine. Clearly, AIDSVAX didn't work. These results were especially disappointing in that, in an earlier trial, the vaccine elicited production of neutralizing antibodies in 99% of vaccinees. Apparently, although antibodies were made, they were unable to prevent infection.

The current best hope for protection is to combine a vaccine similar to AIDSVAX (i.e., a purified HIV envelope protein) with a "vectored" vaccine, consisting of a harmless virus, such as canarypox, that has been genetically engineered to produce HIV proteins. In Phase I and II clinical trials, this approach appeared safe, and elicited both antibody production and activation of killer T cells.

KEEPING CURRENT

Drug therapy of HIV infection is continuously evolving. New drugs are being developed, knowledge of existing drugs is expanding, and new drug combinations are being studied. The following web sites are good sources of very current information:

- **AIDSinfo** (*aidsinfo.nih.gov*). This site, maintained by the U.S. Department of Health and Human Services, has information on treatment guidelines, drugs, vaccines, and clinical trials. Links to other HIV/AIDS-related sites are there too. Content is presented in English and Spanish. You can sign up for e-mail notification of updates.
- **HIV and AIDS Activities** (*www.fda.gov/oashi/aids/hiv.html*). This page on the FDA web site offers the latest information on approved drugs, drug development, and drugs in clinical trials.
- **AIDS Education Global Information System** (*www.aegis.com*). Perhaps the best single web site for information on HIV and AIDS information. The site contains the world's largest HIV/AIDS information base, is continuously updated, and offers chat facilities.

⚡ KEY POINTS

- HIV is a retrovirus that, like all other retroviruses, has RNA as its genetic material.
- HIV uses reverse transcriptase to convert its RNA into DNA.
- HIV uses protease to break large HIV polyproteins into their smaller, functional forms.
- The principal target of HIV is CD4 T cells (helper T lymphocytes). These cells are attacked by HIV because they carry CD4 proteins on their surface, thereby providing HIV with a required point of attachment.
- Because of errors made by reverse transcriptase, HIV can mutate rapidly from a drug-sensitive form into a drug-resistant form.
- HIV infection has three phases. During the initial phase, many patients experience a flu-like acute retroviral syndrome. During the prolonged middle phase, patients are asymptomatic, although CD4 T cells undergo progressive decline. During the late phase, CD4 T cells drop below a critical level (200 cells/μl), rendering the patient vulnerable to opportunistic infections and certain neoplasms.
- HIV replicates rapidly during all phases of HIV infection, including the prolonged phase of clinical latency.
- We have four classes of antiretroviral drugs: nucleoside reverse transcriptase inhibitors (NRTIs), non-nucleoside reverse transcriptase inhibitors (NNRTIs), protease inhibitors, and HIV fusion inhibitors.
- NRTIs suppress HIV replication in two ways: (1) they become incorporated into the growing strand of viral DNA by reverse transcriptase, and thereby prevent further strand growth; and (2) they compete with natural nucleoside triphosphates for binding to the active center of reverse transcriptase, and thereby competitively inhibit the enzyme.
- In order to interact with reverse transcriptase, NRTIs must first undergo conversion to their active (triphosphate) forms.
- All NRTIs can cause lactic acidosis, which can be fatal.
- Zidovudine (an NRTI) can cause severe anemia and neutropenia.
- Didanosine, stavudine, and zalcitabine (all NRTIs) can cause peripheral neuropathy.
- Didanosine (an NRTI) can cause pancreatitis.
- Abacavir (an NRTI) can cause potentially fatal hypersensitivity reactions.
- NNRTIs (e.g., nevirapine) differ from NRTIs in that they are not analogs of natural nucleosides, are active as administered, and cause direct noncompetitive inhibition of reverse transcriptase by binding to its active center.
- NNRTIs frequently cause rash, which can be severe and even life threatening.
- Efavirenz is the only NNRTI recommended for first-line therapy of HIV infection.
- Efavirenz frequently causes adverse CNS effects.
- Protease inhibitors (e.g., saquinavir) are the most effective antiretroviral drugs available.

- Protease inhibitors bind to HIV protease and thereby prevent the enzyme from cleaving HIV polyproteins. As a result, enzymes and structural proteins of HIV remain nonfunctional, and hence the virus remains immature and noninfectious.
- All protease inhibitors pose a risk of hyperglycemia, new-onset diabetes, exacerbation of existing diabetes, fat redistribution, hyperlipidemia, bone loss, elevation of transaminase levels, and increased bleeding in patients with hemophilia.
- All protease inhibitors inhibit cytochrome P450, and can thereby suppress metabolism of other drugs, causing their levels to rise. Accordingly, patients should avoid drugs whose accumulation could lead to serious toxicity. Among these are astemizole, terfenadine, and cisapride (all no longer available in the United States), and triazolam, midazolam, ergot alkaloids, lovastatin, and simvastatin.
- Enfuvirtide, an HIV fusion inhibitor, binds with gp41 on the viral envelope, and thereby blocks entry of HIV into CD4 T cells.
- Enfuvirtide is indicated for HIV infection that is resistant to other antiretroviral drugs.
- The major adverse effects of enfuvirtide are injection-site reactions, which develop in nearly all patients.
- Treatment of HIV infection has four goals: maximal and durable suppression of viral load, restoration and/or preservation of immune function, improvement of quality of life, and reduction of HIV-related morbidity and mortality.
- Resistance to antiretroviral drugs is a major problem. To reduce emergence of resistance, these drugs should never be used alone; rather, they should always be combined with at least one other antiretroviral drug, and preferably two or even three.
- The principal laboratory tests employed to monitor HIV infection and guide therapy are plasma HIV RNA (viral load) and CD4 T-cell counts. Plasma HIV RNA levels indicate the magnitude of HIV replication and predict the rate of CD4 T-cell destruction, whereas CD4 T-cell counts indicate how much damage the immune system has already suffered.
- Plasma HIV RNA is the best measurement for predicting clinical outcome: if HIV RNA is high, the prognosis is poor; if HIV RNA is low, the risk of disease progression and death is greatly reduced. Accordingly, the goal of antiretroviral therapy is to decrease plasma HIV RNA to levels that are undetectable (now defined as less than 50 copies/ml).
- Reducing plasma HIV RNA to undetectable levels does not mean that HIV has been eradicated. It only means there is too little HIV present for us to measure. Nonetheless, patients still harbor HIV and are still infectious. Accordingly, treatment should continue in-definitely and patients should be warned to avoid behaviors that can transmit HIV to others.
- All patients with acute primary HIV disease or advanced (symptomatic) HIV disease should receive maximally effective antiretroviral therapy. The preferred regimen consists of three drugs: one protease inhibitor plus two NRTIs.
- For some patients with chronic asymptomatic HIV disease, it may be appropriate to temporarily postpone antiretroviral therapy.
- In general, the principles that guide antiretroviral therapy in nonpregnant adults also apply during pregnancy. Put another way, women should receive optimal antiretroviral therapy, regardless of their pregnancy status.
- Mother-to-child transmission of HIV occurs primarily during labor and delivery. The risk of transmission can be greatly reduced by HAART that minimizes maternal viral load. Zidovudine should be given to the mother during pregnancy (PO) and labor (IV), and to the infant (PO) for 6 weeks postpartum.
- In general, the principles that guide antiretroviral therapy in adults also apply to children.
- An important reason for changing an antiretroviral regimen is treatment failure, as indicated by (1) failure of plasma HIV RNA to drop to an undetectable level, (2) a rebound in plasma HIV RNA after falling to an undetectable level, (3) continued decline of CD4 T-cell counts, and (4) progression of clinical disease.
- When treatment failure is the result of drug resistance, the preferred response is to change *all* drugs in the regimen. Furthermore, the new drugs should be agents that the patient has not taken before and that are not cross-resistant with drugs the patient has taken before.
- Prophylactic drugs can reduce the risk of infection following accidental exposure to HIV (e.g., from a needle stick). Prophylaxis is most effective when initiated within 1 or 2 hours.
- Because of declining CD4 T-cell counts, individuals with advanced HIV disease are at risk for opportunistic infections (OIs), and hence must take prophylactic antibiotics.
- By elevating CD4 T-cell counts, HAART can restore immune function, and thereby reduce both the risk of OIs and the need for prophylactic antibiotics.
- Among people with AIDS, *Pneumocystis carinii* pneumonia (PCP) is the most common opportunistic infection.
- The preferred regimen for prophylaxis and treatment of PCP is trimethoprim plus sulfamethoxazole.
- Ganciclovir is the drug of choice for cytomegalovirus retinitis, an OI.

Summary of Major Nursing Implications*

NUCLEOSIDE REVERSE TRANSCRIPTASE INHIBITORS

Abacavir
Didanosine
Lamivudine
Stavudine
Tenofovir
Zalcitabine
Zidovudine

Preadministration Assessment

Therapeutic Goals

Treatment has four goals: maximal and durable suppression of viral load, restoration and/or preservation of immune function, improvement of quality of life, and reduction of HIV-related morbidity and mortality.

Baseline Data

All NRTIs. Assess the patient's clinical status and obtain a plasma HIV RNA level and CD4 T-cell count.

Zidovudine. Obtain a hemoglobin value and granulocyte count.

Identifying High-Risk Patients

Didanosine. The risk of pancreatitis is increased by a history of alcoholism or pancreatitis and by use of IV pentamidine.

Zidovudine. The risk of hematologic toxicity is increased by a low granulocyte count; by low levels of hemoglobin, vitamin B_{12}, or folic acid; and by concurrent use of drugs that are myelosuppressive, nephrotoxic, or toxic to circulating blood cells.

Implementation: Administration

Routes

All NRTIs. Oral.
Zidovudine. Oral and IV.

Administration

All NRTIs. **Instruct patients to adhere closely to the prescribed dosing schedule.**

Didanosine. **Instruct patients to take all didanosine formulations 30 minutes before meals or 2 hours after.**

Instruct patients taking buffered didanosine tablets to either (1) chew them thoroughly or (2) manually crush them or disperse them in at least 1 ounce of water.

Instruct patients using enteric-coated capsules to swallow them intact.

Instruct patients taking powdered didanosine to pour the contents of one packet into 4 ounces of water (not fruit juice or any other acid-containing beverage), stir the mixture until the drug dissolves (about 2 to 3 minutes), and then drink the solution immediately.

IV Zidovudine. Administer IV zidovudine slowly (over 1 hour). Do not mix the solution with biologic or colloidal fluids (e.g., blood products, protein solutions). Administer

within 8 hours (if stored at room temperature) or within 24 hours (if stored under refrigeration).

Ongoing Evaluation and Interventions

Evaluating Therapeutic Effects

Plasma HIV RNA. Success is indicated by a reduction in plasma HIV RNA. With HAART, plasma HIV RNA should fall to 1% of baseline within 2 weeks, and reach a minimum by 8 weeks. Ideally, the minimum will be undetectable with sensitive assays.

CD4 T-Cell Counts. As viral load decreases, CD4 T-cell counts may rise, indicating some restoration of immune function.

Minimizing Adverse Effects

Anemia and Neutropenia. Zidovudine can cause severe anemia and neutropenia. Determine hematologic status before treatment and at least every 4 weeks thereafter. In the event of severe anemia (hemoglobin <7.5 gm/dl or down 25% from the pretreatment baseline) or severe neutropenia (granulocyte count <750 cells/μl or down 50% from the pretreatment baseline), interrupt treatment until there is evidence of bone marrow recovery. If neutropenia and anemia are less severe, a reduction in dosage may be sufficient. Some patients may require multiple transfusions. Granulocyte colony-stimulating factors can be used to reverse neutropenia. Epoetin alfa (recombinant erythropoietin) can be given to reduce transfusion requirements in patients with anemia, provided endogenous erythropoietin levels are not already elevated.

Lactic Acidosis. Potentially fatal lactic acidosis can occur with all NRTIs. **Inform patients about symptoms—nausea, vomiting, abdominal pain, malaise, fatigue, anorexia, and hyperventilation—and instruct them to report these immediately.** Diagnosis is done by measuring lactate in arterial blood. If lactic acidosis is present, the NRTI should be discontinued.

Pancreatitis. Didanosine can cause potentially fatal pancreatitis. Monitor patients for signs of developing pancreatitis (elevated serum amylase in association with elevated serum triglycerides, decreased serum calcium, and nausea, vomiting, or abdominal pain). If evolving pancreatitis is diagnosed, didanosine should be withdrawn.

Peripheral Neuropathy. Didanosine, stavudine, and *zalcitabine* can cause painful peripheral neuropathy. **Inform patients about early signs of neuropathy (numbness, tingling, or pain in hands and feet) and instruct them to report these immediately.** Treat pain of severe neuropathy with opioid analgesics. Neuropathy may reverse if these drugs are withdrawn early.

Hypersensitivity Reactions. Abacavir can cause potentially fatal hypersensitivity reactions. **Inform patients of symptoms—fever, rash, myalgia, arthralgia, nausea, vomiting, diarrhea, abdominal pain, pharyngitis, dyspnea, cough—and instruct them to report these immediately.** If a hypersensitivity reaction is diagnosed—or even strongly suspected—abacavir should be discontinued and never used again.

*Patient education information is highlighted as blue text.

Summary of Major Nursing Implications*—cont'd

HIV Transmission. Reduction of plasma HIV RNA may create a false sense of safety. Accordingly, **inform patients that, even when HIV RNA is undetectable, they are still infectious, and hence should avoid behaviors that can transmit HIV.**

Minimizing Adverse Interactions

Zidovudine. Drugs that are myelosuppressive, nephrotoxic, or directly toxic to circulating blood cells can increase the risk of hematologic toxicity. Drugs of concern include ganciclovir, dapsone, pentamidine, pyrimethamine, trimethoprim-sulfamethoxazole, amphotericin B, flucytosine, vincristine, vinblastine, and doxorubicin.

Ribavirin. Ribavirin can increase levels of the active form of *didanosine,* thereby posing a risk of toxicity. Use the combination with caution.

All NRTIs. Giving a combination of NRTIs to a pregnant woman may increase the risk of lactic acidosis. Accordingly, it would seem prudent to avoid these combinations during pregnancy.

NON-NUCLEOSIDE REVERSE TRANSCRIPTASE INHIBITORS

Delavirdine
Efavirenz
Nevirapine

Preadministration Assessment

Therapeutic Goals

Treatment has four goals: maximal and durable suppression of viral load, restoration and/or preservation of immune function, improvement of quality of life, and reduction of HIV-related morbidity and mortality.

Baseline Data

Assess the patient's clinical status and obtain a plasma HIV RNA level, CD4 T-cell count, and liver function tests. Perform a pregnancy test prior to giving efavirenz.

Implementation: Administration

Route

Oral.

Administration

All NNRTIs. Instruct patients to adhere closely to the prescribed dosing schedule.

Delavirdine. Administer with or without food. Advise patients who cannot swallow delavirdine tablets whole to mix them with 3 or more ounces of water. Advise patients with achlorhydria to take delavirdine with an acidic beverage, such as orange or cranberry juice.

Efavirenz. Administer with or without food—but not with a high-fat meal.

Nevirapine. Administer with or without food.

Ongoing Evaluation and Interventions

Evaluating Therapeutic Effects

Plasma HIV RNA. Success is indicated by a reduction in plasma HIV RNA. With triple-drug therapy, plasma HIV RNA should fall to 1% of baseline within 2 weeks, and reach a minimum by 8 weeks. Ideally, the minimum will be undetectable with a sensitive assay.

CD4 T-Cell Counts. As viral load decreases, CD4 T-cell counts may rise, indicating some restoration of immune function.

Minimizing Adverse Effects

Rash. Rash is common and may range from mild to severe to life threatening. If rash is mild, treat with an antihistamine or topical glucocorticoid. If rash is severe or associated with signs of toxic epidermal necrolysis or Stevens-Johnson syndrome (fever, blistering, oral lesions, conjunctivitis, muscle pain, joint pain), the NNRTI should be withdrawn. To minimize risk, use a low dosage for the first 14 days of treatment, and then increase the dosage if rash has not occurred.

Hepatotoxicity. NNRTIs can cause hepatotoxicity, which may be severe. Risk is greatest with nevirapine. Perform liver function tests at baseline and periodically thereafter. Interrupt treatment if tests indicate significant liver injury.

CNS Symptoms. Efavirenz frequently causes CNS symptoms (e.g., dizziness, insomnia, impaired consciousness, drowsiness, vivid dreams, and nightmares). **Inform patients that symptoms typically resolve in 2 to 4 weeks, despite ongoing efavirenz use, and that taking efavirenz at bedtime can minimize CNS effects.** If severe symptoms occur (e.g., delusions, hallucinations, severe acute depression), efavirenz should be withdrawn.

Birth Defects. Efavirenz is teratogenic. **Inform women about the potential for fetal harm and instruct them to use a barrier method of birth control (e.g., condom) in conjunction with a hormonal method (e.g., oral contraceptive).** Perform a pregnancy test prior to treatment.

HIV Transmission. Reduction of plasma HIV RNA may create a false sense of safety. Accordingly, **inform patients that, even when HIV RNA is undetectable, they are still infectious, and hence must avoid behaviors that can transmit HIV.**

Minimizing Adverse Interactions

Nevirapine. Nevirapine *induces* cytochrome P450 and can thereby decrease levels of other drugs. Effects on *protease inhibitors, oral contraceptives,* and *methadone* are of particular concern.

Combining nevirapine with *rifampin,* which also induces P450, can decrease nevirapine levels, and hence the combination is not recommended.

Delavirdine. Delavirdine *inhibits* P450, and can thereby increase levels of other drugs. To avoid toxicity from excessive drug levels, patients must not take *astemizole, terfenadine,* or *cisapride* (all no longer available in the United

*Patient education information is highlighted as blue text.

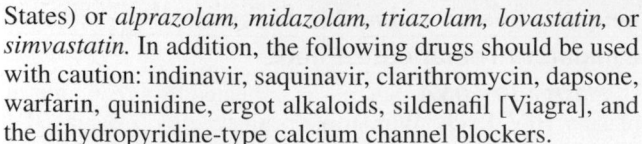

Summary of Major Nursing Implications*—cont'd

States) or *alprazolam, midazolam, triazolam, lovastatin,* or *simvastatin.* In addition, the following drugs should be used with caution: indinavir, saquinavir, clarithromycin, dapsone, warfarin, quinidine, ergot alkaloids, sildenafil [Viagra], and the dihydropyridine-type calcium channel blockers.

Antacids, histamine₂-receptor blockers, proton pump inhibitors, and *buffered formulations* of didanosine can decrease absorption of delavirdine.

Efavirenz. Efavirenz *competes with other drugs for metabolism by P450,* and can thereby increase their levels. To avoid toxicity from excessive drug levels, the patient must not take *astemizole, terfenadine, cisapride, midazolam, triazolam, dihydroergotamine,* or *ergotamine.*

Efavirenz *induces P450,* and can thereby accelerate metabolism of other drugs, including two protease inhibitors: *saquinavir* and *indinavir.* Avoid combined use with saquinavir. Increase indinavir dosage.

PROTEASE INHIBITORS

Amprenavir
Indinavir
Lopinavir/Ritonavir
Nelfinavir
Ritonavir
Saquinavir

Preadministration Assessment

Therapeutic Goals

Treatment has four goals: maximal and durable suppression of viral load, restoration and/or preservation of immune function, improvement of quality of life, and reduction of HIV-related morbidity and mortality.

Baseline Data

Assess the patient's clinical status and obtain a plasma HIV RNA level and CD4 T-cell count. Measure serum transaminases and blood glucose.

Identifying High-Risk Patients

Amprenavir oral solution is contraindicated for pregnant women, children less than 4 years old, patients with renal or hepatic failure, and patients taking disulfiram or metronidazole.

Implementation: Administration

Route

All protease inhibitors are taken orally.

Administration and Storage

All Protease Inhibitors. **Instruct patients to adhere closely to the prescribed dosing schedule.**

Amprenavir. **Inform patients they can take amprenavir without food or with food—as long as the food is low-fat.**

Indinavir. **Instruct patients to administer indinavir (1) with water but on an empty stomach (i.e., 1 hour before a meal or 2 hours after) or (2) with skim milk, coffee,** tea, or a low-fat meal (e.g., corn flakes with skim milk and sugar), **but not with a large meal. Instruct patients to store indinavir at room temperature in the package supplied by the manufacturer.**

Lopinavir/Ritonavir. **Instruct patients to take lopinavir/ ritonavir with food.**

Nelfinavir. **Instruct patients to take nelfinavir with food. Instruct patients to mix the powder formulation with a small amount of water, milk, formula, soy formula, soy milk, or dietary supplement, but not with acidic foods or juices (e.g., applesauce, apple juice, orange juice).**

Ritonavir. **Advise patients to take ritonavir with food. Instruct patients to mix the oral solution with chocolate milk, Ensure, or Advera (within 1 hour of administration) to improve the taste. Instruct patients to store ritonavir refrigerated (2°C to 8°C; 36°F to 46°F) and protected from light.**

Saquinavir. **Instruct patients to take saquinavir hard gelatin capsules with food.**

Inform patients they can take saquinavir soft gelatin capsules with or without food, as long as the drug is combined with ritonavir.

Ongoing Evaluation and Interventions

Evaluating Therapeutic Effects

Plasma HIV RNA. Success is indicated by a reduction in plasma HIV RNA. With triple-drug therapy, plasma HIV RNA should fall to 1% of baseline within 2 weeks, and reach a minimum by 8 weeks. Ideally, the minimum will be undetectable with sensitive assays.

CD4 T-Cell Counts. As viral load decreases, CD4 T-cell counts may rise, indicating some restoration of immune function.

Minimizing Adverse Effects

Hyperglycemia/Diabetes. All protease inhibitors can cause hyperglycemia and diabetes. **Instruct patients to report any symptoms (e.g., polydipsia, polyphagia, and polyuria).** In patients with existing diabetes, monitor blood glucose closely. To detect new-onset diabetes, measure blood glucose at baseline, every 3 to 4 months during the first year of treatment, and less frequently thereafter. Diabetes can be treated with insulin and oral hypoglycemics (e.g., metformin).

Fat Redistribution. **Forewarn patients that all protease inhibitors may cause accumulation of fat on the waist, stomach, breasts, and back of the neck, and loss of fat from the face, arms, buttocks, and legs.** Drug withdrawal may cause symptoms to resolve, but is not recommended.

Hyperlipidemia. All protease inhibitors can elevate cholesterol and triglycerides, thereby posing a risk of cardiovascular events and pancreatitis. Monitoring plasma cholesterol and triglycerides every 3 to 4 months may be wise. If drugs are given to lower lipid levels, two agents—lovastatin and simvastatin—should be avoided.

Increased Bleeding in Hemophiliacs. Protease inhibitors may increase the risk of bleeding in patients with hemophilia. Patients may need higher doses of coagulation factors.

*Patient education information is highlighted as blue text.

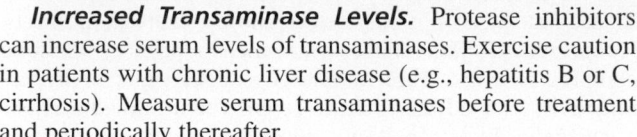

Summary of Major Nursing Implications*—cont'd

Increased Transaminase Levels. Protease inhibitors can increase serum levels of transaminases. Exercise caution in patients with chronic liver disease (e.g., hepatitis B or C, cirrhosis). Measure serum transaminases before treatment and periodically thereafter.

Nephrolithiasis. *Indinavir* can cause nephrolithiasis. Management consists of hydration and interruption of indinavir for 1 to 3 days. **To decrease the risk of nephrolithiasis, instruct patients to consume at least 48 ounces (1.5 L) of water daily.**

Bone Loss. Protease inhibitors may promote bone loss. **To reduce risk, encourage patients to ensure adequate intake of calcium and vitamin D.** Osteoporosis can be treated with bisphosphonates, raloxifene, calcitonin, or teriparatide.

Diarrhea. *Nelfinavir* causes diarrhea in 20% to 32% of patients. Diarrhea can usually be managed with loperamide or some other over-the-counter antidiarrheal drug.

Propylene Glycol Toxicity. *Amprenavir oral solution* contains a large amount of *propylene glycol,* which can accumulate to toxic levels in certain patients. Accordingly, this formulation must not be given to pregnant women, children less than 4 years old, patients with renal or hepatic failure, and patients taking disulfiram or metronidazole. **Advise patients to avoid alcohol.**

HIV Transmission. Reduction of plasma HIV RNA may create a false sense of safety. Accordingly, **inform patients that, even when HIV RNA is undetectable, they may still be infectious, and hence should avoid behaviors that can transmit HIV.**

Minimizing Adverse Interactions

Interactions Resulting from Inhibition of P450. All protease inhibitors inhibit cytochrome P450, and can thereby increase levels of other drugs. To avoid serious toxicity from excessive drug levels, patients must not take *astemizole, terfenadine,* or *cisapride* (all no longer available in the United States) or *triazolam, midazolam, ergot alkaloids, lovastatin,* or *simvastatin.* Additional drugs to avoid are listed in Table 90–6.

Didanosine. Buffered formulations of didanosine decrease absorption of *indinavir* and *ritonavir.* Accordingly, buffered didanosine should be administered 1 or 2 hours apart from these drugs.

Rifampin. Rifampin induces P450, and can thereby reduce levels of the protease inhibitors. Concurrent use with all protease inhibitors should be avoided.

Oral Contraceptives. *Ritonavir, nelfinavir,* and *amprenavir* can reduce levels of ethinyl estradiol, a component of many oral contraceptives. **Advise patients to use an alternative form of birth control.**

Vitamin E. *Amprenavir* formulations contain a large amount of vitamin E. **Warn patients not to take vitamin E supplements.**

St. John's Wort. St. John's wort induces P450, and can thereby reduce levels of protease inhibitors. **Warn patients not to use St. John's wort.**

ENFUVIRTIDE, AN HIV FUSION INHIBITOR
Preadministration Assessment
Therapeutic Goals

Enfuvirtide is indicated for HIV infection that is resistant to traditional antiretroviral drugs. Treatment has four goals: maximal and durable suppression of viral load, restoration and/or preservation of immune function, improvement of quality of life, and reduction of HIV-related morbidity and mortality.

Baseline Data

Assess the patient's clinical status and obtain a plasma HIV RNA level and CD4 T-cell count.

Identifying High-Risk Patients

Use enfuvirtide with *caution* in patients who have pneumonia risk factors: low initial CD4 cell counts, high initial viral load, IV drug use, smoking, and a history of lung disease.

Implementation: Administration
Route

Subcutaneous.

Preparation and Storage

Teach patients to reconstitute powdered enfuvirtide with 1.1 ml of sterile water for injection, and advise them to either (1) inject the solution immediately or (2) store it cold (2°C to 8°C; 36°F to 46°F) for up to 24 hours. Inform patients that powdered enfuvirtide may be stored at room temperature.

Administration

Educate patients on aseptic injection technique, and instruct them to

- Make injections into the upper arm, thigh, or abdomen (but not the navel)
- Rotate the injection site
- Avoid sites where there is an ongoing injection-site reaction or tissue that is scarred or bruised

Instruct patients that, before using stored enfuvirtide solution, they should bring it to room temperature and make sure it is clear, colorless, and free of bubbles and particulate matter.

Ongoing Evaluation and Interventions
Evaluating Therapeutic Effects

Plasma HIV RNA. Success is indicated by a reduction in plasma HIV RNA. Ideally, the minimum level will be undetectable with sensitive assays.

CD4 T-Cell Counts. As viral load decreases, CD4 T-cell counts may rise, indicating some restoration of immune function.

Minimizing Adverse Effects

Injection-Site Reactions. **Inform patients about manifestations of ISRs—pain, tenderness, erythema, induration, nodules, cysts, pruritus, and ecchymosis—and forewarn**

*Patient education information is highlighted as blue text.

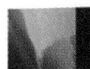
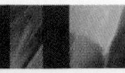

Summary of Major Nursing Implications*—cont'd

them that these occur in nearly everyone. **Inform patients that they can reduce the risk of a severe ISR by rotating the injection site, avoiding sites with an active ISR, and avoiding unnecessarily deep injections. Instruct patients to seek immediate medical attention if a severe ISR occurs or if local infection develops.**

Pneumonia. Enfuvirtide may increase the risk of bacterial pneumonia. **Inform patients about signs of pneumonia—cough, fever, breathing difficulties—and instruct them to report them immediately.** Use enfuvirtide in patients who have pneumonia risk factors.

Hypersensitivity Reactions. Enfuvirtide may cause hypersensitivity reactions, manifesting as rash, fever, nausea,

vomiting, chills, rigors, hypotension, or elevated serum transaminases, or possibly as respiratory distress, glomerulonephritis, Guillain-Barré syndrome, or primary immune complex reaction. **Inform patients about signs of hypersensitivity and advise them to report them immediately.** If a systemic hypersensitivity reaction occurs, enfuvirtide should be discontinued and never used again.

HIV Transmission. Reduction of plasma HIV RNA may create a false sense of safety. Accordingly, **inform patients that, even when HIV RNA is undetectable, they are still infectious, and hence must avoid behaviors that can transmit HIV.**

*Patient education information is highlighted as blue text.

Drug Therapy of Sexually Transmitted Diseases

CHLAMYDIA TRACHOMATIS INFECTIONS
GONOCOCCAL INFECTIONS
NONGONOCOCCAL URETHRITIS
PELVIC INFLAMMATORY DISEASE
ACUTE EPIDIDYMITIS
SYPHILIS
ACQUIRED IMMUNODEFICIENCY SYNDROME
CHANCROID
TRICHOMONIASIS
BACTERIAL VAGINOSIS
HERPES SIMPLEX INFECTIONS
GENITAL AND ANAL WARTS
(CONDYLOMATA ACUMINATA)
PROCTITIS
PEDICULOSIS PUBIS AND SCABIES

Sexually transmitted diseases (STDs) are defined as infectious or parasitic diseases that are transmitted primarily through sexual contact. STDs are very common in the United States and constitute a major public health problem. In 2000, the Centers for Disease Control and Prevention (CDC) logged more than 1 million reports of STDs, including 702,093 cases of genital *Chlamydia trachomatis* infection and 358,995 cases of gonorrhea. According to the CDC, Americans now have a 25% lifetime risk of contracting an STD.

Our objective in this chapter is to describe the principal STDs and provide an overview of their treatment. Table 91–1 presents a summary of the common STDs, their causative organisms, and the drugs of choice for treatment. The basic pharmacology of these drugs is discussed in other chapters.

In May 2002, the CDC released its 2002 "Guidelines for Treatment of Sexually Transmitted Diseases," updating its 1998 guidelines. All treatment recommendations presented in this chapter reflect the new guidelines, which are available online at *www.cdc.gov/std/treatment*.

CHLAMYDIA TRACHOMATIS INFECTIONS

Characteristics

Chlamydia trachomatis is the most common cause of bacterial STD in the United States (Fig. 91–1), infecting about 3 million people annually. The various strains of this organism can cause genital tract infections, proctitis, conjunctivitis, and lymphogranuloma venereum (LGV), as well as ophthalmia and pneumonia in infants. In both men and women, infection is frequently asymptomatic. In women, untreated infection can cause pelvic inflammatory disease (PID), ectopic pregnancy, and infertility. The CDC estimates that chlamydial infections cause sterility in up to 50,000 women each year, primarily from fallopian tube scarring. Because infection may be asymptomatic, and because sequelae can be serious, the CDC now recommends annual screening for all sexually active women under age 25. Screening is also recommended for women over age 25 who have a new sex partner or multiple partners.

Treatment

Adults and Adolescents. For uncomplicated urethral, cervical, or rectal infections in adults or adolescents, two treatments are recommended: (1) a single 1-gm oral dose of *azithromycin* [Zithromax], or (2) 100 mg of *doxycycline* [Vibramycin, others] PO twice daily for 7 days.

Infection in Pregnancy. Preferred treatments for *C. trachomatis* infection during pregnancy are (1) *erythromycin base,* 500 mg PO 4 times daily for 7 days, and (2) *azithromycin,* 500 mg PO 3 times daily for 7 days. Erythromycin *estolate* is contraindicated during pregnancy because of the risk of maternal liver injury. Although doxycycline and other tetracyclines are active against *C. trachomatis,* these drugs are contraindicated because they can damage fetal teeth and bones. Similarly, sulfisoxazole and other sulfonamides are active, but are contraindicated near term because they can cause kernicterus in the infant.

Infants. About half the infants born to women with cervical *C. trachomatis* acquire the infection during the birth process. These infants are at risk for *conjunctivitis* and *pneumonia.* Pneumonia is generally not severe and lasts about 6 weeks. Conjunctivitis does not result in blindness and spontaneously resolves in 6 months. The preferred treatment for both infections is systemic *erythromycin base* or *erythromycin succinate,* 12.5 mg/kg PO 4 times daily for 2 weeks. Although topical erythromycin, tetracycline, or silver nitrate may be given to prevent conjunctivitis, none of these treatments is completely effective.

Children. Although infection in preadolescent children can result from perinatal transmission, sexual abuse is the more likely cause. Because of the legal implications, diagnoses must be definitive. Treatment depends on the age and weight of the child. For children who weigh less than 45 kg, the preferred treatment is oral *erythromycin base* or *eryth-*

TABLE 91–1 ■ Drug Therapy of Sexually Transmitted Diseases

Disease or Syndrome	Recommended Treatment*	Causative Organism(s)
Chlamydia trachomatis Infections		*Chlamydia trachomatis*
Adults and adolescents	Azithromycin, 1 gm PO once *or* Doxycycline, 100 mg PO bid × 7 days	
Children <45 kg ≥45 kg but <8 yr old ≥8 yr old	Erythromycin base/ethylsuccinate, 12.5 mg/kg PO qid × 14 days Azithromycin, 1 gm PO once Azithromycin, 1 gm PO once *or* Doxycycline, 100 mg PO bid × 7 days	
Pregnant women	Erythromycin base, 500 mg PO qid × 7 days *or* Azithromycin, 500 mg PO tid × 7 days	
Newborns: ophthalmia or pneumonia	Erythromycin base/ethylsuccinate, 12.5 mg/kg PO qid × 14 days	
Lymphogranuloma venereum	Doxycycline, 100 mg PO bid × 21 days	
Gonococcal Infections (Gonorrhea)		*Neisseria gonorrhoeae*
Urethral[†,‡] Cervical[†,‡] Rectal[†,‡]	Cefixime, 400 mg PO once *or* Ceftriaxone, 125 mg IM once *or* Ciprofloxacin, 500 mg PO once *or* Ofloxacin, 400 mg PO once *or* Levofloxacin, 250 mg PO once	
Pharyngeal[†,‡]	Ceftriaxone, 125 mg IM once *or* Ciprofloxacin, 500 mg PO once	
Disseminated gonococcal infection in adults	Ceftriaxone, 1 gm IM or IV q 24 h	
Meningitis Endocarditis	Ceftriaxone, 1–2 gm IV q 12 h	
Conjunctivitis	Ceftriaxone, 1 gm IM once	
Newborns Ophthalmia Disseminated infection or scalp abscess	Ceftriaxone, 25–50 mg/kg IM or IV once (max 124 mg) Ceftriaxone, 25–50 mg/kg IM or IV qd × 7 days *or* Cefotaxime, 25 mg/kg IM or IV q 12 h × 7 days	
Children ≥45 kg <45 kg (arthritis, bacteremia) <45 kg (vulvovaginitis, cervicitis, proctitis, pharyngitis, urethritis)	Same as adults Ceftriaxone, 50 mg/kg IM or IV (max 1 gm) × 7 days Ceftriaxone, 125 mg IM once	
Nongonococcal Urethritis		*Chlamydia trachomatis, Mycoplasma genitalium, Ureaplasma urealyticum, Trichomonas vaginalis*
Acute infection	Azithromycin, 1 gm PO once *or* Doxycycline, 100 mg PO bid × 7 days	
Recurrent/persistent	Metronidazole (2 gm PO once) *plus either* erythromycin base (500 mg PO qid × 7 days) *or* erythromycin ethylsuccinate (800 mg PO qid × 7 days)	
Pelvic Inflammatory Disease		*Neisseria gonorrhoeae, Chlamydia trachomatis,* others
Inpatients	Cefoxitin (2 gm IV q 6 h) or cefotetan (2 g IV q 12 h), *either one plus* doxycycline (100 mg IV or PO q 12 h) for 14 days[§]	
Outpatients	Ofloxacin (400 mg PO bid × 14 days) *or* levofloxacin (500 mg PO qd × 14 days), *either one, with or without* metronidazole (500 mg PO bid × 14 days)	

*Recommendations from Centers for Disease Control and Prevention. Sexually transmitted diseases treatment guidelines—2002. MMWR 2002; 51(RR-6):1–80.

†If chlamydia infection has not been ruled out, add either azithromycin (1 gm PO once) or doxycycline (100 mg PO bid for 7 days).

‡For pregnant women, avoid fluoroquinolones and tetracyclines; instead, use a cephalosporin (e.g., ceftriaxone).

§Intravenous therapy with cefotetan, cefoxitin, and doxycycline may be discontinued 24 hours after the patient improves clinically; oral therapy with doxycycline should continue to complete 14 days of therapy.

TABLE 91–1 ▪▪ Drug Therapy of Sexually Transmitted Diseases (continued)

Disease or Syndrome	Recommended Treatment*	Causative Organism(s)
Sexually Acquired Epididymitis	Ceftriaxone (250 mg IM once) *plus* doxycycline (100 mg PO bid × 7 days)	*Chlamydia trachomatis, Neisseria gonorrhoeae*
Syphilis		*Treponema pallidum*
Primary syphilis, secondary syphilis, and early latent syphilis	*Adults:* Benzathine penicillin G, 2.4 million units IM once *Children:* Benzathine penicillin G, 50,000 units/kg IM once (up to a max of 2.4 million units)	
Late latent syphilis or latent syphilis of unknown duration	*Adults:* Benzathine penicillin G, 2.4 million units IM once/wk for 3 wk *Children:* Benzathine penicillin G, 50,000 units/kg IM once/wk for 3 wk (up to a max of 7.2 million units)	
Tertiary syphilis	Benzathine penicillin G, 2.4 million units IM once/wk for 3 wk	
Neurosyphilis	Aqueous crystalline penicillin G, 18–24 million units IV daily for 14 days, administered by continuous infusion or in separate doses of 3–4 million units each q 4 h	
Congenital syphilis	Aqueous crystalline penicillin G, 50,000 units/kg IV q 12 h for the first 7 days of life, followed by 50,000 units/kg q 8 h for the next 3 days *or* Procaine penicillin G, 50,000 units/kg IM once daily for 10 days	
Acquired Immunodeficiency Syndrome (AIDS)	*See* Chapter 90	Human immunodeficiency virus
Bacterial Vaginosis		*Gardnerella vaginalis, Mycoplasma hominis,* various anaerobes
Nonpregnant women	Metronidazole, 500 mg PO bid × 7 days *or* Metronidazole gel (0.75%), 1 full applicator (5 gm) intravaginally qd × 5 days *or* Clindamycin cream (2%), 1 full applicator (5 gm) intravaginally qhs × 7 days	
Pregnant women	Metronidazole, 250 mg PO tid × 7 days *or* Clindamycin 300 mg PO bid × 7 days	
Trichomoniasis	Metronidazole, 2 gm PO once	*Trichomonas vaginalis*
Chancroid	Azithromycin, 1 gm PO once *or* Ceftriaxone, 250 mg IM once *or* Ciprofloxacin, 500 mg PO bid × 3 days *or* Erythromycin, 500 mg PO tid × 7 days	*Haemophilus ducreyi*
Genital Herpes Simplex Virus Infections		Herpes simplex virus
First episode, genital herpes	Acyclovir, 400 mg PO tid × 7–10 days (or longer) *or* Acyclovir, 200 mg PO 5 times/day × 7–10 days (or longer) *or* Famciclovir, 250 mg PO tid × 7–10 days (or longer) *or* Valacyclovir, 1 gm PO bid × 7–10 days (or longer)	
First episode, proctitis, stomatitis, or pharyngitis	Acyclovir, 400 mg PO 5 times/day for 7–10 days (or longer)	
Severe infection	Acyclovir 5–10 mg/kg IV q 8 h for 2–7 days or until clinical improvement, then PO acyclovir to complete at least 10 days	
Recurrent episodes	Acyclovir, 800 mg PO bid × 5 days *or* Acyclovir, 400 mg PO tid × 5 days *or* Acyclovir, 200 mg PO 5 times/day × 5 days *or* Famciclovir, 125 mg PO tid × 5 days *or* Valacyclovir, 500 mg PO bid × 3 days *or* Valacyclovir, 1 gm PO qd 5 days	
Daily suppressive therapy	Acyclovir, 400 mg PO bid *or* Famciclovir, 250 mg PO bid *or* Valacyclovir, 500 mg PO qd *or* Valacyclovir, 1 gm PO qd	

Continued

TABLE 91–1 ▪■ Drug Therapy of Sexually Transmitted Diseases (continued)

Disease or Syndrome	Recommended Treatment*	Causative Organism(s)
Genital Herpes Simplex Virus Infections		
Neonatal herpes	Acyclovir, 20 mg/kg IV q 8 h × 14 days (for skin or mucous membrane infection) or × 21 days (for disseminated or CNS infection)	
Proctitis	Ceftriaxone (125 mg IM once) *plus* doxycycline (100 mg PO bid × 7 days)	*Chlamydia trachomatis, Neisseria gonorrhoeae, Treponema pallidum,* herpes simplex virus
Pediculosis Pubis	Permethrin 1% creme rinse *or* Lindane 1% shampoo *or* Pyrethrins with piperonyl butoxide	*Phthirus pubis* (pubic lice)
Scabies	Permethrin cream (5%)	*Sarcoptes scabiei*
Genital and Anal Warts‖		Human papillomavirus
External genital	*Patient administered:* Podofilox 0.5% solution or gel (topical) *or* Imiquimod 5% cream (topical) *Provider administered:* Cryotherapy with liquid nitrogren or cryoprobe *or* Podophyllin 10%–25% (topical) *or* TCA or BCA 80%–90% (topical) *or* Surgical excision	
Anal	Cryotherapy with liquid nitrogen *or* TCA or BCA (80%–90%) applied to warts *or* Surgical excision	
Vaginal	Cryotherapy with liquid nitrogen *or* TCA or BCA (80%–90%) applied to warts	
Urethral meatus	Cryotherapy with liquid nitrogen *or* Podophyllin 10%–25% (topical)	
Oral	Cryotherapy with liquid nitrogen *or* Surgical excision	

‖TCA = trichloroacetic acid, BCA = bichloroacetic acid.

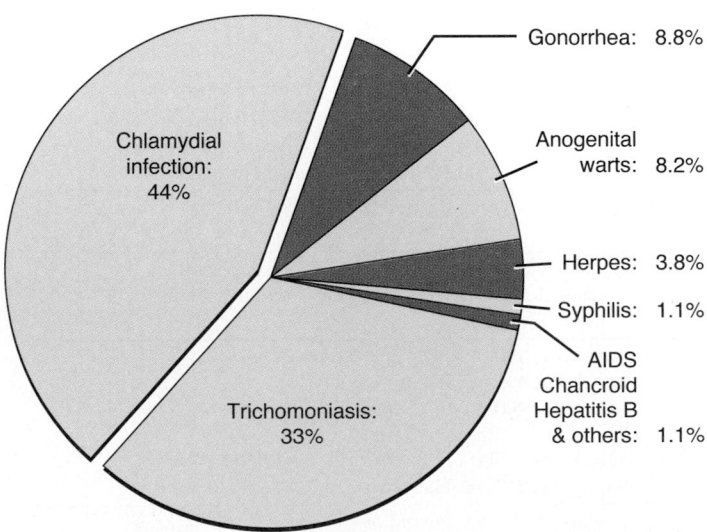

Figure 91–1 ■ Annual incidence of sexually transmitted diseases.

romycin succinate, 12.5 mg/kg 4 times a day for 14 days. For children who weigh 45 kg or more, but are less than 8 years old, the preferred treatment is a single 1-gm oral dose of *azithromycin.* For children at least 8 years old, the preferred treatments are (1) a single 1-gm oral dose of *azithromycin* or (2) 100 mg of *doxycycline* PO twice daily for 7 days.

Lymphogranuloma Venereum. LGV is caused by a unique strain of *C. trachomatis.* Transmission is strictly by sexual contact. LGV is most common in tropical countries, but does occur in the United States, especially in the South. Infection begins as a small erosion or papule in the genital region. From this site, the organism migrates to regional lymph nodes, causing swelling, tenderness, and blockage of lymphatic flow. Tremendous enlargement of the genitalia may result. The enlarged nodes, called buboes, may break open and drain. The treatment of choice for genital, inguinal, and anorectal LGV is 100 mg of *doxycycline* PO twice daily for 3 weeks.

GONOCOCCAL INFECTIONS

Characteristics

Gonorrhea is caused by *Neisseria gonorrhoeae,* a gram-negative diplococcus often referred to as the gonococcus. The incidence of gonorrhea is high: About 650,000 Americans acquire the infection each year. Gonorrhea is transmitted primarily by sexual contact, although it can also be transmitted by contact with infected exudates.

The intensity of symptoms differs between men and women. In men, the main symptoms are a burning sensation during urination and a pus-like discharge from the penis. In contrast, gonorrhea in women is commonly asymptomatic. However, serious infection of female reproductive structures (vagina, urethra, cervix, ovaries, fallopian tubes) can occur, ultimately resulting in sterility. Among people who engage in oral sex, the mouth and throat can become infected, causing sore throat and tonsillitis. Among people who engage in receptive anal sex, the rectum can become infected, causing a purulent discharge and constant urge to move the bowels. Bacteremia can develop in both sexes, causing cutaneous lesions, arthritis, and, rarely, meningitis and endocarditis.

Treatment

Because of antibiotic resistance, treatment of gonorrhea has changed over the years—and undoubtedly will continue to evolve. In the 1930s, virtually all strains of the gonococcus were sensitive to sulfonamides. However, within a decade, sulfonamide resistance had become common. Fortunately, by that time penicillin had become available, and the drug was active against all gonococcal strains. However, in 1976, organisms resistant to penicillin began to emerge. More recently, resistance to tetracyclines and quinolones has begun to appear.

A high percentage of patients with gonococcal infection are co-infected with *C. trachomatis.* Accordingly, when they are treated for gonorrhea, they should be treated for *C. trachomatis* as well (unless the infection has been ruled out). As noted above, the preferred drugs for *C. trachomatis* are *doxycycline* and *azithromycin.*

Urethral, Cervical, and Rectal Infection. Five agents are recommended for these infections: *cefixime* [Suprax], 400 mg PO once; *ceftriaxone* [Rocephin], 125 mg IM once; *ciprofloxacin* [Cipro], 500 mg PO once; *ofloxacin* [Floxin], 400 mg once; and *levofloxacin* [Levaquin], 250 mg PO once. Alternatives include *spectinomycin* (IM), *cefuroxime* (PO), and *gatifloxacin* (PO).

Pharyngeal Infection. Gonococcal infection of the pharynx is more difficult to treat than infection of the urethra, cervix, or rectum. The preferred treatments are IM ceftriaxone and PO ciprofloxacin. Dosages are the same as for urethral, cervical, or rectal infection.

Conjunctivitis. Gonococcal conjunctivitis can be reliably eradicated with ceftriaxone, 1 gm IM once. Treatment also includes washing the infected eye with saline solution once.

Disseminated Gonococcal Infection. Disseminated gonococcal infection (DGI) occurs secondary to gonococcal bacteremia. Symptoms include petechial or pustular skin lesions, arthritis, arthralgia, and tenosynovitis (inflammation of the tendon sheath). Endocarditis and meningitis occur rarely. Strains of *N. gonorrhoeae* that cause DGI are uncommon in the United States. In the absence of endocarditis or meningitis, treatment consists of IM or IV *ceftriaxone,* 1 gm every 24 hours. For patients with endocarditis or meningitis, the preferred treatment is IV *ceftriaxone,* 1 to 2 gm every 12 hours.

Neonatal Infection. Neonatal gonococcal infection is acquired through contact with infected cervical exudates during the birth process. Infection can be limited to the eyes or it may be disseminated.

Gonococcal *neonatal ophthalmia* is a serious infection. The initial symptom is conjunctivitis. Over time, other structures of the eye become involved. Blindness can result. The recommended therapy is IV or IM *ceftriaxone,* 25 to 50 mg/kg administered once.

To protect against neonatal ophthalmia, a topical antibiotic should be instilled into both eyes immediately postpartum—as required by law in most states. Any of three agents may be used: *0.5% erythromycin, 1% silver nitrate,* or *1% tetracycline.* It should be noted, however, that topical antibiotics are not 100% effective. Furthermore, if parenteral therapy is to be used, topical therapy is unnecessary.

In neonates, *disseminated gonococcal infection* is rare. Possible manifestations include sepsis, arthritis, meningitis, and scalp abscesses. There are two recommended treatments: (1) *ceftriaxone,* 25 to 50 mg/kg IV or IM once a day for 7 days (or for 10 to 14 days if meningitis is present); and (2) *cefotaxime,* 25 mg/kg IV or IM every 12 hours for 7 days (or for 10 to 14 days if meningitis is present).

Children. Among preadolescent children, sexual abuse is the most likely cause of gonococcal infection. Vaginal, anorectal, and pharyngeal infections are most common. Because of legal implications, diagnosis must be definitive.

Treatment depends on the weight of the child and the type of infection. For children who weigh less than 45 kg and have localized infection (vulvovaginitis, cervicitis, urethritis, pharyngitis, proctitis), the preferred treatment is a single 125-mg IM dose of *ceftriaxone.* For children who weigh less than 45 kg and have systemic infection (bacteremia, arthritis), the preferred treatment is *ceftriaxone,* 50 mg/kg IV or IV once daily for 7 days. For children who weigh 45 kg or more, treatment is the same as for adults—except that fluoroquinolones (e.g., ciprofloxacin) should probably be avoided.

NONGONOCOCCAL URETHRITIS

Nongonococcal urethritis (NGU) is defined as urethritis caused by any organism other than *N. gonorrhoeae,* the gonococcus. The most common infectious agents are *C. trachomatis* (25% to 40%), *Ureaplasma urealyticum* (about 20%), and *Trichomonas vaginalis* (<5%). NGU is diagnosed by the presence of polymorphonuclear leukocytes and a negative culture for *N. gonorrhoeae.* The infection is especially prevalent among sexually active adolescent girls. The recommended treatment is either (1) *azithromycin* [Zithromax], 1 gm PO once, or (2) *doxycycline* [Vibramycin], 100 mg twice daily for 7 days. For persistent or recurrent NGU, the recommended treatment is *metronidazole* [Flagyl], 2 gm PO once, combined with either *erythromycin base* (500 mg PO 4 times a day for 7 days) or *erythromycin ethylsuccinate* (800 mg PO 4 times a day for 7 days).

PELVIC INFLAMMATORY DISEASE

Acute PID is a syndrome that includes endometritis, pelvic peritonitis, tubo-ovarian abscess, and inflammation of the fallopian tubes. Infertility can result. Prominent symptoms are abdominal pain, vaginal discharge, and fever. Most frequently, PID is caused by *N. gonorrhoeae, C. trachomatis,* or both. However, *Mycoplasma hominis* as well as assorted anaerobic and facultative bacteria may also be present.

Because multiple organisms are likely to be involved, drug therapy must provide broad coverage. Since no single drug can do this, combination therapy is required. For the *hospitalized patient,* treatment can be initiated with either *cefoxitin* (2 gm IV every 6 hours) or *cefotetan* (2 gm IV every 12 hours), combined with *doxycycline* (100 mg IV or PO every 12 hours). After symptoms resolve, IV therapy can be discontinued—but must be followed by oral *doxycycline* (100 mg every 12 hours) to complete a 14-day course of treatment.

Outpatients can be treated with either *ofloxacin* (400 mg PO every 12 hours for 2 weeks) or *levofloxacin* (500 mg PO daily for 2 weeks). *Metronidazole* (500 mg PO every 12 hours for 2 weeks) may also be included. Because PID can be difficult to treat, and since the consequences of failure can be severe (e.g., sterility), many experts recommend that *all* patients receive IV antibiotics in a hospital.

ACUTE EPIDIDYMITIS

Epididymitis may be acquired by sexual contact or nonsexually. Sexually acquired epididymitis is usually caused by *N. gonorrhoeae, C. trachomatis,* or both. It may also be caused by *Escherichia coli.* The syndrome occurs primarily in young adults (under 35 years) and may be associated with urethritis. Primary symptoms are fever accompanied by pain in the back of the testicles that develops over the course of several hours. For patients with gonococcal or chlamydial infection, the recommended treatment is *ceftriaxone* [Rocephin], 250 mg IM once, plus *doxycycline* [Vibramycin, others], 100 mg PO twice daily for 7 days. For patients with infection caused by *E. coli,* the recommended treatment is *ofloxacin* [Floxin], 300 mg PO twice daily for 10 days, or *levofloxacin* [Levaquin], 500 mg PO once daily for 10 days. Testicular pain can be managed with analgesics, bed rest, and ice packs.

Nonsexually transmitted epididymitis generally occurs in older men and men who have had urinary tract instrumentation. Causative organisms are gram-negative enteric bacilli and *Pseudomonas.* Ofloxacin can be used for treatment.

SYPHILIS

Syphilis is caused by the spirochete *Treponema pallidum.* The incidence of syphilis increased during the 1980s but has steadily declined throughout the 1990s. In the United States, about 120,000 people are infected each year. Fortunately, *T. pallidum* has remained highly responsive to penicillin, the drug of choice for treatment.

Characteristics. Syphilis develops in three stages, termed primary, secondary, and tertiary. *Treponema pallidum* enters the body by penetrating the mucous membranes of the mouth, vagina, or urethra of the penis. After an incubation period of 1 to 4 weeks, a primary lesion, called a chancre, develops at the site of entry. The chancre is a hard, red, protruding, painless sore. Nearby lymph nodes may become swollen. Within a few weeks the chancre heals spontaneously, although *T. pallidum* is still present.

Two to 6 weeks after the chancre heals, secondary syphilis develops. Symptoms result from spread of *T. pallidum* via the bloodstream. Skin lesions and flu-like symptoms (fever, headache, reduced appetite, general malaise) are typical. Enlarged lymph nodes and joint pain may also be present. The symptoms of secondary syphilis resolve in 4 to 8 weeks—but may recur episodically over the next 3 to 4 years.

Tertiary syphilis develops 5 to 40 years after the initial infection. Almost any organ can be involved. Infection of the brain—neurosyphilis—is common, and can cause senility, paralysis, and severe psychiatric symptoms. The heart valves and aorta may be damaged. Lesions may also occur in the skin, bones, joints, and eyes. The risk of neurosyphilis is increased in individuals who are infected with HIV.

Infants exposed to *T. pallidum in utero* can be born with syphilis. Signs of congenital syphilis include sores, rhinitis, deafness, and severe tenderness over bones.

Treatment. *Penicillin G* is the drug of choice for all stages of syphilis. The form and dosage of penicillin G depend on the disease stage. *Early syphilis* (primary, secondary, or latent syphilis of less than 1 year's duration) is treated with a single IM dose (2.4 million units) of benzathine penicillin G. *Late syphilis* (more than 1 year's duration) is also treated with IM benzathine penicillin G, but the dosage is increased (2.4 million units once a week for 3 weeks). *Neurosyphilis* requires more aggressive therapy. The recommended treatment is 18 to 24 million units of penicillin G daily for 14 days, administered by continuous infusion. For *congenital syphilis,* two regimens have been recommended: (1) IV penicillin G, 50,000 units/kg every 12 hours for the first 7 days after birth followed by the same dose every 8 hours for 3 more days; or (2) IM procaine penicillin G, 50,000 units/kg once daily for 10 days. *Syphilis in pregnancy* should be treated with penicillin G, using a dosage appropriate to the stage of the disease.

How should patients with *penicillin allergy* be treated? For *nonpregnant* patients, either *doxycycline* or *tetracycline* may be used. Dosages for *early syphilis* are (1) doxycycline, 100 mg PO twice daily for 2 weeks, or (2) tetracycline, 500 mg PO 4 times a day for 2 weeks. Dosages for *late syphilis* are the same as for early syphilis, except that treatment lasts 4 weeks instead of 2. If the patient is *pregnant,* the U.S. Public Health Service recommends that she go through a penicillin-allergy desensitization protocol to permit penicillin use, rather than substituting another drug for penicillin.

ACQUIRED IMMUNODEFICIENCY SYNDROME

AIDS is caused by the human immunodeficiency virus (HIV). The pathophysiology and treatment of HIV infection are discussed in Chapter 90.

CHANCROID

Chancroid, also known as soft chancre, is caused by *Haemophilus ducreyi.* Transmission is primarily by sexual contact. The infection is characterized by a painful, ragged ulcer at the site of inoculation, usually the external genitalia. Regional lymph nodes may be swollen. Multiple secondary lesions may develop. Although primarily a tropical disease, chancroid has become an important STD in the United States. There are four recommended treatments: (1) *azithromycin* [Zithromax], 1 gm PO once; (2) *ceftriaxone* [Rocephin], 250 mg IM once; (3) *ciprofloxacin* [Cipro], 500 mg PO twice a day for 3 days; and (4) *erythromycin,* 500 mg PO 3 times a day for 7 days.

TRICHOMONIASIS

Trichomoniasis is an STD caused by *Trichomonas vaginalis.* In men, the infection is usually asymptomatic. In women, the infection may be asymptomatic or may cause a diffuse, malodorous, yellow-green vaginal discharge, along with burning and itching sensations. Most infections can be eliminated with a single, 2-gm oral dose of *metronidazole* [Flagyl, others]. This dose can be repeated in the event of treatment failure. Male partners of infected women should always be treated, even if they are asymptomatic. Although some clinicians remain concerned about giving metronidazole during pregnancy, there is no evidence that the drug causes birth defects in humans.

BACTERIAL VAGINOSIS

Bacterial vaginosis results from an alteration in vaginal microflora. Organisms responsible for the syndrome include *Gardnerella vaginalis* (also known as *Haemophilus vaginalis*), *Mycoplasma hominis,* and various anaerobes. The syndrome occurs most commonly in sexually active women, although it may not actually be transmitted sexually. Bacterial vaginosis is characterized by a malodorous vaginal discharge, elevation of vaginal pH (above 4.5), and generation of a fishy odor when vaginal secretions are mixed with 10% potassium hydroxide.

Treatment may be oral or intravaginal. The recommended oral therapy is *metronidazole* [Flagyl], 500 mg twice a day for 7 days. Two intravaginal options are available: (1) *metronidazole* (0.75% gel), 5 gm twice daily for 5 days; and (2) *clindamycin* (2% cream), 5 gm every evening for 7 days.

HERPES SIMPLEX INFECTIONS

Characteristics. Most genital herpes infections are caused by herpes simplex virus type 2 (HSV-2). A few genital infections are caused by herpes simplex virus type 1, the herpesvirus that causes cold sores. Genital herpes is transmitted primarily by sexual contact. In the United States, the infection has reached epidemic proportions, afflicting over 45 million people. About 500,000 new cases occur annually. There is no cure.

Symptoms of primary infection develop 6 to 8 days after contact. In females, blisters or vesicles can appear on the perianal skin, labia, vagina, cervix, and foreskin of the clitoris. In males, vesicles develop on the penis and occasionally on the testicles. Painful urination and a watery discharge can occur in both sexes. Also, the patient may experience systemic symptoms: fever, headache, myalgia, and tender, swollen lymph nodes in the affected region. Within days, the original blisters can evolve into large, painful, ulcer-like sores. Over the next 2 to 3 weeks, all symptoms resolve spontaneously. However, this does not indicate cure: The virus remains present in a latent state and can cause recurrence. Because we can't eliminate the virus, symptoms may recur for life. Fortunately, subsequent episodes become progressively shorter and less severe, and in some cases cease entirely. Transmission of HSV-2 can occur when symptoms are absent as well as when symptoms are present. Use of a condom reduces the risk of transmission.

Neonatal Infection. Genital herpes in pregnant women can be transmitted to the infant. The infant can acquire the virus *in utero* or during delivery. Infection acquired *in utero* can result in spontaneous abortion or fetal malformation. Infection acquired during delivery can cause severe neurologic damage and even death. To protect the infant during delivery, birth should be accomplished by cesarean section if the mother has an active infection.

Treatment. Genital herpes can be treated with three drugs: *acyclovir* [Zovirax], *famciclovir* [Famvir], and *valacyclovir* [Valtrex]. These agents cannot eliminate the virus, but they can reduce symptoms and shorten the duration of pain and viral shedding. Patients with recurrent infection may take these agents every day or just when symptoms appear. Continuous daily administration reduces the frequency and intensity of episodes, whereas episodic treatment simply reduces symptoms once an episode has begun. Dosing information is summarized in Table 91–1.

Suppression of Transmission. Recent data indicate that *valacyclovir* (500 mg once daily) can decrease transmission of genital herpes by 50%. This is the first demonstration that a drug can reduce transmission of this STD—or any STD, for that matter. Unfortunately, treatment is somewhat expensive, costing about $3.50 a day (about $1280 a year). Also, valacyclovir only *reduces* transmission, it doesn't stop it entirely. Accordingly, patients must continue to use condoms, and must abstain from sex at times when the infection is active.

GENITAL AND ANAL WARTS (CONDYLOMATA ACUMINATA)

Genital and perianal warts are caused by human papillomaviruses (HPVs), of which there are 40 types. Although warts caused by most types of HPV are benign, warts caused by a few types have been strongly associated with genital carcinoma. Accordingly, a wart biopsy may be appropriate.

HPV can be transmitted by sexual contact. Individuals with anogenital warts should be warned that they can transmit the infection to sexual partners. Partners of infected individuals should be examined for warts. Use of a condom can minimize the risk of transmission.

Several forms of therapy are used to remove venereal warts. However, no therapy can eradicate the virus. Hence, even after successful wart removal, the virus remains.

Genital warts can be removed in two basic ways: with physical measures or with topical drugs. Physical measures—cryotherapy (freezing), electrodesiccation, laser surgery, and conventional surgery—are much faster than drugs but more painful. Procedures that are suitable for removing warts at specific locations are summarized in Table 91–1.

The drugs used to remove warts can be divided into two groups: (1) agents that must be administered by a physician and (2) agents that can be applied at home. With both groups, application is done repeatedly until the warts disappear. Physician-applied drugs include *10% to 25% podophyllin* [Podocon-25, Podofin], *80% to 90% trichloroacetic acid* (TCA), and *80% to 90% bichloroacetic acid* (BCA). Podophyllin is applied once every 1 to 2 weeks. TCA and BCA are reapplied after erosions from the prior treatment have healed, which usually takes 2 to 4 weeks. Two preparations can be applied at home: *0.5% podofilox* [Condylox] and *5% imiquimod* [Aldara]. Podofilox is applied 2 times a day for 3 consecutive days each week. Imiquimod is applied overnight 3 times a week. All of the drugs used for wart removal act slowly and they all cause irritation. The pharmacology of these agents is discussed in Chapter 101.

PROCTITIS

Sexually acquired proctitis (inflammation of the rectum) results primarily from receptive anal intercourse. Symptoms include anorectal pain, tenesmus (painful straining at stool), and rectal discharge. Usual causative organisms are *N. gonorrhoeae, C. trachomatis, T. pallidum,* and HSV. The preferred treatment is *ceftriaxone* (125 mg IM once) plus *doxycycline* (100 mg PO twice daily for 7 days).

PEDICULOSIS PUBIS AND SCABIES

Pediculosis pubis and scabies are skin infestations caused by lice and mites, respectively. Both infestations produce intense itching, and both can be transmitted by sexual contact. Topical *permethrin* can eliminate both organisms: 1% permethrin [Nix] is used for pubic lice; 5% permethrin [Elimite] is used for scabies. Pediculosis, scabies, and their treatment are discussed fully in Chapter 96 (Ectoparasiticides).

∴ KEY POINTS

All of the drugs used to treat STDs have been introduced in other chapters. Key points for these drugs are presented in those chapters.

Antiseptics and Disinfectants

Antiseptics and disinfectants are locally acting drugs that are toxic to microorganisms. These agents are used to reduce acquisition and transmission of infection. Drugs suitable for antisepsis and disinfection cannot be used internally because of toxicity.

GENERAL CONSIDERATIONS

Terminology

The terms *antiseptic* and *disinfectant* are not synonymous. In common usage, the term *antiseptic* is reserved for agents *applied to living tissue. Disinfectants* are preparations *applied to inanimate objects.* As a rule, agents used as disinfectants are too harsh for application to living tissue. Disinfectants are employed most frequently to decontaminate surgical instruments and to cleanse hospitals and other medical facilities. Most uses of antiseptics are prophylactic. For example, antiseptics are used to cleanse the hands of medical personnel; they are applied to the patient's skin prior to invasive procedures (surgery, insertion of needles); and they are used to bathe neonates. Rarely, antiseptics are employed to treat an existing local infection. However, in most cases, established infections are best treated with a systemic antimicrobial drug.

    Several related terms may need clarification. *Sterilization* indicates complete destruction of all microorganisms. In contrast, *sanitization* implies only that contamination has been reduced to a level compatible with public health standards. A *germicide* is a drug that *kills* microorganisms. Germicides may be divided into subcategories: *bactericides, virucides, fungicides,* and *amebicides.* In contrast to a germicide, a *germistatic drug* is one that decreases the growth and replication of microorganisms, but does not kill them.

Properties of an Ideal Antiseptic

The ideal antiseptic, like any other ideal drug, should be safe, effective, and selective. The preparation should be germicidal (rather than germistatic) and should have a broad spectrum of antimicrobial activity: The drug should kill bacteria and their spores, and also viruses, protozoa, yeasts, and fungi. Effects should have a rapid onset and long duration. Development of microbial resistance should be low. The drug should have no harmful effects on humans: It should not produce local injury, impair healing, or produce systemic toxicity following topical application. Lastly, the drug should not cause stains and should be devoid of offensive odor. No antiseptic has all of these properties.

Time Course of Action

Toxicity to microorganisms is determined in part by duration of exposure to an antiseptic or disinfectant. Some agents act much more quickly than others. For example, ethanol (70% solution) reduces cutaneous bacterial count by 50% in just 36 seconds. In contrast, benzalkonium chloride (at a dilution of 1:1000) requires 7 minutes to produce the same effect. Because such differences in time course exist, effective use of antiseptics and disinfectants requires that healthcare personnel understand the exposure requirements of these agents.

Use of Antiseptics to Treat Established Local Infection

In the past, topical agents were used routinely to treat established local infection. Today, *systemic* anti-infective drugs are the treatment of choice. Systemic agents are preferred for two reasons: they are more effective than topical drugs, and they are less damaging to inflamed or abraded tissue. Experience has shown that antiseptics do little to reduce infection in wounds, cuts, and abrasions. This lack of efficacy is attributed to poor penetration to the site of infection, and to diminished activity in the presence of wound exudates. Although of limited value for *established* local infection, antiseptics are quite useful as *prophylaxis:* When applied properly, antiseptics can help cleanse wounds and decrease microbial contamination.

Using Antiseptics and Disinfectants Most Effectively

The principal value of antiseptics and disinfectants derives from their ability to prevent contamination of the patient by microorganisms present in the *environment;* it appears that antiseptics applied directly to the *patient* contribute relatively little to prophylaxis against infection. A number of clinical studies support this conclusion. In one study, over 5000 preoperative patients were bathed with hexachlorophene. Although this treatment greatly reduced the concentration of surface bacteria, it had no effect on the incidence of postoperative infection. Similarly, in a study of patients who had undergone cardiothoracic surgery, it was found that most postoperative infections were caused by organisms not present at the site of incision. From these studies and others, we can conclude that infections are caused primarily by environmental microorganisms rather than by organisms living on the skin of the patient. Consequently, use of antiseptics by nurses, physicians, and others who contact the patient is of much greater importance than application of antiseptics to the patient. Patients also benefit greatly by the rigorous use of disinfectants to decontaminate surgical supplies and medical buildings.

PROPERTIES OF INDIVIDUAL ANTISEPTICS AND DISINFECTANTS

Antiseptics and disinfectants derive from a variety of chemical families, ranging from alcohols to iodine compounds to phenols. The various antiseptics and disinfectants differ from one another with respect to mechanism of action, time course, and antimicrobial spectrum. In almost all cases, the drugs employed as disinfectants are not used for antisepsis and vice versa. The more commonly employed antiseptics and disinfectants are listed in Table 92–1. For each drug, the table indicates chemical family and clinical use (antisepsis, disinfection, or both).

Alcohols
Ethanol

Ethanol (ethyl alcohol) is an effective virucide and kills most common pathogenic bacteria as well. The drug is inactive against bacterial spores, and its activity against fungi is erratic. Bactericidal effects result from precipitating bacterial proteins and dissolving membranes. Ethanol can enhance the effects of several other antimicrobial preparations (e.g., chlorhexidine, hexachlorophene, benzalkonium chloride).

Ethanol is employed almost exclusively for *antisepsis*. The most frequent uses are hand washing by hospital staff and cleansing the skin prior to needle insertion and minor surgery. Because it has limited activity against bacterial spores and fungi, ethanol is not a good disinfectant.

Optimal bacterial kill requires that ethanol be present in the proper concentration and for sufficient time. The drug is most effective at a concentration of 70%. Higher concentrations are *less* active. To produce 90% kill of surface bacteria, the skin must be kept moist with ethanol for 2 minutes. This extended exposure can be accomplished by using ethanol foam. Exposure is prolonged because evaporation from this formulation is slower than from ethanol solution.

Ethanol should not be applied to open wounds. The drug can increase tissue damage and, by causing coagulation of proteins, can form a mass under which bacteria can thrive.

Isopropanol

Isopropanol (isopropyl alcohol) is employed primarily as an antiseptic. When applied in concentrations greater than 70%, isopropanol is somewhat more germicidal than ethanol. Like ethanol, isopropanol can increase the effects of other antiseptics. Isopropanol promotes local vasodilation and can thereby increase bleeding from needle punctures and incisions. Isopropanol is available in concentrations ranging from 70% to 100%.

Aldehydes
Glutaraldehyde

Glutaraldehyde [Cidex] is lethal to all microorganisms; the drug kills bacteria, bacterial spores, viruses, and fungi. Antimicrobial effects result from cross-linking and precipitating proteins. Glutaraldehyde is used to disinfect and sterilize surgical instruments and other medical supplies, including respiratory and anesthetic equipment, catheters, and thermometers. The drug is too harsh for antiseptic use. To completely elimi-

		Application	
Chemical Category	**Drug**	**Antisepsis**	**Disinfection**
Alcohols	Ethanol	✔	
	Isopropanol	✔	
Aldehydes	Glutaraldehyde		✔
	Formaldehyde		✔
Iodine Compounds	Iodine tincture	✔	
	Iodine solution	✔	
	Povidone iodine	✔	✔
Chlorine Compounds	Oxychlorosene	✔	
	Sodium hypochlorite	✔	✔
Phenolic Compound	Hexachlorophene	✔	
Miscellaneous Agents	Chlorhexidine	✔	
	Thimerosal	✔	
	Hydrogen peroxide		✔
	Benzalkonium chloride	✔	✔

TABLE 92–1 ■ Antiseptics and Disinfectants: Chemical Category and Application

nate bacterial spores, instruments and equipment must be immersed in glutaraldehyde for at least 10 hours. Glutaraldehyde is most active at alkaline pH. However, under alkaline conditions, glutaraldehyde eventually becomes inactive because of gradual polymerization. Consequently, alkaline solutions of glutaraldehyde are active for only 2 to 4 weeks. Glutaraldehyde should be used with adequate ventilation because fumes can irritate the respiratory tract.

Formaldehyde

Formaldehyde kills bacteria, bacterial spores, viruses, and fungi. Like glutaraldehyde, formaldehyde is too harsh for application to the skin. Accordingly, use is limited to disinfection and sterilization of equipment and instruments. For two reasons, formaldehyde is less desirable than glutaraldehyde. First, formaldehyde acts slowly: Destruction of bacterial spores may take 2 to 4 days. Second, because it is more volatile than glutaraldehyde, formaldehyde tends to cause more respiratory irritation.

Iodine Compounds
Iodine Solution and Iodine Tincture

Iodine was first employed as an antiseptic more than 160 years ago. Despite the introduction of numerous other drugs, iodine remains one of our most widely used germicidal agents. The drug is extremely effective, having the ability to kill all known bacteria, fungi, protozoa, viruses, and yeasts. Additional assets are low cost and low toxicity.

The composition of iodine solution and iodine tincture is very similar. Iodine *solution* consists of 2% elemental iodine and 2.4% sodium iodide in water. Iodine *tincture* contains the same amounts of elemental iodine and sodium iodide and also contains 47% ethanol. The ethanol enhances the antimicrobial activity of iodine tincture.

The germicidal activity of iodine tincture and iodine solution is due only to *free* (dissolved) elemental iodine. In both the tincture and the solution, the concentration of free elemental iodine is only about 0.15%. This low figure reflects the poor solubility of iodine. Because only free iodine is active, most of the elemental iodine and all of the sodium iodide present in both iodine tincture and iodine solution do not contribute *directly* to microbicidal activity. However, these components do contribute *indirectly* by serving as reservoirs from which free elemental iodine can be released.

Iodine tincture and iodine solution are employed primarily for antisepsis of the skin, a use for which they are the most effective agents available. When the skin is *intact*, iodine *tincture* is preferred. This preparation is commonly employed to cleanse the skin prior to IV injection and withdrawal of blood for microbial culture. For treatment of *wounds* and *abrasions*, iodine *solution* should be employed. (Because alcohol is an irritant, iodine tincture is less appropriate for application to broken skin.)

Povidone-Iodine

Povidone-iodine is a complex of elemental iodine plus povidone (an organic polymer). Povidone-iodine has no antimicrobial activity of its own. Rather, it serves as a reservoir from which elemental iodine can be released. Free elemental iodine is the active germicide. The concentration of free iodine achieved with application of povidone-iodine is lower than that produced with application of iodine tincture or iodine solution. Hence, povidone-iodine is less effective than these other iodine preparations. Povidone-iodine is employed primarily for prophylaxis of postoperative infection. Additional uses include hand washing, surgical scrubbing, and preparing the skin prior to invasive procedures (e.g., surgery, aspiration, injection). In addition, povidone-iodine is employed to sterilize equipment, although superior disinfectants are

available. The drug is dispensed in a variety of formulations (ointments, solutions, aerosols, gels). It is also available impregnated in swabs, sponges, and wipes. Trade names include ACU-dyne, Betadine, and Operand.

Chlorine Compounds

Chlorine is lethal to a wide variety of microbes. Chlorine is active both as elemental chlorine and as hypochlorous acid, which is formed by reaction of chlorine with water. Chlorine is used extensively to sanitize water supplies and swimming pools. However, because of physical properties that make working with chlorine difficult, chlorine itself is rarely used clinically. Instead, chlorine-containing compounds that release hypochlorous acid are employed.

Oxychlorosene Sodium

Oxychlorosene sodium [Clorpactin] is a complex mixture of hypochlorous acid with alkylphenyl sulfonates. Antimicrobial effects derive from releasing hypochlorous acid. Oxychlorosene is lethal to bacteria, yeasts, fungi, viruses, molds, and spores. The preparation is employed as a topical antiseptic and can be especially useful for treating localized infection caused by drug-resistant microbes. Oxychlorosene is also employed to irrigate and cleanse fistulas, sinus tracts, wounds, and empyemas (pus-filled cavities).

Sodium Hypochlorite

Sodium hypochlorite kills bacteria, spores, fungi, protozoa, and viruses. Undiluted (5%) solutions are employed commonly as household bleach. These concentrated solutions are too irritating for application to human tissue. For antiseptic use, dilute (0.5%) solutions are employed. These preparations can be used to irrigate wounds and to cleanse and deodorize necrotic tissue. To minimize local irritation, solutions of sodium hypochlorite should be rinsed off promptly. A 1% solution can be used to sterilize equipment. Solutions of sodium hypochlorite are unstable and must be prepared fresh before each use.

Phenols

The family of phenolic compounds consists of phenol itself and several phenol derivatives. Following its introduction in 1867, phenol rapidly became both the antiseptic and disinfectant of choice. Today, use of phenol for antiseptic purposes is rare. However, the drug is still employed in some hospitals for disinfection. One member of the phenol family—hexachlorophene—is discussed below.

Hexachlorophene

Actions. Hexachlorophene is *bacteriostatic*, not bactericidal. The drug is quite active against gram-positive bacteria—the bacteria found most frequently on the skin. However, hexachlorophene has little or no effect on gram-negative bacteria. In fact, when used on a regular basis, hexachlorophene encourages overgrowth with gram-negative organisms. (By killing off gram-positive bacteria, hexachlorophene makes conditions more conducive to gram-negative growth.)

Uses. Hexachlorophene is employed most commonly as a hand-washing preparation for healthcare personnel. Although the effects of a single wash are minimal, with repeated use hexachlorophene can significantly reduce the population of cutaneous gram-positive bacteria. This cumulative effect results from residual hexachlorophene retained on the skin. Hexachlorophene has been employed to prepare the skin prior to surgery. However, availability of superior antiseptics (e.g., chlorhexidine) makes this use inappropriate.

Adverse Effects. Hexachlorophene can be absorbed through intact skin and mucous membranes. Absorption through denuded areas can be especially significant. If absorbed in sufficient amounts, hexachlorophene causes central nervous system stimulation. Responses range from confusion to twitching to seizures. Deaths have occurred. To minimize systemic toxicity, hexachlorophene should not be applied extensively to burns, wounds, cuts, or mucous membranes. In addition, total body bathing, especially of infants, should be avoided. For bathing infants, chlorhexidine is safer and more effective.

Preparations. Hexachlorophene is available only by prescription. The drug is dispensed in solution and as a foam. Trade names are pHisoHex and Septisol.

Miscellaneous Agents
Chlorhexidine

Actions and Uses. Chlorhexidine is an important surgical antiseptic. The drug is fast acting and lethal to most gram-positive and gram-negative bacteria. Virucidal activity is lacking. Antibacterial effects are reduced somewhat in the presence of soap, blood, and pus. Chlorhexidine that remains on the skin after rinsing is sufficient to exert continuing germicidal effects. Chlorhexidine is used for preoperative preparation of the skin and as a surgical scrub, hand-wash preparation, and wound cleanser.

Adverse Effects. Chlorhexidine is very safe. Even with routine preoperative use, local adverse effects are rare. Inadvertent IV injection has been reported twice: in one patient, hemolysis occurred; in the other, no ill effects were observed.

Preparations. Chlorhexidine gluconate (0.5%, 2%, 4%) is dispensed in combination with isopropanol (4% or 70%). Trade names include Exidine-2 Scrub, Dyna-Hex 2 Skin Cleanser, Hibistat Germicidal Hand Rinse, and Hibiclens.

Hydrogen Peroxide

Hydrogen peroxide is an excellent disinfectant and sterilizing agent, but is useless as an antiseptic. The entity in hydrogen peroxide solution responsible for antimicrobial effects is the hydroxyl free radical. These free radicals are destroyed when hydrogen peroxide is acted upon by catalase, an enzyme found in all tissues. Hence, contact with tissue terminates hydrogen peroxide's germicidal actions. The only benefit resulting from application of hydrogen peroxide to wounds derives from liberation of oxygen (by the reaction with catalase), which causes frothing that is sufficient to loosen debris and thereby facilitate cleansing. The principal use of hydrogen peroxide is disinfection and sterilization of instruments. A 3% to 6% solution is employed.

Thimerosal

Thimerosal is an organic compound that contains 49% mercury, the active antimicrobial factor. Thimerosal has only weak bacteriostatic and fungistatic properties; it does not kill bacteria or fungi. Antimicrobial actions are reduced in the presence of blood and tissue proteins. Thimerosal is less effective than ethanol. Use on large areas of denuded skin may yield systemic toxicity from absorption of mercury. Poisoning from thimerosal ingestion can be treated with dimercaprol (see Chapter 105). Thimerosal has been employed to irrigate wounds and to prepare the skin prior to surgery. It has also been employed as an antiseptic for the eyes, nose, throat, and genitourinary tract. Trade names are Mersol and AeroAid.

Benzalkonium Chloride

Actions. Benzalkonium chloride (BAC) is an organic quaternary ammonium compound that has antimicrobial and detergent properties. BAC is active against many gram-positive and gram-negative bacteria as well as some fungi, protozoa, and viruses. The drug is relatively inactive against *Mycobacterium tuberculosis, Clostridium,* and other spore-forming bacteria. Germicidal effects result from disruption of membranes, and are enhanced by ethanol. BAC is inactivated by soaps and organic material. BAC is slow acting compared with iodine.

Antiseptic Uses. BAC is employed for preoperative preparation of the skin and mucous membranes; as a surgical scrub; as an antiseptic for abrasions and minor wounds; as a vaginal douche; and for irrigation of the eyes, body cavities, and genitourinary tract. Since BAC is inactivated by soap, all soap must be removed by rinsing with water and 70% alcohol prior to BAC application. Concentrated solutions of BAC can cause severe local damage. Hence, care must be taken to use solutions of appropriate dilution. For several reasons (limited antimicrobial spectrum, lack of rapid action, potential for toxicity, availability of superior agents), there seems to be little to recommend BAC for antiseptic use.

Disinfectant Use. Immersion in BAC solution is employed for sterile storage of instruments and supplies. Adsorption of BAC onto porous material can significantly reduce the concentration of BAC in solutions. To ensure continuing efficacy, solutions should be changed (or at least replenished with BAC) on a regular basis.

Preparations and Dosage. BAC is dispensed in concentrated (17%) and dilute (1:750) solution. Trade names include Benza and Zephiran. Recommended dilutions are 1:750 (for application to intact skin and to minor wounds and abrasions); 1:2000 to 1:5000 (for application to mucous membranes and diseased or seriously damaged skin); and 1:750 to 1:5000 (for storage of instruments and supplies).

HAND HYGIENE FOR HEALTHCARE WORKERS

Effective hand hygiene is the single most important factor in preventing the spread of infection in healthcare settings. Each year, an estimated 2 million patients in the United States acquire an infection while in a hospital; about 90,000 of them die as a result. Patients can also acquire infections in other settngs, including clinics, dialysis centers, and long-term care facilities. In all of these places, the leading cause of infection spread is the transfer of pathogens from one patient to another on the hands of healthcare workers (HCWs). Accordingly, the best way to reduce new infections in these settings is to improve hand hygiene.

Traditionally, HCWs cleaned their hands with soap and water. Unfortunately, this technique has several drawbacks: it takes considerable time, requires a sink and handwashing supplies, and promotes skin irritation and dryness. As a result, compliance tends to be poor.

In October 2002, the Centers for Disease Control and Prevention (CDC) issued new guidelines designed to improve hand-hygiene practices among HCWs and to reduce transmission of pathogenic microorganisms to patients and personnel in healthcare settings. A central recommendation in the guidelines is the use of *alcohol-based handrubs,* rather than soap and water, for routine hand antisepsis. There are four reasons for this recommendation:

■ *Accessibility*—Handrubs don't require a sink or towels, and hence are more accessible than washing with soap and water.

■ *Time savings*—Using a handrub is much faster than washing with soap and water. All you do is apply the handrub to the palm of one hand, and then rub your hands together until they are dry. The CDC estimates that, during an 8-hour shift, an ICU nurse would save about 1 hour by using a handrub instead of soap and water.

- *Lessened skin damage*—Today's alcohol-based handrubs contain emollients and moisturizers, and hence don't irritate or dry the skin like soap and water do.
- *Greater efficacy*—Alcohol-based handrubs reduce the number of bacteria on the skin more effectively than does washing with soap and water.

Studies have shown that, because of these advantages, switching from soap and water to an alcohol-based handrub can significantly improve compliance among HCWs.

It is important to note that alcohol-based handrubs have limitations. First, they can't remove dirt or organic material. Accordingly, when the hands are visibly soiled, soap and water must be used first. Second, alcohol lacks residual killing power. For routine clinical practice, this lack is no concern. However, under certain conditions—including infectious disease outbreaks and performance of invasive procedures—an antiseptic that does have residual effects (e.g., chlorhexidine), should be used.

Specific CDC Hand-Hygiene Recommendations

Major recommendations from the CDC hand-hygiene guidelines are presented below. Each recommendation is categorized on the basis of existing scientific data, theoretical rationale, applicability, and economic impact. The five categories employed are defined as follows:

Category IA—Strongly recommended for implementation and strongly supported by well-designed experimental, clinical, or epidemiologic studies.

Category IB—Strongly recommended for implementation and supported by certain experimental, clinical, or epidemiologic studies and a strong theoretical rationale.

Category IC—Required for implementation, as mandated by federal or state regulation or standard.

Category II—Suggested for implementation and supported by suggestive clinical or epidemiologic studies or a theoretical rationale.

No recommendation/Unresolved issue—Practices for which insufficient evidence or no consensus regarding efficacy exist.

Indications for Handwashing and Hand Antisepsis

- When hands are visibly dirty or contaminated with proteinaceous material or are visibly soiled with blood or other body fluids, wash hands with either a non-antimicrobial soap and water or an antimicrobial soap and water (IA).
- If hands are not visibly soiled, use an alcohol-based handrub for routinely decontaminating hands in all clinical situations described in italics below (IA). Alternatively, wash hands with an antimicrobial soap and water in all clinical situations described in italics below (IB).
- *Decontaminate hands before having direct contact with patients (IB).*
- *Decontaminate hands before donning sterile gloves when inserting a central intravascular catheter (IB).*
- *Decontaminate hands before inserting indwelling urinary catheters, peripheral vascular catheters, or other invasive devices that do not require a surgical procedure (IB).*

- *Decontaminate hands after contact with a patient's intact skin (e.g., when taking a pulse or blood pressure, and lifting a patient) (IB).*
- *Decontaminate hands after contact with body fluids or excretions, mucous membranes, nonintact skin, and wound dressings if hands are not visibly soiled (IA).*
- *Decontaminate hands if moving from a contaminated body site to a clean body site during patient care (II).*
- *Decontaminate hands after contact with inanimate objects (including medical equipment) in the immediate vicinity of the patient (II).*
- *Decontaminate hands after removing gloves (IB).*
- Before eating and after using a restroom, wash hands with a non-antimicrobial soap and water or with an antimicrobial soap and water (IB).
- Antimicrobial-impregnated wipes (i.e., towelettes) may be considered as an alternative to washing hands with non-antimicrobial soap and water. Because they are not as effective as alcohol-based handrubs or washing hands with an antimicrobial soap and water for reducing bacterial counts on the hands of HCWs, they are not a substitute for using an alcohol-based handrub or antimicrobial soap (IB).
- Wash hands with non-antimicrobial soap and water or with antimicrobial soap and water if exposure to *Bacillus anthracis* is suspected or proven. The physical action of washing and rinsing hands under such circumstances is recommended because alcohols, chlorhexidine, iodophors, and other antiseptic agents have poor activity against spores (II).
- No recommendation can be made regarding the routine use of non–alcohol-based handrubs for hand hygiene in healthcare settings (Unresolved issue).

Hand-Hygiene Technique

- When decontaminating hands with an alcohol-based handrub, apply product to palm of one hand and rub hands together, covering all surfaces of hands and fingers, until hands are dry (IB). Follow the manufacturer's recommendations regarding the volume of product to use.
- When washing hands with soap and water, wet hands first with water, apply an amount of product recommended by the manufacturer to hands, and rub hands together vigorously for at least 15 seconds, covering all surfaces of the hands and fingers. Rinse hands with water and dry thoroughly with a disposable towel. Use towel to turn off the faucet (IB). Avoid using hot water, because repeated exposure to hot water may increase the risk of dermatitis (IB).
- Liquid, bar, leaflet, or powdered forms of plain soap are acceptable when washing hands with a non-antimicrobial soap and water. When bar soap is used, soap racks that facilitate drainage and small bars of soap should be used (II).
- Multiple-use cloth towels of the hanging or roll type are not recommended for use in healthcare settings (II).

Surgical Hand Antisepsis

- Remove rings, watches, and bracelets before beginning the surgical hand scrub (II).
- Remove debris from underneath fingernails using a nail cleaner under running water (II).

■ Surgical hand antisepsis using either an antimicrobial soap or an alcohol-based handrub with persistent activity is recommended before donning sterile gloves when performing surgical procedures (IB).

■ When performing surgical hand antisepsis using an antimicrobial soap, scrub hands and forearms for the length of time recommended by the manufacturer, usually 2 to 6 minutes. Long scrub times (e.g., 10 minutes) are not necessary (IB).

■ When using an alcohol-based surgical hand-scrub product with persistent activity, follow the manufacturer's instructions. Before applying the alcohol solution, prewash hands and forearms with a non-antimicrobial soap and dry hands and forearms completely. After application of the alcohol-based product as recommended, allow hands and forearms to dry thoroughly before donning sterile gloves (IB).

Other Aspects of Hand Hygiene

■ Do not wear artificial fingernails or extenders when having direct contact with patients at high risk (e.g., those in intensive care units or operating rooms) (IA).

■ Keep natural nails tips less than 1/4-inch long (II).

■ Wear gloves when contact with blood or other potentially infectious materials, mucous membranes, and nonintact skin could occur (IC).

■ Remove gloves after caring for a patient. Do not wear the same pair of gloves for the care of more than one patient, and do not wash gloves between uses with different patients (IB).

■ Change gloves during patient care if moving from a contaminated body site to a clean body site (II).

■ No recommendation can be made regarding wearing rings in healthcare settings (Unresolved issue).

Administrative Measures Regarding Hand Hygiene

■ As part of a multidisciplinary program to improve hand-hygiene adherence, provide HCWs with a readily accessible alcohol-based handrub product (IA).

■ To improve hand-hygiene adherence among personnel who work in areas in which high workloads and high intensity of patient care are anticipated, make an alcohol-based handrub available at the entrance to the patient's room or at the bedside, in other convenient locations, and in individual pocket-sized containers to be carried by HCWs (IA).

⁞ KEY POINTS

■ Because the various antiseptics and disinfectants require different durations of exposure to be effective, you must know the time course of action of the specific agent you are working with.

■ Although antiseptics can help prevent *development* of a local infection, systemic anti-infective drugs are preferred for treating an *established* local infection.

■ Washing with antiseptics by nurses, physicians, and others who contact the patient will do more to protect patients from infection than will application of antiseptics to patients themselves.

Anthelmintics

CLASSIFICATION OF PARASITIC WORMS

HELMINTHIC INFESTATIONS

    Nematode Infestations (Intestinal)

    Nematode Infestations (Extraintestinal)

    Cestode Infestations

    Trematode Infestations

DRUGS OF CHOICE FOR HELMINTHIASIS

    Mebendazole

    Albendazole

    Thiabendazole

    Pyrantel

    Praziquantel

    Diethylcarbamazine

    Ivermectin

    Bithionol

Helminths are parasitic worms, and *anthelmintics* are the drugs used against them. Helminthiasis (worm infestation) is the most common affliction of humans, affecting more than 2 billion people worldwide. The intestine is a frequent site of infestation. Other sites include the liver, lymphatic system, and blood vessels. Infestation is frequently asymptomatic. However, infestation with some parasites can cause severe complications. Helminthiasis is most prevalent where sanitation is poor. Cleanliness greatly reduces the risk of infestation.

Treatment of helminthiasis is not always indicated. Most parasitic worms do not reproduce within the human body. Hence, in the absence of reinfestation, many infections subside on their own as adult worms die. Since many infestations abate spontaneously, treatment may be optional. In countries where physicians and medication are readily available, drug therapy is definitely indicated. However, in less fortunate locales, several factors—cost of medication, limited medical facilities, and high probability of reinfestation—may render individual treatment impractical. In these places, preventative measures, such as improved hygiene and elimination of carriers, may be the most valuable way to control infestation.

In approaching the anthelmintic drugs, we begin by reviewing classification of the parasitic worms. Next we briefly discuss the characteristics of the more common helminthic infestations. After this, we discuss the drugs of choice for treatment.

CLASSIFICATION OF PARASITIC WORMS

The most common parasitic worms belong to three classes: Nematoda (roundworms), Cestoda (tapeworms), and Trematoda (flukes). Nematodes belong to the phylum Nemathelminthes. Cestodes and trematodes belong to the phylum Platyhelminthes (flat worms).

Nematodes (Roundworms)

Parasitic nematodes can be subdivided into two groups: (1) those that infest the intestinal lumen and (2) those that inhabit tissues. There are five major species of intestinal nematodes. Common names for these organisms are giant roundworm, pinworm, hookworm, whipworm, and threadworm. Official names of these parasites are listed in Table 93–1. Two types of nematodes invade tissues: (1) pork roundworms (responsible for trichinosis) and (2) filariae. The three species of filariae encountered most commonly are listed in Table 93–1.

Cestodes (Tapeworms)

Three species of cestodes infest humans. Common names for these parasites are beef tapeworm, pork tapeworm, and fish tapeworm. Their official names appear in Table 93–1.

Trematodes (Flukes)

Five species of trematodes infest humans. These organisms fall into four groups having the following common names: blood fluke, liver fluke, intestinal fluke, and lung fluke. Official names of the five species belonging to these groups are given in Table 93–1.

HELMINTHIC INFESTATIONS

This section describes the major characteristics of infestation by specific helminths. These infestations can differ with respect to anatomic site and danger to the host. Infestations also differ with respect to the drugs employed for treatment (see Table 93–1 for a summary).

The name applied to an infestation is based on the official name of the invading organism. For example, infestation with the giant roundworm, whose official name is *Ascaris lumbricoides,* is referred to as *ascariasis.*

In the discussion below, the helminthic infestations are grouped in four categories: (1) nematode infestations of the intestine, (2) nematode infestations of extraintestinal sites, (3) cestode infestations, and (4) trematode infestations.

Nematode Infestations (Intestinal)

Ascariasis (Giant Roundworm Infestation). Ascariasis is the most prevalent helminthic infestation. Worldwide, one of every three people is affected. Adult worms inhabit the small intestine. Ascariasis is usually asymptomatic. However, serious complications can result if worms migrate into the pancreatic duct, bile duct, gallbladder, or liver. In addition, if infestation is extremely heavy, intestinal blockage may occur. Be-

TABLE 93–1 ■ Drugs of Choice for Parasitic Worms

Worm Class	Parasitic Organism		Drugs of Choice
	Common Name	Official Name	
Nematodes (roundworms): intestinal	Giant roundworm	*Ascaris lumbricoides*	Mebendazole or pyrantel or albendazole
	Pinworm	*Enterobius vermicularis*	
	Hookworm	*Ancylostoma duodenale, Necator americanus*	
	Whipworm	*Trichuris trichiura*	Mebendazole
	Threadworm	*Strongyloides stercoralis*	Ivermectin
Nematodes: extraintestinal	Pork roundworm	*Trichinella spiralis*	Mebendazole*
	Filariae	*Wuchereria bancrofti, Brugia malayi, Loa loa*	Diethylcarbamazine
		Onchocerca volvulus	Ivermectin
Cestodes (tapeworms)	Beef tapeworm	*Taenia saginata*	Praziquantel*
	Pork tapeworm	*Taenia solium*	
	Fish tapeworm	*Diphyllobothrium latum*	
Trematodes (flukes)	Blood fluke	*Schistosoma* species	Praziquantel
	Intestinal fluke	*Fasciolopsis buski*	
	Lung fluke	*Paragonimus westermani*	
	Liver flukes	*Fasciola hepatica* (sheep liver fluke)	Bithionol† or triclabendazole
		Clonorchis sinensis (Chinese liver fluke)	Praziquantel or albendazole*

*Not approved by the Food and Drug Administration for this indication.
†Available from the Centers for Disease Control and Prevention.

cause of these potential hazards, ascariasis should always be treated. Drugs of choice are *mebendazole, albendazole,* and *pyrantel.*

Enterobiasis (Pinworm Infestation). Enterobiasis is the most common helminthic infestation in the United States. Adult pinworms inhabit the ileum and large intestine. Their life span is approximately 2 months. Although usually asymptomatic, enterobiasis may cause intense perineal itching in some patients. Serious complications are rare. Drugs of choice are *mebendazole, albendazole,* and *pyrantel.* Because enterobiasis is readily transmitted, all family members of an infected individual should be treated simultaneously.

Ancylostomiasis and Necatoriasis (Hookworm Infestation). Hookworm infestation is most common in rural areas where hygiene is poor and people go barefoot. Adult hookworms attach to the wall of the small intestine and suck blood. As a result, infestation is associated with chronic blood loss and progressive anemia. Symptomatic anemia is most likely in menstruating women and undernourished individuals. Nausea, vomiting, and abdominal pain may accompany the infestation. *Mebendazole, albendazole,* and *pyrantel* are the treatments of choice.

Trichuriasis (Whipworm Infestation). Trichuriasis is extremely common, affecting about 1 billion people worldwide. Larvae and adult worms inhabit the large intestine. Mature worms may live for 10 or more years. The disease is usually devoid of symptoms. However, when the worm burden is very large, rectal prolapse may occur. Patients with severe infestation require therapy. *Mebendazole* is the treatment of choice.

Strongyloidiasis (Threadworm Infestation). Strongyloidiasis is common in the southern United States. Larval and adult threadworms inhabit the small intestine. The disease can be very dangerous, although symptoms are usually absent. Mild infestation may cause abdominal pain and occasional diarrhea. Severe infestation can cause vomiting, massive diarrhea, dehydration, electrolyte imbalance, and secondary bacteremia. Death has occurred. Affected individuals should always be treated. *Ivermectin* is now the treatment of choice.

Nematode Infestations (Extraintestinal)

Trichinosis (Pork Roundworm Infestation). Trichinosis is acquired by eating undercooked pork that is infested with encysted larvae of *Trichinella spiralis.* Adult worms reside in the intestine, whereas larvae migrate to skeletal muscle and become encysted. Some encysted larvae live for years; others die and calcify within months. Symptoms of trichinosis include GI upset,

fever, muscle pain, and sore throat. Potentially lethal complications (heart failure, meningitis, neuritis) arise in some patients. *Mebendazole* is the drug of choice for killing adult worms and migrating larvae. However, this agent may not be active against larvae that have become encysted. *Prednisone* (a glucocorticoid) is given to reduce inflammation during larval migration.

Wuchereriasis and Brugiasis (Lymphatic Filarial Infestation). *Wuchereria bancrofti* and *Brugia malayi* are filarial nematodes that invade the lymphatic system. Infestation with either organism can cause severe complications. When infestation is heavy, lymphatic obstruction occurs, resulting in *elephantiasis* (usually of the scrotum or legs). In addition, "filarial fever" may develop. Symptoms include chills, fever, headache, nausea, vomiting, constipation, and lymphadenitis. The drug of choice for killing both filarial species is *diethylcarbamazine.*

Onchocerciasis (River Blindness). *Onchocerca volvulus* is a filarial nematode found in streams and rivers of Mexico, Guatemala, northern South America, and equatorial Africa. The parasite is transmitted to humans by the bite of certain flies. Heavy infestation with *O. volvulus* causes dermatologic and ophthalmic symptoms. Dermatologic manifestations include subcutaneous nodules (filled with adult worms) and persistent pruritic dermatitis. Ocular lesions, caused by the infiltration and death of microfilariae, result in optic neuritis, optic atrophy, and then blindness. The drug of choice for treating onchocerciasis is *ivermectin.*

Cestode Infestations

Taeniasis (Beef and Pork Tapeworm Infestation). Taeniasis is acquired by eating undercooked beef or pork that contains tapeworm larvae. Adult tapeworms live attached to the wall of the small intestine. Infestation is usually asymptomatic. Taeniasis is treated with *praziquantel.*

Diphyllobothriasis (Fish Tapeworm Infestation). Diphyllobothriasis is acquired by ingestion of undercooked fish that is infested with tapeworm larvae. Adult worms inhabit the ileum. Infestation is usually devoid of symptoms. Worms can be killed with *praziquantel.*

Trematode Infestations

Schistosomiasis (Blood Fluke Infestations). The term *schistosomiasis* refers to infestation with blood flukes of any species (e.g., *Schistosoma mansoni, S. japonicum*). Specific snails serve as intermediate hosts

TABLE 93–2 ■ First Choice Anthelmintic Drugs: Target Organisms and Dosages

Generic Name [Trade Name]	Target Organism	Adult Dosage	Pediatric Dosage
Mebendazolel [Vermox]	Giant roundworm Whipworm Hookworm	100 mg bid for 3 days or 500 mg once	Same as adult
	Pork roundworm	200–400 mg tid for 3 days, then 400–500 mg tid for 10 days	Same as adult
	Pinworm	100 mg; repeat in 2 weeks	Same as adult
Albendazole [Albenza]	Giant roundworm Hookworm	400 mg once	Same as adult
	Pinworm	400 mg; repeat in 2 weeks	Same as adult
	Chinese liver fluke	10 mg/kg for 7 days	Same as adult
Triclabendazole* [Fasinex]	Sheep liver fluke	10 mg/kg once	Same as adult
Pyrantel [Antiminith, others]	Giant roundworm	11 mg/kg once (max. 1 gm)	Same as adult
	Hookworm	11 mg/kg (max 1 gm) for 3 days	Same as adult
	Pinworm	11 mg/kg (max. 1 gm) repeat in 2 weeks	Same as adult
Praziquantel [Biltricide]	Beef tapeworm Pork tapeworm Fish tapeworm	5–10 mg/kg once	Same as adult
	Blood flukes	20 mg/kg bid for 1 day	Same as adult
	Intestinal fluke Chinese liver fluke	25 mg/kg tid for 1 day	Same as adult
	Lung fluke	25 mg/kg tid for 2 days	Same as adult
Diethylcarbamazine [Hetrazan]	*Wuchereria bancrofti* *Brugia malayi*	Day 1: 50 mg Day 2: 50 mg tid Day 3: 100 mg tid Days 4–14: 2 mg/kg tid	Day 1: 1 mg/kg Day 2: 1 mg/kg tid Day 3: 1–2 mg/kg tid Days 4–14: 2 mg/kg tid
	Loa loa	Days 1–3: Same as above Days 4–21: 3 mg/kg tid	Days 1–3: Same as above Days 4–21: 3 mg/kg tid
Ivermectin [Stromectol]	Threadworm	200 µg/kg for 1 or 2 days	Same as adult
	Onchocerca volvulus	150 µg/kg every 6–12 months until asymptomatic	Same as adult
Bithionol† [Bitin, Lorothidol]	Sheep liver fluke	30–50 mg every other day for 10 to 15 doses	Same as adult

*Approved only for veterinary use, but is safe and effective in humans.
†Available from the Centers for Disease Control and Prevention.

for these flukes. Schistosomiasis cannot be acquired in the continental United States because the appropriate snails are not indigenous.

Schistosomiasis has an acute and a chronic phase. The acute phase subsides in 3 to 4 months. Symptoms during this phase include lymphadenopathy, fever, anorexia, malaise, muscle pain, and rash. During the chronic phase, schistosomes take up residence in the vascular system, primarily in veins of the intestines and liver. This late infestation can produce intestinal polyposis, hepatosplenomegaly, and portal hypertension. For either the acute or the chronic stage, *praziquantel* is the treatment of choice.

Fascioliasis (Liver Fluke Infestation). Fascioliasis is caused by liver flukes: *Fasciola hepatica* (sheep liver fluke) and *Clonorchis sinensis* (Chinese liver fluke). Both parasites inhabit the biliary tract. Symptoms (anorexia, mild fever, fatigue, aching in the region of the liver) are delayed for 1 to 3 months.

Liver flukes differ in their drug sensitivity. The preferred drugs for use against *F. hepatica* are *bithionol* and *triclabendazole* (a veterinary anthelmintic). The preferred drugs for use against *C. sinensis* are *praziquantel* and *albendazole*.

Fasciolopsiasis (Intestinal Fluke Infestation). Fasciolopsiasis is most common in Southeast Asia. Adult worms inhabit the small intestine. The

disease is usually asymptomatic. However, some people experience ulcer-like pain. Some develop constipation or diarrhea. And, in the presence of massive infestation, bowel obstruction may occur, requiring surgery for clearance. *Praziquantel* is the treatment of choice.

DRUGS OF CHOICE FOR HELMINTHIASIS

The major anthelmintic drugs are considered below. These agents differ from one another in antiparasitic spectra: some agents are active against several worms; others are more selective. Because of these differences, it is important to identify the invading organism so that the most appropriate therapeutic agent can be chosen. Table 93–2 lists the major anthelmintic drugs and indicates the parasites against which each is most effective. Although the discussion that follows is limited to drugs of choice, be aware that additional anthelmintics are available.

Mebendazole

Target Organisms. Mebendazole [Vermox] is a drug of choice for most *intestinal roundworms.* This agent clears infestation with *pinworms, hookworms, whipworms,* and *giant roundworms.* Because of its relatively broad spectrum of action, mebendazole is especially useful for treatment of mixed infestations. In addition to its use against intestinal roundworms, mebendazole is the drug of choice for *pork roundworms,* the cause of trichinosis.

Mechanism of Action. Mebendazole prevents uptake of glucose by susceptible intestinal worms. Lack of glucose results in immobilization followed by slow death. Since the worms die slowly, up to 3 days may elapse between initiating treatment and complete clearance of parasites. Mebendazole does not influence glucose uptake or utilization by humans.

Pharmacokinetics. Only a small fraction (5% to 10%) of orally administered mebendazole is absorbed, and this fraction undergoes rapid metabolism. Consequently, plasma levels of mebendazole remain low.

Adverse Effects. Systemic effects are rare at usual doses, perhaps because the drug is so poorly absorbed. In patients with massive parasitic infestations, transient abdominal pain and diarrhea may occur.

Relatively low doses of mebendazole are embryotoxic and teratogenic in rats. However, these effects have not been observed in dogs, sheep, or horses. Limited experience with mebendazole in pregnant women has shown no increase in spontaneous abortion or fetal malformation. Nonetheless, *it is recommended that pregnant women avoid this drug, especially during the first trimester.*

Preparations, Dosage, and Administration. Mebendazole [Vermox] is available in 100-mg tablets for oral administration. The tablets may be chewed, crushed, or swallowed whole. Dosages are summarized in Table 93–2.

Albendazole

Target Organisms. Albendazole [Albenza] is active against many cestode and nematode parasites, including larval forms of *Taenia solium* and *Echinococcus granulosus.* In the United States, the drug is approved only for (1) parenchymal *neurocysticercosis* caused by larval forms of the pork tapeworm, *T. solium,* and (2) *cystic hydatid disease* of the liver, lung, and peritoneum caused by larval forms of the dog tapeworm, *E. granulosus.* However, despite lack of formal approval, albendazole is considered a drug of choice for infestation with giant roundworms, hookworms, pinworms, and Chinese liver flukes.

Mechanism of Action. Albendazole inhibits polymerization of tubulin, and thereby prevents formation of cytoplasmic microtubules. As a result, microtubule-dependent uptake of glucose is prevented.

Pharmacokinetics. Albendazole is poorly absorbed from the GI tract, owing largely to low solubility in water. Absorption is enhanced by administration with a fatty meal. Following absorption, albendazole is rapidly converted to albendazole sulfoxide, its active form. Albendazole sulfoxide is distributed widely to body fluids and tissues, and is excreted in the bile. The half-life is 8 to 12 hours.

Adverse Effects. Albendazole is generally well tolerated. Mild to moderate *liver impairment* has occurred in 16% of patients, as indicated by elevation of liver transaminases in plasma. Liver function should be assessed before treatment and periodically thereafter. Albendazole is teratogenic in animals and hence *should not be used during pregnancy.* If pregnancy occurs, the drug should be discontinued immediately.

Preparations, Dosage, and Administration. Albendazole [Albenza] is dispensed in 200-mg tablets for oral use. Each dose (for neurocysticercosis or cystic hydatid disease) is 400 mg (for patients >60 kg) or 7.5 mg/kg (for patients <60 kg). The dosing schedule for cystic hydatid disease is 2 doses twice daily with meals for 8 to 30 days. Dosing for neurocysticercosis is done in three consecutive cycles, each consisting of 2 doses twice daily with meals for 28 days followed by 14 days with no drug. Dosages for infestation with giant roundworms, hookworms, pinworms, and Chinese liver flukes are shown in Table 93–2.

Thiabendazole

Target Organisms. At one time, thiabendazole [Mintezol] was the drug of choice for *threadworms.* However, ivermectin is now preferred.

Pharmacokinetics. Thiabendazole undergoes rapid absorption and metabolism. Most of each dose is excreted in the urine as metabolites within 24 hours.

Adverse Effects. The incidence of adverse reactions is high: As many as one third of patients become incapacitated for several hours. The most common effects are GI (anorexia, nausea, vomiting) and neurologic (dizziness, drowsiness) reactions. Because of the potential for reduced alertness, patients should avoid hazardous activities (e.g., driving). Hepatotoxicity with jaundice has been reported. Accordingly, thiabendazole should not be used by patients with liver dysfunction.

Preparations, Dosage, and Administration. Thiabendazole [Mintezol] is available in 500-mg chewable tablets and an oral suspension (100 mg/ml). Patients should be instructed to chew the tablets thoroughly. Gastrointestinal discomfort can be reduced by administering thiabendazole with food. The adult and pediatric dosage for threadworm infestation is 25 mg/kg twice daily for 2 days.

Pyrantel

Target Organisms. Pyrantel [Antiminth, others] is active against *intestinal nematodes.* The drug is an alternative to mebendazole or albendazole for infestations with *hookworms, pinworms,* and *giant roundworms.*

Mechanism of Action. Pyrantel is a depolarizing neuromuscular blocking agent that causes spastic paralysis of intestinal parasites. The paralyzed worms are cleared in the feces.

Pharmacokinetics. Pyrantel is poorly absorbed, and plasma levels remain low. Most of an administered dose is excreted unchanged in the feces.

Adverse Effects. Serious reactions are rare. The most common effects are GI reactions (nausea, vomiting, diarrhea, stomach pain, cramps). Possible central nervous system effects include dizziness, drowsiness, headache, and insomnia.

Preparations, Dosage, and Administration. Pyrantel pamoate [Antiminth, Pin-Rid, Pin-X, Reese's Pinworm] is dispensed in soft-gel capsules (180 mg) and liquid formulations (50 mg/ml) for oral use. The entire prescribed dose should be taken at one time. Dosages for intestinal nematodes are given in Table 93–2.

Praziquantel

Target Organisms. Praziquantel [Biltricide] is very active against *nematodes* (flukes) and *cestodes* (tapeworms). This agent is a drug of choice for *tapeworms, schistosomiasis,* and other *fluke infestations.*

Mechanism of Action. Praziquantel is readily absorbed by helminths. At low therapeutic concentrations, the drug produces spastic paralysis, causing detachment of worms from body tissues. At high therapeutic concentrations, praziquantel disrupts the integument of the worms, rendering the parasites vulnerable to lethal attack by host defenses.

Pharmacokinetics. Praziquantel is rapidly absorbed from the GI tract. The drug undergoes extensive hepatic metabolism. Metabolites are excreted in the urine. The half-life is short (about 1.5 hours).

Adverse Effects. Praziquantel is relatively free of toxicity. Transient headache and abdominal discomfort are the most frequent reactions. Drowsiness may occur, and patients should avoid driving and other hazardous activities.

Preparations, Dosage, and Administration. Praziquantel [Biltricide] is available in 600-mg tablets for oral administration. Tablets should be swallowed intact. Dosages for tapeworm and fluke infestations are presented in Table 93–2.

Diethylcarbamazine

Target Organisms. Diethylcarbamazine [Hetrazan] is the drug of choice for *filarial infestations.* The drug destroys microfilariae of *W. bancrofti, B. malayi,* and *Loa loa.* In addition, it kills adult females of these species.

Mechanism of Action. Diethylcarbamazine has two antifilarial actions. First, the drug reduces muscular activity, thereby causing parasites to be dislodged from their site of attachment. Second, by altering the surface properties of the parasites, the drug renders the organisms more vulnerable to attack by host defenses.

Pharmacokinetics. Diethylcarbamazine is readily absorbed and undergoes rapid and extensive metabolism. Metabolites are excreted in the urine.

Adverse Effects. Reactions caused directly by diethylcarbamazine are minor (headache, weakness, dizziness, nausea, vomiting). Indirect effects, occurring secondary to death of the parasites, can be more serious. These include rashes, intense itching, encephalitis, fever, tachycardia, lymphadenitis, leukocytosis, and proteinuria. Fortunately, these reactions are transient, lasting just a few days—and can be minimized by pretreatment with glucocorticoids.

Preparations, Dosage, and Administration. Diethylcarbamazine citrate [Hetrazan] is dispensed in 50-mg tablets for oral use. The drug is available without charge from Lederle Laboratories. Dosages for filarial infestations are presented in Table 93–2.

Ivermectin

Target Organisms. Ivermectin [Stromectol] is active against many *nematodes.* Currently, the drug has two approved indications: *onchocerciasis* (a major cause of blindness worldwide) and intestinal *strongyloidiasis.* Ivermectin is active against the tissue microfilariae of *O. volvulus* (the cause of onchocerciasis), but not against the adult form. As discussed in Chapter 96, ivermectin can also be used to kill *mites* and *lice,* although these parasites are not approved targets. In addition to its use in humans, ivermectin is used widely in veterinary medicine.

Mechanism of Action. Ivermectin disrupts nerve traffic and muscle function in target parasites. The underlying mechanism is the opening of cell-surface chloride channels, which allows chloride ions to rush into nerve and muscle cells. The resultant hyperpolarization of these cells causes paralysis followed by death. Host cells are not affected because ivermectin is selective for chloride channels in parasites.

Pharmacokinetics. Ivermectin is administered orally and achieves peak plasma levels in 4 hours. Distribution to the central nervous system is poor. The drug is metabolized in the liver and excreted in the feces. Less than 1% of the drug appears in urine. Ivermectin has a half-life of 16 hours.

Adverse Effect: Mazotti Reaction. The Mazotti reaction occurs in patients treated for *onchocerciasis.* Principal symptoms are pruritus (28%), rash (23%), fever (23%), lymph node tenderness (13%), and bone and joint pain (9%). The apparent cause is an allergic and inflammatory response to the death of microfilariae. Mazotti-type reactions do not occur in patients treated for strongyloidiasis.

Use in Pregnancy. Ivermectin is teratogenic in mice, rats, and rabbits. Cleft palate is the most common effect. There are no adequate data on teratogenesis in humans. Until data are available, *ivermectin should be avoided during pregnancy.*

Preparations, Dosage, and Administration. Ivermectin [Stromectol] is available in 6-mg tablets for oral administration. Instruct patients to take the drug with water. For *strongyloidiasis,* the adult and pediatric dosage is 200 μg/kg for 1 or 2 days. For *onchocerciasis* (river blindness), the adult and pediatric dosage is 150 μg/kg, repeated every 6 to 12 months.

Bithionol

Bithionol [Bitin, Lorothidol] is a drug of choice for treating infestation with the liver fluke *F. hepatica.* The drug's most frequent adverse effects are photosensitivity reactions, vomiting, diarrhea, abdominal pain, and urticaria. Leukopenia and toxic hepatitis occur rarely.

The recommended dosage for adults and children is 30 to 50 mg on alternate days for 10 to 15 doses. Bithionol, an investigational drug in the United States, is available from the Centers for Disease Control and Prevention.

∴ KEY POINTS

- Because each anthelmintic drug is active against a limited range of worms, we must select the appropriate drug for the infestation to be treated.
- Because many worm infestations are both asymptomatic and self-limited, drug therapy can be optional. When cost is not an issue, treatment is clearly indicated. However, in countries where healthcare funds are very limited, preventative public health measures directed at improved hygiene and elimination of carriers may be more cost-effective than treating each infested individual.
- With the exception of thiabendazole, the drugs discussed in this chapter are generally devoid of serious adverse effects.

Antiprotozoal Drugs I: Antimalarial Agents

Malaria is a parasitic disease caused by protozoa of the genus *Plasmodium*. With the exception of tuberculosis, malaria kills more people than any other infectious disease. Between 270 million and 490 million people are afflicted, and more than 1 million die each year. Seventy-five percent of deaths occur in Africa, primarily among children under the age of 5. In the United States, about 1200 cases are reported annually.

Large-scale attempts to eradicate the disease have achieved only partial success. Eradication programs have been directed at the malarial parasite as well as the *Anopheles* mosquito, the insect that transmits malaria to humans. Failure to produce complete control has resulted largely from development of drug resistance by both the parasite and the mosquito. The incidence of malaria is rising in regions where it had once been suppressed. There remains a great need for safe, effective, and affordable agents capable of killing the malaria parasite and its mosquito carrier.

In approaching the antimalarial drugs, we begin by reviewing the life cycle of the malaria parasite. After that we discuss the two major subtypes of malaria: falciparum malaria and vivax malaria. Next, we consider basic principles of treatment, focusing on therapeutic objectives and drug selection. Lastly, we discuss the pharmacology of the antimalarial drugs.

LIFE CYCLE OF THE MALARIA PARASITE

In order to understand the actions and specific applications of antimalarial drugs, we must first understand the life cycle of the malaria parasite. As indicated in Figure 94–1, this cycle takes place in two hosts: humans and the female *Anopheles* mosquito. In the human host, the parasite undergoes asexual reproduction. In the mosquito, the parasite undergoes sexual reproduction.

The human phase of the life cycle begins when sporozoites are injected into the bloodstream by a feeding *Anopheles* mosquito. These sporozoites invade parenchymal cells of the liver, where they multiply and transform into merozoites. This process, which takes from 12 to 26 days, depending upon the species of parasite, is referred to as the pre-erythrocytic or exoerythrocytic phase of the life cycle. Upon release from the liver, merozoites infect erythrocytes. Within the erythrocyte, each parasite differentiates and divides, becoming first a trophozoite and then a multinucleated schizont. The schizont then evolves into new merozoites. This process of asexual reproduction takes 2 to 3 days, after which red blood cells burst and release the new merozoites into the blood. These new merozoites then infect fresh erythrocytes, thereby establishing an escalating cycle of red cell invasion and lysis. Each time the erythrocytes rupture, they release pyrogenic (fever-inducing) agents. These substances cause the repeating episodes of fever that characterize malaria. After several cycles of asexual reproduction, a few parasites differentiate into male and female gametocytes.

Sexual reproduction occurs following ingestion of gametocyte-containing blood by a female *Anopheles* mosquito. Within the mosquito, the gametocytes differentiate into mature forms, after which fertilization takes place. The resulting zygote then produces sporozoites, thus completing sexual reproduction.

TYPES OF MALARIA

Malaria is caused by four different species of *Plasmodium*. In this chapter, we limit discussion to the two species encountered most frequently: *Plasmodium vivax* and *Plasmodium falciparum*. Malaria caused by either species is characterized by high fever, chills, and profuse sweating. However, despite similarity of symptoms, these two forms of malaria are very different. They differ most with regard to severity of symptoms, occurrence of relapse, and drug resistance. These and other differences are summarized in Table 94–1.

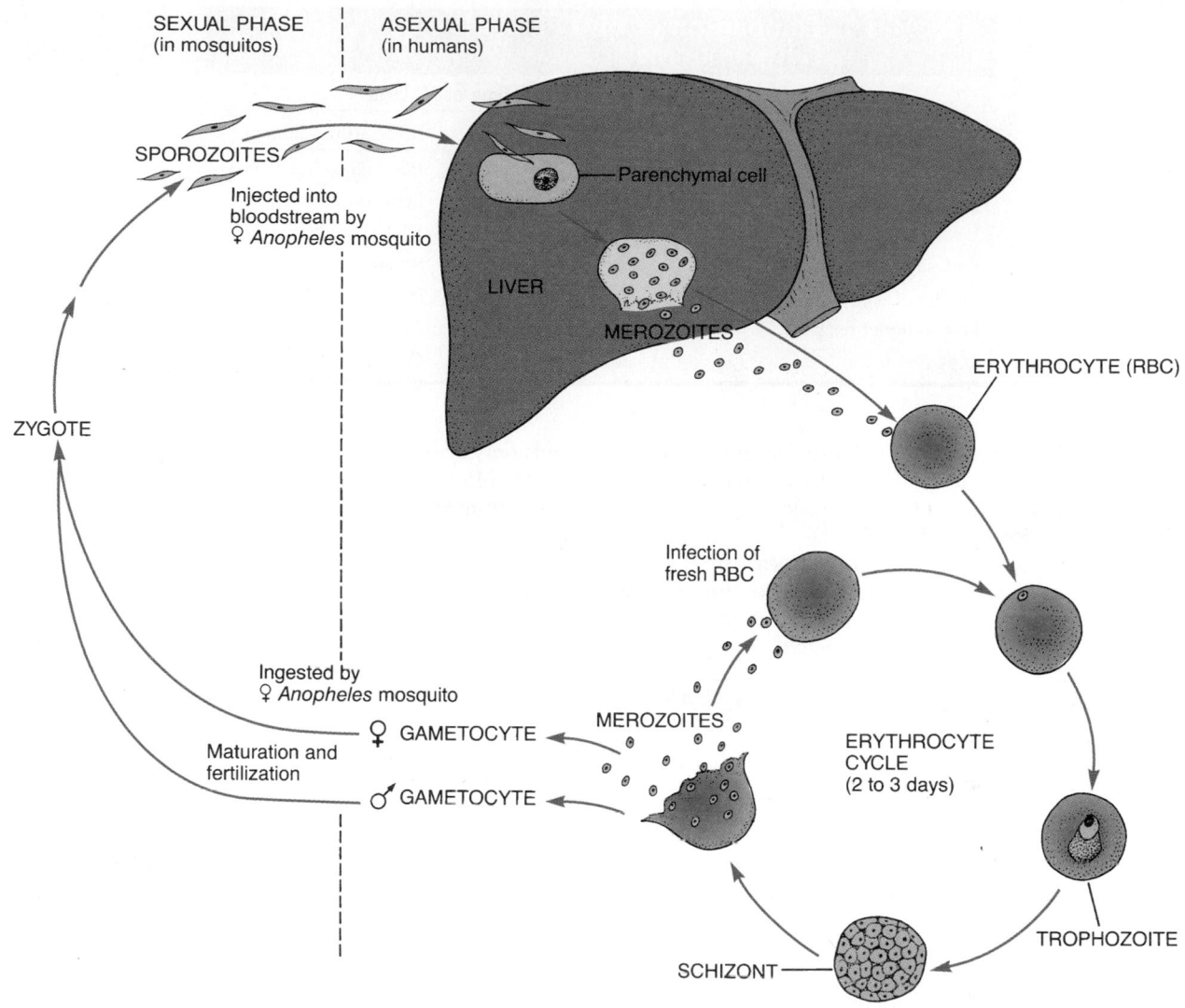

Figure 94–1 ■ **Life cycle of the malaria parasite.**

Vivax Malaria

Vivax malaria, caused by *P. vivax,* is the most common form of malaria. Fortunately, the disease is relatively mild and usually self-limiting. Because drug resistance by *P. vivax* is still uncommon, symptoms can be readily suppressed with medication.

Infection begins when the host is inoculated with *P. vivax* sporozoites. After 26 days, merozoites emerge from the liver and begin their attack on erythrocytes. Symptoms of malaria (chills, fever, sweating) commence as infected erythrocytes rupture, releasing pyrogens and other substances into the blood. Symptoms peak, decline, and peak again every 48 hours in response to cyclic reinfection and lysis of red blood cells. This cycle continues until terminated by drugs or by acquired immunity. Unfortunately, relapse is likely following termination of the acute attack. Relapse is possible because dormant forms of *P. vivax* remain in the liver. These dormant forms periodically evolve into merozoites, emerge from the liver, and start the erythrocytic cycle anew. Relapse becomes less frequent with the passage of time, and, after 2 or more years, ceases entirely. Relapse can be stopped with drugs capable of killing the dormant hepatic parasites.

Falciparum Malaria

Malaria caused by *P. falciparum* is less common than malaria caused by *P. vivax,* but is much more severe. In the absence of treatment, the disease is lethal to about 10% of victims. This infection is made even more dangerous by the emergence of drug-resistant strains of *P. falciparum.* Unlike the symptoms of vivax malaria, which peak every 48 hours, the symptoms of falciparum malaria occur at irregular intervals. The erythrocyte cycle of *P. falciparum* can destroy up to 60% of circulating red blood cells, resulting in profound anemia and weakness. The hemoglobin released from these cells causes the urine to darken, giving rise to the term *blackwater fever.* Falciparum malaria can produce serious complications, including pulmonary edema, hypoglycemia, and toxic encephalopathy, characterized by confusion, coma, and convulsions.

TABLE 94–1 ■ Comparison of Vivax Malaria and Falciparum Malaria		
	Type of Malaria	
Characteristics	Vivax Malaria	Falciparum Malaria
Causative organism	*Plasmodium vivax*	*Plasmodium falciparum*
Frequency of infection	More common	Less common
Latency of symptoms	26 days	12 days
Intensity of symptoms	Mild	Severe
Timing of febrile paroxysms	Every 2 days	Irregular
Probability of relapse	High	None
Drug resistance	Uncommon	Common

When treated early, falciparum malaria usually responds well. However, if treatment is delayed, the disease may progress rapidly to irreversible shock and death. In contrast to infection with *P. vivax,* infection with *P. falciparum* does not relapse. Why not? Because there are no dormant forms of *P. falciparum* in the liver. Hence, once the erythrocytic forms have been eliminated, the patient is free of the infection.

PRINCIPLES OF ANTIMALARIAL THERAPY

Therapeutic Objectives

Drug responsiveness of the malaria parasite changes as the parasite goes through its life cycle. The *erythrocytic* stages are killed most easily, whereas the *exoerythrocytic* (hepatic) stages are more difficult to kill. *Sporozoites* do not respond to drugs at all. Because of these differences in drug sensitivity, antimalarial therapy has three separate objectives: (1) treatment of an acute attack (clinical cure), (2) prevention of relapse (radical cure), and (3) prophylaxis (suppressive therapy). Because sporozoites are insensitive to drugs, therapy cannot prevent primary infection of the liver.

Treatment of an Acute Attack. Clinical cure is accomplished with drugs that are active against erythrocytic forms of the malaria parasite. By eliminating parasites from red blood cells, the erythrocytic cycle is stopped and symptoms cease. For patients with vivax malaria, clinical cure will not prevent relapse, because dormant parasites remain in the liver. However, for patients with falciparum malaria, successful treatment of the acute attack prevents further episodes (unless the patient is re-inoculated by another infected mosquito).

Prevention of Relapse. People infected with *P. vivax* harbor dormant parasites in the liver. In order to prevent relapse, a drug capable of killing these hepatic forms must be taken. The use of drugs to eradicate hepatic *P. vivax* is referred to as radical cure. Since reinfection by a mosquito bite is a virtual certainty as long as one remains in a region where malaria is endemic, radical cure is usually postponed until departure from the region.

Prophylaxis. Persons anticipating travel to an area where malaria is endemic should take antimalarial medication for prophylaxis. Although drugs cannot prevent primary infection of the liver, they *can* prevent infection of erythrocytes. Hence, although the parasite may be present, symptoms of malaria are avoided. Because prophylactic treatment prevents only symptoms but not invasion of the liver, such treatment is often referred to as *suppressive therapy.*

Nondrug measures can help greatly to prevent infection. Since *Anopheles* mosquitoes only bite between dusk and dawn, clothing that covers as much skin as possible should be worn during this time; a diethyltoluamide (DEET)-containing insect repellent should be applied to skin that remains exposed. Sleeping under mosquito netting that has been impregnated with permethrin (an insecticide) further reduces the risk of a bite.

Drug Selection

Selection of antimalarial drugs is based largely on two factors: (1) the goal of treatment and (2) drug resistance of the causative strain of *Plasmodium.* Drugs of choice for treatment and prophylaxis are discussed below and summarized in Table 94–2.

Treatment of Acute Attacks. Chloroquine is the drug of choice for an acute attack of malaria caused by chloroquine-sensitive strains of *P. falciparum* or *P. vivax.* As a rule, a 3-day course of treatment produces clinical cure. For strains of *P. falciparum* that are resistant to chloroquine—and most are—quinine is the drug of choice, combined with either doxycycline, tetracycline, clindamycin, or Fansidar (a fixed-dose combination of pyrimethamine plus sulfadoxine). Malarone, a fixed-dose combination of atovaquone plus proguanil, is an effective alternative to the quinine-based regimens. For strains of *P. vivax* that are resistant to chloroquine, quinine combined with doxycycline is the treatment of choice. Mefloquine is a good alternative.

Prevention of Relapse. The agent of choice for preventing relapse of vivax malaria is primaquine, a drug that is highly active against the hepatic stages of *P. vivax.* For falciparum malaria, no treatment is needed, since relapse does not occur following clinical cure.

Prophylaxis. Selection of drugs for prophylaxis is based on the drug sensitivity of the plasmodial species found in the region to which travel is intended. In regions where chloroquine-sensitive strains are found, chloroquine is the preferred drug for prophylaxis. In regions of chloroquine resistance, either mefloquine, doxycycline, or atovaquone/proguanil may be used. Recommendations regarding preferred drugs for prophylaxis in specific regions of the world are available online at *www.cdc. gov/travel/regionalmalaria/index.htm.*

TABLE 94–2 ■ Drugs of Choice for Malaria*

Therapeutic Objective	Plasmodium falciparum		Plasmodium vivax	
	Chloroquine Sensitive	Chloroquine Resistant	Chloroquine Sensitive	Chloroquine Resistant
Treatment of acute attack	Chloroquine†	Quinine† *plus either* doxycycline, tetracycline, pyrimethamine/sulfadoxine or clindamycin *or* Atovaquone/proguanil	Chloroquine†	Quinine† *plus* doxycycline *or* Mefloquine
Prevention of relapse	Primaquine	Primaquine	NA‡	NA‡
Prophylaxis	Chloroquine	Mefloquine, doxycycline, or atovaquone/proguanil	Chloroquine	Same as for *P. falciparum*

*All drugs are given orally except where noted otherwise.
†For severe attacks, treat parenterally with either quinidine gluconate, quinine dihydrochloride, or artemether.
‡Not applicable. Malaria caused by *P. falciparum* does not relapse following successful treatment of the acute attack.

PHARMACOLOGY OF THE MAJOR ANTIMALARIAL DRUGS

Chloroquine

Actions and Use. Chloroquine [Aralen] is the most generally useful of the antimalarial drugs. This agent is highly active against erythrocytic forms of the malaria parasite. Consequently, chloroquine is the drug of choice for treating acute attacks caused by sensitive strains of *P. vivax* or *P. falciparum*. Chloroquine is also the drug of choice for prophylaxis (suppressive therapy).

Chloroquine is not active against *exoerythrocytic* forms of the malaria parasite. Hence, the drug is unable to prevent primary infection by *P. vivax* or *P. falciparum*. Nor is it able to prevent relapse of vivax malaria, which is caused by emergence of dormant hepatic parasites.

Several mechanisms have been proposed to explain the lethal effects of chloroquine on erythrocytic stages of the malaria parasite. The most likely is that chloroquine prevents the organism from converting heme to nontoxic metabolites. (Heme, a potentially toxic compound, is produced by the parasite as it digests hemoglobin in the host's red blood cells.) Chloroquine concentrates in parasitized erythrocytes, and this may explain the selective actions against erythrocytic forms of *Plasmodium*.

Pharmacokinetics. Chloroquine is rapidly and completely absorbed from the GI tract. A substantial fraction of absorbed drug is deposited in certain tissues (e.g., lung, spleen, liver, kidney). Slow release from these sites helps maintain therapeutic plasma levels. Hence, when used for prophylaxis, chloroquine can be administered just once a week. Excretion is primarily nonrenal.

Adverse Effects. Because the doses required for prophylaxis are low, and because the higher doses required for treatment are taken only briefly, chloroquine rarely causes serious adverse effects. When employed to treat an acute malarial attack, chloroquine may cause visual disturbances, pruritus, headache, and GI effects (abdominal discomfort, nausea, diarrhea). Gastrointestinal effects can be minimized by taking the drug with meals. Because chloroquine concentrates in the liver, it should be used with caution in patients with hepatic disease.

Routes of Administration. Chloroquine may be administered orally or IM. Oral therapy is preferred. Intramuscular administration is employed only when emesis precludes oral treatment or when infection is especially severe.

Preparations and Dosage. *Chloroquine phosphate* [Aralen] is dispensed in tablets (250 and 500 mg) for oral administration. *Chloroquine hydrochloride* (50 mg/ml in 5-ml ampules) is employed for IM injection.

For *prophylaxis* of malaria, the adult dosage is 500 mg of chloroquine phosphate once a week. The pediatric dosage is 8.3 mg/kg once a week. Treatment should commence 1 week before expected exposure to malaria and should continue 4 weeks after leaving the endemic region.

To *treat an acute attack,* the adult dosage is 1 gm of chloroquine phosphate (PO) initially followed in 6 hours by a 500-mg dose. Additional 500-mg doses are given on days 2 and 3.

Primaquine

Actions and Use. Primaquine is highly active against *hepatic* forms of *P. vivax*. Effects against *erythrocytic* forms are less profound. The drug is used to eradicate *P. vivax* from the liver, thereby preventing relapse. Primaquine is similar to chloroquine in structure, and may act by the same mechanism: promotion of heme accumulation to toxic levels within the parasite.

Pharmacokinetics. Primaquine is well absorbed following oral administration. Absorbed drug is rapidly metabolized to products of low antimalarial activity. Metabolites are excreted in the urine.

Adverse Effect: Hemolysis. The most serious and frequent response to primaquine is hemolysis. This reaction develops in patients whose red blood cells are deficient in glucose-6-phosphate dehydrogenase (G-6-PD). Deficiency of G-6-PD is an inherited trait, occurring most commonly in black populations and in darker skinned whites (e.g., Sardinians, Greeks, Iranians, Sephardic Jews). When possible, patients suspected of G-6-PD deficiency should be screened for this trait before treatment. During primaquine therapy, periodic blood counts should be performed. Also, the urine should be monitored (darkening indicates the presence of hemoglobin). If severe hemolysis develops, primaquine should be discontinued.

Preparations, Dosage, and Administration. Primaquine phosphate is dispensed in 26.3-mg tablets and as a powder (5, 25, 100, and 500 gm). Administration is oral. For radical cure (prevention of relapse) of vivax malaria, the usual adult dosage is 26.3 mg/day for 2 weeks. The pediatric dosage is 0.53 mg/kg/day for 2 weeks.

Quinine

At one time, quinine was the only drug available to treat malaria. Today, quinine has been largely replaced by more effective and less toxic agents (e.g., chloroquine). However, quinine still has an important role: treatment of chloroquine-resistant malaria. Quinine occurs naturally in the bark of the cinchona tree. Commercial preparations are derived from this source.

Actions and Use. Quinine is active against erythrocytic forms of *Plasmodium* but has little effect on sporozoites and hepatic forms. Like chloroquine, quinine concentrates in parasitized red blood cells and may be selective against erythrocytic parasites for this reason. Also like chloroquine, quinine kills plasmodia by causing heme to accumulate within the parasites.

The principal application of quinine is malaria caused by chloroquine-resistant *P. falciparum.* Because quinine is not highly active, adjunctive therapy with another agent is required. Drugs employed for adjunctive therapy include doxycycline, tetracycline, clindamycin, and Fansidar (pyrimethamine plus sulfadoxine).

Pharmacokinetics. Quinine is well absorbed from the GI tract, even in patients with diarrhea. The drug is metabolized by the liver, and metabolites are excreted in the urine. Plasma levels of quinine fall rapidly after stopping treatment.

Adverse Effects. At usual therapeutic doses, quinine frequently causes mild *cinchonism,* a syndrome characterized by tinnitus (ringing in the ears), headache, visual disturbances, nausea, and diarrhea. The physician should be notified if these symptoms develop. Because of its adverse effects on vision and hearing, quinine is contraindicated for patients with optic neuritis or tinnitus.

Like primaquine, quinine can cause *hemolysis* in patients whose red blood cells are deficient in G-6-PD. Patients should be monitored for hemolytic anemia. Quinine is contraindicated in the presence of G-6-PD deficiency.

Intravenous administration may cause *hypotension* and *acute circulatory failure.* To minimize risk, IV quinine should be diluted and injected slowly. Patients should be transferred to oral medication as soon as possible.

Quinine has *quinidine-like effects on the heart* and must be used cautiously in patients with atrial fibrillation: By enhancing atrioventricular conduction, quinine can increase passage of atrial impulses to the ventricles, thereby causing a dangerous increase in ventricular rate.

Quinine can cause profound *hypoglycemia.* The mechanism is stimulation of pancreatic beta cells, which results in hyperinsulinemia. Quinine-induced hypoglycemia can be difficult to treat, even with glucose infusions.

Quinine is classified in Food and Drug Administration Pregnancy Risk Category X: the risks of use during pregnancy clearly outweigh any possible benefits. The drug has caused fetal abnormalities, the most common being deafness from damage to the auditory nerve. Quinine can stimulate the uterus, and might thereby induce premature labor. *The drug must not be taken by pregnant women.*

Preparations, Dosage, and Administration. Quinine is available as two salts: *quinine sulfate,* for oral administration, and *quinine dihydrochloride* (no longer available in the United States), for IV administration.

For chloroquine-resistant falciparum or vivax malaria, the adult oral dosage is 650 mg every 8 hours for 3 to 7 days. The pediatric oral dosage is 8 mg/kg every 8 hours for 3 to 7 days.

Pyrimethamine/Sulfadoxine

Therapeutic Use. The combination of pyrimethamine and sulfadoxine, marketed as Fansidar, is used jointly with quinine to treat acute malaria attacks caused by chloroquine-resistant *P. falciparum.* In addition, pyrimethamine is a drug of choice for toxoplasmosis (see Chapter 95).

Mechanism of Action. Pyrimethamine inhibits dihydrofolate reductase, an enzyme that converts folic acid to its active form. Without active folic acid, cells are unable to synthesize DNA, RNA, and proteins. Pyrimethamine rarely disrupts host biochemistry because the concentration of pyrimethamine required to inhibit human dihydrofolate reductase is about 1000 times greater than the concentration needed to inhibit plasmodial dihydrofolate reductase.

The effects of pyrimethamine are potentiated by sulfadoxine, a member of the sulfonamide family. Unlike humans, the malaria parasite is unable to take up preformed folic acid from its environment. Consequently, the parasite must synthesize folic acid of its own. Sulfadoxine inhibits this process. Hence, the combination of sulfadoxine with pyrimethamine produces a *sequential block* in a critical biochemical pathway. In step one, sulfadoxine inhibits folic acid synthesis, thereby reducing folic acid levels. In step two, pyrimethamine prevents conversion of the reduced pool of folic acid into an active form.

Pharmacokinetics. Pyrimethamine is well absorbed following oral administration. The drug is highly bound to plasma proteins, and hence is eliminated slowly. The plasma half-life of the drug is approximately 4 days. Pyrimethamine undergoes limited hepatic metabolism. Metabolites and parent drug are excreted in the urine.

Sulfadoxine is well absorbed following oral administration and undergoes distribution to all tissues. The drug crosses the placenta with ease. Elimination is primarily renal.

Adverse Effects. At the doses employed for treatment of malaria, pyrimethamine produces few adverse effects. However, at high doses, such as those used to treat toxoplasmosis, pyrimethamine can produce symptoms of *folic acid deficiency.* Symptoms result from effects on the bone marrow and the GI mucosa, tissues that have a high percentage of cells undergoing division. Effects on the bone marrow manifest as leukopenia, thrombocytopenia, and anemia. Effects on the GI mucosa manifest as ulcerative stomatitis, atrophic glossitis, pharyngitis, and diarrhea. These responses reverse upon discontinuation of treatment, and can be prevented by giving folic acid or folinic acid.

The principal concern with sulfadoxine is hypersensitivity reactions. Mild reactions, such as rash and drug fever, are relatively common. Rarely, the drug causes *Stevens-Johnson syndrome,* a severe reaction with a mortality rate of about 25%. Symptoms include widespread lesions of the skin and mucous membranes, together with fever, malaise, and toxemia. To minimize risk, sulfadoxine should not be given to patients with a history of hypersensitivity to sulfonamides or to chemically related drugs, including thiazide diuretics, loop diuretics, and sulfonylurea-type oral hypoglycemics (e.g., tolbutamide).

Preparations, Dosage, and Administration. Pyrimethamine and sulfadoxine are available in a fixed-dose combination sold as Fansidar. Tablets contain 25 mg of pyrimethamine and 500 mg of sulfadoxine. To treat an acute attack of chloroquine-resistant malaria, Fansidar is used in conjunction with quinine, and is administered as a single dose on the last day of quinine administration. Fansidar dosages are as follows: adults, 3 tablets; children 9 to 14 years, 2 tablets; children 4 to 8 years, 1 tablet; children 1 to 3 years, one-half tablet; and children under 1 year, one-quarter tablet.

Mefloquine

Actions and Uses. Mefloquine [Lariam] kills erythrocytic forms of *P. vivax* and *P. falciparum*. The mechanism of action is unknown. Mefloquine is a drug of choice for prophylaxis of malaria in regions where chloroquine-resistant *P. falciparum* or *P. vivax* are found. The drug can also be used to treat acute attacks by these parasites. Unfortunately, resistance to mefloquine may emerge rapidly. The mechanism of resistance is not known.

Pharmacokinetics. Mefloquine is well absorbed following oral administration. The drug undergoes hepatic metabolism and is excreted in the bile and feces. Mefloquine has a prolonged half-life, ranging from 1 to 4 weeks.

Adverse Effects. Adverse effects are dose related. At the low doses employed for prophylaxis, reactions are generally mild (nausea, dizziness, syncope). At the higher doses used to treat acute attacks, more intense reactions may occur, including GI disturbances, nightmares, altered vision, and headache. Some of these effects may be indistinguishable from symptoms of malaria.

Toxicity to the central nervous system is a concern. Mefloquine can cause vertigo, confusion, psychosis, and convulsions. The incidence of these neuropsychiatric effects is about 1 in 13,000 at the low doses used for prophylaxis, but increases to 1 in 250 at the doses used to treat an ongoing attack. High-dose mefloquine should be avoided by people with epilepsy or psychiatric disorders. Patients who develop psychiatric symptoms (hallucinations, depression, suicidal ideation) should discontinue the drug immediately and contact their physician for a substitute (e.g., doxycycline, atovaquone/proguanil).

Preparations, Dosage, and Administration. Mefloquine [Lariam] is available in 250-mg tablets for oral administration.

For *prophylaxis,* the adult dosage is 250 mg once a week. Dosing should begin 1 week prior to travel to an endemic region and should continue 4 weeks after leaving.

The adult dose for *acute treatment* of *P. falciparum* or *P. vivax* malaria is 1250 mg (5 tablets) taken all at once with at least 8 ounces of water.

Atovaquone/Proguanil

Activity and Therapeutic Use. The combination of atovaquone plus proguanil, available as Malarone, is highly effective for both the prophylaxis and treatment of malaria caused by chloroquine-resistant *P. falciparum*. Both drugs are active against erythrocytic and exoerythrocytic forms of *P. falciparum*, including strains that are resistant to chloroquine, mefloquine, and pyrimethamine/sulfadoxine. In addition to its use in malaria, atovaquone, by itself, is used to treat *Pneumocystis carinii* pneumonia (see Chapter 95).

Mechanism of Action. Atovaquone and proguanil disrupt two separate pathways in pyrimidine synthesis, and thereby suppress DNA replication. Atovaquone has a unique mechanism: disruption of mitochondrial electric transport. No other antimalarial drug works this way. Proguanil is inactive as administered, but gets converted to cycloguanil, its active form, in the body. Like pyrimethamine, cycloguanil inhibits plasmodial dihydrofolate reductase, and thereby prevents activation of folic acid. In the absence of useable folic acid, *P. falciparum* is unable to make DNA, RNA, and proteins.

Pharmacokinetics. Absorption of atovaquone is low and variable, but can be greatly enhanced by fatty foods. The drug is 99% bound to plasma proteins, has a prolonged half-life (2 to 3 days), and undergoes excretion unchanged in the feces. In contrast to atovaquone, proguanil is extensively absorbed, both in the presence and absence of food. The drug concentrates in erythrocytes and undergoes hepatic metabolism followed by renal excretion. Its half-life is 12 to 21 hours.

Adverse Effects and Interactions. The combination of atovaquone plus proguanil is generally well tolerated. When atovaquone is used alone, the principal adverse effect is rash, which occurs in 20% to 40% of patients. Other reactions to atovaquone include nausea, vomiting, diarrhea, headache, fever, and insomnia. When proguanil is used alone, the most common side effects are oral ulceration, GI effects, and headache. In addition, the drug may cause hair loss, urticaria, hematuria, thrombocytopenia, and scaling of the soles and palms. Proguanil is considered safe for use during pregnancy; the safety of atovaquone has not been established. Proguanil appears devoid of significant drug interactions. In contrast, certain drugs, including tetracycline and rifampin, can reduce levels of atovaquone by as much as 50%.

Preparations, Dosage, and Administration. Atovaquone combined with proguanil is available in tablets formulated for adults and for children. Adult-strength tablets [Malarone] contain 250 mg of atovaquone and 100 mg of proguanil. Pediatric-strength tablets [Malarone Pediatric] contain 62.5 mg atovaquone and 25 mg proguanil.

For *prophylaxis* of malaria, dosing begins 1 or 2 days before entering a malaria-endemic area and continues for 7 days after leaving. The dosage for adults is 1 adult tablet a day. Dosages for children are based on body weight as follows: 11 to 20 kg, 1 pediatric tablet a day; 21 to 30 kg, 2 pediatric tablets once a day; 31 to 40 kg, 3 pediatric tablets once a day; and over 40 kg, 1 adult tablet a day.

For *treatment* of malaria, the dosage for adults is 2 adult tablets twice a day for 3 days. Dosages for children are based on body weight as follows: 11 to 20 kg, 1 *adult* tablet a day for 3 days; 21 to 30 kg, 2 *adult* tablets once a day for 3 days; 31 to 40 kg, 3 *adult* tablets once a day for 3 days; and above 40 kg, 2 *adult* tablets twice a day for 3 days.

To enhance absorption, all tablets should be administered with food or milk.

Halofantrine

Halofantrine [Halfan] is a preferred drug for acute therapy of mild to moderate malaria caused by chloroquine-resistant *P. falciparum* or *P. vivax*. The drug kills the erythrocytic stage of *Plasmodium* species. Its mechanism is unknown. Development of resistance may be a problem. Administration is oral and absorption is low and variable, but can be greatly increased by fatty foods. Because absorption is so variable, clinical responses—both therapeutic and adverse—vary as well. Mild side effects include diarrhea, abdominal pain, and pruritus. The adult dosage for an acute attack is 500 mg every 6 hours for three doses (repeated in 1 week for those with falciparum malaria).

Although halofantrine is generally safe, higher doses can be *cardiotoxic*. The drug prolongs the QT interval, and can thereby cause fatal ventricular dysrhythmias. Electrocardiographic monitoring is recommended. Halofantrine should be avoided by patients with cardiac conduction defects and by those taking other drugs that can prolong the QT interval. Because higher blood levels are more dangerous, and because food can promote excessive absorption, halofantrine should be administered at least 1 hour before meals or 2 hours after.

Artemether and Artensunate

Artemether [Artenam] and artensunate are derivatives of artemisinin, a compound isolated from an herbal remedy. All three compounds have antimalarial activity, and all three undergo conversion to an active metabolite: dihydroartemisinin. Artemether, given by IM injection, is a preferred drug for treating severe acute malaria caused by all strains of plasmodia, both chloroquine sensitive and chloroquine resistant. Artensunate, combined with mefloquine, is a preferred oral treatment for acute attacks caused by chloroquine-resistant *P. falciparum*. Both artemether and artensunate may increase the duration of coma, cause neurologic toxicity, and prolong the QT interval. In addition, artemether may cause convulsions and artensunate may cause ataxia and slurred speech. The adult dosage for artemether is 3.2 mg/kg IM as a loading dose followed by 1.6 mg/kg daily for 5 to 7 days. The adult dosage for artensunate is 4 mg/kg/day PO for 3 days, given in combination with oral mefloquine: 750 mg followed in 12 hours by 500 mg. Neither artemether nor artensunate is available in the United States.

Antibacterial Drugs

Tetracyclines. Two members of the tetracycline family—*doxycycline* and *tetracycline*—are used against chloroquine-resistant malaria. Both drugs kill the erythrocytic stage of the malaria parasite, although the rate of kill is slow. Doxycycline is used for prophylaxis and for acute attacks, whereas tetracycline is used for acute attacks only. To treat acute attacks, these drugs are combined with quinine, which acts more quickly than the tetracyclines. All tetracyclines are contraindicated for use by pregnant women and children less than 8 years old. To treat an acute attack, adults take 100 mg of doxycycline bid for 7 days, or 250 mg of tetracycline tid for 7 days. For prophylaxis, adults take 100 mg of doxycycline every day, beginning 2 days before traveling to a malaria-endemic area, and continuing 4 weeks after leaving the area. The basic pharmacology of the tetracyclines is presented in Chapter 82.

Sulfonamides. Like the tetracyclines, sulfonamides act slowly to kill the erythrocytic stage of the malaria parasite. For antimalarial therapy, sulfonamides are combined with pyrimethamine. The combination used most often is pyrimethamine plus sulfadoxine, available under the trade name Fansidar. Fansidar is combined with quinine to treat acute attacks caused by chloroquine-resistant *P. falciparum.* Sulfonamides carry a risk of severe allergic reactions, including potentially fatal Stevens-Johnson syndrome.

Clindamycin. Clindamycin is active against the erythrocytic stage of the malaria parasite. The drug is used as an adjunct to quinine to treat malaria caused by chloroquine-resistant *P. falciparum.* The principal adverse effect of clindamycin is colitis secondary to overgrowth of the bowel with *Clostridium difficile.*

⸪ KEY POINTS

- There are two principal forms of malaria, one caused by *Plasmodium vivax* and the other by *Plasmodium falciparum.*
- Vivax malaria is more common than falciparum malaria, but falciparum malaria is more severe.
- Drug resistance is common with *P. falciparum* and uncommon with *P. vivax.*
- Plasmodia reside in the liver and in erythrocytes. Those in the liver are harder to kill.
- Clinical cure of malaria (i.e., elimination of symptoms) results from killing plasmodia in erythrocytes.
- Vivax malaria relapses after clinical cure (because dormant parasites remain in the liver); falciparum malaria does not relapse.
- Chloroquine is the drug of choice for treatment and prophylaxis of malaria caused by chloroquine-sensitive strains of *P. vivax* and *P. falciparum.*
- Quinine, combined with an adjunctive drug (e.g., doxycycline) is the drug of choice for treatment of malaria caused by chloroquine-resistant *P. vivax* or *P. falciparum.*
- For prophylaxis of chloroquine-resistant malaria, any of three preparations may be used: doxycycline, mefloquine, or atovaquone/proguanil.
- Primaquine, which kills dormant *P. vivax* in the liver, is the drug of choice for preventing relapse of vivax malaria.
- The principal adverse effect of primaquine is hemolytic anemia, which occurs in patients whose red blood cells have a genetically determined deficiency in glucose-6-phosphate dehydrogenase.
- The principal adverse effects of quinine are cinchonism (tinnitus, headache, visual disturbances, nausea, vomiting), hemolytic anemia (as with primaquine), and birth defects.
- High therapeutic doses of mefloquine can cause neuropsychiatric reactions, and hence should be avoided in patients with epilepsy or psychiatric disorders.

Antiprotozoal Drugs II: Miscellaneous Agents

PROTOZOAL INFECTIONS

DRUGS OF CHOICE FOR PROTOZOAL INFECTIONS

Iodoquinol

Metronidazole

Benznidazole and Tinidazole

Pentamidine

Atovaquone

Trimetrexate

Suramin

Melarsoprol

Eflornithine

Nifurtimox

Pyrimethamine

Sodium Stibogluconate

Because of increasing world travel by Americans, and because of increased immigration by individuals from regions where infectious protozoa are endemic (South America, Asia, Africa), the incidence of protozoal infection in the United States is rising. The organisms encountered most frequently are *Entamoeba histolytica, Trichomonas vaginalis,* and *Giardia lamblia.* Infections with most other protozoa (e.g., *Leishmania* species, trypanosomes) are rare in North America. In approaching the antiprotozoal drugs, we begin by discussing the diseases that protozoa produce, after which we discuss the drugs used for treatment.

PROTOZOAL INFECTIONS

Our goal in this section is to describe the major protozoal infections, except for malaria, which is the subject of Chapter 94. Discussion focuses on causative organisms, sites of infection, symptoms of disease, and preferred drug therapy. Causative organisms and drugs of choice are summarized in Table 95–1.

Amebiasis

Amebiasis is an infestation with *Entamoeba histolytica.* In the United States, the disease affects between 2% and 4% of the population. Worldwide, about 10% of the population is infected. The principal site of infestation is the intestine. However, amebas may migrate to other tissues, most commonly the liver, where abscesses may form. Amebiasis is usually asymptomatic. When symptoms are present, the most characteristic are diarrhea, abdominal pain, and weight loss.

Drugs of choice for amebiasis are *iodoquinol, paromomycin, metronidazole,* and *tinidazole.* Iodoquinol and paromomycin are active only against amebas residing in the intestine. Metronidazole and tinidazole are active against amebas that inhabit the intestine, liver, and all other sites. For patients with asymptomatic intestinal infection, therapy with iodoquinol or paromomycin is sufficient. For patients with severe intestinal disease or with liver abscesses, metronidazole is given initially, followed by iodoquinol.

Iodoquinol, metronidazole, and tinidazole are discussed below. Paromomycin is discussed in Chapter 83.

Giardiasis

Giardiasis is an infection with *Giardia lamblia.* In the United States, giardiasis has an incidence of 2% to 10%. Infestation usually occurs by contact with contaminated objects or by drinking contaminated water. The primary habitat of *G. lamblia* is the upper small intestine. Occasionally, organisms migrate to the bile ducts and gallbladder. As many as 50% of affected individuals remain free of symptoms. However, symptoms that are both unpleasant and uncomfortable can develop. These include profound malaise; heartburn; vomiting; colicky pain after eating; and malodorous belching, flatulence, and diarrhea. The pain associated with giardiasis may mimic that of gallstones, appendicitis, peptic ulcers, or hiatal hernia. The treatment of choice is *metronidazole.*

Leishmaniasis

The term *leishmaniasis* refers to infestation by certain protozoal species belonging to the genus *Leishmania.* Worldwide, the incidence of leishmaniasis is estimated at 10 million. The disease is acquired through the bite of sand flies indigenous to tropical and subtropical regions. In the human host, the parasites take up residence inside cells of the reticuloendothelial system.

Leishmaniasis has three different forms: *cutaneous, mucocutaneous,* and *visceral.* The particular form acquired is determined by the species of *Leishmania* involved. The forms of leishmaniasis vary greatly in severity, ranging from mild (cutaneous leishmaniasis) to potentially fatal (visceral leishmaniasis). In *cutaneous* leishmaniasis, a nodule forms at the site of inoculation; later, this nodule may evolve into an ulcer that is very slow to heal. *Mucocutaneous* leishmaniasis is characterized by ulceration in the mucosa of the mouth, nose, and pharynx. Symptoms of *visceral* leishmaniasis include fever, hepatosplenomegaly, liver dysfunction, hypoalbuminemia, pancytopenia, lymphadenopathy, and hemorrhage. Left untreated, the disease is frequently fatal. For all forms of leishmaniasis, *sodium stibogluconate* is the traditional treatment of choice. However, two antifungal drugs—*fluconazole* (given PO) and *amphotericin B* (given IV)—are highly effective alternatives.

Pneumocystis carinii Pneumonia

Pneumocystis carinii pneumonia (PCP) is caused by *Pneumocystis carinii,* an organism that was formerly classified as a protozoan, but is now classified as a fungus. In people with advanced HIV infection (AIDS), PCP is the most common opportunistic infection and the leading cause of death. The treatment of choice for PCP is *trimethoprim plus sulfamethoxazole.* Alternatives include *pentamidine, dapsone, atovaquone,* and *primaquine combined with clindamycin.* The pathophysiology and treatment of PCP are discussed further in Chapter 90 (Antiviral Drugs II: Drugs for HIV Infection and Related Opportunistic Infections).

Toxoplasmosis

Toxoplasmosis is caused by infection with *Toxoplasma gondii,* a protozoan of the class Sporozoa. The parasite is harbored by many animals as well as by humans. Infection is acquired most commonly by eating undercooked meat.

TABLE 95–1 ▪■ Drugs of Choice for Protozoal Infection

Disease	Causative Protozoan	Drugs of Choice
Amebiasis	*Entamoeba histolytica*	Iodoquinol, paromomycin, metronidazole, tinidazole*
Giardiasis	*Giardia lamblia*	Metronidazole
Leishmaniasis	*Leishmania* species	Sodium stibogluconate, amphotericin B
Pneumocystis carinii pneumonia	*Pneumocystis carinii*	Trimethoprim plus sulfamethoxazole
Toxoplasmosis	*Toxoplasma gondii*	Pyrimethamine plus sulfadiazine
Trichomoniasis	*Trichomonas vaginalis*	Metronidazole, tinidazole*
Trypanosomiasis: American (Chagas' disease)	*Trypanosoma cruzi*	Nifurtimox, benznidazole*
Trypanosomiasis: West African (sleeping sickness) Early (hemolymphatic) stage Late (CNS) stage	*Trypanosoma brucei gambiense*	Pentamidine Melarsoprol, eflornithine
Trypanosomiasis: East African (sleeping sickness) Early (hemolymphatic) stage Late (CNS) stage	*Trypanosoma brucei rhodesiense*	Suramin Melarsoprol, eflornithine

*Not available in the United States.

However, toxoplasmosis may also be congenital. Congenital infection can damage the brain, eyes, liver, and other organs. Extensive disease is usually fatal. In immunocompetent adults, infection is usually asymptomatic. However, in immunocompromised hosts, such as those with AIDS, the disease may progress to encephalitis and death. The treatment of choice is *pyrimethamine plus sulfadiazine.*

Trichomoniasis

Trichomoniasis is caused by *Trichomonas vaginalis,* a flagellated protozoan. Trichomoniasis is a common disease, affecting about 200 million people worldwide. The usual site of infestation is the genitourinary tract. Parasites may also inhabit the rectum. In females, infection results in vaginitis. In males, infection causes urethritis. The disease is usually transmitted sexually but can also be acquired by contact with contaminated objects (e.g., toilet seats). Oral *metronidazole* is the treatment of choice. *Tinidazole,* a related drug unavailable in the United States, is at least as effective and better tolerated.

Trypanosomiasis

There are two major forms of trypanosomiasis: African trypanosomiasis and American trypanosomiasis. Both forms are caused by protozoal species belonging to the genus *Trypanosoma.*

American Trypanosomiasis (Chagas' Disease). Chagas' disease is caused by infection with *Trypanosoma cruzi,* a protozoan of the class Sporozoa. The disease is prevalent in South America and the Caribbean, where it affects some 10 million people. The parasites are harbored in the digestive tract of certain blood-sucking bugs, and are transmitted as follows: the bug bites a sleeping person (usually on the face) and also defecates; the parasites, which are contained in the bug's feces, are then forced into the bite wound by rubbing or scratching. An early sign of the disease is swelling and severe inflammation at the site of inoculation. Over time, parasites invade cardiac cells and neurons of the myenteric plexus. Destruction of these cells can cause cardiomyopathy, megaesophagus, and megacolon. Death has occurred, usually secondary to cardiac injury. In its early phase, Chagas' disease can be treated with *nifurtimox.* Unfortunately, neither this drug nor any other is very effective against chronic infection.

African Trypanosomiasis (Sleeping Sickness). African trypanosomiasis, transmitted by the bite of the tsetse fly, is caused by two subspecies of *Trypanosoma brucei: T. brucei gambiense* and *T. brucei rhodesiense.* Trypanosomiasis caused by either subspecies has similar symptoms. Early symptoms, which involve the hemolymphatic system, include fever, lymphadenopathy, hepatosplenomegaly, dyspnea, and tachycardia. Late symptoms, which result from involvement of the central nervous system (CNS), include mental dullness, incoordination, and apathy. As CNS involvement

advances, sleep becomes continuous and death may eventually follow. During the early (hemolymphatic) phase of African trypanosomiasis, *pentamidine* and *suramin* are the agents of choice. (Pentamidine is preferred for disease caused by *T. brucei gambiense,* and suramin is preferred for disease caused by *T. brucei rhodesiense*). During the late (CNS) stage, *melarsoprol* and *eflornithine* are the agents of choice, regardless of the causative subspecies. All four drugs—pentamidine, suramin, eflornithine, and melarsoprol—can produce serious side effects. Treatment is difficult and frequently unsuccessful.

DRUGS OF CHOICE FOR PROTOZOAL INFECTIONS

The major antiprotozoal drugs are discussed below. With the exception of metronidazole, each of these agents is active against only one organism. Although consideration here is limited to drugs of choice, be aware that additional antiprotozoal drugs are available.

Iodoquinol

Actions and Use. Iodoquinol [Yodoxin] is a drug of choice for asymptomatic intestinal amebiasis. In addition, the drug is employed in conjunction with metronidazole to treat symptomatic intestinal infection and systemic amebiasis. In these last two cases, iodoquinol is administered after treatment with metronidazole to eliminate any surviving intestinal parasites. The mechanism of amebicidal action is unknown.

Pharmacokinetics. Only a small fraction (5% to 8%) of oral iodoquinol is absorbed. The fraction absorbed is excreted as metabolites in the urine.

Adverse Effects. Mild reactions occur occasionally. These include rash, acne, slight thyroid enlargement, and GI effects (nausea, vomiting, diarrhea, cramps, pruritus ani). Rarely, prolonged therapy at very high doses has caused optic atrophy with permanent loss of vision.

Preparations, Dosage, and Administration. Iodoquinol [Yodoxin] is available in tablets (210 and 650 mg) and as a powder for oral administration. The usual adult dosage is 650 mg 3 times a day for 20 days. The dosage for children is 10 to 13 mg/kg 3 times a day for 20 days.

Metronidazole

Therapeutic Uses. Metronidazole [Flagyl, Protostat] is the drug of choice for symptomatic intestinal amebiasis and systemic amebiasis. Because most of each dose is absorbed in the small intestine, metronidazole concentrations in the colon remain low, allowing amebas living there to survive. To kill these survivors, metronidazole is followed by iodoquinol, an amebicidal drug that achieves high concentrations in the colon.

Metronidazole is the agent of choice for infection with *T. vaginalis.* The drug is effective against trichomoniasis in males as well as in females.

Metronidazole is the drug of choice for *giardiasis.* Quinacrine, the former drug of choice, is more effective but has been withdrawn from the U.S. market.

Many anaerobic bacteria are sensitive to metronidazole. Antibacterial applications are discussed in Chapter 87.

Mechanism of Action. To be effective, metronidazole must first be converted to a more chemically reactive form. This reactive form interacts with DNA, causing strand breakage and loss of helical structure. The resulting impairment of DNA function is thought responsible for the drug's antimicrobial and mutagenic actions.

Pharmacokinetics. Metronidazole is readily absorbed from the GI tract and undergoes extensive hepatic metabolism. Metabolites and unchanged drug are excreted in the urine.

Adverse Effects. Metronidazole produces a variety of untoward effects, but these rarely lead to termination of treatment. The most common side effects are nausea, headache, dry mouth, and an unpleasant metallic taste. Other common responses include stomatitis, vomiting, diarrhea, insomnia, vertigo, and weakness. Harmless darkening of the urine may occur; patients should be forewarned of this effect. Certain neurologic effects (numbness in the extremities, ataxia, convulsions) occur rarely. If these develop, metronidazole should be withdrawn. Metronidazole should not be used by patients with active disease of the CNS. Carcinogenic effects have been observed in rodents, but there is no evidence of cancer in humans.

Use in Pregnancy. Metronidazole readily crosses the placenta, and is mutagenic in bacteria. However, experience to date has shown no fetal harm following treatment of pregnant women. Nonetheless, it is recommended that metronidazole be avoided during the first trimester, and employed with caution throughout the rest of pregnancy.

Drug Interactions. Metronidazole has disulfiram-like effects, and hence can produce unpleasant or dangerous reactions if used in conjunction with *alcohol.* Accordingly, patients must be warned against alcohol consumption.

Metronidazole inhibits inactivation of warfarin, an anticoagulant. Dosages of warfarin must be lowered.

Preparations, Dosage, and Administration. Metronidazole [Flagyl, Protostat] is available in capsules (375 mg), standard tablets (250 and 500 mg), and extended-release tablets (750 mg); in solution for injection (5 mg/ml); and as a powder (to be reconstituted for injection). For protozoal infections, the oral formulations are used. Antibacterial therapy usually requires IV treatment. Dosages for antiprotozoal therapy are given below. Dosages for antibacterial therapy are presented in Chapter 87.

Amebiasis. The adult dosage is 500 to 750 mg 3 times a day for 10 days. The pediatric dosage is 12 to 17 mg/kg 3 times a day for 10 days. Following treatment with metronidazole, iodoquinol is given for 20 days.

Trichomoniasis. Treatment for adults consists of either (1) a single 2-gm dose or (2) 500 mg twice daily for 7 days. The pediatric dosage is 5 mg/kg 3 times a day for 7 days.

Giardiasis. The adult dosage is 250 mg 3 times a day for 5 days. The pediatric dosage is 5 mg/kg 3 times a day for 5 days.

Benznidazole and Tinidazole

Benznidazole [Rochagan] and tinidazole [Fasigyn] are chemical relatives of metronidazole. Benznidazole is a drug of choice for American trypanosomiasis (Chagas' disease); tinidazole is a drug of choice for amebiasis and trichomoniasis. The adult dosage for benznidazole is 2.5 to 3.5 mg/kg twice daily for 30 to 90 days, and the pediatric dosage is 5 mg/kg twice daily for 30 to 90 days. Dosages for tinidazole are as follows:

- For trichomoniasis—*adults,* 2 gm once or 500 mg twice; *children,* 50 mg/kg (max. 2 gm) once
- For amebiasis—*adults,* 670 mg 3 times a day for 3 days; *children,* 50 mg/kg (max. 2 gm) for 3 days

Although benznidazole and tinidazole are very effective, neither drug is available in the United States.

Pentamidine

Actions. Pentamidine [Pentam 300, Pentacarinat, NebuPent] is active against *P. carinii.* The drug disrupts synthesis of DNA, RNA, phospholipids, and proteins. We do not know if these actions underlie its antiprotozoal effects.

Uses. Pentamidine is given by injection (IM or IV) and by inhalation. Pentamidine injection is used to treat active PCP. *Inhaled* pentamidine is used to prevent PCP in high-risk HIV-positive patients. High-risk patients are those with (1) a history of one or more episodes of PCP or (2) peripheral CD4 lymphocyte counts of less than 200 cells/mm³. In addition to treatment of PCP, pentamidine has been used on an investigational basis to treat leishmaniasis and trypanosomiasis.

Pharmacokinetics. For treatment of active PCP, pentamidine is administered IM or IV. Equivalent blood levels are achieved with both routes. The drug is extensively bound in tissues. Penetration to the brain and cerebrospinal fluid is poor. Between 50% and 65% of each dose is excreted rapidly in the urine. The remaining drug is excreted slowly, over a month or more.

Adverse Effects Associated with Parenteral Pentamidine. Pentamidine can produce serious side effects when given IM or IV. Caution is needed.

Sudden and severe *hypotension* occurs in about 1% of patients. The fall in blood pressure may cause tachycardia, dizziness, and fainting. To minimize hypotensive responses, patients should receive the drug while lying down. Blood pressure should be monitored closely.

Hypoglycemia and *hyperglycemia* have occurred. Hypoglycemia has been associated with necrosis of pancreatic islet cells and excessive insulin levels. The cause of hyperglycemia is unknown. Because of possible fluctuations in glucose levels, blood glucose should be monitored daily.

Intramuscular administration is painful. Necrosis at the injection site followed by formation of a sterile abscess is common.

Some adverse effects can be life threatening when severe. These reactions and their incidences are leukopenia (2.8%), thrombocytopenia (1.7%), acute renal failure (0.5%), hypocalcemia (0.2%), and dysrhythmias (0.2%).

Adverse Effects Associated with Aerosolized Pentamidine. Inhaled pentamidine does not cause the severe adverse effects associated with parenteral pentamidine. The most common reactions are cough (38%) and bronchospasm (15%). Both reactions are more pronounced in patients with asthma or a history of smoking. Fortunately, these reactions can be controlled with an inhaled bronchodilator, and rarely necessitate pentamidine withdrawal.

Preparations, Dosage, and Administration. Pentamidine isethionate *for injection* [Pentam 300, Pentacarinat] is dispensed in 300-mg single-dose vials. For treatment of active PCP, the dosage for adults and children is 3 to 4 mg/kg IV daily for 2 to 3 weeks. Administration must be done slowly (over 60 minutes).

Pentamidine isethionate *aerosol* [NebuPent] is used for prophylaxis of PCP in patients with AIDS. The dosage is 300 mg once every 4 weeks. Administration is performed with a Respirgard II nebulizer by Marquest. Solutions should be freshly prepared.

Atovaquone

Actions and Use. Atovaquone [Mepron] is approved for mild to moderate PCP in patients who cannot tolerate trimethoprim-sulfamethoxazole. Atovaquone is less effective than the trimethoprim-sulfamethoxazole but better tolerated. Benefits appear to derive from inhibition of DNA synthesis secondary to disruption of mitochondrial electron transport in *P. carinii*. As discussed in Chapter 94, atovaquone is also used to treat malaria.

Pharmacokinetics. Atovaquone was initially formulated in tablets, but is now formulated as a suspension. This change was made because absorption of the tablets was poor and erratic. Absorption of the suspension is more complete and is greatly enhanced by food, especially fatty food. Atovaquone is 99% bound to plasma proteins, has a prolonged half-life (2 to 3 days), and is excreted unchanged in the feces.

Adverse Effects and Interactions. The principal adverse effect is rash, which occurs in 20% to 40% of patients. Other adverse effects include nausea (21%), diarrhea (16%), headache (16%), vomiting (14%), fever (14%), and insomnia (10%). Safety for use by young children or by women who are pregnant or breast-feeding has not been established. Atovaquone undergoes extensive protein binding, and hence should not be combined with other drugs that are highly protein bound.

Preparations, Dosage, and Administration. Atovaquone [Mepron] is dispensed as a suspension (150 mg/ml) for oral use. For treatment of *active PCP infection,* the dosage for adults and children older than 13 years is 750 mg twice daily for 21 days. For *prophylaxis of PCP infection,* the dosage is 1500 mg once daily. Because absorption is poor in the absence of food, the drug must be administered with meals.

Trimetrexate

Therapeutic Use. Trimetrexate [Neutrexin], in combination with leucovorin, is indicated for moderate to severe PCP in immunocompromised patients, such as those with AIDS. Leucovorin must be taken with trimetrexate to protect against toxicity (e.g., severe bone marrow depression), which can be life threatening. Because of its potential for toxicity, trimetrexate is not a first-line drug for PCP.

Mechanism of Action. Trimetrexate inhibits dihydrofolate reductase, the enzyme that converts dihydrofolic acid into tetrahydrofolic acid, its active form. In the absence of tetrahydrofolic acid, cells are unable to make DNA, RNA, and proteins, and hence they die.

Selective kill of *P. carinii* is achieved by administering *leucovorin* (folinic acid) along with trimetrexate. Leucovorin protects the host but not *P. carinii.* To protect host cells, leucovorin first undergoes uptake via an energy-dependent, carrier-mediated process. Once inside cells, leucovorin bypasses the metabolic block caused by trimetrexate. Leucovorin does not protect *P. carinii* because the parasite lacks the transport system required for leucovorin uptake.

Adverse Effects. By suppressing synthesis of DNA, RNA, and proteins, trimetrexate can cause serious harm, and even death. Possible effects include bone marrow suppression, hepatotoxicity, nephrotoxicity, and damage to the GI mucosa. Fortunately, when trimetrexate is used properly—that is, in combination with leucovorin—the risk of serious injury is low. Patients should be informed about the protective effects of leucovorin and warned that failure to take the drug could be fatal.

Hematologic toxicity secondary to bone marrow suppression is the greatest concern. To monitor for bone marrow suppression, absolute neutrophil counts and platelet counts should be obtained before treatment and twice weekly during treatment. If hematologic toxicity is detected, the dosage of leucovorin should be increased and the dosage of trimetrexate decreased.

Effects in Pregnancy. Trimetrexate is in Food and Drug Administration Pregnancy Risk Category D: there is a proven risk of human fetal harm. In rats and rabbits, doses lower than those used clinically have been teratogenic and fetotoxic; skeletal, visceral, ocular, and cardiovascular abnormalities have been observed. Women receiving trimetrexate should be warned against becoming pregnant.

Drug Interactions. *Zidovudine and Ganciclovir.* Both drugs, which are commonly used by patients with AIDS, suppress bone marrow function. As a result, both can intensify hematologic toxicity from trimetrexate. Exercise caution if either agent is used concurrently with trimetrexate.

Inhibitors of P450 Enzymes. Trimetrexate is inactivated by cytochrome P450 drug-metabolizing enzymes. Accordingly, drugs that inhibit P450 enzymes can cause trimetrexate levels to rise; toxicity can result. Unfortunately, patients with AIDS, who are likely candidates for trimetrexate therapy, often take drugs that inhibit P450 enzymes. Among these are protease inhibitors (e.g., ritonavir), certain antifungal drugs (e.g., ketoconazole), rifampin, rifabutin, and erythromycin. When any of these drugs is taken concurrently with trimetrexate, additional caution is needed to avoid trimetrexate toxicity.

Preparations, Dosage, and Administration. *Preparation and Storage.* Trimetrexate [Neutrexin], dispensed as a powder, is reconstituted

with 5% Dextrose Injection to a concentration of 0.25 to 2 mg/ml. Preparations that are cloudy or contain a precipitate should not be used. Trimetrexate solutions should not be mixed with leucovorin solutions because a precipitate will form.

Trimetrexate powder is stored at room temperature, protected from light. Reconstituted solutions may be stored for 24 hours at room temperature or under refrigeration.

Dosage and Administration. *Trimetrexate is always used together with leucovorin.* Dosing with both drugs is begun the same day; leucovorin is continued for 3 days after the last dose of trimetrexate. For *trimetrexate,* the adult dosage is 45 mg/m² administered once daily by IV infusion over 60 to 90 minutes. For *leucovorin,* the adult dosage is 20 mg/m² administered 4 times a day by mouth or by a 5- to 10-minute IV infusion. Trimetrexate is given for 21 days and leucovorin for 24 days (i.e., 3 days longer than trimetrexate). In the event of hematologic toxicity, the dosage of trimetrexate should be reduced and the dosage of leucovorin increased. In the event of severe hematologic, hepatic, renal, or mucosal toxicity, trimetrexate should be interrupted.

Suramin

Actions and Uses. Suramin sodium [Germanin, others] is a drug of choice for treating the early phase of East African trypanosomiasis (sleeping sickness); for the late phase of the disease (i.e., the stage of CNS involvement), melarsoprol and eflornithine are preferred. Suramin is known to inhibit many trypanosomal enzymes; however, its primary mechanism of action has not been established.

Pharmacokinetics. The drug is poorly absorbed from the GI tract, and hence must be given parenterally (IV). Suramin binds tightly to plasma proteins and remains in the bloodstream for months. Penetration into cells is low. Excretion is renal.

Adverse Effects. Side effects can be severe, and hence treatment should take place in a hospital. Frequent reactions include vomiting, itching, rash, paresthesias, photophobia, and hyperesthesia of the palms and soles. Suramin concentrates in the kidneys and can cause local damage, resulting in the appearance of protein, blood cells, and casts in the urine. If urinary casts are observed, treatment should cease. Rarely, a shock-like syndrome develops after IV administration. To minimize the risk of this reaction, a small test dose (100 to 200 mg) is administered; in the absence of a severe reaction, full doses may follow.

Preparations, Dosage, and Administration. Suramin sodium [Germanin, others] is available from the Centers for Disease Control and Prevention. The drug is dispensed in 1-gm ampules. Administration is by slow IV infusion. Suramin is unstable, hence fresh solutions must be made daily. The adult dosage is 1 gm IV on days 1, 3, 7, 14, and 21. The pediatric dosage is 20 mg/kg IV on days 1, 3, 7, 14, and 21.

Melarsoprol

Therapeutic Use. Melarsoprol [Arsobal, Mel-B] is a drug of choice for both East and West African trypanosomiasis (sleeping sickness). The drug is employed during the *late* stage of the disease (i.e., after CNS involvement has developed). For earlier stages of the disease, suramin and pentamidine are preferred.

Mechanism of Action. Melarsoprol is an organic arsenical compound that reacts with sulfhydryl groups of proteins. Antiparasitic effects result from inactivation of enzymes. This same action appears to underlie the serious toxicity of the drug. Melarsoprol is more toxic to parasites than to humans because it penetrates parasitic membranes more easily than human cells.

Adverse Effects. Melarsoprol is quite toxic, and adverse reactions are common. Frequent responses include hypertension, albuminuria, peripheral neuropathy, myocardial damage, and Herxheimer-type reactions. Reactive encephalopathy may develop during the first course of treatment. Although fatalities have occurred, they are much less common than in the past.

Preparations, Dosage, and Administration. Melarsoprol [Arsobal, Mel-B] is administered by slow IV injection. The drug is highly irritating to tissues, and hence care must be taken to avoid extravasation. Because of its toxicity, melarsoprol should be administered in a hospital setting. Treatment for adults begins with 2 to 3.6 mg/kg IV daily for 3 days. Seven days later, a second course (3.6 mg/kg IV daily for 3 days) is given. This is repeated once more after 10 to 21 days. Melarsoprol can be obtained through the Centers for Disease Control and Prevention. The drug is not available commercially.

Eflornithine

Actions and Use. Eflornithine [Ornidyl] is indicated for patients with late-stage African trypanosomiasis (sleeping sickness). The drug is highly effective against *T. gambiense* (West African sleeping sickness), but only variably active against *T. rhodesiense* (East African sleeping sickness). In both cases, benefits derive from irreversible inhibition of ornithine decarboxylase, an enzyme needed for biosynthesis of polyamines, which are required by all cells for division and differentiation. Parasites weakened by eflornithine become highly vulnerable to lethal attack by host defenses. Since cells of the host can readily synthesize more ornithine decarboxylase to replace inhibited enzyme, cells of the host are spared.

Pharmacokinetics. Eflornithine may be administered orally or IV. Once in the blood, the drug is well distributed to body fluids and tissues, including the CNS. Eflornithine has a half-life of 100 minutes and is eliminated largely unchanged in the urine.

Adverse Effects. The most common adverse effects are anemia (48%), diarrhea (39%), and leukopenia (27%). Seizures may occur early in therapy but then subside, despite continued treatment. Since IV administration of eflornithine requires large volumes of fluid, fluid overload may develop over the course of treatment. Eflornithine can also cause hair loss. In fact, the drug is now available for topical use to remove facial hair (see Chapter 101).

Preparations, Dosage, and Administration. Eflornithine may be administered PO or IV. The dosage for adults is 100 mg/kg IV 4 times a day for 14 days, followed by 300 mg/kg PO daily for 3 to 4 weeks. Higher doses may be needed in children. Eflornithine is dispensed as a concentrated solution (200 mg/ml in 100-ml vials) and must be diluted for IV infusion. The drug is available only from the World Health Organization.

Nifurtimox

Therapeutic Use. Nifurtimox [Lampit] is a drug of choice for American trypanosomiasis (Chagas' disease). The drug is most effective in the acute stage of the disease, curing about 80% of patients. Chronic disease is less responsive.

Pharmacokinetics. Nifurtimox is well absorbed from the GI tract and undergoes rapid and extensive metabolism. Metabolites are excreted in the urine.

Adverse Effects. Therapy is prolonged, and significant untoward effects occur frequently. Gastrointestinal effects (anorexia, nausea, vomiting, abdominal pain) and peripheral neuropathy are especially common. Weight loss resulting from GI effects may require cessation of treatment. Additional common reactions include rash and CNS effects (memory loss, insomnia, vertigo, headache).

Preparations, Dosage, and Administration. Nifurtimox [Lampit] is dispensed in 100-mg tablets. In the United States, the drug is available only from the Centers for Disease Control and Prevention. The adult dosage is 2 to 2.5 mg/kg 4 times a day for 120 days. For young children (ages 1 through 10 years), the usual dosage is 4 to 5 mg/kg 4 times a day for 90 days. For older children (ages 11 to 16 years), the usual dosage is 3 to 4 mg/kg 4 times a day for 90 days.

Pyrimethamine

Pyrimethamine [Daraprim], combined with sulfadiazine, is the treatment of choice for toxoplasmosis. Pyrimethamine is also important for treating malaria (see Chapter 94). For toxoplasmosis, the adult dosage is 25 to 100 mg daily for 3 to 4 weeks. The pediatric dosage is 0.5 mg/kg twice a day for 2 to 4 days, followed by one-half that dosage for 4 weeks. For adults and children, each dose of pyrimethamine should be accompanied by 10 mg of folinic acid to reduce side effects. In addition, the regimen must include sulfadiazine: for adults, 1 to 1.5 gm 4 times a day for 3 to 4 weeks; for children, 100 to 200 mg/kg/day for 3 to 4 weeks. The basic pharmacology of pyrimethamine is discussed in Chapter 94.

Sodium Stibogluconate

Sodium stibogluconate [Pentostam] is a drug of choice for leishmaniasis. The mechanism of action is unknown. The drug is poorly absorbed from the GI tract, and hence must be given parenterally (IM or IV). Sodium stibogluconate undergoes little metabolism and is excreted rapidly in the urine. Although severe side effects can occur, the drug is generally well tolerated. The most frequent adverse reactions are muscle pain, joint stiffness, and bradycardia. Changes in the electrocardiogram are common and occasionally precede serious dysrhythmias. Liver and renal dysfunction, shock, and sudden death occur rarely. Sodium stibogluconate is dispensed in aqueous solution for IM and IV injection. For leishmaniasis, the usual adult and pediatric dosage is 20 mg/kg/day (IM or IV) for 20 to 28 days. In the United States, the drug is available only from the Centers for Disease Control and Prevention.

KEY POINTS

- The principal protozoal infections seen in the United States are trichomoniasis, giardiasis, and amebiasis.
- Metronidazole is the drug of choice for trichomoniasis, giardiasis, and symptomatic or systemic amebiasis.
- Iodoquinol is the drug of choice for asymptomatic amebiasis.
- Patients taking metronidazole should be warned against consuming alcohol because of the risk of a disulfiram-like reaction.

Ectoparasiticides

ECTOPARASITIC INFESTATIONS
    Scabies (Infestation with Mites)
    Pediculosis (Infestation with Lice)
PHARMACOLOGY OF ECTOPARASITICIDES
    Permethrin
    Malathion
    Crotamiton
    Pyrethrins Plus Piperonyl Butoxide
    Lindane
    Ivermectin

Ectoparasites are parasites that live on the surface of the host. Most ectoparasites that infest humans live on the skin and hair. Some live on clothing and bedding, moving to the host only to feed. The principal ectoparasites that infest humans are mites and lice. Infestation with mites is known as *scabies*. Infestation with lice is known as *pediculosis*. Both conditions are characterized by intense pruritus (itching). With the exception of ivermectin, all of the drugs used for treatment are topical.

ECTOPARASITIC INFESTATIONS

Scabies (Infestation with Mites)

Scabies is caused by infestation with *Sarcoptes scabiei*, an organism known commonly as the itch mite. Irritation results from the female mite burrowing beneath the skin to lay eggs. Burrows may be visible as small ridges or dotted lines. In adults, the most common sites of infestation are the wrists, elbows, nipples, navel, genital region, and webs of the fingers. In children, infestation is most likely on the head, neck, and buttocks.

The primary symptom of scabies is pruritus. Itching is most intense just after going to bed. Scratching may result in abrasion and secondary infection.

Transmission of scabies is usually by direct contact—either sexual or of a less intimate nature. Scabies may also be transmitted through contact with infested linen, towels, or clothing.

Scabies is usually treated with a pesticide-containing lotion or cream. To eradicate mites, the entire body surface must be treated (excluding the face and scalp in adults). To prevent reinfestation, bedding and intimate clothing should be machine washed and dried.

Several drugs can kill mites. *Permethrin* (5% cream formulation) is the drug of choice. This preparation is effective in just one application. *Crotamiton* is a preferred alternative. In

addition, there is evidence that a single oral dose (200 µg/kg) of *ivermectin* [Stromectol] can cure scabies, although the drug is not approved for this indication.

Pediculosis (Infestation with Lice)

Pediculosis is a general term referring to infestation with any of several kinds of lice. The types of lice encountered most frequently are *Pediculus humanus capitis* (head louse), *Pediculus humanus corporis* (body louse), and *Phthirus pubis* (pubic or crab louse). Infestation with any of these insects causes pruritus. Infestations with head, pubic, and body lice differ with regard to mode of acquisition and method of treatment.

Pubic Lice

Pubic lice, commonly known as *crabs* (because pubic lice are shaped like crabs), usually reside on the skin and hair of the pubic region. However, pubic lice may also be found on the eyelashes and other places. As a rule, infestation is transmitted through sexual contact. Consequently, crabs are most common among people who have multiple sexual partners. Two preparations—*permethrin* (1% liquid) and *malathion* (0.5% lotion)—are drugs of choice for eliminating crabs. Alternatives include *pyrethrins with piperonyl butoxide* (gel, liquid, shampoo) and oral *ivermectin* (200 µg/kg once). Infestation of the eyelashes is treated with petrolatum ophthalmic ointment. Clothing and linen should be disinfected by washing in very hot water, followed by machine drying at high temperature.

Head Lice

Head lice reside on the scalp and lay their nits (eggs) on the hair. Adult lice may be difficult to observe. Nits, however, are usually visible. Infestation may be associated with hives, boils, impetigo, and other skin disorders. The head louse is more democratic than the pubic or body louse and can be found infesting people from all socioeconomic groups. Head lice may be transmitted by close personal contact and (perhaps) by contact with infested clothing, hairbrushes, furniture, and other objects. Because humans are the only host for these obligate parasites, infestation cannot be acquired through contact with pets (or any other animals). Treatments of choice are *permethrin* and *malathion*. Both drugs kill adult lice as well as nits. A few days after drug treatment, dead lice (and remaining live lice) should be removed from the hair with a fine-toothed comb. Eradication of head lice does not require shaving or cutting the hair.

Body Lice

Despite their name, body lice reside not on the body but on clothing. These lice move to the body only to feed. Consequently, body lice are rarely seen on the skin. Rather, these insects can be found in bed linens and the seams of garments. Transmission of body lice is by contact with infested clothing or bedding. Body lice are relatively uncommon in the United States, where regular laundering precludes infestation. Infestation is most likely among vagrants and other people whose clothes may not be frequently washed. The majority of body lice can be removed from the host simply by removal of clothing. Those lice that remain on the body can be killed by applying a pesticide; *permethrin* and *malathion* are drugs of choice. Clothing and bedding should be disinfected by washing and drying at high temperature.

PHARMACOLOGY OF ECTOPARASITICIDES

As a rule, ectoparasitic infestations are treated with *topical* drugs. Topical agents are available in the form of creams, gels, lotions, and shampoos. Only one ectoparasiticide— ivermectin—is administered *orally*. Properties of the major ectoparasiticides are summarized in Table 96–1.

Permethrin
Basic Pharmacology

Actions and Uses. Permethrin [Nix, Elimite, Acticin] is toxic to mites, lice, and their ova. The drug kills adult insects by disrupting nerve traffic, thereby causing paralysis. In addition to killing mites and lice, permethrin is active against fleas and ticks. The 1% formulation [Nix] is a drug of choice for lice. The 5% formulation [Elimite, Acticin] is the drug of choice for scabies. As a rule, only one application is required.

Resistance. Permethrin fails to eradicate *head lice* in about 5% of patients. Drug resistance is suspected, although proof is lacking. To manage treatment-resistant head lice, some clinicians are recommending prolonged treatment (several hours rather than the usual 10 minutes) or use of the 5% formulation [Elimite, Acticin] rather than the 1% formulation [Nix]. It should be noted, however, that these practices are controversial.

Pharmacokinetics. Very little (about 2%) of topical permethrin is absorbed. The fraction absorbed is rapidly inactivated and excreted in the urine.

Adverse Effects. Topical permethrin is devoid of serious adverse effects. The drug may cause some exacerbation of the itching, erythema, and edema normally associated with pediculosis. Other reactions include temporary sensations of burning, stinging, and numbness.

Preparations and Administration

Preparations. Permethrin is dispensed in two concentrations: (1) a 1% liquid [Nix] used for lice and (2) a 5% cream [Elimite, Acticin] used for scabies.

Administration. Head Lice. Before applying permethrin (1% liquid) to remove head lice, the hair should be washed, rinsed, and towel dried. Permethrin is then applied in an amount sufficient to saturate the hair and scalp. After 10 minutes, permethrin should be removed with a warm-water rinse. Nits should be removed with a fine-toothed comb that has been dipped in vinegar. If needed, retreatment can be performed in 7 days. However, reapplication is required in less than 5% of cases.

Scabies. The 5% cream [Elimite] is massaged into the skin, from the head to the soles of the feet. After 8 to 14 hours, the cream is removed by washing. Thirty grams is sufficient for the average adult. Only one application is needed.

Malathion

Actions and Uses. Malathion [Ovide] is an organophosphate cholinesterase inhibitor (see Chapter 15). The drug kills lice and their ova. Humans and other mammals are not harmed because an enzyme in their blood converts malathion to nontoxic metabolites. The drug is approved for treatment of head lice. It is also used widely as an insecticide.

Adverse Effects and Interactions. The preparation used topically for head lice is devoid of significant adverse effects. Scalp irritation occurs occasionally. No systemic toxicity has been reported. Likewise, no drug interactions have been reported.

Preparations and Administration. Malathion [Ovide] is dispensed in a 5% lotion. The preparation is applied to dry hair, gently massaged until the scalp is moist, and allowed to dry naturally. (The lotion is flammable because of its 78% alcohol content. Hence, hair dryers and other sources of heat should

TABLE 96–1 ■ Preferred Drugs for Mites and Lice

| Generic Name | Trade Names | Indications | | Dosage Forms | Adverse Effects |
		Scabies (Mites)	Pediculosis (Lice)		
Topical Medications					
Permethrin	Nix		✔	Liquid: 1%	Occasional: burning, stinging,
	Elimite, Acticin	✔		Cream: 5%	itching, numbness, pain, rash, erythema, edema
Crotamiton	Eurax	✔		Cream: 10% Lotion: 10%	Occasional: rash, conjunctivitis
Malathion	Ovide		✔	Lotion: 0.5%	Occasional: local irritation
Pyrethrins plus piperonyl butoxide	RID, others		✔	Gel Liquid Shampoo	Occasional: irritation to eyes and mucous membranes following inadvertent contact
Systemic Medication					
Ivermectin	Stromectol	*	*	Tablet: 200 mg	Rare: hypertension

*Although ivermectin is effective against mites and lice, the drug is not approved by the Food and Drug Administration for treating these infestations.

be avoided until the alcohol has dried.) Eight to 12 hours after application, malathion is washed off with shampoo. Dead lice and ova can then be removed with a fine-toothed comb. Treatment may be repeated in 7 to 9 days if needed.

Crotamiton

Crotamiton [Eurax] is used to treat scabies. The drug is not indicated for pediculosis. This agent has scabicidal actions and may also relieve itching by an independent mechanism. Mild adverse reactions (dermatitis, conjunctivitis) occur occasionally. Crotamiton is available in cream and lotion formulations.

To treat scabies, crotamiton is massaged into the skin of the entire body, starting with the chin and working down. The head and face are treated only if needed. Special attention should be given to skin folds and creases. Contact with the eyes, mucous membranes, and any regions of inflammation should be avoided. A second application is made 24 hours after the first. A cleansing bath should be taken 48 hours after the second application. If needed, treatment can be repeated in 7 days.

Pyrethrins Plus Piperonyl Butoxide

The combination of pyrethrins with piperonyl butoxide is used to remove pubic lice and head lice. Pyrethrins are the components of this preparation that are toxic to lice. The piperonyl butoxide enhances pyrethrins' action by decreasing the ability of insects to metabolize pyrethrins into inactive products. Pyrethrins undergo little transcutaneous absorption and are one of the safest insecticides available. Principal adverse effects are irritation to the eyes and mucous membranes. Accordingly, contact with these areas should be avoided. Pharmaceutical preparations vary in their content of pyrethrins (0.18% to 0.33%) as well as in their content of piperonyl butoxide (2% to 4%). Treatment consists of applying the preparation (gel, liquid, shampoo) to the infested region, followed later by a warm-water rinse. The procedure should be repeated in a week. Nits are removed by combing.

Lindane

Actions and Uses

Lindane [G-well] is absorbed through the chitin shell of adult mites and lice and causes death by inducing convulsions. The drug is also lethal to the eggs. At one time, lindane was a drug of choice for pediculosis and scabies. However, owing to a risk of seizures, the Food and Drug Administration (FDA) now recommends that lindane be reserved for patients who have not responded to safer drugs (e.g., permethrin, malathion). Repeat dosing should be avoided.

Adverse Effects

Irritation. Lindane is irritating to the eyes and mucous membranes. Application to the face should be avoided. If contact occurs, the affected area should be flushed with water.

Convulsions. Lindane can penetrate the intact skin and, if absorbed in sufficient amounts, can cause convulsions. Convulsions can also result from lindane ingestion. Fortunately, convulsions are rare, resulting most often from drug ingestion or from inappropriate administration. If a seizure develops, it can be controlled with an IV barbiturate (e.g., phenobarbital) or with IV diazepam.

The risk of convulsions is highest for infants, children, and patients with pre-existing seizure disorders. Risk is also high for the elderly and for all patients who weigh less than 110 pounds (50 kg). Premature infants are especially vulnerable. Why? Because lindane can penetrate their skin with relative ease, and because limited liver function prevents infants from detoxifying absorbed drug.

To reduce seizure risk, the FDA recommends that lindane *not* be used to treat babies, women who are breast feeding, and anyone who

- Has used lindane in the past few months
- Has not tried a safer medicine for lice or scabies
- Has a seizure disorder or history of seizures
- Has reacted adversely to lindane in the past
- Has open or crusted sores or extensive areas of broken skin in the treatment region
- Has psoriasis or atopic dermatitis

Giving a second treatment too soon after the first increases seizure risk. How soon is too soon? No one knows what a truly safe interval is. Until this is known, patients should wait several months or more before using lindane again.

Preparations and Administration

Preparations. Lindane [G-well] is available in lotion and shampoo formulations. Its concentration in both is 1%.

Administration. Scabies. To treat scabies, a thin layer of lotion is applied to the entire body below the head. No more than 30 gm (1 oz) should be used. The drug is removed by washing 8 to 12 hours later. As a rule, only one application is required. Pruritus may persist because of residual insect products. This itching does not indicate a need for additional treatment. If a second treatment is deemed necessary, several months should elapse before doing it.

Head Lice. To kill head lice and their nits, lindane shampoo (30 to 60 gm) should be worked into dry hair and left in place for 4 minutes. After this, the shampoo should be rinsed off with warm water. Dead nits can be removed with a comb or tweezers. Lindane cream can be employed to treat head lice, but this formulation is less convenient than the shampoo.

Pubic Lice. The affected region should receive the same treatment employed for the removal of head lice. Shampoo is preferred to lotion. One treatment is usually sufficient. Sexual partners should be treated concurrently. Lindane should not be used to treat infestation of the eyelashes by the pubic louse. For this condition, petrolatum ophthalmic ointment is employed.

Body Lice. Body lice can be killed by applying a thin layer of lindane ointment or cream to affected areas. The drug should be washed off 8 to 12 hours after application.

Ivermectin

Ivermectin [Stromectol] is the only oral medication used for ectoparasitic infestations. A single dose (200 µg/kg) is effective against both mites and lice. The drug kills these parasites by disrupting nerve and muscle function—but does not disrupt nerve or muscle function in the host. Although ivermectin is highly effective against mites and lice, it is not FDA approved for this use. The pharmacology of ivermectin is discussed further in Chapter 93 (Anthelmintics).

⁞⁞ KEY POINTS

- Pediculosis (infestation with lice) and scabies (infestation with mites) are usually treated with topical drugs.
- Permethrin is the drug of choice for both mites and lice. The 5% cream [Elimite, Acticin] is for mites; the 1% solution [Nix] is for lice.

Basic Principles of Cancer Chemotherapy

As mortality from infectious diseases has declined, thanks to the development of antimicrobial drugs, cancer has emerged as a leading cause of death. The American Cancer Society estimated that 555,500 Americans died from cancer in the year 2002. Only heart disease kills more people. Among women ages 30 to 74, neoplastic diseases lead all other causes of mortality. Among children ages 1 to 14 years, cancer is the leading nonaccidental cause of death. As shown in Table 97–1, the most common cancers in women occur in the breast, lung, and colon or rectum. In men, the most common cancers arise in the prostate, lung, and colon or rectum.

We have three major modalities for treating cancer: *surgery, radiation therapy,* and *drug therapy.* Surgery and/or irradiation are preferred for most *solid* cancers. In contrast, drug therapy is the treatment of choice for *disseminated* cancers (leukemias, disseminated lymphomas, widespread metastases) along with a few localized cancers (e.g., choriocarcinoma, testicular carcinoma). Drug therapy also plays an important role as an adjunct to surgery and irradiation: By suppressing or killing malignant cells that surgery and irradiation leave behind, adjuvant drug therapy can significantly prolong life.

Anticancer drugs fall into three major classes: *cytotoxic agents* (i.e., drugs that kill cells directly), *hormones and hormone antagonists,* and *biologic response modifiers* (e.g., immunomodulating agents). Of the three classes, the cytotoxic agents are used most often. You should note that the term *cancer chemotherapy* applies only to the cytotoxic drugs—it does not apply to the use of hormones or biologic response modifiers to treat cancer. In this chapter, our discussion of anticancer drugs pertains almost exclusively to the cytotoxic agents.

The modern era of cancer chemotherapy dates from 1942, the year in which "nitrogen mustards" were first used to treat cancer. Since the introduction of nitrogen mustards, chemotherapy has made significant advances. Patients with some neoplastic diseases now have a good chance of being cured (Table 97–2). Cancers with a high cure rate include Hodgkin's disease, Ewing's sarcoma, and acute lymphocytic leukemia. For many patients whose cancer is not yet curable, chemotherapy can still be of value, offering realistic hopes of palliation and prolongation of useful life. However, although progress in chemotherapy has been encouraging, the ability to cure most cancers with drugs remains elusive. At this time, the major impediment to successful chemotherapy is toxicity of anticancer drugs to normal tissues.

Our principal objectives in this chapter are to examine the major obstacles confronting success in chemotherapy, the strategies being employed to overcome those obstacles, and the major toxicities of the anticancer drugs and the steps that can be taken to minimize drug-induced harm and discomfort. As background for addressing these issues, we begin by discussing (1) the nature of cancer itself and (2) the tissue growth fraction and its relationship to cancer chemotherapy.

WHAT IS CANCER?

In the discussion below, we consider properties shared by neoplastic cells as a group. However, although the discussion addresses cancers in general, be aware that the term *cancer* refers to a group of disorders and not to a single disease. The various forms of cancer differ in both phenotype and aggressiveness. In addition, they differ in responsiveness to drugs.

TABLE 97–1 ■ Estimated New Cancer Cases and Deaths, United States, 2002

Type of Cancer	Females		Males	
	New Cases	Deaths	New Cases	Deaths
All types	647,400	267,300	637,500	288,200
Breast	203,500	39,600	1500	400
Prostate			189,000	30,200
Lung and bronchus	79,200	65,700	90,200	89,200
Colon and rectum	75,700	28,800	77,600	24,800
Leukemias and lymphomas	42,200	21,900	49,500	25,600
Endometrium	39,300	6600		
Cervix	13,000	4100		
Ovary	23,300	13,900		
Melanoma of skin	23,500	2700	30,100	4700
Pancreas	15,600	15,200	14,700	14,500
Urinary bladder	15,000	4000	41,500	8600
Kidney	12,700	4400	19,100	7200
Oral cavity and pharynx	10,000	2500	18,900	4900
Stomach	8300	5200	13,300	7200
Esophagus	3300	3000	9800	9600
Liver	5600	5200	11,000	8900
Brain and other CNS	7400	5900	9600	7200
Multiple myeloma	6800	5300	7800	5500
Thyroid	15,800	800	4900	500

Data from American Cancer Society. Cancer Facts & Figures 2002. Atlanta, American Cancer Society, 2002. (Available at *www.cancer.org*)

TABLE 97–2 ■ Some Cancers for Which Drugs May Be Curative

Type of Cancer	Drug Therapy
Hodgkin's lymphoma	Doxorubicin + bleomycin + vinblastine + dacarbazine
Burkitt's lymphoma	Cyclophosphamide + vincristine + methotrexate + doxorubicin + prednisone
Choriocarcinoma	Methotrexate ± leucovorin
Small cell cancer of lung	Etoposide + either cisplatin or carboplatin
Testicular cancer	Cisplatin + etoposide ± bleomycin
Wilms' tumor*	Dactinomycin + vincristine ± doxorubicin ± cyclophosphamide
Ewing's sarcoma*	Cyclophosphamide + doxorubicin + vincristine alternating with etoposide + ifosfamide (with mesna)
Acute lymphocytic leukemia	Vincristine + prednisone + asparaginase + daunorubicin or doxorubicin ± cyclophosphamide

*Chemotherapy is combined with surgery and/or radiotherapy in these cancers.

Characteristics of Neoplastic Cells

Persistent Proliferation. Unlike normal cells, whose proliferation is carefully controlled, cancer cells undergo unrestrained growth and division. This capacity for persistent proliferation is the most distinguishing property of malignant cells. In the absence of intervention, cancerous tissues will continue to grow until they cause death.

It was once believed that cancer cells divided more rapidly than normal cells and that this excessive rate of division was responsible for the abnormal growth patterns of cancerous tissues. We now know that this concept is not correct. Division of neoplastic cells is not necessarily rapid: Although some cancers are composed of cells that divide rapidly, others are composed of cells that divide slowly. The correct explanation for the relentless growth of tumors is that *malignant cells are unresponsive to the feedback mechanisms that regulate cellular proliferation in healthy tissue.* Hence, cancer cells are able to continue multiplying under conditions that would suppress further growth and division of normal cells.

Invasive Growth. In the absence of malignancy, the various types of cells that compose a tissue remain segregated from one another; cells of one type do not invade territory that belongs to cells of a different type. In contrast, malignant cells are free of the constraints that inhibit invasive growth. As a result, cells of a solid tumor can penetrate adjacent tissues, thereby allowing the cancer to spread.

Formation of Metastases. Metastases are secondary tumors that appear at sites distant from the primary tumor. Metastases result from the unique ability of malignant cells to break away from their site of origin, migrate to other parts of the body (via the lymphatic and circulatory systems), and then re-implant to form a new tumor.

Immortality. Unlike normal cells, which eventually die, cancer cells can undergo endless divisions. The underlying cause for this difference is *telomerase,* an enzyme that is active only in cancer cells. Telomerase permits repeated division by preserving *telomeres*—the DNA-protein "caps" found on the end of each chromosome. As normal cells divide and differentiate, their telomerase become progressively shorter. When telomeres have lost a critical portion of their length, the cell is unable to keep on dividing. In cancer cells, telomerase continually adds back lost pieces of the telomere, and thereby preserves or extends telomere length. As a result, cancer cells can divide indefinitely.

Etiology of Cancer

The abnormal behavior of cancer cells results from alterations in their DNA. Specifically, malignant transformation results from a combination of activation of *oncogenes* (cancer-causing genes) and inactivation of *tumor suppressor genes* (genes that prevent replication of cells that have become cancerous). These genetic alterations are caused by chemical carcinogens, viruses, and radiation (x-rays, ultraviolet light, radioisotopes). Malignant transformation occurs in three major stages, called initiation, promotion, and progression. These stages suggest that DNA in cancer cells undergoes a series of small modifications, rather than just one large change. One consequence of malignant transformation is activation of the gene that codes for telomerase.

THE GROWTH FRACTION AND ITS RELATIONSHIP TO CHEMOTHERAPY

The growth fraction of a tissue is a major determinant of its responsiveness to chemotherapy. Consequently, before we discuss the anticancer drugs, we must first understand the growth fraction. In order to define the growth fraction, we need to review the cell cycle.

The Cell Cycle

The cell cycle is the sequence of events that a cell goes through from one mitotic division to the next. As shown in Figure 97–1, the cell cycle consists of four major phases, named G_1, S, G_2, and M. (The length of the arrows in the figure is proportional to the time spent in each phase.) For our

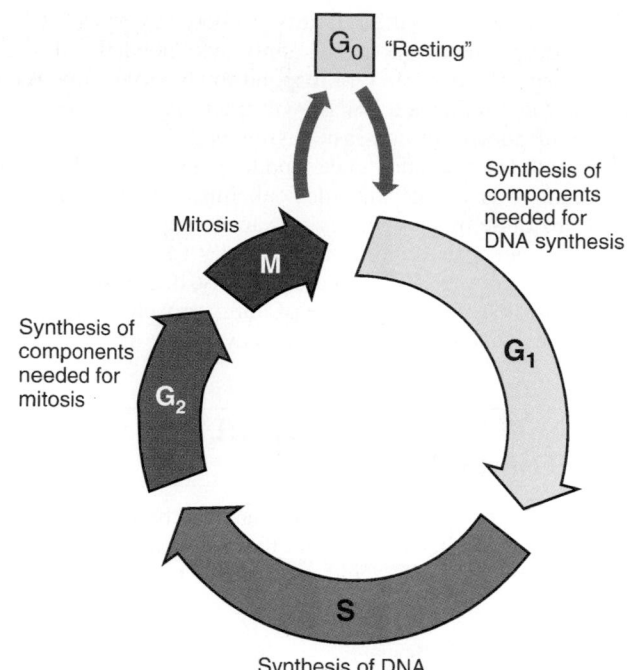

Figure 97–1 ■ **The cell cycle.**

purpose, we can imagine the cycle as beginning with G_1, the phase in which the cell prepares to make DNA. Following G_1, the cell enters S phase, the phase in which DNA synthesis actually takes place. After synthesis of DNA is complete, the cell enters G_2 and prepares for mitosis (cell division). Mitosis occurs next during M phase. Upon completion of mitosis, the resulting daughter cells have two options: they can enter G_1 and repeat the cycle, or they can enter the phase known as G_0. Cells that enter G_0 become mitotically dormant; they do not replicate and are not active participants in the cell cycle. Cells may remain in G_0 for days, weeks, or even years. Under appropriate conditions, resting cells may leave G_0 and resume active participation in the cycle.

The Growth Fraction

In any tissue, some cells are going through the cell cycle, whereas others are "resting" in G_0. The ratio of proliferating cells to G_0 cells is called the *growth fraction*. A tissue with a large percentage of proliferating cells and few cells in G_0 has a *high* growth fraction. Conversely, a tissue composed mostly of G_0 cells has a *low* growth fraction.

Impact of Tissue Growth Fraction on Responsiveness to Chemotherapy

As a rule, *chemotherapeutic drugs are much more toxic to tissues that have a high growth fraction than to tissues that have a low growth fraction.* Why? Because most cytotoxic agents are more active against proliferating cells than against cells in G_0. Proliferating cells are especially sensitive to chemotherapy because cytotoxic drugs usually act by disrupting either DNA synthesis or mitosis—activities that only proliferating cells carry out. Unfortunately, toxicity of anticancer drugs is not restricted to cancers: These drugs are also toxic to *normal tissues* that have a high growth fraction (e.g., bone marrow, GI epithelium, hair follicles, sperm-forming cells).

Having established the relationship between growth fraction and drug sensitivity, we can apply this knowledge to predict how specific cancers will respond to chemotherapy. As a rule, *solid tumors* have a *low* growth fraction, and hence tend to respond poorly. In contrast, *disseminated cancers* have a *high* growth fraction and hence tend to respond well. In practical terms, this means that the leukemias and lymphomas, which are disseminated forms of cancer, represent the majority of cancers that can be successfully treated with cytotoxic drugs. Conversely, and unfortunately, the most common cancers—solid tumors of the breast, lung, prostate, colon, and rectum—are much less responsive to cytotoxic drugs.

OBSTACLES TO SUCCESSFUL CHEMOTHERAPY

Our objective in this section is to examine the major factors that make success in cancer chemotherapy difficult. Foremost among these is the serious and unavoidable toxicity to normal cells caused by currently available cytotoxic drugs.

Toxicity to Normal Cells

Toxicity to normal cells is the principal barrier to success in chemotherapy. Injury to normal cells occurs primarily in tissues whose growth fraction is high (bone marrow, GI epithelium, hair follicles, germinal epithelium of the testes). Drug-induced injury to each of these tissues is discussed in detail below. For now, let's consider injury to normal cells as a group.

Toxicity to normal cells is dose limiting. That is, dosage cannot exceed an amount that produces the maximally tolerated degree of injury to normal cells. Hence, although very large doses of cytotoxic drugs might be able to produce 100% kill of malignant cells, such doses cannot be given because of the very real risk of killing the patient.

Why are cytotoxic anticancer drugs so harmful to normal tissues? Because these drugs lack *selective toxicity.* That is, *they cannot kill target cells without also killing other cells with which the target cells are in intimate contact.* We first encountered this concept in Chapter 79 (Basic Principles of Antimicrobial Therapy). As we noted then, successful antimicrobial therapy has been possible because antimicrobial drugs are highly selective in their toxicity. Penicillin, for example, can readily kill invading bacteria while being virtually harmless to cells of the host. This high degree of selective toxicity stands in sharp contrast to the lack of selectivity displayed by cytotoxic anticancer drugs.

Why have we been unable to develop drugs that selectively kill neoplastic cells? The problem is that neoplastic cells and normal cells are so much alike. To make a selectively toxic drug, the target cell must have a biochemical feature that normal cells lack. By way of illustration, let's consider how penicillin works. This drug kills bacteria by disrupting the bacterial cell wall. Because our cells don't have a cell wall, penicillin can't hurt us. Unfortunately, cancer cells are largely devoid of unique biochemical features that would render them vulnerable to selective attack. However, the recent discovery of telomerase offers hope. Since this enzyme is active in practically all cancer cells, and inactive in normal cells, drugs directed against it may produce the selectivity drugs to date have lacked.

Cure Requires 100% Cell Kill

To cure a patient of cancer, we must eliminate virtually every malignant cell from the body; just one remaining cell can proliferate and cause relapse. For most patients, 100% cell kill cannot be achieved. Factors that make it difficult to produce complete cell kill include (1) the kinetics of drug-induced cell kill, (2) minimal participation of the immune system in eliminating malignant cells, and (3) disappearance of symptoms before all cancer cells are gone.

Kinetics of Drug-Induced Cell Kill. Killing of cancer cells follows *first-order kinetics.* That is, at any given dose, a drug will kill a *constant percentage* of malignant cells, *regardless of how many cells are actually present.* This means that the dose required to shrink a cancer from 10^3 cells down to 10 cells will be just as big, for example, as the dose required to reduce that cancer from 10^9 cells down to 10^7 cells. Hence, with each successive round of chemotherapy, drug dosage must remain the same, even though the cancer is getting progressively smaller. Accordingly, if treatment is to continue, the patient must be able to tolerate the same degree of toxicity late in therapy as he or she could tolerate when therapy began. For many patients, this is not possible.

Nonparticipation of Host Defenses in Cell Kill. In contrast to the antimicrobial drugs, anticancer agents receive very little help from host defenses. Therefore, anticancer agents must produce cell kill almost entirely on their own. There are two reasons why host defenses contribute so little. First, because of their immunosuppressant actions, anticancer drugs seriously compromise immune function. Second, because malignant cells are so much like normal cells, the immune system generally fails to recognize cancer cells as appropriate for attack.

When Should Treatment Stop? We have no way of knowing when 100% cell kill has been achieved. As a result, there is no definitive method for deciding just when chemotherapy should stop. As indicated in Figure 97–2, symptoms disappear long before the last malignant cell has been eliminated. Once a cancer has been reduced to less than 1 million cells, it becomes virtually undetectable; all signs of disease are absent, and the patient is considered in complete remission. It is obvious, however, that a patient harboring a million malignant cells is by no means cured. It is also obvious that further chemotherapy is indicated. However, what is not so obvious is just how long therapy should last: Because the patient is already asymptomatic, we have no objective means of determining when to discontinue treatment. The clinical dilemma is this: If therapy is continued too long, the patient will be needlessly exposed to serious toxicity; conversely, if drugs are withdrawn prematurely, relapse will occur.

Absence of Truly Early Detection

Early detection of cancer is rare. At this time, cancer of the cervix, which can be diagnosed with a Pap test, is the only neoplastic disease capable of truly early detection. All other forms of cancer are significantly advanced by the time they have grown large enough for discovery. The smallest detectable cancers are about 1 cm in diameter, have a mass of 1 gm, and consist of about 1 billion cells (see Fig. 97–2). Detection at this stage cannot be considered early.

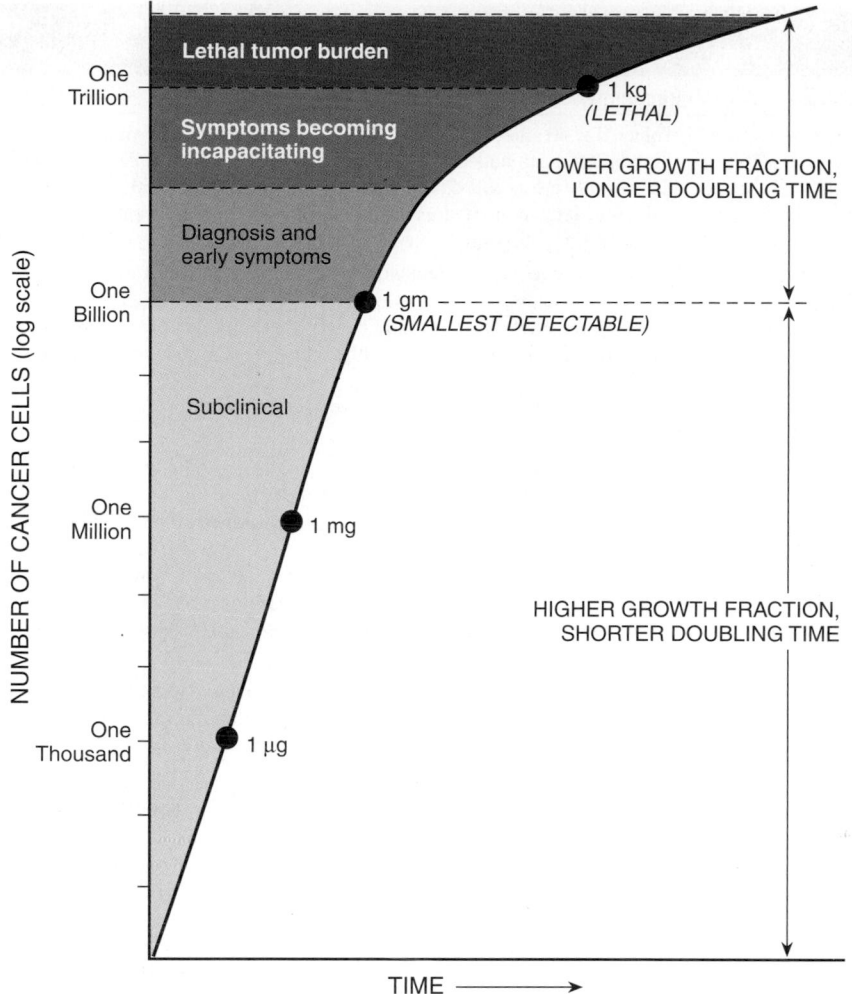

Figure 97–2 ■ **Gompertzian tumor growth curve showing the relationship between tumor size and clinical status.**

Late detection has three important consequences. First, by the time the primary tumor is discovered, metastases may have formed. Second, the tumor will be less responsive to drugs than it would have been at an earlier stage (see below). Third, if the cancer has been present for a long time, the patient may be debilitated by the disease, and therefore less able to tolerate treatment.

Even though *truly* early detection is largely impossible, every effort at *relatively* early detection should be made. Why? Because the smaller a cancer is when treatment begins, the better the chances of long-term survival. Hence, even if a cancer has 1 billion cells when it's detected, that's still far better than a gazillion. The American Cancer Society recommends routine testing for several cancers, including cancers of the prostate, breast, and uterus. Table 97–3 indicates who should be tested, how often, and what test or procedure should be performed.

Solid Tumors Respond Poorly

As noted, solid tumors have a low growth fraction (high percentage of G_0 cells) and are generally unresponsive to cytotoxic drugs. There are two reasons for low responsiveness.

First, G_0 cells do not perform the activities that most anticancer drugs are designed to disrupt. Second, because G_0 cells are not active participants in the cell cycle, they have time to repair drug-induced damage before it can do them serious harm.

Not all solid tumors are equally unresponsive: As a rule, *large tumors are even less responsive than small tumors.* This difference occurs because, as solid tumors increase in size, many of their cells leave the cell cycle and enter G_0, causing the growth fraction to decline. Tumor growth slows, in large part, because blood flow in the tumor core is low, depriving cells of nutrients and oxygen. The decrease in growth fraction in older tumors is a major reason why therapeutic success is more likely when cancers are detected early. Because the rate of growth declines as a tumor gets larger, the tumor growth curve is said to follow *Gompertzian kinetics* (see Fig. 97–2).

The drug sensitivity of a solid tumor can be enhanced by *debulking.* When a solid tumor is reduced by surgery or irradiation, many of the remaining cells leave G_0 and re-enter the cell cycle, thereby increasing their sensitivity to chemotherapy. This phenomenon is known as *recruitment.* Because of

TABLE 97–3 ■ American Cancer Society Recommendations for the Early Detection of Cancer, 2002

Type of Cancer	Recommendation
Breast	Women age 40 and older should have an annual mammogram and an annual clinical breast examination (CBE) by a healthcare professional, and should perform a monthly breast self-examination (BSE). Ideally, the CBE should occur before the scheduled mammogram. Women ages 20–39 should have a CBE by a healthcare professional every 3 years and should perform a BSE monthly.
Colon and rectum	Beginning at age 50, men and women should follow one of the examination schedules below: • A fecal occult blood test (FOBT) every year, *or* a flexible sigmoidoscopy (FSIG) every 5 years, *or*, preferably, both (i.e., a FOBT every year *plus* a FSIG every 5 years) • A double-contrast barium enema every 5–10 years • A colonoscopy every 10 years
Prostate	The prostate-specific antigen (PSA) test and the digital rectal examination should be offered annually, beginning at age 50, to men who have a life expectancy of at least 10 years. Men at high risk—African Americans and men with a family history of one or more first-degree relatives diagnosed with prostate cancer at an early age—should begin testing at age 45. Information should be provided to patients about what is known and what is uncertain about the benefits and limitations of early detection and treatment of prostate cancer, so that they can make an informed decision.*
Cervix	All women who are or have been sexually active or who are 18 and older should have an annual Pap test and pelvic examination. After three or more consecutive examinations with normal findings, the Pap test may be performed less frequently.
Uterus, endometrium	All women should be informed about the risks and symptoms of endometrial cancer, and strongly encouraged to report any unexpected bleeding or spotting to their physician. Annual screening for endometrial cancer with endometrial biopsy beginning at age 35 should be offered to women with or at high risk for hereditary nonpolyposis colon cancer.
Cancer-related checkup	A cancer-related checkup is recommended every 3 years for people 20–39 years old and once a year for people 40 and older. The exam should include health counseling and, depending on the person's age, might include examinations for cancers of the thyroid, oral cavity, skin, lymph nodes, testes, and ovaries, as well as for some nonmalignant diseases.

*In December 2002, the third U.S. Preventive Services Task Force (USPSTF) recommended *against* routine screening for prostate cancer. The USPSTF finds there is good evidence that screening can detect early prostate cancer, but inconclusive evidence that detection improves health outcomes.
Adapted from American Cancer Society. Cancer Facts & Figures 2002. Atlanta, American Cancer Society, 2002. (Available at www.cancer.org)

recruitment, chemotherapy can be very useful as an adjunct to surgery or irradiation even though drugs may have been largely ineffective before debulking was done.

Drug Resistance

During the course of chemotherapy, cancer cells can develop resistance to the drugs used against them. Drug resistance can be a significant cause of therapeutic failure. Mechanisms of resistance include reduced drug uptake, increased drug efflux, reduced drug activation, reduced target molecule sensitivity, and increased repair of drug-induced damage to DNA.

Cellular production of a drug transport molecule, known as *P-glycoprotein,* can confer *multiple drug resistance* upon cells. P-glycoprotein is a large molecule that spans the cytoplasmic membrane and serves to pump drugs out of the cell. Induction of P-glycoprotein synthesis following exposure to

a single anticancer drug produces cross-resistance to many structurally unrelated agents. Several drugs, including calcium channel blockers, have been used investigationally to inhibit the P-glycoprotein pump and reverse multiple drug resistance.

Drug resistance usually results from a change in DNA. Mutation to a drug-resistant form is a spontaneous event and is not caused by the anticancer drugs themselves. However, although drugs do not *cause* the mutations that render cells resistant, drugs do *create selection pressure* favoring the drug-resistant mutants. That is, by killing drug-sensitive cells, anticancer agents create a competition-free environment in which drug-resistant mutants can flourish.

Because the presence of anticancer agents favors the growth of drug-resistant cells, as therapy proceeds, the number of resistant cells will increase. Because resistant cells cannot be killed with drugs, the risk of therapeutic failure becomes greater with each course of treatment. Since patients are usually exposed to drugs over an extended time, therapeutic failure owing to drug resistance is a significant problem.

Heterogeneity of Tumor Cells

Tumors do not consist of a single population of identical cells. Rather, owing to ongoing mutation, tumors are composed of subpopulations of dissimilar cells. These subpopulations can differ in morphology, growth rate, and metastatic ability. More importantly, they can differ in responsiveness to drugs—primarily because of increased resistance. As a tumor ages, cellular heterogeneity increases.

Limited Drug Access to Tumor Cells

Because of a tumor's location or blood supply, drugs may have limited access to its cells. Large solid tumors have poor vascularization, especially near the core. Hence, cells within these tumors are difficult to reach with drugs. Similarly, tumors of the central nervous system (CNS) are hard to reach because most anticancer drugs cannot cross or have difficulty crossing the blood-brain barrier.

STRATEGIES FOR ACHIEVING MAXIMUM BENEFITS FROM CHEMOTHERAPY

Intermittent Chemotherapy

The ultimate goal of chemotherapy is to produce 100% kill of neoplastic cells while causing limited injury to normal tissues—especially the bone marrow and GI epithelium. Intermittent therapy is the primary technique for achieving this goal. When cytotoxic anticancer drugs are administered intermittently, normal cells have the opportunity to repopulate between rounds of therapy. However, for this approach to succeed, one obvious requirement must be met: *Normal cells must repopulate faster than the malignant cells.* If malignant cells grow back faster than normal cells, there can be no reduction in tumor burden between rounds of treatment. The successful use of intermittent therapy is depicted in Figure 97–3.

Combination Chemotherapy

Chemotherapy employing a combination of drugs is generally much more effective than therapy with just one drug. Accordingly, most patients are treated with two or more agents.

Benefits of Drug Combinations

Combination chemotherapy offers three advantages: (1) suppression of drug resistance, (2) increased cancer cell kill, and (3) reduced injury to normal cells (at any given level of anticancer effect).

Suppression of Drug Resistance. Drug resistance occurs less frequently with multiple-drug therapy than with single-drug therapy. To understand why, we need to recall that resistance is acquired through random mutational events. The probability of a cell undergoing two or more mutations, and therefore developing resistance to a combination of drugs, is smaller than the probability of a cell undergoing the single mutation needed for resistance to one drug. Because drug resistance is reduced with combination chemotherapy, the chances of therapeutic success are increased.

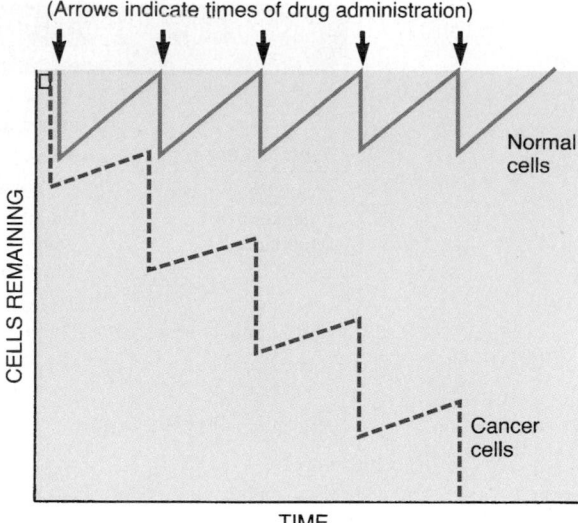

(Arrows indicate times of drug administration)

Figure 97–3 ■ Recovery of critical normal cells during intermittent chemotherapy.
Cancer cells and normal cells (e.g., cells of the bone marrow) are killed with each drug administration. In the interval between doses, both types of cells proliferate. Because, in this example, normal cells repopulate faster than cancer cells, normal cells are able to recover entirely between doses, whereas regrowth of the cancer cells is only partial. As a result, with each succeeding round of treatment, the total number of cancer cells becomes smaller, whereas the number of normal cells remains within a tolerable range. Note that differential loss of malignant cells is possible only if these cells repopulate more slowly than normal cells. If cancer cells grow back as fast as normal cells do, intermittent chemotherapy will fail.

Increased Cancer Cell Kill. If we administer several anticancer drugs, each with a different mechanism of action, we will kill more malignant cells than if we use only one drug. Therapeutic effects are enhanced because the combination attacks the cancer in several ways instead of just one. Greater cell kill is especially likely if a drug-resistant subpopulation of cells is present. The superiority of drug combinations over single-drug therapy is illustrated by the data in Table 97–4.

Reduced Injury to Normal Cells. By using a combination of drugs *that do not have overlapping toxicities,* we can achieve a greater anticancer effect than we could *safely* achieve using any of the agents alone. The data in Table 97–5 indicate why this is so. The table summarizes responses to two drugs—vincristine and cyclophosphamide—when given alone and in combination. Both drugs kill malignant cells, but they act by different mechanisms: cyclophosphamide damages DNA, whereas vincristine blocks mitosis. Furthermore, these drugs have different dose-limiting toxicities: Cyclophosphamide causes *neutropenia,* whereas vincristine causes *neuropathy.* In the table, the intensity of effects is indicated by plus (+) symbols—the more plusses, the more intense the response. With either drug, ++ represents the maximum degree of toxicity that can be tolerated. When administered alone in doses that produce ++ toxicity, each drug produces an anticancer effect of ++ intensity—the greatest therapeutic effect that we

TABLE 97–4 ■ Single-Drug Treatment Versus Combination Chemotherapy

Type of Cancer	Method of Treatment and Drugs Employed	Percentage of Patients with Complete Remission
Acute lymphocytic leukemia of childhood	*Single-Drug Therapy*	
	Daunorubicin	38
	Prednisone	63
	Vincristine	57
	Combination Chemotherapy	
	Prednisone + vincristine	90
	Prednisone + vincristine + daunorubicin	97
Hodgkin's disease	*Single-Drug Therapy*	
	Vincristine	<10
	Prednisone	<5
	Procarbazine	<10
	Mechlorethamine	20
	Combination Chemotherapy	
	Vincristine + prednisone + mechlorethamine + procarbazine	81

Data from DeVita VT, Young RC, Canellos GP. Combination versus single agent chemotherapy: A review of the basis for selection of drug treatment of cancer. Cancer 1975;35:98.

TABLE 97–5 ■ Responses to Cyclophosphamide and Vincristine Alone and in Combination

Therapeutic Regimen	Anticancer Effect	Toxicity	
		Neutropenia	Neurotoxicity
Cyclophosphamide	++	++	0
Vincristine	++	0	++
Cyclophosphamide + vincristine	++++	++	++

can safely achieve with either drug by itself. Now let's consider the effect of combining these drugs, giving each in its maximally tolerated dose. The total anticancer effect of the combination is ++++, twice the effect that could be achieved safely with either agent alone. Because the toxicities of these agents do not overlap, overall toxicity of the combination remains at a tolerable level—although the patient is now exposed to two kinds of toxicity rather than one.

Guidelines for Drug Selection

From the preceding, we can extract three guidelines for selecting drugs to use in combination: (1) each drug should be effective by itself, (2) each drug should have a different mechanism of action, and (3) the drugs should have minimally overlapping toxicities.

Optimizing Dosing Schedules

The administration schedule is an important determinant of treatment outcome. The experiment summarized in Table 97–6 provides a dramatic illustration. In this experiment, two groups of mice were inoculated with cancer cells and then treated with cytarabine. Mice in group I received a *single large dose* of cytarabine on days 2, 6, 10, and 14 after being inoculated with cancer cells. The mice in group II were treated on the same days as the mice in group I, but, rather than receiving one large dose of cytarabine, they were given *eight small doses,* one every 3 hours. By the end of the study, all of the group II mice were cured. In stark contrast, all of the group I mice were dead. Since the two groups had the same disease and were given the same drug, we must conclude that the life-and-death difference was due to the dosing schedules employed.

To understand these results, we need to know two properties of cytarabine: (1) the drug kills cells by disrupting DNA synthesis, and (2) it undergoes rapid inactivation. Because cytarabine acts by disrupting DNA synthesis, it can only affect cells while they are in the S phase of the cell cycle. Because the drug is rapidly inactivated, and because many cells will not be in S phase during the short time before inactivation occurs, many cells will escape injury following each dose. The group I mice died because administration of just one large dose every 4 days did not maintain active drug in the body for a time sufficient to catch all cancer cells as they cycled through S phase. Because the group II mice received multiple doses over a 24-hour period on each of 4 days, the presence of active drug was sustained. Hence, the chance of cancer cells being in S phase while active drug was present was greatly increased, thereby leading to enhanced cell kill with resultant cure.

The message from this experiment is this: Selection of the right drugs for cancer therapy is only one of the requirements for success; those drugs must also be administered according to schedules that will maximize beneficial effects. Dosing schedules are especially critical for drugs that, like cytarabine, act during a specific phase of the cell cycle.

TABLE 97–6 ■■ Effect of Dosing Schedule on Therapeutic Response			
Experimental Group	Dosage Size	Dosing Schedule	Mice Surviving
I	240 mg/kg	1 dose/day*	None
II	15 mg/kg	8 doses/day*	100%

*Cytarabine was administered on days 2, 6, 10, and 14 after mice were inoculated with leukemia cells. See text for further details.

Regional Drug Delivery

By using special techniques for drug delivery, we can increase drug access to tumors, thereby increasing cell kill and reducing systemic toxicity.

Intra-arterial Delivery. Local intra-arterial infusion can be used to treat solid tumors. This technique has the advantage of establishing a high concentration of drug in the vicinity of the tumor while minimizing toxicity to the rest of the body. Specific routes include carotid artery delivery (for brain tumors) and hepatic artery delivery (for liver metastases). Clearly, intra-arterial therapy is suitable only for localized cancers.

Intrathecal Delivery. As noted above, many anticancer agents are unable to cross the blood-brain barrier, and therefore cannot reach malignant cells within the CNS. To enhance therapy of CNS cancers, drugs can be administered intrathecally (by injection directly into the subarachnoid space). This technique bypasses the blood-brain barrier, thereby giving drugs better access to cells within the CNS.

Other Specialized Routes. Anticancer agents can be administered via the portal vein to treat liver metastases, and directly into the bladder to treat bladder cancer. Neoplasms located in the pleural and peritoneal cavities can be treated by direct intracavitary drug administration. As discussed in Chapter 98, carmustine, a drug for brain tumors, is now available in a wafer that is implanted in the brain to kill cancer cells left behind following surgical removal of a tumor.

MAJOR TOXICITIES OF CHEMOTHERAPEUTIC DRUGS

The agents used for cancer chemotherapy constitute our most toxic group of medicines. Serious injury occurs most often to tissues that have a high growth fraction (bone marrow, GI epithelium, hair follicles, and sperm-forming cells). In the discussion below, we consider the more common toxicities of the *cytotoxic* anticancer drugs along with steps that can be taken to minimize harm and discomfort.

Bone Marrow Suppression

Chemotherapeutic drugs are highly toxic to the bone marrow, a tissue with a high proportion of proliferating cells. Myelosuppression reduces the number of circulating neutrophils, thrombocytes, and erythrocytes. Loss of these cells has three major consequences: (1) infection (from loss of neutrophils); (2) bleeding (from loss of thrombocytes); and (3) anemia (from loss of erythrocytes).

Neutropenia

Neutrophils (neutrophilic granulocytes) are white blood cells that play a critical role in fighting infection. In patients with neutropenia (a reduction in circulating neutrophils), both the incidence and severity of infection are increased. Infections that are normally benign (e.g., candidiasis) can become life threatening. There is no question that infection secondary to neutropenia is the most serious complication of cancer chemotherapy. The grim reality of this problem cannot be stressed too strongly.

With most anticancer drugs, onset of neutropenia is rapid and recovery develops relatively quickly. Neutropenia begins to develop a few days after dosing, and the lowest neutrophil count, called the *nadir,* occurs between days 10 and 14. Neutrophil counts then recover in 3 to 4 weeks. Patients are at highest risk during the nadir. Accordingly, special care should be taken to avoid contagion.

With some anticancer drugs, neutropenia is *delayed.* Neutrophil counts begin to fall in 1 to 2 weeks, and reach their nadir between weeks 3 and 4. Full recovery may not occur until after week 7.

Neutrophil counts must be monitored. Normal counts range from 2500 to 7000 cells/mm³. If neutropenia is substantial (absolute neutrophil count below 500/mm³), chemotherapy should be withheld until neutrophil counts return toward normal.

Lack of neutrophils confounds the diagnosis of infection. Why? Because the usual signs of infection (e.g., pus, abscesses, infiltrates on the chest x-ray) depend on neutrophils being present. In the absence of neutrophils, *fever* is the principal early sign of infection.

Patients must be their own first line of defense against infection. They should be made aware of the serious risk they face and should be taught how to minimize contagion. They should be informed that fever may be the only indication of infection and instructed to notify the physician immediately if fever develops. Because infection is commonly acquired through contact with other people, hospitalized patients should be instructed to refuse direct contact with anyone who has not washed his or her hands in the patient's presence. This rule applies not only to visiting friends and relatives but also to nurses, physicians, and all other hospital staff. The normal flora of the body is a major source of infection; the risk of acquiring an infection with these microbes can be reduced by daily examination and cleansing of the skin and oral cavity.

Hospitalization of the infection-free neutropenic patient is controversial. Some physicians feel that hospitalization *increases* the risk of acquiring a serious infection. Why? Because hospitals harbor drug-resistant microbes, which can make hospital-acquired (nosocomial) infections especially difficult to treat. Accordingly, these physicians recommend that neutropenic patients stay at home as long as they remain infection free.

If neutropenic patients *are* hospitalized, every precaution must be taken to prevent nosocomial infection. Patients should be given an isolation room and monitored frequently for fever. Certain foods (e.g., salads) abound in pathogenic bacteria and must be avoided.

When a neutropenic patient develops an infection, immediate and vigorous intervention is required. Specimens for culture should be taken to determine the identity and drug sensitivity of the infecting organism. While awaiting reports on the cultures, empiric therapy with IV antibiotics should be instituted. The drugs selected should cover all likely pathogens. For initial therapy, IV ceftriaxone plus amikacin may be tried.

In recent years, *colony-stimulating factors* have been employed to minimize neutropenia. Two preparations are available: *granulocyte colony-stimulating factor* (G-CSF, filgrastim) and *granulocyte-macrophage colony-stimulating factor* (GM-CSF, sargramostim). Both drugs act on the bone marrow to enhance granulocyte (neutrophil) production. Colony-stimulating factors can decrease the incidence, magnitude, and duration of neutropenia. As a result, they can decrease the incidence and severity of infection as well as the need for IV antibiotics and hospitalization. The basic pharmacology of G-CSF and GM-CSF is discussed in Chapter 53.

Thrombocytopenia

Bone marrow suppression can cause thrombocytopenia (a reduction in circulating platelets), thereby increasing the risk of serious bleeding. Bleeding from the nose and gums is relatively common. Bleeding from the gums can be reduced by avoiding vigorous tooth brushing. Drugs that promote bleeding (e.g., aspirin, anticoagulants) should not be used. When a mild analgesic is required, acetaminophen, which does not promote bleeding, is preferred to aspirin. For patients with severe thrombocytopenia, platelet infusion is the mainstay of treatment. Thrombocytopenia can be minimized by treatment with *oprelvekin* [Neumega], a drug that stimulates platelet production (see Chapter 53).

Caution should be exercised when performing procedures that might promote bleeding. Intravenous needles should be inserted with special care. Intramuscular injections should be avoided if possible. Blood pressure cuffs should be applied cautiously, because overinflation may cause bruising or bleeding.

Anemia

Anemia is defined as a reduction in the number of circulating erythrocytes (red blood cells). Although anticancer drugs can suppress erythrocyte production, anemia is much less common than neutropenia or thrombocytopenia. Why? Because circulating erythrocytes have a long life span (120 days), which usually allows erythrocyte production to recover before levels of existing erythrocytes fall too low.

If anemia does develop, it can be treated with a transfusion or with *epoetin* (erythropoietin), a hormone that stimulates production of red blood cells. Because transfusions require hospitalization, whereas epoetin can be administered at home, epoetin therapy can spare the patient inconvenience. However, epoetin has the drawback of being expensive. In addition, epoetin cannot be used in patients with leukemias and other myeloid malignancies, because it can stimulate proliferation of these cancers. The basic pharmacology of epoetin is discussed in Chapter 53.

Digestive Tract Injury

The epithelial lining of the GI tract has a very high growth fraction, and hence is exquisitely sensitive to cytotoxic drugs. Stomatitis and diarrhea are common. Severe GI injury can be life threatening.

Stomatitis. Stomatitis (inflammation of the oral mucosa) often develops a few days after the onset of chemotherapy and may persist for 2 or more weeks after treatment has ceased. Inflammation can progress to denudation and ulceration, and is often complicated by infection. Pain can be severe, inhibiting eating, speaking, and swallowing. Management includes good oral hygiene and a bland diet. A combination of topical anesthetics and systemic analgesics may be needed to relieve pain. Topical antifungal drugs may be needed to control infection with *Candida albicans.* Inflammation can be reduced with a glucocorticoid and diphenhydramine (an antihistamine). Severe stomatitis may necessitate interrupting chemotherapy.

Diarrhea. By injuring the epithelial lining of the intestine, anticancer drugs can impair absorption of fluids and other nutrients, thereby causing diarrhea. Diarrhea can be reduced with a diet high in fiber (which gives the stool a more firm consistency) and by eating constipating foods (e.g., cheeses).

Nausea and Vomiting

Nausea and vomiting are common sequelae of cancer chemotherapy. These responses, which result in part from direct stimulation of the chemoreceptor trigger zone, can be both immediate and dramatic, and may persist for hours. In some cases, discomfort is so great as to prompt refusal of further treatment.

You should appreciate that nausea and vomiting associated with chemotherapy are much more severe than with other medications. Hence, whereas these reactions are generally unremarkable with most drugs, they must be considered major and characteristic toxicities of anticancer drugs. The emetogenic potential of several agents is indicated in Table 97–7.

Nausea and vomiting can be reduced by premedication with antiemetics. These drugs offer three benefits: (1) reduction of anticipatory nausea and vomiting, (2) prevention of dehydration and malnutrition secondary to frequent nausea and vomiting, and (3) promotion of compliance with anticancer therapy by reducing discomfort. Of the antiemetics in use, *ondansetron* [Zofran] in combination with *dexamethasone* has proved especially effective. Other antiemetics employed during chemotherapy include *granisetron* [Kytril], *metoclopramide* [Reglan], *diphenhydramine,* and *lorazepam* [Ativan].

TABLE 97–7 ■ Emetogenic Potential of Selected Cytotoxic Anticancer Drugs	
Severe	**Moderate**
Cisplatin	Cytarabine
Dacarbazine	Procarbazine
Mechlorethamine	Mitomycin
Streptozocin	Methotrexate (high doses)
Moderately Severe	**Mild**
Cyclophosphamide	Etoposide
Ifosfamide	Fluorouracil
Doxorubicin	Hydroxyurea
Nitrosourea	Bleomycin
Dactinomycin	Vinblastine
	Vincristine
	Chlorambucil
	Methotrexate (low doses)

Combinations of antiemetics are more effective than single-drug therapy. The antiemetic drugs and their use in chemotherapy are discussed further in Chapter 75.

Other Important Toxicities

Alopecia. Reversible alopecia (hair loss) results from injury to hair follicles. Alopecia can occur with most cytotoxic anticancer drugs. Hair loss begins 7 to 10 days after the onset of treatment and becomes maximal in 1 to 2 months. Regeneration begins 1 to 2 months after the last course of treatment.

While alopecia is not dangerous, it is nonetheless very upsetting. In fact, for many cancer patients, alopecia is second only to vomiting as their greatest treatment-related fear. If drugs are expected to cause hair loss, the patient should be forewarned. For patients who choose to wear a hairpiece, one should be selected before hair loss occurs. Hairpieces are tax deductible as medical expenses and are covered by some health insurance plans.

Reproductive Toxicity. The developing fetus and the germinal epithelium of the testes have high growth fractions. As a result, both are highly susceptible to injury by cytotoxic drugs. These drugs can interfere with embryogenesis, causing death of the early embryo. They may also cause fetal malformation. Accordingly, women undergoing chemotherapy should be warned against becoming pregnant. If pregnancy occurs, the possibility of terminating pregnancy should be discussed. Drug effects on the ovaries may result in amenorrhea, menopausal symptoms, and atrophy of the vaginal epithelium.

Cytotoxic drugs can cause irreversible sterility in males. Men should be forewarned and counseled about sperm banking.

Hyperuricemia. Hyperuricemia is defined as an excessive level of uric acid in the blood. Uric acid, a compound with low solubility, is formed by the breakdown of DNA following cell death. Hyperuricemia is especially common following treatment for leukemias and lymphomas (because therapy results in massive cell kill). The major concern with hyperuricemia is injury to the kidneys secondary to deposition of uric acid crystals in renal tubules. The risk of crystal formation can be reduced by increasing fluid intake. If necessary, uric acid levels can be lowered with *allopurinol,* a drug that suppresses uric acid formation (see Chapter 69), or with *rasburicase,* an enzyme that catalyzes uric acid degradation (see Chapter 103).

Local Injury from Extravasation of Vesicants. Certain anticancer drugs, known as *vesicants,* are highly chemically reactive. These drugs can cause severe local injury if they make direct contact with tissues. Vesicants are administered IV, because rapid dilution in venous blood minimizes the risk of injury. Administration is usually by injection (IV push) through a sidearm in a freely flowing IV line. Sites of previous irradiation should be avoided. Extreme care must be exercised to prevent extravasation, because leakage can produce high local concentrations, resulting in prolonged pain, infection, and loss of mobility. Severe injury can lead to necrosis and sloughing, requiring surgical débridement and skin grafting. If extravasation occurs, the infusion should be stopped immediately. Vesicants should be administered only by clinicians specially trained to handle them safely.

Unique Toxicities. In addition to the toxicities discussed above, most of which apply to the cytotoxic anticancer drugs as a group, some agents produce unique toxicities. For example, daunorubicin can cause serious harm to the heart, cisplatin can injure the kidneys, and vincristine can injure peripheral nerves. Special toxicities of individual drugs are considered in Chapters 98 and 99.

Carcinogenesis. Along with their other adverse actions, anticancer drugs have one final and ironic toxicity: These drugs, which are used to treat cancer, have caused cancer in some patients. Cancer results from drug-induced damage to DNA. Cancers caused by anticancer drugs may take many years to appear.

MAKING THE DECISION TO TREAT

From the preceding discussion of toxicities, it is clear that cytotoxic anticancer drugs can cause great harm. Given the known dangers of these drugs, we must ask why such toxic substances are given to sick people at all. The answer lies with the primary rule of therapeutics, which states that the benefits of treatment must outweigh the risks. For most patients undergoing chemotherapy, the conditions of this rule are met. That is, although the toxicities of the anticancer drugs can be very bad, the potential benefits (cure, prolonged life, palliation) justify the risks. However, the desirability of treating cancer with drugs is not always obvious. There are patients whose chances of being helped by chemotherapy are very remote, while the risk of serious injury remains ever present. Because the potential benefits for some patients are small and the risks are large, the decision to institute chemotherapy must be made with care.

Before a decision to treat can be made, the patient must be given some idea of the benefits the proposed therapy might offer. Three basic benefits are possible: cure, palliation, and prolongation of useful life. For treatment to be justified, there should be reason to believe that at least one of these benefits will be forthcoming. If a patient cannot be offered some reasonable hope of cure, palliation, or prolongation of useful life, it would be difficult to justify treatment.

The most important factors for predicting the outcome of chemotherapy are (1) the general health of the patient and (2) the responsiveness of the type of cancer the patient has. General health status can be assessed with the Karnofsky Performance Scale (Table 97–8). A Karnofsky rating of less than 40 indicates the patient is very debilitated and not likely to tolerate the additional stress of chemotherapy. Accordingly, patients with a low Karnofsky rating should receive anticancer drugs only if their cancer is known to be especially responsive.

The responsiveness of some common cancers is indicated in Table 97–9. Patients with highly responsive types of cancer should almost always be treated, regardless of their Karnofsky rating. In contrast, patients with minimally responsive types of cancer should be treated only after careful consideration. It may well be that such patients are better off limiting their problems to the cancer itself, without adding the dangers and discomforts of a course of treatment that has little to offer.

An important requirement for deciding in favor of chemotherapy is that the impact of treatment be measurable. That is, there must be some objective means of determining the cancer's response to drugs. For solid tumors, we should be

TABLE 97–8 ■ Karnofsky Performance Scale

Definition	Percentage	Criteria
Able to carry on normal activity and work; no special care needed	100	Normal; no complaints; no evidence of disease
	90	Able to carry on normal activity; minor signs or symptoms of disease
	80	Normal activity with effort; some signs or symptoms of disease
Unable to work; able to live at home and care for most personal needs; a varying amount of assistance needed	70	Cares for self; unable to carry on normal activity or do active work
	60	Requires occasional assistance; able to care for most needs
	50	Requires considerable assistance and frequent medical care
Unable to care for self; requires equivalent of institutional or hospital care; disease may be progressing rapidly	40	Disabled; requires special care and assistance
	30	Severely disabled; hospitalization is indicated although death not imminent
	20	Very sick, hospitalization necessary; active supportive treatment necessary
	10	Moribund; fatal processes progressing rapidly
	0	Dead

TABLE 97–9 ■ Responsiveness of Some Cancers to Chemotherapy

Responsiveness to Chemotherapy	Type of Cancer	Probable Benefits of Chemotherapy
High	Hodgkin's disease Burkitt's lymphoma Acute lymphocytic leukemia Choriocarcinoma Wilms' tumor Ewing's sarcoma	Cure or substantial prolongation of life
Moderate	Breast cancer Cervical carcinoma Chronic lymphocytic leukemia Bladder cancer Multiple myeloma Prostate carcinoma	Prolongation of life; palliation
Minimal	Colorectal cancer Hepatocellular Melanoma Pancreatic cancer Renal cancer Osteogenic sarcoma	Palliation; minimal prolongation of life

able to measure a decrease in tumor size. For hematologic cancers, we should be able to measure a decrease in the number of circulating neoplastic cells. If we have no way to measure the response of a cancer, then we have no way of knowing if treatment has done any good. If we cannot determine that drugs are doing something beneficial, there is little justification for giving them.

Clearly, not all patients are candidates for chemotherapy. The decision to institute treatment must be individualized. Patients should be informed as accurately as possible about the potential risks and benefits of the proposed therapy. When the decision to treat is made, it should be the result of collaboration between the patient, family, and physician, and should reflect a conviction on the part of the patient that, within his or her set of values, the potential benefits outweigh the inherent risks.

LOOKING AHEAD

Does the future offer hope of developing drugs that can cure people with cancer? This question can be cautiously answered in the affirmative. There is no theoretical reason to believe that cancers are inherently incapable of cure. On the contrary, there is good reason to believe that cancers are, in fact, curable. New insights into tumor biology are suggesting new ways to attack cancer cells. Three potential new approaches are especially exciting: cancer vaccines, angiogenesis inhibitors, and telomerase inhibitors. Custom-made vaccines using the patient's own cancer cells can intensify immune attack against the cancer. Angiogenesis inhibitors may be able to block the growth of new blood vessels into solid tumors, thereby starving the tumor. Telomerase inhibitors offer the possibility of a "magic bullet" that can block the endless proliferation of cancer cells, while leaving normal cells unharmed. These areas of research and others may finally lead to drugs that have the same degree of selective toxicity for cancer as, for example, penicillin G has for gram-positive bacteria. Drugs with this degree of selectivity will offer a cure for neoplastic diseases. It is not completely naive to believe that such drugs will eventually be available.

⠿ KEY POINTS

- Cancer cells are characterized by persistent proliferation, invasive growth, and the ability to form metastases.
- Cancer can be treated with three basic modalities: surgery, radiation therapy, and drug therapy. Drug therapy, in turn, can be divided into chemotherapy (treatment with cytotoxic drugs), hormonal therapy, and immunotherapy.
- Surgery and/or irradiation are the treatments of choice for most solid tumors.
- Drugs are the treatment of choice for disseminated cancers (leukemias, disseminated lymphomas, widespread metastases). Drugs are also used as adjuvants to surgery and irradiation to kill malignant cells that surgery and irradiation leave behind.
- The cell cycle has four major phases: G_1, in which cells prepare to synthesize DNA; S, in which cells synthesize DNA; G_2, in which cells prepare for mitosis (division); and M, in which cells actually divide. Following mitosis, the resulting daughter cells may either enter G_1 and repeat the cycle, or enter G_0 and become mitotically dormant.
- The growth fraction is defined as the ratio of proliferating cells to G_0 cells in a tissue.
- Tissues with a large percentage of proliferating cells and few cells in G_0 have a high growth fraction. Conversely, tissues composed mostly of G_0 cells have a low growth fraction.
- Cytotoxic anticancer drugs are more toxic to cancers that have a high growth fraction than to cancers that have a low growth fraction. Why? Because cytotoxic anticancer drugs are more active against proliferating cells than against cells in G_0.
- As a rule, solid tumors have a low growth fraction, and hence tend to respond poorly to drugs. In contrast, disseminated cancers have a high growth fraction and generally respond well.
- To cure a patient of cancer, we must produce 100% cell kill, which is usually impossible.

- Killing of cancer cells follows first-order kinetics. That is, at any given dose, drugs kill a constant percentage of malignant cells, regardless of how many cells are present.
- Over the course of chemotherapy, cancer cells often become drug resistant, thereby decreasing the chance of success.
- The purpose of intermittent chemotherapy is to allow normal cells to repopulate between rounds of treatment. Unfortunately, if the cancer cells repopulate as rapidly as (or more rapidly than) the normal cells, there will be no reduction in tumor burden with each round of treatment, and hence treatment will fail.
- Multidrug chemotherapy is generally much more effective than single-drug therapy. Why? Because combination therapy can (1) suppress drug resistance, (2) increase cell kill, and (3) reduce injury to normal cells (at any given level of anticancer effect).
- Ideally, the drugs used in combination therapy should have (1) different mechanisms of action, (2) minimally overlapping toxicities, and (3) good efficacy when used alone.
- For drugs that act during a specific phase of the cell cycle, selecting the right dosing schedule is critical to success.
- Toxicity to normal tissues is the major obstacle to successful therapy with cytotoxic anticancer drugs.
- Cytotoxic anticancer drugs injure normal tissue because these agents lack selective toxicity.
- As a rule, serious toxicity occurs to normal tissues that have a high growth fraction (i.e., bone marrow, GI epithelium, hair follicles, and sperm-forming cells).
- Myelosuppression (toxicity to bone marrow) can reduce the number of neutrophils, thrombocytes, and erythrocytes, thereby posing a risk of infection (from loss of neutrophils), bleeding (from loss of thrombocytes), and anemia (from loss of erythrocytes).
- Loss of neutrophils and thrombocytes during chemotherapy is common; significant loss of erythrocytes is rare.
- In patients taking myelosuppressive drugs, neutrophil counts must be monitored. If neutropenia is substantial (absolute neutrophil count below 500/mm³), the next round of chemotherapy should be postponed.
- When a neutropenic patient develops an infection, immediate and vigorous intervention is required. Until lab reports on the identity and drug sensitivity of the infecting organism are available, empiric therapy with IV antibiotics should be instituted.
- Neutropenia can be minimized by treatment with granulocyte colony-stimulating factor or granulocyte-macrophage colony-stimulating factor, both of which act on the bone marrow to increase neutrophil production.
- By injuring the epithelial lining of the GI tract, anticancer drugs often cause stomatitis and diarrhea.
- Many anticancer drugs cause moderate to severe nausea and vomiting, in part by stimulating the chemoreceptor trigger zone.

- Nausea and vomiting can be reduced by premedication with antiemetics. The combination of ondansetron plus dexamethasone is especially effective.
- Anticancer drugs often injure hair follicles, thereby causing alopecia (hair loss). Patients who want to wear a hairpiece should select one before hair loss occurs.
- Anticancer drugs can cause fetal malformation and death. Accordingly, women undergoing chemotherapy should be warned against becoming pregnant.
- Anticancer drugs can cause irreversible male sterility. Accordingly, men undergoing chemotherapy should be counseled about possible sperm banking.

- Chemotherapy can cause hyperuricemia as a result of DNA degradation secondary to massive cell death.
- Renal injury from hyperuricemia can be minimized by giving fluids, allopurinol (a drug that blocks uric acid formation), and rasburicase (an enzyme that catalyzes uric acid degradation).
- Anticancer drugs with vesicant properties can cause severe local injury if the IV line through which they are being administered becomes extravasated.
- Cancer chemotherapy has three possible benefits: cure, palliation, and prolongation of useful life. For treatment to be justified, there should be reason to believe that at least one of these benefits will be forthcoming.

Anticancer Drugs I: Cytotoxic Agents

INTRODUCTION TO THE CYTOTOXIC ANTICANCER DRUGS

The cytotoxic agents constitute the largest class of anticancer drugs. As their name implies, these agents act directly on cancer cells to cause their death. The cytotoxic drugs can be subdivided into seven groups: (1) alkylating agents, (2) platinum compounds, (3) antimetabolites, (4) antitumor antibiotics, (5) mitotic inhibitors, (6) topoisomerase inhibitors, and (7) miscellaneous cytotoxic drugs. We do not discuss each drug in detail. Rather, we focus on selected representative agents. Individual cytotoxic agents are listed in Table 98–1.

Mechanisms of Cytotoxic Action

Table 98–2 summarizes the principal mechanisms by which the cytotoxic anticancer drugs act. As the table shows, most cytotoxic agents disrupt processes related to synthesis of DNA or its precursors. In addition, some agents (e.g., vinblastine, vincristine) act specifically to block mitosis, and one drug—asparaginase—disrupts synthesis of proteins. Note that, with the exception of asparaginase, all of the cytotoxic drugs disrupt processes carried out exclusively by cells that are undergoing replication. As a result, these drugs are most toxic to tissues that have a high growth fraction (i.e., a high proportion of proliferating cells).

Cell-Cycle Phase Specificity

As discussed in Chapter 97, the cell cycle is the sequence of events that a cell goes through from one mitotic division to the next. Some anticancer agents, known as *cell-cycle phase–specific drugs,* are effective only during a specific phase of the cell cycle. Other anticancer agents, known as *cell-cycle phase–nonspecific drugs,* can affect cells during any phase of the cell cycle. About half of the cytotoxic anticancer drugs are phase specific, and the other half are phase nonspecific. The phase specificity of individual cytotoxic agents is summarized in Table 98–1.

    Cell-Cycle Phase–Specific Drugs. Phase-specific agents are toxic only to cells that are passing through a particular phase of the cell cycle. Vincristine, for example, acts by causing mitotic arrest, and hence is effective only during M phase. Other agents act by disrupting DNA synthesis, and hence are effective only during S phase. Because of their phase specificity, these drugs are toxic only to cells that are active participants in the cell cycle; cells that are "resting" in G_0 will not be harmed. Obviously, if these drugs are to be effective, they must be present as neoplastic cells cycle through the specific phase in which they act. This means that these drugs must be present for an extended time. To accomplish this, phase-specific drugs are often administered by prolonged infusion. Alternatively, they can be given in multiple small doses at short intervals over an extended time. Because the dosing schedule is so critical to therapeutic response, phase-specific drugs are also known as *schedule-dependent drugs.*

    Cell-Cycle Phase–Nonspecific Drugs. The phase-nonspecific drugs can act during any phase of the cell cycle, including G_0. Among the phase-nonspecific drugs are the alkylating agents and most antitumor antibiotics. Because phase-nonspecific drugs can injure G_0 cells, whereas phase-specific drugs cannot, phase-nonspecific drugs can increase cell kill when used together with phase-specific drugs.

    Although the phase-nonspecific drugs can inflict biochemical lesions at any time during the cell cycle, *as a rule these drugs are more toxic to proliferating cells than to cells in G_0.* There are two reasons why this is so. First, cells in G_0 often have time to repair drug-induced damage before it can result in significant harm. In contrast, proliferating cells lack time for repair. Second, toxicity may not become manifest until the cells attempt to proliferate. For example, many alkylating agents act by producing cross-links between DNA strands. Although these biochemical lesions can be made at any time, they are largely without effect until cells attempt to replicate DNA. This is much like inflicting a flat tire on an automobile: The tire

TABLE 98–1 ■ Cytotoxic Anticancer Drugs

Generic Name	Trade Name	Cell-Cycle Phase Specificity	Route*	Dose-Limiting Toxicity
Alkylating Agents				
Nitrogen Mustards				
Cyclophosphamide	Cytoxan, Neosar	Phase nonspecific	PO, IV	Bone marrow suppression
Chlorambucil	Leukeran	Phase nonspecific	PO	Bone marrow suppression
Ifosfamide	Ifex	Phase nonspecific	IV	Bone marrow suppression and hemorrhagic cystitis
Melphalan	Alkeran	Phase nonspecific	PO, IV	Bone marrow suppression
Mechlorethamine	Mustargen	Phase nonspecific, but M and G_1 most sensitive	IV, IC, T	Bone marrow suppression
Nitrosoureas				
Carmustine	BiCNU, Gliadel	Phase nonspecific	IV, local	Bone marrow suppression
Lomustine	CeeNU	Phase nonspecific	PO	Bone marrow suppression
Streptozocin	Zanosar	Phase nonspecific	IV	Nephrotoxicity
Others				
Busulfan	Myleran, Busulfex	Phase nonspecific	PO	Bone marrow suppression and lung damage
Temozolomide	Temodar	Phase nonspecific	PO	Bone marrow suppression
Platinum Compounds				
Carboplatin	Paraplatin	Phase nonspecific	IV	Bone marrow suppression
Cisplatin	Platinol-AQ	Phase nonspecific	IV	Nephrotoxicity
Oxaliplatin	Eloxatin	Phase nonspecific	IV	Peripheral neuropathy
Antimetabolites				
Folic Acid Analog				
Methotrexate	Rheumatrex, Trexall	S-phase specific	IV, IM, PO, IT	Bone marrow suppression, oral and GI ulceration
Pyrimidine Analogs				
Capecitabine	Xeloda	Phase nonspecific, but cell must be cycling	PO	Bone marrow suppression, diarrhea
Cytarabine	Cytosar-U, DepoCyt, Tarabine PFS	S-phase specific	IV, SC, IT	Bone marrow suppression
Fluorouracil	Adrucil	Phase nonspecific, but cell must be cycling	IV	Bone marrow suppression, oral and GI ulceration
Floxuridine	FUDR	Phase nonspecific, but cell must be cycling	IA	Bone marrow suppression, oral and GI ulceration
Gemcitabine	Gemzar	S-phase specific	IV	Bone marrow suppression
Purine Analogs				
Mercaptopurine	Purinethol	S-phase specific	PO	Bone marrow suppression
Thioguanine	Generic only	S-phase specific	PO, IV	Bone marrow suppression
Fludarabine	Fludara	S-phase specific	IV	Bone marrow suppression
Pentostatin	Nipent	S-phase specific	IV	Bone marrow suppression, CNS depression
Cladribine	Leustatin	Phase nonspecific	IV	Bone marrow suppression
Antitumor Antibiotics				
Bleomycin	Blenoxane	G_2-phase specific	IV, IM, SC, IP	Pneumonitis and pulmonary fibrosis
Dactinomycin	Cosmegen	Phase nonspecific	IV	Bone marrow suppression, oral ulceration
Daunorubicin	Cerubidine, DaunoXome	Phase nonspecific	IV	Bone marrow suppression, cardiotoxicity
Doxorubicin	Adriamycin, Rubex, Doxil	Phase nonspecific	IV	Bone marrow suppression, cardiotoxicity
Epirubicin	Ellence	Phase nonspecific, but S and G_2 most sensitive	IV	Bone marrow suppression, cardiotoxicity

TABLE 98–1 ▪■ Cytotoxic Anticancer Drugs (continued)

Generic Name	Trade Name	Cell-Cycle Phase Specificity	Route*	Dose-Limiting Toxicity
Antitumor Antibiotics—cont'd				
Idarubicin	Idamycin	Phase nonspecific, but S most sensitive	IV	Bone marrow suppression
Mitomycin	Mutamycin	Phase nonspecific	IV	Bone marrow suppression
Mitoxantrone	Novantrone	Phase nonspecific	IV	Bone marrow suppression
Plicamycin	Mithracin	Phase nonspecific	IV	Bone marrow suppression, bleeding disorders
Valrubicin	Valstar	Phase nonspecific	Intravesical	None
Mitotic Inhibitors				
Vinca Alkaloids				
Vinblastine	Velban	M-phase specific	IV	Bone marrow suppression
Vincristine	Oncovin, Vincasar	M-phase specific	IV	Peripheral neuropathy
Vinorelbine	Navelbine	M-phase specific	IV	Bone marrow suppression
Taxoids				
Docetaxel	Taxotere	G_2-phase specific	IV	Bone marrow suppression
Paclitaxel	Taxol, Onxol	G_2-phase specific	IV	Bone marrow suppression
Topoisomerase Inhibitors				
Etoposide	VePesid, others	G_2-phase specific	IV	Bone marrow suppression
Teniposide	Vumon	G_2-phase specific	IV	Bone marrow suppression
Irinotecan	Camptosar	S-phase specific	IV	Bone marrow suppression and late diarrhea
Topotecan	Hycamtin	S-phase specific	IV	Bone marrow suppression
Miscellaneous				
Altretamine	Hexalen	Mechanism unknown	PO	Bone marrow suppression
Asparaginase	Elspar	G_1-phase specific	IV, IM	None
Pegaspargase	Oncaspar	G_1-phase specific	IV, IM	None
Dacarbazine	DTIC-Dome	Phase nonspecific	IV	Bone marrow suppression
Hydroxyurea	Hydrea	S-phase specific	PO	Bone marrow suppression
Procarbazine	Matulane	Phase nonspecific	PO	Bone marrow suppression
Mitotane	Lysodren	Phase nonspecific	PO	CNS depression

*IA = intra-arterial, IC = intracavitary, IM = intramuscular, IP = intrapleural, IT = intrathecal, IV = intravenous, PO = oral, SC = subcutaneous, T = topical.

can be deflated at any time; however, loss of air is consequential only if the car is moving. Carrying the analogy further, if the flat occurs while the car is stopped, and is repaired before travel is attempted, the flat will have no functional impact at all.

Toxicity

As discussed in Chapter 97, many anticancer drugs are toxic to normal tissues—especially tissues that have a high percentage of proliferating cells (bone marrow, hair follicles, GI epithelium, and germinal epithelium). The common major toxicities of the anticancer drugs, together with management procedures, are discussed at length in Chapter 97. Therefore, as we consider individual anticancer agents in this chapter, discussion of most toxicities is brief.

Dosage, Handling, and Administration

Dosage and Administration. Cancer chemotherapy is a highly specialized field. Accordingly, in a general text such as this, presentation of detailed information on dosage and ad-

ministration of specific agents seems inappropriate. However, you should be aware that dosages for anticancer agents must be individualized and that timing of administration may vary with the particular protocol being followed. Also, because of the complex and hazardous nature of cancer chemotherapy, anticancer drugs should be administered under the direct supervision of a physician experienced in their use.

Handling of Cytotoxic Drugs. Antineoplastic drugs are often mutagenic, teratogenic, and carcinogenic. In addition, direct contact with the skin, eyes, and mucous membranes can result in local injury. Accordingly, it is imperative that healthcare personnel involved in the preparation and administration of these drugs follow safe handling procedures. Risk of injury from contact with parenteral chemotherapeutic drugs can be minimized by using containment equipment and approved technique.

Administration of Vesicants. As discussed in Chapter 97, extravasation of vesicants can cause severe local injury, sometimes requiring surgical débridement and skin grafting. Drugs with strong vesicant properties include carmustine, dacarbazine, dactinomycin, daunorubicin, doxoru-

TABLE 98–2 ■ Actions of Representative Cytotoxic Anticancer Drugs

Drug	Drug Action	Cellular Process Disrupted
Cyclophosphamide	Alkylates DNA, causing cross-links and strand breakage	DNA and RNA synthesis
Methotrexate	Inhibits one-carbon transfer reactions	Synthesis of DNA precursors (purines, dTMP)
Hydroxyurea	Inhibits ribonucleotide reductase	Synthesis of DNA precursors (blocks conversion of ribonucleotides into deoxyribonucleotides)
Thioguanine, mercaptopurine	Inhibits purine ring synthesis and nucleotide interconversion	Synthesis of DNA presursors (purines, pyrimidines, ribonucleotides, and deoxyribonucleotides)
Fluorouracil	Inhibits thymidylate synthetase	Synthesis of dTMP, a DNA precursor
Cytarabine	Inhibits DNA polymerase	DNA synthesis
Bleomycin	Breaks DNA strands and prevents their repair	DNA synthesis
Plicamycin	Binds to DNA	DNA and RNA synthesis
Dactinomycin, daunorubicin	Intercalates between base pairs of DNA	DNA and RNA synthesis
Vinblastine, vincristine	Blocks microtubule assembly	Mitosis
Asparaginase	Deaminates asparagine, depriving cells of this amino acid	Protein synthesis
Topotecan	Inhibits topoisomerase I	Impairs DNA replication
Etoposide	Inhibits topoisomerase II	Prevents resealing of DNA strand breaks

bicin, mechlorethamine, mitomycin, plicamycin, streptozocin, vinblastine, and vincristine. To minimize the risk of injury, IV administration should be performed only into a vein with good flow. Sites of previous irradiation should be avoided. If extravasation occurs, infusion should be discontinued immediately.

ALKYLATING AGENTS

The family of alkylating agents consists of nitrogen mustards, nitrosoureas, and other compounds. Before considering the properties of individual alkylating agents, we discuss the characteristics of the group as a whole. The alkylating agents are listed in Table 98–1.

Shared Properties

Mechanism of Action. The alkylating agents are highly reactive compounds that have the ability to transfer an alkyl group to a variety of cell constituents. Cell kill results primarily from alkylation of DNA. As a rule, alkylating agents interact with DNA by forming a covalent bond with a specific nitrogen atom in guanine (Fig. 98–1).

Some alkylating agents have two reactive sites, whereas others have only one. Alkylating agents with two reactive sites (*bifunctional* agents) are able to bind DNA in two places to form *cross-links*. These bridges may be formed within a single strand of DNA or between parallel DNA strands. Figure 98–1 illustrates the production of interstrand cross-links by nitrogen mustard. Alkylating agents with only one reactive

site (*monofunctional* agents) lack the ability to form cross-links, but can still bind to a single guanine in DNA.

The consequences of guanine alkylation are miscoding, scission of DNA strands, and, if cross-links have been formed, inhibition of DNA replication. Since cross-linking of DNA is especially injurious, cell death is more likely with bifunctional agents than with monofunctional agents.

Because alkylation reactions can take place at any time during the cell cycle, alkylating agents are considered *cell-cycle phase nonspecific*. However, *most of these drugs are more toxic to proliferating cells than to cells in G_0*. Why? Because (1) alkylation of DNA produces its most detrimental effects when cells attempt to replicate DNA, and (2) resting cells are often able to repair damage to DNA before it can affect cell function. Because alkylating agents are phase nonspecific, they needn't be present over an extended time. Accordingly, they can be administered as a single bolus dose.

Resistance. Development of resistance to alkylating agents is common. A major cause of resistance is increased production of enzymes that repair DNA. Resistance may also result from decreased uptake of alkylating agents and from increased production of nucleophiles (compounds that act as decoy targets for alkylation).

Toxicities. Alkylating agents are toxic to tissues that have a high growth fraction. Accordingly, these drugs may injure cells of the bone marrow, hair follicles, GI mucosa, and germinal epithelium. Blood dyscrasias (neutropenia, thrombocytopenia, anemia) caused by bone marrow suppression are of greatest concern. Nausea and vomiting occur with all alkylating agents. Also, practically all of these drugs are vesicants, and hence must be administered IV.

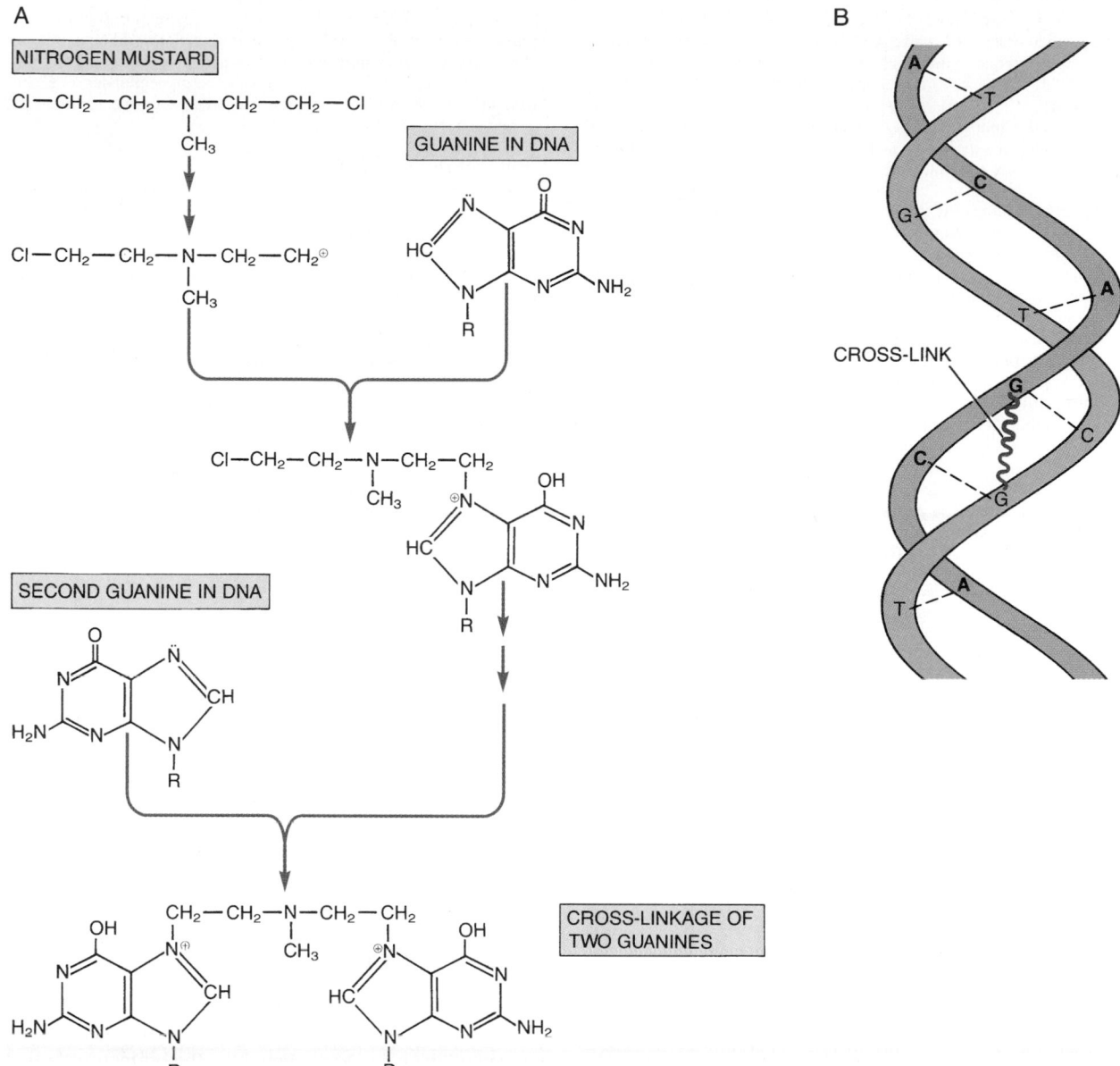

Figure 98–1 ■ **Cross-linking of DNA by an alkylating agent.**
A, Reactions leading to cross-linkage between guanine moieties in DNA. *B,* Schematic representation of interstrand cross-linking within the DNA double helix. (A = adenine, C = cytosine, G = guanine, T = thymine.)

Properties of Individual Alkylating Agents
Nitrogen Mustards

Cyclophosphamide. Cyclophosphamide [Cytoxan, Neosar] is a bifunctional agent active against a *broad spectrum* of neoplastic diseases. Indications include *Hodgkin's disease, non-Hodgkin's lymphomas, multiple myeloma,* and *solid tumors of the head, neck, ovary, and breast.* Of all the alkylating agents, cyclophosphamide is employed most widely.

Cyclophosphamide is a prodrug that undergoes conversion to its active form in the liver. Because activation is required, onset of effects is delayed. In contrast to most other alkylating agents, cyclophosphamide is not a vesicant, and hence can be administered PO as well as IV. Oral doses should be administered with food.

The major dose-limiting toxicity is bone marrow suppression. Severe nausea, vomiting, and alopecia are also common. In addition, the drug can cause acute hemorrhagic cystitis; renal damage can be minimized by maintaining adequate hydration. Other adverse effects include sterility, immunosuppression, and hypersensitivity reactions.

Mechlorethamine. Mechlorethamine [Mustargen], a bifunctional compound, was the first alkylating agent employed clinically. Applications include *Hodgkin's disease* and *non-Hodgkin's lymphomas.* Mechlorethamine is a powerful vesicant and can cause severe local injury. Accordingly, for systemic therapy, the drug must be administered IV. Caution must be exercised to avoid both extravasation and direct contact with the skin. Once in the bloodstream, mechlorethamine undergoes rapid conversion to inactive compounds. The dose-limiting toxicity is bone marrow suppression. Other major toxicities include nausea, vomiting, alopecia, diarrhea, stomatitis, amenorrhea, and sterility.

Chlorambucil. Chlorambucil [Leukeran] is the safest nitrogen mustard available. Bone marrow suppression is the major dose-limiting toxicity. Other adverse effects include hepatotoxicity, sterility, pulmonary infiltrates, and pulmonary fibrosis. Nausea and vomiting are usually mild. Chlorambucil is a drug of choice for palliative therapy of *chronic lymphocytic leukemia*. The drug is also used for palliation of *Hodgkin's disease, non-Hodgkin's lymphomas,* and *ovarian cancer*. Administration is oral.

Melphalan. Melphalan [Alkeran], a bifunctional agent, is generally well tolerated. Bone marrow suppression is the major dose-limiting toxicity. The drug has caused leukemia and may also be mutagenic. Melphalan is not a vesicant. Severe nausea and vomiting are rare. Administration is oral and IV. Melphalan is a drug of choice for palliative therapy of *multiple myeloma,* and is also active against *carcinoma of the ovary and breast*.

Ifosfamide. Ifosfamide [Ifex], a derivative of cyclophosphamide, is approved only for refractory *germ cell tumor of the testes*. Dose-limiting toxicities are bone marrow suppression and hemorrhagic cystitis. The risk of cystitis is minimized by concurrent therapy with *mesna* [Mesnex] and by extensive hydration (at least 2 L of oral or IV fluid daily). Owing to the risk of cystitis, urinalysis should be performed before each dose. If the analysis reveals microscopic hematuria, dosing should be postponed until the hematuria resolves. Additional adverse effects include nausea, vomiting, metabolic acidosis, and central nervous system (CNS) toxicity (confusion, hallucinations, blurred vision, coma). Administration is IV.

Nitrosoureas

The nitrosoureas, which are bifunctional alkylating agents, are active against a broad spectrum of neoplastic diseases. Cell kill results from cross-linking DNA. Unlike most other anticancer drugs, the nitrosoureas are highly lipophilic, and hence can readily penetrate the blood-brain barrier. As a result, these drugs are especially useful against *cancers of the CNS*. The major dose-limiting toxicity is *delayed bone marrow suppression*.

Carmustine (BCNU). Carmustine [BiCNU, Gliadel] was the first nitrosourea to undergo extensive clinical testing and can be considered the prototype for the group. Because of its ability to cross the blood-brain barrier, carmustine is used frequently to treat *primary and metastatic tumors of the brain*. Other indications include *Hodgkin's disease, non-Hodgkin's lymphomas, multiple myeloma, malignant melanoma, hepatoma,* and *adenocarcinoma of the stomach, colon, and rectum*. The principal dose-limiting toxicity is delayed bone marrow suppression; leukocyte and thrombocyte nadirs occur 4 to 6 weeks after treatment. Nausea and vomiting can be severe. Injury to the liver, kidneys, and lungs has been reported.

Administration may be topical or IV. Topical administration is done by implanting a biodegradable, carmustine-impregnated wafer [Gliadel] into the cavity created by surgical removal of a brain tumor. This technique has the obvious benefit of concentrating the drug where it is most needed. When administered IV, carmustine can cause local phlebitis, even though it is not a vesicant.

Lomustine (CCNU). Lomustine [CeeNU] is similar to carmustine in actions and uses. Like carmustine, lomustine crosses the blood-brain barrier and can be used to treat *brain cancer*. The drug is also active against *lymphomas, melanomas,* and *carcinomas of the breast, lung, and colon*. As with carmustine, the major dose-limiting toxicity is delayed bone marrow suppression. Additional toxicities include nausea and vomiting, renal and hepatic toxicity, pulmonary fibrosis, and neurologic reactions. Administration is oral.

Streptozocin. Streptozocin [Zanosar] differs significantly from other nitrosoureas. The drug contains a glucose moiety that causes selective uptake by islet cells of the pancreas. This selective uptake underlies the drug's prin-

cipal indication: *metastatic islet cell tumors*. The major dose-limiting toxicity is kidney damage. Accordingly, renal function should be monitored in all patients. As with other nitrosoureas, nausea and vomiting can be severe. Additional toxicities include hypoglycemia, hyperglycemia, diarrhea, chills, and fever. In contrast to other nitrosoureas, streptozocin causes minimal bone marrow suppression. Administration is IV.

Other Alkylating Agents

Busulfan. Busulfan [Myleran, Busulfex] is a bifunctional agent whose cytotoxic effects are limited almost exclusively to the bone marrow. Because it causes selective attack on the bone marrow, busulfan is a drug of choice for *chronic myelogenous leukemia*. The remission rate is 90% with one course of therapy. Dose-limiting toxicities are bone marrow suppression, pulmonary infiltrates, and pulmonary fibrosis. Other toxicities include nausea, vomiting, alopecia, gynecomastia, male and female sterility, skin hyperpigmentation, cataracts, and hepatitis. Administration is oral and IV.

Temozolomide. Therapeutic Use. Temozolomide [Temodar] is a relatively new drug indicated for oral therapy of adults with *anaplastic astrocytoma* that has relapsed after treatment with preferred agents: procarbazine and a nitrosourea (lomustine or carmustine). Temozolomide can also benefit patients with recurrent *glioblastoma multiforme*. Both of these cancers arise from glial cells in the brain, and both eventually recur despite aggressive treatment. However, even though temozolomide cannot offer cure, it can increase health-related quality of life. The initial dosage is 150 mg/m² once daily for 5 consecutive days, repeated every 28 days. In clinical trials, temozolomide produced partial tumor shrinkage in 27% of patients, and complete shrinkage in 8%. Temozolomide is expensive: A single cycle costs over $1500.

Pharmacokinetics and Mechanism of Action. Temozolomide undergoes nearly complete absorption following oral administration. Food reduces both the rate and extent of absorption. Once in the body, temozolomide undergoes rapid, nonenzymatic conversion to its active form, an alkylating agent known as MTIC. As MTIC, the drug alkylates DNA, and thereby causes cell death. Temozolomide readily crosses the blood-brain barrier to reach its site of action. The elimination half-life is 1.8 hours.

Adverse Effects. The major dose-limiting toxicity is myelosuppression, manifesting as neutropenia and thrombocytopenia. The most common adverse effects are nausea (53%) and vomiting (42%). Both respond well to antiemetic drugs. Other common reactions include headache (41%), fatigue (34%), constipation (33%), and diarrhea (16%). Convulsions may also occur. Patients must not open temozolomide capsules; the drug can cause local injury following inhalation or contact with the skin or mucous membranes.

PLATINUM COMPOUNDS

The platinum-containing anticancer drugs—cisplatin, carboplatin, and oxaliplatin—are very similar to the alkylating agents, and are often classified as such. Like the bifunctional alkylating agents, the platinum compounds produce cross-links in DNA, and hence are cell-cycle phase nonspecific.

Cisplatin

Cisplatin [Platinol-AQ] kills cells primarily by forming cross-links between and within strands of DNA. The drug's principal indication is *testicular cancer*. Other indications include *carcinomas of the ovary, bladder, lung, head, and neck*. The major dose-limiting toxicity is kidney damage, which can be minimized by extensive hydration coupled with diuretic therapy and *amifostine* [Ethyol]. Cisplatin is highly emetogenic; nausea and vomiting begin about 1 hour after administration and persist for 1 to 2 days. Other adverse effects include neurotoxicity, bone marrow suppression, and toxicity to the ear, which manifests as tinnitus and high-frequency hearing loss. Administration is by IV infusion.

Carboplatin

Carboplatin [Paraplatin] is an analog of cisplatin. Cell kill appears to result from cross-linking DNA. The drug's only approved indications are initial and palliative therapy of *ovarian cancer*. Unlabeled uses include *small cell can-*

cer of the lung, squamous cell cancer of the head and neck, and *endometrial cancer.* The major dose-limiting toxicity is bone marrow suppression. Nausea and vomiting occur, but are less severe than with cisplatin. Similarly, nephrotoxicity, neurotoxicity, and hearing loss are less frequent than with cisplatin. Carboplatin is administered by IV infusion. Anaphylactic reactions have occurred minutes after administration; symptoms can be managed with epinephrine, glucocorticoids, and antihistamines.

Oxaliplatin

Actions and Uses. Oxaliplatin [Eloxatin] is a new platinum compound with actions similar to those of carboplatin. Like carboplatin, oxaliplatin produces intra- and interstrand cross-links in DNA. Currently, oxaliplatin is approved only for *colorectal cancer* that has progressed after treatment with first-line therapy (irinotecan plus fluorouracil), and should be used only in combination with fluorouracil (followed by leucovorin to reverse the effects of fluorouracil on normal cells). Investigational uses include *mesothelioma, non-Hodgkin's lymphoma,* and *cancers of the breast, ovary, pancreas, prostate, and lung.* Administration is by IV infusion.

Toxicity. Peripheral Sensory Neuropathy. The major dose-limiting toxicity is peripheral sensory neuropathy, manifesting as numbness or tingling in the fingers and toes and around the mouth and throat. Neuropathy develops in most patients, either early in treatment or after several courses. Neuropathy may impede activities of daily living, such as buttoning clothing, writing, or just holding things. Symptoms are often intensified by exposure to cold. Accordingly, patients should be warned to cover exposed skin before touching cold objects or entering a cold environment. Also, patients should avoid cold liquids and use of ice. Oxaliplatin-induced neuropathy typically resolves after treatment stops, although complete recovery may take several months. Oral gabapentin may reduce or prevent neuropathy.

Other Toxicities. Damage to bone marrow can cause anemia (64%), neutropenia (15% with oxaliplatin alone, 66% when combined with fluorouracil), and thrombocytopenia (41% with oxaliplatin alone, 76% when combined with fluorouracil). Other common reactions are nausea and vomiting (70%), liver abnormalities (46%), diarrhea (41%), fever (36%), abdominal pain (31%), and infection (23%). Alopecia occurs in 2% of patients. Life-threatening anaphylactoid reactions may develop, but are uncommon; epinephrine, glucocorticoids, and antihistamines have been employed for treatment.

ANTIMETABOLITES

Antimetabolites are structural analogs of important natural metabolites. Because they resemble natural metabolites, these drugs are able to disrupt critical metabolic processes. Some antimetabolites inhibit enzymes that synthesize essential cellular constituents. Others undergo incorporation into DNA, thereby disrupting DNA replication and function.

Antimetabolites are effective only against cells that are active participants in the cell cycle. Most antimetabolites are S-phase specific, although some can act during any phase of the cycle (except G_0). To be effective, agents that are S-phase specific must be present for an extended time.

There are three classes of antimetabolites: (1) folic acid analogs, (2) purine analogs, and (3) pyrimidine analogs. Members of each class are listed in Table 98–1.

Folic Acid Analog: Methotrexate

Folic acid, in its active form, is needed for several essential biochemical reactions. The folic acid analogs block the conversion of folic acid to its active form. At this time, methotrexate is the only folate analog employed in cancer chemotherapy. Other folate analogs are used to treat bacterial infections (trimethoprim), malaria (pyrimethamine), and *Pneumocystis carinii* pneumonia (trimetrexate).

Mechanism of Action. As shown in Figure 98–2, methotrexate [Rheumatrex, Trexall] *inhibits dihydrofolate reductase,* the enzyme that converts dihydrofolic acid (FH_2) into tetrahydrofolic acid (FH_4). Since production of FH_4 is a necessary step in the activation of folic acid, and since activated folic acid is required for biosynthesis of essential cellular con-

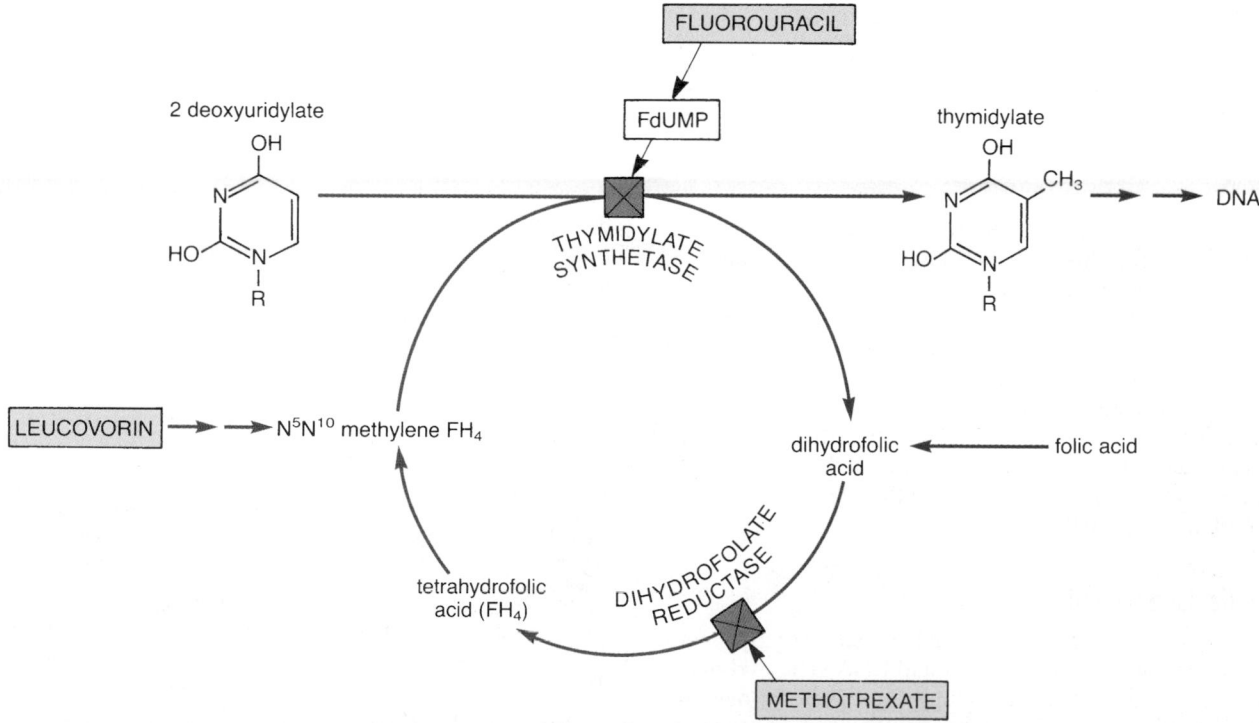

Figure 98–2 ■ **Actions of methotrexate, leucovorin, and fluorouracil.**
(FdUMP = 5-fluoro-2'-deoxyuridine-5'-monophosphate, ⊠ = blockade of reaction.)

stituents (DNA, RNA, proteins), inhibition of FH$_4$ production has multiple effects on the cell. Of all the processes that are suppressed by methotrexate, biosynthesis of thymidylate appears most critical. Why? Because, in the absence of thymidylate, cells are unable to make DNA. Because cell kill results primarily from disrupting DNA synthesis, methotrexate is considered S-phase specific.

A technique known as *leucovorin rescue* can be employed to enhance the effects of methotrexate. Some neoplastic cells are unresponsive to methotrexate because they lack the transport system required for active uptake of the drug. By giving massive doses, methotrexate can be forced into these cells by passive diffusion. However, because this process also exposes normal cells to extremely high concentrations of methotrexate, these normal cells are also at risk. To save them, leucovorin (citrovorum factor, folinic acid) is given. As shown in Figure 98–2, leucovorin bypasses the metabolic block caused by methotrexate, thereby permitting normal cells to synthesize thymidylate and other compounds. Malignant cells are not saved because leucovorin uptake requires the same transport system employed for methotrexate uptake, a transport system these cells lack. It should be noted that leucovorin rescue is potentially hazardous: *Failure to administer leucovorin in the right dose at the right time can be fatal.*

Resistance. Acquired resistance to methotrexate can result from three mechanisms: (1) decreased uptake of methotrexate, (2) increased synthesis of dihydrofolate reductase (the target enzyme for methotrexate), and (3) synthesis of a modified form of dihydrofolate reductase that has a reduced affinity for methotrexate.

Pharmacokinetics. Methotrexate can be administered PO, IM, IV, and intrathecally. For most cancers of the CNS, intrathecal administration is employed. Metabolism of methotrexate is minimal. Most of each dose is excreted intact in the urine. Because elimination is renal, methotrexate can accumulate to dangerous levels in patients with renal insufficiency; hence, the dosage must be reduced to minimize injury.

Therapeutic Uses. *Neoplastic Diseases.* Methotrexate is curative for women with *choriocarcinoma.* The drug is also active against *non-Hodgkin's lymphomas* and *acute lymphocytic leukemia of childhood.* Very large doses coupled with leucovorin rescue have been employed to treat *head and neck sarcomas* and *osteogenic sarcoma.*

Other Indications. Low doses are used for *severe psoriasis* (see Chapter 101). Higher doses are used for severe *rheumatoid arthritis* (see Chapter 69).

Toxicity. The usual dose-limiting toxicities are bone marrow suppression, pulmonary infiltrates and fibrosis, and oral and GI ulceration. Death may result from intestinal perforation and hemorrhagic enteritis. Nausea and vomiting may occur shortly after administration. High doses can cause direct injury to the kidneys. To promote drug excretion, and thereby minimize renal damage, the urine should be alkalinized and adequate hydration should be maintained. Methotrexate has been associated with fetal malformation and death. Accordingly, pregnancy should be avoided until at least 6 months after completing treatment.

Pyrimidine Analogs

Pyrimidines—cytosine, thymine, and uracil—are bases employed in the biosynthesis of DNA and RNA. The pyrimidine analogs, because of their structural similarity to naturally occurring pyrimidines, can act in several ways: (1) they can inhibit biosynthesis of pyrimidines, (2) they can inhibit biosynthesis of DNA and RNA, and (3) they can undergo incorporation into DNA and RNA, and thereby disrupt nucleic acid function. All of the pyrimidine analogs are prodrugs that must be converted to their active forms in the body.

Cytarabine

Cytarabine [Cytosar-U, Tarabine PFS, DepoCyt], also known as *cytosine arabinoside* and *Ara C,* is an analog of deoxycytidine. The drug has an established role in treating *acute myelogenous leukemia.*

Mechanism of Action. Cytarabine is converted to its active form—Ara-CTP—within the body. As Ara-CTP, the drug becomes incorporated into DNA. By a mechanism that is not fully understood, incorporation suppresses further DNA synthesis. Ara-CTP may also impede DNA synthesis by a second mechanism: inhibition of DNA polymerase. Cytarabine is highly S-phase specific.

Resistance. Decreased conversion of cytarabine to Ara-CTP is a major cause of resistance. Other mechanisms include decreased uptake of cytarabine, increased conversion of cytarabine to an inactive product, and increased production of dCTP (the natural metabolite that Ara-CTP competes with for incorporation into DNA).

Pharmacokinetics. Administration may be IV, SC, or intrathecal. Cytarabine is not active orally. The fraction of each dose that is not taken up by cells undergoes rapid deamination in the liver. Metabolites are excreted in the urine.

Therapeutic Uses. The principal indication for cytarabine is *acute myelogenous leukemia.* The drug has been combined with thioguanine and daunorubicin or doxorubicin to treat this disease. Other applications include *acute lymphocytic leukemia, chronic myelogenous leukemia,* and *non-Hodgkin's lymphomas.*

Toxicity. Bone marrow suppression (neutropenia, thrombocytopenia) is the usual dose-limiting toxicity. Nausea, vomiting, and fever may develop, especially after bolus IV injection. Other toxicities include stomatitis, liver injury, and conjunctivitis. High doses may cause pulmonary edema and central and peripheral neurotoxicity.

Fluorouracil

Fluorouracil [Adrucil] is a fluorinated derivative of uracil. The drug is employed extensively to treat solid tumors.

Mechanism of Action. In order to exert cytotoxic effects, fluorouracil must be converted to its active form, 5-fluoro-2′-deoxyuridine-5′-monophosphate (FdUMP). As shown in Figure 98–2, FdUMP inhibits thymidylate synthetase, thereby depriving cells of thymidylate needed to make DNA. Fluorouracil is active only against cells that are going through the cell cycle. However, the drug lacks phase specificity.

Resistance. Potential mechanisms for resistance are (1) decreased activation of fluorouracil and (2) production of altered thymidylate synthetase that has a low affinity for FdUMP. The clinical significance of these mechanisms has not been established.

Therapeutic Uses. Chemotherapeutic use of fluorouracil is limited to solid tumors. The drug is employed for palliative therapy of *carcinomas of the colon, rectum, breast, stomach,* and *pancreas.* In addition to therapy of cancer, fluorouracil is employed topically to treat *premalignant keratoses* (see Chapter 101).

Pharmacokinetics. Administration is IV. Continuous infusion is more effective and less toxic than bolus administration. Fluorouracil is distributed widely and enters the CNS with ease. Elimination is by rapid hepatic metabolism.

Toxicity. The usual dose-limiting toxicities are bone marrow suppression (neutropenia) and oral and GI ulceration. To minimize GI injury (e.g., ulceration of the oropharynx or bowel), fluorouracil should be discontinued as soon as mild reactions (stomatitis, diarrhea) occur. Other adverse effects include alopecia, hyperpigmentation, and neurologic deficits.

Capecitabine

Capecitabine [Xeloda], a prodrug form of fluorouracil, is indicated for oral therapy of metastatic *breast cancer* and metastatic *colorectal cancer*. Once in the body, capecitabine undergoes metabolic conversion to fluorouracil and then to FdUMP, its active form. Consequently, the pharmacology of capecitabine is much like that of fluorouracil itself. Cell kill results from inhibition of thymidylate synthetase. Capecitabine is active only against dividing cells, but is not phase specific. In clinical trials, 20% of patients with breast cancer experienced at least a 50% decrease in tumor size. Severe diarrhea is common and can be dose limiting. Other common side effects include nausea, vomiting, stomatitis, and hand-and-foot syndrome, characterized by local tingling, numbness, pain, swelling, and erythema of the palms and soles. Capecitabine is a teratogen and hence must not be used during pregnancy. The drug can cause leukopenia, but severe myelosuppression is uncommon. Alopecia has not been reported. Postmarketing surveillance has shown that capecitabine enhances the effects of warfarin; to reduce the risk of bleeding, anticoagulant effects should be monitored closely, and warfarin dosage reduced if indicated. The recommended dosage for capecitabine is 1250 mg/m² taken twice daily (after eating) for 14 days, followed by 7 days off. This pattern is repeated as appropriate. In patients with renal impairment, capecitabine can accumulate to toxic levels. If renal impairment is *moderate,* dosage should be reduced 75%; if impairment is *severe,* the drug should not be used.

Floxuridine

Floxuridine [FUDR], like fluorouracil, is converted to FdUMP within the body. Hence, the pharmacologic effects of floxuridine and fluorouracil are nearly identical. Floxuridine is used primarily for *metastatic carcinoma of the colon.* The drug is administered only by intra-arterial infusion.

Gemcitabine

Mechanism of Action. Gemcitabine [Gemzar] is a nucleoside analog that inhibits DNA synthesis. Hence, the drug is S-phase specific. Following uptake by cells, gemcitabine is converted to two active forms: gemcitabine diphosphate and gemcitabine triphosphate. Gemcitabine diphosphate inhibits ribonucleotide reductase, an enzyme needed to form deoxynucleoside triphosphates, which are required for DNA synthesis. Gemcitabine triphosphate undergoes incorporation into DNA, where it inhibits further strand elongation.

Therapeutic Use. Gemcitabine is indicated for *adenocarcinoma of the pancreas* and *non–small cell cancer of the lung.* For pancreatic cancer, the drug may be used as first-line therapy in patients with locally advanced or metastatic disease, and in patients previously treated with fluorouracil. In clinical trials, gemcitabine reduced pain, improved functional status, and prolonged life slightly. The recommended dosage is 1000 mg/m² infused IV over 30 minutes once a week for up to 7 weeks. After a 1-week hiatus, treatment is resumed, but dosing is reduced to one infusion every 3 to 4 weeks.

Toxicity. Although gemcitabine can cause a wide variety of adverse effects, it is fairly well tolerated. Myelosuppression is dose limiting. Nausea and vomiting are common (70%) but usually mild to moderate. Other common reactions include elevation of serum transaminases (75%), proteinuria (45%), hematuria (35%), pain (45%), and fever (41%). Less common reactions include diarrhea, constipation, stomatitis, dyspnea, paresthesias, edema, alopecia, and rash.

Purine Analogs

Like the pyrimidines, the purines—adenine, guanine, and hypoxanthine—are bases employed for biosynthesis of nucleic acids. The purine analogs discussed in this chapter are used primarily in the treatment of cancer. Purine analogs discussed in other chapters are used for immunosuppression, antiviral therapy, and gout.

Mercaptopurine

Mechanisms of Action and Resistance. Mercaptopurine [Purinethol] is a prodrug that undergoes conversion to its active form within cells. Following activation, the drug can disrupt multiple biochemical processes, including purine biosynthesis, nucleotide interconversion, and biosynthesis of nucleic acids. All of these actions probably contribute to cytotoxic effects. Mercaptopurine is S-phase specific. Mechanisms of resistance include reduced activation of the drug and accelerated deactivation.

Pharmacokinetics. Mercaptopurine is administered orally and undergoes erratic absorption. Absorbed drug is distributed widely, but not to the CNS. Extensive metabolism occurs in the liver; an important reaction is catalyzed by xanthine oxidase. Accordingly, for patients receiving allopurinol (an inhibitor of xanthine oxidase), mercaptopurine dosage should be reduced.

Therapeutic Uses. The principal indication for mercaptopurine is *acute lymphocytic leukemia* in children and adults. The drug may also be of some benefit in *acute and chronic myelogenous leukemia in adults.*

Toxicity. Bone marrow suppression (neutropenia, thrombocytopenia, anemia) is the principal dose-limiting toxicity. Hepatic dysfunction, which usually manifests as cholestatic jaundice, occurs in about 30% of patients. Other adverse effects include nausea, vomiting, and oral and intestinal ulceration. Concurrent use of allopurinol increases the overall risk of toxicity. Mercaptopurine is mutagenic, and hence female patients should be warned against becoming pregnant.

Thioguanine

Actions and Uses. Thioguanine acts much like mercaptopurine. Following conversion to its active form, thioguanine inhibits purine synthesis and the interconversion of nucleotides. DNA synthesis is also inhibited. Like mercaptopurine, thioguanine is S-phase specific. The drug is used primarily for *acute lymphocytic and myelogenous leukemias.*

Pharmacokinetics. Administration is oral. Absorption is erratic and incomplete. Thioguanine does not distribute to the CNS. Inactivation is by hepatic metabolism. In contrast to mercaptopurine, thioguanine is not degraded by xanthine oxidase, and hence can be employed concurrently with allopurinol without a dosage reduction.

Toxicity. The usual dose-limiting toxicity is bone marrow suppression. Gastrointestinal reactions (nausea, vomiting, diarrhea) may develop, but these are less severe than with mercaptopurine. Liver injury, manifesting as cholestatic jaundice, may occur.

Pentostatin

Pentostatin [Nipent] is an analog of adenosine. The drug inhibits adenosine deaminase and thereby suppresses synthesis of DNA. Its only approved indication is *hairy cell leukemia* that has not responded to interferon alfa. The major dose-limiting toxicities are bone marrow suppression and CNS depression. Other toxicities include nausea, vomiting, rash, and fever. Administration is by IV bolus or IV infusion. Pentostatin is expensive; the cost to the pharmacist for a single course of therapy is approximately $1400.

Fludarabine

Fludarabine [Fludara] is an analog of adenosine. The drug is approved only for *chronic lymphocytic leukemia.* Following IV infusion, fludarabine undergoes rapid conversion to its active form, 2-fluoro-ara-ATP. Cell kill appears to result from inhibition of DNA replication. Thus the drug is probably S-phase specific. The major dose-limiting toxicity is bone marrow suppression (neutropenia, thrombocytopenia, anemia). Other common toxicities include nausea, vomiting, and chills. When given in especially high doses, fludarabine can cause severe neurologic effects, including blindness, coma, and death. However, neurologic effects are rare (0.2%) at maximal recommended therapeutic doses.

Cladribine

Cladribine [Leustatin] is an adenosine analog with a unique combination of actions. Unlike other purine analogs, which inhibit DNA synthesis only, cladribine inhibits both DNA synthesis and DNA repair. As a result, the drug is active against quiescent cells as well as cells that are actively dividing. Cladribine is highly active against *hairy cell leukemia* and is considered a drug of choice for this cancer. The drug is also active against *chronic lymphocytic leukemia, non-Hodgkin's lymphomas, acute myeloid leukemia,* and *mycosis fungoides.* The major dose-limiting toxicity is myelosuppression.

Very high doses (4 to 9 times normal) have caused acute nephrotoxicity and delayed-onset neurotoxicity. For patients with hairy cell leukemia, cladribine is administered by continuous IV infusion over 7 consecutive days.

ANTITUMOR ANTIBIOTICS

The antitumor antibiotics are cytotoxic drugs that were originally isolated from cultures of *Streptomyces*. In this section, we consider five antitumor antibiotics as well as three of their derivatives. The antitumor antibiotics and their derivatives are used only to treat cancer; they are not used to treat infections. All of these drugs injure cells through direct interaction with DNA. Because of poor GI absorption, they are all administered parenterally (usually IV).

Dactinomycin (Actinomycin D)

Mechanism of Action. Dactinomycin [Cosmegen] is a planar (flat) molecule that kills cells through *intercalation* with DNA. We can understand intercalation by envisioning the stacked base pairs of DNA as having a structure like that of a stack of coins. Having a coin-like shape itself, dactinomycin is able to slip between base pairs of DNA, after which the drug becomes bound to DNA. This process (intercalation) distorts DNA structure. As a result, RNA polymerase is unable to use DNA as a template. Hence, synthesis of RNA and, consequently, proteins is inhibited. Unlike RNA polymerase, DNA polymerase is relatively insensitive to the change in DNA. Consequently, DNA synthesis is not suppressed. Dactinomycin is *phase nonspecific*.

Pharmacokinetics. Administration is by IV infusion. Because of tissue uptake and binding to DNA, dactinomycin is rapidly cleared from the blood. The drug does not cross the blood-brain barrier. Elimination occurs slowly by biliary and renal excretion.

Therapeutic Uses. Major indications for dactinomycin are *Wilms' tumor* and *rhabdomyosarcoma*. Other indications include *choriocarcinoma*, *Ewing's sarcoma*, *Kaposi's sarcoma*, and *testicular cancer*.

Toxicity. Dose-limiting toxicities are bone marrow suppression and oral and GI mucositis. Other toxicities include nausea, vomiting, diarrhea, alopecia, folliculitis, and, in previously irradiated areas, dermatitis. Dactinomycin is extremely corrosive to soft tissue, and hence extravasation will cause severe local injury.

Doxorubicin

Doxorubicin is active against a broad spectrum of neoplastic diseases. Unfortunately, cardiotoxicity limits its utility. Doxorubicin is available in two formulations: conventional [Adriamycin, Rubex] and liposomal [Doxil].

Mechanism of Action. Like dactinomycin, doxorubicin intercalates with DNA, causing distortion of DNA structure. As a result, DNA is unable to function as a template for synthesis of DNA and RNA. Doxorubicin also promotes DNA cleavage by topoisomerase II.

Pharmacokinetics. Doxorubicin is administered by IV infusion and undergoes rapid uptake by tissues. The drug does not cross the blood-brain barrier. Much of each dose is metabolized in the liver. Accordingly, dosage must be reduced in patients with hepatic impairment. Doxorubicin and its metabolites are eliminated primarily in the bile.

Therapeutic Uses. Doxorubicin is active against many neoplastic diseases. The drug is employed to treat solid tumors and disseminated cancers. Specific indications include *Hodgkin's and non-Hodgkin's lymphomas, acute lymphoblastic and myeloblastic leukemias, sarcomas of soft tissue and bone, and various carcinomas*, including *carcinoma of the lung, stomach, breast, ovary, testes, and thyroid*.

Toxicity. Cardiotoxicity. Doxorubicin can cause acute and delayed injury to the heart. Acute effects (dysrhythmias, electrocardiographic changes) can develop within minutes of administration. In most cases these reactions are transient, lasting no more than 2 weeks.

Delayed cardiotoxicity develops months to years after doxorubicin treatment, and manifests as heart failure secondary to diffuse cardiomyopathy (myofibril degeneration). The condition is often unresponsive to treatment. Delayed cardiac injury is directly related to the total cumulative dose: The risk of heart failure increases significantly as the cumulative lifetime dose rises above 550 mg/m^2. Accordingly, the total dose should not exceed this amount.

A relatively new drug—*dexrazoxane* [Zinecard]—can protect the heart from doxorubicin. To do so, dexrazoxane must first undergo conversion to a chelating agent within the body. In this active form, the drug binds intracellular iron, thereby preventing it from interacting with doxorubicin. In clinical trials, dexrazoxane significantly decreased the incidence of doxorubicin-induced heart failure. However, treatment did have two complications: (1) the drug appeared to intensify myelosuppression, and (2) it may have reduced the anticancer effects of doxorubicin. To ensure that the benefits of chemotherapy are not compromised, dexrazoxane is approved only for patients who have already received 300 mg/m^2 of doxorubicin. Furthermore, it is approved only for patients receiving doxorubicin for *breast cancer* (even though doxorubicin is used to treat other malignancies). Why the restriction? Because intensification of myelosuppression may be greater in patients with tumors other than breast cancer.

Recent data indicate that treatment with an angiotensin-converting enzyme (ACE) inhibitor (e.g., ramipril) can improve symptoms of cardiomyopathy. Furthermore, if given early, these drugs may be able to *prevent* cardiac damage.

Other Toxicities. Acute toxicity usually manifests as nausea and vomiting. Because of its vesicant properties, doxorubicin can cause severe local injury if extravasation occurs. In addition, the drug imparts a harmless red color to urine and sweat; patients should be forewarned. The usual dose-limiting toxicity is bone marrow suppression. Neutropenia develops in about 70% of patients. Thrombocytopenia and anemia may also occur. Additional delayed toxicities include alopecia, stomatitis, anorexia, conjunctivitis, and pigmentation in the extremities.

Daunorubicin, Liposomal

Liposomal daunorubicin [DaunoXome] is a new formulation of daunorubicin designed to increase delivery of the drug to tumor cells and decrease its uptake by normal cells. The preparation consists of an aqueous solution of daunorubicin encapsulated within minuscule lipid vesicles (liposomes). When the liposomes are in the vicinity of the tumor, they release daunorubicin over time. Liposomal daunorubicin is administered as a 1-hour IV infusion.

Daunorubicin is nearly identical in structure to doxorubicin, and shares many of its properties. Like doxorubicin, daunorubicin intercalates with DNA and thereby inhibits DNA and RNA synthesis. The drug can act during all phases of the cell cycle, but cytotoxicity is greatest during S phase. The only indication for liposomal daunorubicin is *AIDS-related Kaposi's sarcoma*. As with doxorubicin, the major dose-limiting toxicities are bone marrow suppression and heart failure. In addition, daunorubicin may cause nausea, vomiting, stomatitis, and alopecia. Like doxorubicin, daunorubicin imparts a harmless red color to urine and tears; patients should be forewarned.

Epirubicin

Mechanism of Action and Therapeutic Use. Epirubicin [Ellence], an analog of doxorubicin, is a new IV drug indicated for adjuvant therapy of *breast cancer* following surgical removal of the primary tumor in patients who have axillary node involvement. In one clinical trial, women who received epirubicin, in combination with cyclosporine and fluorouracil, had a 5-year relapse-free survival rate of 63%. Epirubicin is given in repeated 21-day cycles consisting of either (1) 100 mg/m^2 on day 1 only, or (2) 60 mg/m^2 on days 1 and 8. A single cycle costs over $2600, compared with just $500 for equivalent therapy with doxorubicin.

Like doxorubicin, epirubicin intercalates DNA and thereby inhibits synthesis of DNA, RNA, and proteins. In addition, intercalation promotes DNA cleavage by topoisomerase II. Epirubicin is considered cell-cycle phase nonspecific. However, cytotoxicity is maximal during S and G_2 phase.

Pharmacokinetics. Epirubicin is widely distributed following IV infusion. The drug undergoes hepatic metabolism followed by excretion in the bile and urine. Elimination is slowed in patients with liver dysfunction secondary to hepatic metastases or other causes.

Adverse Effects. Epirubicin can cause a variety of serious adverse effects. As with doxorubicin, bone marrow suppression and cardiotoxicity are dose limiting. To reduce the risk of severe cardiac damage, the total cumulative dose should not exceed 900 mg/m^2 (compared with 550 mg/m^2 for doxorubicin). Fortunately, when epirubicin is used for adjuvant therapy, the cumulative dose should be well below the safe limit. In some women, epirubicin has caused irreversible amenorrhea and premature menopause. Extravasation can result in severe local tissue necrosis. In animals, epirubicin is embryotoxic and teratogenic; studies in pregnant women have not been performed. Additional adverse effects include alopecia, nausea, vomiting, mucositis, red discoloration of urine, and increased risk of acute myelogenous leukemia.

Idarubicin

Idarubicin [Idamycin] is a structural analog of daunorubicin and doxorubicin. The drug has one approved indication: *acute myelogenous leukemia* in adults. Cell kill results from intercalation with DNA and subsequent inhibition of nucleic acid synthesis. Idarubicin is most effective during S phase, but is not considered phase specific. Following IV infusion, the drug undergoes rapid and widespread distribution. Elimination is by hepatic metabolism followed by biliary excretion. The principal dose-limiting toxicity is bone marrow suppression. Like daunorubicin and doxorubicin, idarubicin is cardiotoxic, but the maximal cumulative dose has not been determined. Additional toxicities include nausea, vomiting, alopecia, and stomatitis. Idarubicin is a vesicant and can cause severe local injury upon extravasation.

Valrubicin

Mechanism of Action and Therapeutic Use. Valrubicin [Valstar] is a relatively new drug indicated for localized *cancer of the bladder.* Administration is by direct intravesical installation through a urethral catheter. The dosage is 800 mg once a week for 6 weeks. Each dose should be retained for 2 hours. Only 18% of patients have a complete response. Valrubicin is chemically related to doxorubicin and appears to have a similar mechanism of action: intercalation of DNA with subsequent disruption of DNA, RNA, and protein synthesis, along with DNA cleavage secondary to activation of topoisomerase II.

Bladder cancer is highly aggressive, and hence requires appropriately aggressive therapy. The treatment of first choice is bacille Calmette-Guérin (BCG) vaccine, administered directly into the bladder. If BCG fails to eradicate the cancer, surgical resection is the next step. Surgery can prevent metastases and prolong life. Because the response rate to valrubicin is low, the drug should be reserved for patients who have not responded to BCG vaccine, and for whom immediate bladder resection is contraindicated.

Adverse Effects. Side effects of valrubicin are limited to the bladder. The drug is not absorbed from the bladder, and hence systemic effects are absent. The most common local reactions are urinary frequency, dysuria, spasm, hematuria, pain, urinary incontinence, and cystitis.

Mitoxantrone

Mitoxantrone [Novantrone] is a structural analog of doxorubicin and daunorubicin but is less toxic than those drugs. Mitoxantrone appears to act by two mechanisms: (1) intercalation of DNA and (2) promotion of DNA strand breakage secondary to inhibition of topoisomerase II. The drug is cell-cycle phase nonspecific. Principal applications are *prostate cancer* and *acute nonlymphocytic leukemias.* In addition, the drug is used to reduce neurologic disability in people with multiple sclerosis. Mitoxantrone is administered intravenously and undergoes rapid and widespread distribution. Elimination occurs slowly, primarily by hepatic metabolism and biliary excretion. The major dose-limiting toxicity is bone marrow suppression. Other important toxicities—nausea, vomiting, alopecia, mucositis, and cardiotoxicity—are less severe than with doxorubicin. Mitoxantrone imparts a harmless blue-green tint to the urine, skin, and sclera; patients should be forewarned.

Bleomycin

The preparation of bleomycin [Blenoxane] used clinically contains a mixture of glycopeptides. The major components are bleomycin A_2 and bleomycin B_2. Bleomycin is unusual among the cytotoxic agents in that it causes very little bone marrow suppression. However, it can cause severe injury to the lungs. Because myelosuppression is minimal, bleomycin is especially useful in combination chemotherapy. Bleomycin binds to DNA, causing chain scission and fragmentation. The drug is most effective during G_2.

Bleomycin is approved for palliative therapy of a broad spectrum of tumors. Specific indications include *testicular carcinomas* (embryonal cell, choriocarcinoma, teratocarcinoma), *lymphomas* (Hodgkin's, reticulum cell sarcoma, lymphosarcoma), and *squamous cell carcinomas* (head, neck, larynx, cervix, penis, vulva, and skin).

Administration is parenteral (IM, IV, SC, and intrapleural). High concentrations are achieved in the skin and lungs. The drug does not enter the CNS. Most tissues contain large amounts of bleomycin hydrolase, an enzyme that renders the drug inactive. However, cells of the skin and lungs, which are sites of toxicity, lack this enzyme. Most of each dose is excreted unchanged in the urine.

The major dose-limiting toxicity is injury to the lungs, which occurs in about 10% of patients. Injury manifests initially as pneumonitis. In about 1% of patients, pneumonitis progresses to severe pulmonary fibrosis and death. Pulmonary function should be monitored and bleomycin discontinued at the first sign of adverse changes.

Additional toxicities include stomatitis, alopecia, and skin reactions (hyperpigmentation, hyperkeratosis, pruritus erythema, ulceration, vesiculation). Nausea and vomiting are usually mild. Unlike most other cytotoxic anticancer drugs, bleomycin exerts minimal toxicity to bone marrow. About 1% of patients with lymphomas experience a unique hypersensitivity reaction, characterized by fever, chills, confusion, hypotension, and wheezing.

Mitomycin

Mitomycin [Mutamycin] is a prodrug that is converted to its active form within cells. Following activation, it functions as a bifunctional or trifunctional alkylating agent. Cell death is caused by cross-linking DNA with resultant blockade of DNA synthesis. Mitomycin may also induce strand scission. The drug is active during all phases of the cell cycle, but toxicity is greatest during late G_1 and early S phase.

Mitomycin is labeled for *disseminated adenocarcinoma of the stomach and pancreas.* Unlabeled uses include *carcinomas of the colon, rectum, esophagus, lung, breast, cervix, and bladder.*

Mitomycin is administered by IV infusion and is distributed widely, but not to the CNS. The drug is rapidly metabolized by the liver. Metabolites are excreted in the urine.

The major dose-limiting toxicity is delayed bone marrow suppression; nadirs for neutropenia and thrombocytopenia usually occur 3 to 4 weeks after treatment. Other toxicities include nausea, vomiting, stomatitis, alopecia, renal toxicity, and pulmonary toxicity. Mitomycin is a vesicant and can cause severe local injury upon extravasation.

Plicamycin (Mithramycin)

Plicamycin [Mithracin] is a highly toxic drug whose use in cancer chemotherapy is restricted to *testicular carcinoma.* Cell kill results from binding to DNA with subsequent inhibition of DNA and RNA synthesis. The drug is cell-cycle phase nonspecific. Dose-related bleeding is the most serious toxicity. Bleeding results from thrombocytopenia and deficiencies of several clotting factors. Because of the risk of hemorrhage, plicamycin should be used only in a hospital setting. Patients with coagulation disorders and pre-existing thrombocytopenia should not receive the drug. Additional toxicities include nausea, vomiting, stomatitis, renal injury, and disruption of calcium metabolism. Plicamycin is administered IV, and little is known of its fate. Elimination is renal. In addition to management of testicular cancer, plicamycin is used to manage *hypercalcemia of malignancy.* This application is considered in Chapter 70.

Gemtuzumab Ozogamicin

Gemtuzumab ozogamicin [Mylotarg] is a novel drug indicated for patients with CD33-positive *acute myeloid leukemia* (AML). Candidates should be in their first relapse after conventional chemotherapy (e.g., cytarabine plus idarubicin), at least 60 years old, and unable to tolerate further conventional treatment. In clinical trials, gemtuzumab produced complete remission in 30% of patients, about the same response seen with conventional chemotherapy. Treatment consists of two 2-hour infusions (9 mg/m² each) given 2 weeks apart, at a cost of about $12,000.

Gemtuzumab has a unique structure and mechanism. The drug consists of a *monoclonal antibody* (directed against CD33 antigens) coupled with an *antitumor antibiotic* (a derivative of calicheamicin). CD33 antigens are found on the surface of leukemic blasts in 80% of patients with AML, and also on the surface of normal and leukemic myeloid colony-forming cells—but *not* on pluripotent hematopoietic stem cells. The drug works as follows: (1) the antibody portion binds to a CD33 antigen on the cell surface, (2) the resultant complex becomes internalized, and (3) the antitumor antibiotic is released, undergoes conversion to its active form, binds with DNA, and causes strand breakage. The result is cell death.

Principal adverse effects are *acute infusion reactions* and *myelosuppression*. Infusion reactions generally develop after the infusion and resolve in 2 to 4 hours. Manifestations include chills (62%), fever (61%), nausea (38%), vomiting (32%), and hypotension (11%). Pretreatment with acetaminophen plus an antihistamine may help. Because of damage to myeloid colony-forming cells, severe neutropenia and thrombocytopenia occur in 90% of patients. However, because pluripotent hematopoietic stem cells are spared, myelosuppression is reversible. Gemtuzumab is *teratogenic* and *fetotoxic* in laboratory animals, and hence classified in Food and Drug Administration Pregnancy Risk Category D. The drug may also be *hepatotoxic;* hyperbilirubinemia and elevated aminotransferase levels have occurred in a few patients.

MITOTIC INHIBITORS

Mitotic inhibitors are drugs that act during M phase to prevent cell division. There are two groups of these drugs: vinca alkaloids and taxoids.

Vinca Alkaloids

The vinca alkaloids are derived from *Vinca rosea* (the periwinkle plant), hence the group name. *Vincristine* and *vinblastine* are the most important members. These two agents have nearly identical structures and share the same mechanism of action. However, they have quite different toxicities: Vincristine is toxic to peripheral nerves, but does little damage to bone marrow; conversely, vinblastine can cause significant bone marrow suppression, but is relatively harmless to nerves. Vincristine and vinblastine do not share the same indications.

Vincristine

Mechanism of Action. Vincristine [Oncovin, Vincasar] blocks mitosis during metaphase, and hence is M-phase specific. The drug blocks mitosis by disrupting the assembly of microtubules, the filaments that move chromosomes during cell division. To block microtubule assembly, vincristine binds with *tubulin,* the major component of microtubules. In the absence of microtubules, distribution of chromosomes to daughter cells becomes random. Inappropriate allocation of chromosomes is the presumed cause of cell death.

Pharmacokinetics. Because of low and erratic oral absorption, vincristine must be given IV. The drug leaves the vascular system and enters tissues, where it becomes tightly but reversibly bound. Penetration to the CNS is poor. Most of each dose undergoes hepatic metabolism followed by biliary excretion. Only 12% is eliminated in the urine.

Therapeutic Uses. Vincristine is bone marrow sparing. Accordingly, the drug is ideal for combination chemotherapy. Indications include *Hodgkin's and non-Hodgkin's lymphomas,* *acute lymphocytic leukemia, Wilms' tumor, rhabdomyosarcoma, Kaposi's sarcoma, breast cancer,* and *bladder cancer.*

Toxicity. *Peripheral neuropathy* is the major dose-limiting toxicity. Vincristine injures neurons by disrupting neurotubules, structures that are required for axonal transport of enzymes and organelles. Injury to neurotubules results from binding to tubulin, the same protein found in microtubules. Nearly all patients experience symptoms of sensory or motor nerve injury (e.g., decreased reflexes, weakness, paresthesias, sensory loss). Symptoms of injury to autonomic nerves (e.g., constipation, urinary hesitancy) are less common, occurring in 30% to 50% of patients. Because vincristine does not readily enter the CNS, injury to the brain is minimal.

In contrast to most anticancer drugs, *vincristine causes little toxicity to bone marrow.* As a result, the drug is especially desirable for combined therapy with other anticancer drugs.

Vincristine is a powerful irritant and can cause severe local injury if extravasation occurs. Alopecia develops in about 20% of patients. Nausea and vomiting are rare.

Vinblastine

Vinblastine [Velban] is a structural analog of vincristine. The two drugs share the same mechanism of action: production of metaphase arrest through blockade of microtubule assembly. Like vincristine, vinblastine is administered intravenously, does not cross the blood-brain barrier, and is eliminated by biliary and urinary excretion. Indications for vinblastine include *Kaposi's sarcoma, Hodgkin's and non-Hodgkin's lymphomas,* and *carcinoma of the breast and testes.* The major dose-limiting toxicity is bone marrow suppression. (Note that vinblastine differs markedly from vincristine in this regard.) Neurotoxicity can occur, but is much less severe than with vincristine. Additional adverse effects include nausea, vomiting, alopecia, stomatitis, and severe local injury if extravasation should occur.

Vinorelbine

Vinorelbine [Navelbine] is a semisynthetic vinca alkaloid similar in structure and actions to vincristine and vinblastine. The drug is approved only for *non–small cell lung cancer.* Investigational uses include *breast cancer, ovarian cancer,* and *Hodgkin's disease.* Benefits derive from causing metaphase arrest through inhibition of microtubule assembly. Vinorelbine is administered IV, undergoes hepatic metabolism, and is eliminated primarily in the bile. Like vinblastine, and unlike vincristine, vinorelbine can cause profound bone marrow suppression; neutropenia develops in about 50% of patients. Peripheral neuropathy occurs, but is less severe than with vincristine. Vinorelbine can cause interstitial pulmonary changes and adult respiratory distress syndrome, usually within 1 week of treatment; most cases have been fatal. Accordingly, be alert for new-onset dyspnea, cough, hypoxia, and related signs of lung injury. Other adverse effects include alopecia, constipation, nausea, and vomiting, all of which are generally mild to moderate. Like vincristine and vinblastine, vinorelbine can cause local tissue necrosis if extravasation occurs.

Taxoids
Paclitaxel

Actions and Uses. Paclitaxel [Taxol, Onxol], a widely used drug, acts during late G₂ to promote formation of stable microtubule bundles, thereby inhibiting cell division. Paclitaxel (in combination with cisplatin) is approved as first-line therapy for advanced *ovarian cancer* and *non–small cell lung cancer* in patients who are not candidates for potentially curative surgery or radiation therapy. In addition, the drug is approved as second-line therapy for *AIDS-related Kaposi's sarcoma* and as an adjunct to doxorubicin-containing regimens for women with *breast cancer.* Investigational uses include advanced head and neck cancer, adenocarcinoma of the upper GI tract, and leukemias.

Pharmacokinetics. Paclitaxel is administered by 24-hour infusion. The drug undergoes wide distribution, but not to the CNS. Very little is known about how paclitaxel is eliminated; small amounts appear in the urine and bile, but the fate of the remainder is unknown.

Toxicity. Severe hypersensitivity reactions (hypotension, dyspnea, angioedema, urticaria) have occurred during the infusion, probably in response to the vehicle (polysorbate 80) rather than to paclitaxel itself. The risk of severe hypersensitivity reactions can be minimized by performing the infusion slowly and by pretreatment with a glucocorticoid (dexamethasone), histamine$_1$-receptor antagonist (diphenhydramine), and histamine$_2$-receptor antagonist (cimetidine).

The major dose-limiting toxicity is *bone marrow suppression* (neutropenia). Peripheral neuropathy develops with repeated infusions and may also be dose limiting. Paclitaxel can affect the heart, causing bradycardia, second- and third-degree heart block, and even fatal myocardial infarction. Muscle and joint pain have occurred. Practically all patients experience sudden but reversible alopecia, which frequently involves the body as well as the scalp. Gastrointestinal reactions (nausea, vomiting, diarrhea, mucositis) are generally mild.

Docetaxel

Actions, Use, and Source. Docetaxel [Taxotere] is similar in structure and actions to paclitaxel. Like paclitaxel, docetaxel stabilizes microtubules, and thereby inhibits mitosis. Docetaxel has two approved indications: (1) locally advanced or metastatic *breast cancer* that has progressed or relapsed despite prior chemotherapy, and (2) locally advanced or metastatic *non–small cell lung cancer* that has advanced despite prior cisplatin-based therapy. In clinical trials, docetaxel produced objective responses in over 40% of patients with breast cancer. The recommended dosage for breast cancer is 60 or 100 mg/m^2 and the dosage for lung cancer is 75 mg/m^2; both are infused IV over 1 hour every 3 weeks. Like paclitaxel, docetaxel is expensive: The price of a single dose is $1500 to $1900, plus the cost of administration. Docetaxel is manufactured by a semisynthetic process that begins with a compound extracted from needles of the European yew tree.

Toxicity. Significant *neutropenia* develops in virtually all patients. Docetaxel should be withheld if neutrophil counts fall below 1500/mm^3. In clinical trials, death from sepsis occurred in 1% of patients with normal liver function and in 11% of patients with abnormal liver function. Because liver dysfunction increases the risk of death, docetaxel should be avoided if signs of liver disease are present (i.e., plasma aminotransferase activity more than 1.5 times normal and alkaline phosphatase activity more than 2.5 times normal).

Severe *hypersensitivity* can occur. Manifestations include hypotension, bronchospasm, and generalized rash or erythema. Docetaxel should be avoided in patients who reacted strongly to a previous dose or to any drug containing polysorbate 80 (the vehicle docetaxel is supplied in). To reduce hypersensitivity reactions, patients should take an oral glucocorticoid for 5 days, beginning 1 day before each infusion.

Severe *fluid retention* can occur, especially in patients with abnormal liver function. Possible manifestations include generalized edema, dyspnea at rest, cardiac tamponade, pleural effusion requiring urgent drainage, and pronounced abdominal distention (from ascites). As with hypersensitivity reactions, fluid retention can be reduced by treatment with oral glucocorticoids.

Additional common toxicities are anemia, nausea, diarrhea, stomatitis, fever, and neurosensory symptoms (paresthesias, pain).

TOPOISOMERASE INHIBITORS

Topotecan

Mechanism of Action. Topotecan [Hycamtin] inhibits topoisomerase I, an enzyme that relieves torsional strain in DNA by creating *reversible* single-strand breaks. Topotecan binds to the DNA–topoisomerase I complex, and thereby prevents repair of the strand breaks caused by topoisomerase. Cytotoxicity is believed to result from impaired DNA replication. Hence, effects become manifest during S phase of the cell cycle.

Therapeutic Use. Topotecan is approved for *small cell lung cancer* and *metastatic cancer of the ovary* refractory to prior chemotherapy. A single course of treatment consists of 1.5 mg/mm^3 infused IV over 30 minutes on 5 consecutive days. Courses can be repeated after a 16-day hiatus. At least four courses are recommended. Treatment is expensive: Each course costs over $2500 for the drug, plus additional fees for giving the infusions.

Toxicity. Bone marrow suppression is the dose-limiting toxicity. Neutropenia occurs in 98% of patients, thereby posing a risk of serious infection. Anemia and thrombocytopenia are also common, and frequently require transfusion of platelets and red blood cells. Because of myelosuppression, frequent counts of peripheral blood cells should be performed. If the neutrophil count is below 1500 cells/mm^3, topotecan should be withheld. Other side effects include alopecia, nausea, vomiting, diarrhea, stomatitis, abdominal pain, and headache.

Irinotecan

Actions and Uses. Like topotecan, irinotecan [Camptosar] and its active metabolite (SN-38) inhibit topoisomerase I. As a result, DNA replication is impaired. Cytotoxic effects become apparent during the S phase of the cell cycle. Irinotecan is approved for first-line treatment of metastatic *colorectal cancer* (in combination with fluorouracil) and for second-line treatment of colorectal cancer that has progressed despite treatment with fluorouracil alone. Investigational uses include *advanced cancer of the breast, ovary, lung,* and *stomach.* For colorectal cancer, the recommended dosage is 125 mg/m^2 infused IV over 90 minutes once weekly for 4 weeks. In clinical trials, this dosage produced an objective response (complete or partial) in 15% of patients. The average response duration was 5.8 months. Irinotecan is expensive: For a 4-week course of treatment, the price is over $4000 for irinotecan itself, plus the cost of administration.

Adverse Effects. Two types of *severe diarrhea* can occur: early and late. Early diarrhea occurs in 50% of patients; late diarrhea occurs in 88%. Early and late diarrhea differ with respect to cause and treatment. Early diarrhea occurs within 24 hours of infusion onset. The cause is excessive cholinergic stimulation of the GI tract. Accordingly, early diarrhea can be suppressed with IV atropine. Late diarrhea develops 24 hours or more after the infusion. It can be prolonged, causing severe dehydration and electrolyte imbalance, and can thereby pose a threat to life. Late diarrhea should be treated immediately with loperamide. Fluid and electrolytes should be replaced as needed.

Myelosuppression can result in neutropenia (54%) and anemia (61%). Serious thrombocytopenia is uncommon. Sepsis secondary to neutropenia has resulted in death. If the neutrophil count falls below 500/mm^3, irinotecan should be temporarily withheld.

In addition to diarrhea and myelosuppression, irinotecan can cause nausea (86%), vomiting (67%), asthenia (76%), alopecia (61%), abdominal discomfort (57%), anorexia (55%), fever (45%), and weight loss (30%). Less common side effects include stomatitis, dyspepsia, headache, cough, rhinitis, insomnia, and rash.

Etoposide

Etoposide [VePesid, Toposar, Etopophos] is derived from podophyllotoxin, a naturally occurring plant alkaloid. The drug inhibits DNA topoisomerase II, and thereby prevents resealing of DNA strand breaks. The resultant damage to DNA arrests the cell cycle in G$_2$ phase. Etoposide is approved only for *refractory testicular cancer* and *small cell cancer of the lung.*

Administration is PO and IV. Penetration to the CNS is low. Most of the drug is eliminated intact in the urine. Hence, dosages must be reduced in patients with renal impairment.

The major dose-limiting toxicity is bone marrow suppression. Other toxicities include alopecia, peripheral neuropathy, and mucositis. Early adverse effects include nausea, vomiting, diarrhea, and fever. Hypotension can occur with rapid IV administration.

Teniposide

Teniposide [Vumon] is an analog of etoposide and shares that drug's mechanism of action: inhibition of DNA topoisomerase II with resultant DNA strand scission and G$_2$ arrest. The drug's only approved indication is *refractory acute lymphoblastic leukemia of childhood.*

Administration is by slow IV infusion. Most of each dose becomes bound to plasma proteins. Penetration to the CNS is poor. Elimination is by hepatic metabolism and renal excretion.

The major dose-limiting toxicity is bone marrow suppression (neutropenia, thrombocytopenia, anemia). Severe hypersensitivity reactions (urticaria, angioedema, bronchospasm, hypotension) occur in about 5% of patients; symptoms can be suppressed with epinephrine. Secondary leukemias have developed within 8 years of initial drug exposure. Other toxicities include nausea, vomiting, diarrhea, and alopecia.

MISCELLANEOUS CYTOTOXIC DRUGS

Asparaginase

Mechanism of Action. Asparaginase [Elspar] is an enzyme that converts asparagine, an essential amino acid, into aspartic acid. By converting asparagine to aspartic acid, the drug deprives cells of asparagine needed to synthesize proteins. However, not all cells are affected. In fact, toxicity from asparaginase is limited almost exclusively to leukemic lymphoblasts. Why? Because these cells are unable to manufacture their own asparagine, whereas normal cells can. Hence, normal cells are able to replace the asparagine that asparaginase took away, but leukemic lymphoblasts can't. Asparaginase appears to act selectively during G_1.

Pharmacokinetics. Administration is parenteral (IM and IV). Distribution is restricted to the vascular system. The drug does not cross the blood-brain barrier. Asparaginase is inactivated by serum proteases.

Therapeutic Use. The only indication for asparaginase is *acute lymphocytic leukemia*. For induction of remission, asparaginase is usually combined with prednisone and vincristine, and perhaps daunorubicin or doxorubicin.

Toxicity. Asparaginase can cause severe adverse effects. However, the spectrum of toxicities differs from that of other anticancer drugs. By inhibiting protein synthesis, the drug can cause coagulation deficiencies and injury to the liver, pancreas, and kidneys. Symptoms of CNS depression, ranging from confusion to coma, develop in about 30% of patients. Nausea and vomiting can be intense and may limit the dose that can be tolerated. Because asparaginase is a foreign protein, hypersensitivity reactions are common; fatal anaphylaxis can occur, and hence facilities for resuscitation should be immediately available. In contrast to most other anticancer drugs, asparaginase does not depress the bone marrow, nor does it cause alopecia, oral ulceration, or intestinal ulceration.

Pegaspargase

Pegaspargase [Oncaspar] is a modified form of asparaginase that causes fewer hypersensitivity reactions. Otherwise, the drugs are very similar. They have the same mechanism of action (destruction of asparagine) and produce the same spectrum of adverse effects (hypersensitivity reactions, pancreatitis, coagulopathy, and liver and kidney dysfunction). Of the patients who had hypersensitivity reactions to asparaginase, about 30% also have them with pegaspargase. Pegaspargase is indicated only for *acute lymphocytic leukemia*, and only in patients who had a hypersensitivity reaction to asparaginase. Administration is IM or IV.

Hydroxyurea

Mechanism of Action. Hydroxyurea [Hydrea] inhibits DNA replication by suppressing synthesis of DNA precursors. Specifically, the drug inhibits ribonucleoside diphosphate reductase, the enzyme that converts ribonucleotides into their corresponding deoxyribonucleotides. In the absence of deoxyribonucleotides, DNA cannot be made. Hydroxyurea is S-phase specific.

Pharmacokinetics. Hydroxyurea is rapidly absorbed following oral administration. Unlike most anticancer agents, hydroxyurea crosses the blood-brain barrier with ease. Part of each dose is metabolized in the liver. Parent drug and metabolites are eliminated primarily in the urine.

Therapeutic Uses. The principal indication for hydroxyurea is *chronic myelocytic leukemia*. The drug is also used for recurrent, metastatic, or inoperable *carcinoma of the ovary*. In addition, hydroxyurea can relieve symptoms and prolong life in patients with *sickle cell anemia* (see Chapter 103).

Toxicity. The principal dose-limiting toxicity is bone marrow suppression. The drug also causes nausea, vomiting, and dysuria. Neurologic deficits and stomatitis may occur, but these are rare. Hydroxyurea is teratogenic in experimental animals. Hence, like most other anticancer agents, it should be avoided during pregnancy.

Mitotane

Chemistry, Actions, and Uses. Mitotane [Lysodren] is a structural analog of two insecticides: DDD and DDT. For reasons that are not understood, the drug is selectively toxic to cells of the adrenal cortex, both normal and neoplastic. The only indication for mitotane is palliative therapy of inoperable *adrenocortical carcinoma*.

Pharmacokinetics. Mitotane is administered PO. About 40% is absorbed. The drug is distributed widely, but not to the CNS. Because of storage in tissues (primarily fat), active drug remains in the body for weeks after administration has ceased. Elimination is by hepatic metabolism and renal excretion.

Toxicity. The principal dose-limiting toxicities are CNS depression, nausea, and vomiting. Because mitotane injures the adrenal cortex, adrenal insufficiency is likely. Accordingly, patients will require supplemental glucocorticoids, especially at times of stress. Dermatitis is common. Other adverse effects include visual disturbances; orthostatic hypotension; and renal damage, manifested as hematuria, hemorrhagic cystitis, and albuminuria. Mitotane does not cause the toxicities associated with most other anticancer drugs (bone marrow suppression, alopecia, oral and GI ulceration).

Procarbazine

Mechanism of Action. Procarbazine [Matulane] is a prodrug that is converted to active metabolites in the liver. The metabolites cause chromosomal damage and suppress synthesis of DNA, RNA, and proteins. The precise cause of cell death is unknown. Procarbazine is cell-cycle phase nonspecific.

Pharmacokinetics. Procarbazine is readily absorbed following oral administration, but undergoes rapid and extensive hepatic metabolism. Active metabolites are highly lipid soluble and cross the blood-brain barrier with ease. Procarbazine and its metabolites are excreted primarily in the urine.

Therapeutic Uses. The major indication for procarbazine is *advanced Hodgkin's disease*. For this indication, procarbazine is combined with mechlorethamine, vincristine [Oncovin], and prednisone, in the so-called MOPP regimen.

Toxicity. The usual dose-limiting toxicity is bone marrow suppression. Nausea and vomiting may also be dose limiting. Other adverse effects include peripheral neuropathy, CNS depression, secondary leukemias, and sterility, especially in males.

Drug Interactions. Because of its CNS effects, procarbazine should not be combined with CNS depressants (e.g., barbiturates, phenothiazines, opioids). Ingestion of alcohol can induce a disulfiram-like response. Because procarbazine inhibits monoamine oxidase, there is a risk of severe hypertension in response to sympathomimetic drugs, tricyclic antidepressants, and tyramine-rich foods.

Dacarbazine

Actions and Uses. Dacarbazine [DTIC-Dome] is a prodrug that is activated by the liver. Although the precise mechanism of cell kill is unknown, there is evidence for alkylation of DNA, inhibition of DNA and RNA synthesis, and interaction with sulfhydryl groups on proteins. Dacarbazine is considered cell-cycle phase nonspecific. The principal indications for the drug are metastatic *malignant melanoma* and *Hodgkin's disease*.

Pharmacokinetics. Since GI absorption is erratic, procarbazine is administered IV. Penetration to the CNS is poor. Elimination is by hepatic metabolism and renal excretion.

Toxicity. Bone marrow suppression is the usual dose-limiting toxicity. Nausea and vomiting occur in most patients, occasionally requiring cessation of treatment. Other toxicities include a flu-like syndrome, hepatic necrosis, photosensitivity, and burning pain along the injection site.

Altretamine (Hexamethylmelamine)

Altretamine [Hexalen], formerly known as hexamethylmelamine, is indicated for palliative therapy of persistent or recurrent *ovarian cancer*. Altretamine is a prodrug that is converted to active metabolites in the body. The mechanism by which the metabolites act is unknown. Altretamine is well absorbed following oral administration, but undergoes rapid and extensive hepatic metabolism. The metabolites are excreted in the urine. The principal dose-limiting toxicity is bone marrow suppression. However, nausea and vomiting can also limit dosage. Peripheral sensory neuropathy is common. Central neurotoxicity (tremors, ataxia, vertigo, hallucinations, seizures, depression) is less common. Because of peripheral and central neurotoxicity, patients should receive regular neurologic evaluations.

⠿ KEY POINTS

- Cytotoxic anticancer drugs act directly on cancer cells and healthy cells to produce cell kill.
- Cell-cycle phase–specific drugs are effective only during a specific phase of the cell cycle (e.g., S phase, M phase). Accordingly, they are only active against cells that are participating in the cell cycle. Cells in G_0 are spared.
- To be effective, phase-specific drugs must be present as neoplastic cells cycle through the phase in which the drugs act. In practical terms, this means that phase-specific drugs must be in the blood continuously over a long time.
- Cell-cycle phase–nonspecific drugs can affect cells during any phase of the cell cycle, including G_0.
- Although phase-nonspecific drugs can inflict biochemical lesions at any time during the cell cycle, they usually are more toxic to proliferating cells than to cells in G_0. Why? Because (1) G_0 cells often have time to repair drug-induced damage before it can result in significant harm, and (2) toxicity may not become manifest until the cells attempt to divide.
- About 50% of the cytotoxic anticancer drugs are phase specific; the other 50% are phase nonspecific.
- Alkylating agents injure cells primarily by forming covalent bonds with DNA.
- Bifunctional alkylating agents form cross-links in DNA, and thereby prevent DNA replication. Bifunctional agents are more effective than monofunctional agents.
- Because alkylation reactions can take place at any time during the cell cycle, alkylating agents are considered cell-cycle phase nonspecific.
- Cyclophosphamide, the most widely used alkylating agent, is active against a broad spectrum of neoplastic diseases.
- Carmustine (an alkylating agent) is available in a wafer for implantation into the cavity created by surgical excision of a brain tumor. This unique delivery system provides high local concentrations of the drug.
- Antimetabolites are analogs of important natural metabolites, and hence are able to disrupt critical metabolic processes, especially DNA replication.
- Most antimetabolites are S-phase specific.

- Methotrexate, a folic acid analog, prevents conversion of folic acid to its active form. Cell kill results primarily from disruption of DNA synthesis.
- High-doses of methotrexate coupled with leucovorin rescue can be used to treat methotrexate-resistant tumors. This technique can be very dangerous in that failure to give sufficient leucovorin at the right time can be lethal.
- Cytarabine, a pyrimidine analog, undergoes intracellular activation followed by incorporation into DNA, where it acts to inhibit DNA synthesis.
- Fluorouracil, a uracil analog, undergoes intracellular activation, after which it inhibits thymidylate synthetase, thereby depriving cells of thymidylate needed to make DNA.
- Antitumor antibiotics are used to treat cancer, not infections.
- Dactinomycin (Actinomycin D) intercalates DNA, thereby distorting its structure. As a result, RNA polymerase is unable to use DNA as a template, and therefore protein synthesis is disrupted. Interestingly, DNA synthesis is not affected.
- Doxorubicin is cardiotoxic. To reduce the risk of heart failure, the cumulative lifetime dose should be kept below 550 mg/m². The risk can be further reduced with dexrazoxane, a drug that helps protect the heart from doxorubicin. ACE inhibitors also show promise.
- Vincristine and vinblastine block assembly of the microtubules that move chromosomes during cell division. Accordingly, the drugs are M-phase specific.
- Vincristine is toxic to peripheral nerves, but does not significantly suppress bone marrow function. Because it spares bone marrow, vincristine can be safely combined with drugs that suppress bone marrow.
- In contrast to vincristine, vinblastine causes significant bone marrow suppression but is relatively harmless to peripheral nerves.
- Asparaginase converts asparagine into aspartic acid, and thereby deprives cells of asparagine needed to make proteins. Cytotoxicity is limited primarily to leukemic lymphoblasts. Why? Because these cells are unable to manufacture their own asparagine, whereas normal cells can.

Anticancer Drugs II: Hormones, Hormone Antagonists, Biologic Response Modifiers, and Other Anticancer Drugs

---

HORMONES AND HORMONE ANTAGONISTS
Glucocorticoids
Antiestrogens
Aromatase Inhibitors
Drugs for Prostate Cancer
Androgens
Progestins
**BIOLOGIC RESPONSE MODIFIERS:
IMMUNOSTIMULANTS**
OTHER ANTICANCER DRUGS

In this chapter, we continue our discussion of anticancer drugs. Much of the chapter focuses on hormones and hormone antagonists, which are used almost exclusively for breast and prostate cancers. In contrast to the drugs addressed in Chapter 98, many of which are cell-cycle phase specific, the drugs addressed here lack phase specificity. In addition, they generally lack the serious toxicities associated with the cytotoxic agents, including bone marrow suppression, stomatitis, and severe nausea and vomiting. Nonetheless, many of these drugs do have severe toxicities of their own.

Much of the introductory information in Chapter 97 applies to the drugs addressed here. Therefore, if you have not done so already, you should read that chapter now.

HORMONES AND HORMONE ANTAGONISTS

The hormones and hormone antagonists are the least toxic of all anticancer drugs. Because these agents act through specific hormone receptors on target tissues, their actions are highly selective. As a result, these drugs are devoid of the severe cytotoxic effects that characterize most anticancer agents. The hormonal anticancer drugs fall into six basic categories: (1) glucocorticoids, (2) androgens and antiandrogens, (3) estrogens and antiestrogens, (4) aromatase inhibitors, (5) progestins, and (6) gonadotropin-releasing hormone analogs. The principal in-

dications for these drugs are cancers of the breast, endometrium, and prostate. In addition, the glucocorticoids are used against lymphomas and certain leukemias. Trade names, routes of administration, and indications are summarized in Table 99–1.

Glucocorticoids

The basic pharmacology of the glucocorticoids is discussed in Chapter 68 (Glucocorticoids in Nonendocrine Diseases). Discussion here is limited to their the use in cancer.

Glucocorticoids (e.g., *prednisone*) are used in combination with other agents to treat cancers arising from lymphoid tissue. Specific indications are *acute and chronic lymphocytic leukemias, Hodgkin's disease,* and *non-Hodgkin's lymphomas.* Glucocorticoids are beneficial in these cancers because they exert direct toxicity to lymphoid tissues: High-dose therapy causes suppression of mitosis, dissolution of lymphocytes, regression of lymphatic tissue, and cell death. When used acutely, glucocorticoids are devoid of significant adverse effects. However, with prolonged treatment, these drugs can cause a broad spectrum of serious toxicities, including osteoporosis, adrenal insufficiency, increased susceptibility to infection, GI ulcers, fluid and electrolyte disturbances, myopathy, growth retardation, and cutaneous atrophy.

In addition to their use against lymphoid-derived cancers, glucocorticoids are used to manage complications of cancer and cancer therapy. Specific benefits include suppression of chemotherapy-induced nausea and vomiting, reduction of cerebral edema caused by irradiation of the cranium, reduction of pain caused by nerve compression or edema, and suppression of hypercalcemia in steroid-responsive tumors. In addition, glucocorticoids can improve appetite, promote weight gain, and impart a generalized sense of well-being.

Antiestrogens

Antiestrogens are drugs that block estrogen receptors. The only indication for these agents is breast cancer. Benefits derive from depriving tumor cells of the growth-promoting influence of estrogen.

Currently, four antiestrogens are available. Of these, only one—fulvestrant—is a *pure* estrogen receptor antagonist. The

TABLE 99–1 ■ Hormones and Hormone Antagonists

Generic Name	Trade Name	Route	Indications
Glucocorticoid			
Prednisone	Deltasone, others	PO	Acute and chronic lymphocytic leukemias, Hodgkin's and non-Hodgkin's lymphomas
Antiestrogens			
Tamoxifen	Nolvadex	PO	Breast cancer
Toremifene	Fareston	PO	Breast cancer
Raloxifene	Evista	PO	Breast cancer[†]
Fulvestrant	Faslodex	IM	Breast cancer
Aromatase Inhibitors			
Anastrozole	Arimidex	PO	Breast cancer
Letrozole	Femara	PO	Breast cancer
Exemestane	Aromasin	PO	Breast cancer
GnRH Agonists*			
Leuprolide	Lupron Depot, Lupron LA, Viadur	IM, SC, implant	Prostate cancer
Triptorelin	Trelstar	IM	Prostate cancer
Goserelin	Zoladex	SC	Prostate cancer
Androgen Receptor Blockers			
Flutamide	Eulexin	PO	Prostate cancer
Bicalutamide	Casodex	PO	Prostate cancer
Nilutamide	Nilandron	PO	Prostate cancer
Estrogens			
Diethylstilbestrol diphosphate	Stilphostrol	PO, IV	Prostate cancer
Ethinyl estradiol	Estinyl	PO	Prostate cancer
Estrogen Mustard			
Estraumustine	Emcyt	PO	Prostate cancer
Androgens			
Fluoxymesterone	Halotestin	PO	Breast cancer
Testosterone	Generic only	PO	Breast cancer
Testolactone	Teslac	PO	Breast cancer
Progestins			
Medroxyprogesterone acetate	Depo-Provera	PO, IM	Renal and endometrial cancers
Megestrol acetate	Megace	PO	Breast and endometrial cancers

*Gonadotropin-releasing hormone agonists.
†Not approved by the Food and Drug Administration for this use.

other three—tamoxifen, toremifene, and raloxifene—have *mixed* effects on estrogen receptors, causing receptor blockade in some tissues and receptor activation in others. Because they exert both estrogenic and antiestrogenic actions, these three drugs have been labeled *selective estrogen receptor modulators,* or *SERMs*—a term we first encountered in Chapter 59 (Estrogens and Progestins). Hence, although we refer to these drugs as *antiestrogens* when discussing their use in cancer, keep in mind that they can stimulate estrogen receptors as well as block them. Whether estrogen receptors in a particular tissue will be stimulated or blocked depends on the drug being used.

Tamoxifen

Tamoxifen [Nolvadex] is the most widely prescribed drug for breast cancer. This agent is approved for treatment of established disease and for reducing the occurrence of breast cancer in women at high risk. As noted, tamoxifen is a SERM, not a pure estrogen receptor antagonist.

Overview of Actions. Like other SERMs, tamoxifen blocks estrogen receptors in some tissues and stimulates them in others. Receptor blockade underlies the drug's utility against breast cancer. Receptor activation leads to beneficial effects (increased bone mineral density, reduction of low-density-lipoprotein cholesterol, elevation of high-density-lipoprotein cholesterol) as well as adverse effects (increased risk of thromboembolism and endometrial cancer).

Mechanism of Action in Breast Cancer. Tamoxifen blocks estrogen receptors on breast cancer cells, and thereby prevents receptor stimulation by estradiol, the principal naturally occurring estrogen. Estrogen acts on tumor cells to stimulate growth and proliferation. Hence, in the absence of estradiol's influence, the rate of tumor cell proliferation declines.

Tumors regress in size as the rate of cell death outpaces new cell production. Obviously, if tamoxifen is to be effective, target cells must be estrogen-receptor (ER) positive. That is, target cells must possess estrogen receptors.

Use for Treatment of Breast Cancer.

Tamoxifen is a drug of first choice for treating breast cancer. The drug has two treatment applications: (1) adjunctive therapy to suppress growth of residual cancer cells following total mastectomy, segmental mastectomy, and breast irradiation, and (2) treatment of metastatic disease. Efficacy as adjunctive therapy has been evaluated in 55 randomized trials involving more than 37,000 women. The result? Treatment for 1, 2, and 5 years decreased tumor recurrence by 21%, 29%, and 47%, respectively. Benefits were limited almost entirely to women with ER-positive disease.

Use for Prevention of Breast Cancer.

The Food and Drug Administration (FDA) has approved tamoxifen for reducing the development of breast cancer in healthy women at high risk. Approval was based on results of the Breast Cancer Prevention Trial, which enrolled 13,388 otherwise healthy women who had risk factors for breast cancer (e.g., age older than 60, family history of breast cancer, failure to give birth before age 30, a breast biopsy showing atypical hyperplasia). Half of the participants received tamoxifen (20 mg PO daily) and half received placebo. After an average follow-up time of 4 years, daily tamoxifen reduced the incidence of breast cancer by 44%. Unfortunately, tamoxifen *increased* the incidence of endometrial cancer, pulmonary embolism, and deep vein thrombosis. Hence, women considering tamoxifen for chemoprevention must carefully weigh the benefits of treatment (reduced risk of breast cancer) against the risks (increased risk of endometrial cancer and thromboembolic events). According to guidelines issued in 2002 by the United States Preventive Services Task Force, tamoxifen chemoprevention is appropriate only for women at *high* risk, and not for women at lower risk. Specific recommendations for high-risk women in different age groups are as follows:

■ *Age 40 through 49*—Tamoxifen is a good choice, except for women at risk for thrombosis
■ *Age 50 through 59*—Tamoxifen is a good choice, except for women at risk for thrombosis and for women who still have a uterus (the risk of endometrial cancer is higher for women over 50)
■ *Age 60 and above*—Tamoxifen is not recommended (although older women have the highest risk for breast cancer, they also have the highest risk for complications from tamoxifen)

To help determine who is at high risk for breast cancer, the National Cancer Institute has created an internet-based Breast Cancer Risk Assessment Tool. You can access the tool at *www.cancer.gov/bcrisktool*.

Pharmacokinetics.

Tamoxifen is readily absorbed following oral administration. Metabolism by the 3A4 isozyme of cytochrome P450 (CYP3A4) converts some of the drug to *N*-desmethyltamoxifen, an active metabolite. The half-lives of tamoxifen and its metabolite range from 1 to 2 weeks. Because clearance is so slow, once-daily dosing is adequate. Tamoxifen is eliminated in the feces after undergoing extensive metabolism. When treatment is stopped, tamoxifen and its metabolite can be detected in serum weeks afterward.

Drug Interactions.

Drugs that induce or inhibit CYP3A4 can alter the metabolism of tamoxifen. Inducing agents (e.g., phenytoin, carbamazepine) will accelerate metabolism of tamoxifen, thereby reducing its levels. Conversely, inhibitors (e.g., ketoconazole, erythromycin) will retard tamoxifen metabolism, thereby raising its levels.

Adverse Effects.

The most common adverse effects are hot flushes (64%), fluid retention (32%), vaginal discharge (30%), nausea (26%), vomiting (25%), and menstrual irregularities (25%). In women with bone metastases, tamoxifen may cause transient hypercalcemia and a flare in bone pain. Because of its estrogen agonist actions, tamoxifen increases (slightly) the risk of thromboembolic events, including deep vein thrombosis, pulmonary embolism, and stroke.

Perhaps the biggest concern is *endometrial cancer*. Tamoxifen acts as an estrogen agonist at receptors in the uterus, causing proliferation of endometrial tissue. Proliferation initially results in endometrial hyperplasia, and may eventually lead to endometrial cancer. In women taking tamoxifen to *treat* breast cancer, the benefits clearly outweigh this risk. However, in women taking the drug to *prevent* breast cancer, the risk/benefit balance is less obvious.

Dosage and Administration.

The usual dosage for adjuvant *treatment* of breast cancer is 20 mg PO once a day. Larger doses do not increase benefits. Long-term therapy (2 to 5 years) is more effective than short-term therapy. The dosage for *prevention* of breast cancer in high-risk women is 20 mg PO daily for 5 years. There are no data to indicate that extending treatment beyond 5 years increases benefits.

Toremifene

Actions and Use.

Toremifene [Fareston] is a relatively new SERM indicated for metastatic *breast cancer* in women with ER-positive tumors or tumors for which ER status is unknown. The drug is a structural analog of tamoxifen, and shares most of that drug's properties. Like tamoxifen, toremifene has antiestrogenic actions in some tissues, and estrogenic actions in others. In women with breast cancer, toremifene blocks estrogen receptors on tumor cells, thereby depriving them of estrogen's growth-promoting effects. In clinical trials, toremifene was about as effective as tamoxifen: With both drugs, the response rate was about 20%, and median survival time was about 30 months. In a crossover study, most patients who failed to respond to tamoxifen also failed to respond to toremifene. The recommended dosage is 60 mg PO once a day.

Pharmacokinetics.

Toremifene is well absorbed following oral administration. Plasma levels peak in 3 hours. The drug undergoes extensive hepatic metabolism, primarily by CYP 3A4. Metabolites are excreted in the feces. The drug's half-life is prolonged (about 5 days) owing to enterohepatic recirculation. As with tamoxifen, drugs that induce CYP 3A4 will reduce toremifene levels, and drugs that inhibit the enzyme will raise toremifene levels.

Adverse Effects.

Adverse effects are like those of tamoxifen. Hot flushes are the most common reaction, occurring in 35% of those treated. Other common reactions are sweating (20%), nausea (14%), and vaginal discharge (13%). Patients may also experience dizziness (9%), vomiting (4%), and vaginal bleeding (2%). Hypercalcemia may occur in women with bone metastases. There is a small risk of thromboembolic events. Cataracts and elevation of liver enzymes have been reported.

Like tamoxifen, toremifene *stimulates* estrogen receptors in the uterus. As a result, uterine hyperplasia can occur. At this time, we don't know if toremifene increases the risk of uterine cancer. However, given the drug's estrogenic influence, the possibility would appear very real.

Raloxifene

Raloxifene [Evista] is a SERM with actions similar to those of tamoxifen. However, there is one important difference: whereas tamoxifen increases the risk of endometrial cancer, raloxifene does not. Preliminary data indicate that raloxifene can protect against ER-positive breast cancer, although the drug is not yet approved for this use. An ongoing trial—the Study of Tamoxifen and Raloxifene, or STAR—is designed to evaluate just how effective raloxifene really is. If raloxifene proves to be as effective as tamoxifen, it would be an important new weapon in the breast cancer fight. The basic pharmacology of raloxifene, as well as its use in osteoporosis, is discussed in Chapter 70.

Fulvestrant

Actions, Use, and Dosage. Fulvestrant [Faslodex] is a new antiestrogen approved for metastatic ER-positive *breast cancer* in postmenopausal women. Unlike tamoxifen and other SERMs, which block some estrogen receptors and activate others, fulvestrant is a *pure estrogen receptor antagonist*—the first one available. As with other antiestrogens, benefits derive from depriving breast cancer cells of required hormonal stimulation. Fulvestrant is administered IM in the buttock. Dosage is 250 mg once a month, given either as one 5-ml injection or two 2.5-ml injections. The wholesale cost per dose is over $700.

Clinical Trials. In two clinical trials, fulvestrant was compared with anastrozole, an aromatase inhibitor (see below). Study participants were postmenopausal women with locally advanced or metastatic breast cancer that had progressed despite hormonal therapy. The result? Both drugs were equally effective with respect to objective tumor response rates and median time to disease progression. However, duration of response was greater with fulvestrant (16.7 months vs. 13.6 months). At this time, there are no data on how fulvestrant compares directly with tamoxifen.

Pharmacokinetics. Plasma levels peak about 7 days after IM injection, and remain therapeutic for at least 1 month. Steady-state levels are reached after three to six monthly doses. The drug undergoes hepatic metabolism followed by renal excretion. The apparent half-life is 40 days.

Adverse Effects and Drug Interactions. Fulvestrant is generally well tolerated. The most common adverse effects are GI disturbances, hot flushes, headache, pharyngitis, and bone and back pain. Thromboembolism can occur but is uncommon. In contrast to SERMs, fulvestrant poses no risk of endometrial cancer. In clinical trials, injection site reactions (inflammation; mild, transient pain) developed in 7% of women receiving a single 5-ml injection and in 27% of women receiving two 2.5-ml injections. Fulvestrant has no known drug interactions.

Aromatase Inhibitors

The aromatase inhibitors are used to treat breast cancer in *postmenopausal* women. They work by blocking the production of estrogen from androgenic precursors, and thereby depriving breast cancer cells of the estrogen they need for growth. Aromatase inhibitors do not block production of estrogen by the ovaries, and hence are of little benefit in premenopausal women. Recent clinical trials indicate that aromatase inhibitors are more effective than tamoxifen and better tolerated.

Anastrozole

Mechanism and Use. Anastrozole [Arimidex] is now approved for first-line oral therapy of *postmenopausal women* with *early breast cancer* as well as *advanced breast cancer.* Previously, the drug was approved only for advanced breast cancer that had progressed despite use of an antiestrogen (e.g., tamoxifen). Anastrozole works by depriving breast cancer of estrogen. In postmenopausal women, the major source of estrogen is adrenal androgens, which are converted into estrogen by the enzyme *aromatase* in peripheral tissues. Anastrozole inhibits aromatase, and thereby reduces estrogen production. With regular use, the drug lowers estrogen to undetectable levels. In women with estrogen-dependent cancer, estrogen deprivation can arrest tumor growth, and may cause outright cell kill. In clinical trials, anastrozole was not effective in women with ER-negative tumors or in women who did not respond initially to tamoxifen. The recommended dosage is 1 mg PO once a day.

Adverse Effects. Anastrozole is generally well tolerated. In clinical trials, only 3.3.% of patients withdrew because of adverse effects. At a dose of 1 mg, the most common adverse effects are asthenia (16%), nausea (16%), headache (13%), and hot flushes (12%). Other reactions include anorexia, vomiting, diarrhea, constipation, dyspnea, peripheral edema, vaginal hemorrhage, hypertension, and pain (including bone, back, pelvic, and abdominal pain).

Comparison with Tamoxifen. In postmenopausal women with breast cancer, anastrozole is at least as effective as tamoxifen, and causes fewer adverse effects. Data from the Arimidex, Tamoxifen, Alone or in Combination (ATAC) trial indicate that, compared with tamoxifen, anastrozole suppresses tumor growth for twice as long: 11.1 months versus 5.6 months. Regarding side effects, anastrozole is less likely to cause hot flushes, weight gain, or vaginal bleeding—although it may cause more nausea and irritability. In contrast to tamoxifen, anastrozole is devoid of all estrogenic activity, and hence does not promote endometrial cancer or thromboembolic events. Because of this favorable comparison, anastrozole seems likely to replace tamoxifen as the drug of first choice for treating breast cancer in postmenopausal women.

Letrozole

Letrozole [Femara], a selective aromatase inhibitor, is now indicated for first-line therapy of advanced *breast cancer* in postmenopausal women. Previously, the drug was approved for use only after treatment with an antiestrogen (e.g., tamoxifen) had failed. Like anastrozole, letrozole blocks conversion of androgens into estrogens, and thereby deprives breast cancer cells of estrogen's growth-promoting influence. In a recent trial, letrozole (2.5 mg/day) was more effective than tamoxifen (20 mg/day): the objective response rate with letrozole was higher (30% vs. 20%) and the time to tumor progression was longer (9.4 months vs. 6.0 months). Letrozole's most common adverse effects are musculoskeletal pain (21%) and nausea (13%). Reactions that occur in 6% to 9% of patients include headache, arthralgia, fatigue, constipation, dyspnea, cough, vomiting, diarrhea, and hot flushes. Extremely low doses are embryotoxic and fetotoxic in animals. Like anastrozole, and unlike tamoxifen, letrozole poses no risk of endometrial cancer or thromboembolism. No significant drug interactions have been reported.

Exemestane

Mechanism and Use. Exemestane [Aromasin] is indicated for oral therapy of advanced *breast cancer* in postmenopausal women whose disease has progressed despite treatment with tamoxifen. Like anastrozole, exemestane inhibits aromatase, and thereby reduces estrogen levels. A dosage of 25 mg once daily (administered after a meal) reduces circulating estrogen by 85% to 95%. In the absence of sufficient estrogen, estrogen-dependent tumors cannot thrive. In clinical trials, the objective response rate was about 25%.

Pharmacokinetics. Exemestane is rapidly absorbed following oral administration. The drug is widely distributed and cleared by extensive metabolism. Excretion is in the urine and feces. Its half-life is about 24 hours.

Adverse Effects and Interactions. Exemestane is generally well tolerated. The most common adverse effects are fatigue (22%), nausea (18%), hot flushes (13%), depression (13%), and weight gain (8%). Exemestane appears devoid of significant drug interactions.

Drugs for Prostate Cancer
Gonadotropin-Releasing Hormone Agonists

The gonadotropin-releasing hormone (GnRH) agonists suppress production of androgens by the testes. Hence, they can be looked on as indirect-acting antiandrogens. Currently, three GnRH agonists are available: leuprolide, triptorelin, and goserelin. All three are indicated for cancer of the prostate. In addition, leuprolide is used for endometriosis (see Chapter 61).

Leuprolide. Therapeutic Use. Leuprolide [Lupron, Lupron Depot, Viadur] is a synthetic analog of GnRH, also known as *luteinizing hormone–releasing hormone*. Leuprolide is indicated for *advanced carcinoma of the prostate*. Palliation is the primary benefit. For patients with prostate cancer, leuprolide represents an alternative to orchiectomy (surgical castration). Leuprolide may be administered daily (SC), monthly (IM), every 3 months (IM), or once a year (implant).

Mechanism of Action. Cells of the prostate, both normal and neoplastic, are androgen dependent. Leuprolide provides palliation by suppressing androgen production in the *testes*. During the initial phase of treatment, leuprolide *mimics* GnRH. That is, the drug acts on the pituitary to *stimulate* release of interstitial cell–stimulating hormone (ICSH), which acts on the testes to *increase* production of testosterone. As a result, there may be a transient "flare" in cancer symptoms. However, with continuous exposure to leuprolide, pituitary GnRH receptors become desensitized. As a result, release of ICSH declines, causing testosterone production to decline as well. After several weeks of treatment, testosterone levels are equivalent to those seen after surgical castration. Because leuprolide therapy mimics the effects of orchiectomy, treatment is often referred to as *chemical castration*.

It is important to note that leuprolide does *not* decrease production of *adrenal* androgens, which account for about 9% of the androgens in circulation. Hence, even though production of testicular androgens is essentially eliminated, adrenal androgens can provide some support for prostate cancer cells. To offset the effects of adrenal androgens, leuprolide is often combined with an androgen receptor blocker (e.g., flutamide). The androgen receptor blocker has the additional benefit of preventing the symptom flare that can occur early in treatment.

Adverse Effects. Leuprolide is generally well tolerated. Hot flushes are the most common adverse effect, but these usually decline as treatment continues. Impotence and loss of libido may occur. During the initial weeks of treatment, elevation of testosterone levels may aggravate bone pain and urinary obstruction caused by prostate cancer. As a result, patients with vertebral metastases or pre-existing obstruction of the urinary tract may find treatment intolerable. As noted, concurrent treatment with an androgen receptor blocker can minimize these problems.

By suppressing testosterone production, leuprolide may increase the risk of osteoporosis and related fractures. Bone loss can be minimized by consuming adequate calcium and vitamin D, and by performing regular weight-bearing exercise. In addition, a bisphosphonate (e.g., alendronate [Fosamax]) might be used to preserve bone, although bisphosphonates are not specifically approved for leuprolide-induced osteoporosis.

Triptorelin. Triptorelin [Trelstar Depot, Trelstar LA] is a GnRH analog indicated for palliative treatment of *advanced prostate cancer*. The drug has the same mechanism of action and adverse effects as leuprolide, our proto-type GnRH agonist. Triptorelin is administered by IM injection, either once a month (Trelstar Depot), or every 3 months (Trelstar LA).

Goserelin. Goserelin [Zoladex], like leuprolide, is a GnRH analog used for *advanced prostate cancer*. Both drugs share the same mechanism and adverse effects. Administration of goserelin is unique. The drug is formulated as a pellet that is dispensed in a syringe with a 16-gauge needle. The pellet is implanted by SC injection in the upper abdominal wall. Local anesthesia may be used prior to the injection.

Androgen Receptor Blockers

Three androgen receptor blockers are available: flutamide, bicalutamide, and nilutamide. They are indicated only for prostate cancer—and only in combination with either surgical castration (orchiectomy) or chemical castration (GnRH agonist therapy).

Flutamide. Flutamide [Eulexin] was the first androgen receptor antagonist available. The drug is indicated only for *prostate cancer*, and then only in patients taking a GnRH agonist (e.g., leuprolide). Benefits derive from blocking androgen receptors in tumor cells, thereby depriving them of needed androgenic support. In patients taking a GnRH agonist, flutamide serves two purposes: (1) it prevents cancer cells from undergoing increased stimulation during the initial phase of GnRH therapy, when androgen production is increased (see discussion of leuprolide above); and (2) it blocks the effects of adrenal androgens, whose production is not reduced by GnRH agonists. In one trial, patients receiving flutamide plus leuprolide had a mean survival time of nearly 3 years, compared with 2.3 years for those receiving leuprolide alone.

Flutamide is administered orally and undergoes rapid and complete absorption. Most of each dose is converted to an active metabolite on the first pass through the liver. Parent drug and metabolites are excreted in the urine.

The most common adverse effect is gynecomastia. Nausea, vomiting, and diarrhea occur less frequently. Rarely, potentially fatal liver toxicity has occurred. To reduce the risk of serious harm, liver function should be assessed at baseline, monthly during the first 4 months of treatment, and periodically thereafter.

Bicalutamide. Like flutamide, bicalutamide [Casodex] is an androgen receptor blocker used for *advanced prostate cancer* in men undergoing therapy with a GnRH agonist (e.g., leuprolide). The rationale for this combination is explained in the discussion of flutamide. When bicalutamide was used alone in clinical trials, the most common side effects were breast pain (38%) and gynecomastia (39%). When the drug is combined with leuprolide, the most common side effect is hot flushes (49%). The incidence of significant diarrhea with bicalutamide is much higher than with flutamide (6% vs. 0.5%).

Nilutamide. Like flutamide and bicalutamide, nilutamide [Nilandron] blocks intracellular receptors for androgens. The drug is approved for *metastatic prostate cancer* in men who have undergone surgical castration. Benefits derive from blocking the actions of adrenal androgens, which are not reduced by castration. In clinical trials, nilutamide reduced bone pain, prolonged progression-free survival, and increased median survival time. The recommended dosage is 300 mg once daily PO for 30 days followed by 150 mg once daily thereafter. Treatment should begin within 24 hours of castration.

Although nilutamide is structurally similar to flutamide, the drug is not as well tolerated. The most common adverse effects are hot flushes (67%), delayed adaptation to darkness (57%), nausea (24%), constipation (20%), insomnia (16%), and gynecomastia (11%). Other reactions occur less frequently, but are more dangerous. About 2% of patients experience dyspnea secondary to interstitial pneumonitis. If this develops, nilutamide should be withdrawn. About 1% of patients develop hepatitis. To ensure early diagnosis, liver function should be monitored.

Estrogens

Diethylstilbestrol diphosphate [Stilphostrol] and other estrogens are second-line drugs for *prostate cancer.* Benefits derive from suppressing production of androgens, which prostate cells need to thrive. Estrogens suppress androgen production by acting in the pituitary to suppress release of interstitial cell–stimulating hormone (ICSH); in the absence of ICSH, production of androgens by the testes declines. Adverse effects of estrogens include nausea, fluid retention, hypercalcemia, depression, thromboembolic disorders, and gynecomastia. The basic pharmacology of the estrogens is discussed in Chapter 59.

Estramustine

Estramustine [Emcyt] is a hybrid molecule composed of estradiol (an estrogen) coupled to nor-nitrogen mustard (an alkylating agent). The only indication for the drug is palliative therapy of *advanced prostate cancer.* Following oral administration, estramustine becomes concentrated in prostate cells, apparently through the actions of a unique "estramustine-binding protein." Injury to prostate cells appears to result from two mechanisms. First, estramustine acts as a weak alkylating agent. Second, hydrolysis of estramustine releases free estradiol, which suppresses ICSH release by the pituitary, thereby depriving prostate cells of hormonal support.

Adverse effects are caused primarily by free estradiol. Gynecomastia is common. The most serious effect is thrombosis, with resultant myocardial infarction and stroke. Other adverse effects include fluid retention, nausea, vomiting, diarrhea, and hypercalcemia.

Androgens

The basic pharmacology of the androgens is discussed in Chapter 58. Consideration here is limited to their use in cancer.

Therapeutic Use. Androgens are employed for palliative therapy in women with advanced or metastatic *breast cancer.* It should be noted, however, that antiestrogens and aromatase inhibitors are preferred. Androgen therapy should be instituted only if surgery and irradiation are deemed inappropriate. After a delay of several weeks, objective responses are obtained in 50% to 60% of patients. Beneficial effects persist 12 to 14 months. The androgens employed most frequently are *fluoxymesterone* [Halotestin], *testosterone,* and *testolactone* [Teslac].

Adverse Effects. The doses used for breast cancer are high, making virilization a common side effect. Symptoms include clitoral enlargement, proliferation of facial and body hair, deepening of the voice, increased libido, and male-pattern baldness.

The effects of androgens coupled with the effects of osteolytic metastases can result in severe hypercalcemia. Principal dangers are ectopic calcification (especially in the urinary tract) and disruption of calcium-dependent physiologic processes. If hypercalcemia develops, androgen therapy should be temporarily withheld and large volumes of fluids administered. Androgen therapy may resume after calcium levels normalize.

Progestins

Two progestins are employed to treat cancers: *medroxyprogesterone acetate* [Depo-Provera] and *megestrol acetate* [Megace]. Medroxyprogesterone is indicated for *advanced endometrial and renal cancer.* Megestrol is indicated for *advanced endometrial and breast cancer.* In women with metastatic endometrial cancer, progestins promote palliation and tumor regression. About 30% of patients have objective responses. Among those who respond, survival time is increased to about 2 years. This compares with survival times of 6 months among nonresponders. Patients with tumors that test positive for progesterone receptors are more likely to respond. However, the exact mechanism by which progestins suppress tumor growth is unknown. The principal adverse effects of progestins are fluid retention and nonfluid weight gain. Hypercalcemia may occur if bone metastases are present. Progestins are teratogens, and hence should be avoided during the first 4 months of pregnancy. The basic pharmacology of the progestins is discussed in Chapter 59.

BIOLOGIC RESPONSE MODIFIERS: IMMUNOSTIMULANTS

Biologic response modifiers are drugs that alter host responses to cancer. Many of these drugs are immunostimulants, others render cancer cells nonmalignant by causing them to differentiate into nonproliferative forms, and others (hematopoietic growth factors) enable the host to better tolerate the myelosuppressive actions of anticancer drugs (see Chapter 53). In this chapter, all of the biologic response modifiers discussed are immunostimulants. Their trade names, indications, and routes of administration are summarized in Table 99–2.

Interferon Alfa-2a and Interferon Alfa-2b

Interferons are naturally occurring proteins with complex antiviral, anticancer, and immunomodulatory actions. Release of endogenous interferons is triggered by viral infections and other stimuli. Interferons are active against a variety of solid tumors and hematologic malignancies. They are also active against hepatitis B and hepatitis C (see Chapter 89).

Description. Interferon alfa-2a [Roferon-A] and interferon alfa-2b [Intron A] are glycoproteins that contain 165 amino acids. The two drugs, referred to collectively as interferon alfa, are identical except for one amino acid. Commercial production is by recombinant DNA technology.

Mechanism of Action. Anticancer effects are thought to result from two basic processes: (1) enhancement of host immune responses and (2) direct antiproliferative effects on cancer cells. Both processes are mediated by binding of interferons to cell-surface receptors, with resultant increased expression of certain genes and reduced expression of others. Interferons can cause G_0 cells to remain dormant, thereby pre-

TABLE 99–2 ■ Biologic Response Modifiers: Immunostimulants

Generic Name	Trade Name	Route	Indications
Interferon alfa-2a Interferon alfa-2b	Roferon-A Intron A	IM, IV, SC	Hairy cell leukemia, chronic myelogenous leukemia, malignant melanoma, AIDS-related Kaposi's sarcoma*
Aldesleukin (interleukin-2)	Proleukin	IV	Metastatic renal cell cancer
Levamisole	Ergamisol	PO	Duke's stage C colon cancer (combination therapy with fluorouracil)
BCG vaccine	TheraCys, TICE BCG, Pacis	Intravesical	*In situ* bladder cancer

*In addition to these approved indications, interferons have been used to treat many other cancers, including acute leukemias and cancers of the bladder, ovary, and kidney.

venting proliferation. In addition, interferons can cause proliferating cells to differentiate into nonproliferative mature forms.

Antineoplastic Uses. Interferons alfa-2a and alfa-2b are approved for *hairy cell leukemia, chronic myelogenous leukemia, malignant melanoma,* and *AIDS-related Kaposi's sarcoma.* Investigational uses include *acute leukemias* and *cancers of the bladder, ovary,* and *kidney.* Response rates are generally higher with hematologic cancers than with solid tumors.

Pharmacokinetics. Interferon alfa is administered by IM or SC injection. Plasma levels peak in 4 to 8 hours. Inactivation occurs rapidly in body fluids and tissues. No intact drug appears in the urine.

Adverse Effects. Interferon alfa causes multiple adverse effects. The most common is a flu-like syndrome characterized by fever, fatigue, myalgia, headache, and chills. Symptoms tend to diminish with continued therapy. Some symptoms (fever, headache, myalgia) can be reduced with acetaminophen. Other common effects include anorexia, weight loss, diarrhea, abdominal pain, dizziness, and cough. Prolonged or high-dose therapy can cause bone marrow suppression, thyroid dysfunction, alopecia, cardiotoxicity, and neurotoxicity, which can cause profound fatigue and depression.

Aldesleukin (Interleukin-2)

Aldesleukin [Proleukin], also known as interleukin-2 (IL-2), is an immunostimulant used for advanced renal carcinoma. Because severe adverse effects occur often, the drug must be administered in a hospital that has an intensive care facility; a specialist in cardiopulmonary or intensive care medicine must be available.

Description and Actions. Aldesleukin is a large glycoprotein nearly identical in structure and actions to human IL-2. The drug is produced by recombinant DNA technology. Like IL-2, aldesleukin stimulates immune function. Specific responses include enhanced production and cytotoxicity of lymphocytes; increased production of interleukin-1, interferon-gamma, and tumor necrosis factor; and induction of lymphokine-activated killer cell activity. The exact mechanism of antitumor action is unknown.

Therapeutic Use. Aldesleukin is approved only for *metastatic renal cell cancer* in adults. Objective responses occur in about 15% of patients (4% respond completely and 11% partially). The median duration of responses (complete and partial) is approximately 2 years. Investigational uses include *Kaposi's sarcoma, melanoma,* and *colorectal cancer.*

Pharmacokinetics. Aldesleukin is administered by IV infusion and distributes throughout the extracellular space. About 70% of each dose undergoes preferential uptake by the liver, kidneys, and lungs. Renal enzymes convert the drug into inactive metabolites, which are excreted in the urine. The drug's half-life is short—just 85 minutes.

Adverse Effects. Practically all patients experience significant toxicity. The fatality rate is high (4%). Effects seen most frequently are fever and chills (89%), nausea and vomiting (87%), hypotension (85%), anemia (77%), diarrhea (76%), altered mental status (76%), sinus tachycardia (70%), impaired renal function (61%), impaired liver function (56%), pulmonary congestion (54%), dyspnea (52%), and pruritus (48%). Depression may also occur.

Capillary leak syndrome (CLS) is of particular concern. This potentially fatal reaction is characterized by hypotension and reduced organ perfusion (secondary to loss of vascular tone and extravasation of plasma proteins and fluid). Symptoms begin to develop immediately after treatment. CLS may be associated with angina pectoris, cardiac dysrhythmias, myocardial infarction, pronounced respiratory insufficiency, renal insufficiency, GI bleeding, and altered mental status. Because of the risk of CLS, aldesleukin must not be given to patients with cardiac, pulmonary, renal, hepatic, or central nervous system impairment. Careful monitoring is essential.

Levamisole

Actions. Levamisole [Ergamisol] is an immunostimulant. The drug can help restore immune responses that are depressed, but does not enhance responses that are normal. Specific effects include increased antibody formation, increased proliferation and activity of T cells, and increased function of neutrophils, monocytes, and macrophages. The precise mechanism underlying these effects is unknown.

Therapeutic Use. Levamisole, in combination with fluorouracil, is approved only for adjuvant therapy following surgical resection of Dukes stage C *colon cancer.* Although levamisole alone or fluorouracil alone has little effect, the combination produces a 41% decrease in the risk of cancer recurrence and a 33% decrease in mortality (as compared with surgical controls who received no adjuvant therapy).

Pharmacokinetics. Levamisole is administered orally and is rapidly absorbed. The drug undergoes extensive hepatic metabolism followed by urinary excretion. Fluorouracil, which is used together with levamisole, is administered IV.

Adverse Effects. Reactions to levamisole alone are infrequent and mild. In contrast, reactions to levamisole plus fluorouracil can be severe, but these are due primarily to the fluorouracil. The principal dose-limiting toxicity of the combination is bone marrow suppression. The most common responses to the combination are nausea, vomiting, and diarrhea. Other reactions include alopecia, oral and GI ulceration, flu-like symptoms, metallic taste, dizziness, and arthralgia.

BCG Vaccine

Description and Therapeutic Use. BCG vaccine [TheraCys, TICE BCG, Pacis] is a freeze-dried preparation of attenuated *Mycobacterium bovis* (bacillus of Calmette and Guérin). The vaccine is approved for primary and relapsed *carcinoma in situ of the bladder,* both in the presence and absence of associated papillary tumors. However, the vaccine should not be used for papillary tumors alone. To treat bladder cancers, BCG vaccine is administered intravesically (i.e., directly into the bladder through a urethral catheter).

Mechanism of Action. BCG vaccine is a nonspecific immunostimulant. Instillation in the bladder produces a local inflammatory response that, by an unknown mechanism, promotes regression of tumors in the urothelial lining.

Adverse Effects. The most common adverse effects, which result from bladder irritation, are dysuria, urinary frequency, urinary urgency, and hematuria. Urinary status should be monitored closely. The most common systemic reactions are malaise, fatigue, fever, and chills.

Because BCG vaccine consists of live *M. bovis,* therapy carries a risk of systemic infection, including fatal septic shock. Accordingly, the vaccine is contraindicated for (1) immunocompromised patients (e.g., those taking immunosuppressant drugs, those with symptomatic or asymptomatic HIV infection); (2) patients with fever of unknown origin (because it may signify infection); and (3) patients with urinary tract infections (because there is an increased risk of systemic absorption of BCG vaccine).

Because BCG vaccine is infectious, it must be handled using aseptic technique. All materials employed during administration should be disposed of in plastic bags labeled "Infectious Waste." Urine voided within 6 hours of BCG instillation should be disinfected with an equal volume of 5% hypochlorite before flushing.

OTHER ANTICANCER DRUGS

Imatinib

Imatinib [Gleevec], also known as STI571 (for signal transduction inhibitor 571), is an important new drug for oral therapy of *chronic myeloid leukemia* (CML). At this time, imatinib is indicated only for patients who have not responded to interferon alfa, the standard therapy for CML. However, given that imatinib has several advantages over interferon alfa, the new drug is likely to become the treatment of choice. Unfortunately, imatinib frequently causes adverse effects, and may need to be taken indefinitely. Also, the drug is expensive, costing about $2400 per month at the usual dosage (400 mg/day).

In addition to its use against CML, imatinib is under investigation for use against gastrointestinal stromal tumors. As in treatment of CML, benefits derive from inhibiting an abnormal form of tyrosine kinase (see below).

CML and Its Treatment. CML is a cancer in which myeloid cells undergo massive clonal expansion. The disease begins with a chronic phase, progresses through an accelerated phase, and ends with the blast crisis phase. The underlying cause is a genetic abnormality known as the *Philadelphia chromosome,* which is produced by translocation of genetic material between chromosomes 9 and 22. Because of this genetic change, CML cells make an abnormal, continuously active enzyme, called *Bcr-Abl tyrosine kinase.* This enzyme phosphorylates, and thereby activates, as-yet unidentified regulatory proteins, which in turn cause excessive cellular proliferation. The principal treatment options for CML are bone marrow transplantation and drug regimens that include interferon alfa as their major component. Unfortunately, both options have serious drawbacks: bone marrow transplantation is associated with significant morbidity and mortality, and interferon alfa causes multiple adverse effects.

Mechanism of Action and Clinical Effects. Imatinib is a highly specific competitive inhibitor of Bcr-Abl tyrosine kinase. By inhibiting this enzyme, the drug prevents the phosphorylation and resultant activation of regulatory proteins, and thereby suppresses proliferation of CML cells. Imatinib is selective for cells that express Bcr-Abl tyrosine kinase; normal cells are not affected. When tested during the chronic phase of CML in patients who had not responded to interferon alfa, imatinib induced a complete hematologic response in 88% of subjects. Response rates were significantly lower during the accelerated phase, and very poor during blast crisis. At this time, we do not know how long responses to imatinib will persist, nor do we know if the drug prolongs life.

Pharmacokinetics. Imatinib is well absorbed following oral administration. Bioavailability is 98%. In the blood, the drug is highly bound to proteins. Imatinib undergoes extensive metabolism, primarily by hepatic CYP3A4 (i.e., the 3A4 isozyme of cytochrome P450), followed by excretion in the feces. The elimination half-lives of imatinib and its major active metabolite are 18 hours and 40 hours, respectively.

Adverse Effects. Imatinib causes adverse effects in most patients. The incidence and severity of adverse effects is lowest during the chronic phase of CML, higher during the accelerated phase, and highest during blast crisis. However, even though adverse effects occurred often during trials, discontinuation because of them was uncommon: only 1% during the chronic phase, 2% during the accelerated phase, and 5% during blast crisis. Common reactions include nausea (55% to 68%), vomiting (28% to 54%), diarrhea (33% to 49%), rash (32% to 39%), headache (24% to 28%), fatigue (24% to 33%), fever (14% to 38%), and musculoskeletal complaints: muscle cramps (25% to 46%), muscle pain (27% to 37%), and arthralgia (21% to 24%). Fluid retention occurs in 52% to 68% of patients, and may lead to pleural effusion, pericardial effusion, pulmonary edema, or ascites. Neutropenia and thrombocytopenia occur often. Accordingly, complete blood counts should be obtained weekly during the first month of treatment, biweekly during the second month, and periodically thereafter. Hepatotoxicity, as evidenced by severe elevations of transaminases or bilirubin, developed in 1.1% to 3.5% of patients. Imatinib is teratogenic in rats and should be avoided, if possible, during pregnancy. Because imatinib is a relatively new drug, information on long-term toxicity is lacking.

Drug Interactions. Imatinib is a substrate for and competitive inhibitor of CYP3A4, CYP2C9, and CYP2D6. By inhibiting these enzymes, imatinib can raise levels of warfarin and other drugs that are metabolized by them. Drugs that *inhibit* CYP3A4 (e.g., ketoconazole, erythromycin) can raise levels of imatinib. Conversely, drugs that *induce* CYP3A4 (e.g., phenytoin, carbamazepine, St. John's wort) can reduce levels of imatinib.

Comparison with Interferon Alfa. Imatinib has distinct advantages over interferon alfa. The drug is given orally, whereas interferon alfa must be injected. Hematologic responses develop faster with imatinib, and may even occur when interferon alfa has failed. Although imatinib often causes adverse effects, the drug appears better tolerated than interferon alfa.

Bisphosphonates

As discussed in Chapter 70, bisphosphonates (e.g., alendronate, pamidronate) are important drugs for treating osteoporosis and Paget's disease. In addition, evidence indicates that, in women with breast cancer, these drugs can prevent metastases and prolong life. The basic pharmacology of the bisphosphonates is discussed in Chapter 70. Discussion here is limited to their use in cancer.

The anticancer effects of bisphosphonates were discovered somewhat by accident. In women with breast cancer, bisphosphonates were originally employed to suppress bone resorption caused by cancer cells that had metastasized to bone. While using bisphosphonates for this purpose, researchers noted something surprising: Bisphosphonates appeared to reduce the incidence of new bony metastases. Results of a follow-up study confirmed the original observation: In women with breast cancer, treatment with a bisphosphonate reduces metastases to bone and other sites and prolongs survival. These results were obtained using *clodronate,* an oral bisphosphonate available in Europe and Canada. However, other bisphosphonates should also be effective.

How do bisphosphonates suppress metastases? When cancer cells spread to bone, they stimulate the activity of osteoclasts, the cells responsible for bone resorption. In turn, the osteoclasts release growth factors that stimulate the cancer cells, thereby setting up a self-reinforcing cycle. Bisphosphonates interrupt the cycle by inhibiting osteoclast function and blocking tumor adhesion to bone.

Denileukin Diftitox

Therapeutic Use. Denileukin diftitox [Ontak] is an IV drug approved for *cutaneous T-cell lymphoma* (CTCL). In clinical trials, 10% to 16% of patients experienced complete tumor regression, and another 20% to 22% experienced partial regression. Unfortunately, adverse events are very common—and sometimes severe. Denileukin can cause life-threatening hypersensitivity reactions, and hence must be administered in a facility equipped to provide cardiopulmonary resuscitation.

Description and Mechanism of Action. Denileukin is a hybrid molecule consisting of interleukin-2 (IL-2) coupled to diphtheria toxin. The IL-2 portion of the molecule enables it to bind with CTCL cells that have IL-2 receptors. Once the drug is bound, the diphtheria toxin moiety inhibits protein synthesis, causing cell death within hours. Denileukin is produced by recombinant DNA technology.

Adverse Effects. In clinical trials, 21% of patients required hospitalization for adverse events. The incidence of severe or life-threatening reactions was 5%.

Acute hypersensitivity reactions occur in 69% of patients. Prominent symptoms are hypotension (50%), back pain (30%), dyspnea (28%), vasodilation (28%), rash (25%), chest pain (24%), and tachycardia (12%). Management consists of stopping the infusion and, if necessary, administering IV epinephrine, antihistamines, and glucocorticoids.

A *flu-like syndrome* occurs in 91% of patients. Symptoms include fever or chills (81%), asthenia (66%), nausea and vomiting (64%), myalgia (18%), and arthralgia (8%). Diarrhea occurs in 29% of patients, and leads to dehydration in 9%.

Denileukin can cause *vascular leak syndrome,* characterized by hypoalbuminemia, edema, and hypotension. Onset usually occurs during the first or second week of treatment. In clinical trials, 6% of patients required hospitalization for this disorder. Because of vascular leak, hypoalbuminemia occurs in 83% of patients. Serum albumin should be monitored and, if it falls below 3 gm/dl, the next round of treatment should be postponed.

Alitretinoin

Alitretinoin [Panretin] is indicated for topical therapy of *cutaneous lesions* in patients with *AIDS-related Kaposi's sarcoma.* The drug is a retinoid (i.e., a derivative of retinol [vitamin A]) that binds to and activates retinoid receptors. In their active state, these receptors regulate the proliferation and differentiation of cells, both normal and neoplastic. When alitretinoin is added to Kaposi's sarcoma cells in culture, it inhibits their growth.

Alitretinoin is dispensed as a 0.1% gel for topical use. The drug should be applied only to cutaneous Kaposi's sarcoma lesions, not to normal skin. Following application, the area should dry for 3 to 5 minutes before putting clothing over it. Occlusive dressings should be avoided. Treatment is initiated with twice-daily application. Later on, the drug may be applied 3 or 4 times a day, if tolerance permits. Most patients respond in 4 to 8 weeks. However, some respond in only 2 weeks, and others may not respond until 16 weeks.

Adverse effects are limited to the site of application. Local reactions—erythema, scaling, irritation, rash, and dermatitis—occur in 25% to 77% of patients. The incidence of severe reactions is 10%. Other retinoids are known to cause photosensitivity reactions. Although photosensitivity has not been reported with alitretinoin, exposing the treated area to sunlight or sunlamps should nonetheless be minimized. Retinoids are highly teratogenic. Accordingly, women using alitretinoin should avoid getting pregnant (even though systemic absorption of alitretinoin appears to be minimal).

Alitretinoin is expensive: a 60-gm tube costs over $2000. However, this is actually cheaper than other treatments for Kaposi's sarcoma.

Bexarotene

Mechanism and Use. Bexarotene [Targretin] is indicated for oral therapy of *cutaneous T-cell lymphoma* in patients who have been refractory to prior systemic therapy. Like alitretinoin, bexarotene is an analog of vitamin A (retinol) and can activate retinoid receptors. The result is altered regulation of cellular proliferation and differentiation. *In vitro*, bexarotene can inhibit growth of some tumor cell lines. In clinical trials, a dosage of 300 mg/m²/day produced a complete response in 4% of patients, and a partial response (>50% improvement) in 48% of patients.

Pharmacokinetics. Plasma levels peak 2 hours after oral administration. Taking the drug with a high-fat meal increases absorption. Bexarotene undergoes metabolism by CYP3A4 (the 3A4 isozyme of cytochrome P450) followed by excretion in the bile.

Adverse Effects and Interactions. Bexarotene causes lipid abnormalities and other serious side effects. In clinical trials, adverse effects caused 30% of patients to discontinue treatment.

Major *lipid abnormalities* are common. Plasma triglycerides rose to a level 2.5 times above the upper limit of the normal range in 70% of patients. Sixty percent of patients had significant elevations in total cholesterol and low-density-lipoprotein cholesterol. Levels of high-density-lipoprotein cholesterol (good cholesterol) were reduced.

Bexarotene frequently causes headache, asthenia, leukopenia, anemia, infection, rash, and photosensitivity. The incidence of clinically significant hypothyroidism is 30%. Fatal pancreatitis and fatal cholestasis have been reported.

Bexarotene and other retinoids are powerful teratogens. Accordingly, bexarotene is absolutely contraindicated for use during pregnancy. Women taking the drug must ensure pregnancy does not occur.

In theory, drugs that inhibit CYP3A4 can increase bexarotene levels, and drugs that induce CYP3A4 can reduce its levels. Combining vitamin A with bexarotene could result in increased toxicity.

Trastuzumab

Actions and Use. Trastuzumab [Herceptin] is a monoclonal antibody indicated for IV therapy of metastatic *breast cancer.* The antibody may be used alone in women who failed to respond to prior chemotherapy, or in combination with paclitaxel [Taxol] as first-line therapy. All patients must have tumors that overexpress HER2, a transmembrane receptor that helps regulate cell growth. Trastuzumab binds with HER2 and thereby inhibits proliferation and promotes antibody-dependent cytotoxicity. Between 25% and 30% of metastatic breast cancers produce excessive HER2. High numbers of HER2 receptors are associated with unusually aggressive tumor growth.

Clinical Trials. All trial participants had tumors that overexpress HER2. In one trial, treatment with trastuzumab alone produced a complete response in 3% of patients, and a partial response (>50% tumor regression) in 14%. In a second trial, chemotherapy alone (usually doxorubicin plus cyclophosphamide) was compared with chemotherapy plus trastuzumab. The result? Tumor regression (50% or greater) occurred in 29% of women receiving chemotherapy alone, compared with 44% of women receiving chemotherapy plus trastuzumab. The 1-year survival rate was 68% with chemotherapy alone, versus 79% with the combination. In both trials, tumors with the highest HER2 content responded best.

Adverse Effects. The principal concern with trastuzumab is cardiac damage, manifesting as ventricular dysfunction and congestive heart failure.

In clinical trials, the incidence of symptomatic heart failure was 7% with trastuzumab alone, and 28% when trastuzumab was combined with doxorubicin, a drug with prominent cardiotoxic actions. Trastuzumab should be used with great caution in women with pre-existing heart disease. Combined use with doxorubicin and other anthracyclines should generally be avoided. Many patients experience a flu-like syndrome, which also occurs with other monoclonal antibodies. Symptoms include chills, fever, pain, weakness, nausea, vomiting and headache. The syndrome develops in 40% of patients receiving their first infusion, and then subsides with subsequent infusions. In contrast to cytotoxic anticancer drugs, trastuzumab does not cause bone marrow suppression or alopecia.

Postmarketing reports indicate that trastuzumab can cause potentially fatal hypersensitivity reactions, infusion reactions, and pulmonary events. Symptoms include urticaria, bronchospasm, angioedema, hypotension, dyspnea, wheezing, pleural effusions, pulmonary edema, and hypoxia requiring oxygen. Most severe reactions developed in association with the first dose, either during the infusion or by 12 hours after. If symptoms develop during the infusion, the infusion should be stopped. Death occurred primarily in patients with pre-existing pulmonary disorders. Accordingly, patients with compromised pulmonary function should be managed with extreme caution.

Dosage, Administration, and Cost. Treatment consists of a loading dose (4 mg/kg infused over 90 minutes) followed by weekly maintenance doses (2 mg/kg infused over 30 minutes). A 23-week course costs over $13,500.

Rituximab

Actions and Use. Rituximab [Rituxan] is a monoclonal antibody indicated for IV therapy of *low-grade, B-cell non-Hodgkin's lymphoma*. (Low-grade lymphoma is less aggressive than high-grade lymphoma, but more difficult to cure.) Rituximab is directed against the CD20 antigen, which is present on the surface of most normal and malignant B cells. Binding of rituximab recruits components of the immune system, which then cause cell lysis. In one study, rituximab produced a complete response in 6% of patients, and another 42% experienced a partial response (50% or greater reduction in tumor burden). The recommended dosage is 375 mg/m² given by slow infusion once a week for 4 weeks. A 4-week course costs about $11,000.

Adverse Effects. Infusion Reactions. Rituximab can cause severe infusion-related hypersensitivity reactions. Prominent symptoms are hypotension, bronchospasm, and angioedema. More than 70 cases of severe hypersensitivity have been reported, including several fatalities. Management includes discontinuing the infusion and injecting epinephrine.

Tumor Lysis Syndrome (TLS). Rapid and massive death of tumor cells can lead to TLS, characterized by acute renal failure, hyperkalemia, hypocalcemia, hyperuricemia, or hyperphosphatemia. Rarely, the syndrome proves fatal. TLS onset develops within 12 to 24 hours of the first rituximab infusion. The risk of TLS is increased by a high tumor burden. Management includes dialysis and correction of fluid and electrolyte abnormalities.

Mucocutaneous Reactions. Rituximab has been associated with severe mucocutaneous reactions, including Stevens-Johnson syndrome, lichenoid dermatitis, vesiculobullous dermatitis, and toxic epidermal necrolysis. Deaths have occurred. Reaction onset is typically 1 to 3 weeks after rituximab exposure. Patients who experience these reactions should seek immediate medical attention, and should not receive rituximab again.

Other Adverse Effects. Like other monoclonal antibodies, rituximab can cause a flu-like syndrome, especially during the initial infusion. Symptoms include fever, chills, nausea, vomiting, and myalgia. Rituximab causes transient neutropenia, but this does not appear to increase the risk of infection.

Ibritumomab Tiuxetan with Yttrium-90

Description and Use. Ibritumomab tiuxetan (IT), marketed as *Zevalin,* is a compound molecule composed of ibritumomab (a monoclonal antibody) that has been covalently bound with tiuxetan. Like rituximab, IT binds selectively with the CD20 antigen present on most normal and malignant B cells. However, unlike rituximab, which is used alone to treat cancer, IT is first linked with yttrium-90 (Y90), a beta particle–emitting radioisotope. When the IT-Y90 complex binds with cellular CD20 antigens, cell kill results from radiation-induced injury, rather than from injury mediated by ibritumomab itself. Because beta particles have a relatively short path length (about 5 mm), injury is restricted to CD20-containing cells and to neighboring cells within a 5-mm radius. The radioactive drug poses no danger to bystanders. IT-Y90 is the first—and currently the only—anticancer treatment to employ an antibody complexed with a radioactive compound. Like rituximab, IT-Y90 is approved for *low-grade, B-cell non-Hodgkin's lymphoma*. However, because

Special Interest Topic

BOX 99–1 ■■ ANGIOGENESIS INHIBITORS: NO FLOW—NO GROW

Like all other tissues, tumors need blood vessels to provide nutrients and oxygen. To ensure adequate blood flow, tumor cells induce angiogenesis—growth of new blood vessels. Without new vessels, tumors could not grow. In fact, their maximum size would be limited to 2 mm³ (about the size of a pinhead). Because tumors require their own blood supply, drugs that block angiogenesis have the potential to profoundly limit tumor expansion. Furthermore, because angiogenesis inhibitors attack the blood supply, rather than the tumor itself, they should be active against a broad range of cancer types.

The field of angiogenesis inhibition owes much to Dr. Judah Folkman and his colleagues at Harvard Medical School. In 1971, Dr. Folkman discovered tumor-induced angiogenesis, and postulated that inhibitors of the process could cause tumor starvation. For many years, Folkman's lab was unable to find an angiogenesis inhibitor safe enough to use. Then, in 1997, the group reported dramatic results with two new compounds: angiostatin and endostatin. These agents were compared with cytotoxic drugs in mice with three kinds of primary tumors. Initially, both treatments caused tumor regression. However, with repeated rounds of therapy, the tumors developed resistance to the cytotoxic agents. In contrast, after six rounds of antiangiogenesis treatment, the tumors regressed to microscopic size—and then remained dormant a long time. Furthermore, the angiogenesis inhibitors were devoid of adverse effects, in stark contrast to the cytotoxic drugs.

Angiogenesis in Normal Tissues and in Tumors

In normal tissues, angiogenesis occurs during fetal development, growth, wound repair, and the uterine cycle. New blood vessels are derived from endothelial cells—the flat cells that form the inner lining of blood vessels. Angiogenesis has four basic steps:

- Activation of endothelial cells in an existing blood vessel
- Production, by the endothelial cells, of matrix metalloprotcinascs (MMPs), which brcak down thc cxtraccllular matrix of the surrounding tissue
- Proliferation and migration of endothelial cells
- Assembly of the endothelial cells into new blood vessels

This process is tightly regulated by two groups of opposing factors: activators of endothelial cell growth and inhibitors of endothelial cell growth. At least 35 endogenous factors are known to activate endothelial cell growth and migration. Important among these are

- Vascular endothelial growth factor (VEGF)
- Basic fibroblast growth factor (bFGF)
- Epidermal growth factor
- Platelet-derived growth factor
- Placental growth factor
- Interleukin-8
- Tumor necrosis factor-alpha (TNF-alpha)
- Angiogenin
- Angiotropin

Naturally occurring inhibitors of endothelial growth include angiostatin, endostatin, interferons, platelet factor 4, thrombospondin, and three tissue inhibitors of metalloproteinase (TIMP-1, TIMP-2, and TIMP-3).

Tumors can stimulate angiogenesis by releasing growth factors. Two such factors—VEGF and bFGF—are produced by many tumors, and appear important for promoting and sustaining tumor growth. In tumors, a good blood supply is associated with aggressive growth and increased ability to metastasize. Interestingly, MMPs, which break down the matrix that holds cells together, are required for both angiogenesis and metastatic spread.

Angiogenesis Inhibitors in Clinical Trials

More than 30 angiogenesis inhibitors are in clinical trials. These drugs work by four basic mechanisms: (1) inhibition of MMPs, (2) direct inhibition of endothelial cell proliferation and migration, (3) antagonism of angiogenic growth factors, and (4) inhibition of integrin, a protein found on the endothelial cell surface. Specific agents under investigation include *marimastat* (which inhibits MMP), *endostatin* (which directly inhibits endothelial cells), *thalidomide* (which blocks VEGF, bFGF, and TNF-alpha), and *vitaxin* (which blocks integrin). Target diseases include melanoma, Kaposi's sarcoma, malignant glioma, and cancers of the breast, ovary, prostate, colon, and pancreas. Preliminary data indicate that the angiogenesis inhibitors are both safe and effective.

Comparison with Cytotoxic Anticancer Drugs

The angiogenesis inhibitors differ from cytotoxic drugs in four important ways. First, angiogenesis inhibitors are less toxic. Second, angiogenesis inhibitors can be used without interruption. Third, tumor resistance to angiogenesis inhibitors does not develop. Fourth, angiogenesis inhibitors can prolong life without causing tumor regression.

Angiogenesis inhibitors are **safer** than cytotoxic anticancer drugs. Unlike cytotoxic drugs, which attack *all* proliferating cells, angiogenesis inhibitors have limited effects. Accordingly, these agents do not cause myelosuppression, GI ulceration, or hair loss—toxicities that are common with the cytotoxic drugs. However, because of their effects on blood vessels, angiogenesis inhibitors are likely to interfere with wound healing and fetal development, and they may be harmful to growing children. Furthermore, because these drugs are very new, their full range of potential toxicities is unknown.

Angiogenesis inhibitors can be **used continuously.** This is possible because these drugs are harmless to normal cells. Cytotoxic drugs must be used intermittently, so as to permit recovery of normal cells between rounds of treatment.

In long-term preclinical studies, **no tumor resistance** to angiogenesis inhibitors has been observed. By contrast, resistance is common with cytotoxic drugs. Why the difference? Cytotoxic drugs are directed against cancer cells, which are heterogeneous and genetically unstable. As a result, drug-resistant variants can readily evolve and emerge. In contrast, angiogenesis inhibitors are directed at endothelial cells, which are genetically stable, and hence do not evolve into potentially resistant forms.

With angiogenesis inhibitors, the treatment goal is **tumor stabilization,** rather than tumor regression. Although these drugs can block formation of new blood vessels, they do not cause existing vessels to dissolve. Hence, they can block tumor growth, but may not cause an existing tumor to shrink. When cytotoxic drugs are tested, the clinical endpoint is tumor regression. In contrast, when angiogenesis inhibitors are tested, the endpoint is prolongation of life; the tumor may or may not get smaller.

A New Treatment Paradigm

Angiogenesis inhibitors may enable a completely new approach to cancer therapy: long-term maintenance, instead of outright cure. By suppressing growth of new blood vessels, angiogenesis inhibitors can stabilize existing tumors and prevent growth of new ones. With continuous therapy, we may be able to keep the cancer in check indefinitely, even though we can't make it go away. Hence, although treatment may not eliminate the cancer, chronic therapy may still permit a long life. In essence, cancer would become a chronic but treatable disease, much like hypertension or diabetes—diseases that we can manage with drugs, even though we can't cure them. Perhaps the angiogenesis inhibitors will permit cancer patients to live long and otherwise healthy lives, just as drugs have done for patients with these other once-fatal diseases.

---

treatment can be life-threatening, the new drug should be used only after safer alternatives have failed. Therapy with IT-Y90 is expensive: a single course costs about $30,000.

Before patients receive IT-Y90, they are given two small doses of rituximab, 7 to 9 days apart. The contribution of rituximab is twofold. First, it binds with circulating B cells, and thereby greatly reduces their numbers. Second, it occupies nonspecific binding sites that could otherwise attract IT-Y90, and hence would reduce the amount of IT-Y90 available to bind with target cells. For the purpose of diagnostic imaging, the first dose of rituximab is accompanied by a small dose of IT that has been linked to radioactive indium-111.

Adverse Effects. Adverse effects of treatment are due to IT-Y90 itself and to the rituximab given before it. As noted above, rituximab can cause severe infusion reactions. With IT-Y90, hematologic toxicity is the major concern: severe, prolonged cytopenias develop in more than 50% of patients. Counts of neutrophils and platelets reach their nadir 7 to 9 weeks after treatment, and take 3 to 7 weeks to recover. In clinical trials, about 30% of patients developed infection or febrile neutropenia; of these, 7% required hospitalization. Deaths have occurred. Because of its hematologic toxicity, IT-Y90 is contraindicated for patients with (1) lymphoma bone marrow involvement of 25% or more or (2) limited bone marrow reserve (e.g., platelet count <100,000/mm³ or neutrophil count <1500/mm³; history of prior myeloablative therapy).

Thalidomide

Thalidomide [Thalomid] is a drug with complex pharmacologic actions, including the ability to cause severe birth defects. In the United States, thalidomide is approved only for erythema nodosum leprosum, a complication of leprosy. However, the drug has shown promise in other diseases, including several forms of cancer. Anticancer effects have been demonstrated most clearly in patients with multiple myeloma, an incurable cancer of the bone marrow. In addition, thalidomide may be active against plasma cell leukemia and various solid tumors, including renal cell carcinoma, AIDS-related Kaposi's sarcoma, and cancers of the brain, breast, ovary, prostate, and colon. Anticancer effects are thought to derive from (1) effects on the immune system and (2) inhibition of angiogenesis (growth of blood vessels; see Box 99–1). Compared with traditional anticancer drugs, thalidomide is well tolerated. Because thalidomide is a powerful teratogen, patients must comply with a strict set of FDA-mandated safeguards, known as the System for Thalidomide Education and Prescribing Safety, or S.T.E.P.S. The history and pharmacology of thalidomide, as well as the S.T.E.P.S. program, are discussed at length in Chapter 103 (Box 103–1).

Arsenic Trioxide

Actions and Uses. Arsenic trioxide [Trisenox] is approved for *acute promyelocytic leukemia* (APL), a rare form of leukemia in which myeloid cells are blocked from undergoing normal differentiation and apoptosis (programmed cell death). In patients who have relapsed following standard therapy of APL, arsenic trioxide has produced a high rate of complete remission.

The drug appears to work by reversing the blockade on myeloid differentiation and apoptosis, although how this is done is unknown. Pharmacokinetics of the drug have not been studied.

Adverse Effects. Toxicity occurs in most patients. Common side effects include nausea, vomiting, diarrhea, fatigue, edema, hyperglycemia, dyspnea, cough, rash, headache, and dizziness. Leukocytosis (elevation of white blood cell counts) occurs in 50% of patients. Of greater concern, about 23% experience a potentially fatal condition known as APL differentiation syndrome, characterized by fever, weight gain, pulmonary infiltrates, dyspnea, musculoskeletal pain, and pleural and pericardial effusions. Symptoms can be reduced by immediate therapy with high-dose glucocorticoids. Prolongation of the QT interval is common and can lead to life-threatening dysrhythmias. An electrocardiogram should be obtained prior to treatment and at least weekly thereafter. If possible, drugs known to cause QT prolongation should be withdrawn. Among these are class I and class III antidysrhythmics, clarithromycin, daunorubicin, mesoridazine, and thioridazine. Arsenic trioxide has the potential to cause fetal harm, and hence is classified in FDA Pregnancy Risk Category D. In contrast to cytotoxic anticancer drugs, arsenic trioxide does not cause alopecia or mucositis.

KEY POINTS

- All of the hormones, hormone antagonists, and biologic response modifiers used to treat cancer are cell-cycle phase nonspecific, in contrast to many cytotoxic anticancer drugs, which are phase specific.
- In general, the drugs discussed in this chapter lack the characteristic toxicities of the cytotoxic anticancer drugs, including bone marrow suppression, stomatitis, and severe nausea and vomiting. Nonetheless, many of these drugs cause severe toxicities of their own.
- Hormonal anticancer drugs act through specific hormone receptors on target tissues. As a result, their actions are highly selective, and their toxicity to normal cells is generally low.
- Glucocorticoids are toxic to cancers of lymphoid origin (e.g., acute and chronic lymphocytic leukemias, Hodgkin's disease, non-Hodgkin's lymphomas).
- In addition to their use against lymphoid-derived cancers, glucocorticoids are used to manage complications of cancer and cancer therapy. Specific benefits include suppression of chemotherapy-induced nausea

and vomiting, reduction of cerebral edema secondary to irradiation of the cranium, reduction of pain secondary to nerve compression or edema, and suppression of hypercalcemia in steroid-responsive tumors. Also, glucocorticoids can improve appetite, promote weight gain, and impart a generalized sense of well-being.

■ When used acutely, glucocorticoids are devoid of significant adverse effects. However, with prolonged use, these drugs can cause a broad spectrum of serious toxicities, including osteoporosis, adrenal insufficiency, increased susceptibility to infection, and peptic ulcers.

■ Antiestrogens are drugs that block estrogen receptors.

■ Antiestrogens fall into two major categories: (1) pure estrogen receptor antagonists and (2) SERMs, which block estrogen receptors in some tissues, and activate estrogen receptors in others.

■ Tamoxifen, a SERM, is approved for prevention and treatment of breast cancer. Benefits derive from blocking estrogen receptors on tumor cells. The drug is not active against cancers that are ER negative.

■ By activating certain estrogen receptors, tamoxifen increases the risk of endometrial cancer and thromboembolism.

■ Fulvestrant, a pure estrogen receptor antagonist, is approved for treatment of breast cancer, but not for prevention.

■ In contrast to tamoxifen and other SERMs, fulvestrant poses no risk of endometrial cancer, and only a slight risk of thromboembolism.

■ Anastrozole, an aromatase inhibitor, is used to treat breast cancer in postmenopausal women. Benefits derive from preventing production of estrogen from adrenal androgens.

■ For women with breast cancer, anastrozole is more effective than tamoxifen and safer (because it does not pose a risk of endometrial cancer or thromboembolism).

■ Prostate cancer can be treated with gonadotropin-releasing hormone (GnRH) agonists and androgen receptor blockers. Benefits derive from reducing the stimulation of prostate cells by androgens.

■ Leuprolide, a GnRH agonist, has a biphasic mechanism of action. During the initial phase, the drug stimulates release of interstitial cell–stimulating hormone (ICSH) from the pituitary, and thereby increases production of testosterone by the testes. As a result, there may be a transient "flare" in prostate cancer symptoms. With continuous use, the drug suppresses ICSH release, and thereby causes testosterone production to fall. It is important to note that leuprolide does not decrease production of adrenal androgens.

■ Flutamide, an androgen receptor blocker, is used in combination with a GnRH agonist to treat prostate cancer. Benefits derive from (1) preventing cancer cells from undergoing increased stimulation during the initial phase of GnRH therapy, and (2) blocking the effects of adrenal androgens on prostate cells.

■ Interferon alfa benefits cancer patients by enhancing immune responses and by suppressing proliferation of cancer cells.

■ Imatinib is an important new drug for chronic myeloid leukemia. Benefits derive from inhibiting an abnormal form of tyrosine kinase.

■ Angiogenesis inhibitors are experimental drugs that block growth of new blood vessels needed to supply solid tumors with oxygen and nutrients. As a result, tumor growth is arrested.

■ Because angiogenesis inhibitors attack blood vessels rather than specific cancer cells, these drugs should be active against a wide variety of tumors.

Drugs for the Eye

The drugs addressed in this chapter are used to diagnose and treat disorders of the eye. Our primary focus is on glaucoma. Many of the drugs considered here are discussed at length in other chapters. Accordingly, discussion here is limited to their ophthalmologic applications.

DRUGS FOR GLAUCOMA

The term *glaucoma* refers to a group of diseases characterized by visual field loss secondary to optic nerve damage. The most common forms of glaucoma are *primary open-angle glaucoma* and *acute angle-closure glaucoma*. These forms differ with respect to underlying pathology and treatment. With either form, permanent blindness can result.

In the United States, glaucoma is the leading cause of preventable blindness. Of the 120,000 Americans blind from glaucoma, 90% could have saved their sight with timely treat-

ment. Unfortunately, many afflicted persons are unaware of their condition: Of the 4 million Americans with glaucoma, only 50% are diagnosed.

Before discussing glaucoma, we need to review the role of aqueous humor in maintaining intraocular pressure (IOP). As indicated in Figure 100–1, aqueous humor is produced by the ciliary body and secreted into the posterior chamber of the eye. From there it circulates around the iris into the anterior chamber, and then exits the anterior chamber via the trabecular meshwork and canal of Schlemm. If outflow from the anterior chamber is impeded, backpressure will develop, and IOP will rise. Conversely, if production of aqueous humor falls, IOP will decline.

Pathophysiology and Treatment Overview
Primary Open-Angle Glaucoma

Characteristics. Primary open-angle glaucoma (POAG) is the most common form of glaucoma in the United States. About 90% of people with glaucoma have this type. POAG is the leading cause of blindness among African Americans and the third leading cause among whites.

POAG is characterized by progressive optic nerve damage with eventual impairment of vision. Visual loss develops first in the peripheral visual field. As the disease advances, loss occurs in the central visual field. The pathologic process that leads to optic nerve damage is not understood. IOP is often elevated, but it may also be normal. POAG is a painless, insidious disease in which injury develops over years. Symptoms are absent until extensive optic nerve damage has been produced.

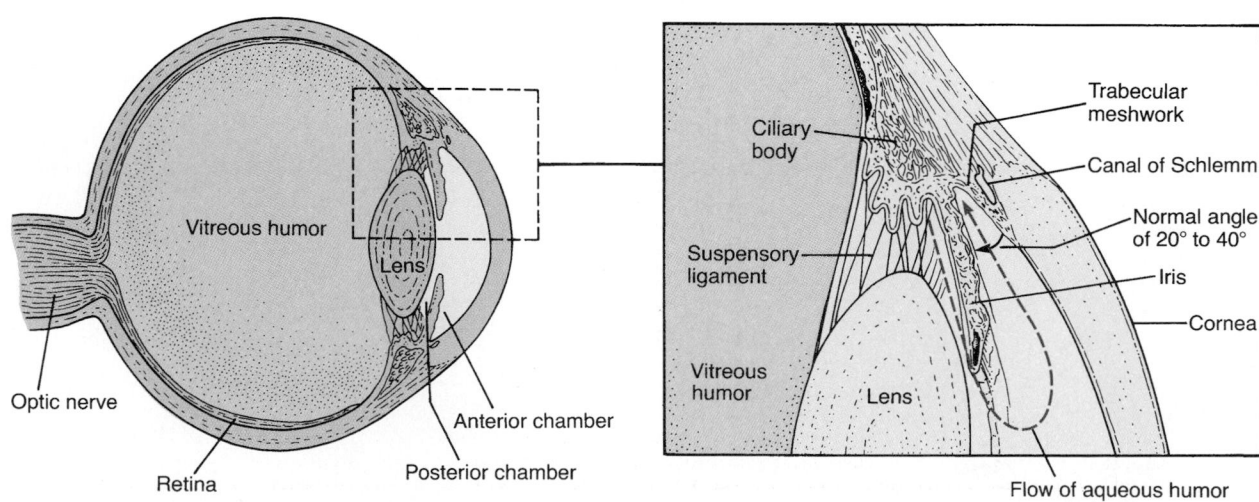

Figure 100–1 ■ **Anatomy of the normal eye.**

Risk Factors. The major risk factors for POAG are

- Elevation of IOP
- Black race
- Family history of POAG
- Advancing age

Of these, elevated IOP is most important. Please note, however, that glaucomatous optic nerve damage can develop even when IOP is normal (i.e., below 20 mm Hg). Furthermore, some individuals can have very high IOP (e.g., 30 mm Hg) with no associated injury to the optic nerve. These individuals are said to have *ocular hypertension*—not glaucoma.

Among African Americans, the incidence of POAG is 3 times higher than among whites. Also, the age of onset is lower and the course of the disease is more aggressive.

Screening. Since POAG is devoid of symptoms (until significant and irreversible optic nerve injury has occurred), regular testing for early POAG is important—especially among individuals at high risk. With early detection and treatment, blindness can usually be prevented. Diagnosis is based on glaucomatous optic nerve atrophy in association with a characteristic reduction in peripheral vision. Individuals with risk factors for POAG should be tested every 2 years up to age 45, and yearly thereafter. Individuals without risk factors should be tested every 4 years up to age 45, and every 2 years thereafter.

Management. Treatment of POAG is directed at reducing elevated IOP, the only risk factor that we can modify. Although POAG has no cure, reduction of IOP can slow or even stop disease progression.

The principal method for reducing IOP is chronic therapy with drugs. Drugs lower IOP by either (1) facilitating aqueous humor outflow or (2) reducing aqueous humor production. As indicated in Table 100–1, the first-line drugs for glaucoma belong to three classes: *beta-adrenergic blocking agents* (beta blockers), *alpha₂-adrenergic agonists,* and *prostaglandin analogs.* Other options—*cholinergic agonists, carbonic anhydrase inhibitors,* and *nonselective adrenergic agonists*—are considered second-line choices. All of the antiglaucoma drugs are available for topical administration, the preferred route. For more than 20 years, the beta blockers (e.g., timolol) have been considered drugs of first choice. However, the alpha₂ agonists (e.g., brimonidine) and prostaglandin analogs (e.g., latanoprost) are just as effective as the beta blockers, and have a more desirable side effect profile. Accordingly, these drugs have joined the beta blockers as first-choice agents. Because drugs in different classes lower IOP by different mechanisms, combined therapy can be more effective than monotherapy. Because all of these drugs are applied topically, systemic effects are relatively uncommon. Nonetheless, serious systemic reactions *can* occur if sufficient absorption takes place.

TABLE 100–1 ■ Topical Drugs for Open-Angle Glaucoma

Class	Drugs	Mechanism	Adverse Effects
First-Line Agents			
Beta Blockers			
Nonselective	Timolol Carteolol Levobunolol Metipranolol	Decreased aqueous formation	Heart block, bradycardia, bronchospasm
Beta₁ selective	Betaxolol		Heart block, bradycardia, hypotension
Alpha₂-Adrenergic Agonists	Apraclonidine* Brimonidine	Decreased aqueous formation	Headache, dry mouth, dry nose, altered taste, conjunctivitis, lid reactions, pruritus
Prostaglandin Analogs	Latanoprost Travoprost Bimatoprost Uniprostone	Increased aqueous outflow	Heightened brown pigmentation of the iris
Second-Line Agents			
Cholinergic Agonists			
Direct acting	Pilocarpine	Increased aqueous outflow	Miosis, blurred vision
Acetylcholinesterase inhibitors	Echothiophate		Miosis, blurred vision
Carbonic Anhydrase Inhibitors	Dorzolamide Brinzolamide	Decreased aqueous formation	Ocular stinging, bitter taste, conjunctivitis, lid reactions
Nonselective Adrenergic Agonists	Epinephrine Dipivefrin†	Increased aqueous outflow	Mydriasis, tachycardia, hypertension

*Apraclonidine is indicated for short-term use only, and hence is *not* a first-line drug for glaucoma.
†Dipivefrin is converted to epinephrine in the eye.

If drugs are unable to reduce IOP to an acceptable level, surgical intervention to promote outflow of aqueous humor is indicated. Two procedures are used: laser trabeculoplasty and trabeculectomy (done with conventional surgical techniques).

Angle-Closure Glaucoma

Angle-closure glaucoma is precipitated by displacement of the iris such that it covers the trabecular meshwork, thereby preventing exit of aqueous humor from the anterior chamber. As a result, IOP increases rapidly and to dangerous levels. This disorder is referred to as *angle-closure* or *narrow-angle* glaucoma because the angle between the cornea and the iris is greatly reduced (Fig. 100–2). Angle-closure glaucoma develops suddenly and is extremely painful. In the absence of treatment, irreversible loss of vision occurs in 1 to 2 days. This disorder is much less common than open-angle glaucoma.

Treatment consists of *drug therapy* (to control the acute attack) followed by *corrective surgery*. A combination of drugs (osmotic agents, short-acting miotics, carbonic anhydrase inhibitors, topical beta-adrenergic blocking agents) is employed to suppress symptoms. Once IOP has been reduced with drugs, definitive treatment can be rendered with surgery. Two surgical procedures are employed: *laser iridotomy* and *iridectomy* performed by conventional surgery. Both procedures alter the iris to permit unimpeded outflow of aqueous humor.

Drugs Used to Treat Glaucoma
Beta-Adrenergic Blocking Agents

Actions and Use in Glaucoma. Six beta blockers—*betaxolol, levobetaxolol, carteolol, metipranolol, levobunolol,* and *timolol*—are approved for use in glaucoma. Administration is topical. These agents cause minimal disturbance of vision and are considered first-line drugs for glaucoma. Formulations and dosages of the beta blockers are summarized in Table 100–2.

The beta-adrenergic blockers lower IOP by decreasing production of aqueous humor by the ciliary body. Reductions in IOP occur with "nonselective" beta blockers (drugs that block beta$_1$ *and* beta$_2$ receptors) as well as with "cardioselective" beta blockers (drugs that block beta$_1$ receptors only).

Beta blockers are used primarily for open-angle glaucoma. These drugs are suitable for initial therapy as well as maintenance therapy. In addition to their use in open-angle glaucoma, beta blockers may be employed in combination with other drugs for emergency management of acute angle-closure glaucoma.

The basic pharmacology of the beta blockers is discussed in Chapter 18.

Adverse Effects. Local. Local effects are generally minimal, although patients commonly complain of transient ocular stinging. Beta blockers occasionally cause conjunctivitis, blurred vision, photophobia, and dry eyes.

Systemic. Beta blockers can be absorbed in amounts sufficient to cause systemic effects. Effects on the heart and lungs are of greatest concern.

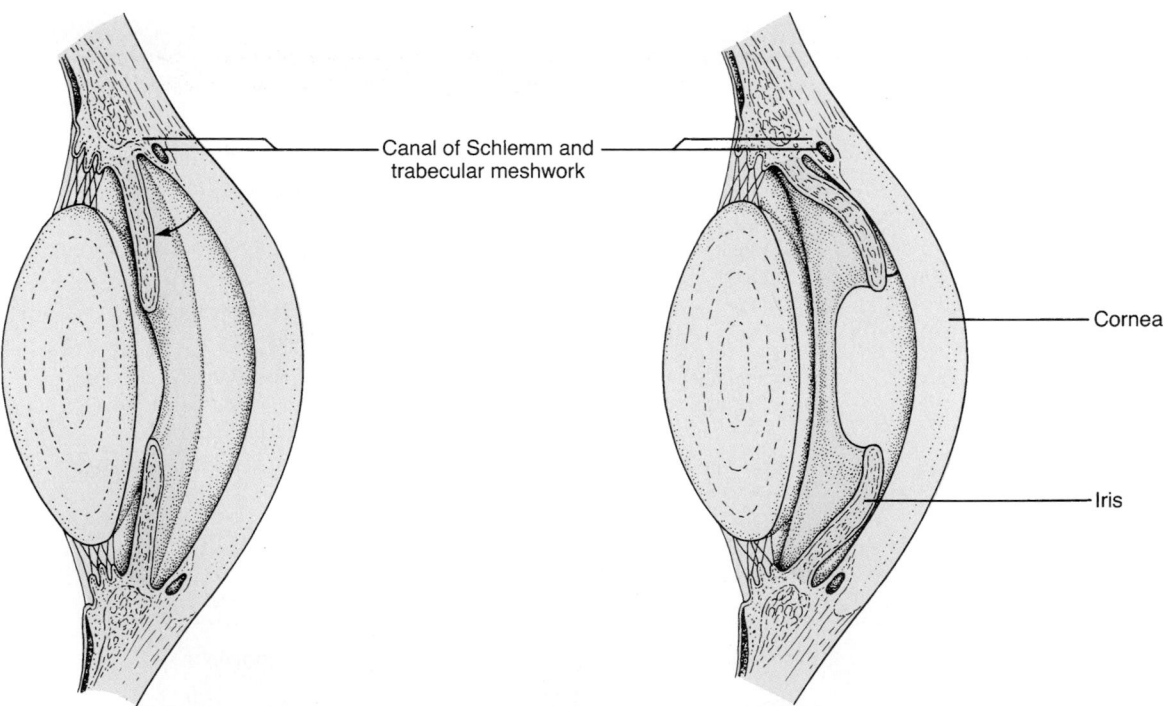

Canal of Schlemm and trabecular meshwork

Cornea

Iris

A   Open-angle glaucoma

B   Angle-closure glaucoma

Figure 100–2 ■ **Comparative anatomy of the eye in open-angle and angle-closure glaucoma.** *A,* Note that the angle between the iris and cornea is open in open-angle glaucoma, permitting unimpeded outflow of aqueous humor through the canal of Schlemm and trabecular meshwork. *B,* Note that the angle between the iris and cornea is constricted in angle-closure glaucoma, thereby blocking outflow of aqueous humor through the canal of Schlemm and trabecular meshwork.

Blockade of cardiac beta$_1$ receptors can produce bradycardia and atrioventricular (AV) heart block. Pulse rate should be monitored. Because of their ability to depress cardiac function, beta blockers are contraindicated for patients with AV heart block, sinus bradycardia, and cardiogenic shock. In addition, they should be used with caution in patients with heart failure.

Blockade of beta$_2$ receptors in the lung can cause bronchospasm. Constriction of the bronchi can occur with "beta$_1$-selective" antagonists as well as with "nonselective" beta-adrenergic blockers—although the risk is greatest with the nonselective agents. Only two ophthalmic beta blockers—betaxolol and levobetaxolol—are beta$_1$ selective, and hence preferred for patients with asthma or chronic obstructive pulmonary disease.

Prostaglandin Analogs

Four prostaglandin analogs are now approved for topical therapy of glaucoma. These drugs are as effective as the beta blockers and cause fewer side effects. Accordingly, they are considered first-line medications for glaucoma. Formulations and dosages are summarized in Table 100–3.

Latanoprost. Latanoprost [Xalatan], an analog of prostaglandin F$_2$ alpha, was the first prostaglandin approved for glaucoma and will serve as our prototype for the group. The drug is applied topically to lower IOP in patients with open-angle glaucoma and ocular hypertension. Latanoprost lowers IOP by facilitating aqueous humor outflow, in part by relaxing the ciliary muscle. The recommended dosage is 1 drop (0.005% solution) applied once daily in the evening. At this dosage, latanoprost produces the same reduction in IOP as timolol twice daily.

Latanoprost is generally well tolerated, and systemic reactions are rare. The most significant side effect is heightened brown pigmentation of the iris. This is most noticeable in patients whose irides are green-brown, yellow-brown, or blue/gray-brown. The effect is rare in patients whose irides are blue, green, or blue-green. Heightened pigmentation stops progressing when latanoprost is discontinued, but does not regress. Topical latanoprost may also increase pigmentation of the eyelid, and increase growth and pigmentation of the eyelashes. Other side effects include blurred vision, burning, stinging, conjunctival hyperemia, and punctate keratopathy. Rarely, the drug may cause migraine.

Other Prostaglandin Analogs. In addition to latanoprost, three other topical prostaglandins are approved for topical therapy of glaucoma. Like latanoprost, these drugs—*travoprost* [Travatan], *bimatoprost* [Lumigan], and *unoprostone* [Rescula]—reduce IOP by increasing aqueous humor outflow. In clinical trials, these agents were at least as effective as timolol, a representative beta blocker. Interestingly, one drug—travoprost—was more effective in African Americans than in non–African Americans. Like latanoprost, these prostaglandins can cause a gradual increase in brown pigmentation of the iris, which may be irreversible. In addition, they may increase pigmentation of the eyelid and growth of the eyelashes. Their most common adverse effect is ocular hyperemia. Less commonly, they may cause blurred vision, eye discomfort, ocular pruritus, conjunctivitis, dry eye, light intolerance, and tearing. Dosages are summarized in Table 100–3.

TABLE 100–2 ■ Beta Blockers Used in Glaucoma

Drug	Receptor Specificity	Formulation	Usual Dosage
Betaxolol [Betoptic]	Beta$_1$	0.25% suspension 0.5% solution	1 drop twice a day 1 drop twice a day
Levobetaxolol [Betaxon]	Beta$_1$	0.5% suspension	1 drop twice daily
Carteolol [Ocupress]	Beta$_1$, beta$_2$	1% solution	1 drop twice a day
Levobunolol [Betagan Liquifilm, AKBeta]	Beta$_1$, beta$_2$	0.25% solution 0.5% solution	1 drop twice a day 1 drop once or twice a day
Metipranolol [OptiPranolol]	Beta$_1$, beta$_2$	0.3% solution	1 drop twice a day
Timolol [Timoptic, Betimol]	Beta$_1$, beta$_2$	0.25% solution 0.5% solution 0.25% gel 0.5% gel	1 drop once or twice a day 1 drop once or twice a day 1 drop once daily 1 drop once daily

TABLE 100–3 ■ Prostaglandin Analogs Used in Glaucoma

Generic Name	Trade Name	Formulation	Usual Dosage
Latanoprost	Xalatan	0.005% solution	1 drop once daily in the evening
Travoprost	Travatan	0.004% solution	1 drop once daily in the evening
Bimatoprost	Lumigan	0.03% solution	1 drop once daily in the evening
Unoprostone	Rescula	0.15% solution	1 drop twice daily

Alpha₂ Adrenergic Agonists

Two alpha₂ agonists are approved for glaucoma. One agent—apraclonidine—is used only for short-term therapy. The other agent—brimonidine—has emerged as a first-line drug for long-term therapy.

Brimonidine. Brimonidine [Alphagan] is the first and only topical alpha₂-adrenergic agonist approved for *long-term* reduction of elevated IOP in patients with open-angle glaucoma or ocular hypertension. The recommended dosage is 1 drop 3 times a day. Effects on IOP are similar to those achieved with timolol (a beta blocker). The drug lowers IOP by reducing aqueous humor production, and perhaps by increasing outflow. In addition to lowering IOP, brimonidine may be able to delay optic nerve degeneration and may protect retinal neurons from death. This possibility arises from the ability of alpha₂ agonists to protect neurons from injury caused by ischemia. The most common adverse effects of brimonidine are dry mouth, ocular hyperemia (engorgement of ocular blood vessels), local burning and stinging, headache, blurred vision, foreign body sensation, and ocular itching. In contrast to apraclonidine (see below), brimonidine does cross the blood-brain barrier, and hence can cause hypotension, drowsiness, and fatigue. Brimonidine can be absorbed onto soft contact lenses. Accordingly, at least 15 minutes should elapse between drug administration and lens installation.

Apraclonidine. Apraclonidine [Iopidine], a topical alpha₂-adrenergic agonist, lowers IOP by reducing aqueous humor production and possibly by increasing outflow. The drug is indicated only for (1) short-term therapy of open-angle glaucoma in patients who have not responded adequately to maximal doses of other IOP-lowering drugs, and (2) preoperative medication prior to laser trabeculoplasty or iridotomy. Side effects include headache, dry mouth, dry nose, altered taste, conjunctivitis, lid reactions, pruritus, tearing, and blurred vision. Apraclonidine does not cross the blood-brain barrier, and hence does not promote hypotension. (Recall from Chapter 19 that activation of alpha₂ receptors in the brain decreases sympathetic outflow to blood vessels, and thereby lowers blood pressure.) For short-term therapy of glaucoma, the dosage is 1 or 2 drops (0.5% solution) 3 times a day.

Pilocarpine (a Direct-Acting Cholinergic Agonist)

Pilocarpine is a direct-acting muscarinic agonist (parasympathomimetic agent). Administration is topical. The basic pharmacology of the muscarinic agonists is discussed in Chapter 14. Consideration here is limited to the use of pilocarpine in glaucoma.

Effects on the Eye. By stimulating cholinergic receptors in the eye, pilocarpine produces two direct effects: (1) *miosis* (constriction of the pupil secondary to contraction of the iris sphincter), and (2) *contraction of the ciliary muscle* (an action that focuses the lens for near vision). IOP is lowered indirectly. In patients with *open-angle glaucoma*, IOP is reduced because the tension generated by contracting the ciliary muscle promotes widening of the spaces within the trabecular meshwork, thereby facilitating outflow of aqueous humor. In *angle-closure glaucoma*, contraction of the iris sphincter pulls the iris away from the pores of the trabecular meshwork, thereby removing the impediment to aqueous humor outflow.

Therapeutic Uses. Although used widely in the past, pilocarpine is now considered a second-line drug for open-angle glaucoma. In addition, pilocarpine can be used for emergency treatment of acute angle-closure glaucoma.

Adverse Effects. The major side effects of pilocarpine concern the eye. Contraction of the ciliary muscle focuses the lens for near vision; corrective lenses can provide partial compensation for this problem. Occasionally, sustained contraction of the ciliary muscle causes retinal detachment. Constriction of the pupil, caused by contraction of the iris sphincter, may decrease visual acuity. Pilocarpine may also produce local irritation, eye pain, and brow ache.

Rarely, pilocarpine is absorbed in amounts sufficient to cause systemic effects. Stimulation of muscarinic receptors throughout the body can produce a variety of responses, including bradycardia, bronchospasm, hypotension, urinary urgency, diarrhea, hypersalivation, and sweating. Caution should be exercised in patients with asthma or bradycardia. Systemic toxicity can be reversed with a muscarinic antagonist (e.g., atropine).

Preparations, Dosage, and Administration. Pilocarpine is available in solution, a gel, and an "ocular system." With all three formulations, administration is topical. Pilocarpine solutions have a relatively short duration of action and must be administered more frequently than the gel or ocular system.

Pilocarpine Solutions. Pilocarpine hydrochloride [Adsorbocarpine, Akarpine, Isopto Carpine, Pilocar, Piloptic, Pilostat] and pilocarpine nitrate [Pilagan] are dispensed in solution for topical application to the conjunctiva. Concentrations range from 0.25% to 10%. For maintenance therapy of open-angle glaucoma, the usual dosage is 1 drop of solution (0.5% to 4%) applied 4 times a day. For patients with acute angle-closure glaucoma, pilocarpine is applied much more frequently (e.g., every 5 to 10 minutes for three to six doses, then 1 drop every 1 to 3 hours).

Pilocarpine Gel. Pilocarpine ophthalmic gel [Pilopine HS] consists of 4% pilocarpine hydrochloride in an aqueous gel base. The preparation has a long duration of action, making once-a-day dosing sufficient. For chronic open-angle glaucoma, the usual dosage is one-half inch of gel applied to the conjunctiva at bedtime.

Pilocarpine Ocular System. The pilocarpine ocular system [Ocusert Pilo-20, Ocusert Pilo-40] consists of a bilayered membrane surrounding a reservoir of pilocarpine solution. The tiny unit is placed in the conjunctival sac, after which pilocarpine is slowly released. A replacement unit should be installed once a week. The ocular system is indicated for chronic open-angle glaucoma. Since the unit may fall out during sleep, patients should check each morning for its presence. Occasionally, the ocular system may migrate to the cornea, causing discomfort and disturbance of vision. Conjunctival irritation may also occur.

Cholinesterase Inhibitors (Indirect-Acting Cholinergic Agonists)

For treatment of glaucoma, two topical cholinesterase inhibitors are available: *echothiophate* and *demecarium*. Both have a long duration of action. The basic pharmacology of these drugs is discussed in Chapter 15. Consideration here is limited to their use in glaucoma.

Effects on the Eye. The cholinesterase inhibitors inhibit breakdown of acetylcholine (ACh), and thereby promote accumulation of ACh at muscarinic receptors. As a result, these drugs can produce the same ocular effects as pilocarpine (i.e., miosis, focusing of the lens for near vision, reduction of IOP).

Use in Glaucoma. The cholinesterase inhibitors are indicated for POAG. However, because of concerns about adverse effects, these agents are not drugs of first choice. Rather, they are reserved for patients who have responded poorly to preferred medications (e.g., beta blockers, apha₂ agonists, prostaglandins).

Adverse Effects. Like pilocarpine, cholinesterase inhibitors can cause *myopia* (secondary to contraction of the ciliary muscle) and excessive pupillary constriction. However, of much greater concern is the association between long-acting cholinesterase inhibitors and development of *cataracts*. Absorption of cholinesterase inhibitors into the systemic circulation can produce typical *parasympathomimetic responses,* including bradycardia, bronchospasm, sweating, salivation, urinary urgency, and diarrhea.

Preparations, Dosage, and Administration. Echothiophate iodide [Phospholine Iodide] is dispensed as a powder for reconstitution to solutions that range in strength from 0.03% to 0.25%. For open-angle glaucoma, the 0.03% solution is commonly employed. Administration into the conjunctival sac may be done once daily, twice daily, or every other day.

Demecarium bromide [Humorsol] is dispensed in sterile solution (0.125%, 0.25%) for topical application to the eye. For initial treatment of open-angle glaucoma, 1 drop is instilled into the conjunctival sac every 12 to 48 hours.

Epinephrine and Dipivefrin

Epinephrine is an adrenergic agonist that stimulates alpha- and beta-adrenergic receptors. Administration is topical. The basic pharmacology of epinephrine is discussed in Chapter 17. Consideration here is limited to its use in glaucoma.

Dipivefrin is a prodrug form of epinephrine. Because of its high lipid solubility, dipivefrin penetrates the cornea more readily than does epinephrine. Once in the eye, dipivefrin is converted to epinephrine by ocular enzymes.

Actions and Uses in Glaucoma. Epinephrine is used for open-angle glaucoma. The drug reduces IOP apparently by increasing aqueous humor outflow. The mechanism by which outflow is enhanced is not fully understood. Epinephrine may be used alone and in combination with other antiglaucoma drugs.

Adverse Effects. Mild reactions—headache, brow ache, blurred vision, and ocular irritation—are relatively common. By contracting the radial muscle of the iris, epinephrine can cause mydriasis (pupil dilation) and thereby can aggravate angle-closure glaucoma. Accordingly, epinephrine is contraindicated for patients with this disorder. In the patient whose lens has been removed, epinephrine can cause an unusual edema of the retina. This reaction is reversible upon discontinuation of treatment. Systemic absorption can cause tachycardia and elevation of blood pressure; caution should be exercised in patients with hypertension, dysrhythmias, and hyperthyroidism (hyperthyroidism sensitizes the heart to stimulation by catecholamines).

Preparations, Dosage, and Administration. Ophthalmic solutions of epinephrine contain one of two salts: *epinephrine hydrochloride* [Epifrin, Glaucon] or *epinephrine borate* [Epinal]. For treatment of open-angle glaucoma, 1 drop of solution (0.25% to 2%) is instilled into the conjunctival sac once or twice daily.

Dipivefrin [Propine, AKPro] is dispensed in a 0.1% solution. For treatment of open-angle glaucoma, 1 drop is instilled into the conjunctival sac every 12 hours.

Carbonic Anhydrase Inhibitors: Topical

Dorzolamide. Introduced in 1995, dorzolamide [Trusopt] was the first carbonic anhydrase inhibitor available for topical administration. The drug is used to reduce IOP in patients with open-angle glaucoma and ocular hypertension. Dorzolamide lowers IOP by decreasing production of aqueous humor. The recommended dosage is 1 drop (2% solution) 3 times a day. Responses are similar to those produced with beta blockers.

Dorzolamide is generally well tolerated. The most common side effects are ocular stinging and bitter taste immediately after dosing. Between 10% and 15% of patients experience allergic reactions, primarily conjunctivitis and lid reactions. If these occur, the patient should stop using dorzolamide and contact the physician. Other reactions include blurred vision, tearing, eye dryness, and photophobia. In contrast to systemic carbonic anhydrase inhibitors, dorzolamide does not produce acidosis or electrolyte imbalance.

In 1999, dorzolamide became available in a fixed-dose combination with timolol. Marketed as *Cosopt,* this combination produces a greater reduction in IOP than either component used alone. The recommended dosage is 1 drop twice a day.

Brinzolamide. Brinzolamide [Azopt] was approved in 1998 for topical treatment of elevated IOP in patients with open-angle glaucoma or ocular hypertension. The drug is as effective as dorzolamide and better tolerated. Like other carbonic anhydrase inhibitors, brinzolamide reduces IOP by slowing production of aqueous humor. The most common adverse effects are bitter aftertaste and transient blurred vision. Brinzolamide causes less ocular stinging and burning than dorzolamide. The recommended dosage is 1 drop (1% solution) 3 times a day.

Carbonic Anhydrase Inhibitors: Systemic

Three carbonic anhydrase inhibitors—*acetazolamide, dichlorphenamide,* and *methazolamide*—are available for systemic therapy of glaucoma. Acetazolamide is the most frequently employed.

Actions and Uses in Glaucoma. The carbonic anhydrase inhibitors lower IOP by decreasing production of aqueous humor. Maximally effective doses reduce flow of aqueous humor by 50%. Administration is oral.

Carbonic anhydrase inhibitors are employed primarily for long-term treatment of open-angle glaucoma. These agents are not drugs of first choice. Rather, they should be reserved for patients who have been refractory to preferred medications (e.g., beta blockers, alpha₂ agonists, prostaglandin analogs). Carbonic anhydrase inhibitors may also be given (in combination with other antiglaucoma drugs) to produce rapid lowering of IOP in patients with angle-closure glaucoma.

Adverse Effects. Systemic carbonic anhydrase inhibitors can produce multiple adverse effects. Effects on the nervous system, which are relatively common, include malaise, anorexia, fatigue, and paresthesias. The sense of malaise causes many patients to discontinue treatment. Reduced appetite, coupled with GI disturbances (nausea, vomiting, diarrhea), may result in weight loss. Carbonic anhydrase inhibitors are teratogenic in animals and should be avoided by women who are pregnant, especially during the first trimester. Additional concerns are acid-base disturbances, electrolyte imbalance, and nephrolithiasis (formation of renal calculi).

Preparations, Dosage, and Administration. *Acetazolamide* [Diamox, Diamox Sequels, Dazamide] is dispensed in tablets (125 and 250 mg) and sustained-release capsules (500 mg) for oral use, and as an injection (500 mg/vial) for IM and IV administration. The usual dosage range is 250 mg to 1 gm/day in divided doses.

Dichlorphenamide [Daranide] is dispensed in 50-mg tablets for oral use. The usual dosage is 25 to 50 mg 1 to 3 times a day.

Methazolamide [GlaucTabs, Neptazane] is dispensed in 25- and 50-mg tablets for oral use. The usual dosage is 50 to 100 mg 2 or 3 times a day.

Osmotic Agents

Four osmotic agents—*mannitol, urea, glycerin,* and *isosorbide*—are employed in the treatment of glaucoma. These preparations render the plasma hypertonic to intraocular fluid and thereby draw water from the eye. The result is a rapid and marked reduction of IOP. The principal indication for osmotic agents is emergency treatment of acute angle-closure glaucoma. Use in open-angle glaucoma is limited to the perioperative period. Glycerin and isosorbide are administered PO; mannitol and urea are administered by IV infusion. Doses for these drugs range from 0.5 to 2 gm/kg. Common side effects are headache, nausea, and vomiting. The use of mannitol for osmotic diuresis is discussed in Chapter 39.

CYCLOPLEGICS AND MYDRIATICS

Cycloplegics are drugs that cause paralysis of the ciliary muscle, and *mydriatics* are drugs that dilate the pupil. Cycloplegics and mydriatics are employed primarily to facilitate diagnosis and surgery of ophthalmic disorders. Agents used to produce cycloplegia, mydriasis, or both fall into two classes: (1) *anticholinergic agents* (muscarinic antagonists) and (2) *adrenergic agonists.*

Anticholinergic Agents

Several muscarinic antagonists (Table 100–4) are employed topically for diagnosis and treatment of ophthalmic disorders. The basic pharmacology of the anticholinergic drugs is discussed in Chapter 14. Consideration here is limited to their ophthalmic applications.

Effects on the Eye

The anticholinergic drugs produce mydriasis and cycloplegia. Mydriasis results from blockade of the muscarinic receptors that promote contraction of the iris sphincter; cycloplegia results from blockade of muscarinic receptors that promote contraction of the ciliary muscle. As discussed below, relaxation of the iris can lead to elevation of IOP.

Ophthalmic Applications

Adjunct to Measurement of Refraction. The term *refraction* refers to the bending of light by the cornea and lens. When ocular refraction is proper, incoming light is bent such that a sharp image is formed on the retina. Errors in refraction can produce nearsightedness, farsightedness, and astigmatism (a visual disturbance caused by irregularities in the curvature of the cornea).

Both the mydriatic and cycloplegic properties of the muscarinic antagonists can be of use in evaluating errors of refraction. Mydriasis (widening of the pupil) facilitates observation of the eye's interior. Cycloplegia (paralysis of the ciliary muscle) prevents the lens from undergoing changes in configuration during the assessment.

Intraocular Examination. Dilation of the pupil with an anticholinergic agent facilitates observation of the inside of the eye. In addition, by paralyzing the iris sphincter, muscarinic antagonists prevent reflexive constriction of the pupil in response to the light from an ophthalmoscope (the hand-held device used to view the eye's interior). Since adrenergic agonists (e.g., phenylephrine) also dilate the pupil, but by a different mechanism, an adrenergic agonist can be combined with a muscarinic antagonist to increase the degree of mydriasis.

Intraocular Surgery. Anticholinergic agents may be employed to facilitate ocular surgery and to reduce postoperative complications. Mydriasis induced by these drugs can aid in cataract extraction and procedures to correct retinal detachment. For these operations, the muscarinic antagonist may be

TABLE 100–4 ■ Muscarinic Antagonists Used for Mydriasis and Cycloplegia

Generic Name	Trade Names	Strength of Solution (%)	Mydriasis Peak (min)	Mydriasis Recovery (days)	Cycloplegia Peak (min)	Cycloplegia Recovery (days)
Atropine	Atropisol Isopto Atropine Atropine Care	0.5, 1, 2	30–40	7–12	60–180	6–12
Cyclopentolate	AK-Pentolate Cyclogyl Pentolair	0.5, 1, 2	30–60	1	25–76	0.25–1
Homatropine	Isopto Homatropine	2, 5	40–60	1–3	30–60	1–3
Scopolamine	Isopto Hyoscine	0.25	20–30	1–3	30–60	3–7
Tropicamide	Mydriacyl Tropicacyl Opticyl	0.5, 1	20–40	0.25	20–35	<0.25

combined with an adrenergic agonist to maximize pupillary dilation. In certain postoperative patients, mydriatics are employed to prevent development of synechiae (adhesions of the iris to neighboring structures in the eye).

Treatment of Anterior Uveitis. Uveitis is an inflammation of the uvea (the vascular layer of the eye). Symptoms include ocular pain and photophobia. Uveitis is treated with a glucocorticoid (to reduce inflammation) plus an anticholinergic agent. By promoting relaxation of the ciliary muscle and the iris sphincter, anticholinergic drugs help relieve pain and prevent adhesion of the iris to the lens.

Adverse Effects

Blurred Vision and Photophobia. The most common side effects of topical anticholinergic drugs are photophobia and blurred vision. Photophobia occurs because paralysis of the iris sphincter prevents the pupil from constricting in response to bright light. Vision is blurred because paralysis of the ciliary muscle prevents focusing for near vision.

Precipitation of Angle-Closure Glaucoma. By relaxing the iris sphincter, anticholinergic drugs can induce closure of the filtration angle in individuals whose eyes have a narrow angle to begin with. Angle closure occurs as follows: (1) partial dilation of the pupil maximizes contact between the iris and the lens, thereby impeding egress of aqueous humor from the posterior chamber, and (2) the resultant increase in pressure within the posterior chamber pushes the iris forward, causing blockage of the trabecular meshwork. Caution must be exercised in patients predisposed to angle closure.

Systemic Effects. Topically applied anticholinergic drugs can be absorbed in amounts sufficient to produce systemic toxicity. Symptoms include dry mouth, blurred vision, photophobia, constipation, fever, tachycardia, and central nervous system effects (confusion, hallucinations, delirium, coma). Death can occur. Muscarinic poisoning can be treated with physostigmine (see Chapter 14).

Phenylephrine (an Adrenergic Agonist)

Adrenergic agonists are mydriatic agents. Pupillary dilation results from stimulation of alpha-adrenergic receptors on the radial (dilator) muscle of the iris. In contrast to anticholinergic drugs, the adrenergic agonists do not cause cycloplegia. Of the adrenergic agents given to induce mydriasis, *phenylephrine* is the most frequently employed. The adrenergic agonists are discussed at length in Chapter 17. Discussion here is limited to the mydriatic use of phenylephrine.

Therapeutic and Diagnostic Applications

The mydriatic applications of phenylephrine are much like those of the anticholinergic drugs. Phenylephrine-induced mydriasis is used as an aid to intraocular surgery, measurement of refraction, and ophthalmoscopic examination. In patients with anterior uveitis, phenylephrine is given to dilate the pupil as part of an overall program of treatment.

Adverse Effects

Effects on the Eye. Like the anticholinergic drugs, phenylephrine can precipitate angle-closure glaucoma secondary to induction of mydriasis. Caution must be exercised in patients whose filtration angle is naturally narrow. Contraction of the dilator muscle may dislodge pigment granules from degenerating cells of the iris. These granules, which appear as "floaters" in the anterior chamber, are usually cleared from the eye within a day. Phenylephrine may also cause ocular pain, corneal clouding, and brow ache.

Systemic Effects. Rarely, topical phenylephrine is absorbed in amounts sufficient to produce systemic toxicity. Cardiovascular responses (e.g., hypertension, ventricular dysrhythmias, cardiac arrest) are of greatest concern. Other systemic reactions include sweating, blanching, tremor, agitation, and confusion.

DRUGS FOR ALLERGIC CONJUNCTIVITIS

Pathophysiology

Allergic conjunctivitis (AC) is defined as inflammation of the conjunctiva in response to an allergen. (The conjunctiva is the delicate membrane that surrounds the eyelids.) AC may be seasonal or perennial (chronic). Primary symptoms are itch-

TABLE 100–5 ■ Topical Drugs for Allergic Conjunctivitis

Class and Generic Name	Trade Name	Concentration	Usual Daily Dosage
Mast-Cell Stabilizers			
Cromolyn sodium	Crolom, Opticrom	4%	1–2 drop q 4–6 h
Lodoxamide tromethamine	Alomide	0.1%	1–2 drops qid
Nedocromil sodium	Alocril	2%	1–2 drops bid
Pemirolast potassium	Alamast	0.1%	1–2 drops qid
H₁-Receptor Blockers			
Emedastine difumarate	Emadine	0.05%	1 drop qid
Levocabastine hydrochloride	Livostin	0.05%	1 drop qid
Mast-Cell Stabilizers/H₁ Blockers			
Azelastine hydrochloride	Optivar	0.05%	1 drop bid
Ketotifen fumarate	Zaditor	0.025%	1 drop q 8–12 h
Olopatadine hydrochloride	Patanol	0.1%	1 drop bid
NSAIDs*			
Ketorolac tromethamine	Acular	0.5%	1 drop qid
Glucocorticoids			
Loteprednol etabonate	Alrex	0.2%	1 drop qid
Decongestants (Vasoconstrictors)			
Naphazoline	Clear Eyes, others	0.012%	1–2 drops up to qid
Oxymetazoline	Visine L.R., OcuClear	0.025%	1–2 drops qid
Phenylephrine	AK-Nefrin	0.12%	1–2 drops qid
Tetrahydrozoline	Visine Allergy Relief	0.05%	1–2 drops qid

*NSAIDs = nonsteroidal anti-inflammatory drugs.

ing, burning, and a thin, watery discharge. In addition, the conjunctivae are usually red and congested.

Symptoms of AC result from a biphasic immune response. Initially, symptoms are caused by release of inflammatory mediators—histamine, prostaglandins, leukotrienes, and kinins—from mast cells. These mediators stimulate mucus production (to cause discharge), activate nerve endings (to cause itching and burning sensations), and promote vasodilation and increase capillary permeability (to cause redness and congestion). These symptoms peak about 20 minutes after allergen exposure and abate 20 minutes later. Following this early response, symptoms typically reappear 6 or more hours later. This late phase is due to recruitment of immune cells—eosinophils, neutrophils, and macrophages—that amplify the inflammatory response.

Drug Therapy

AC can be managed with a variety of topical drugs (Table 100–5). *Mast-cell stabilizers* (e.g., lodoxamide) prevent release of inflammatory mediators. Patients should be informed that benefits take several days to develop, and several weeks to become maximal. In contrast to mast-cell stabilizers, *H₁-receptor antagonists* (antihistamines) can provide immediate symptomatic relief. Some drugs (e.g., azelastine, olopatadine) have two actions: They prevent mediator release from mast cells *and* they block H₁ receptors. Ketorolac, a *nonsteroidal anti-inflammatory drug* (NSAID), reduces symptoms by inhibiting cyclooxygenase, an enzyme required for synthesis of prostaglandins. Like the NSAIDs, *glucocorticoids* (e.g., loteprednol) inhibit production of prostaglandins; in addition, they inhibit production of leuko-

trienes and thromboxane. As a result, these drugs are highly effective. Unfortunately, with prolonged use, they can cause serious adverse effects, including cataracts, eye infection, and elevation of IOP. Accordingly, glucocorticoids are generally reserved for short-term therapy in patients who have not responded adequately to safer drugs. The *ocular decongestants* (e.g., naphazoline, phenylephrine) decrease redness and edema by activating alpha₁-adrenergic receptors on blood vessels, and thereby cause vasoconstriction. Benefits are only symptomatic; these drugs do not interrupt any phase of the immune response. Furthermore, with regular use, rebound congestion is likely.

ADDITIONAL OPHTHALMIC DRUGS

Demulcents (Artificial Tears)

Ophthalmic demulcents are isotonic solutions employed as substitutes for natural tears. Most preparations contain *polyvinyl alcohol, cellulose esters,* or both. Artificial tears are indicated for treatment of dry-eye syndromes and relief of discomfort and dryness caused by irritants, wind, and sun. In addition, demulcents may be used to lubricate artificial eyes. Artificial tears are devoid of adverse effects, and hence may be administered as frequently and as long as desired.

Ocular Decongestants

Ocular decongestants are weak solutions of adrenergic agonists applied topically to constrict dilated conjunctival blood vessels. These preparations are used to reduce redness of the eye caused by minor irritation. The adrenergic agents employed as decongestants are *phenylephrine, naphazoline,* and *tetrahydrozoline.* When applied to the eye in the low concentrations found in decongestant products, adrenergic agonists rarely cause adverse effects. Local reactions (stinging, burning, reactive hyperemia) may occur with overuse. The adrenergic agonists are discussed at length in Chapter 17.

Glucocorticoids

Glucocorticoids (anti-inflammatory corticosteroids) are used for inflammatory disorders of the eye (e.g., uveitis, iritis, conjunctivitis). Administration may be topical or by local injection. Short-term therapy is generally devoid of adverse effects. In contrast, prolonged therapy may cause cataracts, reduced visual acuity, and glaucoma. In addition, there is an increased risk of infection secondary to corticosteroid-induced suppression of host defenses. The glucocorticoids are discussed at length in Chapter 68.

Dyes

Fluorescein is a water-soluble dye that produces an intense green color. This agent is applied to the surface of the eye to detect lesions of the corneal epithelium; intact areas of the cornea remain uncolored while abrasions and other defects turn bright green. Intravenous fluorescein is used to facilitate visualization of retinal blood vessels; IV fluorescein has been employed to help evaluate diabetic retinopathy and other abnormalities of the retinal vasculature. Fluorescein can also be used topically and intravenously to assess flow of aqueous humor. Adverse effects from systemic administration include nausea, vomiting, paresthesias, and pruritus. Severe reactions (anaphylaxis, pulmonary edema, cardiac arrest) are rare.

Rose bengal is applied topically to visualize abrasions of the corneal and conjunctival epithelium. Injured tissue appears rose colored when viewed with a slit lamp. The dye is employed for diagnosis of superficial injury to corneal and conjunctival tissue.

Antiviral Agents

Four drugs—*trifluridine, vidarabine, ganciclovir,* and *idoxuridine*—are used topically to treat viral infections of the eye. The pharmacology and specific applications of these drugs are discussed in Chapter 89.

⠿ KEY POINTS

- The glaucomas are a group of diseases characterized by visual field loss secondary to optic nerve damage.
- In open-angle glaucoma, optic nerve injury develops gradually over years. The cause of nerve damage is not known.
- In angle-closure glaucoma, there is blockage of aqueous humor outflow, which causes an abrupt rise in IOP. In the absence of treatment, irreversible damage to the optic nerve occurs in 1 or 2 days.
- Drug therapy of open-angle glaucoma is directed at reducing elevated IOP, the major risk factor for this disease.
- Angle-closure glaucoma is treated with drugs to rapidly reduce IOP and then with corrective surgery to allow aqueous humor outflow.
- Drugs reduce IOP by either facilitating aqueous humor outflow or reducing aqueous humor production.
- Three drug families—beta blockers, alpha$_2$-adrenergic agonists, and prostaglandins—are considered first-line agents for topical therapy of open-angle glaucoma.
- Timolol and other topical beta blockers lower IOP by decreasing aqueous humor production.
- Topical beta blockers can be absorbed in amounts sufficient to cause bronchospasm, bradycardia, and AV heart block.
- Brimonidine, an alpha$_2$ agonist, lowers IOP by decreasing aqueous humor production, and possibly by increasing aqueous humor outflow.
- Latanoprost and other prostaglandin analogs lower IOP by facilitating aqueous humor outflow.
- Prostaglandins can intensify brown pigmentation of the iris, and pigmentation of the skin around the eye.
- Cycloplegics are drugs that paralyze the ciliary muscle.
- Mydriatics are drugs that dilate the pupil.
- Atropine and other anticholinergic drugs cause cycloplegia by blocking muscarinic receptors on the ciliary muscle and cause mydriasis by blocking muscarinic receptors on the iris sphincter.
- By paralyzing the ciliary muscle, anticholinergic drugs prevent the eye from focusing for near vision.
- By paralyzing the iris sphincter, anticholinergic drugs prevent the pupil from constricting in response to bright light; photophobia results.
- Phenylephrine, an adrenergic agonist, causes mydriasis by stimulating alpha-adrenergic receptors on the radial (dilator) muscle of the iris.

Drugs for the Skin

Our objective in this chapter is to discuss some of the more frequently encountered dermatologic drugs. Most are employed topically; some are given systemically. Before discussing the dermatologic drugs, we review the anatomy of the skin.

ANATOMY OF THE SKIN

The skin is composed of three distinct layers: the epidermis, the dermis, and a layer of subcutaneous fat. These layers and other features of the skin are depicted in Figure 101–1.

Epidermis. The epidermis is the outermost layer of the skin and is composed almost entirely of closely packed cells. As indicated in Figure 101–1*B*, the epidermis itself consists of several layers. The deepest, known as the *basal cell layer* or *stratum germinativum*, contains the only epidermal cells that are mitotically active. All cells of the epidermis arise from this layer. Production of new cells within the basal layer pushes older cells outward. During their migration, these cells

become smaller and flatter. As epidermal cells near the surface of the skin, they die and their cytoplasm is converted to *keratin,* a hard, proteinaceous material. Because of its high content of keratin, the outer layer of the epidermis has a rough, horny texture. Because of its texture, this layer is referred to as the *cornified layer* or *stratum corneum.* By a process that is not fully understood, the surface of the stratum corneum undergoes continuous exfoliation (shedding). This shedding completes the growth cycle of the epidermis.

In addition to germinal cells, the basal layer of the epidermis contains *melanocytes.* These cells, which are few in number, produce *melanin,* the pigment that determines skin color. Following its synthesis within melanocytes, melanin is transferred to other cells of the epidermis. Melanin protects the skin against ultraviolet radiation, which is the principal stimulus for melanin production.

Dermis. The dermis underlies the epidermis and is composed largely of connective tissue, primarily collagen. A major function of the dermis is to provide support and nourishment for the epidermis. Structures found in the dermis include blood vessels, nerves, and muscle. The dermis also contains sweat glands, sebaceous glands, and hair follicles. Sebaceous glands secrete an oily composite known as sebum. Almost all sebaceous glands are associated with hair follicles (see Fig. 101–1).

Subcutaneous Tissue. Subcutaneous tissue consists largely of fat. This fatty layer provides protection and insulation. In addition, the stored fat constitutes a reserve source of calories.

TOPICAL GLUCOCORTICOIDS

The basic pharmacology of the glucocorticoids (anti-inflammatory corticosteroids) is discussed in Chapter 68. Consideration here is limited to their use for disorders of the skin.

Actions and Uses. Topical glucocorticoids are employed to relieve inflammation and itching associated with a variety of dermatologic disorders (e.g., insect bites, minor burns, seborrheic dermatitis, psoriasis, eczema, pemphigus). The mechanisms by which glucocorticoids suppress inflammation and other symptoms are discussed in Chapter 68.

The vehicle in which a glucocorticoid is dispersed (e.g., cream, ointment, gel) can enhance the therapeutic response by helping glucocorticoids penetrate to their site of action. The vehicle may provide additional benefits by acting as a drying agent or an emollient.

Relative Potency. Glucocorticoid preparations vary widely in potency. As indicated in Table 101–1, steroid preparations can be assigned to four groups, which range from low potency to super-high potency. Preparations within each group are of approximately equal potency.

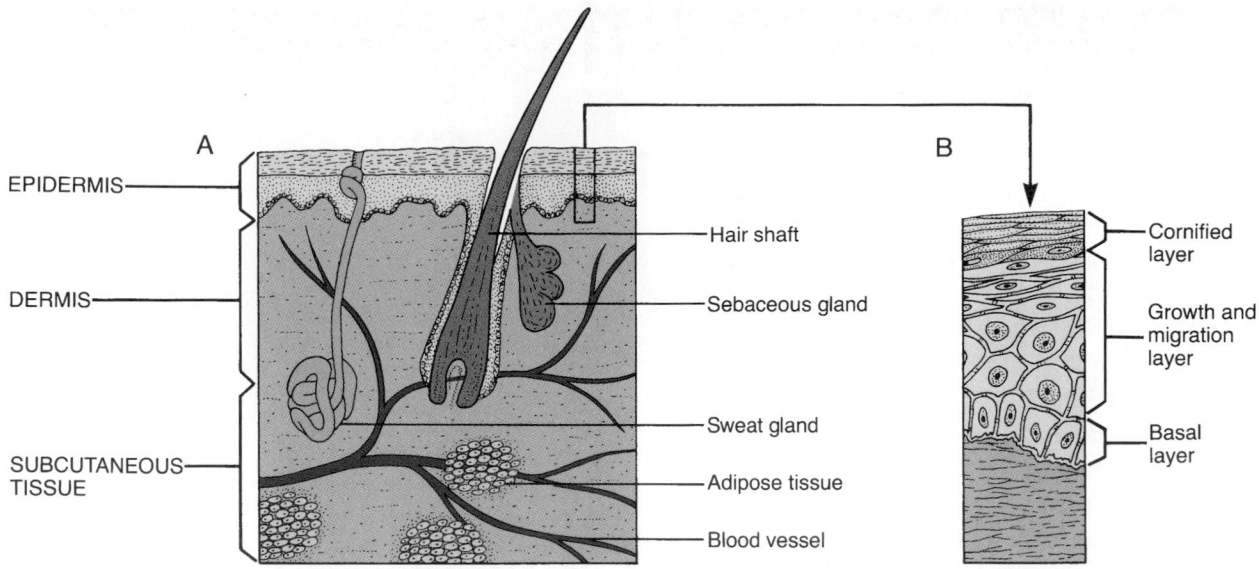

Figure 101–1 ■ **Anatomy of the skin.**
A, Major structures of the skin. *B,* Growth layers of the epidermis.

It is important to note that the intensity of the response to topical glucocorticoids depends not only on the concentration and inherent activity of the glucocorticoid, but also on the vehicle employed and the method of application. Occlusive dressings can enhance percutaneous absorption by as much as 10-fold, thereby greatly increasing pharmacologic effects.

Absorption. Topical glucocorticoids can be absorbed into the systemic circulation. The extent of absorption is proportional to the duration of use and the surface area covered. Absorption is higher from regions where the skin is especially permeable (scalp, axilla, face, eyelids, neck, perineum, genitalia) and lower from regions where penetrability is poor (back, palms, soles). Absorption through intact skin is less than through inflamed skin. As noted, absorption is influenced by the vehicle, and can be greatly increased by use of an occlusive dressing.

Adverse Effects. Adverse effects may be local or systemic. Factors that increase the risk of adverse effects include use of high-potency glucocorticoids, use of occlusive dressings, prolonged therapy, and application over a large surface area.

Local Reactions. Glucocorticoids increase the risk of local infection, and may also produce irritation. With prolonged use, glucocorticoids can cause atrophy of the dermis and epidermis, resulting in thinning of the skin, striae (stretch marks), purpura (red spots caused by local hemorrhage), and telangiectasia (red, wart-like lesions caused by capillary dilation). Long-term therapy may induce acne and hypertrichosis (excessive growth of hair, especially on the face).

Systemic Toxicity. Topical glucocorticoids can be absorbed in amounts sufficient to produce systemic toxicity. Principal concerns are growth retardation (in children) and adrenal suppression (in all age groups). Systemic toxicity is more likely under extreme conditions of use (prolonged therapy in which extensive surfaces are treated with large doses of high-potency agents in conjunction with occlusive dress-

ings). When these conditions are present, the hypothalamic-pituitary-adrenal axis should be monitored. Systemic toxicity of the glucocorticoids is discussed at length in Chapter 68.

Administration. Topical glucocorticoids should be applied in a thin film and gently rubbed into the skin. Patients should be advised not to use occlusive dressings (bandages, plastic wraps) unless the physician tells them to. Tight-fitting diapers and plastic pants can act as occlusive dressings and should not be worn when glucocorticoids are applied to the diaper region of infants.

KERATOLYTIC AGENTS

Keratolytic agents are drugs that promote shedding of the horny layer of the skin. Effects range from peeling to extensive desquamation of the stratum corneum. Two keratolytic compounds—*salicylic acid* and *sulfur*—are considered below. A third agent—*benzoyl peroxide*—is discussed later under *Drugs Used to Treat Acne.*

Salicylic Acid. Salicylic acid promotes desquamation by dissolving the intracellular cement that binds scales to the stratum corneum. Keratolytic effects are achieved with concentrations between 3% and 6%. At concentrations above 6%, tissue injury is likely. Low (3% to 6%) concentrations are used to treat dandruff, seborrheic dermatitis, acne, and psoriasis. Higher concentrations (up to 40%) are used to remove warts and corns.

Salicylic acid is readily absorbed through the skin, and systemic toxicity (salicylism) can result. Symptoms include tinnitus, hyperpnea, and psychologic disturbances. Systemic effects can be minimized by avoiding prolonged use of high concentrations over large areas.

Sulfur. Sulfur promotes peeling and drying. The compound has been used to treat acne, dandruff, psoriasis, and seborrheic dermatitis. Sulfur is available in lotions, gels, and shampoos. Concentrations range from 2% to 10%.

TABLE 101–1 ▪ Relative Potency of Topical Glucocorticoid Preparations		
Potency Class and Drug	**Formulation**	**Concentration**
Super-High Potency		
Betamethasone dipropionate [Diprolene]	Cream, ointment, lotion	0.05%
Clobetasol propionate [Temovate]	Cream, ointment	0.05%
Diflorasone diacetate [Psorcon, Maxiflor, Florone]	Ointment	0.05%
Halobetasol propionate [Ultravate]	Cream, ointment	0.05%
High Potency		
Amcinonide [Cyclocort]	Cream, ointment, lotion	0.1%
Betamethasone dipropionate [Diprosone]	Cream, ointment	0.05%
Desoximetasone [Topicort]	Cream, ointment	0.25%
Diflorasone diacetate [Florone, Maxiflor]	Cream, ointment	0.05%
Flucinolone acetonide [Synalar-HP]	Cream	0.2%
Fluocinonide [Fluonex, Lidex]	Cream, ointment, gel	0.05%
Halcinonide [Halog]	Cream, ointment	0.1%
Triamcinolone acetonide [Aristocort, others]	Ointment	0.1%
Medium Potency		
Betamethasone benzoate [Uticort]	Lotion	0.025%
Betamethasone dipropionate [Diprosone, others]	Lotion	0.05%
Betamethasone valerate [Valisone, Betatrex]	Cream, ointment, lotion	0.1%
Clocortolone pivalate [Cloderm]	Cream	0.1%
Desoximetasone [Topicort]	Cream	0.05%
Fluocinolone acetonide [Flurosyn, Synalar]	Cream, ointment	0.025%
Flurandrenolide [Cordran]	Cream, ointment, lotion	0.05%
Fluticasone propionate [Cutivate]	Ointment	0.005%
	Cream	0.05%
Halcinonide [Halog]	Cream	0.025%
Hydrocortisone valerate [Westcort]	Cream, ointment	0.2%
Mometasone furoate [Elocon]	Cream, ointment, lotion	0.1%
Triamcinolone acetonide [Aristocort, Kenalog]	Cream, ointment, lotion	0.1%
Low Potency		
Alclometasone dipropionate [Aclovate]	Cream, ointment	0.05%
Desonide [DesOwen, Tridesilon]	Aerosol	0.04%
Dexamethasone [Decaspray]	Aerosol	0.04%
Dexamethasone sodium phosphate [Decadron phosphate]	Cream	0.1%
Fluocinolone acetonide [Flurosyn, Synalar]	Cream, solution	0.01%
Hydrocortisone [Cortizone-10, Hycort]	Cream, ointment, lotion	1%

ACNE AND ITS TREATMENT

Acne is the most common dermatologic disease. Over 17 million Americans are affected. Among people ages 11 to 30, about 80% have the disorder. Acne accounts for nearly 20% of all visits to dermatologists.

Pathophysiology

Acne is a chronic skin disorder that usually begins during puberty. The disease is more common and more severe in males. Lesions usually develop on the face, neck, chest, shoulders, and back. In mild acne, *open comedones* (blackheads) are the most common lesion. A comedo forms when sebum combines with keratin to create a plug within a pore (oxidation of the sebum causes the exposed surface of the plug to turn black). *Closed comedones* (whiteheads) develop when pores become stuffed with sebum and scales below the skin surface. In its most severe form, acne is characterized by abscesses and inflammatory cysts. As a

rule, acne begins to resolve after puberty and clears entirely by the early 20s. However, with some people, the disease persists for decades.

Onset of acne is initiated by increased production of androgens during adolescence. Under the influence of androgens, sebum production and turnover of follicular epithelial cells are increased, leading to plugging of pores. Symptoms are intensified by the activity of *Propionibacterium acnes,* a microbe that converts sebum into irritant fatty acids. This bacterium also releases chemotactic factors that promote inflammation. Oily skin and a genetic predisposition are additional contributing factors.

Overview of Treatment

Because acne is a chronic disease, treatment is prolonged. Fortunately, almost all patients respond well. Effective treatment will prevent scarring and limit the duration of symptomatic disease, and will thereby minimize the psychologic effects of having acne.

Nondrug Therapy

Nondrug measures can help minimize lesions, especially in patients with milder acne. Surface oiliness should be reduced by gentle cleansing 2 or 3 times a day. Care should be taken to avoid irritation from vigorous scrubbing or use of abrasives. Oil-based moisturizing products should be avoided. Additional nondrug measures (e.g., comedo extraction, dermabrasion) may be indicated for some individuals. Dietary measures don't help.

Drug Therapy

Drug selection is based on severity of symptoms (Table 101–2). For patients with relatively mild symptoms, topical therapy can suffice. When symptoms are more severe, oral therapy is required. *Mild* acne can be managed with benzoyl peroxide and topical antibiotics. *Moderate* acne can be treated with systemic antibiotics (e.g., tetracycline, erythromycin) and comedolytics (azelaic acid, tretinoin, adapalene, tazarotene). In addition, combination oral contraceptives can be used in young women. The principal agent for *severe* acne is oral isotretinoin.

Drugs Used to Treat Acne
Benzoyl Peroxide

Actions and Uses. Benzoyl peroxide is employed topically to treat mild to moderate acne. Benefits derive primarily from suppressing growth of *P. acnes.* The presumed mechanism is release of active oxygen. In addition to suppressing *P. acnes,* benzoyl peroxide promotes keratolysis (peeling of the horny layer of the epidermis).

Adverse Effects. Benzoyl peroxide may produce drying and peeling of the skin. If signs of severe local irritation occur (e.g., burning, blistering, scaling, swelling), the frequency of application should be reduced.

TABLE 101–2 ▒■ Overview of Drugs for Acne
Mild Acne
Benzoyl peroxide
Topical antibiotics
Clindamycin
Erythromycin
Moderate Acne
Azelaic acid
Topical retinoids
Tretinoin
Adapalene
Tazarotene
Systemic antibiotics
Tetracycline
Minocycline
Doxycycline
Erythromycin
Others
Combination oral contraceptives
Estrostep
Ortho Tri-cyclen
Severe Acne
Isotretinoin, a systemic retinoid

Some formulations contain sulfites, which can cause potentially serious allergic reactions in susceptible persons. The incidence in highest in those with asthma. Otherwise, the incidence is low.

Preparations, Dosage, and Administration. Benzoyl peroxide is available in a variety of formulations (e.g., lotions, creams, gels) for topical use. Concentrations range from 2.5% to 10%. For initial therapy, once-a-day application is recommended. Over time, the frequency of administration can be increased (to a maximum of 3 times a day) as tolerance permits. Patients should be advised to avoid application to the eyes, mouth, and mucous membranes, and to inflamed or denuded skin.

Antibiotics

Topical. Topical antibiotics are indicated for mild to moderate acne. The objective is to suppress growth of *P. acnes.* The antibiotics used most often are *clindamycin* [Cleocin, others] and *erythromycin* [Eryderm, others]. Either drug may be employed alone or in combination with other topical anti-acne drugs (e.g., benzoyl peroxide, tretinoin). With prolonged use, bacterial resistance may develop. Both clindamycin and erythromycin are available in combination with benzoyl peroxide. Clindamycin–benzoyl peroxide is sold as *Benzaclin,* and erythromycin–benzoyl peroxide is sold as *Benzamycin.*

Oral. Oral antibiotics (e.g., tetracycline, minocycline, doxycycline, erythromycin, azithromycin) are indicated when acne is moderate to severe. These agents suppress growth of *P. acnes* and also reduce inflammation directly.

Tetracycline [Sumycin, others] is the traditional treatment of choice. The drug is effective and inexpensive, and has low toxicity. Treatment reduces the population of *P. acnes,* the amount of keratin in sebaceous follicles, and the percentage of free fatty acids in surface lipids. The dosage initially is 1 gm/day in divided doses. Over time, the dosage can be reduced to between 125 and 500 mg/day.

Azithromycin [Zithromax] is an alternative to tetracycline. The drug has a much longer half-life than tetracycline, and hence dosing can be less frequent. Unfortunately, azithromycin is expensive. Accordingly, the drug is generally reserved for patients who are intolerant of or unresponsive to tetracycline and other more commonly used drugs.

Tretinoin

Uses and Mechanisms. Tretinoin [Retin-A, Retin-A Micro, Avita, Renova], a derivative of vitamin A, is a topical drug used for acne and for removing fine wrinkles. Formulations for acne are marketed under the trade names Retin-A and Avita. The formulation for wrinkles, which is nearly identical to one of the formulations for acne, is marketed under the trade name Renova. Tretinoin should not be confused with isotretinoin, an *oral* antiacne medicine (see below).

Acne. Tretinoin is approved for topical treatment of mild to moderate acne. Therapeutic effects can be enhanced by using tretinoin in combination with benzoyl peroxide and oral antibiotics.

Although the mechanism for clearing acne is unknown, tretinoin is thought to help at least in part by increasing the turnover and reducing the cohesiveness of epithelial cells within hair follicles. These actions may promote removal of existing comedones and may suppress formation of new plugs. In addition, by reducing the thickness of the stratum corneum, tretinoin can enhance penetration of other antiacne drugs.

Special Interest Topic

BOX 101–1 ▪▪ FACE TIME WITH BOTOX

Frown ridges got you down? Brow lines make you whine? Don't mind injecting your face with a deadly poison? If you answered "Yes" to these questions, then you may be a candidate for Botox—the hottest thing in cosmetic medicine since the nose job. How hot? In 2001, over 1.6 million Americans underwent Botox treatment, making it the number 1 nonsurgical cosmetic procedure in the United States—and this was *before* the drug was approved for cosmetic use.

Why do people love Botox? Because it makes them look younger. By making facial lines go away. Without surgery. And it's cheaper and less traumatic than a face-lift.

Just what is Botox? Well, Botox is a trade name for *botulinum toxin type A*, a protein produced by the gram-negative bacterium *Clostridium botulinum*. And yes, Botox *is* the same toxin that causes botulism, a potentially fatal condition brought on by eating foods contaminated with *C. botulinum*. (Just in case you're curious: Common signs and symptoms of botulism include double vision, dysphagia, generalized weakness, urinary retention, and respiratory impairment—all without any decrease in mentation. Death results from respiratory arrest secondary to paralysis of the muscles of respiration.) You're probably asking, "Can *Botox* do all of that?" Not really. The doses employed are *much* to small to produce these widespread effects.

How does Botox work? Botulinum toxin type A is a neurotoxin that acts on cholinergic neurons to block release of acetylcholine. Following injection, the drug is taken up by cholinergic nerve terminals where it then inactivates SNAP-25, a protein critical to the function of acetylcholine-containing vesicles. In the absence of SNAP-25, the vesicles are unable to fuse with the terminal membrane, and hence cannot release their acetylcholine. Restoration of neuronal function requires sprouting of new terminals, a process that can take several months. Botulinum toxin blocks transmission at neuromuscular junctions and at cholinergic synapses of the autonomic nervous system.

What are the cosmetic uses of Botox? On April 15, 2002, the Food and Drug Administration (FDA) approved Botox for reducing frown lines, known formally as "glabellar" lines (because they appear on the glabella—the smooth area located between your eyebrows, directly above your nose). At this time, reduction of frown lines is the only cosmetic use approved by the FDA. Nonetheless, Botox is also used widely to soften lines on the forehead and neck, and to diminish "crow's-feet" (lines that form near the outer corners of our eyes when we squint).

Does Botox have any other approved uses? Yes. And they preceded its cosmetic use by more than a decade. In 1989, the FDA approved Botox for two ocular disorders: strabismus (misaligned eye, aka "lazy eye") and blepharospasm (involuntary, intermittent forced closure of the eyelid). Also, in December 2000, the drug was approved for cervical dystonia, a neurologic disorder characterized by painful, sustained contraction of muscles in the neck. Unlabeled uses include spasmodic torticollis (clonic twisting of the head), hemifacial spasms (unilateral contraction of facial muscles in any combi-

nation), overactive bladder syndrome, and hyperhidrosis (excessive sweating) of the armpits and palms.

How is cosmetic Botox applied? With a needle. In the face. To be precise, to reduce frown lines, Botox is injected directly into the small muscles that produce a frown when they contract. Five injections are made, each consisting of 4 units of botulinum toxin in 0.1 ml of fluid. Two injections go into each corrugator muscle and one into the procerus muscle. The whole procedure takes just a few minutes. Discomfort can be reduced by pretreatment with a topical anesthetic cream.

What's the time course of Botox effects? Results are neither instantaneous nor permanent. Rather, muscle paralysis develops slowly—over 3 to 10 days—and then fades within 3 to 6 months. Botox injections may be repeated to maintain cosmetic benefits. However, at least 3 months should separate treatments. At this time, there are no data on the long-term effects of Botox injections.

Does Botox have side effects? Of course—It's a drug, isn't it? The most common side effects are headache, respiratory infection, and a flu-like syndrome. Treatment may also cause facial pain, swelling, and bruising. Swelling and bruising can be reduced by applying ice to the site, and by avoiding alcohol, vitamin E, and aspirin (and related nonsteroidal anti-inflammatory drugs) for the week preceding treatment. There are no data on side effects with repeated use.

Injection into the wrong site (or diffusion from the right site into surrounding tissues) can weaken muscles that were not intended targets, thereby causing multiple undesired effects. Ptosis (droopy eyelids) occurs in about 5% of patients, and can persist for 3 to 6 months. Injections in the lower face can result in drooling, an asymmetric smile, drooping mouth, and biting the inside of the cheek. Injections in the neck can make swallowing difficult and can change vocal pitch. All of these problems can be reduced by taking steps to minimize Botox displacement. Accordingly, for at least 4 hours after the injections, patients should avoid lying down, rubbing the injection site, and washing their hair. Of course, it also helps to have Botox administered by a highly trained expert, preferably a dermatologist or plastic surgeon.

Excessive dosing can cause loss of facial expression. Patients can lose the ability to frown, raise their eyebrows, or squint. This may be fine if you're a professional poker player, but can be a disaster if you're an actor—or just an ordinary person who doesn't want to spend a few months projecting Buddha-like calm (rather than the anger you're really feeling because an incompetent physician froze your face).

Who should *not* use Botox? The drug should be avoided by women who are pregnant or breast-feeding, and by patients who may be allergic to human albumin, a protein found in Botox preparations. In addition, Botox should be avoided by people using aminoglycoside antibiotics or any other agent that has neuromuscular blocking properties. The drug should be used with caution in patients with myasthenia gravis and other neuromuscular disorders that can intensify muscle paralysis. Lastly, Botox should be avoided by people over 65. Why?

Fine Wrinkles. Tretinoin is approved for mitigating (reducing) fine wrinkles, tactile roughness, and mottled hyperpigmentation (liver spots, age spots) in facial skin. Benefits may derive from suppressing genes that code for specific proteases that break down collagen and elastin. In clinical trials, responses to tretinoin were modest. In fact, many patients achieved equivalent effects with a program of comprehensive skin care and sun protection. It is important to note that tretinoin does *not* repair deep, coarse wrinkles and other damage caused by chronic sun exposure. Furthermore, the drug does not eliminate wrinkles, repair sun-damaged skin, reverse photo-aging, or restore the microscopic structure of skin to a more youthful pattern. Lastly, benefits in patients over the age of 50 have not been established.

Adverse Effects. Tretinoin can cause *localized* reactions, but absorption is insufficient to cause systemic toxicity. In patients with sensitive skin, tretinoin may induce blistering, peeling, crusting, burning, and edema. These effects can be intensified by concurrent use of abrasive soaps and keratolytic agents (e.g., sulfur, resorcinol, benzoyl peroxide, salicylic acid). Accordingly, these preparations should be discontinued prior to tretinoin therapy. Skin reactions with two new formulations—Avita and Retin-A Micro—may be less intense than those caused by Retin-A.

Tretinoin increases susceptibility to sunburn. Patients should be warned to apply a sunscreen (sun protection factor [SPF] of 15 or greater) and wear protective clothing. Patients with existing sunburn should not use the drug.

Preparations, Dosage, and Administration. For Acne. For treatment of acne, tretinoin is available under three trade names: Retin-A, Retin-A Micro, and Avita. Products marketed as Retin-A are available in three formulations: cream (0.025%, 0.05%, and 0.1%), gel (0.01% and 0.025%), and liquid (0.05%). Retin-A Micro is dispensed as a 0.1% gel, and Avita as a 0.025% cream. All products are administered topically, usually once a day at bedtime. Before application, the skin should be washed, toweled dry, and allowed to dry fully for 15 to 30 minutes. Tretinoin should not be applied to open wounds or to areas of sunburn or windburn. Contact with the eyes, nose, and mouth should be avoided.

For Fine Wrinkles. Tretinoin [Renova] is available in a 0.05% cream for treating fine wrinkles of the face. Application is done once daily at bedtime.

time. Cosmetics should be washed off before use. Up to 6 months of treatment may be needed to see a response, and treatment must continue to maintain the response.

Adapalene

Adapalene [Differin] is a topical antiacne drug similar to tretinoin. Through actions in the cell nucleus, adapalene modulates inflammation, epithelial keratinization, and differentiation of follicular cells. As a result, the drug reduces formation of comedones and inflammatory lesions. Benefits take 8 to 12 weeks to develop. During the early weeks of treatment, adapalene may appear to exacerbate acne by affecting previously invisible lesions. In clinical trials, 0.1% adapalene gel was as effective as 0.025% tretinoin gel in reducing the total number of comedones, and was more effective than tretinoin in reducing the total number of acne lesions and inflammatory lesions.

Adverse effects are limited to sites of application. The drug is not absorbed, and hence systemic effects are absent. Common side effects include burning (10% to 40%), pruritus or burning immediately after application (20%), erythema, dryness, and scaling. These are most likely during the first 2 to 4 weeks of treatment and tend to subside as treatment continues.

Adapalene increases the risk of developing sunburn and can intensify existing sunburn. Accordingly, all patients should apply a sunscreen and wear protective clothing prior to extended sun exposure. In addition, adapalene should not be used until existing sunburn has resolved.

Adapalene is available in three 0.1% formulations—gel, cream, and solution—for once-daily application in the evening. Application to the eyes, lips, and mucous membranes should be avoided.

Tazarotene

Tazarotene [Tazorac] is a new drug for topical therapy of acne, wrinkles, and psoriasis. Like tretinoin and adapalene, tazarotene is a derivative of vitamin A. For treatment of acne, tazarotene is available in a 0.1% gel and 0.1% cream. The gel or cream is applied to affected areas of the face each evening. The face should be cleaned and dried before application. The most common side effects—itching, burning, and dry skin—occur more often with tazarotene than with tretinoin or adapalene. Like other retinoids, tazarotene sensitizes the skin to ultraviolet light, and hence patients should be advised to use a sunscreen and wear protective clothing. The basic pharmacology of tazarotene is discussed below under *Psoriasis and Its Treatment.*

Azelaic Acid

Azelaic acid [Azelex] is a topical drug for mild to moderate acne. It appears to work by suppressing growth of *P. acnes* and by decreasing proliferation of keratinocytes, which decreases the thickness of the stratum corneum. In clinical trials, topical azelaic acid (20% cream) was as effective as 5% benzoyl peroxide, 0.05% tretinoin, or 2% erythromycin. For severe acne, azelaic acid was much less effective than oral isotretinoin. Adverse effects—which are uncommon and less intense than with tretinoin or benzoyl peroxide—include pruritus, burning, stinging, tingling, and erythema. Azelaic acid may decrease pigmentation in patients with dark complexions. Hence, these people should be monitored for hypopigmentation. Azelaic acid is applied twice daily by gently massaging a thin film into the affected area. Contact with the eyes, nose, and mouth should be avoided. Before application, the skin should be washed and patted dry.

Isotretinoin

Actions and Use. Isotretinoin [Accutane], a derivative of vitamin A, is used to treat *severe nodulocystic acne vulgaris,* a condition for which the drug is highly effective. For most patients, a single course of therapy can produce complete and prolonged remission. Because isotretinoin can cause serious side effects, use is restricted to patients with severe, disfiguring acne that has not responded to more conventional agents, including oral antibiotics. Accutane is highly teratogenic, and hence must not be used during pregnancy.

Isotretinoin has several actions that may contribute to antiacne effects. The drug decreases sebum production, sebaceous gland size, inflammation, and keratinization. In addition, by decreasing availability of sebum, a nutrient for *P. acnes,* isotretinoin lowers the skin population of this microbe.

Pharmacokinetics. Absorption from the GI tract is rapid but incomplete. In the blood, isotretinoin is nearly 100% bound to albumin. The drug undergoes metabolism in the liver and possibly in cells of the intestinal wall. Excretion is by a combination of renal and biliary processes. The drug's half-life is 10 to 20 hours.

Adverse Effects. Common Effects. The most common reactions are nosebleeds (80%), inflammation of the lips (90%), inflammation of the eyes (40%), and dryness or itching of the skin, nose, and mouth (80%). About 15% of patients experience pain, tenderness, or stiffness in muscles, bones, and joints. Among pediatric patients, nearly 30% experience back pain. Less common reactions include skin rash, headache, hair loss, and peeling of skin from the palms and soles. Reduction in night vision has occurred, sometimes with sudden onset. The skin may become sensitized to ultraviolet light; patients should be advised to wear protective clothing or a sunscreen if responses to sunlight become exaggerated. Rarely, isotretinoin causes optic neuritis, cataracts, papilledema (edema of the optic disk), and pseudotumor cerebri (benign elevation of intracranial pressure).

Triglyceride levels may become elevated. Blood triglyceride content should be measured prior to treatment and peri-odically thereafter until effects on triglycerides have been evaluated. Alcohol can potentiate hypertriglyceridemia and should be avoided.

Although the above adverse effects occur frequently, most reverse upon discontinuing the drug.

Rare Effect: Depression. Isotretinoin may pose a small risk of depression and suicide, although proof of a causal relationship is lacking. With some patients, depression developed while taking isotretinoin, resolved when the drug was discontinued, and then recurred when treatment was resumed. Since 1989, at least 12 patients have committed suicide. However, there is no definitive proof that isotretinoin was the cause, and no mechanism for inducing depression has been established. Nonetheless, since the potential consequences of depression are severe, steps should be taken to minimize risk. Accordingly, clinicians should ask patients to report signs of depression (e.g., depressed mood, loss of interest or pleasure) or thoughts of suicide. If these occur, isotretinoin should be withdrawn.

Drug Interactions. Adverse effects of isotretinoin can be increased by *tetracyclines* and *vitamin A.* Tetracyclines increase the risk of pseudotumor cerebri and papilledema. Vitamin A, a close relative of isotretinoin, can produce generalized intensification of isotretinoin toxicity. Because of the potential for increased toxicity, tetracyclines and vitamin A supplements should be discontinued prior to isotretinoin therapy.

Contraindication: Pregnancy. Isotretinoin is teratogenic and must not be used during pregnancy. The drug is classified in Food and Drug Administration (FDA) Pregnancy Risk Category X: the risks of use during pregnancy clearly outweigh any possible benefits. Major fetal abnormalities that have occurred include hydrocephalus, microcephaly, facial malformation, cleft palate, cardiovascular defects, and abnormal formation of the outer ear.

S.M.A.R.T—the System to Manage Accutane-Related Teratogenicity. S.M.A.R.T. is a new and very strict risk management program designed to ensure that (1) no woman starting isotretinoin is pregnant and that (2) no woman taking isotretinoin becomes pregnant. The new safeguards have rules that apply to the physician, the patient, and the pharmacist.

For the Physician. Physicians who want to prescribe isotretinoin must first read a 28-page "Guide to Best Practices" published by the manufacturer, and then must sign a letter of understanding. Certified physicians are given a packet of bright yellow, self-adhesive "Accutane Qualification Stickers" that must be applied to each prescription. The stickers tell the pharmacist that the patient is qualified to receive the drug.

For Female Patients. Each patient must receive oral and written warning about the high risk of fetal harm if isotretinoin is taken during pregnancy.

Pregnancy must be ruled out before the initial prescription, and before each monthly refill. Prior to the initial prescription, *two* negative test results are required. For the monthly refills, only one negative test is required.

Each patient must use *two* effective forms of birth control, even if one of them is tubal ligation or vasectomy of the male partner. In addition, the patient must watch a videotape, provided by the manufacturer, that gives information on contraceptive methods, possible reasons for contraceptive failure, and the importance of using effective contraception while taking teratogenic drugs. Birth control measures must be implemented at least 1 month before starting isotretinoin, and must continue at least 1 month after stopping. Birth control is not required following hysterectomy or for women who commit to total abstinence from sexual intercourse.

Each patient must fill out and sign an informed consent document, designed to reinforce the benefits and risks of isotretinoin use. The prescriber must sign too.

For the Pharmacist. Only those prescriptions that bear an "Accutane Qualification Sticker" can be filled. This restriction applies not only to the original prescription, but to all refills as well. All prescriptions must be presented in person; telephone orders and computerized orders cannot be filled. Prescriptions must be filled within 7 days of the qualification date.

Preparations, Dosage, and Administration. Isotretinoin [Accutane] is dispensed in capsules (10, 20, and 40 mg) for oral administration. The usual course of treatment is 0.5 to 1 mg/kg/day (in two divided doses) for 15 to 20 weeks. If needed, a second course may be given, but not until 2 months have elapsed after completing the first course.

Oral Contraceptives

Two combination oral contraceptives (OCs)—Estrostep and Ortho Tri-Cyclen—are approved for treating acne in young women. Treatment is limited to females at least 15 years old who want contraception, have reached menarche, and have not responded to topical drugs. Acne may take up to 6 months to improve. Benefits derive from the *estrogen* in combination OCs—not from the progestin. Two mechanisms are involved. First, estrogens suppress production of androgens by the ovary. (Recall that androgens promote acne by stimulating production of sebum.) Second, estrogens further reduce androgen availability by increasing production of *sex hormone–binding globulin,* a protein that binds androgens and thereby renders them inactive. Although only two OCs are approved for acne, all combination OCs should be effective. Accordingly, selection among them should be based primarily on tolerability.

SUNSCREENS

Sunlight has multiple effects on the skin. In addition to promoting tanning, solar radiation can cause burns, premature aging of the skin, skin cancer (secondary to DNA damage), and immunosuppression. Sun exposure can also induce photosensitivity reactions to drugs. All of these effects are caused by ultraviolet (UV) radiation.

The dermatologic effects of UV radiation differ for UV radiation in the A range (UVA; wavelengths of 320 to 400 nm) versus UV radiation in the B range (UVB; wavelengths of 290 to 320 nm). UVB radiation causes sunburn and photoaging of the skin (wrinkling, thickening, yellowing, breakdown of elastic fibers). In contrast, UVA radiation, which penetrates much deeper than UVB, can cause immunosuppression, photosensitivity reactions to drugs, and damage to DNA. DNA damage, in turn, leads to premalignant actinic keratoses, basal cell carcinoma, squamous cell carcinoma, and malignant and nonmalignant melanoma. Both UVA and UVB promote tanning.

Benefits of Sunscreens

Sunscreens impede penetration of solar radiation to viable cells of the skin. As a result, they can protect against sunburn, photo-aging of the skin, and photosensitivity reactions to certain drugs (e.g., tricyclic antidepressants, phenothiazines, sulfonamides, sulfonylureas). Unfortunately, *sunscreens provide very little protection against skin cancer:* Regular sunscreen use reduces the risk of squamous cell carcinoma by about 40%, but does not provide any protection against basal cell carcinoma or melanoma.

Compounds Employed as Sunscreens

There are two categories of sunscreens: chemical screens and physical screens. Chemical screens *absorb* UV radiation, whereas physical screens *scatter* UV radiation. At this time, 16 compounds are FDA approved for use as sunscreens.

Chemical Screens. Most (14) of the approved sunscreens are of the chemical type. Almost all of them absorb UV radiation in the B range (see Fig. 101–2). However, only a few absorb radiation in the A range. And only one—*avobenzone*—offers protection against the *full* UVA spectrum. Accordingly, products that contain avobenzone (e.g., Shade UVAGuard, PreSun Ultra, Age Block Daytime Defense Cream) may be superior for protection against cancer, immunosuppression, and photosensitivity reactions to drugs.

Physical Screens. Physical screens act primarily as barriers to the sun's rays. Hence, rather than absorbing solar radiation, they *reflect and scatter* sunlight, thereby preventing penetration to the skin. Only two agents are employed as physical screens: *titanium dioxide* and *zinc oxide.* Preparations containing these compounds are especially useful for protecting limited areas (e.g., nose, lips, tips of ears). In the formulations used today, titanium dioxide and zinc oxide are "micronized." As a result, they are clear when applied to the skin (compared with older formulations, which were white).

Sun Protection Factor

All sunscreen products are labeled with a sun protection factor (SPF). The SPF is an index of protection against UVB radiation. (At this time, there is no test for protection against UVA.)

The SPF is determined by shining UV light on adjacent regions of protected and unprotected skin and recording the time required for erythema (redness) to develop in both areas. The SPF is calculated by dividing the time required for erythema to develop in the protected region by the time required for erythema to develop in the unprotected region. For example, if the unprotected region developed erythema in 15 minutes, and the protected region developed erythema in 150 minutes, the sunscreen would have an SPF of 10 (150 divided by 15). It should be noted that the methods for determining the SPF are not highly precise. Hence, all products labeled with the same SPF may not provide an equal degree of protection.

You should appreciate that the relationship between SPF and protection against sunburn is not linear. That is, an SPF of 30 does not indicate twice as much protections as an SPF of 15. In fact, as the SPF increases, the increment in protection gets progressively smaller. For example, SPF 15 indicates 93% block of UVB, SPF 30 indicates 96.7% block, and SPF 40 indicates 97.5% block. Because SPF values above 30 provide but a small additional benefit, the FDA no longer allows companies to advertise high SPF values (e.g., SPF 50). Instead products with an SPF greater than 30 can only be labeled as SPF 30+.

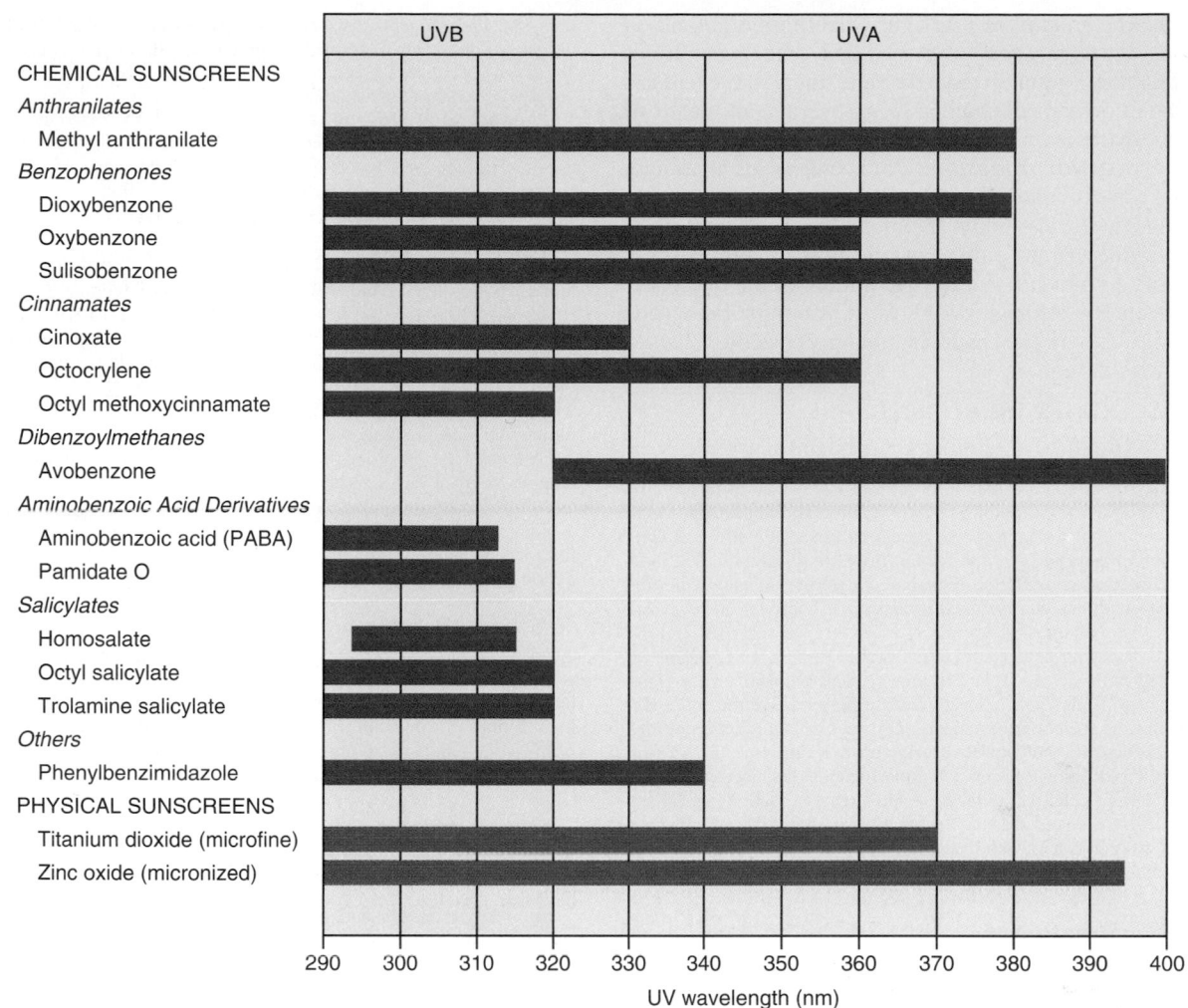

Figure 101–2 ■ Range of UVA and UVB protection offered by FDA-approved chemical and physical sunscreens.

Water and Sweat Resistance

The FDA has defined two degrees of resistance to being washed off in water or by sweating. Products labeled as *water resistant* must retain their SPF for at least 40 minutes of activity. Products labeled as *very water resistant* must retain their SPF for at least 80 minutes of activity.

Adverse Effects of Sunscreens

Contact dermatitis and photosensitivity reactions can occur, especially with products that contain *para*-aminobenzoic acid (PABA) derivatives. PABA-containing products should be avoided by people with allergies to benzocaine, sulfonamides, or thiazides, all of which can cross-react with PABA.

Safe Sunning

To protect against skin damage from sunlight, we should use a sunscreen, protective clothing, and common sense.

Using a Sunscreen Effectively. Sunscreens must be used properly to achieve maximum benefit. The American Academy of Dermatology recommends using a sunscreen with coverage against both UVA and UVB. The SPF should be at least 15. Individuals who burn easily should use a higher SPF.

Protection is greatest when a sunscreen has been allowed to penetrate the skin in advance of exposure to the sun. Accordingly, it is recommended that sunscreens be applied at least 30 minutes prior to going outdoors; sunscreens containing PABA or padimate O should be applied up to 2 hours in advance. The amount applied is an important determinant of protection; 2 mg/cm² is considered adequate. Sunscreens should be reapplied after swimming and profuse sweating; failure to do so reduces the duration of protection. However, it is important to note that reapplication will not extend the period of protection beyond that indicated by the SPF. That is, if treated skin can be expected to burn when sun exposure exceeds 2 hours, no amount of reapplication can prevent burning if the duration of exposure exceeds the limit.

Environmental factors play a part in sunscreen use. The intensity of UVB radiation is greatest between the hours of 10:00 AM and 4:00 PM. Accordingly, the need for a sunscreen is correspondingly high during this time. Ultraviolet radiation can be reflected by painted surfaces, white sand, and snow, thereby augmenting total UV exposure. Accordingly, the contribution of reflected radiation should be considered when choosing a sunscreen. Clouds can filter out UV radiation.

Nonetheless, the amount of UV light reaching the ground on a bright day with thin cloud cover can be as much as 80% of that reaching the ground on days that are sunny and clear. Ultraviolet radiation can penetrate at least several centimeters of clear water; swimmers should be made aware of this fact.

Other Protection Measures. Sunscreens alone cannot completely protect against sun damage. Accordingly, to further reduce risk, you should wear sunglasses, protective clothing, and a wide-brimmed hat. In addition, common sense dictates avoiding sun exposure in the middle of the day, especially between 10:00 AM and 4:00 PM. If you must be outside at these times, stay in the shade as much as possible.

PSORIASIS AND ITS TREATMENT

Pathophysiology

Psoriasis is a chronic inflammatory disorder that follows an erratic course. The initial episode usually develops in early adulthood. Subsequent attacks may occur spontaneously or may be triggered by emotional stress, streptococcal pharyngitis (sore throat), and certain drugs (e.g., propranolol, indomethacin). There is no cure for psoriasis, but symptoms can usually be controlled with medication. Drug-induced remission is common and may last from a few weeks to many years.

Psoriasis has varying degrees of severity. Mild disease manifests as red patches covered with silvery scales; lesions typically appear on the scalp, elbows, knees, palms, and soles. Severe disease may involve the entire skin surface and mucous membranes; patients may develop superficial pustules, high fever, leukocytosis, and painful fissuring of the skin.

Symptoms appear to result from two underlying causes: accelerated maturation of epidermal cells (keratinocytes) and excessive activity of inflammatory cells. There is some evidence that psoriasis is primarily an inflammatory disorder, and that excessive proliferation of keratinocytes is a secondary response.

Overview of Treatment

Drug therapy is directed at two targets: keratinocytes and inflammatory cells. Several drugs suppress proliferation of keratinocytes cells. However, most drugs used for psoriasis suppress activity of T cells and other inflammatory cells.

Drug selection is based on the severity of symptoms. For mild psoriasis, topical glucocorticoids are usually adequate; keratolytic agents (e.g., sulfur, salicylic acid) may be useful adjuncts to steroid therapy. Calcipotriene may also be tried. For patients with moderate symptoms, coal tar or anthralin may be added to the regimen. Topical therapy with tar and anthralin can be enhanced by exposing the skin to UVB light. Treatment options for moderate to severe psoriasis include phototherapy or systemic treatment with methotrexate, acitretin, or alefacept.

Topical Drugs for Psoriasis
Glucocorticoids

In the United States, glucocorticoids are the most commonly used topical drugs for psoriasis. Benefits derive from suppressing the activity of inflammatory cells. Preparations of super-high potency are employed where plaques are thickest. However, super-high-potency agents should not be applied to the face, groin, axilla, or genitalia—because skin in these regions is especially vulnerable to glucocorticoid-induced atrophy.

Tazarotene

Therapeutic Use. Tazarotene [Tazorac] is a vitamin A derivative indicated for topical therapy of mild to moderate psoriasis. Following application to the skin, tazarotene is rapidly converted to tazarotenic acid, its active form. In clinical trials, application of a 0.1% tazarotene gel once daily for 12 weeks produced a significant reduction in lesions in 50% to 70% of patients. Benefits were about equivalent to those seen with 0.05% fluocinonide, a high-potency topical glucocorticoid. Tazarotenic acid stays in the skin long after application of tazarotene has stopped. As a result, benefits may persist for several months.

Adverse Effects. Adverse effects are limited largely to the skin. The most common local reactions (10% to 30%) are itching, burning, stinging, dry skin, and redness. Less common effects (1% to 10%) include rash, desquamation, contact dermatitis, inflammation, fissuring, and bleeding. Tazarotene sensitizes the skin to sunlight. Accordingly, patients should be advised to use a sunscreen and wear protective clothing.

Preparations, Dosage, and Administration. Tazarotene gel [Tazorac] is available in two concentrations: 0.05% and 0.1%. The gel is applied once daily in the evening. No more than 20% of the body surface area should be covered. Wet skin should be dried before application.

Anthralin

Anthralin is indicated only for topical treatment of psoriasis. The drug inhibits DNA synthesis and thereby suppresses proliferation of hyperplastic epidermal cells.

Anthralin may cause local irritation, especially when applied in concentrations above 1%. Erythema (redness) may develop in normal skin adjacent to areas of treatment. Severe conjunctivitis can develop following contact with the eyes. Systemic toxicity has not been documented. Anthralin preparations can stain clothing, skin, and hair.

Anthralin is dispensed in ointments and creams, with concentrations ranging from 0.1% to 1%. In conventional therapy, the drug is applied to lesions at bedtime and allowed to remain in place overnight. Stains can be avoided by wearing old clothing and by covering treated areas with a dressing. Trade names for anthralin products are Anthra-Derm, Drithocreme, Dritho-Scalp, and Micanol.

Tars

Tars suppress DNA synthesis, mitotic activity, and cell proliferation. Coal tar is the tar employed most frequently. Preparations that contain juniper tar, birch tar, and pine tar are also available. Tar-containing products (e.g., shampoos, lotions, creams) are used to treat psoriasis and other chronic disorders of the skin. Tars have an unpleasant odor and can cause irritation, stinging, and burning. They may also stain the skin and hair. Systemic toxicity does not occur.

Calcipotriene

Calcipotriene [Dovonex], an analog of vitamin D_3, is indicated for mild to moderate psoriasis. Responses are equal to those achieved with medium-potency topical glucocorticoids. Improvement may take 1 to 2 months to develop. Benefits may derive from the drug's ability to suppress cell differentiation and proliferation. The most common adverse effect is local skin irritation. Unlike glucocorticoids, calcipotriene does not cause thinning of the skin. At doses twice the weekly recommended maximum of 100 gm, calcipotriene has caused hypercalcemia. Long-term safety has not been established.

Systemic Drugs for Psoriasis
Methotrexate

The basic pharmacology of methotrexate [Rheumatrex] is discussed in Chapter 98 (Anticancer Drugs I). Consideration here is limited to treatment of psoriasis.

Actions and Use in Psoriasis. Methotrexate is a cytotoxic agent that shows some selectivity for tissues with a high growth fraction (i.e., tissues with a large percentage of actively dividing cells). Benefits in psoriasis result from reduced proliferation of epidermal cells. The biochemical mechanisms underlying suppression of cell growth and division are discussed in Chapter 98. Methotrexate is highly toxic and should be used only in patients with severe, debilitating psoriasis that has not responded to safer therapy.

Adverse Effects. Methotrexate is administered systemically, and toxicity can be severe. Death has occurred. Patients should be fully informed of the risks of treatment. Close medical supervision is required. Gastrointestinal effects (diarrhea, ulcerative stomatitis) are the most frequent reasons for interrupting therapy. Blood dyscrasias (anemia, leukopenia, thrombocytopenia) from bone marrow depression are an additional major concern. With prolonged use, even at relatively low doses, methotrexate can cause significant harm to the liver. Accordingly, hepatic function must be monitored; a liver biopsy is the best method for assessing injury. Methotrexate can cause congenital anomalies and fetal death, and hence is contraindicated during pregnancy.

Dosage and Administration. Methotrexate may be administered PO, IM, or IV. Various dosing schedules have been developed. In one schedule, the drug is administered once a week as a single large dose (10 to 25 mg). In an alternative schedule, three smaller doses (2.5 to 5 mg) are administered at 12-hour intervals; this dosing sequence is repeated weekly. Regardless of the schedule chosen, dosages must be individualized.

Acitretin

Acitretin [Soriatane] is the principal active metabolite of etretinate [Tegison], a highly toxic drug that was recently withdrawn. The major difference between the two drugs is pharmacokinetic: Whereas etretinate has a very long half-life (120 days), the half-life of acitretin is much shorter (only 49 hours). Accordingly, acitretin is cleared from the body much faster than etretinate. Although acitretin is less dangerous than etretinate, it still can cause serious harm.

Mechanism of Action. Acitretin acts on epithelial cells to inhibit keratinization, proliferation, and differentiation. These actions probably contribute to its beneficial effects. Benefits may also derive from anti-inflammatory and immunomodulatory actions.

Therapeutic Use. Acitretin is indicated for severe psoriasis, including erythrodermic and generalized pustular types. Efficacy is equivalent to that of etretinate. In clinical trials, the drug produced a 60% to 70% reduction in the severity and area of symptoms. The relapse rate was 40% at 12 weeks after termination of treatment. Because side effects are very common and sometimes severe, acitretin should be reserved for patients who have not responded to safer drugs.

Pharmacokinetics. Administration is oral and absorption is enhanced by food. In the blood, acitretin is 99.9% bound to plasma proteins. The drug undergoes extensive metabolism followed by excretion in the urine and bile. Its half-life is 49 hours. If taken with alcohol, acitretin will be converted to etretinate.

Adverse Effects. Adverse effects are extremely common. Hair loss and skin peeling occur in 50% to 75% of patients. Other dermatologic effects (dry skin, nail disorders, pruritus) occur in 25% to 50% of patients. Mucous membranes are affected, causing rhinitis (25% to 50%), inflammation of the lips (25% to 50%), dry mouth (10% to 25%), nosebleed (10% to 25%), and gingival bleeding, gingivitis, and stomatitis (1% to 10%). Other common reactions include erythematous rash (10% to 25%), bone and joint pain (10% to 25%), spinal hyperostosis (10% to 25%), dry eyes (10% to 25%), and paresthesias (10% to 25%). In addition, acitretin can elevate plasma triglycerides and reduce levels of high-density-lipoprotein cholesterol (good cholesterol). Signs of liver damage (elevation of aminotransferase activity) develop in one-third of patients, but normally resolve when treatment is stopped.

Drug Interactions. Alcohol promotes conversion of acitretin to etretinate, and can thereby greatly prolong the risk of teratogenic effects (see below). Accordingly, women of child-bearing age should be warned against drinking alcohol. Acitretin can reduce the efficacy of progestin-only oral contraceptives, and hence other forms of contraception are preferred. Because acitretin is a derivative of vitamin A, combining it with vitamin A supplements may pose a risk of vitamin A toxicity. Both acitretin and tetracycline can cause pseudotumor cerebri (intracranial hypertension), and therefore combining the drugs is not recommended. In addition, acitretin should not be combined with methotrexate and other drugs that can damage the liver.

Contraindication: Pregnancy. Acitretin is embryotoxic and teratogenic, and therefore must not be used during pregnancy. The drug is classified in FDA Pregnancy Risk Category X: the risks of use during pregnancy clearly outweigh any possible benefits. Major human fetal abnormalities that have been reported include encephalocele (hernia of the brain through a skull defect), reduced cranial volume, facial malformation, cardiovascular defects, absence of terminal phalanges, and malformations of the hip, ankles, and forearms.

Before acitretin is given to women of reproductive age, pregnancy should be ruled out and a method of contraception implemented. Contraception should be initiated at least 1 month prior to treatment and should continue for at least 3 years after treatment has ceased. Women should be thoroughly counseled about the potential for fetal harm. If pregnancy occurs, acitretin should be discontinued immediately, and possible termination of pregnancy should be discussed.

Preparations, Dosage, and Administration. Acitretin [Soriatane] is available in 25- and 50-mg capsules for oral administration. The dosage is 25 or 50 mg once daily, taken with a meal to facilitate absorption. As a rule, administration should cease when lesions have sufficiently resolved.

Alefacept

Alefacept [Amevive], approved in January 2003, is the first biologic therapy for psoriasis. The drug is moderately effective, and has produced prolonged remission in some patients. Alefacept causes few immediate adverse effects, but over time may increase the risk of serious infections and perhaps cancer. Although the new drug is fairly effective, it is also expensive (treatment costs $12,000 or more a year) and inconvenient (treatment requires weekly IV or IM injections along with weekly blood tests), and possible long-term toxicity is unknown.

Actions and Therapeutic Use. Alefacept reduces the number and activity of memory CD4+ T lymphocytes, which are the principal mediators of inflammation in psoriasis. Benefits take about 2 months to develop, and correlate directly with reduced T-cell counts. Alefacept is approved for adults with moderate to severe psoriasis. In one clinical trial, two courses of IV therapy reduced symptom intensity by 50% or more in 71% of patients, and by 75% or more in 40% of patients. Response duration ranged from about 7 months to more than 12 months. Alefacept has not been compared directly with conventional systemic agents (e.g., methotrexate, acitretin).

Adverse Effects. The most common adverse effect was chills, which developed in about 6% of patients receiving alefacept IV (versus 1% of patients receiving IV placebo). Less common effects were pharyngitis, dizziness, cough, pruritus, myalgia, chills, inflammation, and injection site pain.

Alefacept produces a dose-dependent decrease in circulating T cells, and can thereby cause *lymphopenia,* a condition that increases the risk of *infection.* Accordingly, alefacept should be avoided in patients with clinically important infections, and should be used with caution in patients with chronic infection or a history of recurrent infection. If a serious infection develops, the drug should be discontinued. To minimize infection risk, CD4+ lymphocyte counts must be monitored (see below).

Alefacept may increase the risk of *cancer.* In studies with monkeys, the drug was associated with B-cell hyperplasia and B-cell lymphoma. In one clinical trial, the incidence of malignancy was 1.3% in patients receiving alefacept, versus 0.5% in those receiving placebo. Alefacept should be avoided in patients with a history of systemic malignancy, and should be discontinued if malignancy develops.

Drug Interactions. There have been no formal studies on the interaction of alefacept with other drugs. However, common sense dictates that alefacept not be combined with other drugs that can reduce T-cell number.

Monitoring. Counts of CD4+ T cells must be determined at baseline and before each alefacept dose. If the count is below 250 cells/µl, dosing should be postponed. If the count remains below 250 cells/µl for more than 1 month, alefacept should discontinued.

Preparations, Dosage, and Administration. Alefacept [Amevive] is supplied as a powder (7.5 and 15 mg) to be reconstituted with the supplied diluent for IV or IM administration. Dosing is done once a week for 12 weeks. For IV administration, each dose is 7.5 mg, given as a bolus; for IM administration, each dose is 15 mg. If needed, the 12-dose series can be repeated—but no sooner than 12 weeks after completing the first series, and provided T-cell counts are in the normal range. There is no experience with giving a third series.

Cost. Alefacept is expensive. A 12-week IV course (7.5 mg/week) costs about $8400, and a 12-week IM course (15 mg/week) costs about $12,000. If two courses are needed, the cost is doubled. Weekly monitoring of CD4+ T cells can raise the cost by another $8000. In comparison, treatment with oral methotrexate costs only $500 to $800 a year.

Glucocorticoids

Systemic glucocorticoids are effective against psoriasis, but cause Cushing's syndrome and other serious side effects. In addition, psoriasis may worsen when glucocorticoids are discontinued. Most specialists do not use these drugs. If systemic glucocorticoids must be employed, they should be reserved for short-term therapy of patients with severe symptoms.

Phototherapy
Coal Tar Plus Ultraviolet B Irradiation

This procedure involves sequential treatment with coal tar followed by UV radiation. In the first step, affected regions are covered with 1% coal tar ointment for 8 to 10 hours, after which the coal tar is washed off. In the second step, the area is exposed to short-wave UV radiation (ultraviolet B, UVB). This procedure is very safe and produces remission in 80% of patients. Unfortunately, treatment is expensive and time consuming (up to 30 treatments are needed), and patients dislike being coated with smelly coal tar.

Photochemotherapy (PUVA Therapy)

Photochemotherapy combines the use of long-wave UV radiation (ultraviolet A, UVA) with methoxsalen, an orally administered photosensitive drug. Methoxsalen belongs to a chemical family known as psoralens. In response to UVA light shined on the skin, methoxsalen is thought to undergo a photochemical reaction with DNA, resulting in the formation of a DNA-psoralen complex. This alteration in DNA structure is thought to underlie the ability of photochemotherapy to decrease proliferation of epidermal cells. Adverse effects associated with the procedure include pruritus, nausea, and erythema. In addition, the process may accelerate aging of the skin and may increase the risk of skin cancer. Photochemotherapy is indicated for patients with extensive, active psoriasis who have not responded adequately to more conventional therapy. An alternative name for photochemotherapy is *PUVA therapy;* PUVA is an abbreviation derived from *psoralen* and *ultraviolet A.*

OTHER DERMATOLOGIC DRUGS

Drugs for Actinic Keratoses

Actinic keratoses (AKs) are rough, scaly, red or brown papules caused by chronic exposure to sunlight. Lesions typically develop on the face, scalp, forearms, and backs of the hands. A small percentage (0.25% to 1% per year) evolve in squamous cell carcinoma. However, although the *percentage* is small, the *absolute amount* is large: In the United States, nearly half of all skin cancers (about 500,000 cases) began as AKs. AK treatment consists of topical drugs—fluorouracil, diclofenac, and aminolevulinic acid—and physical interventions: cryotherapy, curettage, excision, and laser resurfacing.

Fluorouracil

The basic pharmacology of fluorouracil [Carac, Efudex, Fluoroplex] is discussed in Chapter 98 (Anticancer Drugs I). Discussion here is limited to treatment of dermatologic disorders.

Actions and Uses in Dermatology. Fluorouracil is indicated for topical treatment of *multiple actinic keratoses* and *superficial basal cell carcinoma.* Cytotoxic effects result from disruption of DNA and RNA synthesis. A course of topical treatment elicits the following sequence of responses: (1) mild inflammation; (2) severe inflammation, often with burning, stinging, and vesicle formation; (3) tissue disintegration, characterized by erosion, ulceration, and necrosis; and (4) healing. Although fluorouracil is only applied for 2 to 6 weeks, the events just described may require 3 or more months for completion. Treatment is effective in over 90% of those who can tolerate a full course.

Adverse Effects. Among the more frequent reactions are itching, burning, rash, inflammation, and increased sensitivity to sunlight. Intense, burning pain develops occasionally. Darkening of the skin is rare. Absorption is insufficient to cause systemic toxicity.

Preparations and Administration. Topical fluorouracil is available under three trade names: *Carac* (microspheres in a 0.5% cream), *Efudex* (5% cream, 2% and 5% solutions), and *Fluoroplex* (1% cream and solution). Carac is applied once daily; Efudex and Fluoroplex are applied twice daily. Treatment should continue until a stage-three response (tissue disintegration) develops, usually within 2 to 6 weeks. Complete healing may not occur for another 1 to 2 months.

Diclofenac Sodium

Diclofenac sodium [Solaraze], in a 3% gel, is the first nonsteroidal anti-inflammatory drug (NSAID) approved for topical use. The drug's only indication is AK. Topical diclofenac is better tolerated than fluorouracil, but is less effective and treatment takes longer. In clinical trials, twice-daily application for 60 to 90 days produced complete clearing in 50% of patients. The mechanism underlying benefits is unknown. The most common side effects are dry skin, itching, redness, and rash at the site of application. Diclofenac may sensitize the skin to UV radiation, and hence patients should avoid sunlamps and minimize exposure to sunlight. Systemic absorption is low (10%), and therefore the risk of GI injury is much less than with oral diclofenac and other NSAIDs.

Aminolevulinic Acid Plus Blue Light

Topical aminolevulinic acid [Levulan Kerastick], in conjunction with blue light photoactivation, is a new therapy for AKs of the face and scalp. Treatment takes place in two steps. First, the physician applies a 20% solution of aminolevulinic acid to AK lesions. Fourteen to 18 hours later, the physician photoactivates the drug by exposing lesions to 1000 seconds of blue light, using the Blu-B Blue Light supplied by the manufacturer. In clinical trials, 66% of patients experienced complete clearing by 8 weeks after a single treatment, and 77% of patients experienced clearing of 75% or more. The mechanism underlying benefits is complex and incompletely understood. Local effects—burning, stinging, redness, and edema—occurred in nearly all patients. Because aminolevulinic acid is light sensitive, patients should protect treated areas from exposure to sunlight and bright indoor light prior to blue light exposure. The best protection is a wide brimmed hat; sunscreens won't help.

Drugs for Atopic Dermatitis (Eczema)

Atopic dermatitis, also known as eczema, is a chronic inflammatory skin disease characterized by dry, scaly skin and intense pruritus that often leads to scratching and rubbing, which in turn can lead to erythema, abrasions, rash, erosions with an exudate, and increased susceptibility to skin infection. The underlying cause is abnormal activity of T lymphocytes. First-line therapy consists of moisturizers and topical glucocorticoids. Unfortunately, the glucocorticoids can cause skin atrophy, hypopigmentation, telangiectasis (permanent focal red lesions) and, in high doses, possible systemic effects (e.g., adrenal suppression). If topical glucocorticoids are insufficient, patients may be treated with systemic immunosuppressants. Among these are methotrexate, cyclosporine [Sandimmune], azathioprine [Imuran], and oral glucocorticoids, all of which can cause serious side effects. Recently, two *topical* immunosuppressants—tacrolimus and pimecrolimus—were approved for atopic dermatitis. These drugs represent an alternative to glucocorticoids for topical therapy.

Tacrolimus Ointment

Tacrolimus, an immunosuppressant available as Prograf for preventing organ transplant rejection (see Chapter 65), is now available as an ointment for moderate to severe atopic dermatitis.

Mechanism of Action. Tacrolimus relieves symptoms by attenuating local immune responses. Specifically, the drug suppresses the activity of T cells and decreases the release of inflammatory mediators from cutaneous mast cells and basophils. The result is reduced inflammation.

Pharmacokinetics. Systemic absorption of topical tacrolimus is low, and gets even lower as the skin heals. Absolute bioavailability is less than 0.05%. Blood levels of tacrolimus are usually low.

Adverse Effects. Tacrolimus ointment is generally well tolerated. The most common adverse effects are erythema, pruritus, and burning sensations at the site of application. As the skin heals, these local reactions lessen. In children, tacrolimus may increase the risk of varicella zoster. Tacrolimus increases the incidence of skin cancer in laboratory animals exposed to UV light. To reduce any risk to patients, they should protect treated areas from direct sunlight, and should avoid sun lamps and tanning beds. In mice, tacrolimus increases the incidence of lymphoma. The risk of lymphoma in humans is unknown. Adverse effects associated with *systemic* tacrolimus (nephrotoxicity, neurotoxicity, hypertension, diarrhea, nausea) have not occurred with topical treatment. Unlike topical glucocorticoids, tacrolimus does not cause thinning of the skin.

Preparations, Dosage, and Administration. Tacrolimus ointment [Protopic] is available in two concentrations: 0.03% and 0.1%. Adults may use either formulation; children should use the 0.03% formulation. All patients should apply a thin layer twice daily. Occlusive dressings should be avoided.

Pimecrolimus Cream

Pimecrolimus 1% cream [Elidel] is a topical immunosuppressant approved for mild to moderate atopic dermatitis. The drug is very similar to tacrolimus with regard to mechanism of action, therapeutic effects, and adverse effects. In clinical trials, twice-daily application for 3 weeks reduced signs and symptoms of eczema by 72%. Initial improvement could be seen in 2 days. Pimecrolimus may be less effective than topical glucocorticoids. Although studies comparing pimecrolimus directly with tacrolimus have not been done, clinical efficacy of the drugs appears to be similar. As with tacrolimus, the most common adverse effects are erythema, pruritus, and burning sensations at the site of application, especially during the first few days of treatment. Like tacrolimus, pimecrolimus sensitizes the skin to UV light, and hence patients should use a sunscreen and should limit exposure to natural and artificial sunlight. Systemic absorption of pimecrolimus is minimal; in clinical trials, blood levels were at or below the limit of detection.

Agents Used to Remove Warts

The common wart (*verruca vulgaris*) is a virally induced skin disease that manifests as a hard, horny nodule. Warts may appear anywhere on the body but are most common on the hands and feet. It should be noted that warts are benign lesions and their presence is no threat to health.

Warts may be removed by physical procedures and by application of drugs. The physical methods are freezing, electrodesiccation (destruction with an electric current), curettage (surgical removal with a loop-shaped cutting tool), and laser therapy. Pharmacologic agents include podophyllin, podofilox, imiquimod, trichloroacetic acid, and topical fluorouracil. Three topical drugs are discussed below. All are used for genital warts.

Podophyllin

Actions and Uses. Podophyllin (podophyllum resin) is indicated primarily for condylomata acuminata (venereal warts). The drug is not very effective against common warts, which are caused by human papillomaviruses (HPVs). Podophyllin is a mixture of resins from the May apple or mandrake (*Podophyllum peltatum Linne*). The active ingredient in the resin is *podophyllotoxin,* a compound that inhibits synthesis of DNA and mitosis. These actions eventually lead to cell death and erosion of warty tissue. Formulations employed to remove warts contain 25% podophyllum resin. These preparations are highly caustic and should be applied only by a trained physician. To minimize the risk of toxicity from systemic absorption, the resin should be washed off with alcohol or with soap and water within 1 to 4 hours of its application. Each treatment should be limited to a small surface area and to a small number of warts.

Adverse Effects. Podophyllin can be absorbed in amounts sufficient to cause systemic toxicity. Systemic effects are most likely when the drug is applied to large areas in excessive amounts. Potential systemic reactions include central and peripheral neuropathy, kidney damage, and blood dyscrasias. Podophyllin is teratogenic and must not be used during pregnancy.

Preparations and Administration. Podophyllin [Podocon-25, Podofin] is available in a 25% solution for topical use. Application should be limited to small areas. The drug should not be applied to moles or birthmarks, nor should it be applied to warts that are bleeding or friable (easily crumbled) or that have undergone recent biopsy. When used to remove venereal warts, podophyllin should be washed off 1 to 6 hours after application. Treatment may be repeated at weekly intervals for up to 4 weeks.

Imiquimod and Podofilox

Imiquimod and podofilox represent alternatives to podophyllin for medical treatment of venereal warts. Both drugs can be applied by the patient, and hence are more convenient than podophyllin, which must be applied by the physician.

Imiquimod. Imiquimod 5% cream [Aldara] is indicated for topical therapy of external genital and perianal warts. The drug is available only by prescription, but is intended for application at home. Imiquimod stimulates production of interferon-alpha, tumor necrosis factor, and several interleukins, and thereby intensifies immune responses to HPV, the virus that causes venereal warts. Imiquimod has no direct antiviral effects of its own. Principal adverse effects are erythema, erosion, and flaking at the site of administration. Local itching, burning, and pain may occur too. Imiquimod undergoes minimal absorption, and hence systemic effects are absent. The drug is applied at bedtime and should be washed off in the morning. Application is done 3 times a week for 16 weeks, or until the warts are gone—whichever comes first. A 4-week course costs about $110.

Podofilox. Podofilox [Condylox] is indicated for topical therapy of genital and perianal warts. The drug is available by prescription for application at home. Like podophyllin, podofilox inhibits mitosis. Whether this action underlies beneficial effects (erosion of warty tissue) is unknown. Podofilox is applied twice daily for 3 consecutive days followed by 4 days off. This pattern is repeated 4 times or until the warts are gone—whichever comes first. Patients should wash their hands before and after applying the drug. However, unlike imiquimod, podofilox needn't be washed from the site of application. Treatment frequently causes local inflammation, burning, erosion, pain, itching, and bleeding. These can be minimized by (1) limiting the application area to 10 cm², (2) applying no more than 0.5 gm/day, and (3) avoiding application to normal skin. Podofilox causes more discomfort than imiquimod, but works faster and costs less (about $60 for a 4-week course).

Antiperspirants and Deodorants

Perspiration is produced by two types of sweat glands: *eccrine glands* and *apocrine glands.* The eccrine glands secrete profuse, watery perspiration. The apocrine glands secrete a small amount of fluid rich in organic compounds. The unpleasant odor associated with sweating results from chemical and bacterial degradation of the compounds in apocrine sweat. Eccrine glands contribute to odor by creating a moist environment that favors growth of bacteria. Perspiration odor can be reduced with *antiperspirants* (agents that decrease flow of eccrine sweat) and *deodorants* (antiseptics that suppress growth of skin-dwelling bacteria).

Antiperspirants. The principal compounds employed as antiperspirants are *aluminum chlorohydrate, aluminum zirconium chlorohydrate, aluminum chloride,* and *buffered aluminum sulfate.* These agents can decrease flow of eccrine sweat by 20% to 50%. The reduction in flow is thought to result from

inhibition of sweat production and from partial occlusion of sweat glands. Topical antiperspirants can cause stinging, burning, itching, and irritation. Dermatitis and ulceration occur rarely.

Deodorants. Deodorants inhibit growth of the surface bacteria that degrade components of apocrine sweat into malodorous products; deodorants do not suppress sweat formation. Agents employed as deodorants include *carbanilide, triclocarban,* and *triclosan.* These antiseptics are the active ingredients in deodorant soaps, such as Dial, Lifebuoy, Safeguard, and Zest.

Drugs for Seborrheic Dermatitis and Dandruff

Seborrheic dermatitis is characterized by inflammation and scaling of the scalp and face. Skin of the underarms, chest, and anogenital region may also be affected. Symptoms result from an inflammatory reaction to infection with *Pityrosporum ovale,* a microbe in the yeast family.

Symptoms respond rapidly to topical treatment with *ketoconazole* [Nizoral], a drug with activity against yeast (see Chapter 88). For treatment of seborrhea, ketoconazole is available in cream and shampoo formulations. Concurrent use of topical glucocorticoids can accelerate initial responses. Once the yeast infection has been controlled, remission can be maintained by periodic use of a shampoo that contains a yeast-suppressing drug, such as *ketoconazole* (in Nizoral), *pyrithione zinc* (in Head and Shoulders), or *selenium sulfide* (in Selsun Blue).

Drugs for Hair Loss

Two drugs are available to promote hair growth: minoxidil and finasteride. Minoxidil is applied topically; finasteride is taken orally. Neither drug was originally developed for baldness: Minoxidil was developed for hypertension, and finasteride for benign prostatic hyperplasia.

Topical Minoxidil

Minoxidil is a direct-acting vasodilator used primarily to treat severe hypertension. The drug's basic pharmacology is discussed in Chapter 44. Consideration here is limited to its use against patterned hair loss in men and women.

Formulations and Dosage. Minoxidil for treating baldness is available in two formulations, a 2% solution [Rogaine for Women, Rogaine for Men Regular Strength] and a 5% solution [Rogaine for Men Extra Strength]. The 2% solution may be used by men or by women; the 5% solution is approved only for men. With either solution, the usual dosage is 1 ml applied to the scalp twice a day.

Mechanism of Action. The mechanism by which minoxidil promotes hair growth is unknown. One possibility is that minoxidil causes resting hair follicles to enter a state of active growth. Improved cutaneous blood flow secondary to vasodilation does not seem to be involved.

Clinical Response. Minoxidil can retard loss of hair and stimulate hair growth. Benefits take several months to develop. Unfortunately, response rates have been somewhat disappointing: Only about one-third of patients experience significant restoration of hair to regions of baldness. Hair regrowth is most likely when baldness has developed recently and has been limited to a small area. Responses with the 5% solution are only 50% greater than with the 2% solution. When minoxidil is discontinued, newly gained hair is lost in 3 to 4 months, and the natural progression of hair loss resumes. In some cases, beneficial effects may decline even with uninterrupted treatment.

Adverse Effects. Topical minoxidil is generally devoid of adverse effects. A few patients have reported pruritus and local allergic responses (e.g., rash, swelling, burning sensation). Absorption is low, and hence systemic reactions (e.g., hypotension, headache, flushing) are rare.

Finasteride

Indications and Formulations. Finasteride is an oral drug with two indications: androgenic alopecia (male pattern baldness) and benign prostatic hyperplasia (BPH). For treatment of androgenic alopecia, finasteride is sold in 1-mg tablets under the trade name *Propecia.* For treatment of BPH, the drug is sold in 5-mg tablets under the trade name *Proscar* (see Chapter 103).

Mechanism of Action. Male pattern baldness is caused by dihydrotestosterone (DHT), a powerful androgenic hormone formed from testosterone. In balding men, the scalp has high levels of DHT, which act on hair follicles to induce shrinkage. Finasteride promotes hair growth by inhibiting the enzyme that converts testosterone into DHT. A 1-mg dose reduces serum levels of DHT by 65% after 24 hours. In the prostate gland, levels of testosterone *increase* by sixfold (because conversion of testosterone into DHT has been suppressed).

Clinical Response. Regrowth of hair with finasteride is very modest. The drug has been evaluated in men 18 to 41 years old. Only 50% grew any hair. Furthermore, even when hair growth did occur, the amount was small: One year of treatment with 1 mg/day increased hair count by only 12% (in a 5.1-cm² circle on the scalp, the average hair count rose by 107 hairs, up from a baseline of 867 hairs). In older men taking 5 mg/day to treat BPH, no hair growth has been reported.

Adverse Effects. At the dosage employed to treat baldness (1 mg/day), adverse effects are uncommon. About 4% of men experience reduced libido, erectile dysfunction, impaired ejaculation, and reduced ejaculate volume. Finasteride is a teratogen that can cause genitourinary abnormalities in males exposed to the drug *in utero*. Accordingly, women who are or may become pregnant should not take finasteride, nor should they handle tablets that are crushed or broken.

Eflornithine for Unwanted Facial Hair

Eflornithine is an old drug with a new indication and new formulation. As discussed in Chapter 95, eflornithine has been available since 1990 for *systemic* therapy of African trypanosomiasis (sleeping sickness). Now, the drug is also available in a 13.9% cream, marketed as *Vaniqa* to reduce unwanted facial hair in women. Topical eflornithine acts on cells in hair follicles to inhibit ornithine decarboxylase, an enzyme required for synthesis of polyamines, which in turn are required for cell division and subsequent hair growth.

In clinical trials, eflornithine cream was moderately effective in some women and ineffective in others. All subjects had beards or mustaches that required removal (by shaving, waxing, tweezing, etc.) at least twice a week. Participants were randomized to receive either (1) eflornithine cream twice a week or (2) the vehicle alone (i.e., the cream without eflornithine). What happened? Substantial hair reduction occurred in 40% of treated women in one study and 20% of treated women in another, compared with a 10% response in women receiving the vehicle alone. Among the women who did respond, benefits developed slowly—over 4 to 8 weeks or more—and then faded entirely by 8 weeks after treatment was stopped. It should be noted that eflornithine does not remove facial hair entirely. Rather, it retards hair growth, causes hair to be finer and lighter, and decreases (but does not eliminate) the need for shaving and other hair-removal procedures. Because effects are not permanent, continuous treatment is required.

Very little of topical eflornithine gets absorbed: about 1% of each dose reaches the systemic circulation. Absorbed drug is eliminated intact in the urine. No metabolism occurs.

Eflornithine cream is generally well tolerated, although there is some concern about possible fetal harm. The most common reactions are transient stinging, burning, tingling, or rash at the application site. Although eflornithine absorption is minimal, it may still be sufficient to cause fetal injury. In animal studies, there was no evidence that topical eflornithine is teratogenic or fetotoxic. However, of the 19 pregnancies that occurred during clinical trials, there were four spontaneous abortions and one birth defect (Down's syndrome). Until more is known, avoidance of pregnancy would seem prudent.

Eflornithine is supplied in 30-gm tubes (a 2-month supply) that cost over $40. Applications are made twice daily, 8 hours apart. Women should rub the cream in thoroughly and should not wash the treated area for at least 4 hours. Cosmetics and sunscreens can be applied as soon as the cream dries.

Local Anesthetics

Local anesthetics (e.g., benzocaine, lidocaine, pramoxine) can be applied topically to relieve pain and itching associated with various skin disorders, including sunburn, plant poisoning, fungal infection, diaper rash, and eczema. Selection of a topical anesthetic is based on duration of action, desired vehicle (cream, ointment, solution, gel), and prior history of hypersensitivity reactions. The pharmacology of the local anesthetics is discussed in Chapter 25. Agents available for application to the skin are listed in Table 25–2.

Anti-infective Agents

The skin is subject to fungal, viral, and bacterial infections. Some of these infections respond to topical treatment; others require systemic treatment. *Antibacterial drugs* are discussed in Chapters 80 through 87. *Antifungal* and *antiviral drugs* are discussed in Chapters 88 and 89, respectively. Topical drugs for prophylaxis against infection (antiseptics) are discussed in Chapter 92.

⸬ KEY POINTS

- Topical glucocorticoids are employed to relieve inflammation and itching associated with a variety of dermatologic disorders.
- Preparations of topical glucocorticoids are classified into four potency groups: low, medium, high, and super-high.
- Prolonged use of topical glucocorticoids can cause atrophy of the dermis and epidermis.
- Topical glucocorticoids can be absorbed in amounts sufficient to cause systemic toxicity. Principal concerns are growth retardation and adrenal suppression.
- Keratolytic agents—salicylic acid, sulfur, and benzoyl peroxide—promote shedding of the horny layer of the skin.
- Topical antibiotics, such as clindamycin or erythromycin, help clear mild to moderate acne by suppressing growth of *P. acnes.*
- Oral antibiotics, including tetracycline and azithromycin, are reserved for moderate to severe acne.
- Tretinoin, a derivative of vitamin A, is a topical drug used for acne and for removing fine wrinkles from the face.
- Topical tretinoin increases susceptibility to sunburn. Patients should use a sunscreen (SPF 15 or greater) and wear protective clothing.
- Azelaic acid, a topical drug for mild to moderate acne, appears to work by suppressing growth of *P. acnes* and by decreasing proliferation of keratinocytes.
- Isotretinoin is an oral drug for severe acne.
- Isotretinoin causes multiple adverse effects, including nosebleeds, inflammation of the lips and eyes, and pain, tenderness, or stiffness in muscles, bones, and joints.
- Isotretinoin is highly teratogenic and must not be used during pregnancy.
- Excessive sun exposure can cause sunburn, premature aging of the skin, and skin cancer.
- Sunscreens can protect against sunburn and aging of the skin, but offer little protection against skin cancer.
- To be most effective, a sunscreen product should offer protection against the full range of UVA and UVB radiation.

Drugs for the Ear

In this chapter, we discuss two drugs for two types of ear disorders: otitis media and otitis externa. In preparation, we review relevant anatomy of the ear.

ANATOMY OF THE EAR

The ear has three major divisions: the external ear, middle ear, and inner ear (Figure 102–1). Their primary features are as follows:

- The *external ear* consists of (1) the auricle or pinna (the cartilaginous flap visible on the side of the head that serves to collect sound waves), and (2) the external auditory canal (EAC), a skin-lined tube that directs sound waves from the auricle to the tympanic membrane (eardrum). The surface of the EAC is coated with cerumen (earwax), a hydrophobic substance that blocks penetration of water and helps protect against bacterial and fungal infection.
- The *middle ear* is the chamber that houses the malleus, incus, and stapes—three tiny bones that transmit sound vibrations from the eardrum to the internal ear. The middle ear is bounded laterally by the tympanic membrane, which walls off the middle ear from the external ear. The eustachian tube (auditory tube) connects the middle ear with the nasopharynx, and thereby allows air pressure within the middle ear to equalize with air pressure in the environment. The mucociliary epithelium that lines the eustachian tube sweeps bacteria out of the middle ear into the nasopharynx.
- The *inner ear* consists of the semicircular canals and the cochlea. The canals provide our sense of balance. The cochlea houses the actual apparatus of hearing.

OTITIS MEDIA AND ITS MANAGEMENT

Otitis media (OM), defined as an inflammation of the middle ear, is among the most prevalent disorders of childhood. The condition affects more than 75% of children by the age of 3 years, and about 95% by the age of 12. In the United States, over 5 million cases are diagnosed annually.

Otitis media may result from bacterial infection, viral infection, or noninfective causes. Only bacterial OM responds to antibiotics. Furthermore, most cases resolve spontaneously, making antibiotics largely unnecessary—even when bacteria *are* the cause. Nonetheless, antibiotics are used routinely. In fact, OM is the most common reason for giving these drugs to kids—at an estimated cost of $3.5 billion a year.

Acute Otitis Media: Characteristics, Pathogenesis, and Microbiology

Acute otitis media (AOM) is defined by *inflammation* and *fluid in the middle ear*. Otalgia (ear pain) is characteristic, often causing the child to tug at the ear or just hold it. Other possible symptoms include fever, vomiting, irritability, impaired hearing, sleeplessness, and otorrhea (discharge from the ear, usually purulent [pus containing]).

AOM may be bacterial, viral, or both. In children with full-blown bacterial AOM, the inner ear is filled with purulent fluid, which can cause the tympanic membrane to bulge outward. If the membrane is perforated, otorrhea results. In children with nonbacterial AOM or with mild bacterial AOM, the tympanic membrane does not bulge. Of the two presentations—bulging or nonbulging eardrum—nonbulging is the more common.

It is important to distinguish between AOM, and OM with effusion (OME). As discussed below, children with OME have fluid in the middle ear but no signs of local or systemic illness. Prolonged OME is common following resolution of AOM.

How does AOM develop? As a rule, the process begins with a viral infection of the nasopharynx, which can cause blockage of the eustachian tube, which in turn can cause negative pressure in the middle ear. When the tube opens, causing pressure equalization, bacteria and viruses can be sucked in. If the mucociliary system is sufficiently impaired, it will be unable to transport these pathogens back to the nasopharynx. Otitis media results when bacteria colonize the fluid of the middle ear and/or when viruses colonize cells of the middle-ear mucosa. As indicated in Table 102–1, bacteria are present in 70% to 90% of fluid samples taken from the middle ear of children with AOM, and viruses are present in nearly 50%. The most common bacterial pathogens are *Streptococcus*

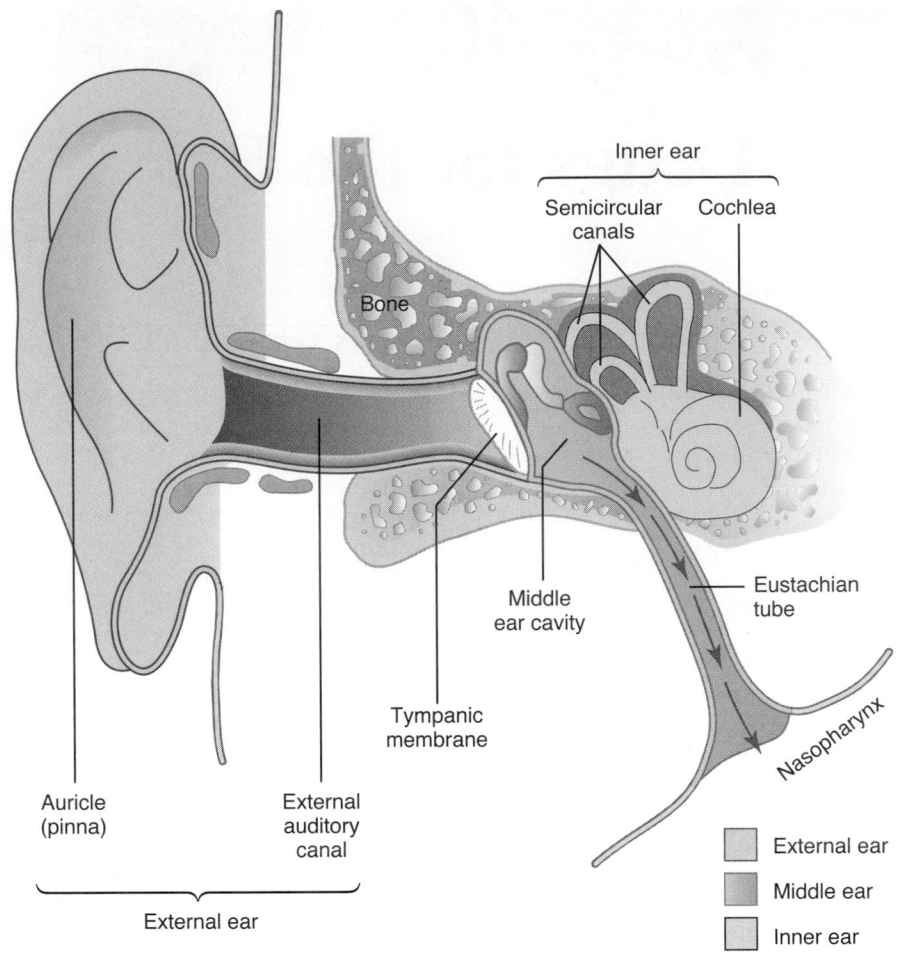

Figure 102–1 ■ Anatomy of the ear.
The *blue arrows* indicate flow of the mucociliary system, which can transport bacteria out of the middle ear.

TABLE 102–1 ■ Primary Pathogens Found in Fluid from the Middle Ear of Children with Acute Otitis Media	
Pathogen	**Children with the Pathogen (%)**
Streptococcus pneumoniae	40–50
Haemophilus influenzae	20–25
Moraxella catarrhalis	10–15
No bacteria found	20–30
Respiratory viruses (with or without bacteria)	48

pneumoniae (40% to 50%), *Haemophilus influenzae* (20% to 24%), and *Moraxella catarrhalis* (10% to 15%).

Treatment of Otitis Media

Management of OM—especially the decision to use antibiotics—is based on clinical presentation. Table 102–2 summarizes management recommendations for specific presentations.

Acute Otitis Media

Treatment of AOM with antibiotics is controversial: Some authorities recommend immediate treatment of all children diagnosed with AOM; others recommend delaying treatment for most children, reserving immediate treatment for selected cases. I believe that the second approach makes more sense. Why? Because the vast majority (81%) of AOM episodes resolve spontaneously within a week. Hence, if antibiotics are prescribed routinely, most recipients will be taking drugs they don't really need. Not only does this generate unnecessary expense, worse yet, it needlessly accelerates emergence of antibiotic resistance.

If we shouldn't treat everyone, whom should we treat? Ideally, we should give antibiotics only to those children who are likely to benefit. The most obvious candidates are children with full-blown bacterial AOM, as indicated by a bulging tympanic membrane. For these children, the treatment of choice is high-dose *amoxicillin* (40 to 50 mg/kg PO twice a day) for 7 days. For children who are allergic to penicillins, good alternatives include azithromycin (PO), cefuroxime (PO), and ceftriaxone (IM).

How should we manage children who have AOM but do not have a bulging tympanic membrane? In the United

TABLE 102–2 ▪ Management of Otitis Media

Clinical Presentation	Recommended Intervention
AOM with bulging eardrum	Immediate treatment with high-dose amoxicillin (40–50 mg/kg PO twice a day for 7 days)*
AOM without bulging eardrum	Prescribe-and-wait strategy (see text)
Recurrent AOM	
Current episode: with bulging eardrum	Immediate treatment with high-dose amoxicillin (see above)
Current episode: without bulging eardrum	Prescribe-and-wait strategy (see text)
Prevention	Vaccination against influenza and treatment of active influenza
	Tympanostomy tube placement in selected patients
	Prophylaxis with antibiotics is *not* generally recommended
Antibiotic-resistant AOM	High-dose amoxicillin-clavulanate (40–50 mg/kg amoxicillin PO twice a day for 7 days) *or*
	Cefuroxime (30 mg/kg PO twice a day for 7 days) *or*
	Ceftriaxone (50 mg/kg IM once a day for 3 days)
OM with effusion	Do not use antibiotics

AOM = acute otitis media, OM = otitis media.
*For children allergic to penicillins, good alternatives to amoxicillin include cefuroxime, azithromycin, and ceftriaxone.

States, these children are usually given antibiotics, even though doing so will not help most of them. In contrast, physicians in the Netherlands follow a *"prescribe-and-wait strategy"* in which parents are given a prescription for antibiotics but are instructed to delay administration for 2 to 3 days, thereby allowing time for AOM to resolve on its own. If there is no improvement within 1 to 2 days (for children younger than 2 years) or within 3 days (for children 2 years and older), then antibiotic therapy is implemented. As part of this strategy, the child is given full-dose acetaminophen [Tylenol, others] to reduce pain and fever, and the parents are informed about (1) the high probability of spontaneous AOM resolution, and (2) the drawbacks of giving antibiotics when they are not needed (needless promotion of resistance and needless exposure of the child to possible adverse effects). In a trial comparing immediate antibiotic therapy with delayed therapy, immediate therapy was only marginally superior at causing AOM resolution, and was no better at relieving pain or distress. Another study showed that parents find the prescribe-and-wait approach acceptable. A major concern with delayed therapy is that it may increase the occurrence of acute mastoiditis (owing to bacterial invasion of the mastoid bone). Fortunately, although delaying treatment does indeed increase this risk, the increase is very small (only 2 extra cases per 100,000 children per year), and hence appears more than balanced by the benefits of avoiding a great deal of unnecessary antibiotic use.

Antibiotic-Resistant Otitis Media

Antibiotic resistance is indicated by persistence of symptoms (fever; earache; otorrhea; a red, bulging tympanic membrane) for 3 or more days despite antibiotic therapy. Major risk factors for developing resistant AOM are

- Attending day care
- Age less than 2 years
- Exposure to antibiotics in the prior 1 to 3 months
- Winter and spring seasons

Over the past 10 to 15 years, the incidence of resistant AOM has greatly increased. Why? Because overuse of antibiotics has favored emergence of resistant pathogens. Resistance among strains of *H. influenzae* and *M. catarrhalis* is limited to beta-lactam antibiotics. The mechanism is production of beta-lactamase, an enzyme that inactivates amoxicillin and certain other beta-lactam antibiotics. In contrast, strains of *S. pneumoniae* are resistant to multiple antibiotics, including erythromycin, trimethoprim sulfamethoxazole, and amoxicillin and other beta-lactam antibiotics. Interestingly, resistance to amoxicillin does not result from beta-lactamase production. Rather, it results from production of altered penicillin-binding proteins (PBPs), whose affinity for amoxicillin is much lower than that of normal PBPs.

How should resistant AOM be treated? The preferred approach is oral therapy with *high-dose amoxicillin-clavulanate*. The clavulanate (clavulanic acid) in the combination inhibits beta-lactamase, and thereby increases activity against resistant *H. influenzae* and *M. catarrhalis*. Using a high dose of amoxicillin increases activity against resistant *S. pneumoniae*. Because the clavulanate in the combination can cause diarrhea, we want to keep its dosage low. This is best accomplished by using *Augmentin ES-600* (600 mg amoxicillin/42.9 mg clavulanate), a formulation that contains less clavulanate per milligram of amoxicillin than any other amoxicillin-clavulanate product. To treat resistant AOM, the dosage is 40 to 50 mg amoxicillin PO twice a day for 7 days. Alternatives to amoxicillin-clavulanate include *oral cefuroxime* (30 mg/kg twice a day for 7 days) and *IM ceftriaxone* (50 mg/kg once a day for 3 days). All three regimens are recommended for (1) children with acute AOM that has not responded to standard antibiotic therapy, and (2) initial therapy of AOM in children with risk factors for resistant infection.

Recurrent Otitis Media

Recurrent AOM can be defined as AOM that occurs 3 or more times within 6 months, or 4 or more times within 12 months. Four management strategies are available: (1) short-term antibacterial therapy, (2) prophylactic antibacterial therapy, (3) prevention and treatment of influenza, and (4) placement of a tympanostomy tube.

Short-Term Antibacterial Therapy. As with nonrecurrent AOM, there is disagreement regarding antibacterial therapy. Some authorities would prescribe antibiotics for each recurrent episode, regardless of its presentation. Others would reserve antibiotics for episodes in which the tympanic membrane is bulging. In both cases, high-dose amoxicillin is the treatment of choice. If resistance is suspected, amoxicillin-clavulanate can be used.

Prophylactic Antibacterial Therapy. Antibacterial prophylaxis is not generally recommended. An analysis of several studies indicates that, for each year of prophylaxis (with sulfisoxazole, trimethoprim-sulfamethoxazole, or amoxicillin), only 1.3 episodes of AOM would be prevented. This small benefit is largely outweighed by the risk of promoting resistance. If prophylaxis *is* elected, it should be conducted only during the head cold season. The preferred drug for prophylaxis is amoxicillin. Why? Because, compared with sulfonamides, amoxicillin is more active against multidrug-resistant strains of *S. pneumoniae.*

Prevention and Treatment of Influenza. As discussed below under *Prevention of Otitis Media,* we can reduce OM occurrence by vaccinating against the influenza virus and by treating active influenza infection. Unfortunately, benefits are seen only during the flu season.

Tympanostomy Tubes. A tympanostomy tube is a small tube that is placed into an incision in the eardrum, thereby permitting drainage and aeration of the middle ear. Tube insertion is performed under general anesthesia and costs about $3000. In children with recurrent AOM, the procedure can significantly reduce AOM episodes. However, benefits are limited to children who experience AOM with a bulging tympanic membrane; the tubes have no effect on recurrence of AOM without a bulging membrane. Complications of the procedure include obstruction of the tube, secondary infection with otorrhea, and premature tube extrusion.

Otitis Media with Effusion

Otitis media with effusion is seen in many children following an episode of AOM. The condition is characterized by fluid in the middle ear but without evidence of local or systemic illness. OME may cause mild hearing loss, but not pain. The condition can persist for weeks to months after AOM has resolved. Antibiotics have minimal effect on OME and should not be used.

Prevention of Otitis Media

In theory, we can prevent OM in three ways: (1) giving antibiotics for prophylaxis of recurrent OM, (2) preventing and treating influenza, and (3) vaccinating against pneumococcal infection. Option 1—antibiotic prophylaxis—is discussed above under *Recurrent Otitis Media.* Options 2 and 3 are discussed immediately below.

Prevention and Treatment of Influenza. As noted, influenza and other viral infections of the respiratory tract predispose children to developing bacterial and viral OM. Accordingly, measures that reduce influenza can reduce OM risk. Two methods are available: (1) vaccination against influenza and (2) treatment of active influenza infection. In one study, children attending day care were vaccinated against influenza. The result was a 36% reduction in diagnosed cases of AOM during the 6-week interval when influenza virus was circulating in the community. In another study, children with active influenza were treated with oseltamivir, a drug with activity against the influenza virus. The result was a 40% decrease in cases of AOM. Although both approaches—immunization and treatment—can be helpful during the flu season, they do nothing to alter AOM risk during the rest of the year.

Vaccination Against Streptococcus pneumoniae. Vaccination with *pneumococcal conjugate vaccine* (PCV) [Prevnar] can slightly reduce the risk of AOM. Although the vaccine is highly active against the strains of *S. pneumoniae* that cause pneumonia and meningitis, it is only moderately active against the strains that cause AOM. In a study involving 37,868 children in Northern California, the benefits of PCV immunization were modest: office visits for AOM were reduced by 7.8%, and the need for tympanostomy tubes was reduced by 24%.

OTITIS EXTERNA AND ITS MANAGEMENT

Otitis externa (OE) is an inflammation of the external auditory canal. The usual cause is bacterial infection, which may be limited to the EAC, or may spread to adjacent tissues. Most cases of OE respond readily to topical drugs.

Acute Otitis Externa
Characteristics, Pathogenesis, and Microbiology

Acute OE, also known as "swimmer's ear," is a bacterial infection of the EAC. The most common pathogen is *Pseudomonas aeruginosa,* which is responsible for 38% of cases. Other common pathogens are *Staphylococcus epidermidis, Staph. aureus,* and *Microbacterium otitidis* (Table 102–3). Patients who have acute OE present with rapid-onset ear pain associated with pruritus, impaired hearing, purulent discharge, and pronounced tenderness of the auricle upon manipulation.

Susceptibility to acute OE is precipitated primarily by two factors: excessive moisture and abrasion. Both facilitate bacterial colonization. Moisture can wash away the protective layer of cerumen. As a result, keratin debris in the EAC is able to absorb water, thereby creating a nourishing medium for bacterial growth. Moisture in the EAC may come from swimming, perspiration, and even high humidity. Abrasion of the epithelium creates a site for bacterial entry. Most often, abrasion results from cleaning the EAC with a cotton swab or some other foreign object (finger, pencil, toothpick, etc.). Abrasion can also be caused by hearing aids and earplugs.

Treatment

Acute OE generally responds well to simple treatment. For most patients, cleaning and use of ear drops will suffice. If the infection is extensive, oral drugs may be needed as well. To facilitate healing, the ear should be kept as dry as possible. Most infections begin to improve in 3 days, and resolve completely by 10 days.

Topical Medications. Acute OE can be treated with a variety of topical medications. A *2% solution of acetic acid* is safe, effective, and cheap. Furthermore, because bactericidal activity results from simply reducing pH, there is no risk of encouraging resistance. A solution of *alcohol plus acetic acid* offers the additional benefit of promoting tissue drying. For many patients, acidification and drying are all that is needed.

If the infection cannot be cleared with acetic acid and alcohol, a topical antibiotic should be employed. Most preparations have three active ingredients: *hydrocortisone, neomycin,* and *polymyxin B.* Hydrocortisone reduces inflammation and edema; neomycin and polymyxin can kill bacterial pathogens. Unfortunately, although these products are effective and inexpensive, they do have drawbacks. Specifically, the neomycin component is ototoxic, and causes local swelling and erythema in about 15% of patients. A relatively new combination—*hydrocortisone plus ciprofloxacin* [Cipro HC Otic]—is an attractive alternative. Ciprofloxacin is highly effective, does not cause local reactions, and is not ototoxic. Principal drawbacks are expense and promotion of resistance to ciprofloxacin itself as well as to other fluoroquinolone antibiotics.

Applying ear drops correctly can improve outcomes and reduce drug-related discomfort. Instillation of cold solutions can cause dizziness, and hence ear drops should be warmed prior to administration. Wiggling the earlobe can facilitate transit of solutions down the EAC. If edema of the EAC is sufficient to impede drug penetration, insertion of a sponge wick can help. Drug solutions are absorbed into the wick, which then delivers them to the epithelium of the entire canal. The wick should be removed every 48 hours to allow cleaning and to determine if further wicking is still needed.

Oral Medications. Oral antibacterial drugs are indicated if the infection extends beyond the EAC to involve the pinna. For *adults, ciprofloxacin* [Cipro] is a good choice. For *children, cephalexin* [Keflex], is preferred. Why? Because, oral ciprofloxacin and other fluoroquinolones can cause tendon rupture in younger patients. Accordingly, these drugs should not be given to patients under the age of 18.

Prevention

The best way to prevent bacterial OE is to keep the natural defenses of the EAC healthy. Ear hygiene can be promoted by following these rules:

- Don't put *anything* in the ear, including cotton-tipped swabs, fingers, pencils, paper clips, toothpicks, liquids, or sprays, all of which can remove cerumen and/or damage the epithelium.
- Dry the EAC after swimming and showering. How? By toweling off and by promoting water drainage (by turning the head to both sides while pulling the auricle in different directions).
- Don't remove cerumen (earwax).
- Don't use earplugs (except when swimming).

Necrotizing Otitis Externa

Necrotizing OE is a rare but potentially fatal complication of acute OE that develops when bacteria in the EAC invade the mastoid or temporal bone. Spread of infection to the skull

TABLE 102–3 ■ Primary Pathogens in Samples From the External Ear of Patients with Acute Otitis Externa

Pathogen	Patients with the Pathogen (%)
Pseudomonas aeruginosa	38
Staphylococcus epidermidis	9.1
Staphylococcus aureus	7.8
Microbacterium otitidis	6.6

base can affect cranial nerves, and spread to the dura mater can cause meningitis and possibly lateral sinus thrombosis. The usual pathogen is *P. aeruginosa.* Patients typically present with progressive severe otic pain, purulent discharge from the ear, and granulation of tissue in the EAC. Necrotizing OE occurs almost exclusively in two groups of high-risk people, specifically, older people with diabetes and people who are immunocompromised, especially those with HIV infection. Most cases can be managed by thorough cleansing of the EAC followed by treatment with antipseudomonal drugs; surgery is rarely needed. All patients should receive antipseudomonal ear drops (e.g., ofloxacin solution). Patients with mild disease should also receive oral ciprofloxacin. Patients with severe disease should receive IV antipseudomonal therapy (e.g., imipenem-cilastatin [Primaxin], meropenem [Merrem IV], or ciprofloxacin). The usual duration of IV therapy is 4 to 6 weeks.

Fungal Otitis Externa (Otomycosis)

In about 10% of patients, OE is caused by fungi and not bacteria. The two most common pathogens are *Aspergillus,* which causes 80% to 90% of otomycoses, and *Candida.* Fungal OE typically manifests as intense pruritus and erythema, with or without pain or hearing loss. As a rule, otomycosis can be managed with thorough cleansing and application of acidifying drops (e.g., 2% acetic acid solution applied 3 to 4 times a day for 7 days). If these measures are inadequate, the patient can apply a solution that contains an antifungal drug (e.g., 1% clotrimazole [Lotrimin] twice daily for 7 days). For infections that still don't respond, *oral* antifungal therapy may be needed. Options include itraconazole [Sporanox] and fluconazole [Diflucan].

⁝⁝ KEY POINTS

- Otitis media (OM), defined as inflammation of the middle ear, is among the most prevalent disorders of childhood.
- Acute otitis media (AOM) is characterized by a combination of inflammation and fluid in the middle ear.
- AOM may be bacterial, viral, or both.
- Routine treatment of AOM with antibiotics is controversial. Why? Because the vast majority (81%) of cases resolve spontaneously.
- If we shouldn't routinely treat every child with AOM, whom should we treat? One approach is to limit *imme-*

diate treatment to children with full-blown bacterial AOM, as indicted by a bulging tympanic membrane.

■ How should we manage children who have AOM but do not have a bulging tympanic membrane? One approach is to follow a "prescribe-and-wait strategy," in which parents are given a prescription for antibiotics but are instructed to delay administration for 2 to 3 days, thereby allowing time for AOM to resolve on its own. If there is no improvement, then antibiotic therapy is implemented. This approach has two benefits: it minimizes the risk of adverse drug effects and it minimizes promotion of drug resistance.

■ When antibiotics *are* used for AOM—either immediately or after waiting—the treatment of choice is high-dose amoxicillin.

■ For children with antibiotic-resistant AOM, the treatment of choice is high-dose amoxicillin-clavulanate.

■ For children who experience recurrent AOM, we can reduce episodes by (1) vaccination against the influenza virus, (2) treatment of active influenza infection, and (3) placement of tympanostomy tubes. Prophylaxis with antibacterial drugs is only moderately effective, and not generally recommended.

■ Otitis media with effusion (OME) is characterized by fluid in the middle ear but without evidence of local or systemic illness. The condition may cause mild hearing loss, but not pain.

■ OME is seen in many children following an episode of AOM, and may persist for weeks to months.

■ Antibiotics have minimal effect on OME and should not be used.

■ Otitis externa (OE) is an inflammation of the external auditory canal (EAC).

■ Acute OE, also known as "swimmer's ear," is a bacterial infection of the EAC.

■ Susceptibility to acute OE is greatly increased by excessive moisture and abrasion of the EAC, both of which facilitate bacterial colonization.

■ In most cases, acute OE can be treated by cleaning and use of ear drops, which may contain 2% acetic acid (which kills bacteria), alcohol (which promotes drying), hydrocortisone (which reduces inflammation and edema), or antibiotics (traditionally neomycin, polymyxin, or both; ciprofloxacin is a new and attractive alternative).

■ If edema caused by acute OE is sufficient to block the EAC, a sponge wick can be inserted to facilitate drug penetration. The wick should be removed every 48 hours to allow cleaning and to determine if further wicking is still needed.

■ If acute OE progresses to the pinna, oral antibiotics should be used. Ciprofloxacin is a good choice for adults, and cephalexin is a good choice for children.

■ The best way to prevent bacterial OE is to keep the natural defenses of the EAC healthy. How? By following these ear-hygiene rules: Don't put anything in the ear (e.g., cotton-tipped swabs, fingers, pencils, etc.); dry the EAC after swimming and showering; don't remove cerumen (earwax); and don't use earplugs (except when swimming).

■ Necrotizing OE is a rare but potentially fatal complication of acute OE that develops when bacteria in the EAC invade the mastoid or temporal bone. The usual pathogen is *Pseudomonas aeruginosa*.

■ Necrotizing OE occurs almost exclusively in people with diabetes (especially the elderly) and in people who are immunocompromised (especially those with HIV infection).

■ Necrotizing OE can be managed by thorough cleansing and use of antipseudomonal drugs. All patients should receive antipseudomonal ear drops (e.g., ofloxacin solution). Patients with mild disease should receive oral ciprofloxacin. And patients with severe disease should receive IV therapy (e.g., imipenem-cilastatin [Primaxin]).

■ In about 10% of patients with OE, the infection is due to fungi and not bacteria. The most common fungal pathogen is *Aspergillus*.

■ As a rule, fungal OE (otomycosis) can be managed by thorough cleansing and application of acidifying drops (e.g., 2% acetic acid solution). If needed, a topical antifungal drug (e.g., 1% clotrimazole) can be used. Unresponsive infections can be treated with an oral antifungal drug (e.g., itraconazole, fluconazole).

Miscellaneous Noteworthy Drugs

DRUGS FOR ERECTILE DYSFUNCTION

Erectile dysfunction (ED), also known as impotence, is defined as a persistent inability to achieve or sustain an erection suitable for satisfactory sexual performance. In the United States, ED affects up to 30 million men, and accounts for 525,000 physician visits each year. ED is commonly associated with chronic illnesses, especially diabetes, hypertension, and depression. The cause may be the illness itself or the drugs used to treat it. Among men with diabetes, the incidence of ED is between 35% and 75%. The risk of ED increases with advancing age. According to the Massachusetts Male Aging Study, among men ages 40 to 70, 52% have some degree of ED, and among men over 70, 67% suffer from ED. Of the men in the 40- to 70-year-old group, 17% report minimal ED, 25% report moderate ED, and 10% report complete ED (i.e., no erection at all). Only 48% report their erections are OK. Treatments for ED include drugs (e.g., sildenafil, alprostadil) and surgical implantation of a penile prosthesis.

Sildenafil

Sildenafil [Viagra] was introduced in 1998 as the first oral treatment for ED. The drug is reliable and easy to use. Benefits derive from enhancing the natural response to sexual stimuli. Sildenafil does not cause erection directly. Although sildenafil is generally well tolerated, it can be dangerous for men taking nitroglycerin and other nitrates, medicines used for angina pectoris.

Sildenafil has been wildly popular. First-year sales were the hottest in pharmaceutical history. By now, tens of millions of men in over 100 countries have used the drug.

The erection-enhancing effects of sildenafil were discovered by accident. The drug was developed as a cardiac medicine, but benefits were minimal. However, in the course of testing, some men noticed a surprising side effect: Their impotence had been cured. The rest, as they say, is history.

Mechanism of Action

Sildenafil causes selective inhibition of cyclic guanosine monophosphate (cGMP)–specific phosphodiesterase type 5 (PDE-5), an enzyme that converts cGMP to guanosine monophosphate. By inhibiting PDE-5, sildenafil enhances the normal erectile response to sexual stimuli (e.g., erotic imagery, fantasies, physical contact). In the absence of sexual stimuli, nothing happens. Here's the sequence of events. Sexual stimuli promote the release of nitric oxide from nerves and blood vessels associated with the corpus cavernosum. Nitric oxide then stimulates production of cGMP, a compound that causes smooth muscle of the corpus cavernosum to relax. As a result, blood rushes into the corpus cavernosum, causing erection. Erection eventually subsides as PDE-5 degrades cGMP. By inhibiting PDE-5, sildenafil can increase and preserve cGMP levels, thereby making the erection harder and more long lasting.

Pharmacokinetics

Sildenafil is well absorbed following oral administration. Bioavailability is about 40%. In fasting subjects, plasma levels peak in about 60 minutes. A high-fat meal slows absorption. As a result, plasma levels peak in 2 hours, and the peak concentration is reduced. Sildenafil is metabolized in the liver, primarily by the 3A4 isozyme of cytochrome P450 (CYP3A4). Both the parent drug and its major metabolite (*N*-desmethyl sildenafil) are biologically active. Both compounds are eliminated primarily in the feces (80%) and partly in the urine (13%). For both compounds, the half-life is 4 hours. Clearance of both is delayed in men older than 65 and in men with hepatic dysfunction or severe renal insufficiency, causing drug levels to rise higher and persist longer.

Sexual Benefits

Men with ED. Sildenafil has been evaluated in over 3700 men (ages 19 to 87) with ED of organic, psychogenic, or mixed-cause origin. At least some improvement in erection hardness and duration was seen in 70% of men taking the drug, compared with 20% taking placebo. Benefits were dose related and persisted up to 4 hours, although they began to fade after 2 hours. Sildenafil was able to help a wide range of patients, including those with ED resulting from diabetes, spinal cord injury, and transurethral prostate resection, as well as ED of no known physical cause.

Men Without ED. Despite anecdotal reports to the contrary, sildenafil has little or no effect on erection quality or duration in men who do not have ED. After all, there's a limit to how good an erection can get. Sildenafil cannot improve on that limit. Any apparent benefits in healthy men are likely the result of a placebo response.

Women. Sildenafil is not approved for use in women, and very little research in women has been done. In a small study involving 17 women who had passed menopause or undergone a hysterectomy, the participants reported that sildenafil improved sexual satisfaction, vaginal lubrication and sensitivity, and the ability to achieve orgasm. However, another study found no benefits beyond those attributable to a placebo effect.

Adverse Effects

Hypotension. At recommended doses, sildenafil produces a small (8.4/5.5 mm Hg) reduction in blood pressure. However, in men taking nitrates (see below), severe hypotension can develop.

Priapism. A few cases of priapism (painful erection lasting more than 6 hours) have been reported. If an erection persists more than 4 hours, immediate medical assistance is required. Left untreated, priapism can damage penile tissue, thereby causing permanent loss of potency. Persistent erection can be relieved by aspirating blood from the corpus followed by irrigation with a solution containing a vasoconstrictor (e.g., epinephrine, phenylephrine, metaraminol).

Other Adverse Effects. The most common adverse effects are headache (16%), flushing (10%), and dyspepsia (7%). Sildenafil may also cause nasal congestion (4%), diarrhea (3%), rash (2%), and dizziness (2%). About 3% of patients experience mild transient visual disturbances (color tinge to vision, increased sensitivity to light, blurring).

Drug Interactions

Inhibitors of CYP3A4. Inhibitors of CYP3A4 (e.g., ketoconazole, itraconazole, erythromycin, cimetidine, saquinavir, ritonavir, grapefruit juice) can suppress metabolism of sildenafil, thereby increasing its levels. Accordingly, these combinations should be used with caution.

Nitrates. Both sildenafil and nitrates (e.g., nitroglycerin, isosorbide dinitrate) promote hypotension, and they both do so by increasing availability of cGMP. If these drugs are combined, life-threatening hypotension could result. Therefore, *sildenafil is absolutely contraindicated for patients taking nitrates.*

Is Sildenafil Safe for Men With CHD?

Reports of adverse cardiovascular events, including at least 130 cardiac deaths, raised concern about the safety of sildenafil in men with coronary heart disease (CHD). However, there was a question as to what caused the adverse events: sildenafil or the sexual activity that sildenafil permitted. When attempting to answer this question, researchers made two important observations: First, giving sildenafil to resting men with severe CHD produced no harmful effects on coronary blood flow or any other hemodynamic parameter. Second, in men with stable CHD performing exercise, sildenafil had no effect on CHD symptoms, exercise tolerance, or exercise-induced ischemia. Taken together, these results suggest that, in men with CHD, sexual activity—and not sildenafil—is the likely cause of ischemic events. However, even though sildenafil itself appears safe for men with CHD, sexual activity may not be. Accordingly, the drug should be used with caution by men with the following conditions:

- Myocardial infarction, stroke, or life-threatening dysrhythmia within the last 6 months
- Resting hypotension (blood pressure <90/50 mm Hg)
- Resting hypertension (blood pressure >170/110 mm Hg)
- Heart failure
- Unstable angina

In addition, *sildenafil should not be used at all by men taking nitroglycerin or any other drug in the nitrate family.*

To reduce the risk of adverse events, candidates for sildenafil therapy should undergo a careful evaluation of cardiovascular function. Those with impaired function should be counseled about the risks posed by sexual activity, and all other moderate to intense physical activity.

Preparations, Dosage, and Administration

Sildenafil [Viagra] is available in 25-, 50-, and 100-mg tablets. The usual dose is 50 mg taken 1 hour before sexual activity. The dosage range is 25 to 100 mg taken 30 minutes to 4 hours before sexual activity. A low dose (25 mg) should be considered for men older than 65, men with hepatic dysfunction or severe renal dysfunction, and men taking drugs that inhibit CYP3A4. Dosing should be done no more than once a day.

Tadalafil and Vardenafil

Tadalafil [Cialis] and vardenafil [Levitra] are new PDE-5 inhibitors similar to sildenafil. Both drugs are approved for treatment of ED in Europe, but are not yet approved for use in the United States. The new drugs are reputed to work faster than sildenafil and cause fewer side effects. However, neither drug has been compared directly with sildenafil—or, for that matter, with the other.

Papaverine Plus Phentolamine

Therapeutic Use. The combination of papaverine (a smooth muscle relaxant) plus phentolamine (an alpha-adrenergic blocking agent) can counteract impotence when injected directly into the corpus cavernosum of the penis. Erection develops within minutes and lasts 2 to 4 hours. In clinical trials, erection suitable for intercourse was produced in 65% to 100% of males whose impotence was of neurologic or vascular origin. For patients who do not respond to papaverine plus phentolamine, addition of alprostadil may help (see below).

Mechanism of Action. Papaverine and phentolamine produce erection by increasing arterial inflow to the penis and decreasing venous outflow. Arterial inflow is augmented by alpha-adrenergic blockade (causing arterial dilation) and by the direct relaxant action of papaverine on arterial smooth muscle. Venous outflow is reduced, probably because relaxation of corporal smooth muscle results in occlusion of the venules that drain the corporal spaces.

Adverse Effects. Priapism (persistent erection lasting more than 6 hours) occurs in about 10% of patients. Development of painless *fibrotic nodules* in the corpus is common. Other adverse effects include *orthostatic hypotension with dizziness, transient paresthesias, ecchymosis* (extravasation of blood into subcutaneous tissue), and *difficulty in achieving orgasm or ejaculation.*

Special Interest Topic

BOX 103–1 ■■ THALIDOMIDE REDEEMED—AND STRICTLY CONTROLLED

On July 16, 1998, the Food and Drug Administration (FDA) finally approved thalidomide for American use—after denying approval nearly 40 years earlier. Because thalidomide is a powerful teratogen, the FDA requires that doctors, pharmacists, and patients follow strict safety rules. At this time, the drug is approved only for erythema nodosum leprosum (ENL), a painful complication of leprosy. However, thalidomide has shown promise in many other diseases, including inflammatory disorders and several types of cancer.

The thalidomide story goes back to the late 1950s, when the drug caused **the most notorious tragedy in pharmaceutical history.** Thalidomide was developed in Germany for use as a sedative, and was sold over the counter in Europe. Many pregnant women took the drug for morning sickness and insomnia. It was not until 1961 that a terrible truth became known: Thalidomide was causing horrific birth defects. Thousands of children were born with stunted, flipper-like limbs (phocomelia). Others suffered deafness, blindness, facial paralysis, brain damage, kidney malformation, and congenital heart disease. Between 1957 and 1961, thalidomide deformed more than 12,000 babies, and killed untold others *in utero.*

Thanks to Dr. Frances O. Kelsey of the FDA, infants in the United States were spared. It was Dr. Kelsey's job to review the application to market thalidomide here. She had just joined the FDA and this was her first assignment. Being concerned about the drug's safety, Dr. Kelsey turned down the application and demanded more studies. Despite pressure from the manufacturer and from her superiors at the FDA, she continued to hold her ground. The drug's teratogenic potential became known before approval was ever granted. In recognition of her courage and dedication, Dr. Kelsey was given the Distinguished Federal Civilian Service Award by President John F. Kennedy.

Thalidomide appears to have **great potential as a therapeutic agent**—far beyond its use in ENL. Responses in cancer have been especially encouraging. In patients with multiple myeloma, an incurable cancer of the bone marrow, thalidomide produced complete remission in 10% of recipients; another 20% or so experienced significant improvement. Furthermore, thalidomide caused fewer adverse effects than traditional anticancer drugs. Early evidence indicates that thalidomide may also help patients with cancer of the prostate, brain, colon, skin, and other tissues. Additional conditions for which thalidomide has shown promise include rheumatoid arthritis, systemic lupus erythematosus (SLE), Crohn's disease (an inflammatory bowel disorder), macular degeneration, chronic host-versus-graft disease, and oral aphthous ulcers associated with AIDS.

Several **pharmacologic actions** may explain therapeutic effects. Of special note are anti-inflammatory and immuno-modulating actions, mediated in part by decreased synthesis of tumor necrosis factor-alpha. In addition, thalidomide suppresses angiogenesis (growth of new blood vessels). This action is thought to underlie benefits in cancer and ENL.

Thalidomide can cause multiple **adverse effects.** Teratogenesis is most important. A single 100-mg dose can cause birth defects. The incidence is nearly 100% when the drug is taken between days 21 and 36 of gestation. Drowsiness occurs in 36% of patients, and can be intensified by other sedative drugs. Peripheral neuropathy—manifesting as limb weakness, incoordination, and tingling in the fingers and toes—develops frequently, and may be irreversible. Other common effects include constipation, orthostatic hypotension, dizziness, dry mouth, and rash.

Thalidomide is available in 50-mg capsules under the trade name *Thalomid.* The wholesale price for a box of 84 capsules is over $600. **Dosing** is done in the evening, preferably at bedtime—and at least 1 hour after eating. The dosages employed for ENL (the only approved application) and some disorders under investigation are as follows:

- *ENL*—100 to 300 mg/day for at least 2 weeks
- *Multiple myeloma*—200 to 800 mg/day for at least 6 weeks
- *SLE*—50 mg/day
- *Crohn's disease*—50 to 300 mg/day
- *Aphthous ulcers*—50 to 300 mg/day

Because thalidomide is a powerful teratogen, all persons who prescribe, dispense, or use the drug must comply with an unprecedented set of FDA-mandated safeguards, known as the **System for Thalidomide Education and Prescribing Safety,** or **S.T.E.P.S.** The objective of S.T.E.P.S. is to ensure full awareness of teratogenic risk, and to implement measures for risk reduction. The program includes the following important provisions:

- Physicians who prescribe thalidomide and pharmacists who dispense it must be registered with the S.T.E.P.S. program.
- Female patients must receive oral and written warning of the risk of birth defects, and must acknowledge their understanding in writing.
- A pregnancy test must be conducted no more than 24 hours before starting therapy. The physician cannot prescribe thalidomide without a written report of a negative test. In addition, pregnancy testing must be done weekly during the first month of treatment, and every 4 weeks thereafter (for women with regular menstrual cycles) or every 2 weeks thereafter (for women with irregular cycles). Thalidomide must be discontinued immediately if pregnancy is detected.
- Female patients must agree in writing to use *two* methods of contraception, a *highly reliable* method (hormonal contraception, tubal ligation, intrauterine device, vasectomy of male partner) and a *reliable* method (cervical cap, diaphragm, latex condom)—beginning 1 month before initiating thalidomide and continuing 1 month after stopping. Contraception is unnecessary for women who (1) have undergone a hysterectomy, (2) are at least 2 years postmenopausal, or (3) chose to abstain from heterosexual intercourse.
- Male patients must receive verbal and written warning of the teratogenic hazards of thalidomide, and must agree to use a latex condom during heterosexual intercourse, even if they've had a successful vasectomy. (We don't know if thalidomide achieves appreciable levels in semen or sperm. Until more is known, precautions for males are prudent.)
- Each box of Thalomid capsules contains a photograph of a thalidomide victim—a baby girl with flipper-like arms and legs. Every time patients reach for a pill, they receive this startling reminder of what thalidomide can do.

Dosage and Administration. For males with psychogenic or neurogenic impotence, erection can be achieved by injecting as little as 0.1 ml of a solution containing 30 mg of papaverine/ml and 1.0 mg of phentolamine/ml. A 1-ml syringe with a 27-gauge or 28-gauge, 3/8-inch needle is used. Injections are made directly into the corpus cavernosum through the lateral aspect of the shaft of the penis. These injections are nearly painless and can be administered by the patient.

Alprostadil (Prostaglandin E₁)

Intracavernous. Like the combination of phentolamine plus papaverine, alprostadil [Caverject, Caverject Impulse, Edex] can produce erection in impotent males when injected directly into the corpus cavernosum. Erection results from increased inflow of arterial blood and reduced outflow of venous blood. Dosages may range from 5 to 40 mg and should be determined in the physician's office. The dosing endpoint is an erection that is sufficient for intercourse, but that does not last for more than 1 hour. Alprostadil should be used no more than 3 times a week and not more than once in 24 hours. Acute adverse effects are penile pain (37%), prolonged erection (4%), and priapism (erection lasting more than 6 hours; 0.4%). Penile fibrosis may develop with continued use.

Transurethral. Alprostadil pellets [Muse], inserted into the urethra, are an alternative to intracavernous injection of the drug. Administration is accomplished by loading a pellet into a small plastic applicator, which is then inserted an inch and a half into the urethra. The procedure is painless. Erection develops 5 to 10 minutes after drug insertion and lasts 30 to 60 minutes. Alprostadil pellets are available in four strengths: 125, 250, 500, and 1000 mg. Dosage should be determined in the physician's office; the objective is to employ the smallest dose required to produce an erection sufficient for intercourse. Alprostadil pellets should be used no more than twice every 24 hours. The most common adverse effect, dull ache in the penis, has an incidence of 11%. Priapism and penile fibrosis, which have occurred with alprostadil injections, have not been reported with the pellets.

Apomorphine

On April 20, 2000, a Food and Drug Administration (FDA) advisory committee recommended approval of apomorphine [Uprima] for ED. Although apomorphine is a derivative of morphine, pharmacologic effects result primarily from activating *dopamine* receptors. If the drug receives final approval, it would become an alternative to sildenafil [Viagra] for *systemic* therapy of ED. Other drugs—alprostadil and papaverine plus phentolamine—are available for *local* therapy. Apomorphine for ED is already available in Canada.

Apomorphine has a different mechanism than sildenafil: Whereas sildenafil acts directly on blood vessels in the penis, apomorphine acts in the brain. Specifically, apomorphine activates dopamine receptors in the paraventricular nucleus of the hypothalamus, and thereby turns on the same neural pathway that mediates psychogenic erection.

Although apomorphine and sildenafil have not been directly compared, available data suggest that sildenafil is more effective and works in a broader population. In clinical trials, men taking apomorphine achieved a functional erection 50% of the time, compared with 35% for those taking placebo. In clinical trials of sildenafil, the drug produced erection 66% of the time, versus 20% for placebo. Furthermore, unlike apomorphine, sildenafil has been proved effective in men whose ED results from an organic cause (e.g., diabetes, prostatectomy, spinal cord injury) in addition to psychologic causes.

The most common side effects of apomorphine are *nausea* and *hypotension.* Nausea is dose dependent and results from activating dopamine receptors in the chemoreceptor trigger zone. (In the past, the emetogenic actions of apomorphine were exploited to treat poisoning.) Some men have required an antiemetic. Like sildenafil, apomorphine can cause hypotension, causing fainting in about 1% of patients. Accordingly, users should avoid driving and other hazardous activities for 2 hours after dosing. Hypotension may exacerbate pre-existing cardiovascular disease; caution is advised. Caution is also needed in men with conditions that predispose to priapism (persistent erection); among these are men with sickle cell anemia, multiple myeloma, and leukemia.

Apomorphine may have significant interactions with *alcohol* and *organic nitrates.* Alcohol increases plasma levels of apomorphine, and can thereby increase the risk of hypotension and syncope. As with sildenafil, combining apomorphine with a nitrate (e.g., nitroglycerin) may increase the risk of hypotension.

Apomorphine is supplied in tablets for *sublingual* administration. If the mouth is dry, it should be moistened with a nonalcoholic beverage before dosing. Advise patients to place a single tablet under the tongue 15 to 25 minutes before anticipated intercourse. If the tablet has not dissolved fully in 20 minutes, the remainder may be swallowed. The recommended initial dose is 2 mg. The maximum dose is 4 mg. Dosing should not be repeated for 8 hours.

Conclusion: Apomorphine appears less effective than sildenafil and causes more adverse effects. Nonetheless, it may benefit men who cannot use sildenafil or don't respond to it.

DRUGS FOR BENIGN PROSTATIC HYPERPLASIA

Pathophysiology and Overview of Treatment

Benign prostatic hyperplasia (BPH) is a common condition that develops in more than 50% of men by age 60 and 90% by age 85. The disorder accounts for 1.7 million physician visits each year and leads to 300,000 prostatectomies. The total annual cost exceeds $2 billion. Although BPH and prostate cancer can coexist, there is no evidence that one disorder predisposes to the other.

Pathophysiology

BPH is a nonmalignant enlargement of the prostate caused by excessive growth of epithelial (glandular) and smooth muscle cells. Overgrowth of epithelial cells causes *mechanical obstruction* of the urethra, whereas overgrowth of smooth muscle causes *dynamic obstruction* of the urethra. In men with BPH, the ratio of epithelium to smooth muscle varies from 1:3 to 4:1—in general, the larger the prostate, the higher the percentage of epithelium. Signs and symptoms of BPH include urinary hesitancy, urinary urgency, increased frequency of urination, dysuria, nocturia, straining to void, postvoid dribbling, decreased force and caliber of the urinary stream, and a sensation of incomplete bladder emptying. There is no direct correlation between symptoms and prostate size. Hence, some men with only moderate enlargement may be highly symptomatic, whereas others with substantial enlargement may have no symptoms.

Treatment Modalities

BPH can be managed in three ways: drug therapy, surgery, and "watchful waiting." Surgical options include transurethral resection of the prostate, transurethral electrovaporization of the prostate, and laser prostatectomy. These procedures are most appropriate for men with severe symptoms or complications (urinary tract infection, uremia due to obstruction, bladder stones). Watchful waiting, which consists of reassurance and annual re-evaluation, is appropriate for men with minimal symptoms.

Drug Therapy

BPH can be treated with *5-alpha-reductase inhibitors* and *alpha₁-adrenergic antagonists.* The goal of treatment is to relieve bothersome urinary symptoms. As discussed below, finasteride and dutasteride may be most appropriate for patients with very large prostates, whereas alpha blockers may be preferred for patients with relatively small prostates.

5-Alpha-Reductase Inhibitors

Finasteride. Finasteride [Proscar] acts in reproductive tissue to inhibit 5-alpha-reductase, an enzyme that converts testosterone to dihydrotestosterone (DHT), the active form of testosterone in the prostate. Treatment reduces levels of DHT in blood by 70% (but does not decrease testosterone levels). By decreasing DHT availability, finasteride promotes regression of prostate epithelial tissue, and thereby decreases *mechanical obstruction* of the urethra. Since the percentage of epithelial tissue is highest in very large prostates, finasteride is most effective in men whose prostates are highly enlarged. Conversely, the drug has little or no effect if the degree of enlargement is small. It should be noted that benefits develop slowly—over a period of 6 to 12 months.

Finasteride is generally well tolerated. However, it does decrease ejaculate volume and libido in 5% to 10% of patients. In addition, gynecomastia (breast enlargement) develops in some men.

Finasteride decreases serum levels of prostate-specific antigen (PSA), a marker for prostate cancer. The expected decline is 30% to 50%. PSA levels should be determined prior to treatment and 6 months later. If PSA levels do not fall as expected, the patient should be evaluated for cancer of the prostate.

Finasteride is available in 5-mg tablets. The usual dosage is 5 mg once a day, taken with or without food. Treatment continues for life.

Dutasteride. Dutasteride [Avodart] is similar to finasteride in most respects. However, there are three significant differences. First, with dutasteride, the reduction in circulating DHT is more complete. Second, dutasteride is harmful to the developing male fetus. Third, dutasteride has an extremely long half-life (about 5 weeks), and hence it takes months to clear the drug once dosing has stopped.

Like finasteride, dutasteride inhibits 5-alpha-reductase, and thereby reduces availability of DHT. However, whereas finasteride inhibits only the form of 5-alpha-reductase found in reproductive tissues, dutasteride also inhibits the form found in the skin and liver. As a result, dutasteride produces a greater reduction in circulating DHT (93% vs. 70%). Whether this translates to a greater clinical response has not been established (dutasteride and finasteride have not been directly compared).

Like finasteride, dutasteride reduces ejaculate volume and libido in some men, and causes a decline in PSA in all.

Animal studies indicate that dutasteride can inhibit development of the external genitalia in the male fetus. Accordingly, the drug is classified in FDA Pregnancy Risk Category X. Dutasteride can be absorbed through the skin, and hence pregnant women should not handle it. Men should not donate blood while using dutasteride or until at least 6 months have passed since stopping it (so as to avoid transmission to women via an infusion).

Dutasteride is available in 0.5-mg capsules. The dosage is 0.5 mg once a day, taken with or without food. As with finasteride, treatment continues indefinitely.

Alpha₁-Adrenergic Antagonists

Alpha₁ antagonists (alpha blockers) relax smooth muscle in the prostate capsule, prostatic urethra, and bladder neck, and thereby decrease *dynamic obstruction* of the urethra. Improvement in symptoms and urinary flow develops rapidly. Because dynamic obstruction is the major contributor to symptoms in patients with relatively mild prostatic enlargement, alpha blockers are preferred to finasteride for these men. To maintain benefits, alpha blockers must be taken lifelong.

Three alpha₁ blockers—*terazosin* [Hytrin], *doxazosin* [Cardura], and *tamsulosin* [Flomax]—are approved for BPH. However, their pharmacology is not identical: Whereas terazosin and doxazosin block alpha₁ receptors in *blood vessels* as well as in the prostate, tamsulosin is selective for alpha₁ receptors in the prostate. By blocking alpha₁ receptors in blood vessels, terazosin and doxazosin promote vasodilation, and can thereby lower blood pressure. In fact, these drugs were developed as antihypertensive agents; their use in BPH came later. Because of their impact on blood pressure, these drugs are especially useful for patients who have hypertension in addition to BPH. In contrast to terazosin and doxazosin, tamsulosin has little or no effect on blood pressure, and hence is of no benefit to people with hypertension.

The alpha₁ blockers are generally well tolerated. For terazosin and doxazosin, principal adverse effects are hypotension, fainting, dizziness, somnolence, nasal congestion, and retrograde ejaculation (secondary to relaxation of smooth muscle in the bladder neck). Like terazosin and doxazosin, tamsulosin can cause retrograde ejaculation. However, because its effects on blood pressure are minimal, tamsulosin is less likely to cause hypotension, fainting, dizziness, or nasal congestion. In contrast to finasteride, the alpha blockers do not reduce levels of PSA.

Dosages for BPH are as follows:

- *Terazosin* [Hytrin]—Start with 1 mg once daily at bedtime and gradually increase to a maximum of 10 mg once daily.
- *Doxazosin* [Cardura]—Start with 1 mg once daily and gradually increase to a maximum of 8 mg once daily.
- *Tamsulosin* [Flomax]—Treat with 0.4 mg once daily, taken about 30 minutes after the same meal (e.g., breakfast) each day.

Note that dosages of terazosin and doxazosin must be titrated, whereas the dosage for tamsulosin is fixed. Titration is done to minimize hypotension.

The basic pharmacology of alpha blockers is discussed in Chapter 18.

Saw Palmetto

Saw palmetto is an herbal preparation that can reduce symptoms of BPH. The product, available as a dietary supplement, is an extract prepared from the dried ripe berries of the American dwarf saw palmetto (*Serenoa repens; Sabal serrulata*), a small palm tree native to the southeastern United States. The active ingredient has not been identified, and commercial products are not standardized. Although published data on saw palmetto are limited, the available literature indicates that the product is effective, reducing urologic symptoms and improving urinary flow. In fact, saw palmetto seems to compare favorably with finasteride, while causing fewer undesired effects. How does palmetto work? No one knows. Possibilities include altered cholesterol metabolism; reduced levels of sex hormone–binding globulin; and antiestrogenic, antiandrogenic, and anti-inflammatory actions. Saw palmetto is discussed further in Chapter 104 (Herbal Supplements).

DRUGS FOR NEONATAL RESPIRATORY DISTRESS SYNDROME

Respiratory distress syndrome (RDS) is the primary cause of morbidity and mortality in premature infants. The underlying cause is deficiency of lung surfactant, a complex mixture of phospholipids and apoproteins that lowers surface tension on the alveolar surface. Consequences of surfactant deficiency include alveolar collapse, pulmonary edema, reduced lung compliance, small airway epithelial damage, hypoxia, and ultimately respiratory failure.

Increased production of cortisol during weeks 30 to 32 of gestation initiates production of lung surfactant. However, surfactant production is not fully adequate until weeks 34 to 36. As a result, the earlier the premature infant is delivered, the greater the risk of RDS. Among infants born during weeks 26 to 28, the incidence of RDS is 60% to 80%; by weeks 30 to 32, the incidence drops to only 20%.

Antenatal Glucocorticoids

When preterm delivery cannot be prevented, injecting the mother with glucocorticoids can accelerate fetal lung maturation, and thereby decrease the incidence and severity of RDS. Glucocorticoids act by stimulating production of fibroblast pneumocyte factor, which in turn stimulates production of surfactant by fetal pneumocytes. Glucocorticoids are effective when used during weeks 24 to 34 of gestation. Beyond week 34, fetal lungs are sufficiently mature that no benefit is gained by giving glucocorticoids. Two regimens are recommended: (1) *dexamethasone*, 6 mg IM every 12 hours for four doses, and (2) *betamethasone*, two 12-mg IM doses, injected 24 hours apart. To be effective, the last glucocorticoid dose should be administered at least 24 hours before delivery, but no more than 7 days before. Routine use of repeat courses should be avoided. The basic pharmacology of the glucocorticoids is discussed in Chapters 57 and 68.

Lung Surfactant

Lung surfactant, administered by direct intratracheal instillation, is indicated for prevention and treatment (rescue therapy) of RDS. Surfactant therapy lowers the surface-tension forces that cause alveolar collapse, and thereby rapidly improves oxygenation and lung compliance and reduces the need for supplemental oxygen and mechanical ventilation. Treatment decreases neonatal mortality by 33%.

In the United States, three preparations of lung surfactant are available: poractant alfa, calfactant, and beractant. At this time, the data are insufficient to recommend any one drug over the others. Initial doses for prevention or treatment of RDS are as follows:

- *Poractant alfa* [Curosurf]—2.5 ml/kg
- *Calfactant* [Infasurf]—3 ml/kg
- *Beractant* [Survanta]—4 ml/kg

Because the effects of a single dose are often transient, dosing may need to be repeated. For poractant alfa, repeat doses should be 1.25 ml/kg—half the initial dose. For calfactant and beractant, repeat doses are the same as the initial dose.

Adverse effects result primarily from the administration process. Bradycardia and oxygen desaturation, which occur secondary to vagal stimulation and airway obstruction, are most common. If these occur, it may be necessary to temporarily suspend administration. Other adverse effects include pulmonary hemorrhage, mucus plugging, and endotracheal tube reflux.

DRUGS FOR CYSTIC FIBROSIS

Cystic fibrosis (CF) is an inherited disorder that results in damage to the lungs, pancreas, and other organs. About 30,000 U.S. citizens have the disease. Thirty years ago, 50% of children diagnosed with CF died before the age of 5. Today, the mean survival is 30 years. Drugs cannot cure CF, but they can reduce symptoms and slow progression of injury.

Pathophysiology of Cystic Fibrosis

The underlying cause of CF is mutation of the gene that codes for a particular type of chloride channel, referred to as the cystic fibrosis transmembrane regulator (CFTR). In cells that have defective CFTRs, the normal transmembrane flow of chloride ions, sodium ions, and water is disrupted. In the lungs, exocrine glands (e.g., pancreas), and other structures, disruption of ion and water flux alters secretions.

Pancreas. Disruption of chloride transport in the pancreas impairs secretion of bicarbonate and digestive enzymes into the small intestine. The immediate result is maldigestion and malabsorption of fats and other nutrients. Absorption of fat-soluble vitamins, especially vitamins A and E, is reduced secondary to malabsorption of fats. Over time, accumulation of digestive enzymes within pancreatic cells leads to cell destruction. At autopsy, the pancreas appears scarred and fibrotic, which led pathologists to name this illness fibrocystic disease of the pancreas—later shortened to cystic fibrosis. Until replacement therapy with pancreatic enzymes became possible, malabsorption of nutrients was the major cause of CF death.

Lungs. Today, destruction of lung tissue is the major cause of morbidity and mortality among patients with CF. In the cells that line the airway, defective CFTRs impair secretion of chloride and enhance reabsorption of water and sodium. As a result, mucus becomes thick and viscous, causing plugging of the airway and promoting chronic bacterial colonization. All patients eventually develop active pulmonary infection; the most common pathogen is *Pseudomonas aeruginosa*. Infection elicits an inflammatory response that is mediated primarily by neutrophils. Accumulation of DNA from dead neutrophils further increases the viscosity of sputum. Over time, chronic bronchitis and associated inflammation cause progressive destruction of lung tissue. In 95% of patients, death from cardiorespiratory failure ultimately ensues.

Reproductive Organs. Among patients with CF, 98% of males and 70% to 80% of females are infertile. In males, the usual cause is obstruction of the vas deferens. In females, the cause appears to be production of thick, sticky cervical mucus, which impedes penetration of sperm.

Drug Therapy

Drugs are used to alleviate symptoms of CF and delay progression of injury to the lungs. Agents employed include pancreatic enzymes, fat-soluble vitamins, antibiotics, dornase alfa, and ibuprofen. Gene therapy is under investigation.

Nutritional Drugs

Pancreatic Enzymes. These enzymes are given as replacement therapy. All preparations contain lipase, protease, and amylase. The most effective formulations deliver the enzymes in enteric-coated microspheres, which are designed to (1) protect the enzymes from stomach acid and (2) ensure dissolution in the duodenum, the site where the enzymes act. Pancreatic enzymes are discussed in Chapter 75.

Fat-Soluble Vitamins. There are four fat-soluble vitamins: A, D, E, and K. Among patients with CF, deficiencies in vitamins A and E are relatively common, whereas deficiency in vitamin K is uncommon and deficiency in vitamin D is rare. Because vitamins are safe and relatively inexpensive, supplementation with all four is done routinely.

Pulmonary Drugs

Inhaled Tobramycin. Tobramycin solution for inhalation [TOBI] is now the treatment of choice for chronic pulmonary infection with *P. aeruginosa.* The dosage is 300 mg every 12 hours in repeating cycles of 28 days on and 28 days off. Inhaled tobramycin improves pulmonary function, reduces the density of *P. aeruginosa* in sputum, and decreases the risk of hospitalization. It is too soon to know if treatment also prolongs life. Unlike IV aminoglycosides, inhaled tobramycin does not cause hearing loss, although it can cause tinnitus (ringing in the ears). Because treatment is prolonged, emergence of resistance is a concern. Inhaled tobramycin is expensive: A year's supply costs over $14,000. The basic pharmacology of tobramycin and other aminoglycosides is discussed in Chapter 83.

Inhaled Dornase Alfa. Dornase alfa [Pulmozyme], a purified preparation of recombinant human deoxyribonuclease, decreases the viscosity of sputum in patients with CF. Dornase alfa is administered by inhalation, using an approved nebulizer. Benefits derive from breaking down extracellular DNA that has accumulated in the lungs secondary to death of neutrophils. With daily use, dornase alfa can improve pulmonary function and decrease infection in some patients. The drug is generally well tolerated. Adverse effects include hoarseness, pharyngitis, laryngitis, rash, chest pain, and conjunctivitis. Dosing is begun at 2.5 mg once daily and may be increased to 2.5 mg twice daily if needed. To remain effective, dornase alfa must be administered every day for life. Unfortunately, treatment is expensive. A year's supply of dornase alfa costs over $12,000. The nebulizer costs another $2000.

Oral Ibuprofen. High-dose ibuprofen can slow progression of pulmonary damage in patients with mild lung disease caused by CF. Benefits derive from suppressing the inflammatory response that underlies destruction of lung tissue. Ibuprofen dosage should be sufficient to produce peak plasma drug levels of 50 to 100 mg/ml. Side effects attributable to ibuprofen include conjunctivitis and epistaxis (nosebleed).

DRUGS FOR SICKLE CELL ANEMIA

Sickle cell anemia (SCA) is an inherited blood disorder characterized by abnormal hemoglobin, chronic anemia, periodic painful episodes, and reduced life expectancy. The underlying cause is a mutation in the gene that codes for hemoglobin (Hb). People who inherit two copies of the gene (one from each parent) produce an altered form of Hb, known as HbS. (People with just one copy are carriers, but do not make HbS.) When HbS is fully oxygenated, there is no problem. However, when HbS gives up its oxygen, molecules of HbS can polymerize, forming long, rigid, rod-like chains. As a result, red blood cells (RBCs) assume a sickle (crescent) shape, and hence cannot pass through tiny blood vessels. As more RBCs get stuck, blood flow stops, thereby depriving tissues of required nutrients and oxygen. The result is severe pain, referred to as a vaso-occlusive crisis. Pain location depends on where vessel blockage occurs (e.g., hands and feet, joints and extremities, abdomen). The crisis may last a few hours to a few weeks. Some patients have 15 or more painful episodes a year, whereas others may have one a year or less. Over time, vaso-occlusive events produce progressive organ damage and premature death. In addition to vaso-occlusive crises, people with SCA suffer from chronic anemia (shortage of RBCs). Why? Unlike normal RBCs, which persist about 120 days, sickled RBCs die in 10 to 20 days. Because RBC loss is unusually rapid, replacements cannot be made fast enough, and hence a chronic shortage results.

Who is vulnerable to SCA? Worldwide, millions of people have the disease. In the United States, about 72,000 people have SCA. Most are African Americans (about 1 in 600 carry two copies of the sickle cell gene, and 1 in 12 carry one copy). In addition, SCA afflicts between 1 in 1000 and 1 in 1400 Hispanic Americans. The disease is not found among white Americans.

Researchers believe that the sickle cell mutation arose in a region where malaria is endemic. There is evidence that, in people with *one* copy of the gene, malaria is less deadly than in people who do not have the gene. As a result, those who carried the gene were more likely to survive, and hence could pass the advantage on to their progeny. Of course, in areas like the United States, where malaria rarely occurs, the gene offers no survival advantage—and, when two copies are inherited, becomes a real threat to survival.

Treatment consists of transfusions, analgesics, glucocorticoids, and hydroxyurea. Blood transfusions help correct anemia and reduce painful episodes. Analgesics and glucocorticoids can alleviate pain. Recently, hydroxyurea has been shown to reduce the incidence and severity of painful episodes and, perhaps more importantly, it has been shown to prolong life.

Analgesics and Glucocorticoids

For patients undergoing an acute crisis, analgesics (and hydration) are the cornerstone of treatment. Unfortunately, most patients generally fail to receive adequate pain relief. If the pain is moderate, a nonopioid analgesic (acetaminophen or a nonsteroidal anti-inflammatory agent) may be sufficient. However, if pain is severe, intensive therapy with an opioid is required. Parenteral (IV or IM) morphine and meperidine have been employed. Patient-controlled analgesia may be especially effective. The basic pharmacology of the opioids is discussed in Chapter 27.

High doses of intravenous methylprednisolone (a glucocorticoid) can shorten the duration of a sickle-cell crisis. The drug should be used together with an opioid, not instead of it. Unfortunately, when glucocorticoids are discontinued, rebound pain may occur. The basic pharmacology of the glucocorticoids is discussed in Chapter 68.

Hydroxyurea

Hydroxyurea [Droxia], a drug developed to treat cancer (see Chapter 98), is now being used against SCA. Treatment can reduce the number of painful events as well as the need for hospitalization and transfusions. Furthermore, it can prolong life.

Mechanism of Action. Hydroxyurea increases production of fetal hemoglobin (HbF), a form of Hb present in infants but not normally present after the sixth month of postnatal life. In patients with SCA, elevation of HbF decreases hemoglobin polymerization, and thereby decreases RBC sickling and prolongs RBC life. The drug also reduces adhesion of RBCs to the vascular endothelium. Precisely how hydroxyurea elevates HbF is unknown.

Clinical Trials. The first major study with hydroxyurea—the Multicenter Study of Hydroxyurea (MSH) in Sickle Cell Anemia trial—was conducted between 1992 and 1995. In this double-blind, randomized, placebo-controlled trial, hydroxyurea produced a 44% reduction in the incidence of painful episodes, a 58% reduction in hospitalizations, and a 34% reduction in transfusions. On the basis of these results, the FDA approved hydroxyurea for reducing painful episodes in adults with SCA. In 2003, results of the MSH Patients' Follow-up trial were published. This trial, which followed patients from the original MSH trial, evaluated the impact of prolonged therapy (up to 9 years) on mortality. The result? Mortality among patients taking hydroxyurea was 40% lower than among those not taking the drug. Furthermore, reductions in mortality were proportional to the extent of HbF elevation and to reductions in painful episodes. It is important to note that hydroxyurea is more likely to benefit patients with severe SCA than patients with moderate or mild SCA. Accordingly, treatment is strongly recommend for the 30% of patients with severe SCA, and is not recommended for the 20% of patients with mild SCA. Whether the drug should be used by the 50% of patients with moderate SCA is unclear.

Adverse Effects. The principal concern is *myelosuppression,* which can reduce neutrophil, platelet, and reticulocyte counts. However, at the doses employed for SCA, myelosuppression has been mild and transient. Nonetheless, frequent monitoring of hematologic status is recommended (see below).

Hydroxyurea can cause *fetal harm,* and hence should be avoided during pregnancy. The drug is classified in FDA Pregnancy Risk Category D.

Among patients receiving hydroxyurea for cancer, a few have developed leukemia. However, it is not clear that hydroxyurea was the cause.

At this time, possible long-term adverse effects are unknown.

Hematologic Monitoring. Hematologic status should be determined every 2 weeks. Acceptable values and values indicating toxicity are as follows:

- *Neutrophils*—acceptable, $\geq$ 2500 cells/mm³; toxic, <2000 cells/mm³
- *Platelets*—acceptable, $\geq$ 95,000/mm³; toxic, <80,000/mm³
- *Hemoglobin*—acceptable, $\geq$ 5.3 gm/dl; toxic, <4.5 gm/dl
- *Reticulocytes*—acceptable, $\geq$ 95,000/mm³ (if Hb is <9 gm/dl); toxic, <80,000/mm³ (if Hb is <9 gm/dl)

Preparations, Dosage, and Administration. For treatment of SCA, hydroxyurea [Droxia] is available in 200-, 300-, and 400-mg capsules. The initial dosage is 15 mg/kg once a day. If blood counts remain acceptable, dosage may be increased by 5 mg/kg/day every 12 weeks—up to a maximum of 35 mg/kg/day. If blood counts indicate toxicity, treatment should be temporarily discontinued. Recovery usually occurs in 2 weeks, after which treatment can be resumed, but at a reduced dosage.

DRUGS FOR HYPERURICEMIA CAUSED BY CANCER CHEMOTHERAPY

Hyperuricemia (elevation of uric acid levels) is a common consequence of cancer chemotherapy. The cause is breakdown of DNA following massive cell death. Two drugs are available for management: rasburicase and allopurinol. Rasburicase, a new drug, accelerates uric acid removal; allopurinol, an old drug, blocks uric acid production.

Rasburicase

Action and Use. Rasburicase [Elitek], produced by recombinant DNA technology, is a form of urate oxidase, an enzyme that converts uric acid into a soluble, inactive product (allantoin). The drug is indicated for management of hyperuricemia in pediatric patients undergoing treatment for leukemias, lymphomas, and solid tumors, when cell lysis caused by chemotherapy is expected to produce a significant increase in plasma uric acid.

Adverse Effects. In clinical trials, the most common reactions were vomiting (50%), fever (46%), nausea (27%), abdominal pain (20%), constipation (20%), diarrhea (20%), and rash (13%). More serious reactions included neutropenia with fever (4%), respiratory distress (3%), sepsis (3%), and mucositis (2%). The most severe reactions, which occurred in 1% of patients or less, were hemolysis, methemoglobinemia, and severe allergic reactions, including anaphylaxis; if any of these reactions occurs, rasburicase should be discontinued immediately and never used again.

Preparations, Dosage, and Administration. Rasburicase [Elitek] is supplied as a powder (1.5 mg/vial) for reconstitution in the diluent provided. When reconstituting, do not vigorously agitate. The recommended dosage is 0.15 or 0.2 mg/kg, infused over 30 minutes, on 5 consecutive days. Start the first infusion 4 to 24 hours prior to the first dose of chemotherapy.

Allopurinol

Allopurinol [Zyloprim] is used to manage hyperuricemia associated with gout and with cancer chemotherapy. Benefits derive from inhibiting xanthine oxidase, the enzyme needed to convert DNA breakdown products (xanthine and hypoxanthine) into uric acid. Allopurinol is discussed at length in Chapter 69 (Drugs for Rheumatoid Arthritis, Osteoarthritis, and Gout).

GAMMA-HYDROXYBUTYRATE FOR CATAPLEXY IN PATIENTS WITH NARCOLEPSY

History. Gamma-hydroxybutyrate (GHB) [Xyrem], also known as sodium oxybate, is a central nervous system (CNS) depressant with a rapid onset and short duration. The drug was originally developed as a surgical anesthetic, but was discontinued owing to serious side effects: profound respiratory depression, coma, and death. In the 1990s, GHB gained notoriety as a drug of abuse: It was used at parties to produce euphoria and disinhibition, and it was administered clandestinely to facilitate rape (see Chapter 38, Box 38–1). As a result, GHB was declared illegal.

Therapeutic Use. In 2002, GHB became the first and only drug approved by the FDA for treatment of *cataplexy* in patients with narcolepsy. Narcolepsy itself, which afflicts about 120,000 Americans, is characterized by fragmented sleep, daytime somnolence, and uncontrollable attacks of sleep during waking hours. In addition, about 60% to 70% of patients experience cataplexy (sudden loss of muscle tone), typically triggered by intense emotion, such as anger, fear, grief, or even amusement. A cataplectic attack may last a few seconds to many minutes, and can range in severity from dropping of the jaw or slumping of the head to buckling of the legs or collapse of the entire body. As discussed in Chapter 35, patients take CNS stimulants (e.g., methylphenidate [Ritalin], dextroamphetamine [Dexedrine]), to promote daytime wakefulness and reduce sudden sleep attacks. GHB is indicated specifically to reduce attacks of cataplexy. Benefits appear to derive from rebound CNS excitement that occurs when the drug's depressant effects wear off. In addition to reducing cataplexy, GHB can improve the quality of nighttime sleep, and can thereby help reduce daytime sleepiness.

Adverse Effects and Abuse. In clinical trials, GHB produced confusion, depression, headache, dizziness, sleepwalking, bedwetting, nausea, and vomiting. In two patients, respiratory depression occurred. The risk of respiratory depression is increased by combining the drug with alcohol and other CNS depressants. Because of its sodium content (a 9-gm dose contains 1.6 gm of sodium), GHB may pose a risk to patients with heart failure. Abuse of the drug could cause physical dependence. Because of its abuse history, GHB is regulated as a Schedule III substance.

Availability. Owing to concerns about adverse effects and abuse, availability of GHB is regulated under a strict and comprehensive risk management program. Provisions include limited distribution, physician and patient education, physician and patient registries, and detailed patient surveillance. Under the program, GHB can be obtained only through a single centralized pharmacy. Before the pharmacy can dispense GHB, the physician must verify that the patient has received instruction on its safe use.

Preparations, Dosage, and Administration. Gamma-hydroxybutyrate [Xyrem] is available in solution (500 mg/ml in 180-ml bottles) for oral use. Patients take two doses each night, one at bedtime and one 2.5 to 4 hours later. At treatment onset, each dose is 2.25 gm (4.5 gm total per night). Dosage can be gradually increased to a maximum of 9 gm total per night. In patients with impaired liver function, the dosage should be halved. Treatment is expensive: at 9 gm per night, the cost is about $740 per month ($8880 per year).

RILUZOLE FOR AMYOTROPHIC LATERAL SCLEROSIS

Amyotrophic lateral sclerosis (ALS, Lou Gehrig's disease) is a neuromuscular disorder characterized by progressive muscle wasting and loss of strength. The underlying cause is degeneration of motor neurons, especially in the outside (lateral) portion of the spinal cord. Why motor neurons degenerate is unknown. Initial symptoms typically include weakness in the hands and legs, muscle cramps, stiffness, and twitching. Over time, the patient becomes weaker and weaker. Eventually, all skeletal muscles, including the muscles of respiration, become paralyzed. Intellectual function, eye movement, bladder function, and sensation are not affected. Most patients die within 3 to 5 years, although some survive for a decade or longer. In the United States, ALS strikes about 5000 people each year. At this time, the disease has no cure.

Riluzole [Rilutek], a glutamate antagonist, is the only drug approved for ALS. In clinical trials, the drug prolonged life or delayed the need for a tracheostomy by 3 to 6 months. However, not only were benefits modest, they were limited to patients whose nerve degeneration began in the *medulla;* riluzole did not help patients whose nerve degeneration began in the *spinal cord.* The reason for this difference is unknown. Riluzole is generally well tolerated. The most common adverse effects are asthenia (decreased strength), GI reactions (nausea, vomiting, diarrhea, abdominal pain), central nervous system effects (dizziness, vertigo, somnolence), and decreased lung function. Riluzole is available in 50-mg tablets for oral administration. The recommended dosage is 50 mg every 12 hours. Increasing the dosage does not increase benefits, but does increase the risk of adverse effects. Riluzole should be taken 1 hour before meals or 2 hours after so as to increase bioavailability.

▪▪ KEY POINTS

- Erectile dysfunction (ED) is defined as a persistent inability to achieve or sustain an erection suitable for satisfactory sexual performance.
- Sildenafil [Viagra] is the first and only oral drug for ED.
- Sildenafil promotes erection by inhibiting PDE-5, the enzyme that converts cGMP to GMP, and thereby causes erection to fade.
- Sildenafil is contraindicated for patients taking organic nitrates because the combination poses a risk of life-threatening hypotension.
- Sildenafil does not increase the risk of cardiovascular events in patients with coronary artery disease—but the sexual activity that sildenafil permits may.
- Symptoms of benign prostatic hyperplasia (BPH) result from (1) mechanical obstruction of the urethra (secondary to overgrowth of epithelial cells), and (2) dynamic obstruction of the urethra (secondary to overgrowth of smooth muscle).
- Finasteride [Proscar] promotes regression of prostate epithelial tissue, and thereby decreases mechanical obstruction of the urethra. Since the percentage of epithelial tissue is highest in very large prostates, finasteride is most effective in men whose prostates are highly enlarged.
- Tamsulosin [Flomax] and other alpha$_1$ blockers relax smooth muscle in the prostate capsule, prostatic urethra, and bladder neck, and thereby decrease dynamic obstruction of the urethra.
- Respiratory distress syndrome (RDS), the primary cause of morbidity and mortality in premature infants, results from a deficiency in lung surfactant.
- When preterm birth is unavoidable, injecting the mother with glucocorticoids can accelerate fetal lung maturation, and can thereby decrease the risk of RDS.
- Lung surfactant—beractant or colfosceril palmitate—is given to preterm infants to prevent or treat RDS.
- Cystic fibrosis (CF) is an inherited disorder that results in damage to the lungs, pancreas, and other organs.

- Inhaled dornase alfa [Pulmozyme] can improve pulmonary function and decrease infection in some patients with CF. The drug decreases the viscosity of sputum by breaking down extracellular DNA that has accumulated secondary to death of neutrophils.
- Inhaled tobramycin [TOBI] is the drug of choice for treating chronic *P. aeruginosa* pulmonary infection in patients with CF.
- High-dose ibuprofen can slow progression of pulmonary damage in CF. Benefits derive from suppressing the inflammatory response that underlies destruction of lung tissue.
- In patients with CF, supplemental pancreatic enzymes promote digestion and absorption of nutrients. All preparations contain lipase, protease, and amylase.
- In patients with sickle cell anemia, hydroxyurea can reduce the number of painful episodes, hospitalizations, and transfusions, and can prolong life. Benefits derive from increasing production of fetal hemoglobin.

- Hyperuricemia secondary to cancer chemotherapy can be managed with two drugs: rasburicase (which accelerates uric acid removal) and allopurinol (which blocks uric acid production).
- In patients with sickle cell anemia (SCA), hydroxyurea can reduce the frequency and intensity of painful episodes; chronic treatment can prolong life.
- At high doses, hydroxyurea can cause severe myelosuppression. However, at the doses employed for SCA, myelosuppression has been transient and mild.
- Gamma-hydroxybutyrate can decrease attacks of cataplexy in patients with narcolepsy.
- Gamma-hydroxybutyrate has significant abuse potential and can cause serious adverse effects (respiratory depression, coma, death). Accordingly, distribution of the drug is strictly controlled.
- In patients with amyotrophic lateral sclerosis (Lou Gehrig's disease), riluzole [Rilutek] can prolong life or delay the need for a tracheostomy by a few months.

Herbal Supplements*

Herbal medicine can be defined as the use of plant-derived products to promote health and relieve symptoms of disease. For millennia, humans have used remedies made from the roots, bark, leaves, fruits, berries, and flowers of indigenous flora. Today, herbal products are used widely in the United States and throughout the world. Some herbal preparations are effective, many are not, and a few can be harmful or even deadly. Unfortunately, it's hard to tell which group a specific product belongs to. Why? Because there's a dearth of reliable data on the safety and efficacy of medicinal herbs, and because these products are exempt from meaningful regulation. As we shall see, herbal products can be manufactured without oversight and sold without a prescription—as long as they are labeled "dietary supplements."

Herbal medicine is the most common form of *alternative medicine,* which can be defined as treatment practices that are not widely accepted or practiced by mainstream clinicians in a given culture. Other names for alternative medicine include *complementary, holistic,* and *integrative medicine.* Alternative medicine encompasses a large and diverse group of theories and practices. Among these are homeopathy, massage, meditation, therapeutic touch, acupuncture, and treatment with high-dose vitamins and herbal remedies. Worldwide, between 70% and 90% of medical practices would be considered alternative medicine compared with conventional practices here.

In the United States, use of alternative medicine is growing significantly. According to a 1998 study published in *JAMA,* 4 out of 10 Americans use some form of alternative medicine. Between 1990 and 1997, visits to alternative medicine practitioners rose 47%—from 427 million to 629 million—thereby exceeding total visits to primary care physicians. In 1997, Americans spent $27 billion out-of-pocket for alternative therapies, which equals their total out-of-pocket expense for physician services.

Like alternative medicine in general, herbal medicine is being used more and more. In 1997, about 33% of Americans took medicinal herbs, for which they spent about $5.1 billion. The growing popularity of herbal medicine may be explained by several factors (Table 104–1). Herbal products are available without prescription, and hence can be purchased without the cost and inconvenience of visiting a prescriber. Furthermore, herbal medicines are frequently cheaper than conventional drugs. Some people like the sense of empowerment that comes from self-diagnosis and self-prescribing. Others may turn to herbal therapy out of anger or frustration with the traditional healthcare system. Still others may distrust conventional medicine or may feel it has failed them. Perhaps the strongest force driving the demand for herbal products is aggressive marketing: In recent years, we have been deluged with advertising in print and on radio and television promising a host of benefits, including enhanced immune function, easy weight loss, clearer thinking, improved memory, better sex lives, and healthier hearts and joints—all by using products touted as "natural," and thus often perceived as safer and more "healthy" than conventional drugs.

Much of our information on herbal products has been amassed by the German Commission E, an expert panel composed of physicians, pharmacists, pharmacologists, and biostatisticians. The commission was established by the German Federal Health Agency (equivalent to our Food and Drug Administration [FDA]) to review and analyze the world literature on plant-based products. Commission E monographs contain information on the chemistry, pharmacology, toxicology, and traditional uses of medicinal herbs, as well as data on clinical trials, epidemiologic studies, and patient case records. These monographs are the most authoritative guide to herbal therapy available today. An English translation, titled *The Complete German Commission E Monographs—Therapeutic Guide to Herbal Medicines,* has been published by the American Botanical Council.

Addresses for some Internet sites dedicated to herbs and other forms of alternative medicine can be found in the list

---

*This chapter was coauthored by Alan P. Agins, Ph.D., and Richard A. Lehne, Ph.D.

TABLE 104–1 ■ Why People Use Medicinal Herbs

- Perception that herbs are safer and "healthier" than conventional drugs
- Sense of control over one's care
- Emotional comfort from taking action
- Cultural influences
- Limited access to professional care
- Lack of health insurance
- Convenience
- Relatively low cost
- Media hype and aggressive marketing
- Recommendation from family and friends

on the inside back cover of this book. The site created and maintained by the Integrative Medicine Service at Memorial Sloan-Kettering Cancer Center is especially good, offering information gleaned from scientific literature. Its web address is *www.mskcc.org/aboutherbs.*

LIMITED REGULATION: THE DIETARY SUPPLEMENT HEALTH AND EDUCATION ACT

Core Provisions

Medicinal herbs are regulated under the *Dietary Supplement Health and Education Act* (DSHEA) of 1994—a bill that exempts vitamins, minerals, and botanical products from meaningful FDA regulation. Under the DSHEA, products that are not already sold as drugs can now be sold as *dietary supplements.* Put another way, if a manufacturer is willing to call its product by another name—"dietary supplement" rather than "drug"—the product can qualify for regulation under the DSHEA, thereby avoiding regulation under the more stringent Food, Drug, and Cosmetic Act. As discussed in Chapter 3, the Food, Drug, and Cosmetic Act requires that conventional drugs—both prescription and over-the-counter agents—undergo rigorous evaluation of safety and efficacy prior to receiving FDA approval for marketing. The DSHEA imposes no such requirements on "dietary supplements." That is, dietary supplements can be manufactured and marketed without giving the FDA any proof they are safe or effective. All the manufacturer needs to do is notify the FDA of efficacy claims. If a product eventually proves harmful or doesn't provide advertised benefits, the FDA does have the authority to intervene—but only *after* the product had been released for marketing. Furthermore, in order to challenge a claim of efficacy, the FDA must file suit in court; the challenge cannot be made through a simple administrative process. As you might guess, the DSHEA was created in response to intensive lobbying from the multibillion-dollar dietary supplement industry, which wanted to minimize government oversight. Clearly, the bill was not designed to benefit the consuming public.

Package Labeling

The DSHEA does impose some restrictions on labeling. All herbal products must be labeled as "dietary supplements." In addition, the label must not claim that the product can be used to diagnose, prevent, or treat disease. In fact, it must state the opposite: *This product is not intended to diagnose, treat, cure, or prevent any disease.* However, the label *is* allowed to make claims about the product's ability to favorably influence *body structure or function.* Put another way, the label can insinuate specific benefits, but can't make overt claims. By way of illustration, labels *can* bear statements like these:

- Helps promote urinary tract health
- Helps maintain cardiovascular function
- Energizes and rejuvenates
- Reduces stress and frustration
- Improves absentmindedness
- Supports the immune system

but labels *can't* bear statements or terms like these:

- Protects against cancer
- Reduces pain and stiffness of arthritis
- Lowers cholesterol
- Supports the body's antiviral capabilities
- Improves symptoms of Alzheimer's disease
- Relieves menopausal hot flushes
- "Antibiotic," "antiseptic," "antidepressant," "laxative," or "diuretic"

If all of this sounds like semantic hair splitting—it largely is. Furthermore, regardless of what the label says, common sense says that people *will* take herbal products to prevent and treat disease.

The DSHEA does not regulate the accuracy of labels. As a result, there is no assurance that a product actually contains the ingredients listed or in the stated amounts. The package may contain ingredients than are *not* listed, or it may *lack* ingredients that *are* listed. Either way, the manufacturer is free to sell the mislabeled product. All the DSHEA does require is the following disclaimer: *This statement* [i.e., the package label] *has not been evaluated by the FDA.*

Adverse Effects

With dietary supplements, as with conventional drugs, the manufacturer is responsible for safety. However, the similarity ends there. Under the DSHEA, a product is presumed safe until proved hazardous. Furthermore, the burden for proving danger lies with the FDA, not the manufacturer. With conventional drugs, opposite logic and regulations apply: Drugs are presumed dangerous until rigorous testing by the manufacturer reveals an absence of serious toxicity. Because of this system, the number of dangerous drugs that reach the market is kept to a minimum. Ask yourself, "Which product would I be more comfortable using—one that has been tested for adverse effects *before* I take it, or one that is evaluated for toxicity only *after* it caused me harm?"

Impurities, Adulterants, and Variability

The DSHEA does not regulate manufacturing of herbal products, and hence impurities and adulterants are common. Also, uniformity among herbal products is generally lacking. As a result, consumers can't know for sure what a preparation really contains. Furthermore, the package label may not help identify the contents. A few examples will illustrate the problem:

- A combination product used to "cleanse the bowel" caused life-threatening heart block. Analysis revealed contamination with *Digitalis lanata,* a plant with powerful effects on the heart.

- Among 125 ephedra products analyzed by the FDA, ephedrine content per dose ranged from undetectable to 110 mg. Also, some products had 6 to 20 additional ingredients.
- Testing of 10 brands of ginseng products revealed a 20-fold variation in ginsenoside content.
- When the California Department of Health Sciences analyzed 243 Asian patent medicines, they found 24 containing lead, 35 containing mercury, and 36 containing arsenic—all in levels above those permitted in drugs. Seven percent of the products were adulterated with undeclared pharmaceuticals, including ephedrine, chlorpheniramine, methyltestosterone, and phenacetin.

Because of inaccurate labeling, product variability, and adulteration, choosing an herbal supplement is largely an exercise in guessing. Perhaps the best approach is to buy a standardized product made by a company you have faith in, and then try the product and see what happens.

Proposed Manufacturing and Labeling Standards

In the spring of 2003, the FDA proposed new standards to regulate the manufacture and labeling of dietary supplements. The standards, referred to as Current Good Manufacturing Practices (CGMPs), are designed to ensure that dietary supplements be devoid of adulterants, contaminants, and impurities, and that package labels accurately reflect the identity, purity, quality, and strength of what's inside. In addition, the label should indicate not only active ingredients but also everything else that may be in the bottle. The CGMPs also mandate that manufacturers establish quality-control procedures, with the objective of preventing mislabeled or underfilled bottles; variations in tablet size, color, or potency; and contamination with drugs, bacteria, pesticides, glass, lead, and other potential contaminants. If adopted, these regulations will go a long way toward correcting existing deficiencies in the DSHEA. Unfortunately, even with the new standards, there is still no assurance that dietary supplements will be either safe or effective.

Comments

Relative to conventional drugs, herbal products and other "dietary supplements" are untested—for both safety and efficacy—and unregulated. Many of these products have constituents that can produce profound pharmacologic effects—both beneficial and adverse. Nonetheless, reliable information on clinical effects is generally lacking. Congress does not allow conventional drugs to be dispensed in the absence of extensive testing, but has made an exception for the supplements. This is both irrational and dangerous. After all, whether you ingest ephedrine in the form of a pill or in the form of *Ma huang,* it's still ephedrine, and it's still going to have powerful effects. Clearly, herbal products should be evaluated and regulated in essentially the same manner as conventional drugs. An editorial in the *New England Journal of Medicine* (1998;339:839–841) addressed this issue with eloquence. Here's the concluding paragraph:

It is time for the scientific community to stop giving alternative medicine a free ride. There cannot be two kinds of medicine—conventional and alternative. There is only medicine that has been adequately tested and medicine that has not, medicine that works and medicine that may or may not work. Once a treatment has been tested rigorously, it no longer matters whether it was considered alternative at the outset. If it is found to be reasonably safe and effective, it will be accepted. But assertions, speculation, and testimonials do not substitute for evidence. Alternative treatments should be subjected to scientific testing no less rigorous than that required for conventional treatments.

ADVERSE INTERACTIONS WITH CONVENTIONAL DRUGS

Herbal products can interact with conventional drugs, sometimes with disastrous results. The principal concerns are increased toxicity and decreased therapeutic effects. Clinicians and consumers should be alert to these possibilities.

For most herbal preparations, reliable information on adverse interactions is lacking. The reason lies with the inherent uncertainties about herbal products: In most cases, the purity and potency of the product is unknown; dosage is not standardized; package labeling is incomplete or inaccurate; and the product may contain multiple ingredients as well as impurities. Hence, if a patient is taking a conventional medication and an herbal supplement, and therapeutic effects are lost or toxicity appears, it is usually impossible to say for sure that the supplement was the cause. Until we can clearly identify interactions, physicians will be unable to avoid them when prescribing. Accurate information on interactions will remain unavailable until herbal products are standardized and labeling is accurate and comprehensive.

A few interactions *have* been identified, including these:

- Several herbal products, including ginkgo biloba, feverfew, and garlic, suppress platelet aggregation, and hence can increase the risk of bleeding in patients receiving antiplatelet drugs (e.g., aspirin) or anticoagulants (e.g., warfarin, heparin).
- Ma huang (ephedra) contains ephedrine, a compound that can elevate blood pressure and stimulate the heart and central nervous system (CNS). Accordingly, ephedra can intensify the effects of pressor agents, cardiac stimulants, and CNS stimulants, and counteract the beneficial effects of antihypertensive drugs and CNS depressants.
- St. John's wort can induce the 3A4 isozyme of cytochrome P450, and can thereby accelerate the metabolism of many drugs, causing a loss of therapeutic effects.

These interactions, at least, can be avoided—provided the prescriber is aware of them, and provided the patient informs the prescriber about herb use. Unfortunately, up to 70% of patients neglect to do so.

ORAL FORMULATIONS

Teas, Infusions, and Decoctions. These preparations are aqueous extracts made from the active portion of a medicinal plant (e.g., roots, berries, leaves, flowers). They are made by steeping the plant component in boiling or cold water and then filtering to remove solid material.

Tinctures and Fluid Extracts. These preparations are made by placing the active portion of a plant in a mixture of water and alcohol. After a few weeks, the solution is filtered or percolated to remove particulate matter. The resulting clear fluid contains both aqueous and fat-soluble constituents. At this stage, the product is considered a tincture. It can be converted to a fluid extract by evaporating off much of the liquid. Tinctures are more potent than teas and infusions, and fluid extracts are more potent than tinctures.

Tinctures and fluid extracts contain up to 60% alcohol, which can be good news and bad news. The good news is that alcohol is a preservative, and hence can extend product shelf life. The bad news is that alcohol can be detrimental for some people, including recovering alcoholics, alcohol-sensitive individuals, and those taking drugs that can block alcohol metabolism, thereby causing accumulation of acetaldehyde, a toxic alcohol metabolite.

Solid Extracts. Solid extracts are simply fluid extracts from which all residual fluid has been removed, either by evaporation or by vacuum distillation. The solid residue is then incorporated into a standard oral formulation (e.g., tablet, capsule). Solid extracts are the most concentrated herbal formulations and are preferred by consumers in the United States.

Glycerites. Glycerites are prepared in the same way as tinctures, but using glycerin instead of alcohol. Glycerites taste better than tinctures, but are usually less potent. In addition, glycerites may have shorter shelf lives.

STANDARDIZATION OF HERBAL PRODUCTS

The concentration of active ingredients in herbal crops can vary from year to year and from place to place. Reasons include differences in sunshine, rainfall, temperature, and soil nutrients. As a result, the potency of herbal products can vary widely.

Variability can be reduced through standardization, a three-step process in which the manufacturer (1) prepares an *extract* of plant parts, (2) analyzes the extract for one or two known active ingredients, and (3) dilutes or concentrates the extract such that the final product contains a predetermined amount of the active ingredient(s). The objective is to achieve therapeutic equivalence from batch to batch made by the same manufacturer, and among batches made by different manufacturers. Table 104–2 lists the concentrations of active ingredients in some standardized preparations.

Standardization has two important benefits. First, it permits accurate dosing. Second, it permits extrapolation of data obtained in clinical trials to the public in general.

Unfortunately, standardization also has drawbacks. The extraction process might destroy active compounds. Further-

more, the process may fail to extract as-yet unidentified active agents, and hence the extract may have a different spectrum of effects than the intact plant. To the extent this is true, historic data obtained with whole plants will lose some value as a basis for helping us understand clinical responses to the standardized extract.

DOSAGE

For reasons that should now be obvious, oral doses of herbal preparations are necessarily imprecise. With conventional drugs, a precise dose is taken (e.g., 20-mg tablet, 2 ml of a 5-mg/ml solution). With herbal products, the dose is less precise—usually *much* less precise. Standardized products offer the best chance for precise dosing. However, even these preparations may contain varying amounts of active ingredients that have not been identified. Furthermore, there is no guarantee that the concentration stated on the label is accurate. With herbal products that have not been standardized, all bets are off.

SOME COMMONLY USED MEDICINAL HERBS

Aloe

Uses. Aloe (*Aloe vera, Aloe barbadensis*) is used primarily for *topical therapy* of skin ailments, including scalds, burns, sunburn, psoriasis, eczema, acne, stings, and abrasions. In addition, topical aloe is used for basic skin and scalp care and to treat sore muscles, cold sores, bruises, sprains, and even arthritis. *Oral* aloe is used to relieve constipation.

Preparations. Commercial processing of the aloe plant yields two products: *aloe gel* and *aloe latex.* Aloe gel, also known as *aloe vera,* is a clear gelatinous material extracted from the inner portion of the aloe leaf. The gel is used for topical therapy only. Aloe latex, a product derived from the layer just beneath the outer skin of the leaf, is taken orally as a laxative.

Actions. Aloe gel contains multiple active ingredients. Among these are monosaccharides (mannose 6-phosphate), polysaccharides (acemannan), salicylic acid, saponins, sterols, and triterpenoids. In addition, the gel contains enzymes: bradykininase and superoxide dismutase. Emollient effects are due largely to the acemannan. Anti-inflammatory and analgesic effects are due in part to bradykininase and superoxide dismutase. The gel promotes healing of burns in part by inhibiting production of thromboxane, a product of arachidonic acid metabolism. Additional benefits of aloe gel derive from mild antimicrobial actions and from moisturizing the skin.

Aloe latex contains aloe-emodin, an anthraquinone. Aloe-emodin has powerful cathartic actions similar to those of senna and cascara.

Effectiveness. *Fresh* aloe gel appears to be effective for minor burns and abrasions. However, some authorities believe that beneficial actions may be lost during storage. There are few well-controlled studies on the topical use of aloe. The laxative efficacy of aloe latex is well established.

Adverse Effects. When applied to the skin, aloe is largely devoid of adverse effects. Hypersensitivity reactions occur on occasion, manifesting as local or generalized erup-

Herb	Amount of Active Agent
Black cohosh	2.5% Triterpene glycosides
Echinacea	4% Phenolic compounds
Feverfew	0.2% Parthenolide
Ginkgo biloba	24% Ginkgo flavenoids, 6% terpenoids
St. John's wort	0.3% Hypericin
Valerian root	1% Valerinic acid

TABLE 104–2 ■ Concentrations of Active Agents in Some Standardized Herbal Preparations

tions. Oral aloe latex can cause severe diarrhea, resulting in profound loss of fluid and electrolytes.

Comments. Although aloe gel is available in many commercial products, the concentration is often low. Furthermore, enzyme activity may not survive processing and storage. Hence, for treatment of minor burns and wounds, the best source of aloe gel may be fresh aloe leaves. (The plant can be grown easily at home.)

Black Cohosh

Uses. Black cohosh (*Cimicifuga racemosa*) has become a popular treatment for acute symptoms of menopause, including hot flushes, vaginal dryness, palpitations, depression, irritability, and sleep disturbance. The preparation may also benefit women with premenstrual syndrome (PMS) and menstrual cramps.

Actions. Benefits of black cohosh derive primarily from suppressing the release of luteinizing hormone (LH) from the pituitary. (Unregulated release of LH has been proposed as an important cause of menopausal symptoms.) Black cohosh has two ingredients that suppress LH release. One ingredient mimics the action of estrogen at receptors in the pituitary; the other acts through an estrogen-independent mechanism. Suppression of LH release correlates with relief of menopausal symptoms. In addition to its effects on LH, black cohosh can relax uterine smooth muscle. This action may underlie relief of dysmenorrhea.

Effectiveness. Black cohosh has been evaluated extensively in Germany, where most studies indicate it can effectively relieve menopausal symptoms. In fact, some studies have shown black cohosh to be as beneficial as estrogen replacement therapy (ERT), the conventional treatment for menopausal symptoms. In contrast to ERT, black cohosh has not been evaluated for long-term use (i.e., beyond 6 months).

There are no published studies on the use of black cohosh for PMS or dysmenorrhea. However, case reports in Germany suggest the herb is effective for both conditions.

Adverse Effects. Years of historic, anecdotal, and clinical experience have led German authorities to proclaim black cohosh safe for routine use. Rarely, a user may get an upset stomach. Due to lack of scientific information on long-term effects in humans, the German Commission E recommends using black cohosh for no more than 6 months. Because of its estrogenic effects, black cohosh should not be taken during pregnancy, especially during the first and second trimesters.

Interactions with Conventional Drugs. Black cohosh may potentiate the hypotensive effects of antihypertensive drugs as well as the hypoglycemic effects of insulin and oral hypoglycemics. Furthermore, owing to its estrogenic actions, black cohosh may potentiate the effects of estrogens used for hormone replacement or contraception, and may reduce the effects of estrogen receptor antagonists.

Comments. Black cohosh has a long history in America. The herb was used by native Americans and later by American colonists. Between 1820 and 1926, it was listed as an official drug in the U.S. Pharmacopoeia. At this time, black cohosh is used widely in Europe and is gaining popularity here.

Users must not confuse black cohosh with blue cohosh (Caulophyllum thalictroides). Although blue cohosh has legitimate uses, including promotion of menstruation and labor, it is much different from black cohosh and potentially more dangerous. Blue cohosh can elevate blood pressure, increase intestinal motility, and accelerate respiration. More importantly, it can induce uterine contractions, and hence should be avoided during pregnancy, except at term. Some commercial products contain both black cohosh and blue cohosh. Women who only want black cohosh should avoid these products.

Echinacea

Uses. Echinacea (*Echinacea angustifolia, E. purpurea, E. pallida*) is used orally and topically. Oral echinacea is taken to stimulate immune function, suppress inflammation, and treat viral infections, including influenza and the common cold. Topical echinacea is used to treat wounds, burns, eczema, psoriasis, and herpes simplex infection. Echinacea was listed in the National Formulary from 1916 to 1950, but fell from favor owing to development of antibiotics and a lack of scientific data to support its use. Nonetheless, echinacea is one of the three best-selling supplements in the United States. Annual sales for 1999 are estimated at $193 million.

Preparations. Active ingredients are present throughout the echinacea plant. Available preparations include dried roots, freeze-dried plants, dry-powder extracts, teas, and tinctures. Preparations made from the roots and leaves are most active.

Actions. Active ingredients in echinacea preparations include cichoric acid, polysaccharides, flavenoids, and essential oils. These ingredients produce antiviral, anti-inflammatory, and immunostimulant effects through a combination of actions, including mobilization of phagocytes, stimulation of T-lymphocyte proliferation, stimulation of interferon and tumor necrosis factor production, and inhibition of hyaluronidase, a proinflammatory enzyme.

Effectiveness. Although echinacea is taken widely to prevent and treat colds, its efficacy is questionable. Recent randomized, placebo-controlled trials designed to evaluate the ability of echinacea to *prevent* colds found no effect on (1) the time to developing an upper respiratory infection (URI); (2) the incidence, duration, or severity of URIs that did develop; or (3) development of experimentally induced URIs. Other recent trials conducted on subjects who already had a URI found echinacea no better than placebo at reducing either the duration or severity of symptoms.

Adverse Effects. Very few adverse effects have been reported. The most common complaint is unpleasant taste. Fever, nausea, and vomiting occur infrequently.

Rarely, echinacea causes allergic reactions, including acute asthma, urticaria, angioedema, and anaphylaxis. At the 2000 meeting of the American Academy of Allergy, Asthma, and Immunology, nearly two dozen cases of echinacea allergy were reported. Individuals with atopy (a genetic tendency toward allergic conditions) appear at increased risk of reacting to echinacea: Of the atopic patients tested, 2 in 10 had a positive skin test, even though they had never taken the herb. Echinacea belongs to the daisy family of plants, whose members include ragweed, asters, chamomile, and chrysanthemums. People allergic to any of these plants are at increased risk of reacting to echinacea.

Because echinacea can stimulate the immune system, it would be prudent to avoid the drug in patients with autoimmune diseases, such as lupus erythematosus or rheumatoid arthritis.

Although short-term exposure to echinacea stimulates immune function, long-term exposure can *suppress* immune function. Accordingly, long-term therapy should be avoided in immunocompromised patients, including those with HIV infection. In addition, prolonged therapy should be avoided in people with tuberculosis and other chronic infections that require optimal immune function for cure.

Interactions with Conventional Drugs. By stimulating the immune system, echinacea can oppose the effects of immunosuppressant drugs. Conversely, by suppressing immune function (in response to long-term use), echinacea can compromise drug therapy of tuberculosis, cancer, and HIV infection.

Feverfew

Uses. Feverfew (*Tanacetum parthenium*) is used primarily for prophylaxis and treatment of migraine. The herb is also used to relieve fever, stimulate menstruation, reduce upset stomach, and suppress inflammation. In addition, it has been applied topically to treat infection and relieve toothache.

Actions. The principal active agent in feverfew is *parthenolide,* a compound found in feverfew leaves. In the past, the antimigraine effects of parthenolide were ascribed to suppression of serotonin release from platelets and leukocytes, and to suppression of inflammation secondary to inhibition of arachidonic acid release. However, recent evidence suggests that parthenolide actually works by blocking the formation of a gene transcription factor required for the activation and proliferation of certain inflammatory cells that are critical to the pathogenesis of migraine.

Effectiveness. Clinical studies and historic evidence suggest that feverfew does indeed benefit patients with migraine. When taken prophylactically, the herb can reduce the frequency and severity of attacks. Unfortunately, feverfew is less effective when taken for treatment. Although the herb *can* abort an ongoing attack, benefits are variable. Furthermore, the doses required are much higher than those needed for prophylaxis. There is no reliable evidence that feverfew can benefit patients with rheumatoid arthritis or other inflammatory conditions.

Adverse Effects. Feverfew is very well tolerated. No serious adverse effects have been reported—although long-term studies of safety are lacking. Mild reactions include abdominal pain, indigestion, diarrhea, flatulence, nausea, and vomiting. Chewing feverfew leaves—a practice that is rare today—can cause oral ulceration, tongue irritation, and swollen lips. Some patients develop *post-feverfew syndrome,* characterized by nervousness, fatigue, insomnia, tension headache, and joint pain or stiffness. Feverfew belongs to the same plant family as echinacea. Accordingly, individuals allergic to ragweed and other members of this family may also be allergic to feverfew.

Interactions with Conventional Drugs. By suppressing release of arachidonic acid in platelets, feverfew can suppress platelet aggregation, and can thereby increase the risk of bleeding in patients taking antiplatelet drugs (e.g., aspirin) or anticoagulants (e.g., warfarin, heparin).

Comments. Parthenolide and related compounds are being studied for their ability to suppress pathologic proliferative processes mediated by nuclear factor-kappa B, a nuclear transcription factor. This transcription factor regulates the activity of multiple genes whose protein products help regulate a variety of processes, including apoptosis (cell suicide), inflammatory reactions, and development of B and T lymphocytes.

Garlic

Uses. Garlic (*Allium sativum*) is used primarily for effects on the cardiovascular system. The herb is taken to reduce levels of triglycerides and low-density-lipoprotein (LDL) cholesterol, and to raise levels of high-density-lipoprotein (HDL) cholesterol. Garlic is also employed to reduce blood pressure, suppress platelet aggregation, increase arterial elasticity, and decrease formation of atherosclerotic plaque. In addition, garlic has been used for antimicrobial and anticancer effects.

Actions. Beneficial effects result from the actions of sulfides in garlic oil. Intact garlic cells contain *alliin,* an odorless amino acid. When garlic cells are crushed, they release allinase, an enzyme that converts alliin into *allicin.* Allicin is the major active agent in garlic oil and the compound that gives garlic its distinctive aroma. In addition to allicin, garlic oil contains *ajoenes* (pronounced AH-ho-weens), biologically active compounds that contribute to beneficial effects.

Garlic lowers cholesterol levels by interfering with cholesterol synthesis in the liver. Several key steps in the synthetic pathway are affected. There is conflicting evidence regarding inhibition of HMG-CoA reductase, the rate-limiting enzyme in cholesterol synthesis and the enzyme the "statin" drugs inhibit.

Antiplatelet effects, which are well documented, result in part from inhibiting thromboxane synthesis. Methylallyltrisulfide is the chemical in garlic believed responsible. In addition, garlic may suppress platelet aggregation by disrupting calcium-dependent processes. Coagulation is also affected by the ajoenes, which have antithrombotic actions and may also stimulate fibrinolysis.

Lowering of blood pressure may be explained by garlic's demonstrated ability to increase the activity of nitric oxide synthetase, the enzyme in blood vessels that makes nitric oxide. Nitric oxide, also known as endothelium-derived relaxant factor, is a powerful vasodilator.

Effectiveness. Garlic can produce favorable effects on blood pressure and plasma lipids. However, benefits depend on the quality of the preparation. When a high-quality preparation is used, garlic can decrease total cholesterol by 6% to 9%, LDL cholesterol by about 11%, and triglycerides by 25%. In addition, garlic can produce a small increase in HDL cholesterol. Garlic can reduce blood pressure substantially: Treatment can decrease systolic pressure by 20 to 30 mm Hg and diastolic pressure by 10 to 15 mm Hg.

The effectiveness of garlic products is determined by their ability to yield allicin. Since both allicin and allinase (the enzyme that makes allicin) are destroyed by heat, cooked garlic is not effective. Benefits of raw garlic are variable. Furthermore, because allicin is inactivated by acid in the stomach, large doses (1 to 2 whole cloves twice daily) are required. Best results are produced with an enteric-coated, dried preparation that contains a specified amount of alliin and allinase. Unfortunately, a German study has shown that only 5 of 18 common garlic products contain allicin in effective amounts.

Adverse Effects. Garlic is generally well tolerated. The most common side effects are unpleasant taste and bad breath.

Rarely, garlic causes heartburn, flatulence, nausea, vomiting, diarrhea, and a burning sensation in the mouth. These effects are most pronounced with raw garlic and in people who don't eat garlic often. Patients suffering from infectious or inflammatory GI disorders should avoid garlic owing to its potential for GI irritation.

Interactions with Conventional Drugs. Garlic has significant antiplatelet effects. Accordingly, it can increase the risk of bleeding in patients taking antiplatelet drugs (e.g., aspirin) or anticoagulants (e.g., warfarin, heparin). Garlic can increase insulin levels, and hence can potentiate the hypoglycemic effects of drugs used for diabetes. Recent evidence indicates that garlic causes a significant reduction in levels of saquinavir, a protease inhibitor used to treat HIV infection.

Comments. Although the effects of garlic on cholesterol levels and blood pressure are modest (compared with conventional drugs), garlic may still benefit patients with mild hypercholesterolemia or hypertension.

Ginger Root

Uses. Ginger root (*Zingiber officinale*) is used primarily to suppress nausea and vomiting caused by motion sickness, morning sickness, and perhaps cancer chemotherapy. Ginger is also taken to improve appetite, calm stomach upset, and reduce flatulence. In addition, ginger has anti-inflammatory and analgesic properties that may help people with arthritis and other chronic inflammatory conditions. Some practitioners use ginger for URIs, although proof of efficacy is lacking.

Actions. The mechanism by which ginger suppresses nausea and vomiting is unclear. A good possibility is blockade of serotonin (5-hydroxytryptamine$_3$, or 5-HT$_3$) receptors located in the chemoreceptor trigger zone of the brain and on afferent vagal neurons in the GI tract. Activation of these receptors triggers emesis. Conversely, blockade of these receptors suppresses emesis. In fact, drugs that block 5-HT$_3$ receptors (e.g., ondansetron [Zofran]) are the most effective antiemetics available. Galanolactone, a major constituent of ginger, can block 5-HT$_3$ receptors *in vitro,* suggesting that receptor blockade may underlie antiemetic effects. Other actions that may contribute to beneficial GI effects include stimulation of intestinal motility, salivation, and gastric mucus production, and suppression of GI spasm secondary to anticholinergic and antihistaminic actions.

The anti-inflammatory effects of ginger have been attributed to inhibiting synthesis of prostaglandins and leukotrienes, which are powerful inflammatory mediators.

Effectiveness. Over the years, enough evidence has been collected to support the benefits of ginger root for prevention and treatment of motion sickness, morning sickness, seasickness, and postoperative nausea and vomiting (in the absence of opioids). For prevention of motion sickness, 940 mg of powdered ginger has been shown more effective than 100 mg of dimenhydrinate [Dramamine], a traditional drug for motion sickness. In patients with rheumatoid arthritis, ginger root appears to reduce pain, improve joint mobility, and decrease swelling and morning stiffness.

Adverse Effects. Ginger is very well tolerated. Severe toxicity has never been reported—although hugely excessive doses have the potential to cause CNS depression and cardiac dysrhythmias.

Ginger should be used with caution during pregnancy. There is evidence that high doses can stimulate the uterus, and might thereby cause spontaneous abortion. However, there are no reports of this ever happening. Nonetheless, prudence dictates limiting intake to usual therapeutic doses (i.e., 1 to 2 gm dried root/day).

Interactions with Conventional Drugs. Ginger can inhibit production of thromboxane by platelets, and can thereby suppress platelet aggregation. Accordingly, ginger can increase the risk of bleeding in patients receiving antiplatelet drugs (e.g., aspirin) or anticoagulants (e.g., warfarin, heparin).

Comments. For suppression of nausea and vomiting, the best source of ginger is the produce section in your local supermarket. Simply peeling the skin and chewing a medium slice (about 1 gm) provides the best and most rapid relief. If this method is too irritating to the mouth and throat (ginger can be extremely hot), you can make a tea by steeping the grated root in boiling water for 10 to 15 minutes. Then just filter and add milk, lemon, honey, or whatever to taste.

Ginkgo

Uses. Ginkgo (*Ginkgo biloba*) is used by many people, both young and old, to improve memory, sharpen concentration, and promote clear thinking. The herb is also used to treat senile dementia and related conditions, including dizziness, vertigo, tinnitus, headache, and mood changes. In addition, ginkgo may help patients with Alzheimer's disease (see Chapter 22). Some people use ginkgo to counteract erectile dysfunction (impotence) induced by antidepressants—especially fluoxetine [Prozac] and other selective serotonin reuptake inhibitors (SSRIs). In men with erectile dysfunction unrelated to antidepressants, ginkgo can reduce the required dosage of anti-impotence drugs. In Germany, extract of ginkgo is a top-selling medicine, with more than 5 million prescriptions filled each year.

Preparations. Medicinal ginkgo is prepared by acetone extraction of leaves from the *Ginkgo biloba* tree. These leaves contain two classes of active compounds: *flavenoids* (ginkgo-flavone glycosides) and *terpenoids* (ginkgolides, bilobalide). *Ginkgo biloba extracts* (GBEs) are standardized to contain 24% flavenoids and 6% terpenoids. Daily oral doses of standardized GBE range from 60 to 240 mg.

Actions. GBE has multiple biologic effects. However, most benefits derive from improved blood flow secondary to ginkgo-induced vasodilation. In the brain, GBE appears to increase blood flow by stimulating synthesis of prostaglandins. Further benefits derive from reducing capillary fragility and scavenging free radicals. (Scavenging free radicals helps protect blood vessels from injury.) GBE also suppresses production of platelet-activating factor (PAF), a mediator of platelet aggregation, bronchospasm, and other processes. Reduced PAF production helps protect against thrombosis as well as bronchospasm and other allergic disorders.

Effectiveness. Numerous studies support the benefits of ginkgo for patients with cognitive impairment secondary to low cerebral blood flow. Ginkgo can stabilize or improve cognitive function in patients with senile dementia, mixed dementias, and Alzheimer's disease. In addition, ginkgo can improve short-term memory in healthy adults as well as in elderly patients with mild to moderate memory impairment.

The impact of gingko on cerebral blood flow can be dramatic, increasing flow by as much as 70% in some patients.

In addition to its effects on cognitive function, ginkgo can improve other disorders caused by reduced blood flow. In patients whose hearing is impaired by low blood flow, ginkgo can improve hearing in 40% of those treated. In patients with occlusive arterial disease of the legs (Fontain stage IIb), ginkgo can improve local blood flow and pain-free walking distance. In patients with diabetes, ginkgo can increase peripheral blood flow by up to 45%.

Ginkgo has produced remarkable benefits in men with SSRI-associated impotence. Improved erection is probably the result of increased blood flow in the corpus cavernosum.

Adverse Effects and Interactions. Ginkgo is generally well tolerated. In some patients, it causes stomach upset, headache, dizziness, or vertigo, all of which can be minimized by increasing the dosage slowly. Ginkgo suppresses coagulation. Accordingly, it should be used with caution in patients taking antiplatelet drugs (e.g., aspirin) or anticoagulants (e.g., warfarin, heparin). There is concern that ginkgo may promote seizures. Accordingly, the herb should be avoided by patients at risk for seizures, including those taking drugs that can lower seizure threshold (e.g., antipsychotics, antidepressants, cholinesterase inhibitors, decongestants, first-generation antihistamines, and systemic glucocorticoids).

Comments. Ginkgo comes from the leaves of *Ginkgo biloba,* which has been documented as the world's oldest tree. At one time, the ginkgo tree grew in many places on the planet, but nearly died out during the Ice Age. The tree did survive in China, where it has been cultivated and respected as a sacred and medicinal plant. Today, the ginkgo tree is grown on plantations around the world, including some in South Carolina. Leaves grown in the United States are dried and shipped to Europe for processing. In Europe, ginkgo is available over the counter and by prescription, and is used by millions.

Goldenseal

Uses. Goldenseal (*Hydrastis canadensis*) has been used to treat bacterial, fungal, and protozoal infections of mucous membranes in the respiratory, gastrointestinal, and genitourinary tracts as well as the oral and sinus cavities. The herb is also given to treat inflammation of the gallbladder and to help correct metabolic sequelae of liver cirrhosis. Goldenseal has a long history of use for skin and eye irritations, and is still employed in some sterile eye washes.

Actions. The active ingredients in goldenseal include *hydrastine, berberine,* and related alkaloids. These alkaloids have multiple pharmacologic effects: they can suppress inflammation of mucous membranes; they have astringent and antiseptic properties; and they can stimulate peristalsis, alter blood pressure, promote hemostasis, and induce secretion of bile.

The antimicrobial effects of goldenseal are incompletely understood. One important action, however, is the ability of berberine, in low doses, to inhibit the attachment of group A streptococci and certain other bacteria to epithelial cells, thereby blocking the initial step of bacterial infection. In patients with colds or flu, additional benefits may derive from weak stimulation of immune function, and from protection against secondary bacterial infection.

Effectiveness. In vitro studies indicate that berberine is bacteriostatic or bactericidal to many common pathogens, including *Staphylococcus, Streptococcus, Chlamydia, Escherichia coli, Pseudomonas,* and *Neisseria.* Although high-quality clinical studies of the antibacterial effects of goldenseal are rare, there is good evidence that it can effectively treat diarrhea caused by *E. coli, Shigella, Salmonella, Klebsiella,* and *Cholera.* In children infected with *Giardia* (a protozoan), berberine is as effective as metronidazole [Flagyl], the conventional drug of choice for this infection. In patients with *Chlamydia trachomatis* infection of the eye, berberine can eradicate the microbe and prevent its return. In addition, there is evidence that goldenseal can suppress growth of *Candida albicans* and other fungi, suggesting it might be used to prevent yeast suprainfection in patients taking antibiotics.

Berberine can be effective in patients with cholecystitis and cirrhosis. Several studies have shown that berberine stimulates secretion of bile and bilirubin. In one study of patients with cholecystitis (inflammation of the gallbladder), berberine caused all symptoms to resolve.

Adverse Effects and Interactions. Goldenseal is relatively nontoxic at therapeutic doses. High doses can cause nausea, vomiting, diarrhea, and stimulation of the CNS. Toxic doses can cause hypertension, convulsions, and death from respiratory failure.

Goldenseal can stimulate the uterus, and hence is contraindicated during pregnancy. We don't know if goldenseal's alkaloids are excreted in breast milk. Until more is known, the herb should be avoided by women who are breast-feeding.

Comments. Goldenseal is among the most popular herbs. Commercial products that are standardized for berberine or hydrastine content are preferred. Goldenseal is often sold in combination with echinacea. The rationale for the combination is relatively sound: goldenseal protects against bacterial infection, while echinacea stimulates the immune system and may protect against common viral infections (colds, flu). Interest in goldenseal increased greatly in the 1990s, when rumors suggested it could mask urine tests for illicit drugs, such as marijuana and cocaine. However, studies indicate that goldenseal has no masking effect.

Kava

Uses. Kava (*Piper methysticum*), also known as *kava-kava* or *awa,* is used to relieve anxiety, promote sleep, and relax muscles. In the United States, the herb is being promoted as a natural alternative to benzodiazepines (e.g., diazepam [Valium]) for treating anxiety and stress.

Actions. The active ingredients in kava are referred to as *alpha-pyrones* or *kava-lactones.* Their precise mechanism of action is unknown. Many researchers suspect that, like benzodiazepines, kava-lactones produce their CNS effects by acting on the gamma-aminobutyric acid (GABA) receptor–chloride channel complex. Another possibility is inhibition of voltage-dependent sodium and calcium channels. Also, kava has local anesthetic and analgesic actions that may contribute to clinical effects.

Effectiveness. Studies conducted in Europe have shown clearly that kava can relax skeletal muscles and relieve both tension and anxiety. As of late 1999, there were no published reports of controlled trials in the United States regarding the impact of kava on anxiety. Interestingly, kava can relax muscles and reduce tension without causing mental clouding. In fact, cognitive function may actually improve. Unlike benzodiazepines, which reduce anxiety rapidly, kava must be taken for weeks before anxiolytic effects develop.

Adverse Effects. Kava is generally well tolerated. However, it *can* cause excessive CNS depression, skin problems, and liver damage.

When taken in high doses, kava has effects like those of alcohol, including excessive CNS depression, impaired vision, and muscle incoordination. Accordingly, kava users should not drive, operate heavy machinery, or engage in other potentially dangerous activities that require good judgment, coordination, and sharp vision.

With prolonged use, kava can cause a skin disorder that resembles pellagra. Symptoms include dry, scaly, flaking skin; reddened eyes; and yellow discoloration of the skin, hair, and nails. The condition takes weeks to months to develop, and resolves after kava is discontinued.

Kava can cause hepatitis, cirrhosis, and even liver failure. Several users have required a liver transplant. Kava users should be informed about signs of liver damage (jaundice, brown urine, fatigue, nausea, abdominal discomfort) and advised to stop kava and undergo liver function tests if these appear. Kava should be avoided by people with existing liver disease. Because of concerns over liver damage, kava sales have been restricted in Germany, Canada, Switzerland, France, and Australia— but not the United States.

Interactions with Conventional Drugs. Because of its CNS-depressant actions, kava can intensify the effects of other CNS depressants, thereby posing a risk of confusion, disorientation, lethargy, and excessive sedation. Accordingly, kava should not be combined with alcohol, benzodiazepines, opioids, barbiturates, and other drugs with CNS-depressant properties.

Because the CNS effects of kava are incompletely understood, it may be that kava has as-yet unknown interactions with a host of CNS drugs, including psychotropic medications (e.g., tricyclic antidepressants, monoamine oxidase [MAO] inhibitors, SSRIs, lithium), centrally acting skeletal muscle relaxants, and drugs for epilepsy and Parkinson's disease.

Comments. Kava has been used for over 3000 years in ceremonial rituals among natives of the South Pacific. Like most (if not all) drugs employed in traditional rituals, kava has mind-altering properties. Because kava has desirable subjective effects, and because it is available freely and without a prescription, the preparation has at least some potential for abuse. In fact, some island countries of the South Pacific have "kava bars" that sell kava tea by the bottle or glass. The extent of recreational kava use in the United States is unknown.

Ma Huang (Ephedra)

The active ingredient in Ma huang (*Ephedra sinica*) is *ephedrine,* a sympathomimetic agent and CNS stimulant. Accordingly, the pharmacology of Ma huang is identical to that of pharmaceutical ephedrine. The basic pharmacology of the sympathomimetic drugs is discussed in Chapter 17.

Uses. Like ephedrine, Ma huang can be used to reduce appetite, increase energy, overcome tiredness, treat narco-

lepsy, relieve bronchospasm, enhance athletic performance, and suppress nasal congestion in people with allergies, influenza, and colds.

Actions. As discussed in Chapter 17, ephedrine is a mixed-acting drug that activates adrenergic receptors in two ways: it (1) binds adrenergic receptors to cause direct activation, and (2) promotes release of norepinephrine, which then binds to and activates adrenergic receptors. As a result of these actions, ephedrine can activate alpha$_1$, alpha$_2$, beta$_1$, and beta$_2$ receptors. Activation of alpha$_1$ receptors causes constriction of arterioles in the skin, mucus membranes, and elsewhere. Activation of beta$_1$ receptors increases heart rate and force of contraction. Activation of beta$_2$ receptors promotes bronchodilation. Activation of adrenergic receptors in the brain causes appetite suppression and CNS stimulation.

Effectiveness. The benefits of ephedrine in relieving symptoms of allergies, colds, and flu are well established. Although ephedrine can relieve bronchospasm in patients with asthma, selective beta$_2$ agonists are preferred. Similarly, although ephedrine can reduce appetite, other drugs (e.g., sibutramine) are preferred. Furthermore, benefits are limited to modest, short-term weight loss. There is no proof that the herb promotes long-term loss. Also, there is little evidence to support use of ephedra to enhance athletic performance.

Adverse Effects. Ephedra is a potentially dangerous product. To date, over 17,000 adverse events have been reported, including the death in 2003 of Steve Bechler, a 23-year-old pitcher for the Baltimore Orioles.

The adverse effects of ephedrine are a direct extension of its pharmacologic actions. Excessive cardiovascular stimulation can result in tachycardia, palpitations, anginal pain, and hypertension. Excessive CNS stimulation can result in agitation, irritability, insomnia, and even psychosis. CNS stimulation can also cause euphoria, and hence can lead to ephedrine abuse. The side effects of ephedrine are dose dependent and minimal at standard doses.

In the mid-1980s, an FDA advisory panel recommended that ephedrine be avoided by patients with heart disease, hyperthyroidism, hypertension, diabetes, or difficulty with urination caused by an enlarged prostate. In addition, the panel recommended that ephedrine not be combined with antihypertensive drugs or antidepressants, including MAO inhibitors. More recently, the FDA made the following recommendations regarding ephedrine-containing supplements:

- Limit the total daily dose to 24 mg
- Limit the duration of use to 7 days (which would preclude using the supplements for weight loss)
- Label many supplements with this warning: "Taking more than the recommended serving may result in heart attack, stroke, seizure, or death"
- Prohibit combined use of ephedrine with caffeine and other stimulants

Following the death of Steve Bechler, the American Heart Association urged that ephedra be banned, arguing that the dangers of using it outweigh any possible benefits.

Interactions with Conventional Drugs. Ephedrine can interact with a wide variety of other drugs. For example, it can potentiate the effects CNS stimulants (e.g., amphetamines, methylphenidate, caffeine, theophylline), beta$_1$ and beta$_2$ agonists, ergotamine, and nasal decongestants. Combined use with MAO inhibitors can cause hypertensive crisis. By raising blood pressure, ephedrine can counteract the effects of antihypertensive agents.

Comments. Attempts to regulate Ma huang have stirred controversy. To the FDA, Ma huang (ephedra) is little more than another formulation of ephedrine. Herbal traditionalists say, "Not so." They point to thousands of years of safe and effective Ma huang use. They also point out that ephedra does not "pack the same punch" as synthetic ephedrine and is often blended with herbs that help counteract or prevent side effects. As with other products that are available without prescription, safe use is ultimately the responsibility of the consumer.

St. John's Wort

St. John's wort (*Hypericum perforatum*) is used widely to relieve depression. For patients with mild to moderate depression, the herb may be as effective as conventional antidepressants. Although side effects are minimal, the herb can interact adversely with many drugs. St. John's wort is discussed at length in Chapter 31 (see Box 31–1).

Saw Palmetto

Uses. Saw palmetto (*Serenoa repens, Sabal serrulata*) is used to relieve urinary symptoms associated with benign prostatic hypertrophy (BPH). The product employed clinically is an extract made from berries of the American saw palmetto, a small palm tree native to the southeastern United States.

Actions. The mechanism by which saw palmetto acts is unknown. However, we do know that saw palmetto extract displays antiandrogenic activity. It has been proposed that compounds in the extract may inhibit the enzyme that converts testosterone into dihydrotestosterone (DHT), the active form of testosterone in the prostate. (This is the same mechanism employed by finasteride [Proscar], the leading conventional treatment for BPH.) In addition to decreasing DHT production, saw palmetto may block DHT receptors. Both actions would suppress DHT-induced proliferation of prostate epithelial cells, and would thereby reduce urinary tract obstruction.

Effectiveness. Numerous placebo-controlled, double-blind studies have been conducted, both in Europe and the United States. With few exceptions, these studies indicate that saw palmetto can relieve urination problems associated with BPH. Taking 320 mg/day for 30 to 90 days can reduce dysuria, nocturia, urinary frequency, and residual volume (postmicturition residue)—although prostate size remains unchanged. Benefits of saw palmetto compare favorably with those of finasteride.

Adverse Effects. Saw palmetto is very well tolerated. Significant adverse effects have not been reported. Rarely, saw palmetto causes upset stomach or headache. High doses may cause diarrhea. Although antiandrogenic effects (e.g., gynecomastia) have not been reported, it may be wise to monitor for them.

Saw palmetto can reduce levels of prostate-specific antigen (PSA), a marker for prostate cancer. As a result, saw palmetto can cause false-negative results on PSA tests. It is important that patients and clinicians appreciate this. All patients should undergo a PSA test before initiating treatment. This is especially important for men who self-prescribe saw palmetto.

Because of its antiandrogenic effects, saw palmetto represents a danger to the developing fetus. (Finasteride is classified in FDA Pregnancy Risk Category X.) Pregnant women should not ingest saw palmetto, and should probably avoid touching it.

Interactions with Conventional Drugs. Because saw palmetto and finasteride may share the same mechanism, combined use may have additive effects. Accordingly, concurrent use is not recommended.

Comments. Because saw palmetto is both safe and effective, urologists frequently recommend it as first-line therapy for BPH. Because saw palmetto reduces urinary symptoms without reducing prostate size, users should continue to see a urologist on a regular basis.

Valerian

Actions and Uses. Valerian root (*Valeriana officinalis*) is a sedative preparation used primarily to promote sleep. In addition, some people take it to reduce restlessness. Valerian may work by increasing the availability of GABA (an inhibitory neurotransmitter) at synapses in the CNS. (Benzodiazepines, which are the major conventional hypnotics, act by potentiating the actions of GABA.) The active ingredient in valerian has not been identified.

Effectiveness. Although valerian has been used for centuries in Europe, China, and other countries, objective evidence of efficacy is limited. In two brief trials, valerian did help people fall asleep, but did not prevent waking during the night. There is some evidence that the hypnotic effects of valerian develop slowly, over a period of days to weeks. In contrast, benzodiazepines promote sleep the first night they are taken.

Adverse Effects. Valerian is generally very well tolerated. Possible side effects include daytime drowsiness, dizziness, depression, dyspepsia, and pruritus. Prolonged use may cause headache, nervousness, or cardiac abnormalities. Because valerian can reduce alertness, users should exercise caution when performing dangerous activities, such as driving or operating heavy machinery. In addition, valerian should be used with caution by people with psychiatric illnesses (e.g., depression, dementia). As with benzodiazepines, there may be a risk of paradoxical excitation and physical dependence. We do not know if valerian enters breast milk or harms the developing fetus. Until more is known, valerian should be avoided by women who are breast-feeding or pregnant.

Interactions with Conventional Drugs. Interestingly, valerian does not seem to potentiate the CNS-depressant effects of alcohol. There are no data on interactions with other CNS depressants (e.g., opioids, benzodiazepines, barbiturates, antihistamines) or with any other drugs that affect CNS function (e.g., antidepressants, antiseizure drugs, centrally acting skeletal muscle relaxants).

Comments. Valerian was used as a tranquilizer throughout World War II and was listed in the U.S. Pharmacopoeia prior to 1945. It was removed from the National Formulary following the introduction of more effective sedatives.

⁙ KEY POINTS

- Herbal medicine can be defined as the use of plant-derived products to promote health and relieve symptoms of disease.
- Herbal medicine is the most common form of alternative medicine, which can be defined as treatment practices that are not widely accepted or practiced by mainstream clinicians in a given culture.
- Medicinal herbs are regulated as *dietary supplements* under the Dietary Supplement Health and Education Act.
- Unlike conventional drugs, dietary supplements can be marketed without any proof of safety or efficacy.
- Under the DSHEA, dietary supplements are presumed safe until proved harmful. Hence, manufacturers don't have to prove their products are safe. Rather, the FDA has to prove they're not.
- Manufacturers can claim that a product favorably influences "body structure and function," but cannot claim that it can be used to diagnose, treat, cure, or prevent any disease.
- The DSHEA does not regulate quality of herbal products, and hence impurities and adulterants are common, and uniformity among herbal products is generally lacking. Also, there is no assurance that a commercial herbal preparation contains the ingredients listed on the label, or in the amounts stated. However, if new regulations proposed by the FDA are put into force, these problems will be corrected.
- Tinctures and liquid extracts are made by steeping the active portion of a plant in a mixture of water and alcohol.
- Some liquid extracts are standardized to contain a specified concentration of one or two active ingredients.
- Herbal products can interact with conventional drugs, sometimes with disastrous results. Be sure to ask patients if they are using medicinal herbs.
- The word *natural* is not synonymous with *safe*. Remember, poison ivy and tobacco are natural, too.

Management of Poisoning

Poisoning is defined as a pathologic state caused by a toxic agent. Sources of poisoning include medications, plants, environmental pollutants, and drugs of abuse. These toxicants may enter the body orally, by inhalation, or by absorption through the skin. Poisoning may be accidental or intentional. Symptoms of poisoning often mimic those of disease; hence, the possibility of poisoning should be considered whenever a diagnosis is made.

Poisonings occur at an estimated rate of 5 million per year. About 5000 deaths result. Approximately 60% of these fatalities are due to ingestion of drugs, either prescription medicines or over-the-counter preparations. The remaining deaths are caused by other chemicals. The *incidence* of poisoning is highest in young children. However, the *mortality rate* in this group is low. Most poisoning-related hospital admissions result from suicide attempts by adults.

FUNDAMENTALS OF TREATMENT

Poisoning is a medical emergency and requires rapid treatment. Management has five basic elements: (1) supportive care, (2) identification of the poison, (3) prevention of further absorption, (4) promotion of poison removal, and (5) use of specific antidotes. These essentials are discussed below.

Supportive Care

Supportive care is the most important element in managing acute poisoning. Support is based on the clinical status of the patient and requires no knowledge specific to the poison involved. Maintenance of respiration and circulation are primary concerns. Measures for support of breathing include in-

sertion of an airway, administration of humidified oxygen, and mechanical ventilation. Volume depletion (resulting from vomiting, diarrhea, or sweating) can compromise circulation. Volume should be restored by administering normal saline or Ringer's solution. Severe hypoglycemia may occur, resulting in coma. Levels of blood glucose should be monitored. For coma of unknown etiology, IV dextrose should be given immediately—even if information on blood glucose is lacking. Acid-base disturbances may occur; determination of arterial blood gases will facilitate diagnosis and management. If convulsions develop, IV diazepam is the treatment of choice.

Poison Identification

Treatment of poisoning is facilitated by knowing the identity and dosage of the toxicant. Efforts to obtain this information should proceed concurrently with medical management.

A history is one means by which a toxic agent may be identified. However, experience has shown that histories taken at times of poisoning are frequently inaccurate. That is, statements about the nature or quantity of poison may be incorrect.

Positive identification can be made using analytic techniques. A gas chromatograph/mass spectrometer can provide qualitative and quantitative information. Analyses can be performed on specimens of urine, blood, and gastric contents. To determine whether poison levels are rising or falling, analyses should be performed on sequential blood samples taken about 2 hours apart.

Prevention of Further Absorption

By reducing the absorption of a poison, we can minimize blood levels, and thereby significantly decrease morbidity and mortality. For ingested poisons, five procedures are available: (1) giving activated charcoal, (2) induction of emesis with syrup of ipecac, (3) gastric lavage and aspiration, (4) whole-bowel irrigation, and (5) catharsis. When poison exposure is topical, surface decontamination is employed. Details of these procedures are discussed in the following section.

Promotion of Poison Removal

Measures that help eliminate poison from the body shorten the duration of exposure and, if implemented before plasma levels have peaked, can reduce the maximal level of poison achieved. By shortening exposure and reducing maximal poison levels, these measures can decrease morbidity and mortality.

Removal of poison can be promoted with drugs and with nonpharmacologic techniques. The drugs used for poison removal act by increasing renal excretion of toxic agents. Nonpharmacologic methods of poison removal include peritoneal dialysis, hemodialysis, and exchange transfusion. Details on methods of poison removal are presented later.

Use of Specific Antidotes

An antidote is an agent administered to counteract the effects of a poison. Examples include naloxone (used to reverse poisoning by heroin and other opioids) and physostigmine (used to treat poisoning by atropine and other anticholinergic drugs). Several specific antidotes are discussed later. Unfortunately, although antidotes can be extremely valuable, these agents are rare: For most poisons, no specific antidote exists. Hence, for most patients, treatment is limited to the general measures described above.

DRUGS AND PROCEDURES USED TO MINIMIZE POISON ABSORPTION

Reducing Absorption of Ingested Poisons

Activated Charcoal

Treatment with activated charcoal is a preferred method for removing ingested poisons from the GI tract. Activated charcoal is an inert substance that adsorbs drugs and other chemicals. Binding of toxicants to charcoal is essentially irreversible. Since charcoal particles cannot be absorbed into the blood, adsorption of poisons onto charcoal prevents toxicity. The charcoal-poison complex is eliminated in the stool. Patients should be advised that charcoal will turn the feces black. Charcoal is nontoxic and there are no contraindications to its use.

Charcoal selectively adsorbs *large molecules* that contain a *carbon atom.* Adsorption of small molecules and molecules that lack a carbon is poor. Among these poorly absorbed molecules are heavy metals, caustics and corrosives, alcohols and glycols, chlorine, iodine, and petroleum distillates.

Because charcoal can adsorb antidotes, and thereby neutralize their benefits, antidotes should not be administered immediately before, with, or shortly after the charcoal.

Activated charcoal has the consistency of a fine powder and is mixed with water for oral administration. The adult dose is 60 to 100 gm. Pediatric doses range from 15 to 30 gm. For poisoning with certain compounds—namely phenobarbital, dapsone, quinidine, theophylline, and carbamazepine—giving sequential doses of charcoal can be beneficial. Charcoal should be administered no later than 60 minutes after poison ingestion.

Syrup of Ipecac

Actions and Uses. Syrup of ipecac induces vomiting, and can thereby remove ingested poison from the stomach. Ipecac promotes emesis by (1) stimulating the chemoreceptor trigger zone of the medulla and (2) irritating the stomach. Vomiting usually occurs 20 to 30 minutes after ipecac administration. The drug's most common side effects are sedation and diarrhea.

Guidelines for Ipecac Use. Although induction of vomiting was common in the past, it is rarely done now. Between 1985 and 1995, ipecac use in cases of poisoning dropped from 15% to only 2.3%. Recently, the American Academy of Clinical Toxicology issued the following guidelines on ipecac use:

- Ipecac should not be used routinely.
- Routine use in the emergency room should be abandoned.
- Ipecac should not be given to patients with seizures or a reduced level of consciousness, or to patients who cannot protect their airways (e.g., those lacking a gag reflex).

- Ipecac should not be administered after ingestion of (1) corrosive acids or bases, (2) hydrocarbons with a high potential for aspiration, (3) substances that could cause a rapid loss of consciousness, and (4) substances that could cause seizures requiring advanced life support within 60 minutes.
- When ipecac *is* used, it should be given within 60 minutes of poison ingestion, and only to patients who are alert, conscious, and have ingested a potentially toxic dose.

Preparations, Dosage, and Administration. Ipecac syrup is dispensed in 15- and 30-ml containers. The drug is available without prescription. Fluid in the stomach increases the effects of ipecac. Hence, administration should be accompanied by an appropriate volume of water. Dosage is a function of age:

- *Children less than 6 months old*—Use only under a physician's supervision
- *Children 6 to 12 months old*—5 to 10 ml followed by 120 to 240 ml of water
- *Children 1 to 12 years old*—15 ml followed by 120 to 240 ml of water
- *Individuals over 12 years old*—15 to 30 ml followed by 240 ml of water

If vomiting does not occur within 20 minutes, dosing should be repeated.

Gastric Lavage and Aspiration

Gastric lavage (irrigation) and aspiration consists of flushing the stomach with fluid and then sucking (aspirating) the fluid back out. The procedure should be done only in life-threatening cases, and only if less than 60 minutes has elapsed since poison ingestion. Specific contraindications to lavage and aspiration include

- Ingestion of caustic agents (owing to the risk of esophageal perforation)
- Convulsions (owing to the risk of injury from the procedure, including aspiration of stomach contents into the lungs)
- Ingestion of high-viscosity petroleum distillates
- Significant cardiac dysrhythmias
- Emesis of blood

Lavage and aspiration is accomplished using a large-bore orogastric tube (No. 36 to 42 French for adults, No. 22 to 28 French for children). Smaller tubes should be avoided because they may not permit removal of solids (food, pills, capsules, tablets) and because their small diameter will impede flow of the lavage fluid. If the patient is comatose, an endotracheal tube with an inflatable cuff should be installed to protect the airway. Because of the anatomy of the stomach, the patient should be placed on the left side with the head down. Prior to initiation of lavage, stomach contents should be aspirated and sent for toxicologic analysis. Lavage may be performed employing tap water or saline solution. Multiple washes are instilled using 150 to 200 ml/wash (for adults and older children) or 50 to 100 ml/wash (for children under 5 years old). Larger volumes should be avoided since they may push stomach contents into the small intestine. Washes should be repeated until the fluid retrieved from the stomach is clear. About 10 to 12 washes are employed.

Whole-Bowel Irrigation

Whole-bowel irrigation is done with a solution of polyethylene glycol that contains balanced electrolytes, available under the trade names CoLyte and GoLYTELY. The solution is administered repeatedly over a 5-hour period, either by mouth or through a nasogastric tube. Rates of administration are as follows:

- For patients ≤ 12 years old: 1.5 to 2 L/hr
- For patients 6 to 12 years old: 1 L/hr
- For patients <6 years old: 0.5 L/hr

The procedure has been effective following ingestion of iron, lithium, and lead, as well as sustained-release products. Whole-bowel irrigation should not be used in patients with ileus, peritonitis, bloody vomitus, or obstruction or perforation of the bowel.

Catharsis

Cathartics can hasten passage of toxicants through the intestine and, in theory, may thereby minimize absorption. However, there are no data to prove that cathartics improve clinical outcome. Hence, although these agents were used widely in the past, they are not recommended today.

Surface Decontamination

Topical exposure to toxicants can cause local and systemic injury. To minimize injury, contaminated clothing should be removed, and the poison should be washed from the victim. The recommended procedure is to alternate soap-and-water washes with alcohol washes. Personnel performing these washes should take precautions to avoid contaminating themselves. If the eyes have been exposed, they should be flushed with water for at least 15 minutes. Shampoo should be employed to remove toxic agents from the hair and scalp.

DRUGS AND PROCEDURES USED FOR POISON REMOVAL

Drugs That Enhance Renal Excretion

Drugs that alter the pH of urine can accelerate the excretion of organic acids and bases. Agents that *elevate* urinary pH (i.e., make the urine more alkaline) will promote the excretion of *acids*. Drugs that *lower* urinary pH will promote the excretion of *bases*. The mechanism underlying these effects is called *ion trapping* (see Chapter 4).

The drugs employed most frequently to alter urinary pH are *sodium bicarbonate* and *ammonium chloride*. Both are administered IV. Sodium bicarbonate renders the urine more alkaline, which decreases the passive reabsorption of acids (e.g., aspirin, phenobarbital), and thereby accelerates their excretion. Ammonium chloride acidifies the urine, and thereby increases the excretion of bases (e.g., amphetamines, phencyclidine). Because of the buffer systems present in blood, sodium bicarbonate and ammonium chloride have a relatively small effect on the pH of blood, while having a large effect on the pH of urine.

Nondrug Methods of Poison Removal

Several nondrug procedures—peritoneal dialysis, hemodialysis, hemoperfusion, and exchange transfusion—can be employed to remove toxicants from the body. Although these procedures are usually of limited value, they can be lifesaving in some situations. Nondrug procedures are most effective when (1) binding of toxicants to plasma proteins is low, and (2) blood levels of toxicants are high (i.e., when distribution of the toxic agent is restricted to the blood and extracellular fluid).

Each of the nondrug methods of poison removal has its benefits and drawbacks. *Peritoneal dialysis* has two advantages: the procedure is relatively simple and it occupies a minimum of staff time. *Hemodialysis,* although more difficult than peritoneal dialysis, is about 20 times more effective. *Hemoperfusion* is a process in which blood is passed over a column of charcoal or absorbent resin. If the affinity of the resin for a particular poison is high, this procedure can strip a toxicant from binding sites on plasma proteins. The principal disadvantage of hemoperfusion is loss of platelets. When binding of a poison to plasma proteins is particularly avid, *exchange transfusion* can be an effective method of removal.

SPECIFIC ANTIDOTES

Heavy Metal Antagonists

The heavy metals most frequently responsible for poisoning are lead, iron, mercury, arsenic, gold, and copper. These metals cause injury by forming complexes with enzymes and other physiologically important molecules. Poisoning may result from environmental exposure, intentional overdose, or therapeutic use of heavy metals.

The drugs given to treat heavy metal poisoning are called *chelating agents* or *chelators*. These agents interact with metals to form *chelates*—ring structures in which the metal and the chelating agent form two or more points of attachment. The chelate formed by mercury and dimercaprol illustrates this concept (Fig. 105–1).

Useful chelating agents have a high affinity for heavy metals, and hence can compete successfully with endogenous molecules for metal binding. By preventing initial binding of metals to endogenous molecules, chelators can prevent injury. By stripping metals that have already become bound, chelators can enhance their excretion.

The selectivity of a heavy metal antagonist is determined by its affinity for specific metals. Some antagonists are selective for only one metal, whereas others can form chelates with several metals. Deferoxamine, for example, binds selectively to iron. In contrast, dimercaprol is relatively nonselective, binding tightly with arsenic, mercury salts, and gold.

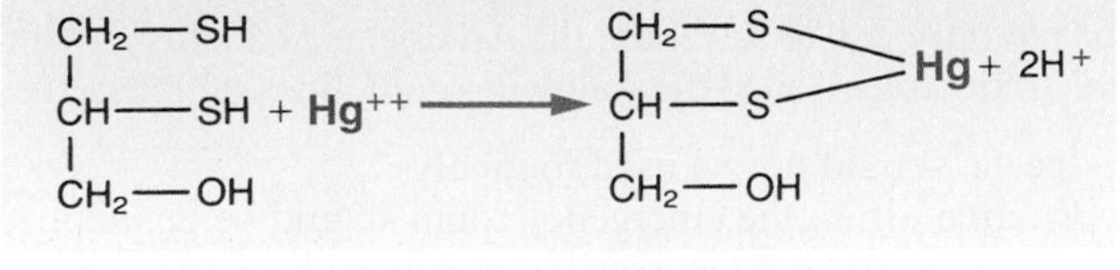

Figure 105–1 ■ **Chelation of mercury by dimercaprol.**

Properties desirable in a heavy metal antagonist include (1) high affinity for a toxic metal, (2) low affinity for essential endogenous metals (e.g., magnesium, zinc), (3) the ability to reach sites of metal storage, (4) high activity at physiologic pH, (5) formation of chelates that are less toxic than the free metal, and (6) formation of chelates that are easily excreted.

Deferoxamine

Actions and Uses. Deferoxamine [Desferal] has a high affinity for ferric iron. The drug chelates free iron and can also strip iron bound to ferritin and hemosiderin. In contrast, iron present in hemoglobin and cytochromes is not affected. Deferoxamine is employed to treat acute and chronic iron toxicity.

Pharmacokinetics. Deferoxamine is poorly absorbed from the GI tract, and hence administration is parenteral. The chelate formed between deferoxamine and iron is excreted primarily in the urine.

Adverse Effects. Deferoxamine is generally well tolerated. Pain may occur at the site of injection. Rapid IV infusion may cause hypotension, tachycardia, erythema, and urticaria. Prolonged therapy may be associated with allergic reactions, abdominal discomfort, leg cramps, fever, and dysuria.

Contraindications. Because deferoxamine is excreted by the kidneys, the drug should not be given to patients with renal insufficiency. Deferoxamine has caused fetal malformations in experimental animals, and therefore is not recommended for pregnant women.

Preparations, Dosage, and Administration. Deferoxamine mesylate [Desferal] is dispensed as a powder to be reconstituted for injection. The drug can be administered by IM injection and by IV or SC infusion. Intramuscular injection is preferred for most patients. Intravenous infusion is usually reserved for patients in shock. The dosage for IM or IV administration is the same. The initial dose for adults and children is 1 gm. This is followed 4 and 8 hours later with 0.5-gm doses. For IV administration, the maximum rate of infusion is 15 mg/kg/hr.

Dimercaprol

Actions and Uses. Dimercaprol [BAL In Oil] binds with arsenic, gold, and mercury. The resulting chelates are excreted in the urine. The drug is used as the sole chelator to rid the body of arsenic, mercury, or gold. In addition, dimercaprol can be combined with edetate calcium disodium (calcium EDTA) to treat poisoning with lead. Since dimercaprol is more effective at *preventing* binding of metals to endogenous molecules than it is at reversing binding that has already taken place, benefits are greatest when the drug is administered early (within 1 to 2 hours of metal ingestion).

Pharmacokinetics. Administration is by deep IM injection. Dimercaprol cannot be used orally. The drug has a short plasma half-life (complete elimination occurs in approximately 4 hours).

Adverse Effects. At recommended doses, dimercaprol is generally well tolerated. Tachycardia and elevation of blood pressure occur frequently; blood pressure returns to baseline within hours. Pain and sterile abscesses may occur at sites of injection. Fever is common in children. High doses produce a broad spectrum of untoward effects.

Chelates formed with dimercaprol are unstable at acidic pH. Hence, if the urine is acidic, heavy metals may dissociate from dimercaprol, resulting in renal toxicity. To protect the kidneys, the urine should be kept alkaline.

Preparations, Dosage, and Administration. Dimercaprol [BAL In Oil] is dispensed in ampules containing 300 mg of the drug in 3 ml of peanut oil. The preparation is administered by deep IM injection. For *mild poisoning with gold or arsenic,* doses of 2.5 mg/kg are administered according to the following schedule: 4 times daily on days 1 and 2, twice daily on day 3, and once daily on days 4 through 13. For *acute poisoning with mercury,* the initial dose is 5 mg/kg. Subsequent doses of 2.5 mg/kg are administered 1 or 2 times daily for 10 days.

Edetate Calcium Disodium (Calcium EDTA)

Actions and Uses. Calcium EDTA [Calcium Disodium Versenate] is used primarily for lead poisoning. The drug combines with lead to form a stable chelate that is excreted in the urine.

Pharmacokinetics. Calcium EDTA may be administered IV or IM. The drug is poorly absorbed from the GI tract, and hence is not administered orally. Elimination is by glomerular filtration. Because calcium EDTA is excreted by the kidneys, the drug should be employed only if urine flow is adequate. If urine flow is insufficient, it should be restored with IV fluids prior to giving the chelator. If anuria develops during the course of treatment, administration should stop.

Adverse Effects. The principal toxicity of calcium EDTA is renal tubular necrosis. Signs include hematuria and proteinuria. Daily urinalysis should be performed to monitor for these effects. If renal toxicity develops, the drug should be discontinued immediately.

Preparations, Dosage, and Administration. Calcium EDTA [Calcium Disodium Versenate] is dispensed in 5-ml ampules containing 1000 mg of drug. Administration may be IV or IM. The IV route is preferred for adults, whereas IM is preferred for children.

For IV use, the contents of 1 ampule are diluted in 250 to 500 ml of 5% dextrose solution or normal saline. Infusion should be done slowly (over 1 hour or more). The adult dosage is 1 gm twice daily for 5 days. After a 2-day hiatus, a second course may be given, if needed.

The IM dosage for children is 35 mg/kg (or less) administered twice daily for 3 to 5 days. After a pause of 4 days or longer, a second course is given.

Penicillamine

Actions. Penicillamine [Cuprimine, Depen] is a breakdown product of penicillin. Commercial preparations are made synthetically. Penicillamine forms water-soluble chelates with copper, iron, lead, arsenic, gold, and mercury. These complexes are excreted in the urine.

Therapeutic Uses. The principal indication for penicillamine is *Wilson's disease,* a disorder of copper metabolism. Individuals with this disease are deficient in ceruloplasmin, a plasma protein that serves as a carrier for copper. Symptoms result from deposition of copper in the liver, brain, kidneys, eyes, and other organs. Penicillamine relieves symptoms by promoting copper excretion. Therapeutic effects may take several months to develop. Additional uses are *rheumatoid arthritis* and *cystinuria.* Beneficial effects in these disorders are not related to chelation of heavy metals.

Pharmacokinetics. Penicillamine is well absorbed following oral administration. Food greatly reduces the extent of absorption. Once absorbed, penicillamine is rapidly excreted in the urine.

Adverse Effects. With prolonged use, penicillamine can cause varied and serious toxicities. Deaths have occurred. The drug should be employed only with close medical supervision. Possible cutaneous reactions include urticaria, maculopapular and morbilliform rash, pemphigoid lesions, and pruritus. Bone marrow suppression can result in leukopenia, agranulocytosis, and aplastic anemia—reactions that can be fatal. Autoimmune and immune complex disorders have been associated with penicillamine. Among these are dermatomyositis, polymyositis, lupus erythematosus, alveolitis, and myasthenia gravis. Renal toxicity may occur.

Contraindications. Penicillamine is contraindicated for patients who have experienced agranulocytosis or aplastic anemia when receiving penicillamine in the past. The drug is also contraindicated for patients with rheumatoid arthritis who also are pregnant or have renal insufficiency.

Preparations, Dosage, and Administration. Penicillamine [Cuprimine, Depen] is dispensed in 125-mg capsules and 250-mg tablets for oral use. For Wilson's disease, the usual dosage is 250 mg 4 times a day. Doses should be administered 1 hour before meals and at bedtime. Dosage is adjusted on the basis of untoward effects and urinary copper content. Treatment is long term.

Succimer

Actions and Uses. Succimer [Chemet] binds avidly with lead, mercury, and arsenic. Binding is less avid with copper and zinc. Binding to iron, calcium, and magnesium is minimal, and therefore succimer presents no risk of depleting these essential minerals. Succimer is our most effective drug for lowering blood levels of lead in children, its only approved indication. However, recent data indicate that, although succimer can reduce lead levels, benefits are limited to prevention of seizures and death from acute encephalopathy. Treatment does not reverse or prevent the long-term neurologic sequelae of lead poisoning, which are irreversible.

Pharmacokinetics. Succimer is rapidly but variably absorbed following oral administration. The drug undergoes extensive metabolism. Metabolites and parent drug are eliminated slowly in the urine.

Adverse Effects. Adverse effects appear to be mild. About 10% of patients experience GI reactions (nausea, diarrhea, cramps). Other moderate reactions include nasal congestion, muscle pain, and rash. Succimer has caused temporary elevations in serum transaminases, indicating possible liver injury. Accordingly, serum transaminases should be measured before treatment and weekly thereafter. In addition, caution should be exercised in patients with liver disease. In mice, the drug is teratogenic and fetotoxic.

Preparations, Dosage, and Administration. Succimer [Chemet] is dispensed in 100-mg capsules for oral use. For children over 1 year old, treatment consists of 10 mg/kg or 350 mg/m² every 8 hours for 5 days, and then every 12 hours for 14 more days. If needed, the entire course can be repeated after a minimum hiatus of 2 weeks.

Fomepizole

Actions and Uses. Fomepizole [Antizole] is used to treat poisoning by *ethylene glycol,* the principal component of antifreeze. Following ingestion, ethylene glycol undergoes gradual enzymatic conversion into glycolic acid, a toxic acidic metabolite. The result is profound metabolic acidosis, which leads to hyperventilation, coma, seizures, hypertension, pulmonary infiltrates, and renal failure. In the absence of treatment, a lethal dose (100 ml or more) will cause death by multiorgan failure in 24 to 36 hours. Fomepizole protects against injury by inhibiting *alcohol dehydrogenase,* an enzyme required for the conversion of ethylene glycol into its toxic form.

In addition to receiving fomepizole, patients poisoned with ethylene glycol need treatment for metabolic acidosis, acute renal failure, hypocalcemia, and adult respiratory distress syndrome. Treatment options include fluids, sodium bicarbonate, potassium, calcium, and oxygen. If poisoning is severe, patients may require hemodialysis.

Pharmacokinetics. After IV infusion, fomepizole distributes rapidly into total body water. A plasma level of 8.2 to 24.6 mg/L is sufficient to inhibit alcohol dehydrogenase. Fomepizole undergoes hepatic metabolism followed by excretion in the urine. The drug induces hepatic P450 enzymes, and can thereby accelerate its own metabolism. With repeated dosing, a significant increase in metabolism can be seen 30 to 40 hours after the initial dose.

Adverse Effects. Fomepizole is well tolerated. The only common adverse effects are headache (12%), nausea (11%), and dizziness (7%). All other adverse effects (e.g., bradycardia, seizures) are uncommon.

Preparations, Dosage, and Administration. Fomepizole [Antizole] is dispensed as a concentrated solution (1 gm/ml) in 1.5-ml vials. The required dose should be withdrawn from the vial and diluted in at least 100 ml of 0.9% sterile saline or 5% dextrose. Treatment consists of a loading dose (15 mg/kg) followed by four smaller doses (10 mg/kg) given every 12 hours, followed in turn by doses of 15 mg/kg given every 12 hours until ethylene glycol levels drop below 20 mg/dl. All doses are infused IV over 30 minutes. If the patient is also undergoing hemodialysis, fomepizole must be given every 4 hours, rather than every 12.

Other Important Antidotes

Throughout this text we have discussed the toxic effects of various drugs. Where appropriate, we have discussed specific antidotes used for treatment. For example, when discussing the adverse effects of opioids, we also discussed use of naloxone for opioid overdose. Similarly, when discussing heparin toxicity, we discussed the use of protamine sulfate as treatment. The major specific antidotes presented in previous chapters are summarized in Table 105–1.

POISON CONTROL CENTERS

The American Association of Poison Control Centers (AAPCC) defines a poison center as an organization that serves a designated geographic region and provides the following services:

- Poison information
- Telephone management advice and consultation about toxic exposures
- Hazard surveillance to achieve hazard elimination
- Professional and public education in poisoning prevention, diagnosis, and treatment

Poison centers certified by the AAPCC are accessible 24 hours a day; have a specially trained, full-time staff (usually nurses, pharmacists, or both); are directed by a board-certified physician-toxicologist; and are associated with a medical center that has laboratory facilities and personnel needed for the diagnosis and management of poisoning. These centers are accessible by phone and can provide immediate instruction on the management of acute poisoning. In the majority of cases, the information supplied will permit successful treatment at home. By facilitating rapid treatment, poison control centers can decrease morbidity and mortality, and can help reduce the cost of emergency care.

TABLE 105–1 ■ Specific Antidotes Discussed in Previous Chapters

Antidote			
Generic Name	Trade Name	Toxic/Overdosed Substance	Chapter
Atropine		Muscarinic agonists, cholinesterase inhibitors	14
Physostigmine	Antilirium	Anticholinergic drugs	15
Neostigmine	Prostigmin	Nondepolarizing neuromuscular blockers	15
Pralidoxime	Protopam	Organophosphate cholinesterase inhibitors	15
Naloxone	Narcan	Opioids	27
Flumazenil	Romazicon	Benzodiazepines	33
Digoxin immune Fab	Digibind	Digoxin, digitoxin	46
Vitamin K		Warfarin	50
Protamine sulfate		Heparin	50
Glucagon		Insulin-induced hypoglycemia	54
Acetylcysteine	Mucomyst	Acetaminophen	67
Leucovorin	Wellcovorin	Methotrexate and other folate antagonists	98

In 2002, the AAPCC established a national poison hotline: 1-800-222-1222. Dialing this number from any place in the United States will connect you with the *local* poison center. (This system is analogous to dialing 911 from any place in the country to contact local emergency-service providers.) Local poison centers can also be contacted by dialing their individual phone numbers, which are listed in Appendix G.

∴ KEY POINTS

- Management of poisoning has five basic components: supportive care, poison identification, prevention of further absorption, promotion of poison removal, and use of specific antidotes.
- The preferred methods for reducing absorption of ingested poisons are adsorption onto activated charcoal and whole-bowel irrigation. Alternatives include induction of vomiting (with syrup of ipecac) and gastric lavage and aspiration.
- Removal of absorbed poisons can be accelerated by using drugs to enhance renal excretion and by nondrug methods, such as hemodialysis and exchange transfusion.
- For most poisons there is no specific antidote.
- Heavy metal poisoning can be treated with chelating agents.
- Poison control centers offer immediate, expert assistance over the phone.
- Dialing 1-800-222-1222 from any place in the United States will connect you with the nearest poison control center.

Potential Weapons of Biologic, Radiologic, and Chemical Terrorism

BACTERIA AND VIRUSES
Bacillus anthracis **(Anthrax)**
Francisella tularensis **(Tularemia)**
Yersinia pestis **(Pneumonic Plague)**
Variola Virus (Smallpox)
BIOTOXINS
Botulinum Toxin
Ricin
CHEMICAL WEAPONS
Nerve Agents
Sulfur Mustard (Mustard Gas)
RADIOLOGIC WEAPONS
Nuclear Bombs
Attacks on Nuclear Power Plants
Dirty Bombs (Radiologic Dispersion Devices)

TABLE 106–1 ▪ Online Resources for Information on Biologic, Radiologic, and Chemical Terrorism

- *www.bt.cdc.gov*—Bioterrorism information from the Centers for Disease Control and Prevention (CDC)
- *www.fda.gov/oc/opacom/hottopics/bioterrorism.html*—Bioterrorism information from the U.S. Food and Drug Administration (FDA)
- *www.bioterrorism.slu.edu*—Bioterrorism information from the Center for the Study of Bioterrorism at the Saint Louis University School of Public Health
- *www.idsociety.org/bt/toc.htm*—Bioterrorism information from the Infectious Disease Society of America
- *www.apic.org/bioterror/*—Resources on bioterrorism from the Association for Professionals in Infection Control and Epidemiology (APIC)
- *www.hopkins-biodefense.org/*—Information on biologic weapons from The Center for Civilian Biodefense Strategies, an independent, nonprofit organization associated with the Johns Hopkins Bloomberg School of Public Health and the School of Medicine
- *Jama.ama-assn.org/cgi/collection/bioterrorism*—Articles on bioterrorism from *JAMA*
- *medicalletter.com/html/prm.htm#Reprints*—Articles on bioterrorism from *The Medical Letter*
- *www.who.int/ionizing_radiation/a_e/terrorism/en/*—Information on nuclear weapons and dirty bombs from the World Health Organization.
- *www.fda.gov/cder/guidance/4825fnl.htm*—Guidance from the FDA on use of potassium iodide as a thyroid-blocking agent in radiation emergencies.

In fall of 2001, the United States was hit by unprecedented terrorist attacks. On September 11, terrorists hijacked four commercial jets, and succeeded in crashing two into the twin towers of the World Trade Center and one into the Pentagon. In October, anthrax spores were mailed to several locations, causing illness and death. These events have generated great concern about our vulnerability to more such attacks, and our ability to manage the consequences.

In this chapter, we discuss some of the potential weapons of terrorism, focusing primarily on bacteria and viruses. Biotoxins, chemicals (nerve agents and mustard gas), and radiologic weapons are addressed as well. Discussion centers on clinical manifestations and treatment. Prevention is discussed where appropriate.

For more information on the weapons discussed here, or for information on other potential weapons, you can consult the online resources listed in Table 106–1.

BACTERIA AND VIRUSES

Bacillus anthracis (Anthrax)

Bacillus anthracis is the bacterium that causes anthrax, a disease with three major forms: inhalational, cutaneous, and gastrointestinal. Our discussion focuses on inhalational and cutaneous anthrax. Gastrointestinal anthrax is not discussed because this form is unlikely to result from a terrorist attack.

Of the microbes that might be used by terrorists, *Bacillus anthracis* is among the most dangerous. In October 2001, spores of *B. anthracis* were mailed to several locations in the United States, causing 22 confirmed or suspected cases of anthrax and five deaths. This experience served to heighten concerns regarding the feasibility of terrorist groups using aerosolized bioweapons to stage large-scale attacks.

Microbiology

Bacillus anthracis is an aerobic, gram-positive bacterium. Its name derives from *anthrakis,* the Greek word for coal (in recognition of the black skin lesions that characterize cutaneous infection). *Bacillus anthracis* can exist as spores (which are dormant) or as actively growing bacteria. Infection is acquired when the *spores* enter a host. Ports of entry are skin lesions and the respiratory and GI tracts. In the presence of nutrients (amino acids, nucleotides, glucose), which are

TABLE 106–2 ■ Therapy of Inhalational Anthrax in the Limited Casualty Setting

Patient Group	Initial Intravenous Therapy	Follow-up Oral Therapy	Duration
Adults	Ciprofloxacin, 400 mg every 12 hr *or* Doxycycline, 100 mg every 12 hr *and* All patients should get 1 or 2 additional antibiotics. Options include rifampin, vancomycin, penicillin, ampicillin, imipenem, chloramphenicol, clindamycin, and clarithromycin. Do not use penicillin or ampicillin alone.	When clinically appropriate, switch to oral antibiotics: Ciprofloxacin, 500 mg twice daily *or* Doxycycline, 100 mg twice daily	For all patients: Treat 60 days total (IV and PO combined)
Children	Ciprofloxacin, 10–15 mg/kg every 12 hr, but no more than 1 gm/day *or* Doxycycline (for young children) >8 yr and >45 kg: 100 mg every 12 hr >8 yr and ≤45 kg: 2.2 mg/kg every 12 hr ≤8 yr: 2.2 mg/kg every 12 hr *As with adults, all patients should get 1 or 2 additional antibiotics.*	When clinically appropriate, switch to oral antibiotics: Ciprofloxacin, 10–15 mg/kg every 12 hr, but no more than 1 gm/day *or* Doxycycline (for young children) >8 yr and >45 kg: 100 mg every 12 hr >8 yr and ≤45 kg: 2.2 mg/kg every 12 hr ≤8 yr: 2.2 mg/kg every 12 hr	
Pregnant	Same as nonpregnant adults	Same as nonpregnant adults	

abundant in the blood and tissues of the host, the spores germinate and transform into mature bacteria. The mature forms grow and divide rapidly until the nutrient supply is depleted, after which they cease dividing and produce more spores. The mature bacteria cannot survive long outside the host. In contrast, the spores can remain viable in the environment for decades. Anthrax is not transmitted from person to person.

Clinical Manifestations

Inhalational Anthrax. Infection begins with deposition of anthrax spores in the alveolar space, followed by transport to regional lymph nodes, where germination occurs. Clinical latency can range from 2 days to 6 weeks. Injury results when mature bacilli release toxins, which cause hemorrhage, edema, and necrosis. Once the concentration of toxin has reached a critical level, antibiotics cannot prevent death, even if they kill all circulating bacilli.

Development of symptoms occurs in two stages. Initial symptoms—fever, cough, malaise, and weakness—may be relatively mild. In the second stage, which develops 2 to 3 days later, there is a sudden increase in fever, along with severe respiratory distress, septicemia, hemorrhagic meningitis, and shock. Interestingly, although the infection originates in the lungs, true pneumonia rarely occurs. Even with treatment, the mortality rate can be high: In the U.S. outbreak of 2001, 45% of victims died.

Cutaneous Anthrax. Symptoms begin 1 to 7 days after exposure to anthrax spores. Areas with cuts or abrasions are most vulnerable, but injury can develop at any site where spores land. The initial lesion is a small papule (solid raised area) or vesicle (fluid-filled raised area) associated with localized itching. Within 2 days, the lesion enlarges and evolves into a painless ulcer with a necrotic core. Seven to 10 days after symptom onset, a black eschar (scab-like structure) forms—but then dries, loosens, and sloughs off by day 12 to 14. In most patients,

the lesions resolve without complications or scarring. However, if *systemic* infection develops, the outcome can be fatal. In the absence of antibiotic therapy, about 20% of people with cutaneous anthrax die. Fortunately, death among treated patients is rare.

Treatment

Inhalational Anthrax. Given the rapid course that inhalational anthrax follows, early therapy with antibiotics is essential. Any delay can reduce the chance of survival. Initial IV therapy is preferred to initial oral therapy. However, if there are mass casualties, IV therapy may be impossible, owing to limited supplies and personnel. Ideally, treatment should start with *IV ciprofloxacin* or *IV doxycycline*. Because the strain of *B. anthracis* may be resistant to these drugs, one or two other IV antibiotics should be added to the regimen. When clinically appropriate, the patient can be switched to oral ciprofloxacin or doxycycline, without additional antibiotics. The duration of treatment—IV plus oral—is 60 days. Specific regimens for adults, children, and pregnant women are presented in Table 106–2 (for limited casualty settings) and Table 106–3 (for mass casualty settings).

Cutaneous Anthrax. Cutaneous anthrax is treated with oral antibiotics. The preferred drugs are *ciprofloxacin* and *doxycycline*. Dosages for adults, children, and pregnant women are the same as those given in Table 106–2 for follow-up oral therapy of inhalational anthrax. Duration of treatment is 60 days. It should be noted that treatment is unlikely to prevent cutaneous lesions, but *will* prevent systemic complications.

Postexposure Prophylaxis

For prophylaxis following exposure to aerosolized anthrax spores, authorities recommend the same oral regimens used for inhalational anthrax in a mass casualty setting (see Table 106–3). Drug use should continue for at least 60 days.

TABLE 106–3 ■ Therapy of Inhalational Anthrax in the Mass Casualty Setting

Patient Group	Preferred Initial Oral Therapy	Alternative Oral Therapy (if Strain Is Proved Susceptible)	Duration
Adults	Ciprofloxacin, 500 mg every 12 hr	Doxycycline, 100 mg every 12 hr Amoxicillin, 500 mg every 8 hr	60 days for all patients
Children	Ciprofloxacin, 10–15 mg every 12 hr, but no more than 1 gm/day	≥20 kg: amoxicillin, 500 mg every 8 hr <20 kg: amoxicillin, 13.3 mg/kg every 8 hr	
Pregnant	Ciprofloxacin, 500 mg every 12 hr	Amoxicillin, 500 mg every 8 hr	

Anthrax Vaccine

Currently, only one anthrax vaccine is licensed in the United States. This product—Anthrax Vaccine Adsorbed (AVA)—is intended for use by the military, and is not available to civilians. AVA is an inactivated, cell-free preparation made from an avirulent strain of *B. anthracis.* The immunization schedule consists of three subcutaneous injections given 2 weeks apart, followed by three more injections given at 6, 12, and 18 months. Annual booster shots are recommended thereafter. The most common side effects are muscle and joint aches (20%); headache (20%); local redness, tenderness, or itching (10%); fatigue (10%); nausea (5%); and chills and fever (5%). Serious allergic reactions occur rarely (less than 1 in 100,000).

Francisella tularensis (Tularemia)

Tularemia, also known as "rabbit fever" and "deer fly fever," is a potentially fatal disease caused by *Francisella tularensis,* one of the most infectious bacteria known. Inoculation with as few as 10 of these microbes can cause disease. Infection can be acquired through the skin, mucous membranes, GI tract, or lungs. Terrorists trying to spread tularemia would most likely deliver the bacteria as an aerosol. Tularemia cannot be transmitted from person to person.

Clinical Manifestations. Symptoms of tularemia develop in 3 to 5 days. Initially, patients present with an acute flu-like illness, characterized by fever (38°C to 40°C), headache, chills, rigors, body aches, sneezing, and sore throat. Pneumonia and pleuritis can develop in the ensuing days to weeks. In the absence of treatment, tularemia can progress to respiratory failure, shock, and death.

Treatment. Tularemia responds well to antibiotics. The treatment of choice is *IM streptomycin* (15 mg/kg twice a day for 10 days). *Gentamicin* (5 mg/kg IM or IV once a day for 10 days) is the preferred alternative. If there is a mass outbreak, oral therapy with doxycycline or ciprofloxacin is recommended. Individuals who have not yet developed symptoms may benefit from prophylactic use of oral doxycycline or ciprofloxacin.

Yersinia pestis (Pneumonic Plague)

Plague is a potentially fatal disease caused by *Yersinia pestis,* a gram-negative bacillus. The disease has two principal forms: *bubonic* (characterized by tender, enlarged, and inflamed lymph nodes) and *pneumonic* (characterized by inflammation of the lungs). Bubonic plague is acquired through the bite of a plague-infected flea, and *cannot* be transmitted from person to person. Rarely, an individual with bubonic plague develops secondary pneumonic plague, which *can* be transmitted person to person (by coughing). *Primary* pneumonic plague is acquired by inhaling aerosolized *Y. pestis.* The source of the aerosol could be a person with pneumonic plague, or it could be a biologic weapon. From the perspective of a potential bioterrorist, *Y. pestis* is attractive for several reasons: The microbe is readily available worldwide, culturing large quantities is relatively easy, the bacterium can be aerosolized for wide dissemination, pneumonic plague can be spread from person to person, and the fatality rate is high.

Clinical Manifestations. Symptoms of primary pneumonic plague usually develop 2 to 4 days after inhaling aerosolized *Y. pestis.* Patients typically present with high fever, cough, dyspnea, and hemoptysis (expectoration of blood or blood-stained sputum). Gastrointestinal symptoms—nausea, vomiting, diarrhea, and abdominal pain—may also be present. In the absence of treatment, the infection rapidly progresses to respiratory failure and death.

Treatment. Antibiotics can be lifesaving, provided they are given early (before or shortly after symptom onset). Treatments of choice are (1) *streptomycin,* 15 mg/kg IM twice daily for 10 days, and (2) *gentamicin,* 5 mg/kg IM or IV once daily for 10 days. Preferred alternatives, all given IV, are doxycycline, ciprofloxacin, and chloramphenicol. In a mass-casualty setting, which may preclude IV or IM administration, oral therapy with doxycycline (100 mg twice daily) or ciprofloxacin (500 mg twice daily) is recommended. There is no vaccine for prevention of pneumonic plague.

Variola Virus (Smallpox)

Smallpox is a serious, contagious, life-threatening disease caused by the *variola virus,* a member of the genus *Orthopoxvirus.* The only natural reservoir for the virus is humans. We have no specific treatment for smallpox, but we *can* prevent the disease by vaccination, given either before exposure to the virus or within a few days following exposure. Because smallpox is highly contagious and because the fatality rate is high (30%), the disease represents a grave threat as a weapon of terrorism.

Thanks to a global vaccination program, begun in 1967, endemic smallpox has been eradicated. The last case in the United States occurred in 1949, and the last case on the planet occurred in Somalia in 1977. Because the threat of smallpox had been eliminated, routine vaccination was discontinued—in 1972 for Americans, and by 1982 for the rest of the world.

Ironically, the successful elimination of smallpox has set the stage for its potential return as a weapon of terrorism. That is, if we hadn't eradicated natural smallpox, then vaccination would still be ongoing. As a result, the population would have immunity, making smallpox useless as a weapon.

Pathogenesis and Clinical Manifestations

Variola virus enters the body through mucous membranes of the respiratory tract, usually as a result of virus inhalation. Initial exposure is followed by an asymptomatic incubation period (usually 12 to 14 days), which is followed in turn by the prodromal phase (2- to 4-day duration), manifesting as high fever, malaise, prostration, headache, and backache. Viral invasion of the oral mucosa and dermis then leads to characteristic eruptions. Small red spots develop in the mouth and on the tongue, and then evolve into sores that break open, releasing large amounts of virus into the mouth and throat. Around the same time, a bumpy skin rash develops, starting on the face and then quickly spreading over the entire body. Within 1 to 2 days, the bumps become vesicular (fluid filled), and then pustular (pus filled). About 8 or 9 days after the rash began, the pustules begin to form a crust and then a scab. By 3 weeks after the rash began, the scabs fall off, leaving a characteristic pitted scar.

About 30% of people with smallpox die, usually during the second week of illness. The most likely cause is toxemia associated with circulating immune complexes and soluble variola antigens.

Transmission

Natural smallpox is transmitted person to person. It is not transmitted by insects or animals. Transmission occurs primarily by touching an infected person or by inhaling aerosolized droplets expelled from the oropharynx. Smallpox can also be acquired by contact with contaminated clothing or bedding. The disease is somewhat contagious during the prodromal phase, but most contagious from the onset of rash through scab formation. After all scabs fall off, infectivity is gone.

If used as a weapon of terrorism, variola virus would most likely be disseminated as an aerosol. Because the virus is fragile, at least 90% of the amount released into the environment would become inactive within 24 hours.

Treatment

There is no proven treatment for smallpox. However, research with newer antiviral drugs is ongoing. One such agent—*cidofovir*—shows promise. Topical *idoxuridine* may benefit patients with corneal lesions. Antibiotics should be used to treat secondary bacterial infections.

Smallpox Vaccine

Vaccination is the only way to prevent smallpox. In addition to conferring protection when done *prior to* viral exposure, the vaccine confers protection when given within a few days *after* exposure. Since 1972, vaccination has been limited to the few scientists and medical professionals who do research on smallpox and related viruses. However, owing to concerns about bioterrorism, the U.S. government is reinstituting a vaccination program. Under the plan, military personnel and hospital smallpox-response teams will be immunized first, followed by police officers, firefighters, and general healthcare workers. Vaccination of the general public will be last. Except for people in the military, vaccination will be voluntary.

At this time, smallpox vaccine is not available to the general public—nor is it recommended. However, in the event of a terrorist attack, prophylactic immunization will be provided.

Description. Smallpox vaccine is a suspension of live *vaccinia virus,* a virus that belongs to the same family as variola virus, but does not cause smallpox. The formulation in current use, known as *Dryvax,* is prepared from the lymph of calves that have been inoculated with vaccinia virus. A new vaccine, containing vaccinia virus that had been grown in monkey kidney and human fibroblast cells, should be available in 2004.

Efficacy. Vaccination *before* exposure to variola virus prevents smallpox in about 95% of vaccinees. Vaccination within 3 days *after* exposure also confers significant protection, greatly reducing symptoms in some people, and preventing them entirely in others. Benefits of vaccination 4 to 7 days after exposure are uncertain.

Duration of Protection. Successful primary vaccination produces a high level of immunity for 5 to 10 years, with decreasing immunity thereafter. Successful revaccination may confer protection for 10 to 20 years, and perhaps even longer. People who were vaccinated in 1972 or earlier probably have little or no protection now.

Administration. Smallpox vaccine is administered by a unique method known as *scarification,* which introduces the vaccine through multiple skin punctures. Administration is *not* by SC, IM, or IV injection. The vaccine is given with a bifurcated (two-pronged) needle that is dipped into the vaccine solution. When removed from the solution, the needle retains a droplet of vaccine between its prongs. The administrator then pricks the skin several times (2 or 3 times for primary vaccination; 15 times for revaccination). The resulting punctures should be superficial—but deep enough to allow a trace of blood to appear after 15 to 20 seconds. Vaccinations are made in the upper arm. To prevent spread of the vaccine, which contains live viruses, the site should be covered with sterile gauze or a semipermeable membrane.

Interpreting the Response. Successful vaccination is indicated when the following events take place. Within 3 to 4 days, a red, itchy bump appears. During the first week, the bump becomes a blister, fills with pus, and then starts to drain. During the second week, the blister begins to dry and develops a scab. In the third week, the scab falls off, leaving a small scar. Reactions to primary vaccination are stronger than reactions to revaccination.

Adverse Effects. The smallpox vaccine carries considerable risk. Past experience suggests that, if 1 million people were vaccinated, 1000 would experience a serious adverse effect, 14 to 52 would develop a life-threatening condition, and 1 or 2 would die. Nonetheless, although vaccination carries significant risk, the risk of smallpox infection is far greater. Accordingly, anyone exposed to variola virus, regardless of health status, should be offered the vaccine.

Mild Effects. In addition to the local reactions that signal a successful immune response, vaccination can cause local inflammation, along with swelling and tenderness in regional lymph nodes. Transient symptoms typical of viral illness (fever, headache, muscle aches, fatigue) are also common.

If the vaccination site is not well covered, vaccinia virus can be transferred to other areas—usually the face, eyelids, nose, mouth, or genitalia—as well as to other people. Transfer to the eyes can cause sight-threatening keratitis. Fortunately, most lesions heal spontaneously.

Moderate to Severe Effects. Serious reactions to smallpox vaccination include eczema vaccinatum, generalized vaccinia, progressive vaccinia, postvaccinial encephalitis, and fetal vaccinia. (The terms *vaccinatum* and *vaccinia* in the names of these disorders simply refer to the cause: vaccinia virus.)

Eczema vaccinatum occurs when infection with vaccinia virus is superimposed on a pre-existing skin condition, usually eczema or atopic dermatitis. As a rule, the disorder is mild and self-limiting. However, in some people it can be life threatening.

Generalized vaccinia is a widespread vesicular rash that resembles smallpox. The cause is transient viremia with localization in the skin. Although the condition is generally self-limiting, it can be severe in the immunocompromised patient.

Progressive vaccinia, also called *vaccinia necrosum,* is a rare but often fatal condition that develops almost exclusively in patients who are immunodeficient. The condition is characterized by progressive necrosis at the inoculation site, often associated with metastatic vaccinial lesions at distant sites (skin, bones, and viscera).

Postvaccinial encephalitis—inflammation of the brain—is rare but dangerous. This complication occurs roughly 2 to 12 times per million vaccinations. The fatality rate is 15% to 25%, and 25% of survivors suffer brain damage.

Fetal vaccinia is a very rare but serious infection of the fetus, manifested by skin lesions and internal organ involvement. The condition can lead to premature birth, or fetal or neonatal death. Fetal vaccinia can result from exposure to vaccinia virus at any stage of pregnancy. Accordingly, women who are pregnant should not be given the vaccine. Women who were recently vaccinated should wait at least 4 weeks before attempting to become pregnant.

Possible Cardiac Effects. Some recent vaccinees have developed cardiac problems—specifically, myocarditis (inflammation of the heart muscle), pericarditis (inflammation of the pericardium), myocardial infarction (heart attack), and angina pectoris (ischemic cardiac pain). However, a definite link between vaccination and these disorders has not been established. Until more is known, routine vaccination should be withheld from people with established heart disease (heart failure, angina, myocardial infarction, cardiomyopathy), and from those with three or more cardiovascular risk factors (see Table 106–4 below).

Management of Adverse Effects. Two agents—*vaccinia immune globulin* (VIG) and *cidofovir* [Vistide]—can be used to treat severe reactions to smallpox vaccine. However, neither preparation is approved for this application.

VIG is a solution that contains immunoglobulins from people vaccinated with vaccinia virus, and hence should contain antibodies directed against the virus. However, therapeutic effects have not been established in controlled trials. There is some evidence that VIG can benefit those with eczema vaccinatum or generalized vaccinia, and possibly those with progressive vaccinia. In contrast, the preparation offers no benefit to those with postvaccinial encephalitis, and may actually *increase* corneal damage in those with vaccinial keratitis. VIG is administered IM into the buttocks or anterolateral thigh. The dosage is 0.6 ml/kg, repeated every 2 to 3 days as needed. VIG is available only from the Centers for Disease Control and Prevention (CDC).

Cidofovir is an antiviral drug with one approved indication: cytomegalovirus retinitis in patients with AIDS. However, in animal studies, the drug also showed good activity against vaccinia virus. Accordingly, some authorities recommend that it be given to patients with severe vaccination complications, including progressive vaccinia, generalized vaccinia, and eczema vaccinatum. The pharmacology of cidofovir is discussed in Chapter 89 (Antiviral Drugs I: Drugs for Non-HIV Viral Infections).

Who Should NOT Be Vaccinated? Certain conditions (e.g., eczema, atopic dermatitis, immunodeficiency, pregnancy) increase the risk of a serious reaction to smallpox vaccine. Accordingly, people who have these conditions, or who live with someone who does, should not be vaccinated—unless, of course, they have been exposed to the smallpox virus, in which case the risk of infection would far outweigh the risk of the vaccine. Table 106–4 gives a full list of medical conditions and other factors that contraindicate routine vaccination.

TABLE 106–4 ■ Medical Conditions and Other Factors That Contraindicate Routine Smallpox Vaccination*

- History of eczema or atopic dermatitis
- Active skin conditions, including burns, herpes, severe acne, psoriasis, chickenpox, or shingles (delay vaccination until lesions heal)
- Immunodeficiency (caused by HIV infection, primary immunodeficiency disorder, or use of immunosuppressive drugs, including glucocorticoids, many anticancer drugs, and drugs used to prevent transplant rejection)
- Pregnancy (or plans to become pregnant within 1 month of vaccination)
- Breast-feeding
- Allergy to the smallpox vaccine or any of its components (polymyxin B, streptomycin, chlortetracycline, neomycin)
- Age less than 18 years (and especially less than 1 year) or greater than 65 years
- Moderate or severe short-term illness (delay vaccination until illness resolves)
- Inflammatory eye disease with ongoing use of steroid eye drops
- Heart conditions, including heart failure, angina, myocardial infarction, and cardiomyopathy
- Three or more cardiovascular risk factors: hypertension, high cholesterol, diabetes, cigarette use, first-degree relative with early heart disease (i.e., before the age of 50)

*Routine vaccination should be avoided in people with these conditions. However, vaccination *is* indicated following exposure to the smallpox virus.

BIOTOXINS

Botulinum Toxin

Botulinum toxin, produced by *Clostridium botulinum,* is the most potent poison known. Just 1 gm, if evenly dispersed and inhaled, could kill more than 1 million people. When used as a weapon of terrorism, the toxin could be delivered as an aerosol or could simply be put into food.

Cosmetic use of botulinum toxin is discussed in Chapter 101 (Box 101–1, *Face Time with Botox*).

Mechanism of Action. How does botulinum toxin work? It blocks release of acetylcholine from cholinergic neurons. The toxin is taken up by cholinergic nerve terminals, where it then inactivates SNAP-25, a protein critical to the function of acetylcholine-containing vesicles. In the absence of SNAP-25, the vesicles are unable to fuse with the terminal membrane, and hence cannot release their acetylcholine into the synaptic space. Restoration of neuronal function requires sprouting of new terminals, a process that can take several months. Botulinum toxin blocks transmission at neuromuscular junctions and at cholinergic synapses of the autonomic nervous system.

Clinical Manifestations. Botulinum toxin poisoning is characterized by symmetric, descending flaccid paralysis, beginning 12 to 72 hours after exposure and persisting for weeks to months. Classic symptoms are double vision, blurred vision, drooping eyelids, slurred speech, dry mouth, difficulty swallowing, and muscle weakness that descends through the body, starting with the shoulders, and then progressing to the upper arms, lower arms, thighs, calves, and feet. Death results from paralysis of the muscles of respiration.

Treatment. Treatment consists of prolonged supportive care and immediate infusion of botulinum antitoxin. Supportive care, which may be needed for several months, includes fluid and nutritional therapy plus mechanical assistance of ventilation. Botulinum antitoxin, produced in horses, should be given as soon as botulism is diagnosed. The antiserum, which contains neutralizing antibodies, can minimize further nerve damage, but cannot reverse damage that has already set in. In the United States, botulinum antitoxin is available only through state and local health departments, which get the antitoxin from the CDC. The recommended dosage is 10 ml (the contents of one vial) diluted 1:10 in 0.9% saline and administered by slow IV infusion.

Ricin

Ricin is a toxin present in castor beans, which are produced by *Ricinus communis,* the castor-bean plant. The toxin is manufactured by extraction from the "mash" left behind when castor beans are processed to make castor oil. When purified, ricin can be formulated as a powder, pellet, or mist, or it can be dissolved in water or weak acid.

Mechanism of Action. Ricin promotes injury by disrupting protein synthesis. How? Ricin is an enzyme that catalyzes the inactivation of ribosomes, which are required for protein synthesis. Inhibition of protein synthesis leads to cell death and related tissue injury.

Clinical Manifestations. Symptoms of poisoning depend on the route of administration:

- *Inhalation*—Within a few hours of inhaling ricin mist or powder, the victim can experience coughing, tightness in the chest, difficulty breathing, nausea, and muscle ache. A few hours later, the airway may become severely inflamed and edematous, making breathing extremely difficult. Cyanosis and death can follow.
- *Ingestion*—Swallowing a significant dose can cause gastric and intestinal hemorrhage, associated with vomiting

and bloody diarrhea. In time, the liver, spleen, and kidneys may fail. Death can occur within 10 to 12 days of ingestion.

- *Injection*—Injection of ricin can lead to severe symptoms and death. However, this is obviously not a route that terrorists can use.

Treatment. Management of poisoning is purely supportive. We have no antidote for ricin.

CHEMICAL WEAPONS

Nerve Agents

Nerve agents are "irreversible" organophosphate cholinesterase inhibitors. By inhibiting cholinesterase, these agents increase the concentration of acetylcholine at neuromuscular junctions, cholinergic synapses in the central nervous system (CNS), and all autonomic synapses that employ acetylcholine as a transmitter. Toxic doses produce a state of cholinergic crisis, characterized by excessive muscarinic stimulation and depolarizing neuromuscular blockade. Treatment consists of (1) mechanical ventilation using oxygen, (2) giving *atropine* to reduce muscarinic stimulation, (3) giving *pralidoxime* to reverse inhibition of cholinesterase (primarily at neuromuscular junctions), and (4) giving *diazepam* to suppress convulsions. Specific nerve agents that might be used for a terrorist attack include *soman, tabun, sarin,* and *cyclosarin*. All are volatile at room temperature. However, nerve agent vapors are denser than air, and hence tend to accumulate in low-lying areas. The toxic effects of nerve agents as well as the use of pralidoxime for treatment are discussed at length in Chapter 15 (Cholinesterase Inhibitors and Their Use in Myasthenia Gravis) under the heading "Toxicology" in the section *"Irreversible" Cholinesterase Inhibitors.*

Sulfur Mustard (Mustard Gas)

Properties. Sulfur mustard (bis[2-chloroethyl]sulfide), also known as mustard gas, is an alkylating agent and vesicant (chemical blistering agent). However, the precise relationship between alkylation of DNA (as well as other cellular components) and production of blisters is unclear. Physically, sulfur mustard is a lipophilic, oily liquid that can be vaporized at high temperatures. For use as a weapon of terrorism, sulfur mustard could be vaporized into the air or released into the water supply. Injuries from sulfur mustard can be severe, but the fatality rate is low. When used as a weapon in World War I, sulfur mustard killed less than 5% of its victims.

Clinical Manifestations. Symptoms of toxicity depend on the dose, the tissue involved, and the duration of exposure. As a rule, symptoms are delayed, usually taking 2 to 24 hours to develop. Effects on specific tissues are as follows:

- *Skin*—Dermal contact causes pain, redness, swelling, and blisters (small to very large) within 4 to 48 hours, depending on the dose. Areas where the skin is warm, moist, and thin are most vulnerable.
- *Eyes*—The eyes are exquisitely sensitive to sulfur mustard. Moderate exposure can produce irritation, pain, swelling,

and tearing in 3 to 12 hours. Severe exposure can cause corneal burns, necrosis, severe pain, and blindness, which may last up to 10 days.

- *Respiratory tract*—Symptoms appear 2 to 24 hours after inhalation of sulfur mustard. Mild exposure can cause runny nose, sneezing, hoarseness, sinus pain, and a dry barking cough. Severe exposure can cause hemorrhage and necrosis of lung tissue, evidenced by coughing up blood.
- *GI tract*—Ingestion of sulfur mustard can cause nausea and vomiting, diarrhea, and abdominal pain. Symptoms typically develop within a few hours and resolve within 24 hours.
- *Bone marrow*—Very high doses cause bone marrow depression, resulting in neutropenia and thrombocytopenia.

Treatment. Management centers on rapid decontamination, supportive care, and drug therapy. People exposed to sulfur mustard should undress immediately and wash three times with soap and water. Those with significant airway damage may need intubation. Severe skin burns are treated by irrigation, débridement, and application of topical antibiotics; burn-related pain can be controlled with an opioid analgesic. Exposed eyes should be irrigated; other treatments include use of cycloplegic-mydriatics, application of topical antibiotics, and application of petroleum jelly to prevent burned lids from sticking. Granulocyte colony-stimulating factor can be used to stimulate neutrophil production by bone marrow.

RADIOLOGIC WEAPONS

Nuclear Bombs

Nuclear bombs present an *immediate* threat from the blast itself and a *delayed* threat from radioactive fallout. Immediate harm is produced in four ways:

- The explosion and its shock wave damage buildings, people, and everything else they reach.
- Intense heat causes injury directly and by igniting fires.
- Intense light damages eyesight.
- Ionizing radiation causes acute radiation syndromes and radiation sickness, characterized by nausea, vomiting, diarrhea, fatigue, dehydration, inflammation, skin burns, hair loss, and ulceration of the mouth, esophagus, and GI tract. Symptoms develop over days to weeks. Among those who survive, radiation exposure increases the risk of cancer.

Radioactive fallout, mainly *iodine-131,* poses a delayed risk. Specifically, it poses a risk of thyroid cancer. A nuclear explosion creates a radioactive cloud that can spread fallout over a large area. Contamination of humans can result from inhaling fallout, touching contaminated objects, or ingesting contaminated water and food. Once in the body, iodine-131 becomes concentrated in the thyroid gland, where it can cause thyroid cancer. The risk of cancer can be reduced by ingesting potassium iodide, which blocks uptake of radioactive iodine by the thyroid. To be effective, potassium iodide must be taken soon after exposure. If taken 48 hours after exposure, the drug is useless. Each dose protects for about 24 hours, and

hence dosing must be repeated daily until the threat of fallout has passed. Daily dosages recommended by the Food and Drug Administration are as follows:

- *Age up to 1 month:* 16 mg
- *Age 1 month to 3 years:* 32 mg
- *Age 3 years to 18 years:* 65 mg
- *Age 18 years and older:* 130 mg
- *Females who are pregnant or lactating, regardless of age:* 65 mg

Potassium iodide tablets designed for blocking radioactive iodine uptake are available only through state and federal agencies, and should be used only when public health officials confirm that iodine-131 has been released.

Attacks on Nuclear Power Plants

Terrorists could attack a nuclear power plant, either with a bomb or by using sabotage to cause meltdown of the radioactive core. In either case, a large amount of radiation could be released. Please note, however, that an attack would *not* cause a nuclear explosion. People in the immediate area could suffer severe radiation exposure, resulting in acute radiation syndrome or radiation sickness (see above). As in a nuclear blast, release of iodine-131 could pose a risk of thyroid cancer (see above).

Dirty Bombs (Radiologic Dispersion Devices)

A dirty bomb is a device that uses a conventional explosive (e.g., dynamite) to disperse radioactive material that has been formulated as a powder or tiny pellets. Resultant radioactive contamination could be external or internal (owing to inhalation, ingestion, or absorption through a wound). However, it is important to appreciate that the primary danger from a dirty bomb is the blast itself, not the radiation. Why? Because the sources of radiation likely to be used are not very dangerous, and because dispersal of radiation would be limited to a small area. The risk of cancer is very low. Persons exposed to a dirty bomb blast should remove their clothes as soon as possible, and should decontaminate their skin by showering. A dirty bomb will not release iodine-131, and hence taking potassium iodide would be of no benefit.

⁙ KEY POINTS

- Anthrax is a potentially fatal disease caused by *Bacillus anthracis,* a bacterium that produces spores that can remain viable in the environment for decades.
- Anthrax infection is acquired when spores enter the body, typically through the skin or through mucous membranes of the respiratory tract.
- Anthrax is not transmitted person to person.
- *Inhalational* anthrax is characterized by severe respiratory distress, septicemia, hemorrhagic meningitis, and shock. About 45% of victims die, even when treated.
- Lesions of *cutaneous* anthrax are characterized by a black eschar (scab-like structure), that eventually

dries, loosens, and sloughs off. Most cases resolve without complications or scarring.

- For initial therapy of inhalational anthrax, treatments of choice are IV ciprofloxacin and IV doxycycline, combined with one or two additional IV antibiotics.
- Drugs of choice for cutaneous anthrax are oral ciprofloxacin and oral doxycycline.
- Anthrax vaccine is available for military personnel, but not for civilians.
- Tularemia is a potentially fatal disease caused by *Francisella tularensis,* one of the most infectious bacteria known.
- Tularemia can be acquired through bacterial invasion of the skin, mucous membranes, GI tract, or lungs.
- Tularemia is not transmitted person to person.
- Tularemia is characterized by pneumonia and pleuritis that can progress to respiratory failure, shock, and death.
- Tularemia responds well to antibiotics. The treatment of choice is IM streptomycin.
- Pneumonic plague is a potentially fatal disease caused by *Yersinia pestis.*
- Pneumonic plague is acquired by inhaling aerosolized *Y. pestis,* and can be transmitted person to person.
- Pneumonic plague is characterized by high fever, cough, dyspnea, and hemoptysis (expectoration of blood or blood-stained sputum). In the absence of treatment, the infection rapidly progresses to respiratory failure and death.
- Treatments of choice for pneumonic plague are streptomycin (IM) and gentamicin (IM or IV).
- Smallpox is a serious, contagious, potentially fatal disease caused by variola virus, whose only reservoir is humans.
- Worldwide vaccination has eliminated naturally occurring smallpox. The last case occurred in Somalia in 1977.
- Variola virus enters the body through mucous membranes of the respiratory tract.
- Smallpox is characterized by (1) eruptions on the mouth and tongue that release virus into the oropharynx and (2) pustules on the skin that release the virus on the body surface.
- Natural smallpox is transmitted person to person, primarily by touching an infected individual or by inhaling aerosolized droplets expelled from the oropharynx.
- There is no proven treatment for smallpox.
- Smallpox vaccine, consisting of live vaccinia virus, confers protection when given before exposure to variola virus and when given within a few days after exposure.
- Smallpox vaccine is administered by scarification, a technique that introduces the vaccine through multiple superficial skin punctures.
- Successful primary vaccination with smallpox vaccine produces a high level of immunity for 5 to 10 years. People vaccinated in 1972 and earlier probably have little or no protection now.
- Smallpox vaccination carries significant risk: Past experience suggests that, if 1 million people were vacci-

nated, 1000 would experience a serious adverse effect, 14 to 52 would develop a life-threatening condition, and 1 or 2 would die.

- Although smallpox vaccination carries risk, the risk of smallpox itself is far greater. Accordingly, anyone exposed to variola virus should be offered the vaccine.
- Routine smallpox vaccination is contraindicated by a number of conditions, including eczema, atopic dermatitis, immunodeficiency, pregnancy, and heart disease.
- Botulinum toxin, produced by *Clostridium botulinum,* is the most potent poison known.
- Botulinum toxin acts on cholinergic nerve terminals to cause prolonged blockade of acetylcholine release.
- Poisoning with botulinum toxin is characterized by symmetric, descending flaccid paralysis, coupled with disturbed vision, drooping eyelids, slurred speech, dry mouth, and difficulty swallowing. Death results from paralysis of the muscles of respiration.
- Treatment of botulinum toxin poisoning consists of immediate infusion of botulinum antitoxin plus prolonged supportive care.
- Botulinum antitoxin can minimize further nerve damage, but cannot reverse damage that has already occurred.
- Ricin is a toxin present in castor beans (which are used to make castor oil).
- Ricin causes injury by inhibiting protein synthesis.
- When ricin is *inhaled,* it causes inflammation and edema of the airway, thereby making breathing extremely difficult. Cyanosis and death can follow.
- When ricin is *ingested,* it causes gastric and intestinal hemorrhage, associated with vomiting and bloody diarrhea. In time, the liver, spleen, and kidneys may fail.
- Management of ricin poisoning is purely supportive. There is no antidote.
- Nerve agents cause "irreversible" inhibition of cholinesterase, and thereby increase the concentration of acetylcholine at neuromuscular junctions, cholinergic synapses in the CNS, and all autonomic synapses that employ acetylcholine as a transmitter.
- Nerve agents produce a state of cholinergic crisis, characterized by excessive muscarinic stimulation and depolarizing neuromuscular blockade.
- Treatment of nerve agent poisoning consists of mechanical ventilation using oxygen, and giving atropine (to reduce muscarinic stimulation), pralidoxime (to reverse inhibition of cholinesterase), and diazepam (to suppress convulsions).
- Sulfur mustard (mustard gas) is an alkylating agent and vesicant that can injure any tissue that it reaches.
- Symptoms of sulfur mustard toxicity include large skin blisters, corneal burns, hemorrhage and necrosis of lung tissue, GI disturbances, and neutropenia and thrombocytopenia (secondary to bone marrow depression).
- Management of sulfur mustard poisoning consists of rapid decontamination, supportive care, and drug therapy.

■ A nuclear bomb presents an immediate threat from the blast itself (including acute radiation sickness) and a delayed threat from radioactive fallout.

■ Iodine-131 in fallout poses a risk of thyroid cancer.

■ The risk of thyroid cancer can be reduced by ingesting potassium iodide, which blocks uptake of iodine-131 by the thyroid. To be effective, potassium iodide must be taken soon after exposure to iodine-131, and dosing must be repeated every 24 hours until the threat of fallout has passed.

■ A terrorist attack on a nuclear power plant could cause the release of large amounts of radiation, including iodine-131, but would not cause a nuclear explosion.

■ A dirty bomb is a device that uses a conventional explosive, such as dynamite, to disperse radioactive material.

■ The primary danger from a dirty bomb is the blast itself, not the radiation.

■ A dirty bomb will not release iodine-131, and hence taking potassium iodide is not indicated.

Guide to Gender-Related Drugs

The purpose of this guide is to help you locate gender-specific drug content, which is scattered throughout the book. Chapter numbers are in **bold** type and page numbers are in parentheses.

Pronunciation of Generic Names of the Top 200 Prescribed Drugs in 2002

The drugs selected for this appendix—representing the top 200 prescribed drugs in 2002—are those identified by *RxList: The Internet Drug Index*, located at *www.rxlist.com/top200. htm*. Because some drugs are prescribed by trade name as well as by generic name, the list of top 200 hundred drugs contains a number of duplicates. We have eliminated those duplicates, and hence our list has fewer than 200 entries.

acetaminophen (ə-se″tə-min′o-fen)
acyclovir (a-si′klo-vēr)
albuterol (al-bu′tər-ol)
alendronate (ə-len′dro-nāt)
allopurinol (al″o-pūr′ĭ-nol)
alprazolam (al-pra′zo-lam)
amitriptyline (am″ĭ-trip′tə-lēn)
amlodipine (am-lo′dĭ-pēn″)
amoxicillin (ə-mok″sĭ-sil′in)
amoxicillin/clavulanate (ə-mok″sĭ-sil′in/klav′u-lə-nāt)
amphetamine mixed salts (am-fet′ə-mēn″)
aspirin (as′pĭ-rin)
atenolol (ə-ten′ə-lol)
atorvastatin (ə-tor″və-stat′in)
azithromycin (az-ith″ro-mi′sin)
benazepril (ben-a′zə-pril)
bisoprolol/hydrochlorothiazide (bis″o-pro′lol/ hi″dro-klor″o-thi′ə-zīd)
budesonide (bu-des′ə-nīd)
bupropion (bu-pro′pe-on)
buspirone (bu-spi′rōn)
captopril (kap′to-pril)
carbidopa/levodopa (kahr″bĭ-do′pə/le″vo-do′pə)
carisoprodol (kar″i-so-pro′dol)
carvedilol (kahr′və-dil″ol)
cefprozil (sef-pro′zil)
celecoxib (sel″ə-kok′sib)
cephalexin (sef″ə-lek′sin)
cetirizine (sə-tir′ĭ-zēn)
ciprofloxacin (sip″ro-flok′sə-sin)
citalopram (si-tal′o-pram)
clarithromycin (klə-rith″ro-mi′sin)
clindamycin (klin″də-mi′sin)
clonazepam (klo-naz′ə-pam)
clonidine (klo′nĭ-dēn)
clopidogrel (klo-pid′ə-grel)
conjugated estrogens (es′trə-jen)
conjugated estrogens/medroxyprogesterone (es′trə-jen/ med-rok″se-pro-jes′tər-ōn)
cyclobenzaprine (si″klo-ben′zə-prēn)

desloratadine (des″lə-rat′ə-dēn)
desogestrel/ethinyl estradiol (des″o-jes′trəl/eth′ĭ-nəl es″trə-di′ol, es-tra′de-ol)
diazepam (di-az′ə-pam)
diclofenac (di-klo′fen-ak)
digoxin (dĭ-jok′sin)
diltiazem (dil-ti′ə-zəm)
divalproex (di-val′pro-eks)
doxazosin (dok″sa′zo-sin)
doxycycline (dok″se-si′klēn)
enalapril (ə-nal′ə-pril)
esomeprazole (es″o-mep′ra-zōl)
estradiol (es″trə-di′ol, es-tra′de-ol)
ethinyl estradiol/norethindrone (eth′ĭ-nəl es″trə-di′ol, es-tra′de-ol/nor-eth′in-drōn)
famotidine (fam-o′tĭ-dīn)
fenofibrate (fen″o-fi′brāt)
fexofenadine (fek″so-fen′ə-dēn)
fluconazole (floo-kon′ə-zōl)
fluoxetine (floo-ok′sə-tēn)
fluticasone (floo-tik′ə-sōn″)
folic acid (fo′lik as′id)
fosinopril (fo-sin′o-pril)
furosemide (fu-ro′sə-mīd)
gabapentin (gab″ə-pen′tin)
gemfibrozil (jem-fib′ro-zil)
glimepiride (gli-mep′ĭ-rīd)
glipizide (glip′ĭ-zīd)
glyburide (gli′būr-īd)
hydrochlorothiazide (hi″dro-klor″o-thi′ə-zīd)
hydrocodone (hi″dro-ko′dōn)
hydroxyzine (hi-drok′sə-zēn)
ibuprofen (i″bu-pro′fən)
insulin NPH (in′sə-lin)
insulin lispro (in′sə-lin)
ipratropium (ip″rə-tro′pe-əm)
irbesartan (ir″bə-sahr′tan)
isosorbide mononitrate (i″so-sor′bīd)
lansoprazole (lan-so′prə-zōl)
latanoprost (lə-tan′o-prost″)
levofloxacin (le″vo-flok′sə-sin)
levonorgestrel/ethinyl estradiol (le″vo-nor-jes′trel/ eth′ĭ-nəl es″trə-di′ol, es-tra′de-ol)
levothyroxine (le″vo-thi-rok′sēn)
lisinopril (li-sin′o-pril)
loratadine (lə-rat′ə-dēn)
lorazepam (lor-az′ə-pam)
losartan (lo-sahr′tan)

meclizine (mek'lĭ-zēn)
medroxyprogesterone (med-rok"se-pro-jes'tər-ōn)
metaxalone (mə-taks'ə-lōn)
metformin (mət-for'min)
methylphenidate (meth"əl-fen'ĭ-dāt)
methylprednisolone (meth"əl-pred-nis'ə-lōn)
metoclopramide (met"o-klo'prə-mīd)
metoprolol (met"o-pro'lol)
metronidazole (met"ro-ni'də-zōl)
minocycline (mĭ-no-si'klēn)
mirtazapine (mir"taz-ə-pēn)
mometasone (mo-met'ə-sōn")
montelukast (mon"tə-loo'kast)
mupirocin (mu-pir'o-sin)
naproxen (nə-prok'sən)
nifedipine (ni-fed'ĭ-pēn)
nitrofurantoin (ni"tro-fu-ran'to-in)
norethindrone/ethinyl estradiol (nor-eth'in-drōn/eth'ĭ-nəl
    es"trə-di'ol, es-tra'de-ol)
norgestimate/ethinyl estradiol (nor-jes'tĭ-māt/eth'ĭ-nəl
    es"trə-di'ol, es-tra'de-ol)
nortriptyline (nor-trip'tə-lēn)
nystatin (ni-stat'in)
olanzapine (o-lan'zəpēn)
omeprazole (o-mep'ra-zōl)
oxybutynin (ok"se-bu'tĭ-nin)
oxycodone (ok"se-ko'dōn)
pantoprazole (pan-to'prə-zōl)
paroxetine (pə-rok'sə-tēn)
penicillin VK (pen"ĭ-sil'in)
phenytoin (fen'ĭ-to-in")
pioglitazone (pi"o-glit'ə-zōn)
potassium chloride (po-tas'e-əm)
pravastatin (prav'ə-stat"in)
prednisone (pred'nĭ-sōn)
promethazine (pro-meth'ə-zēn)
propoxyphene (pro-pok'sĭ-fēn)
propranolol (pro-pran'ə-lol)
quetiapine (quê-ti'ə-pēn)
quinapril (kwin'ə-pril")
rabeprazole (rə-bep'ra-zōl)

raloxifene (ral-ok'sĭ-fēn)
ramipril (rə-mi'pril)
ranitidine (rə-nĭ'tĭ-dēn)
risedronate (ris-ed'rə-nāt")
risperidone (ris-per'ĭ-dōn)
rofecoxib (ro"fə-cok'sib)
rosiglitazone (ro-sig-lit'ə-zōn)
salmeterol (sal-met'ər-ol)
sertraline (sər'trə-lēn)
sildenafil (sil-den'ə-fil")
simvastatin (sim'və-stat"in)
spironolactone (spi"rə-no-lak'tōn)
sumatriptan (soo"mə-trip'tan)
tamoxifen (tə-mok'sĭ-fən)
tamsulosin (tam-soo'lo-sin)
temazepam (tə-maz'ə-pam)
terazosin (tər-a'zo-sin)
tetracycline (tet"rə-si'klēn)
timolol maleate (ti'mo-lol)
tolterodine (tol-ter'ə-dēn)
topiramate (to-pi'rə-māt)
tramadol (tram'ə-dol")
trazodone (tra'zo-dōn)
triamcinolone (tri"am-sin'ə-lōn)
triamterene/hydrochorothiazide (tri-am'tər-ēn/
    hi"dro-klor"o-thi'ə-zīd)
trimethoprim/sulfamethoxazole (tri-meth'o-prim/
    sul"fə-məth-ok'sə-zōl)
valacyclovir (val"a-si'klo-vir)
valdecoxib (val"də-kok'sib)
valsartan (val-sahr'tan)
venlafaxine (ven"ləfak'sēn)
verapamil (və-rap'ə-mil)
warfarin (wor'fər-in)
zolpidem (zōl-pi'dem)

Pronunciation guide: primary stress ('), secondary stress ("), ə (sofa),
ā (mate), ē (beam), ī (bite), ĭ (bit), ō (home).
Drug list adapted from *www.rxlist.com/top200.htm* (accessed June 19, 2003).
Drug pronunciations from *www.dorlands.com* (accessed June 19, 2003).

Weights and Measures

VOLUME EQUIVALENTS

1 milliliter	= 0.034	fluid ounce
	= 0.271	fluid dram
	= 16.2	minims
1 liter	= 1000	milliliters
	= 33.8	fluid ounces
	= 2.11	pints
	= 1.06	quarts
	= 0.26	gallon
1 cubic centimeter	= 1	milliliter
1 minim	= 0.062	milliliter
1 fluid dram	= 3.70	milliliters
	= 60	minims
1 fluid ounce	= 29.6	milliliters
	= 2	tablespoons
	= 8	fluid drams
1 teaspoon	= 5	milliliters
1 tablespoon	= 15	milliliters
	= 3	teaspoons
1 cup	= 237	milliliters
	= 8	fluid ounces
	= 16	tablespoons
1 pint	= 473	milliliters
	= 16	fluid ounces
	= 2	cups
1 quart	= 946	milliliters
	= 32	fluid ounces
	= 2	pints
1 gallon	= 3785	milliliters
	= 128	fluid ounces
	= 4	quarts

MASS EQUIVALENTS

1 milligram	= 0.0154	grain (apothecaries')
	= 1000	micrograms
1 gram	= 15.4	grains (apothecaries')
	= 0.0322	ounce (apothecaries')
	= 0.0353	ounce (avoirdupois)
	= 0.257	dram (apothecaries')
1 grain (apothecaries')	= 64.8	milligrams
	= 0.0021	ounce (apothecaries')
	= 0.0023	ounce (avoirdupois)
	= 0.0167	dram (apothecaries')
1 dram (apothecaries')	= 3.89	grams
1 ounce (apothecaries')	= 31.1	grams
1 ounce (avoirdupois)	= 28.4	grams
1 pound (avoirdupois)	= 454	grams
	= 0.454	kilogram
	= 16	ounces (avoirdupois)
1 kilogram	= 2.20	pounds (avoirdupois)

TEMPERATURE CONVERSION

$(\text{Celsius degrees} \times 9/5) + 32 = \text{Fahrenheit degrees}$
$(\text{Fahrenheit degrees} - 32) \times 5/9 = \text{Celsius degrees}$

Laboratory Reference Values

PART I. HEMATOLOGY

		Conventional Units	SI Units*
Acid hemolysis test (Ham)		No hemolysis	No hemolysis
Alkaline phosphatase, leukocyte		Total score 14–100	Total score 14–100
Cell counts			
Erythrocytes			
Males		4.6–6.2 million/mm³	$4.6–6.2 \times 10^{12}$/L
Females		4.2–5.4 million/mm³	$4.2–5.4 \times 10^{12}$/L
Children (varies with age)		4.5–5.1 million/mm³	$4.5–5.1 \times 10^{12}$/L
Leukocytes			
Total		4500–11,000 mm³	$4.5–11.0 \times 10^{9}$/L
Differential	*Percentage*	*Absolute*	*Absolute*
Myelocytes	0	0/mm³	0/L
Band neutrophils	3–5	150–400/mm³	$150–400 \times 10^{6}$/L
Segmented neutrophils	54–62	3000–5800/mm³	$3000–5800 \times 10^{6}$/L
Lymphocytes	25–33	1500–3000/mm³	$1500–3000 \times 10^{6}$/L
Monocytes	3–7	300–500/mm³	$300–500 \times 10^{6}$/L
Eosinophils	1–3	50–250/mm³	$50–250 \times 10^{6}$/L
Basophils	0–1	15–50/mm³	$15–50 \times 10^{6}$/L
Platelets		150,000–400,000/mm³	$150–400 \times 10^{9}$/L
Reticulocytes		25,000–75,000/mm³ (0.5–1.5% of erythrocytes)	$25–75—10^{9}$/L
Coagulation tests			
Bleeding time (template)		2.75–8.0 min	2.75–8.0 min
Coagulation time (glass tubes)		5–15 min	5–15 min
D-Dimer		<0.5 µg/ml	<0.5 mg/L
Factor VIII and other coagulation factors		50–150% of normal	0.5–1.5 of normal
Fibrin split products (Thrombo-Welco test)		<10 µg/ml	<10 mg/L
Fibrinogen		200–400 mg/dl	2.0–4.0 g/L
Partial thromboplastin time (PTT)		20–35 sec	20–35 sec
Prothrombin time (PT)		12.0–14.0 sec	12.0–14.0 sec
Coomb's test			
Direct		Negative	Negative
Indirect		Negative	Negative
Corpuscular values of erythrocytes			
Mean corpuscular hemoglobin (MCH)		26–34 pg/cell	26–34 pg/cell
Mean corpuscular volume (MCV)		80–96 µm³	80–96 fL
Mean corpuscular hemoglobin concentration (MCHC)		32–36 gm/dl	320–360 g/L
Erythrocyte sedimentation rate (ESR)			
Wintrobe			
Males		0–5 mm/hr	0–5 mm/hr
Females		0–15 mm/hr	0–15 mm/hr
Westergren			
Males		0–15 mm/hr	0–15 mm/hr
Females		0–20 mm/hr	0–20 mm/hr
		20–165 mg/dl	0.20–1.65 g/L
Haptoglobin		26–185 mg/dl	260–1850 mg/L
Hematocrit			
Males		40–54 ml/dl	0.40–0.54 volume fraction
Females		37–47 ml/dl	0.37–0.47 volume fraction

Table continued on following page

PART I. HEMATOLOGY *Continued*

	Conventional Units	SI Units*
Hematocrit (*continued*)		
Newborns	49–54 ml/dl	0.49–0.54 volume fraction
Children (varies with age)	35–49 ml/dl	0.35–0.49 volume fraction
Hemoglobin		
Males	14.0–18.0 gm/dl	2.17–2.79 mmol/L
Females	12.0–16.0 gm/dl	1.86–2.48 mmol/L
Newborns	16.5–19.5 gm/dl	2.56–3.02 mmol/L
Children (varies with age)	11.2–16.5 gm/dl	1.74–2.56 mmol/L
Hemoglobin, fetal	<1.0% of total	<0.01 of total
Hemoglobin A_{1c}	3–5% of total	0.03–0.05 of total
Hemoglobin A_2	1.5–3.0% of total	0.015–0.03 of total
Hemoglobin, plasma	0–5.0 mg/dl	0–0.8 μmol/L
Methemoglobin	30–130 mg/dl	4.7–20 μmol/L

PART II. BLOOD CHEMISTRY

For some procedures the reference values may vary depending on the method used.

	Conventional Units	SI Units*
Alanine aminotransferase (ALT, SGPT), serum	1–45 U/L	1–45 U/L
Aspartate aminotransferase (AST, SGOT), serum	1–36 U/L	1–36 U/L
Base excess, arterial blood, calculated	0 ± 2 mEq/L	0 ± 2 mmol/L
Beta-carotene, serum	60–260 μg/dl	1.1–8.6 μmol/L
Bicarbonate		
Venous plasma	23–29 mEq/L	23–39 mmol/L
Arterial blood	18–23 mEq/L	18–23 mmol/L
Bile acids, serum	0.3–3.0 mg/dl	3–30 mg/L
Bilirubin, serum		
Conjugated	0.1–0.4 mg/dl	1.7–6.8 μmol/L
Total	0.3–1.1 mg/dl	5.1–19 μmol/L
Calcium, serum	9.0–11.0 mg/dl	2.25–2.75 mmol/L
Calcium, ionized, serum	4.25–5.25 mg/dl	1.05–1.30 mmol/L
Carbon dioxide, total, serum or plasma	24–30 mEq/L	24–30 mmol/L
Carbon dioxide tension (P_{CO_2}), blood	35–45 mm Hg	35–45 mm Hg
Ceruloplasmin, serum	23–44 mg/dl	230–440 mg/L
Chloride, serum or plasma	96–106 mEq/L	96–106 mmol/L
Cholesterol, serum or EDTA plasma		
Desirable range	<200 mg/dl	<5.18 mmol/L
LDL cholesterol	60–180 mg/dl	600–1800 mg/L
HDL cholesterol	30–80 mg/dl	300–800 mg/L
Copper	70–140 μg/dl	11–22 μmol/L
Corticotropin (ACTH), plasma, 8:00 AM	10–80 pg/ml	2–18 pmol/L
Cortisol, plasma		
8:00 AM	6–23 μg/dl	170–635 nmol/L
4:00 PM	3–15 μg/dl	82–413 nmol/L
10:00 PM	<50% of 8:00 AM value	<0.5 of 8:00 AM value
Creatine, serum		
Males	0.2–0.5 mg/dl	15–40 μmol/L
Females	0.3–0.9 mg/dl	25–70 μmol/L
Creatine kinase (CK), serum		
Males	55–170 U/L	55–170 U/L
Females	30–135 U/L	30–135 U/L
Creatine kinase MB isoenzyme, serum	0.0–4.7 ng/ml	0.0–4.7 μg/L
Creatinine, serum	0.6–1.2 mg/dl	50–110 μmol/L

Table continued on opposite page

PART II. BLOOD CHEMISTRY *Continued*

	Conventional Units	SI Units*
Estradiol-17-beta, adult		
Males	10–65 pg/ml	35–240 pmol/L
Females		
Follicular phase	30–100 pg/ml	110–370 pmol/L
Ovulatory phase	200–400 pg/ml	730–1470 pmol/L
Luteal phase	50–140 pg/ml	180–510 pmol/L
Ferritin, serum	20–200 ng/ml	20–200 µg/L
Fibrinogen, plasma	200–400 mg/dl	2.0–4.0 g/L
Folate, serum	1.8–9.0 ng/ml	4.1–20.4 nmol/L
Erythrocytes	150–450 ng/ml	340–1020 nmol/L
Follicle-stimulating hormone (FSH), plasma		
Males	4–25 mU/ml	4–25 U/L
Females	4–30 mU/ml	4–30 U/L
Postmenopausal	40–250 mU/ml	40–250 U/L
Gamma-glutamyltransferase (GGT), serum	5–40 U/L	5–40 U/L
Gastrin, fasting, serum	0–110 pg/ml	0–110 ng/L
Glucose, fasting, plasma or serum	70–115 mg/dl	3.9–6.4 mmol/L
Growth hormone (hGH), plasma, adult, fasting	0–6 ng/ml	0–6 µg/L
Haptoglobin, serum	20–165 mg/dl	0.20–1.65 g/L
Insulin, fasting, plasma	5–25 µU/ml	36–179 pmol/L
Iron, serum	75–175 µg/dl	13–31 µmol/L
Iron binding capacity, serum		
Total	250–410 µg/dl	45–73 µmol/L
Saturation	20%–55%	0.20–0.55
Lactate		
Venous whole blood	5.0–20.0 mg/dl	0.60–2.2 mmol/L
Arterial whole blood	5.0–15.0 mg/dl	0.6–1.7 mmol/L
Lactate dehydrogenase (LD), serum	110–220 U/L	110–220 U/L
Lipase, serum	10–140 U/L	10–140 U/L
Lutropin (LH), serum		
Males	1–9 U/L	1–9 U/L
Females		
Follicular phase	2–10 U/L	2–10 U/L
Midcycle peak	15–65 U/L	15–65 U/L
Luteal phase	1–12 U/L	1–12 U/L
Postmenopausal	12–65 U/L	12–65 U/L
Magnesium, serum	1.8–3.0 mg/dl	0.75–1.25 mmol/L
Osmolality	286–295 mOsm/kg water	285–295 mmol/kg water
Oxygen, blood, arterial, room air		
Partial pressure (Pao$_2$)	80–100 mm Hg	80–100 mm Hg
Saturation (Sao$_2$)	95%–98%	95%–98%
pH, arterial blood	7.35–7.45	7.35–7.45
Phosphate, inorganic, serum		
Adult	3.0–4.5 mg/dl	1.0–1.5 mmol/L
Child	4.0–7.0 mg/dl	1.3–2.3 mmol/L
Potassium		
Serum	3.5–5.0 mEq/L	3.5–5.0 mmol/L
Plasma	3.5–4.5 mEq/L	3.5–4.5 mmol/L
Progesterone, serum, adult		
Males	0.0–0.4 ng/ml	0.0–1.3 mmol/L
Females		
Follicular phase	0.1–1.5 ng/ml	0.3–4.8 mmol/L
Luteal phase	2.5–28.0 ng/ml	8.0–89.0 mmol/L
Prolactin, serum		
Males	1.0–15.0 ng/ml	1.0–15.0 µg/L
Females	1.0–20.0 ng/ml	1.0–20.0 µg/L
Protein, serum, electrophoresis		
Total	6.0–8.0 gm/dl	60–80 g/L
Albumin	3.5–5.5 gm/dl	35–55 g/L
Alpha$_1$ globulin	0.2–0.4 gm/dl	2–4 g/L
Alpha$_2$ globulin	0.5–0.9 gm/dl	5–9 g/L
Beta globulin	0.6–1.1 gm/dl	6–11 g/L
Gamma globulin	0.7–1.7 gm/dl	7–15 g/L

Table continued on following page

PART II. BLOOD CHEMISTRY *Continued*

	Conventional Units	SI Units*
Pyruvate, blood	0.3–0.9 gm/dl	0.03–0.10 mmol/L
Rheumatoid factor	0.0–30.0 IU/ml	0.0–30.0 KIU/ml
Sodium, serum or plasma	135–145 mEq/L	135–145 mmol/L
Testosterone, plasma		
Males, adult	300–1200 ng/dl	10.4–41.6 nmol/L
Females, adult	20–75 ng/dl	0.7–2.6 nmol/L
Pregnant females	40–200 ng/dl	1.4–6.9 nmol/L
Thyroglobulin	3–42 ng/ml	3–42 μg/L
Thyrotropin (hTSH), serum	0.4–4.8 μIU/ml	0.4–4.8 mIU/L
Thyrotropin-releasing hormone (TRH)	5–60 pg/ml	5–60 ng/L
Thyroxine, free (FT$_4$), serum	0.9–2.1 ng/dl	12–27 pmol/L
Thyroxine (T$_4$), serum	4.5–12.0 μg/dl	58–154 nmol/L
Thyroxine-binding globulin (TBG)	15.0–34.0 μg/ml	15.0–34.0 mg/L
Transferrin	250–430 mg/dl	2.5–4.3 g/L
Triglycerides, serum, after 12-hr fast	40–150 mg/dl	0.4–1.5 g/L
Triiodothyronine (T$_3$), serum	70–190 ng/dl	1.1–2.9 nmol/L
Triiodothyronine uptake, resin (T$_3$RU)	25%–38% uptake	0.25–0.38 uptake
Urate		
Males	2.5–8.0 mg/dl	150–480 μmol/L
Females	2.2–7.0 mg/dl	130–420 μmol/L
Urea, serum or plasma	24–49 mg/dl	4.0–8.2 nmol/L
Urea nitrogen, serum or plasma	11–23 mg/dl	8.0–16.4 nmol/L
Viscosity, serum	1.4–1.8 times water	1.4–1.8 times water
Vitamin A, serum	20–80 μg/dl	0.70–2.80 μmol/L
Vitamin B$_{12}$, serum	180–900 pg/ml	133–664 pmol/L

PART III. URINE CHEMISTRY

For some procedures the reference values may vary depending on the method used.

	Conventional Units	SI Units*
Acetone and acetoacetate, qualitative	Negative	Negative
Albumin		
Qualitative	Negative	Negative
Quantitative	10–100 mg/24 hr	0.15–1.5 μmol/day
Aldosterone	3–20 μg/24 hr	8.3–55 nmol/day
Delta-aminolevulinic acid (delta-ALA)	1.3–7.0 mg/24 hr	10–53 μmol/day
Amylase	<17 U/hr	<17 U/hr
Amylase/creatinine clearance ratio	0.01–0.04	0.01–0.04
Bilirubin, qualitative	Negative	Negative
Calcium (regular diet)	<250 mg/24 hr	<6.3 mmol/day
Catecholamines		
Epinephrine	<10 μg/24 hr	<55 nmol/day
Norepinephrine	<100 μg/24 hr	<590 nmol/day
Total free catecholamines	4–126 μg/24 hr	24–745 nmol/day
Total metanephrines	0.1–1.6 mg/24 hr	0.5–8.1 μmol/day
Chloride (varies with intake)	110–250 mEq/24 hr	110–250 mmol/day
Copper	0–50 μg/24 hr	0–0.80 μmol/day
Cortisol, free	10–100 μg/24 hr	27.6–276 nmol/day
Creatine		
Males	0–40 mg/24 hr	0.0–0.30 mmol/day
Females	0–80 mg/24 hr	0.0–0.60 mmol/day
Creatinine	15–25 mg/kg/24 hr	0.13–0.22 mmol/kg/day

PART III. URINE CHEMISTRY *Continued*

	Conventional Units	SI Units*
Creatinine clearance (endogenous)		
Males	110–150 ml/min/1.73 m²	110–150 ml/min/1.73 m²
Females	105–132 ml/min/1.73 m²	105–132 ml/min/1.73 m²
Cystine or cysteine	Negative	Negative
Dehydroepiandrosterone		
Males	0.2–2.0 mg/24 hr	0.7–6.9 μmol/day
Females	0.2–1.8 mg/24 hr	0.7–6.2 μmol/day
Estrogens, total		
Males	4–25 μg/24 hr	14–90 nmol/day
Females	5–100 μg/24 hr	18–360 nmol/day
Glucose (as reducing substance)	<250 mg/24 hr	<250 mg/day
Hemoblobin and myoglobin, qualitative	Negative	Negative
Homogentisic acid, qualitative	Negative	Negative
17-Hydroxycorticosteroids		
Males	3–9 mg/24 hr	8.3–25 μmol/day
Females	2–8 mg/24 hr	5.5–22 μmol/day
5-Hydroxyindoleacetic acid		
Qualitative	Negative	Negative
Quantitative	2–6 mg/24 hr	10–31 μmol/day
17-Ketogenic steroids		
Males	5–23 mg/24 hr	17–80 μmol/day
Females	3–15 mg/24 hr	10–52 μmol/day
17-Ketosteroids		
Males	8–22 mg/24 hr	28–76 μmol/day
Females	6–15 mg/24 hr	21–52 μmol/day
Magnesium	6–10 mEq/24 hr	3–5 mmol/day
Metanephrines	0.05–1.2 ng/mg creatinine	0.03–0.70 mmol/mmol creatinine
Osmolality	38–1400 mOsm/kg water	38–1400 mOsm/kg water
pH	4.6–8.0	4.6–8.0
Phenylpyruvic acid, qualitative	Negative	Negative
Phosphate	0.4–1.3 grams/24 hr	13–42 mmol/day
Porphobilinogen		
Qualitative	Negative	Negative
Quantitative	<2.0 mg/24 hr	<9 μmol/day
Porphyrins		
Coproporphyrin	50–250 μg/24 hr	77–380 nmol/day
Uroporphyrin	10–30 μg/24 hr	12–36 nmol/day
Potassium	25–125 mEq/24 hr	25–125 mmol/day
Pregnanediol		
Males	0.0–1.9 mg/24 hr	0.0–6.0 μmol/day
Females		
Proliferative phase	0.0–2.6 mg/24 hr	0.0–8.0 μmol/day
Luteal phase	2.6–10.6 mg/24 hr	8–33 μmol/day
Postmenopausal	0.2–1.0 mg/24 hr	0.6–3.1 μmol/day
Pregnanetriol	0.0–2.5 mg/24 hr	0.0–7.4 μmol/day
Protein, total		
Qualitative	Negative	Negative
Quantitative	10–150 mg/24 hr	10–150 mg/day
Protein/creatinine ratio	<0.2	<0.2
Sodium (regular diet)	60–260 mEq/24 hr	60–260 mmol/day
Specific gravity	1.003–1.030	1.003–1.030
Random specimen	1.003–1.030	1.003–1.030
24-hour collection	1.015–1.025	1.015–1.025
Urate (regular diet)	250–750 mg/24 hr	1.5–4.4 mmol/day
Urobilinogen	0.5–4.0 mg/24 hr	0.6–6.8 μmol/day
Vanillylmandelic acid (VMA)	1–8 mg/24 hr	5–40 μmol/24 hr

*Système International d' Unités (International System of Units).
Adapted from O'Toole MT (ed). Miller-Keane Encyclopedia and Dictionary of Medicine, Nursing, and Allied Health, 6th ed. Philadelphia, WB Saunders, 1997:1843–1845, 1847–1848.

Commonly Used Abbreviations

ac	before meals (*ante cibum*)	DMARD	disease-modifying antirheumatic drug
ACE	angiotensin converting enzyme	DNA	deoxyribonucleic acid
ACh	acetylcholine	DPI	dry-powder inhaler
ad lib	freely as desired (*ad libitum*)	DS	double strength
ADHD	attention-deficit/hyperactivity disorder	ECG (EKG)	electrocardiogram
ADL	activities of daily living	ECT	electroconvulsive therapy
ADP	adenosine diphosphate	EEG	electroencephalogram
AED	antiepileptic drug	EKG (ECG)	electrocardiogram
AIDS	acquired immunodeficiency syndrome	F	Fahrenheit
ALT	alanine aminotransferase (formerly known as SGPT)	FDA	Food and Drug Administration
		FEV	forced expiratory volume
AMI	acute myocardial infarction	FFA	free fatty acid
AMP	adenosine monophosphate	g (gm)	gram
ANA	antinuclear antibodies	G-6-PD	glucose-6-phosphate dehydrogenase
ARB	angiotensin II receptor blocker	GABA	gamma-aminobutyric acid
ARC	AIDS-related complex	GERD	gastroesophageal reflux disease
ASA	acetylsalicylic acid (aspirin)	GFR	glomerular filtration rate
AST	aspartate aminotransferase (formerly known as SGOT)	GI	gastrointestinal
		gm (g)	gram
ATP	adenosine triphosphate	GMP	guanosine monophosphate
AV	atrioventricular	gr	grain
bid	two times a day (*bis in die*)	GTP	guanosine triphosphate
bin	two times a night (*bis in nocte*)	GU	genitourinary
bol	bolus	h, hr	hour
BP	blood pressure	H_2RA	histamine$_2$-receptor antagonist
BPH	benign prostatic hyperplasia	HAART	highly active antiretroviral therapy
BUN	blood urea nitrogen	HBGM	home blood glucose monitoring
C	Celsius (centigrade)	HDL	high-density lipoprotein
CABG	coronary artery bypass graft	HIV	human immunodeficiency virus
CAD	coronary artery disease	HRT	hormone replacement therapy
cAMP	cyclic adenosine 3′,5′- monophosphate	hs	at bedtime (hour of sleep; *hora somni*)
CAT	computerized axial tomography	HSV	herpes simplex virus
CBC	complete blood count	IBD	inflammatory bowel disease
cc	cubic centimeter (milliliter)	ICP	intracranial pressure
CCB	calcium channel blocker	IDDM	insulin-dependent diabetes mellitus
CDC	Centers for Disease Control and Prevention	IM	intramuscular, intramuscularly
CHF	congestive heart failure	INR	international normalized ratio
CMV	cytomegalovirus	IOP	intraocular pressure
CNS	central nervous system	IPV	inactivated polio vaccine
COMT	catechol-*O*-methyltransferase	ISA	intrinsic sympathomimetic activity
COPD	chronic obstructive pulmonary disease	IU	international unit
COX	cyclooxygenase	IUD	intrauterine device
CPK	creatine phosphokinase	IV	intravenous, intravenously
CSF	cerebrospinal fluid	kg	kilogram
CTZ	chemoreceptor trigger zone	KVO	keep vein open
CVA	cerebrovascular accident	L	liter
DBP	diastolic blood pressure	LD	lethal dose
DC	direct current	LDL	low-density lipoprotein
DKA	diabetic ketoacidosis	LGV	lymphogranuloma venereum
dl	deciliter (100 ml)	LSD	D-lysergic acid diethylamide

m	minim	PO	by mouth (*per os*)
MAC	minimum alveolar concentration; *Mycobacterium avium* complex	PPD	purified protein derivative (tuberculin)
		PPI	proton pump inhibitor
MAO	monoamine oxidase	PR	by the rectum (*per rectum*)
MAOI	monoamine oxidase inhibitor	PRN	as needed (*pro re nata*)
MAP	mean arterial pressure	PT	prothrombin time
MBC	minimum bactericidal concentration	PTCA	percutaneous transluminal coronary angioplasty
mcg (μg)	microgram		
MDI	metered-dose inhaler	PTT	partial thromboplastin time
MEC	minimum effective concentration	PVC	premature ventricular complex
mEq	milliequivalent	qd	every day (*quaque die*)
MHc	major histocompatibility complex	qh	every hour (*quaque hora*)
mg	milligram	qid	four times a day (*quater in die*)
MI	myocardial infarction	qod	every other day
MIC	minimum inhibitory concentration	RA	rheumatoid arthritis
ml	milliliter	RBC	red blood cell (erythrocyte)
mM	millimole	RDA	recommended dietary allowance
MMR	measles, mumps, rubella	REM	rapid eye movement
mOsm	milliosmole	RNA	ribonucleic acid
MRI	magnetic resonance imaging	SA	sinoatrial
ng	nanogram	SAARD	slow-acting antirheumatic drug
NGU	nongonococcal urethritis	SBP	systolic blood pressure
NIDDM	non–insulin-dependent diabetes mellitus	SC (SQ)	subcutaneous, subcutaneously
NNRTI	non-nucleoside reverse transcriptase inhibitor	SGOT	serum glutamic-oxaloacetic transaminase (now known as AST)
npo	nothing by mouth (*nil per os*)	SGPT	serum glutamic-pyruvic transaminase (now known as ALT)
NRTI	nucleoside reverse transcriptase inhibitor		
NSAID	nonsteroidal anti-inflammatory drug	sl	sublingual
OC	oral contraceptive	SLE	systemic lupus erythematosus
OD	right eye (*oculus dexter*)	SPF	sun protection factor
OPV	oral polio vaccine	SQ (SC)	subcutaneous, subcutaneously
OS	left eye (*oculus sinister*)	SR	sarcoplasmic reticulum; sustained release
OTC	over-the-counter	SSRI	selective serotonin reuptake inhibitor
OU	both eyes (*oculus uterque*)	stat	immediately
PABA	*para*-aminobenzoic acid	STD	sexually transmitted disease
pc	after meals (*post cibum*)	SVT	supraventricular tachycardia
PCP	*Pneumocystis carinii* pneumonia	TIA	transient ischemic attack
PEFR	peak expiratory flow rate	tid	three times a day (*ter in die*)
PET	positron emission tomography	UTI	urinary tract infection
pg	picogram	VLDL	very-low-density lipoprotein
PG	prostaglandin	VSM	vascular smooth muscle
PID	pelvic inflammatory disease	WBC	white blood cell (leukocyte)
PMS	premenstrual syndrome		

Techniques of Drug Administration

Linda A. Moore, M.S.N., Ed.D., R.N.

Type of Administration	Technique to Use

Oral

Liquids

General Considerations

1. Perform any required dilution using appropriate liquid. Avoid liquids that can reduce drug absorption (e.g., milk will decrease absorption of tetracyclines).
2. Measure using medicine cup or device supplied with medication.
3. Pour medication away from label/directions.
4. Read amount at bottom of meniscus (see diagram).

30 ——
20 ——
15 ——
10 ——
5 ——

Read volume here
at eye level

5. Do not leave patient before medication is taken.

Infants

Do not mix medication with formula or juice in bottle (you cannot be sure of amount taken if all of the liquid is not swallowed).

Nasogastric Tube Administration

1. Ensure correct location of the tube.
2. Follow directions for diluting (e.g., Metamucil becomes thick rapidly and should be mixed at time of administration, not before).
3. Follow with sufficient liquid to clear the tube (stay within fluid restrictions).

Tablets, Capsules

1. If possible have the patient in a sitting position to facilitate swallowing.
2. Check requirement for administration with food or liquids (e.g., medications that irritate often need to be given with food; some medications may have decreased absorption with food).
3. Provide proper liquid for swallowing (stay within fluid restrictions, or, if patient needs increased fluids, this is a good time to provide extra fluid).

Chewable Tablets

Be sure tablet is completely chewed before it is swallowed.

Sublingual and Buccal

Sublingual

1. Place tablet under tongue, and instruct patient to hold it there until dissolved.
2. Swallowing of residual should then occur.

Buccal

1. Instruct patient to hold medication between gums and cheek until it is dissolved.
2. Residual can then be swallowed.

Rectal (Suppository)

1. Patient is to lie in left lateral Sims' position.
2. Nurse to wear gloves during procedure.
3. Lubricate suppository and glove fingertip with water-soluble lubricant.
4. Insert suppository when rectal sphincter is relaxed (see diagram).

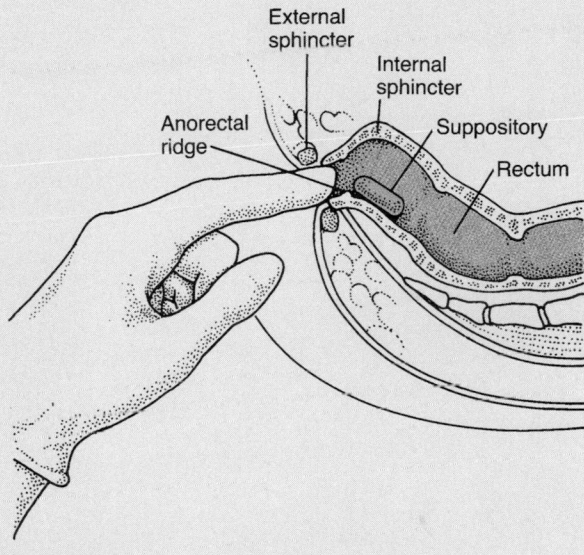

5. Instruct patient as to length of time to retain medication (about 20 to 30 minutes for defecation stimulation and about 60 minutes for systemic absorption).

Vaginal

1. Wear gloves during procedure.
2. Insert foam or suppository into vagina.
3. Instruct patient as to length of time to remain lying down.

Topical

1. Wear gloves when applying *any* topical ointment.
2. Apply with applicator, gauze, or gloved hand.
3. Apply a thin layer by patting, not rubbing.
4. Take care to protect the patient's clothing.
5. Certain medications require plastic wrap to increase absorption (e.g., nitroglycerin ointment).

Otic

1. Medication should be at body temperature.
2. Patient should lie on side with appropriate ear up.

3. Instill drops toward auditory canal wall, not on eardrum. Procedure varies for adults and children. *Adults:* The auricle is pulled back and posteriorly. *Children:* The auricle is pulled down and posteriorly (see diagram).

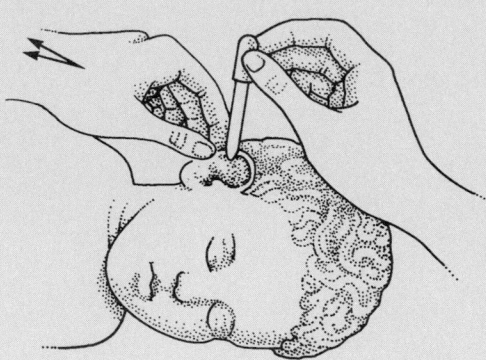

4. Rest hand administering drops lightly against the patient's head to prevent injury from dropper should the patient suddenly move.
5. After instillation, the patient should remain in this position for about 15 minutes.

Optic

1. Have patient lying on back with eyes facing up.
2. Do not touch tip of dropper to patient or to any object.

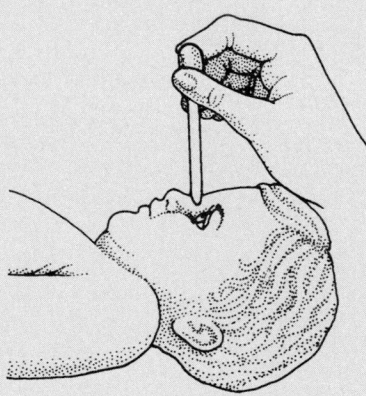

3. Have tissues available to blot any overflow from eyes (use separate tissue for each eye).
4. Rest hand instilling drops on patient's forehead to stabilize dropper and to prevent injury due to sudden patient movement.
5. Instill drops into conjunctival pouch while patient looks upward (see diagram).
6. To decrease systemic absorption, light pressure may be applied to lacrimal sac for about a minute.
7. *Ointment* is applied as a thin "ribbon" along inner aspect of lower lid. Do not touch tube to eye or other surface.

Intradermal

1. Select an appropriate site. (Usual sites for *skin testing* are shown in the diagram below.)

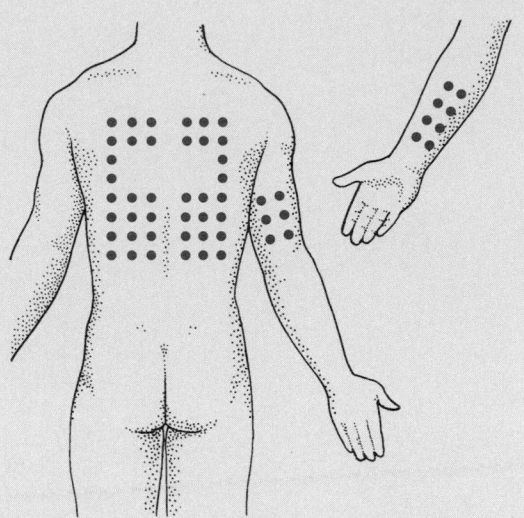

2. Use a short-bevel (26-gauge, ⅜-inch) needle.
3. Amount of medication is limited to 1 ml or less.
4. If skin testing is being done, have emergency medication (epinephrine) available.
5. With bevel of needle pointed up, inject medication into layers of the skin (see diagram).

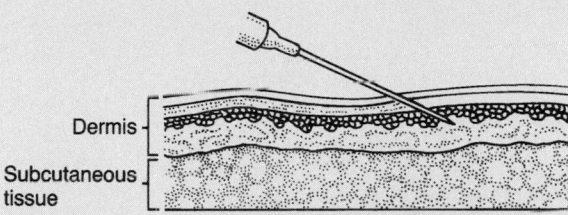

6. Use dry wipe to wipe area following injection.

Subcutaneous

1. Select a needle size (usually 25 to 27 gauge, ½ to ⅝ inch).
2. Select a site that has adequate subcutaneous tissue and that is away from bony prominences, major nerves, and blood vessels (see diagram below).

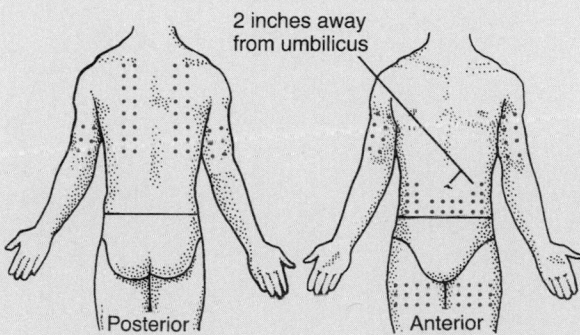

3. Angle of needle insertion depends on size of the individual. Obese people will require needle inserted at 90° angle, whereas very thin people will require pinching of the skin, with insertion at a 90° angle to the pocket pinched. Individuals who are neither fat nor very thin require a 45° angle for needle insertion (see diagram below).

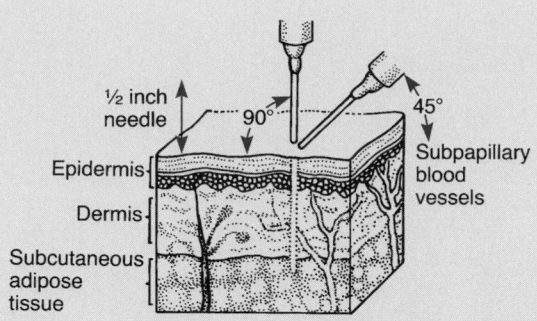

4. Aspiration for blood depends on substance being injected. Follow protocol.
5. Do not rub most SC injection sites.

Intramuscular

1. Select a needle length appropriate to size of patient. The needle should be long enough to reach to the middle of the muscle. Measure the circumference of the arm and select appropriate needle length. The average person requires a 1½- to 2-inch needle. Muscular males require 2- to 3-inch needles or as long as 3 to 5 inches in some cases.
2. Select technique of injection.
   a. *Standard*—insert needle at 90° angle to the muscle after area is cleaned.
   b. *Z-track method*—pull tissue to one side, insert needle, inject medication, and allow tissue to return to original position as needle is removed. (Used for medications that damage tissue and as method to decrease pain of injection.)
3. Select site of injection:
   a. *Dorsogluteal*—to locate, draw a diagonal line between the superior iliac spine and the greater trochanter of the femur (see diagram below). Patient should be prone with toes turned inward. *Do not use this site for children less than 2 years of age or for children who are emaciated.*
   b. *Ventrogluteal*—to locate, place palm of hand over the greater trochanter of the femur with thumb pointing to patient's abdomen, index finger placed over the anterior iliac spine, and middle finger spread back toward the iliac crest. The V-shaped area between the fingers is the ventrogluteal site. Direct needle toward largest muscle mass (see diagram below).

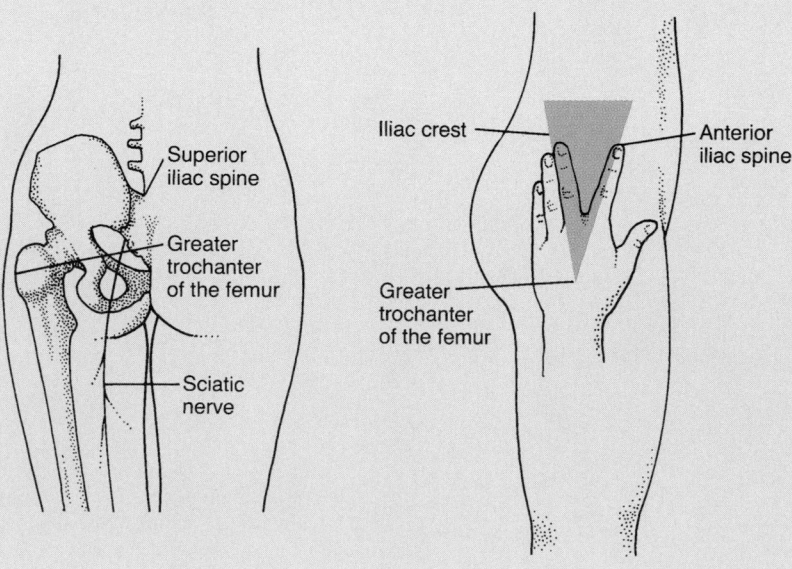

c. *Anterolateral thigh*—area is one third the distance from the greater trochanter to the knee and is between the midline of the anterior and lateral thighs (see diagram below). *This is a good site for infants and children.*

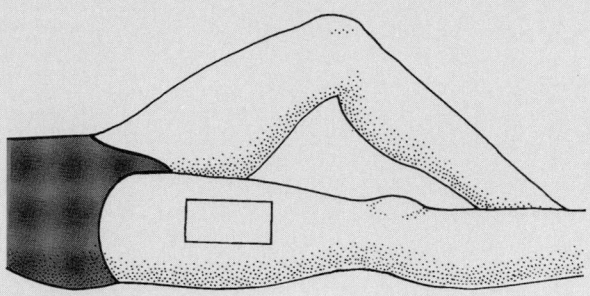

d. *Deltoid*—area is bordered above by 2 fingerbreadths below the acromion process and below by 2 fingerbreadths above the insertion of the deltoid (see diagram). Injection site must be in lateral aspect of the arm.

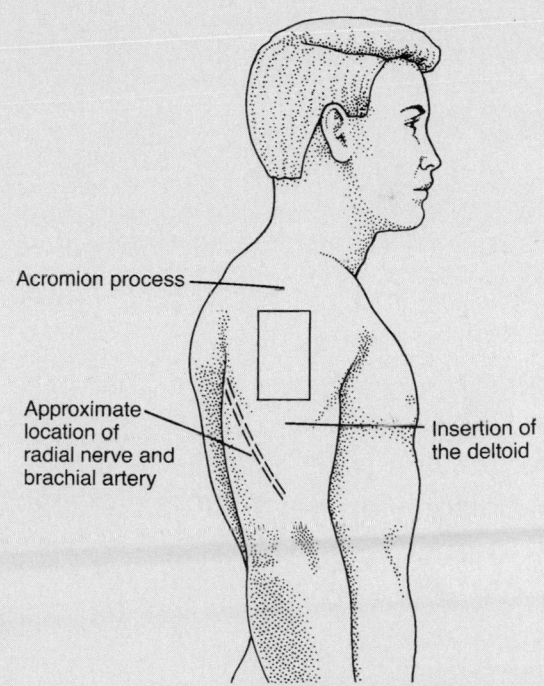

Acromion process

Approximate location of radial nerve and brachial artery

Insertion of the deltoid

4. Insert needle at 90° angle. Aspirate to be sure the needle is not in a blood vessel. Inject slowly. Withdraw needle, and apply pressure to site.

Intravenous

1. Only clinicians with specific training should inject medication intravenously.
2. Medications can be administered into a continuous IV or a heparin lock designed for intermittent administration. Be sure medication is compatible with solution being infused. Check for infiltration prior to administering medication.
3. Do not administer medications that have precipitates or discoloration.
4. Dilute according to directions. Certain medications are not to be diluted. Be sure to check specifics.
5. If "piggybacking" medication, set drip rate for proper infusion time. Note drop rate on IV tubing package.
6. Tape IV line securely but with some flexibility in the tubing.
7. Check IV frequently for correct infusion rate. Discontinue when complete dose has been delivered.
8. Record the name of the medication and volume of fluid administered.

Poison Control Centers in the United States

The American Association of Poison Control Centers (AAPCC) defines a poison center as an organization that serves a designated geographic region and provides the following services:

- Poison information
- Telephone management advice and consultation about toxic exposures
- Hazard surveillance to achieve hazard elimination
- Professional and public education in poisoning prevention, diagnosis, and treatment

Certified poison centers are accessible 24 hours a day; have a specially trained, full-time staff (usually nurses, pharmacists, or both); are directed by a board-certified physician-toxicologist; and are associated with a medical center that has laboratory facilities and personnel needed to diagnose and manage poisoning. In the list below, AAPCC-certified regional poison centers are shown in **bold** type. The list was updated in January 2003. Additions and deletions made since then can be found online at *www.aapcc.org.*

Dialing the following number from any place in the United States will connect you with the *local* poison control center:

National Poison Hotline: 1-800-222-1222

ALABAMA

Alabama Poison Center
2503 Phoenix Drive
Tuscaloosa, AL 35405
Emergency Phone: (800) 222-1222

Regional Poison Control Center
Children's Hospital
1600 7th Avenue South
Birmingham, AL 35233
Emergency Phone: (800) 222-1222

ALASKA

Oregon Poison Center
Oregon Health Sciences University
3181 SW Sam Jackson Park Road, CB550
Portland, OR 97201
Emergency Phone: (800) 222-1222

ARIZONA

Arizona Poison & Drug Info Center
Arizona Health Sciences Center, Room 1156
1501 North Campbell Avenue
Tucson, AZ 85724
Emergency Phone: (800) 222-1222

Banner Poison Control Center
Good Samaritan Regional Medical Center
1111 E. McDowell
Phoenix, AZ 85006
Emergency Phone: (800) 222-1222

ARKANSAS

Arkansas Poison & Drug Information Center
College of Pharmacy, University of Arkansas for Medical
 Sciences
4301 W. Markham, Mail Slot 522-2
Little Rock, AR 72205
Emergency Phone: (800) 222-1222
TDD/TYY: (800) 641-3805

CALIFORNIA

California Poison Control System–Fresno/Madera Division
Children's Hospital Central California
9300 Valley Children's Place, MB 15
Madera, CA 93638-8762
Emergency Phone: (800) 222-1222
TDD/TYY: (800) 972-3323

California Poison Control System–Sacramento Division
University of California, Davis, Medical Center
2315 Stockton Boulevard
Sacramento, CA 95817
Emergency Phone: (800) 222-1222
TDD/TYY: (800) 972-3323

California Poison Control System–San Francisco Division
University of California, San Francisco, Box 1369
San Francisco, CA 94143-1369
Emergency Phone: (800) 222-1222
TDD/TYY: (800) 972-3323

California Poison Control System–San Diego Division
University of California, San Diego, Medical Center
200 West Arbor Drive
San Diego, CA 92103-8925
Emergency Phone: (800) 222-1222
TDD/TYY: (800) 972-3323

COLORADO

Rocky Mountain Poison & Drug Center
1001 Yosemite Street, Suite 200
Denver, CO 80230-6800
Emergency Phone: (800) 222-1222
TDD/TYY: (303) 739-1127

CONNECTICUT

Connecticut Poison Control Center
University of Connecticut Health Center
263 Farmington Avenue
Farmington, CT 06030-5365
Emergency Phone: (800) 222-1222

DELAWARE

The Poison Control Center
Children's Hospital of Philadelphia
34th & Civic Center Blvd
Philadelphia, PA 19104-4303
Emergency Phone: (800) 222-1222
TDD/TYY: (215) 590-8789

DISTRICT OF COLUMBIA

National Capital Poison Center
3201 New Mexico Avenue, NW, Suite 310
Washington, DC 20016
Emergency Phone: (800) 222-1222
TDD/TYY: (800) 222-1222

FLORIDA

Florida Poison Information Center–Jacksonville
655 West Eighth Street
Jacksonville, FL 32209
Emergency Phone: (800) 222-1222
TDD/TYY: (800) 222-1222; (800) 282-3171 (FL only)

Florida Poison Information Center–Miami
University of Miami, Dept. of Pediatrics
P.O. Box 016960 (R-131)
Miami, FL 33101
Emergency Phone: (800) 222-1222

Florida Poison Information Center–Tampa
Tampa General Hospital
P.O. Box 1289
Tampa, FL 33601
Emergency Phone: (800) 222-1222

GEORGIA

Georgia Poison Center
Hughes Spalding Children's Hospital
Grady Health System
80 Jesse Hill Jr. Drive, SE, P.O. Box 26066
Atlanta, GA 30335-3801
Emergency Phone: (800) 222-1222
TDD/TYY: (404) 616-9287 (TDD)

HAWAII

Hawaii Poison Center
1319 Punahou Street
Honolulu, HI 96826
Emergency Phone: (800) 222-1222

Rocky Mountain Poison & Drug Center
1001 Yosemite Street, Suite 200
Denver, CO 80230-6800
Emergency Phone: (800) 222-1222
TDD/TYY: (303) 739-1127

IDAHO

Rocky Mountain Poison & Drug Center
1001 Yosemite Street, Suite 200
Denver, CO 80230-6800
Emergency Phone: (800) 222-1222
TDD/TYY: (303) 739-1127

INDIANA

Indiana Poison Center
Methodist Hospital
Clarian Health Partners
I-65 at 21st Street
Indianapolis, IN 46206-1367
Emergency Phone: (800) 222-1222
TDD/TYY: (317) 962-2336 (TTY)

ILLINOIS

Illinois Poison Center
222 S. Riverside Plaza, Suite 1900
Chicago, IL 60606
Emergency Phone: (800) 222-1222
TDD/TYY: (312) 906-6185

IOWA

Iowa Statewide Poison Control Center
St. Luke's Regional Medical Center
2910 Hamilton Boulevard Lower A
Sioux City, IA 51104
Emergency Phone: (800) 222-1222

KANSAS

Mid-America Poison Control Center
University of Kansas Medical Center
3901 Rainbow Blvd., Room B-400
Kansas City, KS 66160-7231
Emergency Phone: (800) 222-1222
TDD/TYY: (913) 588-6639 (TDD)

KENTUCKY

Kentucky Regional Poison Center
Medical Towers South, Suite 847
234 East Gray Street
Louisville, KY 40202
Emergency Phone: (800) 222-1222

LOUISIANA

Louisiana Drug and Poison Information Center
University of Louisiana at Monroe
College of Pharmacy, Sugar Hall
Monroe, LA 71209-6430
Emergency Phone: (800) 222-1222

MAINE

Northern New England Poison Center
22 Bramhall St
Portland, ME 04102
Emergency Phone: (800) 222-1222
TDD/TYY: (877) 299-4447; (207) 871-2879 (ME only)

MARYLAND

Maryland Poison Center
University of Maryland at Baltimore
School of Pharmacy
20 North Pine Street, PH 772
Baltimore, MD 21201
Emergency Phone: (800) 222-1222
TDD/TYY: (410) 706-1858 (TDD)

National Capital Poison Center
3201 New Mexico Avenue, NW, Suite 310
Washington, DC 20016
Emergency Phone: (800) 222-1222
TDD/TYY: (800) 222-1222

MASSACHUSETTS

Regional Center for Poison Control and Prevention Serving Massachusetts and Rhode Island
300 Longwood Avenue
Boston, MA 02115
Emergency Phone: (800) 222-1222
TDD/TYY: (888) 244-5313

MICHIGAN

Children's Hospital of Michigan Regional Poison Control Center
4160 John R. Harper Professional Office Bldg, Suite 616
Detroit, MI 48201
Emergency Phone: (800) 222-1222
TDD/TYY: (800) 356-3232 (TDD)

DeVos Children's Hospital Regional Poison Center
1300 Michigan, NE, Suite 203
Grand Rapids, MI 49503
Emergency Phone: (800) 222-1222
TDD/TYY: (800) 222-1222

MINNESOTA

Hennepin Regional Poison Center
Hennepin County Medical Center
701 Park Avenue
Minneapolis, MN 55415
Emergency Phone: (800) 222-1222
TDD/TYY: (800) 222-1222; (612) 904-4691 (TTY)

MISSISSIPPI

Mississippi Regional Poison Control Center
University of Mississippi Medical Center
2500 N. State Street
Jackson, MS 39216
Emergency Phone: (800) 222-1222

MISSOURI

Missouri Regional Poison Center
7980 Clayton Rd, Suite 200
St. Louis, MO 63117
Emergency Phone: (800) 222-1222
TDD/TYY: (314) 612-5705

MONTANA

Rocky Mountain Poison & Drug Center
1001 Yosemite Street, Suite 200
Denver, CO 80230-6800
Emergency Phone: (800) 222-1222
TDD/TYY: (303) 739-1127

NEBRASKA

The Poison Center
Children's Hospital
8200 Dodge Street
Omaha, NE 68114
Emergency Phone: (800) 222-1222

NEVADA

Oregon Poison Center
Oregon Health Sciences University
3181 SW Sam Jackson Park Road, CB550
Portland, OR 97201
Emergency Phone: (800) 222-1222

Rocky Mountain Poison & Drug Center
1001 Yosemite Street, Suite 200
Denver, CO 80230-6800
Emergency Phone: (800) 222-1222
TDD/TYY: (303) 739-1127

NEW HAMPSHIRE

New Hampshire Poison Information Center
Dartmouth-Hitchcock Medical Center
One Medical Center Drive
Lebanon, NH 03756
Emergency Phone: (800) 222-1222

NEW JERSEY

New Jersey Poison Information and Education System
University of Medicine and Dentistry at New Jersey
65 Bergen Street
Newark, NJ 07107-3001
Emergency Phone: (800) 222-1222
TDD/TYY: (973) 926-8008

NEW MEXICO

New Mexico Poison & Drug Info Center
Health Science Center Library, Room 130
University of New Mexico
Albuquerque, NM 87131-1076
Emergency Phone: (800) 222-1222

NEW YORK

Central New York Poison Center
750 East Adams Street
Syracuse, NY 13210
Emergency Phone: (800) 222-1222

Finger Lakes Regional Poison & Drug Information Center
University of Rochester Medical Center
601 Elmwood Avenue, Box 321
Rochester, NY 14642
Emergency Phone: (800) 222-1222
TDD/TYY: (585) 273-3854 (TTY)

Long Island Regional Poison and Drug Information Center
Winthrop University Hospital
259 First Street
Mineola, NY 11501
Emergency Phone: (800) 222-1222
TDD/TYY: (516) 924-8811 (Suffolk Co.); (516) 747-3323 (Nassau Co.)

New York City Poison Control Center
New York City Bureau of Labs, 455 First Avenue, Room 123, Box 81
New York, NY 10016
Emergency Phone: (800) 222-1222
TDD/TYY: (212) 689-9014 (TDD)

Western New York Poison Center
Children's Hospital of Buffalo
219 Bryant Street
Buffalo, NY 14222
Emergency Phone: (800) 222-1222

NORTH CAROLINA

Carolinas Poison Center
Carolinas Medical Center
5000 Airport Center Parkway, Suite B
Charlotte, NC 28208
Emergency Phone: (800) 222-1222

NORTH DAKOTA

Hennepin Regional Poison Center
Hennepin County Medical Center
701 Park Avenue
Minneapolis, MN 55415
Emergency Phone: (800) 222-1222
TDD/TYY: (800) 222-1222; (612) 904-4691 (TTY)

OHIO

Central Ohio Poison Center
700 Children's Drive, Room L032
Columbus, OH 43205
Emergency Phone: (800) 222-1222
TDD/TYY: (614) 228-2272 (TTY)

Cincinnati Drug & Poison Information Center
3333 Burnet Avenue
Vernon Place—3rd Floor
Cincinnati, OH 45229-9004
Emergency Phone: (800) 222-1222
TDD/TYY: (800) 253-7955

Greater Cleveland Poison Control Center
11100 Euclid Avenue
Cleveland, OH 44106-6010
Emergency Phone: (800) 222-1222

OKLAHOMA

Oklahoma Poison Control Center
Children's Hospital at Oklahoma University Medical Center
940 N.E. 13th Street, Room 3510
Oklahoma City, OK 73104
Emergency Phone: (800) 222-1222
TDD/TYY: (405) 271-1122

OREGON

Oregon Poison Center
Oregon Health Sciences University
3181 SW Sam Jackson Park Road, CB550
Portland, OR 97201
Emergency Phone: (800) 222-1222

PENNSYLVANIA

Penn State Poison Center
Pennsylvania State University
The Milton S. Hershey Medical Center
500 University Drive
MC H043, PO Box 850
Hershey, PA 17033-0850
Emergency Phone: (800) 222-1222
TDD/TYY: (717) 531-8335 (TTY)

Pittsburgh Poison Center
Children's Hospital of Pittsburgh
3705 Fifth Avenue
Pittsburgh, PA 15213
Emergency Phone: (800) 222-1222

The Poison Control Center
Children's Hospital of Philadelphia
34th & Civic Center Blvd
Philadelphia, PA 19104-4303
Emergency Phone: (800) 222-1222
TDD/TYY: (215) 590-8789

PUERTO RICO

San Jorge Children's Hospital Poison Center
Calle San Jorge #252
Santurce, Puerto Rico 00912
Emergency Phone: (800) 222-1222

RHODE ISLAND

Regional Center for Poison Control and Prevention Serving Massachusetts and Rhode Island
300 Longwood Avenue
Boston, MA 02115
Emergency Phone: (800) 222-1222
TDD/TYY: (888) 244-5313

SOUTH CAROLINA

Palmetto Poison Center
College of Pharmacy
University of South Carolina
Columbia, SC 29208
Emergency Phone: (800) 222-1222

SOUTH DAKOTA

Hennepin Regional Poison Center
Hennepin County Medical Center
701 Park Avenue
Minneapolis, MN 55415
Emergency Phone: (800) 222-1222
TDD/TYY: (800) 222-1222; (612) 904-4691 (TTY)

TENNESSEE

Middle Tennessee Poison Center
501 Oxford House
1161 21st Avenue South
Nashville, TN 37232-4632
Emergency Phone: (800) 222-1222
TDD/TYY: (615) 936-2047 (TDD)

Southern Poison Center
University of Tennessee
875 Monroe Avenue, Suite 104
Memphis, TN 38163
Emergency Phone: (800) 222-1222

TEXAS

Central Texas Poison Center
Scott and White Memorial Hospital
2401 South 31st Street
Temple, TX 76508
Emergency Phone: (800) 222-1222

North Texas Poison Center
Parkland Memorial Hospital
5201 Harry Hines Blvd.
Dallas, TX 75235
Emergency Phone: (800) 222-1222

Southeast Texas Poison Center
The University of Texas Medical Branch
3.112 Trauma Building
Galveston, TX 77555-1175
Emergency Phone: (800) 222-1222

South Texas Poison Center
The University of Texas Health Science Center–San Antonio
Department of Surgery, Mail Code 7849
7703 Floyd Curl Drive
San Antonio, TX 78229-3900
Emergency Phone: (800) 222-1222

Texas Panhandle Poison Center
1501 S. Coulter
Amarillo, TX 79106
Emergency Phone: (800) 222-1222

West Texas Regional Poison Center
Thomason Hospital
4815 Alameda Avenue
El Paso, TX 79905
Emergency Phone: (800) 222-1222

UTAH

Utah Poison Control Center
410 Chipeta Way, Suite 230
Salt Lake City, UT 84108
Emergency Phone: (800) 222-1222

VERMONT

Northern New England Poison Center
22 Bramhall Street
Portland, ME 04102
Emergency Phone: (800) 222-1222
TDD/TYY: (877) 299-4447

VIRGINIA

Blue Ridge Poison Center
Jefferson Park Place
1222 Jefferson Park Ave.
Charlottesville, VA 22903
Emergency Phone: (800) 222-1222

National Capital Poison Center
3201 New Mexico Avenue, NW, Suite 310
Washington, DC 20016
Emergency Phone: (800) 222-1222
TDD/TYY: (800) 222-1222

Virginia Poison Center
Medical College of Virginia Hospitals
Virginia Commonwealth University Health System
P.O. Box 980522
Richmond, VA 23298-0522
Emergency Phone: (800) 222-1222

WASHINGTON

Washington Poison Center
155 NE 100th Street, Suite 400
Seattle, WA 98125-8011
Emergency Phone: (800) 222-1222
TDD/TYY: (206) 517-2394 (TDD); (800) 572-0638 (TDD WA only)

WEST VIRGINIA

West Virginia Poison Center
3110 MacCorkle Ave, S.E.
Charleston, WV 25304
Emergency Phone: (800) 222-1222
TDD/TYY: (304) 388-9698

WISCONSIN

Children's Hospital of Wisconsin Poison Center
PO Box 1997, Mail Station 677A
Milwaukee, WI 53201-1997
Emergency Phone: (800) 222-1222
TDD/TYY: (414) 266-2542

WYOMING

The Poison Center
Children's Hospital
8200 Dodge Street
Omaha, NE 68114
Emergency Phone: (800) 222-1222

ANIMAL POISON CONTROL CENTER

ASPCA
Animal Poison Control Center
1717 South Philo Road, Suite 36
Urbana, IL 61802
Emergency Phone: (888) 426-4435

Canadian Drug Information

Alfred J. Rémillard, PharmD, BCPP

INTERNATIONAL SYSTEM OF UNITS

In an attempt to standardize the large number of different units used worldwide and thus improve communication, the Système International d'Unités (International System of Units; SI) was recommended in 1954. In 1971, the mole (mol) was adopted as the standard for designating the amount of substance present, and the liter (L) was adopted as the standard for designating volume. The World Health Organization recommended the adoption of SI units in 1977. However, Canada had already implemented an equivalent system in 1971.

In therapeutics, the major change caused by adopting the SI was to express drug concentrations present in body fluids in molar units (e.g., mmol/L) rather than in mass units (e.g., mg/L). This allows a better comparison between the pharmacologic and pharmacodynamic effects of different drugs, since these properties are relative to the number of molecules (e.g., mmol) of drug present rather than to the number of mass units (e.g., mg).

DRUG SERUM CONCENTRATIONS

Many drugs have known therapeutic or toxic levels that are monitored in patients to ensure safety and efficacy. In Canada, clinical laboratories report these levels in SI units. Levels traditionally reported as milligrams per milliliter (mg/ml) can be converted to millimoles per liter (mmol/L) using the conversion factor (CF) for that specific drug:

$$CF = 1000/\text{molecular weight of the drug}$$

To convert from micrograms per milliliter to SI units, the following equation is used:

$$\mu g/ml \times CF = \mu mol/L$$

To convert from SI units to micrograms per milliliter, the following equation is used:

$$\mu mol/L/CF = \mu g/ml$$

Table H–1 lists some important drugs for which therapeutic or toxic levels have been established. For most of these drugs, the levels presented are trough (minimum) values, which are measured in blood samples drawn just prior to the next dose. For the aminoglycosides and vancomycin, two levels are listed: a trough level and a peak (maximum) level. Levels must remain between the peak and trough to ensure efficacy of these drugs and at the same time to minimize toxicity.

CANADIAN DRUG LEGISLATION

Two acts form the basis of the drug laws in Canada, the Food and Drug Act and the Controlled Drugs and Substance Act. The responsibility for administering these acts rests with the Therapeutic Products Directorate (TPD) at Health Canada.

The Food and Drug Act (1927), accompanied by the Food and Drug Regulations (1953, 1954, 1979), reviews the safety and efficacy of drugs before they are marketed, and the legislation determines whether the medicine is prescription or nonprescription. The Act controls the requirements for good manufacturing practices, labeling, distribution, and sale, including advertising of the drug.

Prescription Drugs (Schedule F)

All drugs that require a prescription, except for narcotics and controlled substances, are listed in Schedule F of the Food and Drugs Regulations. Prescriptions for Schedule F medications may written (including facsimiles) or transmitted orally (i.e., telephone order directly to the pharmacist) by a medical practitioner, dentist, or veterinary surgeon. The prescription can be refilled as often as indicated by the physician. The symbol Pr must appear on all manufacturing labels. Individual provinces (or states in the United States) can legislate more restrictive control and require a prescription for a medication classified by the TPD as a nonprescription drug (e.g., digoxin).

The Controlled Drugs and Substance Act (1997) establishes the requirements for the control and sale of narcotics, controlled drugs, and substances of abuse in Canada. The Controlled Drugs and Substance Act lists eight schedules of controlled substances. Assignment to a schedule is based on potential for abuse and the ease with which illicit substances can be manufactured in illegal laboratories. The degree of control, the conditions of record keeping, and other regulations depend on the specific schedule. For example, Schedule I, which includes the narcotic agents, requires written orders only and no repeat orders are allowed. Some provinces require prescriptions for certain narcotics such as morphine, to be written on a triplicate prescription form with one copy to be sent to the practitioner's regulatory body. The symbol Ⓒ must appear on the labels of controlled products, while the letter N is printed on the label of all the narcotic agents. Schedules I through IV are defined below; Schedules V through VIII are not yet finalized.

- Schedule I: opium poppy and its derivatives (e.g., morphine, heroin); methadone; coca and its derivatives (e.g., cocaine)

TABLE H–1 ▪▪ Therapeutic Serum Drug Concentrations

Drugs	SI Reference Interval	SI Unit	Conversion Factor	Traditional Reference Interval	Traditional Reference Unit
Acetaminophen	13–40	μmol/L	66.15	0.2–0.6	mg/dl
Acetylsalicyclic acid	7.2–21.7	μmol/L	0.0724	100–300	mg/dl
Amikacin*	—	—	—	15–25†; <8‡	μg/ml
Amitriptyline	430–9000§	mmol/L	3.605	120–250§	ng/ml
Carbamazepine	17–42	μmol/L	4.233	4–10	μg/ml
Desipramine	430–750	nmol/L	3.754	115–200	ng/ml
Digoxin	0.6–2.8	nmol/L	1.282	0.5–2.2	ng/ml
Disopyramide	6–18	μmol/L	2.946	2–6	μg/ml
Gentamicin*	—	—	—	6–10†; <2‡	μg/ml
Imipramine	640–1070§	nmol/L	3.566	180–300§	ng/ml
Lidocaine	4.5–21.5	μmol/L	4.267	1–5	μg/ml
Lithium	0.4–1.2	mmol/L	1.0	0.4–1.2	mEq/L
Netilmicin*	—	—	—	6–10†; <2‡	μg/ml
Nortriptyline	190–570	nmol/L	3.797	50–150	ng/ml
Phenobarbital	65–170	μmol/L	4.306	15–40	μg/ml
Phenytoin	40–80	μmol/L	3.964	10–20	μg/ml
Primidone	25–46	μmol/L	4.582	6–10	μg/ml
Procainamide	17–34§	μmol/L	4.249	4–8§	μg/ml
Quinidine	4.6–9.2	μmol/L	3.082	1.5–3	μg/ml
Theophylline	55–110	μmol/L	5.55	10–20	μg/ml
Tobramycin*	—	—	—	6–10†; <2‡	μg/ml
Valproic acid	300–700	μmol/L	6.934	50–100	μg/ml
Vancomycin*	—	—	—	25–40†; <10‡	μg/ml

*Aminoglycosides (amikacin, gentamicin, netilmicin, tobramycin) and vancomycin are not reported in SI units because of the variability of their molecular weights.
†Peak drug level.
‡Trough drug level.
§Drug level reported as the total of the parent drug and its active metabolite.

- Schedule II: cannabis and its derivatives (e.g., marijuana, hashish)
- Schedule III: amphetamines, methylphenidate, lysergic acid diethylamide (LSD), methaqualone, psilocybin, mescaline
- Schedule IV: sedative-hypnotic agents (e.g., barbiturates, benzodiazepines); anabolic steroids

The Controlled Drugs and Substance Act also provides for the nonprescription sale of certain codeine preparations. The content must not exceed the equivalent of 8 mg codeine phosphate per solid dosage unit or 20 mg/30 ml of a liquid, and the preparation must also contain two additional nonnarcotic medicinal ingredients (usually acetylsalicylic acid or acetaminophen and caffeine). These preparations may not be advertised or displayed and may be sold only by pharmacists. Some provinces restrict the amount that can be sold at any given time.

Nonprescription Medications

Currently there are three categories of nonprescription medications that govern their sale. Restricted Access Nonprescription Drugs are "kept behind the counter" and are available for sale directly from the pharmacist only. Examples include insulin, glucagon, ipecac, loperamide, and nitroglycerin. This restriction is to assure that patients are not self-diagnosing medically serious diseases such as diabetes mellitus or angina and to help ensure proper use of the medicines through appropriate counseling by the pharmacist. The second category, Pharmacy Only Nonprescription Drugs, are sold only through pharmacies and include most antihistamines and the low-dose ulcer medicines. It is expected that, if clients have questions, they could easily consult with the pharmacist. The third category includes nonprescription products that can be sold at any retail outlet. In general, these products are provided with adequate instruction to permit self-treatment. Examples are nicotine gum and patches, aspirin, ibuprofen, and some low-dose "cough and cold" preparations.

Proposed Changes to National Drug Schedules

As previously mentioned, individual provinces have enacted their own legislation controlling the sale of both prescription and nonprescription products. This has led to inconsistency and confusion for both the healthcare practitioner and the consumer. As a result, the National Association of Pharmacy Regulatory Authorities endorsed a proposal for a national drug scheduling model. This model will align the provincial drug schedules so that the conditions for the sale of drugs would be consistent across the country. The harmonized model includes all classes of medications—narcotics, controlled substances, prescription medications, and nonprescription medications—which are assigned to one of the following four categories:

- Schedule I: all prescription drugs, including narcotics and controlled substances
- Schedule II: Restricted Access Nonprescription Drugs (see *Nonprescription Medications* above)
- Schedule III: Pharmacy Only Nonprescription Drugs (see *Nonprescription Medications* above)
- Unscheduled Drugs: those drugs not assigned to the above categories, which can be sold at any retail outlet

The national drug schedule is in various stages of implementation across the provinces.

New Drug Development in Canada

The process for approving a new drug in Canada is very similar, if not identical, to the process in the United States. The same drug data that are required for approval by the Food and Drug Administration in the United States are required by the TPD in Canada. The principal difference between Canada and the United States is one of nomenclature: Once preclinical testing is completed, the manufacturer in Canada applies for a Preclinical New Drug Submission, versus an Investigational New Drug in the United States. At the end of clinical testing, the manufacturer in Canada seeks a New Drug Submission (NDS), versus a New Drug Application in the United States.

After all the information on a new drug has been submitted—including results of preclinical and clinical testing, method of manufacturing, packaging, labeling, and results of stability testing—the pharmaceutical company receives a Notice of Compliance (NOC) from the TPD, and the drug enters the market.

Although data collection for a new drug is thorough, there is no guarantee that all adverse reactions are known, especially when the drug is used concurrently with other drugs. Also, long-term effects are not fully appreciated. For these reasons, postmarketing surveillance plays a major role in monitoring new drugs. The Canadian Adverse Drug Reactions monitoring program has undergone extensive expansion in recent years. The manufacturer and all healthcare practitioners must immediately report any new clinical findings, unexpected adverse effects, or therapeutic failures to the TPD.

Patent Laws

Patent laws in Canada continue to evolve. In 1969, the Patent Act was changed to include compulsory licensing. This new provision allowed generic drug companies to manufacture and distribute patented drugs in Canada, provided that a minimal 4% royalty fee was paid to the patent holder. This system was introduced to help control drug prices. Unfortunately, the system caused a decline in revenue to "innovative" pharmaceutical companies, with a resultant decline in research on

new drug development. After much debate, and retroactive to June 1987, the Patent Act was amended to give patent holders market exclusivity either (1) for 7 to 10 years or (2) until the 17-year patent (from date of filing) expires, whichever comes first. The Patent Act was then further amended to "make Canada's intellectual property legislation more in line with that of the major industrialized countries."

In response to provisions of the North American Free Trade Agreement (NAFTA) and the General Agreement on Tariffs and Trade (GATT), Bill C-91 was introduced in 1993. This bill (1) eliminated compulsory licensing and (2) extended patent protection on brand-name drugs to 20 years, thereby making Canadian patent laws consistent with those of the United States and other industrialized nations. Section 14 of Bill C-91 called for a parliamentary review of legislation in 1997. A special committee reviewed the impact of Bill C-91 on such factors as drug prices, drug research and development, and job creation. No changes to the legislation were made.

In order to respond to concerns arising from changes in the Patent Act, a Patented Medicine Prices Review Board was created. Its mandate is to (1) ensure that prices of patented medicines are not excessive and (2) report on the ratios of research and development expenditures relative to sales for individual patentees and for the pharmaceutical industry as a whole.

SOME IMPORTANT CANADIAN DRUG TRADE NAMES

For a list of common drug trade names used in Canada, go to *evolve.elsevier.com/Lehne/*.

REFERENCES

Bachynsky J. Nonprescription drugs in health care. *In* Nonprescription Drug Reference for Health Professionals. Ottawa, Canadian Pharmaceutical Association, 1996.

Evans WE, Schentag JJ, Jusko WJ (eds). Applied Pharmacokinetics: Principles of Therapeutic Drug Monitoring. Spokane, WA, Applied Therapeutics, Inc., 1992.

Health Protection and Drug Laws. Ottawa, Health and Welfare Canada, Canadian Publishing Center, 1988.

Health Protection Branch. Information Newsletter 1991(798).

Johnson GE, Hannah KJ, Zerr SR. Pharmacology and the Nursing Process, 3rd ed. Philadelphia, WB Saunders, 1992.

Mailhot R. The Canadian drug regulatory process. J Clin Pharmacol 1986;26:232.

McLeod DC. SI units in drug therapeutics. Drug Intell Clin Pharm 1988;22:990.

Subcommittee of Metric Commission Canada, Sector 9.10. SI Manual in Health Care, 2nd ed. Ottawa, Health and Welfare Canada, 1982.

Sullivan P. CMA to support increased patent protection for drugs but will attach strong qualifications. CMAJ 1992;147:1669.

To the Year 2000: The Changing Roles of Nonprescription Medicines and the Practice of Pharmacy. Ottawa, Nonprescription Drug Manufacturers Association of Canada, 1992.

Major Drug Classes and Their Prototypes

The prototypic drugs in this list are classified in two ways: (1) by *pharmacologic family* (e.g., beta-adrenergic blockers), and (2) by *therapeutic family* (e.g., drugs for angina pectoris). Since a single drug may belong to multiple therapeutic families (in addition to its single pharmacologic family), a drug may appear in the list more than once. Propranolol, for example, appears four times: first as a prototype for its pharmacologic family (beta-adrenergic blockers), and later as a prototype within three therapeutic families (antidysrhythmic drugs, drugs for angina pectoris, and drugs for hypertension).

PERIPHERAL NERVOUS SYSTEM DRUGS

Muscarinic Agonists

Bethanechol

Muscarinic Antagonists

Atropine

Cholinesterase Inhibitors

Neostigmine (reversible inhibitor)

Neuromuscular Blockers

Competitive (Nondepolarizing)
Tubocurarine
Depolarizing
Succinylcholine

Ganglionic Blockers

Trimethaphan

Adrenergic Agonists

Epinephrine

Alpha-Adrenergic Blockers

Prazosin

Beta-Adrenergic Blockers

Beta$_1$ and Beta$_2$ Blockers
Propranolol

Selective Beta$_1$ Blockers
Metoprolol

Indirect-Acting Antiadrenergics

Adrenergic Neuron Blockers
Reserpine
Centrally Acting Alpha$_2$ Agonists
Clonidine

CENTRAL NERVOUS SYSTEM DRUGS

Drugs for Parkinson's Disease

Dopaminergic Drugs
Levodopa (increases dopamine [DA] synthesis)
Carbidopa (blocks levodopa destruction)
Amantadine (promotes DA release)
Pramipexole (DA receptor agonist)
Selegiline (inhibits monoamine oxidase B)
Entacapone (inhibits catechol-*O*-methyltransferase)
Centrally Acting Anticholinergic Drugs
Benztropine

Drugs for Epilepsy

Phenytoin
Carbamazepine
Valproic acid
Ethosuximide
Phenobarbital
Diazepam (IV)

Drugs for Alzheimer's Disease

Tacrine (cholinesterase inhibitor)

Drugs for Migraine

Nonsteroidal Anti-inflammatory Drugs
Aspirin
Selective Serotonin Receptor Agonists
Sumatriptan
Ergot Alkaloids
Ergotamine

Local Anesthetics

Ester-type Local Anesthetics
Procaine
Amide-type Local Anesthetics
Lidocaine

General Anesthetics

Inhalation Anesthetics
Halothane
Isoflurane
Nitrous oxide
Intravenous Anesthetics
Thiopental
Ketamine
Droperidol plus fentanyl [Innovar]

Opioid (Narcotic) Analgesics and Antagonists

Pure Opioid Agonists
Morphine
Agonist-Antagonist Opioids
Pentazocine
Pure Opioid Antagonists
Naloxone

Antipsychotic Agents

Traditional Antipsychotics
Chlorpromazine (a low-potency agent)
Haloperidol (a high-potency agent)
Atypical Antipsychotics
Clozapine

Antidepressants

Tricyclic Antidepressants
Imipramine
Selective Serotonin Reuptake Inhibitors
Fluoxetine
Selective Norepinephrine Reuptake Inhibitors
Reboxetine
Monoamine Oxidase Inhibitors
Phenelzine
Atypical Antidepressants
Bupropion

Drugs for Bipolar Disorder (Manic-Depressive Illness)

Lithium
Carbamazepine
Valproic Acid

Drugs for Anxiety and Insomnia

Benzodiazepines
Diazepam (for anxiety)
Triazolam (for insomnia)
Barbiturates
Secobarbital
Nonbenzodiazepine-Nonbarbiturates
Buspirone

Central Nervous System Stimulants

Amphetamines
Amphetamine sulfate
Amphetamine-like Drugs
Methylphenidate
Methylxanthines
Caffeine

DIURETICS

High-Ceiling (Loop) Diuretics

Furosemide

Thiazide Diuretics

Hydrochlorothiazide

Potassium-Sparing Diuretics

Spironolactone
Triamterene

DRUGS THAT AFFECT THE HEART, BLOOD VESSELS, AND BLOOD

Drugs That Affect the Renin-Angiotensin-Aldosterone System

Angiotensin-Converting Enzyme (ACE) Inhibitors
Captopril
Angiotensin II Receptors Blockers
Losartan
Selective Aldosterone Receptor Blockers
Eplerenone

Calcium Channel Blockers

Agents That Affect the Heart and Blood Vessels
Verapamil
Dihydropyridines: Agents That Act Mainly on Blood Vessels
Nifedipine

Drugs for Hypertension

Diuretics
Hydrochlorothiazide
Spironolactone
Beta-Adrenergic Blockers
Propranolol
Metoprolol
ACE Inhibitors
Captopril
Enalapril

Angiotensin II Receptor Blockers
  Losartan
Calcium Channel Blockers
  Verapamil
  Nifedipine

Drugs for Angina Pectoris

Organic Nitrates
  Nitroglycerin
Beta Blockers
  Propranolol
  Metoprolol
Calcium Channel Blockers
  Verapamil
  Nifedipine

Drugs for Heart Failure

ACE Inhibitors
  Captopril
Diuretics
  Hydrochlorothiazide
  Furosemide
Inotropic Agents
  Digoxin (a cardiac glycoside)
  Dopamine (a sympathomimetic)
Beta Blockers
  Metoprolol
Aldosterone Receptor Blocker
  Spironolactone

Antidysrhythmic Drugs

Class I: Sodium Channel Blockers
  Quinidine (Class IA)
  Lidocaine (Class IB)
Class II: Beta Blockers
  Propranolol
Class III: Drugs That Delay Repolarization
  Bretylium
Class IV: Calcium Channel Blockers
  Verapamil
Others
  Adenosine
  Digoxin

Drugs Used to Lower Blood Cholesterol

HMG-CoA Reductase Inhibitors (Statins)
  Lovastatin
Bile-Acid Sequestrants
  Cholestyramine
Others
  Nicotinic acid
  Ezetimibe

Anticoagulant, Antiplatelet, and Thrombolytic Drugs

Anticoagulants
  Heparin (parenteral)
  Warfarin (oral)
Antiplatelet Drugs
  Aspirin (a cyclooxygenase [COX] inhibitor)
  Ticlopidine (an ADP receptor antagonist)
  Abciximab (a glycoprotein IIb/IIIa receptor antagonist)
Thrombolytic Drugs
  Streptokinase
  Alteplase (tissue-type plasminogen activator)

Hematopoietic and Thrombopoietic Growth Factors

Hematopoietic Growth Factors
  Epoetin alfa (erythropoietin)
  Filgrastim (granulocyte colony-stimulating factor)
Thrombopoietic Growth Factors
  Oprelvekin

ENDOCRINE DRUGS

Drugs for Diabetes

Insulin Preparations
  Regular insulin (insulin injection)
  Lispro insulin
  Lente insulins
  Insulin glargine
Sulfonylureas
  Tolbutamide
Meglitinides
  Repaglinide
Biguanides
  Metformin
Alpha-Glucosidase Inhibitors
  Acarbose
Thiazolidinediones
  Rosiglitazone

Drugs for Thyroid Disorders

Drugs for Hypothyroidism
  Levothyroxine (T_4)
Drugs for Hyperthyroidism
  Propylthiouracil

Estrogens

  Conjugated estrogens [Premarin]
  Estradiol

Progestins

  Medroxyprogesterone acetate
  Norethindrone

Contraceptive Agents

Combination Oral Contraceptives
Ethinyl estradiol plus norethindrone
Progestin-Only Oral Contraceptives
Norethindrone
Long-Acting Contraceptives
Subdermal progestin implant [Norplant]
Depot medroxyprogesterone acetate
Drugs for Emergency Contraception
Levonorgestrel alone
Ethinyl estradiol plus levonorgestrel (the Yuzpe Regimen)

Uterine Stimulants and Relaxants

Uterine Stimulants (Oxytocics)
Oxytocin
Ergonovine
Uterine Relaxants (Tocolytics)
Magnesium sulfate

ANTI-INFLAMMATORY, ANTIALLERGIC, AND IMMUNOLOGIC DRUGS

Immunosuppressants

First-Line Agents
Cyclosporine
Tacrolimus
Glucocorticoids
Prednisone

Antihistamines (H₁ Antagonists)

First-Generation H₁ Antagonists
Diphenhydramine
Second-Generation (Nonsedating) H₁ Antagonists
Fexofenadine

COX Inhibitors (Aspirin-like Drugs)

First-Generation Nonsteroidal Anti-inflammatory Drugs (NSAIDs) (COX-1 and COX-2 Inhibitors)
Aspirin
Ibuprofen
Second-Generation NSAIDs (Selective COX-2 Inhibitors)
Celecoxib
Drug That Lacks Anti-inflammatory Actions
Acetaminophen

Glucocorticoids

Hydrocortisone
Prednisone

DRUGS FOR BONE AND JOINT DISORDERS

Drugs for Rheumatoid Arthritis

Nonsteroidal Anti-inflammatory Drugs
Aspirin (a first-generation NSAID)
Celecoxib (a COX-2 inhibitor)

Glucocorticoids
Prednisone
Disease-Modifying Antirheumatic Drugs
Methotrexate
Hydroxychloroquine

Drugs for Osteoporosis

Antiresorptive Agents
Conjugated equine estrogens [Premarin]
Raloxifene (selective estrogen receptor modulator)
Alendronate (bisphosphonate)
Calcitonin-salmon nasal spray
Bone-Forming Agents
Teriparatide

RESPIRATORY TRACT DRUGS

Drugs for Asthma

Anti-inflammatory Drugs: Glucocorticoids
Beclomethasone (inhaled)
Prednisone (oral)
Anti-inflammatory Drugs: Others
Cromolyn
Zafirlukast (leukotriene modifier)
Bronchodilators: Beta₂-Adrenergic Agonists
Terbutaline (inhaled, short acting)
Salmeterol (inhaled, long acting)
Albuterol (oral)
Bronchodilators: Others
Theophylline (methylxanthine)

GASTROINTESTINAL DRUGS

Drugs for Peptic Ulcer Disease

Antibiotics (for Helicobacter pylori)
Metronidazole plus tetracycline plus bismuth subsalicylate
H₂-Receptor Antagonists
Cimetidine
Proton Pump Inhibitors
Omeprazole
Mucosal Protectants
Sucralfate
Muscarinic Antagonists
Pirenzepine
Antacids
Aluminum hydroxide/magnesium hydroxide
Drugs for NSAID-Induced Ulcers
Misoprostol

Laxatives

Bulk-Forming Agents
Methylcellulose
Surfactants
Docusate sodium
Stimulant Laxatives
Bisacodyl

Osmotic Laxatives
Magnesium hydroxide

Antiemetics

Serotonin Antagonists
Ondansetron
Dopamine Antagonists
Prochlorperazine
Metoclopramide
Glucocorticoids
Dexamethasone
Cannabinoids
Dronabinol
Benzodiazepines
Lorazepam

DRUGS FOR INFECTIOUS DISEASES

Penicillins, Cephalosporins, and Other Drugs That Weaken the Bacterial Cell Wall

Penicillins
Penicillin G
Cephalosporins
Cephalothin
Others
Imipenem
Vancomycin

Bacteriostatic Inhibitors of Protein Synthesis

Tetracyclines
Tetracycline
Macrolides
Erythromycin
Others
Clindamycin

Aminoglycosides (Bactericidal Inhibitors of Protein Synthesis)

Gentamicin

Fluoroquinolones

Ciprofloxacin

Sulfonamides and Trimethoprim

Sulfisoxazole
Trimethoprim
Trimethoprim-sulfamethoxazole [Bactrim]

Drugs for Tuberculosis

Isoniazid
Rifampin
Pyrazinamide
Ethambutol

Antifungal Agents

Amphotericin B
Ketoconazole

Antiviral Agents: Drugs for Non-HIV Viral Infections

Purine Nucleoside Analogs
Acyclovir
Drugs for Hepatitis B and C
Interferon alfa
Ribavirin
Drugs for Influenza
Influenza vaccine
Amantadine (for influenza A only)
Oseltamivir (for influenza A and B)

Antiviral Agents: Drugs for HIV Infection

Nucleoside Reverse Transcriptase Inhibitors
Azidothymidine
Non-nucleoside Reverse Transcriptase Inhibitors
Nevirapine
Protease Inhibitors
Saquinavir
HIV Fusion Inhibitors
Enfuvirtide

ANTICANCER DRUGS

Cytotoxic Drugs

Alkylating Agents
Cyclophosphamide
Platinum Compounds
Cisplatin
Antimetabolites
Methotrexate
Fluorouracil
Mercaptopurine
Antitumor Antibiotics
Doxorubicin
Mitotic Inhibitors
Vincristine
Taxoids
Paclitaxel
Topoisomerase Inhibitors
Etoposide
Others
Asparaginase

Hormones and Hormone Antagonists

Androgens
Testosterone
Gonadotropin-Releasing Hormone Analogs
Leuprolide
Androgen Receptor Blockers
Flutamide
Estrogens
Diethylstilbestrol diphosphate

Antiestrogens
Tamoxifen (a selective estrogen receptor modulator)
Aromatase Inhibitors
Anastrozole
Progestins
Medroxyprogesterone acetate
Glucocorticoids
Prednisone

Biologic Response Modifiers: Immunostimulants

Interferons
Interferon alfa-2a
Others
Aldesleukin
Levamisole

Index

Note: **Boldface** page number indicate prototypes, other important drugs, and major topics. *Italic* page number indicate figures. Page numbers followed by "t" indicate tables. Page numbers followed by "b" indicate special interest topics. Trade names appear in SMALL CAPITAL LETTERS followed by the generic name in parentheses; check for further information under the generic name.